UNIT I

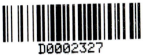

Introduction to Maternal and Neonatal Nursing

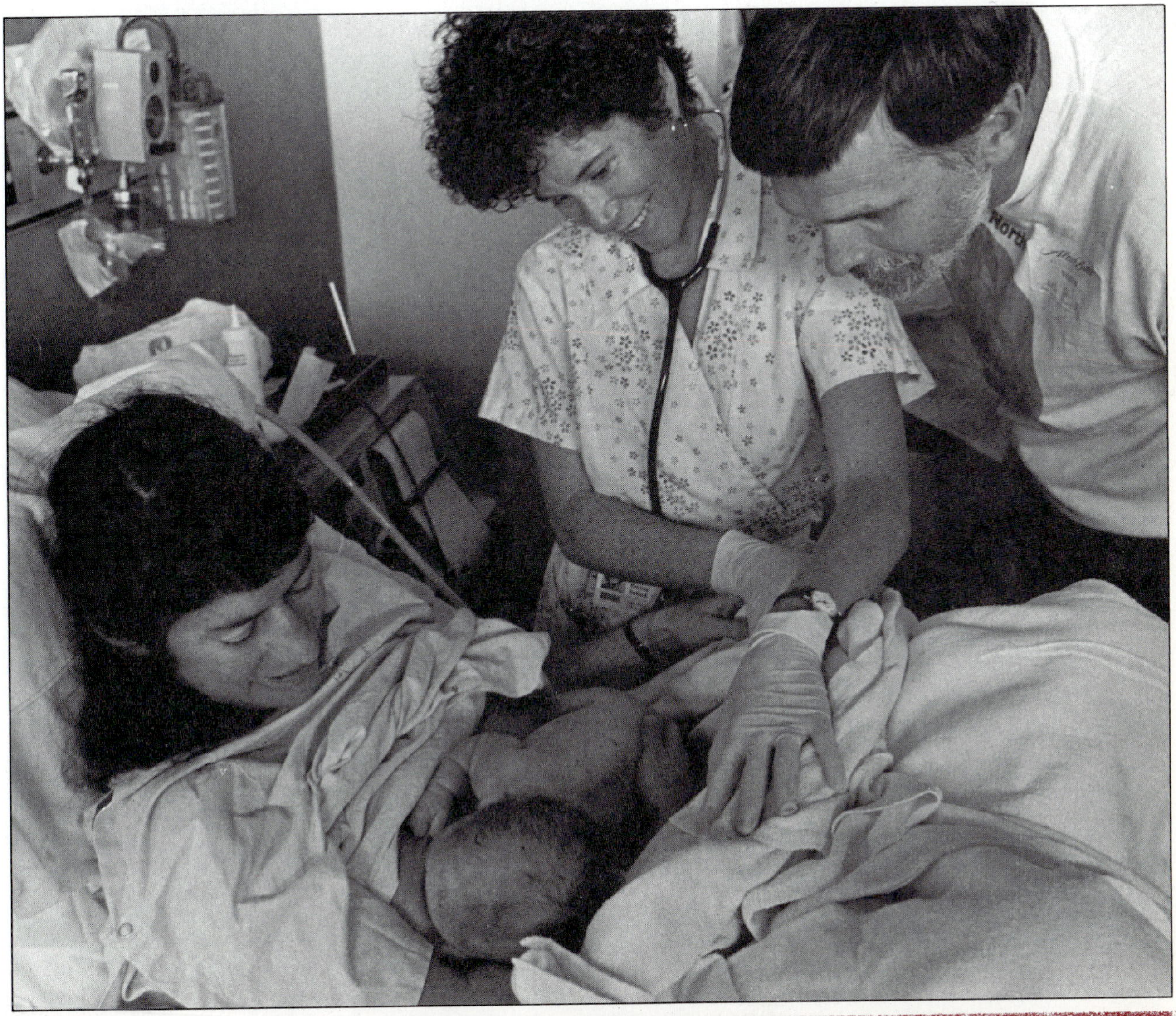

CHAPTER 1

Contemporary Maternal and Neonatal Care

Learning Objectives

After studying the material in this chapter, the student will be able to:

- Outline historical trends affecting the development of perinatal care in the United States.
- Identify social and economic trends affecting the current organization of perinatal care.
- Define family-centered perinatal nursing.
- Discuss the major principles underlying the philosophy of family-centered perinatal care.
- Discuss the nurse's role in establishing and maintaining family-centered perinatal care for childbearing families.

Key Terms

diagnosis-related group (DRG)
family-centered perinatal care
neonatologist
nurse midwife
perinatal period
perinatologist

The knowledgeable maternity or perinatal nurse understands the evolution of health care patterns and the influence of a variety of factors on contemporary delivery of perinatal health care. Awareness of historical, social, and economic trends allows the nurse to anticipate how changes will affect professional practice. Promotion of the well-being of childbearing families is the ultimate goal of quality perinatal care.

Historical Practices in Perinatal Care

Women have cared for other childbearing women throughout much of human history. Many ancient cultures of the world did not develop written language and relied only on oral transmission of knowledge. Therefore, birth practices have been lost or can be reconstructed only by examining current "primitive" practices (Goldsmith, 1984). The roots of perinatal care in the Western world are also ancient; the first recorded obstetric practices are found in Egyptian records dating back to 1500 BC. Practices such as vaginal examination and the use of birth aids are referred to in writings from the Greek and Roman empires. Much information was lost in the Dark Ages. Advances in medicine made during the Renaissance in Europe led to the modern "scientific" age of obstetric care.

Significant discoveries and inventions by physicians in the 16th and 17th centuries set the stage for scientific progress. Inventions included the obstetric forceps, first devised by Peter Chamberlen (1560–1631) and modified by William Smellie (1697–1763). Francois Mauriceau (1637–1709) noted that postpartum or "childbed" fever was an epidemic disease that plagued Europe. In the 19th century, Semmelweis concluded that postpartum fever was spread by contamination from the hands of physicians who were caring for many women without observing elementary hygienic practices. Early work of physicians and scientists in Europe is reflected in common terms in contemporary practice, such as Hegar's sign (softening of the lower segment of the uterus during pregnancy) and Nägele's rule (a method for calculating estimated dates of birth).

Maternity Care in America, 1700 to 1950

When colonists came to North America, they brought traditional English birth practices. Attendance by other women during childbirth and the "lying-in period" of several weeks are examples. Less crowded environments, the relative absence of epidemic disease, and more healthful and plentiful food sources resulted in healthier women. Pregnancies and births had more successful outcomes in America.

Beliefs about high maternal mortality during childbirth among colonial women have been exaggerated. Maternal deaths related to childbirth were relatively rare. Women had children over an extended period. The average age of a woman at first birth was 22 years. Births typically occurred every 2 to 3 years until conception was no longer possible. On the other hand, the childhood mortality rate was high. Colonial families in which seven or eight children were born were likely to see two or three die before the age of 10. This mortality rate was still lower than that in England. A child in the American colonies had a 75% to 85% chance of surviving to 21 years of age. In London, one sixth of all recorded deaths occurred among children under the age of 6 years (Wertz & Wertz, 1989).

Midwifery Care

Birth practices in the 1700s and 1800s were largely the province of midwives, who were women experienced in attending births and who often had many children of their own. They usually were taught through apprenticeship with other midwives. Sometimes midwives were sanctioned and given semiofficial status by local religious leaders, who testified to their good character and their abstention from such heretical practices as witchcraft. In the English tradition, midwives were regarded not as part of the medical establishment but as a separate profession with a unique role. In some cases, the midwife was also a "doctoress," one skilled in herbal remedies and practical care of the ill and injured. Formal training and licensure for "doctoring" in America were not required until the mid-19th century (Wertz & Wertz, 1989).

The Emergence of Obstetric Medicine

Physicians and male midwives began to replace female midwives after 1800. Interestingly, this occurred more rapidly in America than in England. After 1750, increasing numbers of men received medical education in Europe and returned to America to practice. These physicians brought a knowledge of scientific advances not available to female American midwives. Physicians were eager to establish a professional practice with some status in society. Despite the fact that physician or male midwife practice was not superior, the practitioners came to be regarded as more able birth attendants. Physicians and male midwives were increasingly sought after by middle- and upper-class families.

Trained physicians remained rare for some time. Both female midwives and physicians continued to practice in America until the early 1900s. Midwives were still called for uncomplicated births, with physicians called in for complicated deliveries. Some physicians established schools of midwifery with the intention of supporting this model of collaborative practice. Large numbers of men applied for midwifery training, resulting in the new profession of male midwifery. This may have been because early American schools were profit-making enterprises and were not government-supported as were European schools of midwifery. Women were less likely to be able to afford training and may have resisted the notion of being trained by men about practices already known to women. Victorian beliefs about appropriate activities for women were beginning to be felt at this time. These beliefs would restrict women's opportunities for participation in training programs of any kind.

Increasing numbers of men trained as midwives reinforced the existing trend toward training men as physicians. By the late 19th century, midwifery had been absorbed into medical training as a specialty all physicians could practice. In 1847, Simpson introduced chloroform for use during childbirth. The increasing popularity of analgesia for childbirth contributed to the consolidation of physician control over most maternity care. Midwife attendance at birth among the middle class virtually disappeared by the late 1800s. This set the stage for the next major change in maternity care in America—the shift from home to hospital birth in the early 20th century (Wertz & Wertz, 1989).

The Shift to Hospital Care for Childbirth

Before 1900, fewer than 5% of births in the United States occurred in hospitals. Only destitute or extremely ill women were cared for in "lying-in" hospitals. Crowded conditions, lack of skilled nursing care, and the predominance of patients already at risk for illness contributed to high morbidity and mortality among postpartum women and their newborns in hospitals. Hospital policies and procedures were developed to minimize the risk of infection on obstetric wards. Practices included the use of surgical aseptic techniques for all procedures and routine separation of mothers and neonates with the establishment of traditional newborn nurseries (Fig. 1-1). Hospitals developed training programs for nurses, which ensured an acceptable level of nursing care. Student nurses supervised by graduate nurses assumed the nursing care of hospitalized patients. Most graduate nurses provided in-home "private duty" nursing as employees of families. Only rarely were these nurses employed by physicians.

The increasing organization of medicine in the United States resulted in many changes in the American way of birth. Hospitals, built in part with an influx of federal funds, opened and provided a centralized setting for physician practice. Legislation outlawing midwifery practice was passed in many states in the early part of the 20th century. Hospital-based physician care was believed to be superior. This, compounded by the economic pressures of the Great Depression of the 1930s and the resulting sharp decline in the birth rate, caused a decline in the practice of in-home delivery by female midwives. The practice of private duty nursing in the home for childbearing women also became less prevalent at this time.

The hospital setting provided support for the physician's increasingly technologic approach to obstetrics. Gradually the hospital became the setting of choice for childbirth.

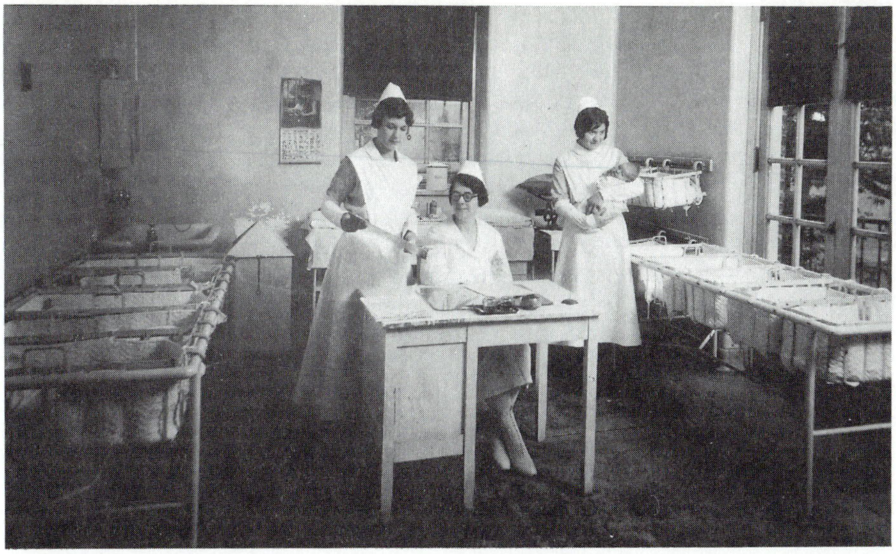

Figure 1-1.
Example of a newborn nursery in 1927. (Photo courtesy of the Archives and Special Collection on Women in Medicine, Medical College of Pennsylvania, Philadelphia, PA.)

Advances in analgesia and anesthesia increased safety and comfort for many women. Advances in operative and life-support techniques allowed intervention for mothers and neonates not dreamed possible at the beginning of the century. However, maternal and infant mortality rates did not decline significantly. The slow improvement in these rates was due primarily to preventable public health problems, such as poor nutrition and infectious diseases.

High maternal and infant mortality rates among indigent women were the impetus for the first federal involvement in maternity care. The Sheppard-Towner Act of 1921 provided funds for state-managed programs in maternal–child health. However, despite evidence that maternal and infant mortality declined sharply under these programs, the bill was repealed in 1930 because of opposition from organized medicine.

Federal involvement in maternal–child health continued during the Depression. A national commission determined that maternal–child health services should be a national priority. In 1935, Title V of the Social Security Act was amended to provide funding for maternal–child health programs. Title V programs targeted women and children most in need. Today's programs, such as Maternal and Infant Care Programs, emphasize comprehensive prenatal and infant care in public clinics.

Other charitable programs evolved to provide services to indigent women. Nurse midwifery began in the United States as a result of these efforts. The Maternity Center Association was founded in 1918 in New York City. It provided care to poor women and children and began training public health nurses in midwifery in 1932. The Frontier Nursing Service, established in 1925 by Mary Breckinridge, provided care for families in a remote area of Appalachia. Nurse midwifery training began there shortly before World War II. Because of these two programs, nurse midwives became the primary care providers for many impoverished families during the 1930s. This pattern continues today.

By the 1950s, the practice of obstetrics in the United States was controlled primarily by physicians. Nurse midwifery practice was concentrated in indigent populations. The hospital was the predominant setting for childbirth. Virtually all nurses caring for childbearing families were employed by hospitals. By 1970, more than 90% of births in the United States were attended by physicians and occurred in hospitals (Wertz & Wertz, 1989).

Consumerism in Perinatal Care

In the late 1950s, a coalition of consumers, health care professionals, and childbirth educators recognized that standard practices in obstetric care did not acknowledge birth as a normal family event. This movement was inspired by the writings of Lamaze, Dick-Read, and others. Some practices were perceived as unnecessary and unsafe for normal healthy mothers and infants. Activist groups began to press for changes in standard obstetric practices. The first practices to be challenged were the routine use of analgesics and anesthesia for childbirth. Routine exclusion of fathers and other family members from labor and delivery units was questioned.

The natural childbirth movement, as it was known, grew in strength and popularity. More health professionals and concerned lay people became active throughout the 1960s. Several specialty organizations were formed from the original grass roots coalition. These organizations included the American Society for Psychoprophylaxis in Obstetrics (popularly known as Lamaze), and the International Childbirth Education Association. Their major strategy was to educate expectant parents. Education included discussions about the range of practices in low-risk obstetric care. Parents were encouraged to ask for the type of birth care they wanted within the limitations of safety. Patient rights were explored. The movement relied heavily on knowledgeable consumers demanding family-centered birth care for themselves and others.

The natural childbirth movement was remarkably successful. Changes in obstetric care happened quickly. By the early 1970s, prepared childbirth was a relatively accepted practice in the United States. Routine use of anesthesia in childbirth was on the decline. Birth attendance by fathers and partners was becoming common in many areas of the country (Mathews & Zadek, 1991).

The Emergence of Perinatal Nursing

Skilled nurses on hospital obstetric wards were needed as birth moved from the home setting into the hospital. Before World War II, obstetric nursing was focused on acute care and the prevention of communicable diseases. In general, nursing was a highly restricted role characterized by deference to the physician, a lack of autonomy, and an almost religious dedication to work. This was true for obstetric nursing.

Initially, obstetric nursing services were organized to provide care across all areas—labor and delivery, postpartum, and the nursery. Obstetric care was primarily provided by family physicians (general practitioners) throughout the 1950s and 1960s. As time passed, specialization in both medicine and nursing increased.

Specialty organizations in perinatal nursing were launched. In 1969, the Nurses' Association of the American College of Obstetricians and Gynecologists (NAACOG) was formed. In 1992, this organization changed its name to the Association of Women's Health, Obstetric, and Neonatal Nurses (AWHONN). The Division of Maternal–Child Nursing within the American Nurses Association was begun in 1986. The establishment of clinical journals within perinatal nursing, such as the *Journal of Obstetric, Gynecologic, and Neonatal Nursing* (JOGNN) in 1972 and *American Journal of Maternal Child Nursing* (MCN) in 1976, reflected the evolution of the specialty. Nursing specialization was further consolidated by the practice of nurses working in large federally funded maternal and child health programs. The establishment of programs to educate nurse practitioners in women's health care in the 1960s supported the advancement of perinatal nursing practice. In the hospital setting, intensive neonatal care emerged as a subspecialty in both medicine and nursing.

The Emergence of High-Risk Perinatal Care

Since the 1960s, two new medical specialties, perinatology and neonatology, have profoundly affected the organization and delivery of perinatal care. These medical specialties have influenced the scope of nursing responsibilities in the care of childbearing families.

Perinatology and Neonatology

The field of perinatology emerged in response to research on the treatment of the mother and fetus before and during childbirth. It is a hybrid of neonatology and obstetrics. Advances in the ability to monitor fetal status became a major impetus to the development of perinatology as a subspecialty. These advances include electronic fetal monitoring (EFM), amniocentesis, ultrasound, therapy to treat preterm labor, and most recently, fetal therapy, including fetal surgery (Fig. 1-2*A* and *B*). As perinatology grew, nursing responsibilities for the monitoring and care of high-risk patients grew. Now many hospitals have special prenatal or high-risk perinatal units.

Neonatology, the medical care of high-risk newborns, emerged as a distinct subspecialty in pediatrics. Neonatology became possible in large part because research produced technologic advances in neonatal life-support and life-functioning monitoring. As neonatal research and practice advanced, a range of levels of neonatal care developed. The result was the establishment of transitional care, special care, and intensive care nurseries (Fig. 1-2*C*).

Nursing responsibilities in the monitoring and care of high-risk and sick neonates expanded as the scope of medical treatment increased (see Fig. 1-1). Today, neonatal care is truly an interdisciplinary practice. Contributions of nurses, physicians, respiratory therapists, pharmacists, laboratory scientists, social service workers, clergy, and others collaborate to provide quality care. Some 330,000 newborns are cared for in neonatal intensive care units (ICUs) across the United States each year, most commonly for conditions associated with low birth weight and prematurity (Morrison, 1990).

Terms Describing Specialty and Subspecialty Practice

The terminology used to describe specialty and subspecialty areas in the care of childbearing women and their families tends to be inconsistent. The term *perinatal* technically refers only to the period from 28 weeks of pregnancy through the first 28 days after birth. However, because the field of perinatology typically focuses on the high-risk mother and fetus/newborn, the term is sometimes used to connote high-risk care as well. For example, some graduate nursing programs prepare "perinatal clinical nurse specialists," yet the degree of concentration on high-risk nursing care varies among different programs. A hospital may employ a "perinatal nurse clinician" when, in fact, the facility delivers care primarily to low-risk mothers and newborns. The terms *perinatal health care* and *perinatal nursing* are increasingly used instead of *obstetric* or *maternity* care and *obstetric* or *maternal–newborn nursing*. Throughout this text, the terms maternity nursing and *perinatal nursing* will be used synonymously to describe nursing care for the woman and family throughout pregnancy, labor, and birth and the first 3 months after birth.

Regionalization in Perinatal Care

The emergence of the high-risk specialties of neonatology and perinatology in medicine, and the resulting growth in nursing responsibilities, led to dramatic changes in the organization of health care for mothers and infants. The trend toward regionalization of maternal and newborn care began in the 1960s as an effort to meet the needs of sick newborns. At that time, only a few institutions had the expert staff and facilities needed for intensive neonatal care. Professional groups and health planning agencies drafted long-term plans for regional perinatal care. Between 1975 and 1980, eight regions in the country developed perinatal networks. Regionalization began as a means to ensure widespread access to the rapidly developing high-technology care available at only a few centers.

Regionalized perinatal care is a network of relationships among hospitals providing care to pregnant women and

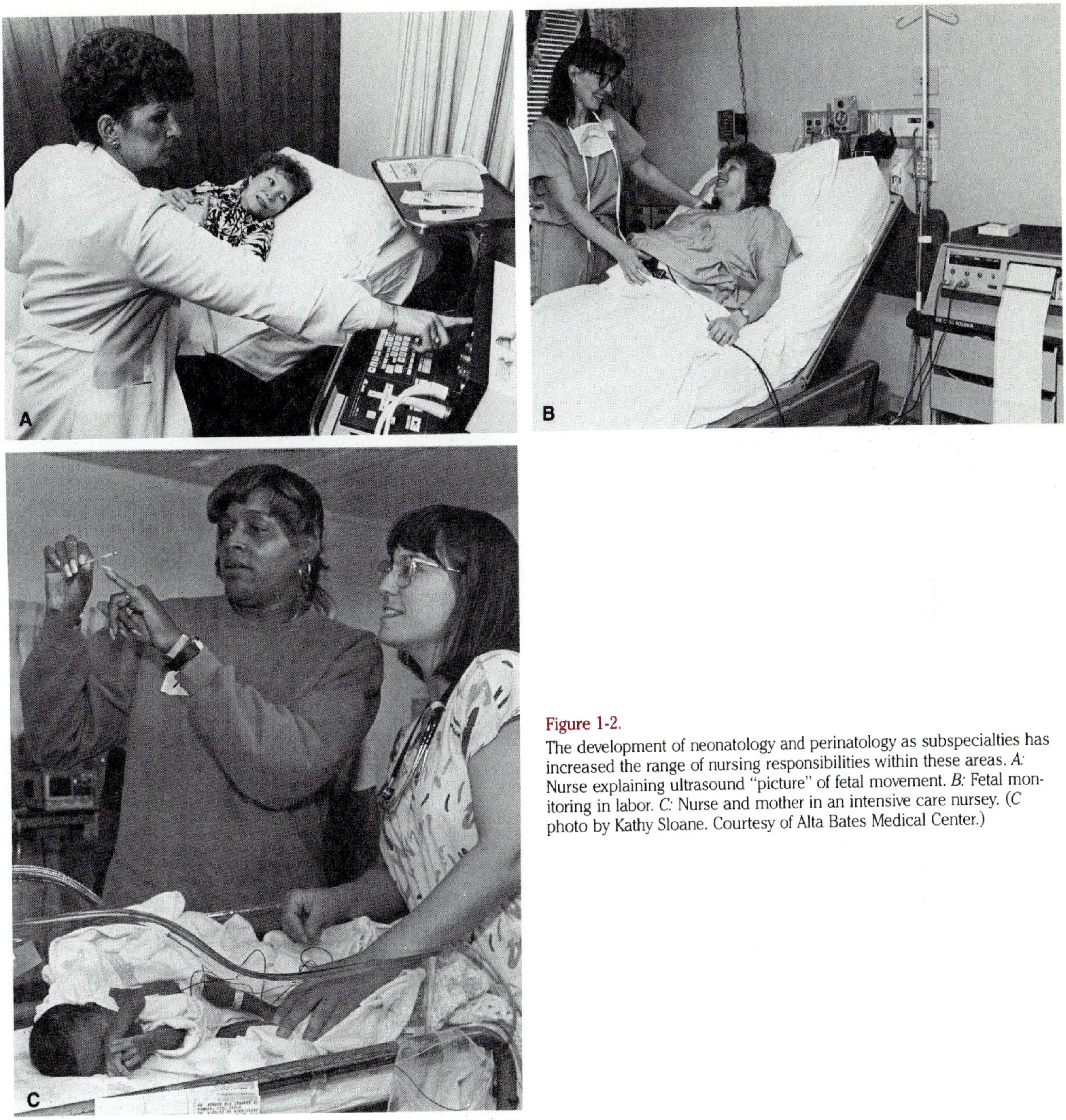

Figure 1-2.
The development of neonatology and perinatology as subspecialties has increased the range of nursing responsibilities within these areas. *A:* Nurse explaining ultrasound "picture" of fetal movement. *B:* Fetal monitoring in labor. *C:* Nurse and mother in an intensive care nursey. (*C* photo by Kathy Sloane. Courtesy of Alta Bates Medical Center.)

newborns. Centers are designated as level I (primary or entry-level care), level II (moderate-risk care), or level III (tertiary or high-risk care). High-risk patients are referred and often transported between hospitals to provide the appropriate level of care. Regionalization resulted in closing low-volume obstetric units and establishing and maintaining specialized education for medical and nursing staff to meet the needs of high-risk pregnant women and newborns. The costs of health care continue to climb and regionalized perinatal care is seen as a means to minimize duplication of services and reduce health care costs.

The overriding goal of regionalized care is to decrease the numbers of pregnant women and neonates at risk. Access to the appropriate level of care is a primary objective of regionalization. However, one drawback associated with regionalized perinatal care may be an emphasis on tertiary care, a tendency to use high-technology approaches excessively while underemphasizing proven "low-tech" practices. Examples include the continuing trend of applying high-risk intervention techniques (such as continuous intrapartum EFM) to low-risk women and the lack of attention to low-technology interventions to improve outcomes, such as preventive health services for childbearing women, health education, and universal access to early prenatal care.

The evolution of perinatal care from ancient times to contemporary patterns of care has shifted from care provided largely by knowledgeable women to care provided by physicians, nurses, and other professionals in hospital settings. Midwifery care in colonial times was followed by the emergence of obstetric medicine, maternity nursing, a shift from home- to hospital-based care, and more recently, the development of specialized high-risk care in the fields of perinatology and neonatology. These factors all have had an influence on the way perinatal care, and specifically perinatal nursing, is currently practiced.

Current Patterns in Perinatal Care Delivery

The developments in the early 20th century in obstetric medicine and nursing contributed directly to the way perinatal health care is organized and delivered today. Prenatal care is delivered largely in outpatient settings, such as clinics and private practices. Birth care is still predominantly delivered by obstetrician-gynecologists and nurses in hospital settings. Certified nurse midwives practice in most states and manage the care of low-risk and moderate-risk women throughout pregnancy, birth, and the interconceptional period.

The vast majority of births in the United States occur in hospitals, with home births estimated to be fewer than 10% of the total. Some nurse midwives attend home births for low-risk women in settings where hospital transfer and admission provisions have been made. Physicians who attend planned home births are rare.

Factors Influencing Delivery of Perinatal Care

Recent years have witnessed a significant change in the delivery of perinatal care in the hospital setting. Changes include the development of alternative birth centers, labor–delivery–recovery (LDR) or labor–delivery–recovery–postpartum (LDRP) rooms, and rooming-in or "mother–baby" units. These options provide alternatives to the more traditional labor and delivery, postpartum, and newborn units. Lengths of hospitalization for childbirth have decreased dramatically, from a routine 10-day stay during the 1950s to the current routine hospitalization of 2 days or less for mothers and newborns without complications.

Postnatal care is often provided on an outpatient basis. Routine follow-up of a normal newborn occurs at about 2 weeks of age, and follow-up care for the mother occurs 4 to 6 weeks after delivery. Settings that provide routine home follow-up for families after birth are uncommon. Routine home visits are usually provided as part of an early discharge program (within 24 hours of birth) for low-risk mothers and newborns. Home visits may also be made by community health nurses for low-income mothers and newborns thought to be at risk in the postpartum period.

Social and Economic Factors

Patterns of perinatal health care delivery are changing rapidly in response to a number of social and economic trends in the United States. The most important factors influencing health care of childbearing families include current economic conditions, technologic advances, and the ethical problems they present; issues of professional accountability and liability; and changes in gender role expectations and family size. The nurse must be knowledgeable about these factors because they directly affect the delivery of perinatal nursing care now and in the future.

The family's ability to pay for care may have a profound impact on the type of perinatal care they receive. Private care providers, such as physicians and nurse midwives, generally practice on a fee-for-service basis. Both are eligible to receive payment from health insurance plans, often called third-party payers. Nurse practitioners in some areas do not receive direct third-party payment but may be reimbursed through a physician practice. Health maintenance organizations (HMOs) or prepaid health plans usually offer a range of comprehensive perinatal care services. They may use nurse midwives and nurse practitioners to a greater extent to deliver primary care to their members. Services provided by public agencies, such as public health departments, clinics, county and city hospitals, and teaching hospitals, often use interdisciplinary health care teams. These teams provide care for socioeconomically disadvantaged "multiproblem" families. Such agencies and institutions depend on federal and state funds to pay costs.

Residential areas of women and their families directly affect the type of perinatal care received. Private care providers, particularly physicians, tend to be concentrated in urban areas rather than rural or remote areas. This maldistribution of physicians has been a major concern of health planners since the 1970s. Families in remote regions may not have a primary care provider available nearby. These families must often travel long distances for hospital care. Nurse midwives and nurse practitioners are increasingly attracted to rural practice, with nearly 20% of nurse practitioners and certified nurse midwives located in medically underserved areas (Lutz, 1991).

Families in lower socioeconomic groups, especially in inner-city areas, may be limited to care in a city or county hospital. State and federal reimbursement regulations may limit their choice of care providers. In many areas of the country, providers are reluctant to provide care to women receiving state or federal health and welfare support. The level of reimbursement from public sources tends to be lower than the reimbursement from private insurance. Often public sources do not adequately cover the cost of treatment. This further restricts options for perinatal care available to poor women and their families and tends to concentrate high-risk populations at public institutions. The ways that social and economic conditions directly affect the health of childbearing families is discussed in greater depth in Chapter 3.

During the last two decades, the United States has experienced a threefold increase in the cost of health and medical care. Various strategies have been tried and have failed to control this explosive cost increase. As costs have soared, the number of people forced to rely on state or federal assistance for health care has risen dramatically. Cutbacks in services may result in less favorable obstetric outcomes among low-income women. A cyclical pattern often results from these cutbacks. Infants and mothers who are at high risk because of poverty conditions require intensive medical services that, in the long run, result in higher health care costs. These and other economic conditions are primarily affecting the delivery of perinatal care and the practice of nursing in this arena.

Cost Containment

Cost containment is a major concern in the field of perinatal care. Although maternity services in hospitals typically break even or lose money, they are regarded as "loss leaders." In other words, these services may not pay for themselves, but they draw other kinds of revenues into the hospital. For example, the increased use of pediatric care facilities, ICUs, operating rooms, or diagnostic units may cover any losses incurred in the short term. Despite this, there are still concerns about the cost implications of some aspects of perinatal care, such as the accelerating use of high technology.

Cost of High Technology. The costs of operating ICUs, especially neonatal ICUs, are extremely high. Neonatal intensive care costs exceed $5 billion a year. Hospital costs of a neonatal ICU hospitalization is between $20,000 and $100,000 on the average (Morrison, 1990). Neonatal intensive care has already become more expensive than coronary artery bypass surgery. The skyrocketing costs of maternal–neonatal intensive care may result in stricter regulation of the establishment and use of high-risk centers. The pressure to manage regionalized perinatal care more efficiently already exists.

Cost and Appropriate Use of Intensive Care. Escalating health care costs may result in part from increasing use of high-technology care. Increased use of intensive care may be a result of patterns of medical education. Physicians are often trained to rely on high-technology practices in teaching centers, and therefore they may continue to do so in private practice. There may also be financial incentives to hospitals to use ICUs because reimbursement rates from insurance carriers are higher for care given in neonatal ICUs than for similar care given in normal neonatal nurseries. However, insurance carriers are beginning to carefully scrutinize services provided in hospitals, and this may affect provider practice habits. The cost and appropriate use of ICUs and high-technology interventions is of concern to the nursing profession. The primary service delivered in perinatal units is specialized nursing care. Therefore, nurses need to actively participate in evaluations of the cost effectiveness and appropriate use of high-technology care.

Prospective Payment. One major strategy for controlling health care costs has been the use of prospective payment. Prospective payment means that payers (federal sources, insurance companies) agree on a certain level of reimbursement in advance for a particular type of care, regardless of the actual costs. This strategy was designed first for Medicare reimbursement in 1987. Level of reimbursement is determined by diagnosis-related groups (DRGs). DRGs related to perinatal care are shown in the accompanying display.

Hospitals or care providers are reimbursed at a particular rate for care delivered to all patients with a given DRG. In this system, there is a financial incentive for the hospital or health care agency to standardize care for similar patients because reimbursement is standardized. For example, in perinatal care, reimbursement for care of all patients with an uncomplicated cesarean delivery would be the same, regardless of the actual length of patient stay. Hospitals that can safely discharge postcesarean patients in 5 days will control costs more successfully than a hospital whose postcesarean patients are discharged on day 7.

Diagnostics-Related Groups (DRGs) in Perinatal Care

The following are DRGs in current use in perinatal care. The numbering system is consistent nationwide and is often used in patient record and billing systems.

370 Cesarean section with complications
371 Cesarean section without complications
372 Vaginal delivery with complications
373 Vaginal delivery without complications
374 Vaginal delivery with sterilization and/or dilation and curettage
375 Vaginal delivery with operative procedures
376 Postpartum diagnosis without operative procedure
377 Postpartum diagnosis with operative procedure
378 Ectopic pregnancy
379 Therapeutic abortion
380 Abortion without dilation and curettage
381 Abortion with dilation and curettage
382 False labor
383 Other antepartum diagnosis with medical complication
384 Other antepartum diagnosis without medical complication
385 Neonatal death or transfer
386 Extreme prematurity with respiratory distress syndrome
387 Prematurity without other complications
388 Prematurity with other complications
389 Full-term neonate with complications

Thus, patient length of stay has become an important factor in controlling health care costs. Reducing length of stay ensures that reimbursement levels received by the hospital are closer to actual costs of delivering care. Shorter lengths of stay also allow for greater patient turnover and higher potential revenue for hospitals.

Studies have shown that nursing interventions are an effective means to reduce patient length of stay while maintaining safe levels of patient care on perinatal units. One study reported that variations in length of stay of patients with cesarean deliveries can be explained by the clinical management of patient care by nurses. This study showed that when nurses reviewed plans of care for patients and worked to prepare patients for timely discharge with use of appropriate services, the hospital saved more than $900/case when compared with conventional nursing care (Cohen, 1991). This form of care, called nursing case management, is discussed in more detail in Chapter 3.

Reimbursement for Nursing Services. Recent economic changes in the health care arena have made reimbursement for nursing services a popular topic of debate within and outside the profession. In most hospitals, nursing services have been grouped together in a category with other miscellaneous services. Nursing services are considered part of the institution's routine operating costs. For this reason, the true cost and cost effectiveness of inpatient nursing services have historically been difficult to determine.

In some areas of perinatal nursing practice, costs and outcomes directly attributable to nursing care can be easily isolated. Nurse midwifery has consistently delivered care equal to or of higher quality than physician care at a lower cost (Jacox, 1988). For some time, nurse midwives have been eligible to receive direct reimbursement by third-party payers. At present, 25 states have legislation to authorize reimbursement to nurse practitioners from private and commercial insurers. Nurse practitioners can receive Medicaid reimbursement in 38 states, and 11 other states plan to have such legislation by 1993 (Pearson, 1992).

Third-party reimbursement mechanisms allow for evaluation of the cost effectiveness of care provided by nurse midwives and nurse practitioners. Similar developments are under way to "cost out" services provided in inpatient settings. At present, services of clinical nurse specialists practicing in designated rural areas can be reimbursed through Medicare (Sullivan, 1992).

Reimbursement for nursing services is seen by many nurse leaders as an essential step in validating the major contribution nursing makes to health care. Direct payment for nursing care further legitimizes professional nursing practice. Nurses will be challenged to develop accurate systems that can account for processes and outcomes in the provision of nursing care.

Technologic Advances and Ethical Considerations

The context of perinatal care is changing rapidly in response to advances in medical technology. The technology of perinatal care has developed dramatically in the last 15 years. Technologic advances include widespread introduction and use of EFM, amniocentesis, the advent of ultrasonography, in vitro fertilization, and most recently, fetal surgery. The appropriate application of technology in care is a central concern to the perinatal nurse (see the accompanying display). These technologies are discussed in this text.

Advances in technology create new opportunities for saving and enhancing the quality of life. However, each technologic advance also presents risks to the provision of safe and humane care. Ethical dilemmas can be described as situations in which the patient's rights and the professional's obligations conflict. Such situations are particularly common in perinatal care because the well-being of both the pregnant woman and the fetus must be considered. Although ethical dilemmas confront nurses in all specialties, the juxtaposition of life and death characteristic of birth highlights moral questions.

For instance, the issue of abortion has been debated for centuries. More recently, the question of whether a pregnant woman has the right to refuse treatment for herself or her fetus has become an issue, now that procedures such as cesarean delivery and fetal surgery can be performed. When such situations arise, nurses often have little time to consider the ethical and legal issues and make a decision. Many hospitals have established ethics committees as a forum for discussing, analyzing, and evaluating approaches to ethical dilemmas.

Nurses in perinatal care are likely to be involved in caring for individuals and families who will be directly affected by technologic advances. Both legal and ethical concerns will arise. Nurses need to consider carefully the implications of the care they deliver. The individual nurse must identify areas of practice that challenge her personal beliefs.

Appropriate Use of Technology in Nursing Care

In the past two decades, advances in technology have resulted in the availability of new equipment and procedures for use in the assessment of patients. Until scientific documentation validating these advances is available, nursing care must be based on proven methods. Guidelines, policies, procedures, and protocols must be developed for use of technology such as electronic fetal monitoring, pulse oximetry, and hemodynamic monitoring in the care of women and neonates. The Committee on Practice supports innovation that involves the use of technologic advances in the nursing assessment of patients. The use of such equipment and procedures, however, does not replace "hands-on-care" of the patient by the nursing staff. Nursing process must remain the foundation for the provision of nursing care.

Approved by the Committee on Practice, AWHONN—The Association of Women's Health, Obstetric, and Neonatal Nurses, September 1991. Reprinted by permission.

The perinatal nurse must also distinguish between true ethical positions and personal preferences. This exploration allows nurses to avoid imposing personal value systems on others.

Professional Accountability and Liability

Increased attention to professional accountability and liability in health care directly affects the perinatal nurse. As a professional, the nurse is accountable for nursing actions and may be held liable for performing activities in a careless, uninformed, or unprofessional manner. Liability results from placing the patient at risk, even if the nurse follows a physician's order. Physicians, and increasingly nurses, are finding that their professional practice is open to scrutiny and may be legally challenged by consumers of health care. Current perinatal care takes place within a social context in which both medical miracles and medical malpractice are equally likely to occur.

In many legal cases, consumers expect the "perfect" birth experience and newborn outcome. When the unexpected happens, parents may look to the courts. This reality leads to "defensive" health care. Procedures may be done for fear of potential litigation should something go wrong. One example of this problem may be seen in the practice of cesarean delivery. Older, more affluent women who had private insurance and delivered in private hospitals were 20% more likely to have a cesarean delivery than were clinic and uninsured patients, regardless of risk status (Taffel, Placek, & Kosary, 1992). Some believe that this pattern reflects physician concern that older, more affluent patients are more likely to sue, so more aggressive medical interventions are chosen, regardless of objective risk.

The nurse must be aware of legal responsibilities in practice. Contemporary health care requires the nurse practice based on a sound knowledge base, responsible communication and documentation of care, and concerned action in the patient's best interest. Chapter 2 discusses professional accountability and liability in more detail. Throughout this text, legal considerations in perinatal nursing practice will be highlighted.

Changing Gender Roles and Family Structure

Changes in gender role expectations and family structures in the United States contribute to the changing context of perinatal care. Middle-class and upwardly mobile men and women are choosing to have smaller families and to delay childbearing until they are financially established. Women continue to enter the work force, stay in it longer, and return to work sooner after childbirth. More than half the American women in families with children under 5 years of age are employed outside the home. Factors such as increasing incidence of separation and divorce, the lack of high-quality or affordable child care, and the changing expectations of women and men create role strain for many parents (Mercer, 1990).

On the other hand, changes in gender role expectations have positive effects as well. Men and women may choose to become single parents or to remain childless. These options were not socially acceptable for many adults a decade or two ago. Women are pursuing careers in demanding professions and achieving rewarding family lives. Men have become more involved in pregnancy and childbirth in recent years. Although the vast majority of primary caretakers of small children are still women, the number of men taking increased responsibility for daily child care and home management duties is on the rise. In some areas of the country, nurses working in well-baby clinics may see either the mother or the father bring an infant in for routine health care (Mercer, 1990).

Changes in family functions and gender role expectations are particularly apparent in the updated practices of health care delivery to childbearing families. Examples of changes in practice habits include elimination of routine separation of parents and infants and reversal of the previous near-total exclusion of fathers from childbirth and early parenting. Practices now focus on family needs during childbirth and emphasize the normal, natural aspects of childbearing. Family considerations are of major importance in perinatal nursing practice and will be highlighted throughout this text.

Family-Centered Perinatal Care

Perinatal care providers are challenged to use technologic advances in an effort to prevent or control maternal or neonate complications, while at the same time provide care in a humane environment supporting the childbearing family. A strong influence on the provision of perinatal care is the philosophy of family-centered perinatal care. This philosophy emphasizes the need to meet the psychosocial needs of the family as well as to promote and protect the physiologic well-being of mother and child. Family-centered care is a direct result of the consumer movement in the 1950s advocating less intervention in obstetrics. Childbirth is viewed as a life transition, which for the most part is a natural and healthy event.

Family-centered perinatal care is defined as the delivery of quality health care that focuses on and accommodates both the physical and psychosocial needs of the pregnant woman, the family, and the neonate. Most health care organizations in the United States have formally recognized that family-centered perinatal care is an essential element in providing quality obstetric care.

However, this consensus is meaningless unless this philosophy is integrated into practice. The effectiveness of family-centered perinatal care ultimately rests on the commitment of the individual professionals and their interactions with the families in their care. In fact, the important difference between traditional obstetric care and family-centered perinatal care is *attitudinal*. Family-centered care is based on supporting the integrity of the family while individualizing care to promote individual and family health. Thus, it is possible to use this approach in every setting and for each individual and family. In many areas of the United States, certain elements of family-centered perinatal care have already become standard practice. Examples include father and family member participation in birth and early extended parent–neonate contact. In other areas of the United States, progress has been slower.

It is especially significant that aspects of family-centered perinatal care may still be relatively unavailable to women who develop complications during childbearing. For example, partners may be permitted to remain with the woman during labor and birth in uncomplicated situations, but they may be routinely excluded from the labor and birth room during administration of regional anesthesia or during operative deliveries. Neonates who require more frequent nursing assessments of body temperature may be moved to the newborn nursery for "observation" rather than keeping the neonate in a suitably warm environment at the mother's bedside. There is still a tendency on the part of many care providers to view birth as a medical emergency first. However, if care providers are committed to the values of family-centered perinatal care, taking steps to counteract the stress of medical complications with supportive family-oriented care would seem to be a logical step. Families requiring intensive medical intervention may benefit the most from supportive care. Nursing has participated in making many changes to date and needs to continue to provide leadership in working with other care providers and consumers to implement safe, high-quality, family-centered perinatal care.

Family-centered perinatal care reflects an underlying philosophy about the nature of childbirth and families. This philosophy is consistent with the holistic, person-centered perspective of nursing and therefore easily forms the basis of nursing in perinatal care. However, the family-centered perspective is not limited to nursing care but should extend to all professionals who come in contact with childbearing families. The principles central to the philosophy of family-centered perinatal care are shown in the accompanying display.

Birth Options and Alternatives. Parents and professionals often describe aspects of family-centered care as options or alternatives. This reflects the underlying philosophy that families have the right to make choices related to the prenatal and birth care they receive. The nurse must realize, however, that unexamined and potentially unsafe practices cannot be considered legitimate options in any care setting. The nurse is responsible for assessing possible risks and benefits of birth practices and advising families of any known risks.

Many options can be managed safely in the hospital setting if the nurse objectively evaluates safety needs and takes steps to ensure these needs are met. The nurse must recognize that resistance to change in routine practices may be based more on habit or a desire to control events than on actual risks. The nurse keeps in mind the goal of a healthy woman, newborn, and family and individualizes care toward that goal.

Family Participation in Birth. One of the most widely recognized trends in family-centered perinatal care has been the dramatic change in the level of family participation in pregnancy and childbirth. Attendance by the father or partner at prenatal classes and birth has become common in most parts of the country (Fig. 1-3). Participation of men in the childbirth experience was a rare occurrence only 25 years ago. Increasing interest in active involvement of other family members, such as grandparents and siblings, is more common today.

Principles of Family-Centered Perinatal Care

The family is capable of making decisions about care during the childbearing period, given adequate information and professional support. This principle requires care providers to enter into a partnership with the family, rather than assuming the role of an "authority" on which the family becomes dependent. Education is essential, and families are included in discussions about care and in decision-making.

In most cases, childbirth is a normal, healthy event in the life of a family. This principle focuses on the professional's attention on maintaining the health of the woman and family during the childbearing cycle. Pregnancy and birth are viewed as states of health that may require preventive or supportive care, rather than as illness states that must be "treated." Health maintenance cannot occur without the active participation of the family members themselves, so the professional must emphasize teaching and self-care activities.

Childbirth is the beginning of a new set of important family relationships. This principle requires the professional to organize care in a way that enhances positive interactions among parents, the newborn, and other family members and minimizes strain on family resources. The professional's concern extends beyond physical needs in recognition of the fact that health also has social and psychological dimensions.

McKay, S., & Phillips, C. (1984). Family-centered maternity care. *Rockville: Aspen Publishing. Reprinted with permission.*

Participation of Partners in Vaginal and Cesarean Births. The more traditional roles of men and women are changing. Men are taking a more active participatory role in the birthing and upbringing of their children. During labor, the partner can lend physical and emotional support to the woman. Active involvement of the partner has become the norm in many hospitals and birthing centers today. Childbirth classes now offer support classes for partners to discuss their own needs and concerns related to pregnancy and birth. Partners learn how to be supportive while attending prenatal classes. Even "unprepared" partners can provide effective support to laboring women if they receive supportive nursing care. (See Chapter 18 for a more detailed discussion of preparation for childbirth.)

The father's role as labor coach has been an area of interest to nurse researchers. Unfortunately, the father's labor coach role in childbirth has been overemphasized at the expense of recognizing that labor and birth are significant events for the father in his own right. Fathers respond to

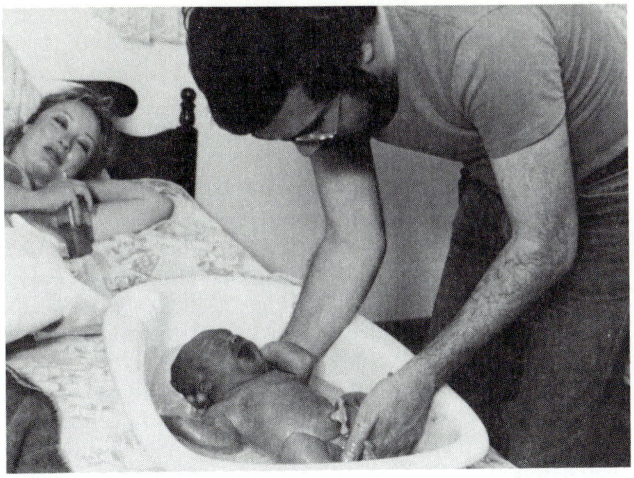

Figure 1-3.
The father bathes his newborn moments after birth in a homelike setting. (Photo by BABES, Inc.)

childbirth in a variety of ways. Some fathers participate willingly and actively support their partners, requiring little assistance from the nurse. Others find this role difficult, preferring the role of passive bystander during the event (May, 1989; Chapman, 1991). Even a "prepared" father may feel inadequate in the role of labor support person. He may lack knowledge about specific ways to increase his partner's comfort. Supporting the father in a role in which he appears to be most comfortable is a primary responsibility of the nurse. This underscores the need for the nurse to be aware of the distinct individual needs of fathers experiencing the pregnancy, labor, and birth.

During the past three decades, participation of partners during cesarean birth has become more common in some parts of the country. During cesarean delivery, the partner is able to support the woman by being with her throughout the procedure. Holding and showing the neonate to the mother for the first time is a joyous event for most couples. Aside from supporting the woman, partners may also experience personal satisfaction and an increase in self-esteem from participating in a cesarean birth (May & Sollid, 1984). Physicians and hospital administrators may oppose and resist couples' desire to share the cesarean birth experience. This opposition stems, in part, from concerns about the emotional distress partners might experience during emergency procedures. Of greater concern is the potential for lawsuits brought by partners who observe events during the procedure. This opposition continues despite the fact that such incidents are extremely rare and remain undocumented in the health care literature.

Support People for Labor and Birth. A major feature of family-centered perinatal care is the presence of a supportive person during labor and birth. This person can either be the father, partner, another family member, a friend, or a trained labor support person, such as a childbirth educator or experienced nurse. The effects of a supportive companion on the progress of labor and birth have been documented. The continuous presence of a support person during labor has been shown to be associated with shorter labors, fewer complications, less need for medical intervention during labor, and more positive maternal perceptions of the birth experience (McNiven, Hodnett, & O'Brien-Pallas, 1992). These benefits may be a result of a reduction in secretion of stress hormones or catecholamines during labor. Catecholamines are thought to impair uterine blood flow. This may result in disruption of labor and birth and may contribute to fetal distress.

Participation of Siblings in Childbirth. Family participation in birth has recently been extended to siblings. Since 1976, many hospitals in the United States have allowed sibling participation at birth in alternative birth settings. This is yet another example of consumer demand for options (Fig. 1-4). Although research has not proved this, no studies have

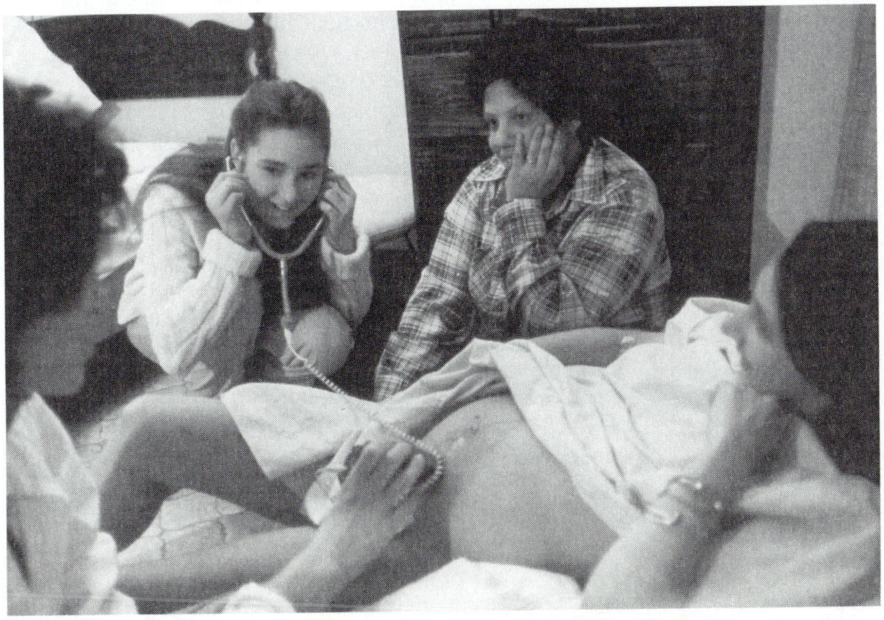

Figure 1-4.
An adolescent listens to the fetal heart beat of her soon-to-be-born sibling as she actively participates in her mother's labor. Participation by siblings in childbirth is gaining popularity across the United States. (Photo by Kathy Sloane.)

documented harmful effects of sibling participation (see the Nursing Research display).

A family's decision to include a child at birth is often based on cultural attitudes, the parents' desires, and the support (or lack of it) by health care providers (Murphy, 1988). Parents who wish to involve the sibling at childbirth view birth as a family event and feel that excluding the older child detracts from family unity. Proponents of sibling participation believe that family bonding may be increased and sibling rivalry may be lessened when the older child is present at the birth. Careful and thorough preparation of siblings who will be present at labor and birth is important. Evidence of preparation of the sibling is required in many settings before the sibling can participate in the birth (Murphy, 1988).

Nursing Research

Sibling Preparation and Adjustment to a Newborn

This study examined whether sibling preparation for the birth of a newborn made a difference in the mother's ability to cope with her children and in the sibling's behavior toward the newborn. Two groups of 20 mothers and their first-born children were included in this study. Mothers were asked to complete an instrument that assessed behaviors most likely to be displayed by children 3 to 5 years of age when confronted with a new sibling. These behaviors included acting younger than their age, crying a lot, eating less at meals, whining, demanding attention, clinging, acting sullen or moody, and having sleep disruptions. Mothers also completed an instrument measuring how well they thought they coped with their child's behavior. Only one group of mothers and children received a specialized sibling preparation class. All children and mothers were tested a month after the birth of the new sibling.

Results of this study suggested that the prepared mothers reported significantly fewer sibling rivalry behaviors in their older child than mothers who did not attend preparation class. Further, mothers of children who received the preparation class were significantly more likely to report that they could cope well with their older child's behavior. Preparation of children and parents for the birth of a sibling may have beneficial effects on family interaction by reducing conflicts between the mother and older child. Including sibling preparation into a family-centered program of perinatal care seems appropriate, based on these findings.

Fortier, J., Carson, V., Will, S., & Shubkagel, B. (1991). Adjustment to a newborn: Sibling preparation makes a difference. *Journal of Obstetric, Gynecologic, and Neonatal Nursing,* 20(1), 73–79.

Extended Early Parent–Newborn Contact. During the 1950s and 1960s, new parents were routinely separated from each other and from their neonates during the hospital stay. This separation occurred primarily because of concerns about infection control and partly because of the large amounts of medication used during labor and birth. Some medications used during labor reduced the responsiveness of women and their neonates in the period immediately after birth.

With the advent of family-centered perinatal care, early parent–newborn contact is becoming standard practice in most settings. Early contact may have benefits for the neonate and parents. During the first hour after birth and again for periods over the first days of life, the neonate is particularly alert and able to absorb and respond to stimulation. Further, some researchers suggested that parents were more receptive to their neonates immediately after birth and that contact during this time would facilitate the process of parent-to-infant attachment.

This phenomenon became popularly known as parent–infant bonding. Bonding was described in a 1981 book by Klaus and Kennell, two pediatricians. There has not been subsequent research to support their conclusions that early parent–neonate contact positively affects attachment. However, the concept of bonding found its way into the popular culture as well as into professional nursing practice. It is not uncommon now to find both parents and nurses who believe strongly that early parent–neonate contact is extremely important for the establishment of positive parenting.

Many parents want to be together with their neonate in the first hours after birth. Often this is an excellent time to assist the mother with first attempts at breastfeeding and to teach both parents about their neonate. However, if early parent–newborn contact is not possible because of maternal or neonatal complications, parents need reassurance that they can make up for this lack of contact. If neonatal intensive care is required, parent–neonate contact needs to be encouraged. Fathers, partners, or other family members should be included if the family wishes (Rempusheski, 1990; Griffin, 1990). Nursing interventions to support the initiation of positive parenting behaviors are discussed in depth in Chapters 21, 28, and 31.

Achievements and Challenges in Family-Centered Care

Considerable progress has been made in achieving some of the goals of family-centered care. Policies restricting participation by fathers and partners in childbirth have been eliminated in many facilities. Many institutions have established alternative birthing rooms or centers. The demand for nurse midwifery services continues to increase as nurse midwives establish themselves in practice across the country. More physicians are willing to discuss "routine procedures" with women and their partners.

However, new problems will arise as advanced technology in obstetric care continues to become available. Some facilities continue to restrict father or partner attendance during certain procedures, such as administration of regional anesthesia or during cesarean birth. These are times that women report they need their partner's support most. Evidence indicates that the time labor and delivery nurses spend in direct supportive contact with women and families may be decreasing because of other demands on nursing time imposed by increasing use of technology in care (McNiven, Hodnett, & O'Brien-Pallas, 1992).

Nurse midwives continue to face opposition and criticism from obstetricians when applying for hospital privileges. Despite evidence that nurse midwifery can provide high-quality, less expensive perinatal care for most childbearing families because most women are obstetrically low risk, practices tend to be limited by lack of support from the medical community (Schlatter, 1991).

Family-centered care is restricted in large part to "normal" childbearing women and their families. Women who may be at risk for complications in childbearing are often told they cannot have certain choices. Often this decision is made by the care provider based on habit rather than an objective evaluation of the risk and benefit of the practice for this particular woman and her family. Sometimes, solving the safety problems can be accomplished more easily than changing the attitudes of a resistant professional.

To make further progress, consumers and concerned providers will need to collaborate. Support of family-centered care by health care professionals is ideal. Nursing can provide leadership in efforts to encourage family-centered practices. The goals of professional nursing practice—the diagnosis and treatment of human responses to actual and potential threats to health—are consistent with the needs of childbearing families.

Several factors influence contemporary perinatal care and the practice of perinatal nursing. Social factors, such as ability to pay for care, maldistribution of health care services, and economic factors, such as the high cost of health care, especially high-technology intensive care, are important. Ethical and legal considerations have a direct effect on the provision of care to childbearing women and their families. Changing family roles and the demand for more family-centered care are important additional factors. Family-centered care is essential in providing comprehensive perinatal nursing care.

Implications for Nursing Care

As perinatal care has evolved and as technology has become more complex, the perinatal nurse has become a specialist, proficient at a high level of skilled care. Concurrently, the consumer is demanding a more humane and family-centered philosophy in perinatal care. The nurse must respond with caring, compassion, and concern for family needs. All these changes require the professional nurse to apply a holistic approach in nursing practice. Effective care is challenging and offers a unique opportunity to use a full range of nursing skills.

Nursing has been at the forefront in acknowledging that people, whenever possible, should be actively involved in their own health care. This person-centered philosophy is particularly evident in nursing practice in perinatal care. Nurses currently provide many of the direct services most valued by families, including primary care giving, prenatal education, sibling preparation, and midwifery, to name a few.

Deficiencies in the current high-technology, high-risk emphasis in medical care can be countered by focusing on humanistic concerns, preventive practice, and the use of effective, less expensive, and less technologically oriented models of care. John Naisbitt, a futurist, pointed out in his book *Megatrends* (1982) that as technology increases, so does the need for intensive human contact. He suggested that a "high-tech, high-touch" philosophy is required with increasing technologic advances. Naisbitt specifically cited nursing as an example of that combination of high-technology expertise and intensive human caring.

Nursing has historically provided the "care" in health care. The practice of nurse midwifery exemplifies a holistic, health-oriented, family-centered approach to perinatal care. Traditional nursing practice in perinatal care has been fragmented to a large extent, often preventing the nurse from caring for women and their newborns together throughout the childbirth experience. Nursing may be too quick to adopt the language and philosophy of high technology. Nurses may eventually lose their ability to assess high-risk from low-risk women using noninvasive methods. Some nurses may fail to develop nursing strategies to prevent and treat undesirable conditions that are within the scope of nursing's responsibility to manage, simply because a medical approach exists. Holistic care contends that the major nursing objective in the care of women and infants is to keep childbirth and infancy as normal as possible. Attention should be focused on discovering how to maximize factors that promote physical, emotional, and spiritual health.

Outstanding examples of the power of proactive nursing research and practice can be seen in the work of some pioneers in perinatal nursing. Andrews (1980) and Roberts and associates (1983) conducted important research on the effects of maternal position and ambulation. Effects on uterine efficiency and on the position of the fetus in the maternal pelvis during labor were studied. Maternal ambulation during labor increased uterine efficiency and helped shorten labor. Use of maternal positioning (sidelying and on hands and knees) during labor was also helpful in correcting for fetal positions that slowed labor progress. This research developed knowledge that enables the nurse to alter the course of labor and birth directly without using invasive means.

More recent examples of this trend include the continuing work of Andrews and Chrzanowski (1990). These researchers conducted a study that suggested women who labor in an upright position have shorter labors with comparable maternal comfort and neonatal safety when compared with women who labor in recumbent positions. Another team of researchers is developing a method that uses auscultation as an alternative to the use of more expensive EFM equipment for assessing fetal well-being (Paine, Benedict, Strobino, Gegor, & Larson, 1992).

Nurses are researching ways to minimize the negative effects and maximize the positive effects of high-technology procedures such as cesarean birth and EFM. In the future, nurses need to take more responsibility for discovering how to prevent the need for such interventions. Controlling health care costs in perinatal care, counteracting the increasingly technologic approaches to medical care, and expanding the scope of nursing research are exciting opportunities and challenges for nurses. Through these activities, nurses can make a significant contribution to improving the quality of care delivered to women, infants, and their families.

The critical passage into parenthood provides the perinatal nurse with a unique opportunity for personal and professional growth. The quality of nursing care contributes directly to how well or how poorly families begin their transition into parenthood. In the practice of family-centered nursing, the nurse's role also extends into the postbirth period. The nurse can act as a liaison with other community resources available to parents. Resources include parenting and counseling services, breastfeeding assistance, well-baby services, and parent education and support groups. Because new families tend to be vulnerable during this transition period, the perinatal nurse's support or lack of support will have a great impact the family's experience in the health care system.

The philosophy and practices of family-centered perinatal care reflect nursing at its best. The role of the nurse in perinatal care involves education, caregiving, advocacy, and the planning and implementation of changes in health care delivery. Nurses are now actively contributing to changes in care by developing and evaluating innovation through clinical practice and research. The quality of birth care in the future depends in large part on how well nurses continue to contribute to this quiet revolution in perinatal care.

Chapter Summary

Social trends have had a dramatic impact on the context of perinatal care and how nursing practice is influenced by these trends. The future certainly holds more technologic development and discoveries that save lives and enhance the quality of life. Unfortunately, developments in medical and health care often hold potential for harm as well as for good. The fact that some recent technologic advances in maternity care have been balanced by the trend toward family-centered, health-oriented care is a hopeful sign.

Developments in technology, including in vitro fertilization, EFM, fetal surgery, and neonatal intensive care have dramatically changed perinatal care and have created, saved, and prolonged lives unimaginable 25 years ago. The changing economic picture in health care has affected services to families. Prospective payment and direct reimbursement for nursing services offer opportunities to deliver more cost-effective care. High costs and heroic medical interventions to save a few conflict with the need for low-cost, widely accessible care for all. Emerging technologies have created ethical questions that consumers and professionals will need to address.

Study Questions

1. *What three historical trends in the United States have directly affected the current organization of perinatal care? What is the nature of their influence?*
2. *What are possible future trends in health care costs?*
3. *What is family-centered perinatal care? Why did it evolve?*
4. *What are the principles that underlie the philosophy of family-centered perinatal care?*
5. *Why is it important to have a supportive person present during labor?*
6. *Why is early parent–newborn contact important?*
7. *What special nursing responsibilities are related to new trends and technologies introduced to current birth practices?*
8. *What is the nurse's role when parents request new or unusual types of care?*

References

Andrews, C. (1980). Changing fetal position. *Journal of Nurse-Midwifery, 25*, 7–10.

Andrews, C., & Chrzanowski, M. (1990). Maternal position, labor and comfort. *Applied Nursing Research, 3*(1), 7–13.

Chapman, L. (1991). Searching: Expectant fathers' experiences during labor and birth. *Journal of Perinatal and Neonatal Nursing, 4*, 21–25.

Goldsmith, J. (1984). *Childbirth wisdom from the world's oldest societies*. New York: Congdon and Weed.

Cohen, E. (1991). Nursing case management: Does it pay? *Journal of Nursing Administration, 21*(4), 20–26.

Griffin, T. (1990). Nurse barriers to parenting in the special care nursery. *Journal of Perinatal and Neonatal Nursing, 4*(2), 56–68.

Klaus, M., & Kennell, J. (1981). *Parent–infant bonding*. St. Louis: C. V. Mosby.

Jacox, A. (1988). The OTA report: A policy analysis. *Nursing Outlook, 35*(6), 262–268.

Lutz, S. (1991, May 13). Practitioners are filling in for scarce physicians. *Modern Healthcare*, pp. 24–30.

Mathews, J., & Zadek, K. (1991). The alternative birth movement in the United States: History and current status. *Women and Health, 17*(1), 39–56.

May, K. (1989). The father role: Is it time to fire the coach? *Childbirth Educator, 2*, 30.

May, K., & Sollid, D. (1984). Unanticipated cesarean birth: From the father's perspective. *Birth, 11*(2), 87–96.

McNiven, P., Hodnett, E., & O'Brien-Pallas, L. (1992). Supporting women in labor: A work sampling study of activities of labor and delivery nurses. *Birth, 19*(1), 3–9.

Mercer, R. (1990). *Parents at risk*. New York: Springer.

Morrison, J. (1990). Preterm birth: A puzzle worth solving. *Obstetrics and Gynecology, 76*(1), 5–12S.

Murphy, S. (1988). *A study of sibling relationships in the perinatal period*. Unpublished doctoral dissertation, University of California, San Francisco.

Naisbitt, J. (1982). *Megatrends*. New York: Warner Books.

Pearson, J. (1992). 1990–91 update: How each state stands on legislative issues affecting advanced nursing practice. *Nurse Practitioner, 16* (1), 11–17.

Paine, L., Benedict, M., Strobino, D., Gegor, C., & Larson, E. (1992). A comparison of the auscultated acceleration test and the nonstress test as predictors of perinatal outcomes. *Nursing Research*, *41*(2), 87–91.

Roberts, J., Mendez-Bauer, C., & Wodell, D. (1983). The effects of uterine contractility and efficiency. *Birth*, *10*(4), 243–248.

Rempusheski, V. (1990). The role of the extended family in parenting: A focus on grandparents of preterm infants. *Journal of Perinatal and Neonatal Nursing*, *4*(2), 43–56.

Schlatter, B. (1991). Nurse-midwifery: The profession and the challenges it faces. *Journal of Perinatal and Neonatal Nursing*, *5*(3), 25–33.

Sullivan, E. (1992). Nurse practitioners and reimbursement. *Nursing and Health Care*, *13*(5), 236–239.

Taffel, S., Placek, P., & Kosary, C. (1992). U.S. cesarean section rates 1990: An update. *Birth*, *19*(1), 21–24.

Wertz, R., & Wertz, D. (1992). *Lying-in: A history of childbirth in America* (2nd ed.). New Haven: Yale University Press.

Suggested Readings

ANA. (1991). *Nursing's agenda for health care reform*. Washington, DC: Author.

Harvey, M. (1992). Humanizing the intensive care unit experience. *NAACOG's Clinical Issues in Perinatal and Women's Health Nursing*, *3*(3), 369–376.

Johnson, S. (1992). Ethical dilemma: A patient refuses a life-saving cesarean. *American Journal of Maternal Child Nursing*, *17*(3), 121–125.

Mathews, J., & Zadek, K. (1991). The alternative birth movement in the United States: History and current status. *Women and health*, *17*(1), 39–56.

Novak, J. (1990). Facilitating nurturant fathering behavior in the NICU. *Journal of Perinatal and Neonatal Nursing*, *4*(2), 68–78.

CHAPTER 2

Conceptual Foundations of Maternal and Neonatal Nursing

Learning Objectives

After studying the material in this chapter, the student will be able to:

- Discuss the advantages of using a conceptual framework in clinical practice.
- Explain the concept of adaptation and discuss why adaptation theory may be useful in caring for childbearing families.
- Explain the nursing process and its relationship to the nursing care plan.
- List nursing diagnoses that may be applicable to the care of childbearing families.
- Describe managed care and explain how it is being used in the care of childbearing families.
- State the importance of teaching as a nursing strategy in perinatal care.

Key Terms

theoretical or conceptual framework
adaptation
nursing diagnosis
collaborative problem
managed care
case management
managed care path
expected outcome

As a health care profession, nursing shares responsibility for the promotion of human health. As a profession, recognition of standards of practice and self-regulation through involvement in professional and specialty organizations must therefore also apply to nursing. Other characteristics of professional status address the knowledge base common to a professional group and the organizing frameworks within which these professionals practice.

This chapter focuses on the use of an identifiable knowledge and theory base in planning and providing nursing care. The use of a systematic approach to practice in perinatal nursing care is described. Although many elements addressed in this chapter are common to all fields of nursing, some have particular importance in the care of childbearing families.

Knowledge and Theory Base for Practice

Nursing practice is based on knowledge and theory about how human beings respond to actual or potential threats to health. This knowledge base and the theories that organize it are constantly changing. Change is part of scientific and professional practice because new knowledge is continually being developed and old methods are continually being reexamined in light of new knowledge. The development of new knowledge in health care is especially dramatic. Health care professionals must update their knowledge base continually to incorporate these changes. The nurse is accountable for maintaining and updating a current knowledge base through continuing study and professional education. As noted in Chapter 1, the scientific advances related to obstetric and perinatal care are proceeding at such a dramatic pace that keeping abreast of the latest developments is a challenge to every professional.

The knowledge and theory base for perinatal nursing

encompasses the physiologic, psychological, developmental, and social aspects of childbearing in the context of the family. "Family" may be defined in many ways. However, from a nursing perspective, care is based on the woman's definitions of family—that is, on whom she identifies as most significant in her life—and not on some "objective" definition. The knowledge base required for perinatal nursing is broad. In the process of giving perinatal care, the nurse may interact with people of all ages, from a variety of cultures, and of varying educational backgrounds and expectations, because family units vary in all those ways.

The knowledge base required for caring for childbearing families is broad. Therefore, the professional nurse must have a way of organizing this knowledge. The nurse looks at families and the health challenges they face in a systematic fashion. The following section discusses the importance of conceptual frameworks and theories in nursing, emphasizing adaptation as a useful organizing principle in perinatal care.

Use of Conceptual Frameworks and Theories

A professional discipline operates from a body of knowledge that is developed and organized in such a way that it can be used by its practitioners. Such bodies of knowledge are usually defined by commonly accepted views or perspectives. Often these perspectives are seen in conceptual frameworks and theories used in practice. These perspectives change over time as the field develops and more knowledge is generated.

For example, medicine has historically operated from a rather narrow biologic perspective on health and illness. This view emphasized the physical sciences and concentrated on biophysical methods of diagnosis and treatment of illness. The medical model has been successful in stimulating research and opening new frontiers of treatment. However, as chronic conditions and diseases of life-style become the dominant health threats, other perspectives integrating behavioral and psychological explanations of illness have begun to gain acceptance in medicine.

Nursing is a young, still rapidly evolving field, and its knowledge base is just beginning to be developed and organized. There is still no one guiding perspective in nursing. Much progress has been made in recent years with a widely accepted definition of nursing and with the identification of *person, health, environment*, and *nursing* as the major domains of interest for nursing. The process of knowledge development in nursing is well under way. Conceptual frameworks and theories are increasingly used in nursing practice as a way to help organize necessary knowledge and provide quality nursing care (Meleis, 1991).

The terms *conceptual framework* and *theory* simply refer to the organizing tools available to the professional. A conceptual framework is defined as a global view of phenomena of interest in a field. A conceptual framework includes *concepts*, which are mental images or ideas, and a set of statements that show how these concepts are linked together. Individual nurses, as they become expert in their practice, often develop their own conceptual frameworks or their own way of looking at women and families.

A theory can be thought of as a more specific and better-defined version of a conceptual framework. A theory is also made up of concepts linked together by statements, but concepts in a theory are well-defined, specific, and usually measurable in some way. In addition, the relationships between concepts in a theory are more precisely and systematically stated. This allows theories to be tested and refined through research. Conceptual frameworks are usually too general and their concepts too vaguely defined to be tested scientifically.

Adaptation: An Organizing Perspective

Throughout this text, *adaptation* is used as an organizing perspective on the childbearing family. Adaptation theory is a widely accepted perspective in psychology and has provided the basis for work on stress and coping, crisis intervention, and other widely recognized areas of research and practice. Nurse theorists have proposed and tested nursing models based on adaptation theory (Roy, 1989). This text uses a conceptual framework focusing on adaptation (St. Louis University School of Nursing, 1979) as a way to help organize the broad and varied knowledge base needed to provide nursing care to childbearing families.

Adaptation is defined here as the capacity to modify behavior and to change the environment, when necessary, to meet needs. Adaptation is a basic characteristic of life. Adaptation is an active process of maintaining optimum conditions over time in relationship to constantly changing demands.

Adaptation occurs in individuals and families and involves physiologic, psychological, sociocultural, and spiritual dimensions. Many life changes require adaptation in most or all dimensions simultaneously. The quality of adaptation is a function of the nature of the stimulus and the dimensions it influences as well as the individual's capacity for change.

The particular characteristics of individual adaptation express the person's uniqueness; thus, human adaptation is endlessly variable. Depending on the resources available to the individual, adaptive responses can be adequate or inadequate, functional or dysfunctional. Health, illness, and survival depend on the quality of adaptation that is possible for the individual or family. Health implies functional or effective responses that result in a dynamic equilibrium, characterized by maximum potential for living and wholeness. Illness implies dysfunctional or ineffective responses that result in disequilibrium, characterized by reduced potential for living and by distress.

To some extent, the individual determines what stimuli will be addressed, the mode of adaptation, and the pace of change. However, in general, the greater the number of changes occurring in a given period of time, the more difficult it is for the individual to adapt. The process itself may be stressful, even when the outcome of adaptation is positive. Previous successful adaptation is likely to expand the individual's repertoire of adaptive responses. Adaptation contributes to flexibility and enhanced ability to meet future demands. In contrast, inability to adapt effectively reduces the individual's resources and compromises well-being. Future adaptation may then become even more difficult.

Adaptation in the Childbearing Family

For several reasons, as will be discussed in later chapters, adaptation is an especially useful organizing perspective when considering the childbearing family. Childbearing and early child rearing are normally periods of concentrated and sometimes intense physiologic and psychological change. The pregnant woman must adapt to hormonal changes followed by pronounced physical and emotional changes. Her partner must also adjust to the woman's changes and to the new expectations and pressures of becoming a parent. The experience of pregnancy touches other family members who must accept the reality of the expected child and the resultant role changes.

The concept of adaptation is a useful organizing perspective not only for clinical practice but also for research and scholarship in perinatal nursing. Many of the nurse scientists whose work appears in the Suggested Readings list for this chapter, and which will be discussed further in upcoming chapters, have made substantial contributions to knowledge about childbearing families. These contributions result from research that has included elements of adaptation theory.

Research and Scholarship

A profession requires vigorous activity by its members in research and scholarship, which are essential to any profession because they build and renew the knowledge base necessary for practice. Research is defined here as the systematic collection, analysis, and reporting of new information. Scholarship is defined as the systematic study, evaluation, and use of existing information. Until recently, most of the knowledge taught in perinatal nursing was knowledge "borrowed" from other disciplines. However, as more nurses prepare to engage in research and scholarship, that trend is changing (Meleis, 1991).

Although large-scale nursing research projects require additional preparation in research methods at the graduate level, nurses in clinical practice are in the best position to identify pressing nursing care problems. Nurses are able to observe and document effects of different types of nursing care in the practice setting. Nurses in practice can also make a significant contribution to the field by systematic analysis and reporting of effects of nursing care in single cases. This is needed because the profession is only beginning to describe and categorize nursing problems or diagnoses. Published case studies enable clinicians to compare interventions and outcomes and to share knowledge that would otherwise not be communicated outside one particular setting. This type of communication and comparison of practice adds to the accumulation of nursing knowledge. Sharing new knowledge enables nurses to develop and test solutions to clinical problems much more rapidly than practicing in isolation (May, 1991).

Perinatal nurses are focusing concerted attention on problems in clinical practice. Emphasis on scholarship and organized research efforts have increased dramatically as staff nurses are encouraged to incorporate new knowledge into clinical care. Nurses in clinical leadership positions in many teaching hospitals are expected to engage in clinical research. Specialty journals now regularly publish scholarly clinical and research articles. Nursing organizations are identifying priority research problems facing nurses in clinical practice (see the accompanying display on the next page).

The process of knowledge generation is especially exciting in perinatal care because the scope of needed knowledge is broad and multifaceted. Throughout this text, nursing research will be highlighted in research displays to acquaint the student with current work in the field.

Professional practice in any field is based on an accepted organized body of knowledge and theory. Nursing has begun to identify and develop the knowledge essential for provision of nursing care. Foundations of practice in perinatal nursing include an understanding of the usefulness of conceptual frameworks in practice. In this text, adaptation theory is emphasized as a particularly useful framework for understanding and addressing the needs of childbearing women and their families. Adaptation as an organizing framework for perinatal nursing and the importance of research and scholarship in professional practice are presented.

Systematic Approaches to Practice

A profession is expected to foster a systematic approach to practice. Systematic practice in the nursing care of women and their families can be seen in the use of the nursing process and its written form, the nursing care plan.

The Nursing Process

The nursing process, the application of the problem-solving process in clinical nursing care, provides a systematic approach to perinatal nursing care. The nursing process focuses the nurse's attention on a logical progression of decisions and actions aimed at resolving specific health problems.

The nursing process has four steps, which are interrelated and may be named or described slightly differently in various texts. The terminology used throughout this book is:

- Assessment
- Nursing Diagnosis
- Planning and Implementation
- Evaluation

The steps in the process are to assess health status, to identify problems that may be in the form of nursing diagnoses or collaborative problems, to plan and implement appropriate nursing care, and to evaluate the effectiveness of that care. The process is circular, with initial assessment, intervention, and evaluation leading to adjustments in care and reassessment of health status. The accompanying display summarizes the activities in each phase of the nursing process.

Research Priorities in Perinatal Nursing, 1988–1995

The Association of Women's Health, Obstetric and Neonatal Nurses (AWHONN), established the following research priorities, which identify areas of particular significance to the specialty, such as the nursing process, interventions, and outcomes of care.

Maternity Nursing

- Prenatal care
- Low birth weight
- Human immunodeficiency virus (HIV)-positive mothers and infants
- Adolescent pregnancy and prepregnancy counseling and care
- Drug and other substance abuse during pregnancy
- Stressors and their effects during pregnancy
- Use of care by pregnant population

Neonatal Nursing

- Low–birth-weight infants and infants in families known to experience high rates of disease, dysfunction, and death
- Promotion of growth and development in all settings, including the hospital and the home
- Short- and long-term consequences of care and parenting
- Evaluation of current and evolving models of home care in terms of quality of patient outcomes and cost of care

Women's Health Nursing

- Prevention of sexually transmitted diseases (STDs) in women, particularly the prevention of HIV-acquired immunodeficiency syndrome (AIDS); and care and support of women and families with STDs
- Psychosocial and physical experience of women in midlife and later years
- Behavioral and environmental factors influencing the health of minority women, including ethnic and cultural minorities and social minorities, such as the homeless and other vulnerable groups
- Women's adaptations to multiple roles and related health outcomes

The Professional Role of Nurses in Delivery of Care

- Context of nursing practice, including constraints and support in the professional environment and effects of malpractice
- Factors affecting recruitment, retention, and attrition
- Alternative educational pathways and new roles for nurses providing care
- Description of role and scope of current nursing practice in various settings
- Dissemination and use of research findings

From the Committee on Research, American Association of Women's Health, Obstetric, and Neonatal Nurses. Reprinted with permission.

Using the nursing process in perinatal nursing is identical to its use in other areas of nursing. However, nurses practice in a wide variety of settings in perinatal care. The pace of movement through the process and the type of information available to the nurse will vary from setting to setting and according to the nature of the health problems encountered.

For instance, during labor and delivery, the processes of assessment, intervention, and evaluation may occur over periods of only minutes as the mother's physiologic status and behavioral patterns change. At birth, nursing assessment and intervention may appear to be nearly simultaneous as the nurse assists the neonate in establishing respiration. The labor and delivery nurse usually has access to the woman's prenatal record. The nurse can often directly observe interactions among family members during assessment of the woman's status. The labor and delivery nurse often sees immediate results of care provided. However, the nurse typically has contact with the family for a period of only hours and may not have the opportunity to evaluate long-term outcomes of care.

In an outpatient setting, such as a prenatal clinic or a home follow-up program, a nurse may have contact with the woman and sometimes with family members over weeks or months. Clinical problem solving will occur over repeated contacts. The nurse may not see immediate results of interventions but may see movement toward long-term goals over time. The clinic or home nurse typically has access to the complete patient record but may not have many opportunities to observe family interaction.

Other nurses working in more specialized clinics, such as prenatal assessment units where amniocentesis or ultrasound tests are done, will have only single contacts with pregnant women and their families. Nursing assessments may be focused on a particular identified problem and may depend heavily on written data collected by others. Nurses in such specialized settings must rely on information in the patient record to evaluate the effectiveness of nursing care.

• • Assessment

Assessment is the initial step in nursing care. *Assessment* includes data collection and analysis. The nurse first collects data in a variety of ways, such as:

Overview of the Nursing Process

Assessment

- Collect data
- Validate data
- Organize data
- Identify patterns

Nursing Diagnosis

- Analyze data
- Formulate nursing diagnoses
- Identify collaborative problems

Planning and Implementation

- Set priorities
- Establish goals
- Determine interventions
- Document the plan of care
- Continue data collection
- Perform nursing interventions
- Document nursing care
- Maintain current plan of care

Evaluation

- Establish expected outcomes
- Evaluate goal achievement
- Identify variables affecting goal achievement
- Modify or terminate plan of care

- Completion of a nursing history
- Interview and observation
- Measurement of vital signs and physiologic indicators
- Review of the patient record
- Use of standardized assessment tools

Standardized assessment tools are becoming available to perinatal nurses to assess the needs of childbearing women and their families in various ways. Usually assessment tools are first used in research and then are demonstrated to be useful in planning and delivering clinical nursing care. Some commonly used assessment tools in perinatal care are listed in Table 2-1. Additional assessment tools to assist in developing appropriate plans of nursing care will be found throughout the text.

• • Nursing Diagnosis

The nurse analyzes data obtained through assessment and identifies patient problems. Patient problems may be thought of as potential or actual health needs for which the pregnant woman and her family see no ready solution without expert assistance that may require nursing or medical care. This process is called *diagnosis*, and the conclusions the nurse draws may include nursing problems that the nurse may appropriately treat as well as possible medical problems that must be referred to a physician or nurse practitioner/nurse midwife for care.

Development and Use of Nursing Diagnoses

The classification of nursing problems into diagnostic categories began in 1973 with the First Conference on Nursing Diagnosis. The work to update and refine nursing diag-

Table 2-1. Examples of Assessment Tools Useful in Maternal Care

Tool	Purpose	Description
Maternal–Fetal Attachment Scale (parent self-report)*	Measures aspects of maternal attachment to fetus A paternal version has been developed and tested	Contains 33 written scales focusing on differentiation of self from fetus, interaction with fetus, attribution of characteristics to fetus, giving of self, and role taking
Brazelton Neonatal Behavior Assessment Scale (BNBAS; completed by professional)†	Assesses social/interactive behavior of newborns from birth to 1 mo May be used to examine early individual differences in infants Has been used in nursing as a strategy for teaching parents about newborn capabilities	Examination guide contains 27 reflex items, 27 behavioral response items, and ratings of infant's predominant states, need for stimulation, and self-quieting activities Typical exam requires 30 min Training is necessary to establish skill in evaluation
Home Observation Measurement of Environment (HOME, birth to 3 y; completed by professional)‡	Identifies aspects of environment that enhance development of infants	Observation of 1 h in home on six subscales focusing on maternal responsiveness and organization of physical (especially play) environment

References for additional information:
*Mercer, R., & Ferketich, S. (1990). Predictors of parental attachment during early parenthood. *Journal of Advanced Nursing, 15*, 268–280.
†Brazelton, T. (1984). *Neonatal Behavioral Assessment Scale* (2nd ed.). Philadelphia, J. B. Lippincott.
‡Lotas, M., Penticuff, J., Medoff-Cooper, B., Brooten, D., & Brown, L. (1992). The HOME scale: The influence of socioeconomic status on the evaluation of the home environment. *Nursing Research, 41*(6), 338–341.

noses continues today. Diagnostic categories in nursing are seen as an important step toward standardization of assessments and the establishment of a common terminology related to actual or potential health needs and appropriate nursing care.

In the past, nursing diagnoses were seen by some as too problem oriented to be a good fit with perinatal nursing. One reason was that nursing diagnoses were too problem oriented to fit the major emphasis on health promotion and disease prevention in perinatal nursing. Nursing diagnoses also did not address the concepts of developmental transition, psychosocial adaptation, or self-care. These concepts are regarded as central to perinatal nursing care. However, nursing diagnoses are becoming an increasingly important part of nursing care, and perinatal nurses are challenged to assist in efforts to make nursing diagnosis work in perinatal care (Henrikson, Wall, Lethbridge & McClurg, 1992).

The term *nursing diagnosis* is used throughout this book. A nursing diagnosis is "a clinical judgment about an individual, family or community response to actual or potential health problems or life processes which provides the basis for definitive therapy toward achievement of outcomes for which the nurse is accountable" (Carpenito, 1991). The accompanying display lists selected nursing diagnoses (part of the list approved in 1992 by the North American Nursing Diagnosis Association) that are of particular use to the nurse in perinatal care.

Collaborative Problems

The diagnostic phase of the nursing process may yield both nursing diagnoses and collaborative problems, as shown in Figure 2-1. Collaborative problems are physiologic complications that have resulted or may result from pathophysiologic, treatment-related, and other situations. Nurses monitor to detect the onset of collaborative problems and work with medicine to determine and implement definitive treatment. The following is a statement of a collaborative problem:

- Potential complication: Sepsis

When the nurse is monitoring for a cluster of complications, the problem may be stated as follows:

- Potential complication of circumcision: Hemorrhage, hypothermia

Differentiation of Nursing Diagnoses and Collaborative Problems

Carpenito (1990) differentiates between nursing diagnoses and collaborative problems, as illustrated in Figure 2-2. Both types of problems may require specific nursing intervention. Throughout this text, nursing diagnoses and collaborative problems (usually in the form of *Collaborative Problem/Potential Complication*) will be discussed for specific groups of patients and will form the bases of nursing care plans. Priorities for any particular patient must be determined by the conditions, the nurse, the woman, and her family. The sample nursing care plans throughout this text will list patient problems for a class of patients in order by clinical priority.

• • Planning and Implementation

Planning for nursing care requires nurses to set priorities within the range of actual or potential health problems they may have identified. The condition of the woman and her family dictates which problems have immediate priority and which ones can be dealt with later. For example, in life-threatening situations the nurse limits assessment and intervention to obtaining data necessary for emergency intervention. More complete assessment is delayed until the woman or neonate is physiologically stable. When a patient is in acute physical or psychological distress, the nurse assesses the cause of the distress and then takes action to reduce the stressor before attempting further assessment.

In most perinatal nursing situations, the patient is not in a life-threatening situation or in acute distress. For this reason, the perinatal nurse must be particularly careful to involve the woman and her family in setting priorities and planning for care. Outside the narrow range of life-threatening situations, the nurse may find the hierarchy of human needs (Maslow, 1943) useful in identifying the priorities for nursing care. This hierarchy organizes needs into five levels: physiologic, safety, love, self-esteem, and self-actualization. Physiologic and safety needs are seen as basic. Maslow theorized that the person will be preoccupied with and motivated by unmet basic needs. Attention will be focused on those basic needs until they are met. As needs are met, the person's attention and behavior are gradually reorganized, and a new, higher need will emerge.

During pregnancy many women and families will experience the needs to feel safe, to maintain the integrity of the love relationship, and to maintain a positive self-image during the dramatic changes childbearing creates in the family system. Priorities for nursing care will depend in large part on how the woman and her family perceive the situation. The plan of care will likely focus on providing information and counseling the woman about ways to meet her needs for love and self-esteem. During childbirth, the woman's needs may be focused more at the physiologic and safety levels. The woman's perceptions of her needs may be unclear or difficult to express, and the nurse must rely on assessment skills to establish priorities for nursing care. The plan of care during this time will *first* be directed at maintaining physiologic integrity and providing for safety needs. Later, attention can be paid to needs for love and security as provided by family members.

An essential aspect of planning care is the establishment of *expected outcomes*. Expected outcomes express what is to be accomplished within a specified time period. Expected outcomes are derived from the problems identified in the diagnostic phase of the nursing process. Expected outcomes will be used to evaluate the effectiveness of care on an ongoing basis. Expected outcomes of care must be stated such that a third party could determine whether or not they match the actual outcomes. Throughout this text, expected outcomes for common health problems will be specified in relation to nursing interventions and will be listed in related nursing care plans for particular groups of women and their family members.

The nurse is responsible for documenting specific health problems, interventions, and expected outcomes for

Nursing Diagnoses Related to the Childbearing Family

Nursing Diagnosis	*Specific Example in Perinatal Care*
Anxiety	Anxiety related to pregnancy changes
Impaired Adjustment	Impaired adjustment related to inadequate support system during early parenting
Hypothermia	Hypothermia related to physiologic immaturity of the newborn
Effective Breastfeeding	Effective breastfeeding
Ineffective Breastfeeding	Ineffective Breastfeeding related to mastitis and maternal pain
	Ineffective Breastfeeding related to poor sucking reflex and neonatal immaturity
Constipation	Constipation related to physiologic changes of pregnancy and iron supplementation
Decisional Conflict	Decisional Conflict related to desire to maintain pregnancy and worsening maternal physiologic condition
Compromised Family Coping	Compromised Family Coping related to multiple strains of high-risk pregnancy treatment
Ineffective Family Coping	Ineffective Family Coping related to parental role overload in caring for triplets
Family Coping: Potential for Growth	Family Coping: Potential for Growth related to additional source of support
Altered Family Processes	Altered Family Processes related to birth of a neonate with a defect
Fatigue	Fatigue related to first trimester of pregnancy
Fear	Fear related to threatened loss of mate from pregnancy complication
Altered Health Maintenance	Altered Health Maintenance related to disruption of routines in early parenthood
Ineffective Infant Feeding Pattern	Ineffective Infant Feeding Pattern related to poverty
High Risk for Infection	High Risk for Infection related to unprotected intercourse with multiple partners
Knowledge Deficit	Knowledge Deficit related to lack of experience in caring for a newborn
Altered Nutrition: Less than Body Requirements	Altered Nutrition (Less than Body Requirements) related to nausea and vomiting in pregnancy
Altered Nutrition: More than Body Requirements	Altered Nutrition (More than Body Requirements) related to cultural beliefs regarding food intake during pregnancy
Pain	Pain related to persistent occiput posterior presentation of fetus during labor
High Risk for Altered Parenting	High Risk for Altered Parenting related to adolescent parenthood and inadequate social support
Altered Role Performance	Altered Role Performance related to demands of new parenthood
Altered Sexuality Patterns	Altered Sexuality Patterns related to physical or psychological changes during pregnancy
Altered Urinary Elimination	Altered Urinary Elimination related to physiologic changes of pregnancy

From North American Nursing Diagnosis Association. (1993). Classification of nursing diagnoses: Proceedings of the tenth conference. *Philadelphia, J. B. Lippincott.*

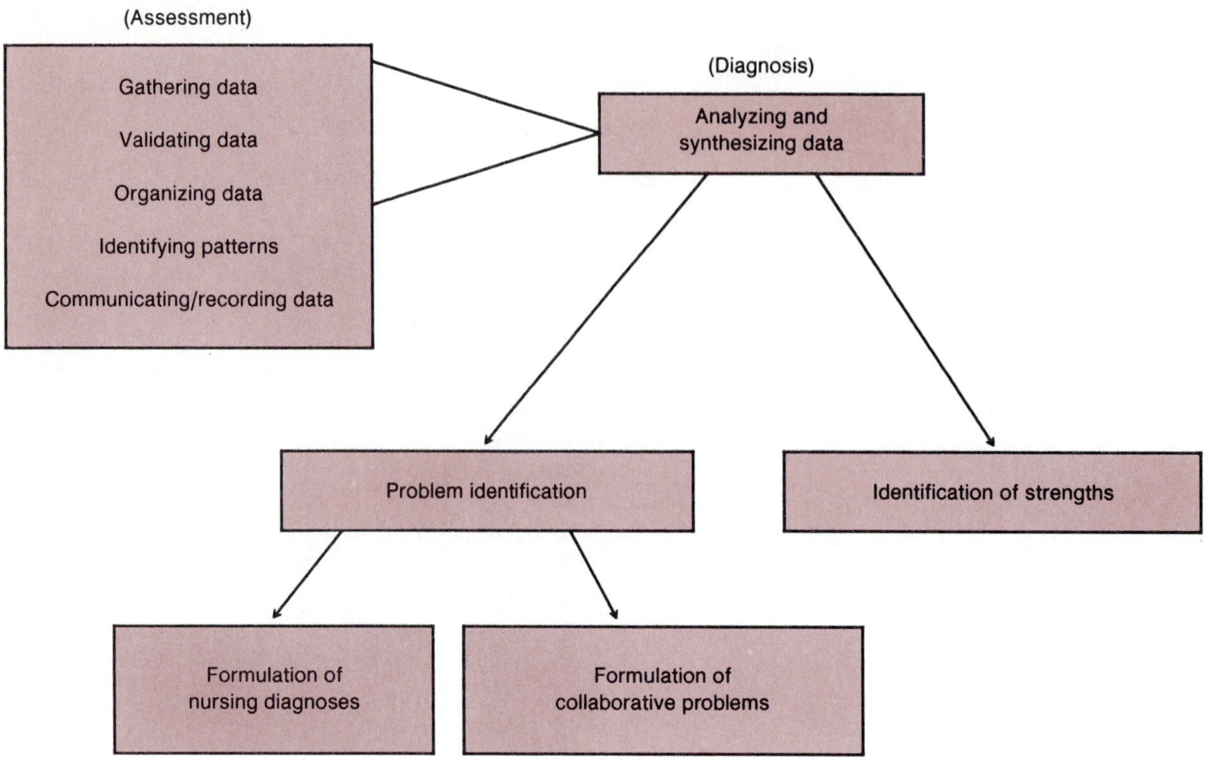

Figure 2-1.
The diagnostic phase of the nursing process, resulting in formulation of either nursing diagnoses or collaborative problems. (From Alfaro, R. [1990]. *Nursing diagnosis and the nursing process: A step-by-step guide* [2nd ed., p. 31]. Philadelphia, J. B. Lippincott.)

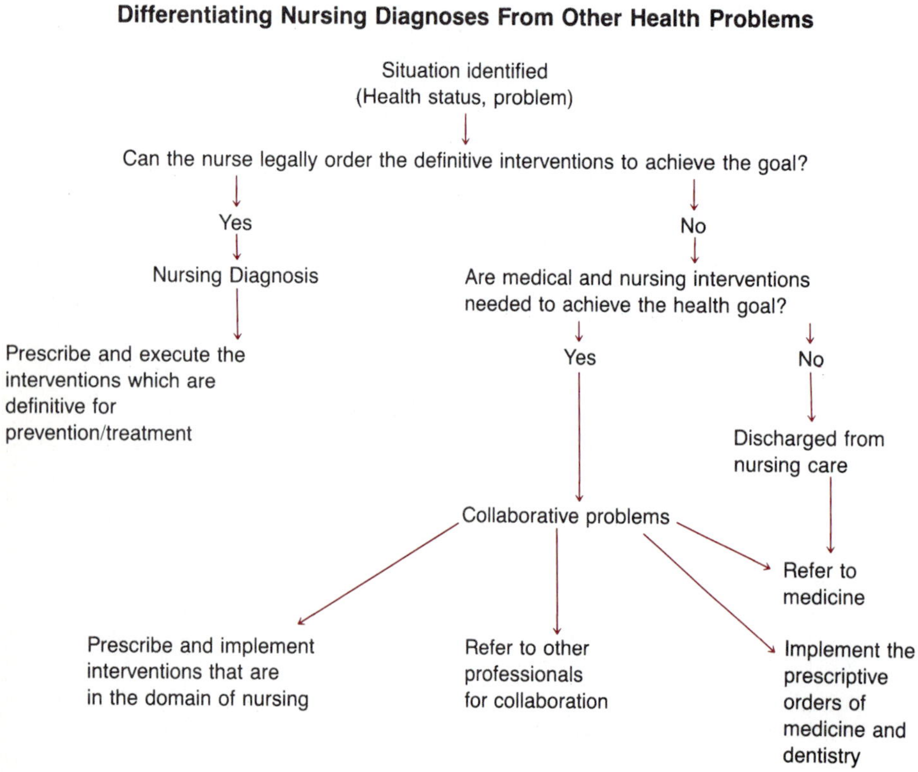

Figure 2-2.
Differentiation of nursing diagnoses from collaborative problems. (From Carpenito, L. J. [1989]. *Nursing diagnosis: Application to clinical practice* [3rd ed., p. 85]. Philadelphia, J. B. Lippincott.)

each problem. This plan of care is usually communicated to colleagues through verbal and written reporting. Some institutions have standardized care plans for groups of patients; the nurse then individualizes these based on the assessment of needs of the woman and her family.

Once a plan of care is established, the nurse implements the plan through interventions directed at priority nursing diagnoses or collaborative problems. Effective nursing intervention requires the nurse to have an accurate understanding of underlying physiologic and psychosocial principles. Skills in monitoring and observation, in administering physical care and comfort measures, and in communicating clearly and sensitively with childbearing women and their families are essential.

Because of the nature of childbearing and the new adaptational demands the process presents for women and their families, perinatal nurses must be especially expert at teaching. Indeed, teaching women and their family members is an essential nursing intervention in perinatal care.

Teaching Women and Their Families for Effective Self-Care

Most childbearing women and their families are healthy. Nursing activities center on providing the family with assistance in managing their own health through the normal psychological and physical transition of pregnancy, childbirth, and postbirth recovery. Teaching women and their families how to care for themselves effectively is a nursing responsibility and must be given appropriate time for planning, implementation, and documentation. Thus, the perinatal nurse must understand principles of adult learning and use them in teaching about self-care.

The nurse plans and implements teaching based on the following considerations:

- Learning needs of the woman and her family members
- Principles of teaching and learning
- Physiologic and psychological condition of the woman, her neonate, and the family
- Sociocultural factors

Learning Needs. The unique learning needs of the woman and her family must be clearly identified for teaching to be effective (Fig. 2-3). The nurse does not assume that all families want or need the same information. Each family member brings a wealth of life experiences to the process of childbearing. The nurse who teaches in rote fashion without considering individual differences will not adequately meet individual learning needs.

Principles of Teaching and Learning. Major principles of teaching and learning are used by the nurse during teaching. The woman's existing knowledge level should be identified before teaching starts. The nurse seeks to create a physical and emotional climate conducive to learning and to offer positive feedback and support. Demonstrations of specific self-care tasks are provided. Perhaps most important, the nurse recognizes signs of readiness for learning and makes full use of teaching opportunities. The Teaching Considerations display includes guidelines for effective parent teaching. Throughout this text, teaching consideration displays will be highlighted for particular situations.

Legal/Ethical Considerations

Documentation of Newborn Discharge Teaching and Legal Liability

The nurse is faced with the task of completing an ever-expanding discharge teaching plan for parents within a diminishing time frame. Parent education is ideally begun in the prepartum period, but it is the nurse's responsibility at the time of discharge to ensure that essential elements of neonatal care and safety have been reviewed and that parents have demonstrated competency in basic newborn care skills. This challenge arises in a period when parents are increasingly willing to litigate when they believe that negligence on the part of health professionals has resulted in the injury or death of their newborn.

Documentation of all aspects of discharge planning and teaching is critical to ensure that no important aspect of parent teaching is overlooked. Such documentation constitutes a legal record for use by the health care facility if a lawsuit is instigated. Although the discharge plan is always individualized, using a formal checklist or teaching plan assists the clinician to use time efficiently. It is essential in today's litigious climate to retain a written record of the areas of newborn care and safety that were covered.

Parents should be provided with written materials that review and reinforce the teaching plan. Parents need to receive telephone numbers of important resources. If a language barrier is identified, a translator should be used and, whenever possible, educational materials should be given to the family in their primary language. These actions will enhance the quality of the discharge plan and reduce legal risks for the practitioner.

Physiologic and Psychological Conditions. Teaching for effective self-care and discharge considers physical and emotional conditions. The presence of pain, physiologic disturbance, fatigue, or worry will affect the family member's ability to learn. A crisis, such as an unexpected complication, will greatly diminish the family's ability to assimilate information. Therefore, information may have to be repeated two or three times before it is understood.

The length of contact the nurse has with the family will also determine the extent and depth of teaching that is possible. Short prenatal visits may preclude in-depth teaching in some settings. Shortened hospital stays have the same effect. In these situations, the nurse identifies and covers

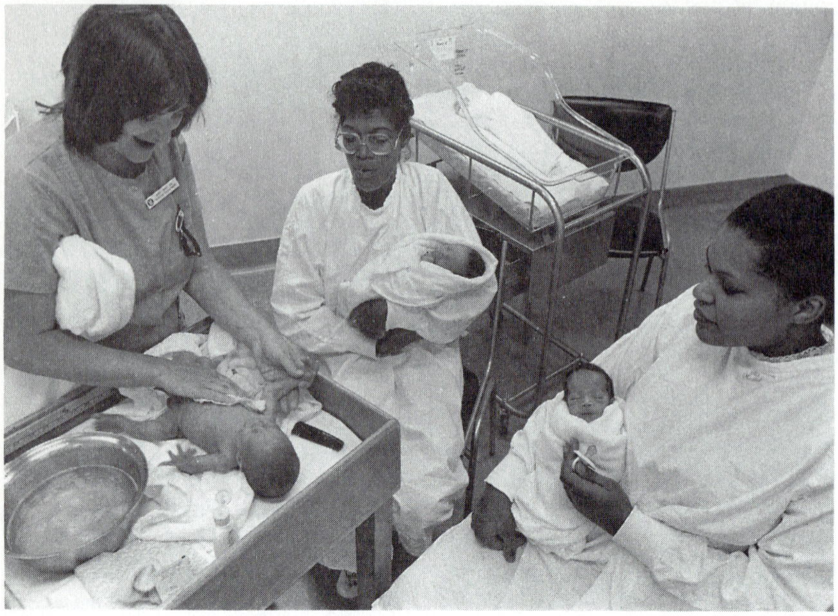

Figure 2-3.
Nurse–parent teaching. The nurse provides valuable teaching about newborn care and parenting as she demonstrates how to bathe and change newborns. (Photo by Kathy Sloane.)

essential points of information and establishes ongoing follow-up with family members so that their learning needs can be met.

Sociocultural Factors. Education, financial status, religious beliefs, and ethnic background are factors nurses must consider before teaching is initiated. It is essential for the nurse to convey recognition of and respect for family values and belief systems. Knowledge of the family members' educational levels will guide the nurse in teaching strategies and the selection of appropriate instructional materials. The nurse should also have knowledge of the family's economic resources to make appropriate recommendations for supplies and equipment.

The nurse recognizes the learning needs of the father and other family members. Although the nurse may have only limited contact with fathers or partners, their needs for emotional support and skillful teaching during the childbearing year are considered. Many men have little or no experience with childbearing and are especially nervous about their ability to care for a small infant. The nurse may use specific strategies to help the father feel more comfortable and to encourage him to express his own learning needs. The nurse should avoid focusing exclusively on the woman and should become familiar with common learning needs of other family members. Teaching can be planned and implemented when opportunities arise.

• • Evaluation

Once interventions have been implemented, the nurse evaluates the effects of interventions by comparing the expected outcomes with outcomes actually observed. Nursing evaluation of actual outcomes may then result in a reassessment and adjustment in the plan of care. Alternatively, the nurse may refocus on other identified problems if care has been successful.

As a professional, the nurse is accountable for examining the effectiveness of the care and for exploring ways in which care can be improved. *Quality assurance programs*, in which records are audited and actual care is evaluated against standards of care, are used by nurses to examine the quality of care. *Clinical research* is another way nurses examine their own practices, either by testing the effectiveness of care or by generating new knowledge on which care can be based.

The Nursing Care Plan

The *nursing care plan* is a detailed written form of the nursing process. The care plan documents the identified health problem, the planned intervention, and the criteria to be used in evaluating the effectiveness of the care. The care plan enables the nurse to communicate the plan of care to others and to document the care delivered. Nursing care plans may also be broken down in various ways, but the underlying principles remain the same. The format used throughout this textbook is shown in the accompanying Format for Nursing Care Plans.

Nursing care plans are a means of communication among colleagues. Care plans are important because nursing has 24-hour accountability for care, and communication must occur among several nurses who will be involved in a particular patient's care. The care plan should be comprehensive and detailed so that any nurse in the setting can use the care plan to organize care. This is especially important in perinatal nursing, where hospitalizations are usually short and much patient teaching must occur before discharge.

Nursing care plans are in widespread use in hospitals today but may be replaced in the next decade by new ways of documenting patient care. One criticism of nursing care plans is that they involve only nursing. Other health professionals, such as physicians, pharmacists, and social workers, do not contribute to formulating the plan and are not

Teaching Considerations

Guidelines for Effective Patient Education

The nurse considers the following points in planning and implementing teaching of new parents:

- In collaboration with the woman and her family members, the nurse identifies the individual learning needs based on an assessment of knowledge and concerns. The nurse sets priorities, by considering what is most important for the woman and her family members to learn and how much time is available to teach it, then teaches the most important information first.
- The nurse provides a comfortable environment. This may mean ensuring privacy and communicating to the woman and her family members that nursing staff are interested and are willing to listen and answer questions.
- The woman and her family members must be given the opportunity to absorb the teaching. If possible, teaching should be reviewed with the family within the day or the next day to see how much was remembered and to answer any questions.
- The nurse must use simple terminology and must verify that the woman and her family members understand the words used; many medical and nursing terms may be new to them.
- Teaching is reinforced with visual aids, whenever possible. Many facilities have audiovisual aids that can supplement or replace some teaching. Printed materials are always helpful because they can augment teaching or provide additional information. However, printed materials must be at an appropriate reading level and in suitable language.
- The nurse includes the family in teaching whenever possible. Family members need most types of information just as much as the woman does.
- Teaching should be documented. It is part of the care the woman and her family received. Charting teaching activities also alerts other staff members to continuing learning needs.

involved in performing and evaluating the care as outlined in it. Because perinatal care is multidisciplinary in nature, this criticism is legitimate.

However, a new development in health care is emphasizing interdisciplinary collaboration in the planning and implementing of health care. This new development is called *managed care*. The benefits of managed care include improved quality of care and control of health care costs. It is of considerable importance to the future of perinatal nursing and is addressed in the next section of this chapter.

In addition to the use and generation of an organized knowledge and theory base, a profession is expected to foster a systematic approach to practice. In nursing this is best exemplified by the nursing process. The nursing process is an agreed on standard of practice that relies on diagnostic categories specific to nursing. The preceding section addressed the nursing process and nursing care plan, emphasizing elements that will be used throughout the text. Teaching is a particularly important form of intervention in perinatal nursing care.

Attention to Quality and Cost of Care

Skyrocketing health care costs and ongoing concerns about maintaining quality of care have set the stage for new developments in health care delivery—managed care and case management. These new trends are already being felt in perinatal care and are certain to be major influences on the organization and delivery of perinatal nursing care into the next century. Both managed care and case management offer new opportunities for nurses to improve the quality of care they deliver. These new modes of care are likely to contribute to controlling costs of health care (see the accompanying display). Managed care and case management are described briefly. Examples of how these systems are already being used in perinatal nursing care are presented.

Managed Care

Managed care is a system that focuses on coordinating the activities of health professionals to address the woman's physical, psychosocial, and family needs effectively and without unnecessary expense. This system of care is implemented at the unit level. To a significant extent, managed care relies on nursing for the planning, implementation, and evaluation of care. Managed care uses a new tool to achieve these goals—new plans of care called managed care paths.

Managed Care Paths

Managed care paths are similar to standardized care plans in that they are developed for particular groups of patients. Managed care paths show the expected progression of the patient from initiation of care through discharge. The managed care path shows important expected outcomes as benchmarks, interventions needed to achieve those outcomes, and specific time frames in which those outcomes should be achieved; a typical format for a managed care path is shown in the accompanying display.

Unlike standardized care plans, the managed care path is used by all care providers to evaluate how a particular patient is progressing. At set intervals (each shift or each day

Nursing Care Plan

The Woman/Neonate With (Statement of Problem)

PATIENT PROFILE This section provides an overview of the clinical situation and background information to help in formulating a plan of care.

History This section provides pertinent information from the patient's health history.

Physical Assessment This section provides pertinent information from the physical assessment that helps in identification of nursing diagnoses and the formulation of a plan of care.

COLLABORATIVE PROBLEMS/POTENTIAL COMPLICATIONS This section lists actual collaborative problems, especially potential complications that must be considered in the nursing plan of care.

Assessment	*Nursing Diagnosis*	*Nursing Interventions*	*Rationale*
This column includes information obtained through the nurses' assessment.	This column lists the nursing diagnoses identified in the clinical situation, based on assessment data. ***Expected Outcome*** This section lists the goals to be achieved and specifies the time frame in which they should be achieved.	This column lists specific nursing interventions to address the nursing diagnoses identified.	This column lists the scientific rationale for interventions.

EVALUATION This section summarizes the outcomes and results of the person's care. It may give information about the next steps to take.

Goals of Managed Care and Case Management

- To facilitate the achievement of expected outcomes by directing the contribution of all care providers toward those outcomes
- To facilitate discharge from professional care after an appropriate interval of care or length of hospital stay
- To promote appropriate (increased or decreased) use of resources
- To promote collaborative practice, coordination of care, and continuity of care
- To promote professional development and satisfaction for care providers

Adapted with permission from the Center for Nursing Case Management (1987), South Natick, MA.

of hospitalization), those responsible for care evaluate each patient's progress and examine factors that may be delaying progress. Some of these factors may not be "controllable," but others may. The care provider then develops a plan for addressing variations in expected progress and documents the plan and its results. Thus, the process of managed care and the use of managed care paths focuses the provider's attention on factors that are controllable and that can be changed to enable achievement of expected outcomes.

In managed care models, care of all patients should be based on managed care paths. The appropriate managed care path may be selected by the professional nurse who assesses the patient on admission; later the managed care path will be individualized by the attending physician and nurses. The managed care path is an integral part of the patient record and may be used for shift change reports, clinical rounds, and consultation meetings. The managed care path helps sequence the processes of care appropriately and can serve as a valuable tool for orienting new care providers, as well as for teaching patients and family members (Giuliano & Poirier, 1991).

Nurses are generally responsible for developing managed care paths and for refining these paths in collaboration

MANAGED CARE PATH

Typical Format for Managed Care Path

Patient Type

Patient Name: ____________________
MD: ____________________
RN: ____________________

Admit date/time: ____________________
CP initiated, date/time: ____________________

Expected length of stay: ____________________
Hospital day: ____________________
Postpartum/postop day: ____________________
Discharge date/time: ____________________

	Day of Delivery	Day 1	Day 2	Day 3
Key Goals **Consults** **Tests/Labs** **Meds** **Treatments** **Teaching** **Equipment** **Diet** **Activity** **D/C Plan**	Care paths will be specific for patient type, ie, cesarean delivery, vaginal delivery, pregnancy-induced hypertension. The entries in each of the columns on the left will be specific to the care needs of that type of patient. The columns across the top, indicating time interval, will usually be in days of hospitalization, but may be customized to show shorter or longer time intervals, depending on expected progress for a typical patient.			

Variation from Expected: (record by date/time)

with physicians, pharmacists, therapists, and others involved in patient care on the unit. Throughout the country, perinatal units are using managed care paths as a method to improve the quality of care while controlling costs. In this text, managed care paths are presented in combination with nursing care plans, where appropriate. As is true with nursing care plans, managed care paths must be individualized for each patient care situation.

Case Management

Case management controls the process of providing care through the actions of a case manager. The case manager plans and coordinates patient care activities so that expected outcomes are achieved within reasonable time frames. Case management may be most useful with high-risk patients with complex and costly health care needs. Increasingly, health care agencies and hospitals are moving toward implementing systems of case management with nurses as case managers. In some systems, the nurse case manager may supervise the work of staff nurses, whereas in others, the nurse case manager also provides some direct care. The nurse case manager is a skilled clinician who is responsible for facilitating use of appropriate resources, evaluating care against established standards, and ensuring that expected outcomes are achieved in a timely and cost-efficient fashion (Sparacino, 1991). Nurse researchers have already begun to evaluate the impact of nursing case management on the quality and cost of patient care. The Nursing Research display cites some cost-saving benefits of managed care. It is clear that managed care and case management will be features of the future health care delivery system, as the federal and states governments, insurers, and health maintenance organizations address the issues of cost and quality in health care.

Managed care and case management offer new opportunities for nurses to improve the quality of care they deliver. Managed care is a system that focuses on coordinating the activities of health professionals to address the woman's physical, psychosocial, and family needs effectively and without unnecessary expense. Managed care uses a new tool to achieve these goals—new plans of care called managed care paths. Managed care paths show the expected progression of the patient from initiation of care through discharge. The managed care path helps sequence the processes of care appropriately and can serve as a valuable tool for orienting new care providers, as well as for teaching patients and family members.

Case management controls the process of providing the care through the actions of a case manager. The case manager plans and coordinates patient care activities so that expected outcomes are achieved within reasonable time frames. The nurse case manager is a skilled clinician responsible for facilitating use of appropriate resources, evaluating care against established standards, and ensuring that expected outcomes are achieved in a timely and cost-efficient fashion. Attention to cost and quality in perinatal care is a major nursing responsibility.

Nursing Research

Early Discharge and Nurse Case-Managed Transitional Care

In response to pressures for cost containment as well as because of consumer demand, hospital stays for childbearing have decreased substantially in recent years, and early discharge is becoming more common, even for families experiencing some perinatal complication, such as cesarean birth or low birth weight.

A team of nurse researchers at University of Pennsylvania (Brooten et al., 1986) demonstrated that very low–birth-weight infants could be safely discharged an average of 11 days earlier with home follow-up by a perinatal nurse specialist acting as a nurse case manager. This nursing case management program of home follow-up resulted in an average savings of $18,506/infant without any increased risk to the infant, such as rehospitalization, acute return visits, or losses in physical or mental growth.

This same team has examined the applicability and effectiveness of this model of nurse case-managed home follow-up on women who experienced unplanned cesarean birth, women with diabetes in the perinatal period, and women who experienced hysterectomies. This model includes telephone contacts, home visits, and telephone availability by nurse specialists, and provides for comparison of normal discharge and early discharge/home follow-up patients on specific expected patient outcomes as well as cost of care.

Brooten, D., Kumar, S., Brown, L. (1986). A randomized clinical trial of early hospital discharge and home followup of very low birth weight infants. *New England Journal of Medicine, 315,* 934–939.

Brooten, D., Brown, L., Munro, B. York, R., Cohen, S., Roncoli, M., & Hollingsworth, A. (1988). Early discharge and specialist transitional care. *Image, 20* 65–68.

Brooten, D. (1988–1992). *Early hospital discharge and nurse specialist followup.* Final report, Grant N5-P01 NR 0185903. National Center for Nursing Research, National Institutes of Health.

Chapter Summary

Perinatal nursing is based on elements of professional practice. These elements include an identifiable knowledge and theory base, a systematic approach to practice, agreed-on standards of practice, documentation of clinical practice, and participation in and support of professional and specialty organizations. The knowledge and theory base of perinatal nursing encompasses the physiologic, emotional, social, and cultural aspects of childbearing within the context of the family and the individual. Family responses to alterations in health status during the childbearing year are considered. A systematic approach to nursing practice is reflected in the nursing process, which focuses attention on assessment of health problems, appropriate nursing interventions, and evaluation of the effectiveness of interventions. Attention to the quality and cost of care is increasingly a nursing responsibility. Nursing will be an integral part of new systems of care delivery, such as managed care and nursing case management. The reality that health care costs must be controlled, or services will be increasingly rationed in the United States, should be a sufficiently strong incentive for nursing to continue to be proactive in the effort to achieve health care reform.

As the field of perinatal nursing changes, new patterns of practice are evolving, such as the increasing use of conceptual frameworks or models to guide practice. Nursing case management is a system of delivering health care to complex patient populations. Many challenges lie ahead as health care costs continue to skyrocket, as indicators of maternal and infant health point to many unmet needs, and as nursing as a predominantly female profession comes to grips with the remaining barriers to full professional practice. Perinatal nursing has been and continues to be a microcosm of the larger nursing profession with all its problems, satisfactions, and rewards.

Study Questions

1. *What is meant by a knowledge and theory base?*
2. *What is meant by a systematic approach to perinatal practice?*
3. *What are the advantages of using a conceptual framework to guide clinical practice? Why is adaptation a useful organizing perspective for perinatal care?*
4. *What are the elements in a complete nursing diagnosis and what is each element designed to communicate?*
5. *What is a managed care path and how is it used?*
6. *What is the difference between a nursing diagnosis and a collaborative problem?*
7. *Why is it essential that patient teaching be documented?*
8. *What is the difference between managed care and nursing case management? Why have these new developments been adopted in the health care system?*

References

Carpenito, L. (1990). *Nursing diagnosis: Application to clinical practice* (3rd ed.). Philadelphia: J. B. Lippincott.

Carpenito, L. (1991). The NANDA definition of nursing diagnosis. In R. Carrol-Johnson (Ed.). *Classification of nursing diagnosis: Proceedings of the ninth conference* (p. 65). Philadelphia: J. B. Lippincott.

Giuliano, K., & Poirier, C. (1991). Nursing case management: Critical pathways to desirable outcomes. *Nursing Management, 22*, 52–58.

Henrikson, M., Wall, G., Lethbridge, D., & McClurg, V. (1992). Nursing diagnosis and obstetric, gynecologic, and neonatal nursing: Breastfeeding as an example. *Journal of Obstetric, Gynecologic, and Neonatal Nursing, 21* (6), 446–456.

Maslow, A. (1943). A theory of human motivation. *Psychological Review, 5*, 370–386.

May, K. (1991). The leader in nursing research. *American Journal of Maternal Child Nursing, 16*(1), 30–33.

Meleis, A. (1991). *Theoretical nursing: Development and progress* (2nd ed.). Philadelphia: J. B. Lippincott.

Roy, C. (1989). The Roy adaptation model. In J. Riehl-Sisca (Ed.). *Conceptual models for nursing practice* (3rd ed.). Norwalk, CT: Appleton and Lange.

Sparacino, P. (1991). The clinical nurse specialist—case manager relationship. *Clinical Nurse Specialist, 5*, 180.

St. Louis University School of Nursing. (1979). *Adaptation: A theoretical base for nursing*. St. Louis, MO: Author.

Eganhouse, D. (1991). Electronic fetal monitoring: Education and quality assurance. *Journal of Obstetric, Gynecologic, and Neonatal Nursing, 20*(1), 16–29.

Krause, K., & Younger, V. (1992). Nursing diagnoses as guidelines in the care of the neonatal ECMO patient. *Journal of Obstetric, Gynecologic, and Neonatal Nursing, 21*(3), 169–177.

Lauver, D. (1992). A theory of care seeking behavior. *Image, 24*(4), 281–288.

Manion, J. (1991). Nurse intrapreneurs: The heroes of health care's future. *Nursing Outlook, 39*, 18–24.

Mercer, R. (1990). *Parents at risk*. New York: Springer.

Morse, J., Anderson, G., Bottorff, J., Yonge, O. L., O'Brien, B., Solberg, S., & McIlveen, K. (1992). Exploring empathy: A conceptual fit for nursing practice? *Image, 24*(4), 273–280.

Symanski, M. (1991). Use of nursing theories in the care of families with high-risk infants: Challenges for the future. *Journal of Perinatal and Neonatal Nursing, 4*(4), 71–77.

Tolentino, M. (1990). The use of Orem's self care model in the neonatal intensive care unit. *Journal of Obstetric, Gynecologic, and Neonatal Nursing, 19*(6), 496–501.

Tulman, L., & Fawcett, J. (1990). Functional status during pregnancy and the postpartum: A framework for research. *Image, 22*(3), 191–194.

Westfall, U. (1992). Nursing chronotherapeutics: A conceptual framework. *Image, 24*(4), 307–312.

Yoder, M. (1993). *Nursing diagnosis vignettes in maternal-child health*. Baltimore: Williams & Wilkins.

Suggested Readings

Brooten, D., Brown, L., Munro, B., York, R., Cohen, S., Roncoli, M., & Hollingsworth, A. (1988). Early discharge and specialist transitional care. *Image, 20*, 65–68.

CHAPTER 3

Challenges in Maternal and Neonatal Nursing

Learning Objectives

After studying the material in this chapter, the student will be able to:

- Discuss current rates of maternal and infant morbidity and mortality in the United States.
- Identify major factors contributing to maternal and infant morbidity and mortality.
- Describe some major challenges facing those engaged in perinatal care.
- List advanced practice roles in perinatal nursing and describe the activities associated with each nursing role.
- Identify factors that will have a dramatic effect on perinatal care and on perinatal nursing in the future.

Key Terms

birth rate	morbidity rate
certified nurse midwife	neonatal mortality rate
infant mortality rate	neonatal period
maternal mortality rate	nurse practitioner

The challenges in perinatal care are considerable. For instance, the number of underserved people is increasing, with women and dependent children overrepresented in the underserved group; health care needs of low-income and minority groups are growing. At the same time, pressure is mounting to reduce health care costs. Escalating malpractice concerns may abate as governmental actions help to moderate liability risks. Concerns about competition and a shrinking middle-class population may continue to fuel opposition to nurse midwifery and nurse practitioner practice from organized medicine. These challenges will determine, to a significant extent, where and how perinatal nurses will practice.

In the midst of rapid change in the health care system, and in the larger society, nurses must maintain a clear vision of the desired future. Perinatal nurses need to concentrate on several goals in an effort to achieve optimal care for childbearing women and their families. These goals include:

- Maintaining an adequate supply of well-prepared nurses to provide expert perinatal care.
- Improving quality through rigorous implementation of standards and scientifically based and compassionate nursing care.
- Ensuring access to nursing and health care by addressing issues such financing, regulation, and discrimination in the health care system.

Provision of Optimal Perinatal Care: An Unrealized Goal

The United States has the highest health care expenditures of any industrialized country. Yet perinatal outcomes to date are not consistent with stated national health goals.

Indicators of Maternal–Infant Health in the United States

Health care is often evaluated by examining numerical data in regard to mortality and morbidity in a given population. Mortality is the death rate in a given population; morbidity is the illness rate. In perinatal care, statistics such as birth rate, maternal and infant mortality and morbidity, and birth weight are major indicators of the health of women and their children.

Birth Rate

Birth rate is reported as the number of live births per 1000 people. Birth rates and death rates in the United States from 1960 through 1990 are presented in Table 3-1. Birth rates steadily declined from peaks in the 1950s to a low from 1975 to 1976 and have shown small increases since that time (National Center for Health Statistics, 1992). There has been a steady increase in the number of first births to women over 30 years of age. This increase probably reflects larger numbers of "baby-boom" children who are delaying their families for financial reasons. Birth rates are typically higher for non-European Americans in the United States.

Birth Weight

Birth weight is an important indicator in perinatal care because low birth weight is often associated with higher infant mortality. The average birth weight for infants born in the United States in 1990 was 3368 g (7 lb 7 oz). A birth weight of less than 2500 g (5 lb 8 oz) is considered to be low birth weight. Low birth weight is more common among non-European Americans, teenagers, and women over 40 years of age. In 1989, low–birth-weight newborns accounted for nearly 7% of all births, a rate that has remained almost unchanged since 1976 (National Center for Health Statistics, 1992).

Maternal and Infant Mortality

Significant improvements have been realized in health outcomes for mothers and infants in the last 50 years, particularly in the last decade. Estimated maternal mortality, expressed as number of maternal deaths per 100,000 live births, has declined steadily in the United States from 21.5 in 1970 to 7.3 in 1990 (see Table 3-1).

However, improvements are slower in the infant mortality rate. This rate is expressed as the number of deaths under 1 year of age per 1000 live births. Between 1950 and 1989, infant mortality dropped from 29.2 to 9.8 deaths per 1000 live births. Provisional data for 1990 estimate the infant mortality rate at 9.1 deaths per 1000 live births. Figure 3-1 displays this decline but also shows that the rate of progress has slowed.

Despite this decreased infant mortality rate, the United States ranks 24th in infant mortality worldwide. Nearly two thirds of the infant deaths in the United States are related to low birth weight. Other contributing factors to infant mortality are congenital anomalies and sudden infant death syndrome. About 10% of infant deaths occur in the first day after

Table 3-1. Summary of Maternal and Infant Health Indicators in United States, 1960–1990

	1960	1970	1975	1980	1985	1990*
Birth Rate						
(Number of live births per 1000 people)						
Total	23.7	18.4	14.6	15.9	15.8	16.3
European American	22.7	17.4	13.8	14.9	14.8	15.3
African American	31.9	25.3	20.7	22.1	21.1	22.0
Maternal Mortality						
(Maternal deaths per 100,000 live births from complications of pregnancy, childbirth, and postpartum)						
Total	37.1	21.5	12.8	9.2	7.9	7.3
European American	26.0	14.4	9.1	6.7	5.1	5.4
African American	103.6	59.8	31.3	21.5	22.2	18.6
Neonatal Mortality						
(Infant deaths per 1000 live births prior to 28 days old, exclusive of fetal deaths [20 wk of gestation to delivery])						
Total	18.7	15.1	11.6	8.5	7.0	5.7
European American	17.2	13.8	10.4	7.5	6.1	5.2
African American	27.8	22.8	18.3	14.1	12.1	11.3
Infant Mortality						
(Infant deaths from birth to 1 y of age per 1000 live births)						
Total	26.0	20.0	16.1	12.6	10.6	9.1
European American	22.9	17.8	14.2	11.0	9.3	8.2
African American	44.3	32.6	26.2	21.4	18.2	17.7

* Provisional data.
From National Center for Health Statistics: Health—United States, 1990. US Government Printing Office, 1992.

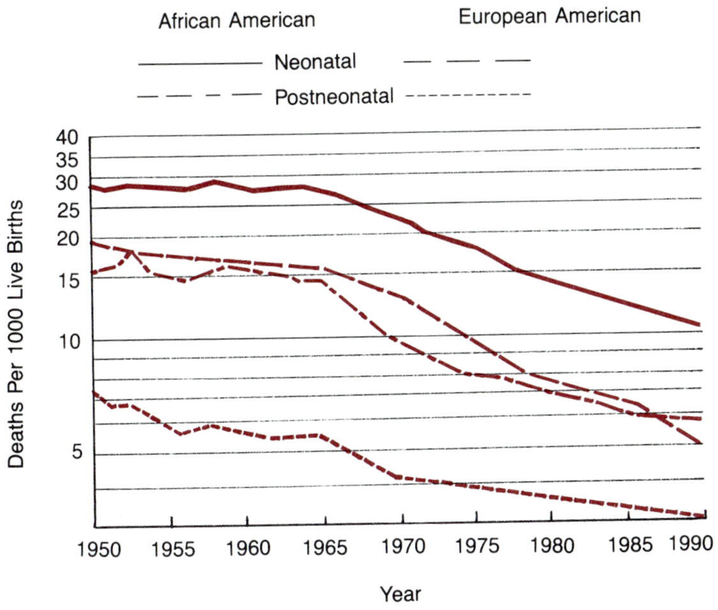

Figure 3-1.
Infant mortality rates in the United States, 1950–1990. (From National Center for Health Statistics, Health—United States, 1991. US Government Printing Office, 1992.)

birth and about 70% in the neonatal period (the first 28 days after birth).

The unfavorable infant mortality rate in the United States may reflect the fact that health care is nationalized in many Western European countries, a factor that increases early prenatal care accessibility. In the United States, early prenatal care and prenatal education do not consistently reach poor women and families most in need. The United States also compares unfavorably with other developed countries in regard to adolescent childbearing. The United States birth rate among adolescents is double that of France, Germany, and the United Kingdom (National Commission to Prevent Infant Mortality, 1988; National Center for Health Statistics, 1992).

The infant mortality rate has fallen in recent decades in all nations. Unfortunately, relative rankings for the United States have worsened, suggesting that other nations are doing a better job at meeting the needs of childbearing families. Indeed, concern is growing in the United States about the availability and quality of services available to women and children. Barriers to early prenatal care for those most in need are increasing (Expert Panel on the Content of Prenatal Care, 1989).

Maternal–Infant Health Concerns in Minority Populations

Progress with improvements in maternal–infant health indicators nationwide continues to be less than optimal. The picture is even more disturbing when indicators in minority populations are examined. There is particular concern about rising rates of low- and very low–birth-weight infants among African Americans and other minorities in the United States (Institute of Medicine, 1985). The National Birth Cohort Study included a survey of 45 cities and showed that infant death rates continue to be higher among African Americans than European Americans, as has traditionally been true. However, the infant death rate is increasing in the African American population. In 32 cities surveyed, the African American infant death rate was more than 50% higher than the European American rate. In 15 cities, the infant death rate among African Americans was double that among European Americans. Rates for some American Indian tribes and for Puerto Ricans were considerably higher than those for European American infants (US Department of Health and Human Services, 1990).

This racial gap in infant survival is thought to be due primarily to rises in the rate of low–birth-weight neonates born to African American women. Among 32 cities surveyed, half showed an increase in the incidence of low birth weight among African American newborns during 1980. African American neonates are at twice the risk for low birth weight than are other newborns. Low birth weight declined from 1970 to 1981 but has remained steady since that time. Adolescent pregnancies, at particular risk for low–birth-weight neonates, are increasing more rapidly among African Americans than European Americans. Poverty is the salient factor here, rather than race. Two thirds of African American women and three fifths of teenagers giving birth in the United States each year are living at or below the poverty level. Their children, most of whom live in the central cities, are as much as 20% behind immunization rates compared to children who live in other places (National Center for Health Statistics, 1992).

African Americans make up 12% of the United States population and comprise the largest minority group. One third live in poverty, a rate three times higher than among European Americans. African American infants are twice as likely to die before their first birthday than their European American counterparts. Maternal well-being is also poorer among African American women. Overweight is a problem for 44% of African American women aged 20 and older compared with 27% of all women. Obesity in women of childbearing age may increase the risk of maternal conditions, such as a diabetes and pregnancy-induced hypertension, and may increase perinatal and neonatal risk (US Department of Health and Human Services, 1990).

Hispanic Americans represent the second largest minority group in the United States, constituting about 8% of the total population. This is a diverse group, and maternal and child health indicators vary substantially among subpopulations. Hispanic American women tend to receive less prenatal care than the total population. In 1987, 13% of Hispanic American mothers had late or no prenatal care compared to 4% of non-Hispanic whites. Nearly 22% had no health insurance compared to 10% of African Americans and 8% of European Americans (US Department of Health and Human Services, 1990).

Asian and Pacific Islander Americans are the third largest minority population. These Americans represent a number of distinct cultures and over 30 different languages. Overall, maternal and infant health indicators vary largely by socioeconomic status and acculturation. However, these groups also face specific health threats from higher rates of infection that may threaten maternal and infant well-being, notably hepatitis B and tuberculosis. The overall carrier rate for hepatitis B in the United States is estimated to be 0.3% of the population compared to nearly 5% of the immigrant Asian population. Both diseases can be spread from mother to infant and from child to child (US Department of Health and Human Services, 1990).

American Indians and Alaska Natives now number nearly 1.6 million people and are the smallest of the minority groups defined by the United States government. Maternal and child health indicators vary by socioeconomic status. It is significant to note that more than 1 in 4 live in poverty and fewer than 8% have college degrees. Particular problems facing women and children in this group include obesity, diabetes, and the consequences of alcohol abuse. In many tribes, 20% or more of the members have diabetes. The incidence of obesity has paralleled the rise in incidence of diabetes. Alcohol abuse is a significant health issue in American Indian culture. As many as 95% of American Indian families may be affected directly or indirectly by a family member's alcohol abuse. The incidence of fetal alcohol syndrome, a collection of congenital problems caused by in utero exposure to alcohol, is five to six times higher in American Indian populations (US Department of Health and Human Services, 1990).

Statistics on maternal and infant mortality indicate that individuals least able to afford private care have the worst obstetric and neonatal outcomes. This raises a serious ethical question. Should the United States continue to invest financial resources in the development of high technology designed to save infants who otherwise would die, when poor maternal and infant health status results in part from socioeconomic need?

National Priorities in Maternal and Infant Health

Nationwide objectives for pregnancy and infant health care were set for the year 1990 by the United States government. Only two of these objectives, reduced infant mortality and reduced neonatal mortality for all races, were met. New health objectives were established in 1990 in a document entitled *Healthy People 2000* (US Department of Health and Human Services, 1990). This document sets broad public health goals for the coming decade. The three principal goals for the next decade are to:

- Increase the span of healthy life for all Americans.
- Reduce health disparities among Americans.
- Achieve access to preventive services for all Americans.

Several areas in the field of perinatal care were targeted. Specific objectives in priority areas of concern are shown in the accompanying display.

Barriers to Optimal Maternity Care

Threats to maternal–infant well-being such as poverty, discrimination, and impaired access to care require attention by professional groups at the national, regional, and local levels. Nurses are the single largest group of health care providers in the United States. Nursing's influence is substantial and could pave the way for eliminating barriers to optimal perinatal care.

Access to Care: The Health Care Nonsystem

Adequate prenatal care is not accessible to all women in the United States. Even when it is accessible, it is not always sought. These facts have direct consequences for maternal and infant well-being. An expectant woman with no prenatal care is three times more likely to have a low–birth-weight neonate. Despite the importance of early prenatal care, nearly 1 in 4 pregnant women in the United States receives no care in the first trimester. A disproportionate number of these women have low income, have less than a high school

Specific Public Health Objectives for Pregnancy and Infant Health in the United States by the Year 2000

- Reduce infant mortality to no more than 7 deaths per 1000 births (a 31% decrease).
- Reduce low birth weight to no more than 5% of live births (a 28% decrease)
- Increase first trimester prenatal care to at least 90% of live births (an 18% increase)
- Reduce teenage pregnancies to no more than 50/1000 teens aged 17 and younger (a 30% decrease)
- Reduce unintended pregnancies to no more than 30% of pregnancies (a 46% decrease)

US Department of Health and Human Services. (September 1990). Healthy People 2000: National Health Promotion and Disease Prevention Objectives.

education, or are adolescent. Although progress was made in increasing early entry into prenatal care during the 1970s, little additional progress has been made in the last decade. A significant factor contributing to this problem is the fact that nearly 14 million women of reproductive age have no insurance to cover perinatal care. Many pregnant women encounter problems in gaining access to available public care because of the confusing requirements and complex array of services (McClanahan, 1992).

Factors related to inadequate prenatal care can be organized into three categories: sociodemographic, attitudinal, and system related. Sociodemographic factors include minority status, poverty, age, and area of residence. Urban-dwelling minority women typically also have low incomes and may have some difficulty obtaining prenatal care services. Rural populations are also likely to be low income and to have little or no close access to care. Increasingly, rural physicians often do not provide obstetric services because of rising malpractice insurance costs and the demands of solo obstetric practice (Bushy, 1990).

Attitudinal factors that influence initiation of prenatal care include an unwanted and unplanned pregnancy, lack of social support and resources, and fear of negative responses from family or care providers. System factors related to inadequate prenatal care include underfunded, understaffed, and crowded care facilities, delays in determining eligibility for public services, and difficulties finding providers who will accept Medicaid reimbursement for obstetric services. In general, problems with obtaining and using prenatal care by those most in need results from patchwork of services, often poorly coordinated, referred to as the health care "nonsystem" (McClanahan, 1992).

Sexism and Racism

Another subtle threat to maternal–infant health is discrimination in care based on gender and ethnicity. More restrictive practices in obstetrics during the 1950s reflected the general view of women as dependent and unable to make decisions about their own care. Organized medicine, like other professions, tended to adopt a sexist ideology growing out of the Victorian Age. Many of the more obvious expressions of sexism in perinatal care have been eliminated as family-centered care has gained greater acceptance.

However, sexist ideology may continue to persist in subtle ways. Sexism may be seen in scheduling prenatal and postpartum clinic hours on the assumption that a woman is available during regular work hours. This scheduling neglects the fact that most women of childbearing age are employed outside the home. Flexible scheduling reflects the need to make perinatal care widely available.

The nurse can observe other signs in the way women are treated as consumers in the health care system. Women with physical complaints are more likely to be regarded as having emotional or stress-related symptoms than are men presenting with the same symptom. Communications between providers and consumers differ both in style and substance depending on the gender of the consumer, with men receiving more factual information and more deference from the provider. A vivid example of this gender-related bias can be seen in the practice of addressing laboring women as "honey" or "dear" instead of by their given names (Hull, 1990; Bergstrom, Roberts, Skillman, & Seidel, 1992).

Racism is another barrier to achieving optimal maternal–infant health care. The poorer health indicators among African Americans and other ethnic minority groups clearly reflect both economic and social disparities. Some of this may be attributable to lingering racial discrimination. A nursing research study that may shed light on this issue is under way in California. It may suggest that low-income African American women can readily describe in detail the discriminatory practices and behaviors they encounter while receiving prenatal care in public agencies. Even when culturally sensitive and appropriate services are established, minority women may be mistrustful because of the long-established pattern of being treated like second-class citizens. This mistrust may result from professionals' negative attitudes about those on public assistance (Norbeck & DeJoseph, 1992).

Perinatal care in the United States is not producing outcomes consistent with national health goals. High rates of infant morbidity and mortality continue when compared to other industrialized countries, especially among those who live in poverty. Data clearly suggest that major threats to health are not being adequately addressed. Problems with access to prenatal care, uncoordinated elements in the health care "nonsystem," and sexism contribute to the unrealized goal of adequate perinatal care in the United States. The challenge of providing adequate care to minority populations at risk for health problems is growing.

Established and Emerging Roles in Perinatal Nursing

Roles and responsibilities change rapidly in health care. Change is certainly evident in the field of perinatal nursing. Regardless of the pace of change in the field, the nurse is responsible for knowing the boundaries of safe practice and for practicing within those boundaries. Professional nursing practice is characterized by its recognition and knowledge of standards of practice. The overall scope of nursing practice is determined in large part by nurse practice acts in each state. However, because practice usually changes more rapidly than legislation, the scope of nursing practice is also governed by community standards. Examples include standards set as policies and procedures in health care agencies or those stated by the Joint Commission on Accreditation of Healthcare Organizations (JCAHO). The nurse is legally held responsible for practicing within the scope of these standards.

Recognition of Standards of Practice

Specialty organizations establish standards specific to particular areas of nursing practice. Specialty organizations are necessary because the scope of knowledge in a profession is too broad across the entire field for effective communication and implementation of appropriate standards. The major points of the Association of Women's Health, Obstetric, and

Major Points From AWHONN Standards for the Nursing Care of Women and Newborns

Standard I: Nursing Practice

Comprehensive nursing care for women and newborns focuses on helping individuals, families, and communities achieve their optimum health potential. This is best achieved within the framework of the nursing process.

Standard II: Health Education and Counseling

Health education for the individual, family, and community is an integral part of comprehensive nursing care. Such education encourages participation in and shared responsibility for health promotion, maintenance, and restoration.

Standard III: Policies, Procedures, and Protocols

Written policies, procedures, and protocols clarify the scope of nursing practice and delineate the qualifications of personnel authorized to provide care to women and newborns within the health care setting.

Standard IV: Professional Responsibility and Accountability

Comprehensive nursing care for women and newborns is provided by nurses who are clinically competent and accountable for professional actions and legal responsibilities inherent in the nursing role.

Standard V: Utilization of Nursing Personnel

Nursing care for women and newborn is conducted in practice settings that have qualified nursing staff in sufficient numbers to meet patient care needs.

Standard VI: Ethics

Ethical principles guide the process of decision-making for nurses caring for women and newborn at all times and especially when personal or professional values conflict with those of the patient, family, colleagues, or practice setting.

Standard VII: Research

Nurses caring for women and newborns use research findings, conduct nursing research, and evaluate nursing practice to improve the outcomes of care.

Standard VII: Quality Assurance

Quality and appropriateness of patient care are evaluated through a planned assessment program using specific, identified clinical indicators.

NAACOG Standards for the Nursing Care of Women and Newborns. (1991). (4th ed.). Reprinted with permission.

Neonatal Nurses (AWHONN) standards are listed in the accompanying display.

A wide variety of roles are available to nurses in the field of perinatal care. In part, this reflects the fragmentation of perinatal care that exists in many settings. It also reflects developments in specialization, such as the continued evolution of the role of the nurse midwife, and the blending of the roles of nurse practitioner and clinical nurse specialist (Gleeson et al., 1990). Increasingly, the scope of practice in perinatal nursing is based on university education and is responsive to rapidly changing delivery system needs.

Nurse Clinicians in Inpatient Perinatal Care

In hospital settings, nurses may have a variety of educational preparation. Educational requirements are dictated by each institution. Although entry-level positions may be available in labor and delivery and newborn nursery areas, often these positions require an internship or an extended orientation period. This is due to the specialized nature of nursing practice and the challenges posed by high-risk perinatal care.

Some facilities continue to maintain separate nursing staff for labor and delivery, for postpartum care of the mother, and for newborn care. Separating the care of the mother and neonate into these arbitrary "phases" tends to create problems in the delivery of comprehensive and well-organized nursing. Nurses may not have extended contact with family members in this model of care. Such staffing arrangements also contribute to nurses' perceiving themselves as specializing in one area or another. Additionally, the division between maternal and newborn nursing care widens with the emergence of neonatology as a medical subspecialty. Many neonatal nurseries are now linked administratively with pediatrics and neonatal intensive care units. Under these circumstances, nurses may regard themselves more as neonatal nurses with less responsibility for direct care of the mother.

As a result of the aforementioned divisions leading to deemphasis of family-centered care, the late 1980s witnessed a new approach to perinatal nursing care. Facilities have implemented "mother–baby" units, in which nurses assume primary care of mothers and their newborns in the postbirth period. The primary nurse is assigned to be responsible for the care of a woman and her family from admission through postbirth follow-up and may even have prenatal contact with the family. This arrangement emphasizes comprehensive nursing care, allows for greater continuity of care, and encourages the nurse to maintain a range of clinical skills across settings (Fig. 3-2).

Blending of Roles: The Advanced Practice Nurse in Perinatal Care

To meet the challenging needs of women, neonates, and their families, a variety of advanced practice roles in perinatal nursing care have evolved. The first advanced practice to develop in perinatal care was the role of the certified nurse midwife (CNM).

The Certified Nurse Midwife

Certified nurse midwives are registered nurses. A CNM must either complete a certificate program or master's degree level educational program recognized by the American College of Nurse Midwifery (ACNM). A certification examination given by that organization entitles the nurse midwife to practice as a CNM. CNMs are prepared to deliver normal gynecologic care. They also provide primary care to women during pregnancy and childbirth and assume care of women and their newborns during the postbirth period. CNMs have expanded practice responsibilities. They may manage labor and birth, prescribe, and perform certain medical and surgical procedures (such as local anesthesia and episiotomy). These activities are within the scope of nurse midwifery practice (Fig. 3-3). CNMs collaborate with physicians in the care of women with complex health problems. If prepared at the master's degree level, CNMs may function as clinical nurse specialists (CNS) in addition to their nurse midwifery practice.

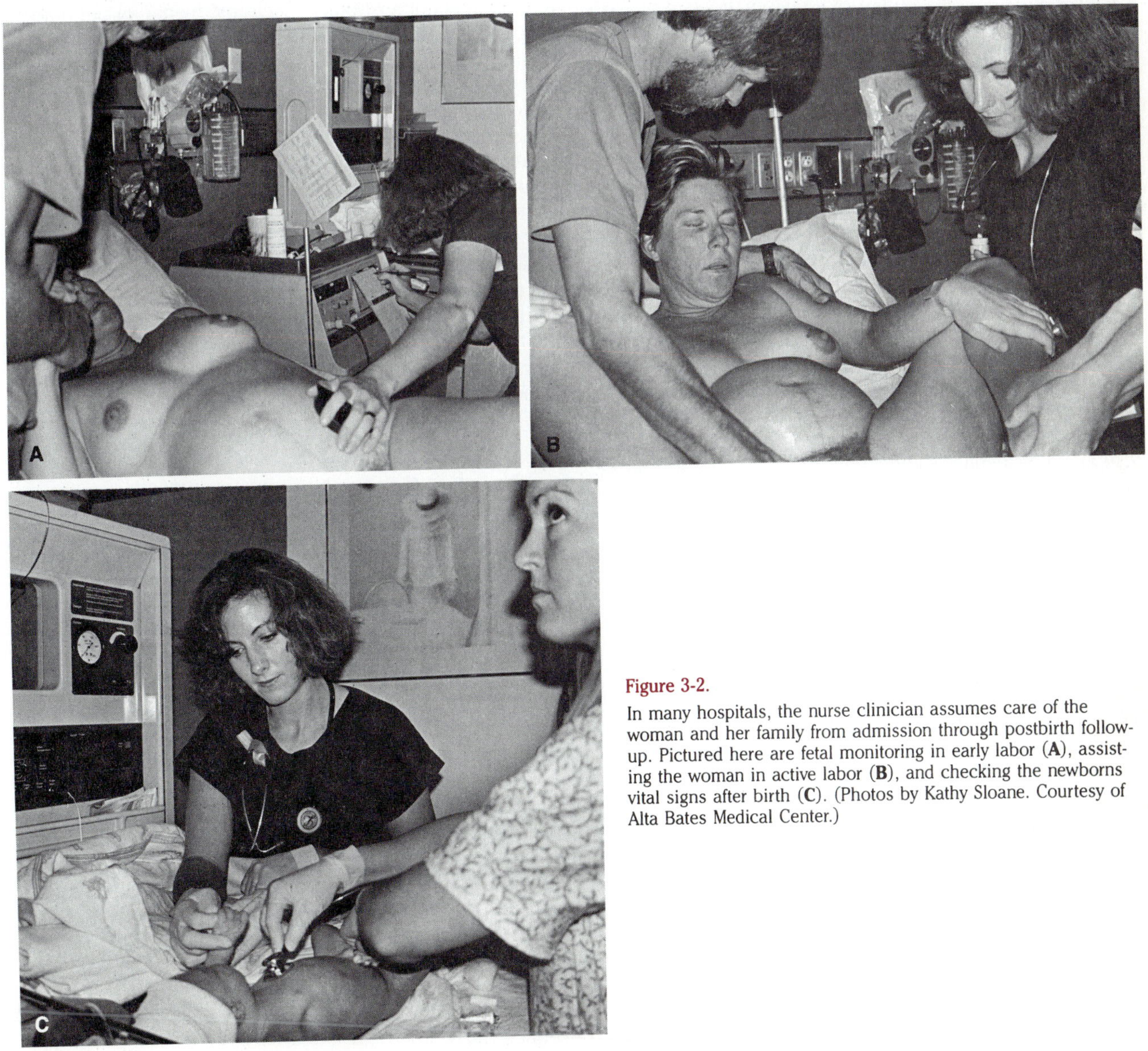

Figure 3-2.

In many hospitals, the nurse clinician assumes care of the woman and her family from admission through postbirth follow-up. Pictured here are fetal monitoring in early labor (**A**), assisting the woman in active labor (**B**), and checking the newborns vital signs after birth (**C**). (Photos by Kathy Sloane. Courtesy of Alta Bates Medical Center.)

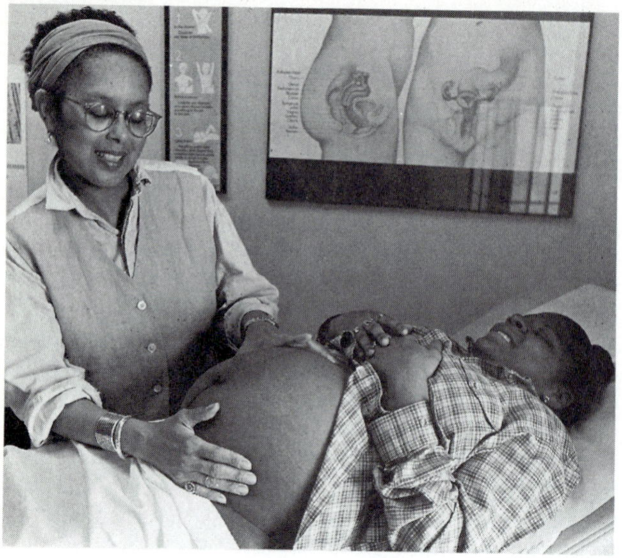

Figure 3-3.
A certified nurse midwife performing a prenatal health assessment on a pregnant adolescent. (Photo by Kathy Sloane. Courtesy of Hill-care Medical Group.)

The Clinical Nurse Specialist

The clinical nurse specialist is a registered nurse who has completed a master's degree program in nursing. Specialized education includes reproductive health and expertise in planning, supervision, and delivery of nursing care to families during the childbearing period. Major responsibilities of the CNS are consultation, family and staff education, and coordination and delivery of nursing care to families requiring intensive nursing support. The CNS may also be engaged in research activities in collaboration with other nurse researchers. These individuals may be based primarily in the inpatient setting but can work across settings to facilitate continuity of care. The CNS may also have primary responsibility for parent education programs, such as prenatal and parenting classes, and support groups. The CNS may care for women or neonates with particular health problems or may work exclusively with high-risk patients and their families.

The Nurse Practitioner in Women's Health

The nurse practitioner (NP) in women's health is a registered nurse with advanced clinical preparation in the provision of primary care to women. This clinical preparation may be obtained in a certificate program or as part of a master's degree in nursing. Graduate programs are more in depth, preparing the nurse to function as a CNS with NP skills. In most cases, NPs must attend programs to meet state requirements for licensure. States often require completion of a certification examination such as the one given by AWHONN. NPs in women's health conduct comprehensive health assessments and manage normal prenatal, postbirth, and gynecologic care in collaboration with physicians and nurse midwives. They diagnose and treat common problems and refer women to physicians according to established protocols.

During the 1990s, the roles of the CNS and the NP are likely to blend. The American Nurses Association has a single Council on Practice, which addresses issues related to advanced practice, emphasizing that advanced practice nurses may care for women and their families in the hospital, the clinic, or the home. Essential elements of advanced practice are similar, regardless of the setting in which care is provided (Gleeson et al., 1990).

Nurse Consultants

Increasing specialization is giving rise to the need for nurse consultants. Nurse consultants are experts in a particular area of practice who establish a private practice to provide consultation to agencies on a fee-for-service basis. For example, nurses are more frequently asked to provide expert review of materials and to act as expert witnesses regarding potential professional liability issues. Other expert nurses consult with corporations that are developing equipment or products to be used in patient care. They may be paid as speakers at continuing education meetings. Still other nurse consultants establish themselves as consultants to publishers of textbooks, electronic media, or periodicals on perinatal health issues. These roles require considerable clinical expertise as well as specialized skills and experience.

The Nurse Scientist in Perinatal Nursing

Perinatal nurses are also engaged in nursing research in increasing numbers. Nurse scientists are employed by schools of nursing, health care agencies, and government. Generally, positions include teaching, administration, and research activities. The desirable educational preparation for a research career in nursing is the doctoral degree; nursing doctoral programs often offer specialization in the study of the family or in women's health. Nurse scientists in perinatal nursing are engaged in the study of health problems facing women and their families (see AWHONN research priorities in Chapter 2).

Innovative Roles in Clinical Nursing Services

Perinatal nursing focuses on providing services to individuals who are healthy and are attempting to prevent health problems during pregnancy and childbirth. Indeed, the strong emphasis on health promotion, self-care, and teaching has contributed to the emergence of the private practice role in nursing. Although nurse midwives and NPs have historically practiced in collaborative arrangements with physicians and other health professionals, some are now choosing to concentrate on an aspect of their practice that is more independent. Specialized educational programs, such as prenatal or breastfeeding education or counseling persons who have concerns about their fertility, are examples of expanded private practice opportunities for nurses in advanced practice.

The options for independent practice for clinical nurses employed in inpatient settings have been more limited. One of the most common ways for perinatal nurses to establish independent practice is through childbirth education. They may teach classes in a particular hospital setting as an independent contractor or in a community on a fee-for-service basis.

However, some unique independent practice arrangements have also developed. Perinatal nurses have established group practices to provide one-to-one postpartum recovery care and home follow-up for families desiring early postbirth discharge. These nurses share on-call time and are paid on a fee-for-service basis. Other nurses have established themselves in private practice as experts in sibling preparation for childbirth. They offer group and private classes for families wanting to teach their older children about childbirth. CNSs have set up practices in collaboration with obstetricians to provide childbirth education, postbirth home follow-up, and parent support groups on a fee-for-service basis.

The field of perinatal nursing will continue to develop in response to the changing social context of childbirth and perinatal care. Many changes in the field will reflect changes in the nursing profession overall. Trends in nursing care will likely include increasing pressure for cost-effective care mandated by prospective payment systems. Nurses will be challenged to create innovative practices in a climate with mounting resistance from other competing professionals.

Innovative practices by perinatal nurses are important to the future development of the specialty. Nurses have tended to undervalue their contribution to health care and have underestimated their ability to provide services beyond the typical nursing roles and practice settings. As nurses develop, expand, and strengthen their clinical practice base, some impediments to full professional practice will continue to confront them.

To meet the challenging needs of women, neonates, and their families, a variety of advanced practice roles in perinatal nursing care have evolved. These roles include the certified nurse midwife, the nurse practitioner, the clinical nurse specialist, the nurse consultant, and the nurse scientist. There is some blurring between these roles, especially between the nurse practitioner and the clinical nurse specialist.

Perinatal Nursing: An Underused Resource

Several barriers prevent the full use of perinatal nursing. These barriers are the same ones facing the entire nursing profession:

- The difficulty of demonstrating the actual cost and value of nursing care in the hospital setting.
- The ongoing struggle to establish and maintain nursing in a decision-making position in planning and implementing health care delivery.
- The problem of recruiting intelligent, career-minded individuals into the field despite relatively low pay and low status.
- The challenging, often extremely difficult working conditions.

However, some factors seem to be more clearly focused in the field of perinatal nursing. These include physician oversupply and maldistribution, professional liability and increasing litigation, sexism in the health care system, and ethical decision-making.

Physician Oversupply and Maldistribution

One factor that may limit the impact of perinatal nursing on the future health of the nation is the projected oversupply of physicians in metropolitan areas. Rural areas continue to be underserved in terms of prenatal and obstetric care (Lutz, 1991). This will have a significant impact on the scope of nursing practice with childbearing families. Will this problem mean changes in CNM and NP practice in perinatal women's health? The answer is likely to be yes. Physician resistance to nursing roles in primary health care is increasing already in metropolitan areas where professionals tend to concentrate and where competition is most acute. In recent years, CNMs have experienced discrimination in obtaining hospital admitting privileges. Some attempts have been made to limit the scope of nurse midwifery practice in several states through legislative changes sponsored by organized medicine.

The crisis in liability insurance has meant that many already underserved populations continue to lose physician providers. Despite the fact that provision of perinatal services by CNMs and NPs remains a logical solution, resistance from individual physicians and from organized medicine still significantly limits nurses practicing in these roles (Jacox, 1987; National Commission to Prevent Infant Mortality, 1988).

Will the physician oversupply in some regions mean that some services now regarded as nursing functions will be absorbed by medicine? Possibly. The next 20 years will be critical. The current debate regarding health care reform is a significant opportunity for nursing to step forward and assume greater responsibility for shaping the health care system of the future (American Nurses Association, 1991). Outcomes will depend in large part on how well nurses demonstrate the value and cost effectiveness of their practice. Individual nurses will need to document and communicate clearly their unique contributions to the health care needs of childbearing families. Research activities need to be undertaken to document the cost effectiveness and appropriateness of nursing interventions. Collectively, nursing must continue to participate in legislative activities. Emphasis on nursing's collaborative rather than subordinate role with medicine will position nursing to meet the future challenges of providing quality health care in a cost-effective manner.

Professional Liability and Increasing Litigation

In recent years the issue of professional liability has become more significant in nursing. Until the 1970s nurses were rarely named in litigation. However, current nursing literature and behavior in the workplace now reflect concerns about the significant legal risk faced by perinatal nurses, especially those practicing in labor and delivery.

Professional liability is defined as responsibility for acts of negligence. In health care, liability concerns the provision of substandard care that results in patient injury. Individual liability includes acts of omission and commission. It includes both failing to do something that should have been done, as well as doing something incorrectly or outside of accepted standards of care. The employer may be liable for employee negligence, even if the employer is without fault in the particular situation in which harm is claimed. Thus, most litigation involving patient claims of injury will name nurses, physicians, and the institution.

Nurses are liable for their own acts, committed either alone or with others; the nurse is generally not liable for the acts of others. However, many lawsuits name both nurses and physicians if the cause of an injury is unclear or both participated in the actions that the patient claims caused the injury. In perinatal nursing, joint actions are common, especially in emergency situations where assessments and interventions happen very quickly (Fiesta, 1991).

Nurses working in labor and delivery are at special risk for litigation for several reasons. First, most lawsuits are based on a claim that the neonate has sustained severe birth injury and will require long-term care. Second, most cases center on a claim that substandard care caused this injury. Cause and effect are often difficult to prove. Evidence of substandard care unrelated to the injury may lead to a decision against the care provider. Finally, labor and delivery nurses are especially vulnerable because of the frequent unavailability of physicians. The labor and delivery nurse is responsible for communicating information to the physician. The physician uses this information to decide about medical care. The time frame between first observation of worrisome signs and actual harm to mother or fetus is often short. Thus, the labor and delivery nurse must be skilled at monitoring, interpreting, and communicating information as well as acting promptly on that information (Fiesta, 1991).

Critical Nursing Errors

Critical nursing errors that consistently appear in cases that come to litigation are listed in the Legal/Ethical Considerations display and are discussed briefly below.

A key legal expectation of the professional nurse is the ability to foresee harm to the patient. Thus, the initial history and examination must be complete so that the nurse may identify risk factors that will influence the process of ongoing nursing care. The nurse must assess the status of the woman and fetus immediately and recognize situations that require additional action, including communication with the birth attendant. The nurse is legally responsible for initiating and maintaining timely and effective communication. This responsibility includes provision of critical information to enable the birth attendant to make reasonable judgments and specific requests for assistance.

Documentation of patient status and the care rendered is another vital nursing responsibility. Critical legal consequences can result from incomplete medical records. The medical record is regarded as the only valid record of events from a legal standpoint. The record must provide evidence that the nurse maintained standards of practice in nursing care. Hospital policies and procedures records are often subpoenaed. This requires the nurse not only to document problems but also to document the actions taken and the effectiveness of those actions.

Legal/Ethical Considerations

Critical Nursing Errors in Cases Involving Litigation

The following errors or omissions may seem unimportant and may not be proved to contribute directly to injury to the patient but may cast enough doubt about clinical care that a judgment against the professional will result.

- Incomplete initial history and physical examination
- Failure to observe and take appropriate action
- Failure to communicate changes in the patient's condition
- Incomplete or inadequate documentation
- Failure to use or interpret fetal monitoring appropriately

Appropriate use and interpretation of fetal monitoring has become a central element in contemporary perinatal nursing practice. Concern about the widespread use of electronic fetal monitoring in low-risk situations continues. However, in the presence of any risk factor, continuous fetal monitoring is standard practice. The nurse is responsible for maintaining appropriate surveillance and for interpreting data on fetal heart rate accurately. This aspect of practice is discussed in detail in Chapter 22.

The most effective way to avoid professional liability in nursing practice is through careful, critical assessment of clinical care against recognized standards. At the institutional level, the process of "risk management" involves setting up standards of practice, standards for professional training, and policies and procedures designed to reduce or eliminate the chances of injury.

However, these measures have been insufficient. The rising incidence of litigation in obstetric care in recent years has caused nationwide concern about the economic and human costs of malpractice and liability. Indeed, obstetrics has become one of the three specialties most susceptible to malpractice litigation. This explosion in litigation against care providers has been recent: 80% of all medical malpractice cases in United States history have been filed since 1975. Almost three quarters of all the obstetrician-gynecologists in the United States have been sued, and nearly 30% have had three or more suits filed against them. One especially unfortunate result of the malpractice crisis has been the rising cost of liability insurance and its effects on access to obstetric care (National Commission to Prevent Infant Mortality, 1988; Lederman, 1991).

All physicians have been affected by extreme increases in liability insurance rates. Unfortunately, this fact has led to unwillingness on the part of some physicians to provide perinatal services because of the risk of lawsuits. The low reimbursement rate by Medicaid is hastening the departure of physicians from obstetric practice. Even though some states have increased Medicaid payments for perinatal care, nearly all states remain below usual charges and insurance payment rates. This gap in access to care cannot be filled readily by other providers, such as CNMs and NPs. They also are saddled with increasing insurance costs and cannot practice without a collaborative arrangement with a physician. More than one third of CNMs deliver care to women and families who have low-income status. Nurse midwives and family physicians deliver two thirds of the health care in rural and inner city areas. Clearly, rising insurance rates and liability concerns will have their greatest impact on health care providers with relatively low incomes (Lederman, 1991).

A few states have enacted legislation aimed at alleviating problems of affordability and availability of liability insurance. These states are attempting to improve access to perinatal care for low-income groups. Examples of such actions include creating state funds to help pay liability insurance premiums for perinatal care providers who practice in underserved areas. State governments may cover malpractice awards against providers in public clinics. Some states are considering reducing the period of time within which malpractice suits can be filed (the statute of limitations). In some states, the statute of limitations begins to apply only when the child reaches the age of majority (usually 18 years of age). This extends the threat of liability over many years (National Commission to Prevent Infant Mortality, 1988).

A full discussion of legal issues in perinatal nursing is beyond the scope of this text. Examples are presented throughout the text in special displays entitled Legal/Ethical Considerations.

Sexism in the Health Care System

A lingering problem facing nurses that may limit the impact nursing has on the health of childbearing women and their families is sexism (O'Rourke, 1989). Sexism is especially evident in perinatal care because most nurses are women and care is provided to pregnant women, largely by male physicians. Small examples can be seen in nurse–physician interactions. For instance, typically nurses are addressed by their first names, yet physicians are addressed by their professional title. Another example of sexism in the health care system is the extent to which nurses are excluded or disregarded as experts in health care (see the Nursing Research display).

Other examples of sexism come from within nursing itself. It is still not unusual for male nursing students and male nurses to experience a subtle form of discrimination in the scope of work experiences available to them in perinatal care. On occasion, hospitals still require nursing instructors to obtain "permission" from physicians for male nursing students to work with laboring or postpartum women in the hospital setting. However, perinatal nurses have an excellent vantage point from which they can identify and work to change problems such as this one.

Nursing Research

Nurses as Experts: A Media Perspective

A nursing study conducted in 1990 examined the degree that nurses were used by health journalists as sources of information. The researchers analyzed the content of 423 articles from major national newspapers. Of the 908 sources directly quoted, nurses (the largest profession in the health care system) were quoted least often, less than 2% of the time. Persons in occupational groups such as physicians, government officials, business people, patients, family members, and other hospital workers were quoted more frequently than nurses. Nurses were almost entirely absent as sources of information, even in stories on topics that depend heavily on nursing, such as the care of AIDS patients.

When it was possible to determine the gender of the journalist by the byline, women accounted for 35% of the writers. Female journalists tended to use a slightly larger percentage of female sources, but they did not seek out nurses or report on nursing any more often than did their male counterparts.

The authors concluded that it is difficult for the nursing profession to have a strong influence in the development of public policy and in decisions about allocation of health care resources when it is virtually unseen and unheard in the public dialogue. Nursing's contribution to improvement in the health care system will continue to be limited if nurses are not considered to be legitimate sources of health information.

Buresh, B., Gordon, S., & Bell, N. (1991). Who counts in news coverage of health care? *Nursing Outlook, 39*(5), 204–208.

Ethical Complexity in Perinatal Care

Because it is usually the nurse who spends the most time with women and their families, ethical issues in perinatal care are difficult and often personally troubling to nurses. The difficulties in sorting out ethical issues may limit the extent to which perinatal nurses engage in dialogue and debate about the care of women as individuals or as a group.

One recurring theme in the literature focuses on the issue of maternal and fetal rights. The concept of the fetus as a person separate from the mother has emerged with advances in technology that allow assessment of fetal well-being and treatment of fetal conditions. Probably the most difficult cases arise when a mode of therapy becomes an accepted practice and a woman refuses it. In recent years, several court cases have resulted in court-ordered cesarean deliveries to protect a potentially viable fetus over the woman's objections to the surgery (Greenlaw, 1990).

These cases have been controversial for two main reasons. First, it is clear that fetal life and well-being do not exist independently of the woman. Second, forced medical treatment of the fetus against the woman's wishes requires that she become a patient against her will. If she is a competent adult, this approach is generally not accepted legally or ethically (Strong & Kinlaw, 1991). It is unclear how far the courts will go to protect a fetus before viability. However, the standard of viability is likely to change, as technologic advances move from experimental treatment to standards of care. The contemporary problems of maternal substance abuse and maternal human immunodeficiency virus infection make ethical challenges even more pressing (Chaukin, Allen, & Oberman, 1991).

Ethical analysis of enforced fetal therapy will continue to be an important issue in perinatal care for some time to come. Both risks and benefits to the fetus and woman must be taken into consideration. Aumann (1988) stated that simplistic approaches to ethical decision-making, that is emphasizing fetal rights, women's rights, parental desires or health care provider's capabilities alone, are inadequate in perinatal nursing. Regardless of the inescapable difficulty of ethical issues in providing care, it is imperative that the professional nurse have a working knowledge of clinical ethics. Recognizing ethical dilemmas, taking an ethical position in relation to nursing care, and acting based on that position are expectations of professional practice. Ethical considerations in perinatal nursing will be highlighted throughout the text in the Legal/Ethical Considerations displays.

Factors that may limit the impact of perinatal nursing in improving the health of women and their families include physician oversupply and maldistribution, increasing concerns about professional liability and litigation, sexism in the health care system, and the ethical complexity inherent in perinatal care. Physician oversupply and maldistribution have created opportunities for nurses in advanced practice, but resistance to those roles inhibits full use of nurses in these roles. Sexism in the health care system and in society tends to limit the extent to which nursing is regarded as a strong and capable force for change. Each of these factors has a specific effect on professional nursing practice and the services nurses provide.

Chapter Summary

Ensuring safe and satisfying childbirth for women in the United States is a top priority. Reduction of maternal and infant morbidity and mortality will require the concerted efforts of all health professions. Factors such as maldistribution of providers and complex legal and ethical concerns make provision of quality health care a continuing challenge. Expanded nursing roles and advancement of clinical nursing practice requires innovative thinking and action to stay abreast with changing health care needs.

The future of perinatal nursing is both challenging and rewarding. It requires creativity, adaptability, a thirst for knowledge, and a commitment to improving human health. Nursing has an opportunity to meet the needs of families at a critical transition point: pregnancy and childbirth. The following quotation from one of the first nursing publications in the area of women's health succinctly describes the challenges that are still ahead: "Providing health care means articulation with the client in a way that maximizes communication and preservation of personhood in a collaborative effort. That we have not achieved this is obvious. That we can is the challenge" (Hawkins & Higgins 1981).

Study Questions

1. *What is meant by the terms maternal morbidity and mortality rate, infant morbidity and mortality rate, and low birth weight?*
2. *How do infant mortality rates in the United States compare with those in other industrialized countries? What are possible reasons for these rates?*
3. *What national priorities in perinatal care are proposed for the year 2000? Why have these been identified as priorities?*
4. *What advanced nursing roles in perinatal care are available? What is the scope of practice for each?*
5. *What standards of care in perinatal nursing have been established? Explain the importance of standards.*
6. *How does nursing have an impact on improving maternal–infant health? What societal factors limit the impact?*
7. *What is the single most important nursing error found in medical record reviews?*
8. *What are potential ethical issues facing perinatal nurses?*

References

ANA. (1991). *Nursing's agenda for health care reform*. Washington, DC: Author.

Aumann, G. (1988). New changes, new choices: Problems with perinatal technology. *Journal of Perinatal and Neonatal Nursing, 1*(3), 1–5.

Bergstrom, L., Roberts, J., Skillman, L., & Seidel, J. (1991). "You'll feel me touching you, sweetie": Vaginal examinations during the second stage of labor. *Birth, 19*(1), 10–18.

Bushy, A. (1990). Rural determinants in family health: Considerations for community health. *Family and Community Health, 12*(4), 29–34.

Chaukin, W., Allen, M., & Oberman, M. (1991). Drug abuse and pregnancy: Some questions on public policy, clinical management and maternal–fetal rights. *Birth, 18*(2), 107–12.

Expert Panel on the Content of Prenatal Care. (1989). *Caring for our future: The content of prenatal care*. Washington, DC: Public Health Service.

Fiesta, J. (1991). Obstetrical liability. *Nursing Management, 22*(5), 17.

Gleeson, R., McIlvain-Simpson, G., Boos, M., Sweet, E., Trzcinski, K., Solberg, C., & Doughty, R. (1990). Advanced practice nursing: A model of collaborative care. *American Journal of Maternal Child Nursing, 15*(1), 9–12.

Greenlaw, J. (1990). Treatment refusal, noncompliance and substance abuse in pregnancy: Legal and ethical issues. *Birth, 17*(3), 152–156.

Hawkins, J., & Higgins, L. (1981). *Maternity and gynecological nursing*. Philadelphia: J. B. Lippincott.

Hull, R. (1990). *Dealing with sexism in nursing and medicine*. NLN Publication (20-2294).

Institute of Medicine. (1985). *Preventing low birthweight*. Washington, DC: National Academy Press.

Jacox, A. (1987). The OTA report: A policy analysis. *Nursing Outlook*, *35*(6), 262–265.

Lederman, R. (1991). Professional liability and obstetrical health care delivery. *Nursing Outlook*, *39*(1), 14–16.

Lutz, S. (1991, May 13). Practitioners are filling in for scarce physicians. *Modern Healthcare*, pp. 24–30.

McClanahan, P. (1992). Improving access to and use of prenatal care. *Journal of Obstetric, Gynecologic, and Neonatal Nursing*, *21*(4) 280–286.

National Center for Health Statistics. (1992). *Health: United States–1990*. Washington DC: US Government Printing Office.

National Commission to Prevent Infant Mortality. (1988). *Infant mortality: Care for our children, care for ourselves*. Washington DC: Author.

Norbeck, J., & DeJoseph, J. (1992). *Predictors of pregnancy complications in lower SES woman*. National Institutes of Health, National Center for Nursing Research, Grant RO 1 NR 01459.

O'Rourke, M. (1989). Generic professional behavior: Implications for the clinical nurse specialist role. *Clinical Nurse Specialist*, *3*(3), 128–132.

Strong, C., & Kinlaw, K. (1991). Maternal rights, fetal harm. *Hastings Center Reports*, *21*(3), 22–33.

US Department of Health and Human Services. (1990). *Healthy People 2000: National Health Promotion and Disease Prevention Priorities*. Washington, DC: US Government Printing Office.

Suggested Readings

Arnold, L., & Grad, R. (1992). Low birth weight and infant mortality: A health policy perspective. *NAACOG's Clinical Issues in Perinatal and Women's Health Nursing*, *3*(1), 1–12.

Balcazar, H., Aoyama, C., & Cai, X. (1991). Interpretive views on Hispanics' perinatal problems of low birth weight and prenatal care. *Public Health Reports*, *106*(4), 420–426.

Bullough, B. (1992). Alternative models for specialty nursing practice. *Nursing and Health Care*, *13*(5), 254–259.

Francis, M. (1992). Eight homeless mothers' tales. *Image*, *24*(2), 111–114.

Holmes, H., & Purdy, L. (1992). *Feminist perspectives in medical ethics*. Bloomington, IN: Indiana University Press.

Johnson, S. (1992). Ethical dilemma: A patient refuses a life-saving cesarean. *American Journal of Maternal Child Nursing*, *17*(3), 121–125.

Manion, J. (1991). Nurse intrapreneurs: The heroes of health care's future. *Nursing Outlook*, *39*(1), 18–21.

McGauhey, P., Starfield, B., Alexander, C., & Ensminger, M. (1991). Social environment and vulnerability of low birth weight children: A social-epidemiological perspective. *Pediatrics*, *88*(5), 943–953.

Shoultz, J., Hatcher, P., & Hurrell, M. (1992). Growing edges of a new paradigm: The future of nursing in the health of the nation. *Nursing Outlook*, *40*(2), 57–61.

Woodring, B. (1991). When being a clinical expert is not enough: Role ambiguity in the maternal-child clinical nurse specialist. *Journal of Perinatal and Neonatal Nursing*, *5*(3), 7–15.

UNIT II

Dynamics of Human Reproduction

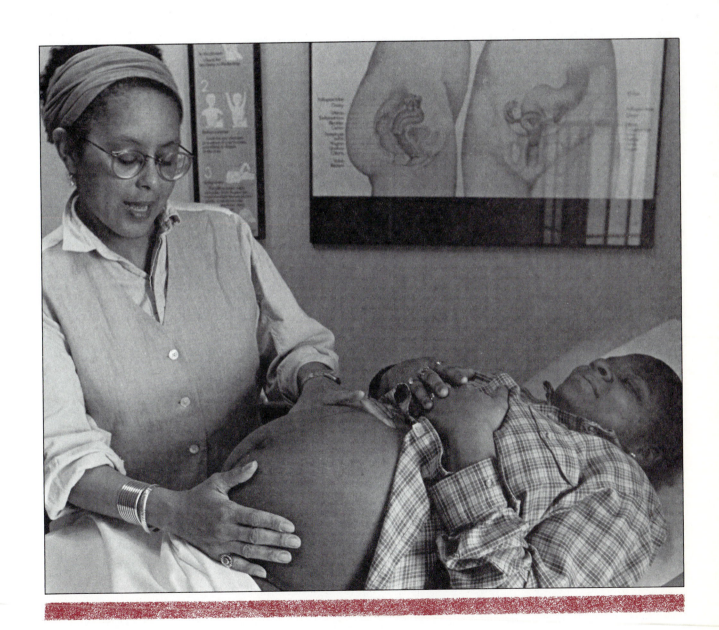

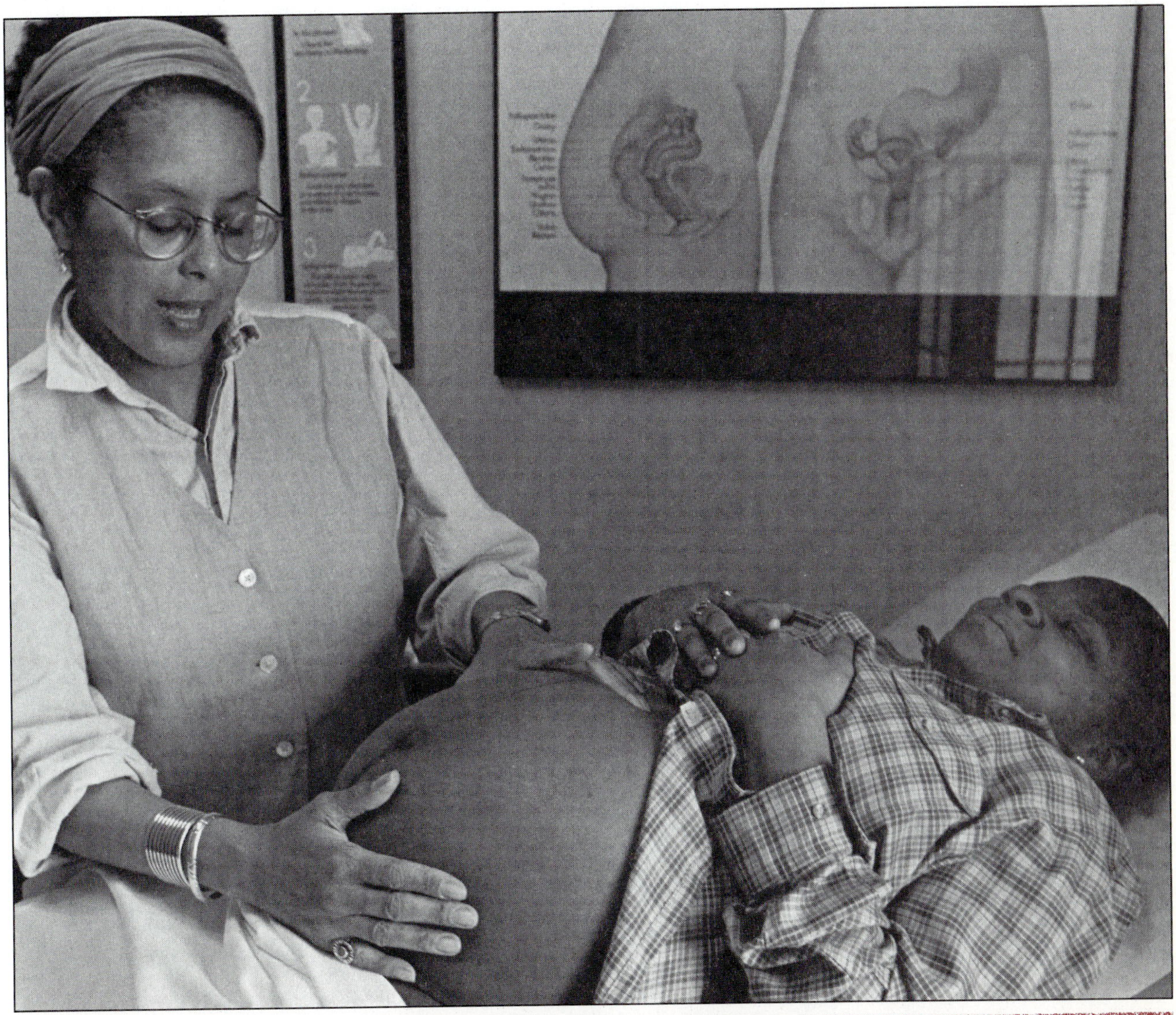

CHAPTER 4

Normal Reproductive Anatomy and Physiology

Learning Objectives

After studying the material in this chapter, the student will be able to:

- Describe the differentiation process in fetal development.
- Demonstrate a basic understanding of the male and female reproductive tracts.
- Identify the structures making up the female internal and external genitalia, and describe their function.
- List the major female hormones and their functions.
- Discuss the menstrual cycle, and identify phases of the cycle and the dominant hormones of each phase.

Key Terms

copulation
endometrium
gonad
gonadotropins
invagination
menarche
menopause
menstrual cycle
menstruation
oocyte
ovary
ovulation
puberty
spermatogenesis
stroma

For most people human reproductive function "comes naturally." However, nurses working with women and their families have two prerequisites: knowledge and confidence. A sound understanding of male and female anatomy gives the nurse confidence in dealing with sensitive issues surrounding reproduction. The nurse may use opportunities to share information and answer questions openly regarding human reproduction. Teaching adolescents about reproduction provides a sense of satisfaction when adolescents respond positively by showing interest and understanding.

Women may be less knowledgeable than men about their sexual anatomy because their organs are concealed. They also may be less comfortable about discussing their sexual anatomy than men and reserve their questions for close friends or health care providers. The nurse's role in health promotion is an ideal way to dispel the myths and misinformation perpetuated by uninformed sources.

This chapter presents the normal anatomy and physiology of the male and female reproductive systems. A discussion of male and female hormones and their importance in maintaining a normal reproductive tract closes the chapter. Although all body systems are exposed to the sex steroids, the male and female reproductive organs are controlled by them. The ebb and flow of hormones play an important role in sexual activity. For conception to occur hormone levels must be sustained at a critical level in the woman.

Sexual Differentiation

The biologic process that determines whether the conceptus is male or female is an amazing one. Each reproductive structure in one sex generally corresponds to a similar structure in the other sex, as shown in Figure 4-1. Reproductive structures in both sexes are homologous; that is, they rise from the same embryonic tissue. In the fifth and sixth weeks of pregnancy, two primitive gonads form. The gonads are considered bipotential, meaning that they can differentiate

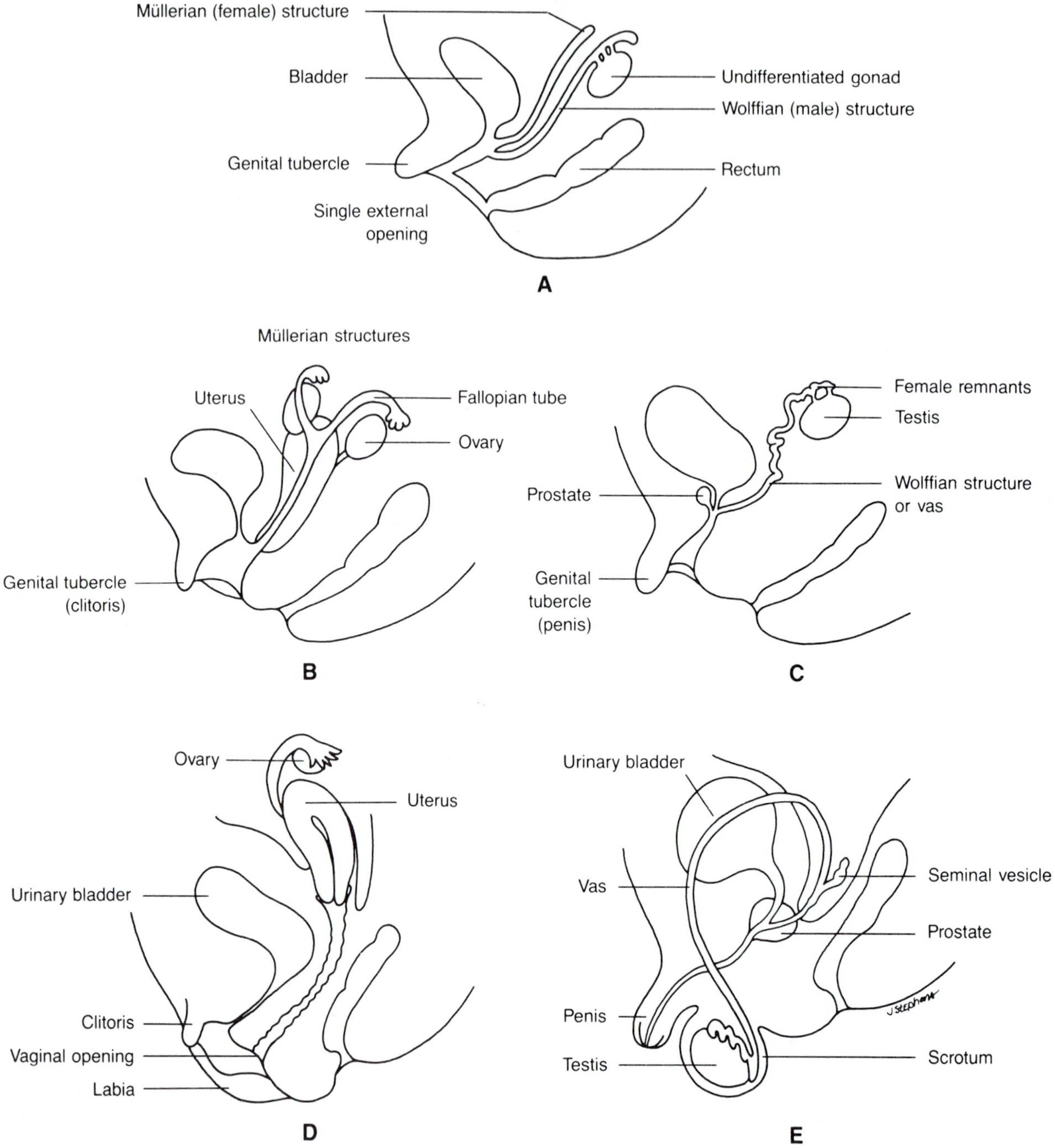

Figure 4-1.
Stages of internal fetal sex differentiation (Childbirth Graphics). (Adapted from Masters, W. & Johnson, V. [1966]. *Human sexual response*. Boston: Little, Brown & Co.)

into either testes or ovaries. Two paired primitive duct systems form in both male and female embryos at this time, the müllerian and the wolffian ducts.

The primitive gonads will develop into testes when H-Y antigen (controlled by the Y chromosome) is present. Without the H-Y antigen the primitive gonads will always develop into ovaries. Fetal androgen must continue to be present in appropriate amounts and at the right times for further development of the male structures from the wolffian ducts. The testes will be formed by the eighth week if the embryo is male and will produce two chemicals: müllerian duct inhibiting factor and androgens. Müllerian duct inhibiting factor causes the müllerian ducts (or female duct system) to shrink and nearly disappear, thus inhibiting formation of the fallopian tubes in the male. The androgens, which are hormones that cause masculinization, consist of testosterone and dihydrotestosterone. Testosterone stimulates the development of the wolffian ducts into the epididymis, vas deferens, seminal vesicles, and ejaculatory ducts. Dihydrotestosterone stimulates the development of the penis, scrotum, and prostate gland.

The differentiation of the primitive gonads into ovaries

does not depend on hormones. The ovaries develop at approximately the 12th week of embryonic life. The müllerian duct system forms the uterus, fallopian tubes, and inner third of the vagina in the female embryo. The wolffian duct system in the female shrinks into tiny remnants because high levels of testosterone are absent.

The external genitals of the male and female embryo begin to differentiate between the seventh and the 14th week of development. A slight amount of testosterone remains in the female embryo, promoting the development of the clitoris, vulva, and vagina. In the male, testosterone causes the shaft of the penis to form by the 12th week of gestation. The penis results from a growing together of the folds that would develop into the labia minora in the female (Fig. 4-2).

The genital tubercle develops into the glans of the clitoris in the female and the glans of the penis in the male. The adult form of these homologous organs is shown in Figure 4-3. The labioscrotal swellings become the outer vaginal lips of the female and the scrotum in the male. Thus, by the 12th to 14th week of gestation, the biologic sex of the fetus has been fairly well established, as shown in Table 4-1.

Although biologically (that is, genetically) sex is determined at conception, for the first 6 weeks of gestation the conceptus remains sexually undifferentiated. The conceptus is neither male nor female. As they develop, the reproductive structures are similar to that of the opposite sex.

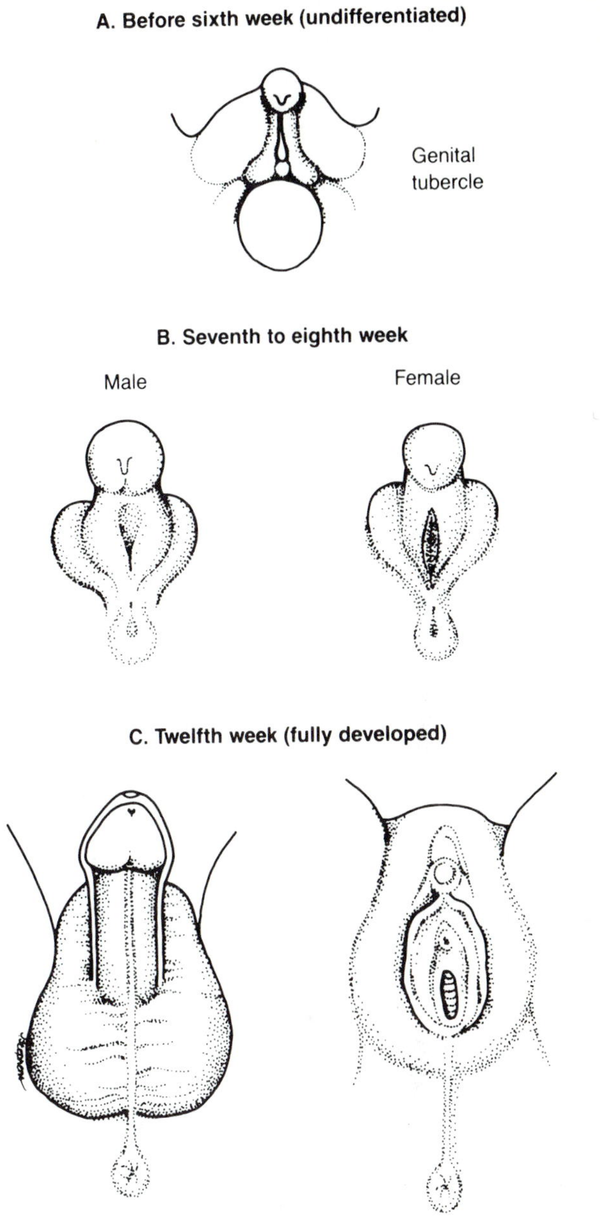

Figure 4-2.
Three stages in the differentiation of the male and female external genitalia. **A**: The undifferentiated stage appears during the second month of gestation. **B**: The differentiated stage occurs at approximately the third month of gestation. **C**: The fully developed stage at birth (Childbirth Graphics).

Structure and Function of the Male Reproductive System

The male reproductive system is composed of structures that enable production, storage, and delivery of sperm. The male reproductive system has external and internal structures.

External Male Genitalia

The male external genitalia include the penis and the scrotum. There also is a characteristic distribution of pubic hair, called the escutcheon. In males the escutcheon is roughly diamond-shaped, with hair growing toward the umbilicus, laterally across the pubic arch, and downward over the thighs. The penis is capable of becoming erect during sexual arousal. Its structure enables placement of sperm near the cervix during sexual intercourse.

Penis

The penis, the male organ of copulation or sexual intercourse, delivers semen into the female reproductive tract. It is elongated, pendant, and consists of a shaft attached anteriorly and laterally to the pubic arch. There is a glans located at the distal end of the penis. Essential parts of the organ are three cylindric columns of cavernosa, or erectile bodies, and the urethra.

The erectile columns that make up the bulk of the penis are two lateral corpora cavernosa and a single corpus spongiosum (Fig. 4-4). The corpora cavernosa are surrounded by an outer longitudinal layer and an inner circular layer of dense fibrous connective tissue called the tunica albuginea. This sheath of tissue controls the distention of the erectile tissue beyond a certain point. The two corpora cavernosa are separated by a layer of fascia and form the anterior portion of the penis.

The corpus spongiosum, similar to its neighboring bodies, surrounds the urethra and is in the median posterior position. The urethra within the corpus spongiosum remains patent during sexual excitement to allow passage of semen during ejaculation. Extending beyond the lower borders of

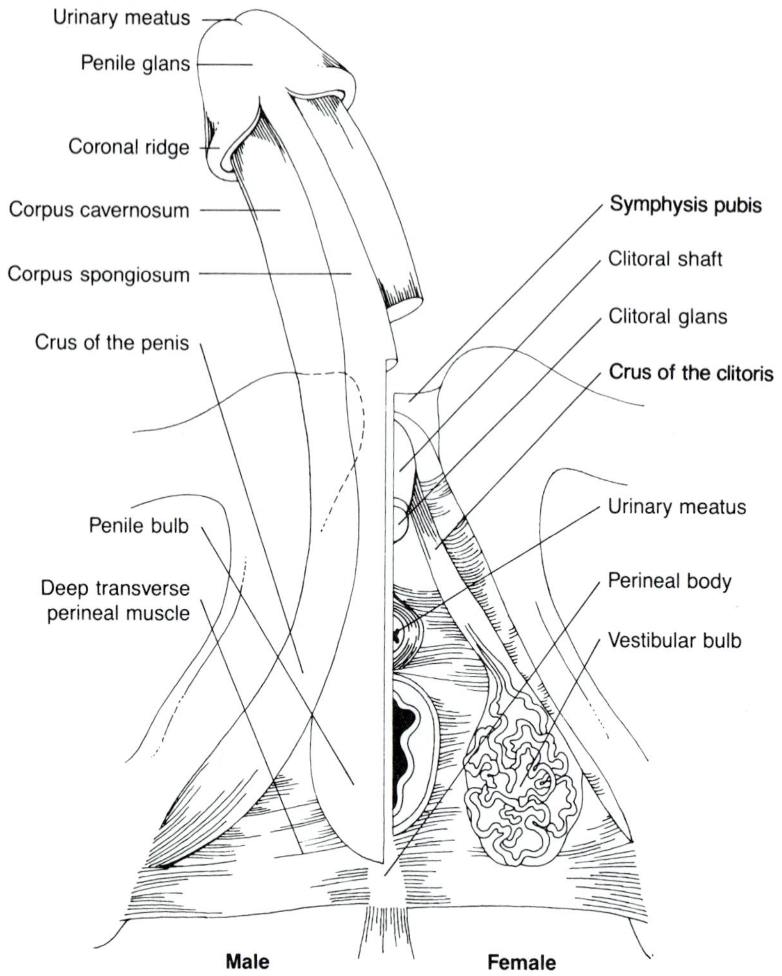

Figure 4-3.
Clitoral and penile structures. This drawing allows comparison of the placement and size of clitoris and penis. Note that the vestibular and penile bulbs are similar in size. The crura of the penis and clitoris also are similar in size, shape, and anchoring site. The pelvic bones of the female are slightly larger than those of the male. The pendulous portion of the penis is vastly larger than its homologue, the clitoral shaft and glans. (After Sherfey, M. J. [1972]. *The nature and evolution of female sexuality* [2nd ed.]. New York: Random House.)

the corpora cavernosa, the corpus spongiosum becomes the glans penis at its distal end.

Supported by fibrous connective tissue, the structure of the penis contains no adipose tissue. It is covered by loose skin. The skin at the neck of the penis behind the glans folds back on itself and forms a cufflike, movable foreskin, or prepuce (Fig. 4-5). The foreskin of the penis can be circumcised or uncircumcised. The skin of the glans is hairless, and its surface contains many highly sensitive nerve papillae.

Sensory impulses to the glans penis are highly organized. Sexual sensations pass through the pudendal nerve, the sacral plexus, the sacral portion of the spinal cord, and up the spinal cord to unidentified areas of the cerebrum. Areas adjacent to the penis also aid in stimulation during sexual intercourse. Signals are sent to the spinal cord from stimulation of the anal epithelium, the scrotum, and perineal structures. (See Chapter 5 for the neurologic bases of the male sexual response.)

Table 4-1. Sexual Development in the Fetus

	Characteristic	Male	Female
Fertilization	Chromosomal complement	XY	XX
6th week	Gonadal development	Testes	Ovaries
	Androgen level	High	Low
8th week	Internal ducts		
	Wolffian	Form vas deferens and associated glands	Degenerate
	Müllerian	Degenerate	Form vagina, uterus, and fallopian tubes
12th to 14th week	External anatomy		
	Genital tubercle	Forms glans of penis	Forms glans of clitoris
	Labioscrotal folds	Form scrotum and lower shaft of penis	Form major and minor labia

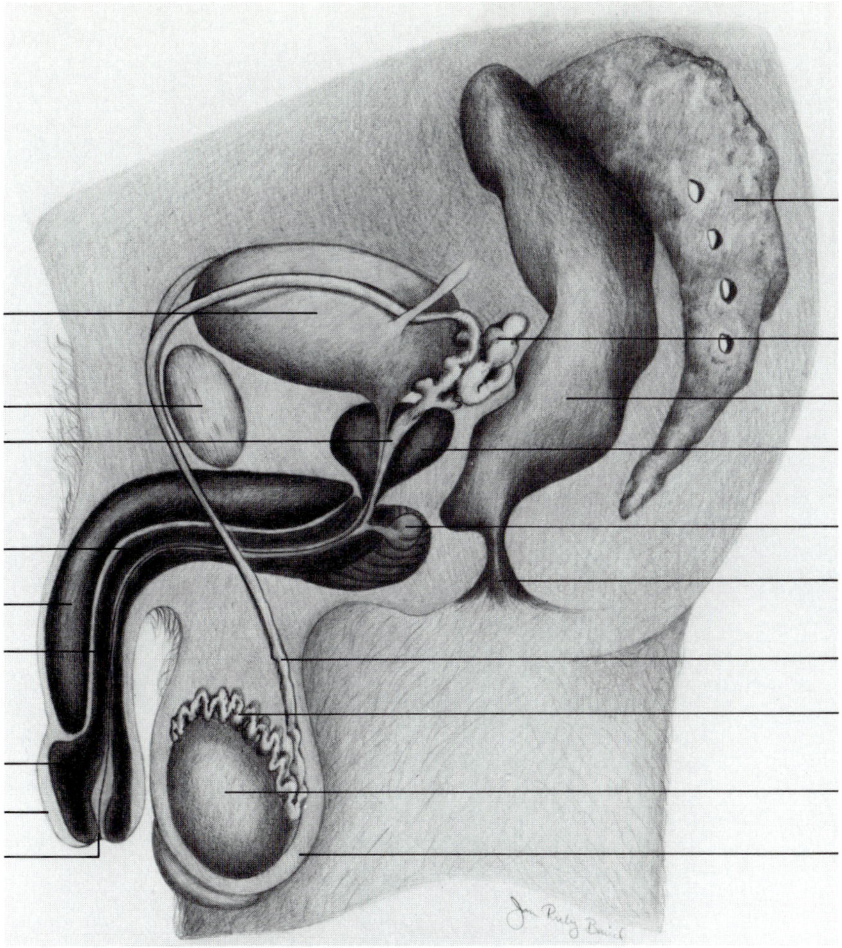

Figure 4-4.
Male reproductive organs. The external genitalia include the penis and the scrotum. All other structures are internal (Childbirth Graphics).

Erectile Tissue

Internally, the cavernous bodies of the penis consist of a spongelike meshwork of lined spaces (venous sinusoids). The sinusoids receive and drain blood through the afferent arteries and efferent veins. These vessels remain collapsed when the penis is flaccid. When sexual excitement occurs, pressure on the fibrous sheets of the corpora cavernosa from blood causes the penis to become stiff and erect. After ejaculation has occurred and sexual excitement subsides, the arteries contract. Blood drains from the cavernous bodies and leaves the penis flaccid. This process is called detumescence. Blood supply to the penis is primarily supplied by the internal pudendal artery and is drained by veins of the same name. (See Chapter 5 for a summary of the male sexual response cycle.)

Scrotum

The scrotum is formed by the invagination (creation of a pouch) of loose skin and fascia originating from the lower abdominal wall. It appears externally as a pouch of skin separated by a median ridge known as the raphe. Secretions emanating from the sebaceous glands in the scrotal skin produce a distinctive odor. The skin of the scrotum is more darkly pigmented than that surrounding it and has a sprinkling of scattered hairs.

During fetal life the skin and subcutaneous fascia were the only epidermal layers that invaginated from the abdominal wall to construct the scrotal sac. To form the covering of the spermatic cord, the remaining layers of the abdominal wall were penetrated by the testes and their ducts, vessels, nerves, and muscle tissue. These structures journeyed from the abdominal cavity into the scrotum during the seventh fetal month. The point where these structures penetrate the abdominal wall is weakened, predisposing men to inguinal hernias.

The subcutaneous fascia of the scrotal wall is made up of involuntary muscle fibers called the tunica dartos. In colder temperatures these muscles contract, causing shrinking and wrinkling of the scrotal wall. This mechanism draws the scrotum closer to the body for additional warmth. The testes contained within the scrotum cannot produce sperm at body temperature. For this reason men who have jobs that require long hours of sitting, such as truck drivers, or who wear tight pants or frequently use a hot tub may experience temporary

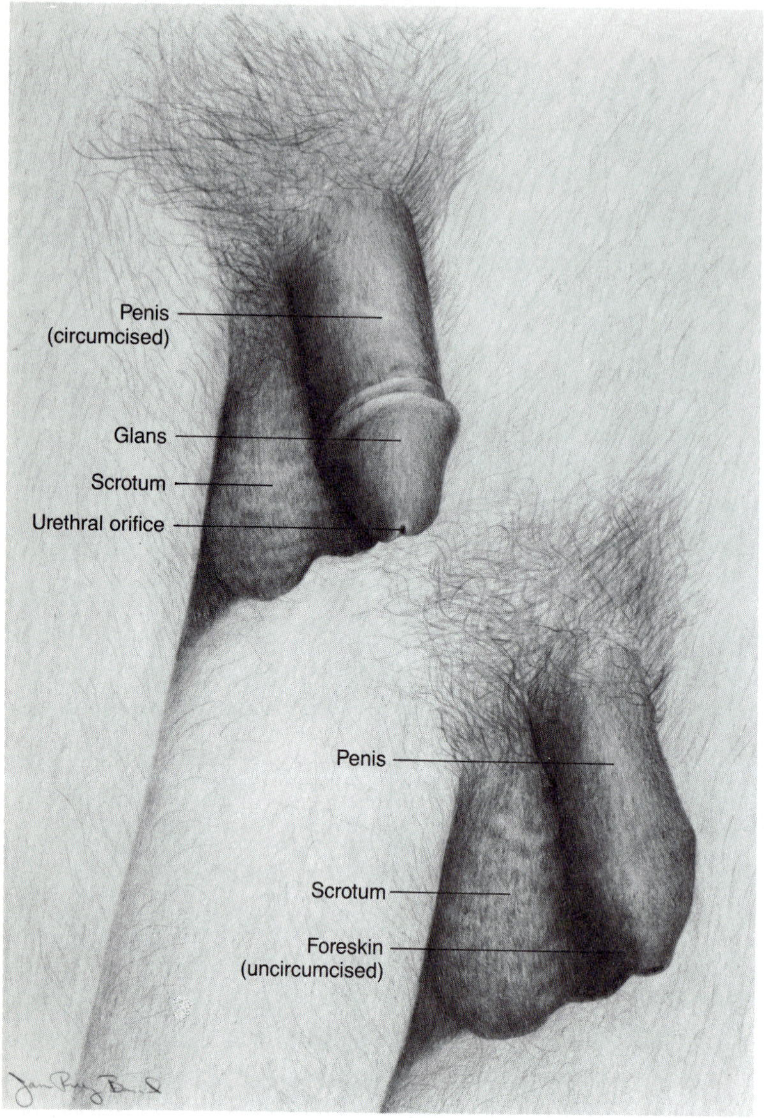

Figure 4-5.
External male genitalia, circumcised and uncircumcised (Childbirth Graphics).

infertility due to the inhibition of spermatogenesis (sperm production) by excessive heat (Speroff, Glass, & Kase, 1989).

Internal Male Reproductive Structures

The male internal genitalia include the testes, seminiferous tubules, a sophisticated ductal system, and accessory glands. These structures function in harmony to enable the mature male to produce viable sperm.

Testes (Gonads) and Seminiferous Tubules

Internally, the scrotum is divided into two sacs by a septum. Each sac contains a single testis. The testis is a solid, ovoid organ approximately 4 cm long and weighing approximately 100 g. It is covered by a thick, fibrous, whitish-appearing coat called the tunica albuginea. Septa pass from the fibrous coat into the interior of the testis, dividing it into approximately 250 lobules (lobuli testis). The septa converge on the posterior border of the testis, where blood vessels, nerves, and the ductus deferens enter and exit. This area is called the mediastinum testis.

Each lobule contains one to three seminiferous tubules, the essential structures of the testes (Fig. 4-6). When unraveled, each tube is approximately 60 cm long. On the inner surface of the tunica albuginea, loose connective tissue enters to fill the spaces between the seminal tubules. Contained in this tissue are Leydig cells. These cells make up the endocrine-secreting tissue that produces testosterone. Cells lining the tubules also are sperm producing (spermatogenic).

Spermatogenesis

Beginning at an average age of 13 years and continuing throughout life, spermatogenesis occurs in all seminiferous tubules. Spermatogenesis results from stimulation of the gonads by the anterior pituitary gonadotropin hormones. Testosterone, one of these hormones, is produced by the

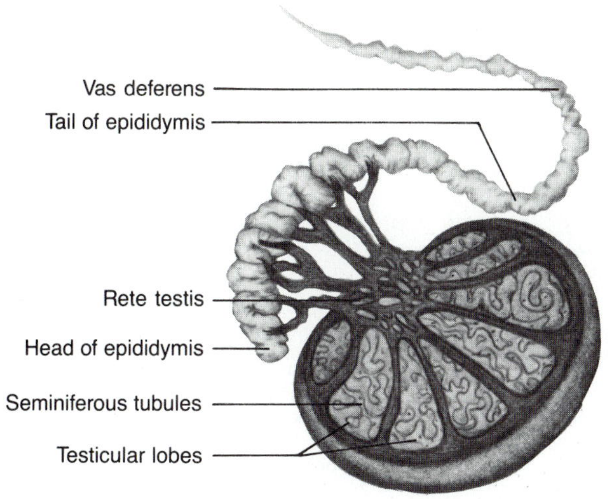

Figure 4-6.
Structure of the testis and epididymis (Childbirth Graphics).

Leydig cells within the seminiferous tubules and is responsible for stimulating the formation of mature, functional sperm.

The first stage of spermatogenesis begins with the growth of spermatogonia into enlarged cells called spermatocytes. The spermatocyte divides by meiosis. No new chromosomes are formed, but the chromosomal pairs separate. Two spermatids are formed, each containing 23 chromosomes. After several weeks of maturing in the epididymis, the spermatids become spermatozoa, or mature sperm.

At all stages of germinal cell division and in the final conversion of spermatocytes into spermatozoa, the developing spermatozoa are in contact with Sertoli cells. These cells are essential in providing a special environment in which the germinal cells develop. Sertoli cells secrete fluid that bathes the germinal cells. They provide fluid within the seminiferous tubule that contains nutrients for the developing and newly formed spermatozoa and secrete müllerian duct inhibiting factor. The entire period of spermatogenesis from germinal cell to sperm takes approximately 75 days.

A mature sperm consists of a head, neck, and tail. Chromosomal material is contained in its head and neck. The tail contains the contractile mechanism for self-propulsion. On the front portion of the sperm is the acrosome. Substances that facilitate the entry of the sperm into the ovum are found here. The centrioles are aggregated in the sperm's neck. The mitochondria that contain the cell's source of energy are arranged in a spiral in its body (Fig. 4-7).

A long tail, an outgrowth of one of the centrioles, extends beyond the body of the sperm. Provided with energy by the mitochondria, the sperm's tail projects the sperm forward on release into the female genital tract. As the tail waves back and forth and moves spirally near its tip, a snakelike propulsion projects the sperm forward at a speed of 20 cm/h.

Although some sperm are stored in the epididymis, most are stored in the vas deferens and its ampulla. Sperm maintains its fertility for several months when stored within the body. With normal sexual activity, prolonged storage does not occur. With excessive sexual activity, sperm may be stored for no longer than 4 hours. Sperm that has been ejaculated and remains at body temperature lives only 24 to 72 hours. Semen stored at low temperatures may have viable sperm for several weeks. Semen frozen at temperatures below −100°C (−212°F) have been preserved successfully for years (Speroff et al., 1989).

Semen

Ejaculated semen, the discharge from the male urethra after orgasm, is composed of fluids from the vas deferens, seminal vesicles, prostate, and mucous glands. Fluid from the seminal vesicles makes up the bulk of semen (60%) and helps to dilute the sperm. Otherwise, sperm cells would have impaired motility due to their sheer number. Seminal fluid is the last to be ejaculated and serves to wash sperm from the ejaculatory duct and urethra. The semen's milky appearance derives from the prostatic fluid. The mucoid consistency comes from secretions of the seminal vesicles and mucous glands.

Ductal System

The production of viable sperm and seminal fluid is not sufficient to ensure male fertility. A complex system of ducts functions to transport and store sperm within the male reproductive system. These are outlined in Table 4-2.

Epididymis

The epididymis is a small, oblong body located beside the posterior surface of the testis. It consists of a convoluted tube 13 to 20 ft long and terminates at its lower pole into the ductus deferens (Fig. 4-8). The epididymis constitutes the beginning of the excretory duct of each testis and stores sperm. Sperm may be maintained within the epididymis for 3 weeks as they mature and become motile.

Ductus Deferens, Seminal Vesicles, and Ejaculatory Ducts

Located on the posterior border of the testis is the ductus deferens. The ductus deferens retraces the upward course through the abdominal wall that the testis took in its embryonic descent. It is a highly muscular channel that can

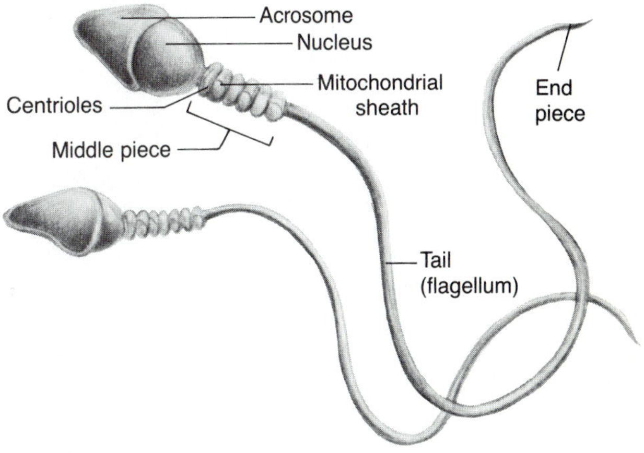

Figure 4-7.
Structure of the sperm (Childbirth Graphics).

Table 4-2. Passage of Sperm Through the Male Reproductive System

Organ	Function
Testes ↓	Produce spermatogenic cells Produce testosterone
Seminiferous tubules	Divide spermatocytes by meiosis
Epididymis ↓	Stores mature spermatozoa Moves sperm along tract by smooth muscle action Contributes secretions to seminal fluid
Ductus deferens ↓	Stores spermatozoa and tubal fluid in its ampulla Carries spermatozoa to duct of seminal vesicle by muscular contraction
Seminal vesicles ↓	Contribute nutrient-laden secretions and prostaglandins to semen Join ductus deferens to become ejaculatory duct
Ejaculatory duct ↓	Extends from junction of ductus deferens and seminal vesicles through prostate gland to prostatic urethra, carrying sperm
Bulbourethral glands (Cowper's glands) ↓	Secrete viscid alkaline fluid, contributing to semen and deacidifying vaginal environment
Prostatic urethra ↓	Counteracts acidity of semen by addition of alkaline secretions to increase sperm motility
Penile urethra (corpus spongiosum)	Allows excretion of ejaculate to exterior
External urethral orifice	Permits exit of semen

be felt as a rigid, almost wirelike structure in the upper part of the scrotum.

Each ductus joins the spermatic cord through the inguinal canal, arching around the ureter to the posterior wall of the bladder. The ductus deferens is joined at this point by short ducts that originate at the seminal vesicles. The seminal vesicles are coiled and branched, producing a sticky secretion that provides a supportive medium for sperm motility. The secretion contains an abundance of fructose and other nutrients, as well as large quantities of prostaglandin and fibrinogen. During ejaculation the sperm emerge from the vas deferens, and the seminal vesicles empty their contents into the ejaculatory duct. Seminal fluid adds bulk to the semen and supplies nutrients to the sperm. It is postulated that prostaglandins aid fertilization by rendering the cervical mucus more receptive to sperm. Prostaglandins also may cause reverse peristaltic contractions of the uterus and oviducts. This action may help to move the sperm toward the ovaries.

Before entering the prostate, the ductus deferens becomes enlarged into the terminal ampulla. This structure stores spermatozoa and tubal secretions. Each ductus joins the short ducts of one of the seminal vesicles to form two ejaculatory ducts. Both ducts traverse the entire length of the

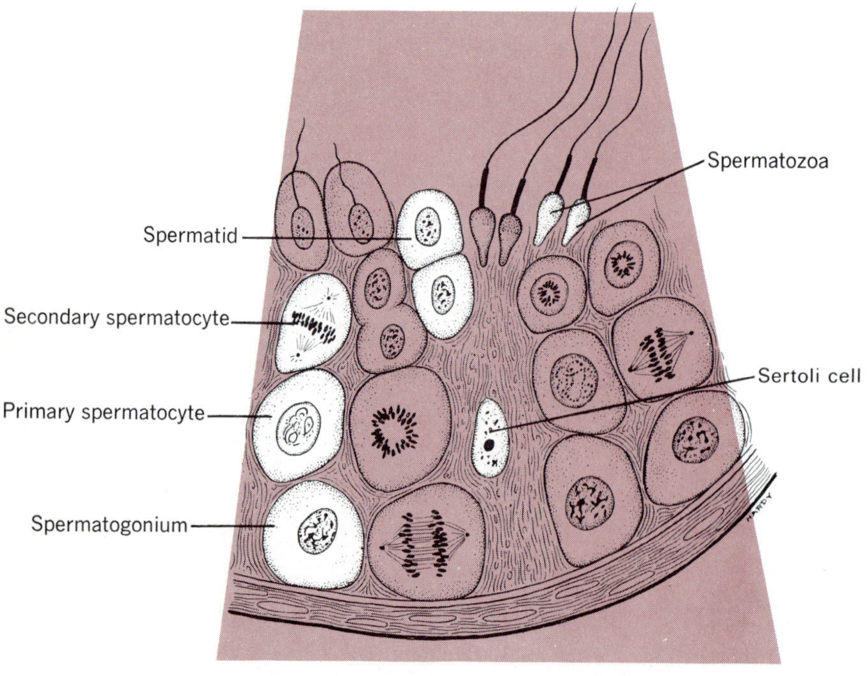

Figure 4-8.
Cross-section of the seminiferous tubule.

prostate. In these ducts the sperm are mixed with seminal and prostatic secretions. If ejaculation does not occur regularly, spermatozoa degenerate, die, and are reabsorbed. Therefore, after a period of prolonged abstinence, the first ejaculation may contain deformed and degenerated sperm.

Ejaculation. When sexual excitement reaches a climax, the smooth and skeletal muscles of the male reproductive system contract. The semen is emptied into the urethra (emission). By a series of rapid, rhythmic muscle contractions, the semen is then forcefully expelled from the penis (ejaculation), and orgasm is experienced. During ejaculation the urinary sphincter at the base of the bladder is closed, so semen cannot enter the bladder, and urine cannot be expelled.

Urethra

The male urethra serves as a passage for urine and semen. It extends from the bladder to the external urethral orifice and consists of three portions. The prostatic portion passes through the prostate and is where the ejaculatory and prostate ducts empty their fluids into the urethra. The membranous portion penetrates the urogenital diaphragm, where it is surrounded by the external urethral sphincter muscle. Finally, the penile urethra passes through the spongy erectile body of the corpus spongiosum. Numerous urethral glands open into this area and are called the urethral lacunae (gland openings). At the penile glans the corpus spongiosum flattens to form the fossa navicularis. The urethra widens at this point and terminates at its slitlike orifice, where semen or urine is passed.

Accessory Glands

The male reproductive system has accessory glands that secrete substances necessary for optimal functioning. The prostate gland and the bulbourethral glands secrete fluids that ensure sperm viability and motility.

Prostate

The prostate gland is fully developed before puberty (the point at which the human becomes functionally capable of reproduction). Full growth is realized only after stimulation from testosterone. The prostate gland surrounds the neck of the bladder and the first 3 cm of the urethra. Approximately the size of a chestnut, the prostate is a solid organ consisting of a median and two lateral lobes. It lies in front of the rectum and can be palpated for size, congestion, and nodularity through the rectal wall.

The prostate gland contains an inner layer of smooth muscle fiber that secretes a thin, opalescent fluid into the urethra. Prostatic fluid is alkaline and contains calcium, citric acid, and other substances. Its alkalinity may be important in counteracting the acidity of the secretions from the ductus deferens and seminal vesicles. The sperm is optimally mobile in an alkaline pH of 6.0 to 6.5.

Bulbourethral (Cowper's) Glands

The two bulbourethral (Cowper's) glands are the size and shape of a pea. They are located in the urogenital diaphragm, which forms the floor of the male pelvis. Ducts of these glands open into the posterior cavernous urethra. The fluid secreted by the glands is clear, viscous, and alkaline. Similar to prostatic fluid, the alkalinity of bulbourethral fluid assists in neutralizing acidic female vaginal secretions. As discussed previously, an acidic pH would be detrimental to sperm survival.

The male reproductive system consists of the testes, or male gonads, which produce sperm; ducts that store or transport sperm; accessory glands that produce secretions constituting the semen; supporting structures; and the penis. The three major functions of the male reproductive system, spermatogenesis, performance of the male sex act, and hormonal regulation of the male reproductive functions, are described. The following section discusses the female reproductive system.

Structure and Function of the Female Reproductive System

The female reproductive system includes internal and external structures governed by a complex pattern of hormonal cycles. The female reproductive system functions to produce ova; to maintain a physiologic environment that allows conception, pregnancy, and birth to progress normally; and to produce breast milk to sustain the neonate.

External Female Genitalia

The external female genitalia include structures that allow penetration by the penis during sexual intercourse. External female genitalia include the vulva, the mons pubis, the clitoris, the labia minora and labia majora, the vestibule, the vaginal opening, and the perineum (Fig. 4-9).

Vulva

Also known as the pudenda, vulva is the term used to designate all externally visible structures in the woman. The vulva extends from the pubis to the perineum, as shown in Figure 4-9.

Mons Pubis

The mons pubis (or mons veneris) is the fatty cushion that lies over the anterior symphysis pubis. After menarche (the onset of menstruation), pubic hair grows over the mons pubis. The characteristic distribution of this hair is called the escutcheon. The female escutcheon occupies a triangular area. The base of this triangle is formed at the upper margin of the symphysis and an apex of hair growing downward over the labia majora and thighs. This secondary sexual characteristic does not necessarily follow a textbook description. In Asian women pubic hair may be sparse and fine, while in African American or other dark-skinned women it is coarse, thick, and curly. Many women have pubic hair growth that resembles the male pattern. It is considered within normal

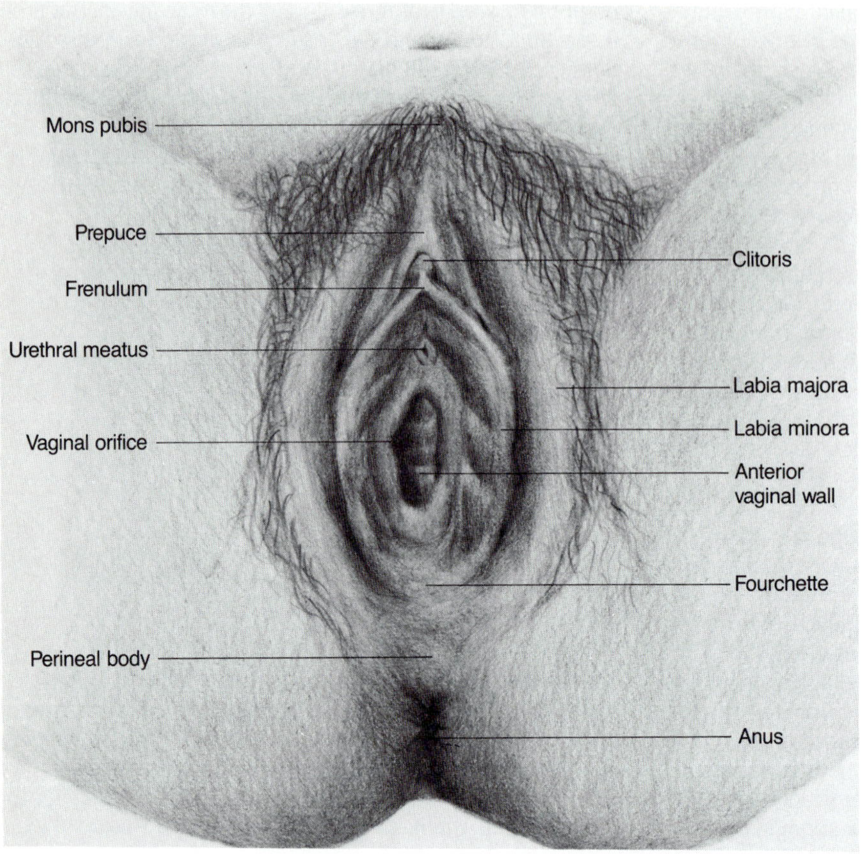

Figure 4-9.
External female genitalia (Childbirth Graphics).

limits for pubic hair in women to grow upward on the abdomen and downward on the thighs.

Clitoris

The clitoris is a small, cylindric, erectile body within the anterior portion of the vulva. It projects between the upper branched lamellae of the labia minora, which form the prepuce that covers the clitoris. Consisting of a glans, a body (corpus), and two crura, the clitoris rarely exceeds 2 cm in length. As shown in Figure 4-10, the glans of the clitoris is a smooth, round bump. It is highly sensitive to touch, because it contains many nerve endings. Erectile tissue and blood vessels lie beneath the top layer of perineal muscles.

The glans of the clitoris has only one known function, which is to focus and accumulate sexual sensations. The clitoral hood often covers the glans. Observing the glans may be difficult unless the hood is retracted and the inner lips of the vagina are parted. The clitoris may vary considerably in size and shape. These factors have little impact on the intensity of sexual arousal in the woman.

Labia Majora

The labia majora are two rounded folds of pigmented adipose tissue covered with skin (see Fig. 4-9). They converge at the mons pubis and extend downward and backward to the posterior commissure. The labia majora measure 7 to 8 cm in length and 2 to 3 cm in width, tapering at their lower borders. These tissue folds form the lateral boundaries of the vulva and are analogous to the scrotum in men.

The labia majora normally differ in appearance from woman to woman, depending on the amount of fatty tissue they contain. After puberty their outer surfaces become covered with curly, dark hair, while their inner surfaces are smooth and hairless. In nulliparous women and in young girls the labia are approximated and conceal the underlying structures. In multiparous women the labia become less full and remain separated. After menopause (the cessation of the menstrual cycle at midlife) they shrink and may disappear.

Labia Minora

When the labia majora are separated, the labia minora are exposed. These two thin folds of skin are devoid of hair and subcutaneous fat but are richly supplied with blood vessels and sensitive nerve endings. Although not as sensitive as the clitoris, both the labia majora and the labia minora contain numerous genital corpuscles. Both the labia minora and labia majora function as major mediators of erotic sensation, contributing to overall sexual stimulation.

Lying within the labia majora, the labia minora extend posteriorly to the fourchette in nulliparous women and blend into the labia majora in multiparous women. Anteriorly, the labia minora converge into two lamellae (thin plates of skin). The lower plate is fused and forms the frenulum of the clitoris, while the upper plate forms the clitoral prepuce.

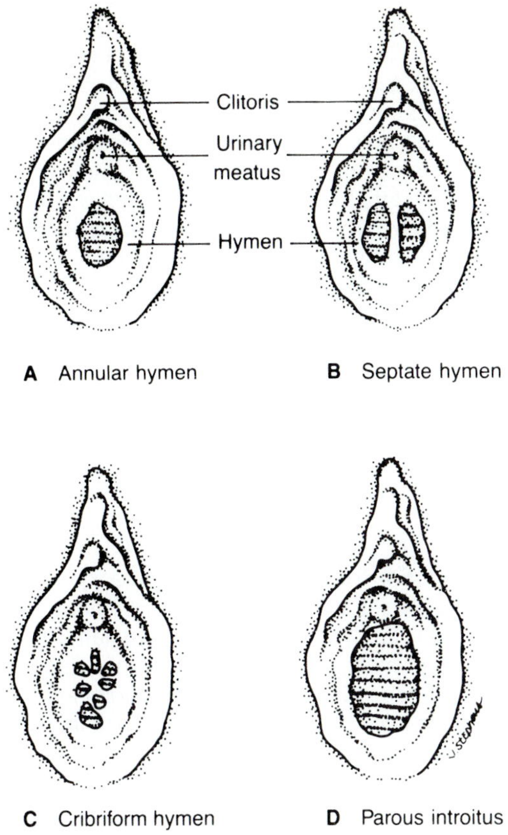

Figure 4-10.
Variations in the hymen (Childbirth Graphics).

Vestibule

The vestibule is an almond-shaped area, bordered by the labia minora, that extends from the clitoris to the posterior fourchette. Lying on either side of the vestibule beneath the mucous membrane are the vestibular bulbs. These structures are elongated masses of vascular, erectile tissue that connect with the clitoris. The vestibular bulbs are homologous to the male corpus spongiosum, the erectile tissue surrounding the male urethra. In the posterior vestibule, the area located between the posterior fourchette and the vaginal opening is called the fossa navicularis. This fossa is normally obliterated by childbirth and is only observable in nulliparous women.

The vestibule contains the openings of six structures. The urethra, the two Skene's ducts of the paraurethral glands, the vaginal orifice, and the two ducts of Bartholin's glands drain into the vestibule, contributing to the overall functioning of the female reproductive system.

Urethra

The female urethra is approximately 4 cm long. It courses downward and anterior to the bladder neck. The urethra terminates in the vestibule of the vagina between the labia minora and approximately 2.5 cm posterior to the glans of the clitoris.

A spongy body of tissue surrounds the urethra. This tissue probably protects it from direct pressure during sexual activity. The area is called the urethral sponge. Located in the urethral sponge are several glands. These are called the paraurethral glands (Skene's glands). Their specific function is unknown.

The urethral meatus is characterized by a vertical slit 2 to 3 mm in length and appears puckered, lying just above the vaginal opening. On either side of the urethral meatus at approximately 5 and 7 o'clock are two small duct openings to the paraurethral glands. They are approximately 0.5 mm in diameter and may not be visible.

Vaginal Opening and Hymen

The opening to the vagina is located at the inferior portion of the vestibule. This opening normally varies greatly in size and shape. The hymen, a fold of mucous membrane, partially covers the vaginal opening and marks the division between the external and internal organs. In virgin women the hymen often is hidden by the labia minora. During the first experience of intercourse, the hymenal membrane is ruptured. Hymenal tags are visible at the vaginal opening. These are called carunculae myrtiformes (hymenal remnants). Variations in the hymen are shown in Figure 4-10. Folklore that treats the rupture, or absence, of a hymen as proof of lost virginity or previous sexual intercourse is fallacious. The hymen may be ruptured during vigorous physical activity or by use of tampons, or it may be congenitally absent (Cunningham, MacDonald, & Gant, 1989).

Bartholin's Glands

Bartholin's glands are 0.5 to 1 cm in diameter. They are located in the lower vestibule, one on either side of the lateral margins of the vaginal orifice. The ducts of Bartholin's glands are 1.5 to 2 cm in length and secrete a clear, odorless mucus. Normally, the Bartholin's glands and ducts are not palpable.

Perineum and Perineal Body

The perineum is the region of the genital area that lies between the vulva and the anus. It is bounded anteriorly by the symphysis pubis, laterally by the ischial tuberosities, and posteriorly by the coccyx. This area contains a complex structure of skin, muscles, fascia, blood vessels, nerves, and lymphatics. Support of this area is primarily provided by the urogenital and anal triangles. In obstetrics the perineal body is referred to as the perineum. The perineal body is composed of muscular structures that provide central support to the perineum. These structures include the levator ani, the bulbocavernous muscle, the superficial and deep perineal muscles, and the external anal sphincter. During delivery these structures may be lacerated.

The primary blood and nerve supply to the perineum is provided by branches of the internal pudendal artery and pudendal nerve. The blood and nerve supply to the vulva, also known as the urogenital triangle, is provided by branches of the internal pudendal artery and pudendal nerve. The perineal branch of the posterior femoral cutaneous nerve and a branch of the ilioinguinal nerve all provide cutaneous innervation to the mons pubis, the labia majora, and most of the perineum.

Internal Female Reproductive Organs

The internal female reproductive organs include the vagina, uterus, fallopian tubes, and ovaries (Fig. 4-11). Optimal functioning of each of these organs is necessary to achieve conception, pregnancy, and birth.

Vagina

The vagina has three functions. First, it serves as the excretory duct of the uterus for its excretions and menstrual blood flow. Second, it is the female organ of copulation. Third, it is the canal for the vaginal birth of a neonate.

To accommodate these functions the vagina is specially structured. It is a musculomembranous tube lined with transverse, corrugated mucosa called rugae, which are pliable and capable of marked distention during childbirth. Normally the vaginal walls lie close together with a small space between them. The anterior vaginal wall is 6 to 7 cm in length, and the posterior wall measures 7 to 10 cm.

At the introitus, or the vaginal opening, there is a perforated fold of pink mucous membrane called the hymen (see previous section on vaginal opening). At its terminal end the vaginal circumference is attached to the uterine cervix. Its posterior wall is attached high on the posterior cervix, accounting for its additional length. As a consequence, a small, pouchlike area called the posterior fornix is formed beneath the cervix. Similar but smaller spaces surrounding the lateral and anterior vaginal attachments are called the lateral and anterior fornices. These areas provide access for vaginal palpation of the uterus and adnexa (area of the oviducts and ovaries), through their thin-walled tissues.

Anatomically, the vagina is located between the bladder and rectum (see Fig. 4-10). The tissue separating the bladder from the vagina is called the vesicovaginal septum. Tissue separating the vagina from the rectum is called the rectovaginal septum. Manual palpation of the bladder and the rectum and ligaments is possible through the thin walls of the vagina. Thus, the vagina permits a clinical assessment of pelvic structures.

Vaginal Environment. The mucosa of the vaginal wall is lined with stratified squamous epithelium. This layer of cells, when stimulated by estrogen, maintains the normal acidic vaginal ecology. Maintenance of this acidic vaginal environment depends on a delicate physiologic balance of hormonal and bacterial action. Döderlein bacilli, more commonly known as lactobacilli, are normal vaginal inhabitants.

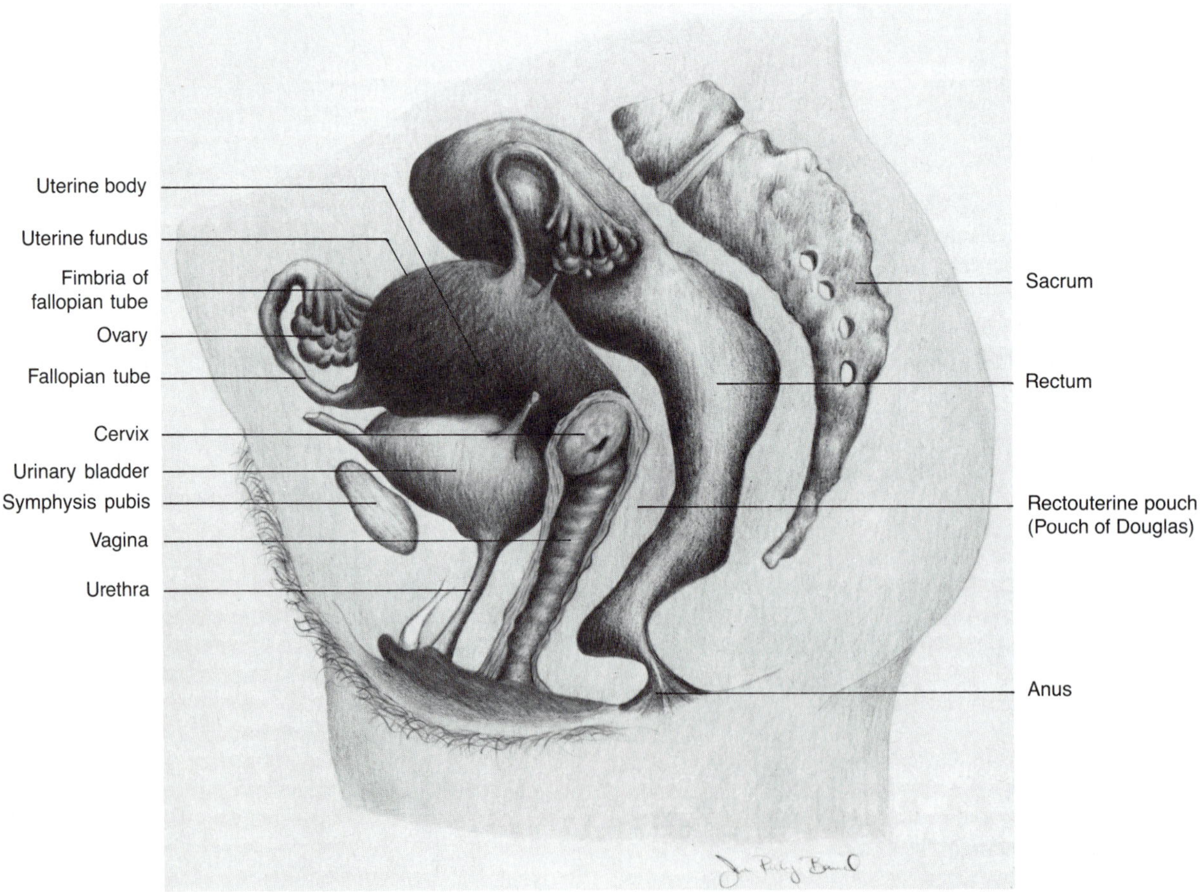

Figure 4-11.
Internal female reproductive organs (Childbirth Graphics).

When estrogen levels are adequate, the squamous epithelium contains an adequate supply of glycogen for lactobacilli to thrive. A by-product of glycogen metabolism by the lactobacilli is lactic acid. This acid maintains the normal 4.0 to 5.0 pH acidic milieu of the vagina.

During pregnancy the vaginal rugae become more pliable to permit additional distention of the vaginal walls. This change allows the vagina to accommodate delivery of the neonate. In preparation for childbirth the vagina becomes increasingly vascular, and its walls grow thicker and longer. An increased amount of white vaginal discharge during the gestational period is normal.

Uterus

The normal uterus is a small, muscular organ (Fig. 4-12). It has several functions, including the following:

- Proliferation of its lining (called the endometrium) once in each menstrual cycle in anticipation of conception and shedding its lining through the process of menstruation when conception does not occur
- Provision of a proliferated endometrium for the implantation of a fertilized ovum
- Nurturing and enhancement of development of a placenta that will provide the means to nourish and support the developing fetus during pregnancy
- Protection of the fetus and contraction during labor to expel the neonate

The nonpregnant uterus is located in the lower pelvis. It lies between the urinary bladder anteriorly and the rectum posteriorly. Shaped like an inverted, flattened pear, the uterus has two anatomic subdivisions. The triangular upper portion of the uterus is called the body or corpus, and the lower portion is called the cervix (Fig. 4-13). The dome-shaped upper segment of the uterine body located between the insertion points of the fallopian tubes is called the fundus uteri or, more commonly, the fundus.

The uterine body is composed of three distinct layers. The uterus has an outer covering of serous peritoneum. A thick middle layer of muscle fiber (myometrium) makes up the bulk of the uterus. The inner mucous layer of glands and stroma (foundation or supporting tissue) attached to the myometrium is called the endometrium. The inner anterior and posterior surfaces of the uterus (or the endometrium) lie in close approximation, forming a mere slit.

The axis of the uterus varies, as shown in Figure 4-14. The uterus is partially mobile, and although the cervix is fixed, the uterine body may move to the front or back. Uterine position may change depending on the position of the woman's body. It normally forms a sharp angle with the vagina, so its anterior portion rests on the superior surface of the bladder. The uterine body is then in a horizontal plane

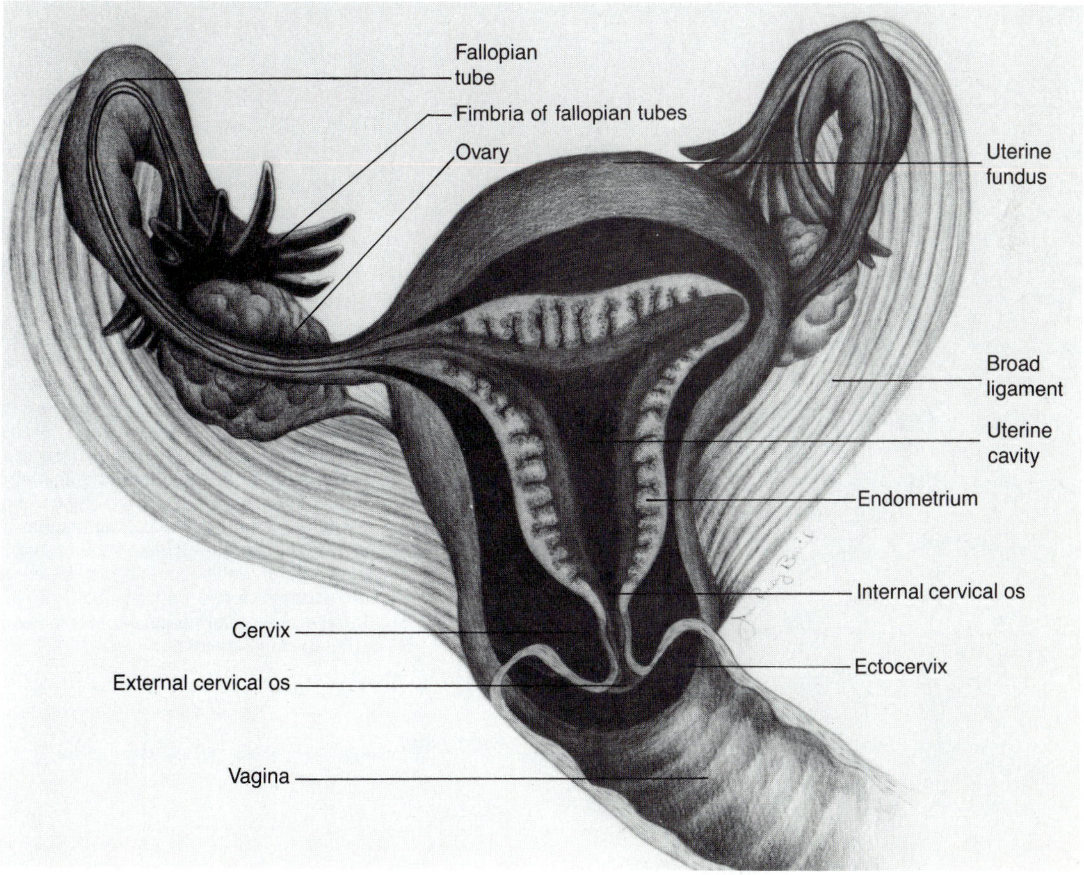

Figure 4-12.
The uterus and broad ligament (Childbirth Graphics).

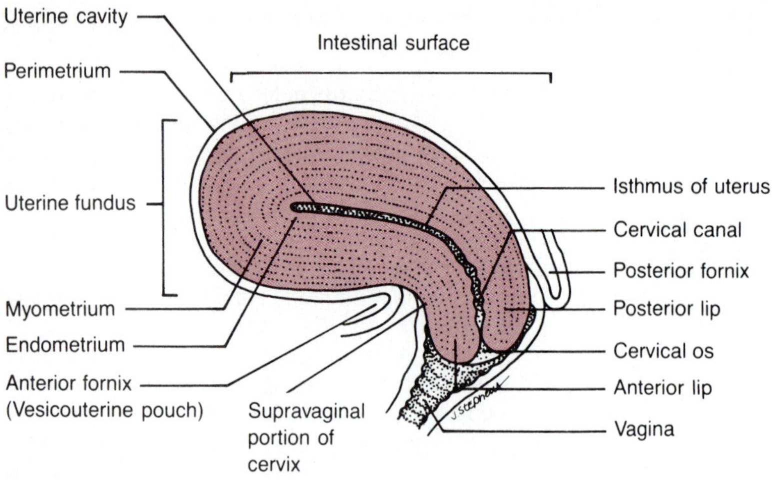

Figure 4-13.
Cross-section of the normal uterus (Childbirth Graphics).

when the woman is standing erect. A bend is created in the area of the isthmus, causing the cervix to face downward. In this position the uterus is said to be anteverted, the most common uterine position. Other less common normal positions include anteversion, retroversion, and lateral version. The anteverted uterus is flexed forward at the isthmus and bends on itself. In retroversion the uterus bends backward on itself. Midline uterine position occurs when the uterus does not bend. Lateral version is the term describing the uterus bending toward one side.

Throughout pregnancy the primary site of uterine growth is in a muscular layer called the myometrium. During the first half of pregnancy, there is a proliferation of new muscle fibers. Under the influence of estrogen, the myometrial cells increase to approximately 200 billion at term. In the latter half of pregnancy, the myometrium normally becomes hypertrophied, and its fibers increase more than tenfold in length. As gestation progresses, the uterine wall thins, becoming soft and easily compressible. These changes accommodate fetal growth and movement. Changes in the uterine musculature also make it possible to palpate the fetus through the uterine wall.

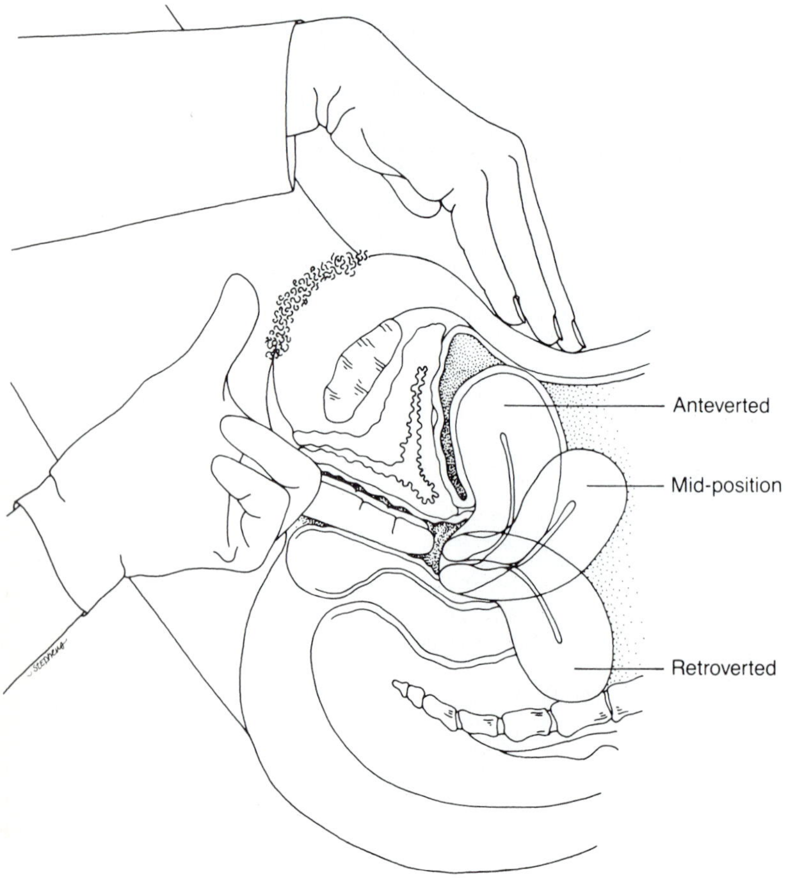

Figure 4-14.
Rotation of the uterus. The anteverted uterine fundus rotates approximately 90 degrees anterior to the long axis of the uterus and can be palpated by the abdominal hand on bimanual examination. In the midline position the long axis of the uterus lies in the same plane as the vagina and will not be palpable on bimanual examination. In the retroverted position the uterus rotates posteriorly to the long axis of the vagina and may be felt through the posterior fornix on bimanual examination or through the rectal mucosa on rectal examination (Childbirth Graphics).

Uterine Cervix

The cervix is the lower end of the uterus. The exterior portion of the cervix visible on speculum examination is called the portio vaginalis cervicis, or the ectocervix. The external cervical os is located at the lower extremity of the ectocervix. Protruding from 1 to 3 cm into the vagina, the ectocervix normally varies in appearance in different women, depending on age, parity, and use of oral contraceptives. Normally the cervix is pink, but it may appear purplish during pregnancy and pale pink after menopause. The cervix is approximately 2 to 3 cm in diameter in nulliparous women and 3 to 5 cm after vaginal delivery.

Cervical tears are common during vaginal delivery. This can cause characteristic changes in the appearance of the cervix. Before childbirth the cervical os is a small, regular opening. After childbirth the os becomes a transverse slit (sometimes described as fish mouthed) that may even divide the cervix into anterior and posterior lips. Severe trauma to the cervix at the time of delivery may cause it to become irregular, nodular, or stellate.

The mucosa of the endocervical canal is lined with a single layer of columnar epithelium. Columnar cells are mucus secreting and in the cervix produce a thick, tenacious, mucoid secretion. If a gland duct becomes occluded, causing its secretions to back up and be retained in the gland, nabothian cysts may form. These are benign, smooth, small, round, yellowish cysts that are frequently seen on the cervix during speculum examination; they require no treatment. Cervical secretion is one ingredient of normal vaginal discharge. During pregnancy the cervical mucus forms a plug within the canal that effectively blocks bacteria and other substances from entering the uterine cavity.

The ectocervix, or that portion of the cervix protruding into the vaginal canal, is covered with the same squamous epithelium that lines the vagina. Because the cervical canal is lined with columnar cells that extend to the cervical os, the point at which the squamous and columnar epithelium meet is called the squamocolumnar junction (Fig. 4-15). In the reproductive years this junction is located at the lower portion of the cervical canal. During pregnancy and in women using oral contraceptives, the junction is located on the ectocervix. In these situations the squamocolumnar junction appears red, bumpy, and symmetric. To the untrained eye the cervix may appear eroded or abnormal because of the presence of exposed ducts of the columnar cells that open onto the cervix. This process usually is normal and is called ectopy (displacement) or ectropion (eversion of an edge or margin).

The squamocolumnar junction also is called the transformation zone, because one type of cell is merging into another, that is, columnar into squamous. The squamocolumnar junction is significant because it is where cervical cancer usually begins. For this reason when Pap smears are performed, cells must be retrieved from the squamocolum-

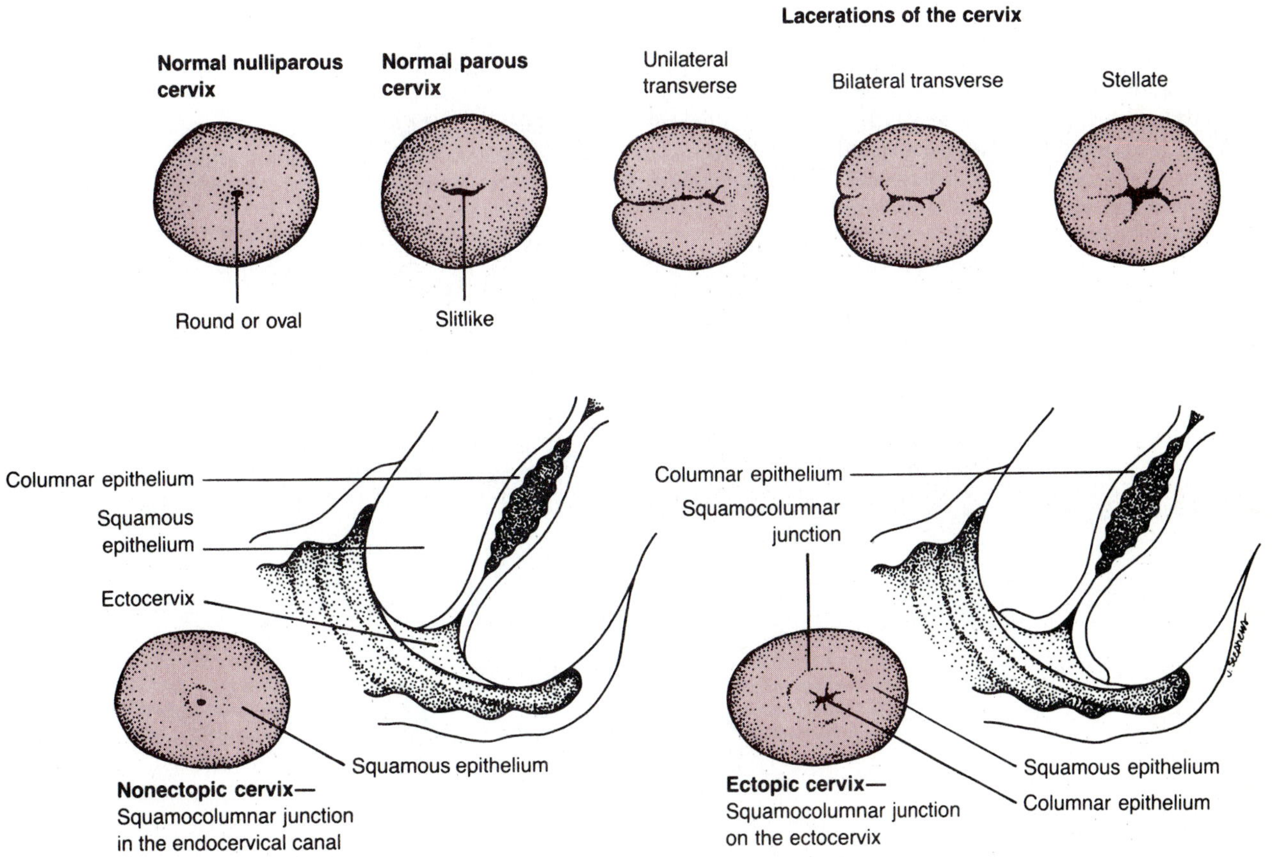

Figure 4-15.
Variations of the cervix and squamocolumnar junction (Childbirth Graphics).

nar junction whether it is located inside the cervical os or on the ectocervix. Specimens received by the cytology laboratory without cells representative of the squamocolumnar junction are of little value for diagnosing early carcinoma, and the patient will have to return for collection of a second specimen (Lichtman & Papera, 1990).

The cervix serves a variety of functions during pregnancy, including retention of the fetus within the uterus, helping to protect the fetus from infection ascending from the vagina, and opening to permit passage of the fetus into the vagina during childbirth. The portion of the uterus above the cervix, the isthmus, also changes to accommodate the fetus and prepare for childbirth.

Isthmus

The isthmus is the area that lies between the uterine body and the cervix. This portion of the uterus is approximately 5 to 7 mm in length, lying above the internal os of the cervix. Its upper limit marks the lower boundary of the corpus. At its lower limit, the isthmus marks the transition from its own mucosa to the mucous membrane of the endocervical canal at its internal os. The isthmus is shown in Figure 4-16 along with the comparative sizes of the uterus at different developmental stages.

The isthmus in its nonpregnant state is unimpressive. During pregnancy the isthmus takes on special significance. As the uterus grows, the isthmus increases in length and becomes soft and compressible. One of the early signs of pregnancy, known as Hegar's sign, is the softening of the isthmus between the uterine body and the cervix. As pregnancy progresses, the isthmus expands to accommodate the growth of the uterus and gradually becomes incorporated into the uterus. During labor the upper uterine segment (the corpus) is firm and hard. The lower uterine segment (the isthmus) is distended and passive. This allows the lower segment and the cervix to dilate and expand during labor, while the upper segment contracts to push the fetus downward.

Ligaments of the Uterus

The supportive ligaments that maintain the position of the uterus are those that extend from either side of the uterus. The uterine ligaments include the broad, round, and uterosacral ligaments.

Broad Ligament. The broad ligament is a winglike transverse fold of peritoneum. It arises from the floor of the pelvic cavity between the bladder and the rectum. The broad ligament effectively divides the pelvic cavity into two compartments, anterior and posterior. The uterus lies within the median portion of the broad ligament and is attached on either side. The free border of the broad ligament contains the fallopian tubes. The outer third portion of the broad ligament forms the suspensory ligament of the ovary, through which the ovarian vessels pass. The dense portion of the ligament is located laterally and is called the cardinal ligament, or transverse cervical ligament.

Round Ligaments. Arising below and anterior to the oviducts, the round ligaments extend from either side of the lateral portions of the uterus. Each is continuous with the broad ligament and extends downward to the inguinal canal. Passing through the inguinal canal, the round ligaments terminate within the upper portions of the labia majora. During pregnancy these ligaments hypertrophy and become larger and longer. As the fetus grows and the uterus enlarges, these ligaments become stretched, causing discomfort to the pregnant woman. Round ligament pain is a common concern during pregnancy.

Uterosacral Ligament. The uterosacral ligaments attach to the cervix and encircle the rectum. These ligaments form the lateral boundaries of the rectouterine cul-de-sac (pouch of Douglas). They support the uterus by the traction they exert on the cervix posteriorly.

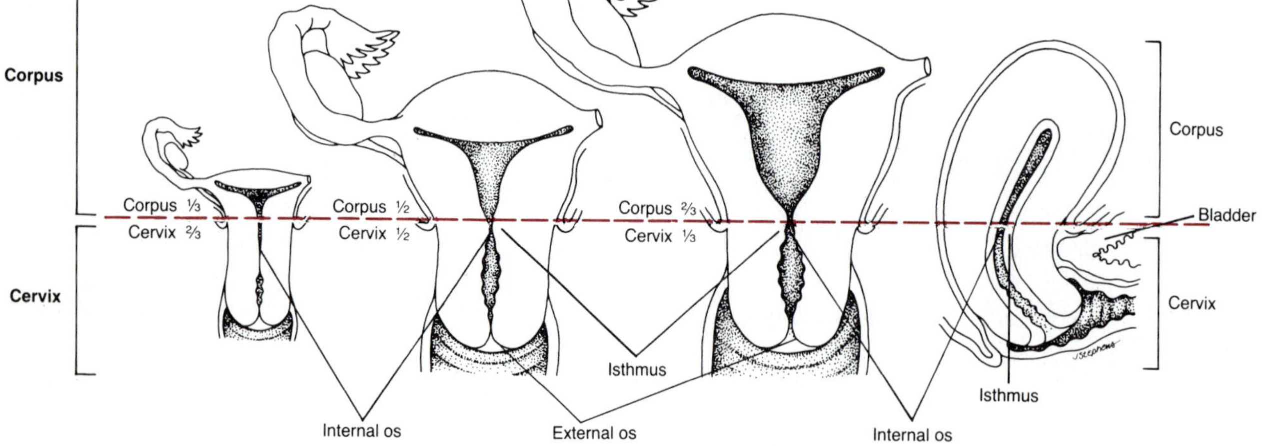

Figure 4-16.

Comparative sizes of prepubertal, adult nonparous, and multiparous uteri, frontal and sagittal sections, and the changing proportions of the cervix and corpus (Childbirth Graphics).

Fallopian Tubes

The fallopian tubes, or oviducts, assist the sperm in reaching the ova and convey the ova into the uterus by means of their ciliated lining (Figs. 4-16 and 4-17). Extending from the superior angles of the uterine corpus to the region of the ovaries, each tube is 8 to 14 cm long. The fallopian tubes are covered with peritoneum and have a lumen lined with mucous membrane. Each tube is divided into four portions:

- The interstitial portion within the uterine musculature, which travels upward and outward from the uterine cavity
- The isthmus, the narrow portion adjoining the uterus, which gradually passes into the ampulla
- The ampulla, which is wider and more tortuous and terminates in the infundibulum
- The infundibulum, a fimbriated, funnel-like opening situated at the distal end of the oviduct that opens into the abdominal cavity

The infundibulum lies close to the fimbria ovarica, which is longer than other fimbriae, forming a shallow gutter to the ovary. These distal openings from each tube connect the pelvic cavity to the outside world. This means that they can become a source of danger when infection travels through the vagina, uterus, and fallopian tubes into the abdomen.

Thickness of the oviduct varies from 2 to 3 mm in diameter at the narrow isthmus to 5 to 8 mm at the widest portion of the ampulla. It has an outer longitudinal and an inner circular layer of smooth muscle tissue. Ciliated columnar epithelium lines the oviducts. In combination with tubal contractions, the movement of the cilia is in large measure responsible for the transport of the ovum through the tube. When ovulation occurs the tubal musculature and its suspensory ligament become increasingly active. They draw the ovary and the flaring end of the tube close together while the fimbriae sweep the ovum into the oviduct.

The fallopian tube is more than just a passageway for the fertilized ovum to reach the uterus. Its lumen must be patent (open) and wide enough to permit the ovum (the largest cell in the body) and the sperm to migrate through it. The fluid contained in the fallopian tube's interior facilitates the conditioning of the ovum for penetration by the sperm. For further discussion of conception and fetal development, see Chapter 12.

Ovaries

The ovaries are paired, almond-shaped organs. They develop and produce ova and secrete steroid sex hormones. Each ovary measures approximately 2.5 to 5 cm in length, 1.5 to 3 cm in breadth, and 0.7 to 1.5 cm in width. One ovary weighs approximately 4 to 8 g.

The ovaries lie on either side of the uterus on the lateral

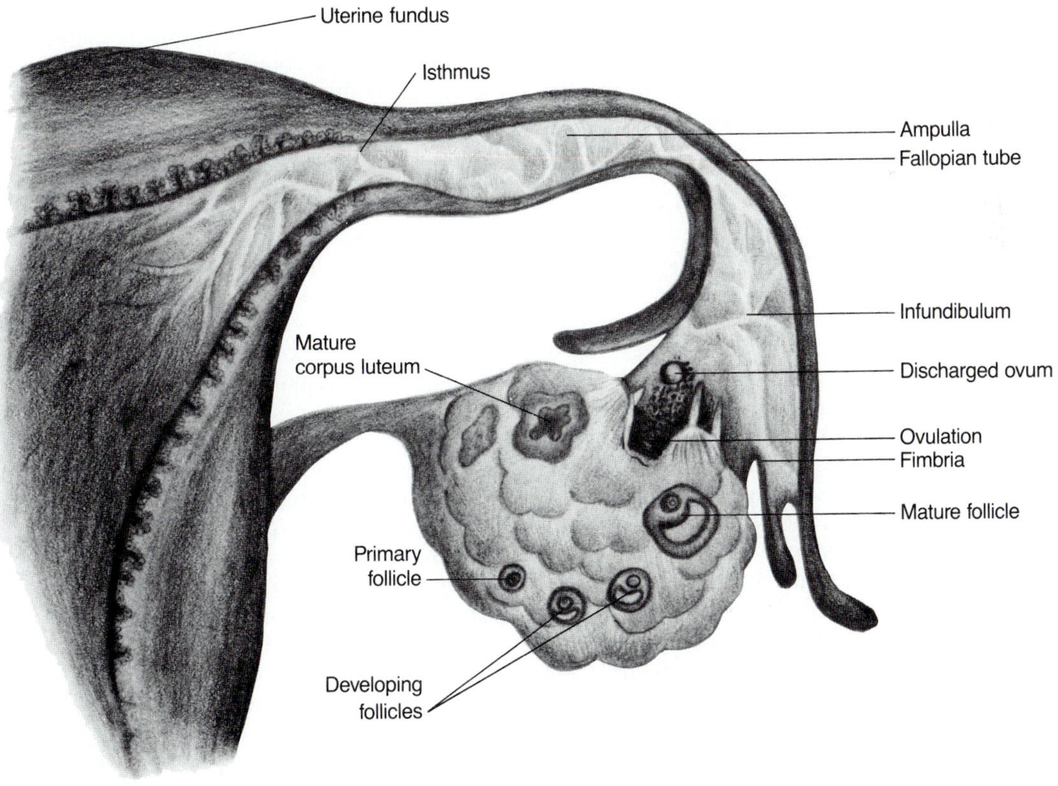

Figure 4-17.
The ovary and fallopian tubes. In response to low levels of blood estrogen the hypothalamus releases FSH, initiating the maturation of an oocyte and increased estrogen production. FSH production decreases as estrogen levels rise and triggers the production of LH, which peaks rapidly and results in ovulation. Following ovulation the empty follicle remains in the ovary and develops into the corpus luteum, which takes over the production of estrogen, particularly progesterone (Childbirth Graphics).

walls of the true pelvis. They are attached by a short fold of tissue called the mesovarium to the posterior broad ligament of the uterus (see Fig. 4-17). Between the folds of this structure the blood vessels and nerves pass to reach the hilus of the ovary. The ovaries also are attached by the ovarian ligament to the side of the uterus and by the suspensory ligament to the pelvic wall.

Covered by columnar epithelium, the mature ovary consists of a cortex and medulla. The medulla, the central portion of the ovary, is made up of supporting tissue (stroma), nerves, blood vessels, lymphatic tissue, and smooth muscle fibers. No ova or follicles are present in this central area.

The cortex is the outer ovarian layer. The ovarian and graafian follicles are located within the cortex. Ovarian follicles in various stages of maturity are numerous during the follicular phase of the menstrual cycle (see Fig. 4-17). On maturation the ova project into the surface of the cortex. They are then called graafian follicles.

Graafian follicles secrete the female hormone estrogen. The maturation of these follicles, particularly the follicle that is destined to ovulate, produces the midcycle spurt of estrogen necessary for ovulation. The remaining follicles degenerate at the stage of development that they have achieved; this is called follicular atresia. After ovulation the cells of the follicle that have ruptured undergo a rapid increase in size and form a yellow body, the corpus luteum. The corpus luteum produces small amounts of estrogen and large amounts of progesterone. These hormonal changes represent the luteal, or second, phase of the menstrual cycle.

The Ovary During the Life Span

The ovary is formed during the process of sex differentiation in the fetus. Ovarian follicles are formed in the fetal ovary in a complex series of events. The cycle of follicle formation, a variable degree of ripening of many oocytes (primitive ova before they have developed fully), and atresia occur. These events are the same as those that occur during adult reproductive life, but full maturity of ovarian function, as evidenced by ovulation, does not take place.

At a point as early as 4 to 6 weeks of fetal life, the fetal ovary begins to synthesize small amounts of estrogen. By 6 to 8 weeks' gestation, the oogonia (the primordial cells from which oocytes originate) begin rapid mitotic multiplication. The oogonia produce 6 to 7 million germ cells by 20 weeks' gestation. This astounding number of germ cells is the maximum number that the ovary will ever contain. The process of egg depletion by atresia begins at about 15 weeks' gestation, as maturation of the oocytes begins.

As a result of follicle maturation and atresia during fetal life, the total number of germ cells is reduced to 1 to 2 million by birth, a loss of 80% of the total number of oocytes. By puberty germ cells number 300,000 to 400,000, many more than would be needed for future reproduction. During the next 30 to 40 reproductive years, these cells will become further depleted as menopause approaches. The typical monthly menstrual cycle of follicle maturation, ovulation, corpus luteum formation, and menstrual bleeding occurs approximately 400 times during the fertile years.

Beginning at about 38 to 40 years of age, ovulation decreases in frequency. The ovarian follicles that remain are less sensitive to gonadotropin stimulation and may not reach maturity. This means that less estrogen is being secreted as fewer follicles ovulate. As more cycles become anovulatory, the estrogen needed to stimulate growth of new follicles decreases. At approximately 50 years of age, the store of germ cells becomes exhausted at menopause (Hacker & Moore, 1992).

Pelvic Blood and Nerve Supply

The uterine artery supplies the major portion of blood to the uterus. It is a large vessel that runs anteriorly over the levator ani muscle to the base of the broad ligament. It courses through the broad ligament and supplies branches to the vagina, uterus, and uterine tubes. The uterine artery anastomoses with the ovarian artery. The internal pudendal artery passes through the pelvis, supplying blood to the perineal region.

Nerves supplying the pelvis consist of somatic motor and sensory fibers. These nerves supply the muscles of the pelvic outlet and skin of the perineum. Pelvic viscera are innervated by autonomic nerve plexuses that supply sympathetic and parasympathetic motor and visceral sensory nerves to the pelvic organs.

Supporting Structures of the Female Pelvis

The female pelvis is uniquely designed to allow for pregnancy and parturition. The supporting structures, including the bony pelvis, the perineum, and the muscles of the pelvic floor, accommodate the amazing growth of the uterus during pregnancy.

Bony Pelvis

The bony pelvis is constructed for strength and stability. It transmits body weight to the lower extremities. In women the pelvis is especially adapted for childbearing. Its dimensions must be adequate to allow delivery of a neonate. When the anterior, posterior, or transverse diameters of the pelvis are insufficient to permit passage of the largest diameter of the neonate's head, cesarean delivery becomes necessary. The bony pelvis usually is measured during vaginal examination.

The pelvis, meaning "basin," is composed of four bones: two innominate bones, the sacrum, and the coccyx. The innominate bones result from the fusion of the ilium, the ischium, and the pubis, as shown in Figure 4-18. The sacroiliac joint fuses the sacrum to the iliac portion of the innominate bones posteriorly, and the symphysis pubis is joined anteriorly. The pelvis is divided into two parts by the linea terminalis, a plane that passes through the sacral promontory, and the upper margin of the symphysis pubis.

The false pelvis is the portion of the pelvis lying superior to the linea terminalis (also called the pelvic brim). The false pelvis varies in size among women and is not of obstetric importance. The true pelvis lies below the linea terminalis and has significance during vaginal delivery. The true pelvis is the first bony canal through which the fetus must pass. Consisting of a part of the ilium, the ischium, the pubis, and the sacrum and coccyx, its bony wall is more complete than that of the false pelvis.

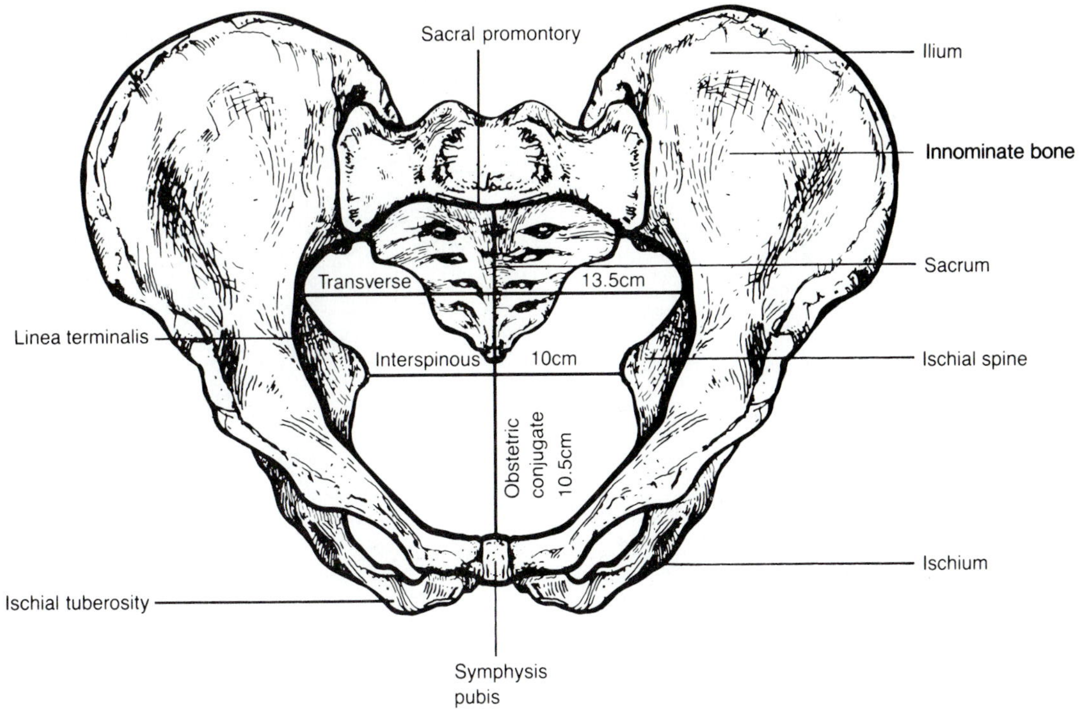

Figure 4-18.
The bony pelvis. Adult female pelvis showing the anteroposterior and transverse diameters of the pelvic inlet and the interspinous (transverse) diameter of the midpelvis. Normally the obstetric conjugate is greater than 10 cm (Childbirth Graphics).

The true pelvis' superior border, the circumference of which marks the pelvic brim, is called the inlet. At its lower circumference, bordered by the tip of the coccyx and the ischial tuberosities and spines, lies the pelvic outlet. The ischial spines are of particular significance because the distance between them (10.5 cm) represents the shortest diameter of the pelvis. If the fetal head cannot pass through the ischial spines during delivery, a cesarean birth will be necessary. The rectum is housed posteriorly in the true pelvis, and the bladder is located anteriorly. The uterus and vagina are located between these two structures.

The pelvic cavity is a curved canal. When the body is in a standing position, the pelvis is in an oblique position relative to the trunk. The plane of the inlet of the true pelvis forms an angle of 60 degrees with the horizontal plane. The anterior spine of the ilium is in the same vertical plane as the top of the symphysis pubis. The pubic arch in women is characteristically at a 90- to 100-degree angle that forms an arch under which the fetal head will pass during vaginal birth.

Pelvic Planes and Diameters. Describing locations in the pelvis is difficult because of its peculiar shape. Variations in the shapes and planes of the pelvis are numerous. Because the size and shape of the individual pelvis are important to the mechanism of labor and its management, awareness of these differences is important. For convenience, four imaginary flat surfaces crossing the pelvis at different levels are conventionally described. These planes are (1) the plane of the pelvic inlet (or superior strait), (2) the plane of greatest dimensions, (3) the plane of least dimensions (midpelvis), and (4) the plane of the pelvic outlet (or inferior strait) (Fig. 4-19). The size and shape of the pelvic inlet (superior strait) determine the type of pelvis—gynecoid (normal), android, anthropoid, or platypelloid, as shown in Chapter 13.

Contents of the Bony Pelvis. The pelvis contains not only the pelvic organs, but also the sigmoid colon, cecum, and ileum. The sigmoid colon continues into the pelvis as the rectum, lying anterior to the sacral promontory. The uterus lies between the rectum and the bladder and divides the pelvis into two pouches, the rectouterine and the vesicouterine (Fig. 4-20). The rectouterine pouch (commonly known as the cul-de-sac of Douglas or the posterior cul-de-sac) is formed by the peritoneum that turns back on itself from the rectum to the posterior wall of the uterus and vagina. In the vesicouterine pouch the peritoneum turns back on itself from the anteroinferior surface of the uterus to the urinary bladder.

The uterine body is located within the pelvic cavity. The fallopian tubes extend laterally from the uterine fundus to the lateral pelvic walls, with the almond-shaped ovaries attached to the broad ligament in close approximation. The ureters and round ligaments also are located on the lateral walls of the pelvic cavity. Fascia, numerous ligaments, muscles, blood vessels, and nerves help to support, nourish, and innervate all the organs located in the pelvic cavity.

Perineum and Perineal Body

The perineum, the region between the thighs and the buttocks, is the most inferior portion of the trunk. It is bounded anteriorly by the pubic arch, laterally by the pubic and ischial rami, and posteriorly by the sacrum and coccyx.

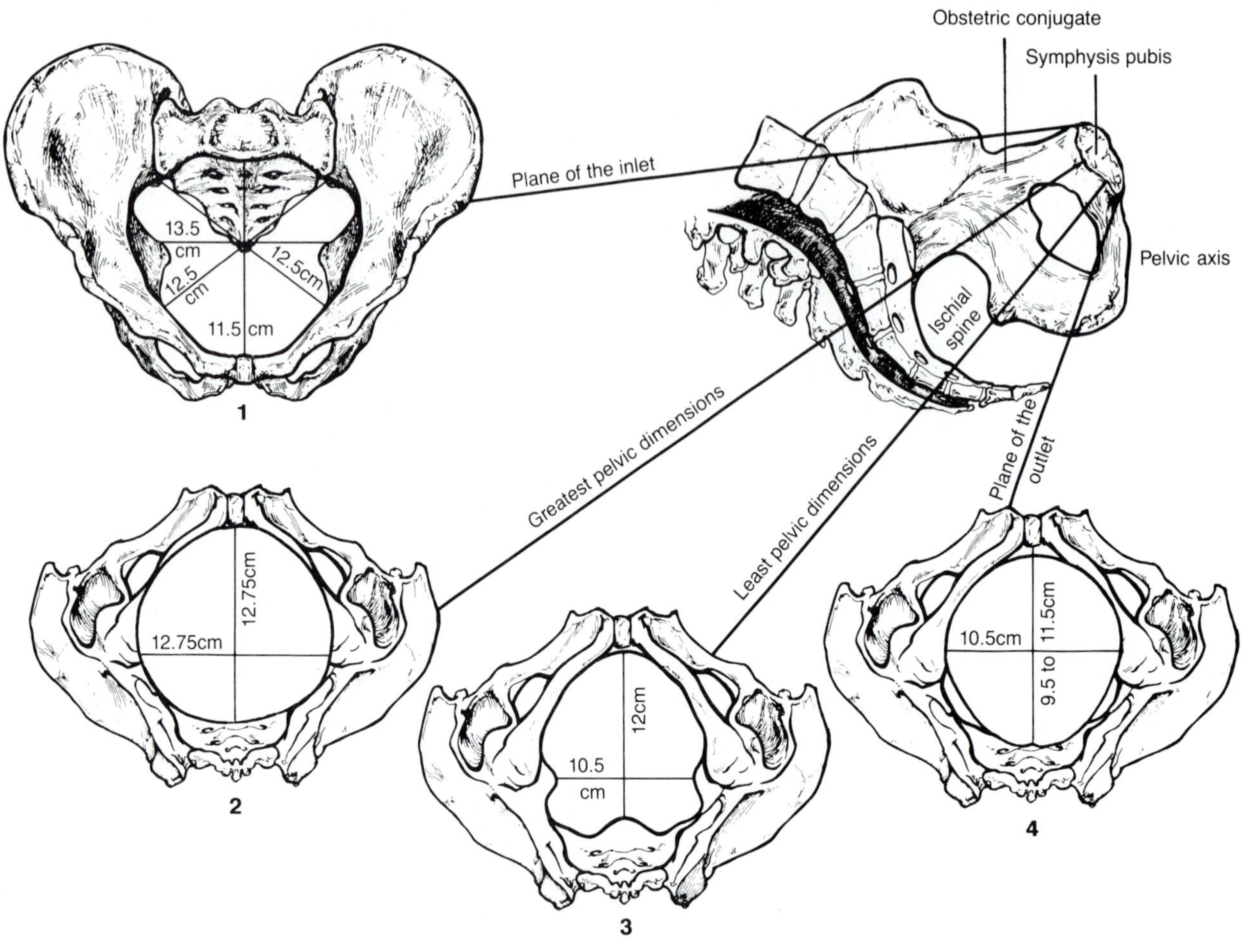

Figure 4-19.

Planes and diameters of the bony pelvis. The cavity of the true pelvis resembles an obliquely truncated curved cylinder with its height greatest posteriorly. Note the curvature of the pelvic axis (Childbirth Graphics).

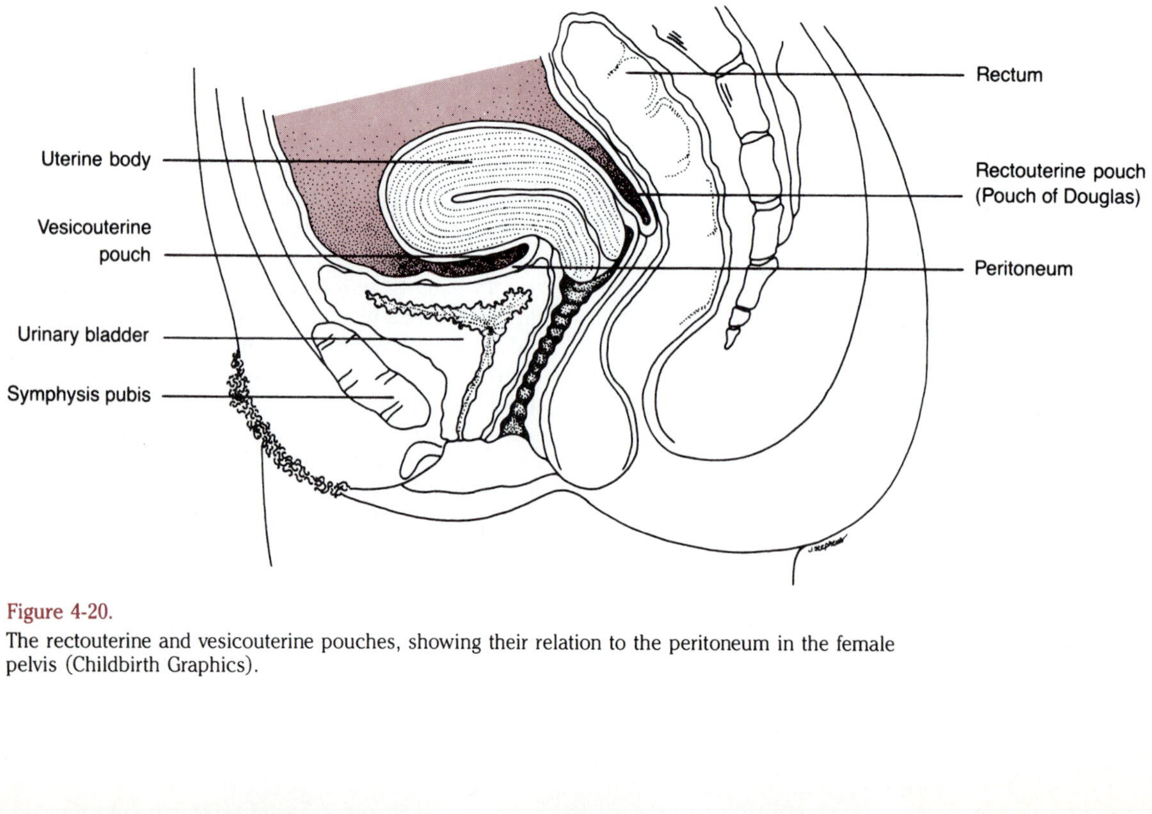

Figure 4-20.

The rectouterine and vesicouterine pouches, showing their relation to the peritoneum in the female pelvis (Childbirth Graphics).

The blood supply to the perineum is provided by branches of the internal pudendal artery and vein. The perineal body is the mass of skin, muscle, and fascia between the vagina and the rectum. In common obstetric practice the perineal body often is referred to as the perineum.

Pelvic Floor Muscles

When the female pelvis is viewed from below, the center of the pelvic floor seems to project downward much like a funnel. The anal canal approximates the center of the pelvis. The two levator ani muscles and the coccygeus muscle make up the pelvic floor, forming a figure eight around the vagina and anus. Because these muscles support the entire pelvic contents, they are of great importance.

The pubococcygeal muscle is constructed in such a way that it can expand enough for childbirth and contract enough to keep the pelvis supported. The presence of the vaginal and anal openings in the pubococcygeal muscle causes an inherent weakness in the muscular structure. During childbirth the pelvic floor muscles are stretched to their limit by passage of the fetus and will rarely regain their previous strength or integrity. Tears in the muscle can occur during birth, and even more damage can be done. Women who practice Kegel exercises to strengthen these perineal muscles after childbirth may have better bladder and vaginal tone then those who do not (see Chapter 15 for an explanation of Kegel exercises). Some protection may be afforded by these exercises against the weakening of urinary control in later years (Lichtman & Papera, 1990).

The urogenital diaphragm reinforces the perineum by surrounding the membranous portion of the urethra with ring-shaped fibers. The medial portion of the pelvic floor and the urogenital diaphragm jointly support the pelvic contents when a woman is standing erect. Support of the urogenital diaphragm is supplied by the superficial transverse perineal, the bulbocavernosus, and the ischiocavernosus muscles. The levator ani and coccygeus muscles are innervated by the sacral plexus (third and fourth sacral nerves). All other perineal muscles are innervated by the perineal branch of the pudendal nerve.

Breasts

Although the breasts are not involved in the actual physiologic process of reproduction, their function in the process of lactation merits inclusion in any discussion of the female reproductive system. The appearance of the breasts (mammary glands) varies from woman to woman. Although the breasts usually are equal in size, one may be slightly larger than the other. The size, shape, and symmetry of the breasts are largely influenced by heredity, hormonal stimulation, and nutrition.

The female breasts are located in the superficial fascia of the pectoral region. They lie over the pectoralis major muscles and are attached to them by a layer of connective tissue. Normally, each breast extends vertically from the second to the sixth rib and laterally from the lateral sternal border to the axilla. The skin of the breasts is similar to skin found on the abdomen. The areola surrounding the nipple has hair follicles on its border. In dark-haired, dark-skinned women the areola will appear dark brown, while in fair-skinned women it will appear pink.

Each breast consists of approximately 20 irregular lobes of secreting tissue, separated by adipose tissue. The amount of fatty tissue present determines the size of the breast. However, breast size has no relationship to the amount of milk produced during lactation. Each lobe has one lactiferous duct that converges to the areola of the nipple. Alveoli are milk-secreting glands contained in each lobe. They appear as grapelike clusters with stems that terminate in the ducts. The alveoli and their adjacent ducts are surrounded by myoepithelial cells. These cells, shaped like quarter moons, are contractile and squeeze milk from the alveoli into a duct that forms a reservoir called the ampulla, or lactiferous sinus, as shown in Figure 4-21. The nursing neonate grasps the nipple and areola in its mouth to compress the ampulla adequately, causing breast milk to flow.

Breasts are present in rudimentary forms in infants, children, and men. In infancy male and female mammary glands are underdeveloped and consist of a few rudimentary ducts lined by epithelium and surrounded by collagenous tissue. During puberty and adolescence the female produces increased amounts of estrogen, which causes the elongation of the mammary ducts and the growth of their epithelium. Fat and fibrous tissue surround the ducts, resulting in the increased size and firmness of the female adolescent breast. The areola and nipple increase in size and become pigmented.

Secondary mammary development occurs when ovulation begins, usually 1 to 2 years after menarche. The effect of progesterone from the luteal phase of the menstrual cycle causes formation of the mammary lobules. During each menstrual cycle, changes occur in the breasts as a result of the concentration of the female hormones estrogen and progesterone in the blood. These cyclic breast changes continue to occur for the remainder of the woman's reproductive years.

In preparation for milk production, marked changes occur in the breast. These changes begin during pregnancy and continue after childbirth by way of a complex sequence of endocrine events. Chapter 11 provides detailed information about breast changes during pregnancy, and breastfeeding is discussed in Chapter 28.

The female reproductive tract consists of the external genitalia, which include the vulva, mons pubis, labia majora, labia minora, vestibule of the vagina and its related structures, and perineum. Internal reproductive structures include the vagina, uterus, fallopian tubes, ovaries, and supporting structures of the female pelvis. The breasts are considered accessory organs. Male and female sexual function depend on a variety of hormonal influences.

Hormonal Control of the Male and Female Reproductive Cycles

Both the male and female reproductive systems are under hormonal control. A hormone is a substance released from special tissue into the bloodstream to travel to distant responsive cells where it exerts its effects. Sex hormones are produced by the endocrine glands and are chemical compounds that produce profound physiologic effects in target organs of the reproductive system.

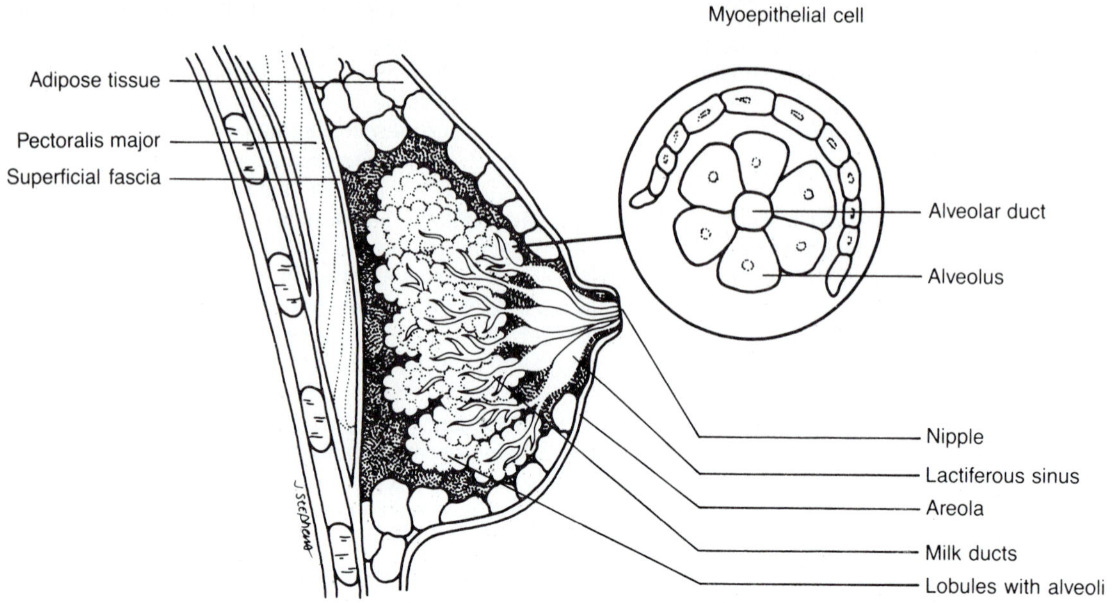

Figure 4-21.

Breast structure and action of the myoepithelial cell during breastfeeding. Under the influence of prolactin, the alveoli secrete milk. When the neonate begins to suck, oxytocin is released and causes the myoepithelial cells to contract and squeeze milk into the ducts during the let-down reflex. The milk flows into the lactiferous sinus, where it collects for immediate use by the neonate (Childbirth Graphics).

Hormones and Glands in Reproductive Functioning

The pituitary and the hypothalamus are primary structures located in the brain that are responsible for the reproductive functions in men and women. Normal reproductive functioning is dependent in large part on the complex interrelationships between hormones and their target organs.

Pituitary Gland

The pituitary gland, known as the hypophysis, is one of the most complex of all endocrine glands. It is a small, pea-shaped structure lying at the base of the brain. The pituitary gland is connected to the hypothalamus by a system of blood vessels and nervous tissue fibers. The general function of pituitary hormones is to stimulate other endocrine glands to produce hormones that, in turn, stimulate the growth and maturation of tissue throughout the body. Its specific role in sexual physiology is to secrete the gonadotropins (hormones that stimulate the gonads) in men and women. The pituitary hormones also stimulate the production of follicle-stimulating hormone (FSH) and luteinizing hormone (LH), which stimulate the sex organs in both men and women, and a third hormone, prolactin, which is responsible for stimulating milk production in the female breast.

Hypothalamus

Even though the hypothalamus occupies only 0.3% of the brain, it receives sensory input from all portions of the central nervous system and performs many essential functions. The hypothalamus is responsible for regulating such body mechanisms as appetite, thirst, water conservation, sleep, autonomic response, and endocrine secretion. Neuroendocrine substances released from neural cells within the hypothalamus stimulate the secretion of growth hormone, thyroid-stimulating hormone, adrenocorticotropic hormone, and the gonadotropins FSH and LH.

Other neural cells within the hypothalamus have characteristics of both nerve and endocrine gland cells. These cells respond to signals from the bloodstream, as well as neurotransmitters within the brain (neurosecretion).

Male Reproductive System

Testosterone is primarily responsible for the distinguishing characteristics of the masculine body. During fetal development the testes are stimulated by chorionic gonadotropin from the placenta to produce moderate amounts of testosterone. During childhood little testosterone is produced. At the age of 10 to 13 years, production of testosterone is greatly increased.

Beginning at puberty the hypothalamus of the young boy stimulates the pituitary gland to produce FSH and LH. The function of FSH is to stimulate the germ cells within the testes of the male to manufacture sperm. The function of LH is to stimulate the production of testosterone in the testes.

Testosterone is responsible for the development of the secondary sexual characteristics in the boy that occur at puberty (see the display on male secondary sexual characteristics produced by testosterone). It is unclear how testosterone causes these changes to occur. It is believed that testosterone stimulates increased production of protein in

Male Secondary Sexual Characteristics Produced by Testosterone

- Growth of penis, scrotum, and testes until approximately age 20
- Prolific hair growth on the body, pubis, face, and chest. (Testosterone may cause a decrease of hair growth on the head if two factors contributing to baldness are present: a predisposition to baldness and a genetic predisposition to the production of more than average quantities of androgenic hormones.)
- Deepening of the voice as a result of hypertrophy of the laryngeal mucosa and enlargement of the larynx
- Thickening of the skin and the secretions of the sebaceous glands, which predisposes to acne
- Increased muscular development as a result of protein deposition in the tissue
- Thickening of the bones as a result of greater quantities of calcium being deposited in the bone matrix

cells of the tissues responsible for development of the secondary sexual characteristics. This stimulus continues until approximately age 50, when it decreases rapidly to become 20% to 50% of the peak value by age 80.

Testosterone and other male sex hormones secreted by the testes, in combination with steroids produced by the adrenal cortex, are collectively called androgens. Androgens produced by the adrenals are much less potent than testosterone and cannot duplicate its function (Guyton, 1991).

Female Reproductive System

The primary hormones of the female reproductive system include estrogen, progesterone, and the gonadotropins FSH and LH. A description of these hormones is given in Table 4-3.

Hormones associated with the female reproductive system serve three important and interrelated functions:

- Satisfaction of sexual desires
- Maturation of the reproductive organs
- Preparation of the reproductive organs for conception, gestation, and childbirth

Levels in the Hormonal System

The female hormone system consists of three separate hierarchies of hormones and activities.

Level 1. The hypothalamus secretes gonadotropin-releasing hormone (GnRH) to the pituitary in response to signals received from higher centers in the central nervous system or from the external environment. Rather than controlling the menstrual cycle, the hypothalamus responds to positive or negative feedback from the ovarian hormones.

Level 2. The anterior pituitary hormones, FSH and LH, are secreted to stimulate the ovary in response to stimulus from the GnRH of the hypothalamus.

Level 3. The ovarian hormones estrogen and progesterone are secreted in response to stimulation from FSH in

Table 4-3. Female Hormones

Hormone	Description
Estrogen	Hormone produced by ovarian follicles, corpus luteum, adrenal cortex, and placenta during pregnancy. It is associated with "femaleness." The three principal types are 1. Estrogen E_1 (estrone)—the estrogen of menopause, oxidized from estradiol. (It is the second most active type, with a relative potency of 10.) 2. Estradiol E_2—the estrogen of reproductive-age women and the most potent type (relative potency 100) 3. Estriol E_3—the estrogen of pregnancy, formed from estradiol and estrone in liver, uterus, placenta, and estrogen precursors from the fetal adrenal gland. (It is the least potent estrogen with a relative potency of 1.)
Progesterone	Hormone secreted by the corpus luteum of the ovary, adrenal glands, and placenta during pregnancy. It is the hormone of the luteal phase of the menstrual cycle and of pregnancy.
Gonadotropins (FSH and LH)	Hormones that, when stimulated by GnRH from the hypothalamus, are released from the anterior pituitary gland to stimulate follicular growth and development, growth of graafian follicle, and production of progesterone
GnRH	Hormone that acts on the pituitary gland to release LH and FSH in response to feedback from the ovarian follicle destined to ovulate
Prolactin	Hormone produced by the pituitary gland, which, in association with estrogen and progesterone, stimulates breast development and formation of milk during pregnancy. (Stress of any kind also can stimulate prolactin release in the nonpregnant woman.)

the follicular phase and from LH in the luteal phase of the menstrual cycle.

Activities of Hormones

The pituitary gland monitors the levels of estrogen and progesterone secreted by the ovaries. When blood levels of these two hormones reach a certain concentration, they are "turned off" by the pituitary.

The neurohormone that controls the gonadotropins LH and FSH is called the GnRH. The neurohormone that controls prolactin (the hormone involved in milk secretion) is the prolactin-inhibiting factor. Not only do these hormones affect the pituitary, but behavioral effects have been associated with several of the releasing factors.

The hypothalamus is sensitive to information about emotional and stressful situations received from the environment by means of the nervous and circulatory systems. It is not uncommon for women to experience menstrual changes during disruptive periods of their lives. For instance women who were in the military and were shipped to war zones overseas during World War II experienced long periods of amenorrhea or other types of menstrual dysfunction. When young women leave home to attend college or to seek employment, they also may experience menstrual problems. Young women at menarche usually experience a year of erratic, heavy, and unpredictable menstrual bleeding due to hypothalamic immaturity.

It was believed for many years that the hypothalamus was the "great regulator" of the hormonal system. This theory has been debunked during the last decade. Research has proved that the ultimate regulator of the female hormonal system is the ovary. More specifically, the growing follicle, destined to ovulate from the ovary and produce increasing amounts of estrogen, is in control (Mishell, Davajan, & Lobo, 1991).

Effects of progesterone, estrogen, and the gonadotropins on the body are described in Table 4-4. The interactions of the structures of the female hormonal system and their effects on the cyclical function of the reproductive system are extremely complex. This interrelationship is known as the hypothalamic–pituitary–ovarian system, and it is responsible for the process known as the menstrual cycle (Guyton, 1991).

Menstrual Cycle

The menstrual cycle is produced by a complex pattern of hormonal fluctuations. The cycle includes the process of maturation of the ova, transport of the ova through the fallopian tube into the uterus, preparation of the uterine lining for conception, and finally elimination of that lining when conception has not occurred. This cycle is repeated for 30 or more years in the life of a physiologically normal female, beginning with the first menstrual period in adolescence through the last at menopause.

Menarche

Menarche refers specifically to the first menstruation and is not the same as puberty. Puberty is the period of transition from childhood to maturity, in which menarche is one major event. Age of menstrual onset in the United States has been declining steadily and is now between 9 and 17 years, with a mean of 12 years. Earlier menarche in this decade is possibly due to better nutrition and health care. Body weight has been suggested as a critical factor in the initiation of growth and the occurrence of menarche.

The usual sequence of events in growth initiation in the female includes three phases, lasting approximately 2 years. Thelarche (the beginning of breast development), pubarche (the beginning of the development of pubic hair), and finally menarche signal physiologic maturation in the female. All major body systems are influenced by the beginning of estrogen secretion. Thus, this hormone plays an essential role in adolescent development (Tuttle, 1991).

In early menarche, menses usually are anovulatory (no ovulation occurs) and may be irregular and heavy. This pattern continues for 12 to 18 months. Thereafter, normal cycles usually occur monthly. There is a correlation between mothers' and daughters' ages at menarche.

Reproductive Cycle

As the female reaches physiologic maturity, the hormonal control of the reproductive cycle becomes well regulated. Control of the female reproductive cycle depends on constant release of GnRH. This in turn depends on the interaction of the releasing hormones, LH and FSH, and the ovarian hormones estrogen and progesterone. Hormonal levels are controlled by a feedback system (Fig. 4-22). The feedback system can be positive (stimulatory) or negative (inhibitory).

The long feedback loop demonstrates efforts of blood levels of target organ hormones to stimulate the hypothalamus to increase the amount of releasing hormones. This in turn triggers the pituitary to increase production of FSH or LH. The short feedback loop indicates negative feedback of the gonadotropins on the pituitary secretion when their levels become too high and need to be lowered. This is accomplished by the inhibitory effects of GnRH in the hypothalamus. Normal menstrual cycles indicate that this system is working harmoniously. Any disruption in the menstrual cycle in the absence of some physical anomaly indicates some disruption in the hormonal system (Mishell, Davajan, & Lobo, 1991).

The menstrual cycle can be considered as two interrelated cycles. One cycle takes place in the ovary. The other cycle takes place in the uterus and is simultaneous with and dependent on the ovarian cycle. This unique mechanism causes the endometrium to prepare for the development of the fertilized egg at the precise time of the ovarian cycle when the egg is present. The ovarian and uterine cycles are summarized in Figure 4-23 and Table 4-5.

Ovarian Cycle

The ovarian cycle refers to the process in which an ovum is matured and expelled into the fallopian tube, and the maturation of another ovum is inhibited until the next cycle. The ovarian cycle has three phases: the follicular phase, ovulation, and the luteal phase.

Follicular Phase. The follicular phase of the ovarian cycle lasts from approximately the fourth to the 14th day. During these 10 days, the ovary is under the influence of FSH

Table 4-4. Influence of Female Hormones on the Body and Menstrual Cycle

Organ/System	Action of Estrogen	Action of Progesterone	Action of Gonadotropins
Uterus	Increases excitability of myometrium Causes proliferation of endometrium Increases amount of cervical mucus Causes uterine growth in pregnancy	Promotes secretory changes in endometrium Decreases amount of cervical mucus and renders it impermeable to sperm Promotes coiling of uterine arteries Promotes deposition of glycogen in endometrium Causes menstruation to occur when conception has not taken place Reaches peak of activity 1 week after ovulation	None
Fallopian tubes	Influence activity of tubal musculature	Decrease tubal contractility in later luteal phase May be important to transport fertilized ovum into uterus	None
Vagina	Causes proliferation and cornification of vaginal epithelium Maintains optimum acidic pH of 3.5–5.5 in vagina	Causes change from cornified superficial cells to intermediate and basal cell predominance	None
Ovaries	Interact with gonadotropins to stimulate growth of ovarian follicle and release of ovum Produce estrogen May be responsible for LH surge at menstrual midcycle	Possibly involved in ovulation	FSH Initiates and stimulates development of ovarian follicles Promotes estrogen production and secretion by ovarian follicles LH Causes final growth of graafian follicle Causes steroidogenesis in conjunction with FSH Stimulates ovary Aids in formation of corpus luteum from ruptured follicles Promotes production of progesterone by the corpus luteum
Mammary glands	Promote development and growth of ductal system, gland buds, and nipples Partially responsible for lobular and alveolar growth and deposition of fatty tissues Promote increased production of prolactin in pregnancy	Promote development of lobules and alveoli during pregnancy in preparation for lactation Cause retention of subcutaneous fluid and swelling of breasts before menstruation	None
Skin	Diminishes sebaceous activity of skin Increases water content of skin	May increase sebaceous activity of skin	None
Cardiovascular system	Increases blood flow Increases amount of angiotensin, factor V, and prothrombin in blood	None	None
Secondary sexual characteristics	Responsible for female contours of fat deposition and axillary and pubic hair	Partially responsible for breast development	None
Thermogenic activity		Increases the basal body temperature approximately 0.4°C–0.6°C after ovulation, identifying luteal function Influences deposition of glycogen in endometrium to furnish nutrients for implantation and support of fertilized ovum	None
Metabolism	Causes sodium and water resorption from kidney tubules Affects calcium metabolism and bone growth	None	None

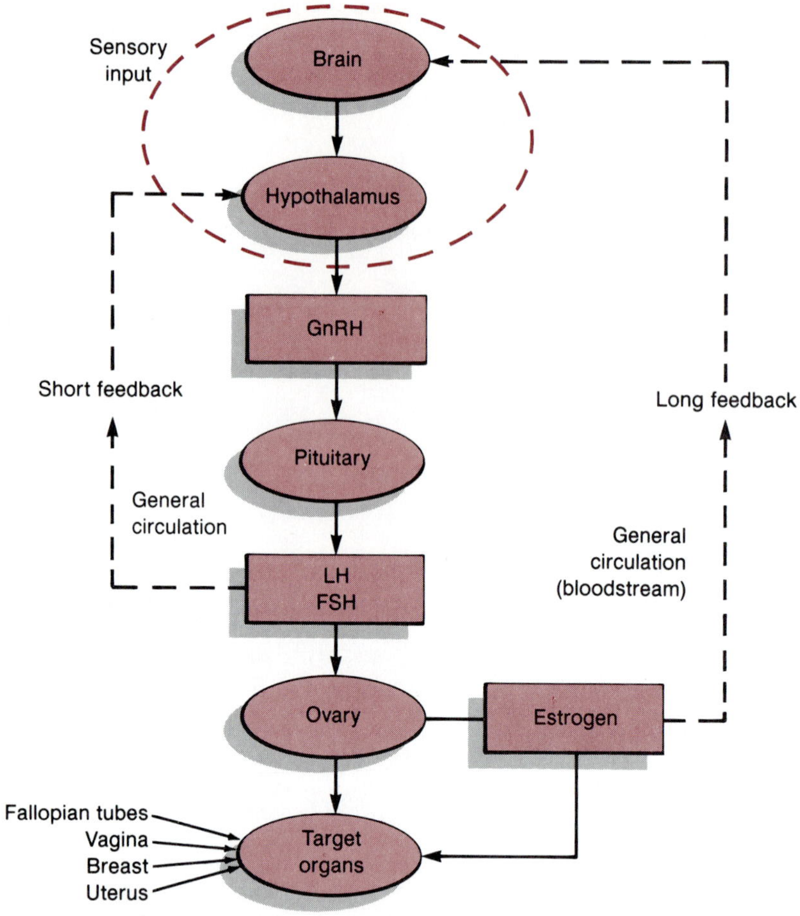

Figure 4-22.
Diagrammatic representation of the neuroendocrine feedback mechanisms.

secreted by the pituitary. Its function is to stimulate a number of ovarian follicles to grow, develop, and produce estrogen. Each follicle contains an egg cell (ovum), but only one is destined to mature fully and to ovulate. Other growing follicles are less receptive to FSH and estrogen stimulation and will have limited growth.

Estrogen is secreted by all the growing follicles. However, the dominant follicle secretes the major portion. When the estrogen level in the bloodstream is high, it exerts a negative feedback effect on the hypothalamus. In turn the hypothalamus signals the pituitary to inhibit its FSH production because the dominant follicle is producing high levels of estrogen. A progesterone surge after day 10 of the cycle stimulates the production of LH. This will suppress the lesser follicles, causing the graafian follicle (the dominant follicle) to mature. On day 14, with the aid of a progesterone spurt, a peak of LH causes the ovum to burst from the surface of the ovary. At this time ovulation is said to have occurred (see Fig. 4-23). Because the number of days necessary for follicle maturation varies, the follicular phase of the cycle causes variation in the length of menstrual cycles from month to month.

Ovulation. Ovulation usually occurs 14 days before the beginning of the next menstrual cycle. The timing of ovulation is important. If conception is desired, the ovum must be fertilized within 1 to 2 days of ovulation while the sperm and ovum are still viable. For couples not desiring pregnancy, it is especially necessary to use contraception during the fertile period.

Ovulation can be detected in approximately 25% of women by lower abdominal discomfort on the side where ovulation has occurred. Called mittelschmerz, this discomfort may be caused by follicular fluid or blood released from the ruptured follicle irritating the peritoneum. Women who experience mittelschmerz may be at an advantaged for planning pregnancy. However, this symptom may not occur during every cycle. Another method of determining ovulation is the daily use of a basal body temperature chart, which shows a shift of body temperature just before ovulation. Use of this method to determine time of fertility is discussed in Chapter 7.

Luteal Phase. The luteal phase of the ovarian cycle begins on approximately the 15th day of the menstrual cycle and ends on approximately the 28th day. As a consequence of the midcycle LH surge that caused ovulation, estrogen levels fall sharply early in the luteal phase. A brief midcycle rise of progesterone initiates the precipitious drop in LH.

After the rupture of the graafian follicle and the release of the ovum, the cells of the empty follicle increase in size. They fill with a yellow pigment called lutein to form the corpus luteum. Under the influence of LH, the corpus luteum begins to produce high levels of progesterone and low levels of estrogen. Capillaries contained within the central cavity of the corpus luteum fill with blood 8 to 9 days after ovulation.

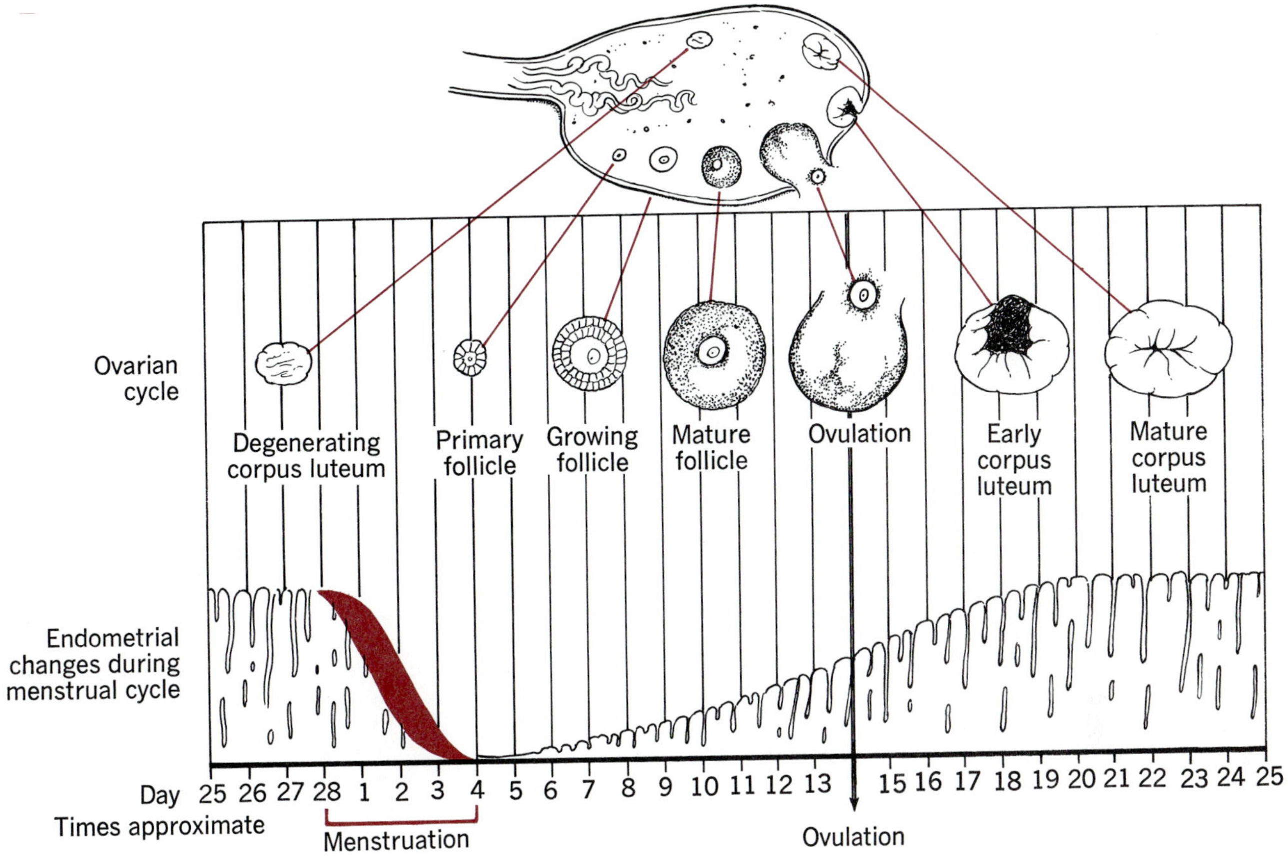

Figure 4-23.
Schematic representation of one ovarian cycle and the corresponding changes in thickness of the endometrium. It is thickest just before the onset of menstruation and thinnest just as it ceases.

Blood levels of estrogen and progesterone reach their peak. Progesterone counteracts the effects of estrogen and suppresses new follicular growth in the ovary.

If the egg is not fertilized, the corpus luteum begins to decline approximately 10 days after ovulation. Levels of FSH start to rise at approximately day 26 to begin early follicular development in the ovary in preparation for the new cycle. The LH concentration becomes so low that it can no longer support the corpus luteum. As the corpus luteum degenerates, its production of estrogen and progesterone falls off rapidly. Progesterone and estrogen reach their lowest levels at this time. As a result, the endometrium begins to shed, and menstrual flow ensues.

When conception has occurred, the corpus luteum is maintained beyond 14 days. This occurs because of the presence of human chorionic gonadotropin (HCG), an LH-like hormone secreted by the implanting blastocyst. The function of HCG is to maintain the growing blastocyst until the placenta is sufficiently developed to take over production of estrogen and progesterone. This occurs at 6 to 10 weeks of gestation.

Endometrial (Uterine) Cycle

The endometrium of the uterus has a parallel cycle, which is simultaneous to and controlled by the ovarian cycle. The endometrial cycle has three phases, the proliferative phase, the secretory phase, and menstruation.

Proliferative Phase. As the ovarian follicles are producing increasing amounts of estrogen, the uterine endometrium is growing in preparation for possible conception. The endometrium grows from 0.5 mm in thickness after menstruation to between 3.5 and 5 mm in thickness. This growth results not only from estrogen stimulation, but also from incorporation of water and amino acids into the stroma, the foundation layer of the endometrium. The stroma contains spiral vessels, which form a loose capillary network below the surface. While there is some actual tissue growth, the major element in achieving endometrial thickness is expansion or "inflation" of the stroma.

Secretory Phase. The secretory phase of the uterine cycle occurs as the corpus luteum is providing support for the ovum in preparation for fertilization. In preparation for implantation the endometrial growth is pronounced. The stroma becomes increasingly edematous, and the spiral vessels are densely coiled and swollen (see Fig. 4-23). This state signals the readiness of the endometrium for implantation of the fertilized ovum.

When fertilization does not occur, HCG is not produced, the corpus luteum degenerates, and levels of estrogen and

Table 4-5. The Menstrual Cycle

← **Estrogen Dominant** ←→ **Gonadotropin Surge** ←→ **Progesterone Dominant** →

Follicular Phase (Ovarian)—Day 2–14

- Rise in FSH levels, beginning day 24, due to estrogen decrease in previous luteal phase
- Early growth of ovarian follicles
- Stimulation of graafian follicle by FSH
- Continued follicular growth with increased production of estradiol, reaching a peak before ovulation
- Stimulation by FSH and estradiol of rapid rise in LH production after day 10 (positive feedback)
- Decline in FSH just prior to ovulation in response to increased estrogen from developing follicle (negative feedback)
- Secretion of estradiol, primarily by follicle that will ovulate
- Increase of preovulatory progesterone production to 2–3 ng/mL
- Atresia of all but dominant ovarian follicle caused by androgen production late in phase

Proliferative Phase (Uterine)—Day 2–14

- Proliferation of endometrium and myometrium
- Increased vascularity, vasodilation, and rhythmic contraction of uterine blood vessels
- Increased uterine motility in nonpregnant uterus in preparation for effect of progesterone after ovulation

Ovulation (Ovarian)—Day 14

- LH surge at midcycle requires estradiol concentration over 200 mg/mL and exposure to estrogen for a minimum of 50 hours
- Rupture of follicle, usually within 24 hours of LH peak
- Ovulation (occurs only if mature follicle [adequate estrogen] is present)
- Modest rise in FSH (may be necessary for normal corpus luteum development)
- High gonadotropin levels, lasting only 24 hours
- Precipitous drop in estrogen, probably due to luteinization of follicle
- Shift from estrogen to progesterone dominance

Luteal Phase (Ovarian)—Day 15–28
Secretory Phase (Uterine)—Day 15–28

- Initial sharp drop of estrogen (time from midcycle LH surge to menses is consistently about 14 days in 90% of women)
- Plasma level of progesterone of 3 mg/mL produced, reliable evidence of ovulation at peak (8–9 days postovulation)
- Formation of corpus luteum (CL) from follicle remnants after ovulation; synthesis by CL of androgens, estrogens, and progesterone
- Stimulation by progesterone growth of endometrium, with coiling, enlargement, and spiraling of arteries in preparation for implantation of fertilized ovum
- With fertilization the CL is maintained, and progesterone production reaches a plateau at 9–13 days after ovulation; implantation occurs 6–8 days after ovulation
- Secretion of human chorionic gonadotropin by the implanting blastocyst (maintains steroidogenesis of CL until the 6th–10th week of gestation, when the placenta takes over)
- Without fertilization, maintenance of CL is maintained by LH for 14 (±2) days
  - Inhibition of LH secretion by high progesterone levels
  - Decrease in estrogen production after degeneration stimulating FSH secretion
- Degeneration, scarring, and eventual disappearance of the CL taking place over a 3-month period
- Rise in FSH levels, beginning day 24, to stimulate early follicular development for the new cycle

Menstrual Phase (Uterine)—Day 1–2

- Menstruation, with sloughing off of the endometrium

progesterone fall. This hormone withdrawal causes the endometrium to become dehydrated and to "deflate." Blood flow in the spiral vessels diminishes, and the cells disintegrate. With this change menstruation begins. Within 13 hours the thickness of the endometrium decreases from 4 mm to 1.25 mm. Menstrual flow ceases in 3 to 4 days.

Menstruation. The length of a normal menstrual cycle is determined by counting from the first day of menstrual flow in one cycle to the first day of menstrual flow in the next. Normally, the menstrual cycle varies between 24 and 34 days, the average interval being 28 days. Duration of menstruation is variable, but 2 to 8 days is considered normal. In most women the duration of flow is consistent from cycle to cycle.

Blood loss during normal menstruation varies from spotting to heavy bleeding. It may be as little as 30 mL or as much as 80 mL. More than 80 mL is considered excessive. Most blood loss occurs during the first 3 days of menstruation, so heavy blood loss usually is not prolonged.

Menstrual discharge contains not only blood, but such substances as endometrial debris, prostaglandins, enzymes, cervical mucus, vaginal cells, and bacteria. Normally odorless, the menses may emit a characteristic odor as a result of the action of bacteria on the discharge. This is especially true when perineal hygiene is less than optimum.

The usual clotting that occurs when bleeding is caused by a cut or other trauma does not occur with menstrual blood. Clotting is prevented during menses by a high level of fibrinolysin, a substance contained in the endometrium. If continued heavy bleeding is sustained, however, fibrinolysin may become depleted, causing clotting of menstrual blood (Hamm, 1991).

Absence of Menstruation

In women who have been experiencing regular, normal menses, the absence of a period may come as a surprise. In sexually active women using contraception sporadically, the lack of menstruation should come as no surprise. Women who use contraception carefully and consistently may attribute lack of menstruation to a physiologic problem.

If a sexually active woman who is healthy and experiencing no temporary physical or emotional problems misses a menstrual period, pregnancy should be assumed until proved otherwise. When pregnancy has occurred, the embryo is well established before the woman even misses her first menstrual period. The physiologic events of pregnancy that occur unnoticed in the interim between the beginning of the last menstrual period and the woman's realization of a missed menses are swift and dramatic. The events surrounding conception are discussed in Chapter 11.

Menopause

The cessation of menstruation at midlife, known as menopause, is a normal part of female reproductive functioning. The ovary exhausts its numbers of oocytes, which have produced the major portion of estrogen during the woman's reproductive years. This loss of ovarian follicle function results in a substantial decrease of estrogen and in turn causes a change in the sex hormone output of the hypothalamus, pituitary, and adrenal glands. Chapter 6 discusses the physiologic processes of menopause, the health implications of menopause for women, and current approaches to health promotion and disease prevention for women throughout the life span.

Reproductive functioning in both sexes is controlled by a complex hormonal system, controlled principally by the pituitary and the hypothalamus. The male reproductive system is primarily mediated by the hormone testosterone. The female reproductive system has a far more complex cycle of hormonal interactions controlling the menstrual cycle.

Implications for Nursing Care

Knowledge of male and female reproductive anatomy and physiology is essential for the provision of safe and effective nursing care to childbearing women and their families. Without knowledge and understanding of these complex systems, it would be difficult to grasp the concepts of the normal menstrual cycle, fertility, contraception, or the important role of the maternal systems on the growth and development of the human fetus.

This information is useful to help adolescents and young adults understand the dynamics of human reproduction and how their bodies function. Knowledge about reproductive functioning is essential for sexual self-care and responsible sexual activity. The nurse can use this information to teach those who are thinking about becoming sexually active or those who already are sexually active.

Using this knowledge, the nurse also can help to identify women and their partners who may be at risk for problems related to conception and maintenance of pregnancy and can refer them for appropriate preventive care. The nurse also can use this knowledge to provide factual information and reassurance to those who may be concerned about their reproductive functioning but who show no evidence of reproductive problems.

Finally, the nurse uses information about normal reproductive anatomy and physiology in the care of women throughout pregnancy, birth, and the postpartum period. Such knowledge is essential in the provision of safe care, because it allows the nurse to recognize deviations from normal anatomy and physiology and to understand appropriate medical and nursing actions.

Chapter Summary

Understanding normal male and female reproductive systems enables the nurse to assist women and their families during the childbearing years and beyond. The development of the reproductive systems during the fetal period shows the parallels between male and female organs. Each reproductive structure in one sex corresponds to a similar structure in the other sex.

Both male and female reproductive systems are composed of external and internal organs. Male external organs include the penis and scrotum, and the internal organs are testes and seminiferous tubules, the ductal system, and accessory glands, which include the prostate and bulbourethral glands. The female reproductive tract consists of the following external organs: vulva, mons pubis, labia majora and minora, vestibule of the vagina, and perineum. Internal structures include the vagina, uterus, fallopian tubes, and ovaries. Breasts are accessory organs.

The male and female generative organs are controlled by the sex hormones. Primary control of this complex system is mediated by the pituitary–hypothalamus axis. Testosterone is the primary male hormone, while the primary female reproductive hormones are estrogen, progesterone, and the gonadotropins, FSH and LH.

The female reproductive system has the capacity for maintaining a complex cycle, known as the menstrual cycle, throughout the first half of adult life. This cycle involves the ovaries and the uterus in a process of preparing for conception, making physiologic changes to support an embryo if conception occurs, and renewing the uterus through the process of menstruation if it does not. The complementary functioning of male and female reproductive systems enables conception, pregnancy, and birth to occur.

Study Questions

1. *How does the embryo differentiate into male and female in the fifth to sixth week of gestation?*
2. *What structures constitute the male internal and external reproductive organs? What are the functions of each structure?*

3. *How does the female external genitalia differ from the male?*
4. *What hormones influence the male and female reproductive systems, and where to do they originate?*
5. *How does the uterus prepare for pregnancy, and what changes occur if conception does not occur?*
6. *What are the phases of the ovarian cycle, including significant hormonal changes in each phase?*
7. *How does the nurse use knowledge about normal reproductive anatomy and physiology during the care of childbearing women and their families?*

References

Cunningham, F., MacDonald, P, & Gant, N. (1989). *Williams obstetrics* (18th ed.). Norwalk, CT: Appleton-Century-Crofts.

Guyton, A. (1991). *Textbook of medical physiology* (8th ed.). Philadelphia: W.B. Saunders.

Hamm, T. (1991). Physiology of normal female bleeding. *NAACOG'S Clinical Issues in Perinatal and Women's Health Nursing*, *2*(3), 289–293.

Hacker, N., & Moore, G. (1992). *Essentials of obstetrics and gynecology* (2nd ed.). Philadelphia: W.B. Saunders.

Lichtman, R., & Papera, S. (1990). *Gynecology: Well woman care*. Norwalk, CT: Appleton and Lange.

Mishell, D., Davajan, V., & Lobo, R. (1991). *Infertility, contraception and reproductive endocrinology* (3rd ed.). Boston: Blackwell Scientific.

Speroff, L., Glass, R., & Kase, N. (1989). *Clinical gynecologic endocrinology and infertility* (3rd ed.). Baltimore: Williams & Wilkins.

Tuttle, J. (1991). Menstrual disorders during adolescence. *Journal of Pediatric Health Care*, *5*(4), 197–203.

Suggested Readings

Cumming, D., Cumming, C., & Kieren, D. (1991). Menstrual mythology and sources of information about menstruation. *American Journal of Obstetrics and Gynecology*, *164*(2), 472–476.

Filicori, M. (1991). Reproductive physiology: Recent advances of clinical interest. *Current Opinion in Obstetrics and Gynecology*, *3*(3), 309–315.

Wurtman, J., Brezezinski, A., Wurtman, R., & Laferrere, B. (1989). Effect of nutrient intake of premenstrual depression. *American Journal of Obstetrics and Gynecology*, *161*, 1228–1234.

CHAPTER 5

Human Sexuality

Learning Objectives

After studying the material in this chapter, the student will be able to:

- Discuss the concept of sexual health.
- Discuss the changes that occur for both women and men during sexual response.
- Explain the four phases of the sexual response cycle.
- Describe how pregnancy results in changes in sexual response in the areas of desire, arousal, and orgasm.
- Identify issues of sexual concern for pregnant couples in all three trimesters and the postpartum period.
- Discuss the basic guidelines for advising couples on the relative risks of intercourse during menstruation, pregnancy, the postpartum period, and breastfeeding.
- Offer specific suggestions to use when approaching sexual problems during pregnancy and postpartum.

Key Terms

cunnilingus
dyspareunia
gender identity
fellatio
homophobia
lesbian
masturbation
orgasm
sexual orientation

Cultural messages sometimes make it difficult to connect the image of parenthood with the idea of sexual desire and activity. Beliefs about pleasure in sexual activity and sexual activity during pregnancy have ranged from complete prohibition to lack of any restriction. The rationale and guidelines for restrictions of sexual activity during pregnancy have been inconsistent.

Many pregnant women and their partners want more information about sexual feelings and behaviors during the childbearing year but are reluctant to initiate discussion with the nurse or physician. Frequently, health professionals do not inquire about a woman's sexual concerns or questions because they lack the education that prepares them to do so comfortably. Both medical and nursing schools traditionally have avoided including human sexuality in their curricula. Progress is being made slowly, along with a current emphasis on total family care. Although medical and nursing programs are adding human sexuality to their curricula, the material taught is not standardized.

This chapter discusses basic information about human sexuality as a foundation for understanding how sexuality may be affected by childbearing and the changes of pregnancy that can inhibit or enhance sexual feelings. Understanding the sexuality of pregnant couples and the relative risks and advantages of sexual activity will provide the nurse with information, suggestions, and support to offer childbearing families.

Developmental Aspects of Sexuality

The roots of sexual well-being begin early in childhood. Children learn about sexuality when learning the names for the parts of their bodies, particularly the genitals, and when learning whether they are boys or girls. The underlying message conveyed by the relative comfort of a parent with sex education comes through to a child in many ways. How parents deal with nudity, masturbation, childhood sexual play, explanations about where babies come from, and preparations for changes associated with puberty will convey an attitude about sexuality and further questioning.

Children by the age of 5 should have a basic understanding of body parts and their functions and a general knowledge of where babies come from. Correct anatomic names should be used. Children should have a firm idea of their own gender and an understanding of the concepts of maleness and femaleness. The exhibition of a child's maleness or femaleness may differ depending on the gender cues given by the adult with whom the child interacts. By ages 6 through 9, children need reassurance that their bodies belong to them and that they have a choice about permitting or refusing physical affection. Children should never be forced to kiss relatives or family friends. They should be taught how to recognize and avoid sexual abuse. By ages 9 through 12, children should know what body changes to expect at puberty. They should understand that each child develops at his or her own rate and should have basic knowledge about the human reproductive system and how it works. Menstruation, masturbation, and "wet dreams" should be understood as a normal part of development. By the ages of 12 to 14, adolescents should know about contraception and avoiding sexually transmitted diseases (Katz & Walsh, 1991).

The most important developmental task of adolescence is the process of identity formation. Part of achieving a growing, separate identity includes acceptance of one's fertility. Acceptance of this aspect of sexuality is necessary to ensure responsible sexual behavior (see Chapters 7 and 9 for discussion of the special reproductive health needs of adolescents). Another important aspect of identify formation is the acceptance of gender identity and sexual identity.

Gender Identity and Sexual Orientation

The development of *gender identity*, that is, the recognition of self as either male or female, has its roots in early childhood. However, its evolution is not complete until adulthood. Gender identity is basic to personality development. *Sexual orientation* is the recognition of self as heterosexual, homosexual, or bisexual. Sexual orientation becomes more clearly defined during adolescence and is usually clearly defined by young adulthood.

During early and middle adolescence (ages 10 to 16), young people normally concentrate heavily on relationships with their peers. They search for their own concept of normalcy and self-identify through comparison with peers of the same gender. The awkwardness of new heterosexual social and interpersonal relationships is not easily bridged for many adolescents. Thus, there is continued need for same-gender friendship and intimacy. Same-gender sexual exploration is normal and acts of fellatio (oral stimulation of the penis) and cunnilingus (oral stimulation of the female genitalia) may occur (Muscari, 1987).

Adolescents may become concerned about their own sexual identity if they feel, or once felt, attracted to someone of the same gender. Society places undue concern on the issue of homosexuality at this age. It is also important to note that adolescents often find it difficult to discuss sexual concerns with anyone. If they become too isolated or alienated from peers and family, they may become suicidal. Therefore, it is vitally important for health professionals to be alert to adolescents' concerns regarding sexual orientation.

Unfortunately, homophobia (the fear or dislike of homosexuals) in contemporary society is a significant factor in the process of acknowledging sexual orientation for many adolescents. Homophobia is driven by the misconception that homosexuals are unstable and abnormal. This misconception may prevent adolescents who are in the process of acknowledging their sexual orientation as homosexual from openly entering into same-gender relationships until well into adulthood (Sanford, 1989). Homophobic or stereotyped thinking about gay or lesbian people may also affect the quality of health care received.

As many as one in ten women identify themselves as lesbian. An increasing number of lesbians desire children and, should pregnancy be achieved, will likely seek perinatal care (Kenney & Tash, 1992). The maternity nurse should be knowledgeable about the special needs of lesbian women during the childbearing years (see Chapter 6 for discussion of the special needs of lesbian women for well-woman care and Chapters 8 and 36 for discussion of the psychosocial needs of lesbian mothers).

Regardless of sexual orientation, sexuality evolves and changes during the adult years, partly in response to psychological maturation and adaptation. Physiologic changes associated with childbearing and aging also affect sexuality. The following sections discuss the physiologic elements of human sexuality and the specific changes in sexuality through the childbearing year.

Physiology of Human Sexual Response

Human beings have a capacity for some level of sexual response early in their development. Male fetuses have the capacity for intrauterine erection, as demonstrated through sonography. There has been no direct observation of clitoral erection or vaginal lubrication in female fetuses; however, these are possible from birth onward. Historic research by Kinsey and his colleagues reported the capacity for orgasm (ie, the state of emotional and physical excitement that occurs at the climax of sexual stimulation) in infants as young as 4 months (Masters, Johnson, & Kolodny, 1992). However, sexual physiologic development is more typically thought to begin with the onset of puberty.

Puberty is the period of life in which functional capacity for reproduction is attained and ends in the attainment of physiologic sexual maturity. Peak growth occurs in reproductive, cardiovascular, and musculoskeletal systems during puberty (see Chapter 4 for discussion of the development and maturation of male and female reproductive systems). On attainment of sexual physiologic maturity, both males and females are capable of sexual response.

Human Sexual Response Cycle

In the 1950s, Dr. William Masters and Mrs. Virginia Johnson began laboratory observations of human sexual response at the Reproductive Biology Research Foundation in

St. Louis. Early observations were made during masturbation (the stimulation of genitals or other erogenous areas by some means other than sexual intercourse), sexual intercourse, and "artificial coition" using a lighted photographic vaginal probe. This classic research resulted in a detailed understanding of the human sexual response (Masters et al., 1992). The sexual response cycle has four phases: the excitement phase, the plateau phase, the orgasm phase, and the resolution. The phases are general descriptions and can vary from person to person and from experience to experience. The transition from phase to phase is not always clearly demarcated. These phases are described briefly here and summarized and illustrated in Table 5-1.

The primary reaction to sexual stimuli in the excitement phase is vasocongestion. This engorgement or vasocongestion may be triggered by direct physical stimulation, a sexually stimulating sight, or an erotic train of thought. The second reaction is myotonia, evidenced by spasms in the hands and feet, facial grimaces, and tensing of extremities or other body parts during orgasm. The physiologic changes that proceed through the sexual response cycle remain basically the same regardless of the type of stimulation used.

The plateau phase is characterized by a degree of sexual arousal that is much higher than the excitement phase and is lower than the threshold level required to trigger orgasm.

Orgasm is a reflex response to a stimulus that is sufficiently effective to reach the threshold level of arousal. The reflex can be thought of as similar to a sneeze. The blood causing the vasocongestion of the erectile tissue is forced back into the bloodstream by the contraction of muscles surrounding that tissue. Ejaculation occurs in this phase.

The resolution phase is the return of the genital organs and body to the unaroused state. If no orgasm has occurred, resolution takes longer because of lingering vasocongestion. If there has been considerable, prolonged excitement, the unrelieved vasocongestion may feel heavy or aching.

Women are capable of being multiorgasmic, meaning that they can repeatedly go through the response cycle to orgasm without the recovery time. To be multiorgasmic, women need consistently effective stimulation. This type of stimulation most frequently occurs with masturbation rather than intercourse.

Men may also experience multiple orgasms if the definition of having two or more climaxes within a short period of time is used. The period between orgasms is longer for men than for women and depends on the length of the refractory period.

Pregnant women and their partners may need information about changes in sexuality during the childbearing year. Understanding the sexuality of pregnant couples and the consequences of sexual behavior will allow the nurse to offer useful information and support. The roots of sexual well-being begin in childhood, and healthy sexual development occurs throughout adolescence and into adulthood. The concepts of gender identity and sexual orientation are important in understanding human sexuality. Although sexual orientation varies among humans, physiologic sexual responses are gender specific. The phases of the physiologic sexual response cycle, ie, excitement phase, plateau phase, orgasm phase, and resolution phase, were presented.

Adaptation to Sexuality During the Childbearing Year

Information on sexuality during the pregnancy and postpartum period is limited, and studies of sexuality during pregnancy have produced conflicting findings. Without further research, it is possible only to say that there appears to be a wide range of normal feelings, sexual desires, frequency of intercourse, sexual enjoyment, and sexual adjustment during the childbearing year. Few studies have collected data from couples. Most have relied on retrospective questionnaires completed only by women. Despite the lack of research on this subject, it is clear that numerous factors affect the sexual relationship during pregnancy. These factors include:

- The sexual pattern before pregnancy, including frequency, enjoyment, comfort, and ability to communicate about sex.
- The meaning of sex to each member of the couple.
- The meaning of pregnancy to each member of the couple, and experiences during previous pregnancies, if any.
- The woman's general state of health during pregnancy.
- Other medical problems that may occur during pregnancy.
- Advice from health care providers regarding sexual activity.
- Whether or not the pregnancy is planned and wanted by both partners.
- Fear of miscarriage or of hurting the fetus through sexual activity.
- Cultural expectations regarding sexual activity during pregnancy.
- Responses of each member of the couple to physical changes in the woman's body.

Sexual Activity and Safety Concerns During Pregnancy

Intercourse and orgasm seem to be safe for most pregnant women throughout pregnancy. There appears to be a small risk of death from air embolism during pregnancy after blowing of air into the vagina during cunnilingus (Guana-Trujillo & Grant-Higgins, 1987). Otherwise, sexual activities do not pose a threat to the healthy pregnant woman.

Because sexual activity can cause uterine contraction and alteration of uterine blood flow, physicians commonly advise women in high-risk pregnancies to abstain from activities that may lead to sexual excitement or orgasm. Women who are likely to be advised to restrict sexual activities include those with the following conditions:

- Premature dilation of the cervix
- Previous threatened abortion

Text continues on page 88

Table 5-1. Summary of Sexual Response Cycle Changes

General Physiologic Changes	Specific Changes in Women	Specific Changes in Men
Excitement Phase		
Excitement phase occurs at the onset of arousal. The stimulation may be physical or psychic. Erotic feelings come through all senses—sight, feel, touch, smell, taste, hearing—and through thought or fantasy.		
Vasocongestion (engorgement—more blood flows into the area than flows out of it) is the primary reaction to stimulation, regardless of technique. *Myotonia* (contraction of various muscle fibers, muscles, and groups of muscles) is the secondary reaction to stimulation, regardless of technique.	*Vaginal lubrication*—primary sign of excitement phase. Lubrication is due to vasocongestion and occurs within 10–30 s of the onset of stimulation. Vaginal lubrication appears as a "sweating" reaction of vaginal lining.	*Erection of the penis*—primary sign of excitement phase. Erection is due to vasocongestion in the penis and occurs within a few seconds, regardless of the nature of the stimulation. A small penis may double in length. The lengthening is less marked in a large penis.
Tachycardia. Heart rate increases in direct proportion to rising tension, regardless of stimulation technique.	*Expansion of inner two thirds of vagina.* Back of vagina begins to balloon out 3.75–4.25 cm in width and 2.3–3.5 cm in length.	*Enlargement of testicles*—owing to engorgement.
Blood pressure elevation occurs in direct proportion to rising tension, regardless of stimulation technique.	*Elevation of cervix and uterus.* Cervix is pulled up and out of the way.	*Elevation of testicles*—owing to shortening of spermatic cords that suspend the testicles in the scrotal sac.
Respiratory rate increases are slight in this phase. *Sex flush* appears as maculopapular rash starting on abdomen and spreading over chest. Time of appearance varies.	*Engorgement of clitoral glans and clitoral shaft.* Degree of swelling is not related to either sexual responsiveness or ability to achieve orgasm. *Separation and flattening of labia majora.* Changes in labia are heightened in multiparous women owing to increased engorgement. *Engorgement of labia minora.*	*Thickening, flattening, and elevation of scrotal sac.*
	Erection of nipples owing to contraction of nipple muscle fibers. Nipples may not erect simultaneously.	*Erection of nipples* occurs inconsistently in men.
	Enlargement of breasts. Areola begins to swell, and pattern of veins on surface of breast becomes more distinct.	
Plateau Phase		
Plateau phase is a more advanced stage of arousal during which the person is actively engaged in sexual activity and stimulation, either alone or with a partner. The entire body is responding with increasing intensity and reaching toward a peak (orgasm).		
Vasocongestion. Engorgement reaches its maximum level during plateau phase. *Myotonia.* Muscle tension in both involuntary and voluntary muscles reaches its maximum level. *Tachycardia.* Recorded rates average from 100–175 bpm.	*Formation of the orgasmic platform.* The primary sign of plateau appears as engorgement and swelling of tissues surrounding outer third of the vagina. As a result of this final engorgement, the diameter of the vaginal opening is reduced. (If a penis is in the vagina at this time, the effect is actually a gripping of the base of the penis.) Appearance of the orgasmic platform does not necessarily mean orgasm is imminent.	*Expansion in diameter of coronal ridge* (at base of glans). The glans may deepen in color to a reddish purple hue.
	Full expansion of inner two thirds of vagina. Back of the vagina is now widely ballooned.	*Enlargement of testicles* by up to 50% occurs.
	Full elevation of cervix and uterus.	*Elevation of testicles.* Testicles now rotate and are positioned in close contact with the perineum. This is a sign that orgasm is imminent.
Blood pressure elevation. Systolic pressure can rise 20–60 mm Hg and diastolic pressure can rise 10–20 mm Hg. *Respiratory rate.* Can become hyperventilation late in phase. *Sex flush* may be more prominent.	*Retraction of clitoris glans* due to shortening of clitoral shaft. Glans seems to be hiding but is still responsive to stimulation. *Engorgement of labia majora* continues to its fullest extent. *"Sex skin" appears in labia minora,* late in plateau phase. The inner lips turn a deep red color. It is a sign of impending orgasm if effective erotic stimulation is continued.	
	Full engorgement of areola. The swelling can be so marked that it masks nipple erection.	*Secretion from Cowper's gland,* often called

Excitement Phase

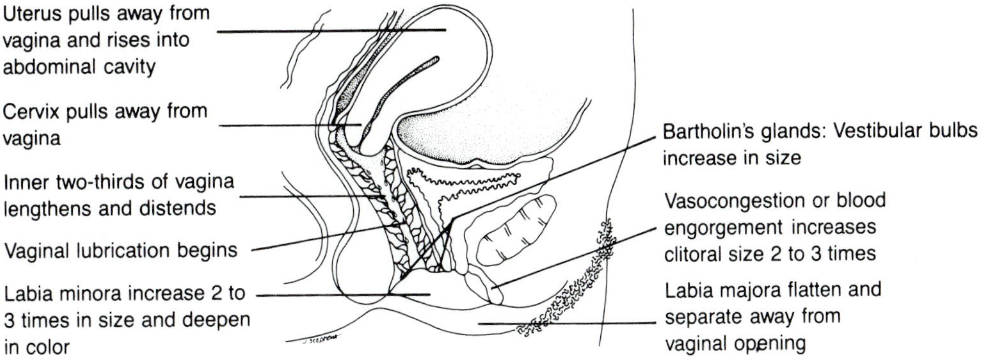

Uterus pulls away from vagina and rises into abdominal cavity
Cervix pulls away from vagina
Inner two-thirds of vagina lengthens and distends
Vaginal lubrication begins
Labia minora increase 2 to 3 times in size and deepen in color
Bartholin's glands: Vestibular bulbs increase in size
Vasocongestion or blood engorgement increases clitoral size 2 to 3 times
Labia majora flatten and separate away from vaginal opening

Female excitement phase

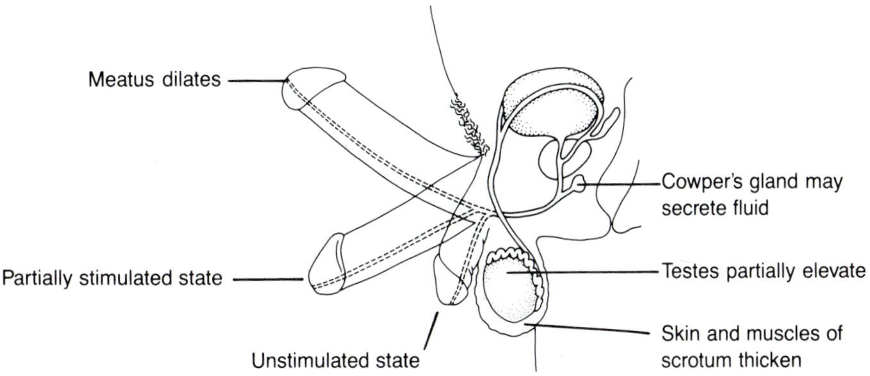

Meatus dilates
Partially stimulated state
Unstimulated state
Cowper's gland may secrete fluid
Testes partially elevate
Skin and muscles of scrotum thicken

Male excitement phase

Plateau Phase

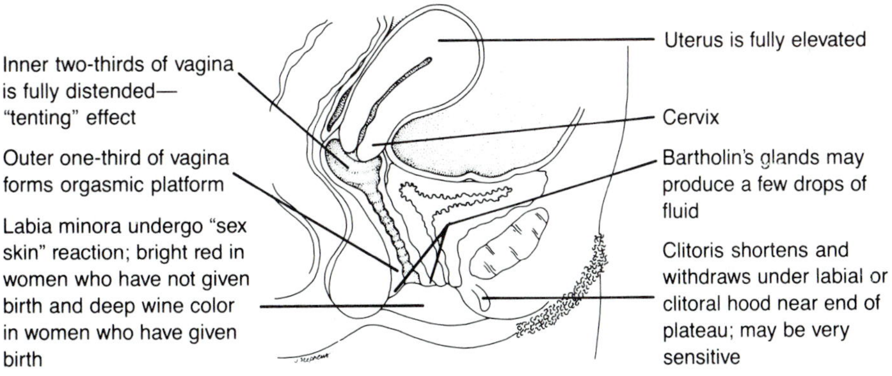

Inner two-thirds of vagina is fully distended—"tenting" effect
Outer one-third of vagina forms orgasmic platform
Labia minora undergo "sex skin" reaction; bright red in women who have not given birth and deep wine color in women who have given birth
Uterus is fully elevated
Cervix
Bartholin's glands may produce a few drops of fluid
Clitoris shortens and withdraws under labial or clitoral hood near end of plateau; may be very sensitive

Female plateau phase

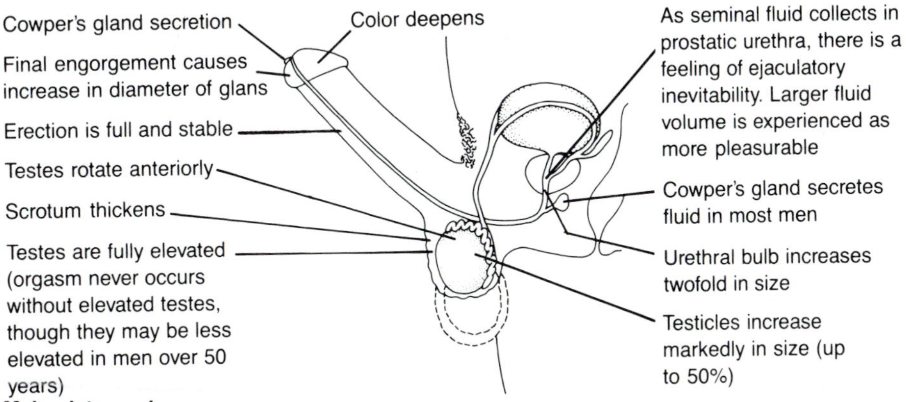

Cowper's gland secretion
Final engorgement causes increase in diameter of glans
Erection is full and stable
Testes rotate anteriorly
Scrotum thickens
Testes are fully elevated (orgasm never occurs without elevated testes, though they may be less elevated in men over 50 years)
Color deepens
As seminal fluid collects in prostatic urethra, there is a feeling of ejaculatory inevitability. Larger fluid volume is experienced as more pleasurable
Cowper's gland secretes fluid in most men
Urethral bulb increases twofold in size
Testicles increase markedly in size (up to 50%)

Male plateau phase

(*continued*)

Table 5-1. Summary of Sexual Response Cycle Changes ***(Continued)***

General Physiologic Changes	Specific Changes in Women	Specific Changes in Men
	Increase in breast size. Change is greater in women who have never breastfed. *Slight secretion from Bartholin's glands* may occur.	preejaculatory fluid. Small amounts of this clear fluid appear at the urethral opening. Live spermatozoa have been observed in this fluid.
Orgasm Phase		
Orgasm is considered the peak or climax of sexual arousal and is intensely pleasurable.		
Vasocongestion is reversed by orgasm. *Myotonia.* Muscles throughout the body tend to contract at orgasm. Face may be contorted, muscles of the neck, arms, and legs frequently contract in a spasm, gluteal and abdominal muscles are often contracted, and carpopedal spasms of the hands and feet may occur. *Tachycardia.* Rates range from 100–180 bpm. *Blood pressure elevation.* Systolic increase from 30–80 mm Hg, diastolic increase from 20–40 mm Hg. *Hyperventilation.* Rates of up to 40 breaths/min.	*Contraction of orgasmic platform.* Usually appears as an initial spasm followed by a series of rhythmic contractions at 0.8-s intervals. The more intense the orgasm, the more contractions will follow. *Rhythmic contractions of uterus* begin at fundus and move like a wave down to the cervix. If orgasm is very intense, uterine contractions may be severe. *Orgasm* occurs even in women with hysterectomies and women who have had the clitoris surgically removed.	*Ejaculation* takes place in two phases. *Emission.* During the first phase, fluid containing live spermatozoa and secretions from the prostate, seminal vesicles, and vas deferens begins to pool in the prostatic urethra as a result of a series of rhythmic contractions of those organs. This signals the stage of ejaculatory inevitability. *Ejaculation.* During the second phase, rhythmic contractions of the urethral bulb and penis at 0.8-s intervals propel the fluid out the end of the penis, since the internal sphincter of the bladder is tightly closed.
	Contraction of anal sphincter at 0.8-s intervals. External urethral sphincter may contract. Cervical os may relax.	*Contraction of anal sphincter* at 0.8-s intervals.
Resolution Phase		
The body begins to return to its preexcitement state. There is often a sense of calm and well-being.		
Vasocongestion. Congested blood is released back into general circulation after orgasm. If there is no orgasm, reversal of vasocongestion may take a couple of hours. *Relaxation.* Muscles feel relaxed; body feels generally rid of tension.	*Rapid disappearance of orgasmic platform.*	*Refractory period.* During this period, the man is physiologically unable to initiate the sexual response cycle. He may feel subjectively aroused during this time and may still have a partial erection, but the pelvic organs need time for the sexual response mechanisms to become operational again. In some men, this period will be no longer than 10 min.
	Loss of erection. Clitoris rapidly returns to normal position (5–10 s).	Loss of erection occurs in two stages. During the first stage, 50% of the erection is rapidly lost. During the second stage, the rest of the erection occurs more gradually.
Respiratory rate, pulse rate, and blood pressure return to normal levels. *Sweating reaction* may occur in which body is covered with a thin film of moisture. *Sex flush* rapidly disappears.	Vaginal walls relax (10–15 min). Cervix and uterus descend to normal position. The cervix rests in a small depression in the vagina called the *seminal pool.* Cervical os remains open for 20–30 min after orgasm. Breast size and nipple erection decrease slowly.	
	Labia minora and labia majora return to normal color and position.	Testicles decrease in size and descend to their preexcited state.

Orgasmic Phase

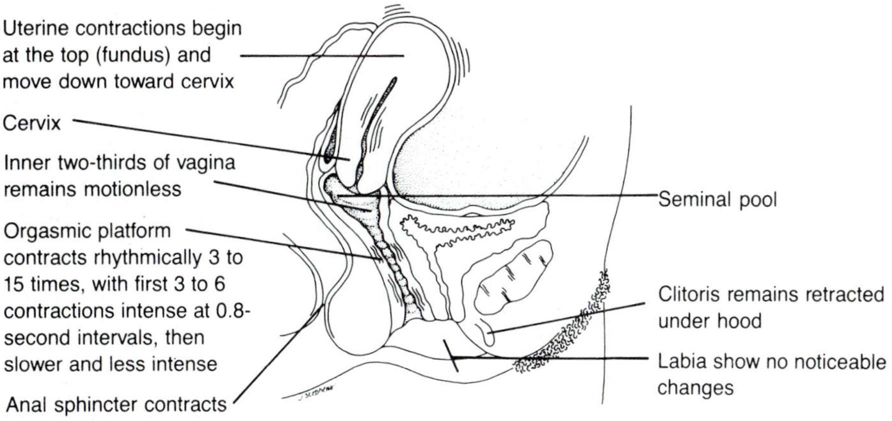

Female orgasmic phase

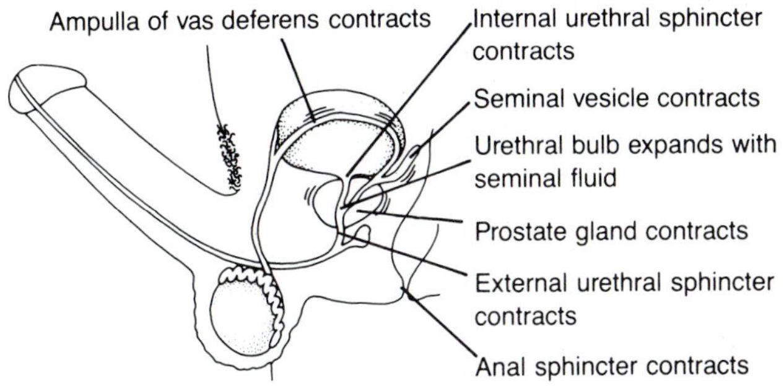

Male orgasmic phase: stage 1

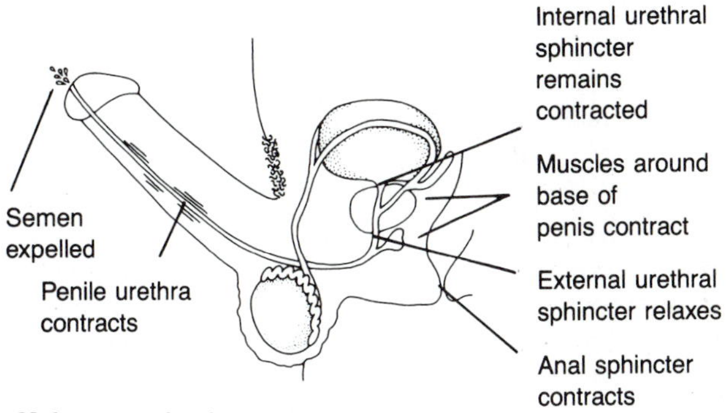

Male orgasmic phase: stage 2

Resolution Phase

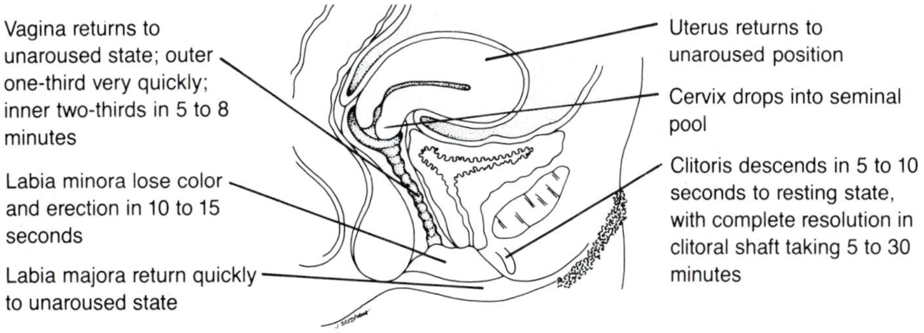

Female resolution phase

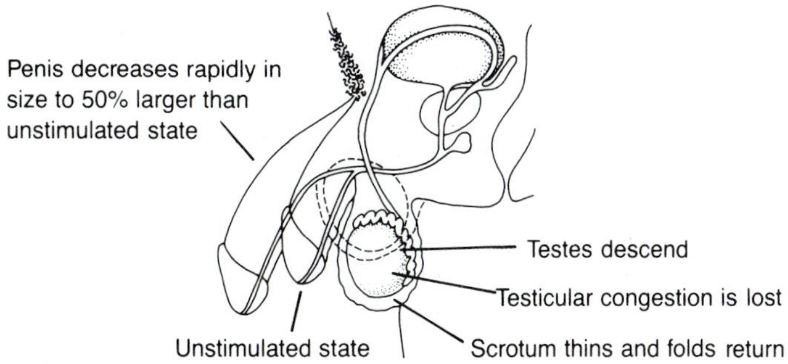

Male resolution phase

- Previous preterm labor
- Multiple gestation
- Possible placenta previa
- Pregnancy-induced hypertension
- Diabetes

Changes in Sexuality During Pregnancy

Variations in sexual interest and activity during pregnancy are difficult to predict in individual women and their partners. The woman's physical status, comfort, and sense of well-being are closely linked to her interest in sexual activity during pregnancy. A classic study by Bing and Colman (1977) identified four typical patterns of interest in sexual activity among women during pregnancy:

- A steady continuous increase in sexual interest throughout pregnancy.
- A decline in sexual increase in the first trimester, a relative increase in the second trimester, and a decline in the third trimester.
- A steady decline in sexual interest throughout pregnancy.
- No changes from the prepregnant state.

For some women, pregnancy is a time of heightened sexual awareness and sensuality, whereas for others, there is either no change or a decline in interest and frequency of sexual activity. Certainly the sexual interest of the partner of the pregnant woman must also be considered. Few studies have systematically included partners in data collection about sexual changes in pregnancy. However, variations also occur in sexual interest among partners of pregnant women (Bogren, 1991). See the Family Considerations display and Chapter 8 for a discussion of psychosocial changes during pregnancy.

The First Trimester

After the sixth or seventh week of pregnancy, nausea and vomiting commonly get in the way of erotic feelings. Sexual activity, or even the thought of it, can be enough to make the nauseated pregnant woman feel that she may vomit. Often women find that their sense of smell is heightened in the first trimester, and any odor may become particularly nauseating or antierotic.

Breast tenderness is common in early pregnancy, and tenderness during arousal can be especially painful. Breast stimulation may have to be stopped altogether. The woman will need to communicate about what kind of touch is pleasurable, if any.

Tiredness and "overdoing things" play a part in curtailing sexual interest. The extent of this physical exhaustion caused by hormonal changes can be surprising to some women. They may feel they can barely wait to get to bed to fall asleep.

Fear of miscarriage creates anxiety that can cause couples to avoid any sexual expression at all, even cuddling. If the woman has previously lost a pregnancy or has noticed any unusual signs in the current pregnancy, she may naturally feel that sex is a threat to the fetus. Her partner may also

Family Considerations

Men's Sexuality During the Childbearing Year

Research suggests a complex relationship centering on a man's personality characteristics, his experience of his own sexuality during the childbearing year, and the quality of his relationships with his mate and his newborn. Marital satisfaction is known to decrease on the birth of the first child, and sexual satisfaction declines. Men are likely to be more distressed about this change, attributing it to childbearing, whereas women are less concerned about the change and are likely to attribute it to other life concerns.

It is clear that men's sexual functioning is closer to the core of their self-concept than appears to be true for women. This decline in sexual satisfaction may have a more significant impact on men. In one study, men who rated their own sexual satisfaction as high during the first trimester of pregnancy appeared to adapt more easily in the postpartum period. Mates of these men were psychologically healthier in the postpartum period themselves and established more positive relationships with their newborns.

Thus, a man's sexuality during the childbearing year seems to be linked with the well-being of his mate and the family overall. Unfortunately, men often regard childbearing as the "kiss of death" for a satisfying sexual relationship. This may be because they equate *change* with *decline.* The nurse working with childbearing couples should take every opportunity to discuss anticipated changes in the couple and sexual relationship. In this way, the nurse can help couples adapt creatively and maintain satisfying levels of intimacy through pregnancy and the first few months after childbirth.

May, K. (1987). Men's sexuality during the childbearing year. Implications of research findings. Holistic Nursing Practice, 1 *(4), 60–66.*

feel this danger. If sexual activity does occur, additional stress, guilt, and anxiety may develop. Health professionals can help relieve this guilt by reassuring the couple that there is no evidence that lovemaking is related to early pregnancy loss when no other complications are present.

The Second Trimester

The tissues around and inside the vagina become engorged due to the increased vascularity and blood volume characteristic of pregnancy. The tissues are swollen and red to purple in color. They remain in this state throughout pregnancy, so the pregnant woman is in a constant state of early physiologic arousal. This arousal level also causes a constant state of extra vaginal lubrication.

During this phase of pregnancy, resolution after orgasm takes longer and is less complete. This adds to the feeling of pelvic congestion and may contribute to cramping and backache. As the second trimester progresses, the woman's body begins to look more pregnant as her abdomen begins to enlarge. This is the time when the "missionary position" (male on top) during intercourse may become uncomfortable because any weight on the breasts or abdomen is painful. At this point, couples may wish to try other positions that prevent any abdominal pressure or deep penetration. The following positions for intercourse may be suggested:

- Sidelying with vaginal entry from behind
- Sidelying facing one another
- Woman sitting up supported by pillow with knees drawn up and resting over the man, who is on his side below her
- Woman on top facing partner's face
- Woman on top facing partner's feet
- Woman standing bent over, entry from behind
- Woman on hands and knees, entry from behind
- Both sitting facing one another with woman's legs over man's legs

Finally, dyspareunia (painful intercourse) may be a problem. This can be caused by a urinary tract infection, problems with lubrication, vaginitis, pressure on the abdomen, or penile thrusting against the cervix. Fetal movement may also decrease interest in sexual activity.

The Third Trimester

By the third trimester, indigestion and heartburn are often major concerns. If the woman lies down flat, these problems often worsen. If hemorrhoids are painful or inflamed, they can also have an inhibiting effect on sexual interest.

The uterus may have one long sustained contraction after orgasm, lasting for a minute or more. For some women, this is an interesting and pleasurable sensation. For others, the sensation may be frightening. They may fear the fetus will be deprived of oxygen or injured during this contraction. Fetal heart rate may slow minimally, but there is no evidence that this is dangerous to the healthy fetus. The resolution phase after orgasm is still incomplete, so the sense of arousal may be constant. Some women complain that no matter how often they masturbate or have intercourse or orgasm, they cannot feel satisfied.

As the pregnant woman becomes larger, she may feel her body is too awkward and enormous for sex, or she may feel like a beautiful, bountiful goddess. Her body image along with her physical state will direct her sexual interest. If she feels too ugly, she may be convinced that her partner finds her ugly too. Quite often, men are awed and delighted by seeing a pregnant woman's body. Sometimes, however, they cannot feel aroused. The man may have his own fears of harming the fetus during intercourse. This fear or his reaction to his partner's extremely womanly body may occasionally inhibit the ability to have an erection.

Fatigue often returns during the third trimester because of the lack of sleep. Fatigue can also result from the physical demands of moving an enlarged body around all day. Last-minute preparations for the newborn may be tiring. Fatigue is often an inhibitor of sexual interest.

Labor and Birth

If the pregnant woman is at term and the cervix is ripe, her care provider may encourage sexual activity, especially orgasm. During sexual arousal, oxytocin is released into the pregnant woman's bloodstream. Breast stimulation in particular stimulates the secretion of oxytocin. This may play an important role in helping the cervix to ripen and dilate in preparation for labor.

There is much variation in the extent to which women experience a connection between the process of labor and birth and their sense of themselves as feminine and sensual. Some women might find any connection between labor and birth and sexual pleasure impossible to understand. Other women describe birth as a powerfully erotic experience of moving sexual energy. Even if a woman could envision herself having an intense sexual experience during birth, she might feel inhibited to express it.

In the early research on father attendance at labor and birth, concerns were expressed about the possible negative effects on the sexual relationship that might result from the man observing his partner as she gives birth (May, 1987). These concerns have not been supported by research and there is no evidence that a healthy sexual relationship is likely to be disrupted in this way. However, there is always the possibility that the visual images of labor and birth may be overwhelming to the partner. Thus, it is important that partners be given a choice about the level of their involvement in labor and birth.

Postpartum Adaptation and Sexual Activity

Physical restoration of the woman after childbirth plays a major part in determining how quickly she is ready to resume sexual activity. By the end of the first week, the cervix is healing. The uterus generally takes 6 weeks to involute to the prepregnant state. Lochial flow generally lasts 2 to 3 weeks. Some women and some partners are bothered by the presence of this discharge; others view it as a natural part of the postpartum experience. The vaginal walls, vulva, and other perineal tissues gradually diminish in size but rarely return to their prepregnant condition. Tears in the vaginal or vulvar tissue may cause a decrease in subsequent orgasmic reaction.

The episiotomy site is generally a cause of concern for many women and their partners. Actual healing of the episiotomy generally takes about 2 weeks. However, it may be as long as 4 months before the scar is elastic enough to permit sexual activity, especially penetration, without pain.

Women are typically advised to wait 4 to 6 weeks after childbirth before resuming sexual activity. This delay allows the woman to be examined during her routine 6-week postpartum check and makes it convenient for her care provider to prescribe contraceptives as needed at that time. Despite this advice, many couples resume sexual activities before this time, often between 3 to 4 weeks after birth. More appropriate advice to couples would be to delay sexual activity until the flow of lochia has stopped, there is no perineal discomfort, and both partners feel psychologically ready.

There is great variation in when couples feel ready to resume sexual activity after childbirth. Some women have a heightened awareness of their bodies and feelings of sexiness in the first weeks after delivery. Other women are just as intensely estranged from their bodies and find the idea of having sex unthinkable (Guana-Trujillo & Grant-Higgins, 1987). It is not uncommon for women to require 6 months to recover physically from childbirth. Some women may not feel ready for sexual activity before that time. Women and their partners need to be informed that it may take a long time before the woman may be comfortably ready to resume sexual activity. If couples do not have this information, the woman may feel inadequate and guilty if she is not interested in sex at the end of the traditional 6-week recovery period, and her partner may feel cheated and neglected.

Besides the process of physical recovery in the woman, many other factors in the postpartum period can interfere with intimacy and resumption of sexual activity among new parents. Fatigue from sleep deprivation, emotional stress, and physiologic changes all decrease interest in sex. The woman may experience some level of mood disturbance or depression in the postpartum period, which can virtually eliminate sexual desire. Some couples report that as soon as they start to make love, the neonate "seems to know" and begins to cry or wants to be fed. No evidence indicates that the newborn is sensitive to parental sexual activity. However, it is possible that, in these cases, the newborn has been rushed through a feeding so that the scene can be set for parents to enjoy themselves, and this results in the neonate's crying.

For couples who have lost newborns through stillbirth or neonatal death, the issue of resuming sexual relations may be prominent. Some couples may feel that sexual expression is a loving act between two grieving partners, which brings respite from painful feelings. Others may feel so depressed that it will be a while before sexual interest returns. Finally, there may be guilt feelings if the parents believe sexual activity may in some way have contributed to complications during pregnancy.

The first resumption of intercourse should be preceded by much touching and caring, open communication between the partners. Sexual encounters that do not involve penetration and perhaps careful exploration with fingers in the vagina should be attempted first. This enables the couple to get an idea what penetration might be like and to check for remaining tender areas. Penile penetration needs to be slow and easy, using plenty of added water-soluble lubrication. If the woman is on top, she may have much more control over the angle and depth of penetration. Even women who have had a cesarean delivery may experience pain during penetration for several months after delivery. This is probably due to the lack of natural lubrication and changes in vaginal and pelvic tissues. Cesarean incisions heal in about 3 months, but special care should be taken to use positions for intercourse that do not put pressure on the incision (see previous section).

Effect of Breastfeeding on Postpartum Sexual Activity

Breastfeeding has many sensual aspects. However, nursing mothers may feel so tired and drained that they are not interested in sexual activity. Some women will feel their needs for body contact and intimacy are met through breastfeeding and do not require additional sensual contact with their partners. Still other women view breastfeeding as a wonderfully sensual experience and some have orgasms while nursing. Partners may be exhilarated by watching the woman breastfeed or may feel jealous that the newborn has priority. The woman may view her breasts as purely functional, whereas her partner may continue to view them as sexual objects. Some partners find the fullness of the partner's breasts to be sexually exciting; others find them to be overwhelming. It is important for women and their partners to understand that all of these responses are normal.

The effect of breastfeeding on sexual desire in women is unclear. Some women do not notice any effect, yet others do. One study found that sexual desire was lower in breastfeeding women than in women who were formula feeding at 6 months postpartum. Among breastfeeding women, weaning brought a quick return to prepregnant levels of sexual desire (Adler & Bancroft, 1988). To the extent that breastfeeding requires extra energy, the woman may feel overburdened and overtired. Such feelings are common inhibitors of sexual feelings. Breastfeeding mothers are also likely to maintain extra body fat as long as they are nursing. This may contribute to body image problems and anxieties about desirability.

Finally, breastfeeding may create minor annoyances that may affect sexual activity. The breasts can leak or spurt milk during arousal and orgasm. Emotional stress is also common among parents in the postpartum period, especially among breastfeeding mothers. If there is any difficulty with breastfeeding or if the newborn is feeding frequently and is difficult to soothe, nerves may become worn thin and sexual feelings are likely to be lost.

Pregnancy causes changes in sexuality, ranging from marked decreases or increases in sexual desire and activity, which can vary as pregnancy progresses. The pregnant woman and her partner will need to maintain open communication and a willingness to experiment to find ways of expressing sexual feelings that are comfort-

able and satisfying for both partners. Postpartum adaptation and breastfeeding also directly affect sexuality. The nurse can provide couples with valuable information and support. The practice of nursing emphasizes holistic perinatal care. The nurse can initiate discussion of sexual matters based on an assessment of the woman's needs and concerns. If the nurse is not interested or able to discuss sexual matters with patients based on self-assessment, the goals of nursing care can still be realized by ensuring that the woman's sexual concerns are sensitively addressed by other providers.

Implications for Nursing Care

Often, human sexuality is left unconsidered throughout the woman's interaction with the health care system. Health care providers may believe women and their families do not have sexual concerns. Care providers may be uncomfortable with the subject of sex themselves or may believe the woman will be offended if the subject is raised. Finally, care providers may believe that discussion of sexual concerns takes too much time or that another care provider will do it. The practice of nursing emphasizes viewing the woman and her family in a holistic fashion. If nursing care fails to include sexuality, then nursing fails in its goals.

Before initiating any discussion with the woman or her partner in regard to sexual well-being, the nurse should first conduct a self-assessment. The nurse's personal comfort and values related to human sexuality will have a major impact on the effectiveness of care provided. Each nurse should look within to see if there is a level of comfort necessary to conduct an assessment of sexual well-being with women and their partners. Not all nurses will be interested in doing so. Self-awareness begins by asking the questions in the accompanying display.

Once the nurse has determined self-readiness to include sexuality in perinatal care, an assessment of the sexual aspects of the woman's life is in order. In this way, sexual functioning is considered as much a part of health in the childbearing years as nutrition, sleep, exercise, and stress management.

Self-Assessment for the Nurse Concerning Sexuality

- How do I feel about providing sexual information, counseling, and support to women and their partners so they can have a better sexual future?
- What is my own concept of sexual adequacy or of what is sexually normal? Will I unintentionally impose that on those for whom I provide care?
- Do I honestly want those for whom I provide care to function better sexually?
- How ready am I for an honest discussion of sexuality?
- How would I feel if I were receiving care, given the same set of circumstances?
- How do I feel about homosexuality, heterosexuality, masturbation, orgasm, unmarried mothers and couples, lesbian mothers, and surrogate mothers?
- What verbal and nonverbal messages do I convey about my sexuality?

Communication About Sexuality

Generally, women want the health professional to initiate discussion about sexuality. Women and their partners usually believe that health professionals should know about sexual matters and will have answers to their questions. However, they may avoid the issue to protect the health professional from embarrassment if they sense the nurse or physician is uncomfortable with the topic of sex.

Because women may not ask direct questions, the nurse does not always know what interest there is in having a discussion about sexual matters. Women may drop hints in the form of jokes or a concern about someone else. A male partner may also drop hints. The nurse learns to listen for cues and to explore the underlying concern.

Language is often a barrier to clear communication about sex. The cultural taboos surrounding the discussion of sexual topics have given rise to countless euphemistic terms, vague generalities, and oversimplifications. Many different levels of terminology can be used to discuss sex, including scientific language, religious language, commonly used terminology, and street language or slang. Health professionals should familiarize themselves with all levels and understand definitions of terms that may be used.

From the woman's choice of words, the nurse should gain an understanding of the terminology the woman prefers. Nurses should use terminology they also find comfortable, but they should recognize that scientific language may not be understood by others.

One way to introduce the topic of sexuality with the pregnant woman would be to say something like: "Many couples have concerns about sexual activity during pregnancy. I'm wondering what concerns you may be having." This line of questioning accomplishes several things. First, it is an open-ended question that prompts the woman to respond with something other than yes or no. Second, it lets the woman know that others have concerns and reinforces that concerns about sexuality are normal. Third, it introduces the topic so that the woman knows that sexuality is a permissible topic to discuss in a health care setting.

Once the topic has been introduced and a concern has been raised, the nurse should systematically assess the nature of the problem and the woman's expectations (see the Assessment Tool). The woman should be encouraged to give specific details of any problem and to describe a typical situation in which the problem occurs. The nurse must clarify each statement that could be misinterpreted. For example, a woman may say "I have so little desire for sex and my partner wants to have sex so frequently." The nurse should

Assessment Tool

Sexual Problem History

I. Description of the current problem (what the woman/couple sees as the problem)

- Ask about the effect on the woman/couple:
  "How does this affect you?"
  "How do you feel about it?"
- Explore the effects on the partner:
  "How does this concern affect your partner?"
  "How has your partner dealt with the problem?"
- Explore the severity:
  "How often do you have this difficulty?"

II. Description of the onset and course of the problem

- Obtain a description of the onset (gradual or sudden, precipitating events) and consequences:
  "When did this start occurring?"
  "What was the situation the first time this occurred?"
- Obtain a description of the course (changes over time; increase, decrease, or fluctuation in severity, frequency, or intensity; relationship of problem to other variables).

III. Identification of the woman's/couple's perception of the factors causing and maintaining the problem

- Ask about psychological, biologic, sociological, and environmental influences that the woman/couple thinks may be contributing factors

IV. Elucidation of previous interventions to deal with the problem and their results

- Ask about previous medical interventions (specialty, date, form of treatment, results, current medications of any kind).
- Ask about other professional or paraprofessional interventions (specialty, date, form of treatment, results). Include questioning that covers alternative treatments, such as biofeedback, special diets, exercise, and so on.
- Ask about self-help (what, when, results).
  "How have you tried to solve the problem up until now?"
- Ask about communication with partner:
  "Have you discussed this with your partner?"
  "What were the results?"

V. Identification of current expectations and goals (specific and general)

- Explore how the woman/couple would like things changed:
  "How would you like the situation to be different?"

first clarify what the term "so frequently" actually means because it may mean anything from three times a day to once a month.

If the woman has no questions or concerns at this time, the nurse can offer information by treating it as a review. The nurse might begin by saying "As you may already know . . . " and then review important information. This approach imparts information and allows the woman to feel safer by not having to reveal a sexual concern or question. Even if the woman has no immediate concerns, this approach will have opened the possibility of discussing sexual concerns in the future.

Even though the nurse may not choose to become expert in counseling women with sexual concerns or problems, caring for childbearing families includes integrating aspects of sexual health promotion into the overall plan of care. Nursing activities that promote sexual well-being in childbearing women and their families include the following:

- Facilitating open discussion of sexual concerns
- Providing information and anticipatory guidance
- Validating normalcy
- Referring women and partners to more intensive therapy for sexual problems, as appropriate

Evaluating the effectiveness of nursing care directed toward promoting sexual well-being is often difficult because the absence of expressed concerns may reflect a state of well-being or an inability to seek help. Thus, it is especially important to create a supportive environment so women can voice concerns and receive appropriate assistance. This is accomplished either through teaching for self-care or through referral.

Chapter Summary

Sexuality is an aspect of human experience beginning in early childhood and extending throughout life. The roots of psychosexual development can be seen in early childhood in the process of establishing gender identity. The process of confirming gender identity and establishing sexual orientation begins with puberty, the attainment of physiologic sexual maturation during adolescence. Research has described the physiologic processes in the human sexual response in women and men. The sexual response cycle consists of four phases: the excitement phase, the plateau phase, orgasm, and the resolution phase.

A woman's sexuality and her sexual relationship with

her partner are usually significantly affected by pregnancy. Nurses can promote sexual health for pregnant women and their partners by anticipating information that will be needed, by confirming the normalcy of changes in sexual patterns, and by facilitating communication about sexual concerns. Generally, sexual activity can continue throughout a healthy, low-risk pregnancy. In particular, couples may need permission to continue their sexual activities or to stop doing something because it does not feel right to them. Often the most helpful thing the nurse can do is to listen to the couple's concerns and to communicate the message that such concerns are as valid as concerns about diet or exercise.

Each couple brings together a unique combination of sexual desires, concerns, behaviors, attitudes, and motivations. Each pregnancy is different and affects each couple differently. Therefore, the nurse who is interested in promoting sexual health must investigate factors that may have a bearing on sexuality. If the woman and her partner feel supported in adapting to their changing couple relationship, their strength and resilience can be significantly enhanced.

Study Questions

1. *What is meant by gender identity and sexual orientation?*
2. *How does homophobia affect the health care received by lesbian women in the childbearing years?*
3. *What are the phases of the human sexual response? What do they involve?*
4. *Under what circumstances may sexual activity be contraindicated during pregnancy?*
5. *In what ways may a woman's interest in sex fluctuate during pregnancy?*
6. *What are the physiologic and anatomic changes occurring during pregnancy that may make intercourse more difficult?*
7. *What positions for sexual intercourse may be more comfortable for the pregnant woman.*
8. *What six factors could affect a couple's sexual relationship during pregnancy?*
9. *When is resumption of intercourse generally considered safe in the postpartum period?*
10. *What effects may breastfeeding have on sexual activity?*

References

Adler, E., & Bancroft, J. (1988). The relationship between breastfeeding persistence, sexuality and mood in postpartum women. *Psychological Medicine*, *18*(2), 389–396.

Bing, E., & Colman, L. (1977). *Making love during pregnancy*. New York: Bantam Books.

Bogren, L. (1991). Changes in sexuality in women and men during pregnancy. *Archives of Sexual Behavior*, *20*(1), 35–45.

Guana-Trujillo, B., & Grant-Higgins, P. (1987). Sexual intercourse and pregnancy. *Health Care for Women International*, *8*(4), 339–346.

Katz, P., & Walsh, P. (1991). *Child development*. Chicago: University of Chicago Press.

Kenney, J., & Tash, D. (1992). Lesbian childbearing couples' dilemmas and concerns. *Health Care of Women International*, *13*(2), 209–219.

Masters, W., Johnson, V., & Kolodny, R. (1992). *Human sexuality* (4th ed.). New York: HarperCollins.

May, K. (1987). Men's sexuality during the childbearing year: Implications of research findings. *Holistic Nursing Practice*, *1*(4), 60–66.

Muscari, M. (1987). Obtaining the adolescent sexual history. *Pediatric Nursing*, *13*(5), 307–310.

Sanford, N. (1989). Providing sensitive health care to gay and lesbian youth. *Nurse Practitioner*, *14*(5), 30–39.

Suggested Readings

Abraham, S., Child, A., Ferry, J., Vizzard, J., & Mira, M. (1990). Recovery after childbirth: A preliminary prospective study. *Medical Journal of Australia*, *152*(1), 9–12.

Bogren, L. (1991). Changes in sexuality in women and men during pregnancy. *Archives of Sexual Behavior*, *20*(1), 35–45.

Kenney, J., & Tash, D. (1992). Lesbian childbearing couples' dilemmas and concerns. *Health Care of Women International*, *13*(2), 209–219.

Glatt, A., Zinner, S., & McCormack, W. (1990). The prevalence of dyspareunia. *Obstetrics and Gynecology*, *75*(3), 433–436.

May, K. (1987). Men's sexuality during the childbearing year: Implications of research findings. *Holistic Nursing Practice*, *1*(4), 60–66.

Nash, J. (1992). Is sex really necessary? *Time*, *139*(3), 47.

Slater, S., & Mencher, J. (1991). The lesbian family life cycle: A contextual approach. *American Journal of Orthopsychiatry*, *61*(3), 372–382.

CHAPTER 6

Women's Health Across the Life Span

Learning Objectives

After studying the material in this chapter, the student will be able to:

- Describe how the factors of sexism and poverty directly and indirectly affect the health and well-being of women.
- Identify the five major causes of death in women.
- Explain breast cancer screening techniques and state how often women should be screened.
- Describe cervical screening techniques and state how often women should be screened.
- Discuss the major mental health concerns affecting women.
- List the most common sexually transmitted diseases in the United States and discuss modes of prevention, detection, and treatment.
- Summarize the major physiologic changes women experience with aging.
- Define menopause and list its signs and symptoms and current treatments.
- Discuss the relationship between menopause and osteoporosis.

Key Terms

cervical intraepithelial neoplasia
cervicitis
fibrocystic breast disease
heterosexism
hormone replacement therapy
mammography
metrorrhagia
osteoporosis
perimenopausal period
vasomotor disturbance

The field of women's health has emerged as an area of specialty practice in nursing. The development of women's health nursing is a natural outgrowth of nursing's historical concern for the welfare of women and their families. As such, it extends concern for women's health and well-being beyond the limits of the childbearing cycle. Women's health nursing focuses on the maintenance and promotion of health in the broader context of women's lives.

The development of the specialty of women's health has paralleled ongoing social discussion about gender roles and sexism and the ways in which they affect health and well-being. The scope of women's health is extensive. This chapter provides an overview of the factors that significantly affect the health of women. Common health concerns faced by women during young, middle, and older adulthood are discussed. Additional readings are suggested for more detailed discussion of women's health issues and health care.

Sexism and Health

Health status and access to quality health care are impossible to separate from the social conditions in which an individual lives. Those who have economic resources and education and who are viewed as more important by virtue of their class or gender have more access to better health care than those who do not. Regardless of individual views about women's roles in contemporary society, it is nevertheless clear that many women face some significant barriers to appropriate and sensitive health care.

To a large extent, the field of women's health developed in response to a health care system that was insensitive and in some cases, sexist, in orientation. Typically, health care of women in the past meant an almost exclusive emphasis on the female reproductive system, a situation that may still persist. Women who have access to regular gynecologic care often do not receive any other form of preventive health care. In fact, the only health care many women receive is care provided during pregnancy, in relation to contraception, or routine gynecologic examinations. Women today can expect to live one third of their lives after menopause. Thus, it is important for preventive health care and health maintenance practices to focus on women across the life span, rather than focusing exclusively on the reproductive years.

Screening for other health issues or concerns is generally not a part of gynecologic care. Unfortunately, women often do not receive, nor do they expect to receive, information and assistance with other kinds of health concerns. Thus, a woman's most frequent and consistent form of health care may focus entirely on conditions that only affect the reproductive system. Women may receive gynecologic care from a male physician, and may not perceive the care provider as being sensitive to their needs. They may be subtly or openly discouraged from asking questions about their care.

At the societal level, sexist attitudes affect the nature and provision of health care and social welfare services. For example, research dollars spent by the National Institutes of Health (NIH) for investigating health problems of major importance to women historically lag far behind funding levels for the study of other conditions. Priorities for research were determined by men whose interests and concerns were considerably different from those of women. Research funding on diagnosis and treatment of conditions such as osteoporosis, breast and ovarian cancer, and heart disease in women is widely acknowledged now to have been inadequate over the last 40 years.

Women and Their Health Care

Today, women are at risk because diagnostic and treatment practices may be inadequately developed. Further, women have been systematically excluded from many large-scale clinical trials. Because treatments were not tested on women, the effects on women are unclear. Even when women were included in clinical trials, the research findings have often not been carefully analyzed regarding the effect gender has on the results. A new set of research priorities at the NIH emphasizes women's health issues; however, it will be decades before the gender gap in health science research is closed (Woods, 1992).

In the past, many believed health problems that received the most emphasis at the federal level were those of concern to powerful, generally middle-aged European American men. The emphasis on the prevention and treatment of heart disease is an example.

Although it is not widely recognized by the lay public, the leading cause of death of women between ages 35 and 55 is coronary heart disease. Further, the consequences of heart disease for women are more severe than for men. Half of women but only 30% of men die within a year of a heart attack. Current screening and diagnostic practices are specifically designed for men. Many women who present with symptoms suggestive of heart disease are managed as if their problems are psychosomatic in nature. Women are far more likely to be misdiagnosed in the early stages of heart disease than their male counterparts. Many suggest that this is because virtually all treatment modalities for heart disease were developed and refined using male populations, and thus diagnostic and treatment procedures are less effective in women. Only in the 1980s was the diagnosis and treatment of coronary heart disease in women officially identified as a major federal priority for research (US Department of Health and Human Services, 1991).

Obesity and diets high in fat may predispose postmenopausal women to heart disease and cancer of the breast and uterus. If so, many women are at risk. More than 25% of American women between the ages of 20 and 74 are considered overweight, with obesity most common among African American women and lower-income women. However, obesity in women, especially that resulting from pregnancy weight gain, has received little scientific attention. Methods to prevent and treat obesity in women have only limited success.

Women are now threatened by problems once common only in men. Deaths from lung cancer among women have increased 600% in the last 30 years, and the rate is now comparable to that in men. However, the future looks even more dismal because adolescent girls are now three times more likely to begin smoking than their male counterparts. Public health efforts to curb smoking have until now largely been targeting men (US Department of Health and Human Services, 1991).

Women suffer from other health problems in disproportionate numbers compared to men. Women are 15 times more likely to develop autoimmune disorders (rheumatoid arthritis, lupus erythematosus). Women are more likely than men to experience problems related to chemical abuse. Female alcoholics experience greater morbidity and mortality than do male alcoholics. Probably this results from the concentration of alcohol in body fat and the poor access to residential treatment for pregnant women and women with dependent children. Women are more likely to abuse prescription drugs than are men. The use of illegal drugs among women is increasing. Women are twice as likely to experience depression than men and are five times more likely to be victims of abuse and violence in the home. At least 1 in every 200 adolescent girls develops an eating disorder and 10% to 15% of these will die from the disorder (US Department of Health and Human Services, 1991).

The health needs of women deserve more systematic attention and greater emphasis in research and treatment programs than they have received to date. If women are likely to receive health care that is less than optimal, minority and lesbian women are at even greater risk. The effects of racism, sexism, and heterosexism (the assumption that all individuals are or ought to be heterosexual) are evident. The design and provision of culturally appropriate health care to meet the needs of all women are significant challenges.

Lesbian Women: Consequences of Heterosexism

Women in general experience difficulty in obtaining sensitive and appropriate health care. Lesbian women face similar problems. Their status is even more of an issue because their sexual orientation places them at risk for insensitive and inappropriate care. Approximately 5% of all women are exclusively lesbian as adults although probably most lesbian women have been sexually active with men at some point in their lives.

Lesbian women require the full scope of health care

offered to heterosexual women. Estimates suggest that 50% to 70% of lesbian women wish to become mothers. Lesbian women face a choice regarding self-disclosure of their sexual orientation to health care providers (Hitchcock & Wilson, 1992). Perceived or actual negative responses from health care providers contribute to delays in seeking health care or in reluctance to self-disclose. Stereotyped thinking and reactions to lesbian women undermine the effectiveness of interactions with health care professionals. Insensitive health care can result in barriers to accurate understanding of the woman's health care needs (Stevens, 1992). For example, questions about marital status, sexual intercourse, and birth control can be phrased in a heterosexist fashion (that assumes all women are heterosexual). Such questions will result in inaccurate information and convey an exclusionary message. (See Chapter 8 for a discussion of health care for lesbian women during pregnancy.)

Women in the Workplace

Sexism and heterosexism at the societal level have a direct effect on the well-being of women and their families. More women are in the workplace than ever before. However, child care services are not considered essential. Pay for women workers still is not equal to payment for comparable work done by male workers. The vast majority of those living under the federal poverty line are women and children, yet job training or education programs specialized for the needs of women with dependent children have not been implemented nationwide (Curry, 1991). This section examines the effects of workplace and poverty on the health status of women.

Increasing numbers of women have been entering the workplace steadily since World War II. This trend is expected to continue. Over 50% of women with children under 5 years of age and 75% of women with school-age children work outside the home. The numbers of women in the professions and other highly paid employment groups are increasing dramatically. Women now hold 40% of all executive, administrative, and management positions.

However, wages earned by women still lag significantly behind those earned by men. Women earn only 70 cents for every dollar earned by men. Although this can be explained by the still prevalent opinion that the work done is not of comparable value, the facts belie this view. Women with higher educational achievement at the college level still earn less than their male classmates in their first position after graduation. This wage differential is often never eliminated (Aburdene & Naisbitt, 1992).

Women may attain less occupational status and remain in positions that have high levels of stress and relatively low levels of decision-making power. Working conditions for predominantly female occupational groups, such as nurses, secretaries, and teachers, are often pressure filled and demanding while allowing the individual worker little flexibility in terms of work flow, work location, and schedule.

Environmental protections in the workplace are an increasing source of concern to many women (Fig. 6-1). Women may be exposed to an increasing number of workplace hazards. Environmental risks may include exposure to

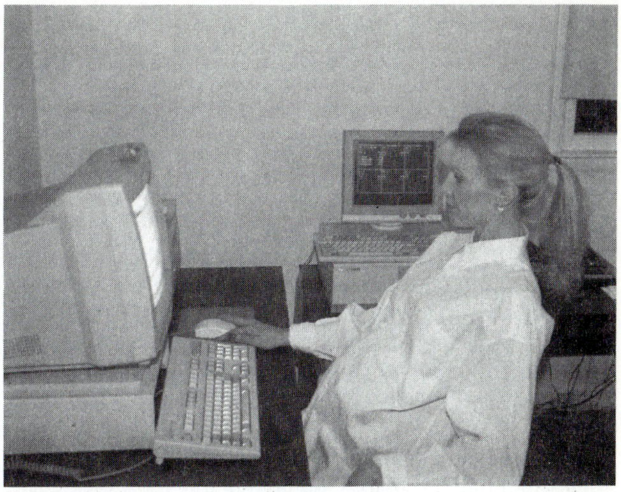

Figure 6-1.
Women are often exposed to environmental hazards in the workplace. These hazards may put them at reproductive risk or at more general health risks because of the physically and emotionally stressful nature of the work.

any of the more than 500 agents now thought to threaten reproductive health. Potentially hazardous exposures include lead, vinyl chloride, polychlorinated hydrocarbons, and solvents used in manufacturing; exposure to electromagnetic fields generated by computer display terminals and copying machines; and drugs such as anesthetic agents and antineoplastic medications. Rather than ensuring that adequate environmental protections are in place for all workers of reproductive age, some manufacturers have prevented women from working in highly paid jobs because of the risks associated with fetal exposure to teratogens. At times, manufacturers permitted women to hold jobs at risk only after they were sterilized (Bernhardt, 1990).

Women may be at risk because they strive to maintain a high level of productivity in physically demanding jobs under less than healthy circumstances. For instance, women may work longer into pregnancy and return to work in physically challenging positions sooner after childbirth than is advisable. This is often due to economic constraints or concerns about job security. The level of physical activity in "women's jobs" typically is underestimated; work in nursing, transportation, and manufacturing is often extremely taxing physically (Muller, 1990).

Workplace health risks require care providers of women to carefully assess the woman's occupational status in regard to health concerns. The effects of the workplace on health may be subtle. However, the effects of underemployment or unemployment and the resulting poverty are having an increasingly serious effect on the health and well-being of women.

Women and Poverty in America

The health status of low-income women and their children in the United States has become a major concern. In the United States, nearly 80% of the poor are women and children. The poorest children are now between the ages of 1 month and 5 years of age. The fastest growing group of homeless are single women with children. Older women are also at risk. Among the elderly poor, 75% are women (Curry, 1991). This phenomenon has been called "the feminization of poverty."

Many families in the United States (especially women with dependent children) are now as vulnerable as they were during the Great Depression. The number of one-parent families has doubled in the last 15 years, and the number of never-married female heads-of-households has increased six times during the same period. One quarter of children today live with only one parent. One third of children living in families headed by women under the age of 30 live in poverty. The median income of these young families has decreased 26% between 1973 and 1986, a decline similar to that experienced during the Great Depression (Curry, 1991). Many women are members of the "working poor." They maintain employment and therefore are not eligible for public assistance, but they earn too little to afford health insurance or health care services.

Poverty and the associated social conditions have a huge impact on the health and well-being of women. At a time when poverty is growing, support for public assistance and health care programs is threatened by the need to reduce federal spending. The growing number of women living and raising children in poverty will have significant consequences on the health of future generations.

Women's health is an emerging specialty in nursing. It emphasizes attention to factors that affect health and well-being of women throughout their lives, not simply in terms of their reproductive status. The past three decades has seen exclusion of women from much biomedical research, as well as inadequate attention to health concerns of particular importance to women. Women face barriers to appropriate and sensitive health care in terms of sexist and heterosexist policies and practices. Women also suffer disproportionately from the consequences of poverty and economic discrimination. The health care system of the future must consider these factors in providing care for *women instead of simply care* of *women.*

Major Health Concerns of Women

The major health concerns facing women regardless of age are those arising from the hazards of modern life: coronary heart disease, cancer of the lung and reproductive organs, and accidental injury. In-depth discussion of these health problems is beyond the scope of this book. The following section discusses health threats unique to women or that disproportionately affect women.

Cancer in Women

Cancer has become a significant health concern for women of all ages. The most common cancers in women are cancer of the breast, lung, colon and rectum, cervix, uterus, and ovary (Fig. 6-2). Incidence of lung cancer as a direct consequence of smoking has increased dramatically in women over the last 30 years. Cancer of the breast and reproductive organs is also increasing.The following section discusses cancers of the female reproductive system.

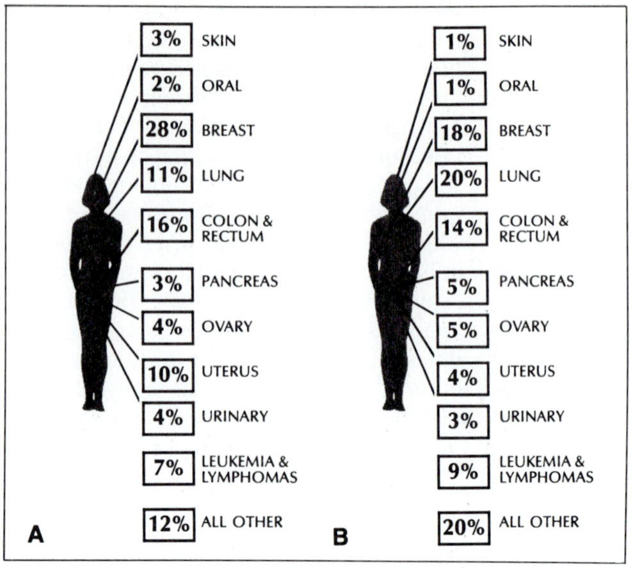

Figure 6-2.
Cancer incidence and death in women (1992 estimates) by site. *A:* Cancer incidence. *B:* Cancer deaths. (From American Cancer Society (1992). *Cancer facts*. New York: American Cancer Society.)

Breast Cancer

One in nine women in the United States will be diagnosed with breast cancer at some time in her life. Incidence is increasing, and the reasons for this are unknown. Of those who develop breast cancer, 80% have no known risk factors (see the accompanying display). Breast cancer is second only to lung cancer as a cause of cancer deaths in women. In 1991, an estimated 45,000 women died of breast cancer (Romans, 1991).

Cancer can develop in the ductal system or in the epithelial layer of the lobe. (See Chapter 4 for a discussion of the anatomy of the breast.) Lesions are described as either invasive (infiltrating) or in situ (noninvasive). The most common site for breast cancer is the upper outer quadrant of the breast; 50% of lesions are found here. These lesions are likely to metastasize to the axillary lymph nodes. About 20% of breast lesions are found in the region directly under and around the nipple; these lesions can metastasize to the mammary lymph nodes.

Early detection is the best predictor of a woman's prognosis in breast cancer. Of women seeking medical care for a breast lump of 1 month's duration that has been diagnosed as malignant, half will already have axillary node involvement, or spread of the cancer. Of women with a breast lump of 6 months' duration that has been diagnosed as malignant, two thirds have axillary node involvement. Spread of the disease is believed to progress primarily through the bloodstream, with the primary metastatic sites being the mammary and axillary lymph nodes, lungs, bone marrow, liver, brain, and bone (Nettles-Carlson, 1989).

Women at Risk for Breast Cancer

The following factors are thought to be associated with a higher risk of breast cancer:

- Age more than 40
- White
- History of cancer in one breast
- Family history of premenopausal bilateral breast cancer
- History of fibrocystic breast disease with atypical hyperplasia
- Living in urban areas of North America and Northern Europe
- History of primary cancer in ovary or endometrium
- Low socioeconomic class
- Single
- First full-term pregnancy after age 35
- Oophorectomy
- Early menarche
- Late menopause
- Diet high in fat and protein

There are several systems for classifying the anatomic extent of cancer. The TNM Classification System is often used in describing breast malignancies (see the accompanying display). In this the system, the T refers to the extent of the primary tumor, the N refers to involvement of lymph nodes, and the M refers to the extent of metastasis.

Treatment options and prognosis are based on staging and grading. Staging determines the size of the tumor and the existence of metastasis, and grading refers to the classification of the tumor cells. Grading is assigned a numeric value ranging from 1 to 4. Grade 1 tumors closely resemble the tissue of origin in structure and function, whereas Grade 4 tumors do not. Grade 4 tumors are poorly or undifferentiated tumors. They tend to be more virulent and less responsive to treatment.

Etiologic and Predisposing Factors

The cause of breast cancer is as yet unknown. Breast cancer occurs only in females after menarche. This suggests that the changes produced in the female breast by hormonal cycles may be a factor in the development of abnormal cellular growth.

The only procedure demonstrated to reduce mortality is a combination of screening with mammography and breast examination. Because 90% of breast cancer occurs in women over age 40, screening is especially important in this group.

Diagnosis

Screening for breast cancer includes breast self-examination (BSE) and periodic screening with mammography and clinical breast examination by a health professional. Guidelines for breast cancer screening are:

- BSE monthly
- Annual breast examination by a health care professional
- Baseline mammogram between ages 35 and 40
- Mammogram every 1 to 2 years for women between the ages of 40 and 50, and every year thereafter

Breast Examination. BSE is of considerable importance because 95% of breast lumps are discovered by women themselves. Women are advised to perform BSE monthly, yet only about 30% of women do so regularly (Wyper, 1990). The Teaching Considerations display outlines the process of BSE.

When teaching women to perform BSE, the nurse should reinforce that the goal is not to determine "normal" from "abnormal," but rather to alert the woman to changes in her breasts that may require further examination by the health care provider. Women often say they do not know what they are feeling—that "everything feels lumpy." The nurse can stress that BSE is intended to identify *changes*. With practice, the woman will be able to recognize if the breast feels similar or different over time.

TNM Classification System

T* Subclasses

Tx: tumor cannot be adequately assessed

T0: no evidence of primary tumor

TIS: carcinoma in situ

T1, T2, T3, T4: progressive increase in tumor size and involvement

N† Subclasses

Nx: regional lymph nodes cannot be assessed clinically

N0: regional lymph nodes demonstrably normal

N1, N2, N3, N4: increasing degrees of demonstrable abnormalities of regional lymph nodes

M‡ Subclasses

Mx: not assessed

M0: no (known) distant metastasis

M1: distant metastasis present, specify site(s)

Histopathology

G1: well-differentiated grade

G2: moderately well-differentiated grade

G3, G4: poorly to very poorly differentiated grade

** T, Primary tumor.*
† N, Regional lymph nodes.
‡ M, Distant metastasis.
From the American Joint Committee on Cancer. (1992). Manual for staging of cancer. *Philadelphia: J.B. Lippincott.*

Teaching Considerations

Breast Self-Examination

The nurse can use the following points in teaching women about breast self-examination (BSE).

Three procedures are necessary for a complete examination. They are inspection before a mirror, inspection and palpation in the shower, and palpation while lying down. The woman should perform the examination at the same time each month. An ideal time is 7 to 10 days after the onset of her menstrual period, when swelling is reduced in the breasts. The postmenopausal woman should select a day of the month on which she will easily remember to do BSE.

Inspection in a Mirror

The woman stands in front of a mirror for inspection, and performs the following steps (see panels A and B). With her arms at her sides, the woman looks for

- Changes in the size and shape of breasts
- Changes in the skin: dimpling, puckering, scaling, redness, swelling
- Changes in the nipple: inversion, scaling, discharge, erosion, nipples pointing in different directions.

Holding her arms over her head, she inspects closely, using the mirror to observe for masses, breast symmetry, or puckering. Pressing her hands firmly on her hips, the woman bows slightly forward (panel C). She inspects in the mirror for lumps or pulling of the skin. Each breast should be a mirror image of the other. If the woman detects a lump in a breast, she should check the other side to see if it feels the same. If so, this is undoubtedly normal tissue. She examines the entire breast, using the circular or grid motion as in the shower. The woman then gently squeezes the nipple of each breast between the thumb and index finger to check for signs of discharge or bleeding.

Inspection and Palpation in the Shower

Some women find it easier to examine their breasts when their hands are soapy. With one hand behind the head, the woman examines her other breast with the flat portions (not the tips) of the fingers of her second hand (panel D). The woman should use either a grid motion (following imaginary lines on the breast dividing it into sections and palpating each section before moving on to another) or a circular motion (moving around the breast systematically in concentric circles, ending with palpation around the nipple). She then should reverse the procedure to examine the second breast. The entire breast should be examined each month. Breast tissue that extends into the axilla should be palpated, as well as the area around and under the nipple.

Palpation Lying Down

Lying flat on her back (panel E), with her right hand under her head and a pillow or towel under her right shoulder, the woman uses her left hand to gently feel her right breast, using concentric circles to cover the entire breast and nipple. She then repeats this process on the left breast.

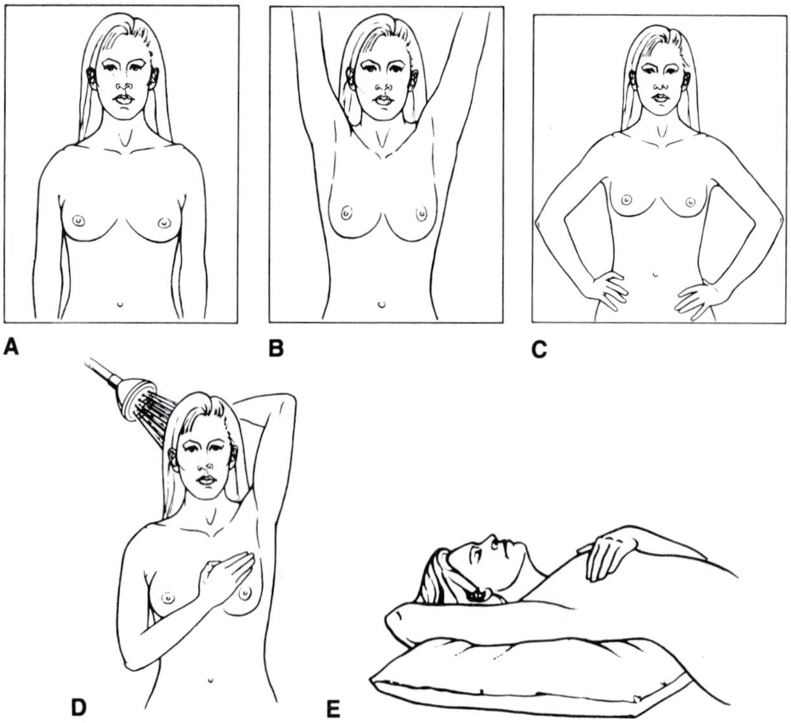

An ideal time to perform BSE is 5 to 7 days after the onset of menses in women of reproductive age. Postmenopausal women should select a day that will be easily remembered each month on which to perform BSE.

Clinical breast examination by a health care professional should occur each year and immediately on identification of a breast lump by the woman herself. If the lump appears to be suspicious to the health care provider, additional testing may be advised. Generally, a biopsy will be recommended if a breast lesion is identified. If the lump is cystic (fluid filled), a needle aspiration may be performed. A needle biopsy will often be performed on fluid or solid tissue. Needle biopsies cannot conclusively rule out the presence of cancerous cells. If the lump is thought to be solid, the woman may be referred for either ultrasound examination of the breast or mammography.

Mammography. Mammography is an x-ray image of the soft tissue of the breast. It is useful in detecting lesions too small to be felt and for making a differential diagnosis of a breast lesion (Fig. 6-3). Mammography is less effective in identifying lesions in denser breast tissue characteristic of younger women; ultrasonography may be more commonly used in this group.

One of the challenges facing the field of women's health care is the infrequent use of recommended breast cancer screening procedures. A recent survey revealed that only 31% of women age 40 or older were following recommended screening guidelines. Of those who had had a mammogram, 75% reported that their care provider had recommended it. The remainder reported they had sought screening on their own. However, of those women who had never had a mammogram, nearly half reported that their care provider had not yet advised them to receive a mammogram. The findings of the study suggest that a minority are following accepted screening guidelines (Romans, Marchant, Pearse, Gravenstine, & Sutton, 1991).

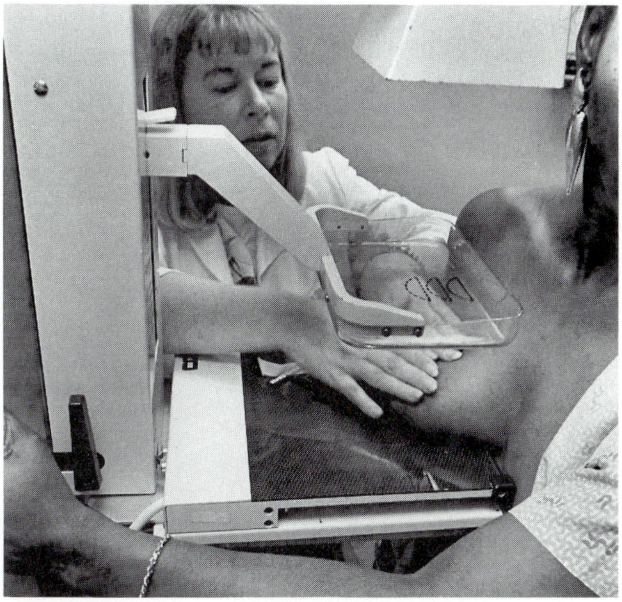

Figure 6-3.
Mammography is an effective means to screen for breast cancer and to assist in early diagnosis. Unfortunately, women may not receive appropriate encouragement from care providers to have routine mammography after age 35. (Photo by Kathy Sloane.)

Research to address the infrequent use of cancer screening practices among women has identified a variety of barriers. Barriers related to health professionals themselves include lack of time for explanations and performing examinations, lack of confidence in the effectiveness of screening procedures, and pressure of other client problems. System-related barriers include the cost of screening and accessibility of services. Barriers related to the woman herself include beliefs about the usefulness of screening, personal risk of having the disease, and fear of developing the disease (Lauver, 1992). It is clearly a nursing responsibility to increase women's knowledge and understanding of the importance of breast cancer screening and to work to improve access and acceptability of those services.

Treatment

Current treatment modalities for breast cancer include surgery, chemotherapy, and radiation therapy. Treatment depends on the stage of the disease and may vary regionally depending on cancer treatment protocols at various institutions. In general, surgical excision of all involved tissue will be performed. Various surgical procedures have been developed; these are summarized in the following display.

In addition to surgery, radiation and chemotherapy are generally recommended when the disease involves lymph nodes of the axilla. Breast cancer can metastasize to the lungs, brain, liver, and bone. In these cases, combinations of radiation, chemotherapy, and hormone therapy may be recommended to stop the spread of the disease.

Cervical Cancer

Cervical cancer is a disease that can be identified early and treated successfully. The first stage of the disease includes precancerous conditions that have been called cervical dysplasia or cervical intraepithelial neoplasia (CIN). Newer terminology for labeling cervical findings, called the Bethesda Classification System, may be used in some settings. This classification system refers to the precancerous condition as squamous intrepithelial lesion (SLE), and rates the severity of the condition as low grade or high grade.

In the population of women receiving cervical cancer screening, approximately 1% to 3% appear to have this precancerous condition. The prevalence of this condition appears to be increasing, with rates of 18 to 20/1000 cases in women ages 15 to 19, and 28 to 30/1000 in women aged 20 to 24. Once it has progressed to the cancerous stage, cervical cancer can be limited to a well-defined site (known as carcinoma in situ) or can be invasive (Lichtman & Papera, 1990).

Etiologic and Predisposing Factors

The specific cause of cervical cancer is unknown. Risk factors include early age at first coitus (less than 20 years of age), and having more than three sexual partners (see the accompanying display). There is growing evidence that increases in cervical dysplasia (presence of abnormal cell growth) and cervical cancer are related to the spread of

Surgical Procedures in Treatment of Breast Cancer

The following surgical procedures may be used in the treatment of breast cancer. The selection of the procedure depends on the size and location of the lesion, the extent to which surrounding tissue is involved, and the woman's preference for treatment.

- **Radical mastectomy**. Removal of entire breast, skin, major and minor muscles, lymph nodes of the axilla, and surrounding fatty tissue. This procedure was the first to be used but is used less frequently today because of extensive mutilation and consequences for arm range of motion with loss of pectoral muscles.
- **Modified radical mastectomy**. As above, but the pectoralis major muscle is preserved. This is the most frequently used procedure.
- **Simple mastectomy**. Removal of breast preserving underlying muscles. A variation may be the subcutaneous mastectomy in which skin and nipple are preserved, allowing for eventual reconstruction.
- **Partial mastectomy**. Removal of the lesion and surrounding tissue, including lymph nodes. A variation may be the lumpectomy in which only the lesion and a band of surrounding normal tissue are removed. These procedures are generally used when cancer is diagnosed early, the lesion is compact and well defined, and when the woman is strongly opposed to more extensive and mutilating procedures.
- **Lumpectomy**. Removal of the lesion and 3 to 5 cm of tissue on either side. Other breast tissue and skin is retained.

Women at Risk for Cervical Cancer

The following factors are thought to be associated with a high risk of cervical cancer:

- Early age at first coitus (less than 20 years of age)
- Multiple sexual partners
- First pregnancy at an early age
- High parity
- History of sexually transmitted diseases
- Smoking
- African American ancestry
- Intercourse with men who have had venereal disease or prostatic cancer

human papillovirus (HPV) and other sexually transmitted organisms, including *Treponema pallidum* (causes syphilis), *Neisseria gonorrhoeae* (causes gonorrhea), *Chlamydia trachomatis*, and *Trichomonas* species. Other risk factors include smoking, which may affect the immune response, and race—the incidence of invasive cervical cancer is twice as high in African American women than in European American women (Lichtman & Papera, 1990).

Diagnosis

The major tool in the early diagnosis of cervical cancer is the Papanicolaou (Pap) smear. The Pap smear is a screening test that identifies precancerous or cancerous changes in cervical cells.

Cervical Screening: Pap Smear. The Pap smear is an effective screening tool to reduce morbidity and mortality from invasive cervical carcinoma. The Pap test involves removal of cells from a region of the cervix called the squamocolumnar junction. In this region, there is an area called the transformation zone in which there is a predominance of immature and rapidly dividing cells(see Chapter 4). These cells may reflect early or precancerous changes when exposed to carcinogens.

Adolescents are at greatest risk for cervical pathology because of the prominence of the squamocolumnar junction on the outside of the cervix. This makes the transformation zone, an area of rapidly dividing cells, more accessible to pathogens. As women mature, the sqamocolumnar junction regresses within the endocervical canal, and is thus somewhat more protected (Fig. 6-4).

The American College of Obstetricians and Gynecologists advises that all sexually active women receive a Pap smear annually. The American Cancer Society advises that, after having a normal Pap smear for 2 consecutive years, a woman should have a Pap smear every 3 years until age 65 (Ginsberg, 1991). As a result of the effectiveness of early diagnosis and treatment, cervical cancer is now considered largely a preventable disease.

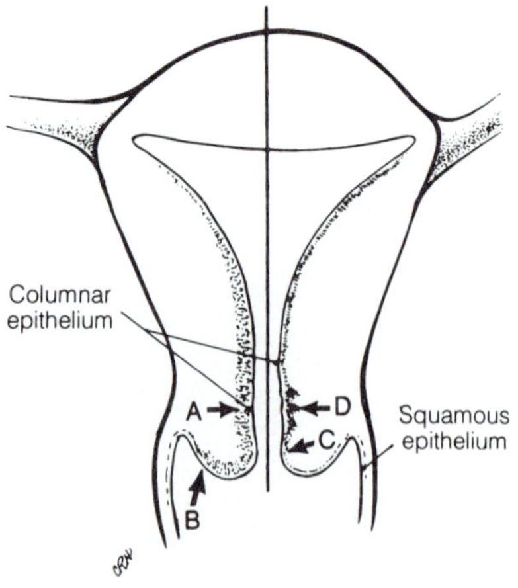

Figure 6-4.
Location of the squamocolumnar junction in menarchal (*A*), menstruating (*B*), menopausal (*C*), and postmenopausal (*D*) women. (From Porth, C.M. [1994]. *Pathophysiology: Concepts of altered heatlth states*, 4th ed. Philadelphia: J.B. Lippincott.)

Follow-up of abnormal Pap smears generally includes repeat Pap smears to identify if the condition will resolve spontaneously. If smears repeated at a 3-month interval continue to show abnormal cells, colposcopy (a procedure that magnifies and delineates cervical abnormalities more clearly) may be performed. Biopsies of areas that appear to be suspicious will often be done at that time.

Treatment

Treatment of precancerous or cancerous lesions of the cervix include cryotherapy, laser conization of the cervix, and on occasion, hysterectomy. Cryotherapy (freezing the top 5 mm of tissue), laser conization (excising a cone of tissue around the os of the cervix), and the LLETZ procedures (large loop excision of the transformation zone) are aimed at removing precancerous or cancerous tissue to prevent its spread. Hysterectomy may be necessary if disease is advanced.

Ovarian Cancer

Ovarian cancer is the leading cause of death from gynecologic cancers, primarily because the disease is diagnosed and treated later than other forms of cancer. Ovarian cancer is often diagnosed after the disease has progressed because the symptoms are nonspecific, and no cost-effective screening method has been discovered.

Etiologic and Predisposing Factors

Ovarian cancer is most common in North American and European populations. Most ovarian cancers appear at or after menopause, with 20% occurring in women under 40 years of age. Risk factors are thought to include nulliparity, menopause before age 45, breast cancer, and a high fat diet (see the accompanying display). No specific cause has been identified, but current theories suggest that ovulation may damage the capsule of the ovary, thus making it more vulnerable to cellular change and abnormal cell growth.

Diagnosis

Symptoms may include vague abdominal or pelvic discomfort or swelling, and abnormal bleeding. No screening test for ovarian cancer is currently available. In many cases, ovarian abnormalities can be identified on the basis of bimanual examination. Definitive diagnosis is made using ultrasound and laparoscopic examination.

Treatment

Treatment for ovarian cancer is based on the extent of the disease and the involvement of other organs. Treatment modalities include radiation, chemotherapy, and surgery. Women with cancer only involving the ovaries (without metastasis) have long-term survival rates of 60% to 70%. Unfortunately, less than 25% of women diagnosed with ovarian cancer are in this category; most do not survive beyond 5 years of diagnosis (Lichtman & Papera, 1990).

Women at Risk for Ovarian Cancer

The following factors are thought to be associated with a high risk of ovarian cancer:

- White, of European or North American origin
- Women at menopause or after menopause age
- Family history of ovarian cancer
- Nulliparity or low parity
- Late childbearing
- Menopause before age 45
- History of breast cancer
- High fat diet

• • Implications for Nursing Care

Nursing care for the woman with cancer of the reproductive system spans the period from identification of the lesion and diagnosis through treatment and recovery. A full discussion of nursing care of the woman with reproductive cancer is beyond the scope of this chapter; the reader is referred to more comprehensive references listed in the Suggested Readings list at the end of the chapter. However, several critical points are discussed here.

• • Assessment

The nurse is often in a position to identify women who are at risk for cancer through a careful assessment and history. Risk factors were listed in earlier displays in this chapter. Women with a family history of cancer or who have other risk factors should receive information about appropriate screening procedures. The nurse stresses the importance of routine breast and cervical screening and encourages women to be consistent with BSE. A variety of patient education materials are available that explain BSE; these should be used when appropriate.

The American Cancer Society has developed an educational program called "Taking Control." The program combines diet, exercise, and general tips that people can follow to reduce their risk of developing cancer. Nurses in women's health care can use such tips in their teaching (see the accompanying display).

The nurse may also identify breast lumps or possible signs of pelvic abnormalities in women who present for routine health care. The nurse should explain that careful follow-up of any breast lump, change in vaginal discharge, vaginal bleeding, or pelvic discomfort is important and to ensure that the woman receives an appropriate referral to a women's health specialist.

• • Nursing Diagnosis

The following are nursing diagnoses that may be applicable in the care of a woman with suspected or diagnosed cancer of a reproductive organ.

- Fear related to the possibility of cancer
- Decisional Conflict related to treatment options

Teaching Considerations

Ten Steps of Cancer Prevention

The nurse can use the following points in teaching patients about cancer prevention:

Protective Factors

- Increase consumption of fresh vegetables (especially those of the cabbage family). (*Rationale:* Fresh vegetables increase fiber and vitamin intake.)
- Increase fiber intake. (*Rationale:* High fiber diets reduce risk of developing certain cancers, such as breast, prostate, and colon cancers.)
- Increase intake of vitamin A. (*Rationale:* Vitamin A reduces the risks of some cancers, such as esophageal, laryngeal, and lung.)
- Increase intake of foods rich in vitamin C. (*Rationale:* Citrus fruits and vegetables may protect against cancer of the stomach and esophagus.)
- Practice weight control. (*Rationale:* Obesity is linked to cancers of the uterus, gallbladder, breast, and colon.)

Risk Factors

- Reduce the amount of dietary fat. (*Rationale:* A high fat diet increases risk of developing breast, colon, and prostate cancers.)
- Reduce intake of salt-cured, smoked, and nitrate-cured foods. (*Rationale:* Moderation in consumption of these foods is recommended; they have been linked to cancers of the esophagus and stomach.)
- Stop cigarette smoking. (*Rationale:* Smokers are at risk for lung cancer.)
- Reduce alcohol intake. (*Rationale:* Drinking large amounts of alcohol increases the risk of liver cancers. Heavy drinkers who smoke are at a greater risk for cancer of the mouth, throat, larynx, and esophagus.)
- Avoid overexposure to the sun. (*Rationale:* Overexposure to the sun increases the risk of skin cancer. Protective clothing or use of a sunscreen reduces the risk.)

Modified from the Taking Control Program of the American Cancer Society.

- Situational Low Self-Esteem related to body image and reaction of sexual partner
- Ineffective Family Coping related to diagnosis of cancer

• • Planning and Implementation

Once a diagnosis has been established, the nurse then follows up to make sure that the woman understands the proposed treatment plan and has all the information necessary to make an informed decision about her care. A diagnosis of reproductive cancer affects virtually every aspect of a woman's life. Thus, nursing care must attend to the physiologic and psychosocial adaptations demanded of the woman and her family in this situation. In many settings, education of the woman and her family about the treatment alternatives and the usual course of recovery is a nursing responsibility.

The nurse is usually responsible for assessing the woman's psychological adaptation to her diagnosis and treatment. In the event that mastectomy or hysterectomy is required, the nurse must carefully assess the woman's response to the loss. Care must be taken to allow a normal grieving period. The nurse must be sensitive to the needs of the woman's sexual partner, and plan carefully for how to include the partner in care. The nurse tactfully assesses the woman's sexual situation and listens to concerns. Based on the woman's readiness, the nurse can help her make plans for a comfortable resumption of sexual activity.

Expected Outcomes

- The woman demonstrates understanding of her diagnosis and the proposed treatment plan.
- The woman participates in her care plan.
- The woman's family members discuss stressors related to the woman's treatment and recovery.
- The woman adheres to recommended treatment and follow-up plans.

• • Evaluation

The nurse plans for appropriate follow-up after discharge and through the recovery period. Community resources such as the American Cancer Society's "Reach for Recovery" breast cancer program can be invaluable in providing practical information and support for the woman as she begins to resume activities of daily living. The nurse stresses the importance of routine medical monitoring of the woman's condition, and the need for adherence to ongoing treatment plans.

Mental Health Concerns

The health and well-being of women are often significantly impaired by mental health concerns that go unrecognized or untreated. For example, women experience eating disorders and depression at significantly higher rates than men. The following section highlights these particular health concerns.

Eating Disorders

Eating disorders, such as anorexia and bulimia, are significantly more common in women than in men. The incidence of anorexia and bulimia among adolescents and young women has been estimated to be as high as 20% in some populations (Love & Seaton, 1991).

Anorexia is a condition of extreme weight loss because of inadequate food intake, and is defined as weight loss to a level of 15% or more below expected weight for height and age. Virtually all (95%) cases occur in middle-class, European American families, although it may occur in preadolescent girls as well. The onset may be sudden or gradual over a number of years, and is marked by a distorted body image of being "fat." Signs of starvation such as amenorrhea, hair loss, hypothermia, and hypotension may appear (Fig. 6-5). Approximately 9% of all cases result in premature death from deterioration of the heart muscle, opportunistic infections, and suicide.

Bulimia is differentiated from anorexia by the occurrence of episodes of binge eating (eating of extraordinarily large amounts of food) and the subsequent use of self-induced vomiting, cathartics, laxatives, diuretics, and overexercise are used to control body weight. Generally, individuals are believed to be bulimic if they experience at least two episodes of binge eating per week for a period of 3 months or more. Changes is body weight are likely to be less dramatic than in anorexia.

Incidence of bulimia is estimated at 1% to 5% among adolescents. Some suggest it may be as high as 20% in some populations. Complications include erosion of dental enamel, esophageal tears, and irritated gums and salivary glands secondary to vomiting.

Etiologic and Predisposing Factors

Strong social pressures to be "thin"and "attractive" create significant emotional tension for many young women. As a result, some women develop patterns of dysfunctional eating, overexercise, or engage in compulsive eating behaviors. Eating disorders are more common in affluent, European-American families; this trend suggests that social expectations and an emphasis on physical appearance may place these adolescents at particular risk.

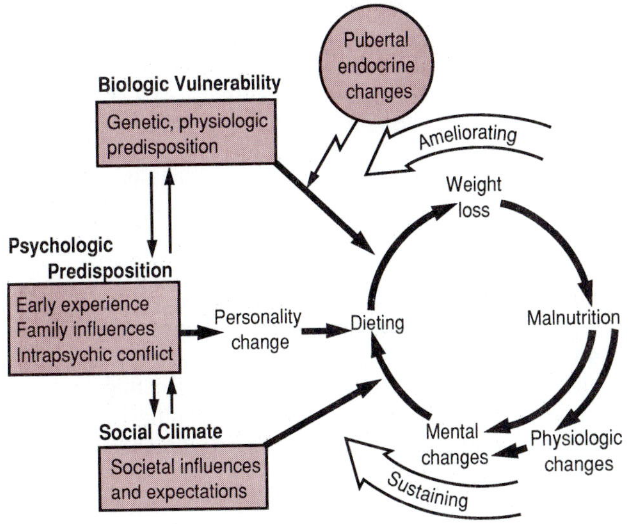

Figure 6-5.
A theoretical model for understanding the multiple factors associated with anorexia nervosa. (Reprinted with permission from: Lucas, A. R. [1981]. Toward the understanding of anorexia nervosa as a disease entity. *Mayo Clinic Proceedings, 56*, 258.)

Diagnosis

Diagnosis of eating disorders requires a comprehensive psychiatric-mental health evaluation. However, signs of disordered eating can be identified based on observation of eating behaviors and physical signs and symptoms. Clinical manifestations of eating disorders are listed in Table 6-1.

Treatment

Treatment for these conditions is often difficult. Denial of the condition by the young woman and her family members interferes with early identification and treatment. Treatment to date is limited to intensive counseling and use of antidepressant therapy. Nurses may be in a particularly important position to identify women at risk and to help them find appropriate assistance. Nurses, usually female, also have to confront the same societal pressures in many cases. It is important for nurses to be knowledgeable about the signs of disordered eating patterns and the forms of treatment available to women with these conditions in their community.

The physical and emotional consequences of eating disorders are considerable. Anorexia can result in life-threatening debilitation and death if untreated. Less dramatic conditions can still be emotionally destructive as young women place more and more emphasis on thinness and invest their physical appearance with such importance (White, 1991). If eating disorders go unrecognized and untreated into adulthood, they can result in eventual fertility problems and chronic dental and digestive problems.

Depression

Depression in women occurs at a rate twice as high as men and is most common between 25 and 44 years of age. One in four women will experience some symptoms of significant depression during her lifetime, and 7 million women in the United States have clinically significant depression.

Etiologic and Predisposing Factors

Factors that contribute to a woman's sense of helplessness and lack of control in her life may increase her vulnerability to this disorder. Depression may also be a result of unresolved sexual trauma: one study estimated that two thirds of women who were victims of intimate violence, either as children or adults, developed clinically significant depression (Mackey, Sereika, Weissfeld, Hacker, Zender, & Heard, 1992).

Diagnosis

Diagnosis of depression requires a psychiatric-mental health evaluation. However, signs of depression can be identified by other care providers through careful assessment. Signs of significant depression include:

- Strong negative affect and feelings of hopelessness over a period of weeks.

Table 6-1. Clinical Manifestations of Eating Disorders

Manifestation	Anorexia Nervosa	Bulimia Nervosa
Physical	Disturbed body image Weight loss of at least 15% of original weight Absence of known physical illness Absence of three consecutive menstrual cycles Yellow-tinged skin (hypercarotenemia) Lanugo (fine body hair) possibly due to prolonged malnutrition Deterioration of teeth, mucous membranes, hair, nails, loss of muscle mass, and dependent edema Fatigue, hypotension, and bradycardia, as weight continues to drop	Recurrent episodes of rapid consumption of large amounts of high-calorie food, usually in less than 2 h Inconspicuous eating Termination of eating episodes by sleep, social interruption, or abdominal pain or self-induced vomiting Repeated attempts to reduce weight by severe, restricted diets, self-induced vomiting, or use of cathartics or diuretics Frequent weight fluctuations of more than 10 lbs coinciding with binges and fasts No known physical illness
Emotional	Intense fear of becoming obese Feelings of fatness even when emaciated Coldness, indifference, anxiety, anger, and withdrawal Being out of touch with own emotions Fear of sexual maturity, feeling of incompetence in dealing with a changing body and new social and emotional requirements	Fear of not being able to stop eating voluntarily Before binge eating: anxiety, helplessness, anger, depression, sense of futility, inability to meet others' expectations, or elation and joy During and after the binge-purge behavior: guilt, repulsion, self-disgust, or excitement, increased energy, and stimulation Tension (the *A*ntecedent) drives bulimic adolescents to the *B*ehavior of binging and purging, which relieves the tension and produces euphoria or an almost sexual release followed by calmness and a sense of relaxation (*C*onsequence)
Cognitive	Constant preoccupation with food, and refusal to maintain body weight above a minimum for age and height Negative attitude about self and own achievements Irrational beliefs (eg, must be perfect in everything) Attempts to be in control of all aspects of own life	Self-deprecating thoughts after binge eating Refusal to acknowledge inner stress or adjustment difficulties Denial of underlying emotional problem(s)
Social	Low self-esteem Isolation and alienation from significant others Other behavior including excessive exercising, compulsive weighing of oneself, and food rituals	Low self-esteem Family dynamics that involve power struggles, dependence, enmeshed roles, or identities History of other impulsive behavior (eg, shoplifting, alcohol or drug abuse, suicide attempts, and self-mutilation)

From Jackson, D.B., & Saunders, R.B. (1993). *Child health nursing: A comprehensive approach to the care of children and their families.* Philadelphia: J. B. Lippincott.

- Excessive sleeping or eating, or conversely, inability to sleep or eat.
- Withdrawal from usual daily activities and social contacts.
- Lack of energy (Hauenstein, 1991).

Depression in adolescence may be a significant contributing factor to substance abuse, eating disorders, and suicide. Depression in adult women interferes with work and family and is a significant factor in substance abuse.

Treatment

Depression can be successfully treated with appropriate psychiatric counseling and antidepressant medications. Treatment of psychiatric-mental health specialists is essential to prevent progression of this disorder. The reader is referred to the Suggested Readings list for a more complete discussion of treatment alternatives.

Intimate Violence and Rape

Violence against women is a significant social and health concern. As many as 4 million women each year in the United States are raped. Each year, one woman in ten is physically abused by the man with whom she lives. One third of women have experienced an attempted or actual rape, and a similar number of women report that they were sexually assaulted as children. A rape is reported every 12 minutes in the United States. Women are ten times more likely to be victims of violence and sexual abuse than men. Experts agree that the reported incidence of intimate violence and rape significantly underestimates actual incidence (Sampselle, 1991).

Etiologic and Predisposing Factors

Violence is overwhelmingly likely to come at the hands of an individual the woman knows or with whom the woman is intimate. Societal factors that perpetuate this problem include attitudes that devalue women, that reflect masculine entitlement and control, and that view a woman as property (Sampselle, 1991).

Diagnosis

Women who are victims of intimate violence usually suffer both physical and emotional consequences of the assault. Responses of women may vary according to the nature of the assault. Battered women may present themselves for care of injuries but attribute them to falls or other accidents. Assessment protocols must include matter-of-fact questions about whether the woman has ever been hit by a member of the family. If the woman is psychologically ready to seek help, she may respond.

Usually battered women have low self-esteem and a pervasive sense of guilt that somehow they deserve mistreatment. This prevents many women from acting in their own defense and leaving the abusive relationship. Often, it is impossible to provide assistance to move the woman to a safe environment until she is ready to take that initiative (Bohn, 1990). See Chapter 13 for assessment practices related to victims of intimate violence.

Treatment

Specialized services are needed to deal with the immediate reaction and those that will follow in the weeks and months afterward. Immediate care for the woman who has been sexually assaulted must be sensitive and suited to the crisis nature of the situation. In many communities, sexual assault teams are on call in emergency rooms and police stations. The team members are skilled in the initial psychological and physical evaluation of the woman's condition. Because of the potential for legal action, physical evidence of the assault must be precise. Evidence includes a detailed account of visible injuries and a precise recording of the woman's report. Careful collection of vaginal, cervical, and rectal specimens, testing for sexually transmitted diseases (STDs), and pregnancy prevention (use of oral contraceptives as postcoital prevention, see Chapter 7) may be needed if penetration was accomplished.

Immediate care must support the woman's sense of safety and security. She should not be made to wait for care or to wait alone. Privacy should be encouraged. Follow-up contact must be arranged, and referrals for psychological support and counseling are essential.

In most metropolitan areas, women's shelters are available that provide a safe place for women who are victims of intimate violence. The location of such shelters is often kept confidential so that the abusive partner cannot locate the shelter or contact the woman unless she chooses to be contacted. In most cases such shelters can accommodate the woman's children if necessary. It is an important nursing responsibility to ensure that specialized services for women who are victims of violence are available and publicized in the community. (See Chapter 15 for further discussion of care of battered women during pregnancy.)

Implications for Nursing Care

Mental health conditions such as eating disorders, depression, and intimate violence have a significant and negative impact on the health and well-being of women. The ongoing care and treatment of these problems is outside the scope of women's health nursing and requires referral to those specializing in psychiatric-mental health nursing. However, the nurse in women's health is in an excellent position to identify women who are at risk for these problems and provide anticipatory guidance and referral when needed. The reader is referred to the Suggested Readings list for additional sources of information on nursing care of women who are victims of intimate violence and rape.

Only recently have major health concerns of women been identified as national health care priorities in the United States. Major causes of morbidity and mortality in women include coronary heart disease; cancer of the lung, breast, and reproductive organs; substance abuse; and intimate violence. Screening techniques exist for breast and cervical cancer. Effective use of screening techniques can result in prevention of some diseases that affect women. Treatment modalities for cancer of the female reproductive tract have improved, and survival increases with each decade.

Other major health concerns in women include conditions that have both an emotional and physical component such as eating disorders, depression, and intimate violence. Women are disproportionately at risk for these conditions. Screening practices may not be widely applied in many settings, and women who could benefit from treatment may be overlooked. The high incidence of these conditions is associated with sexist attitudes. With increased sensitivity to women and their health care needs, health care providers can have a significant impact on morbidity and mortality in women.

Common Health Concerns in Adolescence and Young Adulthood

The psychosocial, behavioral, and physiologic characteristics of adolescence and young adulthood predispose women to a unique set of health concerns. Although some of these concerns do also extend into middle and later adulthood, many are first encountered early in adult life. It is important to understand that most conditions affecting the health and well-being of women are overlaid with a complex set of cultural meanings about female sexuality and womanhood. Thus, the significance of these conditions will depend in part on the individual woman's social, psychological, and cultural experience.

Physiologic and Psychosocial Aspects of Maturation

Although girls become physiologically mature early in adolescence, psychological maturity typically is not reached until the early twenties. Adolescents typically regard themselves as invulnerable. They may not be able to anticipate consequences of their actions. Strong peer pressures to be attractive and to "fit in" generally lead to concerns about sexual activity, physical appearance, and being normal.

High-risk behaviors, such as alcohol and drug use and sexual experimentation, are common and place young women at risk for a variety of health problems (Fig. 6-6). By high school, two thirds of American adolescents have experienced at least one episode of sexual intercourse. Regular gynecologic care is important after onset of sexual activity.

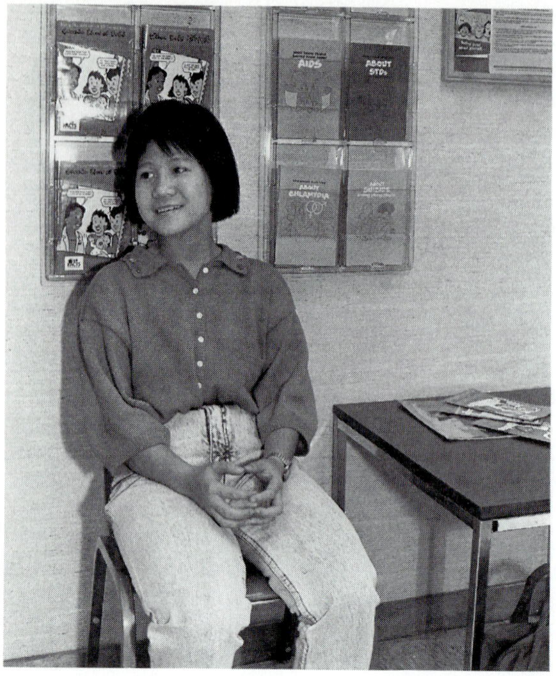

Figure 6-6.
A variety of information is available to the adolescent who may inquire about sexually transmitted diseases and contraceptive care. (Photo by Kathy Sloane.)

Nursing Research

Measuring Safe Sex Behaviors

The purpose of this study was to refine an instrument, the Safe Sex Behavior Questionnaire, for use in assessing sexual behavior in adolescents and young adults. A team of nurse researchers developed the instrument based on available knowledge about motivation for safe sex behavior, risky sexual practices, and the effect of assertiveness on safe sexual behavior. The instrument has 27 items that ask individuals to report frequency of risky behavior, assertiveness, use of condoms, avoidance of body fluid contact, and anal sex homosexual practices. The instrument was first tested on a sample of 89 sexually active college freshmen, most of whom were European American and heterosexual, and half of whom were male. A second test of the instrument was conducted with a sample of 178 sexually active college freshmen. Findings suggested that the Safe Sex Questionnaire was a reliable and valid way to assess self-reported sexual behavior in college-age populations. The investigators are continuing to refine the instrument to make it more suitable for use in other populations, including younger adolescents, minority groups, and older adults.

DiIorio, C., Parson, M., Lehr, S., Adame, D., & Carlone, J. (1992). Measurement of safe sex behavior in adolescents and young adults. *Nursing Research, 41*(4), 203–207.

However, health problems encountered in adolescence, especially those related to sexuality, are likely to frighten adolescent and young adult women. Young women may delay seeking health care because they deny the existence of symptoms, are fearful of gynecologic care, or lack ready access to appropriate and sensitive care (Muller, 1990).

Adolescents are especially vulnerable to pregnancy and STDs. If they take the initiative to attempt to prevent pregnancy on their own, they are likely to first use withdrawal or condoms. However, often they do not use these methods consistently. If they receive appropriate contraceptive care, they are likely to prefer oral contraceptives. Thus, without the use of condoms, they still remain at risk for STDs. The Nursing Research display discusses recent research on "safe sex." Adolescents are at highest risk of all age groups for pelvic inflammatory disease (PID) as a result of genital infection. Adolescent and young adult women also experience a wide range of gynecologic conditions that affect health and well-being.

The following section highlights conditions of the reproductive system that may be significant health concerns for adolescent and young adult women.

Menstrual Conditions

Conditions related to the menstrual cycle are a significant factor in the perceived well-being of many women of childbearing age. Common cultural beliefs about menstruation may limit women's physical activities during menses, such as exercise, bathing, or sexual intercourse. Other beliefs about menstruation reflect negative attitudes toward women, such as those suggesting that women are generally incapacitated or may be unpredictable during this time. However, increasingly menstruation is regarded as a normal physiologic process. Characteristics of normal menstruation are discussed in Chapter 4. The following section highlights common menstrual conditions.

Dysmenorrhea

Painful menstruation affects as many of 50% of women. It is the single most common cause of lost work or school days among young women. Pain is usually associated with ovulatory cycles rather than anovulatory cycles. Symptoms typically include pelvic pain on the first day of the menses and may be accompanied by nausea, vomiting, and diarrhea.

Etiologic and Predisposing Factors

Although a precise cause is not known, current theories center on increased secretion of or increased sensitivity to prostaglandins in affected women. Dysmenorrhea is classified either as primary (no organic cause) or secondary (associated with another condition causing dysmenorrhea).

Secondary dysmenorrhea generally begins after 20 years of age. It is often associated with endometriosis, PID, cervical stenosis (narrowing of the cervical os), and fibroid tumors.

Diagnosis

Dysmenorrhea is typically diagnosed on the basis of the primary symptom, pain on the first day of menses, in the absence of any other identified physical problem. Another cause of pain associated with menstruation is endometriosis. Because this condition can have implications for future fertility, a young woman with severe dysmenorrhea should be evaluated to rule out endometriosis (see section below).

Treatment

Some women find that over-the-counter preparations are sufficient for pain control. Women with more pronounced symptoms may require prescription medications. Prostaglandin synthetase inhibitors (ibuprofen, naproxen sodium, mefenamic acid) or inhibition of ovulation with oral contraceptives is generally effective in reducing or eliminating pain. Moderate exercise is sometimes helpful in reducing the severity of menstrual cramps and pain. Application of heat to the lower abdomen with baths or heating pads and resting with the knees drawn up to the chest may reduce discomfort and pain.

Premenstrual Syndrome

Premenstrual syndrome (PMS) is a cluster of symptoms presenting in a cyclic pattern during the luteal phase of the menstrual cycle and extending to or through the menses. Symptoms include headache, breast swelling and tenderness, nausea, edema, cravings for sweets or salt, insomnia, anxiety, depression, irritability, and forgetfulness.

Etiologic and Predisposing Factors

Extensive studies have failed to demonstrate a clear relationship between hormonal fluctuations and symptoms. Because symptoms are often ill-defined and may involve multiple organ systems, it is unlikely that the condition has a single cause. No clear predisposing factors have been identified, although extensive research is now under way. It is estimated that as many as 50% of women with normal reproductive function experience at least one of the symptoms listed above. Some studies have reported a higher incidence of PMS in women over 30 (Lichtman & Papera, 1990).

Diagnosis

Since the cause of this condition is not known, diagnosis begins with the woman charting her symptoms in relation to her menstrual cycle and other life events in an effort to identify a pattern (see the Assessment Tool). This is done in an effort to identify a pattern. If the woman's symptoms do not cluster during the luteal phase of the menstrual cycle, an evaluation of alternative psychological causes for her symptoms may be necessary, since many women who complain of PMS have a depressive disorder unrelated to menstrual functioning.

Treatment

Treatment for PMS centers on three recommendations: stress reduction, health promotion, and symptom management. Thus, a recommended course of treatment may include lifestyle changes such as exercise and stress management (see the accompanying Teaching Considerations display). Building up the body's natural defenses may be recommended through use of vitamin B_6, vitamin E, and magnesium, and dietary changes.

Emotional support for the woman with PMS symptoms may be as important as other aspects of treatment. The nurse should recommend that the woman explore self-help groups and self-help literature. Empathetic listening and a nonjudgmental attitude may be the nurse's most effective tools to help women combat the stress that can result from premenstrual symptoms (Lichtman & Papera, 1990).

Amenorrhea

Amenorrhea is the absence of menstrual cycles. Primary amenorrhea is defined as no menstrual cycle within 4 years of onset of puberty (noted by development of secondary sex characteristics). The average age of menarche (onset of menstrual cycles) is 13 years. After menarche is established, regular monthly menstrual cycles may not occur for 2 to 3 years. By age 16, 95% of adolescent females have menstruated.

Etiologic and Predisposing Factors

Causes of primary amenorrhea include pregnancy, endocrine disorders, and psychosocial stress. Secondary amenorrhea is an absence of periods for at least 3 months in a woman who had been menstruating. Causes of secondary amenorrhea include pregnancy, endocrine disorders, menopause, excessive exercise and very low body fat, increased stress, and oral contraceptive use.

Diagnosis

Primary amenorrhea requires a complete assessment to determine the cause (Fig. 6-7). A full gynecologic examination is necessary to rule out pregnancy, congenital obstructions of the uterus, absence of internal female reproductive organs, and endocrine imbalance. Secondary amenorrhea also requires a complete assessment. The potential causes are more delimited since the woman's menstrual cycle is known to have functioned normally in the past.

Treatment

Treatment depends on identification of the underlying cause. Primary amenorrhea as a result of congenital problems is often not treatable. Secondary amenorrhea as a result of endocrine disorders may be amenable to hormonal therapy. When excessive exercise and stress are thought to be the cause, the woman will be advised to increase caloric intake, decrease physical activity, and use stress management techniques to see if normal menstrual functioning returns. If it does not, a complete evaluation is indicated. Amenorrhea after use of oral contraceptives is common and generally resolves within a year after oral contraceptive use is stopped (Lichtman & Papera, 1990).

Endometriosis

In endometriosis, implants of endometrial tissue are found outside the uterine cavity. This condition affects about

Assessment Tool

Diary for Evaluation of PMS Symptoms

NAME ____________________

YEAR ____________________

Grading of Symptoms:
0—*No Symptoms* 2—*Moderate Symptoms*
1—*Mild Symptoms* 3—*Severe Symptoms (i.e., Disabling)*

DAY OF CYCLE	1	2	3	4	5	6	7	8	9	10	11	12	13	14	15	16	17	18	19	20	21	22	23	24	25	26	27	28	29	30	31
DATE																															
MENSES																															

PSYCHOLOGICAL SYMPTOMS

Depression																															
Anxiety																															
Irritability																															
Lethargy																															
Insomnia																															
Forgetfulness																															
Confusion																															

PHYSICAL SYMPTOMS

Swelling																															
Breast Tenderness																															
Abdominal bloating																															
Palpitations																															
Weight gain																															
Constipation																															
Headache																															
Rhinitis																															

PAIN SYMPTOMS (Usually NOT associated with PMS)

Menstrual cramps																															
Painful intercourse																															
Pelvic pain																															
Backache																															

Morning weight (lb)																															

From Chihal, H. J. (1990). *Premenstrual syndrome: A clinic manual* (2nd ed., pp. 80–81). Dallas: Essential Medical Information Systems.

10% to 12% of childbearing women. Endometrial implants may be found in the gastrointestinal tract, ovary, uterine ligaments, and the pelvic peritoneum.

Etiologic and Predisposing Factors

The cause of endometriosis is unknown. A common theory traces implantation from reflux of endometrial cells through the fallopian tubes during menstruation. The disease is generally progressive, with symptoms becoming more pronounced over time. For this reason, and because the condition may interfere with conception, many women are not diagnosed with endometriosis until their late 20s or early 30s.

Diagnosis

Symptoms largely depend on the location of implants and may include progressive dysmenorrhea, dyspareunia, premenstrual spotting, and painful defecation. Symptoms result from bleeding of the implants in response to the menstrual cycle and subsequent formation of adhesions and cysts. Bleeding sites in the fallopian tubes can cause scarring and adhesions and infertility.

Too often, young women are told that dysmenorrhea is normal, especially when other female family members also have this symptom. Thus, endometriosis can progress during adolescence and have a significant effect on future fertility. A complete evaluation of dysmenorrhea and related symptoms should be conducted, regardless of the young woman's age.

Although careful documentation of symptoms and bimanual examination may suggest the presence of endometrial implants, definitive diagnosis of endometriosis can be made only by direct visualization of the implants through laparoscopy.

Teaching Considerations

Self-Care in Premenstrual Syndrome

The nurse can use the following points in teaching women with premenstrual syndrome:

- Exercise regularly.
- Get plenty of sleep (usually 7 to 8 hours or as needed).
- Use relaxation techniques to reduce symptoms.
- Develop friendships that will be supportive.
- Increase foods rich in vitamins B_6, E, and magnesium.
- Eat plenty of fresh vegetables.
- Eat protein-rich foods and complex carbohydrates.
- Eat small meals.
- Drink plenty of water.
- Avoid salty foods, sweets, caffeine, and chocolate.

Treatment

Treatment focuses on arresting the progression of the disease, symptom control, and preservation of fertility (if desired). Hormonal therapy with oral contraceptives, or androgens (Danazol) to suppress ovarian function may be advised. This may result in atrophy of the endometrial implants. Symptoms may be reduced with the use of nonsteriodal antiinflammatory drugs (NSAIDs) such as ibuprofen, as well as analgesics.

Endometrial implants can be reduced or removed through laser surgery. In cases where pain (dysmenorrhea or dyspareunia) is significant and not well controlled and when conception is not desired, a hysterectomy with bilateral salpingo-oophorectomy may be recommended.

Implications for Nursing Care

Menstrual conditions can be a significant cause of distress and worry for some women. An important nursing responsibility in the women's health setting is obtaining an accurate health history that pays particular attention to menstruation and related symptoms. The nurse is in an excellent position to identify women who may require additional gynecologic evaluation based on a description of their symptoms.

Once a diagnosis is made, the nurse may be responsible for explaining the condition, its cause, and alternative treatment methods. It is important that the woman have sufficient information with which to make treatment decisions appropriate to her. The woman may find it helpful to discuss the implications of the condition and its treatment with the nurse. This may be especially important if the woman has negative attitudes associated with menstrual conditions, or she believes others have such attitudes. The nurse can be a careful and sensitive listener, and help the woman avoid unnecessary anxiety and self-blame over menstrual conditions.

When conditions associated with future fertility problems are diagnosed, such as untreatable amenorrhea or endometriosis, the nurse must be especially sensitive to the woman's concerns in this area. For some women the risk of reduced fertility is a serious threat to her hopes and plans. For others, it may be a relatively minor concern.

The nurse plays an important role in helping women manage symptoms related to menstrual conditions. If medications are recommended, the nurse is responsible for educating the woman in regard to safe use. The nurse should consider presenting the woman with a range of other safe and effective self-care techniques and encouraging the woman to experiment and find a combination that works well for her. This strategy reinforces the woman's role in her own care and enables her to adapt her self-care regimen as changing circumstances require.

The reader is referred to the Suggested Readings list at the end of the chapter for more information on self-care for menstrual conditions.

Conditions Affecting the Breast, Uterus, and Ovary

The reproductive organs may exhibit changes that produce worrisome symptoms and may prompt the woman to seek health care. The following sections addresses benign conditions that affect the breast, cervix, uterus, and ovary.

Cyclic Changes in the Normal Breast

The female breast responds to hormonal changes in the body throughout the reproductive years. Benign conditions of the breast can also develop, and these must be distinguished from more serious conditions.

Women may experience breast swelling and tenderness 3 to 4 days before the onset of menses or for a longer period during the menstrual cycle. These cyclic changes cease after the onset of menopause. Women may have concerns about breast swelling and tenderness. They may palpate lumps or thickening in the breasts on self-examination.

Women may also develop benign fatty tumors of the breast called fibroadenomas. These tumors often develop in women in their early twenties and are usually found by accident. They generally do not produce any symptoms. Evaluation of the tumor by a health professional is *always* indicated. However, fibroadenomas are not associated with any increased risk of breast cancer or other breast disease and generally do not require treatment.

Fibrocystic Breast Disease

Fibrocystic breast disease (FBD) is a common disorder characterized by palpable irregularities in breast tissue that fluctuate with the menstrual cycle. Incidence of this condition may occur in 50% of all women. Pain and tenderness may occur and may become progressively worse until menopause.

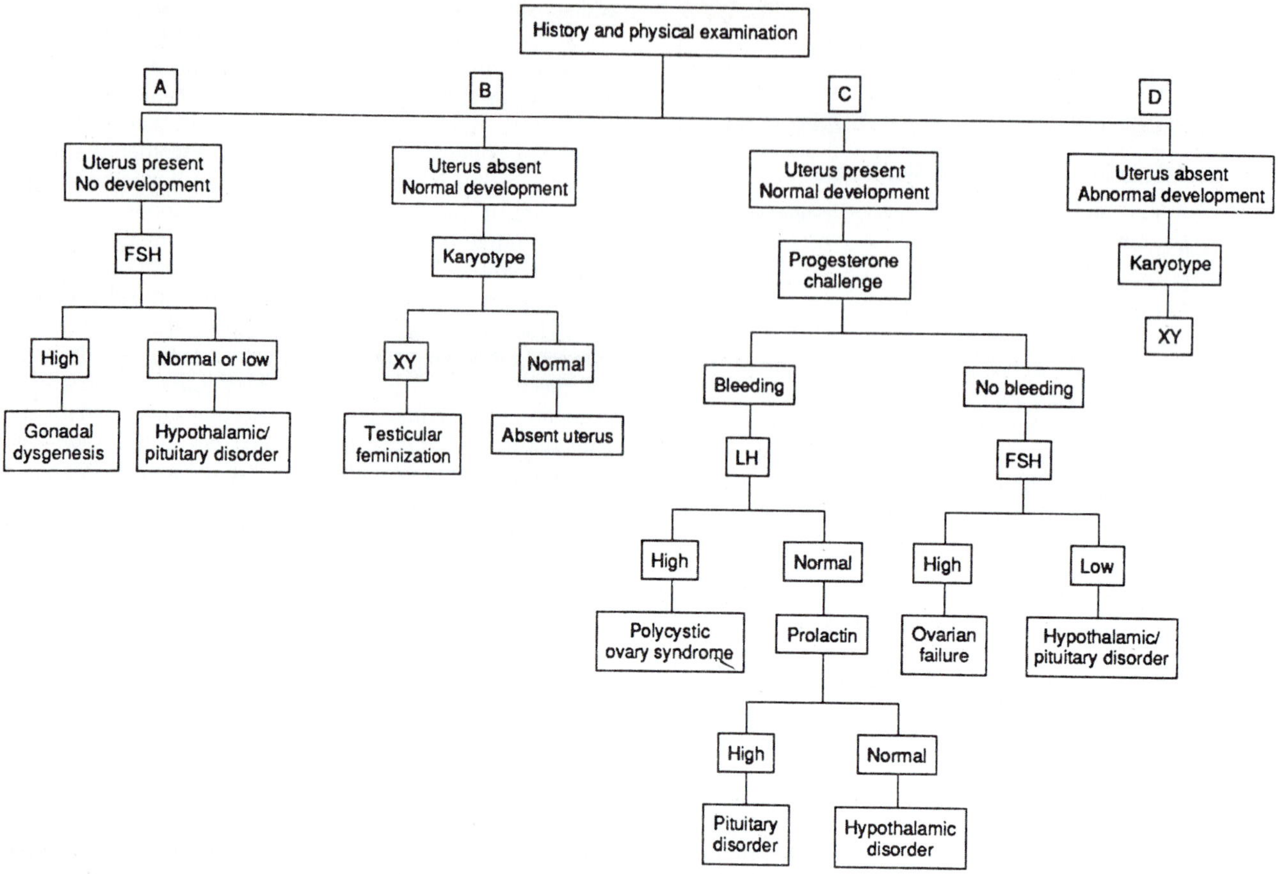

Figure 6-7.

Flowchart for evaluation of primary amenorrhea. Evaluation is indicated if menses are absent by age 16 with normal development, by age 14 without development, or by 4 years after onset of puberty. Section A diagrams the most common situation. Section B diagrams a congenital anomaly. Section C presents an evaluation similar to that for secondary amenorrhea (after a negative pregnancy test). Section D shows an unusual circumstance in which the patient has either an enzyme defect or absent gonads that prevented normal male development. FSH, follicle-stimulating hormone; LH, luteinizing hormone. (From: Oski, F. A., DeAngelis, C. D., Feigin, R. D., & Warshaw, J. B. [1990]. *Principles and practice of pediatrics*. Philadelphia: J.B. Lippincott.)

Etiologic and Predisposing Factors. The cause of fibrocystic breast disease is not known. Peak incidence is reported in women aged 40 and older and is more common in nulliparous women. There is conflicting research evidence about the relationship between caffeine intake and fibrocystic breast disease, and no link has been clearly established (Norwood, 1990).

Diagnosis. FBD has several forms; if atypical cells are identified by needle aspiration, careful and ongoing screening for breast cancer is indicated (Norwood, 1990). Of major concern is the difficulty of early detection of breast cancer in women with nodular and fibrocystic breasts. Women with FBD who perform routine BSE are likely to require more frequent evaluation. Women with certain forms of FBD do appear to be at increased risk for the development of breast cancer and require close professional follow-up.

Treatment. Pain and tenderness can be managed with analgesics initially. However, because the disease is often progressive, other measures may be advised. Oral contraceptives are useful in reducing FBD symptoms in many women. Other measures to reduce symptoms may include limiting sodium intake and the use of a mild diuretic before menses to reduce swelling and tenderness. Research about the effect of dietary caffeine and vitamins on FBD symptoms has been inconclusive to date. However, some women may prefer to limit caffeine intake if there is a chance it may diminish symptoms. In the most severe cases, medications including danazol and bromocriptine, both hormone inhibitors, may be prescribed for 6-month intervals to reduce symptoms (Norwood, 1990).

Other Reproductive Organ Conditions

Conditions producing worrisome symptoms affecting the cervix, uterus, and ovary may arise during early adulthood. These conditions, while generally benign, must be evaluated to verify that more serious conditions, such as cancer or endometriosis, are not causing symptoms. The following section discusses cervicitis and uterine and ovarian masses.

Cervicitis

Cervicitis is a general term referring to inflammation of the epithelial cells of the squamocolumnar junction (see Fig. 4-15). Cervicitis can be caused by a variety of sexually transmitted organisms. The most common cause is *C. trachomatis*, followed by HSV and *Trichomonas vaginalis*. Symptoms of cervicitis may include vaginal discharge, pain, or dysuria. Women often are asymptomatic and diagnosis is made on cervical examination. Treatment is specific for the causative agent. Close observation by repeated Pap smear 3 months after initial diagnosis is generally indicated. Cervicitis is associated with a higher risk for cervical cancer. Thus, careful follow-up with Pap smears every 3 to 6 months may be recommended (see the previous section on cervical cancer).

Uterine and Ovarian Masses

Most abnormal masses in the ovary and uterus are benign growths. Ovarian cysts occur as a result of disturbances in the normal menstrual cycle. They often occur at the site of the corpus luteum. Ovarian masses may cause lower abdominal discomfort associated with the menstrual cycle but often are asymptomatic and found only on bimanual examination. Ultrasound diagnosis may be used to confirm clinical findings. Most cysts resolve without treatment. However, if symptoms such as pain and irregular menstruation are pronounced, laparoscopic surgery may be recommended to rule out other ovarian problems and remove the ovarian lesion.

Uterine masses are usually benign fibroid tumors, which are overgrowths of uterine muscle and connective tissue. Symptoms may include lower abdominal pain, dysmenorrhea, and metrorrhagia (abnormal bleeding between menses). Generally, no treatment is required. However, close observation and more frequent pelvic examinations are advisable. Most uterine masses shrink after menopause. However, abnormal uterine bleeding may be a problem and may lead to chronic anemia.

Implications for Nursing Care

The nurse plays an important role in identifying women who may have symptoms that suggest conditions such as FBD, cervicitis, and pelvic masses. Women who experience breast discomfort or pain or vague pelvic symptoms should be encouraged to seek gynecologic evaluation.

Women diagnosed with benign conditions still may experience considerable worry and distress from these conditions. The nurse must have accurate and current information about the relationship between benign conditions and more serious conditions such as cancer of the breast or reproductive tract. Nursing interventions are aimed at providing accurate information about the condition and appropriate treatment and follow-up. The nurse can help alleviate anxiety by providing information while underscoring the importance of regular checkups to monitor the condition.

Pelvic Infections

A significant source of morbidity in women results from pelvic infections, including those of the urinary and reproductive tracts. This section addresses urinary tract infections (UTIs), vaginal infections, PID, and toxic shock syndrome. The most common of these are UTIs, which affect 20% of women at some point in their lives.

Urinary Tract Infections

UTI is defined as the presence of bacteria in the urinary tract, as demonstrated by bacteriuria (bacteria in the urine). Traditionally, 100,000 or more bacterial colonies per milliliter of urine is the indicator for a UTI. However, if clinical symptoms are present, lower bacteria counts are significant.

Asymptomatic bacteriuria is a condition in which there is laboratory evidence of a UTI, but the woman reports no symptoms. This condition is especially significant during pregnancy (see Chapter 16) but is not thought to predispose healthy women to more serious infection and is often not treated.

Cystitis is a relatively common condition in which the infection is limited to the bladder and involves only the superficial lining of that organ. Interstitial cystitis is a rare condition, more common in women over the age of 30, characterized by urinary frequency and urgency, decreased bladder capacity, and pinpoint hemorrhages of the bladder mucosa. Pyelonephritis is less common than cystitis but is more serious. It is a systemic infection that may lead to sepsis and renal damage.

Etiologic and Predisposing Factors

The most common organisms found in UTI are *Escherichia coli*, *Klebsiella* species, and *Proteus* species. Factors contributing to the incidence of UTI are:

- Voluntary suppression of the urge to void
- Relative incompetence of the urinary sphincter, as reflected in a history of bedwetting or stress incontinence
- Pregnancy
- High parity
- Lower socioeconomic status
- Sexual activity

The first three factors include conditions that contribute to stasis of urine, compression of the ureters, and enhanced access of organisms to the urinary tract. The latter two factors may reflect higher risk of infectious exposure, poor physical health, and inadequate nutrition. Symptoms and treatment of the condition depend on the extent of the infection (Lichtman & Papera, 1990).

Diagnosis

Cystitis is generally associated with dysuria, frequency, urgency, and a low-grade fever. Laboratory analysis of urine will show bacteriuria, increased white blood cell counts, and occasionally hematuria.

Interstitial cystitis is associated with pain, urgency, dyspareunia, and disruption of sleep with frequent urination. Diagnosis is made by exclusion if symptoms persist in the absence of bacteriuria.

Pyelonephritis is characterized by sudden onset of symptoms, which are more systemic in nature. The woman may present with chills, high fever, flank pain, nausea, and vomiting. Suprapubic and costovertebral angle tenderness is usually present. If cystitis is also present, urinary frequency and urgency may occur.

Treatment

Treatment of cystitis generally includes a course of sulfisoxasole, ampicillin, or nitrofurantoin. Women should be advised to avoid caffeine (which exacerbates frequency and urgency), to keep fluid levels up, and to avoid anorectal contamination by wiping from front to back after voiding.

There is no known cause for interstitial cystitis and no effective treatment has been found. The condition can be debilitating and supportive therapy to relieve symptoms is a priority (Lichtman & Papera, 1990).

Treatment for pyelonephritis may include hospitalization. Intravenous fluids and antibiotic therapy are instituted even before culture and sensitivity tests have been completed. After the results of the urinalysis are received, antibiotic therapy may be changed. Antibiotics commonly used include cephalexin, sulfisoxasole, ampicillin, and nitrofurantoin. Usually after 3 to 4 days of treatment, symptoms subside dramatically (Lichtman & Papera, 1990).

Vaginal Infections

Several organisms are normal inhabitants of the vagina, and they may cause vaginal infection under certain conditions. Prevention of vaginal infections can depend on common health practices, as well as on specialized treatment for recurring infections. Measures to prevent vaginal infections of all types are shown in the Teaching Considerations display.

Teaching Considerations

Preventing Vaginal Infections

The nurse can use the following points in teaching women to prevent vaginal infections and limit their severity:

- The genital area should be kept dry by wearing 100% cotton underwear.
- Clothing tight in the crotch and hips should be avoided.
- Sleeping without underwear is helpful.
- Wiping after defecation should always be from front to back. This reduces fecal contamination of the vagina.
- Sanitary napkins and tampons should be changed frequently; barrier contraceptives should be worn no more than 30 hours at a time. Use of vaginal spermicides may provide some protection from vaginal infection.
- Intercourse should be avoided or condoms should be used when infection is present. Any sexual activity causing pain or abrasion of the vagina should be avoided.
- Irritants to the vulvar and vaginal area should be avoided, including harsh deodorant or perfumed soaps or sprays.
- Vaginal douches may alter the normal pH of the vagina and predispose to infection.

Bacterial Vaginosis

Bacterial vaginosis (previously called nonspecific vaginitis) is the most common form of vaginal infection in the United States. Incidence may range from 10% to 25% of women of childbearing age.

Etiologic and Predisposing Factors. The main cause is an increase or overgrowth of normal vaginal anerobes, in many cases accompanied by *Gardnerella vaginalis*. The cause of this overgrowth is not clearly understood. A contributing factor may be trauma to the vaginal tissue during sexual intercourse.

Diagnosis. Symptoms of bacterial vaginosis include vaginal odor (often described as "fishy"), increased vaginal discharge, and less frequently, itching. Diagnosis is made by microscopic examination of a wet mount preparation of a sample of vaginal discharge suspended in normal saline. The appearance of "clue cells" (squamous epithelial cells with bacterial overgrowth) is diagnostic of bacterial vaginosis. Cultures of the discharge are generally not required.

Treatment. Treatment of bacterial vaginosis has traditionally been prescription of metronidazole (Flagyl) orally for a 7-day course. This medication is contraindicated during the first trimester of pregnancy because of potential teratogenic effects. Newer treatment is prescription of metronidazole (Flagyl) vaginal cream and clindamycin (Cleocin) vaginal cream daily for 7 days. Treatment of sexual partners is generally not indicated (Lichtman & Papera, 1990).

Moniliasis (Candida albicans)

Moniliasis (*Candida albicans* or candidiasis or yeast infection) is the second most common form of vaginal infection. *C. albicans* is a normal inhabitant of the mouth, intestines, and vagina in 25% to 50% of women. Infection is caused by overgrowth. The causes of this overgrowth are not well understood (Lichtman & Papera, 1990).

Etiologic and Predisposing Factors. A number of factors are thought to predispose women to this infection, including use of broad-spectrum antibiotics, uncontrolled diabetes, pregnancy, use of corticosteroids, obesity, and immunosuppressed states, including human immunodeficiency virus infection (HIV). Women often have recurring monilial infections, and may identify individual factors that seem to result in infection, such as stress, use of certain feminine hygiene products, missed menstrual cycles, or the use of oral contraceptives.

Diagnosis. The most common symptom of moniliasis is severe vulvar and vaginal itching. Vaginal discharge may vary from a white, curdy vaginal discharge, to a thin watery discharge with a yeasty or musty smell. Microscopic examination of a wet mount preparation of vaginal discharge shows yeast hyphae (filaments) and spores. A culture is the most reliable diagnostic test but it is costly and it takes several days to get the results.

Treatment. Treatment of moniliasis includes use of vaginal suppositories or creams containing nystatin, miconazole nitrate, clotrimazole, or other antifungal agents. Recurrent infections may indicate the sexual partner is also infected. Men can carry the organism in folds of penile skin. Treatment of the sexual partner may be helpful in reducing recurrent infections (Lichtman & Papera, 1990). Women with recurring monilial infections may be encouraged to initiate self-treatment with prescribed antimicrobials once they can consistently and accurately recognize their symptoms.

Pelvic Inflammatory Disease

PID is a condition that results from infection ascending through the genital tract into the fallopian tubes and sometimes into the peritoneal cavity. PID is usually caused by the progression of an STD that itself may have been asymptomatic in its early stages. However, once such an infection ascends into the pelvic region, it can cause bleeding, inflammation, inflammation, scarring, and adhesions, which can result in blockage of the fallopian tubes and resultant infertility.

Etiologic and Predisposing Factors

The organisms most frequently associated with PID are the sexually transmitted organisms *Chlamydia* species and *N. gonorrhoeae*. (See the section on STDs later in this chapter.) PID is most common in young, sexually active women with multiple sexual partners or those with an intrauterine device.

Diagnosis

Symptoms of PID include acute bilateral cramping pain in the lower abdomen, fever, purulent vaginal discharge, dysuria, nausea and vomiting, and abnormal vaginal bleeding. Women with HIV may present first with symptoms of PID. A small proportion of women with PID will be asymptomatic.

Diagnosis includes laboratory tests to determine the infectious organism, as well as ultrasound examination of the pelvis. In some cases, laparoscopic examination is used to determine the location and extent of the infection and to obtain cultures from the fallopian tubes.

Treatment

Treatment for PID generally requires hospitalization. Intravenous administration of antibiotics, and supportive care for the most severe symptoms will be needed. After the acute infection is treated, follow-up evaluation may be advised if the woman has concerns about tubal damage. PID and subsequent tubal damage is the single most frequent cause of female infertility (Lichtman & Papera, 1990).

Toxic Shock Syndrome

Toxic shock syndrome (TSS) is a rare but serious multisystem disorder. It is characterized by acute onset of disease in at least three organ systems (gastrointestinal, muscular, renal, hepatic, hematologic, and central nervous systems).

Etiologic and Predisposing Factors

Toxic shock syndrome is thought to be caused by toxins produced by *Staphylococcus aureus*. The disorder has been associated with use of tampons and barrier methods of contraception. Extended obstruction of the cervix by use of a tampon, diaphragm, or contraceptive sponge may increase the risk of TSS. This may allow the organism to reproduce in the vagina and to enter the circulatory system through the uterine lining. Incidence of TSS is estimated to be 8.9 cases per 100,000 menstruating women, with a mortality rate of less than 3%. The incidence of cases in the United States has decreased since 1980, probably in response to widespread education about the condition and changes in tampon design and use. Recommendations for reducing the risk of TSS include those in the Teaching Considerations display.

Teaching Considerations

Tampon Use

The nurse can use the following points in teaching women who use tampons:

- Tampon use should be avoided by adolescents, postpartum women, women with staphylococcal infections, women with a history of toxic shock syndrome, and during light flow (at the beginning and end of the menstrual period).
- Tampons should be used only during times of moderate to heavy flow.
- Women should wash their hands before inserting anything into the vagina.
- Tampons should be handled carefully so they are not exposed to infectious surfaces.
- Women should read and follow the guidelines for tampon use included in the tampon packaging.
- Superabsorbent tampons should not be used.
- Tampons should be changed frequently—every 1 to 3 hours.
- Pads rather than tampons should be used at night.
- Tampon use should be discontinued if the following symptoms occur: vomiting, profuse watery diarrhea, high fever, weakness, rash, sore throat, headache, and muscle ache. A health care professional must be contacted immediately.

Diagnosis

Early symptoms of TSS include a high fever, vomiting, profuse watery diarrhea, headache, and muscle ache. The disease progresses to hypotensive shock within 48 hours, development of a profuse rash, and increasing disorientation. There is no specific diagnostic test for this condition, although a tentative diagnosis can be made on the basis of presenting symptoms. TSS can be life-threatening if not diagnosed and treated promptly (Lichtman & Papera, 1990).

Treatment

There is no specific treatment for TSS. Intensive care is required and aimed at specific symptoms and organ systems involved. Intravenous fluids and the use of vasopressor medications to prevent hypovolemic shock is central to treatment. Women with TSS generally recover within 10 days. However, long-term health consequences may result, including gangrene as a result of cyanosis of the extremities, muscle weakness, cold intolerance, and loss of memory (Lichtman & Papera, 1990).

Sexually Transmitted Diseases

STDs are a group of infections transmitted primarily through sexual contact. Knowledge about STDs has increased over the last two decades at an astounding rate. More than 20 organisms that cause STDs have now been identified.

STDs are more common in young, urban-dwelling, low-income groups. Incidence of most STDs is increasing in the United States. Each year, approximately 12 million cases of STD occur in the United States; this is believed to be a conservative estimate since underreporting continues to be a major problem.

It is extremely common for an individual infected with one disease to have one or more other infections at the same time. The damage done by superimposed infections is cumulative and results in more harmful consequences than would any one infection alone (Tillman, 1992). In general, severity of symptoms and disease is greater in women than men. This is probably because early symptoms in women may be subtle, thus contributing to a delay in diagnosis and treatment.

Specific treatment is available for many but certainly not all STDs. Prevention through safe sexual practices is a major priority in the field of women's health. Abstinence is the only sure protection against STDs. Careful selection of sexual partners and use of condoms and other barrier methods of contraception are also effective prevention strategies. The following section discusses the cause, symptomatology, and treatment of the STDs most commonly seen in women's health care settings. For discussion of the consequences of STDs in pregnancy, see Chapter 16.

Chlamydial Infection

Genital infections caused by *C. trachomatis* are the most prevalent of STDs in the United States. Rates of infection decline with age; adolescents may have infection rates as high as 30%, with infection becoming less common among women in their twenties and thirties. Chlamydia can cause a range of other types of infections. These include PID in women, nongonococcal urethritis in men, and conjunctivitis and pneumonia in the newborn through perinatal transmission.

Etiologic and Predisposing Factors

Chlamydia shows an affinity for the squamocolumnar junction of the cervix. There is speculation that chlamydia may have a role in the initiation of cervical cancer, since it is frequently present in women with CIN and preterm labor (Centers for Disease Control, 1990). In the Third World, this organism causes an endemic infection of the eye, called trachoma, which causes blindness. Transmission in this case is thought to be child to child, but it is unclear if the origin of infection is the genital tract.

Diagnosis

Women with chlamydial infections are often asymptomatic. If symptoms are noted in women, they include mucopurulent vaginal discharge, intermenstrual bleeding, postcoital bleeding, and diffuse low abdominal pain. Men are more likely to have symptoms of painful urination.

Chlamydial infection is impossible to distinguish from gonorrhea on the basis of clinical signs. Further, chlamydial infection frequently coexists with gonorrhea, so concomitant testing for gonorrhea is standard. Diagnosis of chlamydia is made by cervical culture.

Treatment

Treatment includes the use of tetracycline or doxycycline. A follow-up culture is necessary to ensure efficacy of treatment. Sexual partners should be tested and treated because reinfection is common (Csonka, 1990). Undiagnosed chlamydial infections in women can lead to PID and subsequent fertility problems.

Herpes Genitalis

Herpes genitalis virus (herpes simplex virus or HSV) has become a major STD. Two strains of the virus have been identified:

- Type 1 (HSV-1), usually acquired in the first year of life, with active infections seen through lesions of the oral mucosa.
- Type 2 (HSV-2), generally acquired during sexual activity, with lesions typically in the genital area.

Both types are now seen in both areas of the body, presumably because of changing sexual practices.

Infection of the genital tract with either type of HSV progresses through two stages, the primary episode and recurrent episodes. The primary episode of the disease is characterized by fever, malaise, and muscle ache. Genital symptoms may include itching, vaginal or urethral discharge, dysuria, and inguinal lymphadenopathy. Blisterlike, extremely painful lesions appear on the genitalia within hours or days of exposure. Generally symptoms subside in 5 to 7 days, and lesions are often healed in 2 to 3 weeks.

Recurrent episodes occur because the virus lays inactive in cells of the nervous system for long periods of time and can be reactivated. Recurrent episodes are generally shorter, lasting 8 to 12 days, and may be triggered by a variety of events, including illness, menstruation, or pregnancy, but the cause is unknown. Recurrence may be heralded by a prodromal periods that may include mild tingling or itching at the site of a herpetic lesion. Symptoms are generally less severe than in a primary outbreak, although women generally have more severe symptoms overall than men. However, women may be asymptomatic during a recurrence if lesions are only present in the cervix or posterior vagina.

Etiologic and Predisposing Factors

The herpes virus is spread through intimate, usually sexual contact. The virus enters the body through a mucosal surface such as the mouth, cervix, or conjunctiva, or through small cracks in the skin. The infection is most common in European Americans between the ages of 15 and 35 years. Those with multiple sexual partners who do not use condoms are at significantly greater risk.

Diagnosis

Diagnosis is generally made on the basis of clinical symptoms. Testing to verify the diagnosis can be done using a Pap smear, ELISA (enzyme-linked immunosorbent assay), and cultures. Some individuals are found to have HSV but do not report lesions and report no history of the primary outbreak. This explains how individuals can acquire and transmit the disease without knowing they are infected. It is thought that these individuals' immune systems resulted in a relative lack of symptoms. It is believed that most transmission occurs through contact with active or healing lesions (Csonka, 1990).

Treatment

There is no treatment and no cure for HSV infection. Oral acyclovir, an antiviral agent, has been shown to decrease severity of symptoms and decrease the time during which the virus is shed. It is also used as suppressive therapy in patients with frequent recurrent outbreaks. Use of acyclovir ointment to speed healing of lesions may be recommended. Prevention of secondary infection by careful genital hygiene is essential. Women should be advised to abstain from sexual activity when lesions are present. Teaching Considerations are given in the accompanying display. Because of the increased risk of HIV infection associated with the presence of HSV genital ulcers, safe sexual practices should be used at all times (Centers for Disease Control, 1990).

Trichomoniasis

Trichomoniasis is a common type of vaginal infection that is sexually transmitted. The incidence of this infection may reach as high as 30% depending on the population studied. Although this is a sexually transmitted infection, its effects are limited to the vagina. It does not become systemic and is not a known cause of infertility.

Etiologic and Predisposing Factors

This STD is caused by trichomonas, a single-celled motile organism that thrives in wet environments. The incidence

Teaching Considerations

Self-Care for Genital Herpes

The nurse can use the following points in teaching women about genital herpes:

- Herpes is transmitted mainly by direct contact; abstinence is required for a brief period.
- Control of the condition will not require a major life-style change. Intercourse is avoided during treatment, but hand-holding and kissing are permissible.
- Women can be reassured that they can have children; their obstetricians need to know that they have the condition so they can be monitored appropriately.
- Conscientious hygienic practices of cleanliness (hand washing, perineal cleanliness) must be practiced. The patient should wear loose, comfortable clothing, eat a balanced diet, and get adequate rest and relaxation.
- Lesions should be washed gently with mild soap and running water and lightly dried.
- Prolonged exposure to the sun should be avoided, since it seems to cause recurrences (and skin cancer).
- Occlusive ointments, strong perfumed soaps, or bubble baths should be avoided.
- Medications must be taken as prescribed; follow-up appointments with health care personnel should be kept, and recurrences, which are not as severe as the initial episode, reported.
- The patient is encouraged to join a group to share solutions and experiences and hear about newer treatments. Information can be obtained from HELP (Herpetics Engaged in Living Productively), 260 Sheridan Avenue, Palo Alto, CA 94306.
- Usually precautions are unnecessary in the absence of active lesions.
- Lesions away from the mouth or perineum can be covered with a dressing and an impermeable cover during intercourse; such lesions are infrequent.
- For a partner with no history of genital herpes, a condom should be used.

From Smeltzer, S.C., & Bare, B.G. (1992). Brunner and Suddarth's textbook of medical-surgical nursing *(7th ed.). Philadelphia: J. B. Lippincott.*

of this infection peaks before age 35, although it is seen in older women (Lichtman & Papera, 1990).

Diagnosis

Trichomoniasis may be asymptomatic, acute, or chronic. Acute infection is characterized by a yellow green, frothy vaginal discharge often with a foul odor, inflammation of the vulva, and itching. Diagnosis can be made by microscopic examination of a smear using a wet mount that shows multiple motile organisms with white blood cells (a sign of inflammation) or by identification of characteristic features of the infection on a Pap smear.

Treatment

Treatment generally includes prescription of metronidazole for the infected woman and her sexual partner. The organism can survive in penile skin folds and this may be a source of repeated infections in the female partner. Intercourse should be avoided or condoms used until the course of antibiotics is completed. The woman may find that vinegar douches help to alleviate symptoms before and during treatment and may help in preventing reinfection.

Condyloma Acuminatum (HPV)

Condyloma acuminatum, also known as genital tract human pappilloma virus (HPV) infection or genital warts, is a common STD in the United States. Incidence of this infection has increased dramatically in the last two decades, with 50 cases reported per 100,000 population. There are more than 50 types of HPV, and a number of these are associated with malignancies of the reproductive tract in women (Csonka, 1990).

Etiologic and Predisposing Factors

The virus is transmitted through sexual contact. Infectivity of this virus is high, with 50% to 70% infection rates found in sexual partners of infected individuals (Netting & Kaufman, 1990). Individuals with multiple sexual partners and who engage in intercourse without condoms are at increased risk.

Diagnosis

Symptoms of HPV include the development of soft, gray, wartlike lesions in the genital area. Some women who report symptoms of recurrent vaginal infections unresponsive to treatment may have microscopic lesions. These lesions may not be detected by clinical inspection (Deitch & Smith, 1990).

Diagnosis may be made on clinical appearance alone or with the help of a Pap smear or biopsy. Condyloma should be differentiated from other lesions, which may be malignant. Careful cervical screening is necessary because of the association of HPV with precancerous changes in the cervix.

Treatment

Treatment of HPV focuses on reducing or removing the condyloma and preventing reinfection. Cryotherapy, laser therapy, or topical application of a compound called podophyllin may remove the growths or significantly reduce their size. Sexual partners should be screened for infection and treated as needed. Condoms are protective against HPV and should be used by all infected women and those with infected partners.

Gonorrhea

Gonorrhea is caused by the bacteria *N. gonorrhoeae*. Incidence of the disease declined during the 1970s and 1980s. However, with the emergence of penicillin- and tetracycline-resistant strains of the organism, incidence may again be on the rise.

Etiologic and Predisposing Factors

Gonorrhea is transmitted by sexual contact. Risk factors for this infection include low socioeconomic status, urban residence, early onset of sexual activity,and multiple sexual partners. More males than females are diagnosed with this infection, in large part because symptoms are usually pronounced in men whereas women may be asymptomatic (Lichtman & Papera, 1990).

Diagnosis

Definitive diagnosis of gonorrhea is made on the basis of cultures from the urethra, cervix, or rectum. Because gonorrhea is often asymptomatic in women, cervical cultures for this infection are routinely done as part of the gynecologic examination. When symptoms do occur in women, they include vaginal discharge, intermittent vaginal bleeding, and menorrhagia (excessive bleeding at the time of menstruation). In contrast, symptoms in men, usually acute dysuria and urethral discharge, are pronounced.

Treatment

Treatment for gonorrhea usually includes ceftriaxone, or in some cases, penicillin, amoxicillin, or ampicillin. In nearly half of diagnosed cases of gonorrhea, superimposed chlamydial infection must also be treated. Gonorrheal infection does not confer immunity, and reinfection is possible. Women who are treated for gonorrhea must be advised to encourage sexual partners to be screened and treated as needed.

Because symptoms may be mild or nonexistent in women, the disease may progress untreated for some time. The most common complication of gonorrhea in women is PID. PID is the spread of an infection into the uterus, fallopian tubes, and peritoneal cavity, causing bleeding, scarring, and pain. Untreated gonorrhea can also progress into the disseminated form of the disease, which can cause joint disease, hepatitis, and pericarditis (Lichtman & Papera, 1990).

Syphilis

Syphilis is a sexually transmitted and complex systemic disease. Because the symptoms may be subtle, infected individuals may not seek care until the disease is far advanced. The natural course of the disease is divided into early and late stages. The early stages of the disease are characterized by the development of nonspecific symptoms such as malaise, weight loss, and slight fever. A painless ulcer called a chancre develops at the site of entry of the organism, often on the vagina or vulva. Multiple chancres may develop and heal spontaneously. The lack of pain at the site of the chancre distinguishes this symptom from ulcers produced by HSV, which are painful. Diagnosis of syphilis can be made on the basis of serologic tests at this point when the chancre appears.

Between 2 and 12 weeks after the initial infection, the infected individual develops more systemic symptoms, including fever, adenopathy, hair loss, and red bronze macular lesions on the palms and soles. Widespread organ system changes can result in hepatitis, arthritis, meningitis, nephritis, and cranial nerve palsies. If untreated, the disease will progress into a latent but still infectious phase.

Approximately 30% of those who remain untreated will develop the late stage of syphilis. This stage is a slowly progressive chronic disease that can affect the cardiovascular and neurologic systems. Late stages of syphilis can lead to death. However, generally even late stages of the disease are responsive to treatment (Tillman, 1992).

Etiologic and Predisposing Factors

Syphilis is caused by the spirochete *T. pallidum*. The disease was well controlled through widespread use of penicillin and mandatory reporting in the years after World War II. However, incidence in the United States has climbed steadily in recent years. Between 1986 and 1990, the number of reported cases doubled to a total of 49,000, including 1747 cases of congenital syphilis in infants of infected mothers. Epidemiologists believe that three unreported cases of syphilis occur for each reported one.

Diagnosis

Diagnosis is made on the basis of blood tests, such as the Venereal Disease Research Laboratories (VDRL), rapid plasma reagin (RPR), or the fluorescent treponemal antibody absorption (FTA-ABS) test. The VDRL and RPR are nonspecific tests for syphilis; false positive results on these tests can be caused by infectious mononucleosis, autoimmune diseases such as lupus erythematosis and arthritis, and pregnancy. The FTA-ABS is a more specific test for syphilis. For this reason, this test may be used to confirm a positive VDRL or RPR test.

Treatment

The preferred treatment for syphilis is intramuscular or intravenous penicillin. Infection does not confer immunity, so reinfection can occur. Women should be advised to avoid sexual activity until serologic evidence indicates the disease has been successfully treated. The woman should be encouraged to advise sexual partners that they should be tested.

HIV and AIDS

HIV and the resulting disease, AIDS, are infections spread by contact with body fluids. Transmission usually occurs during sexual contact or needle-sharing among intravenous drug users. A full discussion of the disease and current therapy is beyond the scope of this chapter. The following section focuses on the implications of the epidemic for women and the field of women's health (see Chapter 16 for a discussion of care of the pregnant women with HIV).

Women are now the fastest growing category of infected individuals (Osborn, 1990/91). HIV and AIDS disproportionately affect minority and low-income women. Over 70% of infected women are minorities; 51% are African American and 20% are Hispanic American. Women with AIDS are significantly younger than men with the disease, and most infected women are of childbearing age (Osborn, 1990/91).

For many women, their sexual partner is their only source of personal and economic security. Asserting their personal right to protect themselves through use of condoms and safe sexual practices may conflict with basic survival needs. By 1990, more than 3 million women worldwide were infected with HIV (Chin, 1990). The relative incidence of infection in women has been steadily increasing since the epidemic began. Between 1981 and 1989, only 9% of reported AIDS cases were women. However, by 1990, women accounted for 11.5% of new cases.

The national and international response to the HIV and AIDS epidemic has not been as tailored to the needs of women as it might have been. Public health measures early in the epidemic concentrated only on infection in pregnant women. Until recently, information about infection rates among women could be obtained only through studies focusing on the perinatal aspects of HIV transmission. Specialized services for HIV-infected women were available in many communities only if the women were pregnant (Smeltzer & Whipple, 1991).

Etiologic and Predisposing Factors

Risk factors for HIV infection include unsafe sexual practices, needle sharing, and presence of other STDs. The latter appears to allow a portal of entry for the virus through inflammation and lesions caused by other STDs. Prevalence of HIV is three to five times higher in individuals with ulcerative STDs (such as herpes simplex virus, syphilis, HPV) than those without ulcerative disease (Anderson, 1989).

The major mode of transmission in women is unprotected heterosexual intercourse with infected men. The incidence of HIV infection among lesbian women is thought to be very low, with the major risk arising from intravenous drug users who share needles (Chu, Buehler, Fleming, & Berkelman, 1990).

Diagnosis

Antibody assays of serum are used to determine HIV antibody status. The ELISA is the standard initial test for the presence of HIV antibodies. False positive ELISA tests can be a result of autoimmune disease or a history of multiple pregnancies or multiple transfusions. False negative ELISA tests can result from blood testing either after infection but before serum antibodies appear or late in the disease. An initial reactive ELISA test is followed by the Western blot test.

Relatively little is known about the specific manifestations of the infection in women. In many cases, women are diagnosed with possible HIV infection on the basis of clinical symptoms. The following symptoms, called gynecologic clinical markers, may suggest the presence of HIV infection in women:

- Protracted herpes simplex infections
- Recurrent vaginal candidiasis

- Widespread condylomata
- Advanced cervical dysplasia
- Fulminating PID (Tinkle, Amaya, & Tamayo, 1992).

Women with advanced symptomatic HIV may present with opportunistic infections such as *Pneymocystis carinii* pneumonia, candidiasis of the esophagus and lungs, and disseminated tuberculosis. After women are diagnosed with HIV, there is some evidence that they become sick faster and die sooner than men. The reason for this is unclear, although it is probable that failure to recognize female-specific patterns of symptoms contributes to late diagnosis and treatment (Hankins, 1990).

Treatment

At this time, no treatment for HIV or AIDS is available. A variety of treatments are being tested in laboratories and clinical trials worldwide. Antiviral agents have been shown to inhibit the ability of the virus to replicate in laboratory research, and are now being used on an experimental basis. The most commonly used antiviral agent is zidovudine (AZT). AZT has been shown to improve the immunologic condition of people with AIDS. Various drugs to prevent the onset of opportunistic infections are also being investigated.

Supportive care for women with HIV and AIDS presents a significant nursing challenge. A full discussion of this area of nursing practice is beyond the scope of this chapter; the reader is referred to the Suggested Reading list for source materials on this subject.

Nurses will need to play an important part in shaping care for HIV-infected women in the future. Worldwide, women with HIV infection are usually those with the least power to make decisions regarding to their own health. Smeltzer and Whipple (1991) note that "women who may have HIV infection or AIDS need to be regarded by society and treated by health care professionals as individuals in their own right rather than merely potential infectors of their children and their sexual partners (p. 255)." Nurses must be aware that public policy, public health measures, and provision of clinical services have largely ignored the needs of women infected with HIV.

Implications for Nursing Care

The growing health problems associated with STDs place a significant responsibility on nurses in women's health care settings. Symptoms that may be the result of vaginal or sexually transmitted infection are frequently the reason women seek health care. Thus, the nurse must be well informed about risk factors, as well as diagnostic and treatment procedures for STDs.

• • Assessment

Nurses play an important role in identifying women who are at risk for STDs by taking a thorough health history. The nurse should be alert for factors that put women at risk, the most notable of which are intercourse without the use of condoms and multiple sexual partners. Women who report any vaginal or pelvic symptoms or whose male partners report urinary symptoms should be carefully evaluated and screened for STDs.

• • Nursing Diagnosis

The following nursing diagnoses may be applicable in the care of the woman with suspected or documented sexually transmitted infection:

- Fear related to diagnosis of STD
- Ineffective Family Coping related to suspicion and anger regarding STD infection
- Personal Identity Disturbance related to shame and stigma associated with STD
- Ineffective Individual Coping related to possible diagnosis of untreatable STD
- High Risk for Infection related to unsafe sexual practices

• • Planning and Implementation

The nurse is often responsible for explaining the diagnosis and treatment alternatives to the woman with an STD. The nurse must be able to impart information in a nonjudgmental and supportive fashion. It is important that the woman understand the treatment plan and the need for her sexual partners to be screened and treated.

In some cases, STDs are readily treated and may not be a cause for serious concern. In those situations, priorities in nursing care should be teaching women how to prevent reinfection and stressing the importance of safe sexual practices. The nurse can assist the woman in dealing with emotional responses to the diagnosis of an STD, and help her problem-solve with regard to her sexual partners and avoiding reinfection. A sensitive, accepting, and matter-of-fact attitude on the part of the nurse will often help the woman to put this experience in perspective.

Some women diagnosed with an STD face a much more difficult situation. Some must accept a chronic condition that may not be easily treatable. Others will be forced to come to grips with the terrifying realization that they are infected with HIV. In these cases, the nurse should be familiar with the ongoing treatment plan and be certain to link the woman with resources that may be available in the community for long-term support and assistance.

Expected Outcomes

- The woman with an STD states its implications for her health and that of her sexual partners.
- The woman with an STD describes the importance of the treatment plan.
- The woman with an STD seeks follow-up evaluations as recommended.
- The woman with an STD uses available services appropriately for ongoing care.

• • Evaluation

The nurse evaluates the woman's response to the proposed plan of care and modifies the plan as needed. When time and resources allow, the nurse should follow up to verify that treatment has been successful, that the woman's sexual partners have been advised to seek screening and treatment, and that the woman is using self-care strategies to avoid reinfection. Unfortunately, this level of careful follow-up may not be possible in many cases.

Common health concerns of adolescent and young adult women often center on emotional aspects of their lives, including their sexuality and reproductive functioning. Menstrual functioning may be a significant concern to young women. Young women are at risk for infections and STDs. The numbers and incidences of STDs are increasing dramatically among women and are considered epidemic in some communities. Women most at risk are urban dwelling and of low income, that is, women who may have difficulty gaining access to appropriate health care. In many cases, women with STDs may be asymptomatic, and diagnosis and treatment may be delayed with serious consequences. The single greatest cause of female infertility is PID as a consequence of sexually transmitted infections. STDs are also associated with greater risk for life-threatening conditions such as HIV and cervical and ovarian cancer. A major nursing priority is the education of women about human sexuality and how to prevent common health problems from negatively affecting women's health long into adulthood.

Common Health Concerns in Middle and Older Adulthood

Although common health concerns in middle and older adulthood may include conditions that arise earlier in life, major health concerns of adult women tend to be related to physiologic and psychosocial changes associated with aging. The following section highlights conditions likely to occur later in life, most notably menopause.

Aging is inevitable; it is a natural biologic process that begins at birth. The most apparent signs of the aging process in middle-aged and older women are physical changes. However, psychosocial changes are also part of the process.

A variety of factors, including genetics, life-style, diet, disease, and environmental factors, contribute to the rate and quality of aging. Health care behaviors can help to minimize the negative effects of much of the aging process.

Psychosocial Adaptation in Aging

Emotional and physical well-being are profoundly influenced by the process of aging. Women may be prone to negative attitudes about aging, especially if they have placed great emphasis on their physical appearance or on the childbearing and childrearing role or if changes in family structure (such as launching children, losing a spouse) overwhelm the ability to cope. Positive mental attitude appears to be a significant predictor of women's well-being in midlife and beyond. Active involvement in meaningful activities and an organizing "meaning for life" are important factors in keeping women active and healthy. A willingness and ability to accept the changes associated with middle and later adulthood and to perceive them as normal and positive may help women cope with the emotional and physical challenges associated with aging (Aber, 1992).

Physiologic Adaptation in Aging

The aging process affects virtually all physiologic processes in the body. Although menopause is the most frequently noted change in midlife women, other physiologic changes may have significance for an individual woman's health and well-being.

Musculoskeletal and Skin Changes

Muscles lose their elasticity and power when increased amounts of fibrous tissue replaces muscle tissue. This process begins in the late twenties. Changes in stamina and muscle strength may be noticeable in the thirties and forties. These changes increase in pace after age 50 when body muscle is replaced by fat. The body becomes softer and less firm, and body weight generally increases.

Musculoskeletal changes contribute to a variety of physical sensations and mild complaints. Backache and back pain may become more frequent as abdominal muscles gradually lose tone. Muscle cramps in the extremities at night or after exercise become more common. Tolerance for temperature change is reduced.

Changes in the skeletal system include increasing bone brittleness and arthritis (Fig. 6-8). Vertebral atrophy in the older woman may result from osteoporosis, a process in which bones gradually become demineralized, leaving them brittle and prone to breakage. The rate of bone loss in women becomes greatest after age 50. Pain and stiffness may result from the onset of arthritis. This is more common in women than men and may become more pronounced after age 60.

Changes in the composition of facial and body skin causes wrinkles and sagging because of loss of subcutaneous fat. Women who smoke and who have experienced unprotected exposure to the sun are more susceptible to wrinkles than those who do not. Sun exposure contributes to the development of skin cancer or melanoma later in life. Graying and coarsening of head and body hair is a normal process. Development of more pronounced facial hair on the upper lip, chin, and neck is common. Drying of skin, hair, and nails also is a normal finding.

Sensory Changes

As people age, their acuity of smell, taste, sight, and hearing deteriorates. By the mid twenties, hearing loss begins and increases over the life span. Functional hearing loss is present in more than half of those over age 65 (Fig. 6-9*A*). With aging, the lenses become more rigid and the pupillary response less efficient (Fig. 6-9*B*). The visual field decreases and more light is needed to see well. At about age 40, near vision may deteriorate as ocular muscles become slower to accommodate. By age 65, approximately half of all people have a visual acuity of 20/70 or less, and over 90% of those 65 or older wear corrective lenses (Lichtman & Papera, 1990).

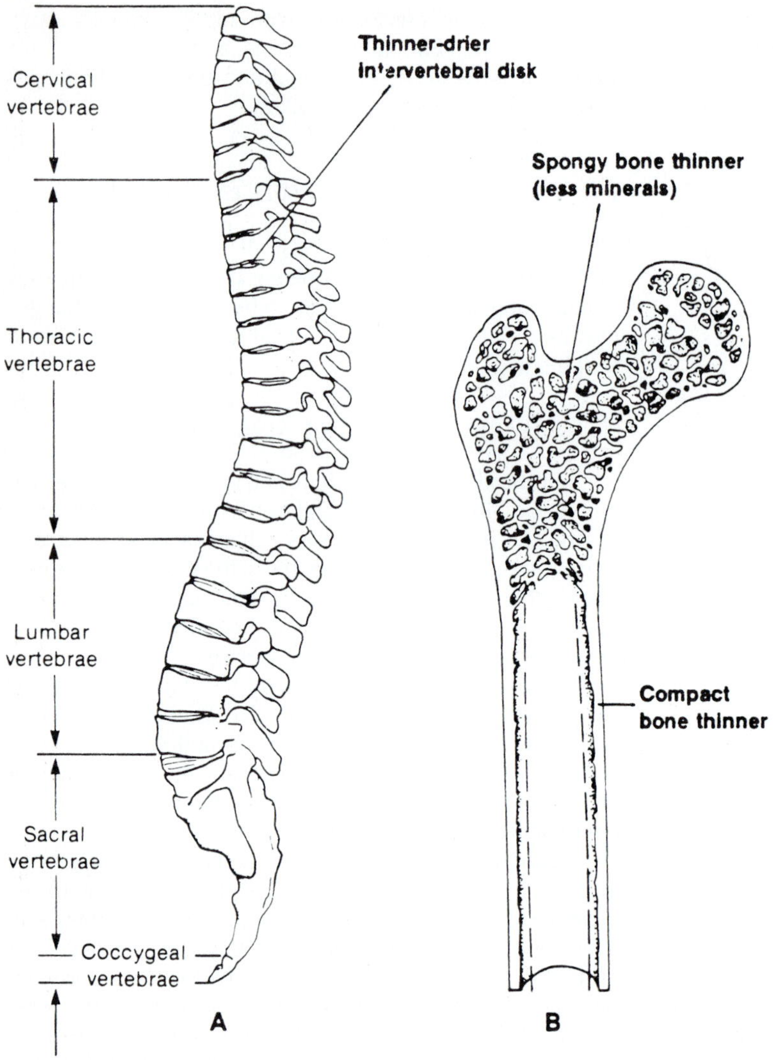

Figure 6-8.
Aging changes in bones.

Cardiovascular Changes

Cardiac output decreases by 30% between the ages of 25 and 65 years. Progressive loss of elasticity and an increase in calcium deposits in the arteries lead to decreased distensibility of blood vessels, which may contribute to increased blood pressure. Women appear to benefit from some hormonal protection from cardiovascular disease during their productive years, but this protection disappears after menopause. Cardiovascular changes are compounded by hypertension, smoking, obesity, and hereditary factors. High blood pressure and elevated cholesterol levels become more common in women after age 50. Rates of hypertension and elevated cholesterol levels in women exceed rates in men by age 65 (Lichtman & Papera, 1990).

Gastrointestinal and Genitourinary Changes

Absorption, motility, and enzyme secretion are reduced in the intestines with age. The weight of the liver decreases 20% after age 50, causing slowing of liver metabolism. Gastric production of hydrochloric acid is decreased with age. Constipation is a frequent complaint of older adults. It may be caused by a lack of fiber in the diet, inadequate fluid intake, lack of physical activity, or chronic laxative ingestion.

Urinary symptoms are common in older women. The number of nephrons in the kidney is reduced with aging. The functional capacity of the kidneys declines. Nocturnal frequency and urinary incontinence may be sources of distress in older women.

Pelvic Relaxation

Pelvic muscles and supporting structures atrophy with age (Fig. 6-10). This may result in problems associated with progressive pelvic relaxation. The outcome may include the development of cystocele (an outpouching of the anterior vaginal wall caused by the bladder), rectocele (an outpouching of the posterior vaginal wall caused by the rectum), or prolapse of the uterus into the vagina. Pelvic relaxation may contribute to urinary incontinence, backache, and problems with bowel elimination.

Endocrine Changes

The most notable change in endocrine function associated with aging is menopause. However, significant changes in thyroid and pancreatic function also occur. Abnormal

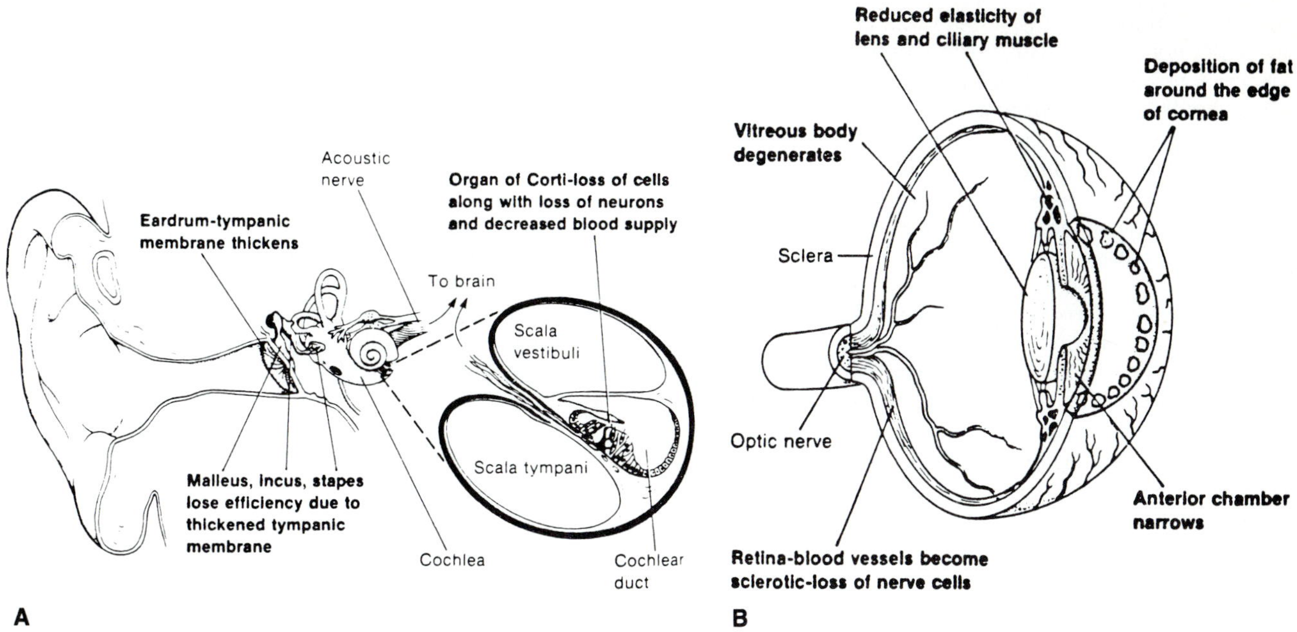

Figure 6-9.
Aging changes in hearing (*A*) and vision (*B*).

carbohydrate metabolism (diabetes) becomes increasingly common. However, late adult onset of diabetes does not carry with it the risk of serious complications associated with onset in childhood or early adulthood.

Menopause

Menopause, or the cessation of the menstrual cycle, is a clear sign that the reproductive period of a woman's life has ended. The average age at which women experience menopause in the United States is 51 years. However, for most women menopause is more a process than a distinct event. Most women begin to notice changes in their menstrual cycle several years before menses completely stop. This transition, often called the perimenopausal period or the climacteric, may last 3 to 5 years. The age of onset of menopausal changes is determined by a variety of factors, including genetic and nutritional factors (Freeman, 1992).

Etiologic and Predisposing Factors. The precise physiologic mechanism that causes natural cessation of ovarian function is not known. The decline and cessation of ovarian function appears to trigger declining estrogen levels. Decreases in circulating estrogen inhibit the feedback loop controlling normal reproductive endocrine functioning of the hypothalamus and pituitary gland. As a result, levels of serum gonadotropins (follicle-stimulating hormone and lu-

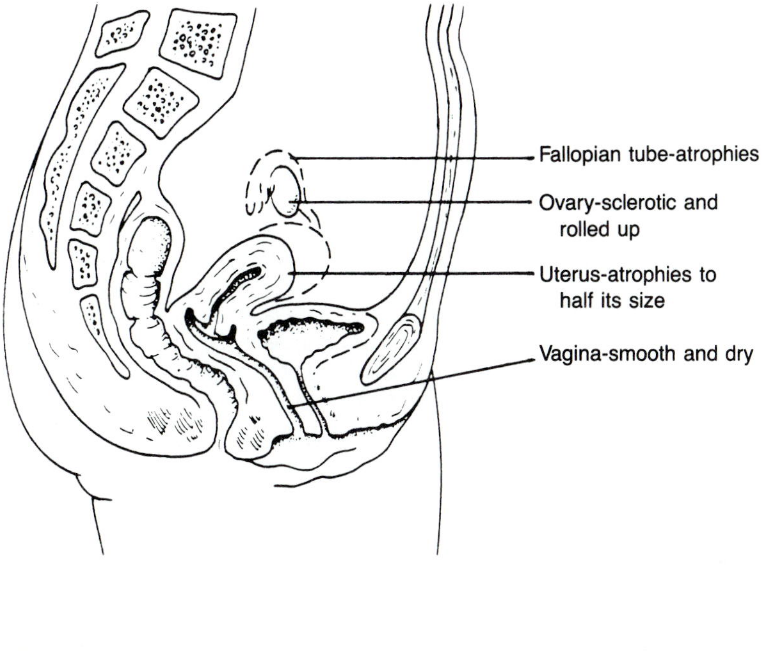

Figure 6-10.
Aging changes in the female reproductive system.

teinizing hormone) increase (see Chapter 4). The rise in these hormones along with declining serum estrogen levels are responsible for most of the signs and symptoms experienced by perimenopausal women. Eventually, estrogen levels diminish to a point where menstruation stops. Women who have bilateral salpingo-oophorectomy (removal of both ovaries and fallopian tubes) will undergo an abrupt premature or iatrogenic menopause because of the loss of ovarian hormone secretion.

Diagnosis. Various physical changes occur during the perimenopausal period. The major change of the perimenopausal period is a gradual decrease in amount and duration of menstrual flow. Cessation of menstrual flow is accompanied by atrophy of all internal reproductive organs. Atrophy of the vaginal epithelium is associated with vaginal dryness, pruritus, and dyspareunia. External genitalia also atrophy. The labia become thinner, pubic hair thins or disappears, and breasts lose their firmness and become more pendulous (Freeman, 1992).

A characteristic symptom of menopause is vasomotor disturbance. This symptom, often called "hot flash/flush" includes a sensation of heat in the face and neck, followed by marked sweating over the upper body. Vasomotor disturbances may be momentary or last as long as 10 minutes. A variation may be experienced in the form of night sweats. The etiology of this symptom is unknown. However, it is assumed to be related to drops in estrogen levels and rises in serum gonadotropin levels. Vasomotor disturbance is among the most common of perimenopausal symptoms. Approximately 75% of women will experience this symptom. Most women will experience hot flashes over a period of a year, but 25% of women will continue to have flashes for up to 5 years. This symptom may occur more frequently at night and may be a cause for significant sleep disturbance. Emotional changes in menopausal women may actually be attributed to sleep deprivation as much as to hormonal changes (Freeman, 1992).

Women may experience nonspecific symptoms associated with menopause, such as palpitations, apprehension, irritability, depression, and mood swings. These complaints are more common in the period just preceding cessation of menses. Generally they decline during the 1 to 2 years following cessation of menses. Vasomotor disturbance, sleep deprivation, and negatively perceived changes in sexual functioning may contribute to nonspecific symptoms.

Treatment. Menopause is a natural physiologic change, and as such does not require medical treatment. However, some conditions associated with menopause may require medical treatment, including abnormal bleeding, troublesome menopausal symptoms, and osteoporosis (discussed in the following section).

Abnormal bleeding in the perimenopausal period may become a significant problem. Bleeding may occur because of uterine masses, or because of endometrial hyperplasia, a precursor to endometrial cancer. If the results of endometrial biopsy are worrisome, or if bleeding and pelvic discomfort are significant, hysterectomy may be considered.

Hysterectomy is the second most frequently performed major surgical procedure in the United States, and as such it affects many women. Women may have significant concerns about hysterectomy in terms of their identity and functioning as a woman. They may associate the procedure with declining health and vitality. Women may also have concerns about what hysterectomy may mean for relationships with their male partners (see the accompanying Nursing Research display).

Treatment for menopausal symptoms through the use of hormone replacement therapy may be recommended. However, the use of it primarily for the treatment of menopausal symptoms is controversial. Some argue that menopause has been "medicalized" and the associated symptoms are a natural part of life that may not require treatment.

Nursing Research

Men's Views About Hysterectomies and Women Who Have Them

This exploratory study examined men's views about the effect of hysterectomy on women and on their relationships with women who had them. Semistructured interviews were conducted with 25 men ranging in age from 18 to 60, most of whom were middle class and educated beyond high school.

Results showed that men know little about hysterectomy, but they had negative attitudes about the procedure and believed that the surgery had negative effects on women. Men generally believed that hysterectomy had a significant negative effect on womens' self-image and sexuality. Men believed that women felt incomplete after the surgery, had diminished sexual drive, and felt less attractive sexually. Men believed that the loss of childbearing capacity was a significant loss to most women. The men who were interviewed believed that the procedure had a negative effect on relationships, largely because of the woman's lack of confidence and general emotional lability as a result of the surgery.

The investigator concluded that men are poorly informed about the procedure and are likely to presume negative effects on women when probably none exist. This preliminary study raises questions about the extent to which misinformation about hysterectomy is present in the general population and may suggest a clear direction for nursing intervention with women anticipating hysterectomy and their partners.

Bernhard, L. (1992). Men's views about hysterectomy and women who have them. *Image, 24*(3), 177–179.

Hormone Replacement Therapy. Hormone replacement therapy or estrogen replacement therapy has been available for the prevention of troublesome menopausal symptoms and the prevention of serious postmenopausal conditions since the 1960s. Replacement therapy reduces the incidence and severity of vasomotor disturbance, vaginal atrophy, postmenopausal bone loss, and cardiovascular heart disease in postmenopausal women. The American College of Obstetricians and Gynecologists currently recommends use of replacement therapy for prevention of osteoporosis and cardiovascular disease in menopausal women (Bowman, 1990).

Hormonal replacement may be administered on a cycle, such as some oral contraceptives, or on a continuous dosage basis. For women who have not had a hysterectomy, progestin is generally added to estrogen to prevent the development of endometrial hyperplasia and endometrial carcinoma.

Hormonal replacement therapy has potentially harmful side effects. It can increase the risk of uterine cancer and thrombosis, including cerebrovascular and cardiovascular accidents. For this reason, women on replacement therapy are advised to discontinue use of hormones and seek medical advice if they experience headaches, visual changes, signs of thrombophlebitis, chest pain, or any vaginal bleeding.

Osteoporosis

Osteoporosis is the process of prolonged and excessive bone loss that is only partially replaced by new bone formation. Loss of estrogen secretion in postmenopausal women is now recognized as a major factor in the development of osteoporosis. During the first 20 years after menopause, 75% or more of bone loss occurs. Bone loss begins as early as the twenties when trabecular bone (the honeycombed interior) is lost from the vertebrae. After menopause, cortical bone (hard, outer covering) is lost twice as fast in women than in men.

Etiologic and Predisposing Factors. Factors contributing to the development of osteoporosis are listed in the accompanying display. Of particular importance are risk factors that can be ameliorated by self-care in the areas of diet, substance use, and exercise (Lichtman & Papera, 1990).

Dietary factors can contribute to the development of osteoporosis. A diet poor in calcium may be a significant risk factor. Caffeinated drinks and coffee as primary sources of liquids increase the risk of calcium loss through urinary excretion. The high salt content of "junk foods" that are excreted along with calcium through urinary excretion triggers the release of parathyroid hormone. This hormone removes calcium from the bones to restore appropriate blood calcium levels.

Smoking is associated with earlier menopause and an increased risk of osteoporosis. Blood levels of smokers are lower than those of nonsmokers. It is unclear whether this is because of a direct effect of smoking on bone density or whether it is a reflection of other life-style factors, such as reduced physical activity. Alcohol use inhibits calcium absorption in the intestines and may interfere with the liver's ability to activate vitamin D, an essential ingredient for the absorption of calcium.

Lack of weight-bearing exercise plays a significant part in the development of osteoporosis. Bones grow larger and stronger in response to the stresses of muscle pull and weight bearing. Thus, women who do not exercise sufficiently are at risk for an increased rate of bone loss.

Women at Risk for Osteoporosis

The following groups of women are at increased risk to develop osteoporosis, based on the predisposing factors noted.

Hormonal Predisposition

- Women who have had an early menopause
- Women who had surgical removal of ovaries at an early age
- Women with endocrine disorders (hyperparathyroidism, hyperthyroidism, Cushing syndrome, kidney disease, diabetes, and rheumatoid arthritis).

Genetic Predisposition

- Women who have a family history of osteoporosis
- Women of European, Chinese, or Japanese heritage
- Women of fair complexion and small body size

Dietary or Behavioral Predisposition

- Women who smoke cigarettes
- Women with poor eating habits that do not provide the calcium needed to ensure healthy bones and who ingest caffeine and alcohol regularly
- Women with milk intolerance or allergies or who are vegetarians
- Women who are immobilized for long periods of time or who are extremely sedentary

Diagnosis. Women thought to be at risk for osteoporosis may be advised to have bone mass measurements at the onset of menopausal symptoms. Careful measurement of height may be important in the care of postmenopausal women at risk for osteoporosis. Loss of height as a consequence of vertebral compression and the development of the characteristic "dowager's stoop" (a marked forward curvature of the upper thoracic and cervical spine) may be the first sign of significant bone loss. Unfortunately, the first diagnosis of osteoporosis is often made when a women is treated for a bone fracture as a result of minimal trauma. The most common fractures are those of the wrist and vertebrae, followed by the hip.

Treatment. Treatment of osteoporosis at present includes the use of thyrocalcitonin, etidonate diphosphonate (agents which inhibit bone reabsorption), sodium fluoride (which stimulates osteoblast activity), and hormone replacement therapy. Unfortunately, treatment is not usually effective in preventing vertebral compression and bone fractures after bone loss is advanced.

Implications for Nursing Care

Sensitive nursing care of women in the middle and later adult years must consider the influence of psychosocial and physiologic aspects of aging. The nurse assesses the woman's perceptions about aging, physical changes, loss of reproductive capacity, and her social and psychological environment. The negative attitudes about aging common among women may have detrimental effects on a woman's ability to age in a healthy and satisfying way.

The nurse assists the older woman in establishing priorities for her own health. In collaboration with other care providers, the nurse then formulates a plan of care in collaboration with the woman herself to ensure that these priorities are met. The nurse can assist the older woman in promoting and maintaining optimal health by stressing exercise, a healthy diet, and maintenance of a positive attitude about life. It is important that the nurse emphasize health care as a partnership. Through health teaching, the older woman receives information she needs to make informed decisions about her own health and carry out recommended treatment plans for health problems.

Conditions arising earlier in life may continue to be concerns in middle and older adulthood, but major health concerns of adult women tend to be related to changes associated with aging. Aging is a natural biologic process that affects physiologic and psychological health and begins with birth. It affects every body system. A variety of factors contribute to the rate and quality of aging. The most significant aging change is menopause, the cessation of the menstrual cycle. The average age for experiencing menopause in the United States is 51 years. The precise physiologic mechanism causing menopause is unknown; however, the process triggers a decline in estrogen levels. Loss of estrogen secretion in postmenopausal women is recognized as a major factor in the development of osteoporosis. Osteoporosis is the process of prolonged and excessive bone loss that is only partially replaced by new bone formation. Hormone replacement therapy has been available since the 1960s; however, its use remains controversial.

Chapter Summary

Women's health is an emerging specialty in nursing, based on a commitment to health promotion, maintenance, and restoration through care centered on women's needs. Responsibility is shared by women and health care providers. Nurses are in a key position to ensure that women receive sensitive and appropriate care and information to make informed choices about their own health. The goal of women's health care is to empower women to assume greater control over their health and their health care.

The nurse can have a significant impact on health care of women and childbearing families. Nurses can provide information to adolescent and young adult women about their health care concerns and help them gain access to appropriate and sensitive health care. Education about the normal functioning of the female body and health promotion and disease prevention practices is a nursing care priority.

Women often have misinformation about their bodies and health risks. The nurse needs up-to-date information about common health problems and available diagnostic and treatment methods. It is essential that the nurse be able to communicate this information in a form that is meaningful to the woman.

As young women become sexually active, it becomes even more important that they receive regular and appropriate health care. All sexually active adolescent females should receive an annual physical examination with pelvic examination, Pap smear, and contraceptive counseling. The nurse plays and important role in explaining why these services are important in terms of health promotion and disease prevention. During gynecologic checkups, the nurse also is responsible for providing support, explanations, and reassurance. Unless the young woman understands the rationale for these examinations and feels the environment is supportive and safe, it is unlikely that she will adhere to recommended health maintenance routines.

Women's health concerns change as they mature and their life circumstances change. As women age, they may increasingly feel devalued; this perception can significantly affect the woman's physical and emotional well-being. Health care settings that emphasize reproductive or contraceptive care give the older woman an unintended but nevertheless negative message. The nurse should be aware that ageism is as much a part of contemporary society as sexism.

Provision of women's health care is based on a partnership between the woman and the health care provider. Women are entitled to full explanations about their condition, and to make informed decisions about treatment. In collaboration with the woman, the nurse identifies priority issues and concerns, and plans care to meet the woman's identified health needs. Encouraging women to take increased responsibility for their own health early in life, promoting self-care and disease prevention practices are the hallmark of quality nursing care.

Nurses prepared with specialized knowledge about the health needs of women will make significant contributions to the health and welfare of women and their families.

Study Questions

1. *What are the effects of sexism and poverty on the health and well-being of women?*
2. *What are the leading causes of death in women?*
3. *How well informed are women you know about the leading causes of death? How can women become better informed?*
4. *What techniques are available to screen women for*

breast cancer? How often should those techniques be used?

5. *What techniques are available to screen women for cervical and ovarian cancer? How often should those techniques be used?*
6. *What are three major psychosocial concerns facing women and the potential long-term health consequences? Why are these conditions more common in women than men?*
7. *What are the most common forms of STDs in the United States? How can they be prevented, detected, and treated?*
8. *What are the common physiologic changes women experience in relation to aging? How might men and women perceive these changes differently?*
9. *What is menopause and its associated symptoms and treatment? How are menopause and osteoporosis related?*

References

Aber, C. (1992). Spousal death, a threat to women's health: Paid work as a "resistance resource." *Image*, *24*(2), 95–99.

Aburdene, P., & Naisbitt, J. (1992). *Megatrends for women*. New York: Villard Books.

Anderson, J. (1989). Gynecologic manifestations of AIDS and HIV disease. *The Female Patient*, *14*, 57–68.

Bernhardt, J. (1990). Potential workplace hazards to reproductive health: Information for primary prevention. *Journal of Gynecologic, Obstetric, and Neonatal Nursing*, *19*(1), 53–56.

Bohn, D. (1990). Domestic violence and pregnancy: Implications for practice. *Journal of Nurse-Midwifery*, *35* (2), 86–88.

Bowman, M. (1990). Hormone replacement therapy: A new look at the combination regimen. *The Female Patient*, *15*, 63–67.

Centers for Disease Control. (1990). *Sexually transmitted disease statistics*. Atlanta: US Department of Health and Human Services.

Chin, J. (1990). Current and future dimensions of the HIV/AIDS pandemic in women and children. *Lancet*, *336*, 221–224.

Chu, S., Buehler, J., Fleming, P., & Berkelman, R. (1990). Epidemiology of reported cases of AIDS in lesbians, United States: 1980–89. *American Journal of Public Health*, *80*(11), 1380–81.

Csonka, G. (1990). *Sexually transmitted diseases: A textbook of genitourinary medicine*. New York: Baillere Tindall.

Curry, M. (1991) Women's, children's and family health. In P. Chinn (Ed.). *Health Policy: Who Cares?* Washington, DC: American Academy of Nursing.

Deitch, K., & Smith, J. (1990). Symptoms of chronic vaginal infection and microscopic condyloma in women. *Journal of Obstetric, Gynecologic, and Neonatal Nursing*, *19*(2), 133–138.

Freeman, S. (1992). Management of perimenopausal symptoms. *NAACOG Clinical Issues in Perinatal and Women's Health Nursing*, *2*(4), 429–439.

Ginsberg, C. (1991). Exfoliative cytologic screening: The Papanicolaou test. *Journal of Obstetric, Gynecologic, and Neonatal Nursing*, *20*(1), 39–49.

Hankins, C. (1990). Women and HIV infection and AIDS in Canada: Should we worry? *Canadian Medical Association Journal*, *143*, 1171–1173.

Hauenstein, E. (1991). Young women and depression: Origin, outcome, and nursing care. *Nursing Clinics of North America*, *26*(3), 601–612.

Hitchcock, J., & Wilson, H. (1992). Personal risking: Lesbian self-disclosure of sexual orientation to professional health care providers. *Nursing Research*, *41*(3), 178–183.

Lauver, D. (1992). Addressing infrequent cancer screening among women. *Nursing Outlook*, *40*(5), 207–212.

Lichtman, R., & Papera, S. (1990). *Gynecology: Well woman care*. Norwalk, CT: Appleton and Lange.

Love, C., & Seaton, H. (1991). Eating disorders: Highlights of nursing assessment and therapeutics. *Nursing Clinics of North America*, *26*(3), 677–697.

Mackey, T., Sereika, S., Weissfeld, L., Hacker, S., Zender, J., & Heard, S. (1992). Factors associated with long-term depressive symptoms of sexual assault victims. *Archives of Psychiatric Nursing*, *6*(1), 10–25.

Muller, C. (1990). *Health care and gender*. New York: Russell Sage Foundation.

Netting, S., & Kaufman, F. (1990). Diagnosis and management of sexually transmitted lesions. *Nurse Practitioner*, *15*(1), 20–24.

Nettles-Carlson, B. (1989). Early detection of breast cancer. *Journal of Gynecologic and Neonatal Nursing*, *19*(2), 116–121.

Norwood, S. (1990). Fibrocystic breast disease: An update and review. *Journal of Obstetric, Gynecologic, and Neonatal Nursing*, *19*(2), 116–121.

Osborn, J. (1990/91). Women and HIV-AIDS: The silent epidemic. *SIECUS Report*, *19*, 1–4.

Romans, M. (1991). Report of the Jacobs Institute workshop on screening mammography. *Women's Health Issues*, *1*, 63–67.

Romans, M., Marchant, W., Pearse, B., Gravenstine, B., & Sutton, S. (1991). Utilization of screening mammography—1991. *Women's Health Issues*, *1*, 68–73.

Sampselle, C. (1991). The role of nursing in preventing violence against women. *Journal of Obstetric, Gynecologic, and Neonatal Nursing*, *20*(6), 481–487.

Smeltzer, S., & Whipple, B. (1991). State of the science: Women and HIV infection. *Image*, *23*(4), 253–256.

Stevens, P. (1992). Lesbian health care research : A review of the literature from 1970 to 1990. *Health Care of Women International*, *13*(2), 91–120.

Tillman, J. (1992). Syphilis: An old disease, a contemporary perinatal problem. *Journal of Obstetric, Gynecologic, and Neonatal Nursing*, *21*(3), 209–214.

Tinkle, M., Amaya, M., & Tamayo,O. (1992). HIV disease and pregnancy. Part 1: Epidemiology, pathogenesis and natural history. *Journal of Gynecologic and Neonatal Nursing*, *21*(2), 86–93.

US Department of Health and Human Services. (1991). *Public Health Service Action Plan for Women's Health*. Washington, DC: US Public Health Service.

White, J. (1991). Feminism, eating and mental health. *ANS-Advances in Nursing Science*, *13*(3), 68–80.

Woods, N. (1992). Future directions for women's health research. *NAACOG Women's Health Nursing Scan*, *6*(5), 1–2.

Wyper, M. (1990). Breast self-examination and the health belief model: Variations on a theme. *Research in Nursing and Health*, *13*(2), 421–426.

Suggested Readings

Bernhard, L. (1992). Men's views about hysterectomies and women who have them. *Image*, *24*(3), 177–182.

Boston Women's Health Book Collective. (1992). *The new our bodies, ourselves: A book by and for women*. New York: Simon & Schuster.

Buenting, J. (1992). Health life styles of lesbian and heterosexual women. *Health Care of Women International*, *13*(2), 165–171.

Corea, G. (1992). *The invisible epidemic: The story of women and AIDS*. New York: HarperCollins.

Dahl, R. (1992) Women's mental health care—into the 1990s. *Perspectives in Psychaitric Care*, *28*(4), 29–31.

Dow, K. (1990). Breast cancer and fertility. *NAACOG's Clinical Issues in Perinatal and Women's Health Nursing*, *1*(4), 444–452.

Ellerhorst-Ryan, J., & Goeldner, J. (1992). Breast cancer. *Nursing Clinics of North America*, *27*(4), 821–833.

Gilligan, C., Rogers, A., & Tolman, D. (1991). *Women, girls, and psychotherapy: Reframing resistance*. New York: Haworth Press.

Ginsberg, C. (1991). Exfoliative cytologic screening: The Papanicolaou test. *Journal of Obstetric, Gynecologic, and Neonatal Nursing*, *20*(1), 39–49.

Irvine, D. (1992). Addressing infrequent cancer screening among women. *Nursing Outlook*, *40*(5), 207–212.

Lauver, D. (1992). Addressing infrequent cancer screening among women. *Nursing Outlook*, *40*(5), 207–212.

Lightfoot-Klein, H., & Shaw, E. (1991). Special needs of ritually circumcised women patients. *Journal of Obstetric, Gynecologic, and Neonatal Nursing*, *20*(1), 102–104.

McGrath, E. (1990). *Women and depression: Risk factors and treatment issues*. Washington, DC: American Psychological Association.

Nettles-Carlson, B. (1989). Early detection of breast cancer. *Journal of Gynecologic and Neonatal Nursing*, *19*(2), 116–121.

Norwood, S. (1990). Fibrocystic breast disease: An update and review. *Journal of Obstetric, Gynecologic, and Neonatal Nursing*, *19*(2), 116–121.

Norr, K., McElmurry, B., Moeti, M., & Tiou, S. (1992). AIDS prevention for women: A community-based approach. *Nursing Outlook*, *40*(9), 250–257.

Whipple, B. (1992). Issues concerning women and AIDS: Sexuality. *Nursing Outlook*, *40*(5), 203–207.

Williams, A. (1991). Women at risk: An AIDS educational needs assessment. *Image*, *23*(4), 208–215.

Woods, J., & Shaver, J. (1992). The evolutionary spiral of a specialized center for women's health research. *Image*, *24*(3), 223–228.

Zlotnick, C., & Cassanego, M. (1992). Unemployment and health. *Nursing and Health Care*, *13*(2), 78–80.

CHAPTER 7

Fertility Management

Learning Objectives

After studying the material in this chapter, the student will be able to:

- Discuss trends in contraceptive use among women in the United States.
- Define typical failure rate and discuss three factors affecting method effectiveness.
- List contraceptive methods available in the United States and discuss the effectiveness, the contraceptive action, health benefits, and side effects of each method.
- State the contraindications to oral contraceptive use and link these to the major complications that can occur with this method.
- Discuss special contraceptive needs of women after unprotected intercourse, during the postpartum period, over age 35, and if they are infected with human immunodeficiency virus.
- List and discuss at least four nursing responsibilities in counseling for contraceptive use.
- Discuss the relationship of gestational age to safety of elective abortion.
- Explain the most common causes of infertility and their treatments.
- Discuss two ethical problems related to assisted reproductive technologies.

Key Terms

abstinence
basal body temperature
calendar method
cervical cap
coitus interruptus
diaphragm
dilation and evacuation
endometrial biopsy
fertility
gamete intrafallopian tube transfer
hysterosalpingogram
intrauterine device
in vitro fertilization
postcoital protection
postcoital test
primary infertility
semen analysis
spermicide
sterilization
vacuum curettage
vasectomy

Fertility is the capacity of our bodies to create, nurture, and sustain the earliest lives of our children. It is an astonishing and complex realm of life that exists in a web of personal, social, and cultural contexts. For many women, adapting to their fertility will at certain times mean seeking ways to prevent or postpone pregnancy, whereas for other women fertility itself may be in question. This chapter explores these two distinct but complimentary areas on the reproductive health spectrum. It begins with contraceptive health care and then moves to health care for women and partners experiencing impaired fertility.

Contraception

If a fertile individual has intercourse regularly during one year, the chance of pregnancy occurring is 85%. Couples using a contraceptive method—any method—not only have a better chance of preventing pregnancy and pregnancy-related health problems but also of maintaining or enhancing their good health.

At any given time, almost two thirds of the 58 million women in their childbearing years who are sexually active are at risk for unintended pregnancy. Almost 90% of women aged 15 to 44 who could become pregnant, however, use contraception. Despite the fact that most sexually active women in the United States are trying to postpone childbearing or prevent it altogether, half of all unintended pregnancies occur among those using contraception (Harlap, Kost, & Forrest, 1991). Several factors make pregnancy prevention difficult for American women and couples. These factors include a limited range of methods, limits on access to reproductive health care, and misinformation on method safety and effectiveness. Nurses working in women's health care can play a key role in eliminating many of these problems.

Choosing a Contraceptive Method

Choosing a contraceptive method is often a complex decision. Each individual must weigh many factors simultaneously. Choice will be influenced by childbearing aspirations, sexual behavior, past health, current health practices, and willingness and ability to use the method correctly and consistently. Because women's reproductive years span half their adult lives, changes such as a new sexual partner may lead to choosing a different method.

Among women in the United States intending to have a child sometime in the future, half choose the oral contraceptive (OC) pill. Condoms are the second most frequently chosen reversible method. Among women and men not intending to have future pregnancies, sterilization is the most commonly selected method. In fact, more than one fourth of all women and 10% of men chose sterilization, making it overall the most widely used method in the United States. Women and men of different ages choose differently. For example, 25% of 15- to 19-year-olds report condom use, but only 11% of 30- to 34-year-olds rely on condoms (Harlap et al., 1991).

Deciding which contraceptive is best is highly personal. Each woman needs the opportunity to discuss her fears and questions. These discussions should include factors such as:

- Method cost
- Dependence of the method on the health care system
- Effect of the method on the partner
- Information and help with a second method
- Teaching in regard to avoiding sexually transmitted diseases (STDs)

After receiving this information, each individual should be able to choose the method or combination of methods most desirable at a given time (see the Nursing Research display). Other considerations important in teaching women and their partners about contraceptives are mechanism of action, method effectiveness, safety, and benefits of the method (Lethbridge, 1991).

Nursing Research

Personal Considerations in Choosing a Contraceptive

Little research has been conducted on the impact of contraceptive use on women's lives and sense of well-being. A study of 30 women using contraceptives between the ages of 19 and 45 used in-depth interviews to develop a description of their experiences with contraceptives. Data were analyzed for descriptive words and themes.

Within the central process of contraceptive self-care, women described three subprocesses: avoiding pregnancy, assigning the burden of contraceptive responsibility, and negotiating with those in control of contraception. The authors concluded that women attended to their contraceptive needs with varying degrees of comfort, diligence, and success. They were influenced by a complex combination of factors such as contraceptive side effects, subjective estimate of the probability of pregnancy, and feelings about becoming pregnant. Further research is needed to explore men's feelings about participation in contraceptive use.

Lethbridge, D. (1991). Choosing and using contraception: Toward a theory of women's contraceptive self-care. *Nursing Research, 40*(5), 276–280.

Method Effectiveness

Often when discussing method choice, the first question a woman asks is how well does a given method work to prevent pregnancy. Three factors control the effectiveness of any method:

- Inherent attributes of the method that contribute to its effectiveness when used correctly
- Characteristics of the user
- Reliability of research reports on method effectiveness

The lowest expected failure rate is the number of pregnancies that occur among couples who use the method consistently and correctly. The typical failure rate is the number of pregnancies that occur among users who do not report perfect use but who use the method for a full year. Table 7-1 shows failure rates for contraceptive methods currently in use in the United States.

In counseling patients, nurses must clearly state which type of rates are being discussed. For some methods, such as sterilization, a method with inherently high efficacy (not reliant on the user), there is little difference between these two failure rates. For other methods, such as the diaphragm, differences may be substantial. Method effectiveness over several years is important. However, research seldom reports use longer than the first year (Hatcher, Stewart, & Trussell, 1990).

Women must understand that effectiveness rates do not protect the individual user and that only correct use of the contraceptive protects from pregnancy. Women also should be advised that using two methods in combination dramatically lowers the risk of accidental pregnancy and that methods that work over a long time, such as hormonal implants and injections and intrauterine devices (IUDs), are associated with fewer failures.

Safety and Benefits

Several issues must be considered by each individual to determine contraceptive method safety. First, each woman needs to know that having a full-term pregnancy carries more health risks than any contraceptive method. Thus, taking any steps to avoid pregnancy will preserve a woman's health. Second, methods themselves cause few life-threatening complications, illnesses, or death. Third, most methods cause side effects that are not hazardous, but for some users, may prevent consistent use. Fourth, each individual's past and present health and behaviors influence method risks.

A safe contraceptive may also preserve and enhance the user's general and reproductive health by providing noncontraceptive benefits. Barrier methods, for example, offer some protection against STDs, and oral contraceptives decrease menstrual cramps, allowing some women to be more productive during menstruation than if they were not using this method.

Table 7-1. Contraceptive Failure Rates, United States—1990

Method	Percent of Women Experiencing an Accidental Pregnancy in the First Year of Use: Lowest Expected* (1)	Typical† (2)	Lowest Reported‡ (3)
Chance	85	85	43.1
Spermicides	3	21	0.0
Periodic abstinence		20	
Calendar	9		14.4
Ovulation method	3		10.5
Symptothermal	2		12.6
Postovulation	1		2.0
Withdrawal	4	18	6.7
Cap	6	18	8.0
Sponge			
Parous women	9	28	27.7
Nulliparous women	6	18	13.9
Diaphragm	6	18	2.1
Condom	2	12	4.2
IUD		3	
Progestasert®	2.0		1.9
Copper T 380A	0.8		0.5
Pill		3	
Combined	0.1		0.0
Progestogen only	0.5		1.1
Injectable progestogen			
DMPA	0.3	0.3	0.0
NET	0.4	0.4	0.0
Implants			
NORPLANT® (6 capsules)	0.04	0.04	0.0
NORPLANT®-2 (2 rods)	0.03	0.03	0.0
Female sterilization	0.2	0.4	0.0
Male sterilization	0.1	0.15	0.0

Reproduced with the permission of the Population Council, from Trussell, J., Hatcher, R., Cates., W., Stewart, F., & Kost, K. (1990). Contraceptive failure in the United States: An update. *Studies in Family Planning, 1*(1), 52.

* Lowest expected failure rate refers to the estimated rate of accidental pregnancy during the first year of use in couples who use the method consistently and perfectly.

† Typical failure rate refers to the estimated rate of accidental pregnancy among couples who use the method in a typical fashion (occasionally inconsistently or incorrectly).

‡ Lowest reported failure rate refers to the lowest failure rate reported in the literature on contraceptive methods.

Assessment for Initiating Contraception

All women need their general health evaluated before they begin using contraceptive methods that require medical prescription. Assessment will guide counseling for appropriate choices. The evaluation should include the following elements:

- Health history—preexisting major or chronic illnesses, nutritional status, and health behaviors, including medication and substance use.
- Family health history—inherited diseases, particularly cancers and cardiovascular illnesses.
- Menstrual history—menarche, cycle characteristics, problems.
- Obstetric history—including plans for future childbearing.
- Sexual history.
- Contraceptive history—previous methods, problems, questions.
- Social and employment history—circumstances that may impede or promote particular contraceptive method use, exposure to toxics, emotional stresses.
- Physical examination—blood pressure; weight and height; examination of head and neck; thyroid size; breast examination for detecting masses and teaching breast self-examination; abdominal examination of liver size, tenderness, and nodes; abdominal tenderness or masses; examination of extremities to evaluate peripheral circulation, varicosities, edema, bruising.
- Pelvic examination—assessment of external genitalia; speculum examination to view the cervix, vagina, vaginal discharge; bimanual examination, including palpation of the uterus to determine its size and position; examination of the cervix; palpation of ovaries for size and tenderness; rectovaginal examination.
- Laboratory tests—hemoglobin and hematocrit; urinalysis for glucose; rubella screening; Papanicolaou smear; screening for syphilis, gonorrhea and chlamydia; microscopic examination if a vaginal infection is suspected.

Contraceptive Methods

The following section summarizes methods currently available in the United States and Canada, from abstinence to voluntary sterilization. Each method's characteristics, actions, side effects, benefits to general health and contraceptive health, risks, instructions for users, and implications for nursing care are included.

Abstinence

Abstinence is usually defined as refraining from penis-in-vagina intercourse. Deliberately choosing to abstain should be seen as a normal, common, and acceptable choice for heterosexual women of all ages. A wide array of sexual expression such as hugging, kissing, massage, and masturbation offer pleasure and intimacy. Information on the numbers of women and men who choose abstinence as a contraceptive method are not available, but in a 1988 survey of American women aged 15 to 44, about 5% stated they had not had intercourse in the previous 3 months (Mosher & Pratt, 1990b).

Mechanism of Action and Method Effectiveness

Abstinence acts as a contraceptive by virtually eliminating the possibility that sperm can enter the woman's reproductive tract and cause conception. If practiced strictly, abstinence is completely effective in preventing pregnancy.

However, if practice is inconsistent, pregnancy can occur from unprotected intercourse. For this reason, the woman choosing abstinence should consider having other backup methods available.

To use this method effectively, women may need to learn to avoid situations where pressure to engage in sexual activity may be high. Women may also need to learn how to state clearly and in a convincing fashion, what activities they will and will not allow. For these reasons, abstinence may be easier for older women who have greater self-confidence and may be a challenge for younger women and adolescents, for whom peer pressure is often strong.

Safety and Benefits

Abstinence carries no health risk. It is totally effective in preventing pregnancy and protects against STD transmission. The method has been integrated into many human immunodeficiency virus (HIV) prevention programs aimed at adolescents (see the accompanying Teaching Considerations display). Research on program effectiveness is needed.

A period of abstinence may be recommended for health problems such as:

- Known or suspected STD
- Postoperative pain
- Pelvic pain
- After myocardial infarction
- Sexual therapy
- High-risk pregnancy

Coitus Interruptus

Throughout history men have used coitus interruptus (withdrawal). It remains popular in many parts of the world today. In the United States, 2% of those using contraception report using coitus interruptus as their primary method. This is about the same percentage using IUDs or natural family planning. Although withdrawal is frequently dismissed as an ineffective and unsatisfactory method, it is relatively effective and for some couples may enhance sexual pleasure. For couples having unanticipated coitus, or who are not using any other method, coitus interruptus may be the only method available. In the United States, evidence suggests that coitus interruptus is most often chosen by individuals using contraception for the first time and by those who have tried a wide variety of other methods (Mosher & Pratt, 1990b).

Mechanism of Action and Method Effectiveness

Coitus interruptus prevents ejaculation in or near the introitus. After sexual foreplay, when the man feels he is about to ejaculate, he removes his penis from the vagina. Ejaculation occurs away from the vagina and external genitalia. Often, during sexual foreplay and minutes before ejaculation, a few drops of seminal fluid, which contains semen, will leak from the urethra. Wiping this off before coitus is begun may aid in preventing sperm entry into the vagina, although the sperm content of this preejaculatory emission is uncertain.

Little research has been reported on the effectiveness of coitus interruptus, but estimates are that about 18% of couples will have an accidental pregnancy in the first year of using coitus interruptus (Mosher & Pratt, 1990b). One reason this method has not been studied is that it is completely within the individual's control; thus, users have no contact with health care personnel. Also, individuals and couples may use this method sporadically or in addition to other methods. These practices confound estimates of withdrawal's unique success or failure rates.

Safety and Benefits

Coitus interruptus is a safe method with no health risks to users or partners. Its advantages include availability, cost, and personal control. This method is easy to learn and use, requiring no devices. Withdrawal may enhance sexual pleasure for couples interested in exploring nonvaginal orgasm. Compared to using no method, coitus interruptus offers reasonable contraception.

Although no health problems result directly from the method itself, coitus interruptus does have some risks. It offers no protection against STDs or HIV infection. Interruption of the excitement phase of the sexual cycle may diminish pleasure for one or both partners.

The man must be able to control ejaculation. This may be difficult for adolescents because orgasm may be too rapid. Either partner may feel anxious about the man's ability to withdrawal early enough for the method to work. Finally, women who have unexpected sexual encounters who plan to use this method will need to persuade partners to use it. It may be necessary to teach the man how the method works. Women choosing this method also need to consider the possibility that postcoital contraception may be needed if the method is not strictly followed (see the accompanying Teaching Considerations display).

Teaching Considerations

Using Sexual Abstinence

The nurse can use the following points when teaching women about using sexual abstinence:

- High-pressure situations should be avoided.
- You have personal rights in social relationships.
- Decisions should be made in advance about which sexual activities you will permit. Discuss those with your partner.
- Tell your partner, clearly and in advance, what activities you will *not* allow.
- If you say no, say it like you mean it.
- Learn about other birth control methods and have a backup method accessible.
- Learn about postcoital contraception should you have intercourse when unexpected.

Teaching Considerations

Using Coitus Interruptus

The nurse should use the following points in teaching couples about coitus interruptus as a contraceptive method:

- Before beginning lovemaking, partners should talk about how to combine coitus interruptus with sexual pleasuring.
- Before inserting the penis into the vagina, all fluid at the tip of the penis should be wiped off because it may contain some sperm.
- When the man feels almost ready to ejaculate, he should remove his penis from the vagina and ejaculate *away* from the vagina.
- If semen (fluid from the penis) may have come in contact with the inside or outside of the vagina, the woman should contact her family planning clinic to find out about "morning after" birth control.

Natural Family Planning

Menstrual cycle charting combined with abstinence during the fertile period of the menstrual cycle is called natural family planning or periodic abstinence. Four distinct methods can be practiced: calendar, temperature, mucus, or symptothermal. All four methods center on self-awareness of the natural changes of the menstrual cycle, particularly ovulation. Of the 18% of American women choosing natural family planning, three fourths use the calendar method (Harlap et al., 1991). Method effectiveness depends on the user accurately predicting when ovulation will occur or detecting that it has happened, and on the user and her partner abstaining from intercourse during the woman's fertile period.

Mechanism of Action

The *calendar method* works on three assumptions about the menstrual cycle:

- Ovulation occurs on day 14, plus or minus 2 days *before* the onset of the next menses.
- Sperm remain viable for 72 hours.
- The ovum survives 24 hours after ovulation.

To begin to use this method, a woman keeps a record of the length of each menstrual cycle over at least 8 consecutive months. Day 1 of each cycle is always the first day of bleeding. After recording several cycle lengths, the woman can calculate the span of "fertile days," the time she has the highest chance of pregnancy if she has intercourse. The calculation is as follows:

- Note the shortest and longest number of days in the recorded cycles.
- Look at the shortest cycle and subtract 18 days from the total days in it. The *earliest* fertile day is the difference between these numbers. For example, if the shortest cycle lasted 22 days, then on day 4 of the cycle the user will begin to abstain from intercourse.
- Determine the *last* fertile day by subtracting 11 days from the total days of the longest cycle. For example, if the longest cycle has lasted 28 days, the last fertile day is day 17.
- Abstinence would be used from day 4 to 17 of all menstrual cycles.

Basal body temperature recordings also predict ovulation by following natural changes in body temperature before and after ovulation occurs (Fig. 7-1). Progesterone secreted in large amounts after ovulation causes this temperature rise. To use this method, the woman takes her basal body temperature (BBT) every morning for 5 minutes before rising, at about the same time. Special BBT thermometers (manual or electronic) are recommended because they measure tenths of degrees, not two tenths like regular fever thermometers. The thermometer may be used either orally, rectally, or vaginally.

- Each temperature is recorded on a special calendar sheet, and the daily dots are connected to form a pattern over the month. After about 6 months, BBT records can start on day 6 of each cycle because ovulation rarely occurs earlier than that.
- After *3 consecutive days* of temperatures at least 0.2°F or higher than the previous six daily temperatures have been noted, it is likely that ovulation has occurred (see Fig. 7-1).

The "safe" days for intercourse are from the evening of the third day of temperature rise (after ovulation) until menstrual bleeding occurs again. The "risky" days for intercourse start as menstrual bleeding stops (usually day 3 to 4) until the evening of the third consecutive day of temperature increase.

Cervical mucus changes occur in a recognizable pattern throughout the menstrual cycle. Mucus characteristics change because of the dominance of either estrogen before and at ovulation or dominance of progesterone after ovulation. After menstrual flow has stopped, the next 2 to 4 days are "dry," that is, the cervix does not produce mucus. As ovulation approaches, mucus reflecting enhanced fertility appears. It is abundant, flowing, clear, and slippery, resembling raw egg white. After ovulation, mucus is thick, cloudy, and pasty for a few days, and then dry days return for the 7 to 12 remaining days of the cycle.

Normal cervix characteristics of position, consistency, and openness of the os can be felt with two fingers. These changes result from estrogenic or progestational influence. During fertile periods, the cervix is higher in the pelvis, open, soft, and wet; during infertile periods, the cervix is lower in the pelvis, closed, firm, and dry. Women may choose to combine mucus and cervical checks; however, the mucus changes are considered more reliable for contraceptive effectiveness.

The *symptothermal method* combines the various charting techniques. The most common combination is the cer-

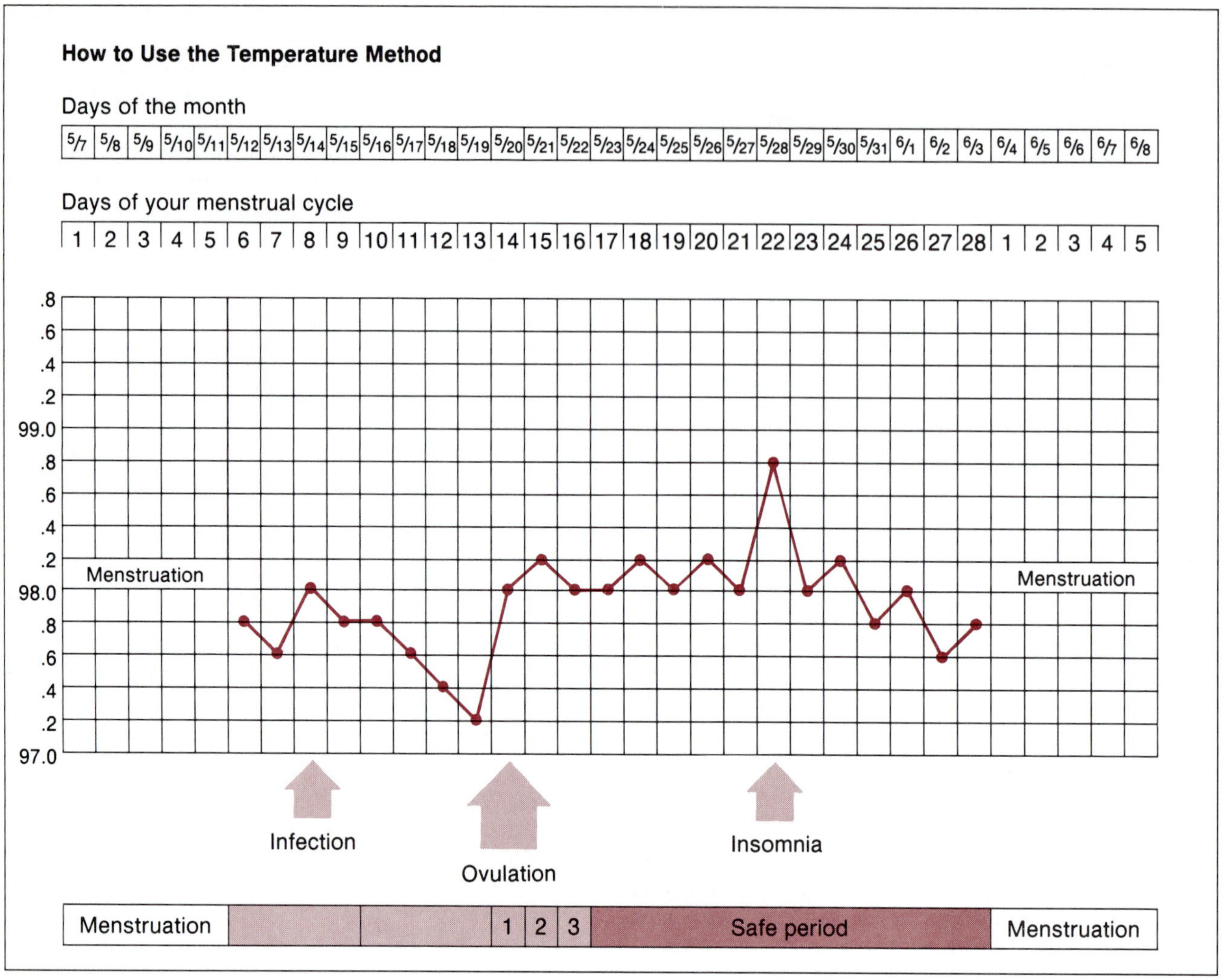

Figure 7-1.

Basal body temperature is measured with a special basal body thermometer at the same time every day, preferably every morning before rising. The temperature is recorded on a graph. The result is a curve with two distinct phases, one high and one low. The temperature remains high during the second phase. It falls a day or so before menstruation. Ovulation occurs within a range of 4 days before to 2 days after the temperature rises. Anything else that may make the temperature rise is noted. Infection and insomnia are examples on the graph above. Safe days for intercourse will be from 3 days after the sudden drop in temperature until 3 or 4 days after the period is over.

vical (symptoms) and temperature (thermal). Couples using this method safely engage in intercourse only if one key condition from each method has occurred: 4 days must pass after the last slippery mucus is noted, and 3 days must elapse after the BBT rise.

Method Effectiveness

During the first year of use, failure rates for typical use are 20% for the calendar method and 10% for the other methods. Effectiveness rates can be improved with limiting intercourse to only the days *after* the fertile period. The proportion of user failures resulting from improper teaching is unknown; taking risks during the fertile period is believed to account for most unintended pregnancies (Nofzinger, 1988).

Safety and Benefits

These methods carry no inherent risks but offer no protection against STDs or HIV infection. Women with irregular or anovulatory menstrual cycles or without the predictable temperature or mucus patterns will find these methods less successful. For all except the mucus method, literacy is necessary. BBT recording may be complicated for women working at night or a variety of shifts. Cervical mucus or digital examination may be unacceptable. Success also depends on access to a trained natural family planning teacher because most health care professionals have not had sufficient education to teach the technique. Nurses assisting women in choosing these methods should have contact with local counselors for referral.

Health benefits include avoidance of drugs and devices

and becoming aware of one's fertility cycle. This knowledge is helpful for planning pregnancy. After initial intensive teaching, women can use the methods independently, with minimal financial cost. For some individuals these are the only personally or religiously acceptable methods for fertility control.

Barrier Methods

Putting a barrier between sperm and ovum is one of the oldest and most natural ways to prevent pregnancy. A barrier can be placed either into the vagina or over the penis. This section begins with vaginal barriers—diaphragms, caps, sponges, and the new female condoms, and concludes with male condoms. Spermicides will be included because they are often used with a barrier method (see the accompanying Teaching Considerations display).

Vaginal Barriers

The vagina, with the cervix at its inner end, opening to the uterine body, is well adapted to promoting pregnancy. With sexual excitement, for example, the upper third of the vagina expands, and vaginal secretions increase. Cervical mucus helps to guide sperm into the cervical os. In view of these vaginal dynamics, it may seem surprising that barrier methods can be successful.

Diaphragms, caps, and sponges provide similar effectiveness and noncontraceptive benefits, including some protection against STDs. Slight differences in how they are used may make one option more appealing than another to individual women. About 5% of women choose the diaphragm, with a smaller percentage of women under age 25 and slightly higher over 30 years of age. No estimates are available on percent of women using sponges or the cervical cap (Hatcher et al., 1990). Diaphragms and caps must be fitted by a clinician who also teaches users how to insert and remove the device. Sponges and spermicidal gels can be purchased over the counter. These three devices are illustrated in Figure 7-2.

Diaphragms are dome-shaped rubber cups with a flexible spring rim inserted by the woman to cover the cervix (see Fig. 7-2*A*). One side of the rim is tucked behind the cervix and the other fits snugly up against the pubic bone. The rim keeps the diaphragm in place by pressing out against the vaginal walls.

Because the fit cannot be exact, the diaphragm does not seal the cervix from the vagina and thus could allow semen entry to the cervical canal. To add to its contraceptive action, spermicidal gel or cream is put into the dome, which should inactivate any sperm that get around the edge of the diaphragm. Spermicides are biochemically active for a limited time—generally 2 hours once placed in vagina. The diaphragm actually works in two ways: as a shield for the cervix and as a reservoir for spermicide. Women using diaphragms should be instructed to put additional spermicidal gel in the vagina for subsequent acts of intercourse, but they should leave the diaphragm in place. Women should not douche after intercourse because this washes away the spermicidal protection.

Cervical caps are cup-shaped soft rubber devices that fit

Teaching Considerations

Using Barrier Methods in Contraception

The nurse can use the following points when teaching women about using barrier methods of contraception:

- The method should be used every time intercourse is likely to occur.
- The woman should wash her hands before inserting a contraceptive device into the vagina.
- The sponge, cap, or diaphragm with spermicide must be in place before the penis enters the vagina. After the woman inserts the device and before intercourse begins, she should check once more with her fingers to make sure the cervix is completely covered.
- The sponge, cap, or diaphragm should be left in place at least 8 hours after intercourse.
- If the woman is using a diaphragm and has intercourse more than once, she should leave the diaphragm in place but put additional spermicidal gel in her vagina.
- After removal, the diaphragm or cap should be washed in soap and water, dried, and stored in its case to prevent damage to the latex.
- Diaphragms and caps should last at least a year. Sponges should be discarded after use.
- Women using barrier methods should learn the danger signs for toxic shock syndrome and should call their health care providers immediately if they have these signs.
- If either partner experiences vaginal or penile irritation, a different brand of spermicide should be used.
- The woman should not douche after intercourse because this can wash away the spermicide.
- The woman should keep a written record of her menstrual periods; if she misses one, she should have a pregnancy test.
- Condoms should be used along with other barrier methods. This combination increases protection from unintended pregnancy and STDs.

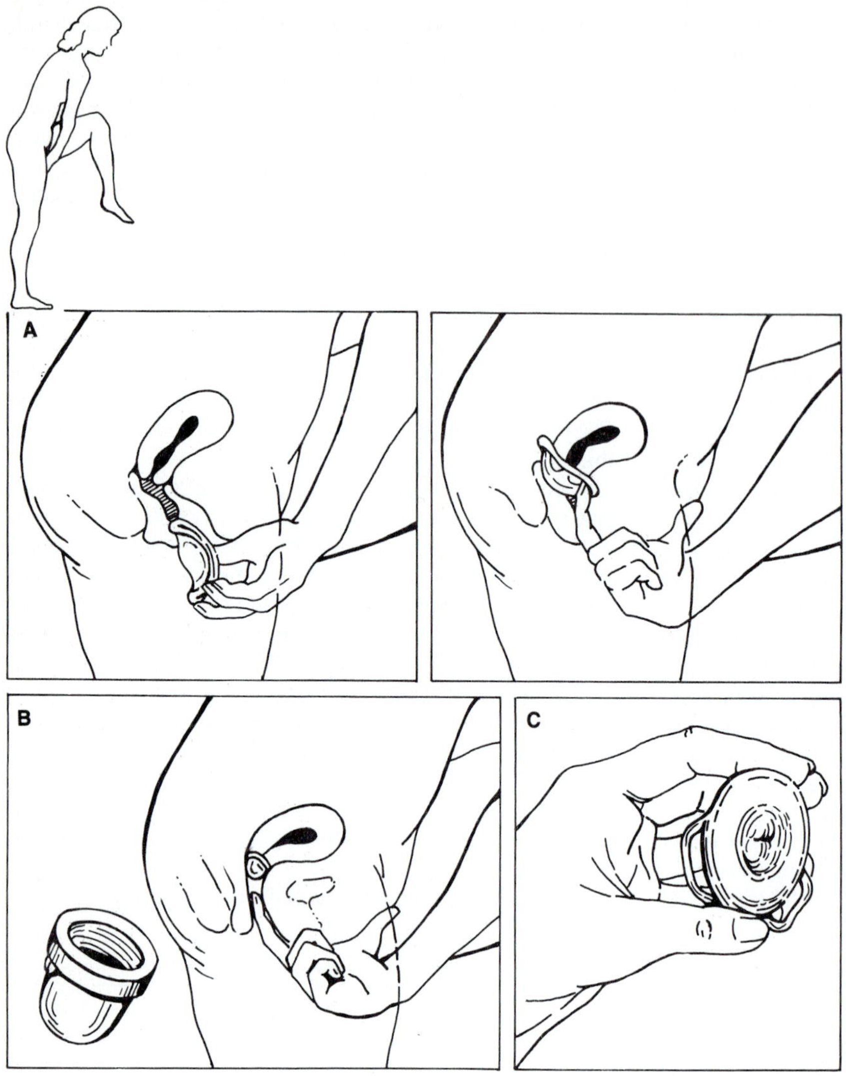

Figure 7-2.
Vaginal barriers used in contraception. The woman may use the same standing position for insertion of all of these devices. *A:* Diaphragm use: (*left*), insertion; (*right*), fit of diaphragm over the cervix. *B:* Cervical cap use: (*left*), cervical cap; (*right*), fit of cervical cap over cervix. *C:* Vaginal sponge provides both a physical and chemical barrier.

directly over the cervix and are held in place by a seal formed between its firm, flexible rim and the surface of the cervix (see Fig. 7-2*B*). Only one model, the Prentif Cavity Rim Cervical Cap, is currently available in the United States. Although this method has been widely used in the past in Europe, it is seldom used there now. It was not until 1988 that cervical caps received initial Food and Drug Administration (FDA) approval for use in the United States. The cap works much like the diaphragm, blocking sperm entry to the cervix and acting as a container for a small amount of spermicide. It can remain in place for 48 hours, provides protection regardless of the number of times intercourse occurs, and does not require additional spermicide (Hatcher et al., 1990).

The *contraceptive sponge* currently available is a disposable polyurethane pillow that contains 1 g of the spermicide, nonoxynol-9. It is one size with a concave dimple on one side that allows it to fit closely over the cervix (see Fig. 7-2*C*). The other side has a polyester loop attached to help with removal. This product has been available in the United States since 1983. The sponge releases spermicide, traps sperm, and also presents a barrier to sperm.

Before it is inserted, the sponge must be moistened with water to activate the spermicide. Once inserted it works for up to 24 hours no matter how many times intercourse occurs. The sponge should remain in place at least 8 hours after intercourse. After removal, the sponge should be checked to be sure it has not been torn. If so, any pieces remaining in the vagina should be removed and discarded.

Mechanism of Action and Method Effectiveness

Vaginal barrier methods have two mechanisms of action. First, they form a physical barrier to prevent sperm from entering the cervix. Second, they are either used with or contain spermicide, which kills sperm while still in the vagina.

Although the typical user failure rate of vaginal barriers is 18% in the first year of use, this high rate must be carefully interpreted when counseling a patient considering these methods. Successful use depends on two important and distinct factors: the natural fertility of the woman and her correct and consistent use of the method. Consistent use has been directly linked to the quality of teaching a new user receives and the teacher's attitude about the method. For example, in a study of more than 2000 women who chose the diaphragm and received thorough counseling and follow-up contact with the clinic, the pregnancy rate after a year of use was 3%. Studies that report far higher failure rates may not eliminate inconsistent users who become pregnant while not actually using the method (Hatcher et al., 1990).

Safety and Benefits

The only serious health problem that vaginal barriers can cause is toxic shock syndrome (TSS). This rare but serious illness occurs during or immediately after menstruation and is caused by a reaction to *Staphylococcus aureus* toxins released in menstrual blood. The annual incidence of this syndrome in the United States is 4 to 14 cases per 100,000 menstruating women. In 99% of reported cases, the women had used tampons. It is unclear whether using a vaginal barrier actually increases a woman's risk of TSS. Sponges have been implicated because 13 cases of TSS occurred among sponge users in the United States during the first year they were available (Mosse & Heaton, 1990). To avoid this risk, all women using vaginal barriers should be reminded that they should wash their hands before inserting a contraceptive device into the vagina. Women should be taught the symptoms of TSS (see the accompanying display).

Vaginal barrier methods have few additional risks, other than side effects, which occur infrequently. They are:

- Local skin irritation caused by sensitivity or allergy is the most frequent problem for all three methods. The reaction may be to the spermicide or the material of which the barrier is made. Partners may also have a local reaction. Changing brands of spermicide or diaphragm or switching to another type of barrier may solve the problem.
- Difficulty removing the device occurs more often with the sponge and cap than the diaphragm. The sponge may tear, requiring a pelvic examination to remove pieces.
- Foul vaginal odor and discharge occur if the barrier is inadvertently left in place more than a few days. Removal eliminates the odor.
- Urinary tract infections have been reported more often for diaphragm users than for users of other types of contraception. The reasons for this are not clear but may relate to the diaphragm's rim pressing against the urethra or bladder neck, causing local trauma. Diaphragm users also seem to have vaginal colonization with *Escherichia coli*. This organism is commonly found on the perineum but is pathogenic in urine. If a woman develops recurrent cystitis during diaphragm use, another barrier or another method may be a healthier choice.

All vaginal barrier methods afford some protection from STDs, largely because of the combined physical barrier with the chemical action of spermicide. Once a woman has received careful fitting and instructions for use, barrier methods afford independence from the health care system and are entirely under the woman's control. These methods do not involve participation of partners. This may be an attractive and important benefit for some women. Relative to other methods, barrier methods are safe, with no known systemic side effects. Used in combination with condoms, barrier methods provide effective protection against unintended pregnancy and STDs.

Signs of Toxic Shock Syndrome

The nurse should be aware that women who use barrier methods of contraception and those who wear tampons may be at risk for toxic shock syndrome. Women should be advised to contact their health care provider immediately if they should develop any or all of these signs:

- Sudden, high fever
- Vomiting or diarrhea
- Dizziness and faintness
- Sore throat and aching muscles
- A rash similar to a sunburn or peeling of skin on hands and feet

Vaginal Contraceptive Pouch

A relatively new contraceptive in the United States is a latex sheath designed as a woman's equivalent to the male condom. It has received provisional approval by the FDA. The sheath is closed at one end. The closed end is inserted into the vagina and placed in front of the cervix (Fig. 7-3). The sheath has two flexible plastic rings, one at the closed end and the other at the open end to hold it in place against the cervix and over the labia.

Mechanism of Action and Method Effectiveness

The mechanism of action of the vaginal contraceptive pouch relies on the fact that the entire vagina is lined with latex. If the sheath dislodges during intercourse, sperm would still be prevented from entering the cervix because the sheath would still cover the penis. The pouch can be inserted at any time before sexual activity and should be removed and discarded after ejaculation has taken place. Preliminary reports from a clinical trial with 80 users over 6 months indicate a pregnancy failure rate comparable to condoms—about 15%. Like the condom, most of these pregnancies occurred because of inconsistent or incorrect use of the pouch (Hatcher et al., 1990).

Safety and Benefits

Two important benefits occur with the use of the vaginal pouch. First, this is an additional female-controlled contraceptive choice. Second, the pouch promises excellent protection against bacterial and viral STDs because it is made of a thicker latex than male condoms. Testing is in progress to determine whether it will, as hoped, be a barrier to HIV infection. Risks are minimal, as with all barrier methods. Allergy to the material or discomfort from the rings might occur.

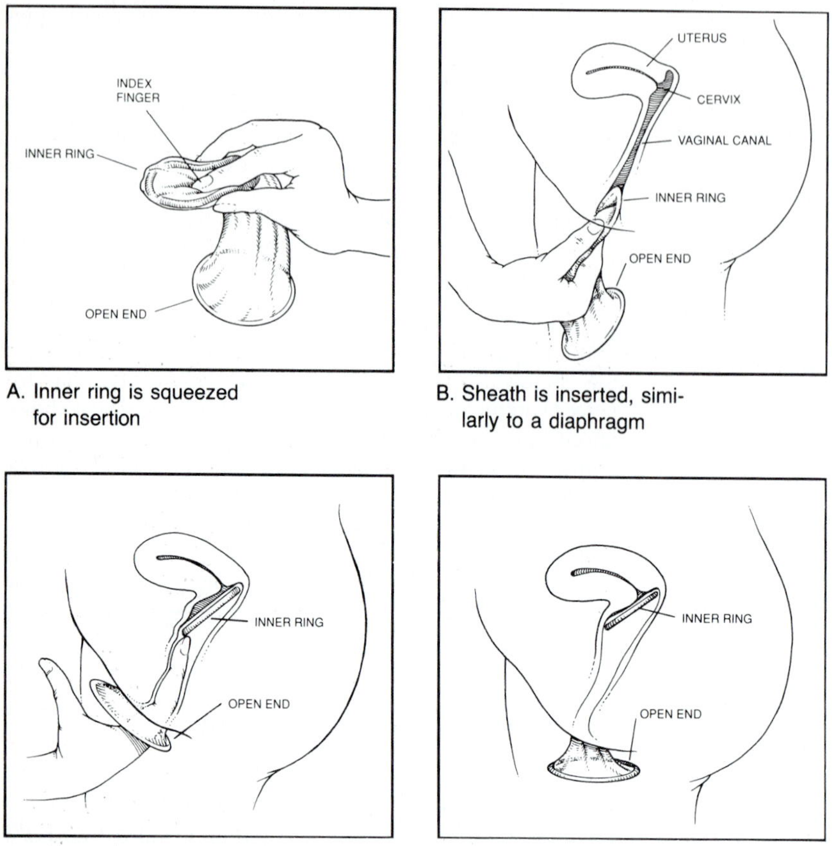

A. Inner ring is squeezed for insertion

B. Sheath is inserted, similarly to a diaphragm

C. Inner ring is pushed up as far as it can go with index finger

D. Vaginal pouch in place

Figure 7-3.

Vaginal pouch insertion and positioning. *A:* The inner ring is squeezed for insertion. *B:* The sheath is inserted similarly to a diaphragm. *C:* The inner ring is pushed up with the index finger as far as it can go. *D:* The vaginal pouch in place. (Courtesy of the Wisconsin Pharmacal Company. Reproduced with permission.)

Condoms

Condoms are a safe and reliable way for men and women to live with their fertility and sexuality. Available since the 1930s, latex condoms have become increasingly popular because they provide one of the only preventive measures against HIV transmission. Condom use for contraception rose 40% in the United States from 1982 to 1988, moving from 6.7% to 9% of all those using contraception. For single women the condom was the second most popular choice (Harlap et al., 1991). For many additional couples condoms are used with another method or if a regular method is not available. Condoms are the most affordable barrier method. Many family planning clinics dispense them at no cost because of their multiple benefits.

Mechanism of Action and Method Effectiveness

When placed over the erect penis, a condom prevents sperm from entering the vagina. Most condoms are made of very thin latex (less than a millimeter thick) or processed animal collagenous tissue. Once the sheath is unrolled over the penis, a firm rubber rim holds the condom in place at the base of the penis (Fig. 7-4). Condoms are made in only two lengths, but a variety of shapes, colors, and styles are available. Some condoms are lubricated with nonoxynol-9 spermicide.

The typical first-year failure rate for condoms is 12%. Effectiveness depends almost exclusively on consistent use. The most frequent error users make is not to use one. Condoms can break occasionally or slip off after erection has subsided, adding to the risk of accidental pregnancy. Condoms lubricated with spermicide should offer added protection against pregnancy and STDs. To date, no reports compare failure rates for condoms with or without spermicidal lubrication.

Safety and Benefits

The risks and complications of condom use are relatively rare; they include:

- Allergy of either partner to latex or the lubricating material.
- Erection may be inhibited for some men.
- Natural skin condoms do not protect against STDs.
- Women whose partners decline or refuse to use condoms face a difficult decision: they must either decline to participate or engage in intercourse or other sexual acts risking pregnancy or STDs.

Side effects of condom use may be a significant barrier to continued use. The major complaint of condom users is that the condom reduces penile glans sensitivity; however, if very thin condoms are used (to enhance perceived sensitivity) they may easily break. Vaginal or penile friction from

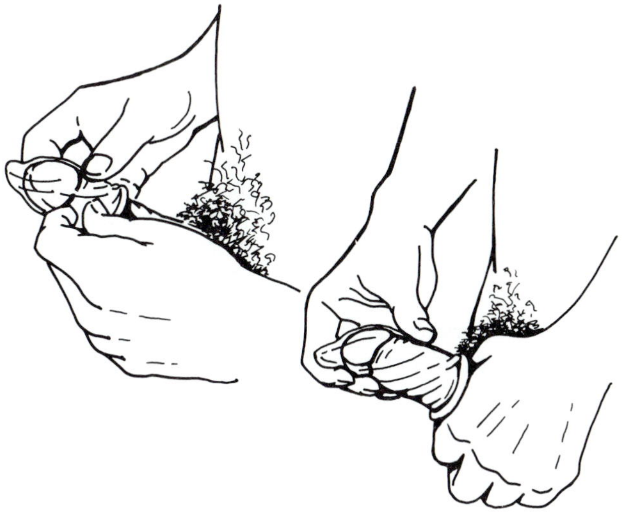

Figure 7-4.
The condom is unrolled onto the erect penis, leaving space at the tip for ejaculate.

the condom may cause local irritation or discomfort to either partner. Interrupting foreplay to put the condom on may be psychologically or emotionally unpleasant.

Besides protecting against pregnancy, this method has additional advantages. Condoms are inexpensive and accessible (stocked in stores, in vending machines, and at clinics). Users do not require a medical examination. Condoms encourage male participation in contraception and STD prevention. By diminishing the risk of STDs for women, they indirectly contribute to preventing cervical cancer (by preventing human papilloma virus transmission). Condoms also reduce the risk of pelvic inflammatory disease (PID; see Chapter 6). Postcoital discharge of semen from the vagina, which may be an annoying aftermath of intercourse for some women, is avoided (see the accompanying Teaching Considerations display).

Teaching Considerations

Using Condoms in Contraception

The nurse should use the following points when teaching women and their partners about condom use:

- A condom should be used *every* time the couple has intercourse.
- The condom should be put on the erect penis *before* the penis comes in contact with the woman's genitals.
- The male should leave 1/2 inch of empty space at the tip by pinching the tip of the condom as it is rolled on the penis.
- The condom should be rolled all the way to the base of the erect penis.
- Male partners should wait until the vagina is naturally well lubricated to insert the penis covered by the condom because a condom can tear if the vagina is dry.
- If extra lubrication is desired, petroleum-based products (such as Vaseline) should not be used because they can damage the condom. Contraceptive foam or gel or water-soluble jelly should be used instead.
- For extra protection, another birth control method can be used in addition to the condom.
- After intercourse, the penis should be withdrawn while it is erect by holding on to the condom rim to prevent spilling.
- The used condom should be discarded. New condoms should be stored in their packages in a cool place. Even body heat may cause the rubber to weaken. Properly stored, they will last up to 5 years.

Vaginal Spermicides

Although fewer than 1% of women choose this method, many may use it as a backup or as an adjunct to increase the effectiveness of another method such as the condom (Mosse & Heaton, 1990). Spermicides share many of the advantages of barrier methods. Spermicides can be purchased without a prescription or medical examination, are relatively inexpensive, cause no major health consequences, and offer limited protection against STDs because they kill many infection-causing organisms.

Mechanism of Action and Method Effectiveness

All spermicidal preparations consist of two components. The first is an inert base or carrier (foam, jelly, cream, or tablet) that ensures dispersion in the vagina. The second is a chemical that kills sperm and other organisms. In the United States, although two spermicidal products are available, nonoxynol-9 is found in nearly all products. The ability to destroy cell walls accounts for the chemical sperm destruction, as well as destruction of gonorrhea and chlamydia organisms. However, viruses and other intracellular organisms appear to be less susceptible to spermicidal destruction. For this reason, spermicides cannot be relied on to provide complete protection from STDs.

All spermicidal products become activated rapidly when exposed to body warmth in the vagina. It is important to note that they are short acting, becoming inactive an hour after application. One application of any of the spermicides provides contraception for only one coital ejaculation.

Typical user failure rate in the first year of using spermicides is 20%. The major reason for this high failure rate is inconsistent use. Differences in effectiveness among foam, suppositories, or creams have not been reported (Hatcher et al., 1990).

Safety and Benefits

No severe adverse reactions have been reported for currently available products. Theoretically, absorption of the spermicides through the vaginal walls could have systemic effects. Animal studies, but not human studies, report liver damage when large vaginal doses are administered. If pregnancy occurs, no teratogenic effects have been found for offspring of spermicide users.

Side effects of spermicides include skin irritation of the vulva or penis caused by sensitivity or allergy to one or both agents in the preparation. In addition, taste of the chemicals may interfere with pleasure of oral sex, and the effervescence of foaming tablets or melting suppositories in the vagina may cause an unpleasant sensation. Insertion may be awkward or messy and the spermicide may leak out of the vagina after coitus.

Teaching Considerations

Using Spermicide Contraception

The nurse should use the following points when teaching woman and their partners about the use of spermicide contraception.

Before Intercourse

- The woman should always have a supply of the product available.
- The woman should read the package instructions to be sure of the time period the product needs to become effective before intercourse.

For Insertion

- The woman should wash her hands with soap and water before use.
- When using foam, the container should be shaken at least 20 times, then the nozzle should be used to fill the applicator. When using jelly or cream, enough should be squeezed from the tube to fill the applicator completely.
- For both foam and creams, the applicator should be inserted into the vagina as far as it will comfortably go. Then the plunger should be pushed fully into the applicator to release the spermicide deep into the vagina.
- When using a suppository, the suppository should be unwrapped and pushed with fingers into the vagina as far as possible so it rests next to the cervix. The woman should wait the time the product instructions indicate for effectiveness before intercourse.
- A new application of spermicide is essential for protection each time intercourse occurs.
- Using a condom improves spermicide effectiveness.

Spermicides are available at relatively low cost in most pharmacies and are safe. A woman can choose and use this method without involving her partner in the decision or actual use (see the accompanying Teaching Considerations display). Spermicides can be easily kept at hand for unexpected sexual intimacy. If a partner is using a condom and it breaks, spermicide can be quickly inserted afterward to try to kill sperm in the vagina. Spermicides provide lubrication and may add to pleasure during intercourse. If a woman is using oral contraceptives and forgets to take one or two pills, a spermicide should be used for a week after the missed pills to bolster uncertain oral contraceptive action. Spermicides offer limited protection against some STDs (Hatcher et al., 1990).

Oral Contraceptives

Often called birth control pills, or simply "the pill," OCs are the most popular reversible method of contraception in the United States, with 30% of those using contraception choosing it. OCs contain either a combination of synthetic estrogen and progesterone or progesterone alone. This discussion concentrates on the hormonal combination pills because they are used more widely.

Oral contraceptives are taken daily from day 1 of the menstrual cycle through day 21. During the next 7 days, either no pill or a placebo is taken. OCs contain doses thought to be the lowest possible to maintain high effectiveness and low rates of side effects. Both estrogen and progesterone have potential to cause a wide variety of side effects in some users.

Currently, two types of estrogen are used in doses ranging from 20 to 50 μg in each pill. Progestin, a derivative of progesterone, is available in five compounds, which differ in their properties and their bioactivity. The hormones are combined in one of two ways. The first way is called monophasic, and the user takes 21 pills of identical dose. Multiphasics, on the other hand, have three different combinations of estrogen and progesterone to take during the 3 weeks of pill use. A wide variety of pill formulations are available.

Mechanism of Action and Method Effectiveness

Oral contraceptives alter the menstrual cycle in a number of ways, primarily preventing pregnancy by preventing ovulation. OCs deliver doses of estrogen and progesterone *higher* than the lowest natural amount in the cycle, but *lower* than the natural surges in the cycle. The result of this low but constant dose through the first 21 days of the cycle suppresses follicle-stimulating hormone (FSH). The ovary does not undergo ovulation. Additional effects of the pills include:

- Blocking the function of luteinizing hormone (LH) in activating ovulation.
- Inhibiting implantation by altering the quality and thickness of the endometrial lining.
- Making cervical mucus hostile to sperm transport.
- Slowing ovum transport in the fallopian tube.

For OCs to work, they must be taken daily to maintain the steady blood level of hormones that block ovulation. Used correctly, this is an effective method. During the first year that women use OCs, the typical failure rate is 3%, and for users younger than age 22, the failure rate is slightly higher—4.7%. Effectiveness does not differ between multiphasic and monophasic combined formulations. Despite this effectiveness, however, 25% of women discontinue OC use after a year. The major reason women cite is side effects. Many family planning practitioners recommend that new users receive instructions for alternative methods because of the high discontinuation rate. Having a supply of a second contraceptive method is advisable (Mosse & Heaton, 1990).

Effectiveness may be decreased depending on interactions of OCs and some medications. Anticonvulsants and some antibiotics, for example, directly decrease the amount of estrogen circulating in the blood. This hormonal change decreases the contraceptive action of OCs. If a woman who uses OCs takes a medication that itself has the side effect of nausea or vomiting, the woman may not be able to take or absorb her daily dose of OC.

Safety and Benefits

For healthy women under 35 years of age who do not smoke, oral contraceptives are generally safe. Compared with childbearing, the risk of death is far smaller from taking OCs than having a term birth—1 in 63,000 versus 1 in 14,300. Rarely, however, oral contraceptives can cause serious health risks. The major risks are cardiovascular, but liver disease and possibly breast cancer also must be considered.

The most important complications are circulatory disorders, including hypertension, myocardial infarction, cerebral vascular accidents, and deep vein thrombosis, which occur because estrogen causes increased coagulability and clot formation. About 5% of OC users will develop mild hypertension, which disappears within a few weeks of stopping pill use. Women using OCs must periodically have their blood pressure taken. The risk of myocardial infarction and cerebrovascular accidents is also increased slightly (Mosse & Heaton, 1990).

Women must be counseled about the danger signs of OC use, including:

- Abdominal pain (severe)
- Chest pain (severe), cough, difficulty breathing
- Headache (severe), weakness, or numbness
- Eye problems, including severe visual disturbances ("flashes," "spots")
- Severe leg pain in calf or thigh

Women should be advised to seek immediate care if any of these symptoms develop.

The circulatory health risks of OC use are serious, but the occurrences are rare. Circulatory complications can be prevented to a large extent by careful patient selection and counseling so that women with health risks either do not use this method or have frequent clinical evaluation for safe use. The relationship between use of OCs and cancer of the reproductive tract is as yet unclear.

Both beneficial and negative side effects occur for some women who use OCs. Beneficial side effects include decreased menstrual cramping and amount of flow and regular cycles. Some women experience decreased premenstrual syndrome symptoms. OCs offer protection against PID because of thick, hostile cervical mucus, decreased tubal and uterine motility, and decreased menstrual blood, which acts as a culture medium for pathogens. OCs also may offer some protection against ovarian cysts and against ovarian and endometrial cancer. These conditions are rare; however, pill users have lower rates of these forms of cancer than women who have never used the pill.

Oral contraceptives may also play a role in preventing pregnancy after unprotected sexual intercourse. Contraceptive methods are imperfect, sexual behavior is unpredictable, and unfortunately, sexual assault occurs. Therefore, women will need access to contraception after unexpected, unprotected sexual intercourse. The risk of accidental pregnancy is high, particularly if intercourse has taken place at midcycle. Taking a large dose of OCs soon after the event effectively disrupts the endometrial lining and alters tubal transport of the fertilized ovum, preventing implantation.

For women needing this one-time contraception, a regimen can be prescribed by the care provider, which is 99% effective in preventing pregnancy: 1 mg progestin (norgestrel) and 100 mg estrogen (equivalent to 2 tablets of Ovral) within 12 to 24 hours after intercourse and again 12 hours after the first dose. Treatment may cause nausea, and if vomiting occurs, the health care provider should be notified. The woman's period should begin in 2 to 3 weeks, and if it does not, a pregnancy test is indicated.

To summarize, the safety of OCs depends on each woman considering her overall health and the potential benefits and risks oral use will have for her. This information must be weighed against the health risks of other methods and the risk that pregnancy would pose for the individual.

No method is as dependent on instructions for self-care as oral contraceptives because effectiveness depends on taking the pills correctly (see the accompanying Teaching Considerations display). Two essential features of OC use for counselors to emphasize are starting each pack as scheduled and taking the daily pill at the same time. The dose of hormones is so low that it must be delivered at the same time and begun correctly, at the onset of menses, to completely prevent ovulation.

Nurses often have primary responsibility for instructing OC users. Verbal instructions should be reinforced with written handouts. Because of the complexity of the instructions and widespread functional illiteracy, a recent recommendation is that the reading level for patient package inserts be lowered from a twelfth grade to fifth grade level (see the Nursing Research display).

NORPLANT Implants

Besides the OC pill, hormones can be delivered to the bloodstream through a subdermal implant. In 1991, NORPLANT, the first subdermal hormonal implant, received FDA approval for marketing in the United States. NORPLANT offers women the first new approach to contraception in many years. It consists of six soft Silastic rods filled with powdered levonorgestrel (Fig. 7-5). This synthetic progesterone is effective up to 5 years.

Teaching Considerations

Using Oral Contraceptives

The nurse should use the following points when teaching women about oral contraceptive use:

- A backup method such as foam or condoms should be used during the first week of pill use, if the woman forgets to take pills, runs out, or stops taking them because of danger signs.
- The provider will tell the woman when to start the first pack. It will either be *on the first Sunday after her period begins* or *on the first day of her period.*
- The woman should take one pill at the same time each day.
- When the pack is empty, the woman starts a new pack *the next day.* She should not skip any days between packs, unless so instructed by her care providers.
- The woman should check her birth control pill pack each day to be sure she took her pill on the previous day.
- If the woman has light bleeding between periods, it may be caused by taking the pill at a different time or forgetting a pill. She should keep taking them and call her clinic or doctor if she has concerns.
- *If she misses a pill,* she should take it as soon as she remembers.
- If she misses two pills in a row in the first 2 weeks of the pack, she should take two pills on the day she remembers and two pills the next day. *She should use her backup method for 7 days.*
- If she misses two pills during the third week, misses three pills in a row at any time, she should follow these special instructions:
  - If she started her pills on *Sunday,* she should continue taking a pill each day until the following Sunday. On the second Sunday, she should throw away the pack and start a new one. She should use her backup method for 7 days.
  - If she started her pills on the *first day of bleeding,* she should throw out the rest of the pack and start a new pack. She should use her backup method for 7 days.
- Periods are usually shorter and lighter with pills. A drop of blood or a spot may be a period.
- If she misses one period, she should call her care provider. Sometimes, even if a woman takes the pills perfectly, she may miss one period. But if she forgot pills and missed a period, she may be pregnant.
- If she misses *two* periods in a row, she should have a pregnancy test immediately.
- The woman should learn the *danger signs associated with oral contraceptive use* and call her care provider immediately if she experiences any of them.

Mechanism of Action and Method Effectiveness

After local anesthesia has been given, the match stick-sized rods are inserted through a half-inch incision in the skin by a trained nurse practitioner or physician. The rods are usually placed on the inside surface of the nondominant arm. The levonorgestrel "leaks" out of the porous rods into the circulation at about 35 μg/day. This is a small fraction of the daily dose of progestin in most OCs. NORPLANT prevents pregnancy in the following three ways:

- A steady blood level of progesterone inhibits ovulation in about 50% of cycles.
- Cervical mucus becomes hostile to sperm penetration.
- The endometrium becomes hypotrophic, inhibiting implantation.

Based on 20 years of experimental use, NORPLANT prevents pregnancy in the first year of use for 99% of users. Hormonal release begins immediately after insertion. Contraceptive protection begins 24 hours later. By the fifth year of use, the failure rate is 4%, which is comparable to that for OCs. Once the rods are removed, ovulation returns promptly (Sharts-Engel, 1991).

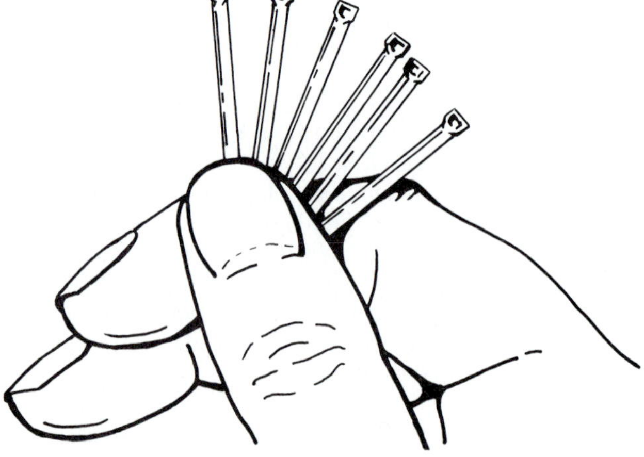

Figure 7-5.
The six-capsule NORPLANT system.

Nursing Research

Readability of Contraceptive Instructions for Users

Written instructions for contraceptive users are only helpful when read and comprehended. This study analyzed and compared commercial package inserts and generic informational materials developed in several family planning settings for level of readability. Materials covered oral contraceptives, diaphragms, foam and suppositories, and condoms.

Results indicated a wide range of readability levels, from grade 4 for one oral contraceptive generic pamphlet to grade 15 for another package insert. Overall, individuals who rely on only package inserts for any method would have to read at least at grade 9 level.

The authors suggested that nurses working with women whose literacy is limited should develop generic materials, so that women do not need to rely on commercial package inserts, which may be incomprehensible. Generic materials should focus on information the user truly needs to know and be culturally specific. Other suggestions included developing alternative methods for instruction such as audiotapes and videotapes.

Swanson, J., Forrest K., Ledbetter, C., Hall, S., Holstine, E., & Shafer, M. (1990). Readability of commercial and generic contraceptive instructions *Image, 22*(2), 96–99.

Safety and Benefits

Information on risk comes from experimental use by thousands of women in other countries. No risks to women's health after 5 years of use have been reported. No reports have evaluated effects of longer use. No risks to the fetus if a pregnancy occurs during NORPLANT use have been reported. Until studies in the United States have been completed in the mid 1990s, American women must consider risk information incomplete. Women should receive information regarding use of barrier methods because NORPLANT confers no protection against STDs, and they should be advised of danger signs (see the accompanying display).

Two types of complications may occur: surgical and long term. Surgical risks include infection, reported to occur less than 1% of the time, up to 3 months after insertion and, rarely, hemorrhage and rod extrusion. Removal may prove difficult if scars and adhesions form after rods have remained in place several years. Reports are not yet available about removal problems in the United States, and few reports from earlier foreign studies demonstrate removal problems (Sharts-Engel, 1991).

Complications requiring removal are rare, particularly if users are carefully selected. Pregnancy is rare; however, detecting it may be complicated because menses are disrupted. Women should be alert to signs of pregnancy and have access to pregnancy testing.

Most healthy women who desire long-term pregnancy spacing can consider this method. In fact, compared with OCs, NORPLANT users avoid the risks and side effects associated with the estrogen in pills. For some women, this method is advantageous for their overall health and satisfaction with the method. Every woman considering this method should receive thorough preinsertion information and counseling on method actions, side effects, risks, benefits, and the insertion procedure. Often counseling will be a nursing responsibility and has been found to be key to user satisfaction.

Absolute contraindications of NORPLANT use include:

- Active thrombophlebitis
- Unexplained genital bleeding
- Suspected pregnancy
- Active liver disease or tumor
- Known or suspected breast cancer

NORPLANT is both long acting and reversible. After counseling and insertion, visits to a health care provider would only be needed for problems and periodic health maintenance. The method is convenient, requires no self-care, and is relatively private because the rods are not visible (but they can be felt through the skin).

Postprocedural side effects include mild tenderness for 24 hours and bruising at the insertion site that takes 1 to 2 weeks to resolve. Also, just as the action of NORPLANT is similar to progestin in OCs, the side effects are similar and include irregular bleeding, headaches, acne, weight change, and breast tenderness. By far the most frequent problem is alteration in menstrual bleeding, with 70% of users reporting changes during the first year of use. Most often the pattern includes no cyclic bleeding, with spotting occurring as often as two to three times a week. A small percentage of women have no bleeding whatsoever. The manufacturer claims that

Danger Signs for NORPLANT Users

The nurse should advise the woman using NORPLANT implants of the following danger signs, and that she should contact her health care provider if she experiences any of the following:

- Pain that gets stronger where the NORPLANT was placed
- Pus or bleeding from the insertion site
- NORPLANT rod coming through the skin
- Heavy vaginal bleeding
- Sudden irregularity in periods after a regular cycle had been established
- Strong abdominal pain

bleeding irregularities diminish by the third year of use (Sharts-Engel, 1991).

Injectable Progestin

For some women, periodically receiving an injection of a long-acting progestin may be a convenient and safe choice. At this time, one product, Depo-Provera, medroxyprogesterone acetate, is available in the United States although it is not approved by the FDA for contraceptive use. The manufacturer has, however, recently requested that FDA reevaluate Depo-Provera for marketing as a contraceptive. It has been used in more than 80 countries for over 20 years and is relatively inexpensive. It is administered by a nurse, or in other countries, by a trained health care worker.

Mechanism of Action and Method Effectiveness

A dose of 100 to 150 mg is given intramuscularly every 3 months. The progestin has the same effects on ovulation, cervical mucus, and the endometrium as NORPLANT, but takes up to 2 weeks after the injection to provide contraception. In a year of use, the typical failure rate is 1%, according to World Health Organization reports from studies of thousands of users in developing countries (Mosse & Heaton, 1990).

Safety and Benefits

Controversial animal research findings have kept Depo-Provera from being approved as a contraceptive in the United States. The two findings are adverse fetal effects and increased risk of cancer in the endometrium and breast. Neither has been found in human beings (Mosse & Heaton, 1990). A major drawback of injecting this preparation is that its actions cannot be reversed. Thus, if a user wishes discontinuation because of side effects, a desire to change method, or return to fertility, she must wait until the last dose clears from her body. Contraindications are the same as for NORPLANT.

Depo-Provera offers highly effective contraception and requires only one visit to a health facility four times a year. Its action actually continues for about 4 weeks beyond the 12-week recommended injection schedule, offering a "grace period" if the user cannot receive the scheduled dose. Because users do not need any supplies at home, it is a relatively private method choice. It is also relatively inexpensive and covered by health insurance.

Any intramuscular injection of medication carries a small risk of local irritation, inadvertent nerve damage, or tissue reaction to the medication. Depo-Provera has not been reported to cause any specific local reactions to the injection. Allergic reactions to these agents occur rarely. As with other progestin preparations, menstrual bleeding changes are the most common side effect. Menstrual cycles will be replaced with irregular spotting. Delayed return of fertility may continue for 6 to 12 months, with the mean interval of 10 months to return of fertility. Occasionally headaches, weight gain, and depression occur, but the rates of these problems are not known, nor can women who may be at risk for these problems be identified before receiving this medication.

Intrauterine Device

With a success rate similar to OCs, the IUD is an excellent choice for selected women, but few women choose this method. In 1988, 1% of contraceptive users, or 0.7 million women, reported using this method. Two reasons account for this small number. First, only two IUDs are currently marketed in the United States because of product liability concerns of the manufacturers. This concern grew from serious complications caused by an earlier IUD, the Dalkon Shield. Thousands of women developed PID and subsequent sterility as a direct result of using it. Lawsuits filed by previous users against the manufacturer resulted in settlements costing over $6 million, and the Dalkon Shield was taken off the market. Second, evidence of risk of PID with current IUDs has been contradictory, causing some clinicians to discourage IUD use. In the last 3 years, research indicates no increased risk for PID if IUD users are carefully selected. Both IUDs require sterile technique for insertion by a trained physician or practitioner (Hatcher et al., 1990).

The Copper T380 is T shaped and made of plastic, with barium added to create radiographic visibility. Both arms are wrapped with fine copper wire. A thin polyethylene "string" extends from the vertical stem (Fig. 7-6). At insertion the horizontal arms are folded down into the inserter barrel, and the string is cut long enough to extend into the vagina, about 5 cm. This IUD is effective for up to 6 years.

The Progestasert is also T shaped and made of a polyethylene, with barium added. In addition, the vertical stem contains a reservoir of 38 mg of progesterone. It has a string attached to the end of the vertical stem. It is effective for a year. Users of both IUDs should periodically check that the IUD remains in place by inserting a finger into the vagina to locate the string. A woman must be advised to check the location of the string after each period and any time she has abnormal cramps during a period. If she cannot feel the string, she should notify her care provider. She must also be advised not to try to remove the IUD herself but to have it removed by her care provider.

Mechanism of Action and Method Effectiveness

The exact way that IUDs prevent pregnancy is not completely understood. Although the IUD is placed in the uterus, it also alters fallopian tube function. IUD actions include:

- Sperm immobilization during migration through the uterus.
- Ova moving faster than normal through the fallopian tube because the IUD alters normal peristalsis.
- Endometrial lining discouraging implantation because the IUD causes a local inflammatory response and increased uterine production of prostaglandins.
- The copper in the IUD competing with zinc and altering endometrial cell growth.
- The endometrium becoming hostile to implantation.

With a typical user failure rate of 0.8% in the first year of use, the Copper T380 has one of the lowest failure rates of any reversible contraceptive. Progestasert has a failure rate of 2% in the first year of use. Accidental pregnancies occur less

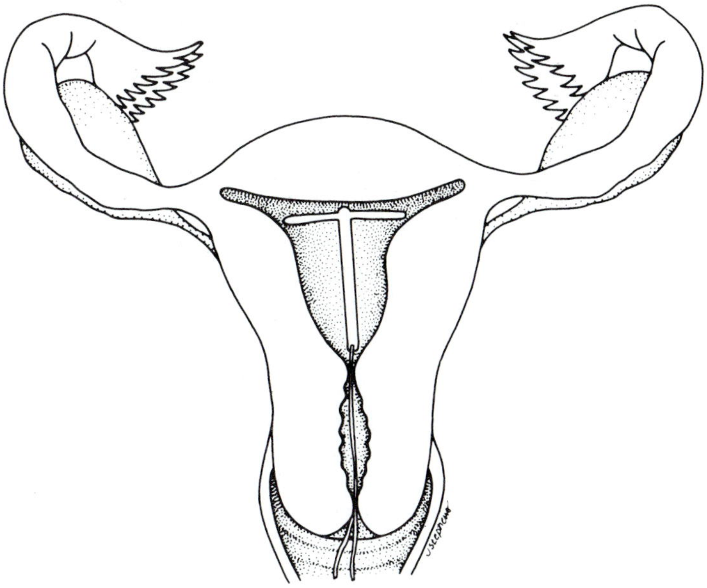

Figure 7-6.
Placement of an intrauterine device within the uterus with strings extending from the cervical os (Childbirth Graphics®, Waco, Texas).

often among older IUD users, reflecting the natural decline of fertility with advancing age. Occasionally, an IUD will be expelled either completely or partially from the uterus. Expulsions, either undetected, or partial, account for one third of all pregnancies among IUD users (Mosher & Pratt, 1990b).

Safety and Benefits

Most complications associated with IUD use can be avoided if two conditions are met: skilled insertion and a user who has not had recurrent STDs or PID. Complications include vasovagal response to insertion or removal, perforation of the cervix or uterus, pregnancy, and PID. Danger signs are listed in the accompanying display.

Any woman who has previously experienced syncope caused by painful insertion procedures should either not have an IUD or should have paracervical anesthesia for the insertion to minimize the painful sensation. For nulliparous women, dilating the cervix even a few millimeters may trigger this response. If it occurs, the procedure must be halted, rescheduled, and a paracervical block used.

Perforation of the cervix or uterus happens in about 1 in 2500 users. The IUD that perforates the cervix may be manipulated back into the uterus and either removed or allowed to remain. Oral antibiotics are given. If the IUD has perforated the uterus, is located in the abdomen (seen by ultrasound or x-ray examination), and is not causing pain, it may be left alone or surgically removed. If any signs of bowel obstruction or pelvic infection occur, the IUD must be surgically removed.

The IUD should be removed to avoid pelvic infection if pregnancy is confirmed. However, removal causes spontaneous abortion 25% of the time. About 5% of pregnancies with a Progestasert IUD in place are ectopic, which is far higher than the ectopic rate for all pregnancies.

Pelvic inflammatory disease is another serious complication associated with IUD use. Diagnosis of PID is often difficult because symptoms are vague and laboratory confirmation of intrauterine infection is practically impossible. Treatment depends on the severity of symptoms (see Chapter 6). The device should be removed and antibiotics begun immediately, along with another contraceptive method. Moderate symptoms warrant intravenous antibiotics and possibly hospitalization; severe symptoms require hospitalization (see Chapter 6).

Side effects of IUD use include cramping and pain, spotting and bleeding, and problems with the device string. During menstruation, some women have painful cramps, which may be relieved with ibuprofen. As many as 15% to 40% of users have IUDs removed because of pain.

Menstrual flow is heavier for Copper T users and lighter for Progestasert users. The heavier flow usually does not

Danger Signs Associated with Intrauterine Device Use

The nurse must be aware of the following danger signs associated with IUD use and should advise women to contact their health care provider if they experience any of these signs:

- Late period (may mean pregnancy), abnormal spotting, or bleeding
- Abdominal pain, pain with intercourse
- Exposure to sexually transmitted infection, abnormal vaginal discharge
- Poor general health, fever, chills
- String shorter or longer in length or cannot be felt.

continue beyond the initial 3 months of use and is not a health problem, unless the user has anemia. If bleeding is irregular and occurs beyond the first 3 months of use, the user should be evaluated for pregnancy, infection, or other sources of bleeding (Mosse & Heaton, 1990).

The benefits of IUD use include long-term, continuous, and reliable contraception that requires minimal user effort. In addition, IUD use is not associated with sexual behavior and is private because the string is seldom felt during vaginal intercourse. The Progestasert also decreases dysmenorrhea and the quantity of menstrual flow (see the accompanying Teaching Considerations display).

Sterilization

Sterilization is a unique form of contraception. It results in a permanent biologic and social change. By surgically altering either the fallopian tubes in the woman or the vas deferens in the man, effective sterilization ends an individual's ability to have children. Because of its permanence, sterilization is ideal for some but inappropriate for other individuals. This method remains controversial. Historically, some groups of women have been coerced into having sterilization, yet others who desire it have been denied the procedure. For example, in the 1960s, several court-ordered cases of sterilization of mentally retarded women occurred. At present in most states, women covered by Medicaid who are under age 21 cannot have sterilization paid for by Medicaid.

Sterilization has become the most widely used contraceptive method throughout the world. In the United States, almost one fourth of women who use contraception use sterilization. Among 35- to 44-year-olds, almost half of those using contraception use sterilization (Harlap et al., 1991). Vasectomy is performed about half as often as tubal ligation. Although both methods should be considered permanent, reversing sterilization is possible, but pregnancy may not result.

Mechanism of Action and Method Effectiveness

Female sterilization is accomplished by blocking the fallopian tubes, thus preventing sperm and ova from uniting. Several methods are used, including ligation, occlusion with rings, or electrocauterization. All of these procedures require either a small abdominal incision, called laparotomy, or access through a laparoscope, which allows visualization and surgical procedures of the pelvic organs. The laparoscope is inserted into the abdomen through a small puncture, thus avoiding a surgical incision. This method requires elevating the uterus with a vaginally inserted instrument to move the uterus into view through the laparoscope. Manipulation adds the risk of uterine perforation. Both procedures require either general, epidural, or local anesthesia. If sterilization is done during the postpartum hospitalization, laparotomy is generally used.

Male sterilization or vasectomy operates on the same principle and results in either occlusion or excision of a small portion of both vas deferens (Fig. 7-7). After the procedure, sperm cannot travel out of the vas and instead are reabsorbed. Semen volume and contents remain unchanged. The surgery is done as an outpatient procedure, using local anesthesia. Through a small incision on each side of the scrotum, the vas deferens is located and a small portion is cut or cauterized. A few weeks after the vasectomy the man has a sperm count performed to ensure that no sperm remain in the vas deferens. This confirms that sterility has been achieved.

Sterilization is the most effective method of all. The failure rate after tubal sterilization is less than 4 in 1000 women, and after vasectomy 2 in 1000 men. Up to 50% of failures result from surgical error; having the tubes grow back together happens only rarely (Mosse & Heaton, 1990)

Safety and Benefits

For any individual who has decided not to have future pregnancies, sterilization is an effective, low cost, safe choice. Long-term benefits include permanent pregnancy prevention, and for some, enhanced sexuality, resulting from the elimination of the risk of unplanned pregnancy.

Two groups of risks are associated with sterilization: surgical and long term. Sterilization presents surgical risks of infection of the incision, hemorrhage, errors in the procedure, injury to adjacent organs, and reaction to the anesthesia. These complications each occur infrequently and vary with the type of procedure and expertise of the clini-

Teaching Considerations

Using Intrauterine Devices

The nurse should use the following points when teaching women about IUD use:

- All women need instructions emphasizing the danger signs associated with IUD use (see Danger Signs display). They should receive a card noting the date of insertion, the name of the device, and a telephone number for emergencies and questions.
- During the first 3 months, the woman should check often to get used to locating the string; expulsion of IUDs occurs most often in this time period.
- After 3 months, the woman should check the location of the string after each period and any time she has abnormal cramps during a period. If she cannot feel the string, she should notify her health care provider.
- The woman should keep a record of her periods. If she misses a period, she may be pregnant and should have a pregnancy test.
- The woman must be cautioned not to try to remove the IUD herself. If she wants it removed at any time, this can be done by her health care provider.

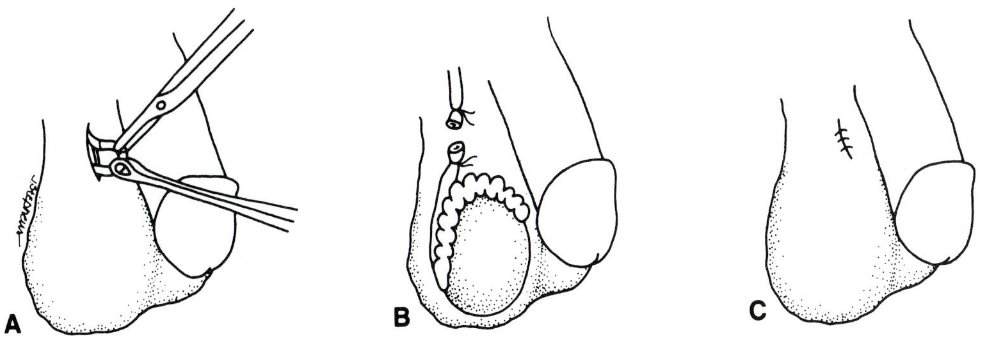

Figure 7-7.
Vasectomy. *A:* Local anesthetic is injected, and a small incision is made in both scrotal sacs. The vas deferens is pulled through the incision in each. *B:* The vas deferens is cut and tied or coagulated. *C:* The incisions are closed (Childbirth Graphics®, Waco, Texas).

cian. About 1% of sterilization procedures result in a complication.

Long-term risks include feelings of regret or loss, decreased libido, desire for reversal, or increased risk of ectopic pregnancy. Attempts to surgically reverse vasectomy and tubal sterilization can be done, but because fallopian tubes and vas deferens are delicate and complex, reversal may not be successful. Estimates of pregnancy rates after reversal in both sexes range from 40% to 90%. The higher success rates are associated with shorter time from sterilization to reversal. Ectopic pregnancy occurs from 4% to 60% of the time in an accidental pregnancy after sterilization because of spontaneous regrowth of the tubes or incomplete occlusion during the procedure (Mosse & Heaton, 1990). Ectopic pregnancy is a medical emergency. In addition to the risks associated with this method, users are not protected from STDs and should consider combining sterilization with a barrier method.

Special Contraceptive Considerations

Some women have special requirements for contraceptive care. This section addresses contraception for HIV-infected women, adolescents and contraception, and elective termination of pregnancy or elective abortion. The contraceptive needs of postpartum women are addressed in Chapter 28.

Contraception for HIV-Infected Women

At present, most methods should be available to HIV-infected women. Ideally, barriers such as condoms or the vaginal pouch should be used as protection against acquiring other STDs for the woman and for partner protection. Barriers might be combined with oral contraceptives, an IUD, a second barrier, withdrawal, or abstinence for enhanced protection. The prescription of NORPLANT for HIV women is controversial. There is the possibility that women may be coerced into using this method by otherwise well-intended providers who want to see a highly effective, provider-controlled method used by HIV-infected women. This method would almost guarantee that the risk of a pregnancy, and thus a newborn with HIV, would be prevented. However, it does nothing to prevent transmission of HIV or other STDs.

Sterilization is controversial for similar reasons. On one hand, women with HIV are entitled to freely choose to continue being fertile. On the other hand, many health care professionals find it difficult to condone a woman choosing to take any chance of giving birth to a neonate with a fatal disease.

An even more complex issue is therapeutic abortion for HIV-positive women. Although HIV-infected women who become pregnant are routinely counseled to strongly consider and undergo abortion, many clinics will not perform such abortions, and the woman may have difficulty finding a setting to have the procedure done. Research investigating HIV-positive women's decisions and rationales for coping with an unanticipated pregnancy finds that many continue to term (Stuntzner-Gibson, 1991). Nurses may be the primary contraceptive counselor for women with HIV infection and as such should examine their own views and feelings on these complex issues to offer truly patient-centered and nonjudgmental care.

Adolescents and Contraception

About 5 of every 10 unmarried 15- to 19-year-olds in a 1988 American survey reported having been sexually active at least once. One in 10 of all women in this age group become pregnant each year. Of sexually active adolescents, almost 80% report using some method of contraception (Enmans, 1992). The most popular method is oral contraceptives, followed by condoms. Although these findings are positive, several challenges exist for health care providers who work with adolescents needing contraception.

Many adolescents initiate sexual relationships before initiating contraceptive use. In fact, half of all adolescent pregnancies occur in the first 6 months after intercourse is initiated. Reasons adolescents give for not using contraception are they did not expect to have intercourse and that they did not think they could become pregnant. Other reasons include fears that contraceptive methods are dangerous, fears that parents would discover contraceptive use, and feelings of embarrassment about communicating with anyone about sexual concerns. Among adolescents who practice contraception, about one third become pregnant while using a method. Reasons for this problem are using unreliable methods, switching methods, and not using methods correctly or consistently (Enmans, 1992). Adolescent sexuality is discussed in Chapter 9.

A variety of factors affect when and how well adolescents seek and use contraception. Research has revealed several social and developmental factors that interact as determinants of contraceptive use:

- Frequency of sexual intercourse
- Perceived probability of pregnancy
- Outcome of sexual activity
- Length and degree of intimacy in heterosexual relationship(s)
- Traditional values and religiousness
- Support by significant others (Jay, DuRant, & Litt, 1989)

Adolescents have a pressing need for information on sexuality and contraception. All adolescents need to understand that the only absolute method of contraception is abstinence. Choosing abstinence is a positive choice that all providers should reinforce. Adolescents not choosing abstinence must first recognize that they are vulnerable to pregnancy. Once they have reached this milestone, some adolescents may begin to practice contraception.

Research indicates that the nature of the interaction between the health care provider and teenager, combined with her sexual behavior and social and psychological status, influence contraceptive method compliance. The clinical setting and personnel involved also influence compliance. Ensuring confidentiality is primary, but long waits for obtaining an appointment or an impatient receptionist may also keep adolescents away (Enmans, 1992). The following strategies have been suggested for improving adolescent use of their chosen method:

- The health care provider should attempt to establish a good relationship with the adolescent and consider the possibility of noncompliance.
- Instructions for method use should be emphatic, structured, and written.
- A contact person's name and telephone number at the clinic should be clearly given to each adolescent to use if questions arise between clinic visits.
- Careful and individualized follow-up should be planned, such as a written note sent to the teen if she misses an appointment.
- Correct and consistent method use should be reinforced with praise and encouragement.
- Method use problems should be discussed, recognizing that any use of contraception takes effort and demonstrates that the adolescent is taking personal responsibility for sexuality.

Elective Abortion

As long as condoms break, pills are forgotten, sexual assault occurs, and appointments for contraceptive care are difficult to arrange, abortion will be needed to back up contraceptive methods. Women have also historically used abortion to voluntarily control fertility. Although contraception represents prevention of a problem, abortion offers one of several options for dealing with an actual pregnancy. Historically, abortion has carried enormous risk, including death. Because of fears of complications, abortion was ruled illegal in the United States at the end of the 19th century. Illegal abortions continued, however, and only in 1973, with the landmark Supreme Court decision in *Roe v. Wade* was abortion again legalized. New restrictions have recently been enacted (July 1992) by the Supreme Court ruling in the *Casey v. Planned Parenthood of Pennsylvania* case. The restrictions include a 24-hour waiting period from counseling until the procedure, with mandatory notification of at least one parent for women under 18 years old.

Today, because legalized abortions are performed in clinics and hospitals by physicians, the health risks are minimal. For example, the risk of death from a first trimester abortion is 1 in 100,000 procedures compared with 8 in 100,000 live births (Mosse & Heaton, 1990). Although the risks are now minimal for most women, abortion services are not uniformly available. Abortion has and will probably always arouse controversy for women, families, and health care providers.

In the United States almost half of women reporting an unintended pregnancy will choose abortion. Among pregnant adolescents, almost half of all those under 16 years of age elect abortion. It is important to note also that 91% of women seeking abortion report either using a contraceptive method or having discontinued use only in the previous 3 months, indicating that success with even the most effective contraceptive methods is not easily achieved by many women (Harlap et al., 1991).

Mechanism of Action and Method Effectiveness

Abortion procedures vary with gestational age, but all require surgical treatment, usually done in a day surgery unit or clinic. All women considering abortion should receive individual counseling to assist in decision-making. Nurses have an important role in this care. The following techniques are used:

- Vacuum curettage
- Dilation and evacuation
- Labor induction

Up to 13 weeks' gestation, *vacuum curettage* is the method of choice. The speculum is inserted into the vagina, and the cervix is cleansed. Paracervical anesthesia may be given. The cervical canal is dilated gently by inserting a series of tapered metal rods that increase progressively in size. Once the canal is open to about 1.5 cm, a plastic cannula is inserted into the uterine cavity. The contents are aspirated with negative suction within 3 to 5 minutes. After the vacuum aspiration, many providers gently scrape the uterine cavity with a curet (a sharp metal, spoonlike instrument) to ensure that the uterus is completely empty.

Dilation and evacuation is generally used between 13 and 16 weeks' gestation. Some providers use this procedure up to 20 weeks' gestation. It is performed in the same manner as the vacuum curettage but requires greater cervical dilation and a larger aspirator cannula because the products of conception are larger.

After 16 weeks of gestation, *labor induction* abortion can be carried out with several agents that stimulate uterine contractions or cause fetal death. Prostaglandins stimulate uterine contractions and are given either as a vaginal suppository every 12 hours or as an intraamniotic infusion once. The suppositories frequently cause nausea, vomiting, diarrhea, and slight temperature rise. Prostaglandin may be combined with either hypertonic saline or hypertonic urea. Hypertonic saline, 20% solution, is injected into the amniotic sac. This is feticidal, and labor usually ensues within 24 hours. Giving intravenous oxytocin shortens labor. Saline carries significant maternal risk of severe electrolyte imbalance if it moves accidentally from amniotic fluid to the vasculature. Hypertonic urea is used in the same manner as saline but carries less maternal risk.

Second trimester abortion requires overnight hospitalization. Preparatory cervical dilation with an osmotic dilator known as laminaria is usually necessary. Once placed in the cervical canal, the laminaria absorbs body fluids, expands, and over 12 hours gradually dilates and softens the canal. Cervical lacerations occur less frequently when a laminaria is used.

Inducing early abortion with an oral medication instead of a surgical procedure has been investigated in Europe and appears to be highly effective. The drug, RU-486, is a progesterone antagonist that disrupts implantation and causes complete abortion in over 90% of women who receive it. It can only be used only up to 3 weeks after missing a period. This treatment would eliminate surgical risks, be convenient and private, and would cost about the same as vacuum curettage. Long-term risks are unknown because it has only been used since about 1988. It is not available in the United States at present (Harlap et al., 1991).

Safety

Safety is directly linked to early pregnancy diagnosis, prompt decision-making, and having the procedure done as early as possible. Additional factors include a healthy woman, a highly trained clinician, use of laminaria, the woman's understanding of danger signs and self-care, and availability of 24-hour follow-up services.

During vacuum curettage and dilation and evacuation, complications may occur. As with any use of anesthesia, the woman may react adversely to the anesthetic agents. Vasovagal shock may occur from dilating the cervix, particularly if paracervical anesthesia is not used. The cervix may be lacerated if dilation is forceful or in second trimester abortions with induced labor. The cervix or uterus may be perforated during aspiration or the scraping. Perforation occurs in fewer than 1 in 1000 procedures, but the likelihood increases with later gestational age (Mosse & Heaton, 1990).

After any elective abortion procedure, other complications are possible. The most frequent complication is retained blood clots in the uterus from the aspiration. The woman will have cramps, and the uterus will be tender and slightly enlarged on examination. The treatment is either repeating the curettage or having the woman take ergometrine, which causes sustained uterine contractions. This, in turn, will completely eliminate the blood clots. Infection may occur, but generally is easily treated with antibiotics. Continuing pregnancy may occur because of incomplete evacuation of the uterus. This occurs in less than 1% of women having an abortion; in these cases, signs of pregnancy will persist.

Hemorrhage occurs rarely after abortions performed before 13 weeks' gestation. Hemorrhage occurs more often after late abortions when the placenta is retained for more than an hour after termination. Disseminated intravascular coagulation (DIC) may result and is more frequent after saline inductions.

A woman should be advised to return for care if she experiences fever, severe or prolonged cramps, or heavy or prolonged bleeding (beyond 1 to 2 weeks); she should be provided with information about how to contact a counselor to talk about her emotional response to the experience. Routine follow-up examinations are often scheduled at 3 weeks, and the woman should be advised to avoid intercourse and tampon use until that time. See the Teaching Considerations display for additional measures.

Elective abortion may raise issues of values and reli-

Teaching Considerations

Self-care After Elective Abortion

The nurse should use the following points in teaching women about self-care following elective abortion:

- The woman may have mild to moderate cramping for several days. If so, she can take mild nonasprin pain medication.
- Most women have light bleeding for 1 to 2 weeks, with spotting lasting up to 4 weeks. The woman should use sanitary napkins, not tampons.
- The woman's next period should be in 4 to 6 weeks.
- The woman's breasts may be sore for a few days. If they produce milk, she should wear a tight-fitting bra. Milk should disappear in 1 to 2 days.
- The woman may take a shower, sponge bath, and shampoo as soon as she desires.
- She may return to her normal activities the day after the procedure. She should try to get extra rest during the next week.
- Emotions after abortion vary considerably. Most people say they feel relieved. The woman should be instructed to contact her health care provider is she wants to talk to a counselor about any emotional problem.
- The woman should wait until after her checkup at 3 weeks to begin sexual intercourse and tampon use again.
- The woman should be alert to these *danger signs*, and call her health care provider if she experiences any of these: fever over 100°F (37.7°C), severe or prolonged cramps, or heavy or prolonged bleeding.

gious beliefs for anyone. Nurses employed in a setting in which elective abortions are performed must reflect on their own attitudes and positions to decide if participation in this care would be personally congruent and professionally satisfying. In general, nurses who choose not to care for women undergoing elective abortions can negotiate within their work setting to avoid such assignments. However, should complications result from an elective abortion procedure, the nurse is professionally bound to provide life-sustaining care to any patient should that be required, regardless of the circumstances.

Implications for Nursing Care

Nurses often provide initial care for women and their partners seeking contraceptive methods. A careful assessment of the woman's health history, her goals for contraception and protection against STDs, and her life-style will assist the nurse in identifying methods that suit the woman's needs. An important part of nursing care is education about proper contraceptive techniques and safety issues associated with their use. Women and their partners also will benefit from a discussion of how a contraceptive method fits into their pattern of sexual intimacy. This is an especially important aspect for the nurse to consider when working with women whose sexual patterns are not necessarily predictable.

Evaluation and follow-up of contraceptive care is also often an important nursing responsibility. Careful evaluation of the woman's physical adjustment to a contraceptive method is needed to prevent exacerbation of undesirable side effects. Discussion with the woman, and her partner if possible, about how they view the method selected gives an opportunity to help solve any problems. This process of "troubleshooting" is critical to prevent user failures and the likely consequence of unintended and unwanted pregnancy.

At various times in their reproductive years, most sexually active women and their partners may decide to limit their fertility. Choosing to use contraception may mean a private decision and action, discussion with partners, or interaction with the health care system. Selecting and using a method involves balancing method health benefits, side effects, risks, and personal style. The nurse must use information gathered in a careful health history to identify contraceptive methods that will meet the woman's needs, personal values, and life-style. A variety of contraceptive methods are available to women today. Many, such as barrier methods, require some advanced planning, but they also confer added protection against STDs. Other methods, such as OCs, IUDs, and implants, do not require planning and preparation for sexual intimacy, but likewise do not provide any protection against STDs, and may present particular risks of their own to some women.

Infertility

Most people assume they are fertile, but only when a pregnancy occurs is fertility a fact. For an estimated 2 million women and couples in the United States, pregnancy will either require medical help or not be possible (Mosher & Pratt, 1990a). The following discussion reviews the incidence, causes, diagnosis, and treatments for infertility. In addition, the discussion highlights ethical and legal issues posed by emerging technologies for women, their families, and health care providers.

The discussion concludes with a description of the crucial role of nurses in psychosocial support for women and families adapting to this health problem. Nurses offer essential continuous support through months and even years of complex diagnosis and treatment. Recently, nurse researchers have begun to map the complex responses of individuals and couples to the diagnosis and treatment for infertility (Blenner, 1990; Hahn, 1991; Olshansky, 1988; Sandelowski, 1986; Woods, Olshansky, & Draye, 1990).

Infertility must be distinguished from decreased fertility or impaired fecundity. Infertility is the inability of a couple to conceive after 12 months of intercourse without contraception. For an individual, infertility means either that a woman cannot conceive or that a man is not able to impregnate a woman. Infertility does not describe individuals who choose not to attempt conception or persons who have chosen to be sterilized. Decreased fertility means that circumstances may impede conception but not prevent it. For example, if coitus takes place infrequently, conception may take longer than expected, but it will occur naturally. Impaired fecundity is a measure of both difficulty in conceiving and difficulty (or danger) in carrying a pregnancy to term. Thus, this term includes infertility.

Two types of infertility may occur. *Primary infertility* means the couple has never conceived despite unprotected intercourse over 12 months. *Secondary infertility* means the couple has previously conceived but is subsequently unable to conceive within 12 months of unprotected intercourse.

Incidence of Infertility in the United States

The number and percent of infertile couples has steadily decreased over the past 25 years, from 11%, or 3 million married couples in 1965, to 8% or 2.4 million couples in 1988. Infertility is directly related to age. Of women aged 15 to 19 in 1988, 2% were infertile; for women aged 35 to 39, 24% reported infertility. Women and couples of color are 1.5 times as likely as whites to have infertility (Mosher & Pratt, 1990a).

Overall, about 30% of infertile married couples seek treatment of infertility at some time in their lives. In the last decade, about 1 million couples used some form of fertility care each year, and an estimated 150,000 persons are diagnosed as infertile each year. Those with primary infertility are twice as likely as those with secondary infertility to seek care, and older women seek care more often than younger women. Although the proportion of women of color who are infertile is larger than that among European Americans, the percentage who seek care is 5% smaller (Mosher & Pratt, 1990a).

Although the number of women and couples who are infertile has been declining, the demand for services has risen sharply. In 1972, for example, 900,000 physician visits occurred for infertility care. By 1987, about 2 million visits took place. Several reasons account for this increase:

- More couples have primary versus secondary infertility.
- More physicians offer infertility services.
- Social milieu favors discussion of infertility; media awareness has increased.
- New reproductive technologies are evolving.
- Availability of children for adoption is declining.

Causes of Infertility

Often complex and not well understood, infertility results from either a problem for the woman (40% of the time) or for the man (40% of the time). About 10% of the time both partners have a problem, and for another 10%, the cause is not identified.

Female Infertility

Three factors explain most infertility in women—problems in ovulation, blocked or scarred fallopian tubes, and cervical factors. Additional less frequent causes of female infertility include:

- Endometriosis
- Congenital anomalies of the reproductive tract, including exposure to diethylstilbestrol (DES) in utero
- Overproduction of prolactin
- Strenuous exercise
- Exposure to chemicals and radiation
- Genetic abnormalities in embryos
- Illnesses such as cancer and their treatments
- Iatrogenic factors such as surgical scarring in the abdomen
- Immunologic abnormalities causing antibodies to sperm

Ovarian Factors

Ovarian dysfunction is caused by incorrect signals from the hypothalamus or pituitary to the ovary. This dysfunction leads to anovulation, the complete absence of expulsion of the mature ovum from the ovary, or oligoovulation, irregular and infrequent ovulation. In either case, conception cannot occur. Additionally, the ovary itself may not produce sufficient amounts of progesterone to prime the uterine lining (endometrium) for embryo implantation. An estimated 15% of women with infertility have ovarian dysfunction (Speroff, Glass, & Kase, 1989).

Tubal Factors

Three major causes of damaged fallopian tubes include previous PID, tubal pregnancy, and pelvic or tubal surgery. A fourth cause, IUD use, remains controversial.

Sexually transmitted diseases are the leading cause of preventable infertility. They cause PID in the reproductive tract. If these infections are not treated, they may leave scars in the fallopian tubes, damage the lining of the tubes, or block the movement of the ova and sperm in the fallopian tubes. Twenty percent of cases of infertility in the United States are caused by STDs.

The most frequent infection leading to tubal damage is from *Chlamydia trachomatis*. Ironically, this bacteria causes no notable symptoms for the infected woman (see Chapter 6). This organism alone causes 25% to 50% of all PID in women, and half of the cases of male urethritis and epididymitis. Gonorrhea acts similarly to chlamydia, but affects fewer individuals. Women who get either of these infections have a 10% risk of developing PID, and of women with PID, 10% to 20% become infertile. With three episodes of infection, the likelihood of infertility is 55% to 75% (Speroff et al., 1989).

Ectopic pregnancy occurring in a fallopian tube causes direct mechanical damage, and surgical repair causes scarring in the tube. Tubal function may be either partially or completely impaired. Pelvic surgery may result in adhesions or scarring adjacent to or in one or both fallopian tubes. Mechanical and functional damage can result.

The relationship of IUDs, PID, and subsequent infertility has been controversial. It may be that the IUD sets up a "sterile" inflammatory response that might reduce resistance to infectious organisms. Thus, a woman who has an IUD in place and then contracts an STD may develop PID more readily than if she were not using an IUD.

Cervical Factors

About 5% to 10% of infertility results from abnormal cervical mucus or mucus–sperm interaction. Normal midcycle mucus facilitates passage of motile spermatozoa, and as cervical crypts fill with the mucus at midcycle, some sperm lodge in the crypts and are gradually released. Mucus hostile to sperm may result from inadequate estrogen, vaginal or cervical infection, acid mucus, or the presence of sperm antibodies in the mucus.

Male Infertility

The only factor definitively linked with male infertility is abnormal formation, number, or motility of sperm. Often no specific cause for these conditions is identified. Additional causes of male infertility include varicocele (varicosity in the testicle); hypospadias or other congenital anomalies of the reproductive tract; retrograde ejaculation, impotence; chemical agents or excessive heat; infections; and immune disturbances of the sperm.

Sperm Abnormalities

The vast majority of infertile men have either faulty sperm production (spermatogenesis), abnormally formed sperm, or sperm with impaired motility. Abnormal semen characteristics result from changes in hormonal levels; genetic abnormalities such as retrograde ejaculation; and from drug use, exposure to occupational and environmental toxins, infection, or surgery. If testicles are exposed to only slightly elevated temperatures, for example in an industrial occupation, sperm maturation may be impaired. Smoking further alters sperm motility and cell formation.

Varicocele. Whether varicocele impedes fertility is controversial. The possible mechanism responsible for disturbed spermatogenesis is that blood pooled in veins increases the testicular temperature, or decreases oxygenation of the testis, which in turn kills the sperm or speeds up sperm production abnormally. Causes of varicocele are also unknown.

Identification and Treatment of Infertility

Wrestling with the realization that something as natural as pregnancy may be impossible often triggers complex emotions. Although individual responses are highly variable, some commonalities seem to occur. Many women experience fluctuations of emotions during the menstrual cycle, feeling hopeful as ovulation approaches and sad or despairing with onset of the menstrual flow. In addition, many women and men have a deep sense of failure because their bodies have not performed a basic function. Closely allied is the sense of loss of control.

Identifying oneself as infertile comes slowly. Perhaps, accepting oneself as infertile might block participating in an investigation of causes and the search for a cure (Woods et al., 1990). Entwined with the emotional work of coping with accepting infertility comes coping with the medical regimens required to seek answers. The following section briefly describes the standard evaluation for men and women desiring confirmation of the infertility, clarification of cause, and treatment.

Assessment

After a year of unsuccessful attempts to conceive, individuals and couples are considered infertile. With the recognition of infertility comes the first in a series of difficult choices for the infertile couple.

For those who do seek evaluation of their fertility, gynecologists provide 80% of the basic evaluation and treatment. Because infertility may be complex, infertility teams are becoming prevalent. Members of the team might include a gynecologist specializing in reproductive endocrinology, a urologist, a genetic counselor, a psychologist, and a clinical nurse specialist.

Although each procedure is designed to evaluate one aspect of reproductive function, fertility evaluation must consider the couple as a unit. The components of the assessment will include for each individual:

- Complete health history that includes occupation, substance use, nutrition, exercise, emotional status
- Family health history
- Gynecologic and sexual history
- Physical examination with attention to secondary sex characteristics and structural abnormalities
- Basic laboratory testing (Jaffe & Jewelewicz, 1991)

Diagnostic Procedures

Thorough evaluation requires several procedures, and for many couples, the testing is time consuming and costly. The order of testing moves from simple to complex, as listed in Table 7-2. Tests include hormone testing, semen analysis, menstrual cycle mapping, cervical mucus evaluation, postcoital test, endometrial biopsy, hysterosalpingogram, and laparoscopy. Table 7-2 outlines the purpose and nature of each of these tests.

Treatments for Infertility

Treatment for specific causes of infertility are available. Many therapies are complex, require repetitive attempts, and have only limited success. Because women are the primary

Table 7-2. Infertility Diagnostic Tests

Test	Purpose	Method
Hormone testing (women: prolactin, thyroid, adrenal, LH, FSH; men: LH, FSH, and testosterone)	To determine normal endocrine functioning	Blood Urine (LH, FSH)
Semen analysis	To determine normal sperm count, motility and morphology, and normal pH and viscosity of semen	Masturbated sperm sample
Menstrual cycle mapping	To determine normalcy of menstrual patterns over 6 mo period; to track ovulatory and anovulatory cycles	Basal body temperature
Cervical mucus evaluation	To determine qualities of cervical mucus, which reflect normal functioning: elasticity (spinnbarkheit), presence of cells, debris, organisms	Cervical mucus
Postcoital test (women)	To test receptivity of cervical mucus to sperm penetration	Cervical mucus (1–2 d before ovulation) immediately after intercourse
Endometrial biopsy	To determine if cyclic development of endometrium is normal	Suction biopsy of uterine lining
Hysterosalpingogram	To determine if fallopian tubes are patent	Injection of radiopaque dye through cervix, with serial x-rays to track dye through cervix, uterus, and tubes
Laparoscopy	To permit direct observation of ovaries, tubes, and uterus	Insertion of lighted scope into abdomen under general anesthesia

FSH, follicle-stimulating hormone; LH, luteinizing hormone.

subjects for many of the therapies, some commentators have expressed concern that women are more directly at risk for emotional and physical trauma induced by these technologies. Women seem to bear a greater degree of guilt when their bodies do not produce a pregnancy (Olshansky, 1988; Woods et al., 1990).

Female Infertility Treatment

As with diagnosis, treatment ranges from simple to complex depending on the causes. About 80% of infertility care consists of medical and surgical procedures. Treatment focuses mainly on problems in altered ovulation and tubal dysfunctions. This section discusses treatments including stimulating ovulation with fertility drugs, treating infections, and removing scars from fallopian tubes.

New and controversial assisted reproductive technologies—in vitro fertilization (IVF), gamete transfer, and artificial insemination—are available for selected infertile women and men if the standard therapies fail. These procedures are also discussed.

Ovarian Dysfunction. Most disorders of ovulation are treated with fertility drugs, which alter hormonal interplay and stimulate ovulation. These medications have been successful in many cases and have become standard therapy. In fact, if infertility is caused only by lack of ovulation, a couple can expect their chance of conceiving to match the general population after drug therapy. However, the side effects may have implications for the woman and her partner (see the accompanying Family Considerations display).

Two drug treatments used over the past 25 years are clomiphene citrate and Perganol combined with human chorionic gonadotropin (see the accompanying display). Women must be fully informed of the side effects, risks, costs and benefits of these agents. Several other hormonal agents are available, but experience with them is still evolving (Taymor, 1990). Ovarian stimulation with these drugs is also the first step in several new assisted reproductive technologies, such as IVF, described below.

Tubal Dysfunction. If infection is diagnosed during the infertility evaluation, antibiotic therapy will successfully eliminate the problem. Unfortunately for many women, infection occurs before infertility is realized. In that case, microsurgery or laser surgery removes scarring or blockage of the tube, thus restoring tubal function. Two major complications of surgical repair are scarring from the microsurgery or laser itself and ectopic pregnancy after tubal surgery. Ectopic pregnancies occur at alarmingly high rates after such procedures, reported as high as 4% to 38% (Speroff et al., 1989). If tubal dysfunction is not treatable and is the only cause of infertility, IVF may offer hope for some women and couples.

Male Infertility Treatment

Male infertility generally is related to problems in production of normal sperm. Relatively few treatment modalities are available for male infertility compared with those available to treat female infertility.

Family Considerations

Clomiphene-Induced Mood Swings

A qualitative study of 25 couples treated for infertility was conducted to explore personal and interactional experiences while on clomiphene therapy. Of the 50 individuals interviewed, 14 women had taken clomiphene; of these women, 9 experienced mood swings. Their experiences regarding mood swings were described in three phases over time: unawareness of the relationship between mood swings and the drug, gaining awareness of that relationship, and managing the mood swings. Couples in this study named these mood swings "the Bambi-Hitler syndrome"; women reported this as causing altered perceptions and a distorted sense of reality.

This study suggested that mood swings may be more prevalent than is commonly acknowledged by health professionals. Mood swings may pose some situational distress for couples. This may exacerbate already high levels of stress in couples being treated for infertility. Certainly, further study with larger samples should assess the prevalence of clomiphene-induced mood swings. Anticipatory guidance in regard to possible drug side effects may be an important aspect of nursing care for families undergoing infertility treatment.

Blenner, J. (1991). Clomiphene-induced mood swings. Journal of Obstetric, Gynecologic, and Neonatal Nursing, *20(4), 321–327.*

Sperm Abnormalities. Although identification of abnormalities in sperm and semen are relatively simple, few medical treatments exist for correcting these problems. Technologic advances have, however, made artificial insemination a highly successful treatment, particularly for the 25% of men with no identified cause for their sperm production or function (Amar, 1991).

Intrauterine insemination with a concentrated sample of the partner's sperm can be used for male infertility. This procedure can also be used for women with cervical mucus that is hostile to sperm or if the cervical canal is abnormal. Insemination occurs close to ovulation and is simple and usually easily tolerated. Success rates, however, are low (Taymor, 1990).

Varicocele. For the 20% to 40% of infertile men with testicular varicocele, the varicocele can be surgically corrected by ligating the varicose vein. This treatment remains controversial because it may not improve impaired spermatogenesis.

Medications to Induce Ovulation

Medication

Clomiphene citrate (Clomid)

Purpose and Action

Clomid correct anovulations; increases FSH and LH, which stimulates follicle growth

Administration

Daily, 50 to 100 mg orally for 5 days

Side Effects

Vasomotor flushes (10%); abdominal bloating or pain (5%); and breast soreness, visual symptoms, headache (each less than 2%)

Disadvantages and Complications

Multiple pregnancies, almost entirely twin (5%); long half-life; 50% is cleared by 5 days, thus 50% is present after ovulation; no increase in spontaneous abortion or congenital anomaly rate

Effectiveness

After three cycles of use, ovulation in 80% of users; pregnancy in 40% of those who ovulate

Medication

Human menopausal gonadotropin (Perganol) contains combined FSH and LH with human chorionic gonadotropin (HCG)

Purpose and Action

Perganol directly stimulates ovarian follicle growth; usually reserved for failed clomiphene treatment, whereas HCG affects ovulation

Administration

Daily injections (it is inactive orally) or 6 to 12 days of Perganol; one injection of HCG to stimulate ovulation

Side Effects

None

Disadvantages and Complications

Costs about $1000/cycle; invasive route of administration; requires frequent ultrasound and serum estrogen measurements to monitor follicle growth; intercourse or intrauterine insemination must be scheduled; multiple pregnancy rate is 20% to 25% with associated fetal loss and premature birth; ovarian hyperstimulation syndrome (1%) causing ascites, hemorrhage, and ovarian damage, may be life threatening

Donor Insemination. If all of the previously described treatments are unsuccessful or not applicable, donor insemination is an available option. Donor insemination has been used successfully for years in the United States and is becoming increasingly sought by lesbian women as well as heterosexual women and couples. The treatment involves monitoring ovulation by urinary LH testing and timing insemination to coincide with ovulation. If infertility is due to sperm factors, pregnancy usually occurs after five to seven cycles of properly timed inseminations. The incidence of spontaneous abortion and genetic defects appears to be lower than for the general childbearing population. This may be attributed to careful donor sperm selection.

Donor selection criteria and screening have been rigorously established in the last decade. All donors should be tested for HIV infection; all semen specimens are cryopreserved (frozen and stored) to recheck for HIV after 6 months. If the donor remains HIV negative, the sample is used. Guidelines prohibit mixing donor and any other (ie, partner) samples to keep paternity clearly separate. Whether the woman or couple using the sample should have access to nonidentified donor health information remains controversial. The question of commercial monetary gain for donors is also a highly debated issue. In addition, some infertile women and couples are selecting donors known to them. This raises new and complex issues of parental rights for the donor or the psychological impact of being a donor with knowledge of, but limited or no contact with, the offspring (Hahn, 1991).

In vitro fertilization has recently become accepted as a treatment for male infertility because fertilization can occur with a small number of motile sperm. IVF is, however, less successful if the cause of infertility is the male factor rather than the female factor.

Technologic advances in infertility treatments offer promise for male problems. For example, micromanipulation, or retrieving and placing sperm in particularly advantageous locations in the woman's reproductive tract for fertilization, is being studied. This technique permits sperm to be put into the zona pellucida or directly into the cytoplasm of the ovum in the woman's body.

Assisted Reproductive Technologies

About 10% to 15% of couples who have not achieved a pregnancy or living neonate with the conventional treatments previously discussed may pursue more complex, expensive, and demanding therapies. Some hold promise of conception and birth. This section briefly reviews the three currently available assisted reproductive technologies: IVF; gamete intrafallopian tube transfer (GIFT); and IVF with donor egg and gestational carrier. Procedures, risks, success rates, and controversial issues are discussed for each.

In Vitro Fertilization

More than 15,000 neonates have been born worldwide since IVF was introduced in 1978. Today, over 200 clinics in the United States offer this option. The four phases of the procedure are ovarian hyperstimulation, oocyte retrieval, oocyte insemination, and embryo replacement (Congress of the United States, 1988).

Mechanism of Action. Ovarian hyperstimulation involves the same medications and monitoring used for ovarian dysfunction. The difference is, however, that 10 to 20 oocytes develop at one time. Using vaginal ultrasound guidance, all mature oocytes are retrieved directly from the ovarian follicles under local anesthesia. The procedure takes about 30 minutes and is usually easily tolerated. The oocytes are then transferred immediately to a special culture. A semen sample is obtained and the washed sperm are mixed with the oocytes. Fertilization should occur 18 to 24 hours later, and incubation continues until about the two- to eight-cell division stage. Three or four embryos are transferred through the cervix and placed into the uterus through a small catheter. If more than four embryos are successfully fertilized, they are frozen (cryopreserved) and stored for later use if the current procedure fails.

Method Effectiveness. Success for IVF is difficult to measure because of a variety of definitions of success. Some reports consider any pregnancy a success; others count births of live neonates as success. In 1990, only 19% of patients using IVF achieved pregnancy, and 14% had a delivery. Spontaneous abortion occurred for 22%, which is the expected rate for all childbearing women. On average, after one stimulation cycle, a woman has a 10% chance of a viable neonate. Thus, most couples will need to repeat IVF (Hahn, 1992).

Safety and Benefits. Problems resulting from IVF include a large number of multiple pregnancies, which is not surprising given the placement of three to four embryos. In 1988, 19% of deliveries were of multiple gestation, with associated increased rates of premature birth. The four-stage procedure carries some risks. The side effects of ovulatory drugs have been discussed. Using aspiration to retrieve the eggs could lead to trauma to pelvic and abdominal organs; the catheter for transfer could damage the endometrium; and one or more of the embryos could implant in the fallopian tubes, causing ectopic pregnancy (Speroff et al., 1989).

Gamete Intrafallopian Tube Transfer

Gamete intrafallopian tube transfer was developed in 1984. This technique assists women and couples with normal fallopian tube function whose infertility is unexplained.

Mechanism of Action and Method Effectiveness. GIFT has four steps:

- Ovarian hyperstimulation.
- Gamete transfer in which four oocytes are retrieved and mixed immediately with sperm from a semen sample.
- Placement of the oocyte/sperm mixture into the fimbriated end of each fallopian tube using a laparoscope.
- Support of the endometrium for implantation through administration of progesterone to ensure normal endometrial development.

Clinical pregnancy rates for 135 clinics reported for 1990 was 29% of 3700 GIFT procedures. Almost 900 births occurred (22% of the pregnancies), and spontaneous abortion and multiple gestation rates were similar to IVF rates. The pregnancy and birth rate successes are thought to be better for GIFT than IVF because incubation and embryo development in the natural location of the fallopian tube is better than in the laboratory (Mosher & Pratt, 1990a).

Safety and Benefits. The safety and benefits associated with GIFT are comparable to those of IVF.

Legal and Ethical Implications

For either IVF or GIFT, using oocytes from a woman with normal ovaries has recently become possible. This provides another means of fertility for some women who cannot produce viable oocytes. Involving a third person in reproduction raises serious issues for all three adults and most of all for the children who are created. Legal safeguards are of paramount importance, but issues have not been legally clarified.

Another extension of the IVF process involves the use of a surrogate. Women with either impaired uterine function or a disease that could be life threatening during pregnancy, such as severe heart disease, can consider this option. Surrogate mothers have not been widely used because the procedure raises several psychological and legal issues needing clarification and research. For example, would the genetic mother or the gestational carrier be the child's actual parent? Or, a wealthy woman could "hire" and pay a woman of lower income to bear her child for a fee that would be substantial for her. Our legal system remains undecided and untested on how to define the rights of the gestational mother. At this time the rights of the gestational mother remain subordinate to the rights of the genetic mother or couple.

Human Responses to Assisted Reproductive Technology

The array of reproductive options may hold hope for many infertile couples. One nursing study of seven couples using assisted technologies found several common themes in their experiences:

- A driven quality in the couple's pursuit of a conception.
- Difficulty stopping treatments before they were sure they had tried everything possible.
- Marital and sexual disruption.
- Cyclic pattern of hope as a new treatment cycle began and despair if the treatment failed repeatedly.

Olshansky (1988) concluded that "serious emotional stresses are created in response to high technology treatment." Nurses must develop and test models of interventions based on this understanding to improve the quality of life for couples as they undergo months of treatments (see the accompanying display).

The Experience of Infertility Diagnosis and Treatment

Multiple diagnostic tests, invasive procedures, and repeated, complex treatment may induce stress, fatigue, or a sense of isolation for some individuals. Nurses working with individuals with infertility must examine the effects of the medical regimens, assisting couples with healthy adaptation during the months and years of care. Several nurse researchers have contributed to understanding men and women's experiences.

One study (Blenner, 1990) concluded from interviews with 25 married infertile couples that couples pass through discrete stages in treatment. These stages were:

- Dawning awareness that fertility cannot be assumed.
- Facing the new reality by confirmed diagnosis of infertility.
- Having hope and determination that treatment will result in conception.
- Intensifying treatment—making it a central life focus.
- Spiraling down when no treatment appears to be successful.
- Letting go or going through the motions of treatment.
- Quitting treatment and grieving the loss of fertility.
- Shifting focus to other areas of life or toward adoption.

Identifying Blenner's stages may help couples anticipate and cope with the long-term nature of infertility care. Often couples may move back and forth among these stages before resolving their feelings about their infertility.

Another study of the coping methods of 24 women during a year of diagnosis and treatment found decreases in the sense of mastery over life, self-esteem, and support from their partners. After a year of infertility treatment, women had either overcome infertility and had become pregnant, were working toward circumventing infertility through treatment, or were reconciling themselves to infertility and were seeking adoption or deciding to live child free (Davis & Dearman, 1991).

At present, only 50% of infertile couples achieve a pregnancy (Hahn, 1992). For many couples, infertility treatment is the central focus of their lives for several years. Stopping too soon may mean not trying another treatment that might prove successful. For many couples, the cost of therapy exhausts personal resources.

Some couples may be waiting for providers to advise stopping, but for many physicians and nurses, the quest for conception is also consuming and may seem achievable. This attitude, however, may prevent the provider from even discussing the option of halting treatment. For other couples and individuals, coming to terms with infertility requires mourning the potential loss of conception, pregnancy, and parenthood. Questions that might help infertile individuals as they decide whether to proceed or stop include:

- Is further treatment worth the pain, expense, and disruption?
- Is adoption or childless living becoming an acceptable option?
- Is treatment costing so much that other goals are sacrificed?
- If it is not yet time to stop, when will it be?

Two questions that those involved in infertility care need to consider about the services they provide involve access

Nursing Approaches to Helping Infertile Women

Preserving self-esteem can be fostered through:

- Acknowledging the validity of women's experiences and emotional responses
- Minimizing the interference of infertility treatment with other sources of esteem, such as work
- Offering mutual participation and promoting control in the health care system by offering choices, encouraging vacations, scheduling tests and treatments in a flexible fashion, sharing knowledge, and supporting a woman's decision to stop treatment.

Promoting access to social resources reflects the importance of positive affect and affirmation in infertile women's lives. Social resources can be enhanced through:

- Preserving emotional ties to family and friends by providing them with information about infertility, its treatment, and how to help
- Helping infertile women share their experience with others, especially other women
- Permitting and acknowledging that one's partner may be at a different place emotionally and may also need support in working through feelings related to infertility
- Lobbying for health policies that include third-party payment for infertility services

Finally, facilitating the use of coping methods that reduce distress can occur through:

- Balancing direct coping methods (such as problem solving) with indirect coping methods (such as avoidance and withdrawal)
- Expanding support networks to include others experiencing infertility, such as through RESOLVE, to deflect support demands from spouses
- Integrating attention to emotional care and physical care in infertility clinics

From Woods, N., Olshansky, E., & Draye, M. (1990). Infertility: Women's experiences. Health Care for Women International, 12, *188.*

and cost (see the Legal/Ethical Considerations display). These questions directly determine who seeks and gets health care for prevention and treatment of infertility in the United States. Preventive measures such as screening and care for STDs is widely accepted and financed. Some diagnostic testing such as semen analysis is relatively inexpensive, but a thorough evaluation and conventional treatment for ovarian drug treatment is estimated at $9000/woman in 1992 and is successful only about 30% of the time. IVF and GIFT are not covered by many private insurance plans or Medicaid. In 1992, an estimated $1.7 billion was spent on infertility diagnosis and treatment. Debate over federal financing of advanced technologies remains controversial in light of the cost of health care needs for the nation. Without federal funding, low-income women and men will most likely not have the choice of sophisticated diagnostic methods and treatments (Gennaro, Klein, & Miranda, 1992).

Legal/Ethical Considerations

Access to High Technology Infertility Services

The high cost of artificial reproductive technology has become a topic of growing concern as costs of health care continue to escalate. The costs of such services are now beginning to approximate the other costly services provided in intensive care units; however, infertility services are not lifesaving services. Future discussions about rationing of health care services will certainly include the topic of high technology infertility services.

Another issue of concern is the fact that not all individuals have equal access to infertility services. Those who can afford to pay or whose insurance carriers will cover the costs of such services can hope to realize their goal of conception. However, infertile individuals who are not insured or who rely on public assistance programs do not have access to these services. Health care providers will need to consider the reality that health care is rationed based on the ability to pay. Nurses who work with women during their childbearing years will need to become informed about the issues of access to infertility services and be prepared to help families make appropriate decisions about their own fertility status. Decisions about rationing of care will not become easier in the next decade, and nurses are likely to be closest to those whom decisions most directly affect.

Gennaro, S., Klein, A., & Miranda, L. (1992). Health policy dilemmas to high technology infertility services. Image, *24(3), 191–194.*

Implications for Nursing Care

At every step of the diagnostic and treatment process, the nurse has a key role in providing current and correct information, anticipatory guidance, and emotional support. Assessment of individual coping and stress is ongoing. Most couples would benefit from professional counseling, particularly if a couple is divided about choice of treatment options or is considering options involving a donor.

Perhaps the single most important intervention for the nurse is assisting individuals with decision-making because the "succession of decisions facing all infertile couples is a major source of stress" (Sandelowski, 1986). Another intervention is providing anticipatory guidance for the variety of diagnostic testing both partners may require. Many of these tests may involve embarrassment or a sense of intrusion. Recognizing that many people feel a loss of control, the health team's philosophy and strategies should be truly family centered. Treatment timetables and choices should be mutually decided on by the woman, her partner, and the health care team.

For many women and couples, infertility is a *potential* loss rather than a real loss of a pregnancy and a neonate. Resolution may be more difficult because it is an unrecognized loss, "socially unspeakable"; there are no social rituals or social support for failure to conceive (Menning, 1988). Discontinuing infertility treatment may also trigger grief as individuals attempt to separate from the elusive, exhausting hope of childbearing.

Because our society is strongly pronatalist, couples may feel negative social pressure if they do not have a child. Nurses working with couples after they discontinue infertility efforts must validate their choice to be childless or their desire to seek adoption.

Although research is under way to investigate responses of women and men to infertility, usually studies are limited exclusively to middle and upper class white married couples. Determining perceptions and experiences of women and couples of color and less economically advantaged individuals is clearly needed. The experiences of parents who have had a child because of successful infertility treatment have not been evaluated. It would be of interest to know how parent–child relationships are affected if donor insemination or oocyte placement has been used. Finally, models of specific nursing interventions must be tested, refined, and evaluated.

Nurses provide essential reproductive health care to patients adapting to and managing their own fertility. The basis for nursing assessment and care is respect for each individual's beliefs and values about the body and the desire to prevent or postpone pregnancy.

Women and couples who find pregnancy a distant hope adapt to a health problem with significant emotional impact. For those who seek assistance to conceive, a wide array of promising and rapidly developing diagnostic and treatment technologies awaits them. Along with hope, these technologies raise difficult choices and questions for infertile individuals and health care providers. Such issues as treatment effectiveness, emotional and financial cost for complex procedures, and equal access to care influence the decision-making process. In addition, assisted reproductive technologies require serious consideration of parental rights, psychological outcomes, and the social place of childless individuals.

Nurses work with couples and individuals continuously through the often arduous process of achieving parenthood. Nurses are in a position to provide emotional support and to assess how the woman and her partner are coping with the stressors. These interventions should lead to optimal emotional adaptation, regardless of whether the outcome is helping the couple achieve the hoped-for pregnancy or helping them to move to acceptance, resolution, and a new life.

Chapter Summary

The process of controlling fertility is complex, and one that brings most women to the health care system for assistance at one point or another in their lives. For some, the issue is safe, affordable, and comfortable contraception. Others require assistance in determining their own reproductive potential and enhancing that potential, if possible.

Nurses are involved in virtually every aspect of fertility care. Nurses are in a unique position to provide women and their partners with accurate information about their options and to help them sort out the right choice from the many available to them. More important, nurses are able to help women and their partners toward healthier and more productive lives by guiding them toward choices that are right for them. By doing so, nurses have a direct and positive effect on the health status of women and their families.

Study Questions

1. *What three factors influence choosing a contraceptive?*
2. *What are the advantages and disadvantages to coitus interruptus?*
3. *After choosing one of the four methods of natural family planning, explain how and why it works?*
4. *What are the similarities and differences among the three female barrier methods of contraception?*
5. *What are three health benefits of oral contraceptives? What are three major complications of oral contraceptives?*
6. *What are the basic diagnostic tests included in an infertility work-up? Describe them and discuss the appropriate times for performing these tests?*
7. *What are the common causes of infertility for men and women and the treatment available for each?*
8. *What is known about the emotional aspects of infertility, particularly how it affects the lives of those experiencing it?*
9. *What specific nursing interventions can be used to assist women and couples in decision-making during infertility evaluation?*
10. *What are three ethical issues for couples or individuals choosing donor-assisted technology?*

References

Amar, L. (1991). Male infertility. In C. Garner (Ed.). *Principles of infertility nursing*. Boca Raton, FL: CRC Press.

Blenner, J. (1990). Passage through infertility treatment: A stage theory. *Image*, *22*(3), 153–158.

Congress of the United States (1988). *Infertility: Medical and social choices*. Washington, DC: US Government Printing Office.

Davis, D., & Dearman, C. (1991). Coping strategies of infertile women. *Journal of Obstetric, Gynecologic, and Neonatal Nursing*, *20*(3), 221–224.

Enmans, J. (1992). Teens and contraception: Encouraging compliance. *Contraception Report*, *11*(6), 4–7.

Gennaro, S., Klein, A., & Miranda, L. (1992). Health policy dilemmas related to high technology infertility services. *Image*, *24*(3) 191–194.

Hahn, S. (1992). Caring for couples considering alternatives in family building. In C. Garner (Ed.). *Principles of infertility nursing*. Boca Raton, FL: CRC Press.

Harlap, S., Kost, K., & Forrest, J. (1991). *Preventing pregnancy, protecting health: A new look at birth control choices in the United States*. New York: The Alan Guttmacher Institute.

Hatcher, R., Stewart, F., & Trussell, J. (1990). *Contraceptive technology* (15th ed.). New York: Irvington Publishers.

Jaffe, S., & Jewelewicz, R. (1991). The basic infertility investigation. *Fertility and Infertility*, *56*(4), 599–613.

Jay, M., DuRant, R., & Litt, I. (1989). Female adolescents' compliance with contraceptive regimens. *Nursing Clinics of North America*, *36* (3), 731–746.

Lethbridge, D. (1991). Choosing and using contraception: Toward a theory of women's contraceptive self-care. *Nursing Research*, *40*(5), 276–280.

Menning, B. (1988). *A guide for the childless couple* (2nd ed.). New York: Prentice Hall.

Mosher, W., & Pratt, W. (1990a). *Fecundity and infertility in the United States: 1965–1988*. Washington, DC: US Department of Health and Human Services.

Mosher, W., & Pratt, W. (1990b). *Contraceptive use in the United States: 1973–1988*. Washington, DC: US Department of Health and Human Services.

Nofzinger, M. (1988). *Signs of infertility: The personal science of natural birth control*. Nashville: MND Publications.

Olshansky, E. (1988). Responses to high technology infertility treatment. *Image*, *20*(3), 128–132.

Sandelowski, M. (1986). Sophie's choice: A metaphor for infertility. *Health Care for Women International*, *7*(2), 439–442.

Sharts-Engel, N. (1991). Levonorgestrel subdermal implants (NORPLANT) for long-term contraception. *American Journal of Maternal Child Nursing*, *16*(4), 232–236.

Speroff, L., Glass, R., & Kase, N. (1989). *Clinical gynecologic endocrinology and infertility* (4th ed.). Baltimore: Williams & Wilkins.

Stuntzner-Gibson, D. (1991). Women and HIV disease: An emerging social crisis. *Social Work*, *36*(1), 22–28.

Taymor, M. (1990). *Infertility: A clinician's guide to diagnosis and treatment*. New York: Plenum Publishing.

Woods, N., Olshansky, E., & Draye, M. (1990). Infertility: Women's experiences. *Health Care for Women International*, *12*(3), 179–185.

Suggested Readings

Blenner, J. (1991). Health care providers' treatment approaches to culturally diverse infertile patients. *Journal of Transcultural Nursing*, *2*(2), 24–27.

Dunnington, R., & Estok, P. (1991). Potential psychological attachments formed by donors involved in infertility technology—another side of infertility. *Nurse Practitioner*, *16*(11), 41–48.

Harris, B., Sandelowski, M., & Holditch-Davis, D. (1991). Infertility and new interpretations of pregnancy loss. *American Journal of Maternal Child Nursing*, *16*(4), 217–224.

King, J. (1992). Helping patients choose an appropriate method of birth control. *American Journal of Maternal Child Nursing*, *17*(2), 91–95.

Jarret, M., & Lethbridge, D. (1990). The contraceptive needs of midlife women. *Nurse Practitioner*, *15*(2), 34–39.

James, C. (1992). The nursing role in assisted reproductive technologies. *NAACOG Clinical Issues in Perinatal and Women's Health Nursing*, *3*(2), 328–334.

Lasker, J., & Borg, S. (1987). *In search of parenthood: Coping with infertility and high-tech conception*. Boston: Beacon Press.

Lethbridge, D. (1991). Coitus interruptus as a method of birth control. *Journal of Obstetric, Gynecologic, and Neonatal Nursing*, *20*(1), 80–85.

Lommel, L., & Taylor, D. (1992). Adolescent use of contraceptives. *NAACOG Clinical Issues in Perinatal and Women's Health Nursing*, *3*(2), 199–208.

Low, M. (1992). Personal values and contraceptive choices. *NAACOG Clinical Issues in Perinatal and Women's Health Nursing*, *3*(2), 192–198.

Lynaugh, J. (1991). The death of Sadie Sachs. *Nursing Research*, *40*(2), 124–125.

Nathanson, C., & Becker, K. (1985). The influence of client-provider relationships on teenage women's subsequent use of contraception. *American Journal of Public Health*, *75*(1), 33–38.

Rosenberg, M., Davidson, A., Chen, J., Judson, F., & Douglas, H. (1992). Barrier contraceptives and sexually transmitted diseases in women: A comparison of female-dependent methods and condoms. *American Journal of Public Health*, *82*(5), 669–674.

Tucker, S. (1991). The sexual and contraceptive socialization of black adolescent males. *Public Health Nursing*, *8*(2), 105–112.

UNIT III

Adaptation in the Prenatal Period

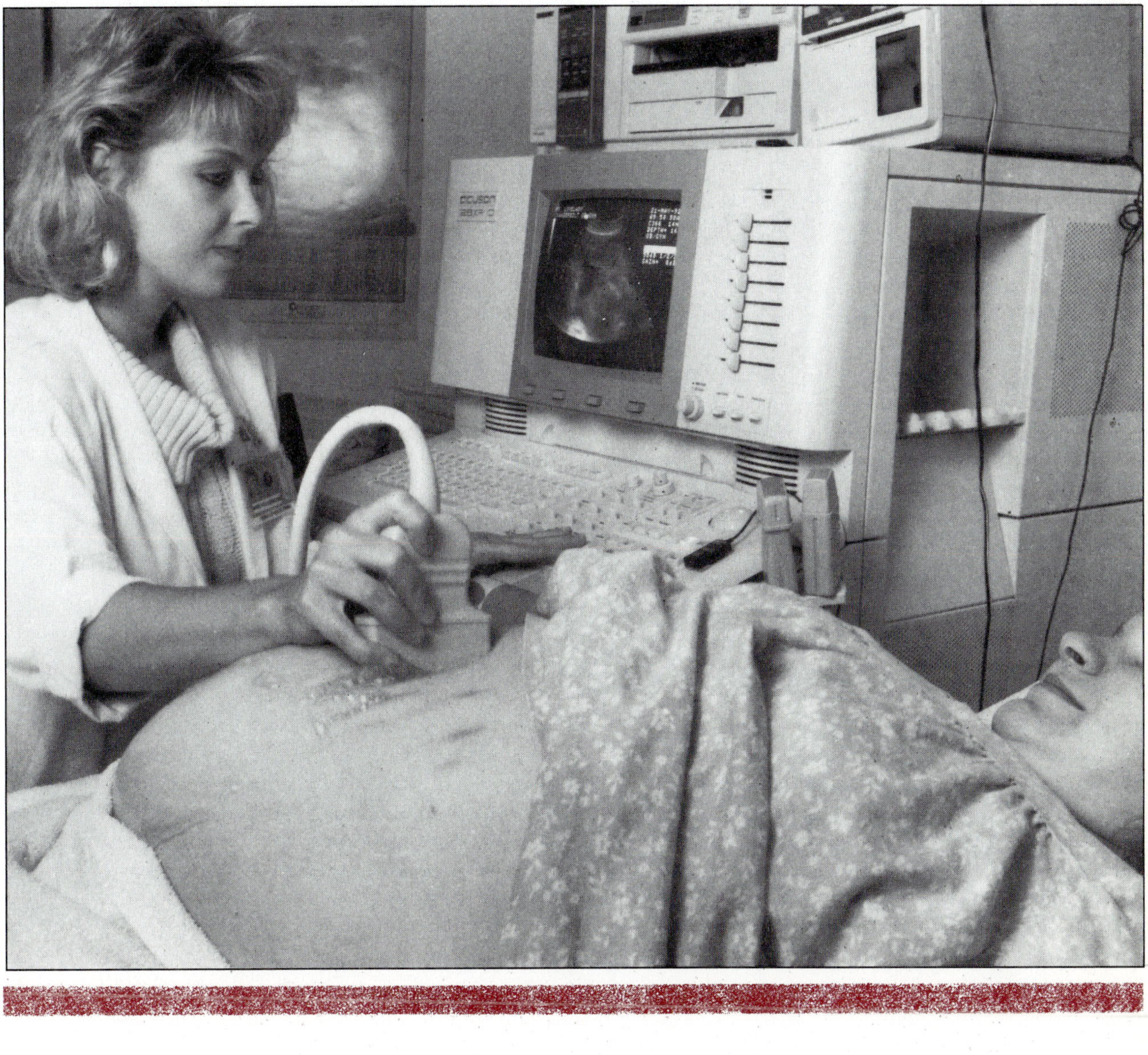

CHAPTER 8

Individual and Family Adaptation to Pregnancy

Learning Objectives

After studying the material in this chapter, the student will be able to:

- Identify major social factors that influence decisions about childbearing.
- Describe how birth practices may vary across cultures.
- Discuss nursing strategies for assessing cultural variations in birth practices.
- Explain basic functions and developmental tasks of the childbearing family.
- Describe the crisis potential of pregnancy and explain why family crises may occur during pregnancy and how they can be prevented.
- List maternal and paternal tasks during pregnancy and discuss their significance for healthy individual and family adaptation.
- Identify common maternal and paternal responses to pregnancy and suggest nursing interventions.

Key Terms

acculturation
attachment
cognitive processes
couvade syndrome
cultural relativism
developmental task
ethnocentrism
maturational crisis
situational crisis

Childbearing has strong psychological and social meanings in human culture. These meanings affect human health. The strong consumer movement for family-centered maternal care, as discussed in Chapter 2, arose in part because these important issues were ignored too long in traditional obstetric care (Mathews & Zadek, 1991). The improved obstetric outcomes noted even among high-risk women cared for by nurse midwives and nurse practitioners may result in part from the delivery of more sensitive and culturally appropriate care.

Pregnancy and childbirth are events that touch nearly every aspect of the human experience: biologic, psychological, social, and cultural. Individual adaptations to childbearing on each of these levels may be different. Variations in age, health, socioeconomic status, and cultural background of the woman and her family will influence health care needs. These differences result in a wide range of individual and family needs for information and assistance during the childbearing year.

Despite this tremendous natural variation, recurring themes or patterns can guide the nurse in providing sensitive and effective care. This chapter discusses the definition, structure, and function of families and how they necessitate adaptations. Major social, cultural, and psychological patterns describe how people adapt to the childbearing experience. The study of these patterns spans several disciplines, including sociology, anthropology, and psychology.

The Childbearing Family

Much research continues to be directed at understanding how individuals and families accommodate a pregnancy and eventually a newborn into their lives. Studies about the quality of adaptation to pregnancy and its impact on later family adjustments have been undertaken. Two major concerns face clinicians providing care during pregnancy.

First, the quality of a woman's psychosocial adaptation to pregnancy is related to her physical health during the childbearing year. Second, problems in the family unit during pregnancy may contribute to later family problems and deterioration in other family relationships.

Definition of Family

The family is the fundamental unit of all human societies, the unit responsible for reproduction and socialization of their young. Some common functions are shared by all families. Family structure—that is, who is considered a member of the family and what each member's roles and responsibilities are—varies widely among and within cultures. How the term *family* is defined reflects this variability in structure. No single standard definition is final. The following are some currently accepted definitions of family as used by social scientists.

- A family is a social system made up of two or more interdependent persons who remain united over time and mediate individual needs with demands of the larger society.
- A family is a group of interacting and interdependent personalities.
- A family is a group of individuals related by blood, marriage, or adoption, residing in the same household, sharing a common history, and interacting with each other on the basis of their roles in the group.

All of these definitions center on the idea that a family is composed of at least two interacting individuals bound together by emotional or social ties. An unmarried pair of adults sharing a household may be considered a family under the first two definitions but not the third.

One problem in defining family is that each individual's view tends to be based on his or her own experience. For instance, some people may consider neighbors, housemates, or even household pets as "members of the family" and interact with them on that basis. Some may believe that couples not bound by blood or marriage cannot be defined as a family. Others may believe that the presence of children is what distinguishes a family from other groups.

For the purposes of scientific writing, it is important to select a working definition of family and use it consistently. Because pregnancy and childbirth are usually considered major family events, identifying the woman's definition of family and providing care on that basis is essential. A woman's family, whatever that means to her, is most often her primary support during the childbearing year. Her family environment will have a direct influence on her emotional and physical health. This is where the neonate will be nurtured and raised. To better provide family health care, the nurse must have some understanding of the common variations in contemporary family structure and function.

Family Structure

Family structure refers to the arrangement of members and their roles. If asked to describe the typical American family structure, many would probably describe a family with a husband, a wife, and two children. This "typical" family was featured prominently in television and fiction during the 1950s. The typical family was portrayed as European American and middle class, with a father who worked to support the family, a mother who was a homemaker and cared for the children, and children who behaved well and stayed out of trouble. This tranquil view of the family probably reflected the nation's need to return to stability and traditional values after the disruption of World War II. Indeed, that view of the "typical" American family is based more on media portrayal than on reality. American families have always been more varied than that stereotypical image suggests (South & Tolnay, 1992).

During the 1950s, the birth rate increased dramatically (called the baby boom). Political, social, and economic changes during the 1960s focused attention on long-ignored aspects of American society, such as racism, sexism, and political dissent. These issues seemed to be in direct conflict with this complacent view of the family. Many people, especially the young middle class who attended college in record numbers in the 1960s, began to explore and debate sensitive issues related to the family. Relevant issues included women's roles, abortion, birth control, overpopulation, divorce, and social justice.

This reexamination of the American family led to the recognition that family structures in the United States were far more diverse than the predominant view of the 1950s. Not only was the two-parent household, with father as breadwin-

Family Structures Encountered by the Perinatal Nurse

Nuclear family: Group made up of parents and dependent children living in a single family residence, separate from family of origin. The nuclear family is the most common family unit in the United States.

Kin network or extended family: Group made up of two or more nuclear family units that provide mutual support.

Single-parent family: An adult head-of-household with one or more dependent children. This structure is becoming more common in the United States.

Nuclear dyad: Couple living without children in single-family residence.

Reconstituted or blended family: Arrangement in which remarried adults are raising children from previous marriage and/or from current marriage.

Three-generation family: Arrangement in which one or more grandparents and adult children and grandchildren live together. This arrangement is especially common among immigrants from Asia and Central and South America and other minority groups.

ner and mother as homemaker, not universal, it was also, in fact, becoming less common. New structures continued to emerge through the 1980s. The accompanying display lists family structures the perinatal nurse is likely to encounter.

Family Function

The family carries out certain functions or tasks essential to the survival of the individual as well as the larger society. Family functions center around meeting individual human needs while maintaining some sense of order and predictability in social interaction. In general, families work as cooperative groups to achieve the goals listed in the accompanying display, Basic Social Functions of the Family.

Maslow's hierarchy of needs (Fig. 8-1) suggests that basic physiologic needs must be met before the individual can reach his or her fullest potential. A comparison might be drawn with family functions. A family that is unable to meet its members' basic needs for food, shelter, safety, and security is unlikely to be able to meet higher needs. The individual may be deprived of affiliation and affection, socialization, or recreational or religious activities. On the other hand, a family in which basic needs are readily met is likely to have more resources to devote to higher needs.

Because family structures vary, not every family unit will engage in all of these higher functions. Societies are structured so that basic human needs are most often met within the family. Other social institutions, such as churches, schools, and government agencies, are created to augment family resources in certain areas, but the primary responsibility for these functions still lies with the family unit.

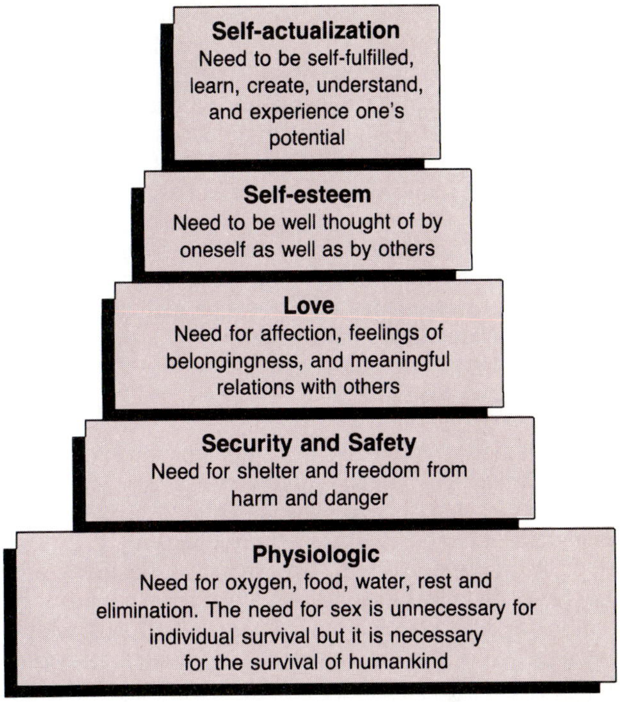

Figure 8-1.
Maslow's hierarchy of needs. (From Maslow, A. (1970). *Motivation and personality*. New York: Harper and Row.

Adaptational Demand

Developmental Tasks

As the family adapts to pregnancy, it must accomplish certain developmental tasks in preparation for birth and childrearing. The display, Developmental Tasks of the Childbearing Family, lists these tasks. The accomplishment of these tasks during pregnancy lays the groundwork for the later, more complex adaptations required when the newborn is added to the family unit.

Basic Social Functions of the Family

- Provision of basic needs for food, shelter, safety, and security
- Provision of stable sexual relationships for the adult
- Fulfillment of affection, love, and affiliation
- Reproduction
- Conferring roles and status
- Socialization of the young
- Provision of recreational needs
- Provision of religious and spiritual needs

Developmental Tasks of the Childbearing Family

- Acquiring knowledge and plans for the specific needs of pregnancy, childbirth, and early parenthood
- Preparing to provide for the physical care of the expected newborn
- Adapting financial patterns to meet increasing needs
- Defining evolving role patterns
- Adjusting patterns of sexual expression to accommodate pregnancy
- Expanding communication to meet present and future emotional needs
- Reorienting relationships with relatives
- Adapting relationships with friends and community to take account of the realities of pregnancy and the anticipated newborn
- Maintaining a health morale and philosophy of life

Adapted from Duvall, E. (1985). Marriage and family development. *Philadelphia: J.B. Lippincott.*

The nurse can observe families as they work to achieve these tasks during pregnancy. Each task requires some reorganization in current patterns of activity and interaction. The adjustments required of families during pregnancy are major and take considerable amounts of time and energy to accomplish. If a family is unable to reorganize itself to meet these developmental requirements, unmet needs will begin to mount and the family's coping mechanisms may become overwhelmed. The nurse must be able to recognize individuals and families who are beginning to experience problems in adapting to pregnancy and intervene early to promote optimal individual and family health.

Coping with Crisis

Some degree of change during pregnancy is unavoidable. That change is often required over a short period of time. Social scientists and clinicians have described pregnancy as a time of crisis, that is, an unsettling event that leads to a state of disequilibrium. A pregnancy, especially a first pregnancy, is unlike other previous life experiences. It brings with it stressors to which the couple involved must adapt. Some stressors can be described as frequent stressors. These types of stressors happen with enough regularity that they might be expected to affect most families. Other stressors may be unanticipated, such as complications of pregnancy or unexpected personal and family losses. The combination of frequent and unanticipated stressors experienced by each family is unique. Whether or not these stressors produce a crisis in the family greatly depends on factors present to balance stressors.

Balancing factors include the individual's or family's ability to perceive realistically the stress in the situation and the use of coping mechanisms to reduce and adapt to that stress. The expectant parents first respond to stress by using coping patterns that have been successful in the past. If these are successful, a crisis does not result. Often, however, previously successful coping patterns are not adequate for the demands of pregnancy, and a crisis can result (Lewis, W., 1988). Successful resolution depends on:

- How realistically the situation is perceived
- The individual's and family's precrisis level of functioning
- The range of coping patterns available
- Past success or failure in dealing with crisis, anxiety, and stress
- The resources available to the individual and family
- The ability to mobilize and use those resources

Crises are by their nature of limited duration. Because individuals and families cannot continue with high levels of anxiety and stress, they will adapt in whatever way possible to reduce the distress to tolerable levels. The crisis potential in the process of family adaptation to pregnancy is shown in Figure 8-2.

Crisis can be seen as a turning point. A crisis is dangerous because if adaptation is not successful, the potential exists for further deterioration in the individual's status and psychological regression. A crisis is an opportunity because if adaptation is successful, there is potential for considerable psychological growth and maturation.

Crises can be categorized in one of two ways, either situational, arising from a change in events or life circumstances, or maturational (or normative), arising from internal changes in the individual or family, associated with normal growth and development. Most often pregnancy is regarded as a maturational crisis (Mercer, 1990). Childbearing is a predictable event in most people's lives and is regarded in society as an important part of the transition to adulthood. However, pregnancy can also be a situational crisis. Other unexpected problems, such as maternal complications or a financial setback, can result in a situational crisis for an expectant family.

The crisis potential of pregnancy may be heightened if one partner feels that the other cannot understand and meet his or her needs adequately. Pregnancy changes something that partners usually take for granted and consider stable—their characteristic ways of relating to each other. The process of reorganizing relationships—forming new attachments, loosening old ones—is basic in human interaction. This process takes on new significance during the childbearing year.

Prenatal Attachment

In each person's life, much of the joy and sorrow revolves around attachments or affectionate relationships—making them, breaking them, preparing for them, and adjusting to the loss of attachments. Attachment and loss are an intrinsic part of the childbearing experience. The process of parent–newborn attachment has received much scientific and clinical attention. This work has most often focused on the discovery of steps in the process of attachment, the identification of factors that enhance or inhibit the formation of parent–newborn attachment, and the investigation of how clinicians can influence the process. Attachment, loss, and grief are discussed in Unit 5, in the context of postpartum and neonatal nursing care.

Attachment usually refers to a strong affiliation with another, based on a long period of mutual stimulation and response, more like the process of "staying in love." The earliest use of the term typically referred to the newborn's tie to the parent or caretaker. However, current use also includes the parent's emotional tie to the newborn (Mercer, 1990).

Women are usually aware of the growing fetus for 20 weeks or more before birth and know that the fetus is there for an even longer period. They usually demonstrate some investment in a relationship with the fetus by the middle trimester. This is true even in high-risk situations in which the woman is herself at physical risk because of the pregnancy (Mercer, Ferketich, May, DeJoseph, & Sollid, 1988). Evidence of the growing maternal–fetal attachment can be seen in maternal behavior during pregnancy. The pregnant woman may interact with the fetus either by talking or by interpreting movements. She may try to stimulate or stop fetal movement by changing positions and activities.

How the pregnant woman views the fetus varies considerably across cultures. Some groups in Southeast Asia believe that the fetus should receive tender, loving care and be taught about life almost from the moment of conception. Other groups, including many in Western countries, do not consider the fetus fully human until fetal movement has

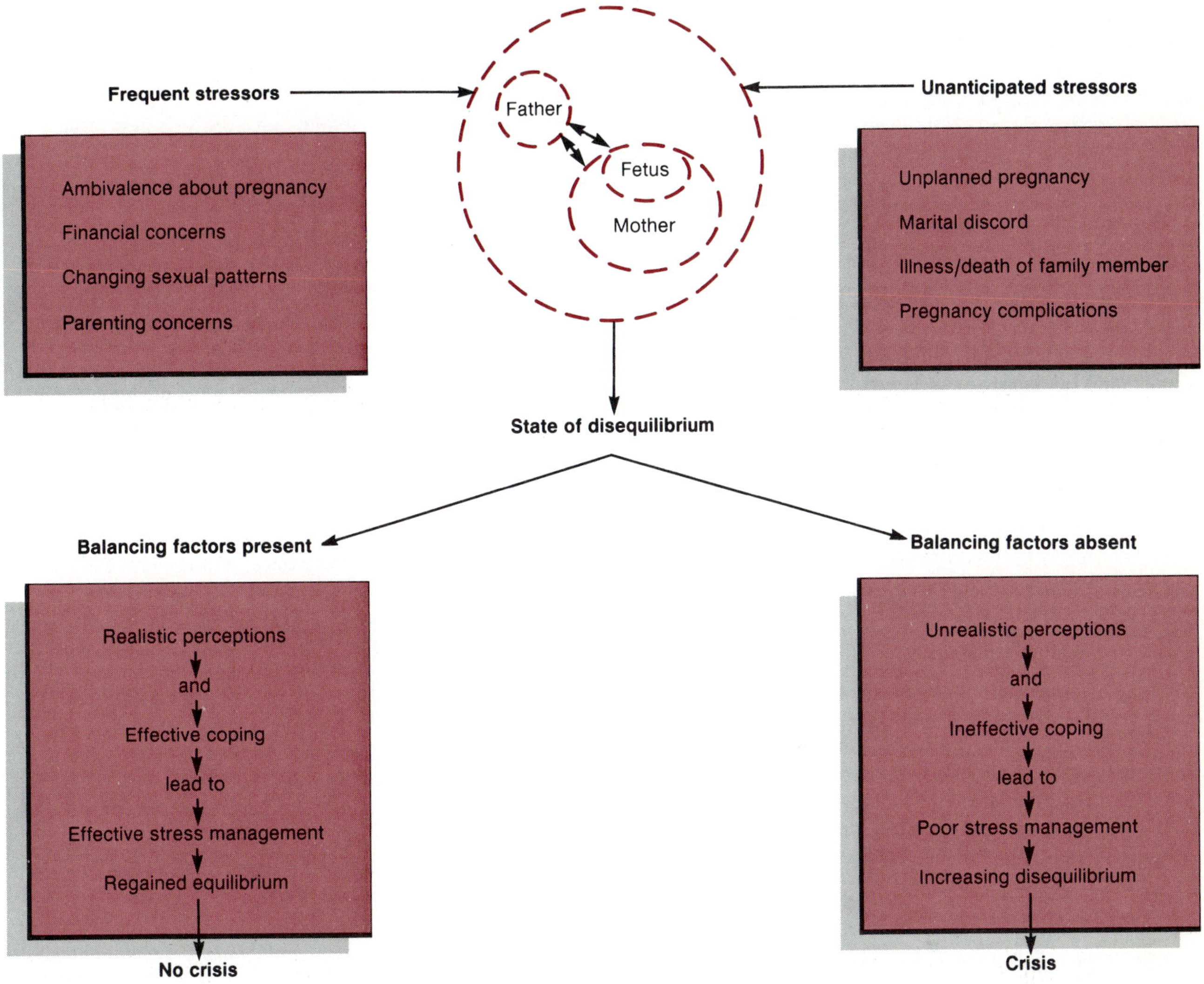

Figure 8-2.
Family adaptation during pregnancy: potential for crisis. (Adapted from Donaldson N. [1981]. The postpartum follow-up clinician. *Journal of Obstetric Gynecologic, and Neonatal Nursing, 10*[4], 249.)

occurred. Cultural beliefs will influence how prenatal attachment develops.

Prenatal maternal attachment is influenced to some extent by the biologic and hormonal changes caused by the pregnancy itself. An example is the nesting behavior of mammals. Hormonal influences trigger behaviors like nest building shortly before labor begins. Prenatal attachment in human beings cannot be explained entirely on that basis because fathers also appear to demonstrate attachment to the fetus during pregnancy (Mercer et al., 1988).

Research on paternal prenatal attachment has begun only recently. Findings appear to be similar in many ways to those among mothers. However, fathers may express their attachment to the fetus more through their involvement in activities related to the pregnancy than in interaction with the fetus. In part, this is because they have to "go through" the pregnant woman to interact with the fetus; the father's experience of fetal life is always "one step removed."

The pregnant woman and her partner together may engage in attachment behavior. Parents may use pet names for the fetus and may "play games" with the fetus in three-way interaction. The pregnant woman may try to stimulate fetal movement so the partner can feel it. Often parents will talk about the personality of the fetus and draw conclusions about sex and temperament from these early interactions (see the Nursing Research display).

Nurse researchers began to explore how to assess prenatal attachment more systematically in the 1980s and to consider what significance, if any, prenatal attachment has for the quality of later parent–newborn interaction. Tools have been developed to measure prenatal attachment, and some studies have suggested that high levels of prenatal attachment may be associated with more positive maternal perceptions of the neonate after birth (Cranley, 1981; Muller, 1992).

A major goal of perinatal nursing care is to help families make the healthiest adjustment to the normal stresses of the childbearing year. Definitions of family vary, and the nurse should identify the woman's own definition of family before planning care. Various contemporary structures of the family meet necessary basic family functions. Adaptation demands include developmental tasks, coping with pregnancy as a crisis, and beginning the process of parent-to-fetus attachment. Continuing research provides knowledge on which nursing care can be based.

Social Aspects of Childbearing

Childbearing is inherently a social process. The woman, her partner, and her family exist as members of a social group. As such, their behavior affects and is affected by those around them. Decisions about childbearing are strongly influenced by social factors, such as knowledge of sexuality and contraception, gender role expectations, and sociocultural norms.

Social Factors Influencing Childbearing Decisions

In most Western countries, the decision about whether or not to risk pregnancy is a most significant one, ultimately affecting many lives. Pregnancy usually marks a person's entry to the parental role. As such, this decision has lifelong implications. Many factors determine whether a person behaves in ways that risk pregnancy, consciously decides to have a child, or chooses to remain childless.

Knowledge of Human Sexuality

Deciding whether or not to bear children requires a sound knowledge base. In the not-too-distant past the topic of sexuality was forbidden in polite company. The mid to late 1800s, known as the Victorian Age, were characterized by sexual repression and a strong sense of modesty. Women of good character and children were considered to be pure and innocent. Women were believed to have little or no capacity for sexual response and were viewed as inferior to men both physically and intellectually. The need for sex education was considered useless and inappropriate for females and superfluous for the more sophisticated male.

This attitude prevailed until the 1920s. Influenced by new social and economic freedom for women, sexual attitudes during the Jazz Age became increasingly less inhibited. Information on birth control and marriage manuals with detailed descriptions of sexual techniques were widely published. The work of Sigmund Freud stressed the psychological importance of sexuality in motivating human behavior in both health and disease. After World War II, Alfred C. Kinsey, a zoologist from Indiana University, began his revolutionary inquiry into human sexual behavior, opening a floodgate of research on this once taboo topic. Kinsey's work was modified and advanced by such leading sex researchers as William Masters and Virginia Johnson. The belief that to understand the complexities of human sexuality a person must understand sexual anatomy and physiology as well as psychological and sociologic factors became widely held (Wertz & Wertz, 1989).

Despite efforts to increase knowledge of human sexuality, controversy still exists regarding mandatory sex education for school-age children. Proponents of mandatory sex education claim that a sound knowledge base would decrease adolescent pregnancies and the spread of sexually transmitted diseases in that population. Opponents believe that making formal sex education mandatory usurps the role of parents as educators and decreases the authority of local school officials to determine curricular content. There is considerable disagreement in the scientific community about the relationship between sexual activity and sex education. Further research is needed.

Availability of Contraceptive Options

The dramatic development in contraceptive options since the 1960s has directly affected the way people make decisions about childbearing. Contraceptives have created the opportunity for decision-making in this area. In realistic terms, throughout most of human history, parenthood (more particularly, motherhood) could not be chosen; childbear-

Nursing Research

Parents' Awareness of Their Fetus in the Third Trimester

An exploratory study of 26 couples was conducted to examine what parents know about their fetus, as reflected in their day-to-day experiences during pregnancy. Couples were interviewed, using these questions as a guide to elicit parents' perceptions: What do you know about your baby now? What does your baby do? What behaviors have you noticed? How do you know that? When does the baby do that?

Four different levels of parental awareness were identified. These levels did not necessarily develop sequentially, but sometimes coexisted. They were: awareness of the fetus as an idea, awareness of the fetus' presence, awareness of specific unborn fetal behavior, and awareness of the fetus' interactive ability.

The process of prenatal attachment is a combination of interacting maternal and paternal styles of interpreting cues and assigning meanings. This study suggested that parental development of sensitivity to the newborn begins prenatally and that this may be part of the process of parent-to-newborn attachment.

Stainton, M. (1990). Parents' awareness of their unborn infant in the third trimester. *Birth, 17*(2), 92–96.

ing was simply a predictable consequence of intercourse. Although techniques for contraception have been recorded throughout history, only in the last 50 years has contraception been reliable enough to allow people to choose the timing of pregnancy (Wertz & Wertz, 1989).

Contemporary Male and Female Roles

The nature of socially acceptable sex roles plays a large part in decisions about childbearing. Male and female adult sex roles in Western culture are still defined predominantly in terms of parenthood. Many young adults in the United States still hold childbearing as a positive value and intend to become parents at some time. This orientation toward parenthood may be more evident in women than in men. Women tend to be socialized throughout life in nurturing functions, with the expectation of motherhood. Men are socialized primarily toward a productive occupational career and only secondarily toward future fatherhood (Tiedje & Collins, 1989; Bozett & Hanson, 1991).

Even though sex roles still reflect an orientation toward parenthood, there are now competing social roles, especially for women. The costs and benefits of parenthood, especially motherhood, may be evaluated in terms of occupational roles. The modern family in America relies heavily on the earnings of the female partner employed outside the home. More than 50% of women in families with children under 5 years of age were employed outside the home in 1991, and this trend shows no evidence of weakening. Childbearing, however, typically interrupts a woman's earning power, at least temporarily, and lost income and career development usually cannot be recovered (South & Tolnay, 1992).

Women continue to be primarily responsible for management of the home and for providing or arranging for child care, even when they are also employed outside the home. This may be changing in some segments of the population. Some middle-class couples are now exploring more equal participation by the father in child care. In other cases fathers assume the primary responsibility for taking care of young infants. These arrangements may result in some financial sacrifice and loss of occupational advancement for the father. However, these changes affect only a small minority of adults of childbearing age at this time.

Peer, Partner, and Family Influences

Pressures from a partner or peers can persuade a person to risk pregnancy even when the individual is not ready to do so. Peer pressure often influences an adolescent to initiate sexual activity. In couple relationships, pressure to become pregnant may be used as a way to test or force a partner into commitment.

Family pressures may influence childbearing practices. The family continues to be the basic societal unit to perpetuate the species and socialize the young. Although childless-by-choice marriages are increasingly common and accepted, pressures on adults to bear children are still strong. Parents may expect to be provided with grandchildren. Friends and siblings who have children often try to persuade others to follow their example. Finally, with the increasing life expectancy in Western countries, the fear of growing old and being alone may be an influential factor in the decision to bear children.

Socioeconomic Influences

Socioeconomic status, usually described in terms of occupation, education, and income, may reflect values and life-styles that directly affect decisions about procreation. This can be seen in part in the differential birth rate among socioeconomic groups in the United States. Middle-class Americans are restricting their family size to two children more consistently than lower- or upper-class groups. It is interesting to note that the differences in contraceptive use and family size between social classes are becoming smaller. More couples are deferring marriage until their middle or late twenties and delaying the first birth for several years after marriage. Concerns about overpopulation, environmental pollution, or global warfare may lead some couples to delay, limit, or avoid childbearing, while motivating others to start families sooner. Some couples will delay pregnancy until adequate financial resources are available. Others feel that if they wait to become financially secure before starting a family, they will never start one.

Concepts of reproductive decisions are, in large part, products of society, socioeconomic class, and culture. Pregnancy and childbearing have specific social significance. Decisions about childbearing may be regarded as important or of little consequence. Social factors that influence reproductive behavior and decisions about pregnancy and birth need to be considered. Important factors include knowledge of sexuality; the availability of contraceptive options; the nature of socially acceptable gender roles; influences from peers, partners, and family; and socioeconomic conditions.

Cultural Aspects of Childbearing

Culture is defined as a system of goals, beliefs, attitudes, and roles that change but tend toward stability. Culture is shared by a distinct human group, transmitted by that group, and learned by succeeding generations. The culture of any particular group consists of its technology, its social structure and norms, and its belief systems. Culture develops in response to the unique psychological and physical environmental conditions experienced by a given group. Thus, cultural norms both shape human behavior and are shaped by it in a continuous process of social interaction.

The more central an event is to human existence, the more highly developed cultural practices are likely to be around that event. Events that mark changes in status tend to be particularly important; these types of events involve many unknowns and potential physical risk. Pregnancy and childbirth, as human events of individual and social importance, are reflected in the practices of the wider culture (Fig. 8-3). Practices related to pregnancy and childbirth tend to be highly developed and associated with strong and persistent beliefs (Kay, 1982).

As people of different cultural backgrounds come to-

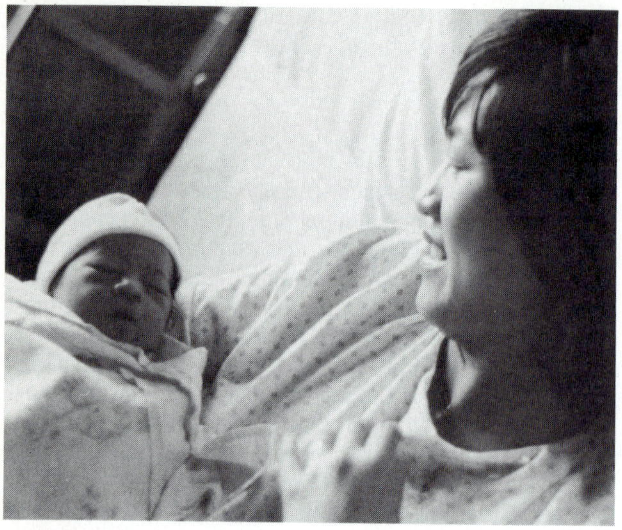

Figure 8-3.
Cultural beliefs dictate how women and their families view childbearing and care for their newborns. (Photo by BABES, Inc.)

gether, the process of acculturation occurs. In this process, some beliefs and practices are modified or dropped in favor of practices of the dominant culture, whereas other practices or beliefs are retained or change more slowly. How quickly individuals or groups become acculturated depends on many factors. Opportunities for learning in the new setting, the extent to which the dominant culture discriminates against minorities, and the amount of physical and cultural difference between two groups affect the process of acculturation.

Generalizations about cultural groups are often oversimplifications. Therefore, generalizations are likely to provide little information about any particular individual from that group. Individuals vary tremendously in their traditionalism or modernism, even within the same cultural group. Even generalizations true on a global level may not be useful in explaining behavior for a given individual.

Cultural and Socioeconomic Differences

There is a strong tendency for socioeconomic patterns to be mistaken for cultural patterns. For example, writings in sociology in the 1960s described a pattern of female-headed households among African Americans as a cultural tendency toward matriarchy. However, more careful examination showed that this was true only among African Americans in the lowest socioeconomic levels. As socioeconomic status increased, the number of of female-headed households decreased (TenHouten, 1970). In other words, female-headed households are no more common among African Americans than among European Americans of equivalent socioeconomic status. Despite the fact that this has been known for more than 20 years, it is still a widely held assumption that this cultural difference exists between African Americans and European Americans.

This type of misconception arises in large part because ethnic minorities tend to be poorer than European Americans overall and are overrepresented among the very poor. Thus, ethnic minorities have fewer opportunities for education and upward mobility. The economic gap accentuates differences and soon the assumption is made that observed differences are cultural in origin.

Ethnocentrism and Cultural Sensitivity in Health Care

The overwhelming majority of nurses and other health care providers in the United States are European American, middle class, and well educated. They have been socialized to the dominant cultural practices surrounding pregnancy and birth and take for granted that these practices are desirable. They may regard other sets of beliefs and practices as deviant or questionable.

Ethnocentrism, or the practice of judging cultural beliefs or practices by standards from another culture, is a common human behavior. By its very nature, culture is taken for granted and rarely examined by those within it. People of every culture tend to assume that their ways are the only reasonable ones. This kind of judgment can complicate interactions with women and their families and undermine the effectiveness of health care.

Cultural relativism is the practice of judging the customs of a particular culture by standards that are consistent with the values of that culture. Culturally sensitive health care does not require professionals to become experts in cultural differences in health practices. However, it does require professionals to acknowledge belief and value systems different from their own. These differences should be considered when delivering care to childbearing women and their families.

Cultural Patterns in Pregnancy and Birth

Prenatal care as practiced in Western countries is unique, reflecting the view that pregnancy is a condition that requires medical observation. Many cultures regard pregnancy as a normal state, and women seek the help of a healer only if problems arise. Women from other cultures often present themselves for prenatal care late in pregnancy.

Most cultures view pregnancy and birth as a period of increased vulnerability and risk, not as an illness. Many culturally prescribed birth practices appear to be aimed at decreasing risk by protecting the woman and the fetus from harmful influences. Cultural beliefs about the relative risks of pregnancy, the intrapartum period, and the postpartum period also differ. For instance, the traditional Chinese custom of "doing the month"—in which the mother stays in the house, rests, and avoids activities other than caring for the newborn—reflects the underlying cultural belief that the postpartum period constitutes a time of vulnerability. In contrast, the dominant American view is that childbirth is the period of highest risk, and the postpartum period is perceived as a less vulnerable time (Kay, 1982).

Balance as a Cultural Value

A recurring theme in many cultures is the notion of maintaining a balance in the woman's physical, emotional, and spiritual nature during pregnancy. Anthropologists refer to humoral pathology, the belief that a balance between intrinsic body qualities, such as heat and cold or moisture and dryness, is essential for good health during the childbearing year. If one of these qualities is diminished through childbirth, practices are aimed at restoring the balance. Balance is considered a value in emotional and spiritual matters in many cultures. Strong emotions are sometimes thought to "mark" or threaten the fetus. A pregnant woman may attempt to avoid certain types of thoughts, emotions, or interactions for this reason.

Self-Care Activities and Cultural Beliefs

Cultural variations tend to cluster around activities as self-care practices during pregnancy and the postpartum period. Examples include diet, activity and rest, maternal emotions, and preparation for birth and for parenthood. It is beyond the scope of this chapter to discuss these variations in detail, even as they relate to the most prevalent cultural groups in the United States. Furthermore, a listing of cultural practices for a particular group is basically a generalization that may or may not be useful in clinical care. However, a brief discussion of cultural variations in pregnancy and birth practices will help to sensitize the reader to areas where dominant and subcultural beliefs may differ.

Dietary Customs. Most cultures encourage the pregnant woman to maintain a diet considered normal for that culture. Food taboos are common, usually reflecting a cultural belief that certain foods are unclean. Fears that ingesting certain foods will produce undesirable physical characteristics in the newborn are common. Food cravings are considered normal among pregnant women in many cultures. Satisfaction of the woman's craving may be seen as vital to the well-being of the fetus.

Foods may also be considered important in maintaining a physical balance in the pregnant or newly delivered woman. Asian and Mexican practices emphasize the importance of "hot" foods after childbirth as a way to restore health and prevent complications arising from the loss of body heat through birth (Kay, 1982). For a detailed discussion of dietary needs in pregnancy and the postpartum period, see Chapters 17 and 35.

Activity and Rest. Most cultures encourage a pregnant woman to maintain normal activities but avoid strenuous work. Some encourage increased rest during pregnancy. Norms for sexual activity during pregnancy are more variable, ranging from no change to strict prohibitions of sexual intercourse through the second half of pregnancy.

The postpartum period is often characterized by more restrictions on activity. Most cultures encourage a period of rest, some as long as 40 days. During this time, the woman may be confined to her home, often to her bed. Some cultures regard the postpartum woman as unclean, prohibiting her participation in religious activities. When this is the case, there is usually provision for a ritual cleansing for both mother and infant at the end of the confinement period.

Preparation for Birth

Preparations for the actual birth may include intensive preparation of the house. Actual physical preparation of the pregnant woman through specific exercises, religious practices, or diet may be stressed. However, some cultures view preparation in advance of the event as potentially dangerous. Advance preparation, or even referring to the fetus by name, may be seen as tempting fate, or "the evil eye." This could make the woman and fetus vulnerable to evil influences (Kay, 1982).

Birth Practices

Birth practices vary widely. Cultural norms about who attends labor and birth, what positions and activities are healthy and acceptable for the laboring woman, and practices involving the placenta and umbilical cord appear on a continuum. Most cultures encourage other female members of the family to be present at birth. A few traditional cultures include the father or other men (Bozett & Hanson, 1991). Many groups encourage use of tonics, teas, or certain foods during or just before labor. This is done to prevent a state of imbalance in the woman. In American culture the custom of prohibiting food and drink in labor started in the middle of the 20th century with the use of general anesthesia. Today, although methods of anesthesia have improved, food and drink are still largely prohibited (Broach & Newton, 1988).

Expression of pain during labor varies considerably from culture to culture. Some cultures, notably Arab and some Hispanic groups, consider crying, moaning, and other verbal expressions of pain as normal. Others, including many Asian groups, have a tradition of stoicism, and responses to pain are subtle (Kay, 1982).

Cultural practices surrounding the umbilical cord and placenta also vary. Some groups follow specific practices in cutting the cord and caring for the umbilical stump, which may be seen as a vulnerable area. Folk practices of binding the umbilicus with "belly bands" or binders are common among southern African Americans and Mexican Americans. Some cultures view the cord as spiritually related to the infant. For example, traditional Japanese practices include preserving the cord and keeping it in the family home (Perry, 1982).

Preparation for Parenthood

Culture dictates the nature of preparation for the parental role. Women are usually socialized clearly to expect to become mothers. Many cultures begin preparation for parenthood through sibling caretaking of younger children, usually by the older daughters. Lifelong preparation for motherhood may be reinforced by religious beliefs or traditions emphasizing the importance of motherhood. A dramatic example of this influence may be seen among Mormons who believe that marriage and children ensure parents of a high place in heaven. Mormon families with six children or more are not unusual. This contradicts the prevailing practice among Americans to limit births to two or three.

In many cultures, there appears to be little preparation for fatherhood (Bozett & Hanson, 1991). However, so-called primitive cultures usually have some male rituals related to birth and fatherhood. These rituals are called "ritual couvade" and often involve dietary restrictions or a set of behaviors mimicking the woman in labor and birth. Anthropologists described these rituals in great detail in the early part of this century. These rituals were believed to be a form of sympathetic magic aimed at warding off evil influences from the vulnerable woman and fetus. The father-as-labor-coach role, which has become common in the United States, has some similarities to this practice.

Cultural Variations in the United States

As individuals and families leave their countries of origin and come to the United States, traditional practices and practices of the larger American culture may blend, conflict, or coexist. The following section provides a brief discussion of practices related to pregnancy and birth among common ethnic groups in the United States. Some variations may appear to be cultural but actually are a reflection of socioeconomic conditions in which many minority groups live.

These generalizations do not apply to all individuals. They are presented here only to increase an awareness of cultural variations related to pregnancy and birth. In clinical practice, the soundest approach is to ask what the woman considers normal practice during pregnancy, birth, and the postpartum period. (See the Implications for Nursing Care section later in this chapter for some useful questions.) Observation of family behavior is necessary to plan appropriate nursing care. The accompanying display offers suggestions for assessing cultural practices.

Cultural Practices in Childbearing

What is the meaning and value of reproduction in this culture?

How is pregnancy viewed? Is it a state of illness, vulnerability, or health?

What responsibilities do the parents have as a result of pregnancy?

Is birth seen as a normal process or as being related to illness and danger?

Is birth considered a public or private event? Who should be present?

What practices govern diet and food preparation before birth?

What practices govern the pregnant woman's activity level and the types of activities acceptable during pregnancy and labor?

What precautions are important for the woman and neonate after birth?

When is the newborn accepted into the family?

What type of help is acceptable after birth and from whom?

What kinds of behaviors are expected of the mother, father, and other family members in relation to the newborn?

Affonso, D. (1979). Assessing cultural perspectives. In A. Clark & D. Affonso (Eds). Childbearing: A nursing perspective. *Philadelphia: F.A. Davis.*

African Americans

African American women tend to view pregnancy as a normal healthy state. Their experience of pregnancy may be strongly influenced by social factors, such as the couple relationship, economic pressures, and whether or not the pregnancy was intended. Although single motherhood is not a desirable situation, children born to single mothers are usually cherished and are not stigmatized. Children of adolescents are often raised by the grandmother as her own. In a descriptive study of 19 African American grandmothers, Flaherty, Facteau, and Garver (1987) found that the adolescent mothers were expected to make daily care decisions concerning the infant. Decisions about medical care, however, were most frequently made by the grandmother.

Southern African American women may engage in a practice called pica, or the eating of clay, laundry starch, or other substances generally considered nonnutritive. This is most likely a learned behavior characteristic of lower socioeconomic groups, in which African Americans are overrepresented. (See Chapter 17 for further discussion of pica.) Other dietary practices may include avoidance of "acid" or "strong" foods during pregnancy to prevent having a "hard-to-manage" newborn. The woman's behavior during labor may be subdued and stoic to avoid drawing undue attention to herself. Her response to pain, on the other hand, may be verbal and pronounced. Occasionally, an African American woman may express a wish or preference for lighter-skinned children. This is likely to be a reflection of more overt discrimination against African Americans with distinct Negroid features.

Southeast Asian Americans

Since 1975, the United States has resettled approximately 750,000 Southeast Asian refugees, three quarters of whom are Vietnamese (D'Avanzo, 1992). Those who immigrated in the early 1970s tended to be middle class and well educated. Immigrants who arrived later were more likely to be poor, less educated, new to Western culture, and to have spent time in refugee camps before arriving in this country. These immigrants include Cambodian, Laotian, and Hmong people. Most of these immigrants are young and of childbearing age (D'Avanzo, 1992).

The strong cultural tradition of politeness and deference to authority in Southeast Asian cultures may be reflected in a tendency to avoid eye contact and social physical contact such as shaking hands and the touching of shoulders. Answering questions affirmatively, regardless of true feelings, is a cultural pattern. Southeast Asians may hold Catholic, Buddhist, Confucian, or spiritualist beliefs that influence childbirth practices. In general, there is a commitment to stoicism. Women may consider crying out or complaining to be shameful, especially in the presence of a man. This may result in unexpectedly imminent births unless the nurse is alert.

Squatting may be the preferred position for birth. The woman is taught to conserve body heat during childbirth and in the postpartum period. The nurse can provide warmed extra blankets and drinking water without ice. Bathing after childbirth may be considered risky for the woman. Women may eat only "hot" traditional foods from home during the early postpartum period. The woman's activities may be restricted for 40 to 60 days, with other female relatives assuming household and infant care responsibilities (Mattson & Lew, 1992).

Mexican Americans

Mexican Americans are the second largest minority group in the United States. Most Mexican Americans and Mexican immigrants are of childbearing age. The fertility rate of this group is 50% higher than that of any other ethnic group in the United States (US Department of Health and Human Services, 1990).

Women of Mexican descent tend view to pregnancy as a natural condition requiring no medical care under usual circumstances. The woman and fetus are considered vulnerable to outside bad influences. The woman may wear a cinta (a belt with keys attached) or a muneco (a knotted cord around the abdomen) to prevent complications. Women may avoid drinking milk and may stay physically active to help prevent the development of a large fetus and a difficult delivery. An interesting study by Cummins, Scrimshaw, and Engle (1988) found that a majority of low-income Mexican American women in the study group viewed cesarean birth in a positive light rather than the negative view held by some other cultures.

Female family members are often present during labor and birth. Among more traditional couples, the father rarely participates. In more modern or more acculturated families, the father may be an active participant. Attitudes about breastfeeding tend to vary in this population. For example, some women may believe colostrum to be unclean and will not breastfeed until the second day after birth. Mexican American women may observe a 40-day resting period after birth called *la cuarentina*. During this time, dietary and activity restrictions apply, including a prohibition on sexual intercourse. The infant's umbilicus may be bound to prevent *mal aire* (bad air) from entering. Consequently, Mexican American mothers may resist allowing the umbilicus to air dry. The nurse should be alert to this possibility and provide information about cleanliness, frequent changing of binding, and appropriate fit to prevent infection (Coreil & Mull, 1990).

Filipino Americans

Because of the long-standing relationship between the United States and the Philippines, Filipino Americans may demonstrate a range of traditional and Western practices. Western medicine is generally well accepted. Traditional practices may be maintained in certain areas, such as the woman's activity level and diet patterns during the prenatal and postpartum periods. Hot, spicy, or salty foods may be avoided during pregnancy, and satisfying food cravings may be seen as important in preventing premature birth. Women are encouraged to decrease their activity during pregnancy and especially during the postpartum period. This may be misinterpreted as laziness or noncompliance by hospital staff.

Politeness, ease in social interaction, and deference to family authority, particularly the woman's mother, may create misunderstandings between staff and the family. The woman may smile pleasantly and indicate that she understands certain instructions, but later will not follow staff recommendations, instead adhering to traditional ways as encouraged by her mother. This reflects an effort to avoid contradicting the nurse directly. Women are socialized toward motherhood at an early age, and the extended family is seen as having an important role in child care (Asperilla, 1986).

Asian Americans

Large populations of Asian Americans can be found in metropolitan areas on each coast. Practices among Asian Americans range from fairly traditional Asian practices to near-total adoption of American patterns. Asian Americans are more concentrated on the West Coast and have attained the highest median income and educational level of any minority group in the United States. Cultural norms place a high value on deference and politeness, emotional reserve, conformity, and allegiance to family. More traditional families may show strong male dominance, and the extended family may be important in daily life.

The birth of a male child may confer high status on the mother. Western medicine tends to be well accepted. Pregnancy is viewed as a state of health requiring little change in normal activities. Childrearing habits in Japan greatly encourage dependence on the mother, who is expected to satisfy neonatal needs immediately and to maintain close contact with the neonate. Similar patterns may be seen to a lesser extent among Japanese American women.

Chinese American customs related to childbearing vary according to the length of time the parents' families have been in the United States. Educational level also affects beliefs about pregnancy and childbearing. Beliefs in the value of maintaining physical and spiritual balance during pregnancy and the postpartum period may be present. Herbal teas may be used as tonics during pregnancy, and certain foods may be avoided. A prime example of the importance of balance in maintaining health is the custom of "doing the month." This is a period of 40 days after birth when the woman is advised to stay in the house, rest, and avoid unnecessary activity. The woman may avoid contact with water during this period. This avoidance reflects a belief that the postpartum woman has an excess of cold in her body and is vulnerable to arthritis and other body aches later in life if she becomes chilled during the postpartum period (Kay, 1982).

Arab Americans

Arab immigrants are estimated to number 3 to 4 million in the United States. Arab Americans may adhere to either Christianity or Islam but have common cultural practices. Childbearing is a major role for women, whose domain is primarily the home and family. Infertility in a married woman is considered grounds for divorce in some Arab countries. Male children are highly valued. The sex of the newborn may appear to be more important to parents than the newborn's health. The husband is involved in all aspects of his wife's care, and often the woman will defer to him in decisions about her own care. Arab women are expected to be modest and deferential. It is considered normal for Arab women to moan and cry during labor, yet few request analgesia.

Advance preparation for the birth and the neonate is avoided for fear of attracting the "evil eye." Compliments about the neonate are avoided for the same reason. A traditional mistrust of written agreements may present difficulties when informed consent for medical procedures is being obtained. Trust is more readily placed in verbal agreements, especially with others of similar background. Arab families thrive on a high level of interaction and cohesiveness. Visiting by the extended family during the postpartum period is considered an obligation. Children are included in all aspects of family life, and women may have a strong desire to have older children greet the neonate in the hospital (Meleis & Sorrell, 1981).

Pregnancy and Childbirth in the "American" Culture

Two opposing trends characterize childbirth in America: the trend toward increasing medical and technologic intervention in childbirth and the consumer movement toward family-centered childbirth. From a cultural perspective, these opposing trends characterize a typically "American" approach to childbirth. This approach places an emphasis on technologic intervention to ensure a positive outcome and an emphasis on a family-centered approach with participation by family members, especially fathers.

High standards of living, widespread access to health care, and the high value placed on educational and occupational advancement also contribute to a pattern sometimes called "the premium birth/baby syndrome." Because middle-class couples expect to have a small family, they do everything in their power to ensure a good outcome of pregnancy and birth. This involves getting into good physical shape before trying to conceive, getting early prenatal care, taking every available class, and observing every possible precaution. This pattern may include disdain for those who fail to take advantage of current technology and to eliminate unhealthy practices, such as smoking, during pregnancy. Unfortunately, this perspective can lead to intense self-doubt and guilt if expectations for a "good birth" and a healthy newborn are not met. This may be true even if the outcome was not preventable.

The American way of birth seems as foreign to people outside the United States as non-American ways do to health professionals here. Care should be given without letting ethnocentrism blind actual needs and concerns of childbearing women and their families. Whether or not a particular birth practice is rational or normal is not the issue. The issues for the professional must always be: Is it safe? Is it feasible? Is it important to the woman? The nurse must evaluate cultural practices in the light of these questions. If they can be answered affirmatively, there usually is no sound reason not to support the wishes of the woman and her family. This is true even if the chosen practices do not fit with the nurse's own belief system.

Culture exerts a major influence on childbearing practices. Cultural aspects of childbearing involve acculturation and cultural relativism. Ethnocentrism must be not be an issue in care. Generalizations do not apply to all members of a culture. Individual roles develop within the cultural context and must be considered in assessment and provision of health care. Cultural practices in pregnancy and birth are likely to reflect concepts of risk and vulnerability, self-care, and preparation for birth and parenthood.

Psychological Aspects of Childbearing

Childbearing involves complex psychological changes for women and their family members. This section addresses factors that affect individual adaptation to childbearing, maternal and paternal tasks of pregnancy, and adaptations required by other family members.

Individual Development and Adaptation

A major factor influencing the psychological impact of pregnancy is the individual's own maturity and readiness for this transition. Readiness for childbearing is defined as the ability to adapt to the demands and complete the tasks of pregnancy, childbirth, and parenthood. Psychosocial readiness and physiologic readiness for childbearing are not the same thing. This is evidenced by the many social problems encountered by adolescents who bear children. A person might be said to have achieved psychosocial readiness for childbearing if he or she has the following characteristics:

- The capacity to establish and maintain intimate relationships
- The ability to give to and care for another human being
- The ability to learn and to adjust patterns of daily life
- The ability to communicate effectively with others
- An established gender identity and sexual orientation

However, individuals themselves often have additional criteria that they see as important factors in psychosocial readiness for childbearing. Adults in social groups where contraception and planning of first pregnancies are common may consciously focus on and think about these issues more than adults in social groups where conception is not usually controlled or planned. For example, a middle-class, well-educated couple may think of establishing careers and a comfortable household and having time as a couple before feeling ready for the first child. A couple from a lower-class minority group may see those goals as out of reach and may perceive pregnancy and childbirth more as an inevitable consequence of life as a couple.

However, some criteria for readiness are generally recognized by most adults. In our culture most children are born to women in relatively stable monogamous relationships with male partners. Therefore, both men and women often cite the existence of a stable couple relationship as a major factor in readiness for childbearing. Financial security tends to be an important factor—one that may be mentioned more often by men than women. This probably reflects the fact that the "breadwinner" function is a large part of the traditional male sex role in Western society. The attainment of personal goals may be an important benchmark; these goals will vary and may range from finishing high school and getting a job to successfully taking over the family business.

Motivations for Childbearing

People do not always make a clear, conscious decision for pregnancy or parenthood. The pros and cons of parenting, with its expectations and life changes and the necessity of taking on a permanent new life role, are not always considered. Often the decision to risk pregnancy is based more on emotional responses in a particular situation than on rational thought and a life plan.

With so many influences on contraceptive and childbearing decisions, it is rare for persons to be fully aware of their own motivations to bear a child. Some motivations can be classified as healthy and individuals may be aware of them. For example, there is the simple desire of a couple in an emotionally satisfying relationship to have a family. Some people may be aware of a desire to share a part of themselves with the world or to leave a legacy for the future. Some may feel childbearing is part of the adventure or challenge of life, a pathway toward achieving their own potential. For others, parenthood is a desirable status, one that permits them to share experiences with parents, peers, and siblings. Some may feel incomplete as adult members of society without children.

Other motivations for childbearing are considered less healthy and reflect unresolved problems. Often the people concerned are unaware of these motivations or refuse to acknowledge them. These motivations are more common among adolescents and reflect their psychosocial immaturity (Poole, 1987). Such motivations may include having a child to save a faltering relationship, to provide a source of affection and security, or to replace a loss (such as a miscarriage, death of a significant other, or some personal failure). Others may choose childbearing as a means to prove sexual ability or fertility. Beginning a family may provide a means to escape an unhappy home life or work situation.

Impact of Childbearing on Adult Roles

Pregnancy and childbirth signal the acquisition of a new role, that of father or mother. Roles are learned through formal and informal means, and the socialization to function in major roles begins in childhood. Girls are often encouraged to learn to care for younger children and to meet and anticipate the emotional needs of others. They tend to be socialized in preparation for their future roles as mothers. Boys are less often socialized as future fathers but that may be changing as sex roles change in Western countries. Much learning about the parent roles is indirect. Children observe their parents and the examples provided by other family members. As new parents, individuals commonly mimic parenting behaviors they observed as children.

Childbearing and Women's Roles

Pregnancy and childbirth have significant psychological and physical effects on women. These changes are irreversible. Women carry the fetus in their bodies and have a relationship with the developing fetus through pregnancy and childbirth that changes them physically and emotionally. A woman can never "not know that she is a mother," even if she relinquishes her neonate.

Childbearing has major social implications for women as well. The changes in women's roles in the last two decades have been dramatic. The role of wife and mother in the home was considered the norm in the 1950s among the middle class. Pregnancy often signaled a departure from other roles and a refocusing of attention on childbearing and home management. Women in lower socioeconomic classes did not have the luxury of giving up paid employment. They often continued to be employed in traditional semiskilled or unskilled women's jobs while rearing their children. However, as more women moved into the job force and into nontraditional work roles, childbearing gradually became a function that was added to other responsibilities rather than substituted for them.

Women are likely to report more overall change and more change in their personal lives after the first birth than do their partners. Even if she is employed outside the home, major responsibility for childrearing and home management decisions typically fall to the woman. Thus, raising children constitutes a second or even a third "full-time job" for many women, added to outside employment and home management.

Even though this state of affairs is clearly not healthy for women or families over the long term, sex roles are slow to change in some areas. The man's share of household management and childrearing responsibilities still tends to be less than half. This is true even among men who say they believe in sexual equality and want to participate more in home life. Thus, pregnancy and the first birth often mean a shift to a more traditional division of labor than may have existed in a couple relationship before.

This shift occurs for several reasons. First, men tend to be socialized to expect that they do not know enough to care for a neonate. As a result, they do not expect to participate. Although they may not know any more than their male partners, women are socialized to expect that they should know how to care for a newborn. This pattern persists throughout childrearing. Breastfeeding, which is gaining in popularity, requires the woman to be engaged in most direct caretaking. Although maternity leave is a common option for women, paternity leave is still rare in the United States. Thus, from a financial standpoint, women are encouraged to stay home for some period of time after birth, whereas men are not. This period of primary child care responsibility sometimes delays the man's skill development in this area and further contributes to the pattern in which women assume major child care and home management responsibilities after the first birth.

Childbearing and Men's Roles

Childbearing creates changes in men's roles, although the changes are usually not as apparent as those experienced by their female partners. Men may father children and never know that they have done so. They experience childbearing as if they were "one step removed," at least in the biologic sense. However, fatherhood has always introduced important changes in men's lives. More attention is now being paid to the experience of fatherhood than ever before.

Men are not socialized to delve into the emotional aspects of their lives and their relationships. The typical male role in Western countries is to deny, or at least avoid, emotional responses except in certain acceptable "male" arenas. These may include competition, sports, protection of family, and occupational strivings. The primary role for adult men is their occupational role. For many men, that role changes little with the birth of a child although men often will report that they feel "more responsible" and compelled to be a better provider after they have a child. It is only recently that men have been expected to take a more active role in pregnancy, birth, and early parenting. As yet, we know little about the long-term consequences of this role change on fathering behavior. More research in the area of men's roles in childbearing and childrearing is needed.

Men tend to report less overall change in their lives and less personal change with parenthood than do their female partners. This perhaps is to be expected given the fact that pregnancy is a biologic event for women, whereas men can only observe this biologic shift. Men tended to express more negative response to any change in sexuality in the couple relationship than their female partners (May, 1987). This may suggest that the sexual relationship is of more significance to men in the couple relationship. Even fairly predictable changes in sexuality caused by childbearing may cause more stress for the father. This might in part be explained by the fact that the primary source of support and nurturance for most men is their spouse, and the sexual relationship may be the main way in which they feel cared for and loved.

One important aspect of childbearing that touches men's views of themselves is the notion of having responsibility for a child. Men often see the father role as a great responsibility—their tie to the future and their link to the past. Having a child to "carry on" may be important, even if it is not a male child to carry the family name. The notion of having a child to carry on the family traditions or to provide an enjoyable future for an aging grandparent is often important to men as they anticipate and experience fatherhood.

Childbearing and the Couple Relationship

Childbearing has a profound effect on the couple as a unit. The couple's response depends on how the pregnancy is viewed. Pregnancy may signal the initiation into full family status for the couple or the beginning of hard times, stress, and unmet emotional needs. A research project that followed couples through pregnancy and into the first year of parenthood found that the way in which couples fared in the transition to parenthood depended in part on their typical style of interaction and the amount of time they spent together (Lewis, J., 1988; Lewis, W., 1988). Partners who showed a greater tendency toward mutuality (or "coupleness") in their relationship coped with the transition to parenthood better if their life-style and the division of labor supported that mutuality. For example, a flexible work schedule that allowed the man to spend more time with his new family contributed to the sense of "coupleness," making the transition easier. A rigid work schedule, on the other hand, could make it more difficult to maintain the couple relationship after birth. However, couples who tended toward more separateness in their relationship during the pregnancy were more satisfied after the birth if their situation reinforced this separateness while still allowing some tasks to be shared.

This same study showed that communication patterns were affected by these shifts in role behaviors and by each partner's sense of self. Practical issues such as the mother's and newborn's physical status and fatigue level also affected communication in the couple. The partners tended to perceive the same event or milestone differently. A period of worry for one might be a period of happiness for the other. This difference in perception not only reflects a shift in how the couple communicates about their experience but also indicates that the process of becoming a family is different for each member, even if they live and experience the process together.

Maternal Adaptation to Pregnancy

Pregnancy is a time when women literally begin to share themselves and their bodies with another being. This relationship will continue for many years of motherhood. This event naturally produces many profound changes in the ways a woman views herself, her body, her relationship with the child's father, and her future with her as-yet unknown offspring.

The perinatal nurse must be knowledgeable about the processes involved in maternal adaptation to pregnancy. This will enable the nurse to provide appropriate emotional support, supply needed information, and help expectant women to anticipate events and prepare for future needs. The following section highlights some aspects of expectant motherhood and discusses maternal tasks of pregnancy.

The Expectant Mother

The miracle of a woman's ability to conceive and bear children has been a major theme in art and literature throughout human history. The theme of the pregnant woman as being unusually powerful and in harmony with nature is repeated in ancient mythology and in nearly all cultures.

Western culture has devoted much scientific attention to the physical and psychological processes of pregnancy. Early psychoanalytic thought, emerging during the restrictive Victorian era, reflected both the fascination with and the fear of the woman's ability to create life. This conflict was clear in the societal view of expectant motherhood during that era. The word pregnant was not used in polite company. Instead, women were said to be indisposed and in a period of confinement. Expectant mothers were rarely if ever seen in public in the latter half of pregnancy. They were considered to be unusually frail and vulnerable.

However, as women's roles changed in the years before and after World War II, pregnancy gradually became a more natural part of a woman's life. The baby boom of the 1950s reinforced this normalization of pregnancy as women in record numbers were conceiving and bearing children. Maternity clothes, once limited to one or two outfits handmade to last throughout pregnancy, took on a new look, as the manufacturing of maternity clothes became a thriving business. The prepared childbirth movement, with its strong grassroots origins, brought pregnancy even more into public view. Women began keeping paid positions later into pregnancy. Pregnant women appearing in public places were no longer regarded as unusual (Wertz & Wertz, 1989).

The women's movement of the 1960s and 1970s continued this normalization process. Pregnancy began to be viewed as a state of health that should not interfere with a woman's activities. Conventional prenatal and birth care practices began to be challenged. Decisions about perinatal care became increasingly seen as matters that a woman should control (Mathews & Zadek, 1991).

There is also a growing recognition among care providers that not all pregnant women are heterosexual. Lesbian women are increasingly likely to want children. They face unique challenges, including how to conceive, where to find a care provider sensitive to their unique concerns, and how to elicit support from family members and others regarding the pregnancy (Kenney & Tash, 1992). Little research has been conducted to date on the process of psychological adaptation to pregnancy among lesbian women. Thus, it is important for the perinatal nurse to consider ways in which the needs of the pregnant woman in a same-sex relationship are similar and different from those of a single pregnant woman or those of women in heterosexual relationships. (See the section on lesbian childbearing later in this chapter.)

Maternal Tasks of Pregnancy

Several developmental tasks that reflect healthy maternal adaptation to pregnancy and provide a basis for the acceptance of the maternal role have been identified. These tasks are often discussed within a framework of trimesters of pregnancy. This occurs because some concerns are more pressing at one point in pregnancy than another. The biologic nature of pregnancy provides some predictable sequences of events. The knowledgeable nurse is able to recognize that tasks overlap. Maternal tasks may emerge in different ways at various points in pregnancy. Distinctions between completion of one task and the beginning of another are not clear-cut.

Accepting the Pregnancy

Even if they have been actively trying to conceive, women often are surprised to realize that they may be pregnant. Some women may ignore or not even notice early symptoms. They may not seek confirmation of pregnancy until after several missed menses. Others delay confirmation because they are unwilling to hear definite news one way or the other. Recent advances in home pregnancy testing enable women to confirm their own pregnancy with high levels of accuracy before a second period is missed.

A woman's initial response to the news that she is pregnant may be shock, joy, delight, anger, or a combination of these feelings. Typically, if the pregnant woman's response is a happy one, she will announce the news to her partner fairly soon. If her initial response is more negative or if she anticipates that his response will be negative, she may wait for several days or weeks before disclosing the news.

In most cases, regardless of whether or not the woman planned the pregnancy, she experiences some early ambivalence. She may feel the timing is not right and can find many reasons why she should not be pregnant. An early nurse researcher in perinatal nursing, who first outlined maternal tasks, described this as the "someday, but not now" phenomenon (Rubin, 1970).

Accepting pregnancy requires the woman to first accept the reality of pregnancy and the fact that her body will become the vehicle for supporting another life. The woman may first view the fetus as an intruder. This reflects a normal egocentric reaction to this remarkable experience. The woman's behavior is typically self-centered, attending to her own needs and concerns first. The fetus is a separate being, yet it is part of her. Accepting the fact of pregnancy on an intellectual level is a first step. The woman must then acknowledge the pregnancy on an emotional level as *her* pregnancy.

Establishing a Relationship With the Fetus

For the woman to establish a relationship with the fetus, she must come to perceive it as a being separate from herself. However, a risk in this process is that the woman will see the fetus as separate and intrusive. If the fetus remains an alien presence and a threat to her selfhood, the woman will not nurture and protect it. Psychologically, this risk is avoided by the process of incorporation.

Incorporating the Fetus

As the woman accepts the pregnancy and begins to adjust to the physiologic and emotional changes it produces, she gradually comes to see the pregnancy and the fetus as part of herself. She begins to see herself as pregnant and, as such, deserving of special attention. The woman may begin wearing maternity clothes far earlier than is actually necessary, an announcement to the world that she is pregnant. Self-absorption allows the woman to incorporate the fetus and the pregnancy as part of herself, without experiencing a significant threat to her self-concept. Once this is accomplished, the woman can allow herself to view the fetus as a separate being with whom she is beginning to establish a relationship.

Separating the Fetus From Self

The process of identifying the fetus as a separate being usually begins with the increased uterine growth and sensations of fetal life in the second trimester. Some women may begin this process earlier. Separation begins as the woman identifies the fetus as a separate being with its own boundaries and selfhood, but still a valued part of her and dependent on her. The woman comes to think of the fetus as a fantasized infant; she may begin to daydream about the infant, and engage in conversations and interactions with the fetus. This signals the beginning of maternal–fetal attachment, as the woman invests herself emotionally in a relationship with the fetus.

This process of separating fetus from self while forming a growing attachment continues throughout pregnancy. In the last weeks of the third trimester, the physical discomforts and the feelings of "being tired of being pregnant" signal a tipping of the scale. The pregnant woman is now ready to give up the pregnancy, separate physically from the fetus through childbirth, and welcome her newborn.

Adjusting to Changes in Self

Another set of maternal tasks of pregnancy is related to the changes the woman experiences in her emotions, attitudes, and body. These changes include physical and emotional changes, as well as changes in the couple relationship.

Physical Changes. The pregnant woman must adjust to multiple physical changes, such as changes in perceived body size, in mobility, in body function, and in emotional investment in physical appearance. These adjustments begin almost immediately after conception. The rapid physiologic alterations of early pregnancy are felt more than seen. Hormonal fluctuations, the subtle abdominal growth, and breast swelling may combine to produce a negative response to her own body. Women often are concerned that others understand they are pregnant and "not just getting fat." Later, when more pronounced physical changes are noticeable, the woman also has to adapt to the limitations of a larger, heavier body. She will most likely experience a sense of increased vulnerability and physical awkwardness.

Some women welcome these physical changes as part of pregnancy. Others dislike them intensely. Many women will avoid cameras and mirrors; others appear to be fascinated with their changing bodies and have more pictures taken of themselves pregnant than at any other time. Most women accept their pregnant bodies with some regret and some pleasure. Women who have a large investment in their physical appearance and their trim bodies may have more difficulty accepting these changes. Generally, however, acceptance is not stressful enough to disrupt maternal adaptation to the pregnancy overall. Concerns about body image persist through pregnancy and into the postpartum period.

Emotional Changes. Emotional changes have come to be associated with pregnancy just as closely as unusual food cravings and maternity clothes. Expectant mothers exhibit a degree of emotional lability. This type of emotional response would be regarded as pathologic in the nonpregnant woman. Rapid and dramatic mood swings may be a result of hormonal fluctuations or may simply reflect elevated anxiety levels. Mood swings usually occur in response to some environmental cue. The woman may respond with great happiness to a kind word and later be reduced to tears by a stranger's stare. Such mood swings can be confusing to the woman and to family members.

Another characteristic emotional change of pregnancy is increasing anxiety. Fears about her own physical vulnerability and that of the fetus create anxiety. The pregnant woman may worry about the anticipated pain and work of childbirth and changes in her relationship with her partner. Another source of increasing anxiety is the fact that pregnancy signals a transition to motherhood with its responsibility and long-term commitment. The pregnant woman must, in a sense, rediscover who she is. The woman's status with friends, relatives, even her own mother, changes with pregnancy. She will need to renegotiate these relationships in terms of her future motherhood.

One outlet for this increased anxiety during pregnancy may be through fantasies and dreams. Women often report having strange, sometimes bizarre fantasies and dreams about the infant and birth process. Highly erotic dreams are not uncommon. Such dreams may reflect processing of unconscious fears and conflicts and are regarded as a normal side-effect of the pregnant woman's emotional adaptation to pregnancy.

Adjusting to the Changing Couple Relationship

Another maternal task of pregnancy is to adjust to the changes pregnancy causes in her relationship with her mate. The couple's relationship changes because both partners are changing. Their anticipated future together is also changing. Research has found that both positive and negative changes occur in the marriage relationship as a result of pregnancy (Saunders & Robins, 1987; Tomlinson, 1987). The woman experiences shifts in her usual emotional responses to her partner. Two areas are particularly important: increases in her dependence on her mate and shifts in her sexual relationship.

Increases in Dependence. The pregnant woman becomes more dependent on others, particularly her mate, for physical and emotional support. Signs of dependence tend to vary. There may be extreme worry about her partner when they are separated, an increased impatience with activities and interests that do not include her, and reliance on the partner for physical help at home.

Experienced perinatal nurses have observed that adaptation to pregnancy and motherhood is most successfully achieved when a pregnant woman herself is "mothered." In a sense, the woman's needs for affection, attention, and support must be met before she can give to her neonate. Reassurance of support from her partner and friends becomes extremely important (Fig. 8-4). This is true for women who, at other times in life, are independent and self-reliant. The single pregnant woman with little economic security and without the support of a family will probably experience extremely high levels of stress. Her needs for support may not be met if she is living alone without a circle of close friends.

Changes in the Sexual Relationship. Although most women feel an increased need for love and affection during pregnancy, the desire for sexual activity during pregnancy varies among women. Sexual desires and activities can vary even in the same woman at different times during pregnancy. These physiologic and psychological changes are discussed in detail in Chapter 5.

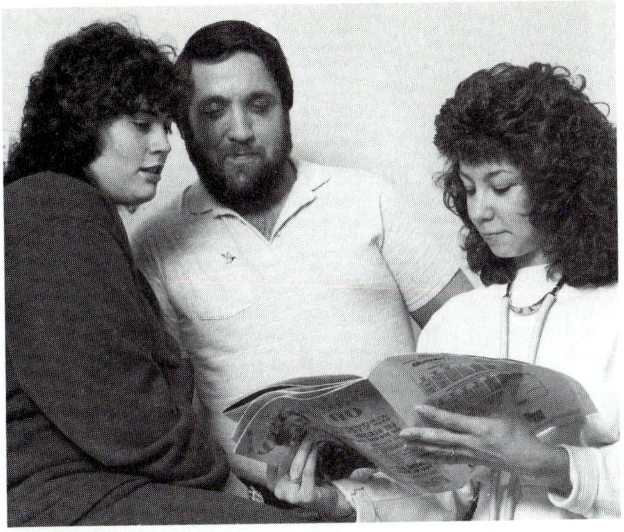

Figure 8-4.
Support from her partner is an important factor in healthy maternal adaptation to pregnancy. Here a husband and wife both listen to a description of fetal growth. (Courtesy of the Department of Medical Photography, Children's Hospital of Buffalo, NY.)

Changes in the woman's desire for sexual activity tend to have a "ripple effect" in the relationship. Her decreased interest may cause her partner's interest to decline. This may cause her to worry about her attractiveness, making her even more uncomfortable and concerned. The woman may worry that sexual activity will have a harmful effect on the pregnancy or the fetus. She may discourage her partner's interest for that reason. Women in relationships with established open communication about sexuality are likely to have less difficulty with changes in sexual activity. Women who are unaccustomed to discussing sexual matters with their partners are likely to have greater difficulty in adapting to these changes.

Preparing for Birth and Early Motherhood

The process of maternal adaptation to pregnancy is completed as the woman prepares herself to experience labor, to give birth, and to take on the maternal role. Although this process occurs to some extent throughout pregnancy, the woman begins preparation in earnest in the last trimester (Bliss-Holtz, 1988). Preparation for childbirth is institutionalized to some extent through prepared childbirth classes, baby showers, and physical preparation of the nursery. The woman may engage in a flurry of activity in the last weeks of pregnancy, sometimes called "nesting behavior." She will hurry to finish preparing the neonate's layette or clean the entire house in preparation for the newborn. Folk wisdom suggests that nesting behavior signals that labor will begin soon. There is no scientific proof that this is true; however, experienced labor and delivery nurses have observed that women often come into labor tired, having had a burst of energy and activity a day or two before they went into labor.

Resolving Fears About Childbirth. A woman typically has fears and worries about the process of labor and birth. These fears are understandable. The primipara who has not experienced the process of childbirth fears the unknown. The multipara may know what can go wrong and exactly what to anticipate. A woman often has fears about how she will respond to the pain and work of labor, about losing control emotionally and physically, and about whether she and her newborn will survive. Some of these fears can be resolved with information and reassurance from care providers. A supportive partner can help, but ultimately the woman must cope with fear in her own way (Fig. 8-5).

Accepting the Maternal Role. Accepting the maternal role occurs when a pregnant woman internalizes the maternal role in preparation for actually enacting the role with her newborn. The processes that take place during the attainment of the maternal role are discussed in greater depth in Unit 5. The woman begins the process of learning the maternal role during pregnancy at the same time that she begins to attach to her fetus. The nurse needs to understand that each process affects and is affected by the other. Anticipatory socialization into the maternal role occurs with input from a variety of sources. The pregnant woman fantasizes about herself and her infant, observes other mothers and chooses behaviors to mimic or avoid, and engages in role play as she cares for other children. This will help the pregnant woman prepare for the maternal role. With the birth of the neonate, the woman continues the process of maternal role attainment. The role has been attained when the woman feels a sense of comfort and competence as a mother.

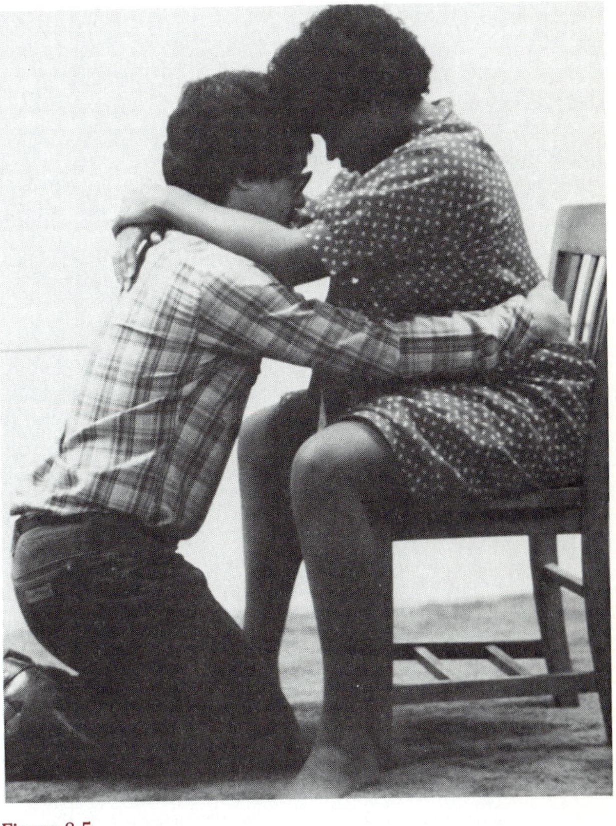

Figure 8-5.
Couple rehearsing labor. Rehearsing with her partner how she will cope with labor helps the pregnant woman prepare for childbirth. (Photo by BABES, Inc.)

Situational Factors Affecting Maternal Adaptation

Certain situational factors affect the woman's adaptation to pregnancy. Some of these are of particular importance to the perinatal nurse because they also may have a significant impact on the woman's health during the childbearing year. These factors include single parenthood, high-risk pregnancy, and the woman's developmental status.

Partnered Versus Unpartnered Status. Little is known about the experience of the single mother. Women who have less social support and perceive a troubled relationship with the father of the newborn experience higher rates of perinatal complications. They have higher stress than other women, but the differences may have more to do with socioeconomic or psychological distinctions than with an unmarried or unpartnered status itself. Tilden (1983), a nurse researcher who did early work on this topic, identified some areas of concern during pregnancy that are uniquely different for single mothers. Single mothers had more difficulty making a decision to keep a pregnancy because they had to choose to be a solo parent and could not count on partner support. Single mothers experienced some stress and uncertainty in deciding how to disclose the news of their pregnancy to friends and family and whom to tell. The single mother had to take legal issues into consideration, such as who would care for the neonate if something happened to her; whom to list as father of the infant on birth records; and what arrangements, if any, should be made to allow the father contact with the infant. Single mothers had to enlist social support. This was necessary to substitute for the support of a partner and to replace family support, which was sometimes withdrawn after pregnancy was announced.

Tilden's research suggested that the first and second trimesters were particularly stressful for single mothers because of the unique issues they faced. These findings point to the need for specialized supportive care for women who choose to become single mothers.

Subsequent Pregnancies. Nursing research has identified some important differences between women's experiences of first and subsequent pregnancies. The multipara experiences all of the changes pregnancy brings. In addition, she must cope with the demands of older children and concerns about how the arrival of the newborn will affect her relationships with them (Walker, Crain, & Thompson, 1986). The multipara is often older, may have less energy, and may require a longer time to recover from physical stress. She may have specific fears about labor and birth based on previous experiences. The multipara may complain that her partner is not as excited about this pregnancy and does not treat her as special. She may perceive this as a lack of support. Health care providers may tend to assume that the multipara knows what to expect and assume she may not have as many questions. Sometimes an "experienced mother" is given less time during prenatal visits because of this false assumption. It is important to recognize that an experienced mother will have many questions. Each pregnancy is unique. Past experiences may be totally different from those in the present pregnancy. The multipara needs special assistance in planning how to prepare her older children for the arrival of the newborn. Arranging for help to permit adequate rest and time to be with the neonate after it arrives should be encouraged (Fig. 8-6).

High-Risk Pregnancy. Although about 20% of all pregnancies in the United States are labeled high risk, relatively little attention to date has been given to the woman's experience of high-risk pregnancy. The woman whose pregnancy comes to be labeled high risk must accomplish the same tasks of pregnancy, but she faces additional challenges as well. The reality of a high-risk pregnancy and birth results in a physical threat to the well-being of the woman and the fetus. Treatment regimens designed to reduce physiologic risk may increase her psychological stress and uncertainty about outcomes even in the best of circumstances.

The woman and her partner may have difficulty resolving ambivalence and establishing a relationship with a fetus who may not be healthy and may not survive. Concerns about the welfare of the mother and fetus predominate. The couple may curtail their sexual relationship completely and find that they talk about nothing but the latest laboratory reports or the status of the fetus. New developments in prenatal assessment may provide parents with more information but may not necessarily reassure them about the outcome of the pregnancy (Kemp & Page, 1987).

An at-risk pregnancy may also have widespread effects on the family as a whole. The pregnant woman may be on

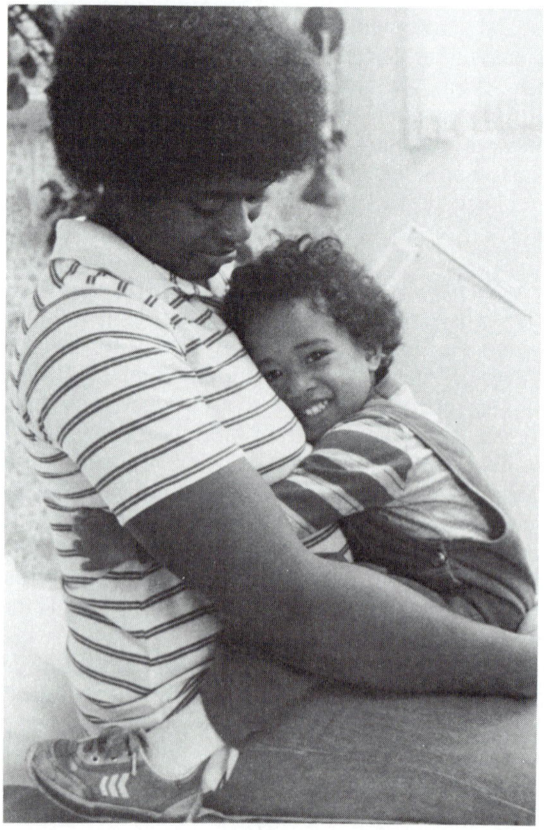

Figure 8-6.
The multipara must prepare herself to care for and love two children. (Photo by BABES, Inc.)

bed rest for weeks, without reliable household help. Her family not only loses her contributions in the home but also her income if she was employed outside the home. Older children in the family may not understand why family routines are disrupted. They may become more difficult for the mother to handle. All of these factors further complicate the process of maternal adaptation in a high-risk pregnancy and may create a situation with high crisis potential.

Sexual Orientation: Lesbian Women and Pregnancy. Lesbian women are increasingly likely to want children and perinatal care that is sensitive to their unique concerns. Research suggests that lesbian women are most likely to seek the assistance of a health care provider to achieve pregnancy through donor insemination (Harvey, Carr, & Bernheine, 1989). Lesbian pregnant women are generally careful to select a care provider who is knowledgeable about lesbian sexuality and unlikely to be "heterosexist" in attitude.

Little research has been conducted on the process of maternal adaptation to pregnancy in lesbian women. However, it is clear that traditional modes of assessment, including questions about marital status, sexual history, and social support, are oriented toward use with heterosexual women. Although the developmental tasks of pregnancy are likely to be similar, the lesbian woman faces unique obstacles and challenges. Thus, nursing assessment should be adapted (see the Assessment Tool display). The perinatal nurse needs to strive toward the use of inclusive language, for example, partner rather than spouse or husband, and to avoid making assumptions about a woman's gender orientation without information.

Developmental Variations in Maternal Adaptation

The pregnant woman's own developmental status significantly affects how she adapts to pregnancy. Most first pregnancies occur among women in their early to middle twenties. However, both adolescent females and first-time pregnant woman over 35 years of age are increasing in number. These developmental variations are discussed in Chapters 9 and 10, respectively.

Paternal Adaptation to Pregnancy

Relatively little is known about the process of paternal adaptation to pregnancy. Expectant fatherhood has only recently become a topic of interest in social science and health research. The following section reviews current knowledge about expectant fatherhood, highlighting some areas of particular importance to the perinatal nurse. In this chapter, as throughout the book, the term "father" refers to the male who participates in the pregnancy in a biologic and psychological sense. Virtually no research has been conducted on the experiences of men who are "social" fathers. These are men who participate in pregnancies for which they are not biologically responsible or men who know they have fathered a child but abandon their female partner and psychologically cut themselves off from the pregnancy.

The Expectant Father

Before the 1960s, there was no clearly defined role for expectant fathers in Western society, other than providing emotional and financial support for the pregnant woman. Published research before 1960 tended to focus on abnormal psychological reactions among expectant fathers. Clinical depression and unusual sexual behavior were studied. However, this focus changed with the advent of the prepared childbirth movement.

The prepared childbirth movement of the 1960s most often involved well-educated, middle-class couples who saw participation by the father as an important aspect of the childbearing experience. These consumers pressured hospitals and health professionals to change policies that prevented fathers from participating in normal childbirth. Gradually, research about expectant and new fatherhood appeared in scientific journals. Most research focused on the effects of participation by the father on the course of labor and on later parent–neonate interaction. Not until later was attention directed toward exploration of the experience of expectant fatherhood itself. Nurse researchers played an important part in generating knowledge in this area.

There are still large gaps in our knowledge about expectant fatherhood. Little attention has been paid to the experience of men from ethnic and lower socioeconomic groups. Most recent research has been done with middle-class, well-educated, European American fathers; their experiences of expectant fatherhood are likely to be different from those of minority and lower-class fathers in important ways. Other aspects of expectant fatherhood that need further exploration are differences between the responses to pregnancy of first-time and experienced fathers as well as single expectant fathers and the responses of expectant fathers to high-risk pregnancy.

Paternal Tasks of Pregnancy

Paternal tasks of pregnancy are similar in many ways to those described for pregnant women. Like their female counterparts, fathers experience psychological and sometimes physical changes as pregnancy progresses. However, the father's response to pregnancy is primarily psychological, without the biologically induced changes women experience. Although it is convenient to examine paternal adaptation by trimesters of pregnancy, the nurse should realize that the time frame of trimesters may not fit as well for partners as it does for women.

For instance, men experience fewer benchmarks of pregnancy than their partners and probably will feel them later. The woman feels her body changing dramatically in the first trimester. The expectant father can only see that she is gaining a little weight and may be sleeping more. The expectant mother typically feels fetal movement long before the father can feel it. Furthermore, not all events of pregnancy will have the same meaning for men. Feeling fetal movement or participating in prenatal classes may be mildly positive experiences for some men. Others may be thrilled by these "peak experiences," depending on their overall outlook on the pregnancy. Therefore, the nurse should recognize there may be more variation in men's experiences of pregnancy,

Assessment Tool

The Lesbian Childbearing Experience

Developmental Task	Assessment Question
Acceptance of the pregnancy by others	What is the impact of this pregnancy on the couple's family, social network, and support system? What is the legal relationship of the biologic father to this newborn? Does the partner intend to have a long-term legal or social relationship as coparent?
Binding-in	How was the pregnancy achieved? If by donor insemination, what was the partner's role? Is the couple aware of the sperm donor's physical characteristics? Were they matched with the mother? the partner? Was a sex selection method used with donor insemination? Is there a sex preference for the newborn by the couple? How will the couple's social network and support systems view the sex of the neonate? What is the mother's image of the unborn child? the partner's?
Safe passage	What health screening criteria were used for donor sperm selection? Does the couple feel safe to disclose their relationship to the birth attendants? How can the nurse assist in ensuring a positive labor and delivery experience for the couple?
Self-giving	What are the costs and benefits (emotional, economic, sociolegal) of this neonate to the couple? How does the partner replenish the pregnant woman's emotional and physical reserves?
Maternal role development	Who will the mother use as a role model? How is the pregnant woman's mother involved with the pregnancy?
Coparent role development	How is this pregnancy affecting the partner's life and relationship with the mother? How does the partner plan to be involved in the pregnancy, birth, and infant care? What does the partner wish to be called by the child?

Wismont, J., & Reame, N. (1989). The lesbian childbearing experience: Assessing developmental tasks. *Image, 21*(3), 140.

both in the nature and in the pace of change over time. The nurse should take care not to assume that expectant fathers are all alike.

Accepting the Pregnancy

Most men are proud and happy when a pregnancy is announced. Many will communicate pleasure and happiness about the pregnancy to their partner. Often this is an important reassurance for the woman because she is likely to be experiencing some reservations about the pregnancy.

A pregnancy typically does not feel "real" for the man until the physical changes in his partner are apparent. Sometimes the pregnancy does not become a reality for the expectant father until he can feel or hear fetal life. Intellectually, he may know his partner is pregnant, but he can forget that fact because the pregnancy is not yet a central part of his life (Jordan, 1990). He may feel increasing anxiety about the long-term future commitment and financial demands of parenthood, but this reflects acceptance on a cognitive level. The expectant father may not feel an emotional investment in the pregnancy until much later. How readily the man accepts pregnancy on an emotional level depends in large part on how ready he feels for it (May, 1982c).

Men experience ambivalence about pregnancy just as women do, perhaps more so. This may be because men are not socialized to anticipate parenthood to the extent that women are in our society. Men are at a further disadvantage because they do not feel the profound physical and physiologic changes of pregnant women. These changes reinforce the reality of pregnancy for the woman and help her to resolve her ambivalence.

Furthermore, men often will not discuss their reservations about a pregnancy with their partners, in part to spare their partner additional emotional pain. Complaining about a pregnancy they helped create is also regarded as unmanly by many men.

Expectant fathers often have no one else with whom they can discuss such matters, so they are left to resolve these feelings on their own. During the process of resolving doubts about a pregnancy, an expectant father will usually maintain some emotional distance from the pregnancy. He may resist efforts of others to involve him more, until he can overcome his ambivalence. A man who feels relatively ready for pregnancy may need only a few days for this process. A man faced with a pregnancy for which he was totally unprepared may spend much of the pregnancy attempting to adjust (May, 1982a).

Pregnancies seem to catch more men by surprise than one might expect. In one study of 20 expectant couples, more than half the men reported that the pregnancy was unplanned, whereas their partners reported the opposite (May, 1982c). Despite the effect unreadiness for pregnancy might have on the amount of emotional support an expectant father may be able to give his partner, prenatal records often fail to include any information about the man's readiness for pregnancy. Any information recorded usually is collected from the woman rather than first-hand from the man.

Establishing a Relationship With the Fetus

Establishing a relationship with the fetus appears to be a somewhat different process for the expectant father than for the expectant mother. The pregnant woman's relationship with the fetus is direct and personal, reinforced by physical sensations. The man's relationship is more indirect until late in pregnancy. One of the major indicators of the man's growing relationship with the fetus is his involvement in pregnancy and preparation for birth. To some extent, this has been institutionalized by the current widespread acceptance of participation by the father in childbirth.

The prepared childbirth movement resulted in the evolution of the expectant father's role as "labor coach." The United States is unique among Western countries in its acceptance of and emphasis on active participation by the father in childbirth. This trend was welcomed by many men and their partners. It encouraged a level of participation in pregnancy and birth for the father, unheard of in the 1950s and early 1960s.

One negative consequence of the prepared childbirth movement is the assumption that all expectant fathers want to be involved in pregnancy and birth. By the 1970s, over 90% of expectant fathers were attending prenatal classes and childbirth in some areas of the country. Men who chose *not* to be actively involved were sometimes regarded with concern and suspicion by health professionals.

Becoming Involved in the Pregnancy

Research has clearly indicated many variations in the type of involvement in pregnancy that men find most comfortable for themselves and their partners (May 1982a; Jordan, 1990). Some men are comfortable being highly emotionally invested in the pregnancy and exploring the changing emotional impact the pregnancy has on them. Often these men see themselves as "full partners" in the experience. They welcome participation in prenatal classes and childbirth because it allows them to share the experience with their spouses.

Other men may see their role in pregnancy as more task oriented. They may take responsibility for some aspects of the pregnancy, such as keeping the partner on her prenatal diet plan, making purchases for the newborn, or remodeling their living quarters. Men who are more comfortable in this style of involvement may prefer the more traditional sex role expectations of the husband and father. Men who see themselves as managers may also be comfortable with prenatal classes and involvement in childbirth as the coach.

Others are not comfortable with emotional or active participation in the pregnancy. They may adopt a quiet observer stance. Sometimes men who prefer to watch from the sidelines are those who may still be resolving their own ambivalence about a pregnancy. Some men are quiet and less participatory by nature and are uncomfortable in a more active role. Often their female partners know they are pleased to be expectant fathers and feel supported. Some pregnant women may feel they have to explain the expectant father's apparent uninvolvement because it does not seem to fit the typical pattern (May, 1982b). The type of involvement the man chooses and the extent of his involvement in the pregnancy experience appear to depend on a number of factors.

Sociocultural Factors. The prepared childbirth movement and its emphasis on the father's role as labor coach has generally been well accepted by middle-class American families. Most middle-class men fully expect to be actively involved in pregnancy and preparation for childbirth. On the other hand, the male sex role among minority and lower socioeconomic groups tends to be more traditional. Men in these groups have been slower to adopt this type of participation. This is especially true among lower-class Hispanic and Asian American men. The division of labor between the sexes is particularly distinct in these groups. Men from these groups may tend to adopt a more task-oriented involvement. This is consistent with their view of the husband and father role.

Personality Factors. The man's personality type influences his level of involvement in pregnancy. Men with highly masculine personalities (a strong need for dominance, high assertiveness, and a strong orientation toward activity rather than toward interpersonal interaction) may feel uncomfortable with close involvement in pregnancy. Pregnancy is inherently a feminine arena; men with traditionally masculine self-concepts may feel out of place. These men may tend to be more distant from the pregnancy or may concentrate on concrete physical preparations.

On the other hand, some men have personalities more balanced between masculine and feminine traits (a strong need for affiliation, high empathy with others, and a strong orientation toward interpersonal interaction). Personalities of this kind are called androgynous personalities. Research has suggested that men with androgynous personalities are more comfortable with emotional involvement in pregnancy as full partners. They may be more sensitive and effective labor support people, and more nurturant caregivers with infants and small children.

The Woman's Preferences About Paternal Involvement. The expectant woman may determine to a large extent how involved her partner may become in the pregnancy. In a sense, the woman may function as a gatekeeper. If she wants her partner to be highly involved in pregnancy and child care, he is likely to be involved. However, if the woman wants to keep pregnancy and childbirth experiences more to herself, the male partner will be less likely to be actively involved.

Adjusting to Changes in Self

Pregnancy typically triggers a range of emotional responses among expectant fathers. The man's self-concept begins to shift, taking on the new dimensions of the paternal role. He begins to rediscover himself as an adult and must decide what it means to him to become a father. Certain themes are common as the expectant father adjusts to changes in himself.

Feelings of Increased Responsibility. Men frequently report that their partner's pregnancy heightens their own sense of responsibility. Often this is expressed in concern about financial security. Men may take on additional work to provide more income for their family. Men from minority or lower socioeconomic groups may feel this increased responsibility most acutely because their traditional view of their role of husband and father is strongly oriented toward providing for the family. If they are unable to do so, they may experience self-doubt and shame.

Men may become increasingly concerned about their own and their partner's personal safety. Expectant fathers report being hesitant to take ordinary chances (such as a career change, fishing or camping trips) because there is now "someone else" to think about. Often men will also be more protective of their partners and their homes at this time (Jordan, 1990).

Concerns About Fathering Ability. Most men express some worry about their own ability to be good fathers. This concern may stem from their own experiences of being fathered. If they had a nurturant, available father, men are able to pattern their behavior after their father's. But many men had fathers who were somewhat emotionally distant and were not involved in childrearing. This pattern was the norm throughout most of the years after World War II. Thus, many men now are starting their own families without a positive role model on which to pattern their behavior. They only know they do not want to be the type of father they had (Russell, 1986).

Pregnancy Symptoms in the Male. Men can experience a physical response to their mate's pregnancy. The couvade syndrome is a constellation of symptoms much like those that women experience. Symptoms include weight gain or weight loss, digestive disturbances, particularly morning nausea, fatigue, headache, and backaches. Couvade symptoms are more likely to occur in early pregnancy and tend to diminish as pregnancy progresses. They are fairly common, with 25% to 65% of expectant fathers experiencing some physical symptoms associated with their partner's pregnancy (Clinton, 1986; Strickland, 1987).

Couvade symptoms may result from a combination of stress, anxiety, and empathy for the pregnant spouse. They are usually harmless or, at most, only minor discomforts. In rare cases, a father experiences physical symptoms that become disabling. This signifies a more serious emotional disturbance, and intensive psychological evaluation is indicated. Occasionally, an expectant father exhibits the delusion that he is, in fact, pregnant. This extremely rare condition, known as pseudocyesis, requires psychiatric care.

Adjusting to Changes in the Couple Relationship

Pregnancy profoundly influences the man's relationship with his partner. Each member of the couple is changing, often in seemingly different ways. The man may be surprised at the emotional changes in his partner and may experience her increasing introspection and self-centeredness in a negative way. Some men find their partner's growing preoccupation with pregnancy fascinating. Others see this preoccupation as annoying and a little boring. A major step in the man's adaptation to pregnancy is learning how to adjust to his changing partner to meet her needs while at the same time maintaining satisfaction and security in the relationship.

Sharing the Partner's Attention. Pregnancy may be the first time the man has ever felt that he had to share his partner's attention. He may have to resolve feelings of rivalry with the newborn and learn to put some of his own emotional needs "on hold." This process is directly related to his own maturation as an adult. If he is insecure about his importance in his partner's life, this adjustment may be threatening and may lead to discord. Failure to make this adjustment can signal future problems in his adjustment to parenthood because caring for an infant requires the parent to sacrifice some of his own needs and derive some satisfaction from doing so. However, the process of learning to put his own needs aside can contribute to his own personal development. He learns to put other priorities above his personal needs and to prepare himself for the future demands of parenthood.

Changes in the Sexual Relationship. Changes in the couple's sexual relationship are almost inevitable during pregnancy. These changes occur because of the physical, physiologic, and emotional impact of pregnancy on the woman. This requires the expectant father to adjust to a changing intimate partner. (See Chapter 5 for a discussion of sexuality during pregnancy.) Men appear to be more sensitive to and more bothered by changes in the sexual relationship than are their partners. If the pregnancy has had a distinctly negative effect on a couple's sexual life, the man will probably feel the loss more acutely. His satisfaction with life overall will tend to suffer more (May, 1987).

Preparing for Labor, Birth, and Early Fatherhood

Preparation for birth is most apparent late in pregnancy. Prenatal classes in almost every community prepare fathers for their support role in labor and birth. Sometimes men may come to regard the birth as a testing ground and worry that they may not measure up to their partner's or their own expectations as a labor coach. Men have many fears about their partner's well-being throughout the labor process. They worry about how they will react to their partner's pain and whether she and the neonate will survive.

Most men have little or no experience in caring for newborns and realize that they have much to learn. However, this important aspect may be neglected, in part because of the overemphasis on preparation for labor and birth. If newborn care classes are available and designed to accommodate fathers easily, many men will attend and view them as valuable. Again, this depends on how involved the man expects to be in newborn care. Some men realistically see themselves as rather uninvolved until their children are older. Therefore, they will prepare less during pregnancy.

Situational Factors Affecting Paternal Adaptation

Some situational factors seem to influence paternal adaptation to pregnancy. Little research has been done to date in these areas and current literature may provide limited information. The nurse must keep in mind that nursing diagnoses and interventions with men in these situations will be based solely on assessment of the man's individual situation.

High-Risk Pregnancy. Men normally worry about the well-being of their partner and the fetus during pregnancy. When complications of pregnancy develop, these fears are greatly intensified. Again, the expectant father may have no one with whom he can discuss these concerns except his partner. Most men are unwilling to burden their partners in this way.

If the woman's condition requires hospitalization or bed rest, the man must then manage the household affairs, his job, and his worry about his partner and their fetus. He may worry that his partner and fetus are going to die, even if the risk is remote. He may feel torn between staying with his partner, staying with older children, and fulfilling work responsibilities. The father may not think to ask for help that might be available or may underestimate the problems of finding child care and household help (May, 1993).

Subsequent Pregnancies. Little is known about the differences between paternal adaptation to first pregnancies and adaptation to later ones. Some fathers may have an easier adjustment in subsequent pregnancies because they know what to expect, whereas others may be more fearful because of problems during the first pregnancy. A subsequent pregnancy is more complicated because relationships with the older child must be renegotiated. Often fathers assume more responsibility for caretaking of the older child during pregnancy. This allows the mother to be involved with the newborn. Some fathers may tend to become less involved with a subsequent pregnancy because the novelty and thrill may be lessened. They believe their partner needs their support less. However, this is often not the case and multiparas often complain they are not being treated as special during pregnancy. They miss their partner's active and obvious support.

Developmental Variations in Paternal Adaptation

The man's own developmental status has a profound influence on his adaptation to pregnancy. Paternal adaptation in adolescents and older men is discussed in Chapters 9 and 10, respectively.

Adaptation of Other Family Members to Pregnancy

Pregnancy not only causes shifts in the relationship in the couple but also creates changes in other family relationships. Ties with other family members may become closer because the burdens and rewards of parenthood can now be shared. The future addition of a new family member and changes in the family's daily routines are examples of adaptational demands on families.

Siblings

Sibling adaptation to pregnancy will vary according to the child's developmental level. The areas in which the sibling is likely to experience the most change during pregnancy include maternal appearance; parental behavior; and home environment, particularly sleeping arrangements.

Children under 2 years of age are usually unaware of pregnancy. They do not understand explanations about the future arrival of a new brother or sister. They may, however, pick up and respond to the emotional atmosphere in the household, particularly around the time of birth and shortly thereafter. Children from 2 to 4 years of age may only respond to obvious changes in the mother's body and behavior. They may not remember from month to month why the changes are occurring. However, changes in the physical environment may be disruptive for them. For this reason, if the child's sleeping arrangements must be changed to accommodate the newborn, these changes should be initiated well before the mother leaves home for the birth.

Children aged 4 and 5 often enjoy listening to the fetal heartbeat. They may be interested in learning about fetal development at a level appropriate to their age (Fig. 8-7). They understand that the newborn will be a brother or sister but usually have unrealistic expectations about having a ready-made playmate. Children at this age may sense a shift in the mother's attention. They may resent her physical limitations, such as the mother's inability to lift and hold them or to engage in roughhousing late in pregnancy (Fortier, Carson, Will, & Shubkagel, 1991).

School-age children aged 6 through 12 take a keen interest in the "hows" and "whys" of pregnancy and birth. They have many questions and may welcome age-appropriate books and pictures about birth. Often they plan elaborate welcomes for the neonate and they want to be able to help when the newborn comes home. Children of this age may express interest in being present at the birth and may enjoy preparing for participation in the event.

The responses of adolescents to pregnancy depend in large part on their developmental status. Younger adoles-

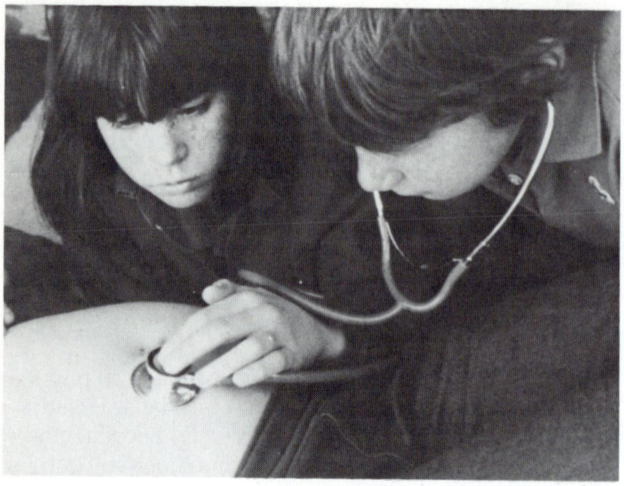

Figure 8-7.
School-age children are fascinated by hearing fetal heart tones and feeling fetal movement. (Photo by BABES, Inc.)

cents may be uncomfortable with the obvious evidence of their parents' sexuality. They may be negative and embarrassed about the changes in their mother's appearance. Adolescents may be fascinated and repelled by the process of birth. Girls may not want to be present at birth because of their own fears, whereas boys may be more interested.

Middle and older adolescents (ages 14 to 19), in the process of loosening their ties to their parents and families, may be somewhat indifferent to the changes associated with pregnancy, unless these interfere with their own activities and independence. They may respond in a more adult fashion by imagining themselves in the parent role and offering support and help.

Preparing the sibling for birth and the arrival of the newborn can make for a smoother adjustment. Research to date has not shown that sibling preparation during pregnancy eliminates sibling rivalry and adjustment problems after the birth. However, there may be positive effects in terms of the older child's behavior (Fortier et al., 1991). Most parents choose to prepare children in some way during pregnancy in an effort to ease the older child's adjustment to changes in the household. Preparation must be carried out at the child's level of understanding and in response to readiness to learn.

Grandparents

One especially important area that changes in response to pregnancy is the relationship with parents, who are soon to become grandparents. Expectant parents often find that their relationship with their own parents, particularly the mother's parents, whether actual or only remembered, seems to become more important and positive during pregnancy (Cronenwett, 1985). For women, and perhaps for men, the first pregnancy signals true adult status and the beginning of a new, more equal kind of relationship with parents. Grandparents are often the first people told about a pregnancy. New parents recognize that the tie to the future represented by the fetus is of special significance to grandparents.

The adjustment grandparents themselves must make is complex. The pregnancy may be a painful reminder of their own advancing age, or it may rekindle their own energy for life and create a sense of hopeful expectation (Fig. 8-8). Grandparents are often unsure how much they should be involved in preparing for and caring for a newborn. Most grandparents are aware that childbearing and childrearing practices have changed dramatically since they were young. Thus, they may think they have nothing to offer the new family. Others may interfere in the family's affairs and may create more strain in the young couple's life. To offer assistance, many institutions and community groups are establishing classes designed to help grandparents adjust to their new roles. These efforts provide current information about birth and childrearing so grandparents can be more effective sources of support for young families.

"We can have ex-spouses and ex-jobs but not ex-children" (Rossi, 1968). This comment points to the irrevocable nature of the psychological change resulting from childbearing. Even when a newborn is placed for adoption and there is no further contact between the newborn and the natural parents, the parents may feel a lifelong pull toward their unknown child. Maternal tasks of pregnancy involve accepting the pregnancy, establishing a relationship with the fetus, incorporating the fetus, separating the fetus from self, adjusting to changes in self, adjusting to the changing couple relationship, and preparing for birth and early motherhood. Paternal tasks include accepting the pregnancy, establishing a relationship with the fetus, becoming involved in the pregnancy, adjusting to changes in self, adjusting to changes in the couple relationship, and preparing for labor, birth, and early fatherhood. There are also developmental variations in adaptations. (See Chapter 36 for discussion of the psychological adjustments required during pregnancy and the transition to parenthood.)

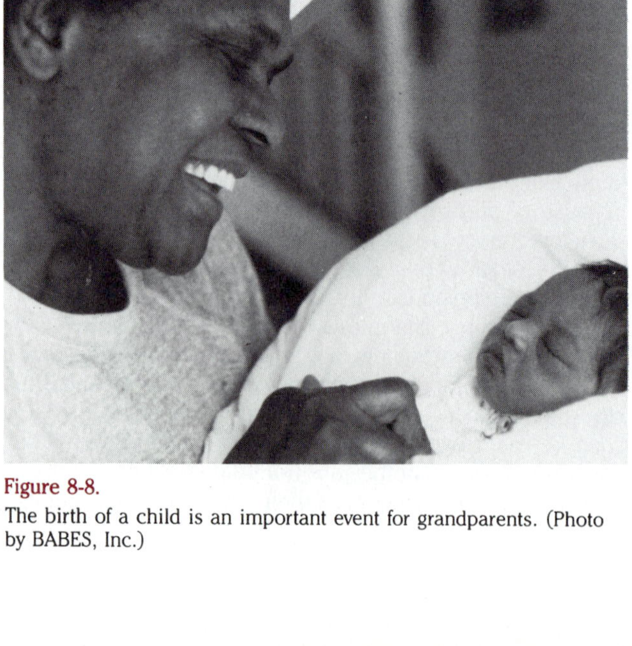

Figure 8-8.
The birth of a child is an important event for grandparents. (Photo by BABES, Inc.)

Implications for Nursing Care

The nurse assumes a variety of roles in meeting the social, cultural, and psychological needs of women and their families during pregnancy. Nurses often function as teachers, role models, counselors, or resource persons, as well as clinicians. Nursing care is aimed at promoting healthy adaptation and preventing and reducing stress caused by the many individual and family adjustments required during pregnancy. In many instances, the nurse is the only health professional to have repeated and extended contact with the woman and her family throughout pregnancy.

Cultural practices related to birth are important because women and their families value these practices. If a woman believes she is in danger of becoming ill because she took a shower during her postpartum hospitalization, she may be at risk because of that very belief. Thus, cultural practices have important implications for the provision of nursing care.

A nurse cannot reasonably hope to become an expert on every cultural group and its birth practices. Even if she could, knowledge of cultural practices might not be helpful in individual cases because of the uneven rate of acculturation and because of the natural variability even among people of the same cultural group. However, the nurse can be open and interested in learning about the pregnant woman's concerns and needs in relation to traditional practices, treating these practices with respect. By so doing, the nurse demonstrates respect for the pregnant woman and her family and facilitates the transition to motherhood.

Most pregnant woman and their partners adjust well to pregnancy. They have functional support systems, communicate their love and concern about each other, and need only encouragement, anticipatory guidance, and factual information from the nurse to maintain equilibrium during the prenatal period. However, some pregnant women and their families are at psychosocial risk. In these cases, the astute nurse is in an excellent position to identify psychosocial problems early, intervening before individual and family functioning begins to deteriorate.

The material in this chapter provides only the basis for a deeper exploration of the psychological and emotional tasks for expectant mothers and fathers and their families as they move through pregnancy, birth, and early parenthood. Units 3 through 5 discuss the nursing care required to support families through the childbearing year. However, some points in this chapter have particular importance for the delivery of clinical nursing care.

Assessing Psychosocial Factors

Some basic information about psychosocial factors is usually reflected in the routine assessment forms used in clinical practice: age, sex, marital status, race, socioeconomic status, educational level, and language barriers are usually noted. However, some important variables are often ignored. Readiness for pregnancy is one of these. Whether the pregnancy was planned and wanted should be noted, as well as the partner's response to the timing of the pregnancy and the responses of any other important family members. If a pregnant woman's significant others are not happy about a pregnancy, the nurse should be aware that the woman may be at increased emotional risk. This woman most likely will require additional support. However, if pertinent information is not obtained or documented, the nurse cannot anticipate problems and help the childbearing family to cope with potential problem areas. This underscores the importance of a family assessment in perinatal care.

Cultural assessment is an area often neglected in prenatal nursing assessment. This type of assessment may be difficult because of language barriers or differences in customary patterns of interpersonal interaction. Strategies the nurse can use to avoid communication barriers that may arise from cultural differences are listed in the accompanying display. The display that appears earlier in the chapter under Cultural Aspects of Childbearing lists specific ques-

Strategies for Avoiding Cultural Barriers in Communication

Approach

- Consider whether a direct approach is acceptable or whether direct questions are embarrassing or offensive.
- Take time to engage in some social interaction to show respect and gain confidence and knowledge.
- Safeguard the woman's sense of modesty.
- Avoid discussing matters related to her care when outsiders are present.

Customs

- Recognize that all human behavior is influenced by cultural patterns. Never assume that a practice is unimportant.
- Learn the significance of practices and facilitate them whenever possible.
- Learn the rationale for unusual practices and incorporate them whenever possible into your plan of care. When they cannot be incorporated, for reasons of safety or practicality, find out whether there are alternatives that would be acceptable to the woman.

Language

- Never assume that the woman understands you if English is her second language. Arrange for translation when possible.
- Obtain written patient information sheets in other languages that you encounter frequently.
- Avoid using American slang and medical jargon.
- Speak slowly and quietly.

Stern, P., Tilden, V., & Maxwell, E. (1980). Culturally induced stress during childbearing: The Filipino American experience. Issues in Health Care for Women, 2, *67.*

tions useful in assessing cultural variations to plan culturally sensitive nursing care.

A sample assessment tool designed to assist the nurse in assessing parental adaptation to pregnancy is shown in the display, Assessment/Intervention for Parental Adaptation to Pregnancy. Maternal and paternal tasks are discussed as they change with pregnancy, expected parental responses are noted, and nursing interventions are suggested. If the nurse detects slow progress or difficulties in adaptation in a particular area, that area should be assessed in greater detail.

Planning Psychosocial Approaches

The planning of appropriate psychosocial and cultural approaches to care must include the woman and members of her family. Other health professionals are often involved as well. Often childbearing women have a variety of psychosocial needs that complicate their health care. Thus, the nurse will need to plan for appropriate referrals to and coordination with social workers, nutritionists, and community agencies. This will ensure that the resources available to the woman and her family are effectively used.

Education is a major part of assisting parents and their families in adjusting to the demands of pregnancy. The nurse can reassure the woman that her emotional responses, although confusing and strange to her, are actually expected changes of pregnancy. Teaching the woman some ways to keep these changes from intruding too much into her daily life is an example of teaching that encourages adaptation to pregnancy. Women may welcome information about their family members' adaptation to pregnancy. They tend to know little about what is "normal" behavior for expectant fathers and siblings.

Most nursing intervention in the area of psychosocial care can be called "watchful waiting." This includes observing how women and their families are adjusting and then filling in with needed information, encouragement, and anticipatory guidance. "Watchful waiting" is also designed to alert the nurse to situations that require more intervention. The nurse is able to take steps to reduce rising stress levels in a family in which adjustments are becoming more difficult. The goal of these more focused interventions is to prevent individual and family crises.

Reducing Stress and Crisis Potential

A single stressful event may not by itself lead to a crisis, but a combination of stress factors can suddenly overwhelm an individual's coping mechanisms. Part of comprehensive nursing care is the systematic assessment of stress factors in the pregnant woman's life. This assessment should be done early in pregnancy. It should be updated as the pregnancy progresses or as the woman's life situation changes.

If a pregnant woman or her family is experiencing high levels of stress that may precipitate a crisis, four specific nursing interventions may be useful:

- Encouraging positive coping behavior
- Providing support
- Manipulating environmental stressors
- Providing anticipatory guidance

Encouraging Positive Coping Behaviors. The nurse can help the woman clarify sources of stress and review the coping patterns that have worked in the past. The nurse may also suggest new ways of coping with pregnancy. Examples include encouraging the woman to attend prenatal classes or support groups, seeking out an experienced friend for support, or acquiring needed information about specific concerns (see the Teaching Considerations display).

Providing Support. The nurse can be helpful by communicating availability and concern. This can be done by calling the pregnant woman between prenatal visits to see how she is getting along. Another helpful approach is listening in an unhurried and receptive fashion during prenatal visits. Appropriate and caring reassurance from a professional is a powerful, although sometimes underused, way to reduce stress.

Manipulating Environmental Stressors. The nurse may be able to identify environmental stressors that can easily be reduced or eliminated. Arranging for a more convenient prenatal visit schedule that allows for child care at home and involvement by the father is one approach. Another is helping the woman to plan travel so that long car rides or crowded conditions on public transportation are avoided. Assisting the family to plan for household assistance after childbirth is a concrete intervention designed to reduce environmental stress for the expectant family.

Providing Anticipatory Guidance. The nurse may help reduce stress levels by anticipating learning needs and

Text continues on page 194

Teaching Considerations

Reducing Stress Levels

The nurse may recommend the following points in teaching parents how to reduce stress:

- Walking for exercise is an excellent way to avoid excessive fatigue and may help to even out mood swings.
- Spending time with other parents of small children and talking with them about the "good" and "bad" parts of parenthood may help in alleviating fears and dispelling unrealistic expectations.
- Taking a little more time with her personal appearance early in pregnancy may help to maintain the woman's self-confidence and reduce negative reactions to normal physical changes.
- Taking time to have fun alone as a couple or with friends early in pregnancy may provide needed opportunities for talking about concerns and giving and receiving support.

Assessment Tool

Interview Guide for Assessing Parental Adaptation to Pregnancy

(This guide should be used at the first prenatal visit and updated throughout the perinatal period.)

Mother's Name ______________________ **Age** ______________________

Father's Name ______________________ **Age** ______________________

Married: Yes __ No __ **Length of Time Married** __ **Number of Children** __

Pregnancy Planned: Yes __ No __ **Gravida** __ **Para** __ **Abortion:** Elective __ Spontaneous __

Stillbirths __

History of birth defects, prematurity, or illness in infants or family: ______________________

Current health status: Mother ______________________

Father ______________________

Other children ______________________

Have they any close friends, relatives, or organizations that they can talk with or turn to for support? Yes ______ No __ Name two: ______________________

Interview Questions

1. How does the woman feel about being pregnant? ______________________
2. Has anything happened in the past or is there a current condition that is causing the client concern? ______________________
3. What effect does the client believe this pregnancy will have on her future lifestyle? ______________________
4. What has been the expectant father's reaction to the pregnancy? ______________________
5. What child-rearing practices were used by the woman's parents when she was a child? ______________________
   a. Which of these child-rearing practices will the couple use with their child? ______________________
   b. Which practices will they avoid? ______________________
6. What does the couple do when faced with a serious problem? ______________________
7. Do they plan to attend childbirth education classes? Yes __ No __
   Why? ______________________
8. Does the expectant father plan to be with the woman during labor and delivery? Yes __ No __
9. Does the woman plan to have rooming-in? Yes __ No __
10. How much physical help do they expect
    a. During pregnancy: ______________________
    b. After pregnancy: ______________________
    c. Who supplies this help? ______________________
11. To what extent will this pregnancy and the infant alter the couple's plans for:
    a. Career and employment: ______________________
    b. Education: ______________________
    c. Lifestyle: ______________________

Additional Comments ______________________

Note

Risk for crisis should be considered to be increased if:

1. The mother experiences any pregnancy complications
2. There is a probability of multiple birth
3. Mother or infant requires transfer to a high-risk center
4. There is continued stress that has not been alleviated
5. The client or family has no support systems

(continued)

Assessment Tool *(Continued)*

Assessment/Intervention for Parental Adaptation to Pregnancy

Tasks	Expected Behavior	Nursing Intervention	Possible Signs of Maladaptation
First Trimester: Maternal Adaptation			
Incorporation of intruding fetus	Ambivalence: "Not me, not now" response. May forget about pregnancy for short periods	Stress normalcy of ambivalence, encourage discussion of feelings. If pregnancy is unplanned and ambivalence strong, assess whether patient should consider terminating pregnancy.	Strong, intense resistance to pregnancy.
Acceptance of pregnancy by self, partner	Informs partner of pregnancy; anticipates partner's response. Negative or ambivalent response usually stressful and worrying.	Give anticipatory guidance about partner response to and needs in early pregnancy. Encourage participation by partner in early prenatal visit.	
Adjustment to change in self:			
Emotional changes	Increasing introversion, narcissism, dependence, mood swings; changes in sexual patterns.	Discuss time-limited, hormonal nature of changes; emphasize meeting woman's own needs. Identify and suggest appropriate reading materials.	
Physical changes	Concern about signs and symptoms (weight gain, breast tenderness, nausea, fatigue)	Give anticipatory guidance about kind and duration of expected symptoms and practical comfort measures.	Disabling physical symptoms
Sexual changes	May report decreased interest in sexual activity and fears about intercourse during pregnancy.	Teach about physiologic causes of shifts in sexual patterns; give guidelines for intercourse during pregnancy.	
First Trimester: Paternal Adaptation			
Adjustment to news of pregnancy	Surprise, joy, or anger, depending on whether or not pregnancy was planned and intended	Stress normalcy of response. Encourage discussion of feelings.	Anger, suggestions for therapeutic abortion, "it's *her* problem"
Acceptance of pregnancy	Ambivalence. May forget pregnancy for long periods.	Stress normalcy of response; point out that many men get more interested later in pregnancy.	
Adjustment to changes in partner			
Emotional changes	Recognition of emotional changes and increasing needs.	Reinforce importance of giving partner extra support; give anticipatory	Anger at partner's emotional needs

(continued)

Assessment Tool *(Continued)*

Assessment/Intervention for Parental Adaptation to Pregnancy *(continued)*

Tasks	Expected Behavior	Nursing Intervention	Possible Signs of Maladaptation
		guidance about changes and duration. Give specific examples of ways to help: helping her eat well, helping with heavy work, giving extra affection.	
Physical/sexual changes	Acceptance of changes in sexual relationship	Explain physiologic causes of changes. Encourage expression of feelings. Counsel about alternative methods of sexual expression.	Unwillingness to accept temporary sexual changes.
	Fears about partner's physical vulnerability	Counsel about pregnancy as state of health; give guidelines for intercourse in pregnancy.	
Adjustment to changes in self:			
Emotional changes	Increasing sense of responsibility; fears about ability to be good father.	Encourage discussion of feelings and concerns, especially with other men.	
Physical changes	May exhibit physical symptoms: weight gain or loss, nausea, fatigue	Explain nature of physical changes in positive light as sign of involvement; give practical suggestions for comfort.	Disabling physical symptoms
Second Trimester: Maternal Adaptation			
Separation of fetus from self; beginning attachment to fetus	Wonder, joy in response to quickening; pet naming of fetus, interactions with fetus.	Encourage "tuning in" to fetal movements; discuss fetal capacities for hearing, responding to interaction and maternal activity.	Quickening experienced as unpleasant; avoidance of maternity clothes.
Acceptance of fetus by others	Increasing need for contact with mother or maternal figure; dreams/fantasies about others' response to child.	Encourage discussion of changing relationships with family and friends.	
Adjustment to changes in self:			
Emotional changes	Tendency to focus on fetus and "leave out" partner; increasing dependence and demands on partner.	Emphasize partner's need for nurturance, reassurance. Encourage open communication with partner.	Denial of any need for change in couple relationship.
Physical changes	Increasing feelings of well-being; more energy. Wearing maternity clothes;	Discuss symptoms and causes; give anticipatory guidance about future	Total avoidance of sexual contact with partner. Avoidance of weight gain;

(continued)

Assessment Tool *(Continued)*

Assessment/Intervention for Parental Adaptation to Pregnancy *(continued)*

Tasks	Expected Behavior	Nursing Intervention	Possible Signs of Maladaptation
	grief work about loss of figure. Avoidance of some activities for self-protection; concerns about sexual relationship.	changes. Encourage discussion of concerns.	strong distress about pregnant figure.
Preparation for maternal role	Mimicry and role playing in maternal role; observing other women; accepting and rejecting behaviors as suitable for themselves. Grief work for roles being relinquished.	Discuss preparations for birth; parenthood. Encourage making early plans. Identify and suggest appropriate reading on parenthood.	
Second Trimester: Paternal Adaptation			
Establishment of relationship with fetus	Excitement at feeling/hearing fetal life; "getting into" pregnancy.	Facilitate partner hearing/feeling fetal life; discuss fetal capabilities (hearing, responding to activity, stimulation).	Continued strong ambivalence and emotional distancing. Uneasiness; anger about fetal movements.
Adjustment to changes in self:			
Preparation for paternal role	Increasing sense of self as father; increasing introspection, reflection on own father.	Encourage discussion of future role as father, plans for involvement in birth and care-taking. Encourage discussion of plans, expectations with partner.	Strong resistance to participation in preparations; continued inability to think about self as father.
Adjustment to changes in partner:			
Emotional changes	Accepting her increasing dependence; protectiveness of her increasing vulnerability. Learning to share her attention with fetus.	Discuss changes in couple relationship during pregnancy and early parenthood. Emphasize need for expression of affection and open communication.	Continued anger at partner's emotional changes.
Physical/sexual changes	Surprise, uneasiness, or enjoyment of partner's pregnant figure; gradual acceptance of changes. Concern over sexual changes in relationship.	Encourage discussion of sexual concerns. Encourage affectionate holding, reassurance of partner. Reinforce guidelines for safe, comfortable sexual activity during pregnancy.	Strong expressions of displeasure with partner's body, sexual relationship.
Third Trimester: Maternal Adaptation			
Preparation for birth and separation from fetus.	Eagerness for pregnancy to end; fears about labor and birth; disturbing birth dreams.	Stress normalcy of fatigue and fears. Focus teaching on preparation for labor and birth, expectations and worries. Give anticipatory	Denial of fears about childbirth. Unrealistic expectations about birth.

(continued)

Assessment Tool *(Continued)*

Assessment/Intervention for Parental Adaptation to Pregnancy *(continued)*

Tasks	Expected Behavior	Nursing Intervention	Possible Signs of Maladaptation
		guidance about hospital policies. Review signs and symptoms of labor and "danger signs." Assess plans for labor support; encourage presence of second support person if appropriate.	
Preparation for early motherhood: acceptance of maternal role	Nesting behavior (preparing home and self for infant); fantasies about motherhood and child; concerns about ability to be good mother.	Discuss preparations for baby; advise against overdoing physical preparations causing excessive fatigue. Encourage attendance at infant care classes. Focus teaching on infant care, feeding methods. Identify and suggest appropriate reading. Discuss expectations and plans for father involvement in care-taking; plans for teaching father infant care skills.	Lack of preparation for infant.
Adjusting to changes in self:			
Emotional changes	Increasing sensitivity and anxiety	Provide reassurance and encouragement.	
Physical changes	Impatience with physical discomforts and awkwardness. Increasing feeling of physical vulnerability.	Give practical suggestions for easing discomforts. Reassure that discomforts are temporary.	
Adjustment to changes in couple relationship	Acceptance of increasing dependence on partner, increasing need for reassurance. Decreasing sexual activity.	Encourage joint activities; stress normalcy and temporary nature of changes. Encourage alternative forms of affection: holding, massage, and so on.	
Third Trimester: Paternal Adaptation			
Preparation for birth	Fears about labor and birth; worries about well-being of partner and child, about ability to support partner.	Stress normalcy of worries. Review signs and symptoms of labor and "danger signs," hospital admission procedures. Assess comfort with labor coach role and reassure as needed. Stress that help in labor	Denial of fears or unrealistic expectations about birth.

(continued)

Assessment Tool *(Continued)*

Assessment/Intervention for Parental Adaptation to Pregnancy *(continued)*

Tasks	Expected Behavior	Nursing Intervention	Possible Signs of Maladaptation
		will be available. Encourage presence of second support person if appropriate.	
Preparation for early fatherhood.	Nesting behavior, purchasing items for baby. Questions about infants; concerns about ability to be good father.	Encourage attendance at infant care classes. Focus teaching on infant care, feeding methods, anticipated changes in household routine. Identify and suggest appropriate reading.	Absence of involvement in preparations.
Adjustment to changes in couple relationship:			
Sexual changes	Concerns about decreasing sexual activity; worries about future sexual relationship.	Stress normalcy; suggest alternative means of sexual expression. Give anticipatory guidance about slow return to normalcy after infant comes.	Continued anger and unwillingness to accept changes in sexual patterns.

providing information about expected events. Examples of anticipatory guidance for the expectant family might be reassuring a pregnant woman that morning nausea usually decreases after the first trimester or explaining to a father that many men do not feel involved in pregnancy until the last weeks. Reassuring the father that he still will likely feel a strong bond with the newborn later may be an effective approach. Even if the parents seem to have a considerable amount of information already, they often welcome discussion with a knowledgeable nurse about what they might expect. If these steps do not seem to meet the woman's need for support, the nurse should consider consultation with the physician and other members of the health care team. If appropriate, referral to more specialized counseling and psychiatric services may be needed.

The nurse will need to rely on interpersonal skills to assess the outcomes of nursing interventions with childbearing families. The effectiveness of care may be reflected only in long-term outcomes, such as healthy parent and family adaptation to the childbearing process.

Chapter Summary

Individual and family adaptation to pregnancy is a complex process that requires extensive psychological, physical, and social adjustments over a fairly brief period of time. Adaptation lays the groundwork for the later transition to parenthood. Thus, adaptation to pregnancy is important to the long-range health of childbearing women and their families. Early assessment and intervention may prevent or greatly reduce later family problems.

Understanding a particular woman's response to pregnancy or her behavior in labor is impossible without some knowledge about what the pregnancy means to her, what she believes is normal and healthy behavior, and what she believes can be harmful to her. More importantly, the nurse cannot plan an effective course of care for a woman without this knowledge.

Many factors influence individual decisions about reproductive behavior and childbearing. The individual's readiness for parenthood, motivations for childbearing, and view of what is acceptable male and female behavior often influence reproductive decisions. Once pregnancy occurs, the ease or difficulty of the adjustment to it are determined in large part by the individual's sex, age, and developmental status. Cultural norms will also have an impact on individual behavior.

Pregnancy is a time of increased vulnerability to crisis. Maternal and paternal responses to pregnancy tend to show fairly predictable patterns that assist the nurse in the assessment and diagnosis of actual or potential difficulties in adaptation. Through psychosocial and cultural assessment, the nurse may be able to anticipate family problems and strengths within the context of perinatal nursing care.

The adequacy of the information derived from a thorough assessment can determine whether the subsequent nursing care is appropriate and effective in promoting the health of childbearing women and their families. Because of repeated contacts with pregnant women and their partners, the nurse can play a central role in assessing individual and family adaptation to pregnancy. The nurse focuses on intervening in ways appropriate to the identified level of need. Providing support to individuals and families during pregnancy is a major nursing responsibility. Successful nursing interventions contribute directly to the psychological and physical well-being of expectant parents and their families.

Study Questions

1. *What are basic functions of families? In what ways can some functions occur outside the family unit?*
2. *How can pregnancy can be a crisis for some individuals and families?*
3. *What social factors might influence a person's decision about whether or not to risk pregnancy?*
4. *What characteristics might be considered important in determining a person's psychosocial readiness for pregnancy?*
5. *What cultural variations in birth practices have you seen or heard about in your clinical setting?*
6. *How would you assess cultural beliefs and practices? How would you adjust your care to maintain safety and deliver culturally sensitive nursing care?*
7. *What are the parental tasks of pregnancy for mothers and fathers?*
8. *Discuss common parental concerns for each trimester of pregnancy and outline appropriate nursing interventions.*

References

Asperilla, P. (1986). Cultural characteristics of the Filipino: Origins and influences. *Journal of the New York State Nurses Association, 17*(1), 16–20.

Bliss-Holtz, V. (1988). Primipara's prenatal concern for learning infant care. *Nursing Research, 37*(1), 20–24.

Bozett, F., & Hanson, S. (1991). *Fatherhood and families in cultural context*. New York: Springer.

Broach, J., & Newton, N. (1988). Food and beverages in labor. Part I: Cross-cultural and historical practices. *Birth*, 15(2), 81–92.

Coreil, J., & Mull, J. (1990). *Anthropology and primary health care*. Boulder: Westview Press.

Clinton, J. (1986). Expectant fathers at risk for couvade. *Nursing Research, 35*(5), 290–296.

Cranley, M. (1981). Roots of attachment: The relationship of parents with their unborn. *Birth Defects: Original Article Series. 17*(6), 59–65.

Cronenwett, L. (1985). Parental network structure and perceived support after birth of the first child. *Nursing Research, 34*(6), 347–350.

Cummins, L., Scrimshaw, S., & Engle, P. (1988). Views of cesarean birth among primiparous women of Mexican origin in Los Angeles. *Birth, 15*(3), 164–168.

D'Avanzo, C. (1992). Bridging the cultural gap with Southeast Asians. *American Journal of Maternal Child Nursing, 17*, 204–207.

Flaherty, M., Facteau, L., & Garver, P. (1987). Grandmother functions in multigenerational families: An exploratory study of black adolescent mothers and their infants. *Maternal-Child Nursing Journal, 16*(4), 61–69.

Fortier, J., Carson, V., Will, S., & Shubkagel, B. (1991). Adjustment to a newborn: Sibling preparation makes a difference. *Journal of Obstetric, Gynecologic, and Neonatal Nursing, 20*(4), 73–78.

Harvey, S., Carr, C., & Bernheine, S. (1989). Lesbian mothers: Health care experiences. *Journal of Nurse Midwifery, 34*(3), 115–119.

Jordan, P. (1990). Laboring for relevance: Expectant and new fatherhood. *Nursing Research, 39*(6), 11–15.

Kay, M. (1982). *Anthropology of human birth*. Philadelphia: F. A. Davis.

Kemp, V., & Page, C. (1987). Maternal self-esteem and prenatal attachment in high-risk pregnancy. *Maternal-Child Nursing Journal, 16*(6), 195–200.

Kenney, J., & Tash, D. (1992). Lesbian childbearing couples' dilemmas and decisions. *Health Care of Women International, 13*(2), 209–219.

Lewis, J. (1988). The transition to parenthood: 1. The rating of prenatal marital competence. *Family Process, 27*(6), 149–152.

Lewis, W. (1988). The transition to parenthood: 2. Stability and change in the marital structure. *Family Process, 27*(7), 273–278.

Mathews, J., & Zadek, K. (1991). The alternative birth movement in the United States: History and current status. *Women and Health, 17*(1), 39–56.

Mattson, S., & Lew, L. (1992). Culturally sensitive prenatal care for Southeast Asians. *Journal of Obstetric, Gynecologic, and Neonatal Nursing, 21*(1), 48–54.

May, K. (1993; in press). The impact of maternal activity restriction during pregnancy on the expectant father. *Journal of Obstetric, Gynecologic, and Neonatal Nursing.*

May, K. (1987). Men's sexuality during the childbearing year: Implications of recent research findings. *Holistic Nursing Practice, 1*(4), 60–65.

May, K. (1982a). Three phases in the development of father involvement in pregnancy. *Nursing Research, 32*(6), 377–383.

May, K. (1982b) The father as observer. *American Journal of Maternal Child Nursing, 7*(6), 319–321.

May, K. (1982c). Factors contributing to readiness for fatherhood: An exploratory study. *Family Relations, 31*(5), 353–357.

Meleis, A., & Sorrell, L. (1981). Arab American women and their birth experiences. *American Journal of Maternal Child Nursing, 6*(8), 171–176.

Mercer, R. (1990). *Parents at risk*. New York: Springer.

Mercer, R., Ferketich, S., May, K., DeJoseph, J., & Sollid, D. (1988). Further exploration of maternal and paternal fetal attachment. *Research in Nursing and Health, 11*(1), 83–87.

Muller, M. (1992). A critical review of prenatal attachment research. *Scholarly Inquiry in Nursing Practice, 6*(1), 5–22.

Perry, D. (1982). The umbilical cord: Transcultural care and customs. *Journal of Nurse Midwifery, 27*(4), 25–30.

Poole, C. (1987). Adolescent pregnancy and unfinished developmental tasks of childhood. *Journal of School Health, 57*(7), 271–276.

Rossi, A. (1968). Transition to parenthood. *Journal of Marriage and the Family, 30*(6), 26–32.,

Rubin, R. (1970). Cognitive style in pregnancy. *American Journal of Nursing, 70*(2), 502–505.

Russell, G. (1986). Primary caretaking and role sharing fathers. In M. Lamb (Ed.). *The father's role: Applied perspectives*. New York: Wiley.

Saunders, R., & Robins, E. (1987). Changes in the marital relationship during the first pregnancy. *Health Care of Women International, 8*(5/6), 361–367.

South, S., & Tolnay, S. (1992). *The changing American family: Sociological and demographic perspectives*. Boulder: Westview Press.

Strickland, O. (1987). The occurrence of symptoms in expectant fathers during the first pregnancy. *Nursing Research, 36*(3), 184–186.

TenHouten, W. (1970). The black family: Myth and reality. *Psychiatry, 33*(2) 145–150.

Tiedje, L., & Collins, C. (1989). Combining employment and motherhood. *American Journal of Maternal Child Nursing, 14*(1), 29–33.

Tilden, V. (1983). Perceptions of single vs partnered adult gravidas in the midtrimester. *Journal of Obstetric, Gynecologic, and Neonatal Nursing, 12*, 40–44.

Tomlinson, P. (1987). Spousal differences in marital satisfaction during transition to parenthood. *Nursing Research, 36*(4), 239–242.

United States Department of Health and Human Services. (1990). *Healthy people 2000: National health promotion and disease prevention priorities*. Washington: US Government Printing Office.

Walker, L., Crain, H., & Thompson, E. (1986). Mothering behavior and maternal role attainment during the postpartum period. *Nursing Research, 35*(6), 352–357.

Wertz, R., & Wertz, D. (1989). *Lying-in: A history of childbirth in America* (2nd ed.). New Haven: Yale University Press.

Suggested Readings

Colman, L., & Colman, A. (1991). *Pregnancy: The psychological experience*. New York: Noonday Press.

Conley, L. (1990). Childbearing and childrearing practices in Mormonism. *Neonatal Network, 9*(3), 41–48.

Conner, G., & Denson, V. (1990). Expectant fathers' responses to pregnancy: Review of the literature and implications for high risk pregnancy. *Journal of Perinatal and Neonatal Nursing, 4*, 33–36.

Faller, H. (1992). Hmong women: Characteristics and birth outcomes, 1990. *Birth, 19*, 144–148.

Gentry, S. (1992). Caring for lesbians in a homophobic society. *Health Care of Women International, 13*(2), 173–180.

Green, N. (1990). Stressful events related to childbearing in African American women: A pilot study. *Journal of Nurse Midwifery, 35*(4), 231–236.

Kulig, J. (1990). A review of the health status of Southeast Asian refugee women. *Health Care of Women International, 11*(1), 49–63.

Monahan, P., & DeJoseph, J. (1991). The woman with preterm labor at home: A descriptive analysis. *Journal of Perinatal and Neonatal Nursing, 4*, 12–16.

Pakizegi, B. (1990). Emerging family forms: Single mothers by choice—demographic and psychosocial variables. *Maternal-Child Nursing Journal, 19*(1), 1–19.

Sachs, B., Poland M., & Giblin P. (1990). Enhancing the adolescent reproductive process: Efforts to implement a program for black adolescent fathers. *Health Care of Women International, 11*(4), 447–60.

Thompson, M., & Peebles-Wilkins, W. (1992). The impact of formal, informal and societal support networks on the psychological well being of black adolescent mothers. *Social Work, 37*(4), 322–328.

Wismont, J., & Reame, N. (1989). The lesbian childbearing experience: Assessing developmental tasks. *Image, 21*(3), 140–146.

CHAPTER 9

Adolescent Childbearing and Parenting

Learning Objectives

After studying the material in this chapter, the student will be able to:

- Describe the incidence of adolescent pregnancy and parenting.
- Discuss the developmental tasks of adolescence.
- Identify factors that contribute to high rates of adolescent pregnancy and parenting.
- Describe the implications of pregnancy and parenting for adolescents and their society.
- Relate poverty and limited life options to the cycle of adolescent pregnancy and parenting.
- Discuss nursing implications related to adolescent childbearing.

Key Terms

biologic maturation	life options
culture of poverty	narcissism
developmental tasks	risk behaviors

Adolescent sexual activity and adolescent pregnancy are major health problems in the United States and Canada. The United States maintains the highest incidence of adolescent pregnancy when compared with other westernized countries; 1 million American adolescent pregnancies result in approximately 500,000 births and 400,000 induced abortions each year. The Children's Defense Fund (1990) reports that each day 7742 American adolescents initiate sexual activity, and 2795 adolescent women become pregnant.

Although the rates in other developed countries continue to decline, rates in the United States have leveled off and declined minimally since 1976. The largest difference between the United States and other developed countries is in the incidence of childbirth and abortion among adolescents younger than 15 years. The birth rate among American women who are 14 years is 5 in 1000, four times higher than that of Canada, which reports the next highest rate (Wadhera & Silins, 1990).

This chapter provides an overview of the complex subject of adolescent childbearing and parenting. Developmental stages of adolescence and factors contributing to high rates of adolescent pregnancy and parenting are identified. Nursing implications are discussed in relation to adolescents and their families and the communities in which they live.

Adolescence as a Developmental Stage

Adolescents are in the process of moving from childhood to adulthood. This prolonged maturational period is a phenomenon of modern developed countries (Mercer, 1979). Adolescents are occupants of a territory that has lost the safety and security of childhood but has not achieved the productive and rewarded status of adulthood.

The age at which biologic maturation occurs (ie, growth and the development of primary and secondary sexual characteristics and the physiologic capacity to initiate pregnancy) has declined significantly during the last century. Biologic

May: MATERNAL AND NEONATAL NURSING, 3rd. ed. © 1994 J.B. Lippincott Company.

> ### *Developmental Tasks of Adolescence*
>
> The specific developmental tasks of adolescence include the following:
>
> - Establishing independence from the family while maintaining interdependence
> - Attaining an adult identity and integrating gender identity, a personal value system, and a vocational or career identity

maturation can begin as early as 8 and as late as 18 years and can reach completion anywhere from 15 to 25 years of age. Unfortunately, biologic maturity does not necessarily correlate with cognitive and psychosocial maturation (McAnarney & Hendee, 1989a).

The progression to adulthood is marked by phases during which adolescents achieve increasing levels of psychosocial and cognitive development. The three phases of adolescence generally fall within particular chronologic periods: early (12 to 14 years), middle (15 to 16 years), and late (17 to 20 years). Successful progress through these phases permits adolescents to complete their developmental tasks (Holt & Johnson, 1991), which are listed in the accompanying display.

Early Adolescence: Ages 12 to 14

During early adolescence, rapid growth and the development of secondary sexual characteristics may occur. This can result in a disturbance in the adolescent's self-image as attempts are made to incorporate these bodily changes. The adolescent relates primarily to the same age peers and compares self with others within this group. Exploratory sexual behavior may occur with friends of the same or opposite sex.

The adolescent uses concrete operational thinking that focuses on the present and is egocentric in nature. Early adolescents have a rich fantasy life and may believe they are the focus of others' thoughts and attention. They may have role models of the opposite sex who may be the focus of fantasy or "crushes." Early adolescents may be argumentative with parents because they are attempting to separate from the family. They generally rebound or regress back to a need for parental contact and control at times, and psychological maturation occurs through this process of separation and regression (McAnarney & Hendee, 1989a; Mercer, 1979).

Middle Adolescence: Ages 15 to 16

Physiologic growth and the complete development of primary and secondary sexual characteristics may be completed during this period. Middle adolescents continue their efforts to disengage and establish independence from parents; they usually become involved in heterosexual relationships at this time. Sexual experimentation may occur in group or couple situations. The middle adolescent uses peers to share experiences, to avoid social isolation, and to try out adult roles.

The middle adolescent may become increasingly self-centered or narcissistic with a deep appreciation of beauty and nature. Creativity and a flair for the dramatic may become evident, and emotions may be labile. The middle adolescent tends to overestimate his or her own power to influence events and may believe in what has been called the "personal fable of invincibility." While testing the limits of that power, they may engage in high-risk behaviors. Cognitively, middle adolescents begin to use deductive reasoning and problem solving. They begin to link current actions to future educational or job opportunities. However, under pressure, middle adolescents tend to regress to previous cognitive levels of concrete thinking and an inability to anticipate future consequences (McAnarney & Hendee, 1989a; Mercer, 1979).

Late Adolescence: Ages 17 to 20

The late adolescent is characterized by the ability to maintain stable, mutual, reciprocal relationships. The importance of family is acknowledged, but more important relationships are developed with significant others (Fig. 9-1). Chosen life tasks and goals are acquiring shape. Late adolescents still have some uncertainty with regard to social roles, but they are more clearly defined and articulated than during middle adolescence. Late adolescents demonstrate a stable pattern of functions and interests and extend their independence. Generally, conflict with family members diminishes during this phase.

Sexual identity usually is firmly established during late

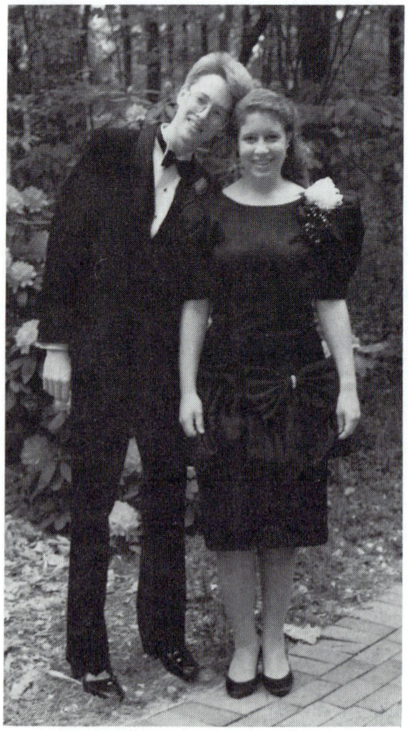

Figure 9-1.

In late adolescence, important relationships are developed with significant others. Movies, parties, and dances are part of this ritual. (From Jackson, D. B., & Saunders, R. B. (1993). *Child health nursing: A comprehensive approach to the care of children and their families* (p. 371). Philadelphia: J. B. Lippincott) adolescence. The late adolescent's mental functioning is stable and future oriented. He or she is able to view problems and consequences of behavior in a comprehensive fashion, and behavior becomes more predictable (McAnarney & Hendee, 1989a; Mercer, 1979).

Adolescents in developed countries are in the process of developing from childhood to adulthood. They vacillate between these periods of development psychosocially. Chronologic phases are called early (12 to 14), middle (15 to 16), and late (17 to 20) adolescence. Physiologic growth and development of secondary sexual characteristics and sexual identity affect self-image and peer and heterosexual relationships. Relationships with the family change and develop as the adolescent goes through the three phases.

Factors Contributing to Adolescent Pregnancy

Many factors have been shown to contribute to early sexual activity and resulting adolescent pregnancy and parenting. The most important contributing factors are socioeconomic status, early sexual activity and contraceptive use, perceived limited life opportunities, family characteristics, developmental status, and substance use and abuse.

Sociodemographic Factors

The adolescent birth rate is strongly influenced by sociodemographic factors. Poverty is a strong influence; poverty and minority status are frequently linked. Pregnancy rates among African American adolescents are higher than those in the European American populations, although this difference is virtually eliminated when economic status is controlled. Nevertheless, minority groups are disproportionately represented among the poor in the United States; thus, the incidence of adolescent pregnancy also is disproportionately high in these groups.

Although African American adolescent women account for only 14% of the adolescent population, they are more than twice as likely to get pregnant, three times as likely to give birth, and five times as likely to raise their children as single parents when compared with European American adolescents (Frager, 1991a). In a sample of 4061 urban adolescent men, adolescent fathers were almost three times more likely to be African American than European American (Hanson, Morrison, & Ginsburg, 1991).

Hispanic American and Native American adolescents are at the next highest risk for adolescent pregnancy and parenting. A study of Mexican American and European American adolescents indicated Mexican-born Hispanic Americans had the lowest rate of early intercourse and the highest rate of early births. European Americans had the highest rate of early intercourse and the highest rate of induced abortions (Aneshensel, Becerra, Fielder, & Schuler, 1990).

In some cultures marriage for women is common during adolescence. In many cases the husband is an older adult. The role of women is generally defined around parenting and homemaking but may include other activities to supplement the family income. In this particular circumstance adolescent pregnancy and parenting may not result in the negative sequellae observed in American society.

These figures provide some insight into the possible resolutions of adolescent pregnancy. American adolescents choose to terminate the pregnancy, complete the pregnancy and give the newborn up for adoption, or complete the pregnancy and retain responsibility for the newborn. The family or significant others play an important role in pregnancy resolution decisions (see the display on making decisions about adolescent pregnancies). Current estimates of the rate at which teenagers are retaining responsibility for their newborns range from 90% to 96% (Castiglia, 1990a; Rothenberg & Sedhom, 1990). Consequently, a small number of adolescents (4% to 10%) are opting for adoption; these usually are European American women who are in advantaged social situations and have higher educational goals and achievement (Farber, 1991; Hardy & Zabin, 1990).

Family Considerations

Making Decisions About Adolescent Pregnancies

Families play an important role in decisions about adolescent pregnancy. Decisions about abortion, adoption, or parenting affect the adolescent woman, her partner, and their immediate and extended families. The family's expectations and desires, the adolescent's own beliefs and attitudes, medical factors, and the timing of the decision affect the resolution.

Working class or middle class families may be more likely to recommend abortion or adoption, while single parent families and those from lower socioeconomic groups may be more likely to accept the inevitability of adolescent parenthood. Adolescents are in a difficult position. While they may fear family conflict when the news of the pregnancy is shared, they generally come to rely on their own families as a major source of advice and guidance. Support may be offered by other adults, but the adolescent's parents are likely to be the key support.

Farber, N. (1991). The process of pregnancy resolution among adolescent mothers. Adolescence, *26(103), 696–716.*

Sexuality and Contraceptive Use

The number of sexually active male and female adolescents is rising in every age and sociodemographic group but especially among younger adolescents. Approximately 42% of women aged 15 to 19 are sexually active (Brindis, 1990a), and approximately 60% of men in this age group are sexually active (Sonenstein, Pieck, & Ku, 1991). Research suggests that male African Americans have more partners than male Hispanic and European Americans. Generally, American adolescents delay seeking contraception for an average of 1 year after becoming sexually active. This delay, compounded by poor contraceptive use, lack of accurate contraceptive knowledge, and lack of financial and physical access to contraception, clearly puts sexually active adolescents at risk. All of these factors are linked to an increased incidence of adolescent pregnancy and parenting (Frager, 1991a; Thomas, Mitchell, & Devlin, 1990). Recently, an increase in the use of condoms at first sexual intercourse has been reported by urban males and females, with approximately 50% reporting condom use (Sonenstein et al., 1991). However, whether condom use is consistent is difficult to determine, and even isolated episodes of unprotected intercourse put the adolescent at risk.

These risk factors must be considered in relation to the overall climate toward sexuality in the United States. Societal ambivalence toward sexuality presents adolescents with conflicting messages. The national media flaunt sexuality and rarely present desirable role models who abstain from sexual intercourse or practice responsible sexual activity. This translates into a message that sexual abstinence is not valued and places those who abstain in a socially undesirable minority group. Television networks rarely carry contraceptive advertising or cover any discussion of the consequences of sexual activity likely to attract the attention of adolescents. Unfortunately, younger adolescents are much more likely to accept the "realism" of images portrayed on television (Brindis, 1990a). Lack of clear societal messages about appropriate sexual activity and responsible contraceptive use may reinforce the adolescent's tendency to deny that they are at risk for an unwanted pregnancy.

Limited Life Opportunity: The Culture of Poverty

The culture of poverty imposes pessimistic attitudes about opportunities for educational and vocational advancement on adolescent women and men. These adolescents may turn to pregnancy and parenting to achieve the adult status in their communities that they so desperately seek (Castiglia, 1990a; Castiglia, 1990b). In urban centers the culture of poverty is compounded by an acceptance or even an expectation of early sexual activity associated with the urban cultural context. Young adolescents who experience overcrowding, disorganized relationships, involuntary sexual observations and contacts, limited cognitive function, and an underdeveloped sense of identity may readily engage in early, unprotected sexual activity. Early academic failure and negative attitudes about school also are more prevalent among disadvantaged groups, and these factors are associated with early pregnancy.

Family Characteristics

Characteristics of the family of origin are strongly linked to the risk of early sexual activity and resulting pregnancy. Among adolescent women, a disturbed mother–daughter relationship, a seductive father–daughter relationship, hostility and distancing in the parents' marriage, and absent, ineffectual, or unemployed fathers are believed to increase the likelihood of pregnancy (Thomas et al., 1990). In a conflictual and disinterested family environment, adolescent women may use pregnancy to establish a sense of independence from the family (Holt & Johnson, 1991). Peer and familial factors, such as devaluing of education, low educational expectations, poor parental education, and single-parent families, increase the likelihood of adolescent males becoming fathers (Hanson et al., 1989). Generally, adolescents whose families did not provide structure and support, who did not set limits on problem behavior, and who failed to provide consistent guidance have been at highest risk for pregnancy and parenting (McAnarney & Hendee, 1989a). The Nursing Research display discusses other factors in adolescent risk taking.

Developmental Status

Some authors suggest that adolescent pregnancy and parenting are associated with low cognitive recognition of future consequences of sexual activity, high impulsiveness, and a high need for short-range gratification (McAnarney & Hendee, 1989a; Thomas et al., 1990). These behaviors generally are characteristic of the early and middle stages of adolescence.

Others suggest that adolescents may see pregnancy and parenting as a way to establish independence from conflicted or disinterested family members (Holt & Johnson, 1991). Despite the common assumption that promiscuity is widespread in adolescence, research has shown that adolescents typically engage in long-lasting monogamous relationships. Therefore, risk may come not from contact with many sexual partners, but from unprotected intercourse with one or two partners (Thomas et al., 1990).

Substance Use and Abuse

Although behaviors such as early sexual activity, drug use, and alcohol use are consistent with adolescents' efforts to establish their independence during this developmental stage, these behaviors also put them at risk for pregnancy (Jessor, 1991). As many as one in four teens in the United States, 7 million of those aged 10 to 17, are at high risk from use of drugs and high levels of stress and violence in their daily lives (Dryfoos, 1991).

The average age for initiation of drug and alcohol use is 14, and many adolescents are using more than one drug simultaneously (Adger, 1991). Many of the same factors associated with pregnancy are associated with drug abuse, and this creates a cluster of problem behaviors that has serious health implications for adolescents (Jessor, 1991; McAnarney & Hendee, 1989a).

With the increasingly widespread use of crack cocaine

Nursing Research

Factors Affecting Adolescent Risk Taking

The health status of adolescents has declined in the last 20 years in the United States, primarily because of risk-taking behaviors. This study examined personality factors and social support and their effect on the adolescent's willingness to engage in risk behaviors.

A convenience sample of 187 students (101 males and 86 females) aged 14 to 19 years completed a set of questionnaires during school hours. The questionnaires measured health locus of control or the extent to which individuals feel they have control over their health (known as internal locus of control) or feel health status is controlled by others or by fate (known as external locus of control). The questionnaires also measured social support available to the adolescent and the extent to which the adolescent engaged in risk behavior.

The findings suggest that risk behavior was primarily related to an external locus of control, indicating that adolescents believe other people are responsible for their health and that health is not an individual responsibility. While social support was less clearly related to risk behaviors, younger adolescents did report relying on family members for social support, while older adolescents reported relying on their peers.

Whately, J. (1991). Effects of health locus of control and social network on adolescent risk taking. *Pediatric Nursing, 17*(2), 145–148.

and other drugs among adolescents, there may be an associated exchange of sex for drugs (Brindis, 1990b). In part because of drug activity such as sharing needles, African American and Hispanic American adolescents living in poverty are at greatest risk for developing acquired immunodeficiency syndrome (AIDS) and other sexually transmitted diseases (STDs). Late adolescence combines one of the most sexually active periods in life with one of the most intense periods of drug use (Joseph, 1991).

Poverty is a strong influence on birth rate. Minority groups are disproportionately represented among the poor in the United States, and the incidence of adolescent pregnancy is disproportionately high in these groups. The number of sexually active adolescents is rising in every age group but especially among younger adolescents. Societal ambivalence, especially in the media, presents adolescents with conflicting messages. Family characteristics are strongly linked to the risk of early sexual activity and resulting pregnancy. Developmental status and substance abuse use and abuse also are strongly related to adolescent sexual activity and childbearing. In fact a cluster of problem behaviors has serious health implications for adolescents.

Healthy Adaptation and Adolescent Childbearing Consequences

The already complex process of adaptation to pregnancy and early parenthood is further complicated by the unique demands of adolescent development. Childbearing and childrearing have profound effects not only on the health and well-being of adolescents, but also on their children, their families, and society.

Physiologic Adaptation

The challenge of physiologic adaptation during adolescent pregnancy and parenting is most significant for adolescent women. Although most authorities agree that the physiologic problems for adolescent women are diminished by early, effective prenatal care, many adolescents deny, ignore, or incorrectly interpret the signs of pregnancy and consequently seek confirmation and assistance late in pregnancy (Farber, 1991; Morris, 1991). Some of these actions may be related to their developmental stage and their inability to consider long-term consequences of actions.

Inadequate prenatal care (defined as care initiated in the third trimester or the absence of prenatal care) is a problem that crosses adolescent age groups and socioeconomic boundaries but is more prevalent in adolescents younger than 15, those who are African American, and those who are abusing drugs or alcohol (Farber, 1991; Hardy & Zabin, 1990).

Regardless of when prenatal care is initiated, adolescents are thought to be at increased physiologic risk. In the past this was thought to be because of their physiologic immaturity. However, some argue that poor pregnancy outcomes are more likely to be caused by poverty or other health-related problems (Lee & Corpuz, 1988). When the effects of poverty and other sociodemographic factors are controlled, pregnant adolescents are at a risk for morbidity comparable with that for mothers in their 20s and have a lower risk than mothers in their 30s.

Only pregnancy-induced hypertension has been shown to be associated consistently to low maternal age; young (less than 16 years) nulliparous African American women appear to be at increased risk for this condition. Otherwise, complications such as cephalopelvic disproportion and cesarean delivery have not been shown to be associated with low maternal age (McAnarney & Hendee, 1989a).

While significant physiologic changes are normal in pregnancy, they do have an intensified effect on adolescents. Physical changes, such as increases in skin pigmentation, breast development, weight gain, vaginal discharge, nausea and vomiting, constipation, urinary frequency, and sleep disturbances, can have negative effects on adolescents' self-esteem, interactions with peer group members, and developing independence from family members (Mercer, 1979).

Biologic immaturity has health consequences for adolescent pregnant women because it may be confounded by a number of other factors, including maternal minority status, low socioeconomic status, inadequate nutrition, STDs, illicit drug use, smoking, and alcohol abuse (Morris, 1991).

Nutritional Status

Poor nutrition and anemia in adolescents are associated with poverty, minority status, and poor dietary practices. Nutritional status in adolescent pregnant women is especially important because mother and fetus are growing rapidly, creating competition for nutrients (Schneck, Sideras, Fox, & Dupuis, 1990). (Nutritional status among pregnant adolescents is discussed in more detail in Chapter 17.) Unfortunately, many adolescents may have no control over food available to them at home or may have limited access to the food that is available.

Nutritional status also is an issue because of developmental characteristics. Adolescents generally have a tendency to eat foods with limited nutritional value, and they are vulnerable to peer pressure in relation to food choices. They are very active and often skip meals. In addition, they may resist suggestions about proper eating habits at a time when they are trying to establish independence. Because many adolescents also are preoccupied with societal preferences for "thinness," they begin pregnancy underweight and resist weight gain (Schneck et al., 1990). Adolescents' feelings about body image and use of food as a comfort measure also may influence nutritional status; they may diet or overeat in an unsafe fashion during pregnancy.

The average weight gain for nonpregnant adolescents ranges from 8 to 12 lb per year in the 12- to 16-year age groups (Mercer, 1979). Thus, baseline maternal nutritional needs are high enough that achieving additional nutritional intake to ensure a healthy pregnancy may be difficult. Nausea and vomiting, especially persisting late in pregnancy, can complicate the picture (Behrman, Hediger, Scholl, & Arkangel, 1990). Poor nutrition places adolescents at risk for pregnancy-induced hypertension and preterm and low–birth-weight neonates (Nance, 1990).

Sexually Transmitted Diseases

Another challenge to healthy adaptation during adolescent childbearing is the risk of STD. One Canadian report indicated 57% of adolescent women in an urban, low-income group receiving prenatal care presented with STDs (Morris, 1991). STDs such as chlamydia, gonorrhea, and trichimoniasis have been implicated as a cause of preterm birth. Untreated pelvic infections late in pregnancy can increase the risk of postpartum endometritis. STDs have been linked to abnormal cervical cytology (Morris, 1991) and have serious consequences for later fertility if not detected and treated.

Another facet of the problem of STDs among adolescents is the problem of human immunodeficiency virus (HIV) infection. Currently, reported incidence of HIV and AIDS has increased slowly in the adolescent population in the United States, but health care providers believe these reports may underrepresent the true scope of the problem. AIDS in pregnant women can result in significant maternal and newborn morbidity and mortality (Joseph, 1991).

Smoking and Substance Abuse

Smoking and substance abuse complicate physiologic adaptation because these activities are associated with decreased maternal weight gain during pregnancy, decreased nutrient transfer to the fetus, and increased biologic insults (Kelley, Walsh, & Thompson, 1991; Buckley, 1990). Polysubstance abuse also tends to increase other risk behaviors, such as sexual promiscuity and poor dietary habits. Although substance abuse affects all socioeconomic groups, adolescents living in poverty are thought to be more likely to engage in drug use. Cocaine use during pregnancy has been specifically linked to abruptio placentae and maternal seizures, strokes, and cardiac arrests (Kelley et al., 1991; Shaw, 1990).

Psychosocial Adaptation

Although not all adolescents who experience pregnancy are destined to poor outcomes, many continue to fare poorly over time. These young people are faced with unanticipated changes and difficult decisions at a time when they are struggling with the normal difficult developmental challenges of adolescence. The degree to which they are put at psychosocial risk is associated with the quality of health care and support available to them and their own socioeconomic and developmental status.

The younger she is, the more difficulty the adolescent woman has with body image changes, acknowledging the pregnancy, seeking care, and planning for the changes that pregnancy and parenting will bring. These difficulties are due largely to the challenge of adjusting to normal physical and psychological maturation, in addition to coping with the changes of pregnancy (Fig. 9-2). The young adolescent typically has difficulty with anticipating consequences and problem solving, and her tentative feminine identity interferes with her efforts to take on the maternal role. Similar challenges are faced by the young adolescent father. His reliance on concrete thinking and his tentative masculine identity will pose the same problems as he struggles to prepare for future fatherhood.

As adolescents mature, they are more likely to be able to use abstract thinking and problem solving to prepare for birth and parenting, to begin to take on maternal and paternal roles, and to maintain a relationship with one another. Middle adolescents have established more independence and completed more schooling. However, factors such as peer group isolation and societal stigmas associated with early and out-of-wedlock parenting can still make the transition difficult, and even late adolescents may experience negative consequences of early and nonnormative pregnancy and parenting.

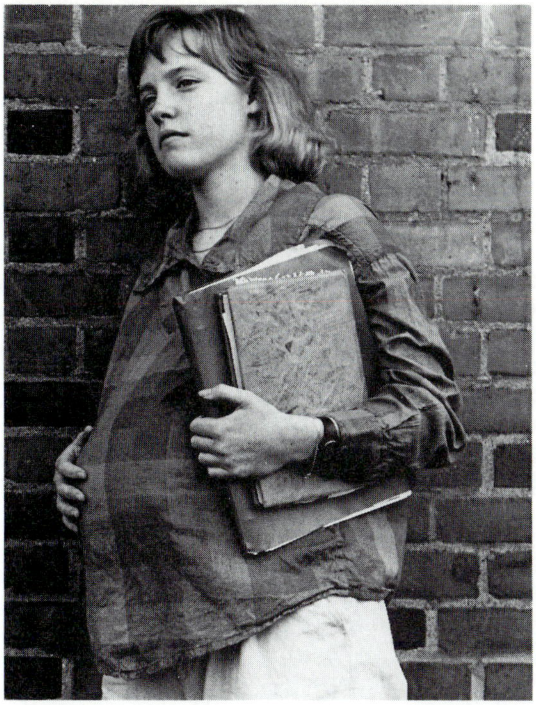

Figure 9-2.

The young adolescent has psychosocial adaptations to make to pregnancy. She has just begun to accept the body image changes that come with adolescence when additional body image adaptations must be made. (From Schuster, C. C., & Ashburn, S. S. (1992) *The process of human development: A holistic life-span approach* (3rd ed., p. 549). Philadelphia: J. B. Lippincott)

Consequences for Adolescent Mothers

While both genders may experience negative consequences from adolescent childbearing, these consequences are more apparent and may be more severe for the young woman. One effect more common among adolescent mothers than their male partners is disrupted school attendance.

Shortened Education

Pregnant and parenting adolescent women are more likely to experience a shortened education than their male partners or their nonpregnant female friends. Slightly less than half the adolescents who drop out of school in the United States cite pregnancy or marriage as the main reason. Lower socioeconomic status, early academic failure, minority status, and negative attitudes about school are associated with dropping out; these factors also are strongly associated with adolescent pregnancy, so educational advancement may be doubly at risk among these adolescents. However, the effect of pregnancy may not always be negative. While pregnancy may exacerbate an already negative school experience, it may provide an alternative to remaining in the school system if enriched school-based services are available and acceptable to the pregnant adolescent (DeBolt, Pasley, & Kreutzer, 1990).

Poverty and minority status also are associated with substandard schools, inadequate social services, and academic failure. Hispanic Americans are more likely to leave school than African Americans, who are more likely to leave than European Americans. Pregnant Hispanic Americans and African Americans also are less likely to seek abortions, because parenting may be seen as an attractive alternative. Thus, adolescent women who are most likely to continue pregnancy are those who are most likely to leave school, to have inadequate social services available to them, and to be living in impoverished circumstances.

Adolescents who maintain their pregnancies and choose to parent cite a variety of factors affecting their decision. Personal factors include an unsuccessful career at school and an expectation that pregnancy and parenting will signal adulthood. Motherhood may be rewarded by their peer group, and they may have role models who have been adolescent mothers (Castiglia, 1990a). Adolescents may intend to complete school but drop out shortly after delivery because of lack of institutional supports. They may maintain high aspirations and have strong institutional and social support but leave when faced with the demands of child care and, not infrequently, a second pregnancy that overwhelms their resources. Some women who drop out of school because of pregnancy further or complete their high school education as late in life as their 20s or 30s, but these women still do not achieve the educational outcomes of their peers who avoided early childbearing (Furstenberg, Brooks-Gunn, & Morgan, 1987).

Although adolescent women may experience many challenges, there also are sources of support. In one study of poor urban women, African American mothers actually had a higher frequency of high school completion than European American mothers (Hardy & Zabin, 1990), and the support of the maternal grandmother or other women in the community may be a factor. Marital status is not necessarily a positive influence on school completion; adolescent women who marry either during pregnancy or after birth have a higher rate of school dropout than those who remain single (DeBolt et al., 1990).

Decreased Vocational Opportunities

The level of formal education is the most important predictor of income and occupation (Grindstaff, 1988). Thus, those who drop out of school because of pregnancy are already at risk. Welfare dependence and poverty are common among adolescents who are parenting (Duncan & Hoffman, 1990). Young mothers often depend on parents or extended family for financial support and housing. Young women may narrow their own horizons by considering parenting as their only viable option (Blinn, 1990). African American adolescents are at great risk, because they face particularly poor economic prospects and career opportunities (Duncan & Hoffman, 1990). Adolescent women who have not completed high school are likely to be underemployed, employed in entry-level jobs, and lacking in job security (Castiglia, 1990a; Grindstaff, 1988). Generally, their jobs are low paying and without such benefits as health care. Adequate, affordable child care also is at a premium (Frager, 1991a).

Single Parenthood and Early Marriage

Marriage does not ensure financial stability, because adolescent couples generally are less able to take advantage of educational and employment opportunities and are likely to be living in impoverished circumstances. The working poor often have incomes below the poverty line and do not qualify for medical aid (including contraception), food aid, or income assistance (Hardy & Zabin, 1990). Families that are excluded from food programs because of low-paying jobs, physical distance from food programs, or illiteracy are at risk for inadequate nutrition. Many adolescent women and their families also live in substandard housing and unsafe neighborhoods (Hardy & Zabin, 1990).

Marriage as a choice among adolescent women varies along ethnic lines, although this is likely to reflect economic rather than purely cultural factors. European American adolescents marry five times more frequently than African American adolescents. In general, however, fewer American adolescents are marrying, and marriage rates decrease as adolescent age increases. There has been a consistent trend since World War II of declining employment opportunities for unskilled urban men, especially among African Americans. Because of this trend, many African American women are choosing to raise their children as single parents because that appears more secure (Duncan & Hoffman, 1990). However, this choice is not an attractive option either, because more than 50% of American families headed by single women live below the poverty line (Frager, 1991a).

Difficult Psychological Adaptation

Psychological adaptation to the demands of pregnancy and early parenting may be a significant challenge for adolescent women. Many young adolescent mothers report depression, worry, and confusion. These feelings may be in response to a sense of lost childhood and social peer isolation. Some women, because they feel trapped, have developed resentment and anger toward their children (Castiglia, 1990a). In single-parent adolescent families, many women have nowhere to turn for support. Some adolescents use family, friends, or boyfriends, but few receive professional counseling (Hardy & Zabin, 1990).

Difficult Adaptation to Parenting

All of these psychosocial factors create challenging parenting situations. In addition, the adolescent's developmental status, marked by emotional immaturity and little ego strength, compounds the problems created by his or her inexperience with parenting. Adolescents need and often seek short-term rewards, such as praise and recognition in relationships; such gratifications are rare when parenting a newborn.

Adolescent mothers generally are less knowledgable about children and their developmental processes (Causby, Nixon, & Bright, 1991). Many adolescents have unrealistic expectations of parenting, including a sense that parenting will be easy, that their newborn will make them feel loved, that plenty of assistance will be available, and that they will get social recognition for being a parent (Browne & Urback, 1989). Expectations and realities are listed in Table 9-1.

When parenting does not meet these romanticized expectations, adolescents may avoid parenting responsibility and try to meet their own needs instead. If their cognitive abilities are still concrete and their problem solving is limited, they may feel overwhelmed by their difficulties, especially in the absence of support.

Support from their male partner, their own families, professionals, and their peer group affects the quality of parenting of adolescent mothers. A supportive male partner seems to influence adolescent mothers by making them more supportive and less punitive with their own children (Seymore, Frothingham, MacMillan, & Durant, 1990). Grandparents, professionals, and peers may assist adolescents to meet their needs, thus permitting them to be more sensitive to their newborn's needs.

Generally, adolescent mothers have been shown to lack sensitivity to their newborns and to interact with them in ways that do not promote optimal infant development. Adolescent mothers tend to establish low levels of verbal interaction with their children and tend to both overestimate and underestimate their children's abilities. They demonstrate less nurturing behaviors and appear to be less tolerant than adult parents (Cooper, Dunst, & Vance, 1991). A recent study suggested that African American and Hispanic American adolescents have demonstrated less affectionate behavior, maintained less physical closeness with their newborn, and vocalized and smiled less during early postpartum feeding when compared with adult mothers from the same ethnic groups (Norr & Roberts, 1991).

This situation is amenable to some level of professional intervention. There is evidence that informal support, the presence of appropriate behavioral role models, and reinforcement of appropriate behavior by others can improve adolescent parenting practices. In addition adolescents generally are interested in learning more about infant development and nutrition and thus may benefit from structured programs with these components (Hutchinson, 1990). Overall, adolescents who participate in parenting programs have better outcomes than those who do not (Causby et al., 1991).

Ineffective Coping Behavior

Adolescent mothers feel significant amounts of stress from the conflict between tasks of early parenthood and developmental tasks of adolescence. Although family members may offer needed support and guidance, they also may contribute to this stress because the adolescent must depend on them while striving for independence. External stressors such as poverty, substandard housing, and unsafe neighborhoods will severely tax the adolescent's ability to cope, because these stressors often are beyond his or her control.

Adolescents frequently feel they must make efforts to reduce their stress levels and may use a variety of coping behaviors. Adolescent mothers appear to use indirect or passive coping strategies, such as avoiding situations, changing the meaning of events, and using distractions such as music (Codega, Pasley, & Kreutzer, 1990). The use of direct coping strategies, such as problem solving, seeking support, and

Table 9-1. Expectations Versus Realities of Adolescent Childbearing

Expectations	Reality
Life With a Newborn	
Life with a newborn will be wonderful.	Life with a newborn isn't wonderful.
The newborn will meet emotional needs.	A newborn doesn't meet emotional needs. The newborn may interfere with the parents' needs.
The parent won't be lonely anymore.	The parent may be even more lonely with the demands and limitations of a newborn.
Parenting	
Parenting is easy (based on babysitting experience). Parents will manage.	Parenting is not easy.
Others will support and help.	Many adolescents are parenting alone. The 24-hour experience is overwhelming. There are few resources for adolescent parents. Some parents are not ready to accept help—education, role modeling, and so forth.
Self-esteem	
Self-esteem will increase with pregnancy and parenthood.	The woman will be self-conscious about her body changes. Society disapproves. Self-esteem actually decreases.
Parent now has a role	Newborn takes attention away from parent.
Relationships	
The pregnant female's parents will be upset, then supportive.	Some have family support. Many "grandparents" reject pregnant daughter and newborn, or they will not support them on adolescent's terms.
Relationship with partner will improve, or he'll "come back."	Some live together or are married. Relationship with partner often is strained. Frequently he leaves.
Peer friendships will continue as they were.	Life is different from that of peers. Adolescent becomes isolated from friends.
Finances	
Somebody will provide welfare.	Welfare is not sufficient. Adolescent parents are unable to manage. Many are not interested in learning to budget.
Some plan to be self-sufficient (ie, finish school, get a job).	Self-sufficiency takes a long time. Often the adolescent doesn't have energy or the organizational skills to continue or reenter school.
Housing	
Adolescents want to live on their own.	Landlords are biased against single mothers, children, and tenants on welfare. Housing may be less available for adolescent parents.
They hope to find housing at an affordable rent.	Much of what is available in housing is inappropriate for young women and young children.
Goals	
Motherhood will make life meaningful.	Life is not made more meaningful by motherhood.
Adolescents tend not to have long-term goals.	Adolescents have difficulty in following through even on short-term goals.

Adapted from Browne, C., & Urback, M. (1989). Pregnant adolescents: Expectations vs reality. *Canadian Journal of Public Health, 80*(3), 227–229.

positive comparisons, has been associated with lower levels of depression and more optimal mother–child interaction.

When coping behaviors of Mexican American and European American middle adolescents were studied, all of the adolescents indicated they used nonprescribed drugs (alcohol or illegal drugs) most of the time to cope. They also described "being close to someone you care about," smoking, and daydreaming as common coping behaviors. European American adolescents in this study used more direct coping behaviors than the Mexican Americans. However, both groups used a high number of passive coping strategies and singled out the importance of maintaining close friends (Codega et al., 1990). African American adolescents also reported seeking closeness of peers and friends, but they more frequently avoided substance abuse, daydreaming, and listening to music (Hutchinson, 1990).

Repeat Pregnancies

Approximately 30% of first-time American adolescent mothers become a parent again within 2 years of their first birth (Seymore et al., 1990). The most significant increase in repeat pregnancy has been in American adolescents age 15 years and younger. Among European American pregnant adolescents, the likelihood of subsequent pregnancies has increased, while among African Americans the risk has declined because of contraceptive use (Hardy & Zabin, 1990).

Generally, adolescent mothers have more children, have them more closely spaced, have more unwanted children, and have more out-of-wedlock births (Nelson, 1990). Variables associated with multiple pregnancies in adolescence include inconsistent contraceptive practices, low educational achievement, weak parental relationships, and marriage during adolescence. Women who remained in school were less likely to have repeat pregnancies, and those who married were more likely to do so (Nelson, 1990). Generally poor economic outcomes are associated with multiple early childbearing and marriage as a result of school dropout and reduced career and vocational opportunities.

Consequences for Adolescent Fathers

Men fathering children with adolescent women are an extremely complex group, more so than are their female partners. For instance these individuals are usually not adolescents. Although 12.6% of women giving birth in 1986 were less than 20 years of age, only 2.7% of the men involved were adolescent fathers (Hardy & Zabin, 1990). Thus, the father role may be performed by the biologic father who may or may not be an adolescent, by a current boyfriend, or by the mother's own father or stepfather who also may be the biologic father as the result of an incestuous relationship (Belsky & Miller, 1986). Although evidence remains anecdotal, there is some indication that very young adolescent mothers often are victims of rape or incest (Wattenberg, 1990).

The question of who the father is also is compounded by problems in access to this individual, either for the purposes of providing services or for obtaining information. Adolescent women's partners often are difficult to identify and access for research purposes, and most of the men studied have been partnered with women treated in specialized clinics. Much of the existing information regarding adolescent fathers has been based on the women's reports about their partners rather than first-hand reports from the men.

The consequences of pregnancy and parenting for these men differ depending on their maturational stage. However, surprisingly, the young adult partners of adolescent women generally fare worse than their younger counterparts. Fathers are, on average, 2 to 4 years older than their adolescent partners. More than 50% of fathers whose newborns are born to European American adolescents were 20 years or older, while only about 25% of those fathering newborns with African American adolescents fell into that category. European American fathers generally are more likely to be older, less likely to be unemployed, and less likely to have fathered a child by another woman than African American fathers (Hardy & Zabin, 1990).

Generally, young adult partners of adolescent mothers have less educational attainment, higher rates of unemployment, and higher arrest rates when compared with adolescent fathers (Wattenberg, 1990). It is unclear whether these men take more financial responsibility to support the adolescent mother and their newborn and thus experience more hardships, or whether these men were already economically and socially disadvantaged at the time the pregnancy occurred.

Shortened Education

High proportions of adolescent fathers are high school dropouts; those who marry first and then conceive have particularly high rates. Consequently, many of these men do not receive high school certification until 20 years or older. Younger males who father a child are more likely to have completed a high school education, possibly because their young age precluded them from assuming family responsibilities.

African American fathers have a higher probability of high school graduation than Hispanic Americans or middle class European Americans (Marsiglio, 1987). Fathers who have cohabited with their adolescent partner and child are less likely to complete high school. It is not clear whether educationally disadvantaged and low-achieving young men become adolescent fathers or whether adolescent fatherhood creates barriers that preclude educational advancement. The outcome in either case is the same.

Decreased Vocational Opportunities

Fathers are expected to provide for their children. Meeting financial responsibilities is difficult in a society in which college or vocational training programs usually are required to obtain employment and jobs paying above the minimum wage (Belsky & Miller, 1986). Many adolescent fathers are unemployed, underemployed, or employed in marginal entry-level jobs that require little specialized training, pay poorly, and offer little opportunity for advancement (Sander & Rosen, 1987; Wattenberg, 1990). Generally, African American adolescents have higher unemployment rates and less income than European American peers.

Concerns Regarding Paternity

Some adolescent fathers have concerns regarding paternity and whether or not they should acknowledge paternity. They may lack well-developed decision-making skills, and their cognitive development may not be sufficiently mature to allow them to consider fully the implications of that decision. There may be some legitimate questioning as to the exclusivity of their relationship with their partners and the possibility that they may not be the biologic father. They may encounter pressure from partners, their families, and their friends to acknowledge paternity (Castiglia, 1990b). On the other hand the adolescent father may wish to acknowledge paternity but may encounter resistance from his partner, her parents, his own parents, and social service personnel who may be hostile and punitive (Wattenberg, 1990).

If the father does not establish paternity, he will have no legal rights to the child but may have to pay child support (see the Legal/Ethical Considerations display). Once adolescent fathers have acknowledged paternity, they must decide whether to marry, cohabit with their partners, or to stay involved with the mother and child in a more informal way.

Difficult Adaptation in the Couple Relationship

It is increasingly rare for adolescent fathers to marry their partners subsequent to a pregnancy. Adolescent fathers usually are involved in relatively stable relationships with their partners over an average period of 2 years, although they may or may not have been exclusively committed to them.

Legal/Ethical Considerations

Adolescent Fathers and Establishing Paternity

An important issue for adolescents facing a pregnancy is the matter of establishing paternity. The legal and health care systems are not consistent in their treatment of this issue. While there may be important advantages to the mother and newborn if paternity is clearly acknowledged, doing so also may jeopardize the ability of the mother to receive certain social services and may weaken the mother's claim as the parent with sole custody should that become an issue.

It is important for the nurse caring for an adolescent couple to be knowledgeable about the issues related to legal acknowledgment of paternity (the usual form is on birth registration or the birth certificate). The nurse should refer the father to counseling or legal aid as appropriate. The nurse should be prepared to act as a community advocate to establish an open simplified system of ensuring that the best interests of all concerned are protected in this matter.

Many adolescent fathers attempt to maintain those relationships in marriage and outside of marriage. Unfortunately, adolescent marriages have a high rate of dissolution. The divorce rate for parents younger than 18 is three times higher than for parents who had their first child when they were older than age 20 (Castiglia, 1990b). The developmental status of the two partners heightens the already significant stresses involved in a new marriage. Their limited identity formation, untried decision-making skills, and immature cognitive judgments make the work of relationship maintenance extremely difficult (Belsky & Miller, 1986). Other family members usually are involved with the young couple, either directly through providing housing and economic support or indirectly by communicating their values and attitudes on the couple and, not infrequently, by actively discouraging the relationship.

Difficult Psychological Adaptation

Many adolescent fathers report feelings of depression and alienation from friends. They are unable to experiment with their lives and to establish adult identities; they feel tied down (Elster & Hendricks, 1986). Some report lack of confidence as fathers, students, and job seekers. They seek support and counseling because they are desperate for help. Adolescent fathers may be at risk for becoming involved in domestic violence, including child abuse or neglect (Castiglia, 1990b; Sander & Rosen, 1987).

Difficult Adaptation to Parenting

Nurturing a newborn requires a certain level of maturity. Psychological readiness for parenting also is an important component in successful adaptation to parenting. Many adolescent fathers lack rational decision-making skills, mature moral and cognitive judgment, and knowledge and realistic expectations about neonatal behaviors. However, these deficits may not have as negative an effect on the quality of fathering as might be expected (Fig. 9-3).

Fathers who do not live with their partners tend to report enthusiasm about their role and ongoing contact with their offspring. They indicate that they provide babysitting, physical care, money for food, and contributions to medical care and clothes. These efforts, however, have been observed to decrease with time and especially toward the end of the first and second years of life (Wattenberg, 1990; Hardy & Zabin, 1990).

Fathers generally request assistance in coping with their parental role. They want information about prenatal care, newborn care, and infant development. Generally, they are worried about being a good father, setting a good example for their children, raising their children, maintaining their health, and ensuring financial stability for their children (Elster & Hendricks, 1986).

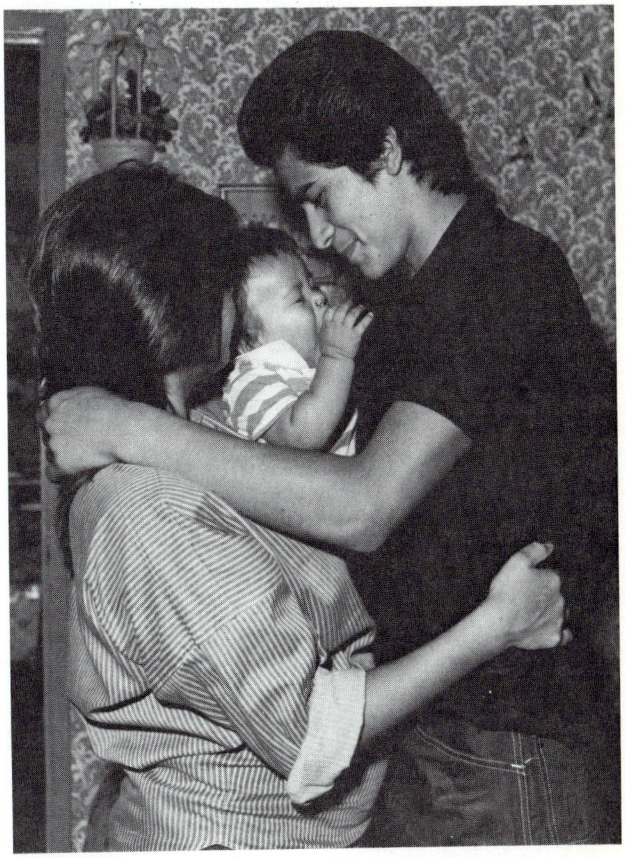

Figure 9-3.
The adolescent father can make a positive adaptation to parenthood with specialized care and adequate social support (Courtesy of Morning Glory Press. Photo by Joyce Young.)

Ineffective Coping Behavior

How adolescent fathers cope is poorly understood, and there is little research. However, there is evidence that most fathers, regardless of minority status, seek advice or assistance with problems from family, most often from an experienced mother. Friends also were indicated as a source of assistance. Few young men indicated that they would seek help from social service agencies. When a small group of fathers was studied, most indicated that they tried to cope directly with problems rather than reduce emotional distress through indirect means such as alcohol; a few redirected their lives away from past social activities. Some fathers did report using alcohol abuse and denial as coping strategies (Elster & Hendricks, 1986).

Consequences for Children of Adolescent Parents

The effects of "children having children" are far-reaching and include all periods of their offsprings' development.

Newborns

Adolescents' newborns are at higher risk for prematurity and low birth weight with concomitant increases in neonatal mortality and morbidity (Lee & Corpuz, 1988). Risks associated with prematurity include respiratory problems, developmental delays, increased incidence of infections, feeding difficulties, and rehospitalization (Damato, 1991). Low birth weight has been associated with increases in congenital anomalies, lower respiratory tract infections, neurologic and developmental delays, rehospitalization rates, and mortality (Gennaro, Brooten, & Bakewell-Sachs, 1991). Along with poor sociodemographic status, risk behaviors such as substance abuse and smoking are believed to be responsible for increased incidence of low–birth-weight neonates seen in adolescent multiparous mothers (Stevens-Simon, Roghmann, & McAnarney, 1990). Risks associated with STDs include increased mortality and morbidity from neonatal infections (Hardy & Zabin, 1990).

Newborn risks resulting from substance abuse during pregnancy include growth retardation, mental retardation, hyperactivity, learning delays, behavioral problems, congenital anomalies, infections, and feeding problems (Buckley, 1990; Peters & Theorell, 1991). The incidence of sudden infant death syndrome is higher among infants of adolescent mothers (McAnarney & Hendee, 1989a; Shaw, 1990).

Any of these factors increases the likelihood of ineffective parenting in a situation in which parents are ill-equipped to deal with the usual challenges of childrearing. Even infants of adolescent mothers who are normal at birth have a higher incidence of rehospitalization during their first year than infants of older mothers (Wilson, Duggan, & Joffe, 1990). Overall, newborns of adolescent mothers experience higher rates of illness and injury. It is unclear whether these outcomes are related to parental age, poor socioeconomic status, and substandard housing or a combination of the three; the latter seems quite likely (Hardy & Zabin, 1990).

Newborns of adolescents also are at risk by virtue of their parents' social disadvantages. Newborns born to married, low-income European American adolescents who were ineligible for food and medical aid were at greater risk for health problems than newborns of African American adolescents who remained single because they were eligible for more social assistance programs (Hardy & Zabin, 1990). Thus, to a certain extent, marriage acted as a disadvantage for some neonates. However, newborns of single mothers face other risks, including loss of legal rights to child support, social security, workers' compensation, armed service benefits, insured health care, and their genetic history when their mothers do not seek legitimization through establishing their paternity (Wattenberg, 1990).

Probably the most subtle but worrisome risk for neonates of adolescent parents is the risk that their development will not be optimal because of limitations in parenting. Infants may be subjected to unrealistic or inappropriate developmental expectations by adolescent parents (Parks & Arndt, 1990). Adolescent parents who are not exposed to effective parenting role models demonstrate less verbal interaction with their newborns and more punitive childrearing attitudes (Castiglia, 1990a; Causby et al., 1991). Consequently, delayed social, emotional, cognitive, and physical development has been identified in some of these infants. Some particularly disadvantaged infants are at risk for abuse and neglect. The social structure of the family, positive relationships with their own mothers, and availability of grandparents to assist with child care can minimize these problems to some extent (Causby et al., 1991).

Preschool and School-Age Children

The pattern of disadvantage among children of adolescent parents continues to be apparent among preschool and school-age children. Some evidence shows that less attentive behavior and verbal interaction with their neonates lead to lower levels of competence at the preschool level (McAnarney & Hendee, 1989a). Adolescents' preschool and school-age children have demonstrated lower developmental scores than those of older parents (Thomas et al., 1990). However, these findings also have been linked to maternal educational attainment and unemployment, which may operate regardless of parental age.

Furstenberg et al. (1987) studied a population of predominantly African American single-parent families and found that preschoolers were substantially more likely to score lower on readiness for school testing when their adolescent mother was single, had not sought further education, and was receiving welfare. Children of welfare recipients with more than one child were more likely to be described as uncooperative, rude, and disobedient but also were more likely to live in unsafe neighborhoods, attend poor quality schools, and encounter negative attitudes toward education from those around them. These factors may be as influential in child behavior as the single factor of maternal age.

Indeed, there is growing evidence that the combination of educational and economic disadvantage and family instability, rather than maternal age, produces this pattern of poor cognitive, social, and emotional development (Baldwin & Cain, 1980). For instance, lower levels of trust, self-esteem, and socialization among children of adolescent mothers may have been related as much to the absence of a father figure as to maternal age (Sander & Rosen, 1987).

Adolescents

The reduced readiness for school, behavioral problems, and lower levels of self-esteem found in preschool and school-age children of adolescent parents might be expected to affect these same children when they become adolescents. In one study of children of low-income African American adolescents followed up 17 years later, there was evidence of massive school failure. Fifty percent of these adolescents had repeated at least one grade, and 61% of them reported they were C or D students. In addition 40% of these adolescents reported disciplinary problems, including school absence, school violence, and school suspension or expulsion (Furstenberg et al., 1987).

Academic failure among these children also was associated with early sexual experience. Adolescent women repeating a grade were twice as likely to have become pregnant as those who had not done so. Young men who had repeated a grade were much less likely to have used contraception. Many of these teens were runaways or had been involved with the law. Sixty percent had used alcohol, and 46% had smoked marijuana (Furstenberg et al., 1987).

This study shows clearly that the risk factors that contributed to their parents' experience with adolescent childbearing were affecting the health and well-being of the next generation. In this group 26% of the adolescent women reported being pregnant. The repetitive cyclical nature of adolescent pregnancy and parenting with its relationship to poverty (Baldwin & Cain, 1980) has implications for the families of adolescents and larger sociocultural repercussions.

Consequences for Families

Often adolescents report they delay informing family members about a pregnancy or suspected pregnancy because they fear their reactions (Farber, 1991). Later in the pregnancy and while parenting, both male and female adolescents usually rely heavily on parents and family for support (Elster & Hendricks, 1986). Although families may be angry and disappointed about the pregnancy, they often offer not only emotional support, but also living space and financial support. Grandparents often are involved in child care while adolescents continue or pursue their education (Parks & Arndt, 1990) (see the Family Considerations display on family involvement in newborn caretaking).

Despite the fact that many families offer support and assistance to adolescent parents, this situation is not without its problems. Clearly, child care issues can be stressful to grandparents who anticipated more independence or who have returned to the work force. Intergenerational differences in views about childrearing also can cause conflicts. Young women's families may demonstrate hostility toward their partners whom they view as responsible. Families may exclude male partners from decision making about the pregnancy and from a parenting role after the neonate is born (Robinson, 1988).

Family Considerations

Family Involvement in Infant Caretaking

Many adolescent mothers live with extended family, such as their own mothers or grandmothers, and maintain contact with the newborn's father. Research to date indicates that adolescents who receive no support with parenting often establish patterns of limited interaction and social stimulation that are inadequate for optimal infant development. However, problems also may arise when an adolescent receives child care assistance from a variety of sources. Child care patterns may be inconsistent, and the adolescent mother may not feel confident in her own knowledge in this regard.

Implications for nursing care include the following:

- The possibility of conflict between the adolescent mother and others' approaches to child care
- A deterioration in the amount and quality of maternal caregiving as the mother relies more on others for assistance
- The potential for the mother's own needs to remain unmet as she struggles to meet her infant's needs
- The need to assess other support people in the environment to determine where positive assistance might be available to the mother

The nurse should assess the availability of alternate caregivers, their knowledge about infant care, and the extent to which nonsupportive interactions may occur. Comprehensive parent education programs may be available for the adolescent mother and father but may not be designed to update the knowledge base of grandparents and other adults. This deficit may be filled readily by involving these other individuals in well-baby visits or through home visiting by nursing personnel.

Families may believe that fathers cannot contribute significantly to their partners' and newborns' support; thus, they may actively discourage young women and their partners from establishing paternity. Paternal grandmothers also may consider the mothers of their grandchildren as unacceptable and discourage their sons from marrying their partners. This may be especially evident when paternal grandparents are trying to protect their sons' schooling, job opportunities, and life chances (Wattenberg, 1990).

Adolescent parents who live with their own families of origin may be impoverished, even when one or more family members are contributing to family support (Hardy & Zabin,

1990). Obviously, families with resources and living space can provide support for their adolescents most easily, which would result in better outcomes (Baldwin & Cain, 1980; Hardy & Zabin, 1990). Families with many children and those dependent on public assistance have the least resources to offer their adolescents who are pregnant or rearing children (Furstenberg et al., 1987).

Consequences for Society

Societies with significant numbers of children born to adolescents living in poverty pay enormous human and financial costs. The cost of adolescent childbearing in the United States in 1985 was over $16 billion. This figure includes only Aid to Families with Dependent Children, Medicaid, food stamps, and direct payment to care providers. Costs that are not included in this estimate are other social services, protective services and foster care, special education, housing, and subsidized day care (Hardy & Zabin, 1990; Frager, 1991a). Other costs incurred are private sector costs underwritten by voluntary agencies, foundations, and families. These cost calculations ignore the human cost in terms of the adults and children who fail to achieve their potential and who recreate the culture of poverty for the next generation.

Adolescent childbearing and parenting have profound effects not only on the health of adolescents, but also on their children, their families, and society in general. Physiologic growth and pregnancy can affect each other adversely. These are compounded by minority and socioeconomic status, nutrition, STDs, and substance abuse. Many childbearing adolescents fare poorly with time, although the outcomes are not always obvious immediately. Adolescent pregnancy has far-reaching concerns for the adolescent mother and father, although mothers have the most negative consequences. The culture of poverty often is recreated for the next generation, and society pays the human and economic costs.

Implications for Nursing Care

As the human and economic costs of adolescent childbearing continue to grow, more nurses are engaging in caring for the large population of adolescents who are at risk for early parenthood. This section focuses on specialized nursing care for the pregnant adolescent and on nursing responsibilities in population-focused care at the local, regional, and national level.

Caring for the Pregnant Adolescent

In many ways the care of the pregnant adolescent and her partner is similar to prenatal care provided to other couples (see Chapters 13 to 15 for a discussion of prenatal care). Aspects of care must be individualized, however, to take into account the unique developmental needs of the adolescent.

• • Assessment

Prenatal Care

The community health nurse often is the first health professional to identify pregnancy in the adolescent. This often occurs when the nurse is providing care for other family members in the community setting. Increasingly, school health nurses may identify pregnancy in young women they encounter in middle or high school. Once the adolescent begins prenatal care, the nurse initiates ongoing assessments.

Many professionals may be involved in the assessment and monitoring of the pregnant adolescent. However, the nurse must have a comprehensive knowledge about her condition and the situation surrounding her pregnancy. The accompanying Assessment Tool lists important data to be obtained or reviewed by the nurse.

In many high-risk settings the nurse serves as a case manager and is responsible for coordinating the services provided for adolescent clients. Nurse midwives and nurse practitioners are ideal health care providers for the pregnant adolescent. The philosophy of family-centered care and their holistic perspective offers the pregnant adolescent a supportive environment that fosters adaptive coping. Furthermore, the adolescent may be less intimidated by a female nurse midwife or nurse practitioner and may more readily develop a trusting relationship with her.

Ongoing prenatal assessments are focused on the early identification of pregnancy complications, such as anemia or pregnancy-induced hypertension. Changing interpersonal relationships with family members or the sexual partner may occur as the pregnancy progresses. Sudden, dramatic crises often arise for the adolescent and may require immediate intervention. The nurse must therefore monitor the young woman's social situation.

Concerns about body image may arise after midpregnancy and can precipitate an emotional crisis. Some adolescents have been known to attempt self-induction of labor (by using drugs or engaging in strenuous activity) to terminate the pregnancy prematurely when weight gain and body changes can no longer be camouflaged.

As the pregnancy advances, the nurse must assess the adolescent's readiness for labor and birth and her knowledge of neonatal care. Even when the adolescent agrees to participate in prenatal education classes, the nurse should determine if she has special needs or concerns regarding childbirth that require additional consideration and support. The nurse also identifies the young woman's support person for labor and evaluates their readiness for the role.

Intrapartum Care

With the onset of labor, the labor and delivery nurse assumes responsibility for the ongoing assessment of the adolescent. The nurse should have a detailed knowledge of the prenatal history, including when prenatal care was started and what special physical or emotional problems and needs the young woman has. The knowledge of special circumstances surrounding pregnancy, such as a history of rape or incest or the absence of family or other support persons in the adolescent's life, is important. The level of

Assessment Tool

Essential Aspects of the Adolescent Assessment

Social and Demographic Information

- Age and developmental stage
- Education and cognitive level
- Circumstances surrounding the pregnancy
  - Planned or unplanned
  - Result of rape or incest
- Identity of father (husband, boyfriend, unknown with multiple sex partners)
- Family constellation and support network
- Place of residence (alone, with father of baby, with family, in shelter for pregnant adolescents)
- Involvement of father of baby
- Financial status
- Cultural background
- Plans for infant (adoption, placement in foster care, keeping infant)
- Previous experience with pregnancy, health care system, and infants

Physical Status

- Nutritional status
- Significant prepregnancy medical problems
- History of physical or sexual abuse
- Presence of sexually transmitted diseases
- Substance use or abuse, chemical dependency

Psychological Status

- Level of self-esteem
- Relationship with father of baby
- Relationship with family
- Feelings about pregnancy
- Body image concerns
- Presence of or previous psychological disorders

Obstetric Status

- Gravidity and parity
- Past obstetric problems
- History of contraceptive use
- Gestational age and estimated date of delivery
- Fetal status
- Presence of or development of obstetric complications

preparation for labor and birth must be evaluated, and any gaps in the adolescent's knowledge should be identified and corrected promptly.

The nurse assesses the adolescent's pain level and tolerance of painful procedures. Plans and desires for pain control should be determined early in the labor process. Maternal and fetal physiologic status is monitored, and the adolescent is assessed for evidence of pregnancy-induced hypertension. The status and reactions of the support person should be assessed and particular attention paid when that individual also is an adolescent.

Postpartum Care

During the immediate postpartum period (24 to 48 hours), the assessment process focuses on monitoring physiologic status. In most cases the adolescent will demonstrate a remarkable recovery of energy resources and physiologic stability. The nurse must determine the level of knowledge regarding self-care, hygiene, newborn feeding practices, and newborn care. Before discharge the nurse must identify the young woman's need for contraceptive information, community referrals, and follow-up care.

If other family members, such as grandparents or the adolescent father of the newborn, will be involved in neonatal care activities, the nurse also must assess their level of knowledge and skill in care. In many cases community health nurses will be involved in ongoing assessments of the adolescent mother after discharge. Assessment of maternal recovery, maternal role attainment, and neonatal growth and development are essential elements of the continuing nursing care. The reader is referred to Chapter 36 for a full discussion of the adaptations that occur in the first postpartum year.

• • Nursing Diagnoses

Nursing diagnoses for the pregnant adolescent, her partner, and family are based on the assessment data obtained by the nurse. Some pertinent diagnoses are listed below:

- Altered Family Processes related to adolescent pregnancy
- Body Image Disturbance related to pregnancy
- Decisional Conflict related to pregnancy and parenting during adolescence
- Altered Nutrition: Less than Body Requirements related to lack of knowledge about pregnancy nutritional needs
- Chronic Low Self-Esteem related to family dysfunction
- Social Isolation related to the reactions of peers and family to pregnancy

• • Planning and Implementation

Prenatal Care

Initial planning of care may begin with community health nurses. When pregnancy is first suspected or identified by the community health nurse, referrals are made for appropriate prenatal care services. Whenever possible, efforts should be made to refer the young woman to a health care agency that provides care especially tailored for adolescent clients. Additional referrals may be made to agencies that offer programs for pregnant adolescents, such as peer-run support groups. The young woman should be encouraged to continue participation in school. If a nurse practitioner or school health nurse is available in the adolescent's school, he or she should be contacted so that coordinated care can be planned and provided.

Additional referrals may be necessary, depending on the adolescent's circumstances, such as evidence of family dysfunction, domestic violence, or substance abuse. If it is determined that the adolescent's living arrangements are inadequate or life-threatening, the nurse may be involved in placing her in a safe shelter or foster care.

Throughout the course of pregnancy, the nurse provides ongoing information about maternal and fetal status and the need for special tests or procedures. When the adolescent demonstrates evidence of health-promoting behaviors, the nurse should provide immediate positive reinforcement and ongoing encouragement. Efforts should be made to establish a trusting relationship with the adolescent and to let her know that the nurse serves as her advocate at all times. The nurse should encourage the active participation of the sexual partner, the primary support person, or family member(s) that the adolescent desires to be involved in her care during pregnancy.

Prenatal education must be geared to the adolescent's educational and cognitive levels. One-to-one teaching sessions may be more effective with very young adolescents (younger than age 15), while older adolescents often enjoy and learn better in groups. Written materials that are disseminated must be appropriate for the adolescents, educational status, and intellectual abilities. Recently, comic-book style educational materials have been created for adolescent clients and those with low literacy skills. Research must be conducted to determine their effectiveness in providing information and changing behavior.

Intrapartum Care

The onset of labor and its associated discomfort may result in maladaptive coping behaviors. The young woman may be unable to cooperate effectively with care and tolerate examinations or invasive procedures, such as injections or the initiation of an intravenous line. The adolescent may use abusive language or physically strike out against health professionals.

The nurse must provide direction and support based on the adolescent's psychological and cognitive level. Close physical contact must be maintained, and adequate pain relief should be provided so that the adolescent can use more effective coping behaviors. All procedures must be explained before they are implemented. The adolescent's questions and concerns should be addressed promptly, and she should be given time to prepare for painful or invasive procedures whenever possible.

Limitations may be placed on inappropriate or abusive behavior. If adolescent friends are present for the labor and birth, they also may need special support and considerations. If they demonstrate inappropriate behavior, they may require firm guidelines to maintain a safe and effective environment for the young woman while she labors. If a close relationship has been established with a nurse in the prenatal clinic, that individual may offer support by visiting the adolescent or telephoning her during labor.

Postpartum Care

The adolescent may exhibit an astounding recovery during the postpartum period. However, she may not be prepared for the slow process of regaining her prepregnancy weight and shape. She may be profoundly disappointed if she is unable to be discharged from the hospital in tight-fitting blue jeans or another prepregnancy outfit that is prized. The nurse must provide support, reassurance, and information regarding the process of physical recovery and permit the adolescent to verbalize her concerns about her body image.

The nurse is responsible for providing essential information about self-care and newborn care activities before discharge. Discharge planning must begin immediately after birth, when the young woman has achieved physiologic stability. Even in the best of circumstances, time to cover a myriad of topics is limited. When other family members will participate in newborn care activities, they must be included in the teaching plan. Referrals should be initiated for follow-up care and ongoing education after the adolescent leaves the hospital.

Support of breastfeeding is an important aspect of nursing care. Unfortunately, many adolescents choose not to breastfeed. Peer pressures, the desire to return to school, concerns about body image, and the time commitment required all contribute to the low rate of breastfeeding in adolescent mothers. Exceptions exist, particularly among Hispanic American adolescents. Cultural traditions and family support encourage breastfeeding in this group of young women.

When bottle feeding is selected as the feeding method, precise instructions must be given to ensure safety. Proper newborn positioning to prevent regurgitation and aspiration must be emphasized and the correct method of formula reconstitution explained when concentrated formula is used. Return demonstrations must be documented in newborn feeding techniques before discharge. As noted previously, written discharge materials must be age and cognitive level specific. Comic books and pamphlets that provide only essential information in simple terms may be most appropriate, depending on the adolescent's abilities. Important resources such as the number of the emergency room, clinic, or telephone hot-lines should be provided. Knowledge about newborn needs and capabilities, as well as early growth and development, should be reviewed, but community follow-up will be essential to build on basic information given before discharge.

Family planning information must be reviewed, and in some settings contraceptives (ie, oral contraceptives, condoms, and foam) may be prescribed before discharge. Because the repeat pregnancy rate is very high during adolescence, special efforts should be made to meet the adolescent's needs for contraception. The risks of HIV and other STDs with sexual activity also must be addressed. With the development of the HIV crisis and the rapid rise in the incidence of STDs among adolescents, the issue of contraception has become more complicated.

Caring for the Adolescent Population at Risk

In view of the enormous long-term human and economic consequences of adolescent childbearing, it may be necessary for maternity nurses to shift their focus from the care of the individual adolescent to caring for the population at risk. This will require a new alliance between maternity nursing

Assessment Criteria in the Socially At-Risk Pregnant Adolescent

The following criteria can be used to identify pregnant adolescents at high social risk who should receive priority for services. Several indicators are needed to place an adolescent in a particular category. Highest priority for services are those in "priority one" status, with mothers in "priority three' status being least in need.

Priority 1

- Evident and physical health needs
- Family history of abuse or violence
- Primary needs* not being met
- No apparent support systems
- 16 years of age or younger
- Second or subsequent adolescent pregnancy
- Drug or alcohol use reported

Priority 2

- Limited support systems
- Some but not all primary needs* being met
- School dropout
- 16 years of age or younger

Priority 3

- Support systems intact
- First pregnancy
- Primary needs* being met
- Self-initiated referral and follow-up possible

**Primary needs are considered to be housing, financial resources sufficient to feed and clothe the mother and infant, access to transportation services permitting use of available community resources, and a plan for the care of the newborn.*

From Jones, M., & Bonte, C. (1990). Conceptualizing community interventions in social service needs of pregnant adolescents. Journal of Pediatric Health Care, *4(4), 193–201 with permission from Mosby-Year Book Inc.*

and community health nursing and will require nursing to turn its attention to social issues, such as discrimination, inequitable distribution of health care resources, and the seemingly intractable problems of poverty and neglect.

The following section describes programs that have been successful in three major areas: delaying sexual activity among adolescents, promoting responsible sexual activity through access to specialized contraceptive services, and promoting pregnancy and parenting outcomes for adolescent mothers, fathers, and their children.

Delaying Sexual Activity

The "just say no" message currently endorsed by governments has been dismissed by most experts as an ineffectual and inappropriate response to adolescent sexuality (Brindis, 1990a; Frager, 1991b). Better alternatives appear to be programs that encourage sexual abstinence and emphasize opportunities for personal and vocational development and life options other than early parenthood. Such programs are complex, and for them to be effective, they must involve adolescents, their parents, community groups, schools, health care professionals, legislators, and the media.

The National Research Council Panel on Adolescent Pregnancy and Childbearing has recommended extensive sex and family life education courses from kindergarten to grade 12. To support these they advocate developing state and federal policies and funding to strengthen such courses. Programs using peer educators and nurses who can serve as health educators have proved effective in delaying sexual activity (Mutter, Ashworth, & Camerson, 1990).

Some states have used a multipronged approach that targeted parents, teachers, church and community leaders, and school children. Such programs have demonstrated a reduction in sexual activity, pregnancy, and birth rates (Brindis, 1990a). Abstinence teaching has received a national focus due to the HIV epidemic and is included in the curricula of almost every state. Mentoring programs in which young people are encouraged to identify with positive role models who influence their behavior have gained momentum, but almost no research has focused on their outcomes. Mentoring usually is used in combination with other interventions (Brindis, 1990c).

Nurses can play an important part in educational programs designed to delay sexual activity. Nurses can teach about sexuality and family life in schools, community clinics, and physicians' offices. Nurses can involve families in the process by teaching them about adolescent development and encouraging them to establish open dialogue and communication at home. Nurses can participate as members of multidisciplinary teams to promote school performance and prevent dropout. Assertiveness training groups can be implemented by nurses or can be promoted by nurses. Assertiveness training can teach adolescents how to avoid coercion by sex partners.

Community health nurses can initiate or work with community health education programs. They can articulate the problems associated with early adolescent sexual activity and attempt to influence community members involved in program development. Nurses who are experts in adolescent health care can write articles for magazines (popular literature) or participate in radio or television programs to raise the community's consciousness about the issue of adolescent sexuality.

At the national level nurses can become political activists and increase national awareness of the importance of sexual abstinence and life option programs for adolescents. Legislators must be provided with cost analyses and other data to support the development of programs for adolescents. Nurses have become skilled in obtaining funding for program development and should continue to lobby for the passage of laws that mandate the creation of innovative, effective programs.

Promoting Responsible Sexual Activity

Other programs seek to promote responsible sexual activity by improving access to and use of contraceptive services for adolescents (McAnarney & Hendee, 1989b). Title X of the Public Health Service Act was enacted to expand family planning services and improve accessibility and services for adolescents. Title X-funded programs have been an important source of contraceptive education for adolescents (Rothenberg & Sedhom, 1990).

Contraceptives are made available through private physicians, family planning clinics, and school-based clinics. Access to school-based clinics have improved adolescent contraceptive behavior. In the United States consent laws vary widely from state to state, but adolescents may give their own consent for family planning in 29 states and the District of Columbia. Many programs report limited success at involving males, and services vary widely because programs are tailored to specific communities (Frager, 1991b).

An extremely successful research-based program offered school class presentations, informal discussions, and individual counseling along with a storefront clinic offering group education, rap sessions, individual counseling, and reproductive health care. The professionals involved were a nurse and a social worker (Zabin et al., 1988). The program was evaluated and demonstrated an improvement in knowledge base, postponement of initial intercourse, male participation, increased contraceptive use in all age groups, and a drop of 26% in conceptions (Frager, 1991b).

Contraceptive education should be included in family life education earlier than the eighth grade. Behavioral counseling should emphasize skill development, interpersonal communication skills, and specific techniques for incorporating life-style changes. Follow-up of adolescents should reinforce effective contraceptive use. Finally, programs should be evaluated to ensure that they are meeting stated objectives.

Nurses play a key role in ensuring access to appropriate and specialized contraceptive services for adolescents. Nurses often are available in the context of physicians' offices, community-based clinics, or school clinics to provide information and debunk myths about birth control and to provide access to birth control. In a clinic or school context, they can offer opportunities for small group discussions or rap sessions.

Nurses can assess the individual adolescent's contraceptive needs, formulate diagnoses, provide contraceptives, teach about appropriate use of contraception, and evaluate the effectiveness and acceptability of the contraception. The nurse also can ensure that cultural beliefs and values about the desirability of contraception and the acceptability of abortion are addressed and that care is provided in a sensitive and nonjudgmental fashion.

Nurses must work with community groups. They must articulate the dangers of STDs, including AIDS, when adolescents engage in unprotected sex. Nurses can and do argue for the importance of accessible, confidential, low-cost family planning services for adolescents. They must collaborate with community leaders to encourage the media to disseminate information about contraception and protected sex among adolescents.

Enhancing Pregnancy and Parenting Outcomes

Programs have been designed to improve pregnancy and parenting outcomes for adolescent mothers, fathers, and their newborns. The Adolescent Health Services and Pregnancy Prevention Act is a federal initiative that was designed to deal explicitly with adolescent pregnancy. The legislation was intended to develop networks of community-based programs to prevent initial and repeat pregnancies among adolescents, to care for pregnant adolescents, and to assist adolescents with developing productive futures. The services to be provided included pregnancy testing, prenatal and postnatal care, family planning and STD screening, sex and family life education, adoption services, and counseling (Rothenberg & Sedhom, 1990).

Ideally, programs should focus on four areas. Initially, early diagnosis of pregnancy and discussion of options, including abortion, should be addressed. Care during the antenatal, intrapartum, early postnatal, and late postnatal period should be coordinated to ensure continuity and appropriateness of services. Economic and social support and activities to improve life options for adolescent parents and improve the cognitive and social development of their children should be in place (Frager, 1991b).

To minimize the risks of adolescent pregnancy and childrearing, care should include the following:

- Prenatal care
- Nutritional counseling and provision of food supplements
- Life-style counseling
- Early intervention or referral for pregnancy complications
- Education and employment counseling
- Psychological counseling when indicated
- Childbirth preparation classes
- Adolescent parenting education programs

For the adolescent who chooses adoption, care and counseling should be provided to ensure her legal rights and to provide emotional support. Multidisciplinary teams should provide family-centered, individualized care. All programs should include evaluation research to document cost-effectiveness and success in terms of reducing the rate of STDs and pregnancy (Frager, 1991b; Rothenberg & Sedhom, 1990).

One successful community program was Serving Pregnant–Parenting Adolescent Needs. The project was supported by a coalition of community agencies and provided group education for adolescents during regularly scheduled prenatal visits. A trained volunteer met with the adolescent each visit and provided ongoing social support. The volunteer also acted as advocate, assisting her to access other health, education, and community agencies. Based on a primary prevention model, the project attempted to identify problems early, so that parenting disorders could be avoided (Jones & Bonte, 1990).

Nurses working in a variety of settings can optimize pregnancy and parenting outcomes for adolescents. If the adolescent chooses to continue her pregnancy, the nurse can provide ongoing assessment, teaching, and emotional support. The nurse can foster family or partner participation in a supportive, accepting environment. The nurse also may provide life-style counseling about such areas as sexual activity and substance abuse.

Nurses can examine existing adolescent pregnancy and parenting programs and assess the adequacy of services. They can then assist in altering existing programs or designing new ones to meet the needs of the community. At the national level nurses should increase awareness of the limited number of adolescent pregnancy and parenting programs.

Lobbying of legislators will raise awareness of the cyclical nature of poverty and adolescent pregnancy and parenting, which results in incalculable costs to society. Efforts can be made to secure dedicated federal funding for adolescent pregnancy and parenting programs. Nurses can seek public and private resources at a variety of levels. With other health professionals, nurses must provide information on existing resources and services. Once committed community resources and strong voluntary community support have been established, politicians and administrators will be more willing to sustain comprehensive funding.

Chapter Summary

Adolescence is a period of adaptation and maturation. Risk behaviors and poverty make adolescents especially vulnerable to the challenges inherent in pregnancy and parenting. This event can prevent optimal development and threaten physiologic and psychological well-being. The costs to adolescents, their offspring, their families, and their society can be enormous. Current programs are focused for the most part on tertiary prevention and often are uncoordinated and inadequate.

Nurses must be prepared to respond on three levels. They must become further involved by encouraging sexual abstinence and developing life options for adolescents. Needs in the areas of contraceptive accessibility and acceptability must be met. Attention should be paid to parenting outcomes in programs designed to reduce the mortality and morbidity associated with adolescent pregnancy and parenting. In addition the focus of nursing must not only be care of individual adolescents and their families, but also should include action at the local, regional, and national level.

Study Questions

1. *Why is the incidence of adolescent childbearing in the United States higher than in other industrialized countries?*
2. *What factors contribute to adolescent pregnancy and parenting? What roles do poverty and ethnicity play in determining outcomes of adolescent childbearing?*
3. *What are the developmental tasks of adolescence? How will pregnancy and parenting interfere with an adolescent's achievement of such tasks?*
4. *What are the implications of adolescent pregnancy and parenting for the offspring of adolescent parents? (Include a discussion of newborns, infants, preschool, and school-age children and adolescents.)*
5. *What are three goals toward which programs targeting adolescents are being directed? How would achievement of these goals affect the health status of childbearing adolescents and their families?*

References

Adger, H. (1991). Problems of alcohol and other drug use and abuse in adolescents. *Journal of Adolescent Health*, *12*(8), 606–613.

Aneshensel, C. S., Becerra, R. M., Fielder, E. P., & Schuler, R. H. (1990). Onset of fertility-related events during adolescence: A prospective comparison of Mexican American and non-Hispanic white females. *American Journal of Public Health*, *80*(8), 959–963.

Baldwin, W., & Cain, V. S. (1980). The children of teenage parents. *Family Planning Perspectives*, *12*(1), 34–39, 42–43.

Belsky, J., & Miller, B. C. (1986). Adolescent fatherhood in the context of transition to parenthood. In A. B. Elster & M. E. Lamb (Eds.), *Adolescent fatherhood* (pp. 107–122). London: Lawrence Erlbaum Associates.

Behrman, C. A., Hediger, M. L., Scholl, T. O., & Arkangel, C. M. (1990). Nausea and vomiting during teenage pregnancy: Effects on birthweight. *Journal of Adolescent Health Care*, *11*(5), 418–422.

Blinn, L. M. (1990). Adolescent mothers' perceptions of their work lives in the future: Are they stable? *Journal of Adolescent Research*, *5*(2), 206–221.

Brindis, C. (1990a). Helping teens wait: Abstinence education. *Family Life Educator*, *9*(1), 11–25.

Brindis, C. (1990b). When teens don't wait: Encouraging contraception. *Family Life Educator*, *9*(1), 26–42.

Brindis, C. (1990c). Reasons to wait: Enhancing life options. *Family Life Educator*, *9*(1), 43–57.

Browne, C., & Urback, M. (1989). Pregnant adolescents: Expectations vs. reality. *Canadian Journal of Public Health*, *80*(3), 227–229.

Buckley, K. (1990). Substance abuse. In K. Buckley & N. Kulb (Eds.), *High risk maternity nursing manual* (pp. 204–218). Baltimore: Williams & Wilkins.

Castiglia, P. T. (1990a). Adolescent mothers. *Journal of Pediatric Health Care*, *4*(5), 262–264.

Castiglia, P. T. (1990b). Adolescent fathers. *Journal of Pediatric Health Care*, *4*(6), 311–313.

Causby, V., Nixon, C., & Bright, J.M. (1991). Influences on adolescent mother-infant interactions. *Adolescence*, *26*(103), 619–630.

Children's Defense Fund. (1990). *S.O.S. America! A children's defense budget*. Washington, DC: Author.

Codega, S. A., Pasley, B. K., & Kreutzer, J. (1990). Coping behaviors of adolescent mothers: An exploratory study and comparison of Mexican-Americans and Anglos. *Journal of Adolescent Research*, *5*(1), 34–53.

Cooper, C. S., Dunst, C. J., & Vance, S. D. (1990). The effect of social support on adolescent mothers' styles of parent-child interaction as measured on three separate occasions. *Adolescence*, *XXV*(97), 49–57.

Damato, E. G. (1991). Discharge planning from the neonatal intensive care unit. *Journal of Perinatal and Neonatal Nursing*, *5*(1), 43–53.

Debolt, M. E., Pasley, B. K., & Kreutzer, J. (1990). Factors affecting the probability of school dropout: A study of pregnant and parenting adolescent females. *Journal of Adolescent Research*, *5*(2), 190–205.

Dryfoos, J. (1991). Adolescents at risk: A summation of work in the field-programs and policies. *Journal of Adolescent Health*, *12*(8), 630–637.

Duncan, G. J., & Hoffman, S. D. (1990). Welfare benefits, economic opportunities, and out-of-wedlock birth among black teenage girls. *Demography*, *27*(4), 519–535.

Elster, A. B., & Hendricks, L. (1986). Stresses and coping strategies of adolescent fathers. In A. B. Elster & M. E. Lamb (Eds.), *Adolescent fatherhood* (pp. 55–65). London: Lawrence Erlbaum Associates.

Farber, N. B. (1991). The process of pregnancy resolution among adolescent mothers. *Adolescence*, *26*(103), 697–716.

Frager, B. (1991a). Teenage childbearing: Part I. The problem has not gone away. *Journal of Pediatric Nursing*, *6*(2), 131–133.

Frager, B. (1991b). Teenage childbearing: Part II. Programs and policies. *Journal of Pediatric Nursing*, *6*(3), 202–205.

Furstenberg, F. F., Brooks-Gunn, J., & Morgan, S. P. (1987). Adolescent mothers and their children in later life. *Family Planning Perspectives*, *19*(4), 142–151.

Gennaro, S., Brooten, D., & Bakewell-Sach, S. (1991). Postdischarge services for low-birth-weight infants. *Journal of Obstetric, Gynecologic, and Neonatal Nursing*, *20*(1), 29–36.

Grindstaff, C. F. (1988). Adolescent marriage and childrearing: The long-term economic outcome, Canada in the 1980's. *Adolescence*, *XXIII*(89), 45–58.

Hanson, S. L., Morrison, D. R., & Ginsburg, A. L. (1989). The antecedents of teenage fatherhood. *Demography*, *26*(4), 579–596.

Hardy, J. B., & Zabin, L. S. (1990). *Adolescent pregnancy in an urban environment: Issues, programs, and evaluation*. Washington, DC: The Urban Institute Press.

Holt, J. L., & Johnson, S. D. (1991). Developmental tasks: A key to reducing teenage pregnancy. *Journal of Pediatric Nursing*, *6*(3), 191–196.

Hutchinson, S. W. (1990). Adolescent mothers' perceptions of new born infants and the mothers' use of coping behaviors: A descriptive study. *Journal of National Black Nurses' Association*, *4*(1), 14–23.

Jessor, R. (1991). Risk behavior in adolescence: A psychosocial framework for understanding and action. *Journal of Adolescent Health*, *12*(8), 597–605.

Jones, E. F., Forrest, J. D., Goldman, N., Henshaw, S. K., Lincoln, R., Rosoff, J., Westoff, C. F., & Wulf, D. (1985). Teenage pregnancy in developed countries: Determinants and policy implications. *Family Planning Perspectives*, *17*(2), 53–63.

Jones, M. E., & Bonte, C. (1990). Conceptualizing community interventions in social service needs of pregnant adolescents. *Journal of Pediatric Health Care*, *4*(4), 193–201.

Joseph, S. C. (1991). AIDS and adolescence: A challenge to both treatment and prevention. *Journal of Adolescent Health*, *12*(8), 614–618.

Kelley, S. J., Walsh, J. H., & Thompson, K. (1991). Birth outcomes, health problems, and neglect with prenatal exposure to cocaine. *Pediatric Nursing*, *17*(2), 130–135.

Lee, K., & Corpuz, M. (1988). Teenage pregnancy: Trend and impact of low birth weight and fetal, maternal, and neonatal morbidity in the United States. *Clinics in Perinatology*, *15*(4), 929–941.

Marsiglio, W. (1987). Adolescent fathers in the United States: Their initial living arrangements, marital experiences, and educational outcomes. *Family Planning Perspectives*, *19*(6), 240–251.

McAnarney, E. R., & Hendee, W. R. (1989a). Adolescent pregnancy and its consequences. *Journal of American Medical Association*, *262*(1), 74–77.

McAnarney, E. R., & Hendee, W. R. (1989b). The prevention of adolescent pregnancy. *Journal of American Medical Association*, *262*(1), 78–82.

Mercer, R. T. (1979). *Perspectives on adolescent health care*. Philadelphia: J.B. Lippincott.

Morris, M. (1991). Adolescent pregnancy. *Journal of Society of Obstetricians and Gynecologists of Canada*, *13*(3), 15–20.

Mutter, G. W. R., Ashworth, C., & Camerson, H. (1990). Canada: Perspectives in school health. *Journal of School Health*, *60*(7), 308–312.

Nance, N. W. (1990). Caring for the woman at risk for preterm labor or with premature rupture of the membranes. In E. J. Martin (Ed.), *Intrapartum management modules: A perinatal education program* (pp. 259–284). Baltimore: Williams & Wilkins.

Nelson, P. B. (1990). Repeat pregnancy among adolescent mothers: A review of the literature. *Journal of National Black Nurses' Association*, *4*(1), 28–34.

Norr, K. F., & Roberts, J. E. (1991). Early maternal attachment behaviors of adolescent and adult mothers. *Journal of Nurse-Midwifery*, *36*(6), 334–342.

Parks, P. L., & Arndt, E. K. (1990). Differences between adolescent and adult mothers. *Journal of Adolescent Health Care*, *11*(3), 248–253.

Peters, H., & Theorell, C. J. (1991). Fetal and neonatal effects of maternal cocaine use. *Journal of Obstetric, Gynecologic, and Neonatal Nursing*, *20*(2), 121–126.

Robinson, B. E. (1988). *Teenage fathers*. Lexington: D.C. Health.

Rothenberg, R., & Sedhom, L. (1990). Teenage pregnancy. In J. N. Nataproff & R. R. Wieczorek (Eds.), *Maternal-child health policy: A nursing perspective* (pp. 131–152). New York: Spring Publishing Company.

Sander, A. H., & Rosen, J. L. (1987). Teenage fathers: Working with the neglected partner in adolescent childbearing. *Family Planning Perspectives*, *19*(3), 107–110.

Schneck, M. E., Sideras, K. S., Fox, R. A., & Dupuis, L. (1990). Low-income pregnant adolescents and their infants: Dietary findings and health outcomes. *Journal of American Dietetic Association*, *90*(4), 555–558.

Seymore, C., Frothingham, T. E., MacMillan, J., & Durant, R. H. (1990). Child development knowledge, childrearing attitudes, and social support among first- and second-time adolescent mothers. *Journal of Adolescent Health Care*, *11*(4), 343–349.

Shaw, P. E. (1990, February/March). Cocaine + adolescence = Perilous pregnancies. *Adolescent Counselor*, 25–29.

Sonenstein, F. L., Pieck, J. H., & Ku, L. C. (1991). Levels of sexual activity among adolescent males in the United States. *Family Planning Perspectives*, *23*(4), 162–167.

Stevens-Simon, C., Roghmann, K. J., & McAnarney, E. R. (1990). Repeat adolescent pregnancy and low birth weight: Methods issues. *Journal of Adolescent Health Care*, *11*(3), 248–253.

Thomas, H., Mitchell, A., & Devlin, M. C. (1990). Adolescent pregnancy: Issues in prevention. *Journal of Preventive Psychiatry and Allied Disciplines*, *4*(2–3), 101–124.

Wadhera, S., & Silins, J. (1990). Teenage pregnancy in Canada, 1975–1987. *Family Planning Perspectives*, *22*(1), 27–30.

Wattenberg, E. (1990, March–April). Unmarried fathers: Perplexing questions. *Children Today*, 27–30.

Wilson, M. D., Duggan, A. K., & Joffe, A. (1990). Rehospitalization of infants born to adolescent mothers. *Journal of Adolescent Health Care*, *11*(6), 510–515.

Zabin, L. S., Hirsch, M. B., Street, R., Emerson, M. B., Smith, M., Hardy, J. B., & Hardy, T. M. (1988). The Baltimore pregnancy prevention program for urban teenagers: 1 How did it work? *Family Planning Perspectives*, *20*(4), 182–187.

Suggested Readings

Bar-Cohen, A., Lia-Hoagberg, B., & Edwards, L. (1990). First family planning visit in school-based clinics. *Journal of School Health*, *60*(8), 418–421.

Cooksey, E. C. (1990). Factors in the resolution of adolescent premarital pregnancies. *Demography*, *27*(2), 207–218.

de Anda, D., Javidi, M., Jefford, S., Komorowski, R., & Yanez, R. (1991). Stress and coping in adolescence: A comparative study of pregnant adolescents and substance abusing adolescents. *Children and Youth Services Review*, *13*, 171–182.

Washburn, P. (1991). Identification, assessment, and referral of adolescent drug abuser. *Pediatric Nursing*, *17*(2), 137–140.

Wuest, J. (1990). Trying it on for size: Mutual support in role transition for pregnant teens and student nurses. *Health Care for Women International*, *11*, 383–392.

CHAPTER 10

Childbearing and Parenting After Age 35

Learning Objectives

After studying the material in this chapter, the student should be able to:

- Describe trends in childbearing for women over age 35 in the United States.
- Discuss the importance of preconception counseling for women planning pregnancy after the age of 35.
- Discuss the impact of aging on reproductive functioning and fertility in women.
- Describe how repeat pregnancy for the older multiparous woman differs from a first pregnancy for the woman over age 35.
- Identify major physiologic complications of pregnancy that are more common with advancing age.
- Discuss how the developmental tasks of pregnancy may differ for both the older primigravida and multigravida.
- List major intrapartum complications for the woman who delays childbearing beyond age 35.
- Describe how advancing age influences postpartum adjustment and maternal role attainment.
- Develop a nursing care plan for the woman over age 35 who is pregnant for the first time.

Key Terms

advanced maternal age	multigravida
anovulatory cycle	multipara
dystocia	nulligravida
fertility	nullipara

The topic of pregnancy and childbirth often engenders mental pictures of a young woman in her early twenties becoming a new mother. However, the excitement and joy surrounding the birth of an infant is experienced increasingly by the mature woman and adds another dimension to maternity nursing. Although most women still begin childbearing in their twenties, first-time pregnancy and parenthood for women over age 35 is increasing. The rate of first births for women age 30 and older increased by 50% through the decade of the 1980s (Fig. 10-1). It is expected to rise, if at a somewhat slower pace into the 21st century (Chen & Morgan, 1991). Advances in reproductive technology have even made it possible for women in their early fifties to consider pregnancy.

In addition, women who have previously given birth may experience repeat pregnancies beyond age 35. More than 250,000 women each year experience a repeat pregnancy after age 35 (Ventura, 1991). These women constitute a diverse group, with different characteristics and responses to pregnancy than women who plan a first birth at an older age. For some women, a late pregnancy represents a planned event to add a final member to the family unit. For others, the pregnancy is unplanned or unexpected. Pregnancy after 35 is still common for women living in poverty who have limited access to family planning services or lack the knowledge and financial resources to limit the number of pregnancies (Arnold & Brecht, 1990).

Nursing care of women who experience pregnancy and childbirth after age 35 is individualized to meet the needs of the specific woman and her family. The conditions surrounding the mature woman's pregnancy must be clearly identified and understood. Whether involved in preconception counseling or prenatal, intrapartum, or postpartum care, the nurse must be knowledgeable about the unique physical risks of later childbearing. The psychological and social impact of delayed childbearing or late, repeat pregnancy on the woman and her immediate family must also be fully understood. The nursing process is used to assess the

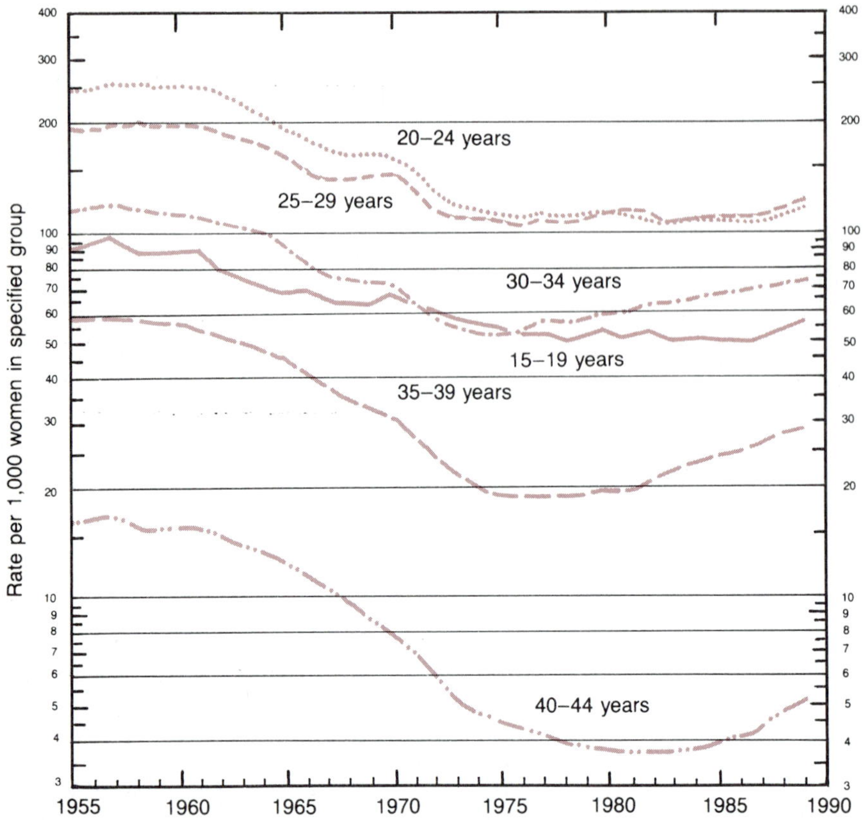

NOTE: Beginning with 1959, trend lines are based on registered live births; trend lines for 1955–59 are based on live births adjusted for underregistration.

Figure 10-1.
Birth rates by age of mother: United States 1955–1989. (Ventura, S. J. [1991]. Advance report of final natality statistics, 1989. *Monthly Vital Statistics Report, 40*[8–5], 3.)

woman and her support unit, identify specific problems and needs, plan nursing interventions, and evaluate the effectiveness of care.

This chapter discusses reasons for delayed childbearing and repeat pregnancy after age 35 and describes the medical and obstetric risks for the woman, fetus, and neonate. Psychosocial aspects of late childbearing and parenting are also explored. Implications for nursing practice are described in relation to the preconception, prenatal, intrapartum, and postpartum periods.

Reasons for Late Childbearing

In general, the number of women giving birth after age 35 is increasing because of the spurt in population growth after World War II. The baby boom generation has made a significant contribution to first births in older women since 1975 and is expected to do so for the remainder of the century (Chen & Morgan, 1991).

Repeat Pregnancy After Age 35

Before reproductive technology permitted the timing of conception, many women experienced repeat pregnancies and childbirth well into their forties. In fact, complications related to grand multiparity remained the leading causes of death for all women until the early decades of the 20th century. They still remain major causes of morbidity and mortality for women in underdeveloped countries. Advances in health care permit older women who live in industrialized nations to extend their childbearing years beyond age 35 with minimal risk.

For most women, however, repeat pregnancy after age 35 is an unplanned event (Jones & Forrest, 1989). For some, pregnancy comes as a total surprise during the early stages of menopause when conception is not thought possible. Contraceptive failures also result in unplanned repeat pregnancies for this group of women. However, poverty and lack of education and knowledge about conception control are the most powerful factors contributing to repeat unplanned pregnancies in women over age 35.

Current social forces have resulted in limited access to family planning clinics for many poor women. A decrease in federal, state, and local funding to women's health programs has reduced the availability of contraceptive services. The lack of private health insurance coverage for nearly 40 million Americans prevents many women from obtaining contraceptive counseling and family planning care (Arnold & Brecht, 1990). Higher repeat pregnancy rates occur for women with less than a high school education, and the number who do not complete the 12th grade is growing. As a result of these factors, second and third pregnancies have increased for women over age 30 (Ventura, 1991).

First Pregnancy in Older Women

Sharp contrasts exist between women who voluntarily delay the first birth and multiparous women who continue to experience pregnancies beyond age 35. Over 50% of women who postpone childbearing until their mid thirties or later in life are white, married, middle class, and college educated (Ventura, 1991; Cunningham, MacDonald, & Gant, 1989). Most have remained continuously employed in careers or professions for 10 years or longer (Blossfeld & Huinick, 1991). In general, they are in good-to-excellent health and maintain life-styles that promote physical and emotional well-being (Mansfield & McCool, 1989).

Undoubtedly the factor most responsible for delayed childbearing in this group of women is their ability to time the first pregnancy. For women in general, fertility control has permitted the pursuit of other life goals before beginning a family. Knowledge that fertility technology permits women to successfully conceive well into their forties or even early fifties has allayed some women's fears about the "biologic clock" winding down. They may feel comfortable postponing childbearing and parenthood. When these factors are coupled with knowledge of contraceptive control and the financial resources necessary to pay for family planning services, women are more likely to delay pregnancy.

Beyond greater reproductive control, the growing participation of women in the educational system may be the most powerful predictor of delayed childbearing (DeWit & Rajulton, 1992). In the past, most women married shortly after completing high school and experienced the birth of the first child within 14 months (Harker & Thorpe, 1992). Extended participation in the educational process delays marriage for women, and the completion of higher education more often results in the pursuit and accomplishment of career goals, further delaying childbearing (Hollander & Breene, 1990).

Research clearly indicates that many women postpone pregnancy while they fully explore the appropriateness of parenthood for them. For many women who delay childbearing, much time is spent considering whether a child or children will complement their lives and add to their fulfillment; quite simply, would parenthood be "right" for them (Barnes, 1991; Winslow, 1987). Another factor that influences the timing of pregnancy is concern about the quality of the marital relationship. Some women delay childbearing and parenting until they have established a mature, stable relationship (Meisenhelder & Meservey, 1987). Additionally, both first marriages and second marriages after divorce occur at an older age.

Fertility problems cause involuntary postponement of pregnancy for some women. It may be years before the precise cause of infertility is identified and treatment is initiated. The woman may find herself in her late thirties or early forties before the first pregnancy occurs.

The reasons for delayed childbearing or repeat pregnancy beyond age 35 are many and varied. Significant changes in role expectations for women, and advances in reproductive technology make pregnancy possible even beyond the decade of the forties.

Reasons for childbearing are not always based on positive psychological and social influences. Many women who are economically and educationally disadvantaged continue to bear children after age 35, when they would prefer to limit family size. The maternity nurse working with mature women must understand and identify the reasons for late childbearing and parenthood to plan and provide appropriate care. At a political level, nurses can make a significant impact on the ability of women to voluntarily choose pregnancy beyond age 35 and limit fertility when so desired. This can be accomplished by becoming knowledgeable about political, economic, and cultural factors influencing later childbearing and supporting changes in the our society and health care system that prevent all women from choosing when to conceive.

Physiologic Risks and Problems Related to Advanced Maternal Age

Preconception Problems

Many women age 35 or older have experienced significant fertility problems before successfully conceiving. It is estimated that approximately one third of women who defer pregnancy until the mid to late thirties will have an infertility problem. The decline in fertility with advancing age has been well documented; however, the mechanism for this decline is unclear. The increased incidence of anovulation with advancing age and the effects of aging on oocytes could act together to cause a decline in fertility (Dicker et al., 1991). There is also a greater likelihood that diseases such as endometriosis will interfere with fertility as the woman enters her thirties. Reproductive damage from exposure to occupational or environmental hazards can accumulate over years and lessen fertility as a woman ages (Shortridge, 1990). In addition, sexually transmitted diseases and pelvic inflammatory diseases have contributed to increases in infertility for women of all ages. For women seeking assistance with conception, in vitro fertilization is also less successful after age 35. Failure rates reach 70% in women after age 37 (Dicker et al., 1991). It is suggested that changes in uterine function and reduced vascularization of the endometrium interfere with successful implantation.

Increased Risk of Spontaneous Abortion

The incidence of spontaneous abortion increases significantly as a woman ages. The rate rises from approximately 10% at age 20 to 18% by the late thirties to 34% in the early forties (Jahoda, Pijpers, Vosters, et al., 1987). Most early abortions after age 35 are due to autosomal trisomies such as trisomy 21. Its incidence is known to increase with older maternal age. The rate of spontaneous abortion is also increased when the embryo is genetically normal in women over the age of 36 (Overbeek et al., 1990). Loss of normal embryos may be due to defects in implantation. Decreasing thickness of the uterine endometrium and decreasing capacity of the endometrium to produce prostaglandins are common sequelae of aging.

Increased Incidence of Chromosomal Abnormalities

There is an strong association between the incidence of Down syndrome (trisomy 21) and advancing age. The frequency of Down syndrome increases from 1 in 885 pregnancies to 1 in 365 pregnancies at age 35, and 1 in 109 pregnancies at age 40 (Cunningham, MacDonald, & Gant, 1989). Other clinically significant trisomies are also related to advancing age in the woman. The effects of paternal age on the incidence of chromosomal abnormalities is less clear. Many experts agree that paternal age makes a modest contribution to chromosomal composition of the embryo after age 40 and becomes a greater consideration after age 53 (Jones & Forrest, 1989). Advanced maternal age is the most common indication for genetic counseling. Chapter 12 contains a more detailed discussion of prenatal diagnosis including amniocentesis and chorionic villous sampling.

Pregnancy Risks and Problems

Diabetes Mellitus. With advancing maternal age there is a rise in the incidence of both preexisting diabetes (type II non-insulin dependent) and gestational diabetes during pregnancy. The rate of diabetes is 64.5/1000 live births among women age 35 or older compared with a rate of 7.4/1000 live births among adolescents (Haines, Rogers, & Leung 1991). Ethnicity may compound the incidence of diabetes in the older woman. O'Brien and Gilson (1987) examined the incidence of gestational diabetes in a sample of Hispanic and Native American women. A high incidence was discovered in this group of women (10%) compared with the incidence of 1% to 3% found in the general population; 55% of the women who tested positive for gestational diabetes were over 30 years of age. Advances in control of carbohydrate intolerance during pregnancy has resulted in improved neonatal outcomes. There is, however, an increased incidence of anomalies and macrosomia even with strict glycemic control in all women.

Hypertension. There is a strong association between advancing maternal age and the development of chronic hypertension and pregnancy-induced hypertension (PIH). Research indicates a twofold to fourfold increase for women over age 35 (Fonteyn & Isada, 1988). The greatest incidence of PIH occurs in primigravidas. The older woman who delays childbearing is therefore more likely to develop PIH than the woman over age 35 who is experiencing a repeat pregnancy. Although maternal risks have been dramatically reduced with early treatment of both chronic hypertension and PIH, the fetus is at increased risk for intrauterine growth retardation. The neonate may require early delivery due to placental insufficiency and is more often small for gestational age.

Multiple Gestation. The incidence of twinning increases with advancing age. The tendency toward multiple ovulation is apparently responsible for this phenomenon. Twins are one third less likely in women 20 years of age than in women between the ages of 35 and 40 (Cunningham et al., 1989). The occurrence of multiple gestation (twins, triplets, quadruplets, and quintuplets) is also increased because of the use of fertility drugs in the older woman. When the older woman experiences a multiple gestation, she is more likely to develop gestational diabetes, preterm labor, and require cesarean birth.

Preterm Labor. The older woman is at increased risk for preterm labor and birth. The reasons for this problem are related to the other common complications experienced among pregnant women after age 35. These factors are listed in the accompanying display. Older women who smoke place themselves at added risk for developing preterm labor. A study done by Wen and colleagues (1990) found that smoking in older women was associated with a greater incidence of preterm labor.

Intrapartum Risks and Problems

Dysfunctional Labor. Labor complications are less well studied among older women than prenatal problems, and data present conflicting findings. Most studies do, however, demonstrate an increase in the incidence of labor dystocia. It is suggested that changes produced by aging in uterine muscle are responsible for ineffective labor patterns. The increased frequency of uterine myomas or fibroids found in the older woman may be responsible for soft- tissue dystocia (Cunningham et al., 1989). Fetal malpresentation and dysfunctional labor are also more common in the multiparous woman over age 35 and are thought to be due to stretching and relaxation of the uterine muscle with successive pregnancies and aging.

Placental Problems. Evidence indicates that women 35 years and older experience an increased incidence of placental previa and abruptio placentae (Cunningham & Leveno, 1990). A major factor in the development of placental

Causes of Preterm Labor and Birth Among Older Women

- Renal disease
- Placenta previa
- Abruptio placentae
- Diabetes mellitus
- Multiple gestation
- Uterine myomas
- Pregnancy-induced hypertension
- Unstable lie—breech presentation

problems appears to be defective vascularization, which occurs with advancing age. The presence of placenta previa is also associated with an increased risk of preterm labor and birth.

Cesarean Birth. The incidence of cesarean birth increases for the older woman. The rate rises to 32% in woman over age 40 compared with a rate of 23% to 25% in the general population (Ventura, 1992). This increase is similar for both nulliparous and multiparous women (Gordon et al., 1991). Possible explanations for this finding include the presence of other problems commonly associated with pregnancy and advanced maternal age (see the previous display). It is suggested that the obstetrician may be more conservative in the management of problems in the older woman and elect cesarean birth to ensure fetal and neonatal well-being (Fonteyn & Isada, 1988).

Maternal and Neonatal Outcomes

Earlier studies of the older pregnant woman found negative maternal, fetal, and neonatal outcomes including late fetal death, an increased incidence of low birth weight and preterm delivery, and greater maternal and neonatal morbidity and mortality (Barkan & Bracken, 1987; Berkowitz, Skovron, Lapinski, & Berkowitz, 1990). Many of these studies did not consider factors that have adverse effects on outcome such as parity, smoking, and socioeconomic status. Recent studies that have controlled for these variables have discovered that age in itself may not have consistently negative effects on the neonate (Cunningham & Leveno, 1990).

Newer studies indicate that healthy women without previous medical or obstetric complications are still more likely to experience both prenatal and intrapartum problems. However, the incidence of neonatal problems approaches that of the general population (Haines et al., 1991). Poor women, grand multiparas, smokers, and those who enter pregnancy with preexisting medical problems continue to experience more adverse maternal and neonatal outcomes.

Women over the age of 35 can now benefit from the tremendous advances in health care, fertility control, and reproductive technology to extend their childbearing years. This can be accomplished with less physical risk and a greater likelihood of positive maternal and neonatal outcomes. The high rate of maternal morbidity and mortality observed in older women was in the past often related to grand multiparity and close spacing between pregnancies. When the pregnancy is planned, preexisting diseases associated with aging are treated before conception, and if the woman receives appropriate prenatal care, perinatal problems can be minimized.

The woman over age 35 may be confronted with significant physiologic risks. Advancing age predisposes the woman to fertility problems, medical complications such as hypertension and diabetes, and increases the risk of conceiving a fetus with Down syndrome. The increased potential for negative outcomes for the woman and her fetus or neonate requires specialized care during the childbearing cycle. The nurse plays a central role in assessing the woman for risk factors, providing patient education, and implementing nursing care geared to the mature woman's unique needs. With appropriate medical and nursing support the woman over age 35 may experience a pregnancy and labor free of significant problems and give birth to a healthy neonate.

Psychosocial Aspects of Childbearing After Age 35

Although many facets of the psychological and social aspects of pregnancy are similar for all women, unique issues exist for older women. The reader is referred to Chapters 8 and 15 for a detailed discussion of the psychological aspects of childbearing and individual and family adaptations to pregnancy. This discussion focuses only on those aspects unique to pregnancy after age 35.

Factors Influencing the Decision to Become a Parent After Age 35

The expectation that a married couple will ultimately have children remains prevalent in our society. Even though an increasing number of couples elect to remain childless, they represent a relatively small percentage of all married couples. Subtle and more obvious pressures to have children influence most married couples to have at least one child during the course of the reproductive years. Many women still view motherhood as an essential aspect of married life.

Although most married couples will eventually have children, the desires to establish a stable relationship and to complete career training or professional goals may delay childbearing for years. Economic considerations and the desire to achieve financial security are other factors that postpone parenthood. Some couples may initially choose to remain childless and then find themselves questioning that decision as they near the end of their reproductive years. A number of them will eventually elect to have children after age 35.

Pregnancy among older single women has also become increasingly common in industrialized nations. Generally older women who choose single parenthood are well educated and economically secure (Ventura, 1991). Motivation for single parenthood in the woman often comes with the realization that she does not wish to marry, or may never marry, yet desires the joys and challenges of childrearing. These women have often made detailed plans and preparations for the pregnancy and childrearing. They also have a strong social support network to help with child care, to provide emotional support, and to provide assistance with unexpected problems.

The reasons for a planned, repeat pregnancy in the woman over 35 are numerous. Some women plan an extended period of childbearing throughout the adult years. A late pregnancy represents a realization of the goal to continue childbearing until menopause. Others follow this pattern because of strong religious or philosophical beliefs about the value of life and the importance of the parenting role for married couples in society. A number of women who have completed childbearing in their twenties now find that they want one last child before menopause occurs. Harker and Thorpe (1992) refer to this as the "last egg in the basket" syndrome. It is also suggested that the anticipated loss of adult children to work, college, or marriage may motivate some women to become pregnant once more.

Readiness for Childbearing and Parenting

Most pregnancies among middle-class, older women are planned and wanted. Psychologically, many of these women feel optimally prepared for the demands of pregnancy and parenthood. They have delayed childbearing until they feel they are emotionally ready. They may spend years reflecting on the pros and cons of a childfree life or parenthood before making the final decision to conceive. In many communities, classes are available and support groups have been formed to help the mature woman and her partner explore issues related to pregnancy after 35.

When the pregnancy is unplanned, psychological issues may be quite different. Whether a first or repeat pregnancy, older women and their mates may feel too old to parent. They may have a circle of friends who have all completed childbearing and may feel "out of step" with them by beginning a new family in their late thirties or early forties. They may be daunted by the prospect of raising an adolescent when they are in their fifties or early sixties, when many people are planning retirement. Parents of adolescent or adult children may fear their children's reaction to the pregnancy and a newborn. Research suggests that adolescent or adult children may experience many negative reactions to a late pregnancy for their mother (Green, Coupland, & Ketzinger, 1990). These couples may need some time to reflect on the consequences of late childbearing and parenting. Even when the decision is made to continue with the pregnancy, many issues may remain unresolved as they approach the birth of the neonate.

Psychological and Developmental Changes for the Older Pregnant Woman

Achieving motherhood may not represent the primary adult developmental landmark for a mature woman. Statistics indicate that the older pregnant woman has probably been employed, at least part-time, for most of her adult life (Ventura, 1989). Parenthood may simply constitute one in a series of major developmental milestones stemming from a fulfilling career and marriage (Hees-Stauthamer, 1985). Career attainment or professional development may radically alter the the meaning and value of motherhood. Unfortunately, few researchers have fully explored these changes in the adult psychological development of women. Results of one study are given in the Nursing Research display.

An important area for further research centers on how pregnancy after age 35 affects the achievement of the developmental tasks of pregnancy described by Rubin (1975) and other researchers.

Acceptance of Pregnancy. The mature, first-time pregnant woman has often planned in great detail for childbearing and parenthood. She is generally excited and happy and seeks confirmation of conception at an early stage of gestation—often within 2 to 3 weeks. If infertility problems have delayed the ability to conceive for years, there may be an initial period of disbelief, followed by happiness and anticipation. If the pregnancy is unplanned, the woman often experiences the same feelings of disbelief, ambiguity, and concern that younger women face. The woman's concerns about her advanced age may make acceptance of the pregnancy even more difficult.

The multigravid woman who becomes unexpectedly pregnant after 35 may also have problems accepting the pregnancy. If childbearing and childrearing were the major focus of the young adult years, the woman may be looking forward to achieving other goals as her children approach maturity. The prospect of having to raise another child may be initially distressing. The older father may also have concerns about his ability to parent at this time in life, and this can contribute to the woman's uncertainty.

Providing Safe Passage. It is well-established that older women often begin the process of providing safe passage in the preconception period (Harker & Thorpe, 1992; Barnes, 1991). Their goal is to achieve the best possible outcome for themselves and their newborns. In an early study of first pregnancy after age 35, Winslow (1987) found that women used three strategies to achieve this task:

- Seeking in-depth information about conception, pregnancy, childbirth, and parenting from a wide variety of formal and informal resources.
- Undergoing genetic screening and ultrasound evaluation to rule out genetic abnormalities.
- Choosing the best possible prenatal services.

For the older multigravid woman, seeking safe passage has not been as well studied. The pioneering investigations conducted by Rubin in the 1970s examined pregnancy for women of all ages, including multiparous women in their thirties. However, her findings cannot be generalized to older multiparous women today. A growing number of women who already have children continue to work during subsequent pregnancies, yet little is known about how they achieve the task of ensuring safe passage under the the double pressures of work and child care. Many women remain employed in strenuous jobs that expose them to fetal teratogens. They are aware of the increased risks to the fetus and seeking safe passage is a critical task for them.

Establishing a Relationship with the Fetus. The mature pregnant woman who has undergone in vitro fertilization or genetic testing may attempt to delay her relationship with the fetus or fetuses due to the possibility of pregnancy loss, elective termination, or an embryo reduction procedure (Farrel, 1989; Morgan & Elias, 1989). However,

Nursing Research

Psychological Experience of the Older Primigravida

To better understand the psychological dimensions of pregnancy in older women, a study was conducted by Winslow to explore the experiences of 12 primigravidas who ranged in age from 35 to 44. All women were interviewed periodically throughout pregnancy and their responses yielded a conceptual framework described as "Pregnancy as a Project." The participants in the study described passing through four phases during the gestational period.

- *Phase One: Planning for the Pregnancy:* choosing the "right time" for the pregnancy; completing career goals; achieving a stable, loving relationship.
- *Phase Two: Seeking Safe Passage:* educating self about pregnancy; ruling out fetal defects; obtaining the best care possible.
- *Phase Three: Accepting the Changing Reality:* accepting changes in life-style and body image; identifying stressors; anticipating birth.
- *Phase Four: Anticipating the Future:* fantasizing about parenthood.

The investigator recommended that nurses identify the specific phase of preparation the older woman is working through before planning care. The nurse can then implement specific nursing actions to support accomplishment of the tasks inherent in each phase. Active listening, encouraging verbalization of concerns and thoughts about pregnancy and parenthood, and providing information appropriate to each phase are essential components of psychosocial support.

Further research is indicated to build on this older study. Cross-cultural studies would be valuable to determine if the experience of the first-time pregnancy for women over age 35 is similar in other ethnic groups.

Winslow, W. (1987). First pregnancy after 35: What is the experience? *American Journal of Maternal Child Nursing, 12*(2), 92.

little research has explored the differences in the development of prenatal attachment that may be influenced by the woman's age and life experiences. One study found that the older career women spent less time engaging in fantasies about the infant or in mental rehearsal for the maternal role (Grace, 1989).

Gaining Acceptance by Others. Whether married or single, a nullipara or multipara, the older woman is often concerned with the reactions of family members, coworkers, and health care providers to the pregnancy. The cultural context in which childbearing occurs will strongly influence the responses of a woman's immediate family and social support group to parenthood after age 35. The reaction of family members, friends, and even health care providers is important for both the physical and emotional well-being of the woman and fetus. Younger children may be unhappy about the prospect of sharing parents with a new sibling. Older children may be shocked or embarrassed by the pregnancy. Adolescents may find the fact that their parents are engaged in sexual activity disconcerting. If significant others believe the woman is too old to begin or continue bearing children, it can have a profound impact on how well the woman copes with pregnancy, childbirth, and the transition to parenthood (Mansfield & McCool, 1989).

Physical and Emotional Changes of Pregnancy. The older pregnant woman typically has a busy life-style by virtue of employment, community activities, or child care responsibilities if she is already a mother. Rubin's finding (1975) that women reduce their level of physical activity and increase the time spent at home near the end of gestation no longer holds true. Nearly 50% of women continue to work during pregnancy today, and 20% of these are employed until the expected date of delivery (Killien, 1990). If the woman over age 35 has been physically active or has made a large investment in her physical appearance for personal or professional reasons, she may find the physical changes of pregnancy disconcerting.

Adjusting to the emotional changes of pregnancy may also be more difficult for the older woman who is pregnant for the first time. Although women normally experience some anxiety during pregnancy, concerns about fetal well-being and significant changes in life-style that will occur with the birth of the newborn may enhance the level of worry. Anxiety often stems from awareness about the tremendous responsibilities inherent in parenting. Research indicates that older women are more aware of the implications of raising a child (Mercer & Ferketich, 1990). If the mature woman is a multigravida, she may have additional concerns about the reaction of siblings or the costs of raising another child.

Giving of Oneself. Rubin (1984) suggests that giving of oneself is the most complex task of pregnancy and childbirth. The older woman who has planned and prepared for pregnancy often begins the process of giving in the preconception period. Life-style and dietary habit changes are made to optimize the chances of creating a healthy fetus and neonate. Older couples often attend early pregnancy classes to enhance their knowledge of health-promoting behaviors.

At the same time, it may be difficult for the older woman

who has a successful career to alter the pace and intensity of work. Multigravid women may feel pulled between the needs of their children and the needs of the growing fetus. Age may complicate this picture by enhancing the normal sensations of fatigue that often accompany pregnancy. The woman over 35 who has delayed childbearing and the busy older multigravida must learn to balance the demands of work and the needs of the fetus. Additional research is needed to understand this process in the mature woman.

Adjusting to the Changing Couple Relationship. Couples who have been together for many years without children will have concerns about how parenthood will change their relationship. Few individuals are truly prepared for the reality, but older couples who have a well structured and organized life-style may have greater difficulty. They may have a hard time believing that "something so small can cause so many changes." Physical and emotional changes that occur during the gestational period may also precipitate changes in the couple's relationship. Pregnant women generally look to their partners for more physical and emotional support during pregnancy. This can lead to the development of anxiety in the older woman who is used to being self-reliant. The husband or partner may also feel discomfort or anxiety when the woman's dependency needs are heightened.

Once the neonate is born, significant disruptions in life-style caused by child care responsibilities, sleep deprivation, fatigue, and body changes can place great strain on the couple relationship. Men today are assuming more responsibility at home, especially when both parents are employed. However, their share of housework still tends to be less than half in most families (Fishbein, 1990). The need to negotiate changes in roles and housekeeping tasks may add to the strain on the couple's relationship. The desire for sexual intimacy often temporarily decreases in the woman after birth, further altering the previous patterns of interaction.

With the many changes that occur with the introduction of a newborn into any household, it is not surprising that two thirds of the women in Mercer's study (1986) reported a change in the couple relationship, including less spontaneous time together and less time to talk or pursue common interests. However, older women less often described problems in mate relations when they were compared with younger women. This may indicate a greater stability and flexibility in the older, more mature couple's relationship.

Postpartum Adjustment and Maternal Role Attainment

Both physical and emotional recovery from pregnancy and birth appear to be influenced by a woman's age (Tulman & Fawcett, 1990). In the landmark study of first-time motherhood by Mercer (1986), older women made slower physical recovery from childbirth and experienced more fatigue. A slower recovery is probably due in part to age as well as the increased incidence of intrapartum complications and the high cesarean birth rate (over 30%) in women over age 40.

First-time older women derive less gratification from the maternal role, expect more of themselves as mothers than do women in their twenties, and experience a significant decrease in self-concept 8 months after birth (Mercer, 1986; Meisenhelder & Meservey, 1987). It is suggested that this may reflect the exacting standards these high-achieving women set for themselves in the mothering role.

Even when the mature first-time mother is highly educated and has completed parenting courses, she may feel less competent in child care skills. This is not surprising. In Mercer's (1986) study, 26% of the women reported having absolutely no experience in caring for young infants. It is also suggested that more education results in higher self-expectations, diminished confidence, and a sense of uncertainty about infant care.

Less confidence in child care skills may be due in part to an absence of role models for the older woman. Many couples today are at great geographic distance from their families, often as a result of employment. The emotional support, practical advice, and teaching of skills that were provided by grandmothers in past generations may be unavailable to new mothers today. In some instances, pregnancy and parenthood occur so late in life (late forties or early fifties) that the maternal or paternal grandparents are no longer living. These factors have significant implications for maternity nurses involved in parent teaching and are discussed in the next section of this chapter.

By contrast, older multigravid women consistently report greater perceived competence in the mothering role (Pridham & Chang, 1992). Froman and Owen (1990) found that mature multiparous women in their study reported more confidence in performing infant care tasks. The greatest challenge for the new mother with other children is often how to meet the needs of all family members while continuing to work outside of the home at least part-time.

The first-time older woman's decreased confidence in infant care skills appears balanced by her perceived competence in meeting the emotional needs of the child. The older woman is usually less bothered by the infant's increased activity level, individuation, and striving for separation that occur during the normal phases of infant growth and development. This is due to her greater maturity, psychological integration, and wisdom that usually come with age and life experience.

Paternal Role Attainment in the Older First-Time Father

Some evidence indicates that men in their thirties may feel more secure in their identity and in the couple relationship, and these factors may aid the first-time father in achieving the paternal role. An older man may share the same insecurities as his partner and feel uncertain about his ability to meet the demands of parenthood. He may also be worried about the responsibilities of parenting a child when he is in his sixties or early seventies.

New fathers are still not as involved in infant care tasks as mothers, even though there have been significant changes in expectations about fathering behaviors (Rustia & Abbott, 1990). The older first-time father may be enthusiastic about a greater role in the child's life but still refrain from performing everyday infant care tasks. On the other hand, older men who have previously been married and took little interest in the care and nurturing of their children may be committed to an active role today. Financial security and the developmental maturity that comes with aging often prompt men who begin new families in midlife to seek a more involved role.

The psychosocial impact of later childbearing and parenthood is still not fully understood. Clearly older women and their partners experience emotional changes and face problems in psychological adaptation that are unique to advanced age when they choose to have children. Yet these have not been clearly identified. Even less research has been conducted to describe the positive aspects of later parenting. Conventional wisdom would indicate that the maturity, wisdom, patience, and personality integration that accompany aging would enhance the ability to successfully parent in our complex society. The generally higher education and socioeconomic status of many older parents may offer the child of older parents additional advantages. The maternity nurse has an excellent opportunity to study these psychological and social factors and support adaptations in all phases of the childbearing cycle—from preconception counseling through the early phases of parenting.

Implications for Nursing Care

The increase in first-time pregnancy and parenting for women after age 35 has created expanding areas of practice for the maternity nurse. New arenas for nursing practice include preconception counseling, infertility treatment, prenatal and parent education, and postnatal support groups for older first-time parents. When nurses provide care in traditional spheres of practice, they must individualize prenatal, intrapartum, and postpartum services to meet the needs of the older woman and her partner. This requires a sound knowledge of the physical and psychosocial factors unique to later childbearing and parenting.

• • Assessment

The nurse should identify special problems related to conception, such as infertility, previous pregnancy loss or termination, or contraceptive failure. Preexisting medical problems such as chronic hypertension and diabetes should be reviewed. The obstetric history of the older multiparous woman is covered in detail. Risk factors such as grand multiparity and previous pregnancy or childbirth complications such as preterm labor or postpartum hemorrhage or the birth of a neonate with genetic abnormalities are also covered.

The nurse may participate in the genetic screening process, which includes obtaining information about inherited disorders, previous pregnancy loss, and for the multiparous woman, the birth of other children with genetic problems. See Chapter 12 for a discussion of genetic testing and counseling.

The childbearing and parenting experience will depend on the woman's life situation and the reasons for the pregnancy. Before the nurse can begin planning appropriate care, whatever the setting for practice, a thorough psychosocial history should be obtained or reviewed. The woman's response to conception, pregnancy, and parenthood should be ascertained. The nurse must determine if this is a first or repeat pregnancy and whether this is a planned or unexpected event.

An ongoing assessment of the woman's emotional status is conducted. Changes in mood and affect are noted and reported. The nurse monitors for psychological responses common in older women and alerts the primary provider should the woman verbalize or demonstrate psychological disequilibrium or distress. Feelings about the normal alterations in body image, changes in role, or the couple relationship should be explored periodically throughout gestation and the postpartum period.

Advanced maternal age labels the woman as high risk and may heighten her level of anxiety. The degree of anxiety and its impact on psychological functioning should be assessed. Other sources of anxiety, such as worries about parenting at a later age or the ability to physically care for a newborn, should be identified. Concerns about the experience of pregnancy, childbirth, and parenting may be less pressing for a multiparous woman but are often replaced by issues surrounding the addition of a new sibling to the family unit, financial considerations, or the prospects of parenting later in life.

It is important to obtain information about the woman's social and cultural background including educational level, type of employment, and plans for work during and after pregnancy. The nurse should determine if the woman is married or partnered. The nurse should attempt to identify the nature and quality of the woman's social support network.

Depending on the setting, the nurse may also be responsible for an assessment of the woman's physiologic systems. Ongoing assessments focus on the identification of complications more commonly observed in women over 35 years of age. If the nurse is involved in preconception counseling, physical assessment often involves an appraisal of reproductive and sexual functioning, contraceptive use, and evaluation of the menstrual cycle. The reader is referred to Chapters 6 and 7 for a complete discussion of the nurse's role in preconception care.

The nurse also conducts an assessment to identify the unique learning needs of the older woman. Most first-time pregnant older women are well educated. They often come to the nurse with an extensive knowledge about conception, pregnancy, and parenthood. First-time pregnant women as well as the older multipara will still require anticipatory guidance and may have gaps in knowledge about specific aspects of childbearing or parenting, which must be identified during ongoing assessment of learning needs. Reviewing the woman's previous experience with child care is a critical aspect of the learning assessment. When the woman has had little or no opportunity to practice infant care skills, the nurse should determine if she has access to resources such as grandparents or friends.

• • Nursing Diagnosis

Nursing diagnoses are often related to the unique psychosocial aspects of childbearing after age 35 and include:

- Anxiety related to change in status, pregnancy, or threats to perceived biologic integrity
- Ineffective Individual Coping related to change in role
- Altered Family Processes related to change in family roles or gain in family member
- Health-Seeking Behavior related to role change or parenthood
- Knowledge Deficit related to lack of previous infant care experience
- Altered Parenting related to new child or lack of extended family
- Altered Role Performance related to new child
- Body Image Disturbance related to pregnancy

• • Planning and Implementation

Planning and implementation of nursing care for the woman after age 35 focus on the following areas:

- Monitoring maternal and fetal physiologic functioning
- Providing emotional support
- Teaching for effective self-care
- Providing accurate information
- Providing anticipatory guidance
- Initiating appropriate referrals

Specific interventions will be based on the specific area of nursing practice. A brief discussion of nursing actions appropriate to the practice setting is presented in the following section.

Preconception Counseling

Ideally, all women should seek preconception counseling, but it is particularly important for the older woman contemplating pregnancy. Once a woman begins preconception counseling, she should be screened for the more common health problems observed in older women such as chronic hypertension, renal disease, diabetes, and endometriosis. She should be apprised of the increasing risks of infertility and fetal genetic disorders with advancing age and how preexisting health problems may affect maternal and neonatal outcomes.

The nurse can begin to explore with the woman life-style and behaviors that positively or negatively influence fertility, pregnancy, and fetal growth and development. The nature of employment should be identified and risks associated with specific work discussed in detail. The role of substance use and abuse in reproductive functioning, conception, and fetal development should also be reviewed. For example, smoking after age 35 is associated with an increased incidence of preterm labor and low–birth-weight infants (Seidman, Ever-Hadani, & Gale, 1990). The nurse clarifies misconceptions and reinforces information provided by the primary health provider. If support groups are available for older couples contemplating parenthood, the woman and her partner can be encouraged to consider participation.

Prenatal Care

Once the pregnancy is confirmed, the nurse collaborates with the woman in plans for prenatal care and appropriate genetic testing. The nurse conducts ongoing physical assessments throughout the gestational period to identify early indicators of pregnancy complications. Because gestational diabetes is a more frequent occurrence in older women, repeat glucose screening may be indicated. Early referral for nutritional counseling and close monitoring of weight gain are also essential to reduce the risk of gestational diabetes. Prenatal fetal assessment (nonstress testing and biophysical profiles) will be initiated when preexisting maternal conditions complicate the pregnancy or problems arise during the gestational period. The nurse often schedules or performs these assessments.

The nurse's affect or emotional tone should be tempered by factors surrounding pregnancy for the older woman. If she is excited and happy about the pregnancy, the nurse should encourage and support these feelings. If an unplanned, repeat pregnancy has occurred after age 35, the nurse must recognize and accept that less positive feelings may be verbalized about the situation. Appropriate referrals should be initiated for counseling and social services as indicated by the woman's emotional status. Additionally, the multipara experiencing a repeat pregnancy who lives in poverty will often require financial assistance and nutritional supplements. The nurse is often responsible for identifying these needs and initiating referrals.

When the pregnancy is unplanned, an empathic and sensitive approach is essential and may encourage the woman to continue prenatal care and to share her concerns and needs with the nurse. Inquiries should be made early regarding the woman's desire for conception control or sterilization after the birth. Grand multiparity and advanced age both place the woman in a high-risk category. This may enhance the woman's level of anxiety even when no specific complications are identified. The nurse must monitor the woman's level of anxiety and initiate appropriate referrals if ineffective coping is identified.

A teaching plan is implemented at the first prenatal visit. Review of health-promoting behaviors that will support early fetal growth and development should be geared to the woman's level of education, previous life experiences, and current knowledge. An important aspect of anticipatory guidance includes a discussion of the minor discomforts of pregnancy and how they are influenced by advancing age. As the pregnancy progresses, the nurse discusses signs and symptoms of preterm labor and PIH with the woman because they are common complications in later childbearing.

The first-time older pregnant woman is usually interested in learning as much as possible about all aspects of childbearing and parenting. Older multiparous women experiencing repeat pregnancy may also desire "refresher" courses about pregnancy, labor, and birth. It should not be assumed that because they are experienced parents, they have all the necessary knowledge.

Psychological changes of pregnancy are addressed throughout the prenatal period. The nurse can play a crucial role in preparing the older woman and her partner for childrearing. In-depth discussion of concerns regarding childbearing and parenting after age 35 are often best accomplished in support groups especially formulated for these first-time parents. Nurses may moderate these groups and guide participants in an exploration of concerns common to older couples (Fig. 10-2).

Intrapartum Care

The first-time older woman often approaches the childbirth experience with high expectations and plans for close collaboration in the birth process. Unfortunately, the higher incidence of labor dystocia and the need for cesarean delivery may result in active management of labor and the need for obstetric interventions, which interfere with these plans. The nurse caring for the older primigravida must monitor her closely for evidence of intrapartum complications, yet remain sensitive to her need for some degree of control and participation in the neonate's birth.

The nurse is often responsible for assessing the progress of labor and documenting findings on the labor graph. The primary health provider should be notified in a timely manner if signs of arrested labor or failure in fetal descent occur. If the older woman presents with signs of vaginal bleeding (placenta previa appears more commonly in some groups of older women) or PIH, the nurse initiates emergency supportive measures until the primary provider arrives. Because the older woman is often well educated and desires as much information as possible about her condition, the nurse should update her about her current status as time permits. Observing principles of family-centered maternity nursing will convey respect and recognition of the woman's birth plan.

The nurse caring for a multiparous woman over age 35 must monitor for additional complications related to her previous childbearing experience. Of particular significance is a prior history of labor dystocia, fetal distress, or postpartum hemorrhage. Although second and subsequent labors are often shorter in duration, if the interval between pregnancies has been prolonged (greater than 8 to 10 years), the labor often resembles the first birth in its duration. The woman may become anxious if the process of labor takes longer than anticipated.

Research indicates that with optimum prenatal care, the healthy older woman can also expect her newborn to be healthy if genetic abnormalities have been ruled out. Because women over 35 are considered high risk, the fetus is monitored more frequently during labor. If maternal complications such as diabetes or PIH have developed during pregnancy, the neonate will be assessed during the postpartum period for evidence of compromise. This may require admission to an observation or special care nursery. The maternity nurse can act as a liaison between the maternal and newborn units until the mother is well enough to visit the neonate. If the woman's partner is available, the nurse should encourage his participation in newborn care until the new mother is able to assume a more active role.

Postpartum Care

The older postpartum woman may require a longer period for physical recovery. If intrapartum problems or a cesarean delivery have complicated the birth, the woman may experience even greater fatigue and physiologic disequilibrium. Ongoing assessment of physiologic status and the level of pain and fatigue is an essential component of nursing care.

The nurse must also assess the perceived quality of the birth experience. Mercer (1986) found that the older woman was more likely to verbalize disappointment in the quality of the experience. This could be due in part to the increased incidence of complications during childbirth, the higher rate of cesarean delivery, and the greater need for control common in older women. The nurse should encourage the woman to verbalize her feelings about the birth to promote psychological adaptation in the postpartum period.

Support of maternal and paternal role attainment requires recognition of the older parent's special needs. If the woman has had little or no experience in the care of newborns, intensive support and teaching are usually required. Interventions are initially aimed at fostering confidence in

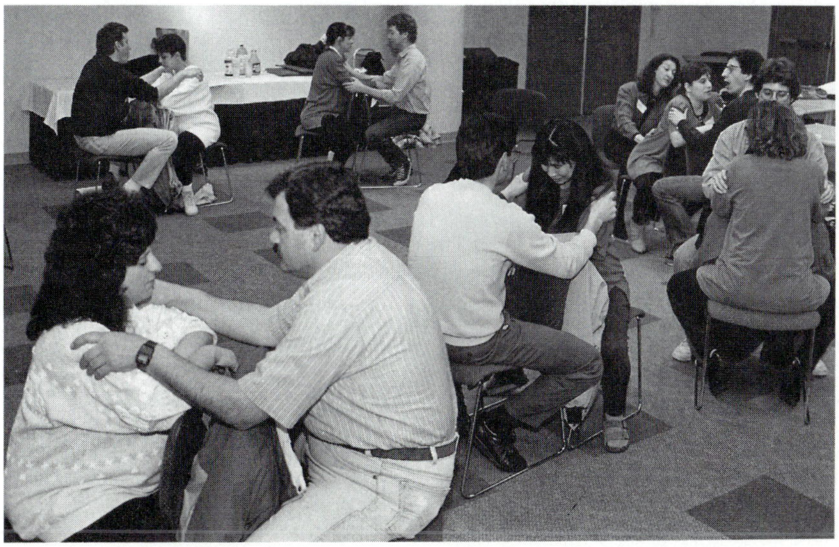

Figure 10-2.
Childbirth classes for first-time parents over age 35 may help the older couple feel more comfortable. (Photo by Kathy Sloane. Courtesy of Alta Bates Medical Center.)

basic skills, including holding, feeding, diaper changing, and safe positioning of the neonate. The partner's expectations and desires regarding infant care should be identified, and he should be included in the teaching. The woman and her partner should also be encouraged to attend child care classes offered in the unit or view videotapes provided for new parents.

In contrast, the multiparous woman may desire a more gradual assumption of infant care activities. Because she has other children, her need to learn infant care skills may be a lower priority (Pridham, Lytton, Chang, & Rutledge, 1991). If the older multipara has primary responsibility for the neonate as well as other children, she may desire time for rest and recuperation before she is discharged from the hospital or birthing unit. It is important for the nurse to identify the woman's wishes in this matter.

Because early discharge is common, ongoing support of parenting skills requires discharge referrals to home health or community nursing agencies in many instances. The nurse should discuss the older woman's desires for follow-up nursing assessment, care, and teaching. This is essential because research indicates that older women take longer to move from the "taking-in" to the "taking-hold" phases identified by Rubin (Ament, 1990) and may not be optimally ready for learning before discharge. The woman should be given information about parenting support groups. Many facilities now offer courses for first-time older parents so that their special concerns and needs can be addressed. The well-educated, career-oriented older primipara may prefer a group setting for the discussion of feelings and exchange of ideas and information (Hampson, 1989).

Discharge teaching covers the same areas of self-care and infant care described in detail in Chapter 29. The nurse should discuss how advanced age may affect the process of recovery in the immediate postpartum period. If preexisting diseases such as chronic hypertension or diabetes exist, the nurse ascertains that appropriate referrals have been made for follow-up medical care.

Postdischarge Care

The most difficult time for the older first-time mother may be after discharge from the hospital. If she is assuming primary responsibility for newborn care and has little or no experience, this can be a most stressful period. Many of these women may lack family support or role models and will require the services of professional nurses to make the adaptation to parenthood. Nurses have developed community-based interventions to assist the older primipara (Tiedje & Collins, 1989). The programs offer a wide range of services including health assessments, education, support groups, housekeeping, and newborn care.

A major focus of support often involves preparation for returning to work. Specific information about selecting appropriate infant day care, continuing breastfeeding while employed, and normal psychological reactions to leaving the infant is provided. The impact of maternal employment on infant growth and development is covered. The research does indicate that employment in itself is not deleterious to the infant's well-being. Critical factors include the woman's desire to work, her satisfaction with her job, and the quality of infant day care.

Many older first-time mothers have been described as high achievers with a past history of success in all areas of life. They may find less gratification in the mothering role than younger women. The community or home health nurse can assist the older woman who has feelings of inadequacy or low self-esteem when she is unable to organize every aspect of her life. Reinforcing the woman's strengths in the new role and praising her accomplishment of neonatal care skills is an important component of this support.

A recent study indicates that women who exhibit the type A behavior pattern, characterized by a competitive, hard-driving work style, may give birth to neonates who have "difficult" temperaments (Parker & Barrett, 1992). The investigators found that women with type A patterns had newborns who cried more often during neurobehavioral assessments in the immediate postbirth period and were rated as more intense and less predictable at 3 months of age. The nurse can play an important role in helping women of less adaptable newborns to cope with their special needs. The woman can be guided to recognize the newborn's cues and to respond appropriately to them. As the new mother achieves greater competence in "reading" the neonate's nonverbal cues, her self-confidence and sense of competence will increase. Research indicates that nursing support until 8 to 12 months after birth can be extremely helpful in facilitating maternal role adaptation (Mercer, 1986).

• • Evaluation

The final phase of the nursing process involves evaluation of the mature woman's responses to nursing care. If successful adaptations have occurred, the woman will conceive and progress through the gestational period. Complications common in older women will be minimized or prevented. The nurse also must evaluate the quality of emotional support and the adequacy of the teaching plan designed to prepare first-time older women for parenthood. When effective strategies have been implemented, the woman and her partner will verbalize satisfaction with the quality of emotional support and information provided by the nurse.

Evaluation continues through discharge from the hospital into the community. With proper nursing guidance, the woman who is an older, first-time parent will demonstrate beginning skill in infant care and will verbalize comfort with the transition to the maternal role. If the woman is a multipara, she will verbalize satisfaction with her decision to bear and parent another child. There will be evidence that the newborn is being successfully integrated into the existing family unit and that the woman and her partner are satisfactorily adjusting to their changing life-style and relationship.

Chapter Summary

Most first-time mothers over the age of 35 are intelligent, well-educated, and successful professionals who approach childbearing and parenting with the highest expectations.

They desire and plan to participate fully in every phase of the pregnancy and to exert control over the experience of labor and birth. The process of parenting is often viewed as a new challenge in an already successful life. They rely on health care providers, especially nurses, to provide information, support, and anticipatory guidance to achieve their goals.

Advanced age, however, brings the possibility of increased physiologic risk for the woman and fetus. The dramatic psychological changes of pregnancy may strain previous coping mechanisms. The childbirth experience may fail to meet expectations. Furthermore, pregnancy and parenting will alter the woman's life-style and, if she is partnered, can disrupt the couple relationship. These factors may not be fully appreciated before conception and may result in significant emotional disequilibrium. Skillful nursing interventions are required to help the older woman and her partner make satisfactory adaptations in all phases of the childbearing cycle.

The multiparous woman over age 35 presents a different set of challenges for the maternity nurse. Although physiologic risk may be increased by a combination of age and parity, psychological adaptation is often much smoother if the pregnancy is desired. Previous childbearing experiences eliminate some of the unknown factors that may cause nulliparous women anxiety. Issues related to first-time parenting are often replaced by concerns about family reintegration and how the newborn will be accepted by siblings.

Because most women with children are employed at least part-time, the older multipara may feel overwhelmed by the demands of work, homemaking, and child care as never before. The nurse can provide guidance regarding time management and describe health-promoting behaviors that reduce fatigue. The greatest challenge for nurses may be nursing care of the older multiparous woman whose unplanned conception is complicated by poverty. Physical, emotional, social, and economic problems may require intensive support throughout the gestational period. Nurses at all levels of practice continue to provide leadership in the development of programs to meet the needs of this special group of women. The greatest probability for improving maternal and neonatal outcomes appears to lie in the realm of political activism. Until all women, particularly the very young and those over age 35, have equal access to reproductive and prenatal health services, these women and their infants will remain at risk for significant morbidity and mortality. All women over age 35 deserve access to quality nursing and health care.

Study Questions

1. *What is the purpose of preconception counseling for the woman over age 35? What is the role of the nurse in this process?*
2. *Why is it important for women over age 35 to receive genetic counseling?*
3. *Why are complications more common during pregnancy for the older woman? What factors increase the risk of pregnancy complications for the woman over age 35?*
4. *What are the essential components of a teaching plan for the older first-time pregnant woman?*
5. *What factors must the nurse consider when caring for the multiparous woman over age 35 who is experiencing an unplanned pregnancy?*
6. *Why is the older first-time mother more likely to verbalize disappointment with her birth experience? How can the nurse optimize the birth experience for the older primigravida when complications arise during labor?*
7. *What strategies can the nurse use to support maternal role attainment for the older first-time mother?*
8. *How do the needs of the older multipara differ from the first-time mother over age 35 in the immediate postpartum period?*
9. *What are the important aspects of care when the nurse provides home health or community health services for the older first-time mother?*

References

Ament, L. (1990). Maternal tasks of the puerperium reidentified. *Journal of Obstetric, Gynecologic, and Neonatal Nursing, 19*(4), 330.

Arnold, L., & Brecht, M. (1990). Legislative issues affecting parenting: An overview of current policies. *Journal of Perinatal and Neonatal Nursing, 4*(2), 24.

Barkan, S., & Bracken, M. (1987). Delayed childbearing: No evidence for increased risk of low birth weight and preterm delivery. *American Journal of Epidemiology, 125*(1), 101.

Barnes, L. (1991). Pregnancy over 35: Special needs. *American Journal of Maternal Child Nursing, 16*(5), 272.

Berkowitz, G., Skovron, M., Lapinski, R., & Berkowitz, R. (1990). Delayed childbearing and the outcome of pregnancy. *New England Journal of Medicine, 322*(10), 659.

Chen, R., & Morgan, S. (1991). Recent trends in the timing of first births in the United States. *Demography, 28*(4), 513.

Cunningham, F., & Leveno, K. (1990). Maternal age and outcome of pregnancy. (Letter to the editor.) *New England Journal of Medicine, 323* (6), 414–415.

Cunningham, F., MacDonald, P., & Gant, N. (1989). *Williams Obstetrics* (18th ed.). Norwalk, CT: Appleton & Lange.

DeWit, M., & Rajulton, F. (1992). Education and timing of parenthood among Canadian women: A cohort analysis. *Social Biology, 39*(1–2), 109.

Dicker, D., Goldman, J., Ashkenazi, J.,(1991). Age and pregnancy rates in in vitro fertilization. *Journal of In Vitro Fertilization and Embryo Transfer, 8*(3), 141.

Farrell, C. (1989). Genetic counseling: The emerging reality. *Journal of Perinatal and Neonatal Nursing, 2*(4), 21.

Fishbein, E. (1990). Predicting paternal involvement with a newborn by attitude toward women's roles. *Health Care for Women International, 11*, 109.

Fonteyn, V., & Isada, N. (1988). Nongenetic implications of childbearing after age 35. *Obstetrical and Gynecological Survey, 43*, 709.

Froman, R., & Owen, S. (1990). Mothers' and nurses' perceptions of infant care skills. *Research in Nursing and Health, 13*, 247.

Gordon, D., Milberg, J., Daling, J., . (1991). Advanced maternal age as a risk factor for cesarean delivery. *Obstetrics and Gynecology, 77*, 493.

Grace, J. (1989). Development of maternal-fetal attachment during pregnancy. *Nursing Research, 38*(4), 229.

Green, J., Coupland, V., & Kitzinger, J. (1990). Expectations, experiences, and psychological outcomes of childbirth. *Birth, 17*(1), 15–24.

Haines, C., Rogers, M., & Leung, H. (1991). Neonatal outcome and its relationship with maternal age. *Australian New Zealand Journal of Obstetrics and Gynaecology, 31*(3), 209.

Hampson, S. (1989). Nursing interventions for the first three postpartum months. *Journal of Obstetric, Gynecologic, and Neonatal Nursing, 18*(2), 116.

Harker, L., & Thorpe, K. (1992). "The last egg in the basket?" Elderly primiparity—a review of findings. *Birth, 19*(1), 23.

Hees-Stauthamer, J. (1985). *The first pregnancy*. Ann Arbor: University of Michigan Press.

Hollander, D., & Breene, J. Pregnancy in the older gravida: How old is old? *Obstetrical and Gynecological Survey, 45*, 106.

Jahoda, M., Pijpers, L., Vosters, R., et al. (1987). Role of maternal age in assessment of risk of abortion. *British Medical Journal, 295*, 1237–1238.

Jones, E., & Forrest, J. (1989). Contraceptive failure in the United States. *Family Planning Perspectives, 21*(3), 103.

Killien, M. (1990). Working during pregnancy: Psychological stressor or asset? *NAACOG Clinical Issues in Perinatal and Woman's Health Issues, 1*(1), 6–13.

Mansfield, P., & McCool, W. (1989). Toward a better understanding of the "advanced maternal age" factor. *Health Care for Women International, 10*, 395.

Meisenhelder, J., & Meservey, P. (1987). Childbearing over thirty. *Western Journal of Nursing Research, 9*(4), 527.

Mercer, R. (1986). *First-time motherhood*. New York: Springer.

Mercer, R., & Ferketich, S. (1990). Predictors of parental attachment during early parenthood. *Journal of Advanced Nursing, 15*, 268.

Morgan, C., & Elias, S. Prenatal diagnosis of genetic disorders. *Journal of Perinatal and Neonatal Nursing, 2*(4), 1.

O'Brien, M., & Gilson, G. (1987). Detection and management of gestational diabetes in an out-of-hospital birth center. *Journal of Nurse-Midwifery, 32*(2), 79.

Overbeek, T., Hop, W., Ouden, M. (1990). Spontaneous abortion rate and advanced maternal age: Consequences for prenatal diagnosis. *Lancet, 336*, July 7, 27.

Parker, S., & Barrett, D. (1992). Maternal type A behavior during pregnancy, neonatal crying, and early infant temperament: Do type A women have type A babies? *Pediatrics, 89*(3), 474.

Pridham, K., & Chang, A. (1991). Transition to being the mother of a new infant in the first 3 months: Maternal problem solving and self-appraisals. *Journal of Advanced Nursing, 17*, 204.

Pridham, K., Lytton, D., Chang, A., & Rutledge, D. (1991). Early postpartum transition: Progress in maternal identity and role attainment. *Research in Nursing and Health, 14*, 21.

Rubin, R. (1984). *Maternal identity and the maternal experience*. New York: Springer.

Rubin, R. (1975). Maternal tasks in pregnancy. *American Journal of Maternal-Child Nursing, 5*(3), 36–39.

Rustia, J., & Abbott, D. (1990). Predicting paternal role enactment. *Western Journal of Nursing Research, 12*(2), 145.

Seidman, D., Ever-Hadani, P., & Gale, R. (1990). Effect of maternal smoking and age on congenital anomalies. *Obstetrics and Gynecology, 76*, 1046.

Shortridge, L. (1990). Advances in the assessment of the effect of environmental and occupational toxins on reproduction. *Journal of Perinatal and Neonatal Nursing, 3*(4), 1.

Tiedje, L., & Collins, C. (1989). Combining employment and motherhood. *American Journal of Maternal Child Nursing, 14*(1), 9.

Tulman, L., & Fawcett, J. (1990). Functional status during pregnancy and the postpartum: A framework for research. *Image, 22*(3), 191.

Ventura, S. (1992). Advance report of new data from the 1989 birth certificate. *Monthly Vital Statistics Report, 40*(S). Washington DC: US Department of Health and Human Services.

Ventura, S. (1991). Advance report of final natality statistics, 1989. *Monthly Vital Statistics Report, 40*(8)(S). Washington, DC: US Department of Health and Human Services.

Ventura, S. (1989). First births to older mothers, 1970–1986. *American Journal of Public Health, 79*(12), 1675–1677.

Wen, S., Goldberg, R., Cutter, G., . (1990). Smoking, maternal age, fetal growth, and gestational age at delivery. *American Journal of Obstetrics and Gynecology, 162*, 53.

Winslow, W. (1987). First pregnancy after 35: What is the experience? *American Journal of Maternal Child Nursing, 12*(2), 92.

Woods, N. F. (1987). Women's lives: Pressures and pleasure, conflict and support. *Health Care for Women International, 18*(2–3), 109.

Suggested Readings

Baird, P., Sadovnic, A., & Yee, I. (1991). Maternal age and birth defects: A population study. *Lancet, 337*, March 2, 527.

Blossfeld, H., & Huinink, J. (1991). Human capital investments or norms of role transition? How women's schooling and career affect the process of family formation. *American Journal of Sociology, 1*, July, 143.

Cnattingius, S., Forman, M., Berendes, H., & Isotalo, L. (1992). Delayed childbearing and risk of adverse perinatal outcome. *Journal of the American Medical Association, 268*(7), 886.

Leyland, A., & Boddy, F. (1990). Maternal age and outcome of pregnancy. *New England Journal of Medicine, 323*(6), 413.

Monahan, P., & DeJoseph, J. (1991). The woman with preterm labor at home: A descriptive analysis. *Journal of Perinatal and Neonatal Nursing, 4*(4), 12.

Ramer, L. (1990). Pregnancy: Psychosocial perspectives. *Prenatal care*, series 2, module 4. White Plains, NY: March of Dimes.

Ventura, S. (1989). First births to older mothers. *American Journal of Public Health, 79*(12), 1675.

Yasin, S., & Beydoun, S. (1988). Pregnancy outcome at greater than 20 weeks in women in their 40s. A case-control study. *Journal of Reproductive Medicine, 3*(1), 209.

CHAPTER 11

Physiologic Adaptations in Pregnancy

Learning Objectives

After studying the material in this chapter, the student will be able to:

- Describe the major physiologic adaptations that occur during pregnancy and recognize their causes.
- Describe the altered physiology of pregnancy to the woman as appropriate.
- Demonstrate an understanding of physiologic adaptations and their effects on the pregnant woman.
- Discuss the normal adaptation of the reproductive organs in pregnancy.
- Identify changes in the endocrine function during pregnancy.
- Explain the actions of the steroid hormones progesterone and estrogen in pregnancy.

Key Terms

collagenous	hyperventilation
diaphoretic	hypervolemia
essential hypertension	interstitial
glomerular filtration rate	ketones
glucocorticoids	metabolite
glucogenesis	neurohumoral substances
homeostasis	nocturia
hygroscopic	precursor
hyperemic	shunt
hyperplasia	sinusoids
hypertrophy	syncytiotrophoblasts

The period from conception to delivery is approximately 40 weeks long. During these weeks the woman's body undergoes complex physiologic changes of such magnitude that many are still not well understood. The fetus grows rapidly and develops into a recognizable human being. This process continues to be one of nature's wonders. The woman, whose body nourishes and sustains the new life, experiences nearly total immersion in its growth and well-being. The growth of the uterus, which makes the woman's pregnancy obvious, is only one of the many transformations that occur during pregnancy. Every system in the woman's body adapts to the demands of the growing fetus. These changes are so dramatic that they would be considered pathologic in the nonpregnant woman. They are the body's adaptive response to the growing fetus' requirements for nutrients, removal of wastes, protection from harm, and space in which to grow.

This chapter discusses the changes produced by pregnancy in the structure and function of the various systems and organs of the body. Because of the dynamic endocrinologic influences that orchestrate these changes, significant hormonal functions are included as each system is addressed. Teaching, counseling, assessment, and patient care of women experiencing symptoms of pregnancy are covered in Chapters 13 through 15.

Adaptations of Body Systems

Adaptation of the Reproductive System

Changes in body systems are most apparent in the reproductive organs (Table 11-1).

Uterus

The uterus is designed for childbearing, and the changes that occur in its structure, position, and function support the all-important physiologic process of replication of human life.

Table 11-1. Summary of Reproductive Tract Adaptations in Pregnancy

Physiologic Changes	Clinical Significance
Uterine Endometrium	
Endometrium, or the uterine lining, proliferates in preparation for ovum implantation.	Estrogen stimulates this process, and when inadequate, the uterine lining is not primed for implantation and early abortion may result.
Glycogen is stored within the endometrium to nourish the blastocyst if conception occurs.	Implantation occurs when levels of estrogen and progesterone are adequate to maintain the endometrium.
Ovaries	
The ovaries are responsible for the formation of the corpus luteum.	Implantation of the blastocyst and development of the placenta is secured by the progesterone secretion. Human chorionic gonadotropin (HCG), by the eighth gestational day, has begun to provide nutrition and hormones to sustain the corpus luteum for 7–10 weeks until the placenta attains full function. HCG may remain in postpartum circulation for 3 days.
Fallopian Tubes	
The fallopian tubes facilitate fertilization of the ovum by the sperm.	With stimulation from estrogen and progesterone, fluid in the oviduct conveys signals that condition the events of sperm capacitation and cleavage in the gametes.
They control timing of egg transport into the uterus.	They provide adequate preparation of the endometrium for implantation of the egg.
Uterine Cervix	
There is increased vascularity, edema, softness, and hypertrophy of the cervical glands.	Estrogen is responsible for cervical changes, and these signs are known as Chadwick's or Goodell's signs. A mucus plug forms in the cervical canal that becomes a barrier to protect the fetus from mechanical or bacterial invasion. In early labor this plug separates and as blood vessels are severed, is expelled as "bloody show."
Breasts	
The breasts increase in size, nodularity, and sensitivity.	Under the stimulation of estrogen and progesterone, the breasts enlarge in size, the nipples enlarge and become dark and erect, and the gland of Montgomery enlarges.
The breast ductal system has intense growth during the first 3 months of pregnancy.	The breasts prepare for lactation.
As pregnancy progresses, the alveolar cells become secretory.	Production of colostrum occurs late in pregnancy, and the breasts continue to enlarge.
Vagina	
The vagina becomes congested and vascularized.	Under the influence of estrogen there is proliferation of vaginal cells that causes the vaginal walls to become thickened, pliable, and distensible in preparation for the passage of the fetal head.
There are increased secretions that are white, thickened, and acidic.	Acidity of the vagina is maintained by lactic acid produced by lactobacilli that favor sperm survival. Acidity also controls growth of pathogens in the vagina (pH 3.5–5.0).
Uterine Growth	
Uterine weight increases from 70 g to 900–1200 g at term.	Estrogen and progesterone stimulate uterine growth and compliance. Progesterone prepares implantation site and inhibits myometrial contractility.
Uterine volume increases from 10 mL to 2–10 L at term (1000 times increase in size).	Uterus becomes palpable: 3 months at symphysis 5 months at umbilicus 9 months at xyphoid process.
Uterus rises into the pelvis at 12 weeks and dextrorotates to the right as it enlarges.	Fetal movement is observed. Uterine growth causes pressure on the right ureter. Weight of the third-trimester uterus on the vena cava and aorta may cause supine hypotensive syndrome.

(*continued*)

Table 11-1. Summary of Reproductive Tract Adaptations in Pregnancy ***(Continued)***

Physiologic Changes	**Clinical Significance**
Uterine Growth (continued)	
Uterus maintains longitudinal position in line with the pelvic axis.	Palpation of fetal growth occurs. Loss of center of gravity occurs as uterus enlarges.
Anterior support is provided by the abdominal wall.	Diastasis recti may occur.
Uterus is less sensitive to contractility until midpregnancy when it becomes more sensitive due to oxytocin stimulation.	Oxytocin causes the myometrium to contract. Contractions early in pregnancy may cause abortion. Preterm birth may be a risk when contractions occur in the second or early third trimester.
In the latter half of gestation the uterus is more susceptible to contractions.	Contractions initiate labor at term. Contractions cause ripening, dilatation, and effacement of the cervix at term.
Braxton Hicks contractions are irregular, sporadic, and nonrhythmic contractions that continue throughout pregnancy.	Estrogen causes stretching and distention of the myometrium. The pregnant woman feels a sensation of painless uterine tightening and pressure. Contractions can be palpated by the examiner. Contractions may be mistaken for labor in the third trimester

Growth

The expansion of the uterus is essential to accommodate the growing products of conception. To achieve this goal, the uterine muscle (myometrium) grows spectacularly and becomes more compliant, and its spiraling muscle bundles uncoil. Its weight increases 20-fold, from 56.7 g (2 oz) in the nonpregnant state to 900 to 1200 g (2 lb) at term. The volume of its cavity increases from 10 mL to 2 to 10 L at term, representing a 1000-fold increase (Fig. 11-1).

Growth of the uterus in the first trimester is more rapid than that of the embryo. Growth of the myometrium is due partly to hyperplasia in early pregnancy but is more directly related to hypertrophy of the existing muscle cells (myofibrils). In conjunction with muscle growth, fibrous tissue accumulates into the outer muscle layer of the uterus, and the amount of elastic tissue increases. These events substantially increase the strength of the uterine wall.

The proportion and density of the myofibrils are highest in the corpus and least in the isthmus; this arrangement is an adaptation for uterine function during normal labor. During labor, contractile forces are strongest in the corpus and are known as *fundal dominance*, whereas contractions in the miduterus are much less forceful. Uterine contractions begin to occur in early pregnancy and continue until delivery. These contractions are painless and usually occur every 5 to 10 minutes but may go unnoticed. These are known as *Braxton Hicks contractions*, named for the obstetrician who described them. These contractions are nonrhythmic, irregular, sporadic, and begin about the sixth week of gestation.

Braxton Hicks contractions are thought to arise from the stretching of the uterine muscle as it grows, and the woman may comment on the sensation of painless uterine tightening and pressure. In late pregnancy uterine contractions also can be felt by the examiner during abdominal palpation. Many women mistake strong Braxton Hicks contractions for true labor. When no cervical dilatation results from these contractions and the pregnancy is full term, the woman is asked to walk or exercise; the disappearance of these contractions is a sign that true labor has not yet begun.

Muscle fibers pull toward the top of the uterus and exert an upward and outward traction on the horizontal and circular muscle bundles of the lower segment during labor. At this time total uterine length decreases, the upper uterine segment thickens, and the lower segment becomes thinned. Late in pregnancy, the uterine wall begins to thin and soften, becoming saclike and pliable. The movement of the fetus can be observed and its body palpated for position and size.

Hormonal stimulus to the growth and compliance of the pregnant uterus results from the release of estrogen and progesterone initially supplied by the corpus luteum and later by the placenta. Estrogen affects myometrial growth through the synthesis of proteins that build contractile muscle. Progesterone is necessary for the preparation of the endometrium for ovum implantation in early pregnancy. Later in pregnancy it renders the smooth muscle quiescent by inhibiting the contractile activity of the myometrium, thereby maintaining the pregnancy.

Oxytocin is a pituitary hormone that stimulates uterine

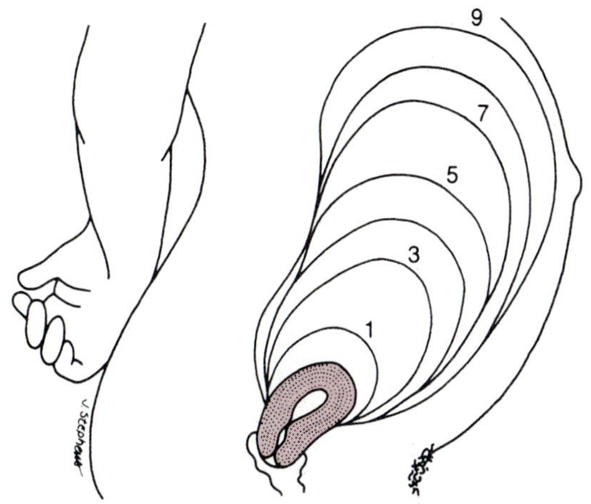

Figure 11-1.
Uterine growth during successive months of pregnancy (Childbirth Graphics).

muscle to contract. Until midpregnancy the uterus is relatively insensitive to the effect of oxytocin, but during the latter half of pregnancy, in preparation for labor and delivery, the uterus becomes increasingly susceptible to contractions. Intravenous administration of exogenous oxytocin will effectively induce labor only in late pregnancy when cervical ripeness has occurred. For the greatest effectiveness, the intravenous dose given to initiate or accelerate labor must be titrated for each woman individually.

Position

As the uterus grows, its shape and position changes. Early in pregnancy it maintains its pear shape, but it becomes more globular (spherical) by 3 months. As the pregnancy continues, the uterus continues to grow, becoming more ovoid. By 12 weeks of pregnancy the uterus has risen into the pelvis, and the uterine fundus can be palpated just above the symphysis pubis.

Early in pregnancy the uterus is more anteflexed (tipped toward the front of the body) than it is in the nonpregnant state. As pregnancy continues, the uterus lifts from the pelvis and becomes dextrorotated, or turned to the right, as a result of pressure from the rectosigmoid located in the posterior pelvis.

As the uterus increases in size, it comes in contact with the abdominal wall and displaces the intestine laterally and superiorly (sideways and up). It maintains a longitudinal position in line with the pelvic axis, as shown in Figure 11-2, and the abdominal wall supports it anteriorly.

In late pregnancy when the pregnant woman lies on her back, the uterus rests posteriorly on the vertebral column, the vena cava, and the aorta. These major blood vessels become compressed between the uterus and the vertebral column, decreasing the blood flow to the brain and uterus. *Supine hypotensive syndrome* (sometimes called vena cava syndrome) may occur, and the woman becomes faint and diaphoretic (see section on cardiac output in this chapter).

Endometrium

The endometrium, or lining of the uterine cavity, is the primary target organ of the estrogen produced by the ovarian follicle and the progesterone produced by the corpus luteum. During the normal follicular phase of the menstrual cycle, estrogen acts on the tissue and glands of the endometrium, producing a typical proliferative pattern. After ovulation, in anticipation of conception, progesterone from the corpus luteum stimulates two important changes in the endometrium. First, glycogen is stored for the nourishment of a blastocyst. Second, endometrial microvilli are modified to ensure contact between the blastocyst and the sustaining endometrial lining. By day 22 of the menstrual cycle, preparation of the endometrial site for implantation of the blastocyst is complete. When progesterone stimulation of the endometrium is insufficient for receiving the blastocyst, either implantation will not occur or an early first-trimester spontaneous abortion will result. Progesterone output that consistently remains low, a condition known as an inadequate luteal phase disorder, is a common cause of infertility and early repeated spontaneous abortion.

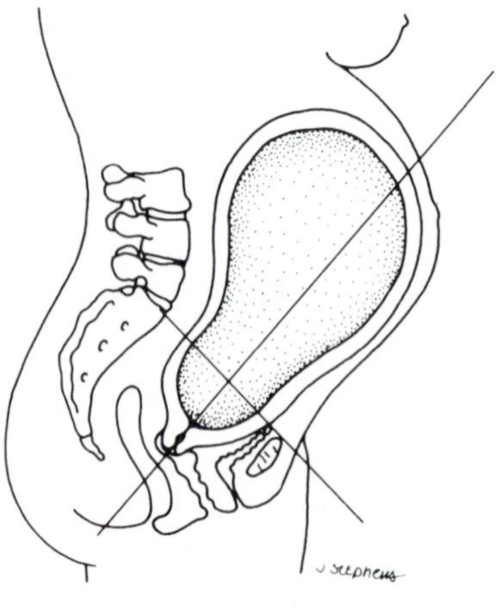

Figure 11-2.
Relationship of the axis of the pregnant uterus to the pelvic axis, showing anterior support of the uterus by the abdominal wall (Childbirth Graphics).

Cervix

During pregnancy the cervix has a dual role. It functions to retain the uterine contents during the prenatal period and then softens, dilates, and effaces to permit eventual delivery. The cervix is structurally quite different from the main body of the uterus. It consists primarily of collagenous tissue. The collagenous tissue is responsible for the rigidity of the cervix and controls the extent to which it will dilate.

Some of the earliest signs of pregnancy are changes in the cervix. As early as 1 month after conception, estrogen stimulation has increased its vascularity, causing it to have a bluish cast known as *Chadwick's sign*. Edema from the increased blood flow gives the cervix its bluish cast and its palpable softness (known as *Goodell's sign*) that are presumptive signs of early pregnancy.

Hypertrophy of the cervical glands occurs to such an extent that they fill approximately one half of the cervical structure and exude enough thick mucus to block the cervical canal. This barrier protects the fetus against mechanical or bacterial invasion from the outside. Called the "mucus plug," it is expelled from the cervix in early labor. As the mucus plug separates from the cervical canal, capillaries are severed and traces of blood are mixed with the mucus, giving it a pinkish color. This "bloody show" is an early sign of labor and is normal.

Fallopian Tubes and Fertilization

When ovulation is complete, the ovum surrounded by the *corona radiata* is expelled directly into the peritoneal cavity. To become fertilized it must find its way into one of the fallopian tubes. Passage into the tube is assisted by the fimbriated ends of the tube around the ovaries. Cilia lining the tubes beat toward the tube opening, assisting passage of the ovum into its lumen.

After ejaculation, sperm are transported through the vagina, cervix, and into the uterus where they are transported to the ovarian end of the fallopian tube. If conception occurs, it usually occurs shortly after entrance of the sperm into the fallopian tube. This achievement only takes 5 to 10 minutes and may be aided by the contractions of the uterus and fallopian tubes initiated by the female orgasm. Approximately one-half million sperm are ejaculated; only 1000 to 3000 successfully reach the ovum.

Meeting of ovum and sperm within the fallopian tube is essential for fertilization. This event is orchestrated in the tube by muscular contractions, the ciliary movements that transport the ovum, and the composition of the ductal fluid. The function of the oviductal fluid is to convey biochemical signals that contribute to sperm capacitation and cleavage in the gametes. The tube temporarily halts the movement of the sperm and ovum while penetration of the egg takes place.

The sperm must open a pathway to the ovum through the many layers of its corona radiata. It is unusual for more than one sperm to enter the ovum. This is because the lattice-type structure of the corona radiata becomes defused and impermeable to other sperm once penetrated by a single sperm.

When fertilization is achieved, the ovum contains 23 male chromosomes and 23 female chromosomes, forming a complete complement of 46 chromosomes. The ovum contains 23 pairs of chromosomes after normal fertilization.

From this time on, the passage of the fertilized ovum into the uterine cavity is rigidly controlled. If the egg reaches the uterine cavity too early, the endometrium may not be prepared completely to receive the fertilized egg (blastocyst stage). If the ovum passes through the fallopian tube too late, the uterine lining may have already begun to break down. On occasion the ovum may be blocked in the lumen of the fallopian tube and may attach to the tubal lining and begin to grow. This condition is called an ectopic or tubal pregnancy.

Vagina

Increased estrogen stimulation during pregnancy causes many changes in the vagina. It becomes increasingly vascularized and congested. Like the cervix, the vaginal walls take on the dark red or violet sheen characteristic of pregnancy (Chadwick's sign). The proliferation of cells and hyperemia of the vaginal connective tissue and its supports cause the vaginal walls to become thickened, pliable, and distensible in preparation for the passage of the fetal head.

Cervical and vaginal secretions become thickened, white, and acidic as a result of the increased glycogen content of the vaginal epithelium. Glycogen is a normal element found within the vaginal environment. It increases as estrogen levels rise. Bacteria normally residing in the vagina (lactobacilli or Döderlein's bacillus) produce lactic acid as a by-product. Maintenance of the normal acidic pH of the vagina and its secretions depends on lactic acid production. During pregnancy high levels of estrogen help to maintain increased vaginal acidity (ranging from a pH of 3.5 to 5.0) and control the growth of the many pathologic bacteria that many inhabit the vagina.

Breasts

Remarkable changes occur in the breasts during pregnancy. As early as the first trimester, the breasts become enlarged and sensitive. The nipples also become larger, darker, and more erectile. The primary areola darkens, while a secondary, less pigmented areola develops around its outer border. The sebaceous glands within the primary areola (Montgomery's tubercles) become hypertrophied.

Growth of breast tissue by cellular proliferation occurs as early as the third or fourth week of gestation. Ductal growth is intense for the first 3 months, after which the lobuloalveolar formation becomes dominant. During the second half of pregnancy the alveolar cells begin to become secretory with a thick, yellowish fluid called colostrum. During the third trimester the blood vessels of the breast dilate, and the breasts become increasingly enlarged. This enlargement in late pregnancy contributes to the change in the pregnant woman's center of gravity.

Hormonal Preparation of the Breasts for Lactation

The ovarian hormones estrogen and progesterone are necessary for breast development. Ductal development depends on the presence of estrogen, growth hormone, and glucocorticoids (adrenal hormones). Development of the lobuloalveolar system requires progesterone, prolactin, and adrenal steroids. Although estrogen and progesterone are responsible for the growth of the ductal and lobuloalveolar systems, they inhibit milk production during pregnancy and the postpartum period and must be withdrawn for lactation to occur. This is accomplished by the loss of the placenta, which is the main source of estrogen and progesterone secretion during pregnancy.

Lactogenesis, the initiation of milk flow, requires fully developed mammary glands. The hormones necessary for milk production include prolactin growth hormones, glucocorticoids, insulin, and parathyroid hormone. These hormones ensure an adequate supply of the necessary amino acids, fatty acids, glucose, and calcium required for milk formation. An essential requirement for lactation, prolactin is secreted by the mother's pituitary gland. The concentration of her blood prolactin level rises from the fifth week of pregnancy until the birth of the infant, when its level becomes ten times that of the normal prepregnant amount.

Prolactin secretion is regulated by hypothalamic control of prolactin inhibitory factor (PIF) and thyrotropin-releasing factor. The suckling of the infant at the breast inhibits the PIF, and prolactin is released. When the concentration of prolactin in the blood is high, the hypothalamus responds by secreting PIF.

Adaptation of the Cardiovascular System

During pregnancy the cardiovascular system exhibits the most profound adaptations of all body systems other than the reproductive system. As pregnancy progresses, the work of maintaining the fetus adds to the metabolic burden of the mother's body. Physiologic changes in the cardiovascular system and their clinical significance are discussed in Table 11-2.

Heart

The position of the heart changes in pregnancy as the growth of the fetus elevates the diaphragm. It is pushed

Table 11-2. Summary of Cardiovascular Adaptations in Pregnancy

Physiologic Changes	Clinical Significance
Mechanical Adaptations	
Cardiac volume increases by 10% (to 75 mL).	Size of the heart on x-ray films increases.
Elevation of the diaphragm from pressure of the uterus displaces the heart to the left and upward.	Changes (murmurs) in cardiac sound that would be considered abnormal in the nonpregnant state occur. Pulmonic systolic murmurs may be heard. Apical systolic murmurs are heard in 90% of pregnant women.
Blood viscosity is lowered, and torsion of the great vessels occurs because of displacement by the enlarged uterus.	Exaggerated splitting of first heart sound and loud third sound may be heard. Diastolic murmurs are abnormal (20% of women have soft, transient murmurs).
Blood Volume Adaptations	
Plasma volume increases by 50% (to 1250 mL), peaking at 30 to 40 weeks. Total plasma albumin decreases from a nonpregnant value between 4.0 and 4.5 g/dL to pregnant value between 3.0 and 3.5 g/dL.	There is significant hydration of maternal tissues. Physiologic anemia from hemodilution occurs.
Cardiac Output Adaptations	
Heart rate increases.	Pulse increases 10 to 15 bpm, reaching maximum in third trimester. Kidney filtration increases. Oxygen transport increases.
Cardiac output increases. The nonpregnant heart pumps 5.0 to 5.5 L/min. This rate is increased 30% to 50% by the end of the first trimester. It increases a further 10% during the last two trimesters when the patient is in the lateral recumbent position.	
The distribution of cardiac output changes.	Maternal–placental circulation in late pregnancy receives blood at a rate of 1,000 mL/min. This is 10% of cardiac output. The following factors decrease uterine blood flow: Uterine contractions Hypertonus, hypertension, hypotension Strenuous exercise Smoking Pathologic states: anemia, placental problems, infarcts, abruption, pregnancy-induced hypertension The following factors increase uterine blood flow: Bed rest Lateral recumbent position
The increase in red cell volume (erythrocytes) is less than one third of the increase in plasma volume.	Packed cell volume (hematocrit) and hemoglobin values fall.
The production of red cells accelerates.	The reticulocyte count increases. With a regular diet (no Iron supplementation), red cell volume increases 18% to 250 mL. With therapeutic iron supplementation, it increases 30% to 400 to 450 mL. Oral supplementation of 60 to 80 mg/d of elemental iron from early pregnancy allows near maximum red cell volume expansion but does not maintain or restore iron stores. Therefore, women with iron stores should receive 30 to 60 mg/day of elemental iron, and those without stores should receive therapeutic amounts of 120 to 240 mg/d.
Of the red cells added to the maternal circulation, 50% (about 600 mL) is lost during delivery and postpartum.	A total of 800 mg of iron is needed during pregnancy to meet maternal and fetal demands (200 mg is excreted during the pregnancy).
Peripheral Circulatory Adaptations	
Total peripheral resistance decreases.	Venous return to the heart increases.
Uteroplacental circulation is a low-resistance system that works as an arteriovenous shunt, decreasing total body vascular resistance by bypassing systemic circulation.	
The uterus presses on pelvic veins and inferior vena cava.	Stagnation of blood in lower extremities may occur.
Blood flow to the skin increases.	Dissipation of fetal heat produces feelings of warmth in the mother. Vascular dilatation of nasal mucous membranes may cause nose bleeds. Increased blood flow to the skin of the hands may cause erythema.

(continued)

Table 11-2. Summary of Cardiovascular Adaptations in Pregnancy (*Continued*)

Physiologic Changes	Clinical Significance
Blood Pressure Adaptations	
Systolic and diastolic pressure is decreased during the first half of pregnancy (5–10 mm Hg) and then rises to nonpregnant levels.	Any rise of 30 mm Hg systolic or 15 mm Hg diastolic pressure above the norm is an abnormal finding. Brachial artery blood pressure varies with the woman's position: Highest: sitting Intermediate: supine Lowest: lateral recumbent
Compression of the inferior vena cava and aorta in third-trimester pregnant women who lie on their backs may cause a decrease in cardiac output.	Supine hypotensive syndrome may occur. Faintness may result from an 8% to 30% decrease in systolic blood pressure. Bradycardia may ensue, and the cardiac output may be decreased by 50%. This can cause a decrease in uterine arterial pressure, which may be deleterious to the fetus if it occurs with hemorrhage or conduction anesthesia during delivery.

upward and to the left, and its apex is moved laterally from the nonpregnant position. This displacement may make the heart appear to be enlarged in its transverse diameter. The heart may actually increase in size to adapt to its increased workload and cardiac output.

Changes in the position and the circulatory dynamics of the heart may cause systolic murmurs as pregnancy proceeds. Apical systolic murmur can be heard in approximately 90% of pregnant women. Diastolic murmurs are heard in approximately 20% of women during gestation. Pulmonic murmurs may be heard at some point in the pregnancy. These murmurs are physiologic and resolve after pregnancy. They are audible in sitting and supine positions and during inspiration and expiration; they become louder as the heart rate increases.

Cardiac Output

The increase in the output of blood from the heart is the most profound change that occurs in the cardiovascular system during pregnancy. The output begins to increase early in the first trimester. It rises rapidly to 30% to 50% above normal during the first 13 weeks of pregnancy. From 30 weeks of gestation to term the cardiac output remains elevated 30% above normal baseline levels.

The physiologic mechanism for increased cardiac output is not well understood. Two possible causes have been identified. The first is the increased amount of circulating estrogen. The second cause is decreased peripheral resistance, which may be a result of the large placental vascular bed acting as a shunt for the blood flowing through it.

The pregnant woman's position has a strong influence on cardiac output, especially during the third trimester when the uterus is greatly enlarged. When the pregnant woman lies on her back (supine), venous return from the lower extremities through the inferior vena cava is obstructed. This results from the pressure of the enlarged uterus on the vena cava. Blood becomes trapped in the extremities, and venous return to the heart is decreased. Cardiac output is compromised, and the blood pressure drops precipitously (Fig. 11-3).

An episode of supine hypotensive syndrome is experienced by approximately 10% of pregnant women near term. When it occurs, the woman appears anxious, becomes lightheaded, is diaphoretic, and will faint if the situation is not reversed. Reversal is accomplished by turning the woman to the lateral (sidelying) position. This quickly removes pressure from the vena cava, allowing cardiac output to increase almost immediately.

Increased venous pressure in the lower extremities may aggravate existing varicose veins or initiate their appearance. As pregnancy progresses, varicosities may become increasingly symptomatic and require specially constructed support stockings that will prevent venous pooling in the lower legs.

Heart Rate

Increased cardiac output is accompanied by an increase in pulse rate. The resting heart rate, or the number of beats per minute, is elevated from the 70 bpm seen in the healthy nonpregnant woman to approximately 78 bpm during the first trimester. At term the pulse increases to 85 bpm. The heart rate returns to normal within 6 weeks after delivery.

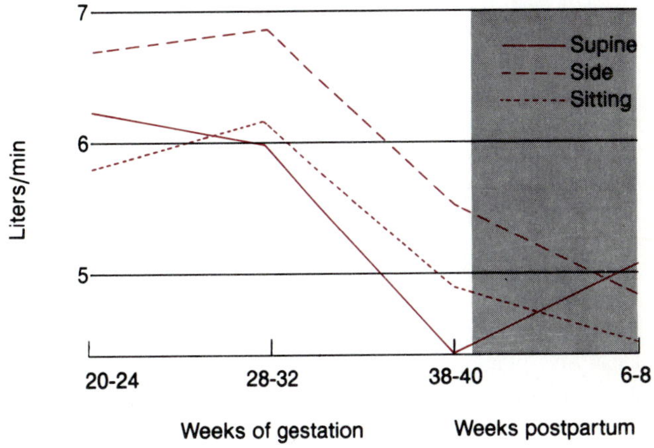

Figure 11-3.
Cardiac output at different stages of pregnancy and postpartum according to patient's position.

Stroke Volume

The stroke volume (amount of blood ejected by the heart per minute) is increased between 13 and 23 weeks of gestation to a maximum of 30% over the normal rate. This may continue unchanged, or it may gradually decrease to prepregnant levels by term. This parameter is difficult to determine, because the woman's position (supine, lateral, or standing) influences the measurement of stroke volume.

Blood Pressure

Changes in blood pressure during pregnancy are minimal in women who were previously normotensive. A slight decrease in blood pressure—the systolic pressure decreasing approximately 2 to 3 mm Hg and the diastolic pressure decreasing about 5 to 10 mm Hg—is considered normal. As term approaches these levels tend to rise to their prepregnant norms.

Blood pressure also is affected by position. It is highest when the pregnant woman is sitting, intermediate when she is supine, and lowest when she lies on her side.

Blood Volume

Blood volume increases dramatically as pregnancy progresses. During the first trimester a slight rise occurs, and by the end of the second trimester blood volume has increased by 50%. This hypervolemia of pregnancy meets the demands of the enlarging uterus and the woman's growing vascular system. Increased blood volume protects the woman and fetus against circulatory insults, including impaired venous return of blood to the woman's heart, and against an anticipated blood loss of approximately 500 mL during delivery.

The increase in the plasma content of the blood during pregnancy occurs earlier and is greater than the increase in red cell mass. The result of the increased ratio of plasma to red cell mass is a decreased hemoglobin or hematocrit. The hematocrit may drop from the average nonpregnant norm of 41% to 37% and the hemoglobin from between 12 and 14 g/dL to 11 g/dL. This is known as physiologic dilutional anemia of pregnancy and is considered normal. After the 13th week of pregnancy, plasma volume ceases to expand while the red blood cell mass continues to rise. As a result hemoglobin concentration increases to more normal levels.

Uterine Blood Flow

Blood flow to the uterus increases dramatically during pregnancy to supply the placenta, myometrium, and endometrium. Blood flow to the nonpregnant uterus is less than 35 mL/min. In early gestation when the uterus and placenta are still relatively small, most of the blood flow is to the myometrium and endometrium. At 10 weeks uterine blood flow is approximately 50 mL/min, and at 28 weeks it is 125 mL/min. This amount gradually increases to between 500 and 1000 mL/min at term.

The placental intervillous spaces must be perfused by the woman's blood to provide nutrients and oxygen to the fetus and placenta and to remove metabolic wastes. The growing fetus creates increased demands for placental blood flow. Uterine blood flow is optimal in the sidelying position and may be impaired in the supine position due to supine hypotension syndrome.

Blood Flow to the Skin

During pregnancy blood flow to the skin increases as pregnancy advances. Capillary blood flow increases, and the veins become more dilated. Resting blood flow to the hands increases seven times, and flow to the feet increases two to three times. Blood flow to the skin may increase to 400 to 500 mL and largely accounts for the total increase in cardiac output. This increase promotes the loss of heat from the skin. However, this heat loss is offset by the increased metabolic rate imposed by the pregnancy.

Adaptation of the Respiratory System

Physiologic changes in the respiratory system and their clinical significance are summarized in Table 11-3.

The major anatomic change in the respiratory system of pregnant women is expansion or flaring of the lower ribs. As a result the subcostal angle widens, and the transverse diameter of the thoracic cage increases approximately 2 cm. The level of the diaphragm rises 4 cm because of the increasing upward growth of the gravid uterus.

Women appear to breathe more deeply during pregnancy. The tidal volume, or the amount of air breathed out during quiet expiration, is 500 mL in nonpregnant women. This amount increases to 700 mL in pregnancy. The respiratory rate remains approximately 16 breaths per minute and may drop slightly at term. Minute volume, the volume of gas expired from the lungs per minute, increases about 37% during pregnancy. Oxygen consumption increases about 14%. Half of the oxygen consumption is used by the embryo and the growing fetus and the rest is consumed by the growing uterus, breast tissue, and increased respiratory and cardiac demands (Fig. 11-4).

Adaptation of the Genitourinary Tract

Renal function changes dramatically during pregnancy. (These changes and their clinical significance are discussed in Table 11-4.) The kidneys handle increased maternal blood volume and metabolic products and act as the primary excretory organ for fetal waste products. The kidneys become heavier and larger as a result of the increased blood volume and enlargement of their interstitial spaces. The length of the kidney increases 1 cm and returns to its normal size after delivery.

Dynamic changes occur in the collecting system of the kidney. The renal calyces, renal pelvis, and ureters dilate during the first trimester, and this change persists for 3 to 4 months postpartum. The maximum expansion of the capacity of the system is reached at term, when 90% of women exhibit ureteral dilatation.

Hypertrophy of the smooth muscle of the ureter and hyperplasia (increased growth) of connective tissue also occur. One of the functions of progesterone is to decrease smooth muscle tone, and its production may contribute to ureteral dilatation. These overall changes contribute to urinary stasis and the risk of increased infection. Decreased peristaltic activity of the urinary system occurs during the first trimester and may persist for 3 to 4 months postpartum.

Table 11-3. Summary of Respiratory Adaptations in Pregnancy

Physiologic Changes	Clinical Significance
Anatomic Changes	
Changes that improve gaseous exchange occur. The lower ribs flare to increase space long before mechanical pressure occurs. They may not return to original position after delivery. The level of the diaphragm rises 4 cm, and the transverse diameter of the chest increases 2 cm.	The movement of tidal air (the volume of air with each breath) increases. More complete expiration is possible.
Hormonal Influences	
Estrogen levels increase.	Estrogen causes decreased pulmonary resistance by increasing the pliability of connective tissue.
Progesterone levels increase.	Progesterone causes decreased pulmonary resistance by relaxing smooth muscle. Minute ventilation increases 37%. Hyperventilation and respiratory alkalosis may occur.
Respiratory center in the brain is sensitive to progesterone, which maintains low serum CO_2 levels. Fetal plasma CO_2 level exceeds that of maternal plasma by 4 to 8 mm Hg	This permits easy passage of CO_2 from fetal to maternal circulation. Dyspnea may occur as a consequence of low CO_2 levels. Its immediate cause is not necessarily related to exercise.
Vocal cords increase in size because of increased circulation due to the influence of progesterone.	The voice becomes deeper.

Hydroureter (retention of water and swelling of the tissue) is common to all pregnancies. It is more marked on the right side, where the ureter lies over the bony brim of the pelvis. Dextrorotation of the uterus, causing pressure on the right side, also may be implicated in the swelling of the ureter on that side. These developments predispose the pregnant woman to urinary tract infection.

The growing uterus displaces the bladder forward and upward. As pregnancy progresses, the bladder mucosa becomes congested with blood (hyperemic). Its walls become hypertrophied as a result of stimulation from estrogen and pressure from the fetus. Decreased drainage of blood from the base of the bladder results in edema of its tissue and renders the bladder more susceptible to trauma and infection during labor and delivery. The effect of progesterone in relaxing the smooth muscle of the bladder wall also increases the bladder's capacity to hold urine. General dilation of the urinary tract during pregnancy not only increases the risk of infection, but makes collection of specimens and evaluation of kidney function tests difficult. A summary of these changes and their clinical significance is given in Table 11-4.

Kidney Function

Changes in the glomerular filtration rate (GFR) and renal plasma flow begin early in gestation and become fully functional by the second trimester. At this time the GFR has increased by 30% to 50%, remaining at this level until term.

Because of increased filtration, laboratory values that measure kidney function are altered. Although the GFR increases, production of serum creatinine or urea nitrogen does not change. This means that the levels of these solutes are decreased from their nonpregnant level of 0.7 and 12.0

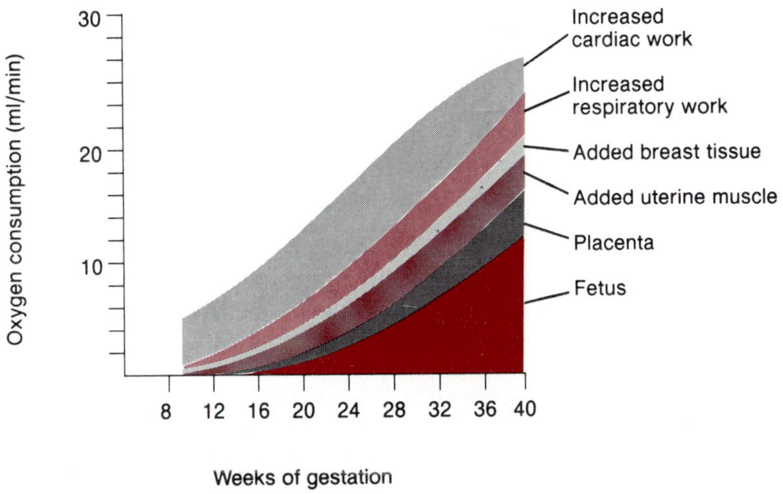

Figure 11-4.
Components of increased oxygen consumption in pregnancy.

Table 11-4. Summary of Genitourinary Adaptations in Pregnancy

Physiologic Changes	Clinical Significance
Mechanical Adaptations	
The uterus enlarges, causing compression of the bladder against the pelvis.	Bladder capacity is reduced, causing more frequent urination.
Enlarged, dextrorotated uterus compresses the ureters as they pass over the pelvic brim, especially on the right side. (The sigmoid colon cushions the left ureter.)	Dilatation of the ureters and renal pelvises occurs. These may contain as much as 200 mL of urine, causing stagnation and increased susceptibility to urinary tract infection (2% of pregnant women suffer from pyelonephritis).
Vesicoureteral reflux may occur.	This may cause changes in 24-hour urine collections (for HCG or estriol testing).
Dilatation of the ovarian vein complex occurs over the right ureter.	Blood drainage decreases.
Base on the bladder is pushed forward and upward from the engaged presenting part of the fetus.	Increased edema and possible trauma may occur. The possibility of infection is increased.
Circulatory Adaptations	
Renal blood flow increases up to third trimester.	Glomerular filtration rate increases 50% (greater in lateral recumbent position and less when standing or sitting). Renal threshold for glucose is lowered (tubules reach maximum of readsorption); glucose is spilled in the urine.
Hormonal Influences	
Under the influence of estrogen, total water retention is 6 to 8 L in late pregnancy, distributed among the mother, fetus, placenta, and amniotic fluid.	Physiologic edema may occur.
Progesterone increases the size of the kidneys.	Sodium and electrolyte loss in the urine (natriuresis) may occur.
Aldosterone secretion from the adrenals and estrogen secretion from the placenta balance progesterone, causing: Dilatation of ureters and renal pelvises Relaxation of bladder and trigone	Readsorption of sodium chloride and water by renal tubules occurs. Volume of urine for secretion does not increase. Urine secretion in late pregnancy decreases; fluid retention increases. Bladder becomes edematous and easily traumatized.
Postural Effects	
Posture affects blood flow and renal function.	When the woman sits or stands there is the following: Decrease in renal blood flow and glomerular filtration rate from pooling of blood in pelvis and legs Decrease in urine volume and secretion Decrease in cardiac output, causing compensatory renal vasoconstriction Water accumulates in the body during the day, causing dependent edema. When the woman is in the lateral position at night, the effect of gravity is removed, distributing fluid throughout the body, with the following effects: Increased kidney filtration, causing nocturia Increased secretion of water and salt
Changes in Nutrient Value of Urine	
The proportion of nutrients in pregnant urine is high	Excretion of folates, glucose, lactose, amino acids, vitamin B_{12}, and ascorbic acid is increased. Higher nutrient content of urine favors rapid growth of urinary bacteria, with greater risk of urinary tract infection.

mg/dL, respectively, to 0.5 and 9.0 mg/dL. When nonpregnant levels of these solutes are found in pregnancy, impaired renal function may be present.

Other solutes are excreted in greater quantities because of the kidneys' increased workload. These include glucose, vitamin B_{12}, folic acid, amino acids, uric acid, and some water-soluble vitamins. Excretion of these nutrients may explain the rapid growth of bacteria in the urine. Excretion of protein is not normally increased. The normal nonpregnant range of 100 to 300 mg of protein in a 24-hour urine collection is applicable to pregnant women.

Glucose in the urine (glucosuria) may not be an abnormal finding in pregnancy. The increased GFR, in conjunction with the decreased capacity of the tubules to reabsorb glucose, may cause one sixth of pregnant women to spill glucose in the urine. However, if glucose is spilled consistently or there is a family history of diabetes mellitus, further diabetes testing is necessary.

Fluid Retention

To supply the demands of the various tissues for water and electrolytes, 6 to 8 L of water is retained in the body during pregnancy. Approximately 4 to 6 L of this fluid passes into the extracellular spaces, causing a physiologic blood volume increase (hypervolemia). The body's volume receptors adapt to the increased fluid load. The excretion of sodium in the normal pregnant woman is similar to that in nonpregnant women. Sodium retention is proportional to the amount of water accumulated during pregnancy. When sodium intake is severely limited in normal pregnancy, decreased kidney function and urine volume may result. Pregnancy outcome may be adversely affected by the practice of reducing sodium intake.

Physiologic edema is normal in pregnancy and usually occurs during the third trimester. Swelling of the ankles and "stiffness" of the fingers signal water accumulation. Ankle edema results from the dependent position of the legs, which favors gravitation of fluid. Because of venous obstruction from the weight of the gravid uterus, blood flow back to the heart is decreased when the woman is supine, stands, or sits. As a result, fluid pools in the lower extremities. When the sidelying position is assumed, three important processes occur: The weight of the gravid uterus is removed from the vessels, venous flow to the heart increases, and kidney function improves. Although lying on either the right or left side will accomplish the first two processes, renal function is further enhanced in the left lateral position. The excessive fluid is mobilized and excreted by the kidneys.

Pregnant women who are retaining fluid are strongly advised to assume a sidelying position several times a day. When edema occurs in conjunction with increased blood pressure, proteinuria, or excessive weight gain, pregnancy-induced hypertension must be suspected, and further assessment and treatment are needed (see Chapter 13).

Adaptation of the Gastrointestinal System

The general performance of the gastrointestinal tract in pregnancy seems sluggish and somewhat impaired. Women commonly have symptoms of nausea, vomiting, heartburn, and constipation. The symptoms are a result of the effects of hormones and a slowed digestive tract. Changes and their clinical significance are discussed in Table 11-5.

Appetite and Food Consumption

There are both quantitative and qualitative changes in the pregnant woman's appetite. Early in the pregnancy, women usually experience a surge in appetite. This tends to decrease as pregnancy progresses. During the first trimester women also may experience nausea, particularly in the morning. These changes are probably a result of hormonal changes.

Some women experience aversions to certain foods, find their senses of taste and smell dulled or enhanced, or crave particular foods or other substances. Craving for and ingestion of substances that are not food items is called *pica*. Women may ingest coal, clay, laundry starch, toothpaste, or any number of other inappropriate substances. The cause of these taste changes and cravings is unknown. Pica is a culturally learned practice (see Chapter 17), but its underlying cause may be related to elevated levels of estrogen and progesterone during pregnancy. Iron deficiency anemia or malnutrition may occur because of a reduction in the intake of necessary nutrients as a result of faulty eating habits.

Mouth

There are few physiologic changes in the mouth during pregnancy, but hyperemia is present, as it is in many areas of the body. Pregnancy gingivitis may result from proliferation of local blood vessels and softening of the gums. A focal vascular hypertrophy of the gums is called *epulis*. The gums appear reddened and swollen and partially cover the upper portion of the teeth. These lesions may bleed excessively if traumatized by a toothbrush or hard objects. The teeth are not affected, and the lesions regress spontaneously during the postpartum period. Their cause is unknown but is probably related to the high levels of estrogen.

Ptyalism is the seemingly excessive production of saliva, particularly in women experiencing nausea. Normally, 1 to 2 L of saliva are produced each day. This amount does not appear to be exceeded by women who experience ptyalism. Women who are suffering from severe nausea may find it difficult to swallow saliva, so that it accumulates and appears unusually copious.

Digestive Tract

As the uterus grows, the stomach and intestines are displaced upward. The motility of the entire alimentary tract is decreased as a result of the action of progesterone on its smooth musculature. The tone of the esophagus is decreased. Small amounts of stomach contents may reach the lower esophagus with increased intragastric pressure and cause heartburn (a condition known as *reflux esophagitis*).

Gastric motility is decreased, as is the production of hydrochloric acid and pepsin. The intestinal transit time of digested food is increased. This facilitates the maximum absorption of nutrients from the *chyme*, a mixture of digested food, digestive secretions, and water found in the stomach and small intestines during digestion of food. Iron is absorbed during the digestive process. In women with iron deficiency anemia or low iron stores, more iron will be absorbed. Another element absorbed readily from the intestinal contents is water. Because the transit time of the chyme in the gut is increased, excessive water is absorbed. The feces become hard and dry, and constipation results. Straining causes increased venous pressure to the rectal vessels, and hemorrhoids may develop or become exacerbated.

Liver and Gallbladder

Significant liver changes are rare in pregnancy. The position of the liver changes during the third trimester, when it is pushed upward and backward toward the right. Its blood flow and metabolic activity are increased, but the liver's volume remains unchanged. The increased metabolic proc-

Table 11-5. Summary of Gastrointestinal Adaptations in Pregnancy

Physiologic Changes	Clinical Significance
Mechanical Adaptations	
Enlarging uterus puts increasing pressure on the stomach and intestines.	Hiatal hernia from partial rupture of the stomach through the diaphragm may occur.
Stomach and intestines are displaced; the appendix is moved upward and laterally.	Constipation and heartburn (pyrosis) are common.
Venous pressure increases below the enlarged uterus.	Hemorrhoids and varicosities may occur.
Hormonal Influences	
Tone and mobility of the smooth muscle of the gastrointestinal tract are lowered. Gastric emptying time increases.	Reflux esophagitis, constipation, and nausea may occur.
Water absorption from the colon increases.	Constipation may occur.
Cholestasis (suppression of bile flow) may occur.	Pruritus (generalized itching of the skin) results from increases retention of bile salts. Cholelithiasis may occur.
Gastric secretion of hydrochloric acid and pepsin decreases (usually after the first trimester).	Indigestion may occur. Peptic ulcers improve because of decreased secretory response to histamines.
Estrogen affects adhesiveness of fibers in collagenous tissue.	Epulis may occur. Swollen, spongy gums bleed easily; condition regresses spontaneously after delivery.
Eating disorders of unknown etiology occur.	Pica is a craving for substances that may or may not be foods, such as clay, laundry starch, soap, toothpaste, plaster.
Saliva production increases (etiology unknown).	Ptyalism is a problem for some women. However, some feel that nauseated women find it difficult to swallow saliva, making it appear excessive.
Dental caries do not increase during pregnancy.	Routine dental care is needed during pregnancy.
Metabolic Adaptations	
Pregnancy has a profound effect on carbohydrate metabolism. Carbohydrates in the form of glucose are the primary energy source for the maternal brain and fetoplacental unit.	Fasting plasma glucose levels drop during pregnancy. Plasma insulin levels show little change until the third trimester, when they rise approximately 30%.
Lipid metabolism in pregnancy causes fat stores to accumulate for periods of fetal growth and lactation.	Approximately 3.5 kg of extra fat is stored by 30 weeks of gestation.
Protein is used by the fetus for growth.	Protein is probably not stored during pregnancy. If inadequate protein is ingested, the pregnant woman's muscle mass may be enlisted as a protein reserve.

esses of the liver are reflected in increased levels of cholesterol, lipoproteins, and triglycerides.

Spider nevi and palmar erythema, usually found in patients with liver disease, are common in pregnancy. They result from increased circulating estrogens rather than altered liver function. These skin changes disappear shortly after delivery.

The gallbladder becomes sluggish during pregnancy. Bile is more viscous from prolonged retention. Incomplete emptying of the gallbladder may cause formation of cholesterol crystals and increase the risk of developing gallstones.

Carbohydrate, Lipid, and Protein Metabolism

Carbohydrates

During pregnancy, carbohydrate metabolism is controlled by glucose levels in the plasma and the metabolism of glucose in the cells. A major source of quick energy for the body, glucose also is the primary energy source for the brain and the fetoplacental unit.

The liver controls the woman's plasma glucose level. The liver not only stores glucose as glycogen, but converts it back to glucose when blood sugar is low. Glycogen is stored in other organs, such as the muscles. However, it can be used only as a local source of energy within these organs because they lack glucagon, a liver enzyme necessary to convert glycogen back to free glucose.

Carbohydrates, which provide 50% of the total energy from the diet, are obtained from starch, sugars, and some animal glycogen. As the carbohydrates are absorbed from the digestive tract, they pass through the portal venous blood into the liver. Here they are converted to glucose or stored as glycogen. After a high carbohydrate meal, plasma glucose rises and stimulates the release of insulin from the beta cells of the pancreas. The blood sugar is reduced when, in response to the effect of insulin, glucose is converted back to glycogen in the liver and muscles. When plasma glucose levels fall too low, the pancreatic hormone glucagon is released. It converts liver glycogen back to free glucose for release into the plasma.

In nonpregnant women fasting plasma glucose is approximately 80 mg/100 mL. In pregnant women it drops to 75 mg/100 mL by 12 weeks of gestation; it drops to 70 mg/100 mL as pregnancy progresses. Plasma insulin levels change little until the third trimester when they rise approximately 30%.

Lipids

Lipid metabolism during pregnancy causes considerable accumulation of fat stores. The plasma lipids most commonly involved during pregnancy are cholesterol, phospholipids, and triglycerides. These lipids promote high levels of fat storage in the woman but appear to have negligible influence on the fetoplacental unit.

It has been calculated that 310 g of extra fat is stored in the woman by the tenth week of gestation, 2 kg by 20 weeks, and 3.5 kg by 30 weeks. After 30 weeks no further fat storage takes place. The stored fat is useful as a source of energy during periods of rapid fetal growth and during lactation.

Protein

Adequate protein intake to permit tissue growth of the fetus and placenta is essential during pregnancy. Whether protein is stored during pregnancy is controversial, but it is generally considered unlikely. During the third trimester, however, 1.2 g of nitrogen is retained in the body daily, and this is equivalent to 7 g of protein. If maternal stores are lacking and inadequate protein is ingested, fetal growth can continue only if protein from the woman's body is used. The pregnant woman's muscle mass can be mobilized by the fetus as a protein reserve when adequate amounts are not available from dietary intake.

Adaptation of the Musculoskeletal System

The principal musculoskeletal changes of pregnancy are the hormonal relaxation of the joints and the adjustments in posture caused by the growth of the uterus (Table 11-6).

As pregnancy advances and the uterus enlarges, the woman's center of gravity is displaced. The upper spine is thrown backward to compensate for the heavy anterior weight of the uterus. Lordosis results and gives the pregnant woman her characteristic stance and gait (Fig. 11-5). Some women also experience aching, numbness, and weakness of the upper extremities. These symptoms are due to the compensatory position of the back, which causes the woman to flex her neck and slump her shoulders anteriorly. This position places stress and traction on the peripheral nerves, causing pain and discomfort. Exaggeration of this position may lead to paresthesia over the ulnar and median nerve, causing motor weakness and tenderness of the muscles of the thumb (carpal tunnel syndrome).

Relaxin, a hormone of pregnancy, is thought to be responsible for the softening and increased mobility of the sacroiliac, sacrococcygeal, and pubic joints. During delivery these joints may flex just enough to allow passage of a fetal head that might otherwise have been unable to negotiate the passage through the maternal pelvis.

The muscles of the abdomen are placed under great stress during the latter half of pregnancy. The vertical muscle located just beneath the skin of the abdomen is called the rectus abdominis. As the uterus grows, a midline lateral separation of the two halves of this muscle may occur, creating a vertical space between them. The width of this space can be palpated when the woman assumes a supine position and places her chin on her chest. A fairly common occurrence in pregnancy, the diastasis is not painful, and unless it is extreme the muscle will return to its normal position after delivery. If the diastasis is extreme, the pregnant uterus may herniate through the muscle opening.

Adaptation of the Integumentary System

Many skin changes occur during pregnancy. Most are benign, and some are reversible. Estrogen affects the skin, as shown in Table 11-7.

Pigmentation

The increased skin pigmentation specific to pregnancy may be striking in some women. Face and body pigmentation resulting from the action of melanocyte-stimulating hor-

Table 11-6. Summary of Musculoskeletal Adaptations in Pregnancy

Physiologic Changes	Clinical Significance
Hormonal Influences	
Joints relax under the influence of relaxin.	Mobility and pliability of sacroiliac, sacrococcygeal, and pubic joints increase in preparation for delivery.
Mechanical Influences	
Weight of the enlarging uterus increases.	Round ligament pain may occur.
Postural changes occur.	Center of gravity shifts, and some women experience backache. Leaning backward to compensate may cause lordosis and back strain.
	Spasm of the uterosacral ligaments may occur.
	Women may experience aching or numbness of upper extremities as a result of anterior slumping of the shoulders and chest.
Diastasis recti may occur.	Uterus may partially herniate through abdominal muscle wall.
Carpal tunnel syndrome may occur.	Paresthesia, motor weakness, and muscle tenderness may be experienced in the wrist and thumb.

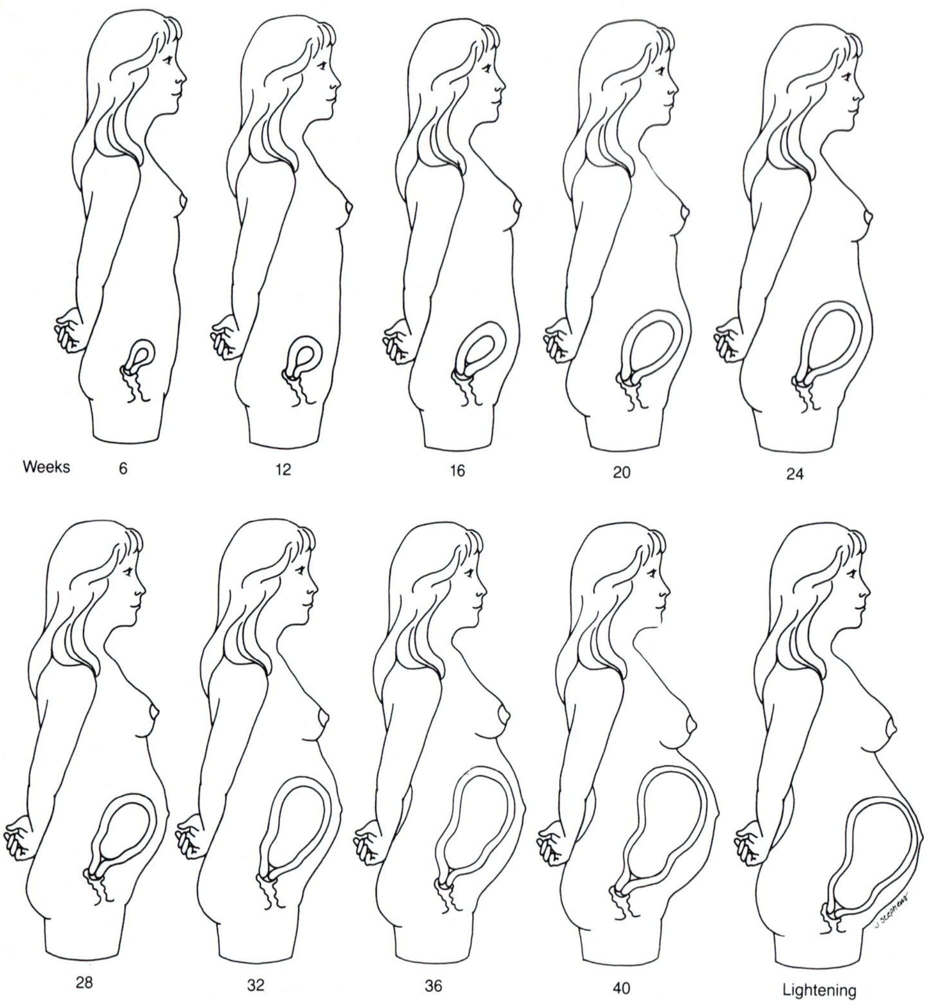

Figure 11-5.

Development of postural changes during pregnancy. Significant postural changes occur as pregnancy progresses, causing accentuated curvature of the lumbar spine. Low back pain, one of the most common complaints of pregnancy, results from the pregnant woman's attempt to maintain her balance by leaning backward (Childbirth Graphics).

mone may occur as early as 8 to 16 weeks of pregnancy. Chloasma gravidarum (the mask of pregnancy) is the brownish pigmentation that appears on the face in a butterfly pattern in 50% to 70% of women. It is usually symmetric and is distributed on the forehead, cheeks, and nose. More common in dark-haired, brown-eyed women, it is progressive during the pregnancy. Women using oral contraception also may experience some increased facial pigmentation.

The nipples, areola, vulva, and thighs may become darker. Linea negra, a dark vertical line, may appear on the abdomen between the sternum and the symphysis pubis. Chloasma may persist after delivery, but the other pigmentation changes usually regress after the postpartum period.

Table 11-7. Summary of Integumentary Adaptations in Pregnancy

Physiologic Changes	Clinical Significance
Hormonal Influence	
Estrogen has decided effects on the skin	In many women the influence of estrogen produces: Increased pigmentation (chloasma, linea nigra) Striae (stretch marks) Spider angiomas (vascular telangiectases) Palmar erythema

Striae

Striae, also known as "stretch marks," are common in pregnancy. They are tears in the connective tissue underlying the skin. They occur in areas such as the abdomen, breasts, buttocks, and thighs where weight gain tends to be rapid. Their appearance is believed to be hormone-related, but it is not known why some women experience numerous striae, whereas others may have very few or none. They appear in approximately 90% of women during the second trimester. They appear as reddish or purplish linear marks (Fig. 11-6) and may cause itching in some women. After delivery they recede to silverish marks but never fully regress. Women have applied various creams and lotions to prevent or reduce their appearance; rarely do they succeed.

Spider Angiomas

Spider angiomas, also known as vascular spiders or vascular telangiectases, are small clusters of thin-walled, dilated capillaries that resemble spiders. They generally appear on the pregnant woman's chest, are thought to be estrogen related, and usually disappear after delivery.

Palmar erythema, or redness of the palms of the hands, frequently occurs in conjunction with vascular spiders. Two thirds of white women and one third of African-American women experience these conditions. Neither is of any clinical significance, and they generally regress after delivery, although they may not completely disappear.

Adaptation of the Endocrine System

The event of conception initiates profound changes in the woman's endocrine system. These changes are essential for the maintenance of pregnancy. A summary of the hormonal changes seen during pregnancy is given in Table 11-8.

When the blastocyst enters the uterine cavity, the corpus luteum of the menstrual cycle (from which the ovum was derived) is transformed into the corpus luteum of pregnancy. Pituitary inhibition of the formation of new ovarian follicles prolongs the life span of the corpus luteum. The progesterone secreted by the corpus luteum ensures that implantation and the development of the placenta can occur. By the eighth day of gestation, concurrent secretion of human chorionic gonadotropin (HCG) has begun to provide nutrition and essential hormones to sustain the corpus luteum for 7 to 10 weeks. Production of HCG declines significantly at this point as the placenta takes over.

The human fetus sustained within the maternal uterus is well protected as it develops from a single zygote into a complex organism consisting of millions of cells. All the needs of the growing fetus—nutrition, removal of wastes, temperature control, and safety—are supplied by the woman. To achieve this ideal situation for fetal maintenance and growth, the woman's physiologic system must increase its normal capacity while maintaining the homeostasis necessary to supply her own needs. This amazing feat is accomplished through the alteration of maternal endocrine function.

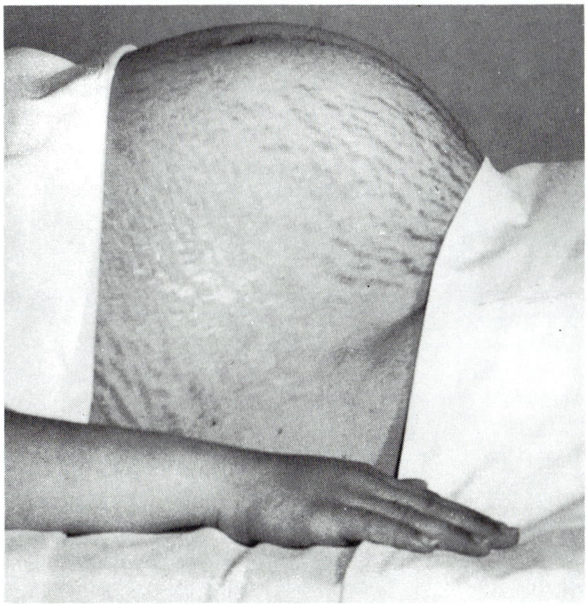

Figure 11-6.
Abdomen of pregnant woman at term, showing striae gravidarum and prominent linea nigra. (From Bookmiller, M. M., Gowen, G. L. [1963]. *Textbook of obstetrics and obstetric nursing*. Philadelphia: W.B. Saunders.)

Steroid Hormones

In nonpregnant women the steroid hormones estrogen and progesterone are produced by the ovaries. During pregnancy this mechanism is shut down; instead, these hormones are synthesized in the maternal–fetal–placental unit and not solely by the placenta as previously believed.

Estrogen

During pregnancy the function of estrogen production is assumed by the placenta, with precursors from the fetal liver and adrenals, in conjunction with androgens (male hormones) from the woman's circulatory system. By 20 weeks of gestation most estrogen excreted in the maternal urine is derived from fetal androgens.

During normal human pregnancy, a hyperestrogenic state of continually increasing proportions exists. This state terminates abruptly after expulsion of the products of conception at delivery. More than 25 different estrogens have been found in the urine of pregnant women. Most are maternal and fetal metabolites of hormones secreted by the placenta. The three classic estrogens of pregnancy—estrone, estradiol, and estriol—all secreted by the placenta, are the best known and studied.

More than 90% of the estrogen excreted in maternal urine is estriol. The concentration of estriol is 1000 times greater in pregnant than in nonpregnant women. It is thought that estriol may function to increase uteroplacental blood flow. Synthesis of normal amounts of estriol depends on an intact fetus and an intact placenta. Estriol secreted by the placenta enters the maternal circulation, is transferred into the amniotic fluid, and is excreted in the urine. When the woman or fetus is compromised, decreased estriol levels may reflect the problem.

Estriol measurements to assess fetoplacental function can be performed on urine, plasma, and amniotic fluid. However, maternal estriol determination is seldom used as a method of determining fetal well-being in high-risk pregnancies. It has been replaced by the simpler, less expensive, and more accurate method of nonstress testing (see Chapter 14).

Functions of estrogens during pregnancy are to ensure the following:

- Uterine growth and enlargement
- Maintenance of uterine elasticity and contractility
- Maintenance of breast growth and its ductal structures
- Enlargement of the external genitalia

Estrogen works in conjunction with progesterone to support pregnancy.

Progesterone

Progesterone production by the placenta does not depend on precursors, perfusion of the uteroplacental unit, or even the presence of a live fetus, because the fetus contrib-

Text continues on page 248

Table 11-8. Summary of Hormonal Influences in Pregnancy

Site of Production	Actions	Clinical Implications
Estrogen (Primarily estriol E_2)		
(Increases 1000-fold during pregnancy) Ovary Adrenal cortex Fetoplacental unit (After the seventh week of gestation, a 50% increase in secretion is ascribed to the placenta.), fetal liver and adrenals (secreted with precursors)	Growth and function of the uterus Hypertrophy of the uterine musculature Proliferation of the endometrium Increased blood supply to the uteroplacental unit	Index of fetal well-being provided by measurement of estriol in urine or amniotic fluid: Decreased level indicates anencephaly; Addison's disease in woman; fetal demise; use of drugs, such as ampicillin, stilbestrol, meprobamate, or glucose in maternal urine Increased level indicates twins, erythroblastosis
	Development of ducts, alveoli, nipples of the breasts	Increased breast size and tenderness
	Enlargement of external genitalia	
	Increased pliability of connective tissue (Tissues become hygroscopic and softer.) Relaxation of pelvic joints and ligaments Stretching capacity of the cervix	Lordosis, backache Tenderness of the symphysis pubis Cervical dilatation
	Decreased gastric secretion of hydrochloric acid and pepsin	Indigestion, nausea, heartburn, decreased absorption of fat
	Increased pigmentation of skin (increased melanocyte-stimulating hormone to pituitary)	Hyperpigmentation: chloasma, darkened genitalia and areola, linea nigra
	Sodium and water retention	Edema, increased plasma volume (physiologic anemia)
	50% increase in clotting potential of blood fibrinogen (factor I)	Increased sedimentation rate Palmar erythema, vascular spiders (angiomas)
	Increased production of estriol in the late third trimester (may stimulate prostaglandin production)	Enhancement of rhythmic uterine contractions; increased vascularity and responsiveness to oxytocin stimulation
	Psychological changes	Emotional lability, possibly changes in libido
Progesterone		
(Increases tenfold in pregnancy) Corpus luteum of the ovary for the first 7 weeks of pregnancy; then maternal–fetal unit	Development of decidual cells in the endometrium	Meets early nutritional needs of the embryo by deposition of glycogen
	Possible role in suppression of the maternal immunologic response to the fetus	
	Decrease in contractility of pregnant uterus	Prevention of premature labor
	Development of lobuloalveolar system of the breasts (secretory character)	Breast tenderness
	Apparent resetting of three hypothalamic centers, causing:	Changes in fat storage, respiration and sensation:
	Extensive fat storage to protect woman and fetus during starvation of strenuous physical exertion	Average storage of 3.5 kg (7.7 lb) of body fat
	Stimulation of the respiratory center; decrease in PCO_2 to facilitate transfer of CO_2 from fetal to maternal blood	Decreases alveolar and arterial P_{CO_2} in woman; hyperventilation
	Increase of 0.2°C (0.5°F) in basal body temperature until midpregnancy; then return to normal	Sensation of being overly warm; increased perspiration
	Stimulation of natriuresis (excess secretion of sodium in urine)	Secretion of aldosterone (sodium saver) to maintain water and electrolyte balance
	Relaxation of smooth muscle	Nausea, reflux esophagitis, indigestion
	Decrease in stomach motility, colonic activity	Delayed emptying with readsorption of water from the bowel, resulting in constipation and hemorrhoids
	Decrease in tone of bladder and ureter; dilatation throughout the system	Stasis of urine, urinary tract infections

(*continued*)

Table 11-8. Summary of Hormonal Influences in Pregnancy (*Continued*)

Site of Production	Actions	Clinical Implications
Human Chorionic Gonadotropin (HCG)		
Placenta, secreted by the syncytiotrophoblasts (appears as early as 8 days after conception; peaks at 60 to 90 days when corpus luteum function is no longer needed to maintain the pregnancy) Peak secretion: 50,000–100,000 mIU/mL/day; (drops to 25,000–50,000 mIU/mL after 4 months of gestation)	Maintenance of the function of the corpus luteum in early pregnancy Possible use in regulating steroid production in the fetus	Possible relationship with nausea Use in pregnancy testing (negative test after 16 to 20 weeks) Use in testing for multiple pregnancies (amount increases) Indication of threatened abortion (amount decreases) Use in diagnosis of trophoblastic disease and ectopic pregnancy (measured by the subunit HCG radioimmunoassay; no cross-reactions with luteinizing hormone)
Human Placental Lactogen (HPL)		
Placenta, syncytiotrophoblasts (detected in the serum of pregnant woman at 6 weeks of gestation; reaches 6000 ng/mL at term)	Action similar to that of growth hormones Anti-insulin effect; sparing of maternal glucose Maintenance of adequate supply of nutrients for the fetus when the women is fasting (amount of HPL secreted correlates with fetal and placental weight)	Increased availability of glucose for fetal use Increased protein synthesis Increased circulating fatty acids to meet increased metabolic needs; conservation of glucose and amino acids for use by the fetus Avoidance of ketosis that might be caused by inadequate maternal glucose intake and that might impair fetal brain development
	Possible effect of the increased incorporation of iron into erythrocytes (currently under study) Stimulation of breast development, casein synthesis, and milk production	Association between high levels of HPL and multiple pregnancies
Prostaglandins		
Maternal–placental–fetal unit (widely distributed in all cells of the body)	Role in cardiovascular changes, cervical ripening, and initiation of labor	Effect on the uterine muscle Prostaglandin E used vaginally or in amniocentesis for second-trimester abortions and in labor induction Possible function in increasing length of gestation
	Synthesis inhibited by anti-inflammatory drugs, such as aspirin and indomethacin	Use of indomethacin to halt premature labor
Prolactin		
Fetal pituitary, maternal pituitary, uterus (elevated blood levels at 8 weeks of gestation, reaching a peak of 200 ng/mL at term)	Sustaining milk protein, casein, fatty acids, lactose, and volume of milk secretion during lactation	Necessity of suckling response for release of prolactin
Thyroid Hormones		
Thyroid gland, with stimulation from adenohypophysis (T_3 decreases until the end of the first trimester, than stabilizes; returns to normal 12 to 13 weeks' postpartum; T_4 increases during pregnancy)	Thyroid enlargement with a 20% increase in function from tissue hyperplasia and increased vascularity	Increase of 25% in basal metabolic rate resulting from metabolic activity of the fetoplacental unit. Increase of protein-bound iodine from 3.6–8.8 to 10–12 U/dL during pregnancy Palpitations, tachycardia, emotional lability, heat intolerance, fatigue, perspiration
Oxytocin		
Hypothalamus to pituitary for release	Stimulates uterine contractions (is not responsible for initial labor, but increases the intensity of contractions) Ferguson's reflex—release of oxytocin by cervical and vaginal distention during labor Stimulates milk let-down and ejection	Uterine involution Role in onset of labor unknown Lactation

utes no precursor. After implantation progesterone is produced by the corpus luteum until 10 weeks of gestation. The function of its secretion is transferred from the corpus luteum to the placenta between the 7th and 11th weeks of gestation. At that time the placenta becomes the major source of progesterone, producing approximately 250 mg/d. At term progresterone levels range from 100 to 200 ng/mL per day.

Progesterone may have a role in suppressing the maternal immunologic response to the fetus and in preventing rejection of the trophoblasts. The question of why the maternal organism does not reject the fetus as a foreign body has been studied for years. When discovered, the answer may dramatically change the field of immunology.

Other better-documented functions of progesterone include the following:

- Development of endometrial decidual cells containing glycogen to meet the embryo's nutritional needs
- Decrease in uterine motility
- Stimulation of the respiratory system
- Relaxation of smooth muscle
- Maintenance of the early corpus luteum

In addition to steroid hormones, the placenta is responsible for secreting essential protein hormones necessary for maintaining pregnancy.

Protein Hormones of the Placenta

Human Chorionic Gonadotropin

HCG is secreted by the syncytiotrophoblasts of the implanting placenta. HCG reaches a maximum level of 50,000 to 100,000 mIU/mL at 10 weeks of gestation. Continued survival of the corpus luteum depends on the presence of HCG. This hormone doubles the growth of the corpus luteum to assure continued adequate secretion of estrogen and progesterone. It also maintains the decidual layer of the endometrium to ensure early placental and fetal tissue development.

By 20 weeks of gestation the HCG levels decrease to 10,000 to 20,000 mIU/mL and remain at this level until term. It has been shown that HCG levels near term are higher in women carrying female fetuses. The reason for this higher level is unknown. Masculine differentiation is a function of HCG because it stimulates the production of androgenic steroids in the early fetal testes.

Sophisticated immunologic and receptor tests are available to detect the presence of HCG in blood or urine. These tests are now standard for the determination of pregnancy. Laboratory tests for HCG are extremely useful and probably life saving for women with ectopic and molar (trophoblastic disease) pregnancies. Levels of serum HCG can be measured in these women to help guide the assessment and management of these conditions.

Human Placental Lactogen

Human placental lactogen (HPL) is also known as human chorionic somatomammotropin. It is secreted by the syncytiotrophoblasts and can be detected in maternal serum as early as week 6 of gestation. The hormone can be measured by radioimmunoassay, and in late pregnancy its levels are higher than that of any other known protein hormone.

Levels of HPL in the maternal circulation are directly correlated with fetal and placental weight. Because HPL is found primarily in the maternal circulation (minute amounts enter the fetal circulation), it is believed that it is metabolized in the maternal rather than the fetal tissues. High levels of maternal HPL are associated with multiple pregnancies. Levels up to 40 g/mL have been found. By the end of pregnancy levels lower than 4 g/mL are considered abnormal.

HPL is important to a number of essential metabolic processes of pregnancy. It facilitates the breakdown of fats to elevate the amount of circulating free fatty acids. These fatty acids are an important energy source for maternal metabolism and fetal nutrition. HPL inhibits the use of maternal glucose and the formation of glucose from noncarbohydrate sources such as protein. HPL also inhibits glucogenesis and the formation of glycogen from amino and fatty acids in the woman. This is called "sparing," and its purpose is to save these products for use by the fetus. HPL also is responsible for increased levels of insulin in the maternal circulation, causing protein synthesis and providing a source of amino acids for use by the fetus.

All these mechanisms help to supply the fetus with the nutrients it needs when the woman is fasting (between meals). If the pregnant woman does not eat sufficient carbohydrates for sustained periods, ketosis develops from the metabolism of fat as an energy source. Fetal development may be impaired by constant exposure to ketones. For this reason caloric intake should not be severely restricted during pregnancy.

Other Hormones

Prostaglandins

Prostaglandins are a group of more than 16 compounds produced and activated in various tissue sites throughout the body. Among the sites pertinent to pregnancy are the myometrium, the amnion, the chorion, and the decidua. Prostaglandins are involved in the cardiovascular adaptation to pregnancy. They also play a major role in cervical ripening and the initiation of labor.

Drugs that inhibit the production or activity of prostaglandins include aspirin and indomethacin. These drugs also have been found to inhibit preterm labor. See Chapter 23 for a complete discussion of prostaglandins' role in labor.

Thyroid Hormones

The thyroid is a butterfly-shaped gland found in the neck just below the cricoid cartilage. The thyroid secretes thyroxine (T_4) and small amounts of triiodothyronine (T_3). Most T_3 results from the conversion of T_4 in other body tissues. In the serum most T_3 and T_4 are bound to proteins. An important protein is thyroxine-binding globulin (TBG). Only the unbound, or free, hormones are biologically active and perform their roles in metabolism, the development of the central nervous system, and general body growth.

Hormone secretion is the result of a negative feedback loop. Elevated estrogen levels lead to greater production of

TBG, which binds more thyroxine. In response the pregnant woman produces more thyroid hormones. However, because most of the new production is bound to TBG, the amount of free T_3 and T_4 remains essentially the same. Basal metabolic rate increases during pregnancy. Most of this increase is not due to the increase in thyroid hormones but rather to the increased oxygen consumption of the woman and her fetus. After delivery the amounts of TBG, T_3, and T_4 return to prepregnancy levels. This process may require 6 to 12 weeks.

Thyroid disorders are more common in women than men; therefore, hypothyroid and hyperthyroid states are seen in pregnancy. The development of the fetal thyroid is generally independent of maternal thyroid function. In most cases the fetal thyroid develops normally even in the presence of maternal disease. However, drugs used to treat the woman may cross the placenta and interfere with the fetal thyroid.

Pregnancy requires multiple physiologic adaptations involving nearly every system of the body. These adaptations begin virtually at the time of conception and continue throughout the pregnancy. The most significant adaptations are those that occur in the reproductive system, including the development of the embryo and the fetus, the growth of the uterus, the shift in hormonal function to support the pregnancy, and the preparation of the breasts for lactation. The cardiovascular and genitourinary systems adapt as the woman's body takes over circulatory, respiratory, metabolic, and excretory functions for the growing fetus. The physiologic adaptations in the gastrointestinal and musculoskeletal systems also are essential to support pregnancy but also may produce some common discomforts of pregnancy. The endocrine system, as the master control system for the body, adapts to take on the specialized functions of maintaining the pregnancy, as well as keeping the maternal metabolic functions optimal for the well-being of the woman and the fetus.

Implications for Nursing Care

Nursing practice is predicated on a strong physiologic knowledge base. This knowledge is especially important for nurses caring for pregnant women in an inpatient and outpatient setting. The body's physiologic adaptations to pregnancy and the major alterations that occur in the pregnant woman's body during the prenatal period are incredible. At no time in a woman's life is her body subjected to such abrupt body changes and symptoms. Most of these adjustments are normal manifestations of the pregnant state and may be easily explained.

Thorough understanding of the underlying physiologic adaptations during pregnancy allows the nurse to assess and diagnose potential or actual problems accurately. This provides the nurse with critical information to implement an optimal plan of care for the pregnant woman.

Chapter Summary

The events involved in the development of a new human life are complex and astounding. Most pregnancies result in a healthy neonate, which is unparalleled accomplishment in view of the fact that fetal deformity or death could result from displacement or malformation of a few cells during early pregnancy. The nurse must help the woman maintain her health and emotional well-being, always taking into account the development and growth of the fetus when any action or decision regarding care of the woman is made.

Study Questions

1. *Why is it important for the nurse to know and understand the physiologic changes that occur in pregnancy?*
2. *What are the major physiologic changes that occur in the body systems?*
3. *What are the symptoms and discomforts of pregnancy that arise from these changes?*
4. *What body system is most affected by pregnancy and why?*
5. *What is the mechanism and treatment of supine hypotensive syndrome?*
6. *What are the possible implications of the decreased motility of the tissues of the urinary tract during pregnancy?*
7. *What are the major hormones of pregnancy, and how do they function?*
8. *Why are women concerned about the skin and body changes that occur during pregnancy?*

References

Blackburn, S., & Loper, D. (1992). *Maternal, fetal and neonatal physiology: A clinical perspective*. Philadelphia: W.B. Saunders.

Cunningham, F., MacDonald, P., & Gant, N. (1989). *Williams obstetrics* (18th ed.). Norwalk, CT: Appleton and Lange.

Gabbe, S., Niebyl, J., & Simpson J. (Eds.). (1992). *Obstetrics: normal and problem pregnancies* (2nd ed.). New York: Churchill Livingstone.

Suggested Readings

Alexander, L. (1987). The pregnant smoker: Nursing implications. *Journal of Obstetric, Gynecologic, and Neonatal Nursing, 16*, 167–173.

Fishbein, E., & Phillips, M. (1990) How safe is exercise during pregnancy? *Journal of Obstetric, Gynecologic, and Neonatal Nursing, 19*, 45–49.

Hofmeyr, G., Marcos, E., & Butchart, A. (1991). Pregnant women's perceptions of themselves: A survey. *Birth, 17*, 205–206.

Pletsch, P. (1991). Prevalence of cigarette smoking in Hispanic women of childbearing age. *Nursing Research, 40*, 103–106.

VanDinter, M. (1991). Pyalism in pregnant women. *Journal of Obstetric, Gynecologic, and Neonatal Nursing, 20*, 206–209.

CHAPTER 12

The Genetic Code and Fetal Development

Learning Objectives

After studying the material in this chapter, the student will be able to:

- Describe the significant events in fetal development.
- Explain how genes are transmitted in families.
- List the major categories of genetic disorders.
- Identify factors that can cause genetic disorders.
- Explain how risk for genetic disorders is assessed.
- Identify groups of women and men who may need referral for genetic counseling and evaluation.

Key Terms

autosome
chromosome
deoxyribonucleic acid
gene
karyotype
meiosis
mitosis
monosomy
pedigree
sex chromosome
teratogen
trisomy
zygote

Environmental and genetic factors affect health before conception and during the prenatal period. It is useful to understand the processes of transfer of genetic information from parents to children, the progression of normal embryonic and fetal development, and the sensitive periods when fetal damage is most likely to occur. This chapter includes an overview of the genetic code, normal fetal development, and the major genetic causes of abnormal fetal development. Nurses armed with this information can assess women and men of reproductive age in an effort to identity those at risk for abnormal fetal development. Nurses can then plan interventions that may reduce this risk by suggesting life-style changes or encouraging more extensive genetic counseling when that is indicated.

The Genetic Code

Genetics is the science of heredity. Genes are the coded sequences of information by which cellular organisms regulate their embryologic development, metabolic functioning, growth, and reproduction. The study of human genetics is becoming increasingly important to the childbearing process. Genetic factors play a role in the etiology of many birth defects and a variety of human diseases.

Genetic information is organized in small cellular structures known as chromosomes. Chromosomes are primarily composed of deoxyribonucleic acid (DNA) and proteins. DNA is a macromolecule composed of three types of chemical units:

- A five-carbon sugar (deoxyribose)
- A phosphate group
- Nitrogen-containing base subunits, of which there are two types: purines and pyrimidines

In DNA there are two purines, adenine (A) and guanine (G), and two pyrimidines, thymine (T) and cytosine (C).

In humans DNA occurs as a double-stranded helix or spiral. Two long chemical chains of DNA molecules are wound around one another. These chains are linked by chemical bonds so that the whole forms a shape like a spiral staircase (Fig. 12-1). The adenine (A) in one strand is bonded to thymine (T) in the other strand, and cytosine (C) in one strand is bonded to guanine (G) in the other strand. All the information needed for the development of an individual human being is carried in the sequence of these four nitrogen base subunits. The genetic code is a series of triplet sequences of the A, G, T, and C nitrogen bases. Each of the 21 amino acids, which are the building blocks of protein, are coded for by a particular combination of three of the nitrogen bases.

The gene, or the unit of hereditary information, is the part of the chromosome that codes for one particular cellular product or outcome. The gene is composed of coding sequences interrupted by noncoding sequences. Each chromosome is thought to contain thousands of genes lined up in a specific sequence. Each gene has a specific location on a particular chromosome. There are thought to be two types of genes. Structural genes control the manufacture of proteins. Regulatory genes control the activity of the structural genes.

Genetic mutations occur when the sequence of the nitrogen bases in a gene changes. These changes can occur in one of three ways:

- One or more of the bases is changed.
- A part of a gene or a whole gene may be lost in the process of chromosome replication or as a result of breakage.
- Additional nitrogen bases may be added to a gene sequence during replication or as a result of translocation.

The consequence of these changes is a misreading of the genetic code. Because each gene codes for a particular cellular product, a coding error can result in no cellular product, an overproduction or underproduction, or production of a cellular product that is structurally abnormal and biochemically inactive or inefficient (Levin, 1987).

Chromosome Structure and Identification

Chromosomes are visible as compact, well-defined structures only during cell division. Therefore, the tissues used to study chromosomes under the microscope must have many viable and rapidly dividing cells. Specially developed tissue culture techniques are used to obtain such cells so that the chromosomes can be studied and photographed. The most common tissues used for chromosome analysis are lymphocytes, skin fibroblasts, and amniotic fluid cells. Other tissues occasionally used to study chromosomes are testicular or ovarian biopsy tissues and bone marrow. After applying one of several different chemical stains, the underlying structure features or bands of the chromosomes are revealed (Fig. 12-2).

The morphology of chromosomes is most easily distinguished during the early parts of the cell division cycle. The prophase and metaphase panels of Figure 12-3 illustrate this. In metaphase, chromosomes observed under the microscope look like Xs and are made up of two identical DNA double helical strands. Each identical DNA strand is called a sister chromatid. These strands are attached to each other by a structure called the centromere (see Fig. 12-2). The centromere divides the chromosome into a short arm region and a long arm region.

The most efficient and accurate way to examine an individual's chromosomal makeup is to make a karyotype. A karyotype is a photograph that shows all the chromosomes of a single cell, arranged by matching pairs from the largest to the smallest. Chromosome analysis involves the microscopic examination of 20 to 30 properly prepared cells. The number of chromosomes in each cell is counted. Approximately five cells are photographed so that the sequence of

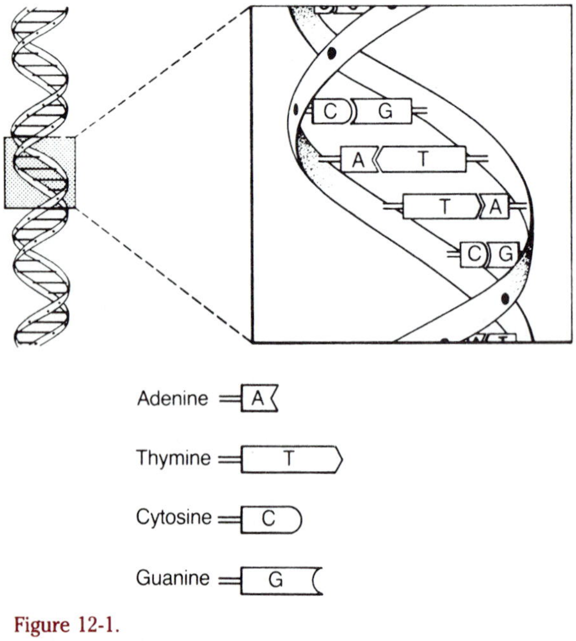

Figure 12-1.
Structure of DNA.

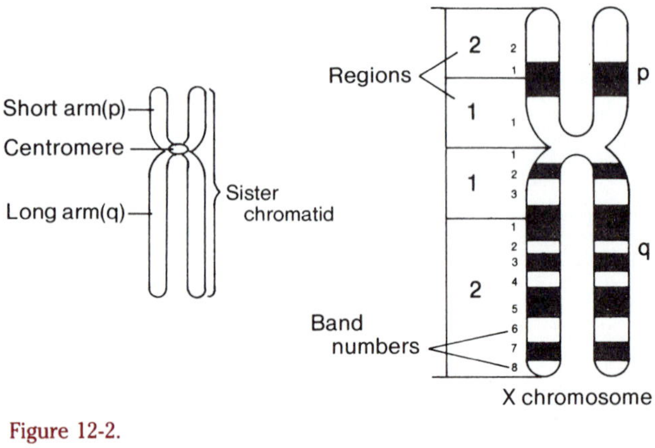

Figure 12-2.
Diagrammatic representation of chromosome structure at mitotic metaphase using chemical stains to differentiate tissue.

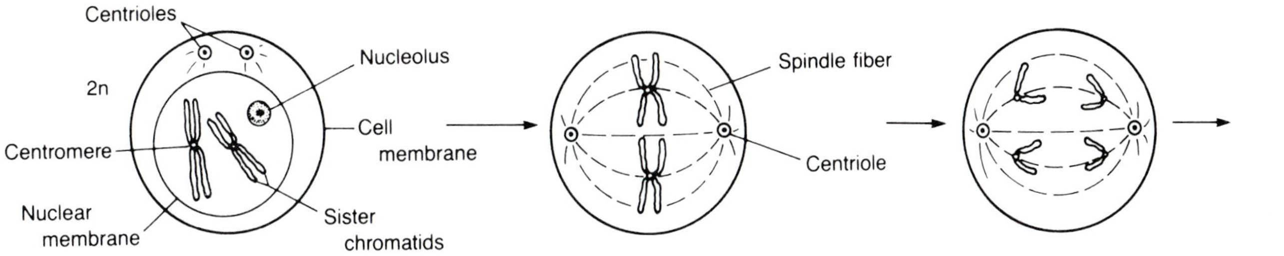

Prophase

Chromosomes are doubled, each consisting of two sister chromatids as they enter prophase. They are joined at the centromere. In late prophase/prometaphase, the nuclear membrane begins to disintegrate; centrioles separate and spindle fiber formation is seen.

Metaphase

Chromosomes line up on metaphase plate and are attached to spindle fibers at their centromere.

Anaphase

Centromeres divide, single-stranded sister chromatids (now chromosomes) are pulled to opposite poles.

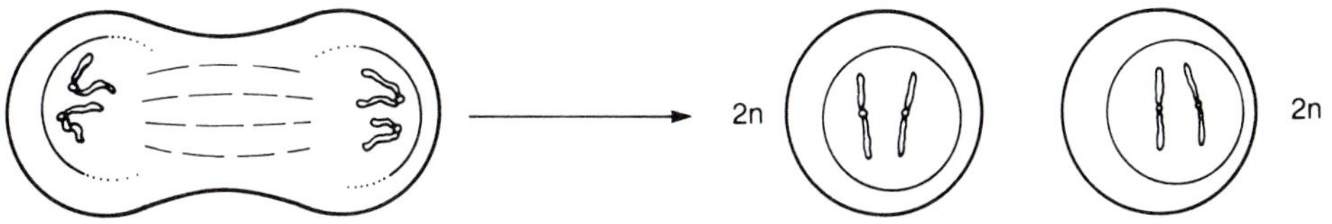

Telophase

Chromosomes reach poles and begin to uncoil and elongate; division furrow is seen at cell membrane; nucleolus and nuclear membrane reform at end.

Cell divides, and new daughter cells enter interphase.

Figure 12-3.
Mitosis shown with one autosomal chromosome pair.

bands can be examined. Numeric changes and structural rearrangements can be identified in this manner.

Classification and Replication of Human Chromosomes

Chromosomes are present in every cell of the body, with the exception of red blood cells, which have no nucleus. On each chromosome genes are arranged in specific sequences and serve as vehicles to transmit genetic information. The number, size, and shape of chromosomes are fixed for all normal members of any species. Somatic cells in the normal human have 46 chromosomes (except for sperm and egg cells or gametes, which have 23). In the cell, chromosomes are arranged in 22 pairs called autosomes. Each autosome is structurally identical to its partner but different from all others. In addition to autosomes, there are two sex-determining chromosomes in each cell, which are labeled X and Y. Normal males have one X and one Y chromosome, and normal females have two X chromosomes. Sperm and egg cells each have 23 chromosomes, one autosome from each pair and one sex chromosome.

The smaller number of chromosomes in sperm and egg cells results from the process of meiosis (Fig. 12-4). During this process genetic material may be exchanged between homologous chromosomes. Thus, each gamete contains half of an individual's genetic information, and the genetic information in each gamete may vary. During fertilization genetic material from two individuals is combined. This process results in genetic variability. New gene combinations may emerge at conception, some of which may be advantageous and some of which may not.

Genes are the coded sequences of information by which cellular organisms regulate their embryologic development, metabolic functioning, growth, and reproduction. Genetic information is organized in small cellular structures known as chromosomes. Chromosomes are primarily composed of DNA and proteins. Genetic mutations occur when the sequence of the nitrogen bases in a gene changes. In the cell, chromosomes are arranged in 22 pairs called autosomes. In addition to autosomes there are two sex-determining chromosomes in each cell, which are labeled X and Y. Normal males have one X and one Y chromosome, and normal females have two X chromosomes. The process of genetic exchange of mate-

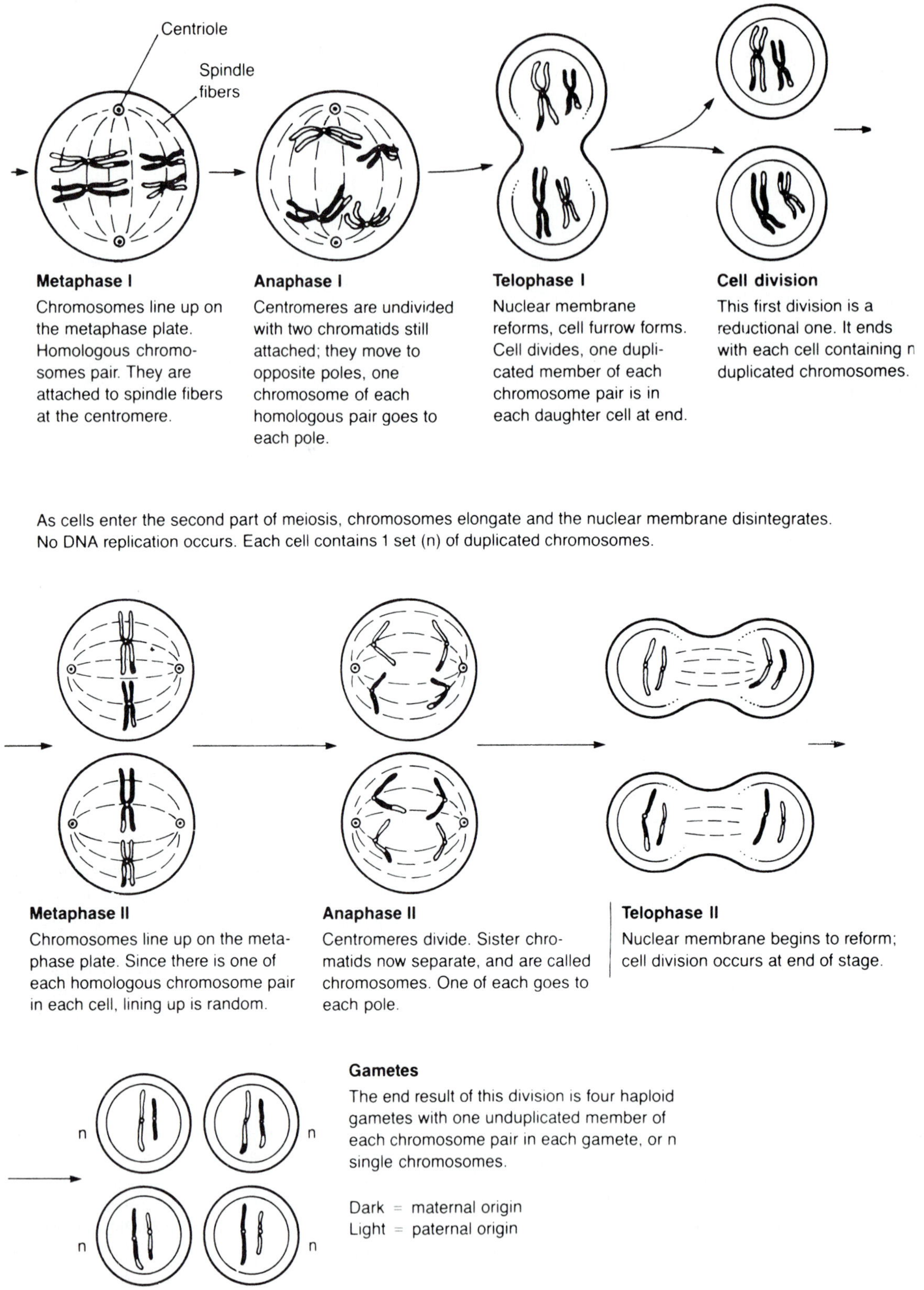

Centriole
Spindle fibers
Metaphase I
Chromosomes line up on the metaphase plate. Homologous chromosomes pair. They are attached to spindle fibers at the centromere.
Anaphase I
Centromeres are undivided with two chromatids still attached; they move to opposite poles, one chromosome of each homologous pair goes to each pole.
Telophase I
Nuclear membrane reforms, cell furrow forms. Cell divides, one duplicated member of each chromosome pair is in each daughter cell at end.
Cell division
This first division is a reductional one. It ends with each cell containing n duplicated chromosomes.
As cells enter the second part of meiosis, chromosomes elongate and the nuclear membrane disintegrates. No DNA replication occurs. Each cell contains 1 set (n) of duplicated chromosomes.
Metaphase II
Chromosomes line up on the metaphase plate. Since there is one of each homologous chromosome pair in each cell, lining up is random.
Anaphase II
Centromeres divide. Sister chromatids now separate, and are called chromosomes. One of each goes to each pole.
Telophase II
Nuclear membrane begins to reform; cell division occurs at end of stage.
n
n
n
n
Gametes
The end result of this division is four haploid gametes with one unduplicated member of each chromosome pair in each gamete, or n single chromosomes.
Dark = maternal origin
Light = paternal origin

Figure 12-4.
Meiosis with two autosomal chromosome pairs.

rial at conception ensures variability in the gene pool of the population.

Fetal Development

With fertilization the process of prenatal development begins and continues for 40 weeks. Prenatal development is divided into three periods:

- The preembryonic period (weeks 1 to 3), involving fertilization of the ovum, development of the conceptus, and formation of the three layers of the embryonic disk
- The embryonic period (weeks 4 to 8), involving rapid growth, tissue differentiation, and formation of all major organs
- The fetal period (weeks 9 to 40), involving growth and development of major body organs and differentiation of organ systems

Substantial developmental changes occur during these three periods. The major events of the first 10 weeks of fetal development are depicted in Figure 12-5. Serious insults during the first 10 weeks are most likely to result in spontaneous abortion.

Preembryonic Period (Weeks 1 to 3)

Fertilization, Cleavage, and Implantation

At conception (day 1) an ovum and sperm, each containing 23 chromosomes, fuse to form the zygote, or fertilized ovum. This is the first cell of the conceptus and contains 46 chromosomes. Each parent has contributed equally to the genetic makeup of this cell. The single-celled zygote divides through the process of mitosis, producing genetically identical daughter cells (see Fig. 12-3). This exact duplication of genetic information is necessary for the differentiation, growth, and biologic maintenance of the organism.

The zygote passes through the fallopian tubes and divides approximately 30 hours after conception into two daughter cells (see Fig. 12-5, stage 2). Subdivisions continue as the original cells result in increasing numbers. This type of cell division is called *cleavage*. By the time the zygote is ready to enter the uterus, it has become a solid ball of 12 to 16 cells called the morula.

Intracellular fluid in the spaces of the morula increases, and a central cavity develops; the conceptus is now called the blastocyst (see Fig. 12-5, stage 3). The blastocyst floats freely in the uterus, nourished by secretions from the uterine lining, called the endometrium. The blastocyst is now comprised of a double layer of cells, called the embryonic disk (see Fig. 12-5, stage 8).

The blastocyst attaches to the uterine lining, usually on the upper lateral wall below the opening from the fallopian tube. The outer cell layer develops fingerlike projections enabling the blastocyst to attach to the endometrium. This process, called *implantation*, occurs within 6 days after conception (see Fig. 12-5, stage 4).

Development of Fetal Membranes and Placenta

During the second week the blastocyst continues to differentiate, forming structures that will become the primitive nervous system (see Fig. 12-5, stage 6). The formation of the placenta and fetal membranes begins at this point. Early uteroplacental circulation begins by maternal blood and endometrial secretions filling spaces, or lacunae, in the outer layer of the blastocyst. Thus, just before week 2 and before the first missed menstrual period, substances in maternal blood can diffuse to the blastocyst. By the end of the second week, the uterine lining at the implantation site has begun to change; it is now called the *decidua* (Fig. 12-6). As pregnancy progresses, the decidua extends to cover the entire lining of the uterus and becomes thickened and extremely vascular.

The fetal membranes (including the chorion, the amnion, and the placenta) develop in the second week of life. The chorion is a layer of cells that develops projections or villi that reach into the decidua (Fig. 12-7). The function of the villi is to allow for diffusion of nutrients from maternal blood and waste products from fetal blood. Small fetal blood vessels form in villi and connect to the fetal heart to allow blood circulation in the primitive embryo.

The amnion forms the wall of the amniotic cavity, and its cells produce amniotic fluid. Continuing growth of the embryo causes it to bulge into the amniotic cavity. As the cavity enlarges, the amnion and chorion fuse.

The placenta is a temporary organ shared by the woman and fetus; it allows exchange of substances by diffusion and active transport between maternal and fetal circulation, as shown in Figure 12-8. Nutrients, oxygen, and fetal waste products diffuse across fetal and maternal membranes. Maternal circulation enters and exits the intervillous spaces by way of uterine blood vessels. Fetal circulation is linked with the placenta and depends on the action of the fetal heart. Maternal and fetal blood do not mix. However, occasional breaks in the chorionic villi do allow leakage of fetal erythrocytes into the maternal circulation.

The placenta has the following functions:

- Respiration: By the process of diffusion, oxygen from maternal blood passes into the placenta and then into fetal blood.
- Nutrition: Carbohydrates, water, fats, proteins, and minerals pass from maternal blood into the fetal system.
- Excretion: End products of fetal metabolism cross the placenta into maternal circulation.
- Protection: The placenta forms a barrier that protects the fetus from many harmful substances.
- Endocrine: The placenta secretes estrogen, progesterone, human chorionic gonadotropin, and human placental lactogen, all of which are important for normal physiologic regulation of pregnancy (see Chapter 4).
- Immunity: Immunity to diseases including smallpox, diphtheria, and measles can be passed to the fetus from maternal antibodies.

Text continues on page 259

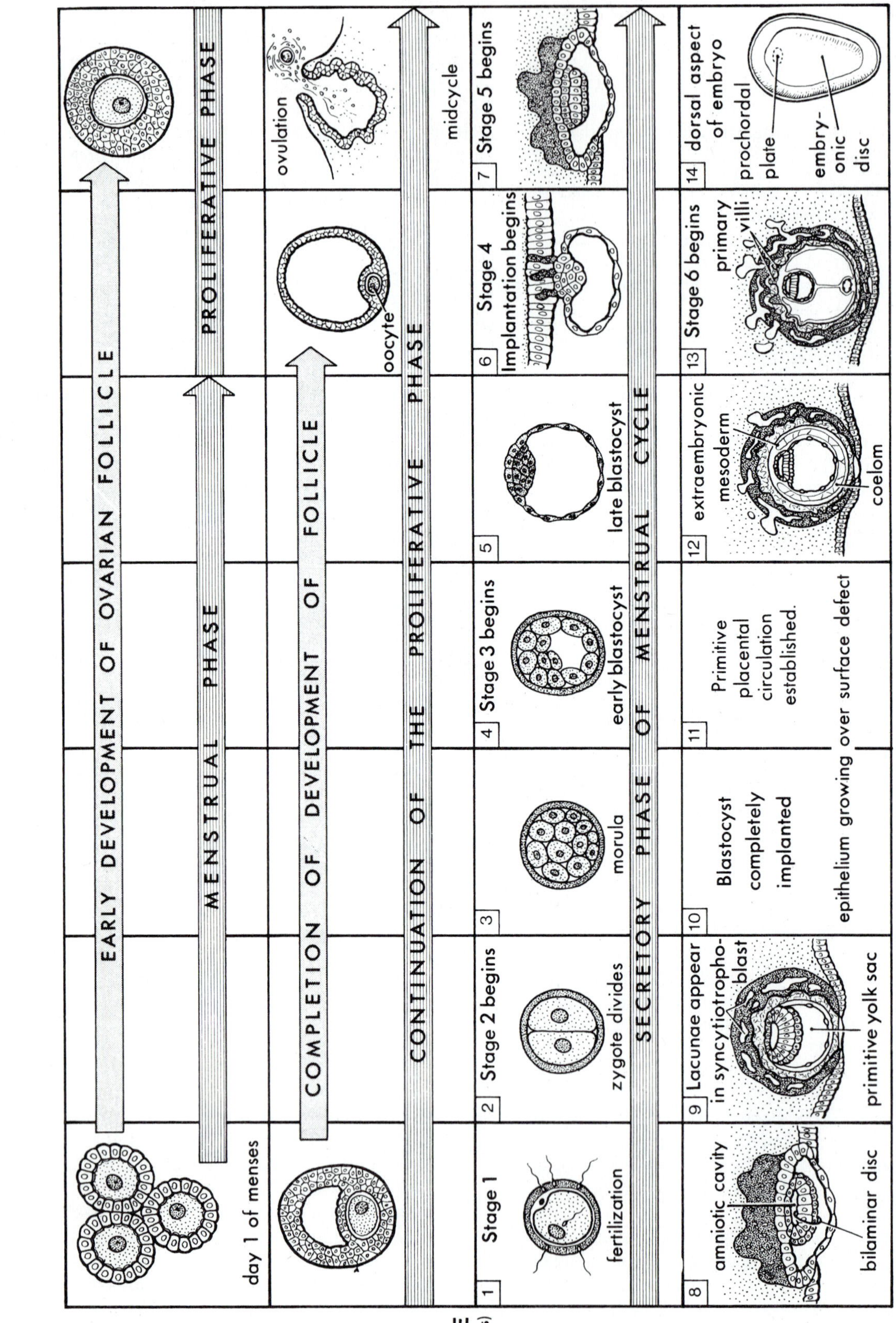

Figure 12-5.
Timetable of human prenatal development, 1 to 2 weeks. (Moore, K. L. [1982]. *The developing human*. Philadelphia: W. B. Saunders.)

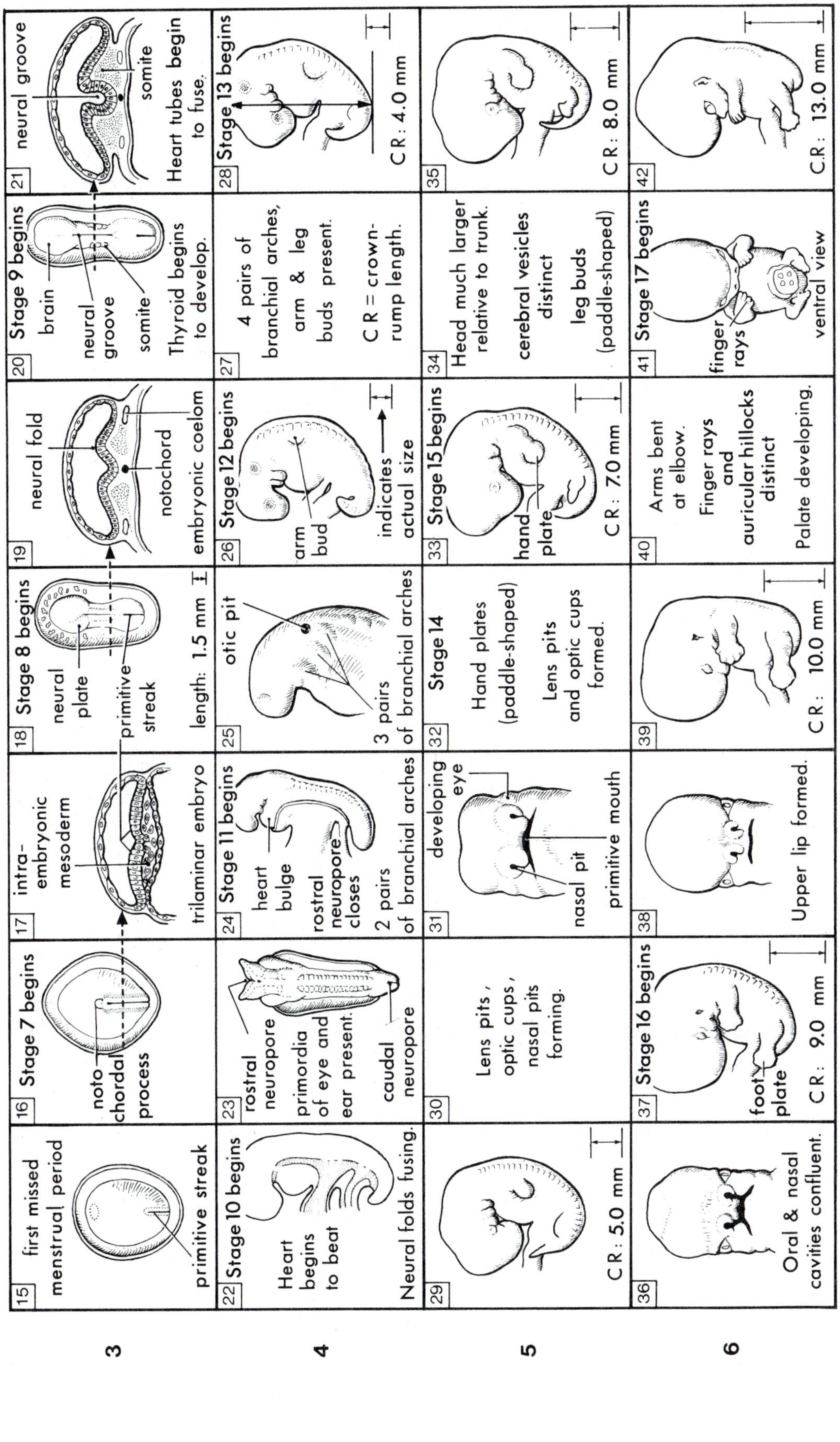

Figure 12-5. *(continued)*

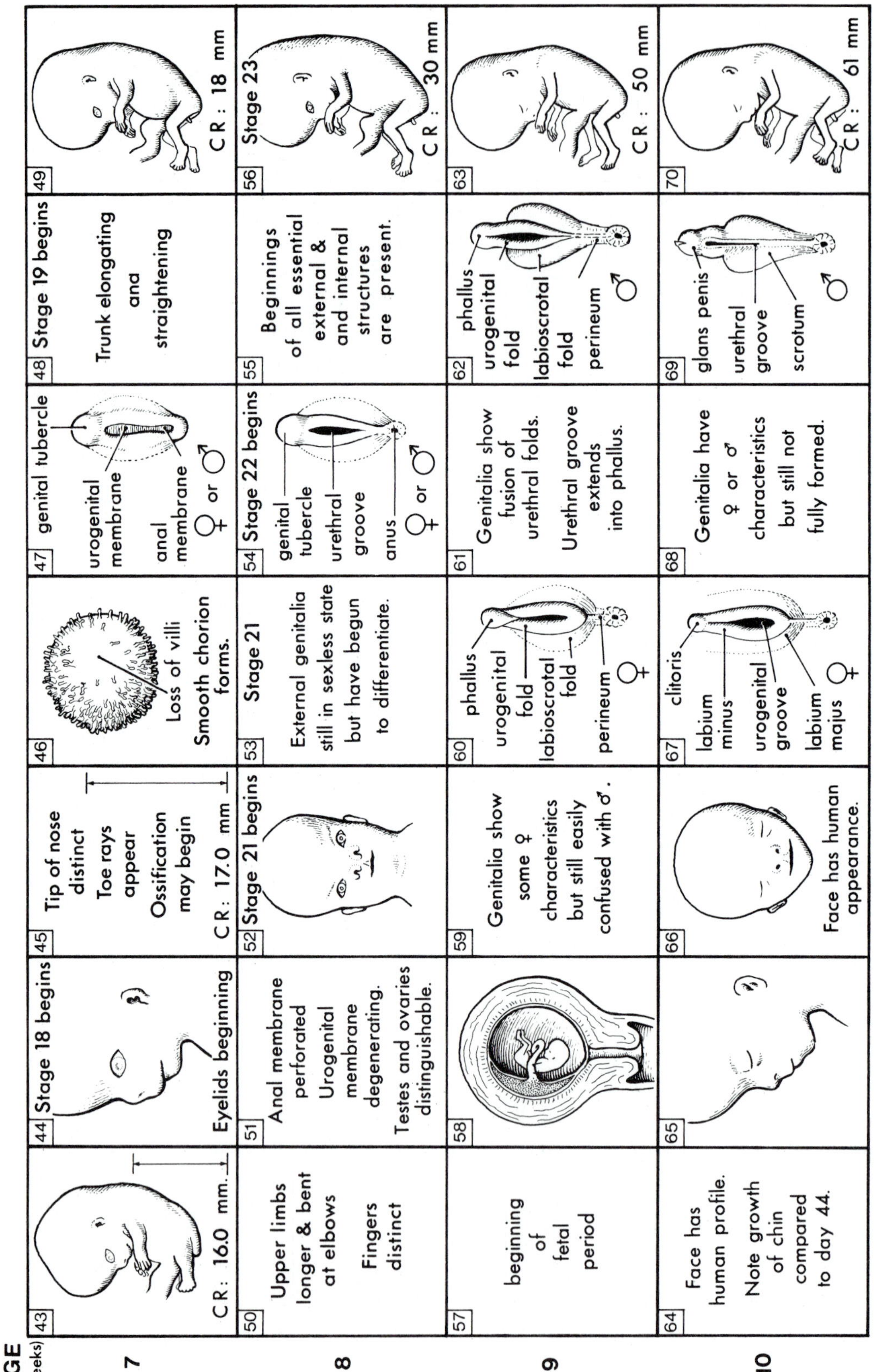

Figure 12-5. (*continued*)

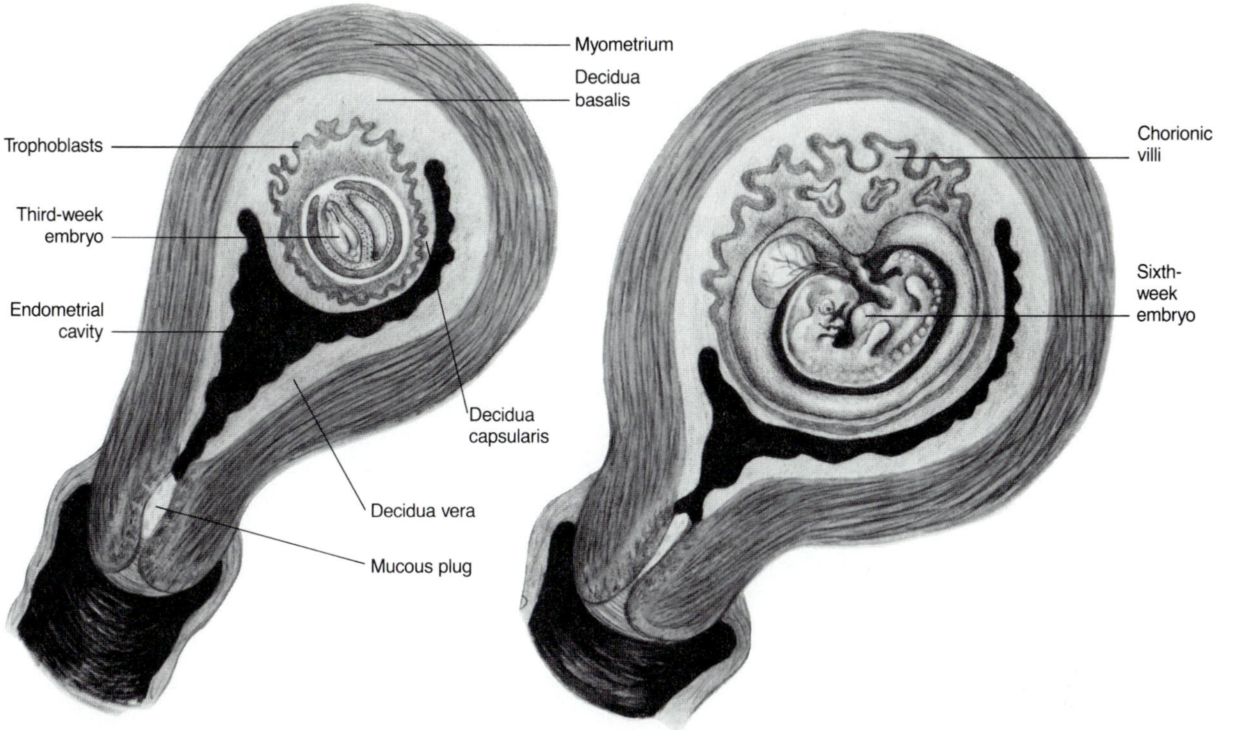

Figure 12-6.
Uterine decidua. Decidua is the name given to the endometrium that envelops the developing ovum. The decidua basalis unites with the chorion to form the placenta. The decidua capsularis surrounds the chorionic sac. The decidua vera is the endometrium of pregnancy that covers all but the blastocyst (Childbirth Graphics®, Waco, Texas).

Placental Transfer

The process of transfer of substances through the placenta is complex. The term "placental barrier" is not completely accurate, because the placenta does permit the ready transfer of a wide range of substances and provides only limited protection to the fetus. The placenta is capable of active or selective transport of some substances. Glucose, calcium, iron, and amino acids are actively transported across placental membranes. Oxygen, carbon dioxide, water, and some electrolytes pass through the placenta by simple diffusion.

Most drugs pass by diffusion through the placenta readily, and many are harmful to the fetus. For this reason all but essential medications should be avoided, especially during the first trimester.

Other substances, such as hormones that have higher molecular weights, pass by diffusion but more slowly. Some immunoglobulins cross from maternal to fetal circulation. Many viruses may cross the placenta and infect the fetus. Larger bacteria rarely affect the fetus, unless the placenta itself is inflamed.

Gastrulation

During the third and final week of the preembryonic phase, the conceptus develops rapidly. Cell layers differentiate (see Fig. 12-5, stage 7) by a process known as *gastrulation*. These cell layers become all the tissues and organs of the embryo. The primitive nervous system begins to develop (see Fig. 12-5, stages 8 and 9) (Moore, 1993).

Normal and Abnormal Events

By the third week of life, the conceptus is approximately 1 mm in length. Major developmental events of weeks 1 to 3 are summarized in the accompanying display. In addition to normal events, abnormal events also may occur during these initial 3 weeks.

Embryonic Period (Weeks 4 to 8)

During this short period of 4 weeks, embryonic development is extremely rapid. All major internal and external organs and organ systems are formed, a process known as *organogenesis*. The embryo changes in shape, and major features of the external body are recognizable by 8 weeks. This stage of growth and development holds the potential for major congenital malformations if the embryo is exposed to teratogens, such as some drugs, chemicals, viruses, and other substances.

During this period the embryo elongates with the formation of a recognizable head and tail. The primitive circulatory system is established. The fetal heartbeat begins and can be detected by ultrasonography by the eighth week. It doubles in size, and its atria and ventricles are visible through the ectoderm. The umbilical cord is now formed. It contains two umbilical arteries and one umbilical vein (see Fig. 12-5, stages 14 and 15). Budlike projections on the surface mark the beginning of limbs. The limb buds are most vulnerable to teratogens at this time.

During the final week of this period, the embryo exhibits

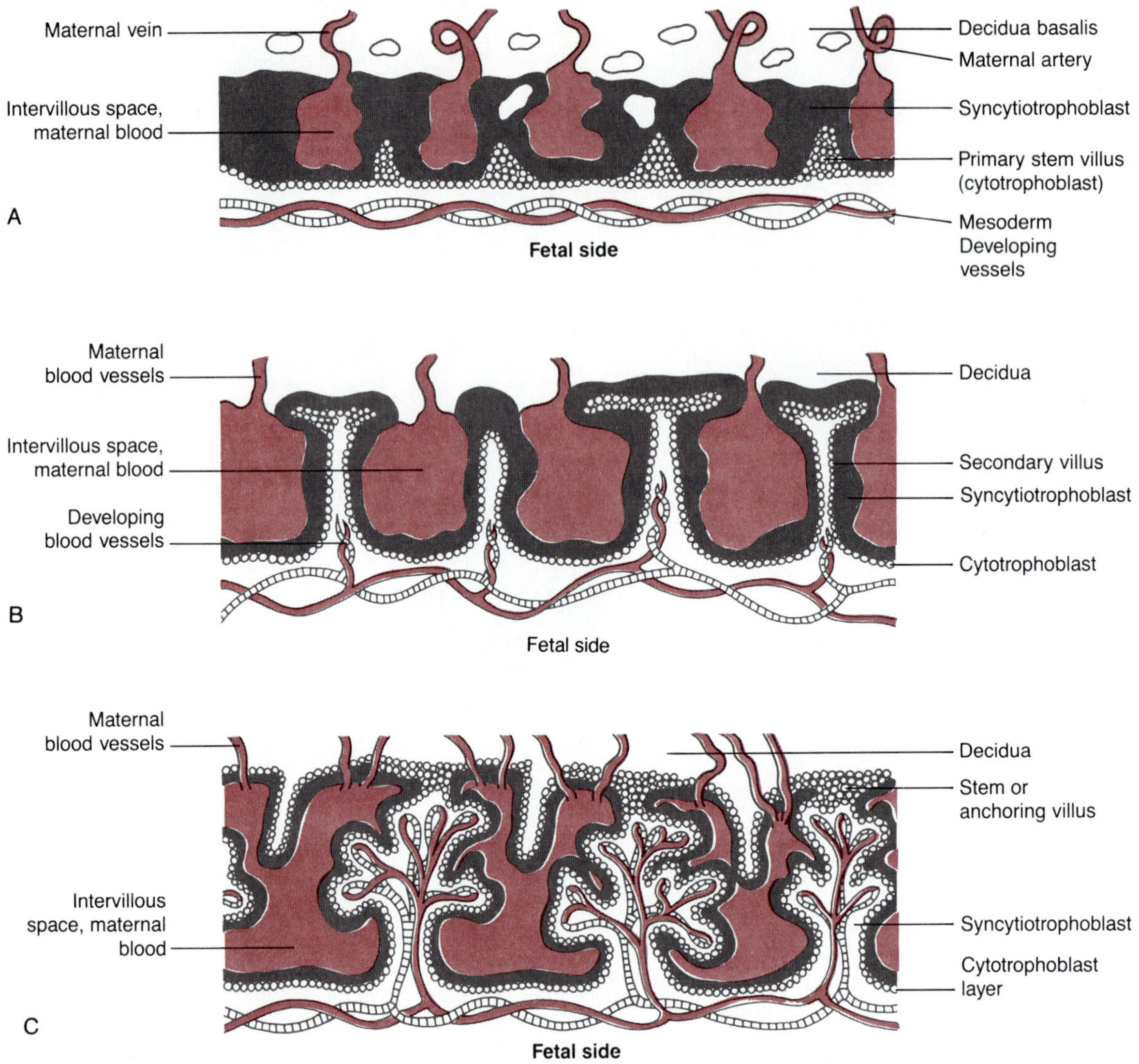

Figure 12-7.

Development of the chorionic villi. *A:* By the second week the primary stem villi consists of a primary stem core made up of cytotrophoblasts, covered by syncytiotrophoblasts. *B:* The mesoderm of the chorion invades the core of each primary villus, which then becomes known as a secondary villus. *C:* By the end of the third week the tertiary villi are formed, and by the end of 4 weeks, tertiary villi cover the entire surface of the chorion (Childbirth Graphics®, Waco, Texas).

definite human characteristics. The head now makes up 50% of the mass of the embryo. Eyelid folds develop, and the eyes continue to move to a frontal position. Fingers and toes are distinct by the end of the eighth week. Sexual differences in the external genitalia can now be seen by the trained eye. The growth in size and complexity of the embryo during this period is quite remarkable (see Fig. 12-5, stages 21 and 22 and Fig. 12-9) (Moore, 1993).

Normal and Abnormal Events

The major events of the embryonic period are summarized in the accompanying display. Major congenital malformations may occur during the embryonic period.

Fetal Period (Weeks 9 to 40)

When the basic organ structures of the embryo have been established and it has recognizable human characteristics, it is called a fetus. During the fetal period the tissues and organs that began their development during the embryonic period continue their growth and differentiation.

The rate of development during this period is most rapid in the first 16 weeks. Male and female external genitalia are not distinguishable at 9 weeks but are fully differentiated at 12 weeks. Production of red blood cells begins in the liver. This function is then assumed by the spleen at 12 weeks. By 16 weeks the kidneys have begun to function, and the fetus begins to swallow amniotic fluid and secrete urine. Fine hair,

Major Events of the Preembryonic Period (Weeks 1 to 3)

Normal Events

Week 1

- Fertilization and formation of the zygote (30 hours)
- Cleavage of the zygote into 12 to 16 blastomeres—the morula (days 2 and 3)
- Formation of the blastocyst (day 4)
- Attachment of the blastocyst (days 5–8)

Week 2

- Formation of the inner cytotrophoblast and outer syncytiotrophoblastic layers (days 7 and 8)
- Invasion of trophoblasts in maternal endometrium and sinusoids (day 8)
- Appearance of the amniotic cavity (day 8)
- Formation of lacunar networks (day 9)
- Establishment of primitive uteroplacental circulation (day 11)
- Formation of primitive chorionic villi (day 13)
- Deciduation of the uterine lining (day 14)
- Development of prochordal plate (day 14)

Week 3

- Formation of blood vessels within the chorionic villi (day 13)
- Gastrulation or conversion of the bilaminar embryonic disk into the three-layered trilaminar disk (day 14)
- Continued development of the chorion with formation of tertiary chorionic villi (days 15–20)
- Development of the neural tube (day 18)
- Formation of somites (day 21)
- Beginning of blood circulation (day 24)

Possible Abnormal Events

- Attachment of the blastocyst in the lower uterine segment rather than in the fundal area can restrict its growth and cause early abortion.
- Abnormal implantation can occur. The blastocyst can contain defective blastomeres, or the trophoblastic cells can develop abnormally. Either can cause spontaneous abortion.
- Ectopic pregnancy can occur. The blastocyst can implant at sites other than the endometrium, leading to an ectopic pregnancy. The most common ectopic sites are the fallopian tubes, accounting for 90% of these pregnancies. Other sites are the pelvis or abdomen. All ectopic implantations cause serious and potentially fatal problems for the woman and often result in spontaneous abortion.
- Maternal infection or a genetic defect may interfere with normal zygote development. Severe damage from teratogens results in spontaneous abortion.
- Chromosomal abnormalities usually result in spontaneous abortions during the first 3 weeks. Estimates are that 50% to 60% of early spontaneous abortions are from such abnormalities. Other causes of early spontaneous abortions are underdevelopment of the endometrium, blighted ovum, and uterine myomas.
- Hydatidiform mole results from excessive invasion of the syncytiotrophoblastic cells in the uterine cavity. The fetus dies, but the trophoblastic cells continue to proliferate and fill the uterine cavity with grapelike clusters.
- If one fertilized ovum splits to form two identical embryos, monozygous twins result. Rarely, splitting on the inner cell mass may be incomplete, resulting in conjoined twins.
- The heart is most susceptible to teratogens between the 19th and 41st days.

called lanugo, forms on the forehead. Fingernails are now formed.

By 20 weeks the fetal body is covered with lanugo. Sebaceous glands begin to secrete sebum, from which vernix caseosa is formed. Vernix is a cheeselike substance that covers the skin of the fetus and protects it from drying and hardening due to exposure to amniotic fluid. Fetal contours are rounder, with increasing deposition of subcutaneous fat. Fetal movements are first felt by the mother between 16 and 20 weeks, and fetal heart tones can be heard with a fetoscope.

The fetus is not yet considered viable. By 24 weeks the fetus may survive outside the uterus, and by 27 weeks survival is more likely, although respiratory function is still quite immature. By 36 weeks the fetus is steadily gaining weight. Vernix has become thick. Survival is likely if born at this point. By 40 weeks the fetus is completely developed. Fingernails and toenails are formed. The testicles of the male fetus have descended into the scrotum. The skull is developed and larger than any other portion of the body (Moore, 1993).

Fetal Circulation

Fetal circulation (Fig. 12-9) is different from that of the newborn and infant. During fetal life the lungs do not function as respiratory organs. The gas exchange function is wholly carried out by the placenta, and blood flow is for nutrition and excretion purposes only. Oxygenated blood flows through veins in the chorionic villi and to the fetus through the umbilical vein. Flow of oxygenated blood from

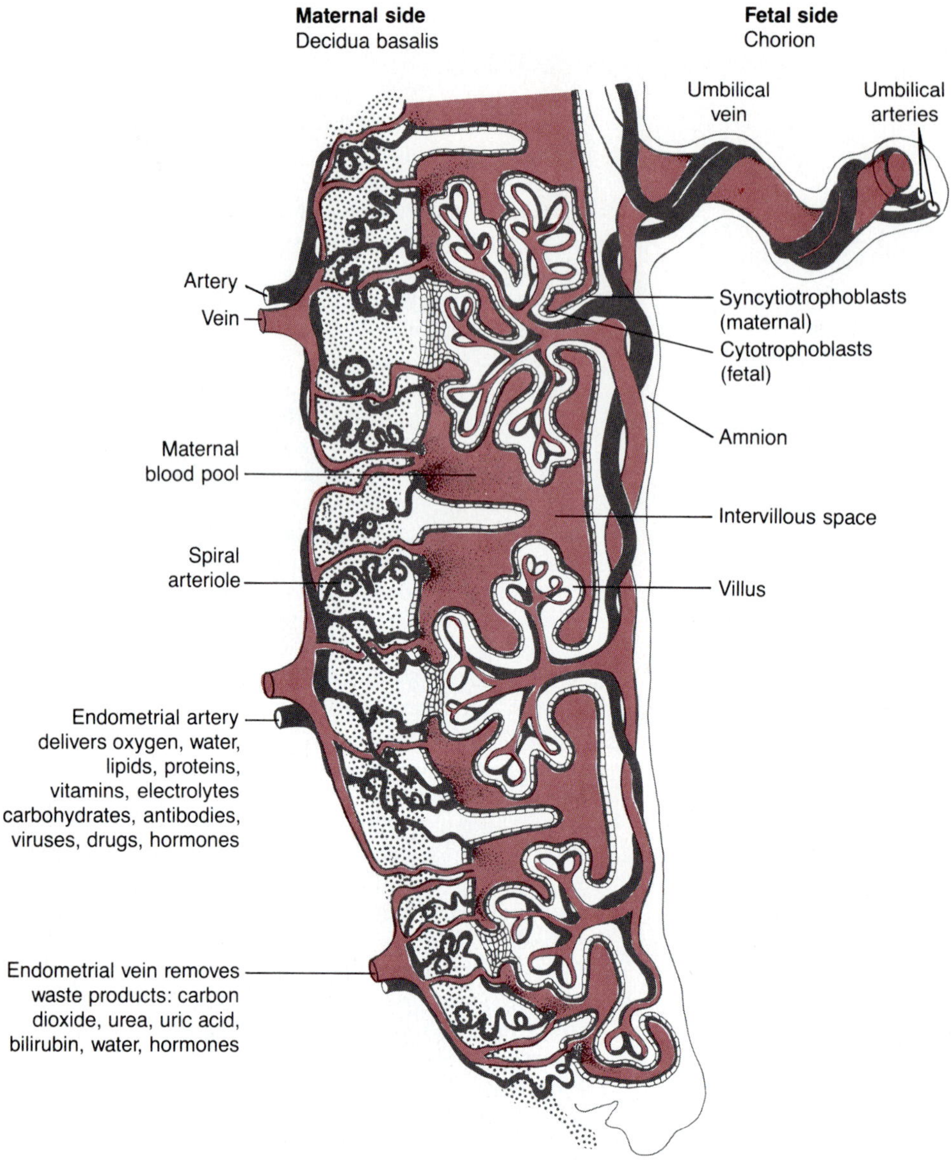

Figure 12-8.
Placental membrane and fetal–maternal exchange (Childbirth Graphics®, Waco, Texas).

the umbilical vein enters the right atrium. Here it mixes with deoxygenated blood returning to the heart from the superior vena cava. Most of this mixture of oxygenated and deoxygenated blood passes through the foramen ovale into the left atrium. (Some passes through the tricuspid valve into the right ventricle and out the pulmonary artery. Most blood in the pulmonary artery passes through the ductus arteriosus and into the aorta. Only a small portion of fetal blood circulates to the lungs.)

Blood in the left atrium mixes with the small amount returning from the lungs through the pulmonary veins. Blood then moves from the left atrium through the mitral valve into the left ventricle and out into the aorta where it mixes with blood from the ductus arteriosus. The blood in the aorta circulates to the upper and lower reaches of the body, as in adult circulation. The umbilical arteries (branching off the internal iliac arteries) carry deoxygenated blood back to the placenta (Danforth & Scott, 1990).

Normal and Abnormal Events

The major normal and abnormal events of the fetal period are summarized in the accompanying display.

Prenatal development is divided into three periods: the preembryonic period (weeks 1 to 3), the embryonic period (weeks 4 to 8), and the fetal period (weeks 9 to 40). The preembryonic period includes fertilization of the ovum and the development of key cell layers, which are the basis of further development. The embryonic period involves rapid growth, differentiation of tissue, and formation of all major organs. The fetal period completes the growth and development of major organs and organ systems.

The placenta is a temporary organ that is shared by the woman and fetus, allowing exchange of substances by diffusion and active transport between maternal and fetal circulation. The placenta provides some protection

Major Events of the Embryonic Period (Weeks 4 to 8)

Normal Events

- Conversion of the flat trilaminar embryonic disk into a C-shaped cylindric embryo
- Formation of the head, tail, and lateral folds
- Formation of the primitive gut by incorporation of the yolk sac into the embryo
- Formation of the lateral and ventral body walls
- Acquisition of an epithelial covering by the umbilicus through the expansion of the amnion
- Establishment of ventral position of the heart and development of the brain in the cranial region of the embryo
- Differentiation of the three germ layers into various tissues and layers that will become established as the major organ systems
- Appearance of the brain, limbs, ears, eyes, and nose
- Development of a human appearance by the embryo

Possible Abnormal Events

- Critical development of organ systems between 4 and 8 weeks of life renders the embryo vulnerable to developmental or environmental influences that may cause malformation:
  - Abnormalities of the genes and chromosomes
  - Alterations of maternal health, such as infection from rubella or herpes
  - Ingestion of teratogenic substances
- During the embryonic period, the risk of mortality is greater than at any other time of life.

Art courtesy of Childbirth Graphics®, Waco, Texas.

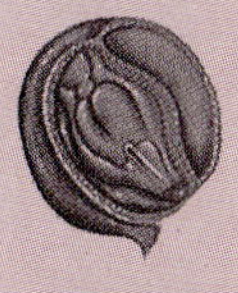
Third week

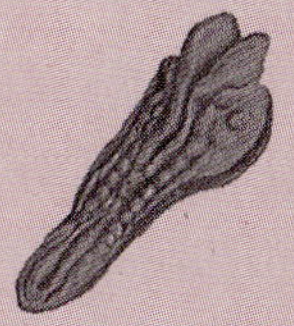
Fourth week

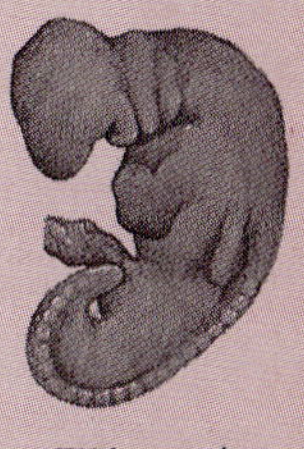
Fifth week

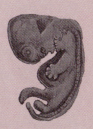

Sixth week

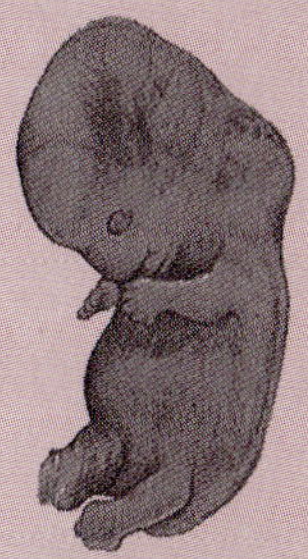
Seventh week

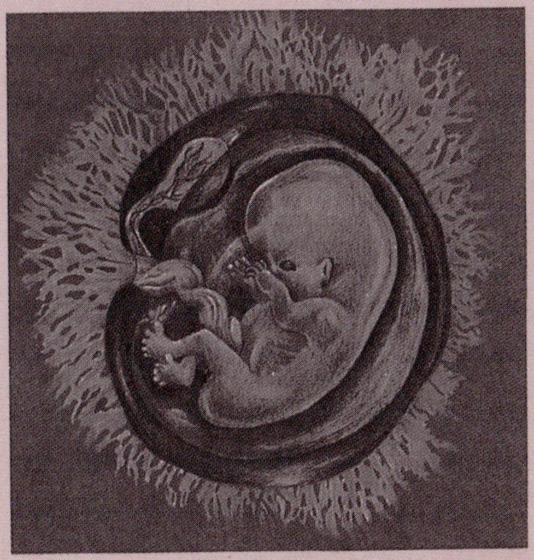
Eighth week

for the fetus, but many harmful substances pass readily from maternal to fetal circulation. The placenta carries out the fetal respiratory function; blood flow through the fetus differs substantially from adult circulation and is for nutrition and excretion purposes only.

Abnormalities in Fetal Development

Most newborns exhibit no observable abnormalities. For those few who are born with abnormalities, the cause often is unclear. Of all malformations 15% to 20% are thought to be genetic, 8% to 10% are a result of environmental factors or maternal disease, and the remaining 65% are of unknown etiology.

Genetic Disorders

The following section discusses genetically based abnormalities.

There are three major categories of genetic disorders: chromosomal abnormalities, single gene inheritance, and multifactorial inheritance.

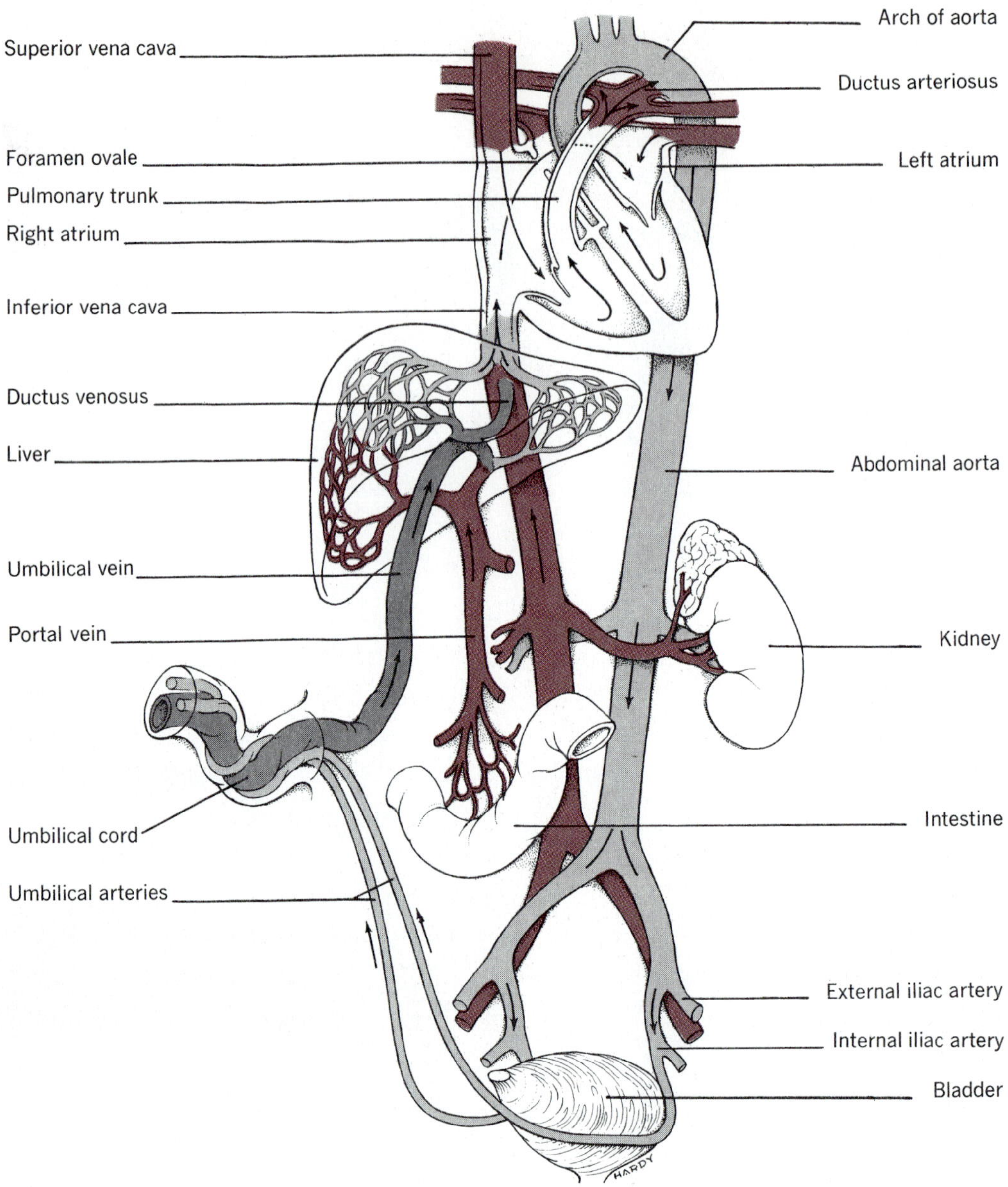

Figure 12-9.

Fetal circulation. By a complex process oxygen passes from the mother's bloodstream through the placenta and into the fetal blood. The course of blood in the fetus is indicated by arrows. Oxygenated blood travels to all fetal organs except the lungs.

Chromosomal Abnormalities

Changes in chromosome number or chromosome structure are a significant cause of spontaneous abortion or fetal wastage during pregnancy. In newborns congenital abnormalities and mental retardation can result from chromosomal abnormalities.

Numeric Abnormalities

A change in the amount of chromosomal material usually has detrimental effects during prenatal and neonatal development. The absence of a single chromosome is called *monosomy* and usually is lethal to the embryo. The presence of an extra chromosome, called *trisomy*, generally is incompatible with life. However, trisomies involving the smaller chromosomes are found in liveborn neonates with congenital defects and mental retardation. Monosomies and trisomies usually are caused by mechanical accidents during meiosis and can involve autosomes or sex chromosomes. Clinical diagnosis usually is made at birth and is confirmed by karyotype analysis.

Autosomal Abnormalities. Numeric abnormalities in autosomal chromosomes include autosomal monosomy, which is rare and usually incompatible with fetal life, trisomy 21 (Down syndrome), trisomy 13 (Patau syndrome), and trisomy 18 (Edwards syndrome). Clinical features of these abnormalities are summarized in Table 12-1. Trisomy 21, or

Major Events of the Fetal Period (Weeks 9 to 40)

Normal Events

Weeks 9 to 12

- Fetal head makes up one-half the fetal body.
- CRL doubles between 9 and 12 weeks.
- Eyelids remain fused.
- Upper limbs develop to normal proportions, while the lower limbs remain less developed.
- Male and female genitalia are recognizable by 12 weeks.
- Production of red blood cells transfers from the liver to the spleen at 12 weeks.

Weeks 13 to 16

- Rapid fetal growth occurs.
- Fetus doubles in size.
- Lanugo begins to grow.
- Fingernails are formed.
- Kidneys begin to secrete urine.
- Fetus begins to swallow amniotic fluid.
- Fetus appears human.
- Placenta is fully formed.

Weeks 17 to 23

- Fetal growth slows.
- Lower limbs become fully formed.
- Fetal body is covered with lanugo.
- Vernix caseosa covers the body to protect the skin from amniotic fluid.
- Fetal movement is first felt by the mother around 20 weeks.
- Fetal heartbeat is first heard with a fetoscope.
- Brown fat forms.

Weeks 24 to 27

- Skin growth is rapid, and skin appears red and wrinkled.
- The eyes open, and eyelashes and eyebrows are formed.
- The fetus becomes viable at 27 weeks.

Weeks 28 to 31

- Subcutaneous fat is deposited.
- If the fetus is born at this time with immature lungs, respiratory distress syndrome may occur.

Weeks 32 to 36

- Weight gain is steady.
- Lanugo has disappeared from the body but remains on the head.
- Fingernails are growing.
- The fetus has a good chance of survival if born during these weeks.

Weeks 37 to 40

- Subcutaneous fat builds up steadily, and fetal contours become rounded.
- Fingernails and toenails are fully formed and extend beyond the ends of the fingers and toes.
- Both testes have descended in the male.
- The skull is fully developed and is larger than any other part of the body.

Possible Abnormal Events

- Mothers who use over-the-counter drugs indiscriminately are more likely to have infants with congenital malformations.
- Withdrawal seizure may occur in infants born to an alcoholic mother, and the newborn may experience fetal alcohol syndrome.
- Inadequate fetal growth may result from intrauterine infections, multiple pregnancies, and chromosome abnormalities.
- Intrauterine growth retardation may result from maternal narcotic use, cigarette smoking, and inadequate prenatal nutrition.
- Fetal growth retardation may result from placental insufficiency caused by such defects as placental infarction.
- Preterm birth is a major threat to survival.

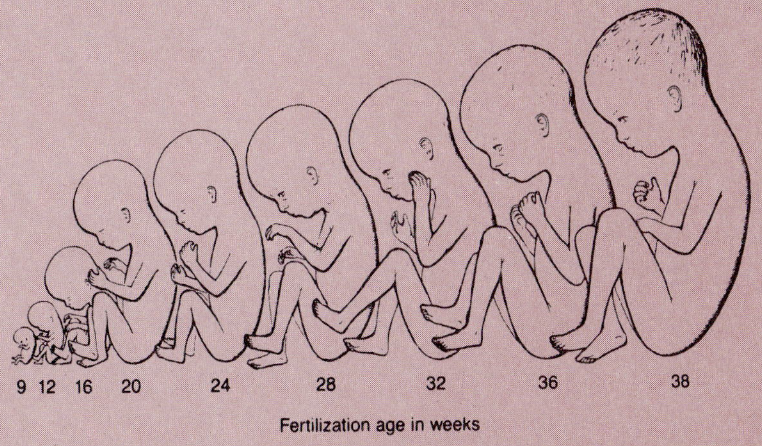

Redrawn from Moore, K.L. (1982). The developing human. Philadelphia: W.B. Saunders.

Table 12-1. Summary of Numeric Chromosomal Abnormalities

Type	Synonym	Incidence	Diagnostic Features at Birth	Prognosis	Detection
Autosomal Monosomy					
		Rare Usually incompatible with fetal survival			
Sex Chromosome Monosomy					
XO	Turner syndrome*	1/10,000 live female births Most common chromosomal abnormality in spontaneous abortions (18%)	Edema of hands and feet Increased incidence of coarctation of the aorta Somatic abnormalities may be few, and condition often is not recognized at birth	Normal intelligence Sterile	Buccal smear for X chromatin bodies may be negative. Endocrine levels are abnormal. Abnormality usually revealed in adolescence by presence of short stature, ovarian streaks, and amenorrhea. Estrogen at puberty may aid development of secondary sex characteristics.
Autosomal Trisomy					
Trisomy 13	Patau syndrome	1/20,000 live births	Microphthalmia (very small eyeballs) Cleft lip Postaxial polydactyly (extra digits) Microcephaly Malformed ears Congenital heart defects Urogenital defects Polycystic kidneys	Severe mental retardation 50% die within first year of life	Karyotype analysis confirms diagnosis.
Trisomy 18	Edwards syndrome	1/8,000 live births	Micrognathia (small jaw) Clenched fist with second and fifth fingers overlapping the third and fourth Rocker-bottom feet Low-set, malformed ears Congenital heart defects	Severe mental retardation in all cases Death usual in first few months	Karyotype analysis confirms diagnosis.
Trisomy 21	Down syndrome	1/800 live births Most common chromosome disorder	Typical round face with flat profile Protruding tongue Epicanthal folds Brushfields' spots (speckling of irises) Simian palm creases	Mild to severe retardation Increased incidence of leukemia Congenital heart defects (40% to 60% of cases) may require surgical correction	Karyotype analysis confirms diagnosis; "older" mother is at higher risk for offspring with this syndrome.
Sex Chromosome Trisomy					
XXX	Triple X syndrome	1/1,000 female births	None	Usually normal intelligence, but slightly increased incidence of mental retardation Fertile, with normal offspring	"Older" mother is at higher risk for offspring with this syndrome. Buccal smears may reveal triple-X karyotype.

(*continued*)

Table 12-1. Summary of Numeric Chromosomal Abnormalities ***(Continued)***

Type	Synonym	Incidence	Diagnostic Features at Birth	Prognosis	Detection
XXY	Klinefelter syndrome	1/1,000 live male births	None—signs usually appear after adolescence	Usually normal intelligence Mild mental retardation does occur Sterile	Feminine characteristics appear in puberty, including gynecomastia. Typically, sufferer is tall and gangly with small testes and underdeveloped facial and body hair. Breast reduction may be advised for psychological and cosmetic reasons.
XYY		1/1,000 live births	None	Rarely, may be associated with some intellectual impairment Fertile	Abnormality may remain undetected until revealed on karyotyping. In persons with XYY syndrome, sperm count may be reduced, and plasma testosterone levels may be high.

*Turner syndrome also can be the result of other chromosomal abnormalities, but these are extremely rare.

Down syndrome, is the most common clinically recognized chromosome disorder. It has an incidence of 1 in every 800 births and occurs whenever an individual is born with an extra number 21 chromosome. In 95% of all cases of Down syndrome, the affected person has three structurally normal number 21 chromosomes instead of two. Affected children often survive and may live into adulthood. The extent of retardation is variable, and special educational programs are beneficial in most cases. Trisomy 13 and trisomy 18 are severe disorders with poor prognoses.

Sex Chromosome Abnormalities. The most common sex chromosome abnormalities are triple X (XXX) syndrome, XXY (Klinefelter syndrome), and XYY syndrome. The only monosomy compatible with life is known XO (Turner syndrome) and is caused by the loss of one sex chromosome. Clinical features of these abnormalities are summarized in Table 12-1. In general the effects of sex chromosome abnormalities are less severe than those of autosomal abnormalities.

Structural Abnormalities

Minor structural variations in parts of the chromosome containing no hereditary information are known to exist. These variations are thought to be benign. However, some structural alterations of chromosomes may lead to birth defects or fetal wastage if a loss or duplication of genes accompanies the structural variation.

Simple duplications or deficiencies arise from breakage or from errors in the reproduction of chromosomes. Translocations arise when chromosomal breakage is followed by an exchange of material either between parts of a single chromosome or among different chromosomes. If no genetic information is lost, the individual is clinically normal and is said to be a balanced translocation carrier. If genetic information is lost during a chromosome translocation, a partial monosomy results. When genetic information is duplicated, a partial trisomy results. The clinical features caused by such an unbalanced chromosome translocation depend on the size and location of the rearrangement.

Deletions of genetic material from an autosomal chromosome usually lead to severe mental retardation and physical abnormalities. For example, cri du chat syndrome arises when an individual is born with a deletion of genetic material from the short arm of the number 5 chromosome. Affected neonates have a characteristic catlike cry; microcephaly, a round face with the appearance of widely spaced eyes that have a downward slant; epicanthal folds; flat nasal bridge; and micrognathia. Severe mental retardation, failure to thrive, and hypotonia are characteristic of this disorder.

Translocations may arise for the first time in an individual, or they may be inherited. Normal balanced translocation carriers have an increased risk of passing an unbalanced amount of chromosomal material to their offspring. Therefore, when a neonate or fetus is found to have an unbalanced translocation, the parents should be offered karyotype analysis and genetic counseling. This helps to determine whether one of them is a balanced translocation carrier. Results allow both parents to be informed of the possibility of increased risk in future pregnancies.

Mosaicism is another genetic abnormality. A mosaic individual is born with two populations of cells, each with a different chromosomal makeup. Such a situation arises after fertilization. During mitosis, an accident in cell division occurs in a single line of cells. The range of clinical symptoms varies. Results of this condition are thought to be related to the percentage of abnormal cells and to the particular body tissues affected.

Causes of Chromosomal Abnormalities

The internal and environmental events that lead to chromosomal abnormalities are not clearly understood. Radiation, drugs, viruses, toxins, and chemicals are known to induce chromosomal damage in certain conditions. However, it is extremely difficult to determine the cause of genetic abnormalities in individual cases. Women exposed to environmental hazards during the first trimester of pregnancy should be referred for genetic counseling to explore the possibility of increased fetal risk.

The most significant predisposing factor for chromosomal abnormalities is increased maternal age. The risk of having a child with Down syndrome increases substantially after age 35. The reason for this correlation between maternal age and this condition is not known. The age of the father has not been found to have a significant effect on chromosomal abnormalities (Snell, 1990).

Single Gene Inheritance

The term single gene traits refers to genetic diseases that are caused by a mutation of a gene at a single site on a chromosome. There are four basic patterns of single gene inheritance:

- Autosomal dominant
- Autosomal recessive
- X-linked dominant
- X-linked recessive

Risks vary with each inheritance pattern. Thus, a pedigree or a pictorial history may be useful. The pedigree is developed during assessment and history taking. It assists in determining which family members need further examination and testing.

Because chromosomes come in pairs (called homologous chromosomes), genes also come in pairs. Genes that are located at the same locus on a pair of homologous chromosomes are called *alleles*. When the genes in a pair are identical, the person is called a *homozygote* for that locus. When genes in a pair are different, the person is a *heterozygote*.

The terms dominant and recessive refer to the clinical expression of a trait in a heterozygous individual. If the presence of a mutant gene is clinically expressed and masks the presence of the normal gene, the mutant gene is called dominant. If the presence of a mutant gene is not clinically expressed and does not mask the presence of the normal gene, the mutant gene is called recessive.

Autosomal Dominant Inheritance

Autosomal dominant disorders are disorders that are clinically expressed when one gene at a given site on an autosomal chromosome is mutant. Most individuals with dominant disorders are heterozygotes, because the mutant homozygous state usually is lethal or severely debilitating. These traits appear in every generation of affected families with no skipping. Male and female offspring are equally likely to be affected.

When a family seeks genetic counseling for a dominant disorder, the pedigree is examined. The diagram may reveal if an affected parent transmitted the mutant gene or whether the mutant gene arose as a new mutation in a genetically normal parent. If both parents are unaffected and the offspring has a new mutation, the recurrence risk of that mutation in subsequent pregnancies is no greater than the risk for the general population. This is because it is unlikely a mutation will occur again in that family. However, the affected offspring has a 50% risk of transmitting the mutant gene in each of its own pregnancies.

A parent who carries a mutant gene for a dominant disorder can transmit either the normal gene or the mutant gene of that gene pair to children (Fig. 12-10*A*). The transmitted gene is selected randomly during meiosis. Thus, in each pregnancy there is a one in two chance that the offspring will inherit the mutant gene and the disorder.

An example of an autosomal dominant disorder is achondroplasia. This is a disorder consisting of short-limbed dwarfism, large head size, and a bulging forehead. This condition can be distinguished from other types of dwarfism by radiologic examination. Most individuals with this condition have normal intelligence and can lead normal lives.

Because it is not unusual for two individuals of very short stature to marry, it may be important for them to determine if one or both of them has this genetic condition, as opposed to the many other forms of short stature. When two achondroplastic individuals mate, one of three outcomes could result. First, there is a 25% chance that their offspring will inherit the mutant gene from each parent. This would result in homozygous achondroplasia, a lethal skeletal disorder. There is a 50% chance that their offspring would have achondroplasia and be heterozygous and a 25% chance that their offspring would inherit a normal gene from each parent and would therefore be of normal height and homozygous (Snell, 1990).

Autosomal Recessive Inheritance

Autosomal recessive disorders are clinically expressed only when both genes at a given location are mutant. In recessive inheritance both parents usually are clinically normal carriers (heterozygotes) of the same mutant gene. Male and female offspring are equally likely to be affected. If partners are biologically related, the likelihood that they carry the same mutant gene is increased.

Individuals who are heterozygous for a mutant gene produce two types of gametes: gametes containing the normal gene and gametes containing the mutant gene. When both parents are carriers of the same mutant gene, one of three outcomes could result. Each of their offspring has a 25% (one in four) chance of inheriting both mutant genes and developing the disease, a 25% (one in four) chance of inheriting two normal genes and being free of the disease, and a 50% chance (two in four) of inheriting one normal and one mutant gene and being a clinically normal carrier (see Fig. 12-10*B*).

Although everyone is believed to carry a few mutant recessive genes in the heterozygous state, the genes responsible for most autosomal recessive disorders are rare. Unless the partners in a couple are blood relatives, the likelihood that both are carriers of a mutant gene at the same locus depends on the incidence of the mutant gene in the population. Examples of autosomal recessive disorders include cystic fibrosis, phenylketonuria, Tay-Sachs disease, oculo-

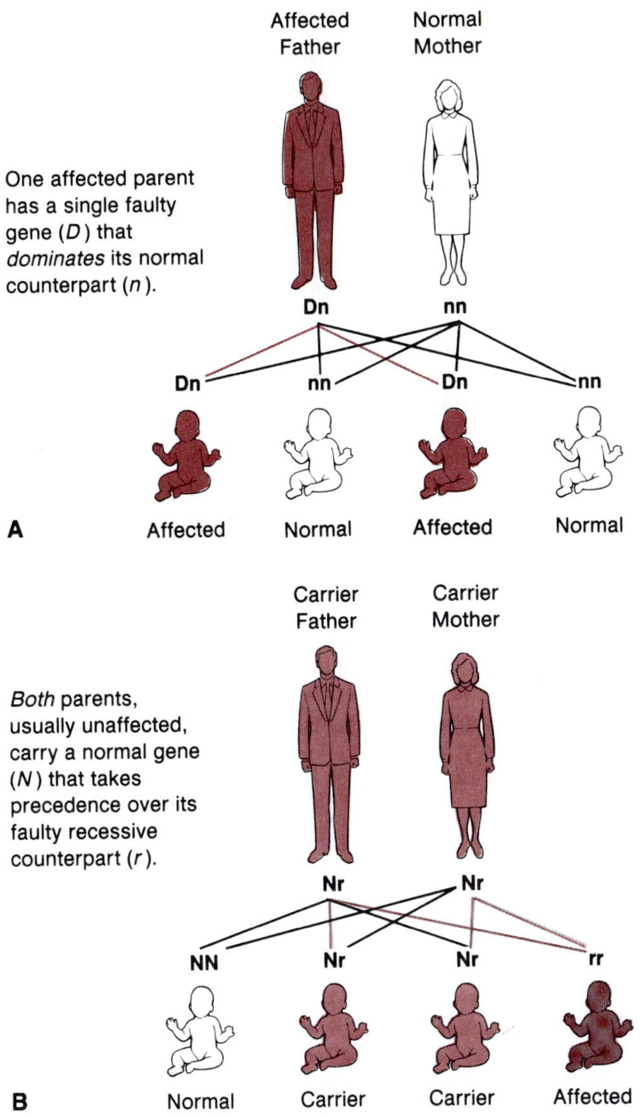

The odds for each child are:

1. a 25% risk of inheriting a "double dose" of *r* genes which may cause a serious birth defect
2. a 25% chance of inheriting two *N*s, thus being unaffected
3. a 50% chance of being a carrier as both parents are

Figure 12-10.
Two types of autosomal inheritance. *A:* Dominant inheritance. *B:* Recessive inheritance. (From Wisniewski, L. P., & Hirschhorn, K. (Eds.). [1980]. *A guide to human chromosome defects.* White Plains, NY: The March of Dimes Birth Defects Foundation. BD:OAS XVI(6).

cutaneous albinism, infantile polycystic kidney disease, and sickle cell anemia.

Cystic fibrosis may be the most common hereditary disorder in the European and European-American populations. Approximately 1 in 20 of these individuals carries the cystic fibrosis gene. In this population the actual incidence of this disorder is 1 in 1600. The carrier rate among African Americans is approximately 1 in 50, and it is even lower in other racial groups. In some cases prenatal diagnosis and carrier detection are possible (Schulman, 1990).

X-Linked Inheritance

Traits that are determined by genes located on the X chromosomes are referred to as X-linked. In relation to X-linked traits, the terms dominant and recessive apply only to females. Females have two X chromosomes and will be symptomatic if they are heterozygous for an X-linked dominant trait but asymptomatic if they are heterozygous for an X-linked recessive trait. Females who are homozygous for an X-linked recessive disorder will manifest disease that often is fatal. Males, on the other hand, having only one X chromosome and one Y chromosome, will always be affected if they inherit an X-linked mutant gene.

Although the X chromosome is involved in sex determination, most of the genes on the chromosome have functions unrelated to sex. Some examples of X-linked recessive disorders are color blindness, hemophilia A and B, Duchenne muscular dystrophy, Lesch-Nyhan syndrome, and glucose-6-phosphate dehydrogenase deficiency (Snell, 1990).

Multifactorial Inheritance in Families

Multifactorial inheritance, the third major category of genetic disorders, is defined as traits and disorders that arise as a result of the interaction of many genetic and environmental factors (Fig. 12-11). Families affected by multifactorial disorders usually cannot be provided with precise counseling about genetic probabilities. Disease can be triggered in two ways: A person may inherit the requisite number of deleterious genes to develop the disorder, or a person may inherit less than the requisite number of deleterious genes, but environmental factors allow for the clinical expression of the disorder to develop.

Some of the more common multifactorial disorders, such as congenital heart disease, club foot, neural tube defects, pyloric stenosis, cleft lip and cleft palate, and congenital hip dysplasia, have a 2% to 5% of recurrence in blood relatives in families in which an infant has been born with one of these conditions.

Teratogenic Abnormalities

Teratogens are agents that cause abnormalities in fetal development. Prenatal exposure to teratogens may cause abortion, intrauterine fetal death, or permanent anatomic, functional, or behavioral abnormalities in the neonate. Teratogens are classified as chemical agents, maternal conditions, or infectious agents.

There are four basic concepts useful in understanding teratogenicity:

- *Dose related response* means that as the amount of exposure increases, the severity of the damage to the fetus increases.
- *Teratogenic threshold* is the amount of exposure required for any observable damage to occur. (For all agents there is a level of exposure that produces no damage, but if exposure levels exceed this threshold, damage will be seen.)
- *Critical periods* are the exposures during certain periods of the prenatal period that are more likely to result

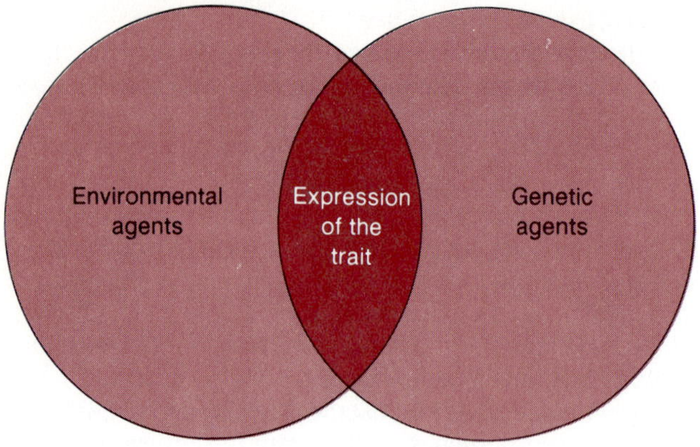

Figure 12-11.
Multifactorial causation.

in damage than at other times. (Exposure during the embryonic period is more likely to result in anatomic malformations, while exposures later in the fetal period may produce behavioral abnormalities.)

- Because of *species variability*, agents shown to be teratogenic in one species may or may not be harmful to another (Beckman & Brent, 1986).

The idea of critical periods is based on embyrologic, fetal, and neonatal developmental periods. Exposure before or during implantation often results in spontaneous abortion. Exposure during organogenesis is most likely to result in anatomic malformations. Exposure during the fetal and neonatal periods is thought to contribute to behavioral abnormalities. The amount and length of exposure, the toxicity of the agent, the time during pregnancy when exposed, and individual genetic susceptibility contribute to the occurrence of fetal damage.

Many chemicals and drugs have demonstrated teratogenic properties; some are listed in Table 12-2. Alcohol, thalidomide, diethylstilbestrol (DES), and cigarettes are some of the most widely known teratogenic agents. Consumption of alcohol creates a risk for fetal alcohol syndrome and cognitive impairment. DES exposure increases the risk for vaginal carcinoma in female offspring and testicular cancer in male offspring. Thalidomide exposure increases the risk of missing or shortened limbs. The effects of cigarette smoking are less clear, but the risk of intrauterine growth retardation appears to be increased in women who smoke 10 or more cigarettes per day (Pletch, 1990).

Heroin has been linked with fetal loss when used early in pregnancy. When used throughout pregnancy heroin is associated with increased maternal–fetal infections and fetal addiction. Cocaine use has been associated with growth retardation and fetal addiction. There is some suggestion that cognitive and behavioral abnormalities occur in offspring with the use of either of these substances. It is difficult to link substance abuse with abnormalities because multiple substance use often occurs (Chasnoff, 1988).

Several maternal conditions and infectious agents have been identified as potentially teratogenic, as listed in the second part of Table 12-2. One of the difficulties in determining the teratogenicity of maternal conditions is separating the effects of the disease from the effects of the treatment.

Prevention of exposure to teratogens is possible and should begin early in pregnancy.

A change in the amount of chromosomal material usually has detrimental effects during prenatal and neonatal development. Numeric abnormalities include monosomies, the absence of one chromosome, and trisomies, the presence of an extra chromosome. These abnormalities usually are caused by mechanical accidents during meiosis and can involve autosomes or sex chromosomes. Other genetic abnormalities include sex chromosome abnormalities, structural abnormalities such as translocations, and single gene dominant or recessive traits, which may involve autosomes or the X chromosome. Fetal disorders also may result from the influence of teratogens.

Implications for Nursing Care

Nurses are in key positions to identify individuals and families at risk for genetic problems. Screening for environmental and genetic risk factors can occur in a variety of settings, such as ambulatory care clinics, maternal and child health clinics, and schools. A genetic history can be a part of health histories taken from individuals of childbearing age.

Good interviewing skills are particularly important in assessing family histories for genetic and environmental exposure risk. For many individuals familial genetic abnormalities, chemical exposure, and drug use are sensitive topics. A nonjudgmental approach and astute listening skills will assist the nurse in obtaining complete information.

Guides such as the following Assessment Tool on Maternal Teratogen Exposure can be incorporated into the health history to screen for environmental risks. For nonpregnant women and for men, preventive measures can be recommended based on risk factors identified. For pregnant women referral to genetic services, including prenatal diagnosis, may be indicated. Programs in the United States and Canada ensure that genetic counseling services are widely available.

Nursing interventions to reduce or prevent hazardous exposure during the childbearing years are most successful when they are individualized to meet the family's needs. Lifestyle changes, such as smoking cessation and alcohol and drug abstinence, are difficult to accomplish. Nurses can intervene to ensure that health promotion programs are available to those who are most at risk. Nurses can work with other health professionals to develop informational materials and programs suited to populations known to be at environmental risk in the community. Finally, nurses can influence public policy to ensure workplace safety with regard to chemical and radiation exposures in populations of childbearing age.

Chapter Summary

This chapter discusses the transfer of genetic information, normal prenatal development, and genetic and environmental mechanisms that may result in fetal abnormalities. Development of the fetus is a complex process. Even though

Table 12-2. Known and Potential Teratogens

Known Teratogenic Chemicals		Potential Teratogenic Maternal Conditions and Infectious Agents	
Agent	**Related Effects**	**Agent**	**Related Effects**
Alcohol	Intrauterine growth retardation; mental retardation; maxillary hypoplasia; reduction in width of palpebral fissures; microcephaly	Cytomegalovirus	Central nervous system damage; intrauterine growth retardation
Anticancer drugs	Drug-specific effects, with wide variation from drug to drug	Diabetes mellitus	Affects various systems; caudal dysplasia or caudal regression syndrome; insulin therapy protects fetus
Anticonvulsants, hydantoins, diones	Orofacial clefts; cardiac and skeletal defects; hydantoin syndrome; trimethadione syndrome; central nervous system anomalies; developmental delay	Endocrinopathies	Effects similar to those of administering the hormone; masculinization of female fetus
Androgenic hormones, progestogenic hormones	Genital malformations; masculinization of female fetus with high doses	Herpes simplex	Central nervous system anomalies; microcephaly; intracranial calcification; eye defects
Aspirin	Heavy use related to low birth weight and bleeding after birth	Phenylketonuria	Fetal death; mental retardation; microcephaly; intrauterine growth retardation
Coumarin anticoagulants	Skeletal defects; nasal hypoplasia; stippling of secondary epiphysis; intrauterine growth retardation; anomalies of eyes, hands, neck, and central nervous system	Rubella virus	Cardiovascular malformations; deafness; mental retardation; cataracts; glaucoma; microphthalmia
Diethylstilbestrol	Masculinization of female fetus; vaginal carcinoma; cervical and uterine anomalies; possible male effects	Syphilis	Maculopapular rash; hepatosplenomegaly; deformed nails; osteochondritis at joints of extremities; congenital neurosyphilis; abnormal epiphyses; chorioretinitis
Lithium carbonate	Cardiovascular malformation; neural tube defects	Toxoplasmosis	Hydrocephaly; microphthalmia; chorioretinitis
Methylmercury	Central nervous system anomalies; Minamata disease; microcephaly; mental retardation; blindness	Varicella-zoster (chickenpox)	Skin and muscle defects; intrauterine growth retardation; limb and eye defects
Radiation	Microcephaly; mental retardation; intrauterine growth retardation	Venezuelan equine encephalitis	Hydroanencephaly; microphthalmia; luxation of hip
Smoking/nicotine	Intrauterine growth retardation; placental lesions		
Thyroid and antithyroid drugs	Hypothyroidism or goiter		
Tetracycline	Hypoplastic tooth enamel; bone and tooth anomalies		
Vitamin A isoretinoin	Urogenital anomalies (large doses); ear, palate, facial, and neural tube defects		
Thalidomide	Limb reduction defects; facial, esophageal, duodenal, and external ear defects; heart or kidney defects		

Adapted from Beckman, & Brent. (1986). Mechanism of known environmental teratogens: Drugs and chemicals. *Clin Perinatol, 13*(3):649–687. Used with permission.

combinations of genetic and environmental factors influence growth and development, fetal development usually is orderly and predictable. Specific causes of abnormalities usually are not known. Complete health histories are essential first steps in identifying the level of risk for individuals and families.

Assisting women and men who are planning pregnancy to adopt healthy life-styles will increase their chances of having a normal pregnancy. Nurses can play an important role in protecting the health status of women and their unborn fetuses. By doing so, the future health and well-being of the next generation can be ensured.

Assessment Tool

Maternal Teratogen Exposure

NAME: ______________________
DATE: ______________________
LMP: __________ EDC: __________

MATERNAL CONDITIONS

1. Have you had any of the following diseases or conditions?

	Yes	No
Diabetes		
Phenylketonuria		
Hormonal or other endocrine problems		
Thyroid disease		
Epilepsy or other convulsive disorder		
Depression		
Cancer or malignancy		
Cardiovascular disease		
Threatened spontaneous abortion		
Severe acne		

2. Did you or are you taking any medication for the condition?
   Medication ______________
   Date (start/stop) ______________

INFECTIOUS AGENTS

3. Have you been exposed to or contracted any of the following?

	Yes	No	Date
Rubella (German measles)			
Herpes simplex			
Varicella zoster (chickenpox)			
Encephalitis (Venezuelan equine)			
Cytomegalic virus			
Toxoplasmosis			
Syphilis			
HIV			

   Were you treated? ______________
   Medication ______________
   Dates (start/stop) ______________

ENVIRONMENTAL

4. Do you live or work in an area where chemicals are present?
   Chemical or type of work ______________
   Dates of exposure ______________
   Note:
   Methylmercury
   Radiation
   Herbicides
   Polychlorinated biphenyls (PCBs)

PRESCRIPTION DRUGS

5. Have you been exposed to or are you taking any of the following drugs or medications?

	Drug Name	Yes	No	Dates
Anticancer				
Anticonvulsants				
Androgenic or progestogenic hormones				
Coumarin anticoagulants				
Diethylstilbestrol (DES)				
Lithium				
Antithyroid drugs				
Tetracyline				
Isotretinoin (Accutane)				

Assessment Tool (*Continued*)

LIFE-STYLE

6. Do you take any over-the-counter or nonprescription medications?
   Aspirin
   Vitamins
   Other
7. Do you drink wine, beer, or alcohol?
   How often ______________________________
   How much ______________________________
   Dates (start/stop) ______________________________
8. Do you smoke cigarettes?
   Packs per day ______________________________
   Dates (start/stop) ______________________________
9. Do you drink coffee, colas, or other caffinated beverages?
   Cups per day ______________________________
   Dates (start/stop) ______________________________
10. Do you use any street or recreational drugs?
   Drug ______________________________
   Dates ______________________________

ATTITUDES

11. Are you familiar with chemicals or drugs that can cause birth defects?
   Discuss . . . .
12. Do you think there is much chance or risk of a baby having birth defects, especially if the mother takes medication, drugs, drinks, etc.
   Discuss . . . .

Reprinted with permission, Dr. Pamela Pletch, University of Wisconsin-Milwaukee.

Study Questions

1. *What is a karyotype? How it is used?*
2. *Why are the first 8 weeks of pregnancy particularly critical?*
3. *What are the primary physiologic developments during the fetal period?*
4. *What kinds of abnormalities are most likely to result from teratogenic exposure during organogenesis?*
5. *What are the major functions of the placenta, and how are these accomplished?*
6. *Why is it important for women who do not yet know they are pregnant to avoid teratogens?*
7. *What are the three main categories of hereditary disorders?*
8. *What is a pedigree? How is it used?*
9. *Who should be referred for genetic counseling?*

References

Beckman, D., & Brent, R. (1986). Mechanism of known environmental teratogens: Drugs and chemicals. *Clinical Perinatology*, *13*(3), 649–687.

Chasnoff, I. (1988) Drug use in pregnancy: parameters of risk. *Pediatric Clinics of North America*, *35*(6), 1403–1412.

Danforth, D., & Scott, J. (Eds.)(1990). *Obstetrics and gynecology* (5th ed.). Philadelphia: J.B. Lippincott.

Filkins, K., & Russon, J. (1990). *Human prenatal diagnosis*. New York: Marcel Dekker.

Levin, B. (1987). *Genes* (3rd ed.). New York: John Wiley.

Moore, K. (1993). *The developing human* (3rd ed.). Philadelphia: W.B. Saunders.

Pletsch, P. (1990). Birth defect prevention: Nursing interventions. *Journal of Obstetric, Gynecologic, and Neonatal Nursing*, *19*(6), 482–488.

Schulman, J. (1990). Treatment of the embryo and the fetus in the first trimester: Current status and future prospects. *American Journal of Medical Genetics*, *35*, 197–200.

Scriver, C., Beaudet, A., Sly, W., & Valle, D. (1989). *The metabolic basis of inherited disease* (6th ed.). New York: McGraw-Hill.

Snell, R. (1990). *Clinical embryology for medical students* (3rd ed.). Boston: Little Brown.

Suggested Readings

Acosta, P., & Wright, L. (1992). Nurses' role in preventing birth defects in offspring of women with phenylketonuria. *Journal of Obstetric, Gynecologic, and Neonatal Nursing*, *21*(4), 270–280.

Bernhardt, J. (1987). Sensory capabilities of the fetus. *MCN: American Journal of Maternal Child Nursing*, *12*(6), 44–46.

Boss, J. (1990). How voluntary prenatal diagnosis and selective abortion increase the abnormal gene pool. *Birth*, *17*(2), 75–80.

Harker, L. & Thorpe, K. (1992). "The last egg in the basket?" Elderly primiparity—A review of findings. *Birth*, *19*(1), 23–31.

Hite, C., & Shannon, M. (1992). Clinical profile of apparently healthy neonates with in utero drug exposure. *Journal of Obstetric, Gynecologic, and Neonatal Nursing*, *19*(4), 305–310.

Janke, J. (1990). Prenatal cocaine use: Effects on perinatal outcome. *Journal of Nurse Midwifery*, *35*(2), 74–77.

Jones, S., & Headrick, E. (1992). Integration of clinical genetics into assisted reproductive technologies: Implications for nursing practice. *NAACOG Clinical Issues in Perinatal and Women's Health Nursing*, *3*(2), 301–312.

Stringer, M., Librizzi, R., & Weiner, S. (1991). Establishing a prenatal genetic diagnosis: The nurse's role. *MCN: American Journal of Maternal Child Nursing*, *16*(3), 152–157.

Zacharias, J. (1990). The new genetics. *Journal of Obstetric, Gynecologic, and Neonatal Nursing*, *19*(2), 122–133.

CHAPTER 13

Nursing Assessment of the Pregnant Woman

Learning Objectives

After studying the material in this chapter, the student will be able to:

- Discuss the various methods used to diagnose pregnancy.
- Explain why early detection of pregnancy is important.
- Differentiate the presumptive, probable, and positive signs of pregnancy.
- Describe the events of the first prenatal visit.
- Explain the importance of the health history in nursing assessment.
- Describe the physical examination, and identify some normal changes of pregnancy.
- Identify the basic laboratory studies performed for early pregnancy assessment and their significance.
- List three symptoms of substance abuse in pregnant women.
- Identify three symptoms of battering in women.
- Describe subsequent assessments of the pregnant woman.

Key Terms

gestation	multipara
gestational age	nulligravida
gravida	nullipara
GTPALM	parity
lightening	primigravida
multigravida	primipara

A great deal of attention during pregnancy is focused on labor and birth, the exciting and dramatic climax to 280 long days of waiting. Equally important events occur during the prenatal period to ensure minimum risk at delivery and maximum health for the woman and her fetus. The value of prenatal care provided in the outpatient setting cannot be overstated. At no other time in life does a healthy woman need health care with such regularity.

Many women today plan for pregnancy. They prepare for the event by maintaining their health at a high level through good nutrition, exercise, and abstinence from cigarettes and drugs. A pregnancy under these ideal conditions has a better chance for healthy growth and development. Prenatal care does not guarantee a normal neonate, but it can identify problems early so that they can be minimized or eliminated.

The intent of this chapter is to acquaint the nurse with the vocabulary of the prenatal period, to explain the techniques used to assess the pregnant woman, to present comprehensive information on the assessment of the woman and fetus, and to present the nursing process as a holistic approach to prenatal care.

Pregnancy Diagnosis

A common saying in the practice of obstetrics and gynecology is that every woman who has been menstruating and misses a menstrual period is pregnant until proven otherwise. Pregnancy must be ruled out in the initial phase of an amenorrhea workup even though the woman insists that she is not pregnant. A good question to ask women who have missed one or more periods is, "Have you been pregnant before?" If the reply is affirmative, the next question is, "Do you feel pregnant now?" If she feels pregnant, there is an 80% chance that she is pregnant. Women who have never been pregnant may be less sensitive or knowledgeable about the early signs of pregnancy.

Women may ask, "How do I know I'm pregnant?" The

woman, nurse, nurse midwife, or physician may use the following means to determine pregnancy:

- Sophisticated pregnancy tests at home or in the health care facility
- Presumptive evidence of pregnancy
- Probable signs of pregnancy
- Positive signs of pregnancy

The earlier pregnancy is diagnosed, the safer it is for the woman and fetus. During the first 12 weeks of pregnancy the vital organ systems of the fetus are developing. Early diagnosis of pregnancy is important for the following reasons:

- It allows the woman wishing to continue her pregnancy to be counseled about potential insults to the developing fetus, such as x-ray exposure, vaccinations, medications, excessive alcohol intake, smoking, over-the-counter and illegal drugs, and occupational or other hazards.
- It enables the woman contemplating abortion to consider her options in early pregnancy. (Abortion is safest for the woman when performed before 12 weeks of gestation.)
- It permits early diagnosis of and intervention in an ectopic pregnancy, a common cause of maternal morbidity and mortality.

Pregnancy Tests

In the last decade pregnancy testing has evolved from the slow and cumbersome biologic testing of animals to sophisticated laboratory tests that can diagnose pregnancy as early as 8 to 10 days after conception. Pregnancy tests analyze maternal blood or urine for the presence of human chorionic gonadotropin (HCG), the hormone produced by the trophoblastic cells of the developing placenta. The test on maternal blood is the earliest to become positive and is the most accurate. However, urine tests are more commonly used and usually are accurate 10 days after conception.

Pregnancy tests available over the counter generally are accurate 14 days after conception and are 97% effective if instructions are followed carefully. However, it is important that negative tests be repeated in 2 weeks to ensure that the test was not done too early to detect urine HCG (Bluestein, 1990). Urine pregnancy tests are not positive signs of pregnancy because conditions other than pregnancy can produce a positive test. Further information on errors in pregnancy tests can be found in the accompanying display.

Sources of Error in Pregnancy Tests

Some factors that influence the results of pregnancy testing follow:

- Careless following of instructions
- Incorrect timing of the test reading
- Use of certain drugs by the woman
- Careless handling of specimens

When pregnancy test results are reported as negative when the woman is in fact pregnant, they are called *false-negative* results. When they are positive and pregnancy has not occurred, they are called *false-positive* results. When either of these errors is suspected, the following causes should be considered:

False-Negatives

- Error in reading
- Test performed too early or too late in pregnancy
- Urine too dilute
- Urine stored too long at room temperature
- Impending spontaneous abortion
- Missed abortion
- Ectopic pregnancy
- Interfering medication

False-Positives

- Error in reading
- Luteinizing hormone cross-reaction (test performed at time of ovulation or in a perimenopausal woman)
- Proteinuria, hematuria
- Persistent corpus luteum
- Recent pregnancy (test performed less than 10 days after abortion or full-term delivery)
- Drug interference (Aldomet, marijuana, methadone, aspirin in large doses, phenothiazine)
- HCG treatment for infertility (injection within preceding 30 days)—affects serum tests only
- Trophoblastic disease (molar pregnancy or choriocarcinoma)
- HCG secreted by malignant tumor (ovary, breast, lung, kidney, gastrointestinal tract, sarcoma, malignant melanoma)

Presumptive Evidence of Pregnancy

Presumptive evidence of pregnancy refers to physical signs and symptoms that suggest, but do not prove, that a woman is pregnant. Pregnancy cannot be diagnosed on the basis of the presumptive signs; it can only be assumed until more concrete data are available. The following signs are considered to be presumptive evidence of pregnancy:

- Abrupt cessation of menses in a healthy woman who previously had predictable menstrual periods suggests pregnancy. In a woman whose menses had been irregular, this symptom would be more difficult to evaluate. Some women experience spotting (light bleeding) during early pregnancy. Women who stop taking birth control pills also may have a variable period of amenorrhea.
- Nausea and vomiting, better known as "morning sickness," occurs in approximately 50% of pregnant women. Symptoms begin between 2 and 6 weeks after concep-

tion and may spontaneously disappear at approximately 12 weeks. Some women continue to experience these symptoms for the duration of pregnancy.

- Bladder irritability occurs early in pregnancy when the enlarging uterus presses on the bladder, causing more frequent urination. As the uterus rises into the abdomen after 12 weeks, this symptom decreases, but it returns late in pregnancy.
- Breast tenderness is one of the earliest symptoms of pregnancy, and nipple tingling is thought to be the first clue to pregnancy for some women. Colostrum may be secreted early in multigravidas.
- Fatigue occurs in early pregnancy in response to increased hormone levels. Women often state they just cannot get enough sleep.

Probable Signs of Pregnancy

The probable signs of pregnancy include objective findings that can be detected by 12 to 16 weeks of gestation. These signs are as follows:

- Enlargement of the abdomen occurs as the fundus of the uterus rises out of the pelvis at 12 weeks of gestation. If other pregnancy symptoms do not corroborate the uterine signs, other causes, such as myomas, pseudocyesis, and neoplasms, need to be ruled out.
- Changes occur in the size, shape, and consistency of the uterus as it progresses from pear-shaped to globular. Later in pregnancy the uterus becomes elongated as it grows upward.
- Braxton Hicks contractions are intermittent painless uterine contractions that occur throughout pregnancy. They may be palpable during the second half of pregnancy.
- Hegar's sign, a softening of the lower uterine segment, may be felt on bimanual examination.
- Chadwick's sign is a purplish hue, seen on speculum examination of the vagina and cervix.
- Increased pigmentation of the skin and striae gravidarum are common manifestations of pregnancy.
- Maternal perception of fetal movement first occurs between 16 and 20 weeks when the woman notices a fluttering movement in the abdomen. If these sensations continue and become stronger daily, pregnancy is likely. By the time movement is felt, the diagnosis of pregnancy usually has been made.
- By 26 to 28 weeks the fetal parts usually can be easily palpated through the abdomen.

Positive Signs of Pregnancy

The following signs are considered diagnostic of pregnancy:

- The fetal heartbeat can be heard and counted separately from the woman's by Doppler stethoscope as early as 10 to 12 weeks.
- The fetus can be recognized by ultrasound as early as 4 weeks after conception using a vaginal probe. Fetal heart motion also can be documented with ultrasound by 6 weeks of gestation.
- Fetal movement can be palpated by a trained examiner after 20 weeks of gestation.

It is important that diagnosis of pregnancy be established as early as possible for the well-being of the mother and the fetus. Pregnancy tests may be performed in the office or in the home. If tests are negative, they should be repeated in 2 weeks. Presumptive evidence does not establish a definite pregnancy but gives an assumption of pregnancy. Probable signs are objective findings that can be detected by 12 to 16 weeks of pregnancy. Positive signs of pregnancy, however, are a fetal heartbeat, ultrasound signs, or fetal movement.

Trimesters of Pregnancy

It has been common practice to divide pregnancy into three equal parts, or *trimesters*. The 9 months of pregnancy are grouped into three periods of approximately 13 weeks each: weeks 1 to 13, 14 to 27, and 28 to 40. The events of pregnancy tend to group themselves into these time periods.

For teaching purposes this division also may be applied to the woman's interests and concerns. Early in her pregnancy the woman may be interested in discussing body changes, the early growth of the fetus, and what she can do to control her nausea and vomiting or the other discomforts of early pregnancy. During the second trimester, the pregnant woman may be more comfortable discussing sexuality, exercise, and nutrition and will experience great excitement when the first fetal movements are felt. The third trimester is a time for anticipation of delivery, discussion of preparations for childbirth and breastfeeding, and touring the labor and delivery suite.

Physical symptoms also seem to group themselves by trimesters. Nausea and vomiting, increased fatigue, and frequent urination are common in the first trimester. The second trimester usually is more comfortable for the pregnant woman both physiologically and psychologically; during the third trimester the woman experiences more discomfort from the growing uterus, increased urination, dependent edema, and sleeping problems. In the latter half of the third trimester, she is anxious for the pregnancy to end. During the third trimester the health care provider must be more alert for signs of complications, such as pregnancy-induced hypertension and gestational diabetes (see Chapter 16 and 27).

Nevertheless, the trimesters are an arbitrary division, not meant to cluster the events of pregnancy rigidly but rather to arrange them for convenience when discussing the progression of events. When reporting or describing a stage of pregnancy or its duration, it is best to use the most precise and accurate information available, which is the gestational age of the fetus.

The First Prenatal Visit

The first prenatal visit is important because at this visit the baseline data on the woman's health and the health of the present pregnancy are collected. A full workup is done, including a complete history, physical examination, and collection of laboratory specimens. Elements of the initial visit are summarized in Table 13-1. Possible pregnancy risk factors also are identified, and a long-term plan of care is formulated to reduce risk to the pregnant woman and her fetus.

During the first prenatal visit, the nurse has the opportunity to set the stage for a continuing relationship with the woman. When prenatal care is initiated at 6 weeks of gestation, the woman may make between 7 and 14 visits during the course of her pregnancy (see the section on prenatal visit schedule later in this chapter). During these weeks the quality of care provided and the support of the nurse will help make the pregnancy a positive growth experience.

The first prenatal visit usually is extended and may take 1 to 2 hours. Although details may vary from one setting to another, the events of this visit generally progress in the following order:

- Orienting the woman to the setting
- Collecting a health history
- Assessing physical status
- Performing a pelvic examination

Table 13-1. Elements of Prenatal Assessment in Initial and Subsequent Visits

Assessment	Rationale
Initial Visit	
Health History: Collect demographic data and detailed health history, present health, and menstrual–obstetric history, present and past pregnancy symptoms or problems.	To obtain data about possible influences (ethnic or cultural factors, work status) and status of present pregnancy (use of drugs, smoking, dietary practices).
Psychosocial Assessment: Assess and record woman's and partner's attitudes toward pregnancy, emotional and financial impact on family, expectations for pregnancy.	To identify women unprepared for life changes associated with pregnancy or who need early referral to additional resources.
Physical Examination: Record height, weight, prepregnant weight, blood pressure, pulse, temperature. Examine body systems: skin, head (eyes, ears, nose, neck, throat), chest (breasts, lungs, heart, back), extremities, abdomen, pelvis (bimanual examination).	To assess maternal health and fetal growth, and to ensure that abnormal findings are promptly identified and treated. Early pelvic examination allows for immediate determination of uterine size or structural abnormalities that may affect pregnancy. However, pelvic examination may be deferred to later visit if necessary for patient comfort; adolescents frequently refuse an initial pelvic examination.
Laboratory Tests: Obtain clean catch blood studies, urine specimen, Pap smear; vaginal and gonorrhea smears, chlamydia culture.	To assess maternal health, identify abnormal findings, and determine presence of vaginal or pelvic infection.
Subsequent Visits	
Pregnancy Status (Ongoing): Assess and record presence of common pregnancy discomforts (nausea, vomiting, backache, constipation, heartburn, headache, varicosities). Assess for abnormal signs (bleeding, lack of fetal movement after quickening, elevated blood pressure, excessive weight gain or loss). Review dietary intake of iron, iron supplementation, 24-hour dietary recall (see Chapter 17). Review weight gain.	To check for symptoms causing maternal discomfort and prescribe care. To check for factors that may inhibit adequate nutrient intake and enable early detection and correction of dietary problems adversely affecting maternal weight gain.
Physical Examination (Ongoing): Check blood pressure, weight, edema, fundal height, fetal heart tones; perform Leopold maneuvers. Date and record when first fetal movements felt.	To rule out presence of hypertension. To monitor growth rate of fetus and confirm gestational age; if uterine fundus is palpated at the umbilicus, pregnancy is confirmed to be at 20 weeks of gestation. First detection of fetal movement usually is at 19–20 weeks in primigravida, 17–20 weeks in multigravida. FHT audible with Doppler at 10–12 weeks and fetoscope at 18–20 weeks.
Laboratory Tests (Ongoing): Perform routine urine dipstick tests for glucose, protein, ketones. Perform complete blood count or Hgb, Hct tests each trimester. Perform Rh antibody screen at 24–28 weeks if Rh negative or previous sensitization. Repeat tests for STDs as indicated. Perform blood glucose screen at 24–28 weeks.	To check for glucosuria (recurring positive urine glucose requires screening for gestational diabetes), proteinuria (possible urinary tract infection, early PIH), ketonuria (indicates inadequate caloric intake). Blood studies will indicate iron deficiency anemia (Hgb of 11 g/dL if other causes have been ruled out). To identify rising antibody titers signaling maternal sensitization. To ensure absence of sexually transmitted infection at time of delivery. To identify gestational diabetes.
Psychosocial Assessment (Ongoing): Assess woman and partner's concerns about physical and emotional changes, plans for meeting learning needs, plans for childbirth; assess maternal perception of fetal movement at each visit.	To identify needs for support, counseling, and anticipatory guidance. To provide referral for childbirth or parenting preparation as needed and desired.
Physical Examination After 38 Weeks of Gestation; assess and record signs of impending labor: lightening, engagement, cervical status.	To document normal progression toward delivery between 38–40 weeks' gestation. Primigravidas experience lightening approximately 2 weeks before delivery; multigravidas usually just before or during labor. Cervical check allows detection of cervical softening, effacement, dilatation, station, and presenting fetal part.

- Collecting specimens for laboratory work
- Identifying risk factors
- Teaching and counseling the patient
- Developing a long-term plan

All these nursing activities are necessary if comprehensive data are to be collected and the woman fully informed.

Orienting the Woman to the Setting

When a pregnant woman first arrives for prenatal care, she is likely to be apprehensive, particularly if it is her first pregnancy. The first person she is likely to meet after registering for her appointment is the nurse. By introducing herself and greeting the woman, the nurse assures her that she is welcome and important. A brief description of the setting, information about its hours of operation, telephone numbers for contacting care providers, and an explanation of what happens during the first prenatal visit is enough for the woman to assimilate at this point.

Collecting the Health History

The setting for collecting the health history should be carefully chosen. It is essential to establish a climate conducive to information sharing. The interview may be described as a conversation with a purpose; an informal conversational style of gathering information is appropriate. This method allows the nurse to guide the discussion and elicit important information, while establishing a relationship with the woman by expressing interest and concern. In addition to providing information about the woman's health, the interview gives the nurse an opportunity to observe her appearance and behavior. Observation can provide valuable information about the woman's feelings about herself and her pregnancy.

The health history is a brief biography and should provide information about the woman's family history, her present and past health, and her social, economic, psychological, and sexual history. Most obstetric settings provide history forms that request data similar to that obtained during a complete medical history, as well as data specific to the woman's reproductive history and her present pregnancy. It is important to know as much as possible about the woman, and such information should be accessible to all members of the health care team. Records necessarily use standardized terminology, and the language used should have the same meaning and value to each professional who consults them. Not only must the information be complete, but the reporting language must be consistent and appropriate as well.

When collecting data, it is helpful to discuss the importance of the information and to explain unfamiliar terminology to the pregnant woman. The health history can be valuable for the nurse and the woman. The following section outlines the information needed to complete the prenatal history. A sample assessment record is shown in the Assessment Tool.

Demographic Data

Information obtained in the demographic portion of the history identifies the woman and her residence, telephone number, age, race, ethnic origin, religion, marital status, and occupation. Important information about the woman may be gained by exploring her replies and observing her behavior. (Information and rationale are listed in Table 13-2.)

Family History

Determining the health status of immediate family members of the pregnant woman and the father of her fetus is necessary to identify specific risks for the woman or the fetus. The family history also serves as a guide for additional diagnostic tests and referrals. Specific diseases, such as diabetes in family members, increases the woman's risk of developing gestational diabetes during pregnancy. A history of pregnancy-induced hypertension among a woman's sisters or mother places her at increased risk for this disease. Fraternal twinning is hereditary and should be noted among the woman's family members. Problems in her mother's obstetric history may suggest the possibility that the pregnant woman was exposed to diethylstilbestrol in utero and thus may have subtle abnormalities of the reproductive tract.

Medical History

The expectant mother's medical history must be reviewed for current or prior medical conditions that may place the pregnancy at risk. Diseases such as diabetes, hypertension, heart disease, or renal disease necessitate referral for high-risk evaluation and management. Previous surgeries involving the reproductive tract must be noted. Drug allergies should be identified and the record marked accordingly.

Infection Screening. Screening the expectant couple for a history of, or possible exposure to, infectious diseases has become an integral part of the prenatal assessment. Sexually transmitted diseases and other illnesses, such as measles and chickenpox, tuberculosis, hepatitis, group B streptococcus (GBS), and human immunodeficiency virus (HIV), should be included in the interview.

Genetic Screening. Identification of inherited diseases and disorders can be diagnosed through prenatal testing and has become an important consideration in obtaining the prenatal history. Failure to identify these risks with the possibility of the birth of an affected infant can have devastating consequences for the family and can result in litigation. One example of a genetic screening guide for the prenatal interview is provided in the accompanying display. For further information see Chapter 12.

Menstrual History. The menstrual history is an important part of data collection, not only for pregnant women but for all female patients. During the reproductive years it is important to know the age when menstruation first occurred (menarche), the regularity of periods, the duration and amount of menstrual flow, whether pain is associated with

Assessment Tool

ACOG Antepartum Record

DATE ____________ Patient Addressograph

NAME ________________________________
LAST FIRST MIDDLE

ID # ____________ HOSPITAL OF DELIVERY ____________

NEWBORN'S PHYSICIAN ____________ REFERRED BY ____________

BIRTHDATE MO DAY YR	AGE	RACE W B O	MARITAL STATUS S M W D SEP	ADDRESS:
OCCUPATION ☐ HOMEMAKER ☐ OUTSIDE WORK ______ ☐ STUDENT Type of Work		EDUCATION (LAST GRADE COMPLETED)		ZIP: PHONE: MEDICAID # / INSURANCE
EMERGENCY CONTACT:				RELATIONSHIP: PHONE:

TOTAL PREG	FULL TERM	PREMATURE	ABORTIONS INDUCED	ABORTIONS SPONTANEOUS	ECTOPICS	MULTIPLE BIRTHS	LIVING

PAST PREGNANCIES (LAST SIX)

DATE MO/YR	GA WEEKS	LENGTH OF LABOR	BIRTH WEIGHT	TYPE DELIVERY	ANES.	PLACE OF DELIVERY	PERINATAL MORTALITY YES/NO	TREATMENT PRETERM LABOR YES/NO	COMMENTS/ COMPLICATONS

PAST MEDICAL HISTORY

	O Neg + Pos.	DETAIL POSITIVE REMARKS INCLUDE DATE & TREATMENT			
			RH SENSITIZED		
DIABETES			TUBERCULOSIS		
HYPERTENSION			ASTHMA		
HEART DISEASE			GYN SURGERY		
RHEUMATIC FEVER			ALLERGIES (DRUGS)		
MITRAL VALVE PROLAPSE			OPERATIONS / HOSPITALIZATIONS (YEAR & REASON)		
KIDNEY DISEASE / UTI					
NERVOUS AND MENTAL			ANESTHETIC COMPLICATIONS		
EPILEPSY			HISTORY OF ABNORMAL PAP		
HEPATITIS / LIVER DISEASE			UTERINE ANOMALY		
VARICOSITIES / PHLEBITIS			INFERTILITY		
THYROID DYSFUNCTION			IN UTERO DES EXPOSURE		
MAJOR ACCIDENTS			STREET DRUGS		
HISTORY OF BLOOD TRANSFUSION			OTHER		
USE OF TOBACCO		# CIGS / DAY PRIOR TO PREG ____ # CIGS / DAY NOW ____ AGE ONSET SMOKING ____ YEARS	USE OF ALCOHOL		# DRINKS / WK PRIOR TO PREG ____ # DRINKS / WK NOW ____ AGE ONSET DRINKING ____ YEARS

INFECTION SCREENING	YES	NO			
			PATIENT OR PARTNER HAVE HISTORY OF GENITAL HERPES?		
HIGH RISK AIDS?			RASH OR VIRAL ILLNESS SINCE LAST MENSTRUAL PERIOD?		
HIGH RISK HEPATITIS B?			HISTORY OF STD, GC, CHLAMYDIA, HPV, SYPHILIS?		
LIVE WITH SOMEONE WITH TB OR EXPOSED TO TB?			OTHER?		

Table 13-2. Demographic Data

Information	Rationale
Address	Obtaining the womans' address offers an opportunity to ask questions about her life-style. In what part of town is her home located? Does she live in a house or an apartment? Does she live alone or with friends, husband, or partner? Will she have trouble getting transportation to prenatal visits?
Age	Age of the pregnant woman is important. Teenagers and women older than 35 are at greater risk for pregnancy complications.
Race or Ethnic Origin	Congenital disorders and chromosome aberrations may be associated with race or ethnicity. Tay-Sachs disease, found in a segment of the Jewish population, is the most common metabolic disorder diagnosed prenatally. Sickle cell disease or trait may be found in the African American population. Culture also may influence a woman's attitude toward prenatal health care practices. There may be taboos related to the genitals, breasts, the use of contraception, or treatment by male health care providers.
Occupation	When a pregnant woman works, it is important to determine the kind of work she performs. Does her job require strenuous activity? Is her job sedentary? Is she exposed to chemicals or other potential teratogens? For example, nursery and elementary school teachers may be exposed to children infected with rubella virus. Pregnant nurses working in newborn nurseries may be exposed to viral shedding from asymptomatic newborns. X-ray or radiation exposure also may present a problem.
Religion	Religious doctrines may influence medical care. Jehovah's Witnesses may refuse medical intervention necessary to maintain health or sustain life. Other religious faiths may prohibit abortion or contraception. The dietary rules of some religions may necessitate adjustments in the recommended nutrition plan to ensure adequate nourishment of the mother and fetus during pregnancy.

menses (dysmenorrhea), and whether uterine bleeding occurs between periods. (Because hormonal contraception produces an artificial menstrual cycle, the history should include only cycles when no hormonal contraception was used.) During the first prenatal visit obtaining a menstrual history is essential to determine gestational age and expected date of delivery (EDD).

Present Pregnancy

The history of the present pregnancy deals with the progress of the pregnancy to date, symptoms being experienced, and the woman's feelings regarding the pregnancy. The following questions will elicit information essential to the nursing assessment and management of the pregnant woman's care (Barger, Lops, & Fullerton, 1988):

Genetic Screening Guide for the Prenatal Interview

The following questions should be asked and recorded during the prenatal interview:

Is the woman older than 35 years of age?

Is the woman of Italian, Greek, Mediterranean, or Oriental descent?

Does anyone in her family or the fetus' father's family have any of the following:

- Neural tube defects
- Down syndrome
- Tay-Sachs disease
- Sickle cell disease or trait
- Hemophilia
- Muscular dystrophy
- Cystic fibrosis
- Huntington chorea
- Mental retardation (If yes, was genetic testing done? What were the results?)
- Other inherited genetic or chronosomal disorders
- A child with birth defects not listed above
- More than three first-trimester spontaneous abortions or a stillbirth

Has the woman used medications or street drugs since her last menstrual period? If yes, what drugs?

- How is her general health? Was a pregnancy test performed? If so, when, and was the result negative or positive?
- Was contraception used before this pregnancy? What kind? Were there side effects? How long was it used, and when and why was it discontinued?
- Was this pregnancy planned? How does she feel about it?
- Has she experienced signs of early pregnancy, such as nausea and vomiting, breast tenderness, or fatigue?
- Has she had any bleeding, spotting, or cramping since her last menstrual period (LMP)?
- What was her prepregnant weight?
- Does she engage in any form of routine exercise?
- Is the father of the fetus involved with the pregnancy? Is he offering support? What is his age, height, weight, and general state of health. Does he have a history of drug use, sexually transmitted diseases, or serious medical problems? What is his occupation?
- Does she smoke or drink alcoholic beverages? If so, how many cigarettes per day? How many ounces of alcohol per day? Does her partner smoke or drink? If so, how much?
- Has she been occupationally exposed to teratogens or

other substances (x-rays, chemicals) that may affect the fetus?

- Has she taken any over-the-counter drugs, street drugs, or prescription drugs since her last period? If so, what is the name of the drug, and when, how often, and how much was taken?
- Has she been exposed to any contagious illnesses since her LMP?
- What are her hobbies? Is there any danger to the pregnancy related to her leisure activities? (Scuba diving, painting, paint stripping, photo processing, and ceramic work using products containing lead are contraindicated during pregnancy.)
- Does she have or care for any cats who may be infected with toxoplasmosis?

Calculating Date of Delivery

The average length of pregnancy, as calculated from the first day of the LMP, is 280 days: 40 weeks, 10 lunar months, or 9 calendar months. The EDD is sometimes also referred to as the estimated date of confinement. The EDD can be calculated by using Nägele's rule.

According to Nägele's rule, the EDD is calculated by adding 7 days to the date of the first day of the LMP and then counting back 3 months (first day of the LMP plus 7 days minus 3 months equals the EDD). For example, if a woman's last normal menstrual period began on February 4, her EDD would be November 11: February 4 + 7 = February 11 − 3 months = November 11 (EDD). Gestational calculators in the form of wheels also can be used to determine the EDD, weeks of gestation, and the estimated length and weight of the fetus for each week of gestation.

Dating Pregnancy When the Last Menstrual Period Is Unknown

When the date of the LMP or conception is not known, a number of parameters can be used to determine the length of gestation:

- Size of the uterus at the first prenatal visit should be reported in terms of weeks of pregnancy (eg, 6 weeks' size).
- Presence of the uterus in the pelvis indicates a pregnancy of *less than* 12 weeks' gestation.
- Presence of the uterus in the abdomen indicates a pregnancy of *more than* 12 weeks' gestation.
- Determine the date of the first positive pregnancy test.
- If Doppler detection of fetal heart tones occurs, gestation is at least 10 weeks.
- Detection of fetal heart sounds with a fetoscope when the uterine fundus is located at the level of the umbilicus indicates a pregnancy of 20 weeks.
- Fetal movement or quickening is felt by 20 weeks of gestation by primigravidas and earlier in multigravidas.
- Ultrasound results on examinations done early in pregnancy (before 26 weeks) are very useful for dating pregnancies (see Chapter 14).

Previous Pregnancies

Pregnancy history can be recorded using the mnemonic GTPALM: G, gravida; T, term pregnancy; P, preterm birth; A, abortion; L, number of living children; M, multiple gestations and births. If a woman has had six pregnancies, four term deliveries, one premature delivery, and one abortion, and has five living children and no multiple gestations, her previous pregnancy history would be reported as 6-4-1-1-5-0. If the premature delivery has resulted in the death of the infant, her history would be reported as 6-4-1-1-4-0.

The history of previous pregnancies provides important data that may be useful in the management of the present pregnancy, especially if problems or complications were experienced. Information obtained from the woman regarding previous pregnancies and births should include the following:

- Length of gestation
- Length of labor
- Type of delivery
- Fetal presentation
- Neonatal outcome, including current health and development of the infant
- Neonatal birth weight
- Complications of pregnancy, labor, delivery, and the postpartum period (Danforth & Scott, 1990)

Assessing Physical Status

Information collected for the health history provides 95% of the data needed to assess patient health. The remaining 5% is obtained from the findings of the physical examination and from laboratory assessments. A physical examination, guided by any information in the history that indicates a health problem, should be performed on all pregnant women at their first visit (Danforth & Scott, 1990).

A complete physical examination should be performed on every pregnant woman. Physical findings will be different from those of the normal, nonpregnant state in the areas of the body where pregnancy changes are most dramatic (Table 13-3). The physical assessment of these areas includes the following:

- Measurement of vital signs, height, and weight
- Examination of mouth, teeth, and gums
- Palpation of thyroid
- Auscultation of maternal heart tones
- Inspection and palpation of the breasts
- Inspection and palpation of the abdomen
- Inspection of extremities
- Measurement of fundal height
- Auscultation of fetal heart tones
- Pelvic examination

Blood Pressure

Blood pressure is taken early in pregnancy to provide a baseline for the evaluation and comparison of readings that may become elevated later in gestation. A systolic increase of 30 mm Hg or a diastolic increase of 15 mm Hg above the baseline blood pressure is a significant abnormal finding.

Height and Weight

Height and weight assessment is important in pregnancy. A woman who has a short, square stature and broad,

Table 13-3. Physical Changes in Pregnancy and Associated Problems

Normal Changes	Related Discomforts	Potential Problems
Head and Neck		
Increased nasal vascularity	Epistaxis (nosebleeds)	
Chloasma (mask of pregnancy)	Cosmetic concern; may persist	
Epulis (gingival growth)	Bleeding gums, difficulty eating and keeping teeth clean	
Ptyalism (excessive secretion of saliva)	Nausea	Malnutrition
Enlarged thyroid gland, increased basal metabolic rate	Palpitations, fatigue	
Chest		
Increased circumference of chest wall	Hyperventilation, dyspnea	
Lateral movement of apex of heart		
Exaggerated splitting of first heart sound, loud third sound		
Systolic murmur in 90% of pregnant women; brachial blood pressure is highest when patient is sitting		Previous undetected cardiac disease
Breasts		
Enlargement of breasts, erection of nipples, darkening of areola, secretion of colostrum	Tenderness, tingling	Enlargement of supernumerary breast tissue in axilla
Abdomen/Pelvis		
Increase in uterine size; rising of uterus from pelvis at 12 to 13 weeks of gestation; decreased bladder tone	Increased frequency and urgency of urination	Nocturia; dysuria; costovertebral angle tenderness; protein, glucose, ketones in urine
Sensation of fetal movement at 18 to 20 weeks of gestation		Absence of fetal movement; lower abdominal pain
Increased white vaginal discharge		Increased risk for vaginal infection due to low pH
Back		
Increased lumbar curvature	Backache	
Extremities		
Palmar erythema	Itching hands	
Pressure on venous circulation of legs	Dependent edema of feet and legs	Varicosities, thrombophlebitis

short hands also may have a small bony pelvis. As pregnancy progresses, she may appear large for dates when in fact this is an illusion created by the shorter distance from pubis to xiphoid. Conversely, a tall woman may appear smaller than her dates because of her long torso.

Prepregnant weight is used to assess sequential and total pregnancy weight gain. Even though a woman's weight gain follows the normal pregnancy curve, nutritional counseling is required to ensure that nutrient intake is adequate to meet the demands of the pregnant woman and the growing fetus. By 20 weeks of gestation weight gain should be 10 pounds; at term the minimum recommended weight gain is 25 pounds (see Chapter 17).

Early loss of weight below the prepregnant level may mean that the woman has experienced significant nausea and vomiting. Referral to a nutritionist is imperative to avoid serious problems, such as dehydration and ketosis.

Weight gain considerably greater than average in late pregnancy (greater than 2.2 lb in 1 week) may indicate overeating or fluid retention. Rapid weight gain caused by fluid retention and protein in the urine (proteinuria) and an elevated blood pressure (as defined above) may indicate that the woman is developing pregnancy-induced hypertension (see Chapter 27). Early nutritional assessment and continued counseling throughout pregnancy are important for a healthy mother and newborn.

Inspection and Palpation of the Breasts

Many physiologic changes occur in the breasts in preparation for milk production. These changes, all considered normal, include the following:

- Breasts enlargement and "lumpiness" because of the growth of the ductal system that produces the milk
- Tenderness and sensitivity of the breasts experienced in the first trimester
- Darkening and enlargement of the areola
- Erection of the nipples and leaking of colostrum late in the first trimester
- Appearance of venous pattern over the breasts
- Striae formation in breasts

Changes in breast tissue make examination difficult, but it is still necessary. Considering that breast cancer will develop in one out of every nine women in the United States, regular breast examination, even during pregnancy, is recommended. Women who practice breast self-examination will notice gradual tissue changes in pregnancy and will be able to identify changes that are not consistent. Women who do not routinely examine their breasts will be less aware of the changes that are occurring.

All pregnant women should have a breast examination as part of their initial physical examination, and those not previously taught breast self-examination should be instructed in the technique (see Chapter 6). Recent lumps or masses; masses that feel hard or fixed; skin changes, such as dimpling, redness, edema, or ulceration; breast pain; nipple retraction or elevation; and rashes are all possible indications of significant breast disease and should be carefully evaluated.

Part of the breast examination during pregnancy should include an evaluation of the nipples for breastfeeding. The areola should be compressed gently just below the nipple to determine if the nipple is everted, flat, or inverted. Women who plan to breastfeed and who have flat or inverted nipples will need to be instructed in preparation measures to correct this before delivery (see Chapter 15).

Inspection and Palpation of the Abdomen

Before the ascent of the uterus from the pelvis into the abdomen early in pregnancy (12 weeks of gestation), a complete abdominal examination can be performed. The abdomen can be inspected, the bowel sounds and aorta auscultated, and the liver, spleen, and bowel palpated and percussed. As pregnancy progresses, the growing uterus fills the abdominal cavity, making external examination of the abdominal organs impossible.

At approximately 12 weeks of gestation, the uterus has grown large enough to rise from the pelvis and become an abdominal organ. After 12 weeks the abdominal examination is performed at each prenatal visit, although for some assessments (eg, fetal lie), the fetus must be large enough for the examiner to palpate fetal parts. Therefore, this portion of the examination is initiated after 26 weeks.

Preparation of the Woman

Correct preparation of the pregnant woman for the abdominal examination will increase her comfort and the efficiency of the examiner. The following steps will accomplish these goals. The abdominal examination and its purpose should be explained to the woman. The woman is asked to empty her bladder. A full bladder places upward pressure on the uterus, causing it to rise higher into the abdomen. Not only does this cause discomfort to the woman, but erroneous measurements can be made when the bladder is mistaken for the uterus.

The woman is helped to assume a comfortable position on the examination table. She should lie on her back with her hands at her sides and her abdomen bared. The head of the table should be elevated slightly, and the woman is asked to flex her knees. This will help ease the tension of the abdominal muscles, allowing easier palpation.

Late in pregnancy, some women become dizzy or faint when lying on their backs. This condition, known as supine hypotensive syndrome, is caused by the weight of the uterus compressing the inferior vena cava and aorta that lie directly posterior to it. The flow of blood back to the heart decreases, cardiac output lessens, and the woman becomes faint. The woman should immediately be turned on her side so that the weight of the uterus will be shifted from the vessels. The woman experiences immediate relief. Supine hypotension syndrome may be prevented by placing rolled towels or a small pillow under the right hip to rotate the weight of the gravid uterus off the central vessels.

Inspection of the Abdomen

The examination is begun by inspecting the skin of the abdomen. With the aid of a good light, the examiner should note the following:

- The presence of scars, rashes, lesions, dilated veins, pulsations, irritation, and the condition of the umbilicus (late in pregnancy it may protrude and become sensitive)
- The presence of a linea nigra, striae, or fetal movement (after 18 to 20 weeks)
- The size, shape, and contour of the uterus

Palpation of the Abdomen

Abdominal palpation permits the examiner to feel fetal parts through the abdominal wall and the uterus late in pregnancy. The examiner should use warm hands and touch the abdomen lightly to reduce reflexive reaction. The examiner keeps the fingers together and uses the palmar surface of the fingers. Smoothly applied pressure is used to palpate the uterus, following the four steps of Leopold maneuvers. (Although Leopold maneuvers are used later in pregnancy, they are described here for flow of the inspection and palpation of the abdomen. Also see the display on Leopold maneuvers.)

Measurement of Fundal Height

Measurement of fundal height provides information about the progressive growth of the pregnancy. The zero line of a centimeter measuring tape is placed on the superior edge of the symphysis pubis and the tape brought over the abdominal curve to the top of the fundus. This is the McDonald measurement (Fig. 13-1). After 20 weeks of gestation the fundal height, measured in centimeters, approximates the weeks of pregnancy. For example, at 20 weeks the uterus is at the umbilicus, and the fundal height measures approximately 20 cm; at 33 weeks the fundal height should approximate 33 cm.

Before 20 weeks of gestation, McDonald's measurements are not accurate, and the uterus is measured in finger breadths above the symphysis or below the umbilicus, rather than in centimeters. At 16 weeks the fundus is located halfway between the symphysis and the umbilicus, approximately three finger breadths above the symphysis. At 18 weeks the fundus is two finger breadths below the umbilicus. Figure 13-1 indicates fundal height at various stages of pregnancy.

Measurement of fundal height provides valuable information on the growth of the fetus and is an important part of the assessment at each visit. When performed by different care providers at each visit, however, measurements may be inconsistent. When measurements are not consistent with the gestational age of the fetus and fetal size cannot be determined by abdominal palpation, further assessment, such as sonography, may be indicated (see Chapter 14).

Auscultation of Fetal Heart Tones

Auscultation of the rate and rhythm of the fetal heartbeat gives an indication of the fetus' general health. The fetal heartbeat can first be heard with a fetoscope at 18 to 20 weeks of gestation; if a Doppler ultrasound device is used,it can be detected as early as 10 weeks of gestation (Fig. 13-2*A*

Leopold Maneuvers

Leopold maneuvers are performed late in pregnancy after the uterus becomes large enough to allow differentiation of fetal parts by palpation.

First Maneuver

Answers the question: *What is in the fundus? Head or breech?*

Finding: *Presentation.* This maneuver identifies the part of the fetus that lies over the inlet into the pelvis. The most common presentations are *cephalic* (head first) and *breech* (pelvis first).

Performing First Maneuver

Facing the woman's head, use the tips of the fingers of both hands to palpate the uterine fundus.

- When the fetal head is in the fundus, it will feel hard, smooth, globular, mobile, and ballotable.
- When the breech is in the fundus, it will feel soft, irregular, round, and less mobile.

The *lie* of the fetus—the relationship between the long axis of the fetus and the long axis of the woman—also can be determined during the first maneuver. The lie is commonly longitudinal or transverse but occasionally may be oblique.

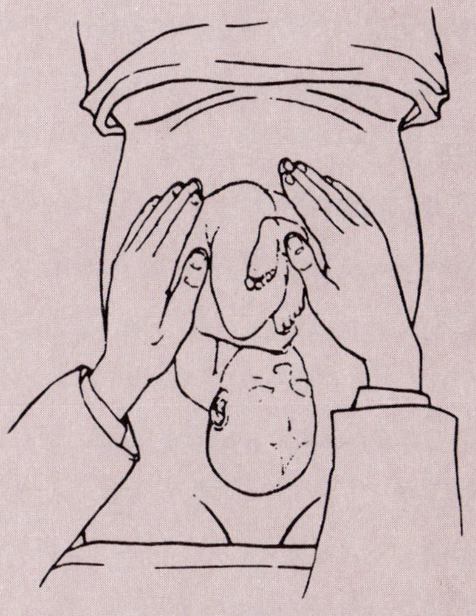

First maneuver.

Second Maneuver

Answers the question: *Where is the back?*

Finding: *Position.* This maneuver identifies the relationship of a fetal body part to the front, back, or sides of the maternal pelvis. There are many possible fetal positions.

Performing Second Maneuver

Remain facing the woman's head. Place your hands on either side of the abdomen. Steady the uterus with your hand on one side, and palpate the opposite side to determine the location of the fetal back.

- The back will feel firm, smooth, convex, resistant.
- The small parts (arms and legs) will feel small, irregularly placed, and knobby and may be actively or passively mobile.

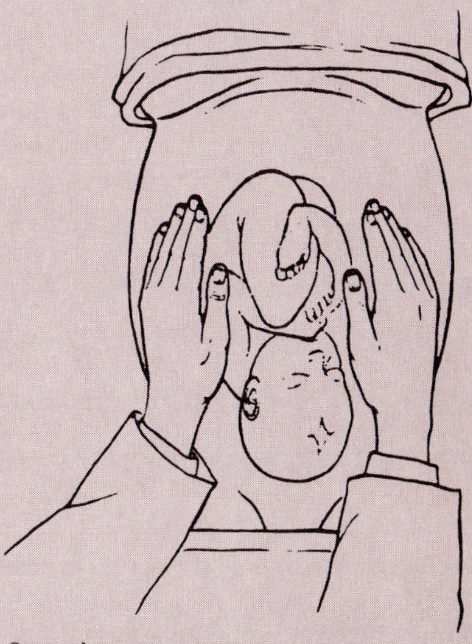

Second maneuver.

(*continued*)

Leopold Maneuvers *(Continued)*

Third Maneuver

Answers the question: *What is the presenting part?*

Finding: *Presenting Part.* This maneuver identifies the most dependent part of the fetus—that is, the part that lies nearest the cervix. It is the part of the fetus that first contacts the finger in the vaginal examination, most commonly the head or breech.

Performing Third Maneuver

Place the tips on the first three fingers of each hand on either side of the woman's abdomen just above the symphysis, and ask the patient to take a deep breath and let it out. As she exhales, sink your fingers down slowly and deeply around the presenting part. Note the contour, size, and consistency of the part.

- The head will feel hard, smooth, and mobile if not engaged, immobile if engaged.
- The breech will feel soft and irregular.

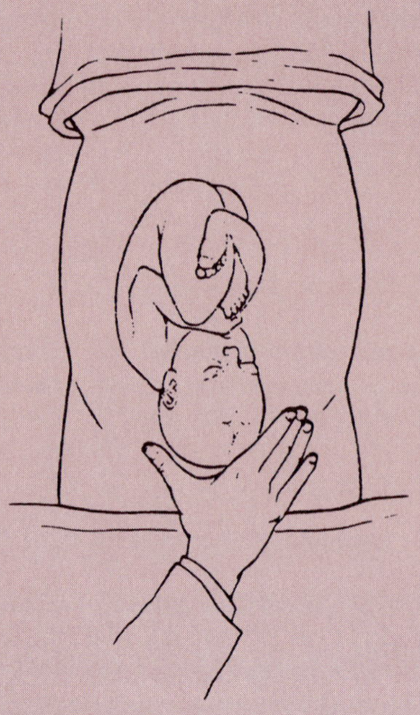

Third maneuver.

Fourth Maneuver

Answers the question: *Where is the cephalic prominence?*

Finding: *Cephalic Prominence.* This maneuver identifies the greatest prominence of the fetal head palpated over the brim of the pelvis. When the head is flexed (flexion attitude), the forehead forms the cephalic prominence. When the head is extended (extension attitude), the occiput becomes the cephalic prominence.

Performing Fourth Maneuver

Face the woman's feet. Gently move your fingers down the sides of the abdomen toward the pelvis until the fingers of one hand encounter a bony prominence. This is the cephalic prominence. If the prominence is on the opposite side from the back, it is the fetus's brow, and the head is flexed. If the head is extended, the cephalic prominence will be located on the same side as the back and will be the occiput. Because this maneuver often causes some discomfort to the woman, it may be deferred.

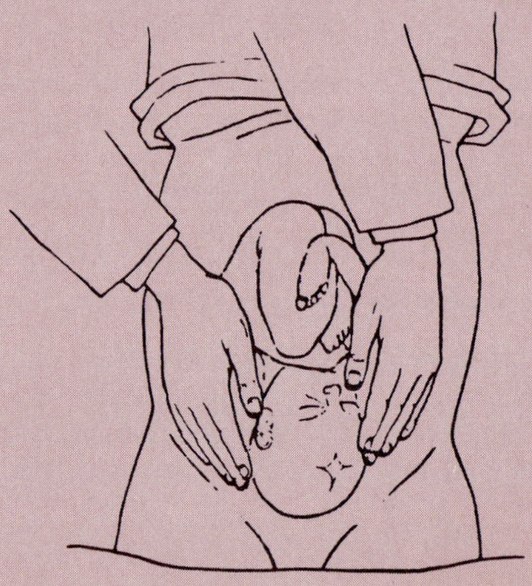

Fourth maneuver.

(Illustrations from Pritchard, J., MacDonald, P. [1980]. Williams' obstetrics (16th ed.). Norwalk, CT: Appleton-Century-Crofts. Reprinted by permission)

and *B*). When the heartbeat is first heard, regardless of the instrument used, the experience of listening to the heartbeat should be shared with the woman and her partner. It may be exciting for them to hear the fetus' heart, and often the pregnancy is validated for them at this time. The point of clearest heart tones for various fetal positions is shown in Figure 13-2*C* and *D*.

The normal fetal heart rate (FHR) is 120 to 160 bpm. When searching for heart tones, the normal rapid beat confirms that the examiner is hearing the fetal heartbeat rather than that of the woman. If the FHR is less than 100 bpm or more than 160 bpm with the uterus at rest, the fetus may be in distress. Regularity of the beat is a normal finding; irregularity is an abnormal finding.

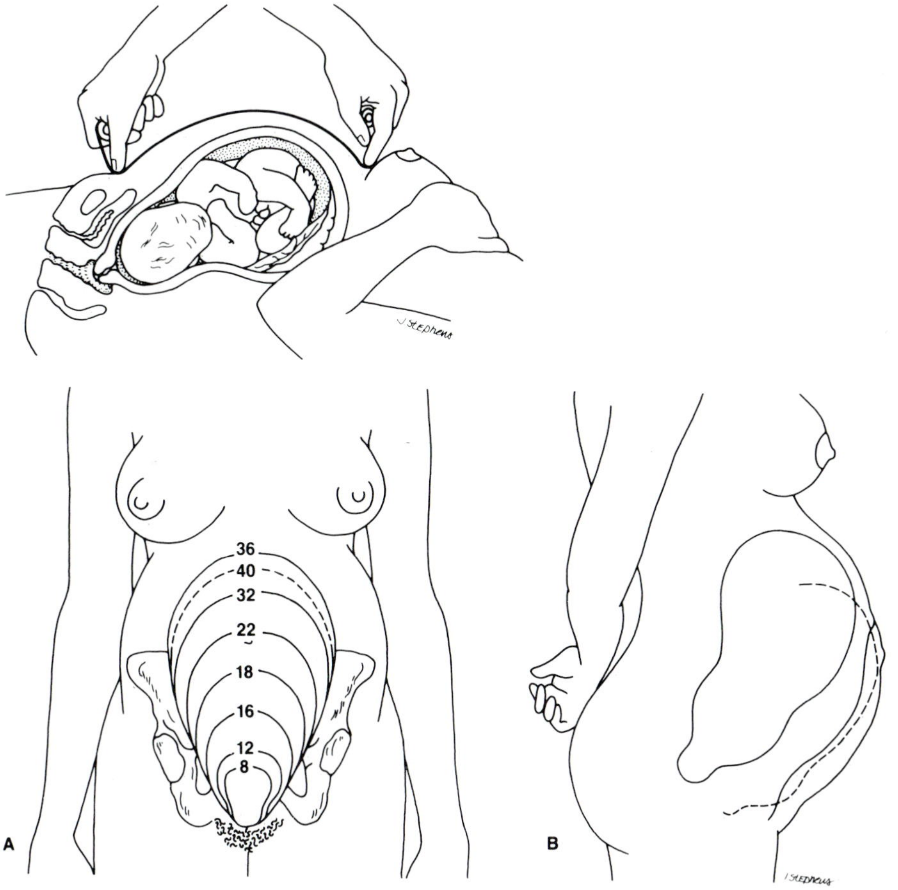

Figure 13-1.
Measurement of fundal height. *Top:* Procedure for measuring fundal height in centimeters (McDonald's measurement). *A:* Fundal height at various weeks of gestation. *B:* Lightening has occurred and the presenting part has settled into the pelvis. Fundal height decreases and the uterus rests anteriorly against the abdominal wall. In lay terms, "the baby has dropped" (Childbirth Graphics®, Waco, Texas).

The loudness of the fetal heart tones depends on the closeness of the fetal back to the pregnant woman's abdomen, as shown in Figure 13-2*C*. The heartbeat will be muffled if the woman's abdominal wall is thick, as it is in obese women or when large amounts of fluid are contained in the amniotic sac, a condition known as hydramnios.

Other sounds heard in the abdomen are funic souffle, caused by the rushing of blood through the umbilical arteries, and uterine souffle, caused by the sound of blood passing through the uterine blood vessels. The former sound is synchronous with the FHR; the latter is synchronous with the maternal pulse.

Failure to hear fetal heart tones may result from the following:

- Defective fetoscope or a noisy environment
- Early pregnancy (the fetus is too small)
- Fetal death (If fetal heart tones were heard previously and fetal movement has ceased, fetal demise is probable.)
- Obesity in the woman
- Hydramnios
- Loud placental souffle that obscures the fetal heart tones
- Posterior position of the fetus (The back of the fetus is facing the woman's back.)

More extensive techniques for assessing fetal well-being are discussed in Chapter 14.

Performing the Pelvic Examination

The pelvic examination is performed after the abdominal examination. It provides a great deal of information about the normalcy of pelvic structures or the problems they might cause, the length of the pregnancy, the presence of infection, and the adequacy of the bony pelvis for delivery of the infant. The examination includes inspection and palpation of the external genitalia, speculum examination of the vagina and cervix, bimanual examination of the uterus and adnexa, and rectovaginal examination. A review of the anatomy of the genital tract (see Chapter 4) will greatly facilitate understanding of the pelvic examination.

Preparation of Equipment

The following equipment is needed to perform a pelvic examination:

- Good light source
- Pair of plastic gloves
- Speculum
- Thayer-Martin media for a gonorrhea culture (if applicable)
- Pap bottle or card carrier with fixative
- Glass slides for the Pap smear
- Glass slides and potassium hydroxide and saline solutions for preparation of a wet mount if vaginal infection is suspected

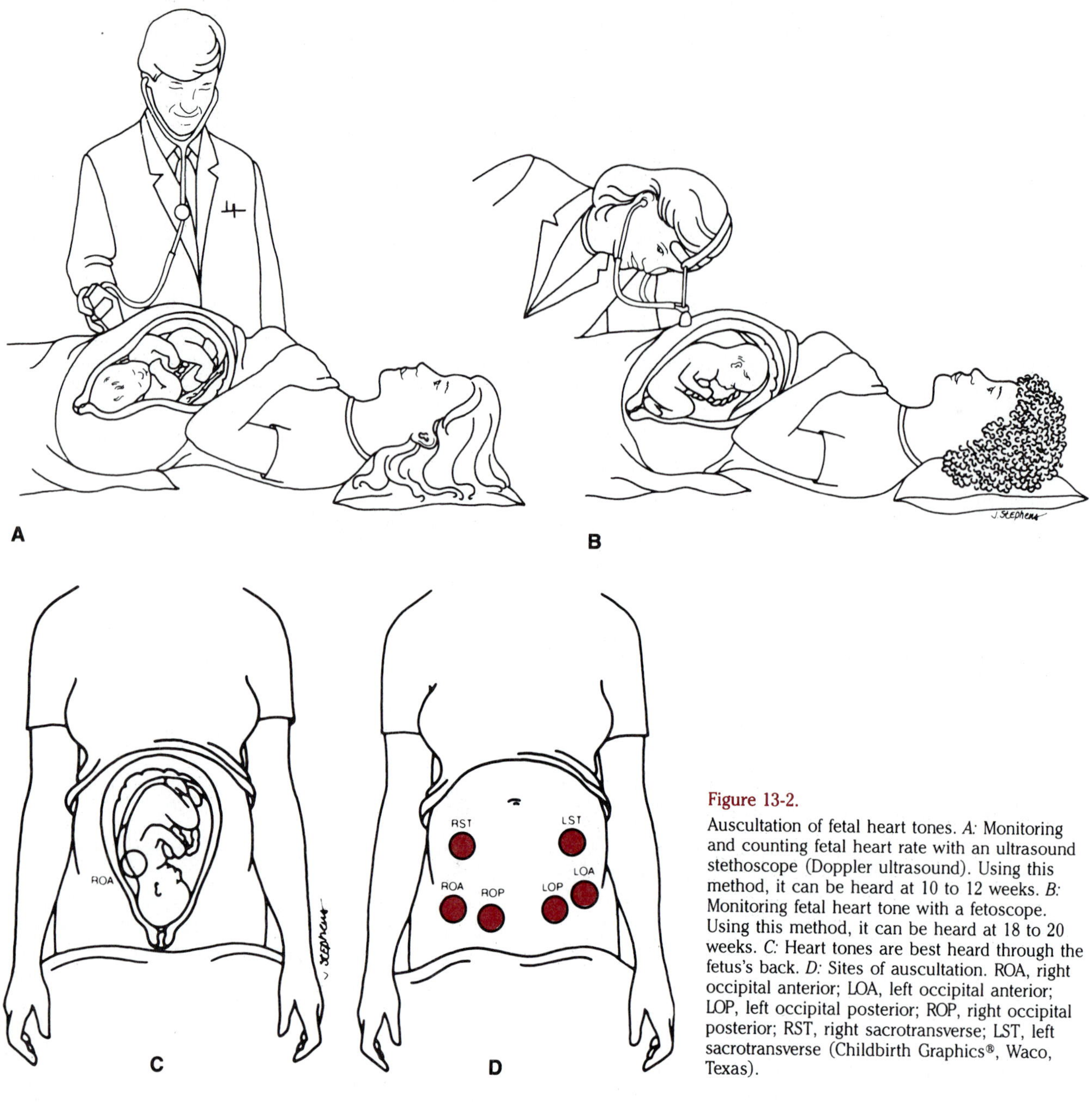

Figure 13-2.
Auscultation of fetal heart tones. *A:* Monitoring and counting fetal heart rate with an ultrasound stethoscope (Doppler ultrasound). Using this method, it can be heard at 10 to 12 weeks. *B:* Monitoring fetal heart tone with a fetoscope. Using this method, it can be heard at 18 to 20 weeks. *C:* Heart tones are best heard through the fetus's back. *D:* Sites of auscultation. ROA, right occipital anterior; LOA, left occipital anterior; LOP, left occipital posterior; ROP, right occipital posterior; RST, right sacrotransverse; LST, left sacrotransverse (Childbirth Graphics®, Waco, Texas).

- Ayre spatula for Pap smear collection
- Sterile cotton swabs to collect secretions for specimens
- Other culture media as needed for specimens collected
- Lubricant, to be used for the bimanual and rectal examinations only

Preparation of the Woman

It is important that the woman's bladder be emptied before she is draped for the examination. A full bladder will cause discomfort during the bimanual examination and will hinder palpation of the uterus for size. The woman should be nude from the waist down, but she may prefer to wear her shoes to protect her feet in the stirrups. She is placed in the lithotomy position with her feet in the stirrups and her buttocks positioned slightly over the edge of the table with her legs spread wide apart (Fig. 13-3). The woman should be instructed to put her arms at her sides or fold them under her breasts. When her head is resting on her elevated arms, the abdominal muscles become taut, and examination is difficult.

The woman should be told what will be happening during the examination and what she may expect to feel as it proceeds. Her experience with pelvic examinations should be explored and reassurance given that procedures will be explained to her. Helping the woman to relax by demonstrating deep, slow breathing often is effective in achieving cooperation.

Some women are helped by seeing the speculum and getting an explanation of its use; however, the opposite might be true for other women. For women interested in seeing their genitals, a long-handled mirror can be provided. In some cases it may be necessary to allow the woman to insert the speculum herself, with direction from the examiner. This

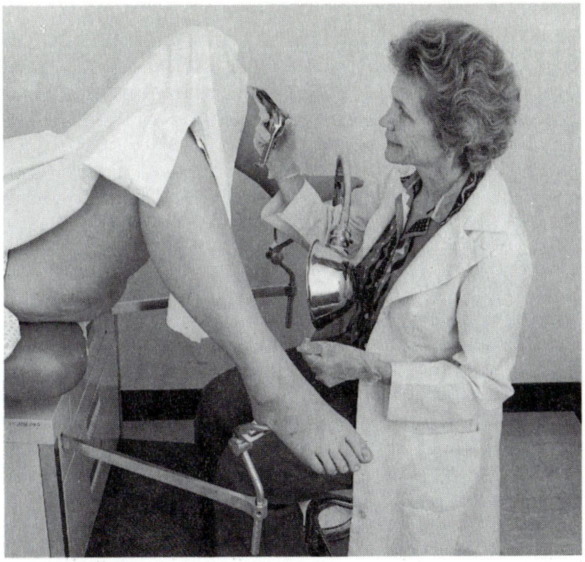

Figure 13-3.
Lithotomy position.

is sometimes helpful with adolescents who are fearful of being hurt. A wide variety of reactions to the examination can occur, and the nurse's attitude will greatly influence the quality of the experience not only in the present examination, but in future ones as well. When the equipment for the pelvic examination is ready and the woman has been prepared, the examination will be performed in the following order:

- Inspection and palpation of the external genitalia
- Speculum examination and specimen collection
- Bimanual examination
- Rectovaginal examination

Inspection and Palpation of the External Genitalia

The first step of the pelvic examination is inspection and palpation of the external genitalia and is especially important during pregnancy (Table 13-4). If abnormalities, such as vulvar varicosities, infection, pediculosis, or hemorrhoids, are found, they can be treated or palliated before labor and delivery. Infections identified in the prenatal period should be treated early to prevent exposing the fetus to infection at birth.

The Speculum Examination

Before the speculum examination, the woman should be questioned about the use of vaginal medication or a douche in the past 24 hours, because vaginal and cervical secretions are washed away or altered by these intrusions. If they have been used recently, collection of the Pap and gonorrhea smears and wet mount slides should be deferred until the next visit. The woman should be cautioned against using medication or a douche before a pelvic examination. She also should be instructed that douching is not recommended during pregnancy.

The speculum is made up of two blades and a handle (Fig. 13-4). Disposable specula made of plastic are in widespread use to minimize the risk of transfer of infections. The posterior blade is fixed, and the anterior blade is movable. Separation of the blades allows visualization of the vagina.

The speculum examination generally is done by physicians or nurses prepared for advanced practice (nurse practitioners, nurse specialists, certified nurse midwives). However, the steps for inspecting and removing the speculum for pelvic examination are outlined in the display, because nurses often are responsible for assisting during the examination.

Specimen Collection. Before the speculum is removed from the vagina, specimens for a Pap smear and screening for sexually transmitted diseases should be collected as indicated. Table 13-5 gives normal and abnormal findings in pregnancy. These tests are described in Chapter 6.

Bimanual Examination

Some of the most vital information from an obstetric or gynecologic physical assessment is obtained during the bimanual examination. As the uterus, ovaries (and their surrounding tissues, the adnexae), pelvic ligaments, and rectum are palpated, a complete picture of the woman's reproductive organs can be drawn.

This examination generally is performed by a physician or advanced practice nurse. Because nurses need to understand the findings of such an examination and may need to explain the process of the examination to the woman, the main points of the bimanual examination are summarized here and in Table 13-6.

During pregnancy the examiner concentrates on findings that provide information about the pregnancy:

- The size of the uterus is noted and described in terms of weeks of gestation (eg, 8 weeks' size).
- The shape of the uterus, its position, its softness or firmness, its location (in the pelvis or abdomen) is noted.
- The condition of the cervical os is assessed: closed or open, soft or firm, thick or thin (the latter condition, known as effacement, is an early sign of labor).
- The presentation (after 27 weeks) of the fetus and the status of its descent into the pelvis in late pregnancy (station) are recorded.

The bimanual examination should never be conducted in the presence of significant vaginal bleeding except by a physician and when immediate emergency care is available. The bleeding may be caused by placenta previa (a placenta lying over the internal cervical os). A finger placed through the os into the placenta may cause the woman to hemorrhage.

Pelvimetry

Pelvimetry is the measurement of the dimensions and proportions of the bony pelvis to assess whether it is large enough to accommodate the delivery of an infant. A normal vaginal delivery can occur only when the bony pelvis is large enough for the largest diameter of the infant, the head, to pass through it. Pelvic measurements can be obtained as part of the bimanual examination. The assessment is subjective, and its accuracy depends on the skill and experience of the examiner.

Table 13-4. Inspection and Palpation of the External Genitalia

Organ or Structure	Action	Normal Findings	Pregnancy Changes	Abnormal Findings
Inspection				
Mons Pubis	Adjust the light, and sit on a stool at the foot of the table facing the woman's perineum. Inspect the external genitals.	Mature secondary sexual characteristics	None	
		Skin covered by inverse triangle of curly hair (female escutcheon)	None	Pediculosis pubis (crab lice) or nits (eggs on hair shafts). Pruritus (itching) excoriation from scratching, folliculitis (infected hair follicle)
Labia Majora		Lie in close opposition in nulliparous women, may gap widely in multiparous ones; feel soft, have moist inner surface	Inner surface drier and skinlike	Pruritus, excoriation form scratching, lesions, vesicles, varicosities, discharge between folds from vaginal infection, Bartholin's gland tenderness, edema, redness
Inspection and Palpation				
	Tell the woman she will be touched. With gloved fingers, separate the labia majora, exposing the labia minora.			
Labia Minora		Hidden under labia majora in nulliparous women, project beyond labia majora in multiparous women; vary greatly in size and shape; feel soft	None in multiparas	Redness caused by vaginal infection or allergic reaction to douches, perfumed soap; wartlike growths, lesions
Clitoris	Observe the clitoris and retract its prepuce.	Small, erectile, highly vascular body, rarely exceeds 2 cm in length, covered by retractable prepuce	None	Clitoral hypertrophy, fixed prepuce that cannot be retracted (may interfere with sexual stimulation), lesions, chancres of sexually transmitted diseases
Urethral Meatus	Spread the labia with the index and second fingers of the gloved hand; inspect the urethra.	Vertical slit with pinkish, puckered appearance	None observable; dilatation of urethral canal due to increased progesterone	Polyps, growths, discharge, caruncle, erythema
Skene's Ducts (on either side of urethra at 4 and 8 o'clock)	Insert the index finger of the right hand 1 inch into the introitus, and gently press upward on the urethra. This is called "milking."	Duct may or may not be observable; no discharge	None	Yellowish-white discharge oozing from Skene's duct (gonorrhea culture needed)
Vaginal Musculature	As the fingers are withdrawn from the vagina, gently spread the vaginal orifice. Holding your fingers steady, ask the woman to cough.	Firm or relaxed muscle tone	More relaxed muscle tone, particularly in multigravidas	Cystocele (prolapse of bladder that protrudes in anterior vagina); rectocele (prolapse of rectum into posterior vagina)

(*continued*)

Table 13-4. Inspection and Palpation of the External Genitalia ***(Continued)***

Organ or Structure	Action	Normal Findings	Pregnancy Changes	Abnormal Findings
Pubococcygeal Musculature	Insert the fingers further into the vagina and ask the woman to tighten her muscles around your finger. (These are the muscles used to stop the stream during urination.)	Tight muscle control	More relaxed muscle tone, particularly in multiparous women	Loss of bladder tone as a result of pregnancy; leaking of urine, especially in older women, when perineal muscle tone is not maintained
Bartholin's Glands	With the fingers in the vagina, sweep them laterally on either side of the posterior fourchette to palpate the Bartholin's glands at 4 and 8 o'clock.	Glands not felt	None	Gland enlargement from infection, usually unilateral, exudate from duct, reddening of skin; may be extremely painful, with patient unable to walk
Perineum (area between the vagina and anus)	Remove the gloved hand from the vagina and use both hands to spread the buttocks apart to observe the perineum and anus.	No lesions; possibly episiotomy scar from previous delivery	None	Lesions, cysts, infection
Anus		Darker skin	None	Hemorrhoids, inflammation, lesions, fissures

If done at all, pelvimetry is delayed until late in pregnancy. It is considered more comfortable for the woman, because the pelvic tissues are softer, and the capacity of the pelvis in relation to the size of the fetus can be more accurately assessed at this time (Danforth & Scott, 1990). The characteristics of the different types of pelves and their measurements are shown in Figure 13-5.

Collecting Specimens for Laboratory Tests

Collection of specimens for laboratory tests during the first prenatal visit is an important part of the assessment of the pregnant woman. The nurse performs an initial assessment of the woman's blood pressure and height and weight. A clean-catch urine specimen is collected so that the dipstick reading is available to the health care provider before the examination. During the pelvic examination, vaginal, gonorrhea, chlamydia, and Pap smears are collected and, along with prenatal blood studies and urine for microscopic examination, are sent to the laboratory (see Chapter 6 for discussion of screening for pelvic infections). In some areas routine pharyngeal and cervical cultures for GBS may be performed once or more during pregnancy to identify women at risk for transmitting that virus to their fetus at delivery (Coleman, Sherer, & Maniscalco, 1992).

Results of these tests are evaluated on the second prenatal visit. The laboratory tests and procedures used to assess the pregnant woman are listed in Table 13-1. If the test results are normal and the woman does not present with later prob-

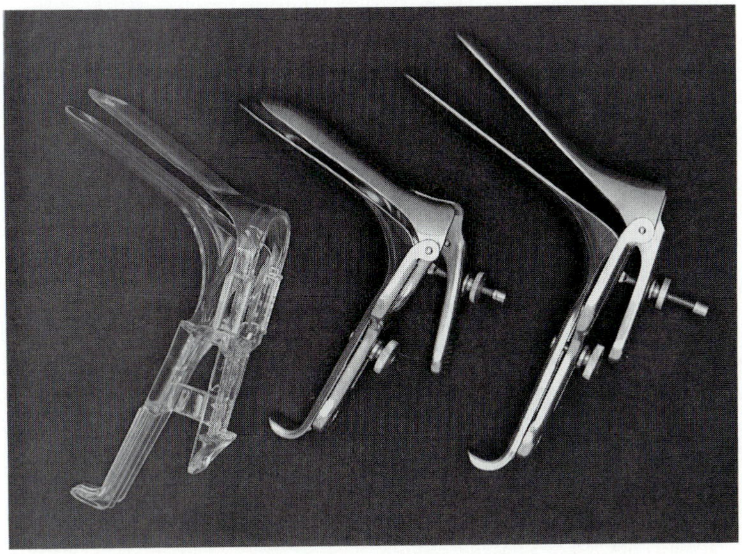

Figure 13-4.
Vaginal specula. The speculum may be made of metal or disposable plastic.

NURSING PROCEDURE
Inspecting and Removing the Speculum for Pelvic Examination

The speculum examination is performed to enable visualization of the vagina and cervix and to permit collection of specimens for laboratory testing. The examination is conducted as follows.

NURSING ACTION	***RATIONALE***
1. Select the speculum appropriate for the woman. Warm it, and lubricate it with warm water. Place the index and middle fingers 1-in into the vagina. Spread the fingers, exerting a downward pressure on the perineal body. Ask the woman to bear down while you insert the closed speculum in an oblique plane until it is beyond the hymenal ring.	To ensure comfortable insertion of the speculum. *Downward pressure* during insertion is extremely important to ensure that the sensitive anterior structures (urethra and clitoris) are not traumatized.

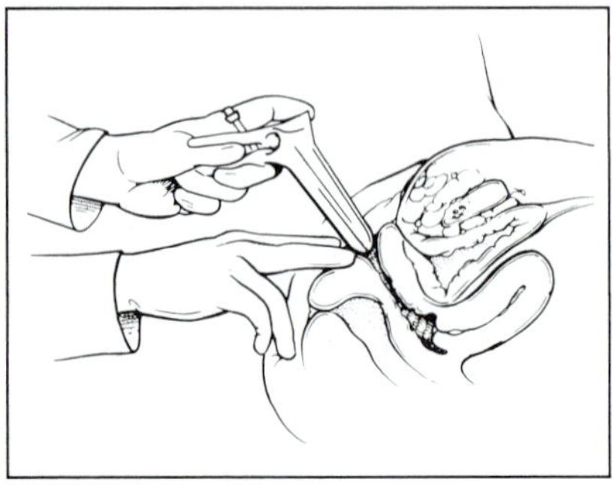

Step 1. Insertion.

2. Withdraw the fingers; turn the speculum to the horizontal plane, and advance it slowly, maintaining downward pressure until resistance is met. The shorter upper blade should be in front of the cervix and is lifted with the thumb lever. Maneuver the speculum so that when the blades are fully opened, the cervix comes into view. If the cervix is not seen, withdraw the speculum approximately halfway, and reinsert it on a different plane. When the cervix is visualized, secure the blades in position.	To ensure visualization of the cervix while maintaining patient comfort during the examination.

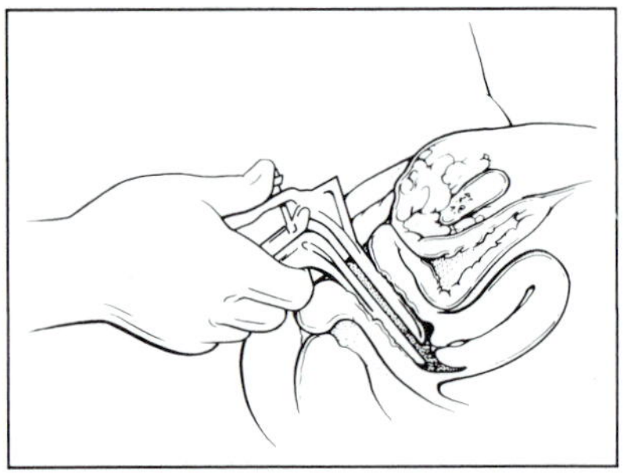

Step 2A. Advance.

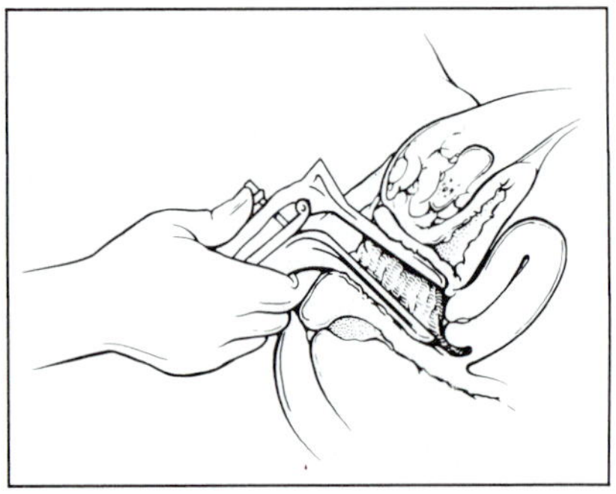

Step 2B. Opening the speculum.

3. With speculum in place, continue inspection of cervix and collection of specimens (see Table 13-5).	To provide information on cervical status, possible pelvic infections.
4. When inspection and specimen collection is complete, loosen the speculum thumbscrew or clamp. Maintaining a downward pressure, rotate the speculum as it is slowly withdrawn. Hold the thumb lightly on the thumbscrew or clamp to allow visualization of the vaginal walls between the blades.	To provide comfort to the woman and to allow the speculum to close gradually as it is withdrawn.

lems, routine monitoring of blood pressure and weight, urine dipstick testing at subsequent visits, and anemia screening every trimester will probably be the only tests required for the duration of the pregnancy. The following tests are used for screening and pregnancy monitoring. When abnormal or inconclusive results are reported, additional tests may be required.

Blood Tests in Prenatal Care

Blood tests provide essential assessment data. Tests include identifying blood group and type, screening for anemia, antibodies, infection, and blood hemoglobinopathies (abnormal forms of hemoglobin [Hgb], such as sickle cell) and diabetes.

Table 13-5. Cervical Inspection and Specimen Collection

Action	Normal Pregnancy Changes	Abnormal Findings
Cervix inspection using speculum 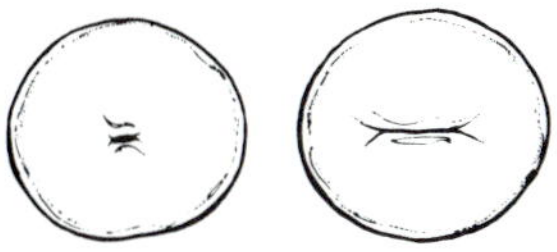 A B	Nulliparous cervical os (A) appears small and round; parous os (B) is splitlike and may have scars from tears during previous delivery. Bluish, friable cervix (breathes easily); white discharge	Dilated os; yellowish, greenish, or foul-smelling discharge at cervical os; inflammation
Cervical specimen collection: Pap smear; gonorrhea, chlamydia, or other cervical smears if infection is suspected	Increased amount of white, normal discharge	Blood from os, lesions, irregular configuration of ectropion
Vaginal specimen collection: Wet mount of saline and KOH to diagnose suspected vaginal infections	Pinkish-blue color rugae	Structural abnormalities, inflammation, lesions, white plaques, contact bleeding

Hemoglobin and Hematocrit. An Hgb or hematocrit (Hct) test is used to detect anemia. An Hgb reading below 10.5 g/100 mL or an Hct below 32% indicates anemia in the pregnant woman. The most common causes of anemia are previous heavy menstrual periods and a diet low in iron. When pathologic causes of anemia have been excluded, iron supplementation and diet counseling are indicated (Barger et al., 1988).

Blood Type. Blood type, Rh, and antibody titer tests identify blood as type O, A, B, or AB and as having Rh factor present or absent. Eighty-five percent of the population has Rh factor present; 15% do not have Rh factor (Danforth & Scott, 1990). When a woman's blood is identified as Rh negative during pregnancy, her mate's Rh factor must be determined. When the father's Rh factor is negative, so is the fetus', and no problems will arise. If, however, the father's blood is Rh positive, the fetus's also may be Rh positive. The combination of an Rh negative mother and an Rh positive fetus may cause the mother's body to react to the blood of the fetus as a foreign protein. This results in the production of antibodies and places the fetus at risk for erythroblastosis fetalis. (See Chapter 16 for more information on this condition.)

To determine whether the Rh negative mother is producing antibodies against her Rh positive fetus' blood, Rh antibody titer tests are performed on the pregnant woman's blood periodically during pregnancy. If antibodies are detected, as indicated by a positive titer, the woman is considered to be at high risk. Although Rh positive is the most common type of blood antibody, other less common types can cause fetal hemolytic disease and can be detected by antibody titer (see Chapter 16).

Rubella Screening. Rubella screening is done to determine whether the pregnant woman has antibodies for rubella (German measles). Past infection can be documented by the presence of antibodies to rubella in her blood. It is very important to counsel women who are not immune to avoid contact with anyone with suspected cases of rubella. If contracted in early pregnancy (the first 12 weeks), the disease may cause grave effects in the fetus, including blindness, deafness, mental retardation, and cardiac defects.

Susceptible women are not immunized during pregnancy because of the attendant risks of infection from the live virus. However, rubella vaccine is given early in the postpartum period to prevent future infection. The vaccine is safe to use in breastfeeding mothers (Barger et al., 1988).

Serology. Serology (the Venereal Disease Research Laboratory and fluorescent treponemal antibody absorption) tests are used to screen and diagnose women with syphilis. The spirochete *Treponema pallidum*, the organism responsible for the disease, crosses the placenta and infects the fetus. When the pregnant woman is treated before 18 weeks' gestation, the spirochete usually is eradicated from fetal tissues, causing minimal or no damage. If the pregnant woman is not treated until after 18 weeks, there may be evidence of a syphilitic infection in the neonate. When untreated, the disease may cause prematurity, intrauterine death, or congenital syphilis (see Chapter 16).

Maternal Serum Alpha-Fetoprotein. This test is used to detect open neural tube defects such as myelomeningocele or open abdominal wall defects such as omphalocele in the fetus by testing maternal serum for an elevated level of this protein. The test should be offered to all women and usually is drawn at approximately 16 to 18 weeks' gestation.

Sickle Cell Screen. This test is used to detect the presence of sickle hemoglobin in women at risk for inheriting the disease. A positive test confirms the presence of the abnormal hemoglobin but does not differentiate the disease

Table 13-6. Bimanual Examination

Procedures	Pregnancy Changes	Abnormal Findings
Remove the glove from the left hand, and lubricate the first two fingers of the right hand. Insert the lubricated finger into the vagina, maintaining *downward pressure.* With the fingers well into the vagina, rotate the hand until the palm is up. The thumb is kept vertical in the midline, while the other two fingers curve out of the way.		
Cervical Examination		
Place the left hand on the abdomen halfway between the symphysis and the umbilicus. Push the vaginal hand forward and backward until each of the fingers is in a lateral fornix with the cervix in between. Palpate the cervix; it should be freely movable.	Cervix 1.5–2.0 cm long; firm until term, then soft, elastic, and thick. External os closed (nullipara) or admits one fingertip (multipara). Internal os closed.	Roughened areas, edema, bleeding, dilatation before term, tenderness with movement; short or irregular length; soft and pliable <37 weeks; internal os open <37 weeks
Uterine Examination		
Determine uterine position by passing the fingers along the front and back of the cervix. With the first two fingers over the cervix, push it upward, lifting the uterus into the abdomen. Palpate the uterus between the vaginal and abdominal hands by moving the uterus from side to side with one finger in the lateral fornices so that the surface of the uterus can be felt.	Shape changes from globular to ovoid. Uterine size depends on age of gestation. Feels softer than nonpregnant uterus. Irregular, painless Braxton Hicks contractions may be felt. Becomes an abdominal organ at 12 weeks.	Tenderness with movement, myomas (fibroids) felt as firm irregularities on its surface. Deviations to either side may be due to pelvic masses or adhesions.
To palpate the adnexa, place the vaginal fingers palm upward in the right lateral fornix and the abdominal hand in the area of the right iliac crest. The hands are brought together and moved together toward the midline. The vaginal fingers will feel the ovaries slip between the fingers while the abdominal hand is pushing them downward. Repeat on the left side. In some women the ovaries are not palpable even in the nonpregnant state.	When the uterus becomes an abdominal organ, the ovaries cannot be palpated.	Tenderness, cystic masses, firm masses, enlargement (normal size 4 × 6 cm)

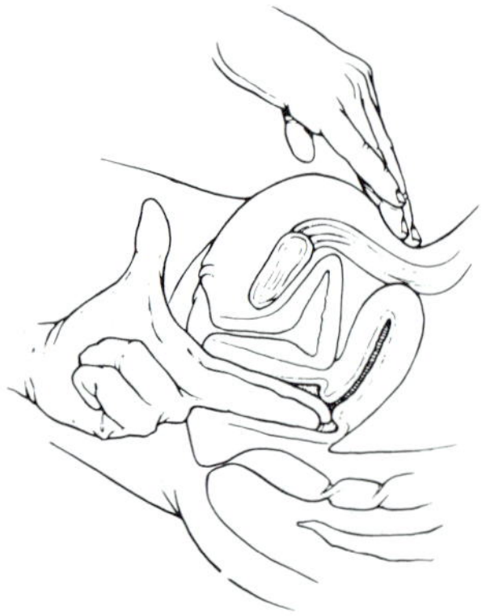

Palpation of the uterus.

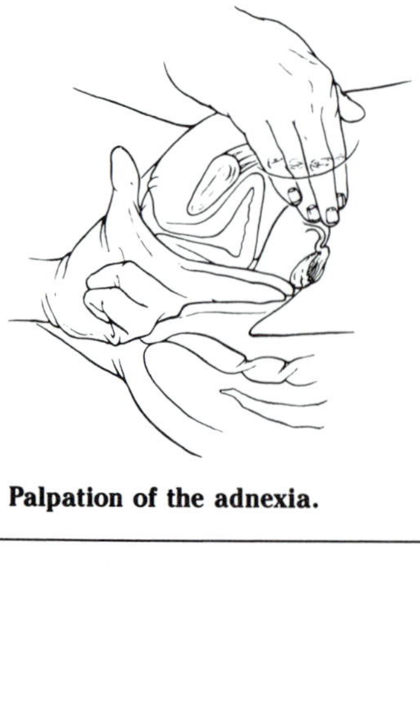

Palpation of the adnexia.

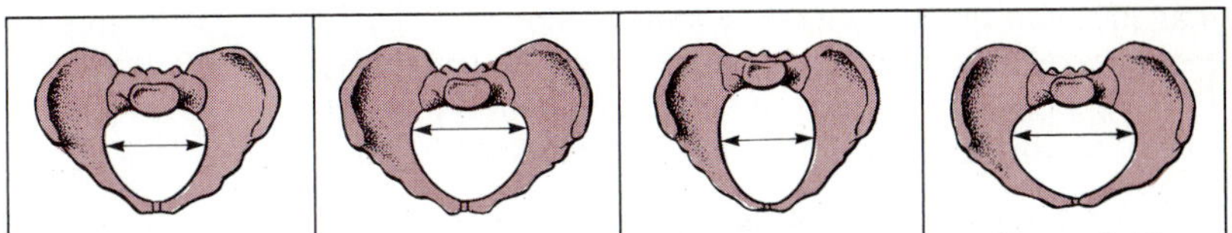

	Gynecoid	Android	Anthropoid	Platypelloid
Bone structure	Medium	Heavy	Medium	Medium
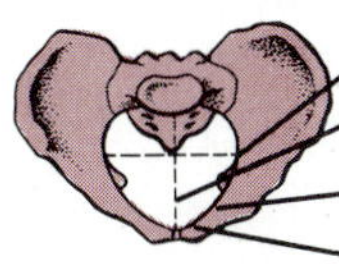 Widest transverse diameter of inlet	12.0 cm	12.0 cm	< 12.0 cm	12.0 cm
Anteroposterior diameter of inlet	11.0 cm	11.0 cm	> 12.0 cm	10.0 cm
Side walls	Straight	Convergent	Narrow	Wide
Forepelvis	Wide	Narrow	Divergent	Straight
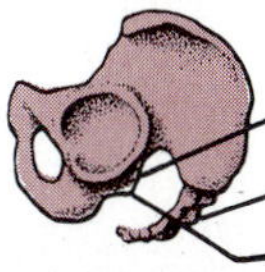 Sacrosciatic notch	Medium	Narrow	Backward	Forward
Inclination of sacrum	Medium	Forward (lower 1/3)	Wide	Narrow
Ischial spines	Not prominent	Prominent	Not prominent	Not prominent
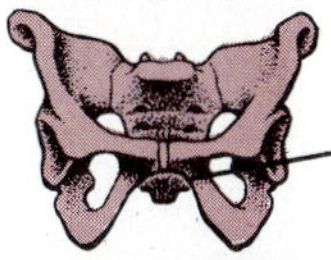 Suprapubic arch	Wide	Narrow	Medium	Wide
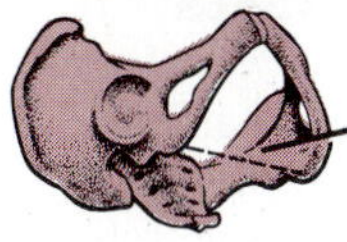 Transverse diameter of outlet	10.0 cm	< 10.0 cm	10.0 cm	10.0 cm

Figure 13-5.
Characteristics of four types of pelves. (Reproduced with permission from Benson, R. C. 1982. *Current obstetric and gynecologic diagnosis and treatment* (4th ed.). Los Altos, CA; Lange Medical Publications.)

state from the more benign carrier state (sickle cell trait). Pregnant women with a positive screen will require further testing, a hemoglobin electrophoresis, to differentiate sickle cell trait (SA) from sickle cell disease (SS). This disease is carried primarily by African American women, who are screened routinely during their first pregnancy (see Chapter 16).

Hepatitis B. Many prenatal clinics also are screening the blood of pregnant women for hepatitis B. During pregnancy this virus has been identified as the most threatening to the fetus and neonate. Inoculation and transmission of hepatitis B infection is through sexual contact and blood or parenteral exposure. Transmission of hepatitis B from mother to infant occurs through blood contact during the intrapartum and postpartum periods. The following women are at most risk for transmitting the virus:

- Women of Asian, Pacific Island, or Alaskan Eskimo descent, whether immigrant or U.S. born
- Women born in Haiti or sub-Saharan Africa
- Women with a history of acute or chronic liver disease or hepatitis
- Women who have undergone repeated blood transfusions
- Women who have frequent occupational exposure to blood in medical or dental settings
- Women who have home contact with a hepatitis B carrier
- Women who have multiple episodes of sexually transmitted disease
- Women who have been rejected as a blood donor
- Women who work or reside in an institution for the mentally retarded
- Women who work in a hemodialysis unit
- Women who exhibit symptoms of fever, headache, anorexia, pharyngitis, or abdominal pain
- Women who are military personnel or foreign travelers
- Women who are heterosexual with multiple partners or with male partners who are bisexual, homosexual, or intravenous (IV) drug users
- Women who use illegal IV drugs

HIV Testing. Most HIV infections in children are a result of transmission of the virus from an infected woman to her fetus or infant. Diagnosis of HIV infection in the woman permits counseling regarding continuation of the pregnancy (see Chapter 16). Early diagnosis also allows for some protection of the fetus through avoidance of invasive procedures that increase the risk of virus transmission. The current recommendation is that all pregnant women be screened for HIV (Fehrs, Hill, & Kerdt, 1991). Women with the greatest risk of the disease belong to one of the following groups:

- Those with evidence of immunosuppression
- Those who have used IV drugs for nonmedical purposes
- Those born in countries where heterosexual transmission is high
- Those who engage in prostitution
- Those who are, or have been sex partners of IV drug abusers, bisexual men, male hemophiliacs, men born in regions where heterosexual contact may play a major role (East and Central Africa, Caribbean), and men who have evidence of HIV infection

Urine Tests in Prenatal Care

Urine collected for testing should always be a midstream specimen. The purpose of urine testing is to detect the presence of urinary tract infection and substances in the urine that may indicate a problem.

Protein should not be present in the urine. Small amounts (traces) may be found when the specimen is contaminated by vaginal secretions or blood. Large amounts of protein may indicate kidney disease or pregnancy-induced hypertension.

Glucose found in the urine on one occasion may indicate the normal stress of pregnancy on the renal threshold. When large amounts appear in the urine on more than one occasion, further testing should be perfomed, as discussed in Chapter 27.

Ketones are products of fat metabolism found in urine only during fasting, after heavy exercise, or when pregnant women cannot maintain food intake because of nausea or vomiting. Because these substances may be deleterious to the fetus, the spilling of ketones should be prevented by adequate nutritional and fluid intake.

Bilirubin is a product of red blood cell destruction. Its presence in the urine suggests liver or gallbladder disease or breakdown of red blood cells.

Blood in the urine (hematuria) suggests urinary tract infection, kidney disease, or vaginal contamination of the specimen.

White blood cells at amounts greater than 4 per high-powered field indicate a urinary tract infection.

Bacteria in the urine (bacteriuria) indicates urinary tract inflammation. A urine culture will diagnose urinary tract infection and identify the organism responsible. A culture is considered positive for urinary tract infection when the colony count exceeds 100,000 (10^5). For laboratory values of the blood and urine tests, see the Appendix.

Diabetes Screening

Screening for gestational diabetes is a standard part of prenatal care for all women. Testing is done at 24 to 28 weeks. Hormonal effects that block insulin use and result in elevated blood glucose are clearly detectable at this time. A blood sample is drawn 1 hour after a 50-g glucose drink is consumed by the pregnant woman. An abnormal result of >135 mg/dL indicates the need for further screening (see Chapter 16).

Group B Streptococcus Screening

Screening for GBS is becoming a standard part of prenatal care in many areas. Because it is a significant cause of perinatal morbidity and mortality (see Chapter 16), routine cervical and pharyngeal cultures for GBS may be obtained during pregnancy. Early identification of women who carry GBS allows for careful intrapartum and postpartum management to reduce the risk of maternal and neonatal infection (Coleman et al., 1992).

The first prenatal visit is important because it establishes baseline data on the woman's and fetus' health. A full workup is done, and the stage is set for a continuing relationship between the woman and her nurse. The first visit is an extended one. The events of that visit progress in this order: orientation, collection of history, physical status assessment, pelvic examination, specimen collection, risk factor identification, teaching and counseling, and developing a long-term care plan.

Subsequent Prenatal Visits

Schedules for return prenatal visits may be adapted to suit the needs of individual women, especially those with physical or emotional problems. However, the usual schedule of visits follows:

- Every 4 weeks until 28 weeks of pregnancy
- Every 2 weeks until 36 weeks of pregnancy
- Every week until delivery

This schedule is in widespread use. However, a recent evaluation of practices in prenatal care suggests that fewer visits may be safe for low-risk women. For this reason prenatal visit schedules such as on the one shown in the accompanying display may be used, depending on the woman's condition (U.S. Department of Health and Human Services, 1989). Data obtained at subsequent visits are summarized in Table 13-1.

Identifying High-Risk Patients

Pregnancy presents a risk of morbidity and mortality over that of the nonpregnant state. High-risk factors, whether the risk is for the woman or the fetus or both, must be identified as early as possible so that appropriate measures can be taken to optimize the outcome of the pregnancy. Many risk scoring systems have been developed to aid in the identification of the pregnancy at risk. Most of these are designed to be completed at specific intervals during pregnancy, such as the first visit and then again at 28 weeks. In reality the pregnant woman must be assessed at every encounter with the health care team for any indication that a complication may be developing.

Schedule for Prenatal Visits

The following schedule has been proposed by the Expert Panel on the Content of Prenatal Care (U.S. DHHS, 1989) as safe and effective for healthy pregnant women. This schedule recommends visits at the following intervals:

- 4 to 6 weeks of gestation
- Within 4 weeks of first contact (nulliparous women only; telephone contact is sufficient for parous women)
- 14 to 16 weeks of gestation
- 24 to 28 weeks of gestation
- 32 weeks of gestation
- 36 weeks of gestation
- 38 to 39 weeks of gestation (38 weeks for nulliparous women, 39 weeks for parous women)
- 40 weeks of gestation
- 41 weeks of gestation

Preterm Delivery

Because the leading cause of neonatal mortality in the United States is prematurity, many health care providers are using preterm delivery risk assessment tools to try to identify the pregnant woman at risk for preterm labor. Unfortunately, such assessment tools have not accurately identified women who will deliver preterm, although they are still in relatively widespread use. (Nursing care of the woman with an at-risk pregnancy is addressed in Chapters 16 and 27.)

Adolescents and Women Older Than 35

Other women who may experience increased risk during pregnancy include adolescents and women older than 35 who are pregnant for the first time. Nursing care of these populations is discussed in Chapters 9 and 10, respectively.

Domestic Violence

Women involved in abusive relationships may be at particular risk during pregnancy. The incidence of battering among pregnant women may be 7% to 10% and is significantly correlated with anxiety, depression, housing problems, and drug and alcohol use (Campbell, Poland, Waller, & Ager, 1992). The financial, social, and psychological stress of an additional family member may precipitate or escalate acts of violence against the pregnant woman. Domestic violence also is discussed in Chapter 6.

The nurse should recognize the following as possible signs of battering in women and should carefully assess the woman's situation:

- Repeated subtle, nonspecific complaints suggesting psychosomatic origins
- Hesitancy, embarrassment, or evasiveness in relating her history, especially of an acute injury
- Overt depression
- Abusive use of alcohol or medications
- History of suicide attempts
- Overly solicitous husband or boyfriend who stays close to the woman and attempts to answer questions directed to her
- Injuries of the head, neck, face, and areas covered by a one-piece bathing suit (during pregnancy, the breasts and abdomen are particular targets of assault)
- Presence of bruises with injuries at several sites in different phases of healing
- Time lag between injury and presentation for care
- Discrepancy between the logic of how the injury happened and the nature of the injury

Nursing assessment of abused women must be conducted privately with assurance of confidentiality. A nonjudgmental, gentle approach is essential, but direct questioning is the most effective way to confirm suspicions of battering. Instruments such as the Abuse Assessment Screen, shown in the Assessment Tool can be used for such assessments. (See Chapter 15 for a discussion of nursing care of battered pregnant women.)

Substance Abuse

The following signs often are associated with substance abuse:

- Late or no prenatal care or poor attendance at appointments
- Poor weight gain or weight loss
- Chronic nasal congestion
- Dilated pupils; habitual wearing of dark glasses
- Elevated or irregular pulse
- Frequent mood swings
- Hostile or violent behavior
- Low self-esteem
- Memory loss
- Severe deterioration in financial or social status
- Evidence of needle use ("tracks")

The nurse noticing a pattern of these signs in a pregnant woman should carefully assess the woman's history. If the woman reports a history of substance use, the nurse should seek assistance in evaluating the woman's condition and readiness for treatment.

Identification of the woman who abuses drugs or alcohol may be difficult due to the reluctance on the part of the user to admit to such practices. The user may fear that disclosure will result in reports to law enforcement or child welfare personnel. In addition these women often do not seek prenatal care. Therefore, opportunities to assess for abuse occur only during the brief stay in the hospital after delivery.

Early identification of substance abuse is essential if treatment is to be offered during pregnancy. While a change in behavior among women who abuse drugs or alcohol may be difficult to achieve, the woman should still be offered counseling, education, and referral to appropriate resources

Assessment Tool

Abuse Assessment Screen

1. Have you ever been emotionally or physically abused by your partner or someone important to you?

YES ☐ NO ☐

2. Within the last year, have you been hit, slapped, kicked, or otherwise physically hurt by someone?

YES ☐ NO ☐

If YES, by whom ____________________

Number of times ____________________

3. Since you've been pregnant, have you been hit, slapped, kicked, or otherwise physically hurt by someone?

YES ☐ NO ☐

If YES, by whom ____________________

Number of times ____________________

Mark the area of injury on a diagram of the body.

4. Within the last year, has anyone forced you to have sexual activities?

If YES, who ____________________

Number of times ____________________

5. Are you afraid of your partner or anyone you listed above?

YES ☐ NO ○

(see the Nursing Research display). One dilemma that arises is the use of drug screening information for purposes other than provision of prenatal care. Further, there is considerable ethical debate about the appropriateness of enforced treatment for maternal substance abuse during pregnancy. The nurse must be aware of the legal and ethical implications of screening for substance abuse during pregnancy (see further discussion of nursing care in Chapters 15 and 16 and the Legal/Ethical Considerations display).

Subsequent prenatal visits are made according to the need of the individual. Fewer visits may be safe for the low-risk woman, while women with physical and emotional problems should be scheduled for more frequent visits. High-risk factors for both the woman and the fetus must be identified as early as possible so that appropriate measures may be taken to optimize the outcome of the pregnancy. High risk categories include women with previous pregnancy complications, adolescents, women older than age 35, women who are physically and emotionally abused, and women who are substance abusers.

Implications for Nursing Care

Prenatal assessment is central to the provision of quality care. The nurse is responsible for informing the woman about her health status based on information gained through the prenatal assessment. When the history and physical examination are completed, the pregnant woman should be assured, when appropriate, that her pregnancy appears to be progressing well. Results of the laboratory studies generally will be available in 3 days, and abnormal findings are followed up as soon as possible. The nurse should reassure the woman (especially if she is an adolescent) that complete physical and pelvic examinations will not be repeated at

Nursing Research

Cocaine Abuse in Pregnancy

A team of nurse researchers reviewed the literature on cocaine abuse in pregnancy from 1982 through 1989. They critiqued the published research, focusing on what is known about obstetric characteristics of women who use cocaine during pregnancy, the outcomes for cocaine-exposed neonates, long-term outcomes for child growth and development, and effectiveness of intervention programs for pregnant women who use cocaine.

The research evidence suggests that, while maternal and neonatal morbidity associated with cocaine use is clear, the specific effects of cocaine are difficult to separate from the effects of other characteristics, such as socioeconomic status, health status, nutritional status, lifestyle, access to prenatal care, psychological and psychiatric problems, and polydrug use. A key problem in many studies of cocaine use in pregnancy is in documenting the type, dose, and frequency of drug use.

Complications often thought to be associated with cocaine use in pregnancy include preterm labor or birth, premature rupture of membranes, and sexually transmitted diseases. The evidence linking placental abruption and hypertension is inconsistent. Neonatal and pediatric complications often thought to be associated with in utero cocaine exposure are fetal distress, low birth weight, neonatal withdrawal, smaller head circumference, and poor motor and state regulation. However, again the research evidence is inconsistent, and these conclusions are muddied by the frequency of polydrug use in the populations studied.

The authors note that the problems in research design and sampling in this area are considerable. While longitudinal research is needed to document effects of cocaine use in pregnancy, it is a huge challenge in this population. Women engaged in drug use often are unlikely to be willing to participate in research projects over time, and the costs of such research are enormous. The authors suggest that more attention should be paid to research that evaluates the cost-effectiveness of early detection, counseling, and drug treatment programs designed especially for women and that can address the particular needs of women during pregnancy.

Lindenberg, C., Alexander, E., Gendrop, S., Nencioli, M., & Williams, D. (1991). A review of the literature on cocaine abuse in pregnancy. *Nursing Research, 40*(2), 69–75.

subsequent visits. They are necessary only if there are special problems or verification of normal progress is needed.

Supplemental iron and prenatal vitamins usually are prescribed. A brief explanation or a handout that contains information on the nutritional needs during pregnancy may be helpful. This is especially true if the woman is unaware of the importance of good nutrition in pregnancy. (Nutritional aspects of pregnancy are further discussed in Chapter 17.)

The nurse also must instruct the pregnant woman about warning signs that require immediate care. If the woman's pregnancy is jeopardized, warning signs will alert her to seek immediate care. Without alarming the woman, the nurse explains to her that if any of the following symptoms occur, day or night, she should call her health care provider or clinic immediately:

- Vaginal bleeding
- Swelling (edema) of the face
- Continuous and severe headache
- Blurring or dimness of vision
- Abdominal pain
- Persistent vomiting
- Chills or fever
- Dysuria (painful urination)
- Fluid from the vagina
- Cessation of fetal movement

Because the first prenatal visit usually is long, it is best to limit the information given the woman to the answers to her own initial questions. She probably will need to ask questions about her care provider and the care that she will receive. The woman's comfort in asking these questions on her initial contact and her impression of the setting may set the tone for future visits. The nurse should answer any questions the pregnant woman has regarding the visit or her care, set a date for her next appointment, and encourage her to call if she has concerns before that time.

During subsequent prenatal visits, when the woman is more comfortable and less distracted, further information about the setting and its resources can be given. Information can be shared about support services, such as childbirth classes, nutritional counseling, dental care, psychological support, referral for food supplements, and other resources. The policies of the facility regarding labor, delivery, and postpartum care can be discussed as the woman indicates interest or as these issues become pertinent. Often the husband or partner cannot participate in the prenatal visits. If the woman has no other support person, it is doubly important for the nurse to spend time with her at each visit, discussing the events of pregnancy, answering questions, providing continuity of support, and assessing psychosocial adaptation (see Chapter 8).

The history-taking and the examination that occurs dur-

> ## Legal/Ethical Considerations
>
> ### Use of Drug Screening Information in Prenatal Care
>
> Prenatal screening for drug use presents the nurse with complex legal and ethical issues. One dilemma that arises is the use of drug screening information for purposes other than provision of prenatal care. For instance in some states, health care providers are expected to report positive tests for illegal drugs to child protective services departments. The benefit to the fetus of reporting illegal maternal drug use during pregnancy is unclear, because in many areas, access for pregnant women to drug treatment programs is extremely limited. Further, enforced treatment and incarceration are not positive alternatives.
>
> The authors argue that reporting prenatal drug use screening information to child protection agencies violates the principles of informed consent and confidentiality in the relationship with the pregnant woman. They conclude that use of this information for diagnostic and treatment purposes is appropriate and that health care providers have a responsibility to work toward better access to drug treatment programs for pregnant women.
>
> *Moseley, R., & Bell, C. (1991). Prenatal screening for illegal drugs: Dilemma for the nurse midwife.* Journal of Nurse Midwifery, *36(4), 245–248.*

ing follow-up prenatal visits are structured to obtain comprehensive information on the physical and emotional condition of the pregnant woman and her developing fetus. When deviation from the normal development occurs, immediate assessment can be made or planned. This process of ongoing assessment and diagnosis will identify a small number of women who, while initially thought to be low risk, will develop complications of pregnancy. The health care provider should be sensitive when explaining to the woman the problems identified, the care that will be provided, and the possible outcomes. When this has been accomplished, the woman is more likely to be able to absorb this information. If the woman feels she has adequate support, she is more likely to feel she can cope with the at-risk situation and do what is necessary to achieve the best possible outcome.

When they come to the health care setting, the woman and her partner are placing their trust in the health care providers. Many times they have specific ideas about what is important in pregnancy management. Some will be interested in childbirth alternatives, and some, for religious or cultural reasons, may be reluctant to participate in certain aspects of prenatal care (such as that involving a male care provider). It may be an important nursing responsibility to ensure that the woman's wishes be recorded so that members of the health care team are aware of her wishes and make their practice conform to the woman's preferences whenever possible (Diamond, 1990).

Based on the information gained through the prenatal assessment (described in this chapter and in Chapter 14), the nurse formulates nursing diagnoses and a plan of care. Nursing care of the expectant family, emphasizing teaching for self-care, is discussed in Chapter 15.

Chapter Summary

Prenatal assessment by the nurse provides baseline data that are valuable in health maintenance during pregnancy and can contribute to a successful outcome. Initial assessment calls for a detailed and meticulously recorded history, a comprehensive physical examination, an array of laboratory tests, and recording of findings. The initial prenatal examination is more than a guide. It establishes the psychophysical basis on which the management of the pregnancy is to proceed.

Prenatal assessment allows the nurse to establish rapport with the pregnant woman. It should be a shared experience involving empathy and mutual interest in a successful outcome. Each of the many steps taken in the prenatal assessment provides the nurse with an opportunity to share his or her knowledge and to explain, teach, and counsel.

Study Questions

1. *What are the advantages of early diagnosis of pregnancy?*
2. *What are the positive signs of pregnancy, and when can they be detected?*
3. *What specific hormone must be present for laboratory diagnosis of pregnancy, regardless of the type of test performed?*
4. *What is the chief objective of prenatal care?*
5. *According to Nägele's rule, what is the woman's EDD if the first day of her LMP was January 16?*
6. *A woman has had three previous pregnancies, one abortion, and one premature delivery, and she has two living children who are not twins. How would this information be recorded using the GTPAL system?*
7. *Why is it important to ask the pregnant woman to empty her bladder before performing an abdominal examination?*
8. *The pregnant woman is at 20 weeks of gestation. Auscultation fails to discern fetal heart tones. What does this signify?*
9. *The pubococcygeal muscle lacks tone on examination. What does this indicate?*
10. *Blood pressure and weight are baseline data used in assessing a pregnant woman's progress. If they appear to be normal, is it necessary to perform blood and urine laboratory tests? If so, why?*
11. *What is the significance of perineal scar tissue discovered when examining a pregnant woman?*

References

Barger, M., Lops, V., & Fullerton, J. (1988). *Protocols for gynecology and obstetric health care*. Orlando: Grune and Stratton.

Bluestein, D. (1990). Should I trust office pregnancy tests? *Postgraduate Medicine*, *87*(6), 57–68.

Campbell, J., Poland, M., Waller, J., & Ager, J. (1992). Correlates of battering during pregnancy. *Research in Nursing and Health*, *15*(3), 219–226.

Coleman, R., Sherer, D., & Maniscalco, W. (1992). Prevention of neonatal group B streptococcal infections: advances in maternal vaccine development. *Obstetrics and Gynecology*, *80*(2), 301–309.

Danforth, D., & Scott, J. (1990). *Danforth's obstetrics and gynecology*. Philadelphia: J.B. Lippincott.

Diamond, J. (1990). Patients' prenatal medical records precis. *Journal of Obstetric, Gynecologic, and Neonatal Nursing*, *19*(6), 491–495.

Fehrs, L., Hill, D., & Kerdt, P. (1991). Targeted HIV screening at a Los Angeles county prenatal/family planning health center. *American Journal of Public Health*, *81*(5), 619–622.

U.S. Department of Health and Human Services (1989). *Caring for our future: The content of prenatal care*. Washington, D.C.: Author.

Suggested Readings

Floyd, R., Zahniser, S., Gunter, E., & Kendrick, J. (1991). Smoking during pregnancy: Prevalence, effects and intervention strategies. *Birth*, *18*(1), 48–54.

Helton, A. (1990). A buddy system to improve prenatal care. *MCN: American Journal of Maternal Child Nursing*, *15*(4) 234–237.

Lindenberg, C., Alexander, E., Gendrop, S., Nencioli, M., & William, D. (1991). A review of the literature on cocaine abuse in pregnancy. *Nursing Research*, *40*(2), 69–75.

Machala, M., & Winer, M. (1991). Piecing together the crazy quilt of prenatal care. *Public Health Reports*, *106*(4), 353–360.

Noel, N., & Yam, M. (1992). Domestic violence: The pregnant battered woman. *Nursing Clinics of North America*, *27*(4), 871–874.

Parker, B., & McFarlane, J. (1991). Identifying and helping battered pregnant women. *MCN: American Journal of Maternal Child Nursing*, *16*(2), 161–169.

CHAPTER 14

Assessment of Fetal Well-Being

Learning Objectives

After studying the material in this chapter, the student will be able to:

- Describe the major modalities used for assessment of fetal well-being and when they are typically used.
- Explain why estimation of gestational age is an important component of prenatal care.
- Explain what information can be gained from amniocentesis, biophysical profile, ultrasonography, Doppler velocimetry, and fetal movement and heart rate studies.
- Explain what information is gained from nonstress testing and contraction stress testing.
- Describe nursing responsibilities related to assessment of fetal well-being.

Key Terms

amniotic fluid index
auscultation acceleration test
biophysical profile
biparietal diameter
contraction stress test
crown–rump length
Doppler velocimetry
lecithin–sphingomyelin ratio
McDonald's measurement
nonstress test
percutaneous umbilical blood sampling
reactivity
ultrasonography
vibroacoustic stimulation

Fetal health largely depends on maternal condition. Nurses who provide family planning advice need to emphasize the importance of being physically healthy, eating a nutritious diet, and avoiding all drugs, including tobacco and alcohol, when planning to conceive. Women who take prescription drugs or have a preexisting health problem should consult with their health care provider before conception.

Attention to optimal maternal health before conception is especially important for women with preexisting disorders that contribute to perinatal problems, such as diabetes mellitus, which is associated with a higher incidence of congenital anomalies, or preexisting hypertension, which is associated with placental insufficiency and intrauterine growth retardation. Evidence supports the role of prepregnancy counseling and care to reduce the risk for congenital anomalies among neonates of diabetic mothers. In addition women with previous children with genetic or structural defects may benefit from evaluation and counseling regarding recurrence risks. Parental chromosomal analysis may be indicated to detect abnormalities that may affect future fetuses. (See Chapter 12 for discussion of genetic screening and counseling.) Knowledge of the ramifications of health problems combined with early prenatal care will help to ensure the well-being of the parents and the neonate.

Assessing Fetal Health

In most situations assessment of fetal health includes monitoring maternal weight gain, uterine growth, fetal activity, and fetal heart rate (FHR) at each prenatal visit. In approximately 20% of all pregnancies further assessment is needed. Indications from the family's health history or the woman's past or present pregnancy history identify the pregnant women in need of further assessment. The prenatal nurse plays an important role in identifying these women, performing many types of assessments, and providing information and support to families. Prenatal assessment of fetal health involves the use of simple, noninvasive techniques that can reassure the health care provider and the expectant parents that the fetus is growing appropriately. When deviations from the norm occur, the nurse's early detection, consultation, and support of the expectant parents may avert or reduce physical and emotional stress.

The following major modalities are used to assess fetal well-being:

- Inspection of uterine growth and auscultation of FHR
- Ultrasonography to estimate gestational age, assess fetal growth, and diagnose intrauterine problems
- Doppler velocimetry to measure vascular resistance
- Assessment of FHR response to changes in oxygenation levels
- Assessment of fetal movement
- Direct assay of amniotic fluid
- Direct assay of umbilical blood

Uterine growth is inspected throughout the prenatal period by measuring fundal height and auscultating FHR. Ultrasonography may be used early in pregnancy to estimate gestational age. This technique can be used later to rule out fetal, placental, or uterine problems. Doppler velocimetry of uterine and umbilical arteries may be used to assess for fetal growth disorders. Fetal movement may be assessed throughout the second and third trimesters. FHR responses to contractions or to fetal movement will be assessed in the second or third trimester if there is a question of fetal status. Direct assay of amniotic fluid through amniocentesis may be performed early in pregnancy for genetic screening. It also may be used later to evaluate fetal maturity or to rule out a complication like intrauterine infection. Direct assay of umbilical blood may evaluate fetal metabolites, blood chemistries or karyotype. The following section discusses these major fetal assessment modalities in more detail as they are likely to be used in each trimester of pregnancy.

Nursing assessment of the fetus begins with a careful, detailed health history of the pregnant woman, the biologic father of the fetus, and the family. The history also should include the maternal menstrual and obstetric history, exposure to teratogens, and the parents' ethnic or racial background.

Objective methods used to assess fetal well-being also are important assessment tools. These include auscultation of FHR, measurement of fundal height, monitoring of quickening and fetal movement, and ultrasonography. The nurse's role in performing these functions is discussed below.

Assessment in the First Trimester

Methods of fetal assessment in the first 13 weeks of pregnancy primarily involve confirmation of the pregnancy and estimation of gestational age. Information collected during these visits will be added to the health history and physical assessment data gathered about the pregnant woman (eg, weight and findings from the bimanual examination of the uterus) to establish a complete data base for the pregnancy.

Fetal Heart Rate

Because fetal heart sounds cannot be heard with a DeLee-Hillis obstetric stethoscope until approximately 20 weeks of gestation, the ultrasound stethoscope, or Doppler ultrasound, provides another method of fetal assessment during the first trimester (Fig. 14-1). The ultrasound stethoscope, or Doptone, is a hand-held, battery-operated device. It uses ultrasound and the Doppler effect to detect motion. The single transducer on the Doptone sends out a continuous beam of high-frequency sound waves. This beam, when directed through to the fetus, is reflected back from fetal tissues. Moving structures or objects, such as the valves of the fetal heart, reflect sound waves at different frequencies; the transducer interprets and translates these into an audible sound, such as the FHR. Gross movements of fetal extremities also can be heard as quick, harsh sounds. The Doptone, like other ultrasound devices, requires the use of gel to improve sound conduction.

Between 10 and 12 weeks of gestation, the FHR can first be heard using the Doptone. It is usually found midline in the suprapubic region. The FHR is normally between 120 and 160 bpm and can be distinguished from the slower maternal heart rate by palpating the woman's pulse at the same time.

Parents may enjoy hearing the FHR. A speaker can be attached to most Doptones, allowing the sound to be amplified into the room. This also can be an opportunity for parents to begin attachment to their newborn. Use of the Doptone during the first trimester has become routine in most prenatal clinics. Although it is not specifically diagnostic of fetal health, it does confirm fetal life.

Ultrasonography

Ultrasonography is a procedure using ultrasound waves to provide imaging of the fetus, placenta, and uterus (Fig. 14-2). Serial sonograms also reflect time-dependent changes in structure. The first scanning methods used a static B-scan, which provided a two-dimensional image in cross-section. Today, real-time (B-scan) ultrasound provides continuous cross-sectional motion pictures of internal structures.

Although more than half of all pregnant women have ultrasound examinations, they should be performed only when there is a specific perinatal indication. During the first trimester ultrasound should be used for the following:

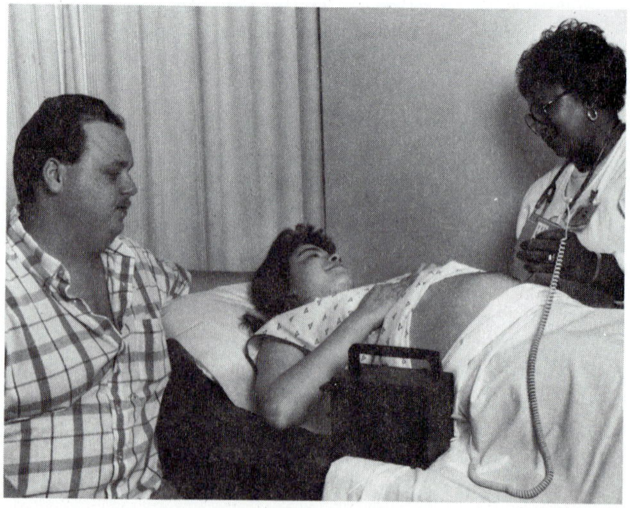

Figure 14-1.
The fetal heart rate is auscultated by use of Doppler ultrasound.

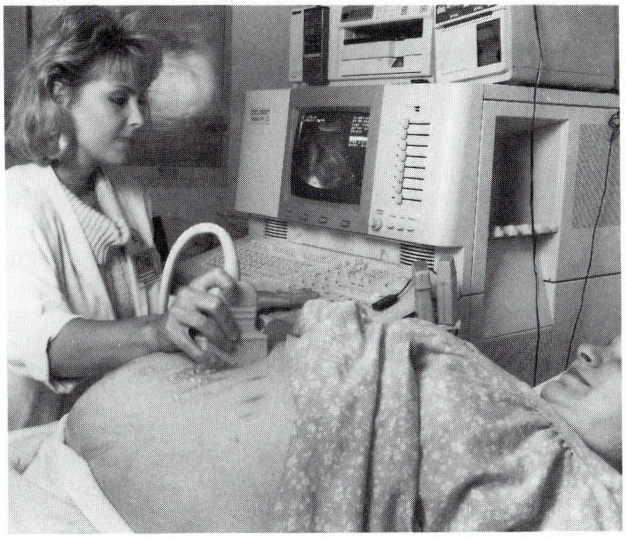

Figure 14-2.
Ultrasound is used in prenatal care.

- Assessment of gestational age
- Evaluation for congenital anomalies
- Diagnostic evaluation of vaginal bleeding
- Confirmation of suspected multiple gestation
- Evaluation of fetal growth
- Adjunct to prenatal testing (amniocentesis, chorionic villus sampling, percutaneous umbilical blood sampling [PUBS])
- Diagnostic evaluation of pelvic mass

The following parameters are measured during ultrasound:

- Location of the gestational sac
- Crown–rump length (CRL; first trimester)
- Presence or absence of fetal life
- Fetal number
- Evaluation of the uterus and adnexal structures
- Presentation (second and third trimesters)
- Estimation of amniotic fluid volume (second and third trimesters)
- Placental location
- Fetal biometry, including biparietal diameter (BPD), head circumference, abdominal circumference, and femur length (second and third trimesters)

As early as 4 weeks after the last menstrual period (LMP), a gestational sac implanted within the endometrial cavity can be detected by a static scanner. Using a real-time scanner, cardiac activity is readily identifiable by 7 weeks after the LMP. Identification of the gestational sac or fetal cardiac activity documents the presence of the fetus.

The most common use of ultrasound during the first trimester is to assess gestational age. Because of the rapid rate of growth in the first trimester, accuracy in dating a pregnancy is believed to be highest between 7 and 13 weeks after the LMP. The CRL of the embryo or fetus is measured using real-time sonography.

Sonographs use a chart of CRLs measured in millimeters to estimate gestational age (Table 14-1). Between 7 and 13 weeks the assessment of gestational age is accurate to within 1 to 3 days with 95% confidence. During the second trimester normal biologic differences in fetal growth contribute to making ultrasound slightly less accurate in assessing gestational age. Fetal measurements, such as BPD, head circumference, femur length, and abdominal circumference, are used to estimate age, rather than the CRL.

Table 14-1. Average Size of Embryo and Fetus by Crown–Rump Length (CRL)

Age	CRL
2 weeks	1.5 mm
3 weeks	2.5 mm
4 weeks	5.0 mm
5 weeks	8.5 mm
7 weeks	20.0 mm

A full bladder may improve ultrasonic resolution in women at 20 weeks of gestation or earlier. The full bladder serves as an anatomic landmark and elevates the uterus out of the pelvis for better visualization. If a full bladder is desirable, women should drink at least 1 L of water 1 to 2 hours before the examination. During the procedure the woman will be placed on her back. It is important to ensure comfort, because the examination could last as long as 30 minutes. Gel is smeared over the abdomen to act as a conductive medium for the ultrasound and to reduce friction from the transducer as it is moved across skin. The procedure is painless, although many women report discomfort from the pressure of a full bladder.

During the first trimester a better image may be obtained by using a vaginal probe. The probe is a smaller transducer designed to be placed at the introitus. The same fetal measures are used whether a transabdominal or transvaginal approach is used.

The nurse should explain to the woman that in most cases she will be able to see an image of her fetus on the machine's monitor. The ultrasonographer can point out identifiable structures, such as the head, extremities, or moving heart valves. Pregnant women usually are delighted to have a first glimpse of the growing fetus. When ultrasound is used as an adjunct to prenatal diagnosis, visualization of the fetus may contribute to the difficult decisions parents face regarding termination or continuation of the pregnancy if a congenital or chromosomal defect is detected. Seeing an image of the fetus may make it more difficult for parents to decide to terminate a pregnancy on the basis of a diagnosed fetal problem. Nurses should be sensitive to these issues and support the parents' decisions about visualization of their fetus using ultrasound. Depending on the care setting, nurses may have growing responsibilities in relation to ordering or performing ultrasound during pregnancy (see the accompanying Legal/Ethical display).

Assessment in the Second Trimester

As the fetus continues to grow, many dramatic changes occur between the 14th and 26th weeks of pregnancy. With the uterus expanding the pregnant woman begins to

Legal/Ethical Considerations

The Nurse's Role in Ultrasound

Ultrasound has become an indispensable diagnostic tool in obstetric and gynecologic care. The traditional nursing role in the care of women undergoing ultrasound evaluations has been limited to education about and preparation for the procedure. Nurses are now being asked to expand their roles in ultrasound evaluations.

Before assuming expanded responsibilities in the performance of ultrasound examinations, nurses should evaluate the scope of practice as defined by their state or area and the regulations of the licensing and accrediting bodies for the agency or institution in which they practice. Relevant issues that should be considered include the type of ultrasound examinations to be performed; educational preparation and clinical practicum under appropriate supervision needed to establish competency, and risk management, liability, and other legal issues.

If this expansion of duties and responsibilities is consistent with one's scope of practice and the regulations of licensing and accrediting bodies, nurses should be provided with the educational content and clinical practicum necessary to achieve competency. The educational content and clinical practicum should be provided before the nurse assumes responsibility for expanded roles in the performance of ultrasound examinations. In addition policies, procedures, and protocols must be developed that direct and guide nurses in the performance of ultrasound examinations.

Approved by the NAACOG Committee on Practice, September 1991.

"show," announcing her pregnancy to the world. In addition the thinner walls of the enlarging uterus combined with the activity of the growing fetus enable the woman to feel fetal movement. These changes will affect the methods of fetal assessment as well.

Assessment of the height of the uterine fundus has long been used to monitor fetal growth and is performed at each prenatal visit after 20 weeks. The uterus is palpated abdominally. The location of the fundus in relation to the symphysis pubis is identified and is referred to as fundal height, expressed in centimeters.

Fundal Height

From 20 weeks of gestation until the end of pregnancy, the fundal height should be measured and recorded on the uterine growth chart at each prenatal visit or weekly if the pregnant woman becomes hospitalized for any reason. This measurement (known as *McDonald's measurement*) is simple to do and is often a nursing responsibility. However, the reliability of the uterine growth chart will be affected if a consistent method of measurement is not used. Accuracy will be less than desired when different examiners are involved. Measurements should always be done with the mother in the same position and having an empty bladder (Engstrom, 1988).

Using a nonstretching but flexible metric measuring tape, the examiner places the zero line of the tape on the superior border of the symphysis pubis. It should then be stretched across the contour of the abdomen at the midline to the top of the fundus. This measurement in centimeters is graphed on the uterine growth chart on the line that corresponds to the number of weeks of gestation, as previously determined. After 20 to 22 weeks of gestation the fundal height in centimeters is expected to approximate the gestational age in weeks.

There should be a consistent increase in uterine size at each visit for a smooth growth curve that indicates adequate interval growth. When the measurement is consistently 1 to 2 cm greater or less than expected, there is usually no cause for concern; individual variation, such as short stature, may be the reason. However, if the measurement has been taken consistently, a discrepancy of 3 cm or more between fundal height and gestational age calls for further evaluation. A discrepancy of uterine size and gestational age also can suggest incorrect dating of the pregnancy. Some other causes of fundal height greater than predicted for gestational age include the following:

- Multiple gestation
- Polyhydramnios
- Fetal macrosomia
- Full maternal bladder

Lower fundal height than expected can indicate the following:

- Abnormal fetal presentation
- Growth-retarded fetus
- Congenital anomalies
- Oligohydramnios

Fetal Heart Rate

During the second trimester assessing the FHR continues to be a part of each prenatal assessment. As the fetus nears 20 weeks of gestation, the fetoscope may be used rather than the Doptone. Use of the fetoscope may lengthen the time necessary to locate and hear the FHR, because the sound produced is soft, similar to that of a watch ticking beneath a pillow. To avoid anxiety to the woman during the search for the heart tone, the nurse should explain that the less sophisticated fetoscope, and not a problem with the fetus, is causing the delay. (See Chapter 13 for a more detailed description of this procedure.)

Fetal Movement and Quickening

An additional parameter used to confirm gestational age is fetal movement or quickening. For most primigravidas fetal movement is first detected between 18 and 20 weeks after the LMP, whereas multigravidas may perceive fetal movement as early as 16 weeks. As the primigravida approaches the midpoint of her pregnancy, she should be advised to expect a light, fluttery feeling that may be fetal movement but is often mistaken for intestinal gas. The pregnant woman should be asked to record the date when she first notices this sensation. (The experienced mother can be advised that she may feel movement earlier than with the first pregnancy, because she is more sensitive to the movement.) The date can then be compared with her LMP to assess the accuracy of the dating of the pregnancy.

Ultrasonography

Ultrasound is used during the second trimester for the following reasons:

- Assess gestational age
- Diagnose multiple gestations
- Assess fetal growth
- Identify congenital abnormalities of the fetus
- Guide procedures, such as amniocentesis and PUBS
- Assess placental location

When gestational age must be verified during the second trimester, ultrasound is used. After 14 weeks of gestation the widest transverse diameter of the fetal head, known as the BPD, is used as a means of assessing gestational age. Ultrasonographers believe that the optimal time for determining gestational age by BPD is between 16 and 20 weeks of gestation. At this time the 90% confidence limits are plus or minus 1 week. After 26 weeks of gestation BPD is not believed to predict gestational age as accurately. The most reliable ways to assess gestational age using ultrasound are CRL measurement between 7 and 13 weeks of gestation and BPD measurement between 16 and 20 weeks. Sonography is recommended at this time as a baseline evaluation for pregnancies that are at risk for complications.

The nurse should review the following clinical parameters for gestational age assessment and compare them to the estimated date of delivery calculated from the LMP:

- Detection of fetal movement
- Audible fetal heart tones
- Fundal height measurement

The accuracy of gestational age estimation by ultrasound is enhanced by early evaluation. When there is concern that the growth of the fetus may be excessive or less than expected, serial or repeated sonograms may be used. They will indicate whether growth is appropriate for gestational age or whether there is evidence of multiple pregnancy or abnormal amounts of amniotic fluid.

Percutaneous Umbilical Blood Sampling

PUBS is a relatively new procedure. It involves the insertion of a needle through the maternal abdomen and amniotic cavity into the umbilical cord at the site of insertion into the placenta (Fig. 14-3). This procedure, which is usually performed in the second or third trimester, also is called cordo-

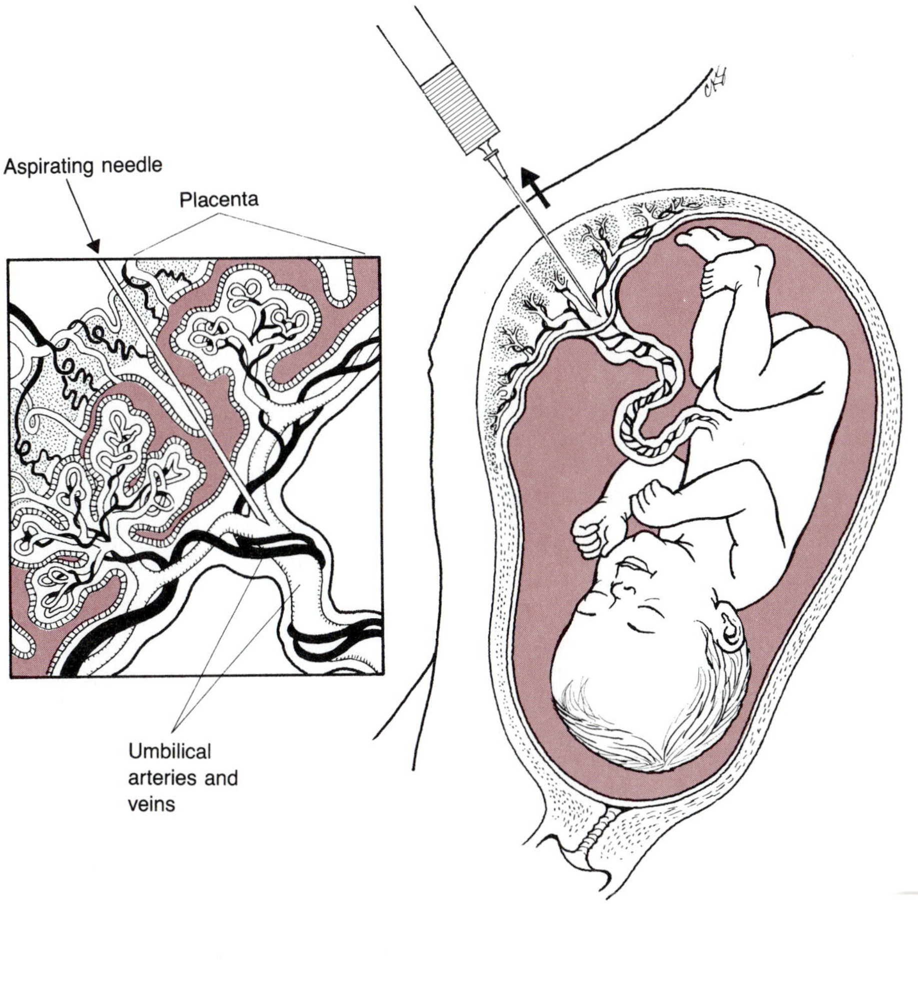

Figure 14-3.
In percutaneous umbilical blood sampling, a fine needle is inserted through the maternal abdomen into the umbilical cord at the site of the insertion of the placenta.

centesis or fetal blood sampling. PUBS is used for a variety of conditions when direct access to the fetal vascular compartment is required. Under direct ultrasound visualization, fetal blood may be aspirated for testing for karyotype, blood chemistries, antibody screening for teratogenic viruses, or blood gases. Once this direct access is obtained, fetal blood transfusions also are possible, as in the case of treatment for Rh sensitization. Complications of the procedure include a 1% to 2% incidence of fetal loss.

Assessment in the Third Trimester

During the last trimester of pregnancy (weeks 28 to 40), fetal growth, FHR, and fetal activity continue to be monitored. The uterine growth curve should continue to show positive interval growth. As the prenatal visits increase in frequency, a continuation of 1 cm/wk growth of fundal height through 36 weeks of gestation is expected. In the primigravida the fetus will begin to descend into the pelvis after 38 weeks, and the fundal height may decrease 2 to 4 cm when "lightening" has occurred. This is considered a normal decrease in fundal height at the end of gestation. At this time the mother will usually report more pressure or weight in her pelvis or lower back but easier breathing because diaphragmatic pressure has decreased.

Fetal Movement

Studies of high-risk pregnancies have reported decreased perinatal morbidity and mortality when fetal activity is monitored by the pregnant woman. Many prenatal health care providers advocate daily maternal monitoring of fetal movement during the third trimester for all high-risk pregnant women. At some time each day, the woman is asked to lie down, preferably on her side, and palpate her abdomen to help detect fetal movement. The nurse often is responsible for instructing women how to use this technique to monitor fetal activity. The accompanying display lists some teaching considerations the nurse can use for maternal monitoring of fetal activity.

Teaching Considerations

Maternal Monitoring of Fetal Activity

The nurse can use the following points in teaching women to assess fetal movement:

- The woman should lie on her side and palpate her abdomen to detect fetal movement.
- Counting continues until ten movements have been felt. Most women report perceiving ten movements in 20 minutes to 2 hours.
- If ten movements have not been felt in 3 hours, the health care provider should be notified. In some cases further fetal heart rate evaluation may be performed.
- Variations in fetal activity and sleep patterns occur, so 3 hours is believed to be adequate time in which to expect ten fetal movements.
- During fetal activity monitoring, the following should be remembered:
  - Fetal activity often increases after meals or light massaging of the abdomen.
  - A short walk may make the fetus more active.
  - The fetus normally has periods of sleep throughout the day, usually lasting 20 minutes.
  - During the last 2 to 3 weeks before delivery, activity normally decreases as the fetal presenting part becomes engaged and there is less room to move around.

Note: When explaining self-monitoring to the mother, the nurse can explain that this is a way the mother may take part in maintaining the health of her baby before it is born. The value of reporting decreased fetal activity cannot be too strongly stressed. Intrauterine fetal death often is preceded by several days of decreased fetal movement.

Ultrasonography

During the third trimester, sonography often is used to determine fetal position and estimate fetal size or amniotic fluid volume. When a sonogram has not been done previously, it is difficult to make an assessment of gestational age at this time. It is helpful to assess fetal growth by comparing previous sonographic measurements with current fetal size. BPD, abdominal circumference, and femur length are the most common measurements taken to estimate fetal weight and interval growth during the third trimester.

Amniotic Fluid Index

Amniotic fluid volume normally increases until approximately 33 weeks' gestation when a slight but consistent decline is noted. Volume decreases slowly until 40 weeks when the rate declines more rapidly (10% to 15% per week after 40 weeks). Extremes of increased and decreased volume are associated with poor perinatal outcomes. Decreased amniotic fluid volume or oligohydramnios is associated with acute and chronic asphyxia and intrauterine growth retardation, presumably due to diminished uteroplacental perfusion, decreased renal blood flow, and subsequent decreased fetal urinary output. Oligohydramnios also may be caused by rupture of the membranes or fetal renal abnormalities. Increased amniotic fluid volume or hydramnios is associated with infants of diabetic mothers and some fetal anomalies. Amniotic fluid volume is best measured by calculation of the amniotic fluid index. This method involves visualization of the amniotic fluid by ultrasound. Measurement of fluid pockets observed in each of the four quadrants of the uterus are added together.

The process of assessing fetal well-being is ongoing throughout pregnancy. Techniques for assessing the fetus include auscultation of the FHR, measurement of fundal height, monitoring the timing of first maternal perception of fetal movement, and ultrasonography. With the exception of ultrasonography, these techniques are standard elements of prenatal care. Performing these assessment and accurately interpreting the findings are major nursing responsibilities.

Monitoring Fetal Well-Being

The field of perinatology has been concerned with maintaining the health of the woman and the growing fetus during the pregnancy. Biophysical tests allow the clinician to "observe" the fetus in utero. Although these tests provide different information, they all indicate in some way whether the maternal–placental–fetal unit is intact and functioning. From this information the clinician can decide whether the pregnancy can safely be continued or whether intervention is indicated.

From a philosophic perspective there are opposing opinions on the use of technology in obstetrics. Proponents cite the many infants who survive because early detection of problems leads to timely medical intervention and management. Those opposed feel that obstetricians and pediatricians begin a process they cannot end. That is, early detection often results in the delivery of a preterm neonate who requires life support systems for an extended time. However, life support does not ensure the recovery of the neonate. The process of life support adds risks that may result in long-term disability. Once the process of life support is begun, the ethical question arises as to who, if anyone, has the right to stop it.

This section discusses the available means of testing for fetal well-being, and the positive aspects are emphasized. The nurse should keep in mind that not all people—parents or clinicians—would agree with this emphasis. Nurses are the members of the health care team most frequently responsible for explaining, and at times performing, the recommended tests. Parents will usually ask the nurse's advice. Nurses must be aware of their own biases and support the family in considering all the factors in their attempt to arrive at the best decision for both the pregnant woman and the unborn.

Amniocentesis

Amniocentesis is the aspiration of fluid from the uterus through an abdominal puncture for the purpose of fluid analysis (Fig. 14-4). This testing may be conducted at any time during pregnancy. When the procedure is advised in the first half of pregnancy (14 to 20 weeks), it is usually for the purpose of studying genetic makeup and determining developmental abnormalities. The procedure is discussed in more detail in Chapter 12. Amniocentesis is done in the third trimester usually for the purpose of determining fetal lung maturity or detecting amnionitis.

Once the fluid is obtained, laboratory testing will depend on the maternal complication. For example, culture

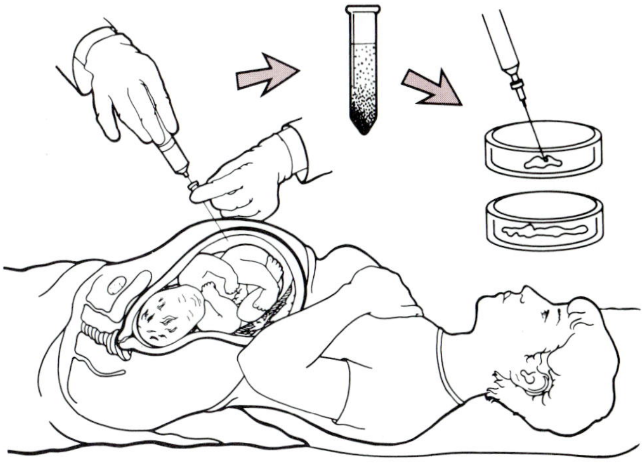

Figure 14-4.
Transabdominal amniocentesis (Childbirth Graphics®, Waco, TX).

and sensitivity tests are performed on the fluid if amnionitis is suspected. Fetal lung maturity tests are indicated with any maternal or potential fetal problem indicating early delivery of the fetus. These include determinations of the lecithin–sphingomyelin (L/S) ratio and tests for the presence of phosphatidylglycerol (PG).

Lecithin–Sphingomyelin Ratio

Because most neonatal morbidity and mortality results from pulmonary immaturity and respiratory distress, reliable indicators of fetal lung maturity are essential in predicting postdelivery status of the neonate. Assessment of the L/S ratio from amniotic fluid is the oldest and most reliable of the tests available today. Lecithin and sphingomyelin are phospholipids produced by the lung tissue. These lipids mix with amniotic fluid in the lung to reduce the surface tension and protect against alveolar collapse. These phospholipids have a detergent quality and are known as surfactants. If an adequate amount of both factors is present at birth, neonatal breathing will result in expanded alveoli. If an inadequate amount is available, varying numbers of alveoli will collapse, and the neonate may develop respiratory distress syndrome (RDS).

Lecithin and sphingomyelin are reported as a ratio. Depending on the laboratory analysis used to determine the amounts of lecithin and sphingomyelin present, different ratios indicate lung maturity. In most centers the ratio 2:1 (ie, twice as much lecithin as sphingomyelin) is used as a level indicating maturity. There is less lecithin than sphingomyelin until 30 to 32 weeks of gestation, and then the concentrations become equal. The amount of lecithin rapidly increases after 35 weeks, while the amount of sphingomyelin remains constant. Thus, laboratory results often are reported as an L/S ratio of, for example, 2 (the constant level of sphingomyelin being understood).

There are two forms of lecithin, stable and unstable. Stable lecithin does not become functional until 35 weeks of gestation. Hypoglycemia, hypoxia, and hypothermia may break down the unstable form of lecithin, increasing the neonate's susceptibility to RDS.

Phosphatidylglycerol

As research has continued on the physiology of fetal lung maturity, many other phospholipids and fatty acids have been identified. The presence of PG and phosphatidylinositol has been found to correlate with fetal lung maturity. PG in particular has become useful when used with the L/S ratio. PG is not present until about 36 weeks' gestation. If the L/S ratio is 2 and the PG is present, there is strong evidence of fetal lung maturity. PG may provide stability that makes the neonate less susceptible to RDS when experiencing hypoglycemia, hypothermia, or hypoxia.

Biophysical Profile and Ultrasonography

Real-time ultrasound also may be used to perform a biophysical profile of the fetus. This procedure involves evaluation of such selected parameters as fetal movement, fetal tone, fetal breathing movements, amniotic fluid volume, and placental maturation. These parameters are assessed and scored numerically. Higher scores provide evidence of fetal well-being, whereas low scores indicate the need for further evaluation (Table 14-2). Biophysical profiles may be used as an adjunct to, or instead of, nonstress and contraction stress testing. Common indications for fetal assessment using biophysical profile include, but are not limited to, the following:

- Hypertensive disorders
- Diabetes mellitus
- Premature rupture of membranes
- Suspected intrauterine growth retardation
- Postdated pregnancy (possible postmaturity)
- Follow-up to nonstress test (NST)

Electronic Fetal Heart Rate Monitoring

Fetal monitors are used frequently during labor to watch for changes in the FHR and pattern. This use of fetal monitors is discussed in Chapters 20 to 22. In this chapter discussion is limited to the use of the electronic fetal monitor (EFM) in evaluating fetal status among pregnant women at risk for fetal stress and intrauterine fetal demise before labor (Fig. 14-5). This type of testing has its own specific procedures and interpretation.

Table 14-2. Biophysical Profile Scoring: Technique, Interpretation, and Recommended Clinical Management

Technique and Interpretation

Biophysical Variable	Normal (Score = 2)	Abnormal (score = 0)
Fetal breathing movement (FBM)	At least one episode of FBM of at least 30-sec duration in 30-min observation	Absent FBM or no episode of >30 sec in 30 min
Gross body movement	At least three discrete body or limb movements in 30 min (episodes of active continuous movement considered as single movement)	Two or fewer episodes of body or limb movements in 30 min
Fetal tone	At least one episode of active extension with return to flexion of fetal limb(s) or trunk; opening and closing of hand considered normal tone	Either slow extension with return to partial flexion or movement of limb in full extension, absent fetal movement
Reactive fetal heart rate (FHR)	At least two episodes of FHR acceleration of >15 bpm and of at least 15-sec duration associated with fetal movement in 30 min	Less than two episodes of acceleration of FHR or acceleration of >15 bpm in 30 min
Qualitative amniotic fluid volume (AFV)	At least one pocket of amniotic fluid that measures at least 1 cm in two perpendicular planes	Either no AF pockets or a pocket <1 cm in two perpendicular planes

Recommended Clinical Management Based on These Results

Test Score Result	Interpretation	Management
10 of 10 8 of 10 (norm fluid) 8 of 8 (NST not done)	Risk of fetal asphyxia extremely rare	Intervention only for obstetric and maternal factors; no indication for intervention for fetal disease
8 of 10 (abnorm fluid)	Probable chronic fetal compromise	Determine that there is functioning renal tissue and intact membranes; if so, deliver for fetal indications
6 of 10 (norm fluid)	Equivocal test possible fetal asphyxia	If the fetus is mature—deliver. In the immature fetus repeat test within 24 h; if <6/10, deliver
6 of 10 (abnorm fluid)	Probable fetal asphyxia	Deliver for fetal indications
4 of 10	High probability fetal asphyxia	Deliver for fetal indications
2 of 10	Almost certain fetal asphyxia	Deliver for fetal indications
0 of 10	Certain fetal asphyxia	Deliver for fetal indications

From Manning, F. A., & Harman, C. R. (1990). The fetal biophysical profile. In R. D. Eden, & F. H. Boehm. *Assessment and care of the fetus: Physiological, clinical, and medicolegal principles.* Norwalk: Appleton & Lange.

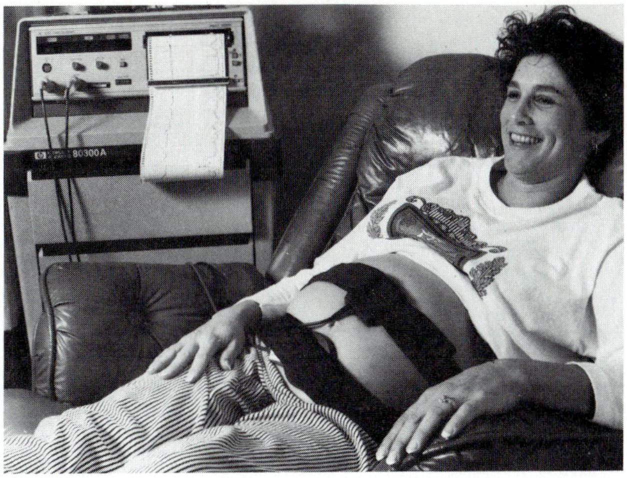

Figure 14-5.
Electronic fetal monitoring.

Nursing Research

Interpretations of Nonstress Tests

A survey of 1000 NAACOG members was conducted to evaluate the accuracy of interpretations of five 20-minute nonstress test strips. Among the 412 (41%) nurses who responded, more than 80% of the answers on each of the five strips were in agreement. The same five strips were interpreted by obstetricians in a previously conducted survey. On only one of the five strips did the degree of agreement among nurses differ from that among physicians; on that strip only 92% of the nurses agreed as to whether the strip was reactive or nonreactive, while 98% of the physicians agreed.

Factors such as clinical experience, clinical training, and the extent of present nonstress test responsibilities were not associated with concurrence on interpretation of the strips. Clinical risk can result when a nonstress test is falsely labeled reactive and needed clinical follow-up is therefore not done; up to 16% of nurses and physicians made this error.

This study showed that nurses as a group performed in a comparable fashion to a group of physicians in accurately interpreting nonreassuring findings on nonstress tests, irrespective of factors such as education, experience, clinical training, and clinical responsibilities.

Chez, B. F., Skurnick, J., Chez, R., Verklan, M., Biggs, S. & Hage, M. (1990). Interpretations of nonstress tests by obstetric nurses. Journal of Obstetric, Gynecologic, and Neonatal Nursing, 19*(3), 227–233.*

Electronic monitors allow observation of the fetus by indicating the response of the FHR to fetal movement or to spontaneous or induced contractions. Contractions "stress" the fetus by interruption of spiral arterial blood flow and subsequent reduction of uterine perfusion. Fetal movement generally produces predictable FHR changes. Variations in FHR in response to contractions or fetal movement may be detectable on the monitor. These variations may distinguish the healthy fetus from the fetus already compromised by any of the following factors:

- Fetal disease
- Placental disease
- Maternal disease
- Cord compression

Nonstress Test

The least invasive test of fetal well-being, the NST, is usually conducted first. The NST indirectly assesses placental respiratory function by observation of the FHR in response to fetal movement. Adequate uteroplacental perfusion is necessary to maintain the integrity of the fetal central nervous system and reflex responses that control the heart rate. The healthy fetus responds to fetal movement with an acceleration (or increase) of heart rate. Different facilities require various schemes and patterns of heart rate accelerations to constitute a "negative" or "reactive" test result. A reactive test indicates healthy placental respiratory function. The most common scheme requires at least two FHR accelerations occurring within a 10-minute period, with each acceleration (increasing heart rate) at least 15 bpm and sustained for at least 15 seconds.

The nurse is almost always responsible for administering the NST (see the accompanying Nursing Research display). The external EFM is applied as described in Chapter 20. The resulting tracing is observed and interpreted. The baseline FHR is identified, and any periodic patterns present are noted. The uterine activity tracing is observed for contractions. The NST is interpreted as reactive or negative for placental respiratory malfunction when the criteria for reactivity described previously are obtained (Fig. 14-6*A*). The FHR should otherwise be *normal*. It is most important to interpret the entire tracing. If an abnormal rate (less than 120 bpm or more than 160 bpm) is noted or decelerations are seen (see Chapter 20 for examples of strips showing FHR decelerations), the test requires follow-up evaluation even if the FHR demonstrates accelerations and the NST itself is reactive.

When performing the NST, the nurse should continue monitoring for at least 40 minutes before the test is interpreted as nonreactive. This is to account for normal periods of fetal sleep. The NST is nonreactive or positive when criteria for reactivity are not met (see Fig. 14-6*B*). It is important to remember that the NST is a screening procedure; thus, a nonreactive test must be followed with further evaluation the same day to determine fetal status. Follow-up tests that may be used include the contraction stress test, described below, or the biophysical profile, described previously.

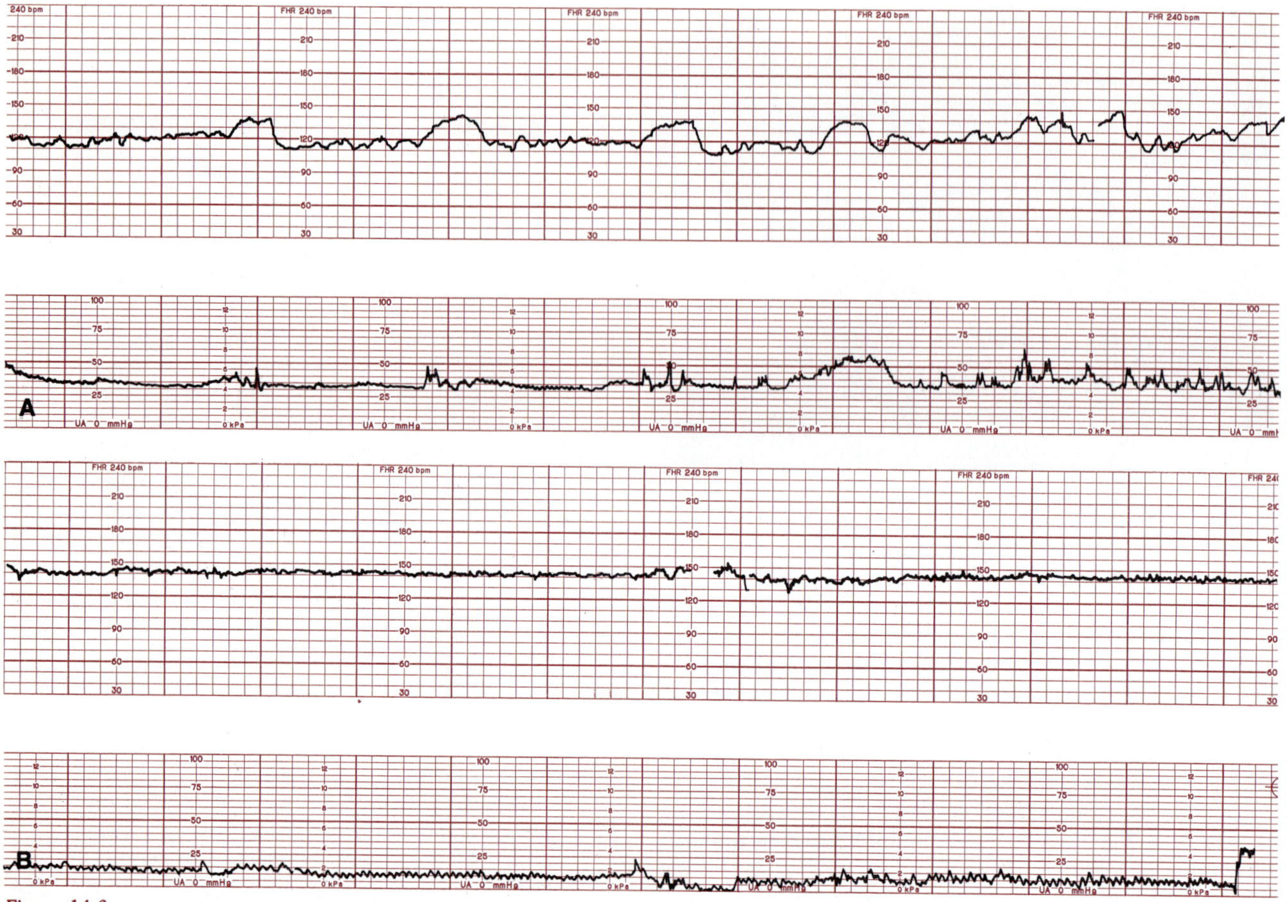

Figure 14-6.
A: Reactive NST. This strip shows a consistent pattern of healthy fetal heart rate (FHR) reactivity to fetal movement. With each fetal movement there is a subsequent increase in FHR. *B:* Nonreactive NST. This strip shows a consistent pattern of absent FHR reactivity to fetal movements. This nonreactivity requires further evaluation to confirm fetal status.

Vibroacoustic Stimulation

Vibroacoustic stimulation is a method often used when the NST is nonreactive. It involves the use of an artificial larynx placed against the woman's abdomen. It emits an auditory stimulus through the woman's tissues to the fetus (Fig. 14-7). When the fetus hears the stimulus, a startle is expected with movement and an FHR acceleration. There has been some concern about the effects of noise on fetal hearing and whether the associated acceleration indicates fetal health. Thus, there is no general consensus on the amplitude and duration of acceleration required to constitute a reactive test. Other modes of assessing FHR changes are being developed. Research on another method is discussed in the Nursing Research display.

Contraction Stress Test

Uterine perfusion through the spiral arteries is decreased during a contraction and thus stresses the fetus with diminished oxygen delivery. The fetus with limited reserve responds with late decelerations and a "positive" contraction stress test (Fig. 14-8*A*). The healthy fetus maintains a normal baseline without decelerations, called a "negative" contraction stress test (see Fig. 14-8*B*). At least three contractions in a 10-minute period must be observed to determine the fetal response to stress. Contractions may be occurring spontaneously with adequate frequency; more often, stimulation will be required by an intravenous oxytocin infusion. This is called the oxytocin challenge test.

Contraction stimulation also can be induced by nipple stimulation. Uterine contractions often can be induced by maternal nipple stimulation. The woman is instructed to rub or roll one nipple gently through light clothing for 2 minutes or until a contraction begins. Stimulation is then stopped and restarted after 2 minutes if by that time the contraction frequency is inadequate. Nipple stimulation and rest periods should be continued intermittently for 2 minutes each. If after 15 to 20 minutes, inadequate contraction frequency is observed, continuous stimulation using one nipple and then two nipples for 10 minutes each should be accomplished. If at any time during stimulation, contraction frequency becomes adequate or hyperstimulation occurs, nipple stimulation should be stopped. If nipple stimulation is unsuccessful, intravenous infusion of low-dose oxytocin is begun at 0.5 mU/min and increased by 0.5 mU/min every 15 minutes until the desired number of contractions is achieved. The goal for

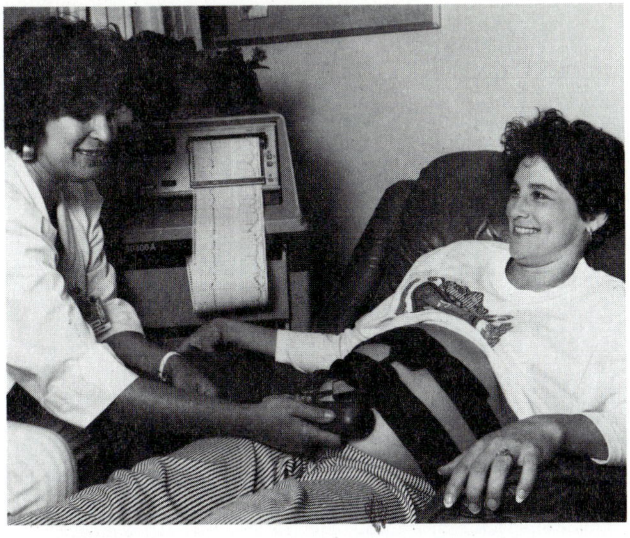

Figure 14-7.
The artificial larynx used for vibroacoustic stimulation.

both methods is to achieve three contractions lasting 40 to 60 seconds each within 10 minutes.

Outcome

Regardless of the type of test performed, the expected outcome is the same. The monitor is placed on the pregnant woman as shown in Figure 14-5. The patient is placed in the lateral recumbent position to prevent vena caval compression. The ultrasound transducer is adjusted to achieve the best possible tracing of the FHR (that is, one without interruptions in the pattern tracing). The tocotransducer is applied as recommended by the monitor manufacturer to obtain an accurate recording of uterine activity. Once a good tracing is achieved and the woman is in a comfortable position, a "baseline strip" is run. This provides a reading of the activity of the uterus and the fetus without intervention or manipulation. The baseline will help determine the need for additional uterine stimulation.

Doppler Velocimetry

Doppler velocimetry is an assessment method that uses the Doppler principle (also used in the ultrasound stethoscope and the EFM ultrasound transducer). It measures velocity waveforms. When used for this purpose, spectra analysis is also used. Two types of instrumentation are now available. The original machine designed for Doppler velocimetry used continuous waveform, which produced a scattered view of data output. Newer machines now incorporate pulsed waveform, which is more focused than continuous waveform.

Both methods require the woman to lie quietly in the recumbent position. A small penlike probe is gently placed against the woman's abdomen and rotated until a clear visual waveform is obtained on the screen (Fig. 14-9*A*). The vessels commonly studied or insonated are the uterine and umbilical arteries. The latter are most often used to assess the fetus for intrauterine growth disorders. The umbilical arterial waveform can be detected first around 15 weeks' gestation and is generally measured and expressed as a systolic to diastolic ratio (S/D). A normal value is 3.0 at 28 to 30 weeks (see Fig. 14-9*B*), which usually decreases with advancing gestation because of a normal fall in resistance in the placental circulation. An absence of diastolic flow is the

Nursing Research

The Auscultated Acceleration Test

The nonstress test (NST) in the most widely used electronic fetal monitoring technique to assess fetal well-being in at-risk pregnancies. However, the NST requires expensive equipment and specially trained personnel and is not regarded as an appropriate universal screening test because of its low sensitivity in predicting perinatal morbidity.

A low-technology screening test, called the auscultated acceleration test (AAT), has been developed by a nurse scientist. This test can be administered by a nurse with a fetoscope in 6 minutes and has been shown to predict normal NST results with more than 90% accuracy.

This study was conducted with 205 women with singleton pregnancies with greater than 34 weeks' gestation. The auscultator listened to the FHR with an Allen-type fetoscope for 2 minutes to establish a baseline FHR. If no acceleration of at least two beats per 5-second period occurred during this initial period, the fetus was externally stimulated using a gentle 5-second shaking motion to stimulate fetal movement. Shaking was repeated once more if no fetal movement occurred in the 2-minute period after the first manipulation. Auscultation continued for an additional 2 minutes for a total of 6 minutes of auscultation. Findings on the AAT were compared to findings on NST, as well as to neonatal outcome data.

The AAT yielded better prediction of poor perinatal outcomes than did the NST; however, the NST was a better predictor of favorable outcomes. Some modifications of the AAT will be necessary to improve its usefulness as a screening test. However, the AAT shows promise as a low-technology prenatal assessment approach, with particular potential for use in areas where technology is scarce and perinatal mortality is high.

Paine, L., Benedict, M., Strobino, D., Gegor, C., & Larson, E. (1992). A comparison of the auscultated acceleration test and the nonstress test as predictors of perinatal outcomes. Nursing Research, *41(2), 87–91.*

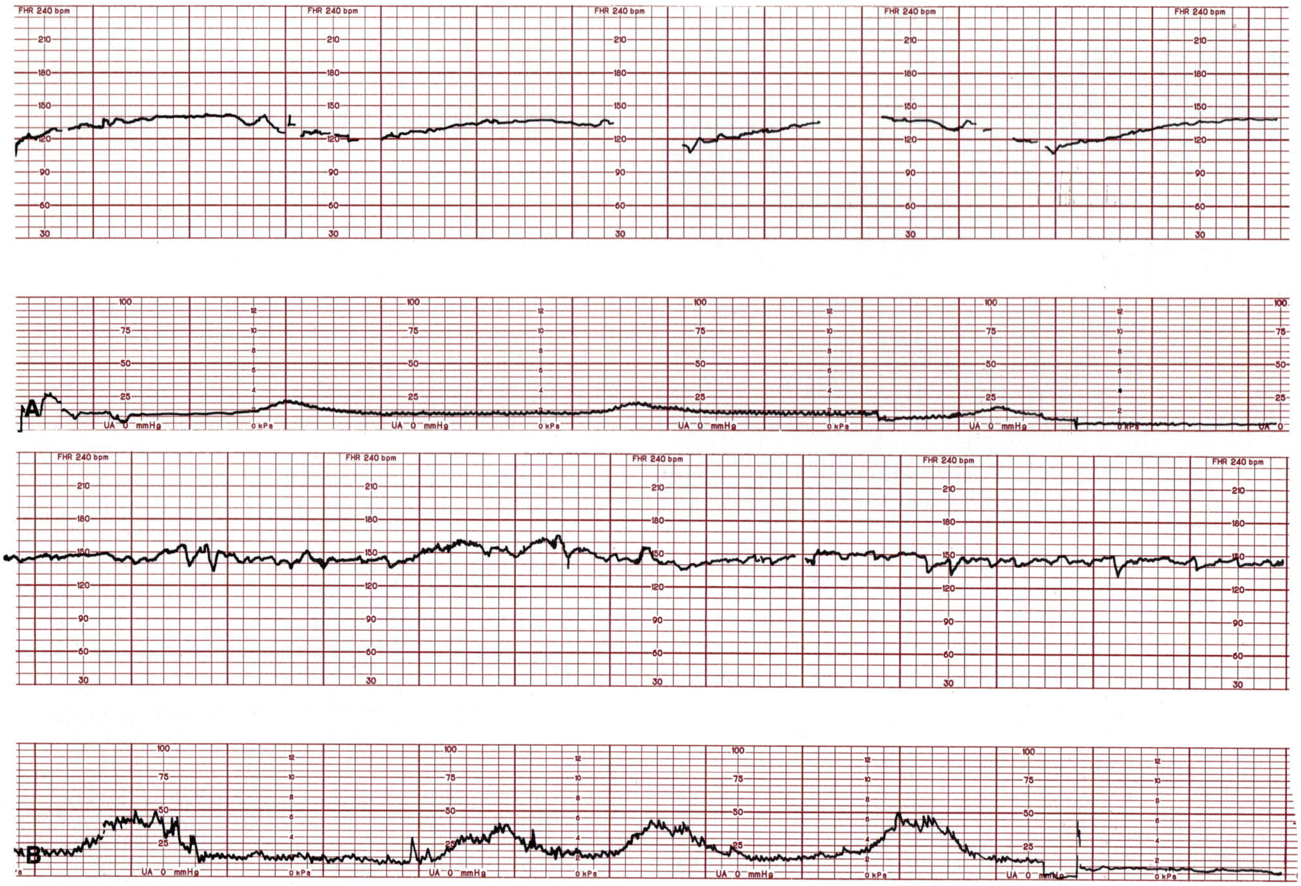

Figure 14-8.

A: Positive CST. This strip shows a pattern of late decelerations in fetal heart rate (FHR) in response to uterine contractions. This suggests the fetus has limited oxygen reserves, and further evaluation is required. *B:* Negative CST. This strip shows no pattern of FHR decelerations in response to uterine contractions. This suggests the fetus has an adequate physiologic reserve at this time.

most extreme form of abnormal Doppler velocimetry (see Fig. 14-9*C*) and is called absent end-diastolic velocity. This finding is associated with intrauterine growth retardation and other poor neonatal outcomes.

Monitoring the well-being of the fetus when there is some question about its condition has become an important emphasis in perinatal care. Techniques such as amniocentesis, the use of ultrasound to construct a biophysical profile of the fetus, NST, contraction stress testing, and Doppler velocimetry are now available to determine whether the fetus has adequate physiologic reserves to grow normally and to cope well with the stress of labor. Increasingly, the appropriate preparation of pregnant women for these tests, conducting them, and interpreting their results are important nursing responsibilities.

Implications for Nursing Care

Ongoing assessment and monitoring of fetal well-being are essential components of prenatal care and have long been major nursing responsibilities in many settings. Such basic assessment techniques as auscultation of FHR and monitoring uterine growth provide essential information about fetal status and the progress of pregnancy. However, new technologic advances have contributed new diagnostic and clinical assessment techniques. With these new techniques come new nursing responsibilities (Fresquez & Collins, 1992).

EFM, especially its application in the prenatal evaluation of fetal status, has had a major impact on nursing practice. For example the nursing skills required for practice have rapidly expanded beyond the standard intrapartum use of EFM to include interpretation of prenatal tests. This rapid expansion in practice responsibilities requires the nurse to update their clinical knowledge continually. The nurse must evaluate innovations in biomedical technology carefully from a nursing perspective by asking questions such as the following: What nursing functions will be changed because of this new technology? What new knowledge and skills are needed? What standardized procedures should be developed and tested? What are the costs of this new technology, and how do they weigh against the benefits? Will the technology generate information that will clearly improve outcomes by reducing risk, or will the procedure generate additional risks?

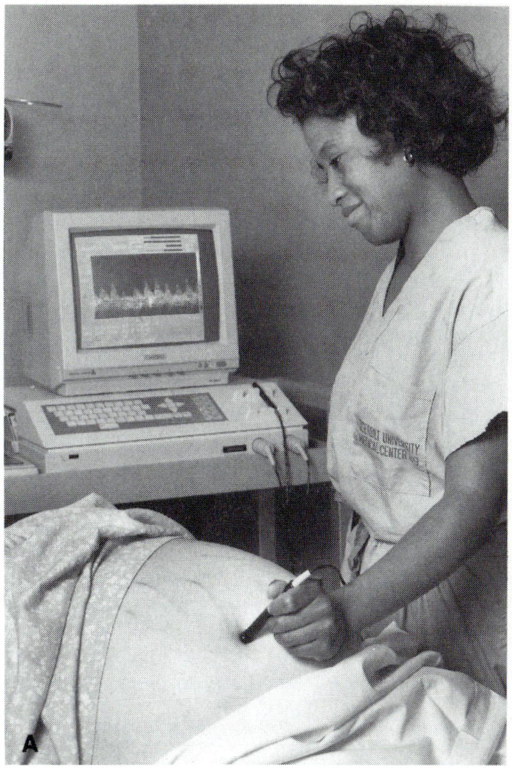

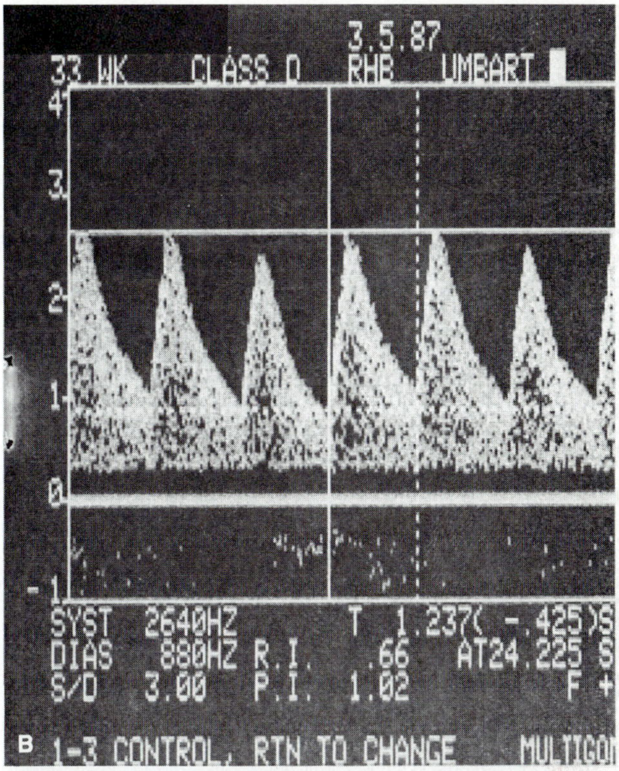

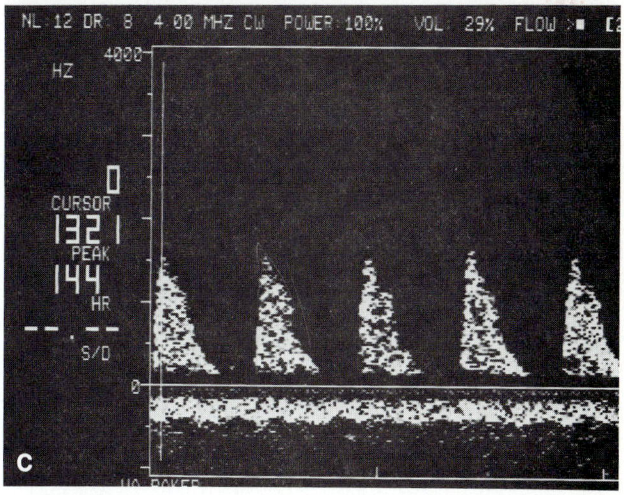

Figure 14-9.

A: The use of Doppler velocimetry in prenatal care. *B:* Normal Doppler velocimetry. *C:* Absent end diastolic velocity.

Finally, the perinatal nurse must constantly keep in mind that "a major challenge to nurses is to balance the impact of instrumentation and monitoring with the primary nurse–patient relationship. Although these techniques augment practice, they should never replace thoughtful analysis and the therapeutic process of human interaction" (Gibes & Angelini, 1987, p. 7).

Chapter Summary

The health status of pregnant women and their fetuses is the most important influence on the future health and well-being of humankind. Nurses in prenatal settings can effectively monitor fetal growth and well-being, teach, and offer anticipatory guidance to pregnant women and their families. To do this the nurse must be knowledgeable about the normal growth of the fetus. Such methods include McDonald's measurements and ultrasonography to assess fetal growth, the normal growth curve of the uterus and its relationship to the pregnant woman's diet, and methods of assessing FHR and fetal responses to changes in oxygenation, such as NST and contraction stress testing. However, technologic advances in this area are occurring rapidly, often outstripping the professional's ability to completely master new technology or consider the ethical and psychological implications. Nurses must continually update their knowledge and understanding and still remain family centered in the care of families who require more intensified fetal assessment.

Study Questions

1. *What two procedures are used to estimate gestational age early in pregnancy? Why is estimation of gestational age an important part of prenatal care?*
2. *How would you instruct a pregnant woman in preparation for ultrasonography?*
3. *A pregnant woman at 32 weeks' gestation is concerned because she has not felt fetal movement for 2 to 3 hours. What would you advise her to do?*
4. *What two tests may be performed on amniotic fluid?*
5. *What are the differences between the NST, the nipple stimulation test, and the oxytocin challenge test?*
6. *How is Doppler velocimetry used, and what are the expected results?*

References

Dauphinee, J. (1987). Antepartum testing: A challenge for nursing. *Journal of Perinatal and Neonatal Nursing, 1*(1), 29–49.

Engstrom, J. (1988). Measurement of fundal height. *Journal of Obstetric, Gynecologic, and Neonatal Nursing, 17*(3), 172–179.

Fresques, M., & Collins, D. (1992). Advancement of the nursing role in antepartum fetal evaluation. *Journal of Perinatal and Neonatal Nursing, 5*(4), 16–22.

Gibes, R., & Angelini, D. (1987). Editorial: Monitoring and instrumentation. *Journal of Perinatal and Neonatal Nursing, 1*(1), 7.

Gregor, C., & Pain L. (1992). Antepartum fetal assessment techniques: An update for today's perinatal nurse. *Journal of Perinatal and Neonatal Nursing, 5*(4), 1–15.

Schulman, H. (1990). Doppler ultrasound. In R. Eden & F. Boehm (Eds.). *Assessment and care of the fetus: Physiological, clinical and medicolegal principles.* Norwalk: Appleton and Lange.

Stewart, L., & Troiano, N. (1991). Perinatal asphyxia: Surveillance of the high risk fetus. *NAACOG Clinical Issues in Perinatal and Women's Health Nursing, 2*(1), 14–34.

Suggested Readings

Goodwin, L. (1992). Home fetal assessment. *Journal of Perinatal and Neonatal Nursing, 5*(4), 33–45.

Harmon, J., & Barry, M. (1989). Antenatal testing-mobile outpatient monitoring service. *Journal of Obstetric, Gynecologic, and Neonatal Nursing, 18*(1), 21–24.

NAACOG. (1991). *Nursing practice competancies and educational guidelines: Antepartum fetal surveillance and intrapartum fetal heart rate monitoring* (2nd ed.). Washington, DC: Author.

Sabey, P., & Clark, S. (1992). Establishing an antepartum testing unit: The nurse's role. *Journal of Perinatal and Neonatal Nursing, 5*(4), 23–32.

Skurnick, J., Chez, R., & Ches, B. (1991). Effect of explicit criteria an nonstress test evaluation by obstetric nurses. *American Journal of Perinatology, 8*(2), 139–143.

CHAPTER 15

Nursing Care of the Expectant Family

Learning Objectives

After studying the material in this chapter, the student will be able to:

- Discuss the importance of individualizing teaching and counseling for each woman or family.
- Explain the rationale for anticipatory guidance, and give an example of how it is used in caring for the expectant family.
- Discuss the importance of making referrals when indicated, and identify situations that require referrals.
- Identify causes, assessment data, interventions, and expected outcomes for the common discomforts of pregnancy.
- Identify symptoms that pregnant women must be taught to report.
- Identify risks related to employment, travel, sports, and exercise during pregnancy.
- Identify the benefits of sports and exercise during pregnancy.
- Teach pregnant women to prepare for breastfeeding.

Key Terms

anticipatory guidance	dorsiflexion
hemorrhoids	lordosis
Homans' sign	toxoplasmosis
pelvic tilt	exercise-talk test
kegel exercises	

The prospects of a smooth pregnancy and the birth of a healthy neonate are aided considerably by early and thorough prenatal care. Because childbearing is an essentially normal process for most women, prenatal care focuses on education aimed at maintaining well-being. Thus, teaching self-care behaviors is a major component of perinatal nursing care.

The nurse is not simply the administrator of another health care provider's orders. The nurse is likely to have more contact with patients and their families than any other health care provider and thus must provide needed teaching. Because of the time spent with women in the obstetric setting, the nurse is in a unique position to assess women's physical and psychosocial needs and decide whether referrals are needed. When answering the many questions that women raise about their pregnancies, their growing fetus, labor and delivery, breastfeeding, and the postpartum period, the nurse contributes directly to the quality of the individual experience and to health outcomes for the entire family.

With knowledge of the needs of the pregnant woman and the many services offered by health care organizations and the community, the nurse can inform pregnant women of the resources available to them. Such intervention, especially early in pregnancy, can significantly enhance perinatal care for the pregnant woman and her family.

The nurse's true value in prenatal care often lies in the ability to develop a trusting relationship with the woman and her family to assess their unique needs and formulate and implement an appropriate plan. By this process the nurse shifts the relationship with the pregnant woman and her family from the trusting realm to the therapeutic realm.

The processes of promoting health maintenance, addressing physical and psychosocial adaptations, providing support for self-care, and helping the woman maintain a healthy life-style during pregnancy are important nursing actions. In addition the nurse is responsible for monitoring the woman's situation for threats to health. All of these actions are based on an assessment of the learning needs and individual circumstances of the pregnant woman and her family, as well as on knowledge about physiologic and psychosocial adaptations to pregnancy.

This chapter focuses on nursing care in the prenatal period, with an emphasis on education. The chapter begins with the concerns encountered during the 9 months of gestation and the nurse's role in anticipatory guidance and education. Nutrition, sexuality, and psychosocial adaptation to pregnancy are discussed in detail in other chapters and addressed only briefly here. This chapter emphasizes teaching and guidance related to exercise, work, travel and leisure, and signs of complications. Objectives of prenatal care are listed in the accompanying display.

• • Assessment

The process of assessment as an essential component of nursing care throughout pregnancy was addressed in Chapter 13. Once the woman's pregnancy has been established, many assessments are made at the first visit and subsequent prenatal visits. Elements of prenatal assessment at the initial visit are the health history (present, menstrual or obstetric, and previous pregnancies), psychosocial assessment (attitudes, emotions, financial impact, and expectations), and complete physical examination. Subsequent visits include continuing assessments to determine how the pregnant woman is adapting physically and psychologically to the pregnancy and if intervention is needed to promote health and prevent complications.

Assessment of the entire family unit may be necessary to provide effective care. The concerns of the father or partner throughout the pregnancy should be within the scope of the nurse's time and attention (Fig. 15-1). The long-term health of the family unit may rest on the degree to which both parents adapt positively to the demands of pregnancy, birth, and the first year of parenting. The process of psychosocial adaptation to pregnancy is discussed in Chapter 8. Some important points are highlighted here, because they relate to the process of identifying needs of the pregnant woman and her family and implementing nursing care to meet those needs.

• • Nursing Diagnosis

Nursing diagnosis in the care of the expectant family tends to focus on identifying learning needs of the pregnant woman and her partner as pregnancy progresses and on supporting self-care behaviors associated with optimal psychosocial and physical adaptation to pregnancy. The following nursing diagnoses reflect possible needs that may arise during the pregnancy:

- Altered Health Maintenance related to physical adaptations to pregnancy
- Anxiety related to anticipated role changes during pregnancy

Objectives of Prenatal Care

In the past, prenatal care focused on the prevention of eclampsia and other maternal correlations of toxemia (now called pregnancy-induced hypertension). In recent years prenatal care has become more concerned with the identification and management of high-risk conditions for the fetus and newborn. A broader, contemporary view of prenatal care, however, sees pregnancy as an opportunity to promote the health and well-being of the family. In addition to assuring the health of the pregnant woman and the birth of a healthy neonate, the objectives of prenatal care apply to the family during the pregnancy and the infant's first year of life.

The objectives of prenatal care for the pregnant woman follow:

- To increase her well-being before, during, and after pregnancy and to improve her self-image and self-care
- To reduce maternal mortality and morbidity, fetal loss, and unnecessary pregnancy interventions
- To reduce the risks to her health prior to subsequent pregnancies and beyond the childbearing years
- To promote the development of parenting skills.

The objectives or prenatal care for the fetus and the infant follow:

- To increase well-being
- To reduce preterm birth, intrauterine growth retardation, congenital anomalies, and failure to thrive
- To promote healthy growth and development, immunizations, and health supervision
- To reduce neurologic, developmental, and other morbidities
- To reduce child abuse and neglect, injuries, preventable acute and chronic illness, and the need for extended hospitalization after birth

The objectives of prenatal care for the family follow:

- To promote family development and positive parent–infant interaction
- To reduce unintended pregnancies
- To identify for treatment behavior disorders leading to child neglect and family violence.

U.S. Department of Health and Human Services. (1989). Caring for our future: The content of prenatal care: A report of the Public Health Service Expert Panel on the content of prenatal care. *Washington D.C.: Author.*

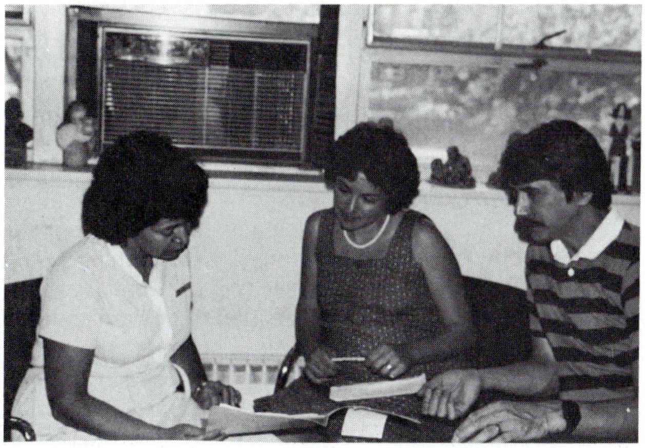

Figure 15-1.
The nurse provides nursing care for the pregnant woman and her partner. Assessment of both the woman and her partner is an important first step for future teaching. (Courtesy of the former Booth Maternity Center, Philadelphia.)

- Pain related to discomforts of pregnancy
- Knowledge Deficit related to health threats in pregnancy
- Health-Seeking Behaviors (information regarding activity, exercise, and breast care) related to pregnancy

While prenatal care usually involves essentially healthy families, the nurse also must be alert for emergence of potential or actual complications so the physician or nurse midwife can be notified. The nurse is responsible for monitoring for potential complications and for teaching the pregnant woman and her family to be aware of the signs and symptoms of these complications.

• • Planning and Implementation

The nurse and the pregnant woman and her family plan and implement care based on identified needs throughout the pregnancy. As pregnancy progresses, the pregnant woman's needs and the needs of her family shift. The nurse will not always be in a position to provide information precisely when the family needs it. The nurse uses knowledge about the kinds of concerns women and their families have at various points during pregnancy to anticipate the needs of the woman and her support person and to help plan and implement appropriate teaching. This provision of the appropriate information to the couple when they are ready to learn about and plan for the future is called anticipatory guidance.

Prenatal classes are a cost-effective way to provide education and anticipatory guidance for pregnant women and their families. Many prenatal classes are available, so all expectant parents should be able to attend some form of prenatal education classes, although some families choose not to attend. Prenatal classes are discussed in more detail in Chapter 18. To meet the needs of individual women and their families, needs must be reassessed and teaching reinforced constantly at individual prenatal appointments.

Promoting Health Maintenance With Informational Support

A family must have certain information to understand the events of pregnancy and to participate in their own care. In addition family members must prepare for the expected changes, share individual concerns, and ultimately experience a positive physical and emotional outcome. The nurse has approximately 7 months to impart this information.

The learning needs of pregnant women and their families vary greatly. Factors such as age, educational level, socioeconomic status, marital status, culture, religion, parity, and perhaps the most important, the interest of the woman and her family will all influence their learning needs. What is taught to one family may be inappropriate for another.

Anticipatory guidance must start with the learner's level of understanding. The nurse must take into account the woman's immediate concerns (see "Trimester Concerns" in the next section). Assessing the woman's social surroundings and history can help to illuminate potential problems. The nurse also must recognize that pregnant women and their family members often see health care providers as authority figures. The family may expect only to be "told" information and may not expect the nurse to discuss and problem-solve with them.

It is more appropriate, however, for the nurse and the family to find solutions by interaction. The nurse brings knowledge of the anatomy, physiology, and psychology of pregnancy and the process of gestation. The family brings its unique understanding of the significance of the pregnancy within their social system. The nurse's task is to promote an exchange of knowledge.

The nurse also should understand that the role of counselor requires an examination of personal biases and perceptions. The nurse should not force the pregnant woman and her family into any particular course of action. The nurse's own beliefs, such as the belief that the father should be actively involved in pregnancy or that all children must be breastfed, must be examined. Steps should be taken to avoid imposing these beliefs on the expectant family. Nurses must realize that even if they have difficulty with the family's decision, the decision is the *family's*. If the nurse wishes to present alternatives for consideration, the alternatives must be compatible with the family's way of life, or they will be disregarded.

Expected Outcomes

- The pregnant woman and her family verbalize an understanding of the nurse as a source of teaching and counseling regarding their concerns during pregnancy.
- The pregnant woman and her family demonstrate learning by maintaining or acquiring useful self-care behaviors.

Addressing Specific Psychosocial Adaptations

The nurse organizes anticipatory guidance and patient teaching during pregnancy around two main issues: trimester concerns and personal concerns. In general the nurse must deal with immediate concerns first and present additional information anticipating other concerns later. The readiness of the woman and her family to learn is the nurse's basic guide to both areas. The remainder of the chapter deals with these issues.

Trimester Concerns

Pregnant women and their family members have different concerns at various stages of pregnancy. The process of psychosocial adaptation to pregnancy in the expectant couple is discussed in detail in Chapter 8, and the Assessment Tool for Assessment/Intervention for Parental Adaptation to Pregnancy in that chapter provides information with which the nurse can address the couple's needs and anticipate future concerns.

In general, time in the first trimester should be devoted to exploring the family's reactions to the pregnancy: how it will change their daily lives, who will be responsible for infant care, and the need for mutual support and sharing of the workload. In the second trimester families are making a transition from acceptance of the pregnancy to preparations for labor and delivery and for the newborn. Discussions should focus on this transition and investigate birth plans and options. In the third trimester concerns turn to the imminent delivery and care of the infant. Couples may tour the labor and delivery rooms and nursery or other facilities they will use (Fig. 15-2). Decisions about infant care practices are a major concern at this time.

The nurse should address the pregnancy as part of the family's total situation. The couple must be allowed to express their doubts, fears, and insecurities. Parents usually know what society expects of them but not what will happen if they alter the typical family structure. For example they may have concerns about others' reactions to having the father stay home with the newborn or about how grandparents will react to modern infant care practices. Beyond anticipating societal pressures, the parents in this instance may need anticipatory counseling to help them adjust to their alteration in roles.

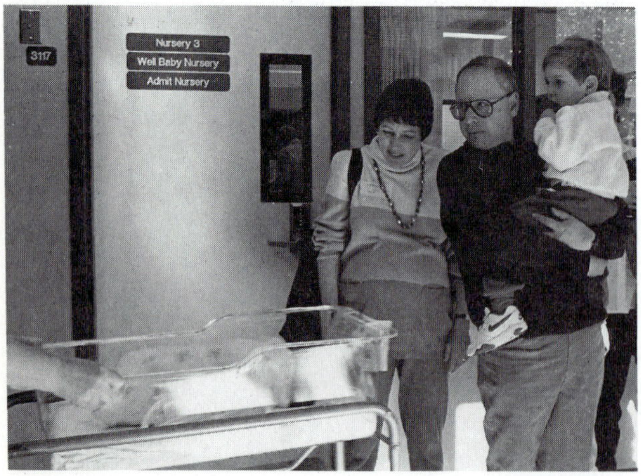

Figure 15-2.
In the third trimester the pregnant woman and her partner are encouraged to tour the facility where their baby will be born. Many couples include their families, as in this tour. (Photo by Kathy Sloane. Courtesy of the Alta Bates Medical Center.)

Delivering the facts about pregnancy is only part of the nurse's job. A challenging and rewarding part of the nurse's role is helping the family to identify their needs, verbalize their feelings and concerns, seek solutions, and work toward goals.

Personal Concerns

The nurse's ability to provide anticipatory guidance is based on knowledge about the transition to parenthood and on assessment of the individual needs of the woman and her family. Age-related, social, and marital issues are some of the issues the nurse will encounter in prenatal counseling.

Age-Related Issues. A woman's age can have a significant impact on her emotional and psychological adaptation to the pregnancy. Pregnant adolescents require an extensive environmental support system. This level of support is necessary to promote optimal health and to enable the pregnant adolescent and her child to reach their psychological and social potential. Because women between 12 and 19 years old vary greatly in their progression through the developmental tasks of adolescence, the pregnant adolescent must be assessed individually. Physical development, attitudes toward health, and interest in or ability to seek prenatal care will all influence the outcome of the pregnancy. Emotional support, financial resources, self-esteem, and ability to formulate personal goals must be assessed. Short- and long-term plans must be developed for each pregnant teenager, with constant reevaluations as the pregnancy progresses (see Chapter 9).

Childbearing women older than age 35 are another population with specific age-related concerns. Generally defined as primiparous women age 35 or older, this group's primary age-related issue is the need for genetic counseling. A couple may refuse genetic counseling or genetic tests; however, the nurse is obligated to raise the subject and must provide families with information about genetic risks. Other age-related issues that may be of concern to the older primigravida are general health status, previous obstetric history, career and life-style interruptions, and changes in the couple's relationship resulting from pregnancy and parenthood (see Chapter 10).

Social and Marital Issues. The nurse will encounter a wide variety of social and marital situations that will require variations in the anticipatory guidance provided to the expectant family. The disappearance of the traditional nuclear family is an ever-present reality today. Single mothers, couples living together but choosing not to marry, second families following divorce, lesbian couples choosing to have children, and three-generation families represent some of the diversity the nurse will encounter. The learning needs in each of these situations will vary greatly.

This variety of social and marital situations is reflected in the support many pregnant women require. A single woman may be concerned about parenting alone or with minimal support from the father of the newborn. If she continues the pregnancy, she must deal with the reality of raising a child alone. Family support may or may not be available to such women, depending on the family's reaction to the pregnancy. Couples who live together and choose not to marry but decide to have children may be concerned about the future of the relationship when the additional responsibility of parenthood is added. All expectant couples with other children are concerned about sibling issues. Newly partnered couples who have children from previous relationships may express concerns about sibling acceptance of a newborn. Almost all expectant families are concerned about additional financial demands.

Thus, the nurse must have a complete and accurate picture of the woman's family situation before appropriate anticipatory guidance and teaching can occur. In addition to the woman's family situation, it is essential that the nurse assess for factors that put the woman at particular psychosocial risk.

Previous Obstetric History. Women who have had previous obstetric complications or losses will bring many anxieties to the current pregnancy. Their concerns may arise from popular myths and misconceptions or from admonitions from previous health care providers. The nurse's role includes obtaining an accurate and detailed health history. An obstetric and gynecologic history, and a social and psychological assessment are needed to ascertain the basis of the woman's concerns. This allows the nurse to formulate appropriate education and counseling plans. These women and their families must be particularly encouraged to call the health care provider when questions and concerns arise.

A woman with a history of one or more spontaneous abortions, late (second-trimester) therapeutic abortions, or a cervical conization may be fearful of spontaneous abortion or preterm labor. Some women verbalize their concerns. Others are afraid to ask questions. Thus, a nurse must be alert for unexpressed concerns when women present with such histories. Occasionally a partner is unaware of the woman's obstetric history, and the pregnant woman may be concerned about maintaining her privacy in that regard. The nurse must ensure confidentiality and not refer to the obstetric history without the woman's approval when the partner is present.

Women with histories of obstetric complications, such as preterm labor, placenta previa, or pregnancy-induced hypertension, will be fearful of recurrences. They must be advised of risks and be reassured of close observation and diagnostic and preventive measures when possible. Families that have experienced the loss of a fetus or neonate or the anxieties of a premature birth will have many concerns during the pregnancy. These families require additional time for sensitive listening and support (Mercer, 1990).

Psychosocial Risk Factors. Pregnant women who suffer from chronic or debilitating diseases and handicapped women will have special concerns. They may wonder about the effects of their disease or medications on the pregnancy and fetus, as well as the effect of the pregnancy on their health status. They may fear alterations in body image and immobility. Pregnant women with chronic disease or handicaps also may worry about their ability to care for an infant, to breastfeed, or to parent a child. Communication with the partner and social and emotional support must be encouraged. Social service referrals may be indicated.

Sometimes women become socially isolated as the result of the absence or indifference of the partner, lack of parental figures or relationship, minimal social contacts, or relocation to a new community. Women who approach pregnancy without social support will require support and assistance from the health care provider. The nurse must be on the alert for these needs and encourage the woman to seek appropriate outlets in social groups, community organizations, or prenatal classes and through social and psychological referrals when necessary.

Referrals

It is not unusual for expectant women and their families to need referrals to other physicians, counselors, or social agencies during the course of the pregnancy. Sometimes the physiologic, psychological, or financial stresses of pregnancy can precipitate a crisis. At other times the changes of pregnancy or the anxieties of additional responsibilities can cause a woman or family struggling with chronic illness or other problems to need help beyond the usual prenatal care and education.

Through nursing assessments the nurse will determine when a family needs a referral for additional assistance. Pregnant women do not always ask for help, so the nurse will have to make suggestions based on knowledge of normal adaptation to pregnancy. This requires the nurse to observe and assess the family's coping mechanisms as the situation changes and as the pregnancy progresses. Offices and clinic facilities that provide prenatal care usually have protocols that can assist the nurse in determining when specific conditions require a referral.

It is essential for the nurse to be aware of resources available in the community. Facilities providing prenatal care usually have referral lists for women with specific needs. Cases can be expected to arise that will not be solved by one telephone call. If a woman or family needs a service that is not supplied by any of the agencies on the list, the nurse must find an agency that does supply it and promptly contact the family to make the referral.

Some women have difficulty entering the health care system for a condition other than pregnancy. They may not follow up on a referral. This is especially true if they are in a state of disequilibrium, are denying the problem, are embarrassed, or think that further care will not do any good anyway. In these situations the nurse can further assist by arranging an appointment (and transportation if necessary) and should find out if the pregnant woman kept the appointment. If a pregnant woman habitually breaks appointments, further assessment is necessary to ascertain the reason. The nurse must carefully document nursing interventions and counseling of the patient to seek additional help.

Counseling Referrals. Certain problems identified during the nursing assessment or reported by the pregnant woman call for a counseling referral. These problems may include marital, sexual, and work-related difficulties; troubles with children; adolescents' difficulties with family or partner; problems with developmental adaptation to pregnancy; and substance abuse or dependency. Psychologists, professional counselors, psychiatrists, community support groups, and crisis-prevention agencies are all appropriate resources.

Nutrition Referrals. The physiologic changes of pregnancy make great nutritional demands on the pregnant woman (see Chapter 17). Clients should be referred to a nutritionist if they begin the pregnancy extremely far under or over their ideal weight, if weight gain during pregnancy is insufficient or excessive, if intake is largely empty calories or is poorly balanced, or if a previously existing nutritional or metabolic disease might be exaggerated by pregnancy. Referral to the Women, Infants, and Children Program should be considered for all patients with reduced income. This program provides low-income women with vouchers that can be used to purchase extra food for themselves and their family (Machala & Miner, 1991).

Adolescents frequently require nutrition referrals for poor eating habits or dieting prompted by concern about their appearance. Families also will benefit from such a referral if low income interferes with eating healthy foods. Nutritionists can give advice about obtaining wholesome food on a limited budget. This is especially valuable when there will be another mouth to feed soon. Women from other cultures may not eat well because they cannot find their customary foods; they should be referred to a nutritionist for assistance.

Social Referrals. When pregnancy places financial burdens on the family that they are unable to handle or work out successfully, a social work referral may be needed. Social workers can help these families deal with the bureaucratic systems that supply food stamps, welfare, and housing; school placement and counseling; and other problems as they arise. Teenagers, single women, and unemployed and low-income women and their families are particularly likely to need to be referred to social workers.

Genetic Counseling Referrals. Health care providers are responsible for informing expectant parents of their genetic risks and of the prenatal genetic diagnostic tests available (see Chapter 12). It is important to inform a couple of the genetic tests available to them, regardless of their age and risk factors. It is the couple's choice to obtain or decline testing. Couples must be given clear and accurate explanations early in the pregnancy so that they can make timely and informed decisions. Health care providers must document the counseling given.

Expected Outcomes

- The pregnant woman and her family use the nurse as a resource person for needed services and information.
- The pregnant woman and her family actively participate in deciding on and implementing health maintenance and promotion activities.

Providing Support During Common Discomforts

One of the characteristics of prenatal care is that the nurse normally is working with a healthy population that requires only guidance about appropriate self-care. During the 9 months of pregnancy, many changes occur in a woman's body as a result of hormonal influences and the body's response and adaptation to the gestational process. The woman and her partner often appreciate changes such as stronger fingernails, hair with fuller body, or larger breasts. Other changes, such as nausea or breast tenderness, are unpleasant for the woman but usually are short lived. Still other changes, such as hemorrhoids or varicosities, usually occur later in the pregnancy and may get worse with time.

Responses to the discomforts of pregnancy vary, depending on the severity of the symptoms, the significance of the symptoms for each woman, and her individual tolerance for discomfort. The nurse's role is to assess completely each specific complaint, reassure the woman, take appropriate nursing actions, and provide the necessary education. Often a pregnant woman will only need reassurance that her discomfort is a temporary and normal phenomenon of pregnancy. Frequently a pregnant woman will need detailed teaching about preventive measures and occasionally will need careful instructions about warning signs to report. Teaching considerations for self-care for common discomforts of pregnancy are listed in the accompanying display.

The following section addresses some common discomforts of pregnancy and provides appropriate nursing interventions, including information that can be provided to the pregnant woman to ensure appropriate self-care. Because the pregnant woman is in the best position to care for herself appropriately, if she is well informed, teaching is a central component of the nurse's care.

Nausea and Vomiting

In the absence of other problems, nausea and vomiting is thought to be related to increased levels of progesterone, increased levels of human chorionic gonadotropin, and decreased gastric secretion of hydrochloric acid and pepsis. It usually resolves spontaneously after the first trimester and occurs in 50% to 80% of all pregnant women. When assessing the pregnant woman with nausea and vomiting, the nurse must differentiate between normal "morning sickness" and hyperemesis gravidarum. The latter is characterized by prolonged vomiting with resulting fluid and electrolyte imbalances. Excessive weight loss, ketonuria, and signs of dehydration may require medical intervention (DiIorio, 1988). Pregnant women should be told to avoid taking over-the-counter antinausea drugs. Vitamin B_6 has been helpful for some women but should be taken only with the advice of the health care provider. The accompanying Nursing Care Plan outlines care of the pregnant woman experiencing nausea and vomiting.

Breast Tenderness

Increasing vascular supply to the breasts in addition to the hypertrophy of breast tissue caused by estrogen and progesterone results in fullness, tingling, and tenderness during pregnancy. Colostrum may be secreted as early as 16 weeks and may be a source of concern to the pregnant woman.

The nurse assesses the pregnant woman for any signs of infection, such as redness, heat, or fever. In the absence of these signs, the woman should be reassured that breast changes are normal and indicate the response of tissues to maternal hormones. A support bra with wide adjustable

Teaching Considerations

Self-Care for Common Discomforts of Pregnancy

The nurse can use the following points in teaching pregnant women appropriate self-care measures for common discomforts of pregnancy.

Nausea and Vomiting

- Eat a high protein snack at bedtime.
- Eat dry crackers before arising.
- Avoid sudden position change.
- Avoid food odors.
- Eat smaller, more frequent meals.
- Get plenty of fresh air.

Urinary Frequency

- Limit caffeine.
- Void when urge occurs.
- Try Kegel exercises.

Breast Tenderness

- Use a comfortable support bra.
- Avoid soap on nipples.

Round Ligament Pain

- Apply local heat.
- Avoid twisting or jerking.
- Change position slowly.
- Lie on your side in a knee to chest position.

Vaginal Discharge

- Avoid panty hose.
- Wear loose cotton underwear.
- Avoid tight pants.
- Keep perineum clean and dry.

Fatigue

- Exercise regularly.
- Take frequent rest breaks.

Headaches

- Practice relaxation exercises.
- Take regular meals and adequate fluid intake.

Constipation

- Exercise regularly.
- Increase fiber in diet.

Leg Cramps

- Keep legs warm.
- Apply local heat.
- Use adequate dairy products in diet.

Backache

- Wear low heeled shoes.
- Exercise regularly.
- Do no heavy lifting.
- Apply local heat.
- Use pelvic tilt exercises.

Varicosities

- Wear support stockings.
- Elevate lower extremities.
- Avoid constrictive clothing.
- Avoid crossing legs.
- Ambulate frequently.
- Wear low heeled shoes.
- Exercise regularly.

Hemorrhoids

- Prevent constipation.
- Use Sitz baths.

Edema

- Rest in lateral position.
- Elevate feet.
- Provide for adequate protein intake.
- Consume ample fluids.
- Use normal salt intake.

straps and a smooth interior should be worn to decrease irritation. A larger size than usual may be necessary. The woman should avoid use of soap on the nipples as this may dry the skin and predispose them to cracking. If colostrum leaks and dries on the nipples, this should be cleansed with warm water only. The importance of routine breast self-examinations during pregnancy should be stressed (see the Teaching Considerations display in Chapter 6). If the patient plans to breastfeed, the nurse may initiate a discussion of breastfeeding preparations, which will begin during the third trimester.

Round Ligament Pain

Stretching of the round ligament caused by uterine growth results in a common complaint of lower abdominal discomfort. Sudden jerking or twisting of the torso also pulls on this ligament, resulting in unilateral or bilateral pain.

Text continues on page 326

Nursing Care Plan

The Pregnant Woman With Nausea and Vomiting

PATIENT PROFILE:

History

KD is a 24-year-old G1, PO at 7 weeks gestation of a planned and wanted pregnancy. She tells the nurse that for the last 2 weeks she has been nauseated almost every morning and vomits after eating in the morning. Nausea and vomiting sometimes persist throughout the day. She states she just isn't interested in eating or drinking, although she "knows it's important for the baby." She asks for a prescription for "something I can take," because she is concerned about the baby's welfare if nausea and vomiting continue.

Physical Assessment

Her stated prepregnant weight was 59.8 kg (132 lb); she now weighs 57.6 kg (127 lb). Her blood and urine laboratory workup from her first prenatal visit are within normal limits. Urine for dipstick is negative for protein and glucose, positive for ketones, and is deep yellow and strong smelling. Skin turgor is normal.

COLLABORATIVE PROBLEMS/ POTENTIAL COMPLICATIONS

- Fluid/electrolyte imbalance
- Hyperemesis gravidarum

(See the accompanying Nursing Alert display.)

Assessment	*Nursing Diagnosis*	*Nursing Interventions*	*Rationale*
KD complains of nausea and vomiting for last 2 weeks. Urine dipstick suggests beginning dehydration and inadequate caloric intake. KD has had weight loss for last 2 weeks.	Altered Nutrition: Less than Body Requirements related to nausea and vomiting. *Expected Outcome* KD regains weight by end of first trimester and continues optimal weight gain. KD states self-care measures help alleviate symptoms.	Assess for possibility of other gastric problems that can cause symptoms.	In the absence of other problems, nausea and vomiting in early pregnancy thought to be related to these physiologic changes in first trimester: • Increased levels of progesterone (decreases gastric emptying time) • Increased levels of HCG • Decreased gastric secretion of hydrochloric acid and pepsin
		Review dietary intake, and encourage KD to increase intake because self-care measures (listed below) reduce symptoms. Advise KD to keep unsalted crackers at bedside, and eat several before arising or moving about. Advise KD to drink fluids between, rather than with, meals; sipping carbonated water may prevent onset of nausea. Advise KD to try spearmint or raspberry tea and 50–100 mg/d of vitamin B to reduce nausea.	Self-care measures are designed to decrease gastric irritability while maintaining intake. KD should try several techniques, because not all work for all women. Inadequate intake can inhibit optimal weight gain.

(*Continued*)

The Pregnant Woman With Nausea and Vomiting
(*Continued*)

Assessment	Nursing Diagnosis	Nursing Interventions	Rationale
		Explain that six small meals with protein snacks (cheese, nuts, and eggs) may be more effective and that foods high in carbohydrates may be better tolerated in the morning.	Low maternal blood glucose can further exacerbate nausea and vomiting.
		Recommend that KD avoid food odors, sudden movements, especially in the morning.	
		Advise that protein snacks, such as yogurt or milk, at night (when awakened by nocturia) may ease morning nausea.	
	Anxiety related to unexpected weight loss and concerns for fetal well-being. ***Expected Outcome*** KD states an understanding of usual course of nausea and vomiting. KD expresses less concern regarding condition on follow up. KD demonstrates an understanding regarding avoidance of medications in pregnancy.	Reassure KD that nausea and vomiting occur in 50% to 80% of women and usually resolve spontaneously after the first trimester. Assess emotional status. Encourage KD to walk outside after meals and other diversions to avoid focusing on symptoms. Caution KD not to use over-the-counter antinausea medications without consulting care provider.	Concern about condition may cause KD to focus unduly on weight loss making her more attentive to symptoms and thus exacerbating them. Over-the-counter preparations are not regarded as safe for use in pregnancy.

EVALUATION

At telephone follow-up 1 week later, KD reports that she is "feeling better" and "able to keep more down" after using recommended self-help measures. At a follow-up clinic visit at 9 weeks of gestation, KD has gained 5 lb (2.2 kg). She reports less nausea in the morning and has not vomited in 3 days, although nausea still occurs at times during the day. Urine dipstick is negative for protein, glucose, and ketones, and is pale yellow in color. KD states she is encouraged, but will call in again if problem worsens. At a routine prenatal visit at 16 weeks, KD has gained a total of 8 lbs 8 oz (3.6 kg) and reports that nausea "suddenly disappeared" several weeks before. Appetite is good and 24-hour diet recall reflects balanced dietary intake.

NURSING ALERT

SEVERE NAUSEA AND VOMITING

If nausea and vomiting are severe or persist beyond early pregnancy, the potential exists for electrolyte imbalance, poor weight gain, and the development of hyperemesis gravidarum (see Chapter 16). When nausea and vomiting develop in early pregnancy, the nurse should evaluate the following parameters to determine if the symptoms are severe enough to require medical therapy:

- Has the woman lost weight in early pregnancy compared with her stated prepregnant weight? Is she behind the expected weight gain for gestational age?
- Is she unable to maintain an adequate nutritional intake on most days (based on 24-hour diet recall) despite the use of self-care measures?
- Is there evidence of beginning dehydration (ketonuria, concentrated urine, poor skin turgor)?

If findings are positive based on these parameters, the nurse should obtain medical consultation to rule out hyperemesis gravidarum and provide supportive therapy, including intravenous rehydration and medical management of symptoms.

If findings based on any of these parameters are positive, the nurse should recommend the pregnant woman be evaluated immediately by her physician or midwife to rule out either one of these serious complications of pregnancy.

The nurse should assess for complications that present with similar symptoms. Corpus luteal cysts and ectopic pregnancies also present with lower abdominal pain and must be ruled out as a possible cause of the symptoms. Pregnant women with impending preterm labor often complain of pressure and heaviness that may be falsely attributed to round ligament pain.

Severe pain with or without bleeding must be reported to the health care provider immediately. The woman should be reassured that mild, occasional lower abdominal pain is normal in pregnancy. She should be advised to avoid sudden jerking or twisting movements, and to apply local heat to the area of discomfort. A sidelying position with the knees drawn close to the chest sometimes provides relief (Brucker, 1988a).

Vaginal Discharge

In the absence of pruritus and foul odor, an increase in white or yellowish discharge is normal in pregnancy. This occurs as a result of an increased production of cervical mucous caused by estrogen and an increased vascularity of the cervical tissues.

The nurse evaluates symptoms to exclude the possibility of vaginal infection, which occurs more frequently during pregnancy. Pruritis, foul odor, spotting, or a change in the color of the discharge from white to yellow may indicate an infection requiring medical intervention (see Chapter 16).

The nurse should provide reassurance that pregnant women normally have increased vaginal discharge. Suggestions for avoiding this complication include wearing cotton underwear, avoiding panty hose and tight undergarments, and keeping the perineal area clean and dry. Tampon use and douching are contraindicated during pregnancy.

Urinary Frequency

Urinary frequency in the first trimester is related to a reduction in bladder capacity from pressure of the enlarging uterus. In the third trimester, the presenting part compresses the bladder, giving rise to the same symptoms. Coughing and sneezing late in pregnancy may cause leakage of urine. This fluid may be confused with rupture of membranes.

The nurse assesses the patient for signs and symptoms of a urinary tract infection, such as dysuria, chills, fever, and costovertebral angle tenderness. In the absence of signs of infection, urinary frequency is a normal finding for the first and third trimesters.

Teaching and counseling should include suggestions to limit caffeinated beverages (which may exacerbate the symptom) and voiding when the urge occurs. This will prevent bladder distension and urinary stasis. Kegel exercises (see the Teaching Considerations display) may help to strengthen pelvic floor muscles and decrease urine leakage. Patients should be taught the signs and symptoms of urinary tract infection and the importance of prompt medical attention if the symptoms occur. Untreated urinary tract infections may progress to pyelonephritis quickly in the pregnant woman, and may predispose her to preterm labor.

Fatigue

Increased demands of the cardiopulmonary system, an increased metabolic rate, and possibly some interaction of the ovarian hormone relaxin result in a common complaint—lack of energy. A need for more sleep during pregnancy is common. The increased demands of work outside the home and care of other children can intensify this problem.

The nurse assesses the woman's situation to rule out any pathologic reason for excessive fatigue. Caloric intake and hemoglobin and hematocrit levels should be noted to ensure that the pregnant woman has adequate nutritional intake and is not anemic. Psychosocial concerns may be manifested through the symptoms of fatigue and excessive need for sleep. The nurse should assess this as a possible underlying cause.

The nurse can reassure the pregnant woman that fatigue is normal and temporary during pregnancy. Regular exercise should be encouraged, coupled with frequent rest periods during the day. If work and home demands are excessive, the woman should be encouraged to explore ways in which household duties can be delegated to others.

Headaches

Headaches are reported by many women during pregnancy. They are probably due to increased circulatory blood volume and heart rate, which cause dilation and distension of the cerebral arteries. Fatigue and emotional tension may also contribute to the development of headaches, as in nonpregnant individuals.

The nurse must determine if the woman's headaches are a normal event of pregnancy or a warning sign of complications. Because headaches commonly accompany elevated blood pressure, the nurse should assess the woman's blood pressure. This is especially true in the second half of pregnancy, when pregnancy-induced hypertension is most likely to develop. In early pregnancy, headaches are generally benign and should resolve with rest. The woman should also

Teaching Considerations

Kegel Exercises

In women the pubococcygeal muscles may be strengthened by Kegel exercises. In 1952 Arnold Kegel developed a series of exercises for women whose pubococcygeal muscles were so slack that they were losing urine when they coughed or sneezed. This may be a problem for older women who lack muscle tone and for pregnant and postpartum women as well.

The steps for the Kegel exercises are as follows:

1. Locate the muscles surrounding the vagina by sitting on the toilet and starting and stopping the flow of urine.
2. Test the baseline strength of the muscles by inserting a finger in the opening of the vagina and contracting the muscles.
3. Exercise A—Squeeze the muscles together, and hold the squeeze for 3 seconds. Relax the muscles. Repeat.
4. Exercise B—Contract and relax the muscles as rapidly as possible 10 to 25 times. Repeat.
5. Exercise C—Imagine sitting in a pan of water and sucking water into the vagina. Hold for 3 seconds.
6. Exercise D—Push out as during a bowel movement, only with the vagina. Hold for 3 seconds.
7. Repeat exercises A, C, and D 10 times each and exercise B once. Repeat the entire series three times a day.

Regular practice of the Kegel exercises can restore muscle tone in approximately 6 weeks. The pelvic floor muscles contract during orgasm, and just like any muscle, they work better when they are in better shape. Thus, there is a sexual benefit when muscle tone improves. Additional benefits from the Kegel exercises may be increased vaginal lubrication during sexual arousal, relief of constipation, increased flexibility of episiotomy scars, and stronger gripping of the base of the penis during intercourse.

be advised that long periods without food can precipitate headaches. Products containing aspirin should be avoided, but regular adult doses of acetaminophen can be used. Any headache that does not respond to this treatment should be evaluated by the health care provider. Likewise, headaches associated with visual changes such as blurred vision should be evaluated immediately (Brucker, 1988a).

The nurse can reassure the patient that headaches are common in pregnancy and should respond to self-care measures. The patient should be reminded to inform the health care provider if these usual self-care measures fail, or if any other signs of pregnancy-induced hypertension are present (see the Teaching Considerations display, Signs and Symptoms to Report, that appears later this chapter). Relaxation exercises may be helpful if headaches are tension-related. The nurse should encourage the woman to rest whenever possible, to eat regular meals, and to avoid taking over-the-counter drugs without first checking with the health care provider.

Constipation

Progesterone has a relaxing effect on the muscles of the gastrointestinal tract and causes a decrease in peristalsis in pregnancy. These changes can result in constipation. In addition, iron supplements commonly prescribed during pregnancy are known to cause constipation. Pressure from the enlarging uterus may have an effect on the colon and rectum. Prolonged episodes of constipation predispose the pregnant woman to hemorrhoids.

The nurse should assess the severity of the problem by documenting the frequency and character of bowel movements. Dietary measures, such as increasing fluid and fiber intake, and regular exercise, such as walking, which will help to stimulate peristalsis, should be encouraged. The woman should be cautioned against using laxatives, mineral oil, or enemas because they may precipitate uterine contractions. If conservative measures fail to establish a normal bowel pattern, an over-the-counter stool softener can be used. The woman should be reminded that she should contact the health care provider before taking any medication (Brucker, 1988b).

Leg Cramps

A disturbance in the body's calcium/phosphorus ratio and excessive or inadequate intake of dairy products may predispose the pregnant woman to leg cramps. Fatigue or muscle strain may also be a causative factor.

The nurse should assess dietary intake for possible causes. Careful examination for signs and symptoms of phlebitis, such as heat, edema, redness, or a positive Homan's sign (pain in the calf when the foot is passively dorsiflexed) is appropriate. If none of these are found, the nurse should review with the woman the proper dietary intake of dairy products to avoid imbalances in the calcium/phosphorus ratio. The woman should be instructed to dorsiflex the foot (point the toes toward the head) when cramping occurs. The woman can be encouraged to apply local heat to sore muscles and maintain regular mild exercise such as walking (Brucker, 1988a).

Backache

Backache is a common discomfort in pregnancy. It occurs as a result of compensatory lordosis (swaying or forward curvature of the back) and muscle strain related to the

Nursing Care Plan

The Pregnant Woman With Backache

PATIENT PROFILE

History

LH is a 35-year-old mother of four, including a set of twins aged 18 months. She is 28 weeks' gestation with a singleton pregnancy. She complains of almost constant lower back discomfort.

Physical Assessment

LH has no costovertebral angle tenderness or urinary symptoms. Blood and urine laboratory tests at 24 weeks were WNL. Weight gain is appropriate for gestation. LH reports no pelvic pressure, uterine irritability, or contractions.

COLLABORATIVE PROBLEMS/ POTENTIAL COMPLICATIONS

- Pyelonephritis
- Preterm labor

(See the accompanying Nursing Alert Display.)

Assessment	*Nursing Diagnosis*	*Nursing Interventions*	*Rationale*
No signs of pyelonephritis, UTI, or preterm labor noted. LH does physically demanding work (mother of four). Hx includes closely spaced pregnancies, including twin gestation.	Pain: backache related to body changes of pregnancy. ***Expected Outcome*** LH states self-care measures provide some relief of symptoms by next follow-up contact.	Assess posture, lifting techniques, and type of footwear. Assess activity and rest periods. Assess for hx of abdominal muscle weakness.	In the absence of other causes, backache probably due to increased weight of growing uterus, which pulls spine forward and changes center of gravity, leading to compensatory lordosis and muscle strain; lack of support from weak abdominal muscles; relaxation of pelvic ligaments and body joints caused by estrogen and relaxin; fatigue and overwork. Increased intercostal respiration and expansion of thoracic cage may contribute to back pain.
		Advise LH to avoid overwork and fatigue with frequent rest periods. Recommend use of massage. Recommend avoiding lifting; sit down and have toddlers climb into lap. Advise application of local heat. Review importance of posture; recommend sitting in tailor fashion on floor or placing foot on low stool while standing to decrease back strain.	Self-care techniques are designed to relieve back strain and promote good posture.

(Continued)

The Pregnant Woman With Backache

(Continued)

Assessment	Nursing Diagnosis	Nursing Interventions	Rationale
		Review warning signs of pyelonephritis and preterm labor.	Backache may mask signs of other pregnancy complications, such as pyelonephritis and preterm labor.

EVALUATION

At telephone follow-up 1 week later, LH reports that she is "not lifting anything and trying to rest more." LH reports backache is "a little better." Nurse reviews self-help measures, and suggests adding use of heating pad to daily rest periods. Nurse inquires about plans for help at home with twins. At a routine prenatal visit at 32 weeks of gestation, LH reports that backache "isn't any worse—maybe a little better." LH reports she "feels like the broad side of a barn" and tires more easily now. LH has made plans to put twins in day care for a few hours each day, beginning next week. LH remains free of signs or symptoms of preterm labor or infection and can state danger signs that require immediate follow-up.

increased weight of the growing uterus pulling the spine forward and changing the center of gravity. Careful assessment for signs and symptoms of pyelonephritis and preterm labor is imperative, since these conditions may present as back discomfort. The pregnant woman with backache is discussed in the accompanying Nursing Care Plan.

Heartburn

Heartburn is a common discomfort of pregnancy, especially in the third trimester. Progesterone relaxes the cardiac sphincter, allowing gastric reflex of stomach contents into the esophagus. In addition, the enlarging uterus displaces the stomach and duodenum in the third trimester.

Reports of heartburn are evaluated to rule out epigastric pain caused by edema of the liver capsule in severe pregnancy-induced hypertension. Other signs of pregnancy-induced hypertension include edema above the waist, especially of the face, elevated blood pressure, headaches, and proteinuria (see Chapter 27).

In the absence of other signs, the nurse should reassure the woman that heartburn is a common discomfort that will disappear after delivery. Aggravating factors such as fried or spicy foods, smoking, and heavy caffeine consumption should be identified and avoided. The woman should be encouraged to eat frequent small meals rather than three large meals each day. She should also avoid lying down after meals or eating large meals before retiring (Brucker, 1988b).

Varicosities

Some pregnant women will be predisposed to varicosities due to a congenital weakness in the vascular walls. The

NURSING ALERT

BACKACHE AS A WARNING SYMPTOM

Backache is a common discomfort of pregnancy. However, it is also a symptom associated with preterm labor and urinary tract infection, two conditions that can threaten maternal and fetal well-being. When a pregnant woman complains of backache, it is imperative that the nurse assess the woman's condition to rule out the presence of preterm labor and urinary tract infection.

The nurse must evaluate the following parameters:

- Is the discomfort intermittent? Is it unrelieved by changes in position or walking (suggestive of preterm labor)?
- Does the woman have any sensation of uterine tightening, cramping, pelvic pressure, increased vaginal discharge, or diarrhea (suggestive of preterm labor)?
- Does the woman have any urinary symptoms (dysuria, frequency beyond that normal for pregnancy, urgency) (suggestive of urinary tract infection)?
- Does the woman have any symptoms of infection (malaise, fever, headache) (suggestive of systemic infection, perhaps pyelonephritis)?
- Is the back pain localized more on the right side, and is it marked at the place where the ribs and spinal column join (possible costovertebral tenderness suggestive of pyelonephritis)?

increase in blood volume and increased pressure from the enlarging uterus are also causative factors in the development of varicosities. Varicosities can arise in the legs, vulva, or anal region (hemorrhoids). Women who are obese and those with jobs that require prolonged standing are more likely to develop this condition.

Any complaint of leg pain by a pregnant woman requires a careful assessment to rule out phlebitis or thrombophlebitis. Edema, redness, heat, or a positive Homan's sign requires immediate medical evaluation.

Varicosities do not resolve during pregnancy, and although they diminish somewhat after delivery, most do not disappear completely. Measures to control discomfort include wearing support hose, avoiding constrictive clothing (such as tight knee-high hose), elevating the legs, wearing comfortable low-heeled shoes, and maintaining regular walking, especially walking for a few minutes every hour if the woman has been sedentary. Hemorrhoids are best prevented and treated by preventing constipation. Sitz baths may provide some relief of hemorrhoid symptoms. The woman should be reminded to consult her health care provider before using any over-the-counter hemorrhoid medications (Brucker, 1988b).

Edema

Normal dependent edema of pregnancy is related to increased sodium and water retention and increased capillary permeability caused by maternal hormones. In addition, increased venous pressure and decreased venous return from the legs predisposes the pregnant woman to edema in the lower extremities.

Since edema, specifically edema above the waist, is one of the signs of pregnancy-induced hypertension, the nurse monitors for other significant signs and symptoms before attributing edema to normal pregnancy changes. Blood pressure should be evaluated. If the woman reports headaches, visual changes, or epigastric pain, she should be seen by a physician immediately.

In the absence of worrisome signs, the pregnant woman should be reassured that dependent edema is a normal phenomenon of pregnancy. She can be encouraged to rest frequently on her side and to elevate her feet to reduce edema. The woman should be advised to maintain a normal intake of salt but to avoid highly salted foods, such as snack foods or processed or canned foods. The woman should be reminded to maintain an adequate protein intake since this will help keep fluid in blood vessels. Maintenance of an adequate daily fluid intake will aid in natural diuresis.

Expected Outcome

- The pregnant woman and family implement and maintain safe and appropriate self-care for common pregnancy discomforts.

Counseling Regarding Threats to Health

Women vary in their knowledge of normal and abnormal occurrences in pregnancy, their attitudes toward obtaining health care, their tolerance for pain and discomfort, and their handling of anxiety when problems are suspected. The nurse assesses the woman's understanding of the physical changes of pregnancy and her motivation to seek health services should a complication arise. Then the nurse and pregnant woman develop a teaching plan that includes the signs and symptoms of potential complications of pregnancy. Some women need only a list of symptoms to report. Others require somewhat detailed explanations. The nurse is responsible for meeting the learning needs of each patient.

Signs and Symptoms to Report Promptly

The following section highlights signs and symptoms that the woman must report at once. Early reporting will lead to early identification of complications. Timely intervention will maximize the chances for a favorable pregnancy outcome. The accompanying display summarizes the signs and symptoms the pregnant woman should report promptly. Complications of pregnancy, such as infections, bleeding, and preexisting medical conditions are discussed in more detail in Chapter 16. The major gestational complications of preterm labor, pregnancy-induced hypertension, and diabetes are discussed in detail in Chapter 27.

Vaginal Bleeding. Any sudden onset of frank, profuse vaginal bleeding should be reported immediately. Such bleeding is different from the light pink spotting that results from a causative action, such as sexual intercourse or a vaginal examination. Vaginal bleeding can be a sign of ectopic pregnancy or threatened abortion in the first trimester, or threatened abortion, placenta previa, or abruptio placentae in the second and third trimesters.

Dizziness. Sudden and extreme dizziness associated with pelvic or uterine pain should be reported immediately. These symptoms may indicate the presence of ectopic pregnancy or abruptio placentae, in which blood is trapped in the abdominal cavity or between the placenta and uterine wall and does not present vaginally.

Preterm Labor Symptoms. Pregnant women should be taught the signs and symptoms of preterm labor (PTL), the name given to labor between 20 and 36 weeks of gestation (see Chapter 27). PTL recognized early and monitored appropriately may be stopped. Even if it cannot be stopped, early detection allows preparations to be made for the birth of a preterm neonate. The nurse should emphasize that any possible symptoms of preterm labor should be evaluated in the health care setting. The woman cannot necessarily recognize contractions at home, and the nurse cannot diagnose the situation accurately over the telephone.

The following symptoms of PTL should be reported to the health care provider immediately:

- Rhythmic tightening (or contracting) of the uterus, as distinguished from irregular Braxton Hicks contractions
- Any constant low abdominal cramping
- Constant low backache

Pregnant women may notice fluid leaking from the vagina and believe it to be urine. It may in fact be urine, but the only way to be sure is to examine it with chemically treated test paper to rule out amniotic fluid leakage. Thus, women must be advised to report any leakage of fluid and seek evaluation.

Teaching Considerations

Signs and Symptoms to Report Promptly

The following signs and symptoms may suggest serious complications of pregnancy. The nurse is responsible for instructing women to report to their health care provider promptly if they develop any of these symptoms.

- Vaginal bleeding—any sudden onset of profuse vaginal bleeding
- Dizziness—sudden extreme dizziness associated with pelvic pain
- Decrease in fetal movements—any abrupt decrease in fetal activity or absence of fetal activity for 8 hours
- Preterm labor symptoms (before 36 weeks of gestation):
  - Tightening of uterus
  - Constant low abdominal pressure or cramping
  - Intermittent or constant low backache
  - Leakage of fluid from vagina
- Pregnancy-induced hypertension symptoms:
  - Generalized edema, especially in face and hands
  - Rapid weight gain over several days or weeks
  - Headaches
  - Visual disturbances (flashing lights, double vision), dizziness
  - Nervousness, irritability
  - Vomiting
  - Epigastric pain (a late and ominous sign)
- True labor symptoms (after 36 weeks of gestation):
  - Rupture of membranes (leaking or gushing of fluid from vagina)
  - Expulsion of pink mucus (mucous plug) from vagina
  - Regular pattern of uterine contractions

Rupture of Membranes. Any sudden gushing or slow leaking of fluid from the vagina must be reported immediately. The amniotic fluid is enclosed in a sac that surrounds and protects the fetus. Once this sac breaks, the fetus can be at risk for infection. Leaking of fluid or rupture of membranes can precede labor in a term pregnancy. Health care providers must ascertain when the leaking begins. Delay of delivery for more than 24 hours after membrane rupture may increase the risk of infection to the fetus.

Pregnancy-Induced Hypertension Symptoms. Early warning signs of pregnancy-induced hypertension will frequently be noted at a prenatal visit (see Chapter 27). Women should be instructed to report any of the signs shown in the display, Signs and Symptoms to Report Promptly. A clinical evaluation is necessary in the presence of any of these symptoms, and the pregnant woman should be advised to go to the health care setting immediately.

Decrease in or Absence of Fetal Activity. Any marked, abrupt decrease in fetal activity or absence of fetal activity for 8 hours should be reported immediately. A significant decrease in fetal activity can be a sign of fetal distress, and cessation of activity could indicate fetal demise. Pregnant women should be taught to attend to fetal activity throughout pregnancy. Mental notes of fetal movements and their pattern allows the woman to recognize a deviation from normal.

Behavioral Threat: Smoking

Smoking is one of the most preventable causes of low birth weight. Approximately 32% of women are smokers at the time of conception, but only 20% to 25% continue to smoke during pregnancy because of concern for the fetus. The effects of smoking on pregnancy are well known by most women and the desire for a healthy infant is the catalyst for a change in lifestyle. Unfortunately, many of these women return to smoking after delivery, perhaps unaware of the harmful effects of passive smoking on the infant.

There are numerous adverse effects of smoking during pregnancy. The most consistent finding is a reduction in birth weight primarily due to intrauterine growth retardation. The rate of preterm delivery is also higher in smokers when compared to non-smokers. The incidence of spontaneous abortion, placental abruption, placenta previa, and bleeding during pregnancy are also increased. Parental smoking after delivery increases the newborn's risk for pneumonia, bronchitis, tracheitis, laryngitis, and otitis media. Sudden infant death syndrome is also higher among infants whose mothers were smokers (O'Connor, Davies, Dulberg, Buhler, Nadon, McBride, & Benzie, 1992).

The nurse is in an excellent position to affect a change in smoking behavior during pregnancy. Posters and pamphlets on the subject can be displayed in waiting areas. All ashtrays should be removed from the waiting room. The staff should act as role models in regard to smoking cessation.

During the initial interview, the nurse should elicit a thorough smoking history, including how long the woman has been smoking, how much she smokes, and if her partner smokes. If the woman has stopped smoking due to knowledge of the harmful effects of smoking on the pregnancy or because of nausea, the nurse can provide positive reinforcement for that decision and counseling to prevent relapse. If the woman is still smoking, the nurse can outline the risks both for her and her fetus. This is done by providing a firm, nonjudgmental message about the importance of cutting down, if not quitting, during pregnancy. It may be helpful to establish a plan for decreasing the number of cigarettes smoked per day, and if possible, to set a date for total cessation.

Whatever progress the woman makes toward decreasing her cigarette consumption should be reinforced. The nurse can be effective in providing the woman with the encouragement she needs to continue to work toward smoking cessation. Family members should also be encouraged to be a support system for the woman. The nurse should inquire at each prenatal visit about her progress. Relapses should be seen as temporary setbacks rather than failures, and as opportunities to resume the plan with new understanding about situations that lead to smoking (O'Connor et al., 1992).

Behavioral Threat: Alcohol and Substance Abuse

A safe level of alcohol consumption during pregnancy has not been clearly established. Therefore the nurse should advise all pregnant women to refrain from alcohol consumption during pregnancy. All pregnant women should be questioned regarding alcohol use during pregnancy at the first prenatal visit.

The woman who abuses drugs or alcohol rarely seeks early prenatal care. She may first present for care very late in pregnancy. The nurse can intervene to minimize the effects of drug use on the pregnant woman and the fetus if the woman comes prenatal care. The woman should be made to feel accepted and should be encouraged to make and keep regular prenatal appointments. If the woman is sexually active, she should be tested periodically for all sexually transmitted diseases during pregnancy. The nurse can encourage the woman to establish and maintain good nutrition and can refer her to supplemental food programs (Chisum, 1990).

If the woman expresses a desire to stop drug use, she should be referred immediately to a center where specialized services are provided for pregnant drug users. She should be advised that abrupt withdrawal from drugs is unsafe during pregnancy, and withdrawal should be overseen by knowledgeable health care personnel. Although some recent court decisions have resulted in enforced drug rehabilitation, the nurse should recognize the ethical implications of such decisions. It is far more likely that positive outcomes for the pregnant woman and her fetus will result from strong, trusting relationships with care providers than from imposed treatment (see the accompanying Legal/Ethical Considerations display).

Family Violence: Battered Pregnant Woman

Domestic violence has become a major health problem in the United States, regardless of socioeconomic status. Estimates vary, but each year at least 2 million women are battered by their intimate partners; this figure may actually be as high as 6 million. Battering during pregnancy probably represents about 10% of those cases (Noel & Yam, 1992).

Available information provides no clear picture of the objective perinatal risks associated with battering during pregnancy. However, the subjective risk perceived by pregnant women in abusive relationships is always high. The woman usually feels helpless and depressed because she cannot break out of the abusive relationship. This is because in most cases there is a history of love and loyalty in the relationship, intensifying the woman's ambivalence. However, the physical risks she faces, as well as the risk to her other children, may precipitate a call for help. Men who batter women often physically or psychologically abuse children as well (Sampselle, Petersen, Murtland, & Oakley, 1992).

If injuries that suggest family violence are recognized, the nurse must interview the woman in a supportive, non-

Legal/Ethical Considerations

Treatment Refusal and Noncompliance in Prenatal Care

The issues of treatment refusal, noncompliance, and maternal use of substances known to be harmful to the fetus are not new to those who provide prenatal care. However, they seem to be more worrisome in recent years, especially with regard to substance use and abuse. Health care providers are increasingly asking questions, such as what are the pregnant woman's rights to engage in behaviors she chooses? What are the professional's obligations when the woman's behaviors pose a threat to the fetus?

In recent years the courts have begun to force pregnant women to undergo specific procedures or to be confined against their will in hospitals or drug rehabilitation centers. Such actions override the principle of autonomy and do not have a sound basis in law. However, such situations are emotional; the system for obtaining court authorization for such actions is skewed in favor of those seeking them. Several states have begun the process of amending their child abuse laws to include action against mothers of neonates found to be drug-exposed in utero. Other states are considering laws requiring drug testing of pregnant women.

Professional organizations, such as the American College of Obstetricians and Gynecologists and the International Childbirth Education Association, have issued statements urging against the use of the legal system to force a pregnant woman to undergo treatment. The nurse must carefully consider the implications of enforced treatment and seek alternative ways to ensure the well-being of the pregnant woman and the fetus.

Greenlaw, J. (1990). Treatment refusal, noncompliance and substance abuse in pregnancy: Legal and ethical issues. Birth, *17(3), 152–156.*

threatening way in a setting that ensures privacy. The nurse should ask the woman gently and directly if she is in a relationship with anyone who threatens or physically hurts her (see the Assessment Tool, Abuse Assessment Screen, in Chapter 13). Many women will respond honestly. Those who cannot will nevertheless have heard the offer of assistance and may accept it at another time (Chez, 1989).

If the woman reports physical abuse, the nurse's first priority is to facilitate care for emotional and physical injuries. This includes assessment of fetal status if the woman expresses concern. The nurse must also remember that documentation should be complete, since patient records may eventually become part of a legal action if required by state law.

The nurse's second priority is to determine the woman's safety. Most female homicide victims in the United States are killed by a husband, lover, ex-husband, or ex-lover. A battered woman is in more danger of being killed by her abusive partner if she leaves him or makes it clear that she is ending their relationship (Parker & McFarlane, 1991).

Unless a woman's injuries require hospitalization, the health care provider usually cannot actively intervene. However, it is important that the health care provider acknowledges that the problem exists, affirms that the abuse is unacceptable and must stop, and informs the woman about the array of community resources available and how she can access them.

The national domestic violence hotline (1-800-333-5723) will provide the woman with information about community resources appropriate to her needs, including bilingual and telecommunication services for the deaf (Chez, 1989). Counseling the woman regarding her situation and assisting her to make a change is beyond the usual scope of maternity nursing practice and is better handled by specialized programs and care providers. However, the nurse can provide significant support by acting as a catalyst for change and by being alert for women who may be at risk. The nurse can also ask about battering when there is reason to ask, and provide support, encouragement, physical comfort, and needed information about available help to women who need it.

Expected Outcomes

- The pregnant woman uses the health care provider as a source of information and guidance in regard to situations that may pose a risk to her health and that of her fetus.
- The pregnant woman abusing substances discusses the importance of reducing use of these substances during pregnancy strives to do so.
- The pregnant woman initiates steps to reduce and eliminate risks.

Promoting a Healthy Pregnancy

Pregnancy is a normal physiologic event and should not require a woman to alter her lifestyle drastically. However, most pregnant women and their partners do wonder whether they can continue their usual activities throughout the pregnancy. This section will examine common concerns about sexuality, employment, travel, leisure activities, and exercise during pregnancy. Guidelines for advising pregnant women and their families will be presented.

Exercise

It is safe for a pregnant woman to continue her usual recreational activities unless she is informed of a specific medical contraindication. If she is proficient in activities requiring strength and agility, she may continue those activities during pregnancy. Modifications may be necessary as the weight of a growing uterus decreases endurance and alters balance. For example, pregnant women should decrease their jogging speed and let their tennis partners dive for the low balls.

Women who are extremely athletic and active generally know the risks of their particular sports. There are a few activities contraindicated in pregnancy because of risks to the fetus. Scuba diving is unsafe because of depth pressures. High-altitude activities are not recommended because of the risks of hypoxia and hypothermia. When in doubt, the woman should ask her health care provider about the safety of her activities.

Normally sedentary women should not take up demanding sports while they are pregnant. This is not the time to learn downhill skiing or wind surfing. It is safe, however, to start an exercise regimen during pregnancy. Exercise carries benefits and risks for all individuals, but there are special considerations for pregnant women. Studies of the effects of exercise on the outcome of pregnancy are limited. The nurse must therefore assess at each woman individually, including her current exercise level and the status of her pregnancy, before providing advice in this area.

Women who have not engaged in any regular exercise before pregnancy should be encouraged to do so during pregnancy. The benefits of exercise include improved fitness and muscle tone, improved sleep, less constipation, increased energy, and a general improvement in the woman's self-image. Swimming and walking at normal speeds are excellent forms of exercise for such women. Initiating a more strenuous form of exercise during pregnancy is not advisable for inactive women, due to the risk of maternal injury.

Women who have been used to regular exercise before pregnancy can usually continue their routine with few exceptions. They should be encouraged to discuss their exercise program with their health care provider early in pregnancy. Moderate aerobic exercise is generally safe, provided the pregnancy is normal. The presence of anemia, multiple gestation, preterm labor, heart or respiratory disease, hypertension, or complications with prior pregnancies make such an exercise program unwise.

Prolonged exercise should be avoided in hot, humid environments. The woman's body temperature should not exceed 40°C (104.0°F). Hot tubs and saunas should not be used during pregnancy. Hyperthermia has been shown to increase the risk of fetal abnormalities.

Pregnant women should be encouraged to monitor their own heart rates during exercise and to avoid overexertion. An easy way to monitor exertional stress is to use the "exercise-talk test." If a woman cannot exercise and talk simultaneously, she is approaching a compromised respiratory or heart rate. Even moderate exercise should not continue to exhaustion, and frequent rest periods are recommended.

Pregnant women should be encouraged to exercise for about 30 minutes three times per week regardless of their exercise level. Some physically fit women will be able to exercise longer. Conditioned runners should reduce their speed as pregnancy progresses, and may need to eliminate running late in pregnancy due to changes in balance and the risk of falls. Cyclists will need to adjust to the change in the placement of the body's center of gravity during the course of pregnancy. Stationary biking requires less balancing and may be safely performed by nearly all women during pregnancy (Jarski & Rippett, 1990).

Sexuality

Pregnancy is characterized by physiologic and emotional changes that can contribute to altered sexual patterns (see Chapter 5 for a detailed discussion). The nurse should provide anticipatory guidance about changes in sexuality during pregnancy, since women may feel uncomfortable asking questions directly.

Employment

Many women comfortably continue working throughout their pregnancies. Two judgments are necessary: is the work environment safe for a developing fetus, and can the pregnant woman carry out work commitments without undue stress and fatigue or physical injury? If a pregnancy becomes complicated, the woman must discuss modifications of work plans with her health care provider. In job safety counseling, the nurse's role is to assist each woman in obtaining information about particular toxic substances or other hazards in the work environment. It may be necessary to support the woman in seeking pregnancy-indicated work transfers. There is some evidence that pregnant women who are not satisfied with their work may experience considerably more job-related psychosocial stress and may experience higher rates of pregnancy complications (Homer, James, & Siegel, 1990). However, the workplace also provides many women with additional resources to promote well-being. The nurse should encourage the pregnant woman to consider how her work may affect her health and well-being, and what changes, if any, may be necessary during pregnancy (Killien, 1990)

Environmental Safety

Pregnant women should not work in environments where they are exposed to hazardous substances. If necessary, the pregnant woman should be transferred to another work area for the duration of her pregnancy. If there is any question about the safety of a particular substance, major medical centers often have teratogen registries that compile information and make it available to the public on request.

Pregnant women need to be particularly careful of substances that have been identified as toxic. These agents include carbon monoxide, mercury, lead, nitro compounds of anesthetic gases, x-rays and radioactive substances, benzene, turpentine, and other industrial cleaning agents. When in danger of exposure to any of these agents, for example, when doing household cleaning, the pregnant woman should be particularly careful about wearing gloves. The area should be well ventilated (Bernhardt, 1990).

One environmental hazard that may easily be overlooked is toxoplasmosis, a parasitic infection caused by *Toxoplasma gondii*. The disease can be acquired through contact with infected cat feces or by eating raw or undercooked meat that has been infected with the organism. Congenital infection can occur when toxoplasmosis is acquired during pregnancy. The pregnant woman who owns a cat should be warned against coming into contact with its waste products. She should avoid emptying or cleaning cat litter boxes and eating raw or undercooked meat. She should be advised to report symptoms of fatigue, muscle pain, or enlarged lymph nodes to her care provider so that diagnostic tests can be performed.

Fatigue and Injury

Pregnant women who continue full-time employment must have adequate breaks to rest and obtain nourishing snacks. Pregnant women employed in positions requiring constant standing and walking or lifting of heavy objects may require transfers to less physically demanding positions. Women performing sedentary jobs should get up and walk around once every hour.

Positions requiring delicate balance, such as scaffold or stepladder work, may pose hazards for the working pregnant woman. She may be unable to safely continue in this type of position as the pregnancy progresses and the growing uterus alters her center of gravity and sense of balance. Women operating heavy equipment or working in jobs where severe injuries are a risk should exercise caution and request transfers when necessary.

Travel and Leisure

There are few absolute restrictions on travel and leisure activities during pregnancy. However, certain precautions are advised to prevent injury to the pregnant woman or fetus.

Travel. The pregnant woman frequently has questions regarding travel during pregnancy. Although each case should be evaluated individually, there are some general guidelines that the nurse can use in providing information.

If there is a history of complications during a prior pregnancy, such as preterm labor, or if complications have developed during this pregnancy, travel should be restricted. Not only can such activity aggravate certain conditions, but there is also the concern about obtaining obstetric care away from home. Whenever travel is necessary during pregnancy, the woman should be encouraged to carry a copy of her medical record with her.

In general, the second trimester is the best time for the pregnant woman to travel. At this time, the woman is usually feeling her best and enjoying a good energy level. Families may want to consider distance from health care facilities in planning a trip. It may not be the best time to do backwoods backpacking, but car camping and day hikes can be considered. On the other hand, experienced backpackers can continue their usual activities, with appropriate adjustments in pack weight and altitudes.

Pregnant women traveling by air should check for any airline restrictions on air travel in late pregnancy. When traveling by air, car, or bus, the pregnant woman should avoid sitting for long periods. A stretch or walk should be scheduled every hour.

Seat Belt Use. The use of safety belts in general is greater among women than men. However, this use may decline during pregnancy because of concern that the restraint itself may increase the chance for fetal injury or death. During the first prenatal visit, the woman should be instructed in the proper placement of safety belts during pregnancy. The lap belt portion of the lap-shoulder belt should be placed under the pregnant woman's abdomen and across her upper thighs. It should be as snug as is comfortably possible. The shoulder restraint should also be as snugly applied as comfort allows. When she is the passenger, the pregnant woman should adjust her sitting position to the restraint so that it crosses at the shoulder without chafing her neck. The shoulder belt should be positioned between the breasts. It should never be slipped off the shoulder since this reduces the effectiveness of the entire restraint system. During long trips, the belt should be periodically readjusted for comfort and position (ACOG, 1991).

The nurse should mention to the expectant mother the future need for an infant restraint system, which may be required by law. During the late second or early third trimester, the nurse should inquire if such a device has been obtained and remind the family that they will need to take their neonate home from the hospital in such a restraint. Most communities have loaner programs for families who cannot afford to purchase infant car seats.

Immunizations. The nurse should be aware of which immunizations are indicated and contraindicated during pregnancy. All pregnant women should be questioned regarding their last tetanus booster and have this protection updated if 10 years have elapsed since their last immunization. In most instances, this is the only immunization routinely given in the prenatal period. Occasionally additional questions may be raised by patients in regard to exposure to a communicable disease or plans to travel to areas of the world where immunizations are necessary. The pregnant woman should consult her physician or nurse midwife about which immunizations are safe during pregnancy.

Dental Care

Assessment of the oral cavity is part of the routine prenatal physical examination. The woman should be advised that gum hypertrophy, tenderness, and even bleeding may accompany a normal pregnancy. Good oral hygiene should be practiced during pregnancy. The woman should inform her dentist that she is pregnant. X-rays should be avoided and any dental care during pregnancy other than routine cleaning can be done after consultation between the dentist and the health care provider. If possible, extensive dental work should be delayed until after delivery. General dental repair and extractions can be done under local anesthetic during pregnancy.

Medications

The nurse should advise the pregnant woman to consult with her health care provider before taking any medication, either prescription or over-the-counter. Because there are some common discomforts of pregnancy that may require use of medication, the nurse should explain what remedies may be safely used during pregnancy. However, there are many medications on the market today about which there is inadequate information in regard to safe use in pregnancy. In general, the health care provider must weigh the risks against the benefits and decide if a drug can safely be used (Briggs, Freeman, & Yaffe, 1990).

Preparation for Breastfeeding

The woman who is interested in breastfeeding should be acquainted with information early in her pregnancy. The earlier she receives information, the more likely it is that she will breastfeed successfully for a substantial period of time (Lawrence, 1989). Preparation for breastfeeding takes place mainly in the third trimester. However, the woman should be examined during the initial physical examination to determine if she has flat or inverted nipples, which may require additional early preparation for successful nursing.

The nurse should inform the woman early in pregnancy about how to care for her breasts so that future problems can be avoided. During pregnancy, the breasts undergo many changes in response to maternal hormones. The nipples also undergo changes to prepare them for nursing. Proper breast care will enhance this process.

The woman should be instructed to avoid washing the nipple and areola with soap, which removes the skin oils. Soap also interferes with the natural acid/alkaline balance. The pregnant woman should avoid scrubbing her nipples, a practice that wears away natural oils, causing the skin to dry and crack. Drying or hardening agents, such as tincture of benzoin, witch hazel, and harsh cleansing agents should also be avoided. Plastic liners in nursing bras or nursing pads should be removed since they produce a warm moist environment for breeding bacteria. Because the skin of the nipple and areola has its own natural lubrication, no additional lubricants should be used.

During the third trimester, the woman can begin routine nipple preparation. Additional layers of keratin can be produced by the skin of the nipples and areola with proper preparation. This keratin layer is a tough, hard, waterproof barrier against bacterial invasion and will help prevent soreness and infection. Techniques for building keratin include:

- Exposure to air and light
- Nipple tug and roll
- Breast massage
- Stimulation during sexual activity

Any type of nipple stimulation can produce uterine activity because of the release of oxytocin from the posterior pituitary. Therefore, women with a history of preterm labor and those at risk for this complication should consult with their health care provider before starting nipple preparation

In the past, some sources advised the pregnant woman to expell colostrum prenatally. However, removal of colostrum is not advisable. Colostrum acts as a barrier to bacteria and viruses. It is also not known if colostrum is continually produced throughout pregnancy, either in terms of quantity or with consistent amounts of its constituent components. Therefore, prenatal removal is not advisable.

If the mother has flat or inverted nipples, she may need

additional preparation during the third trimester to help correct this problem. Milk cups (breast shields) worn inside the bra will exert gentle pressure around the nipple, making the skin more pliable and the nipple easier to grasp. The Hoffman technique involves gentle pulling on opposite sides of the areola which will help the nipple to protrude. Once the nipple has become protractile enough to grasp, the nipple tug and roll can be added to the routine (Lauvers and Woessner, 1989). The accompanying display describes these breast preparation techniques.

True Labor

True labor is unmistakable when it starts abruptly and progresses rapidly. However, not all women experience labor this way. Women in late pregnancy can become discouraged when they experience false labor or when the first stage of their labor is prolonged. Information given in birth preparation classes or in prenatal visits should help the woman distinguish true from false labor (Table 15-1). Frequently the nurse will counsel women by telephone to help them identify their labor signs.

True labor can begin in one of three ways or as a combination of the three. The mucous plug may be expelled from the cervix at the onset of labor as a result of cervical dilatation, appearing as pink mucus from the vagina ("show" or "bloody show"). It can also appear 1 or 2 weeks before the onset of actual labor, however. Rupture of the amniotic membranes may be signaled by a leaking or gushing of fluid. The woman should report the character of the fluid; amniotic fluid is usually clear or slightly blood-tinged. Discolored greenish fluid or frank blood should be reported immediately. When labor does not occur spontaneously after the rupture of membranes at term, many clinicians will choose to induce labor within 12 to 24 hours. Uterine contractions may begin as backache and progress over the abdomen, causing the uterus to become firm. True labor contractions occur at a regular rate and gradually increase in duration, strength, and frequency.

In false labor, contractions generally occur over the abdomen and can sometimes be relieved by walking. Passage of the mucous plug and rupture of ruptures does not occur. False labor consists of Braxton Hicks contractions, which are irregular in duration, strength, and frequency. Occasionally a woman finds false labor so uncomfortable that she is unable to sleep or rest. In such instances a mild sedative may be prescribed (Bonovich, 1990).

Nursing research shows the importance of teaching women to recognize true labor, as indicated in the accompanying display.

Teaching Considerations

Breast Preparation

The nurse can instruct the pregnant woman in two techniques to prepare nipples in the third trimester for breastfeeding. Nipple rolling and the Hoffman technique increase nipple elasticity and help correct flat or inverted nipples; they are described below. The pregnant woman should be advised to practice each technique for 2 to 3 minutes several times a week during the last month of pregnancy.

Nipple rolling: The woman grasps the nipple with the thumb and forefinger and gently rolls the nipple while stretching outward. She gradually moves thumb and forefinger to a new position every few seconds as if around the face of a clock. The woman should be cautioned not to rub or drag fingers over the surface of the nipple, because this can abrade the skin.

Hoffman technique: This technique increases the elasticity of the nipple and may make flat or inverted nipples easier for the newborn to grasp. The woman places thumb or forefinger of one hand or index fingers of both hands on opposite sides of the nipple on the areola. The woman gently pushes fingers apart, stretching the skin. She then lifts the fingers and places them in a new position, as if working around the face of a clock.

Lauvers, J., & Woessner, C. (1989). Counseling the nursing mother. *New York: Avery Publishing Group.*

Expected Outcomes

- The pregnant woman demonstrates appropriate self-care measures in regard to activities such as exercise, employment, environmental exposure, and prevention of fatigue and injury.

Table 15-1. Distinguishing True Labor From Braxton Hicks Contractions

Parameter	True Labor Contractions	Braxton Hicks Contractions
Intervals	Regular	Irregular
Frequency	Gradually increasing	Inconsistent
Intensity	Gradually increasing	Variable
Location	Primarily in the back	Over abdomen
Aggravating or alleviating factors	Intensified by walking	Sometimes relieved by walking
Bloody show	Usually present	Not present
Rupture of membranes	Sometimes present	Not present

Nursing Research

Teaching Women to Recognize the Onset of Labor

According to the labor and delivery records of one 500-bed urban community hospital, 10% to 20% of the pregnant women who come to the hospital with signs of early labor are sent home undelivered. The use of personnel time to assess these women contributes to higher costs and diverts attention of staff from the care of other women and their families. In addition women may spend hours waiting in the hospital before being sent home, using physical and psychological energy that will be needed when active labor begins.

This experimental study compared the use of an educational technique based on active staff involvement with pregnant women to help them understand routine instructions to prepare them to recognize the onset of active labor. Both the experimental subjects ($n = 104$) and control subjects ($n = 104$) received verbal and written instructions on how to recognize and report onset of labor from the time when the woman reached 37 weeks of gestation. Experimental subjects then participated in an exit interview with the nurse investigator who reviewed this information, addressed gaps in knowledge, and gave specific guidance on distinguishing between false and true labor. Results showed a significant decrease in the screening visits made to the labor and delivery floor for labor evaluation by experimental subjects when compared to control subjects, while not substantially increasing the time spent in delivery of clinic care.

Bonovich, L. (1990). Recognizing the onset of labor. *Journal of Obstetric, Gynecologic, and Neonatal Nursing, 19*(2), 141–145.

- The pregnant woman demonstrates appropriate self-care measures in preparation for breastfeeding.

• • Evaluation

Evaluation of prenatal care is usually done on the basis of perinatal outcomes. These include outcomes such as incidence of complications, maternal weight gain, neonatal birth weight, and maternal–neonatal morbidity and mortality. Often referred to as "hard" outcomes, they are easily and routinely measured and are easy to quantify. The quality of nursing care in the prenatal period is directly reflected in these outcomes, as repeated studies have shown (see the Nursing Research display). The fact that prenatal care "works" is hardly questioned. The question more commonly asked in evaluating the effectiveness of prenatal care is not whether it works but when does it work. Most complications still occur in women who have either delayed or no prenatal care because they have inadequate access to health care services (ANA, 1987; Machala & Miner, 1991).

Evaluation of nursing care during pregnancy also should be based on an assessment of outcomes. The extent to which women implement safe and appropriate self-care and use care providers as resources is a reflection of the effectiveness of nursing care. It is not common to systematically document the self-care behaviors of women and their families as they occur. However, this information is needed to evaluate how nursing actions influence self-care, and

Nursing Research

A Buddy System to Improve Prenatal Care

A community approach to encourage early and regular use of prenatal care has proved successful in Houston. The BABY BUDDY program, sponsored by the March of Dimes, has established a partnership between public and private sectors in a community where nearly one third of women in health department clinics received late or no prenatal care and where there was a high infant mortality rate (20.5/1000) and a high low–birth-weight rate (10.6/1000). This program recruits individuals and businesses to donate time, services, or goods to pregnant women receiving prenatal care in a selected clinic. The incentives are donated to pregnant women throughout their pregnancies. The program also includes community education about the importance of prenatal care, a mother's support group, and the active involvement of selected prenatal care clinics.

Analysis shows that the program is working. Women are entering prenatal care because of information they received about the project, and they bring friends and family members to the clinic and the mother's group. Once a woman enters the program, results suggest that she is likely to continue her prenatal care. Further, 32 randomly selected BABY BUDDY mothers were interviewed and were found to have used the information they received and to have shared it with others. The author concludes that this is a model that may be applicable for other health issues for which community outreach, mobilization of effort, and outreach are needed.

Helton, A. (1990). A BUDDY system to improve prenatal care. *MCN: American Journal of Maternal Child Nursing, 15*(4), 234–237.

how self-care influences perinatal outcomes (McClanahan, 1992).

Effectiveness of nursing care is also reflected in what may be referred to as "soft" outcomes. These outcomes include the comfort and ease of family adaptation to pregnancy, the effectiveness with which parents care for themselves, and the extent to which psychosocial risk factors fail to produce actual trauma because they were recognized and counterbalanced by appropriate and supportive care. These outcomes are frequently the result of excellent nursing care, but are difficult to measure. Because of this, nurses are still the invisible providers in prenatal care. Additional research demonstrating the effectiveness of prenatal nursing care in producing positive and documentable outcomes is needed.

Chapter Summary

When working with expectant families, the nurse should assess the meaning and significance of the pregnancy to each family. Each family member carries a previous history as well as current concerns and expectations into the new pregnancy. Individual family members have a variety of learning needs that test the nurse's insights, knowledge, and skills in counseling. The pregnant woman has many rapidly changing needs. For instance, she may need anticipatory guidance about the predictable changes of pregnancy. Otherwise she may not be prepared for the dramatic physical and emotional changes of early pregnancy. Likewise, it may be important for the pregnant woman to know that she probably will be more comfortable in the second trimester. Finally, she and her family will probably benefit from some discussion about the eventful third trimester, when labor and delivery will be uppermost in their minds. Many preparations will be necessary, but it may be useful for her to remember that she may be increasingly uncomfortable and tired.

Although most families share some general concerns associated with pregnancy, many other concerns will be specific to each family. When assessing the family's needs, the nurse uses her knowledge of the physiologic and psychological processes of pregnancy as a framework. The knowledgeable nurse will be able to answer a myriad of questions, using her judgment in deciding how information can best be conveyed to the pregnant woman and her family.

Study Questions

1. *What is an example of information that may be particularly valuable to expectant parents in the form of anticipatory guidance?*
2. *What factors influence a woman's or a family's learning needs in pregnancy?*
3. *What are five reasons why a woman or couple would need a referral? What referrals would be appropriate for these reasons?*
4. *What are five signs or symptoms that a pregnant woman should report at once?*
5. *What clues may suggest a woman has been battered during pregnancy? What is the nurse's course of action when observing such clues?*
6. *A patient has a question about exercising during pregnancy. What points is it important to assess prior to your counseling?*
7. *What is the prenatal preparation for breastfeeding?*

References

American College of Obstetricians and Gynecologists (1991). *Automobile passenger restraints for children and pregnant women.* Technical Bulletin #151. Washington, D.C. : Author.

American Nurses Association (1987): *Access to Prenatal Care: Key to Preventing Low Birth Weight.* Kansas City, MO: Author.

Bernhardt, J. (1990). Potential workplace hazards to reproductive health: Information for primary prevention. *JOGNN, 19,* (1) 53–62.

Bonovich,L. (1990). Recognizing the onset of labor. *JOGNN. 19,* (2), 141–145.

Briggs, G., Freeman, R., & Yaffe S. (1990). *Drugs in Pregnancy and Lactation.* Baltimore: Williams & Wilkins.

Brucker, M. (1988a). Management of minor common discomforts in pregnancy: Part II—Managing minor pain in pregnancy. *Journal of Nurse Midwifery. 33,* (1), 25–29.

Brucker, M. (1988b). Management of minor common discomforts in pregnancy: Part III—Managing gastrointestinal problems in pregnancy. *Journal of Nurse Midwifery, 33,* (2), 67–72.

Chez, R. (1989). Battered pregnant women. *Genesis, 11,* (1), 15–16.

Chisum, G. (1990). Nursing interventions with the antepartum substance abuser. *Journal of Perinatal and Neonatal Nursing, 3,* (4), 26–33.

DiIorio, C., (1988). Management of nausea and vomiting in pregnancy. *Nurse Practitioner, 13,* (5), 23–28.

Homer, C., James, S., & Siegel, E. (1990). Work-related psychosocial stress and risk of preterm, low birthweight delivery. *American Journal of Public Health, 80,* (2), 173–177.

Jarski, R. & Rippett, D. (1990). The risks and benefits of exercise during pregnancy. *Journal of Family Practice, 30,* (2), 185–189.

Killien, M. (1990). Working during pregnancy: Psychological stressor or asset? *NAACOG'S Clinical Issues in Perinatal and Women's Health Nursing, 1,* (3), 325–332.

Lauvers, J., & Woessner, C. (1989). *Counseling the nursing mother.* New York: Avery Publishing Group.

Lawrence, R. (1989). *Breastfeeding—A guide for the medical profession.* St. Louis: C.V. Mosby.

Machala, M., & Miner, M. (1991). Piecing together the crazy quilt of prenatal care. *Public Health Reports, 106,* (4), 353–360.

McClanahan, P. (1992). Improving access to and use of prenatal care. *JOGNN, 21,* (4) 280–286.

Mercer, R. (1990). *Parents at risk.* New York: Springer.

Noel, N., & Yam, M. (1992). Domestic violence: The pregnant battered woman. *Nursing Clinics of North America, 27,* (4), 871–884.

O'Connor, A., Davies, B., Dulberg, C., Buhler, P., Nadon, C., McBride, B., & Benzie, R. (1992). Effectiveness of a pregnancy smoking cessation program. *JOGNN, 21,* (5), 385–392.

Parker, B. & McFarlane, J. (1991). Identifying and helping battered pregnant women. *MCN, 16,* (2)161–169.

Sampselle, C., Petersen, B., Murtland, T., & Oakley, D. (1992) Prevalence of abuse among pregnant women choosing certified nurse-midwife or physician providers. *Journal of Nurse Midwifery, 37,* (4), 269–273.

Suggested Readings

Affonso, D., Mayberry, L., Graham, K, Shibuya, J., Kunimoto, J, & Kuramoto, M. (1992). Adaptation themes for prenatal care delivered by public health nurses. *Public Health Nursing, 9,* (3), 172–176.

Gaffney, K. (1992). Nursing practice model for maternal role sufficiency. *Advances in Nursing Science*, *15*, (2), 76–84.

Husley, T., Patrick, C., & Alexander, G. (1991). Prenatal care and prematurity: Is there an association in uncomplicated pregnancies? *Birth*, *18*, (3), 146–152.

Libbus, M., & Sable, M. (1991). Prenatal education in a high risk population: The effect on birth outcomes. *Birth*, *18*, (2), 78–82.

Pettitti, D., Hiatt, R., & Chin, V. (1991). A outcome evaluation of content and quality of prenatal care. *Birth*, *18*, (1), 21–25.

Weiss, J., & Hansell, M. (1992). Substance abuse during pregnancy: Legal and health policy issues. *Nursing and Health Care*, *13*, (9), 472–479.

CHAPTER 16

Complications of Pregnancy

Learning Objectives

After studying the material in this chapter, the student will be able to:

- Explain the standard medical and nursing care for the woman with hyperemesis gravidarum.
- Identify the major risks associated with placenta previa and nursing actions to reduce risk.
- List the symptoms of ectopic pregnancy and describe appropriate nursing actions when symptoms are identified.
- Describe anticipatory guidance about prenatal care the nurse should provide to the woman diagnosed with multiple gestation.
- Identify maternal risk factors when intrauterine fetal demise complicates pregnancy.
- Describe the consequences of maternal hemoglobinopathy in pregnancy.
- Discuss the major risks associated with thromboembolic disease in pregnancy.
- List the infections known to have teratogenic potential during pregnancy.
- Describe maternal and fetal or neonatal consequences of sexually transmitted disease during pregnancy.
- Discuss commonly abused substances and how their use in pregnancy affects maternal and fetal and neonatal outcomes.

Key Terms

afibrinogenemia
abruption
disseminating intravascular coagulation (DIC)
deep vein thrombosis
ectopic pregnancy
erythroblastosis
gestational trophoblastic disease
hemoglobinopathy
hemolytic disease
hemodynamic stability
hydatidiform mole
hyperemesis gravidarum
hydrops fetalis
intrauterine fetal demise (IUFD)
neonatal abstinence syndrome
placenta previa
postterm pregnancy
pulmonary embolism
Rh immunoglobulin (RhIgG)
sensitization
teratogenic infection

Complications may occur any time during pregnancy. They may result from problems with the pregnancy, preexisting medical problems, infections, or substance use and abuse. Because of the complex connections between maternal problems and the normal physiologic changes that occur during pregnancy, close prenatal surveillance is important. Clinical research has repeatedly found that early and consistent prenatal care results in improved health for the woman and neonate.

The normal physiologic changes that occur in the woman's body during the 9 months of gestation set the specialty of maternity care apart from all other areas in nursing. The objective of prenatal care is to monitor specific parameters with the goal of averting or minimizing problems. To achieve this goal, the nurse must be knowledgeable about the physiology of pregnancy, the numerous changes that normally occur, and the significance of deviations. Nurses prepared to work in high-risk settings can provide guidance and expedite care by monitoring laboratory studies, collecting specimens, and referring patients for special care or treatments. Providing patient support through teaching and encouragement are essential roles for the maternity nurse.

The nurse must be able to translate knowledge into pragmatic teaching that pregnant women will be able to understand. Anticipatory guidance is used to direct teaching about events pertinent to each trimester. This reduces the pregnant woman's fear of the unknown and increases family members' abilities to participate in maintaining their own health. Health teaching offered over time in a positive and informal manner promotes comfort and trust between the nurse and the pregnant woman and her family. Honesty and directness foster confidence and compliance. These principles are especially important when problems arise during pregnancy.

Pregnancy at Risk

Pregnancy is normal until proved otherwise. Because the specialty of obstetrics has closely defined what is normal, all factors outside these parameters are referred to as risk factors. Some of these risk factors, such as genetic susceptibility, hypertension, or anemia, may be identified from the patient's history and physical examination or from laboratory findings. Risk factors that alter the physiologic process of pregnancy may seriously affect the health of the mother and neonate. Maternal problems such as infection and substance use may compromise the quality of the pregnancy and the fetal outcome. Poverty, malnutrition, the fact that a pregnancy is unwanted, and increased maternal age can lead to pregnancy complications. They are also referred to as risk factors.

Most women start their pregnancies expecting a normal prenatal course. As the pregnancy progresses, some women may experience risk factors such as bleeding, inconsistent uterine growth, or anemia. The purpose of prenatal care is to identify the at-risk group of women and initiate early intervention to prevent or alleviate problems.

Rapid technologic advances have changed the practice of obstetrics and maternity nursing. Protocols and screening methods have been devised to identify the woman at risk for pregnancy-related problems. The term "at risk" emphasizes the obstetric approach to prevention, that is, to screen patients, identify problems, and tailor management to promote optimal pregnancy outcome.

The art of maternity care is often overshadowed by the urgency of complications and the marvels of technology. Procedures necessary to facilitate optimal care may be alienating, frightening, and mysterious to the woman and family. The nurse plays the role of mediator and equalizer by translating "high-tech" into humanistic terms. Although this chapter focuses on complications, even when a pregnancy has complications the nurse should be mindful of the ordinary concerns of the family, such as breastfeeding, nutrition, and sibling adjustment. The nurse must maintain the art of caring (see the Family Considerations display).

Because of the growing cost constraints in maternity care, the nurse may need to consider creative ways to provide nursing care to high-risk women and their families, such as through the use of telephone follow-up, home care, and support groups for women who may otherwise be isolated during pregnancy (see the Nursing Research display).

Family Considerations

Needs of the Father in High-Risk Pregnancy

The father is recognized increasingly as being affected by and involved in the experience of pregnancy. Health care providers who are comfortable and supportive of close father involvement in a healthy, low-risk pregnancy may fail to recognize that a high-risk pregnancy places particular stress on most expectant fathers.

A significant stressor for many men is fear of injury to or death of the woman. Even when a man values a pregnancy and desires a child, if the pregnancy is threatened, his first concern will usually be for the well-being of his partner. This is important to remember when discussing relative perinatal risk with the partners of high-risk pregnant women. The nurse should be careful to explain maternal and fetal risk separately and to verify that the man understands the explanations. If the man is confused about the nature of the risk, he may assume that his partner is in greater danger than is in fact the case. For example, when "stress tests" are ordered, the man may assume that tests "stress" his partner in some way and conclude her well-being is threatened. Fathers are at greater risk for misunderstanding and misinformation because they are less likely to receive explanations firsthand from the health care provider.

The nurse can prevent misunderstanding and misinformation by providing clear and careful explanations to the woman and asking her to repeat back the information and offering to speak to the partner directly by telephone, should that be necessary. Although the well-being of the high-risk pregnant woman is of primary concern, the well-being of the couple relationship and the woman's support system should also be a nursing priority.

Gestational Complications of Pregnancy

Gestational complications are specific to pregnancy. This group of disorders represents a wide range of problems, from those that primarily affect maternal physiologic functioning and pose only indirect risk to the fetus, to those that pose direct and life-threatening risk to both the woman and the fetus.

Nursing Research

Prenatal Home Care Services for High-Risk Women

Increasingly high-risk perinatal care is being offered on an outpatient basis, and careful home follow-up is required to ensure maternal and fetal well-being. This type of nursing care has grown rapidly in recent years. However, little published information exists about the types of patient problems these services encounter and what nursing interventions are most commonly used. A study of 9 private and 38 public agencies that provide prenatal home care services to high-risk women were surveyed to determine what types of agencies and services were available.

Findings suggested that the most frequent patient problem identified by the public agencies was home follow-up in adolescent pregnancy. Other frequent patient problems were preterm labor, substance abuse, and poor previous pregnancy outcome. Among private agencies, preterm labor was the most common problem, followed by pregnancy-induced hypertension, teenage pregnancy, and hyperemesis gravidarum. The most commonly used nursing intervention in the public agencies was providing information about nutrition, fetal growth and development, rest and activity, and signs and symptoms of complications. In contrast, private agencies most frequently used nursing interventions in physical assessment of maternal and fetal status, administering medications and fluids, and performing cervical evaluations.

The findings of this study clearly showed the differing needs of pregnant women served by private and public home care agencies. Careful documentation of the services provided and the outcomes achieved is essential if such services are to continue in today's cost-conscious health care system.

Dineen, K., Rossi, M., Lia-Hoagberg, B., & Keller, L. (1992). Antepartum home care services for high risk women. *Journal of Obstetric Gynecologic, and Neonatal Nursing, 21*(2), 121–124.

Complications Involving Maternal Physiologic Alterations

Some gestational complications primarily affect maternal physiologic functioning. They pose direct risk to the woman and fetus because of associated physiologic alterations. The major complications in this category are pregnancy-induced hypertension (PIH) and diabetes mellitus, both discussed in Chapter 27. Hyperemesis gravidarum is another complication that primarily involves alteration in maternal physiologic status.

Hyperemesis Gravidarum

One of the most common and well-known symptoms of early pregnancy is nausea and vomiting, generally called *morning sickness*. This uncomfortable dyad of symptoms occurs in about 70% of all pregnancies. It is often experienced with or without food intake at any time of the day. One or both of the symptoms may continue until about 12 weeks of gestation, at which time they normally disappear or decrease in severity.

In hyperemesis gravidarum, vomiting is severe enough to cause electrolyte, metabolic, and nutritional imbalances. This problem usually begins early in pregnancy.

Etiologic and Predisposing Factors

Many causative factors for nausea and vomiting in pregnancy have been proposed. They include hormonal, histaminic, and psychogenic factors as well as factors related to vitamin use. Current theory postulates that the rapidly increasing levels of human chorionic gonadotropin (hCG) in early pregnancy induce emesis. The validity of this theory is suggested by the fact that women carrying multiple pregnancies and those with hydatidiform moles have extremely high levels of hCG. These women typically experience exaggerated symptoms of nausea and vomiting. However, the theory remains unproven, and the causative factors of the illness have not yet been positively identified.

Diagnosis

Continued nausea and vomiting over time creates a risk of increasing dehydration. When conservative measures of dietary counseling and psychological support do not bring relief or resolution of nausea and vomiting, the following criteria are used to diagnose hyperemesis gravidarum:

- It occurs during the first 16 weeks of gestation.
- It is accompanied by disturbances of appetite.
- It causes alterations in nutritional status, as evidenced by weight loss, electrolyte imbalance, and ketosis with ketonuria.
- It is intractable in nature.

Laboratory studies reveal hemoconcentration in hyperemesis gravidarum. In severe cases, loss of hydrogen, sodium, potassium, and chloride will result in hyponatremia (decreased sodium in the blood) and hypokalemia (decreased potassium in the blood). During pregnancy, gastric acid secretion normally is reduced because of increased estrogen stimulation. This places the pregnant woman at risk for alkalosis rather than the acidosis that usually occurs in an advanced stage of dehydration. Other causes of prolonged nausea and vomiting, such as pancreatitis, hepatitis, and cholecystitis, must be considered.

Treatment

In women who are not seriously dehydrated, hospitalization may be avoided by the administration of intravenous fluids in the outpatient setting. Administration of 1000 mL lactated Ringer's solution corrects dehydration, restores electrolyte balance, and interrupts or relieves the nausea and vomiting cycle. When marked dehydration has occurred, hospitalization is required to correct fluid and electrolyte deficits by intravenous infusion. Treatment should continue until vomiting is controlled.

When hospitalization is required for severe symptoms, treatment goals are to hydrate the patient, establish electrolyte balance, and provide caloric and vitamin supplementation. These goals are accomplished by restricting oral intake and beginning parenteral administration of fluids supplemented with electrolytes and vitamins. Treatment provides rest for the gastrointestinal tract that has become overstimulated by severe vomiting. Patients are generally kept NPO until 48 hours after vomiting ceases.

In some cases, antiemetic drugs may be needed to control vomiting. Because no drugs are approved for this indication, patients needing drug treatment must be informed that only limited information is available regarding the teratogenicity of prescribed drugs. Drugs used to treat hyperemesis gravidarum include phenothiazines such as promethazine, which can be given intravenously or by rectal suppository (Gabbe, Niebyl, & Simpson, 1991).

Maternal, Fetal, and Neonatal Implications

Uncorrected hyperemesis gravidarum can result in severe electrolyte imbalance and possible hepatic and renal damage. The major concern for fetal well-being is uncorrected ketosis, which may result in fetal abnormalities or death in early pregnancy.

Implications for Nursing Care

The distressing nature of the symptoms and the concern the woman and her family may have about the condition and its effects on fetal well-being often cause high levels of stress. Nursing care can be instrumental in helping women cope with hyperemesis.

• • Assessment

Hyperemesis gravidarum insidiously progresses from a mild to a severe state. The nurse can assess the severity of symptoms by using these methods:

- Compare the woman's prepregnant weight with her current weight.
- Compare actual weight gain with the expected weight gain for the appropriate week of gestation.
- Review the woman's dietary intake in the preceding 24 hours.
- Compare the woman's usual eating habits with her current intake.
- Determine whether the woman is ingesting substances that are not foods, such as starch, clay, toothpaste, and so on, which would indicate pica.
- Perform a dipstick urine test for the presence of ketones.
- Examine skin turgor.

• • Nursing Diagnosis

The following nursing diagnoses may be applicable in caring for the pregnant woman with hyperemesis gravidarum:

- Altered Nutrition: Less than Body Requirements related to vomiting and inadequate oral intake
- High Risk for Fluid Volume Deficit related to vomiting and inadequate oral intake
- Fear related to concerns for fetal well-being

• • Planning and Implementation

During hospitalization, nursing care focuses on maintaining patient comfort, monitoring intravenous therapy, and informing the woman about the rationale for interventions. Women should be told that the cause of hyperemesis is unknown. Teaching women that their behaviors have not caused the problem and that symptoms can be expected to subside spontaneously reassures them and reduces stress.

Careful monitoring and recording of the patient's fluid intake and urinary and vomitus output is important to ensure that rehydration is proceeding as expected. Oral hygiene measures are important because the patient's mouth will become excessively dry from lack of oral fluid intake. After vomiting episodes, the mouth should be rinsed. Bed linen or gowns should be changed as necessary.

When vomiting begins to decrease in response to treatment, limited amounts of liquids, such as tea or ice chips, may be offered. Bland foods, such as crackers or toast, may be given at intervals of 2 to 3 hours. Depending on the patient's response to these foods, the diet can be increased gradually until the woman is able to eat a regular diet. During this time, it is also important to provide a quiet and restful atmosphere to promote needed rest and sleep.

During hospitalization, the nurse should be cognizant of the woman's psychological needs. The nurse should reassure the pregnant woman that the threat to fetal well-being is eliminated once dehydration is corrected and nutritional intake resumes.

After intravenous therapy and hospitalization, the patient should be given specific instructions for progressing to oral fluid intake. The nurse should follow up by telephone to assess whether the woman is ready to progress to a more standard diet or whether reevaluation is needed. Appropriate referrals to a social worker, psychologist, or public health nurse may be warranted.

Expected Outcomes

- The woman explains the need for normal hydration and caloric intake for optimal fetal well-being.
- The woman demonstrates signs of normal hydration status (normal urine specific gravity, normal hemoconcentra-

tion, absence of ketosuria) within 6 hours of beginning fluid therapy.
- The woman tolerates adequate oral intake without vomiting.

• • Evaluation

Once the woman's symptoms subside and she is discharged from the hospital, it is important to monitor her closely in the outpatient setting. A single provider of care who is knowledgeable about the woman's history and has established a trusting relationship should be responsible for providing her care consistently. Telephone follow-up can provide information about nutritional intake and symptoms and can offer emotional support to the pregnant woman.

Complications Involving Bleeding

Complications marked by vaginal bleeding are particularly frightening to women and their families. Bleeding complications also present considerable maternal and fetal risk. The following section discusses spontaneous abortion and placenta previa; abruptio placentae is discussed in Chapter 26.

Spontaneous Abortion

Vaginal bleeding occurs in approximately 50% of all pregnancies. Pregnancy loss with early bleeding episodes is a primary concern in the first trimester. Spontaneous abortion is the termination of pregnancy or the expulsion of the products of conception that weigh less than 500 g (17.6 oz) or are not viable. The definition varies from state to state and may specify the maximum number of weeks gestation that constitute nonviability. Spontaneous abortion occurs in about 30% of all pregnancies. Most spontaneous abortions occur before the 16th week, but they may occur into the second trimester.

The pregnant woman is said to experience a *threatened abortion* when slight bleeding persists for several weeks, accompanied by uterine cramping and pain. No cervical dilatation or effacement occurs, and no tissue is passed. If the bleeding persists, little can be done except to advise bed rest for 48 hours. When spontaneous abortion reaches the inevitable stage, the cervix is soft and its os is dilated; bleeding may be profuse, and abdominal cramping begins to resemble the pain of labor.

When the products of conception are only partially expelled, the abortion is said to be *incomplete*. Tissues that remain in the uterus contain portions of the fetal membrane or placenta. Bleeding and cramping continue and become more severe. Prolonged retention of the tissues predisposes the woman to infection. Immediate medical intervention is needed. When the entire products of conception (fetus and placenta) are passed, abortion is considered *complete*. After spontaneous abortion, pain ceases and the bleeding usually stops. Complete abortion is more likely to occur early in gestation.

When the fetus dies in utero but remains, along with the placenta and tissues, in the uterus, a *missed abortion* has occurred. Pregnancy symptoms abate, but amenorrhea continues. When the woman is unaware that a missed abortion has occurred and it is not detected within about 2 months by health care providers, coagulopathy may occur, causing life-threatening illness (see the section in this chapter on intrauterine fetal demise [IUFD]).

Etiologic and Predisposing Factors

Usually the cause for spontaneous abortion is not known. This form of pregnancy loss is more common in older women, leading to speculation that genetic abnormality in the ovum may be a contributing factor. When bleeding occurs in the second and third trimesters, the risk to the woman is much greater.

Maternal factors that can cause abortion are abnormal uterine development, systemic disease, endocrine or nutritional problems, and immunologic deficiencies. Environmental factors, such as drugs, radiation, or trauma, may also play a role in pregnancy loss.

Diagnosis

If any woman experiences vaginal bleeding after pregnancy has been confirmed, spontaneous abortion must be considered the cause unless proved otherwise. If abortion is suspected earlier than 8 weeks' gestation, two serum quantitative hCG tests spaced 48 hours apart will be needed. In a normal pregnancy, the serum level of hCG will double in that time.

When pregnancy is more advanced, the presence of uterine bleeding, uterine contractions, and uterine pain are ominous signs. These signs must be considered as indicative of a threatened abortion, until proved otherwise. Even when these signs are present, the diagnosis of inevitable abortion may be difficult to make. Ultrasound is highly reliable in determining the presence of a viable gestational sac but cannot predict the continued viability of the pregnancy.

Treatment

Early vaginal bleeding generally calls for watchful waiting. Bed rest is often prescribed, but its effectiveness has not been convincingly demonstrated. Symptoms of bleeding and cramping will either subside and cease or worsen, leading to inevitable abortion. When bleeding persists without progression to spontaneous abortion, weekly sonograms are performed to ascertain whether the fetus is still viable.

Many spontaneous abortions occur at home. In spontaneous abortions where the products of conception are contained within an intact sac, complete membranes are present, and bleeding has stopped, no surgical intervention is indicated. Inevitable and incomplete abortions are managed by evacuation of the uterus in the simplest, safest, and most effective manner. Before 12 weeks of gestation, this is accomplished by curettage to ensure that all gestational tissue has been removed from the uterus. The tissue specimen from the evacuation must be carefully examined for completeness. When there is doubt about its completeness or normalcy, it should be sent to the histology laboratory for further examination.

Maternal Implications

Maternal complications of spontaneous abortion are relatively rare but include hemorrhage, infection, and situational depression after pregnancy loss. Several days of rest and emotional support will be needed by most women.

Implications for Nursing Care

Nursing care of the woman experiencing a spontaneous abortion requires sensitivity and a respect for the nature of the family's loss. It is important to focus both on the woman's immediate physiologic and psychological needs, as well as those of her partner (see the Nursing Care Plan for the woman experiencing spontaneous abortion).

Placenta Previa

Growth of the placenta within the uterus normally takes place in the fundal or upper body of the uterus, well away from the lower segment. In placenta previa, the placenta implants and develops in the lower uterine segment, encroaching on or covering the internal cervical os. Lower uterine implantation presents the potential danger of hemorrhage because the placenta may tear away, rupturing blood vessels. The incidence of placenta previa is 1 in 300 pregnancies (Mabie, 1992).

Classification of placenta previa is based on the proximity of the placenta to the cervical os, which is the direct determinant of the risk of hemorrhage to the pregnant woman. Three degrees of placenta previa are recognized (Fig. 16-1):

- Total—the placenta completely covers the internal cervical os.
- Partial—the placenta partially covers the internal os (central).
- Low-lying—the placenta does not reach but is very near the region of the os and may lead to hemorrhage as the cervix dilates.

During labor, the classification of placenta previa may change as cervical dilatation progresses.

Placenta previa should be distinguished from abruptio placentae, which is the sudden separation of the placenta from the uterine wall, regardless of location. Abruptio placentae is life threatening to both the woman and fetus and is more likely to occur in the intrapartum period (see Chapter 26).

Etiologic and Predisposing Factors

The etiology of placenta previa is not known. Factors associated with this complication include:

- Multiparity—80% of cases occur in multiparas
- Prior placenta previa
- Previous cesarean delivery

It is believed that when the development of the vasculature in the uterine fundus is deficient for any reason, the placenta implants at a lower level. The blood supply is more conducive to placental growth under these circumstances. A large, thin placenta may develop in an attempt to increase perfusion. Fetal erythroblastosis and multiple pregnancy may give rise to a larger placenta that may approach a previa condition. Factors that predispose to low placental implantation include previous uterine scarring, the presence of uterine tumors, faulty implantation, and endometritis. Low placental implantation may lead to abnormal fetal presentations because of fetal accommodation to the altered space.

Diagnosis

The cardinal sign of placenta previa is painless vaginal bleeding with no precipitating cause after 24 weeks of gestation. Bleeding occurs without warning. The degree of placental placement over the internal os determines the severity of the bleeding and the onset of the initial episode. In rare cases, bleeding is not present and the presenting symptom is abdominal pain.

The first episode of bleeding usually stops spontaneously and is rarely severe enough to be fatal to the woman or fetus. The amount of bleeding varies, and bleeding may cease for some time after the initial episode. In about 90% of women, however, a subsequent, life-threatening hemorrhage will occur.

Diagnosis of placenta previa is confirmed and is 97% accurate when the location of the placenta is determined by sonography. When the placenta is determined to be normally placed by ultrasound, placenta previa is not the problem and other causes of bleeding must be investigated. When the placenta can be clearly visualized, the radiologist can frequently determine the degree of previa. About 10% of cases are diagnosed incidentally during ultrasound performed for other indications in pregnancy.

Treatment

Treatment of placenta previa is based on gestational age and the amount of bleeding. About 25% of women with placenta previa will complete 36 weeks of gestation and have a planned cesarean birth before the onset of labor. Women at 24 to 37 weeks of gestation who are not actively bleeding and who have hematocrit values greater than 30 mg/dL require careful monitoring and waiting. In this case, it is important to be prepared with matched blood for transfusion in the event significant hemorrhage occurs.

Absolutely no vaginal or rectal examinations are done unless in a setting in which immediate emergency cesarean delivery can be accomplished. This is because digital stimulation or penetration of the cervix can cause tearing of the placenta and immediate life-threatening hemorrhage. Typically, if such examination is necessary, it is done in the inpatient setting with a "double setup" procedure, meaning all preparations have been made for emergency surgery (see Chapter 26).

Controversy exists regarding the need for hospitalization or home care for women who are not bleeding. If home care is chosen, the woman must have 24-hour access to prompt emergency transport in case of hemorrhage. If contractions occur, the woman is likely to be hospitalized and magnesium sulfate therapy to stop labor may be initiated, although this treatment is also controversial (Mabie, 1992). If massive hemorrhage occurs, cesarean delivery is the only means to control bleeding.

Maternal, Fetal, and Neonatal Implications

The major risk to both the woman and fetus is uncontrolled hemorrhage. The fetus may be premature if cesarean delivery is required. Excessive bleeding at delivery is common, and abnormal placental adherence (placenta ac-

Nursing Care Plan

The Woman Experiencing Spontaneous Abortion

PATIENT PROFILE

History

L.K. is a married 26-year-old G1/P0 at 10 weeks' gestation. She has not used contraceptives for 6 months with the intention of achieving pregnancy in the next year. L.K. has had no unusual symptoms to date. Husband is pleased about pregnancy; accompanied her to first prenatal visit. L.K. presents at clinic with her husband for unscheduled visit. She reports having begun uterine "cramps" and bleeding at 6 AM this morning; has saved sanitary napkin "in case it was important that you see it."

Physical Assessment

L.K.'s vital signs are within normal limits. She appears anxious and distressed. Vaginal examination suggests inevitable abortion with presence of tissue and blood in vagina. Nurse verifies that L.K. is Rh negative and initial antibody titer done on confirmation of pregnancy was negative.

COLLABORATIVE PROBLEMS/POTENTIAL COMPLICATIONS

- Spontaneous abortion
- Infection
- Incomplete abortion
- Anemia

(See the accompanying Nursing Alert display.)

Assessment	*Nursing Diagnosis*	*Nursing Interventions*	*Rationale*
L.K. and husband are tearful at physician advice that abortion is probably inevitable. L.K. asks nurse if "jogging this weekend" was the cause.	Grieving related to pregnancy loss. ***Expected Outcome*** L.K. and her husband will demonstrate normal signs of grief and regret.	Offer emotional support and advice about convalescence. Explain expected progress of bleeding over next 24 hours. Recommend several days of rest and schedule return follow-up telephone appointment in 6 weeks.	Parents should take time to recover and acknowledge their loss, as well as to recover from physical stress.
		Reassure couple that maternal behavior not related to bleeding.	L.K. may incorrectly link her behavior with spontaneous abortion.
L.K. asks about whether "Rh is going to be a problem," recalling teaching regarding Rh-negative status.	Health Seeking Behaviors related to preventing maternal sensitization.	Arrange for administration of RhIgG as ordered.	Leakage of fetal blood into maternal circulation is possible.
	Expected Outcome L.K. receives RhIgG prophylaxis as ordered in a timely fashion.	Reinforce L.K.'s behavior and previous teaching as appropriate.	RhIgG is given to prevent maternal sensitization and the resulting complications in future pregnancies.
L.K. asks about when "we can try again."	Health Seeking Behaviors related to sexual activity and contraceptive needs.	Advise use of barrier contraceptive until 6-week checkup.	Early conception before maternal physical and psychological recovery may predispose to later problems.
	Expected Outcome L.K. and her husband can explain rationale for convalescence, contraceptive use, and follow-up with provider as scheduled.	Explain need to avoid infection and allow reestablishment of normal menstrual cycle.	Vulnerability to uterine infection is increased at this time.

(*Continued*)

The Woman Experiencing Spontaneous Abortion

(Continued)

Assessment	Nursing Diagnosis	Nursing Interventions	Rationale
	L.K. will remain free of signs of post-SAB complications at follow-up assessment.	Review signs of infection and reinforce need for prompt medical attention should symptoms appear.	
		Advise iron supplementation, increased dietary intake of iron.	Iron stores may be depleted by tissue growth in early pregnancy and bleeding during SAB.
		Review symptoms of hemorrhage.	Post-SAB hemorrhage is rare but can be serious.

EVALUATION

At telephone follow-up 2 weeks after her spontaneous abortion, L.K. reports that she is "feeling fine"; vaginal bleeding stopped 10 days post-SAB and no signs or symptoms of infection are reported. L.K. returned to work 1 week after SAB without difficulty. L.K. expresses regret at the loss, and some tearful episodes, although they are decreasing in frequency now. L.K. reports her husband had been sad and concerned, but likewise he is "feeling more like himself every day." She and her husband have not had intercourse yet ("we haven't really felt like it"), but are planning to go away this weekend and, laughing, L.K. reports she thinks they will be "needing the condoms." L.K. expresses confidence that they will be able to achieve another pregnancy "later this year." She confirms her telephone follow-up appointment at 6 weeks to talk with the nurse about when to discontinue contraception.

creta, see Chapter 26) is not unusual. Maternal transfusion may be necessary if significant hypovolemia occurs with prenatal hemorrhage or for excessive blood loss at the time of delivery.

Implications for Nursing Care

In the prenatal setting, the nurse may be responsible for explaining to the woman and her family the need for activity restriction, avoidance of any activity that may stimulate the cervix or uterus, and the necessity for access to emergency transportation. The nurse must verify that the woman understands the importance of returning to the hospital if any vaginal bleeding occurs. The nurse instructs the woman not to allow any vaginal or rectal examination except by her own care provider.

The nurse is in a position to provide support for the woman and her family in regard to the stresses associated with this condition. The possibility of hemorrhage and maternal or fetal compromise is extremely frightening. The nurse can assist the family in dealing realistically with this threat by taking appropriate self-care actions.

Intrapartum nursing care is discussed in Chapter 26.

Complications Resulting from Abnormal Embryologic Growth

Some conditions are a direct result of abnormal embryologic growth and place the woman at increased risk. In the case of ectopic pregnancy, implantation occurs outside the uterus and is a serious complication with considerable maternal risk. Another condition, gestational trophoblastic disease, is characterized by abnormal cellular growth in the product of conception which, rather than developing into an embryo, develops into a malignancy that mimics pregnancy. The following section discusses these conditions.

Ectopic Pregnancy

In ectopic (sometimes called tubal) pregnancy, the fertilized ovum implants outside the cavity of the uterus—in the fallopian tube in 95% of the cases. Other rare implantation sites are the abdomen, cervix, ovary, and the uterine wall. Ectopic pregnancy is occurring with increasing frequency, currently in 1 of every 200 pregnancies. This condition can be life threatening, presently responsible for 10% of maternal mortality (Gabbe et al., 1991).

NURSING ALERT

SIGNS AND SYMPTOMS OF POSTSPONTANEOUS ABORTION COMPLICATIONS

The woman experiencing a spontaneous abortion (SAB) is at risk for infection and hemorrhage. Conventional obstetric care may provide for a single follow-up visit at 6 weeks after an SAB. The nurse is responsible for verifying that the woman understands signs and symptoms of complications and that she will seek treatment herself, should signs and symptoms occur.

Signs of abnormally heavy bleeding/hemorrhage include:

- Bleeding that requires changes of four sanitary pads or more per day 3 to 4 days after bleeding begins
- Bleeding that resumes in the absence of heavy physical activity after cessation of bleeding for 5 days or more

Signs of post-SAB infection include:

- Fever and chills within 10 days of SAB
- Pelvic or abdominal pain, back pain
- Change in smell of bloody discharge from fleshy to foul odor

Etiologic and Predisposing Factors

A variety of factors can contribute to an ectopic pregnancy. If the fallopian tube has been damaged, passage of the fertilized ovum is either impeded or prevented. The increase in ectopic pregnancy can be accounted for by the growing number of reproductive-aged women who have pelvic inflammatory disease (PID) or have had tubal surgery for infertility (see Chapter 7). All of these can lead to tubal adhesions and delays in ovum transport.

Diagnosis

If the embryo implants and grows in the small lumen of the fallopian tube, the tube quickly distends beyond its capacity, causing abdominal pain. The tube is highly vascular during pregnancy. If the fallopian tube ruptures, hemorrhage is rapid and life threatening. When ectopic pregnancy occurs, the woman usually experiences symptoms of bleeding and pelvic pain soon after the first missed period. She may still be unaware of the pregnancy.

Rupture of the fallopian tube generally causes sudden, acute, and localized abdominal pain. Internal hemorrhage causes syncope and referred shoulder pain caused by phrenic nerve irritation. Any bleeding or abdominal pain in the first 8 weeks after a missed menstrual period must be considered a symptom of possible ectopic pregnancy. Hemorrhage can be life threatening and prompt emergency medical care is essential (see the accompanying display).

Diagnosis before tubal rupture is desirable but may be difficult because symptoms and physical findings mimic other diseases, such as appendicitis. Once pregnancy is confirmed, bimanual findings of pelvic pain and tenderness, with or without bleeding, suggests ectopic pregnancy. Serial blood tests for hCG usually demonstrate abnormally low levels, indicating disrupted pregnancy progress. Transvaginal ultrasound may be useful to document absence of an intrauterine gestational sac, but ectopic pregnancy cannot be visualized using ultrasound (ACOG, 1990).

Treatment

Once unruptured tubal pregnancy is confirmed, surgical intervention is usually needed. The choice of procedure depends on the woman's desire to preserve the fallopian tube, the degree of tubal damage, and the condition of the other tube. Salpingostomy, or removal of the conceptus, leaves the tube intact but scarred. Removing the damaged segment may be possible, or the entire tube may be removed. Unfortunately, regardless of surgical approach, 10% to 20% of women will have a repeat ectopic pregnancy, and only half will later have a viable intrauterine pregnancy (Gabbe et al., 1991).

Maternal Implications

Ectopic pregnancy represents a significant risk to the pregnant woman. If hemorrhage is diagnosed and treated early, recovery is generally complete. The choice of surgical approach will have an impact on the woman's future fertility and is often significant for the woman and her family.

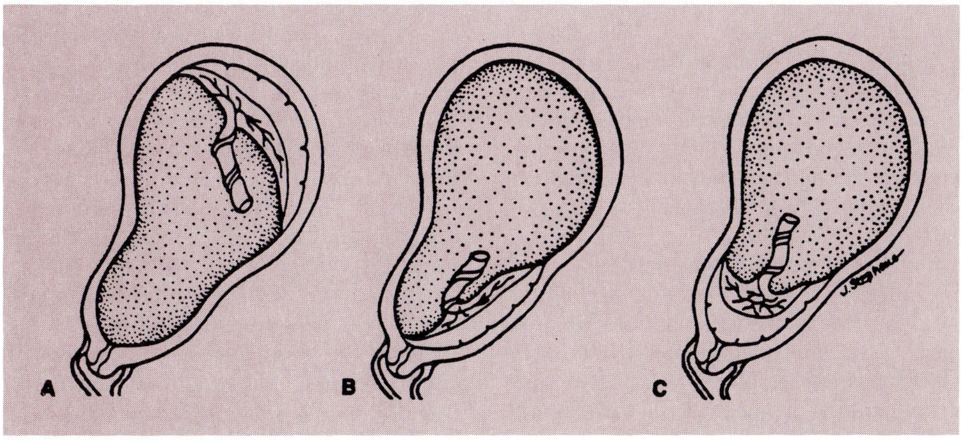

Figure 16-1.

Placental positions. *A:* Normal position. *B:* Partial placenta previa. *C:* Total placenta previa (Childbirth Graphics).

Signs and Symptoms of Possible Ectopic Pregnancy

The nurse should recognize that women with a history of pelvic inflammatory disease are at risk for ectopic pregnancy. A major risk of ectopic pregnancy is internal hemorrhage. Any woman who complains of the following symptoms suggestive of internal hemorrhage after a missed menstrual period must be evaluated on an emergency basis:

- Vertigo and syncope with abdominal pain
- Shoulder pain (likely referred from phrenic nerve irritation from intraperitoneal blood)
- Increasing pulse rate and anxiety

Implications for Nursing Care

In a prenatal health care setting, the nurse may be instrumental in identifying women who are at risk for ectopic pregnancy. A history of pelvic infection, intrauterine device (IUD) use, or tubal surgery should alert the nurse to the risk. The symptoms of amenorrhea, abdominal pain, spotting, and the presence of a pelvic mass located in the area of the adnexa make immediate referral for medical intervention imperative. These symptoms signal an emergency situation.

The nurse should refer the woman to a physician immediately when there is the slightest suspicion of an ectopic pregnancy. When the woman has been informed by the care provider that she has an ectopic pregnancy, the nurse should be available to talk with the woman to help her understand what is happening and to explain the course of treatment. When possible, the nurse should visit the woman after the operative procedure to offer support as needed.

Gestational Trophoblastic Disease

Gestational trophoblastic disease is an alteration of early embryonic growth. This condition causes placental disruption, rapid proliferation of abnormal cells, and embryonic destruction. Gestational trophoblastic disease occurs in about 1 in every 1000 pregnancies in the United States, and in most cases is benign, referred to as hydatidiform mole. In about 10% of cases, the growth is malignant and is known as choriocarcinoma (Gabbe et al., 1991).

The mole, which is a placental tumor, develops after a pregnancy has occurred. For unknown reasons, the embryo dies in utero but the placenta continues to grow rapidly. The trophoblastic cells continue to grow, become aggressive, and form an invasive tumor. The tumor (mole) is characterized by proliferation of placental villi that become edematous and form grapelike clusters. Blood vessels are absent; a fetus and amniotic sac are not found within the uterus.

Etiologic and Predisposing Factors

Genetic abnormalities occurring at the time of fertilization appear to be responsible for trophoblastic disease. The major manifestation of the disease is exaggerated proliferation of early placental cells called trophoblasts.

Diagnosis

Diagnosis of trophoblastic disease is often made on the basis of abnormally high levels of hCG, a hormone produced by placental cells. Symptoms include severe nausea and vomiting, PIH before 24 weeks' gestation, and vaginal bleeding. Diagnosis is confirmed through serial serum hCG elevations and the characteristic ultrasound appearance of molar growth.

Treatment

As soon as the diagnosis of gestational trophoblastic disease is made, the uterus should be evacuated by suction (vacuum) curettage. After curettage, the woman is monitored regularly for hCG levels to ensure that no molar tissue remains. hCG levels are obtained at weekly intervals, and in uncomplicated cases, the hCG value should return to prepregnant levels by the 10th to 14th week after evacuation. To ensure long-term remission of growth, hCG levels are monitored once a month for a year. Treatment for choriocarcinoma includes chemotherapy and careful surveillance for recurrence of the condition (Gabbe et al., 1991).

Maternal Implications

Gestational trophoblastic disease is readily treated and presents no significant threat to maternal well-being. Pregnancy is contraindicated during the first year after treatment for gestational trophoblastic disease. The high levels of hCG associated with it could stimulate the growth of any remaining molar tissue. Birth control pills are not the method of choice for contraception because they suppress pituitary luteinizing hormone, which may interfere with hCG monitoring.

Implications for Nursing Care

In a prenatal setting, the most important contribution the nurse can make to the assessment of the woman with this condition is history taking and the physical examination. Molar pregnancy is relatively rare. However, a history of amenorrhea, the presence of symptoms described, and the physical finding of an adnexal mass should alert the nurse to inform the physician immediately.

Women with molar pregnancy and their families need to understand and deal with the possible consequences of the disease. A long and tedious course of treatment is often necessary. The nurse can discuss the many issues surrounding pregnancy loss, recognition that the pregnancy was abnormal, and the need to postpone a subsequent pregnancy. The woman will need to be able to discuss her grief, anger, or fear. Fifteen percent of patients with hydatidiform mole will progress to choriocarcinoma. Therefore, the nurse should carefully explain the symptoms that may indicate exacerbation of the mole. These include irregular vaginal bleeding, persistent secretion from the breasts (galactorrhea), hemoptysis, and severe and persistent headaches. The latter three symptoms may suggest spread of the disease to other organs.

Complications Affecting Fetal Growth and Duration of Gestation

Some complications of pregnancy primarily affect the fetus in terms of limiting fetal growth and threatening well-being. The major complications in this category are premature rupture of membranes and preterm labor and birth, discussed in Chapter 27. The following section discusses the complications of cervical incompetence, multiple gestation, hemolytic disease of the fetus or neonate, postterm pregnancy, and IUFD.

Cervical Incompetence

Cervical incompetence is defined as the inability of the cervix to maintain a pregnancy to term because of a structural or functional defect. This occurs in less than 1% of all pregnancies, and 90% of women with this condition have had multiple pregnancy losses.

Etiologic and Predisposing Factors

The most frequently associated factor with cervical incompetence is previous cervical trauma from procedures. Examples of such procedures include dilation (for elective abortion or diagnostic dilation and curettage) or cone biopsy for cervical dysplasia. This condition is occasionally caused by congenital malformations or decreased collagen in the cervix.

Diagnosis

Cervical incompetence is diagnosed by the presence of cervical dilation, painless uterine contractions, and at times rupture of membranes during the second trimester of pregnancy (Golan, Barnan, & Vexler, 1989). An accurate obstetric history is important in the diagnosis of this condition because the history may help confirm diagnosis if previous cervical trauma and the woman reports previous pregnancy losses.

Treatment

There are two approaches to treatment of cervical incompetence: watchful waiting and the placement of a cervical cerclage. Watchful waiting may involve recommending the woman limit her physical activity, a restriction on orgasm and intercourse (sometimes called vaginal rest), and frequent assessment of cervical status.

Placement of a cerclage or a pursestring suture may be used to maintain cervical closure (Fig. 16-2). The procedure is performed between 12 and 20 weeks in the presence of a congenital cervical problem; it may be done in the second trimester when the cervix appears normal, but dilation has begun and membranes have not ruptured. After cerclage, the woman is generally advised to maintain modified bed rest and vaginal rest. Use of cerclage is controversial because no randomized prospective studies have documented clear benefits of this treatment in prolonging gestation.

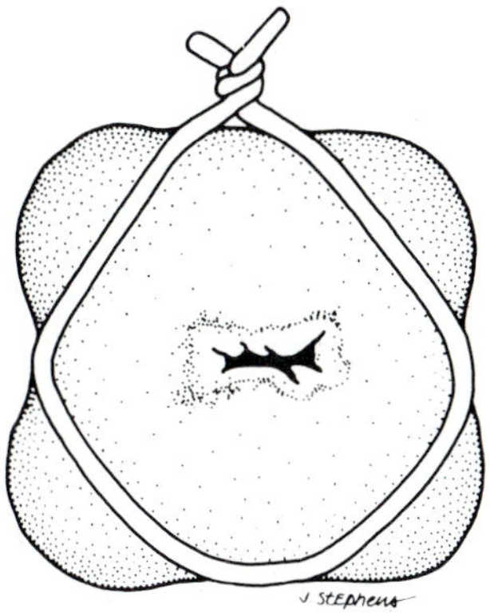

Figure 16-2.
A cross-section of an incompetent cervix showing a cerclage suture in place. The suture is removed at term to allow cervical dilation and delivery (Childbirth Graphics).

Maternal, Fetal, and Neonatal Implications

Maternal implications of cervical incompetence center on the treatment selected. There is some risk of maternal infection from cervical cerclage, and the suture may become displaced, requiring resuturing. The woman should be advised to watch for signs of infection (pain, fever, changes in vaginal discharge).

Weekly bimanual examinations will be needed to check for cervical status. The cerclage is generally removed in the outpatient setting at 37 to 39 weeks of gestation; labor usually ensues soon after removal. If treatment is unsuccessful, there is a risk of fetal loss or preterm birth.

Implications for Nursing Care

The woman with cervical incompetence may have experienced previous pregnancy losses as a result of this condition. Thus, the nurse must be sensitive to the concerns the woman and her family may have as treatment begins. The nurse is generally responsible for advising the woman and her family about self-care activities, such as modified bed rest, vaginal rest, and the need for weekly surveillance of cervical status. An important nursing responsibility is providing emotional support and anticipatory guidance about what the woman can expect in terms of treatment and outcome. The woman may require assistance and anticipatory guidance to plan for activity restriction.

Multiple Gestation

Twins produced from a single ovum are called monozygotic or identical twins. Those produced by separate ova are called dizygotic or fraternal twins. The incidence of 1 in 200 births of monozygotic twins is the same throughout the world. The prevalence figure for fraternal twins is influenced by heredity, with rates varying among families and groups. In the United States, 1% of all births are twins, and two thirds are fraternal (Gabbe et al., 1991). Triplets and higher multiple gestations occur through either monozygotic or dizygotic processes.

Etiologic and Predisposing Factors

Identical twins develop genetically from the splitting of a monozygote. In human beings, the splitting occurs before the 15th day of conception. After this time, splitting cannot occur because of the advanced development of the embryo. In monozygotic twinning, two embryos develop from the identical genetic material of one sperm and one egg. Therefore, monozygotic twins are always of the same sex and are said to be mirror images of each other. These twins have two umbilical cords and may have one or two sets of fetal membranes, but share a common placenta. Almost all placentas of monozygotic twins have blood vessel communication between the twins, a major risk factor for their growth (Gabbe et al., 1991).

Fraternal twins develop from two ova that are fertilized at the same time by two different sperm. Although from the same genetic pool, fraternal twins have separate gestational sacs and placentas and develop as differently as other siblings. The incidence of multiple gestations has increased in recent years in the United States because of the increased use of fertility treatment, which stimulates multiple ovulations.

Diagnosis

Multiple gestation should be suspected if:

- Uterine size is larger than expected for gestational age
- Hydramnios or unexpected anemia develops
- Auscultation suggests more than one fetal heart
- Pregnancy has occurred after ovulation stimulation or in vitro fertilization

Definitive diagnosis is made by ultrasound. Multiple gestational sacs can be identified by ultrasound as early as 6 weeks after a missed menstrual period (Gabbe et al., 1991).

Treatment

In addition to the usual monitoring of prenatal care, special attention to the following aspects of care is imperative.

- Evaluation of cervical status and blood pressure weekly because preterm labor and PIH are more common in twin gestation
- Prevention of maternal anemia by dietary and iron supplementation
- Evaluation of the hemoglobin and hematocrit at 28 and 36 weeks
- Use of serial ultrasound evaluations to evaluate fetal growth and development, as growth retardation occurs in up to half of multiple gestations
- Percutaneous sampling of umbilical cord blood if twin–twin transfusion is suspected (see section below)
- Administration of nonstress testing to assess fetal response twice a week after 32 weeks
- Use of tocolytic therapy prophylactically although this treatment is controversial
- Evaluation of fetal lung maturity prior to 37 weeks if delivery appears necessary
- Use of prescribed bed rest or daily rest period for women at risk for hypertension to increase uterine perfusion

Maternal, Fetal, and Neonatal Implications

Maternal implications of multiple gestation are primarily related to the likelihood of other complications, such as PIH, which may require treatment. There is also a high probability that delivery will be by planned cesarean section, thus increasing maternal risk slightly over that associated with vaginal birth.

Perinatal morbidity and mortality resulting from twin births is as high as 14%. The greatest mortality results from premature birth. Additional factors contributing to neonatal morbidity are growth retardation, hydramnios, congenital anomalies, and cord accidents (ACOG, 1989a).

In monozygotic twins, direct communication of fetal blood vessels may occur, resulting in a "transfusion syndrome." When this happens, one fetus, called the recipient twin, is large, edematous, and polycythemic. The donor twin remains small and anemic because its blood is being shunted to its sibling. If the small twin survives, it will require postdelivery transfusion. The transfusion syndrome increases the probability that both twins will suffer permanent, debilitating consequences. If the donor twin dies in utero, the surviving twin (recipient) will develop normally. After death, the donor twin becomes progressively compressed in utero and assumes a fossil-like configuration known as fetus papyraceus.

The fetal and neonatal risks associated with gestation greater than two fetuses are markedly increased. The major risks associated with these multiple gestations are IUFD of one or more fetuses from unknown causes, intrauterine growth retardation, and prematurity.

Implications for Nursing Care

Nursing care of women with multiple pregnancies should be focused on monitoring prenatal events and maintaining optimum maternal health. Prenatal care of a woman with a twin pregnancy requires knowledge of the problems that may arise and an alertness to early signs of problems. The nurse should ensure that the following priorities are addressed in the woman's care:

- Discussion of the demands of multiple gestation and plans for how the family can adapt during pregnancy and after delivery
- Evaluation of the support system and discussion of self-care practices to deal with stress
- Counseling related to nutritional needs to avoid anemia and provide adequate intake for fetal growth and maternal maintenance
- Instruction on signs and symptoms of preterm labor and PIH (see Chapter 27) with specific steps the woman should take if symptoms develop
- Assistance with birth plans and decisions about breastfeeding and infant care in the postpartum period

Hemolytic Disease of the Fetus or Newborn

The term hemolytic disease means that red blood cell destruction is abnormally accelerated. During pregnancy, this destruction of red blood cells in the fetus may occur if fetal and maternal blood types are incompatible and if these different blood types come into direct contact with each other.

The most frequent and mildest type of hemolytic disease results from ABO blood incompatibility. A more severe, but rare disease results from Rh incompatibility.

Etiologic and Predisposing Factors

To understand the potential problems for a woman and fetus with different blood types, a review of blood groups is important. There are four major blood groups in the ABO system: A, B, AB, and O. Each type has its own distinct protein or antigen on the cell surface. Type A has the A antigen, B has the B antigen, AB has both antigens, and O contains no antigen. If individuals receive a transfusion of a different blood type from their own, an immune response occurs. The individual will produce an antibody (IgG or IgM) directed at the foreign blood antigen.

During pregnancy, fetal red blood cells enter the maternal circulation through the placenta as early as the eighth week of gestation in 15% to 40% of women. In theory, if they are a different blood type from the woman's, her immune system recognizes this and produces either IgG or IgM molecules. This process of developing antibodies to fetal blood is called maternal sensitization. Only IgG molecules can cross the placenta. If this takes place, the antibodies bind to the antigen in fetal red blood cells, and destroy the cell membrane, a process called lysis, which results in destruction of the blood cell.

ABO incompatibility is common, but generally does not pose much threat to the fetus. Major effects are seen in the neonatal period, primarily as hyperbilirubinemia (described in Chapter 33). Rh incompatibility is rare, but it has more severe effects on fetal well-being as described below.

Rh hemolytic disease occurs when the woman is Rh negative and the fetus is Rh positive. Rh is a genetically determined factor present in red blood cells. A complex system, the Rh factors appear to have three loci—C, D, and E—within the cells. These factors are so closely linked that they behave in an integrated fashion, as if they were one gene. There are several different sets of notations for the Rh factors. The most familiar is the D designate or the Du factor. This means that if a person is D positive, the D factor is present on the surface of the red blood cells. Rh(D) negative denotes the absence of the D factor on the red blood cells.

When a pregnant woman is Rh negative, she has no D antigen on the surface of her red blood cells. If the blood of her fetus is Rh positive, the mother may become sensitized. Less than 0.5 mL of Rh-positive blood gaining access to the maternal circulation will sensitize the woman to fetal blood. The first exposure causes a maternal response with IgM antibodies. These antibodies are large molecules that are unable to cross the placenta. In conjunction with high levels of circulating corticosteroids and a tendency toward immunologic tolerance during pregnancy, IgM antibody offers protection against sensitization. However, with repeated transplacental hemorrhages, the woman's body will respond by forming IgG antibodies, which cross the placenta and enter the fetal circulation. The IgG antibodies coat the Rh-positive fetal red blood cells, causing hemolysis. A diagram of this process is shown in Figure 16-3.

In most cases, the woman becomes sensitized in her first pregnancy but because IgM does not pass to the fetus, fetal red blood cells are not lysed. However, if she has a subsequent pregnancy and does not receive preventive therapy, her fetus may develop erythroblastosis fetalis (described below).

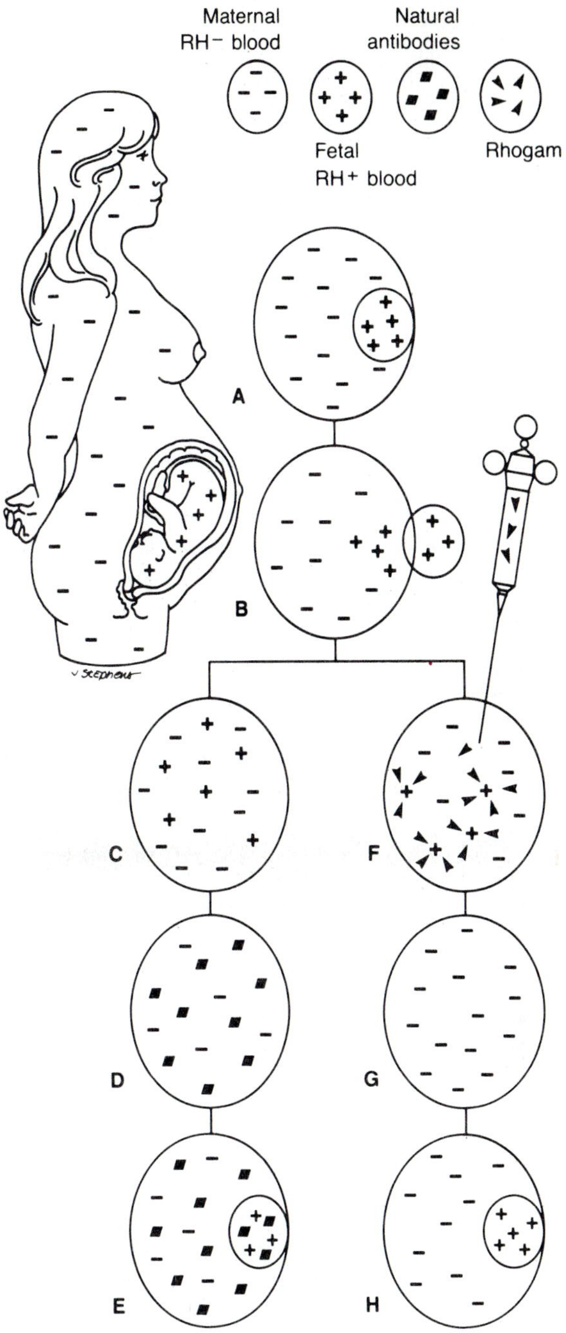

Figure 16-3.

Rh disease and its prevention. *A:* When a primapara has Rh-negative blood and the father's blood is Rh positive, the blood of the fetus may also be Rh positive. *B:* When the Rh-positive neonate is delivered, small amounts of its blood may escape into the maternal circulation. *C:* Immune globulin (RhIgG) is not administered to the mother, so Rh-positive blood cells remain in her circulatory system. *D:* The mother's natural antibodies are released to destroy the foreign Rh-positive cells and she becomes permanently sensitized. *E:* During a subsequent pregnancy with an Rh-positive fetus, the woman's body contains antibodies against her fetus. Erythroblastosis fetalis may result. *F:* To avoid this potentially fatal disease in the fetus, immune globulin should be given after the first pregnancy. Once sensitization takes place, it can never be reversed, even with immune globulin. *G:* An injection of immune globulin after the first pregnancy causes destruction of the Rh-positive cells in the mother's blood and prevents maternal sensitization. *H:* In a subsequent pregnancy with an Rh-negative neonate, the maternal blood is free from anti-Rh negative antibodies (Childbirth Graphics).

Diagnosis

On the first prenatal visit, all pregnant women are tested for blood type, Rh factor, and the presence of antibodies as reflected in an antibody titer (indirect Coombs' test). About 15% of the population is Rh negative. If the pregnant woman is Rh negative with no antibodies detected, and the father's blood type is unknown or is positive, the fetus is assumed to have Rh-positive blood. Thus, these women are candidates for therapy to prevent sensitization of their blood.

If there is evidence of maternal sensitization as reflected in a serum antibody titer greater than 1:16 early in pregnancy, additional assessments of fetal well-being will be performed. These would include amniocentesis to evaluate optical density of amniotic fluid. Amniotic fluid will become clouded by bilirubin components in the presence of fetal hemolysis. Serial amniocentesis and ultrasound evaluations will be performed to evaluate fetal growth patterns and to rule out fetal anomalies. Fetal activity and heart rate monitoring may be used to assess fetal well-being (see Chapter 14). However, severe hemolytic disease is becoming less common because of the development of Rh immunoglobulin (RhIgG) that can prevent maternal sensitization.

Treatment

Hemolytic disease of the fetus or newborn caused by ABO incompatibility cannot be prevented. However, the disease is usually mild and becomes evident in the neonatal period and is responsive to phototherapy (see Chapter 33).

If maternal sensitization has occurred, the woman's antibody titer is carefully monitored during pregnancy. Titers do not correspond with the severity of disease and fetal risk. Thus, careful fetal surveillance will be instituted. At times, a planned early delivery may be needed to prevent further fetal deterioration. If fetal compromise becomes severe between 23 and 32 weeks (before delivery is possible), intrauterine fetal transfusion may be performed to correct anemia. Transfusion is accomplished by amniocentesis and the placement of a catheter into the fetal peritoneal cavity. About 80% of fetuses receiving intrauterine transfusion survive; maternal complications from the procedure are rare (Scott, 1990).

Rh Immunoglobulin. During the 1960s, microbiologists learned that when an antigen and its corresponding antibody are injected simultaneously, the individual does not become sensitized to the antigen. Research has shown that injection with RhIgG within 72 hours of maternal exposure to antigens protected against sensitization in the woman (Burrow & Ferris, 1988). Theoretically, this method of prophylaxis is almost 100% effective. The effect lasts about 3 months. The accompanying display shows the standard doses of RhIgG and indications for its use.

RhIgG Use

Rh immune globulin (RhIgG) should be given to Rh-negative women in a variety of circumstances to prevent Rh sensitization.

The standard 50 μg dose should be given:

- As prophylaxis in an unsensitized pregnant woman at 28 weeks of gestation,
- After an induced or spontaneous abortion,
- During amniocentesis to prevent maternal sensitization from possible transplacental hemorrhage during the procedure.

The standard 300 μg dose should be given:

- Within 72 hours after a term or premature delivery.

Maternal, Fetal, and Neonatal Implications

There are no physiologic implications of hemolytic disease of the fetus or newborn for the pregnant woman. However, concern and uncertainty about fetal status and the stressors of close perinatal surveillance can be trying for women and their families. This is especially true if problems in previous pregnancies have resulted in fetal compromise or fetal loss.

Implications are notable for the fetus or newborn. Maternal sensitization to ABO incompatibility occurs most often if the maternal blood group is O. The natural antibody response for the O blood type is to produce IgG antibodies that can affect the fetus. Fortunately, fetal red blood cell destruction is usually minimal. Instead, the problem is delayed until the neonatal period. ABO incompatibility results in 60% of all hemolytic disease in the newborn. Characteristically, it appears during the first 24 hours as mild hyperbilirubinemia, as discussed in Chapter 31.

Rh incompatibility may result in mild hemolytic disease and fetal anemia, or the more severe form, called hydrops fetalis. This condition is characterized by severe anemia, cardiac decompensation, cardiomegaly, and hepatosplenomegaly. Because of liver and heart dysfunction, progressive edema results in ascites and generalized edema, referred to as hydrops fetalis. When the disease progresses to this point, intrauterine transfusion may not help. There is significant risk of fetal or neonatal death (see Chapter 33 for discussion of care of the neonate with erythroblastosis fetalis).

Implications for Nursing Care

Although incidence of Rh incompatibility is declining as a result of Rh immunoglobulin therapy, nurses still play an important role in prevention and treatment of this condition. The following section addresses nursing care of the woman with Rh incompatibility.

• • Assessment

With the availability of RhIgG for prevention of Rh disease, nurses have a primary responsibility to assess women at risk and to explain preventive treatment. If a women is Rh negative, she should receive information about the benefits of receiving RhIgG therapy with each pregnancy, regardless of its outcome. Patient education is a challenge because sensitization is a complex process to explain in terms understandable to the woman and her family.

• • Nursing Diagnosis

The following nursing diagnoses may be applicable in the care of the pregnant woman with a blood incompatibility:

- Fear related to threat to fetal well-being
- Health-Seeking Behaviors related to maternal actions to ensure appropriate prophylactic treatment
- Ineffective Family Coping: Compromised related to invasive diagnostic and treatment procedures for severe fetal anemia

• • Planning and Implementation

Nurses in prenatal settings must ensure that all Rh negative women receive initial antibody screening and repeat screening at 28 weeks of gestation. If the woman's titer is negative, prophylactic administration of RhIgG according to physician order at that point is a nursing responsibility. Women who receive RhIgG treatment during pregnancy should be retested for presence of antibodies early in each subsequent pregnancy.

In addition to education about Rh sensitization, nurses can help each Rh-negative woman assume personal responsibility for her health. Women should be encouraged to carry evidence of their blood type and of RhIgG administration on a wallet card.

After delivery, Rh and antibody testing will be done again for both the woman and the neonate. If the neonate is Rh positive and the woman is still antibody negative, she should receive postpartum administration of RhIgG within 72 hours. This ensures that the immune globulin enters the maternal circulation in time to counteract any effect from fetal-to-maternal transfusion, which is assumed to happen during any normal vaginal delivery (Gabbe et al., 1991)

Expected Outcomes

- The woman explains the potential risks of Rh incompatibility to the fetus and herself.
- The woman explains the rationale for diagnostic and treatment procedures.
- The woman with Rh incompatibility takes steps to ensure she receives appropriate treatment with each pregnancy.
- The woman who is carrying a fetus with erythroblastosis fetalis and her family seek assistance from the health care team in coping with the stressors imposed by diagnosis and treatment.

• • Evaluation

The nurse is responsible for evaluating whether at-risk women are receiving appropriate information about screening and treatment activities. Explanations about the nature of immunologic disorders will need to be tailored to the woman's level of understanding. If fetal status becomes compromised, the nurse monitors the woman's physiologic and psychosocial responses to ongoing diagnosis and treatment. The high level of concern and worry generated by aggressive medical management may threaten the family's ability to cope. The nurse should be prepared to provide the necessary emotional support and anticipatory guidance, evaluating the adequacy of the plan of care on a regular basis.

Postterm Pregnancy

Postterm pregnancy refers to any pregnancy that continues beyond 42 weeks of gestation (294 days). The terms postdate and postmaturity are also used. Postmaturity is identified by specific characteristics that can be found on physical and neurologic examination of the neonate. Therefore, postmaturity cannot be diagnosed until after the delivery (Chapter 33 discusses neonatal assessment and care for postmaturity).

Postmaturity, which occurs in 10% of pregnancies exceeding 43 weeks, poses known risks to the woman and the fetus. Accurate dating of the pregnancy is important and, as with preterm labor, attempts should be made to correlate the last menstrual period (LMP) and clinical uterine size with support from sonography. Pregnancy can be dated most accurately when dating is begun early.

Etiologic and Predisposing Factors

No cause or predisposing factors have been identified for postterm pregnancy. Causes now under investigation include imbalance in hormonal control of pregnancy and deficiencies in maternal and fetal adrenal corticosteroid production, which are thought to influence onset of labor.

Diagnosis

Postterm pregnancy can be diagnosed only if accurate determination of pregnancy dating has occurred. Ideally, the woman has regular menstrual cycles and will remember the date of her LMP. If not, ultrasound examination done as early as possible aids in estimation of gestational age (see Chapter 14 for fetal assessment). Other clinical findings early in pregnancy that will aid in the subsequent diagnosis of postterm pregnancy include identification of quickening at 20 weeks, consistent uterine size with dates, and auscultation of fetal heart tones by Doppler at 12 weeks.

Treatment

Medical management must balance the risks and benefits of watchful waiting with the risks and benefits of induction of labor. Two factors are key in this decision: evaluation of fetal health and cervical status and readiness for labor. Fetal well-being is established by daily maternal counts of fetal movement, and either stress testing, nonstress testing, or biophysical profile every 3 to 5 days after 41 completed weeks of gestation (see Chapter 14). Cervical examination to assess position, effacement, and dilatation will be performed weekly. No specific guidelines for management exist, and each woman's situation must be evaluated individually to determine the best medical course of action.

Maternal, Fetal, and Neonatal Implications

Many women express anxiety and frustration if pregnancy extends beyond the due date, which has been anticipated for weeks. If assessment of fetal well-being is needed, women must face the inconvenience, cost, and risks of testing. In addition, women with prolonged pregnancy may require induction of labor and, if that fails, cesarean delivery. Both of these procedures are associated with increased maternal morbidity.

Four potential problems contribute to increased fetal and neonatal morbidity in prolonged gestations (ACOG, 1989b). First, oligohydramnios may occur as the normal decrease in amniotic fluid begins by 37 weeks and continues to decrease from 1000 mL of fluid to 250 mL by 42 weeks. Decreased amniotic fluid is associated with umbilical cord compression and fetal hypoxia.

Second, meconium passage occurs in 25% of postterm pregnancies, twice as high as the rate in term pregnancies, probably due to transient fetal distress. With decreased amniotic fluid, fetal or neonatal aspiration of thick meconium-stained fluid may increase the risk of neonatal aspiration syndrome.

Third, macrosomia, or birth weight over 4500 g (9 lb, 14 oz), occurs in 2% to 10% of postterm neonates. These fetuses are subject to asphyxia and difficult vaginal birth. Shoulder dystocia occurs at almost twice the rate in postterm pregnancies as in neonates appropriate for gestational age.

Finally, placental function peaks at 37 weeks and declines slowly until 42 weeks. Thus, continuation of pregnancy places the fetus at risk for placental insufficiency and growth retardation in about 10% of prolonged pregnancies. The neonate appears growth retarded and fragile. The skin is stained by meconium, and the fingernails are long. The neonate often has hypoglycemia and temperature instability (see Chapter 33).

Implications for Nursing Care

When testing for fetal well-being begins, the nurse needs to reassure the pregnant woman. The woman is anxious to deliver and is concerned for the health of her fetus. Testing requires frequent visits to the health facility, blood tests, and fetal monitoring. Without being caused undue anxiety, the woman needs to understand the importance of keeping these appointments. The woman should be given anticipatory guidance about what tests are to be performed, why they are necessary, and what the anticipated outcome will be.

When the woman has not delivered by the end of the 42nd week, she will be admitted to the hospital for induction of labor (see Chapter 23 on labor induction). The nursing emphasis in labor induction is on close monitoring of oxytocin drip, on maintaining uterine contractions at a safe level, on supporting the woman, and on closely monitoring fetal well-being, with continuous internal fetal monitoring being preferred.

The procedure for induction of labor is the same as that discussed in Chapter 23 for oxytocin intravenous infusion. If there is any indication of fetal distress during induction, the neonatal team should be present at delivery. Because meconium aspiration is the most common problem, any evidence of meconium-stained fluid calls for laryngoscopic examination of the vocal cords for evidence of aspiration. A high cesarean delivery rate can be expected because of failed induction secondary to cephalopelvic disproportion, an unripe cervix, or fetal distress. After delivery, the neonate should be observed for signs of hypoglycemia, respiratory distress, and seizures.

Intrauterine Fetal Demise

The attendant medical and psychological stressors of IUFD are extremely traumatic to the woman and her family. Not only does the long-awaited fetus die, but the woman must undergo the process of labor and birth and postpartum recovery. If the fetus remains in the uterus for some time after death has been confirmed, the woman is placed at additional physical and emotional risk.

Categorization of fetal death is determined by the point in gestation when death occurs. Missed abortion refers to fetal death before 20 weeks of gestation not followed by spontaneous abortion. After 20 weeks of gestation, the term fetal death syndrome may be used when labor does not begin within 48 hours of death.

In 75% of cases of IUFD, the woman will experience spontaneous onset of labor within 14 days of the estimated time of fetal death; this percentage increases to 89% by 21 days. An extended period of waiting is particularly stressful to the woman and her family. Fetal death may result in feelings of anxiety, depression, or guilt. It is difficult for the family to grieve their loss until the actual delivery takes place.

Etiologic and Predisposing Factors

It is frequently impossible to determine the cause of IUFD, but it is often associated with severe and poorly controlled maternal diabetes mellitus, PIH, erythroblastosis fetalis (Rh disease), abruptio placentae, and umbilical cord compression (ie, true knots). An increasing cause of IUFD is crack cocaine use. Fetal death in this situation appears caused by disruption in placental perfusion.

Diagnosis

Diagnosis of fetal death usually begins with the woman's observation that fetal movement has stopped. Diagnosis is confirmed when the fetal heart rate cannot be found by electronic fetal monitoring and fetal heart movement is not visualized by ultrasonography.

Treatment

Treatment of IUFD includes induction of labor if it does not occur spontaneously within 3 weeks of the estimated time of fetal death. Close monitoring of maternal coagulation studies is necessary to detect early signs of hypofibrinogenemia and disseminated intravascular coagulopathy (DIC). Medical management of IUFD and nursing implications are described in Table 16-1.

Maternal Implications

When pregnancy is prolonged 5 or more weeks after fetal death without spontaneous onset of labor, the woman is at increased risk of hypofibrinogenemia or DIC. Fibrinogen levels begin to drop 3 weeks after fetal death. At this time, fetal tissue degeneration begins and thromboplastin is released into the amniotic fluid and absorbed into the maternal circulation. Thromboplastin levels rarely increase to the point of endangering the woman until 5 weeks after fetal death, when the risk of DIC is approximately 25%. Hemorrhage resulting from DIC may be life threatening (see Chapter 26).

Table 16-1. Medical Management of Intrauterine Fetal Demise

Medial Management	Rationale	Diagnostic Studies	Nursing Interventions
Confirmation of diagnosis	Medical intervention is not appropriate until after 3 wk of fetal death.	Ultrasound	Offer support to grieving woman and her partner (if present). Make arranagements for woman to be escorted home after diagnosis is confirmed if she is alone.
Scheduling of weekly visits	To monitor for early signs of disseminated intravascular coagulation (DIC)	Weekly hemoglobin, hematocrit, and fibrinogen level tests (if fibrinogen levels drop to 200 mg/dL, delivery is indicated)	Keep woman informed of need for close surveillance of her blood levels and signs of bleeding.
After 3 weeks, collection of blood coagulation studies every 6 h	Woman is at greater risk for DIC.		Obtain type and crossmatch for 2 U whole blood. Order cryoprecipitate and fresh-frozen plasma for emergency use.
Induction of labor	Low fibrinogen levels increase DIC risk and hemorrhage.	Discuss need for induction of labor with woman and answer questions.	
Induction options: • Cervical dilators (ie, Dilapan) placed in cervix 12 h before induction • Prostaglandin gel applied to cervix • Prostaglandin E_2 suppository inserted high in posterior vaginal fornix • Oxytocin infusion	To speed cervical ripening or dilatation or to initiate labor		Assure woman that a nurse will be with her throughout procedure. Obtain type and crossmatch for 2 U whole blood. Order cryoprecipitate and fresh-frozen plasma for emergency use. If prostaglandin to be administered, premedicate with acetominophen, an antiemetic (Compazine), and antidiarrheal agent (Lomotil) to reduce side effects of drug. Assist with insertion of cervical dilators or prostaglandin suppository, informing woman about what is happening and why. Establish an IV line with Ringer's lactate or similar solution.
Amniotomy and insertion of transcervical pressure catheter between amnion and uterine wall	To permit accurate monitoring of uterine pressure and reduce risk of uterine rupture		Collect equipment and assist with placement of intrauterine pressure catheter if being used to monitor uterine forces. Place an external pressure monitor when amniotomy cannot be performed. Coagulation studies are collected every 4 h. Ensure collection of blood specimen and expedite its transport to the laboratory. Monitor vital signs every 2–4 h.
Prescription of analgesic	To decrease patient discomfort from uterine contractions		Offer patient ordered analgesic.
Delivery of fetus			Encourage partner to support patient during labor and delivery. Support couple and assist in their grieving process and its resolution. After delivery, fetus should be cleaned, wrapped in a blanket, and given to parents to hold. They may prefer to be left alone at this time. Refer the couple to a parent support group if they desire.

Implications for Nursing Care

Nursing care for the woman and family experiencing IUFD may be a significant factor in promoting physiologic safety, healthy coping, and eventual adaptation to the loss. It is imperative that the nurse address the physiologic, psychosocial, and spiritual needs of the woman and her family.

• • Assessment

The nurse may be responsible for ongoing assessment of laboratory findings to detect early coagulopathies and DIC. The woman usually goes to a laboratory for periodic coagulation studies. The results are sent to the clinic or the office of the physician or midwife. The woman's physical and emotional status is assessed during visits to the physician or midwife until the onset of labor occurs or the planned induction is implemented. The nurse reviews signs of coagulopathy with the woman, including:

- Vaginal bleeding
- Bruising
- Development of petechiae
- Bleeding of gums
- Hematuria
- Oozing from venipuncture sites

On admission to labor and delivery, the nurse assesses the woman's physiologic status, the progress of labor, and level of discomfort. The woman is monitored for evidence of coagulopathy.

• • Nursing Diagnosis

The following nursing diagnoses may be applicable when IUFD occurs:

- Fear related to pain during labor and delivery
- High Risk for Altered Body Temperature: Hyperthermia related to prostaglandin administration
- Diarrhea related to prostaglandin administration
- Grieving related to death of anticipated child
- Ineffective Family Coping related to stress associated with fetal death

• • Planning and Implementation

Caring for a couple who have experienced IUFD is one of the most emotionally demanding situations the maternity nurse must face. Nursing responsibilities include providing physical and emotional support for the woman and her partner or family through labor and birth, monitoring maternal physiologic status for signs of complications associated with the IUFD, and induction of labor. (See Chapter 25 for a Nursing Care Plan for the Family Experiencing Fetal Demise.)

Nursing care is focused on supporting the progress of labor, providing adequate analgesia, and assisting with the administration of anesthesia (see Table 16-1). If coagulopathies develop, the nurse may be responsible for administering blood or blood components. Because the fetus does not have to be considered when planning pain control strategies, larger doses of analgesia may be given. It is strongly recommended that the woman be awake during the birth of the fetus so that the birth is experienced and remembered as "real." The woman may wish to see and hold the neonate after it is born. She should be alert enough to follow through with these plans.

The nurse administers appropriate medications to treat common side effects of prostaglandins if they are used to stimulate labor. Premedication to prevent hyperthermia, vomiting, and diarrhea is essential before the first dose of prostaglandins is given. The nurse explains the purpose of the medications and the anticipated side effects of prostaglandin administration.

Expected Outcomes

- The woman verbalizes satisfaction with the level of pain control achieved through analgesia or anesthesia.
- The woman maintains normal body temperature during prostaglandin administration.
- The woman demonstrates normal gastrointestinal function during induction of labor.
- The family exhibits normal range of emotions related to IUFD.
- The family members hold the neonate after it has been cleaned after delivery, if desired.

• • Evaluation

The nurse evaluates the woman's responses to medical management once the process of labor begins. The adequacy of treatment for prostaglandin side effects is particularly important. The woman can experience pronounced hyperpyrexia, vomiting, and diarrhea, resulting in significant fluid loss. The nurse must perform ongoing evaluations to detect evidence of dehydration.

The nurse also evaluates the progress of labor once prostaglandin suppositories or oxytocin is administered. When interventions do not achieve expected outcomes, the nurse alters the plan of care to reflect the development of new problems. Appropriate actions are taken to resolve unanticipated problems or complications.

The loss of a viable fetus through intrauterine death is a traumatic experience. It is both physically and psychologically taxing. The consequences of IUFD include both coagulation disorders and significant side effects related to the induction of labor if spontaneous contractions fail to occur. The nurse is responsible for the physical and emotional support of the woman and her family during the period of waiting before birth and after the onset of labor. Humane, sensitive care must be provided while monitoring the woman's physiologic status and dealing with physiologic complications related to IUFD.

Gestational complications present a range of maternal, fetal, and neonatal consequences. Complications vary from those that require comfort interventions to conditions that pose life-threatening risks to the woman and her fetus. Hyperemesis gravidarum is a frustrating and distressing condition for most women. Medical and nursing actions generally provide relief. Other conditions, such as spontaneous abortion and IUFD present health care providers with the challenge of preserving maternal physiologic well-being in the midst of a distressing and emotionally draining experience for the woman and her family. In most cases, complications in pregnancy, such as postterm pregnancy and multiple gestation, require careful ongoing assessment to identify problems and correct them. Some conditions, like ectopic pregnancy and placenta previa, provide no warning and require the nurse to readily identify danger signs and mobilize appropriate medical and nursing care.

Medical Conditions Complicating Pregnancy

Preexisting medical conditions in the pregnant woman may complicate pregnancy and may have deleterious consequences for maternal and neonatal outcomes. The most significant of these high-risk conditions—diabetes mellitus, hypertension, and cardiac disease—are discussed in Chapter 27. The following section discusses problems of maternal origin that have a significant impact on perinatal outcomes, such as anemia and hemoglobinopathies and thromboembolic disease. Table 16-2 summarizes information about additional conditions that may complicate pregnancy but are rarely major sources of morbidity and mortality. These conditions include asthma, neurologic disorders, and cancer in pregnancy.

Anemia

Anemia is the most common hematologic problem in pregnancy. The cause of anemia is often difficult to establish. It has been estimated that 56% of all pregnant women have some degree of anemia, the percentage varying according to geographic location and socioeconomic grouping. Anemia may be caused by a number of conditions in pregnancy, which result from nutritional deficiency, hemolysis, or blood loss (Gabbe et al., 1991; see the accompanying display).

The normal physiologic changes of pregnancy cause increases in blood volume and red blood cell production. A total of 750 to 1000 mg of absorbed iron or the equivalent of 4 U or more of transfused blood is needed to meet the increased iron needs of pregnancy. During the second trimester, a drop in hemoglobin and hematocrit levels can be expected. This results from a 50% increase in plasma volume. Normal retention of intracellular fluid and increased plasma volume cause physiologic hemodilution during pregnancy. Consequently, anemia in pregnancy is defined as a hemoglobin value of 11 g/dL or less during the second and third trimesters (Table 16-3). This low figure reflects the hemodilutional effect.

Hemoglobin levels are influenced by the following additional factors:

- Rate of erythrocyte breakdown and iron reutilization by the bone marrow
- Dietary intake of iron (inadequate diets may provide only 10 to 18 mg of iron daily; the normal requirement during pregnancy is 30 to 60 mg of elemental iron)
- Ability of the gastrointestinal tract to absorb iron (normally only about 10% of intake is absorbed, but this increases to 20% when iron deficiency exists)

The pregnant woman generally does not develop symptoms of anemia unless the hemoglobin level is less than 6 to 7 g/dL, when high output cardiac failure may occur. Less severe anemia, from 8 to 10 g/dL, causes no problems for the pregnant woman but is associated with preterm birth. Some studies have reported low birth weight and fetal death to be associated with less severe anemia. The reason for these associations is unclear, and it may be that these outcomes are a result of other negative environmental factors that also tend to cause severe anemia (Williams & Wheby, 1992).

Iron Deficiency Anemia

Iron deficiency anemia is the most common medical complication of pregnancy. Two thirds of women of childbearing age have evidence of insufficient iron stores. Of these women, 5% will have insufficient hemoglobin production because iron stores are depleted. Many women begin pregnancy slightly anemic. The physiologic demands of pregnancy exacerbate the condition significantly (Williams & Wheby, 1992).

Etiologic and Predisposing Factors

Iron deficiency anemia results from reduced hemoglobin production caused by depletion of iron stores. Depleted iron stores may result from inadequate dietary intake of iron, malabsorption, blood loss, closely spaced pregnancies, or hemolysis.

Diagnosis

Screening for the presence of anemia during pregnancy is routine. A complete blood count (CBC) is performed at the first prenatal visit and again at 28 and 36 weeks of gestation. Additional blood testing is performed if low hemoglobin levels are found. A peripheral blood smear for erythrocyte morphology and a CBC should be performed.

Iron deficiency anemia is usually diagnosed by microcytic (immature) red blood cells that are hypochromic (insufficient hemoglobin). However, in pregnancy, serum ferritin is a more accurate test for iron deficiency anemia than is serum hemoglobin. A serum ferritin level of less than 35 μg/L indicates inadequate iron stores. This is strongly suggestive of iron deficiency anemia. If the serum ferritin level is higher, other causes of anemia must be investigated (Gabbe et al., 1991).

Treatment

Treatment for iron deficiency anemia most often focuses on increasing dietary intake of iron-rich foods. Supplemental iron and vitamins are required. Because iron absorption is pH dependent, women are advised to take the iron tablet with a source of ascorbic acid to enhance duodenal absorption of iron. Supplements of iron and vitamin C are standard treatment for iron deficiency anemia; however, they should never be considered a substitute for good nutrition. The usual recommended dosages for supplementation are:

- Ferrous sulfate, 325 mg orally, three times a day
- Vitamin C, 500 mg orally once daily (Gabbe et al., 1991)

Supplemental iron may cause gastrointestinal upset accompanied by either constipation or diarrhea. To minimize this reaction, the pregnant woman is advised to take the iron preparation with or after meals. This is true especially in early pregnancy when there is a tendency for nausea. However, maximum absorption occurs when iron is taken with orange juice between meals. This method of administration may be easier to initiate after the first trimester. It is important

Table 16-2. Some Medical Conditions and Their Implications for Pregnancy

Condition	Treatment/Modification in Pregnancy	Maternal, Fetal, and Neonatal Implications	Nursing Implications
Asthma			
Chronic inflammatory condition characterized by inflammation and spasm of bronchial tissue.	Most drugs (steroids, theophylline) safe in pregnancy. Doses may be increased because of increased maternal blood volume. Serum theophylline levels should be done weekly.	Disease usually does not affect pregnancy. Severe episodes (status asthmaticus) can cause fetal hypoxia. Upper respiratory infections should be treated aggressively.	Monitor patient compliance with regimen. Check blood glucose if patient uses glucocorticoid (beclomethasone dipropionate) inhaler. Local or regional anesthesia for delivery recommended; some analgesics may cause bronchospasm.
Seizure Disorder			
A range of chronic conditions that result in seizures.	Continue drug therapy. Anticonvulsants have teratogenic potential, but risk of seizures is greater fetal threat. Doses may be altered because of alterations in absorption in pregnancy.	Potential for seizures exists until therapeutic drug levels are reestablished in pregnancy. Possible fetal anomalies with anticonvulsants: microcephaly, facial clefts, limb anomalies.	Advise woman to avoid situations that may stimulate seizures (ie, sleep deprivation). Anticipate serial ultrasounds to evaluate fetal status. Advise against breastfeeding; drugs are present in breast milk.
Cancer			
Most frequent types in childbearing-age women are cancer of breast and cervix and lymphoma. Cancers may progress rapidly during pregnancy, if hormonally sensitive cell types.	Chemotherapy and radiation have high incidence of abortion in first trimester and may cause malformations in second trimester. Chemotherapy may be safe in late pregnancy.	Effects of cancer treatments must be balanced against risk to fetal development and postponing treatment. Postponing treatment may not be an option in rapidly progressing disease.	Team management required with expertise on oncology treatment as well as perinatal risks.
Rheumatoid Arthritis			
Autoimmune condition in which joints become inflamed, causing fatigue, pain, and progressive loss of joint function.	Treatment (salicylates, NSAIDs) generally unchanged in pregnancy. Woman may choose to reduce use of salicylates if inflammation and pain are minimal in pregnancy.	May be remission of symptoms in pregnancy. Maintenance of exercise regimen is important, but use of non–weight-bearing modes may be advised. Continued use of salicylates during pregnancy associated with low risk of fetal anomalies.	Encourage use of nonpharmacologic self-care measures (local heat, rest, and flexibility exercise) and use of salicylates as needed.
Systemic Lupus Erthymatosis (SLE)			
Autoimmune condition with a wide range of inflammatory symptoms, including nephritis, joint inflammation, neuropathies, depression.	Pregnancy does not exacerbate disease. Use of prednisone as prevention for exacerbation not effective. During exacerbations, prednisone and low-dose acetylsalicylic acid may be prescribed.	Risk of abortion, stillbirth, preterm labor, and low birth weight increased. Risk of exacerbation of disease in postpartum period increased. Neonatal lupus and congenital heart anomalies rare but may occur in severe cases. If maternal renal involvement, increased risk of poor perinatal outcomes.	Care will require close coordination with specialists in immunologic disorders. Educate about need to avoid exposure to infection, stress, fatigue. Woman should recognize signs of preterm labor and urinary tract infection and understand need for prompt evaluation.
Multiple Sclerosis			
Condition in which myelin sheath of nerve fibers is destroyed. Muscle weakness, neurologic changes, fatigue with marked loss of sensation and muscle strength during exacerbations.	Condition generally does not worsen with pregnancy. No modifications needed.	Exacerbation may occur in postpartum period. Maternal activity and fatigue may be affected as body weight increases.	Encourage planning for assistance with household tasks and child care in postpartum period. Anticipatory guidance about physical demands of early parenting may be needed.

(continued)

Table 16-2. Some Medical Conditions and Their Implications for Pregnancy ***(continued)***

Condition	Treatment/Modification in Pregnancy	Maternal, Fetal, and Neonatal Implications	Nursing Implications
Glucose-6-Phosphate Dehydrogenase (G6PD) Deficiency			
Female-linked genetic disorder that predisposes red blood cells to lysis when exposed to oxidizing drugs (salicylates, acetominophen, phenacetin, some sulfa drugs).	Condition not affected by pregnancy, except if complicated by anemia. Iron and folic acid supplementation recommended.	No implications except for increased risk of maternal anemia. Many women unaware of condition until unexplained episodes of jaundice are linked to use of oxidizing drugs.	Advise patient of risk of hemolysis and anemia from use of oxidizing drugs. Coordinate with care provider and pharmacy to provide patient with choices for minor discomforts and treatment of infection.

NSAID, nonsteroidal antiinflammatory drug.

to explain that the iron in the pills is not fully absorbed and that it is normal for the feces to become dark green or black.

Maternal, Fetal, and Neonatal Implications

The severity of anemia determines the risk to the woman and the developing fetus. Severe iron deficiency anemia (hemoglobin level less than 6 g/dL) may be associated with an increased risk of maternal cardiac failure, poor maternal wound healing, low neonatal birth weight, prematurity, and IUFD. Less severe anemia (8 to 10 g/dL) does not generally adversely affect the fetus because of active iron transport across the placenta even when maternal iron stores are low. Subtle maternal complications, such as delayed wound healing, infection, and postpartum hemorrhage, may occur with moderate anemia.

Mild anemia of 11 g/dL poses no threat to the woman or fetus. However, it is an indication that the nutritional state of the woman is less than optimal. When the woman intends to breastfeed, it is important for her hemoglobin level to be maintained at 12 g/dL or above. This ensures that her body will be provided with the nutrients and oxygen required for successful breastfeeding (see Chapter 17 for further discussion of nutrition and screening.)

> ### *Causes of Anemia*
>
> The nurse should recognize that anemia in pregnancy can be caused by any one of the following factors:
>
> - Nutritional deficiency
>   - Iron deficiency
>   - Folate or B_{12} deficiency
> - Blood loss
> - Hemolysis
>   - Congenital
>   - Sickle cell anemia, thalassemias
>   - G6PD deficiency
>   - Acquired HELLP syndrome
> - Bone marrow suppression

Implications for Nursing Care

Nursing care of the pregnant woman with anemia relies on careful assessment of the woman's physiologic status. It is important to determine the woman's understanding of her condition and her ability to carry out recommended medical and self-care practices.

• • Assessment

The nurse should assess the laboratory results of all women receiving prenatal care, identifying those who require additional clinical evaluation of anemia. Women diagnosed with iron deficiency anemia should be seen by the nurse or nutritionist for the purpose of evaluating dietary intake. Evaluation of the diet for the previous 24 hours will provide a baseline for planning a diet that includes more iron-rich foods. Chapter 17 contains more detailed nutritional information regarding dietary assessment in relation to anemias of pregnancy.

• • Nursing Diagnosis

The following nursing diagnoses may be applicable in the care of the pregnant woman with iron deficiency anemia:

- Altered Nutrition: Less than Body Requirements related to inadequate intake of iron-rich foods
- Constipation related to iron supplementation

• • Planning and Implementation

Women with iron deficiency anemia must be informed of the self-care measures necessary to correct the condition. Depending on the health care setting, the nurse may develop a dietary plan with the assistance of a dietician. Referral of low-income women to the Women, Infants, and Children Supplemental Food Program is important.

The pregnant woman with iron deficiency anemia should be advised to increase dietary intake of iron-rich foods as an adjunct to iron replacement therapy. As a general counseling rule, the redder the meat and the greener the vegetable, the

Table 16-3. Anemia in Pregnancy: Month-Specific and Trimester-Specific Hemoglobin (Hgb) and Hematocrit (Hct) Cutoffs

Gestation (wks)	12	16	20	24	28	32	36	40
Trimester	1	2	2	2	3	3	3	term
Mean Hgb (g/dL)	12.2	11.8	11.6	11.6	11.8	12.1	12.5	12.9
5th percentile Hgb values (g/dL)	11.0	10.6	10.5	10.5	10.7	11.0	11.4	11.9
Equivalent 5th percentile Hct values (%)	33.0	32.0	32.0	32.0	32.0	33.0	34.0	36.0

From Centers for Disease Control (1989). *CDC guidelines for anemia in children and childbearing-age women.*

richer it is as a source of iron. Vitamin C, a nutrient essential for the optimal absorption of iron, is abundant in dark green fresh vegetables and citrus fruits. Vitamin C is chemically unstable and readily breaks down when heated. Therefore, fresh, uncooked vegetables are an important source of vitamin C. Sufficient quantities of vitamin C must be eaten each day to fulfill daily requirements because it is a water-soluble vitamin. Excess amounts are excreted in the urine and are not stored in the body.

The nurse will need to discuss the importance of iron therapy. The woman should be informed that unabsorbed iron will be excreted in the feces, causing a green or black coloration. The pregnant woman should understand that taking each pill between meals with orange juice or another food rich in vitamin C will enhance absorption. If gastric upset occurs with this approach, the woman should take iron after eating, but should avoid use of antacids, which will block absorption of iron. Iron supplementation may cause constipation. This is easily remedied by increasing dietary intake of fruits, vegetables, and fluids.

Most prenatal vitamins contain supplemental iron. Therefore, if the woman is taking one vitamin daily, she may only need to take two iron tablets. The woman should be encouraged to continue this supplementation through the first month postpartum to aid in rebuilding iron stores.

Expected Outcomes

- The pregnant woman with iron deficiency anemia participates in dietary counseling.
- The pregnant woman explains self-care measures to decrease gastric upset and constipation associated with iron supplementation therapy.
- The pregnant woman explains the rationale and importance of iron supplementation therapy during pregnancy.

• • Evaluation

The body responds to supplemental iron in about 7 to 15 days by increasing its production of young red blood cells (reticulocytes). When the woman has taken the recommended dose of iron, the red blood cell response can be measured in about 2 weeks by an elevation in the percentage of reticulocytes. This is reported by the laboratory reticulocyte count. An early response validating iron ingestion is shown in an increase of reticulocytes from the normal of 0.5% to 1.5% to 3% to 4% at 2 to 4 weeks after therapy has been initiated. A repeat hematocrit after 4 weeks of therapy should also show an increase if mineral supplementation is being taken as prescribed.

Relaying information about improvements in laboratory values to the pregnant woman may be helpful in motivating her to continue treatment. If no improvements in reticulocyte count or hematocrit are found 4 weeks after therapy is begun and the pregnant woman reports she has been taking the prescribed supplements, another cause of anemia should be investigated.

Folic Acid Deficiency

Folic acid deficiency is discussed in Chapter 17.

Hemoglobinopathies: Sickle Cell Anemia and β-Thalassemia

Hemoglobinopathies are conditions characterized by the presence of abnormal hemoglobin; they are usually genetic conditions. Two hemoglobinopathies with special significance in pregnancy are sickle cell anemia and β-thalassemia.

Sickle cell disease (sickle cell anemia) is a genetic disorder limited to African Americans. It is transmitted to the offspring by either the father or mother (heterozygous form) or by both parents (homozygous form). The term sickle cell disease originates from the characteristic abnormal sickle shape of the circulating red blood cells of affected persons. Approximately 8% of African Americans in the United States suffer from sickle cell trait, and 0.3% have sickle cell disease.

Sickle cell disease is characterized by lifelong anemia, chronic illness, and abdominal and joint pain. These symptoms are caused the red blood cells being distorted into a crescent shape by the presence of abnormal hemoglobin, a process called sickling. Crises can occur when these blood cells clog capillaries and cause stagnation in areas such as the spleen, bone marrow, and placenta.

β-Thalassemia is a genetic disorder that affects the cellular structure of hemoglobin. Several types of thalassemia have been identified, with β-thalassemia being the type most frequently encountered in the United States. It is most commonly found in people of Mediterranean or Asian (especially Chinese) origin and in people of African ancestry, including West Indians and American blacks. β-Thalassemia major is the term used to refer to inheritance of the gene from both parents (homozygous form); β-thalassemia minor refers to the heterozygous form that results from inheritance of one abnormal gene from either parent.

Etiologic and Predisposing Factors

Both sickle cell anemia and β-thalassemia are inherited conditions. If only one gene is inherited, the individual is said to have the trait. This individual may have no clinical symptoms or only mild clinical symptoms of hemoglobinopathy. If the individual inherits genes for the condition from both parents, the individual is said to have the disease and is likely to have moderate to severe symptoms.

Diagnosis

Pregnant women with sickle cell or β-thalassemia trait may appear to be anemic, based on hemoglobin and hematocrit studies. Additional specific blood work is needed to diagnose each condition. In the outpatient prenatal setting, initial laboratory assessment is performed to specifically define the hemoglobinopathy. Iron and folate stores and reticulocyte counts are assessed, and screening for hemolysis is completed.

Treatment

Treatment of anemia secondary to hemoglobinopathy centers on dietary counseling and folic acid supplements. Iron therapy is not necessary because iron deficiency is not a characteristic of these diseases. Frequent monitoring for infection is indicated to facilitate immediate treatment and decrease maternal morbidity. Women with hemoglobinopathies are at greater risk for infection.

There is no current standard treatment for pregnant women with sickle cell trait or sickle cell disease. The pregnant woman and her family may require genetic counseling. The father of the fetus should be tested to determine the relative risk of the fetus being born with sickle cell disease. The pregnant woman with sickle cell disease is followed prenatally in a high-risk clinic or private practice where her condition is closely supervised. When infection or other problems arise, the woman is hospitalized immediately.

The pregnant woman with β-thalassemia minor requires no specific treatment, and the pregnancy is generally not affected by the condition. However, there may be concern about the genetic inheritance of the fetus. If the father of the fetus is also diagnosed as having β-thalassemia minor (trait), the fetus is at risk for developing severe disease. This fetus has a 25% chance of having the disease (homozygous disease), a 50% chance of having the trait (heterozygous disease), and a 25% chance of being unaffected. It is possible to diagnose fetal β-thalassemia prenatally through fetoscopy and specialized fetal blood sampling at 16 to 20 weeks of gestation. Risk to the fetus from this procedure ranges from 5% to 10%.

The pregnant woman with β-thalassemia major requires high-risk care because the condition puts her at risk for other pregnancy complications. Transfusions and special treatments to avoid iron overload are generally needed.

Maternal, Fetal, and Neonatal Implications

Women with sickle cell disease experience higher rates of spontaneous abortion, stillbirths, neonatal deaths, and premature labor. One third to one half of all known pregnancies terminate for these reasons. The cause of the perinatal loss is unknown. Placentas from these births exhibit no damage from sickling or infarcts. No increase in congenital anomalies is reported although intrauterine growth retardation is common.

Anemia is the cardinal finding (100%) in pregnant patients with sickle cell disease. The anemia becomes increasingly severe as pregnancy progresses. About 10% to 20% of affected women have acute crises during pregnancy. Crises may occur at any time during the perinatal period.

Pregnancy places women with sickle cell anemia at particular risk for infection. Infection accounts for 50% to 60% of the morbidity experienced during pregnancy. Common infections include urinary tract infection (UTI), pneumonia, and postpartum endometritis. These problems are especially severe in these women and result from stagnation of oxygenated red blood cells in the viscera, which leads to deoxygenation and sickling. A vicious cycle ensues and may lead to crises. Cardiomegaly, congestive heart failure, and pulmonary infarction may occur. A maternal mortality rate of 25% demonstrates the seriousness of sickle cell disease.

Women with β-thalassemia minor and sickle cell trait may never exhibit any symptom but anemia, which is chronic and may be profound, depending on the percentage of abnormal hemoglobin present. Spontaneous abortions and infections are the primary concern for pregnant women who carry the β-thalassemia trait. Most trait carriers have uneventful pregnancies.

Women with β-thalassemia major and sickle cell disease are at significantly increased risk for complications. Women with β-thalassemia major are at increased risk for spontaneous abortion, infection, and PIH. Risk to the fetus is not increased, except that which results from the development of these maternal complications.

Implications for Nursing Care

Although hemoglobinopathies are relatively rare in pregnant women, prenatal care must be specifically tailored to their special needs to ensure optimal outcomes. The nurse can play an instrumental role in this specialized care.

• • Assessment

Initial history taking by the nurse will identify women with a hemoglobinopathy (disease or trait). This is accomplished through the patient's knowledge of its existence or through a family history of disease. When a pregnant woman is unaware that she has a hemoglobinopathy and is told that she is carrying this trait (and possibly transmitting it to her neonate), she will need sensitive and empathic support. Although the disease may not disrupt her health or life, she must be aware of its possible ramifications.

During the prenatal period, the nurse should carefully assess the pregnant woman through the interim history, physical findings, and symptoms. Signs of UTI, of chest colds that might progress to pneumonia, and of pulmonary congestion should be identified early and quickly and appropriately treated.

The initial patient history should document problems or

complications that have been, or are being, experienced by the woman. Interim histories should routinely include queries about even the most minor health problems.

• • Nursing Diagnosis

The following nursing diagnoses may be applicable for use in caring for the pregnant woman with a hemoglobinopathy:

- Fear related to increased risk of fetal death or complication
- Fatigue related to anemia and stresses of illness
- Altered Nutrition: Less than Body Requirements related to need for adequate dietary intake of folic acid and iron
- High Risk for Infection related to complications from hemoglobinopathy
- Decisional Conflict related to continuing pregnancy with genetic risk for the fetus

• • Planning and Implementation

As soon as the trait for hemoglobinopathy is diagnosed in the pregnant woman, the couple should be offered genetic counseling and be encouraged to have the father screened. If he also has the trait, the fetus has a 25% chance of having the disease. Referral to genetic counseling is imperative for couples who may pass on the trait or the disease to their offspring.

Because the woman generally is not ill, normal prenatal activities, counseling, and classes are continued. The necessity for increased rest should be stressed. Special arrangements may be necessary to provide additional help at home with daily activities and child care.

Nurses have an important role in teaching women about their pregnancies, in helping them to maintain optimal health through nutrition counseling, and in monitoring signs of problems. The nurse can intervene in the following ways:

- Ensuring that genetic counseling is made available
- Encouraging frequent prenatal visits for ongoing monitoring
- Obtaining urine cultures once a month, whether or not the woman is symptomatic
- Teaching the woman the importance of taking her daily dose of folic acid
- Assisting with hospital admission when necessary
- Counseling the couple in family planning methods and permanent sterilization or abortion, if requested

Expected Outcomes

- The pregnant woman diagnosed with a hemoglobinopathy explains the nature of the risk to herself and her fetus and measures to reduce that risk.
- The pregnant woman with a hemoglobinopathy uses appropriate self-care measures to avoid fatigue, stress, and infection.
- The pregnant woman with a hemoglobinopathy uses the prescribed dietary regimen and nutritional supplements.
- The pregnant woman with a hemoglobinopathy follows up on genetic counseling in a timely fashion to allow for an informed decision regarding continuation of pregnancy.

• • Evaluation

The nurse is able to evaluate the woman's response to high-risk perinatal care. The nurse should evaluate the extent to which the woman understands her condition and the self-care measures required to maintain optimal health. The nurse must stress the importance of ongoing evaluation of maternal and fetal physiologic status as pregnancy progresses.

Perinatal care for women with hemoglobinopathies is a particular challenge because it requires health care providers to maintain careful surveillance for complications. Complications are not all preventable. However, quality perinatal care will enable the nurse and the pregnant woman to identify situations requiring medical intervention quickly before complications become serious. If complications arise, the nurse is responsible for evaluating the woman's response to changes in the medical and self-care regimen, altering the plan of care as indicated.

Thromboembolic Disease

Thromboembolic disease, especially deep vein thrombosis (DVT), is a rare condition. However, if it occurs, it carries with it life-threatening implications. Thromboembolic disease is characterized by the formation of an abnormal clot in a venous vessel.

Etiologic and Predisposing Factors

During pregnancy and parturition, women are five time more likely to experience venous thromboembolic events than are nonpregnant women. Fortunately, this problem occurs only in 1 of every 1000 pregnancies, and in 2 of every 1000 postpartum women. Women who require cesarean delivery are at increased risk.

Three factors predispose childbearing women to thromboembolic problems. First, during pregnancy, the blood coagulation mechanisms create a hypercoagulable state that is most pronounced in the early postpartum period. Second, venous stasis occurs because venous return from the legs is impeded by the enlarging uterus. Finally, vascular tone is decreased by the action of progesterone.

Diagnosis

Classic symptoms of DVT are leg pain, tenderness, swelling, and localized warmth. However, only 50% of patients will have these symptoms. Many women who have these symptoms do not, in fact, have the condition. The best diagnostic test available is Doppler ultrasound, which can identify even small clots in veins (Bachman, 1990).

Treatment

The mainstay of treatment for thromboembolic disease is anticoagulation therapy. It is begun at the time of diagnosis up until 4 to 12 weeks postpartum. Heparin is the only agent safe for this use in pregnancy because it does not cross the placenta. The usual regimen is subcutaneous injection of 10,000 U every 12 hours. Partial thromboplastin time (clotting time) must be checked weekly to ensure a safe therapeutic effect has been achieved. Bed rest is usually recommended, either in the hospital or at home. Use of elastic support stockings has not been shown to improve outcomes in these patients (Bachman, 1990).

Maternal, Fetal, and Neonatal Implications

The most serious implication of thromboembolic disease during pregnancy is the risk of maternal pulmonary embolism and death. There is no specific threat to the fetus, except through the threat to maternal well-being. Anticoagulant therapy presents the risk of excessive anticoagulation for the woman, as evidenced by bleeding gums, nose bleeds, and hematuria.

Implications for Nursing Care

The nurse can identify women at risk for DVT through a careful history of previous clotting problems or a history of DVT. Women at risk because of long periods of inactivity should be advised to do leg exercises at regular intervals and to avoid wearing restrictive clothing on the legs.

The woman with confirmed DVT during pregnancy will require assistance with self-administration of heparin and recognizing signs of excessive anticoagulation. Women must know the danger signs of pulmonary embolism and have access to emergency transportation. The nurse can provide teaching and emotional support to women and their families who must live with the anxiety that this threat may cause (see the Teaching Considerations display).

Planning for intrapartum and postpartum care for the woman with DVT is a complex process. It will include consideration of intravenous heparin administration, frequent coagulation studies, and avoidance of the lithotomy position or any position that encourages venous stasis. Postpartum care will include replacing heparin with oral anticoagulant (coumarin) that will be continued prophylactically for 2 to 3 months. Again, weekly partial thromboplastin times should be obtained. The woman should be advised that oral contraceptives are contraindicated while she is taking anticoagulant medication. Estrogen alters blood coagulability and places the woman at risk for excessive bleeding. Breastfeeding is safe on this medical regimen. However, the woman should be advised to avoid nipple cracks, which could lead to excessive bleeding.

Maternal medical conditions may complicate pregnancy with deleterious consequences for maternal, fetal, and neonatal outcomes. Anemia, the most common hematologic problem in pregnancy, affects about 56% of all pregnant women to some degree. Of these, iron deficiency anemia is the most common. Screening pregnant women for anemia is routine. Anemias are treated with dietary adjustments and supplemental iron and vitamins. Two hemoglobinopathies of significance in pregnancy are sickle cell anemia and β-thalassemia. Thromboembolic disease, although rare in pregnancy, is life threatening. The woman must be taught signs and symptoms to report immediately.

Teaching Considerations

Signs and Symptoms of Pulmonary Embolism

The nurse can use the following points in teaching the pregnant women with thromboembolic disease. These women must recognize the symptoms of pulmonary embolism and be instructed to seek emergency medical assistance should any of the following occur:

Symptoms

- Sudden onset of dyspnea accompanied by sweating, pallor
- Confusion
- Cough with or without hemoptysis
- Chest pain
- Confusion or fear of imminent death
- Sensation of pressure in bowel or rectum

Signs

- Tachycardia and systemic hypotension
- Friction rub and evident atelectasis on chest auscultation
- Increased jugular vein pressure
- Gallop heart rhythm
- Unexplained fever

Pulmonary embolism can be minor if only a small vessel is occluded or quickly lethal if a major vessel is blocked. The nurse's first priority if a woman reports any of these symptoms is to ensure that emergency medical care and cardiorespiratory support are mobilized immediately.

Infections in Pregnancy

Infections are a major source of perinatal morbidity and neonatal mortality. Thus, the maternity nurse must be knowledgeable about the range of infections that have implications for maternal, fetal, and neonatal well-being. The following section focuses first on infection as a general threat to health and then addresses specific kinds of infections, including systemic infections, such as hepatitis, tuberculosis and teratogenic infections, as well as infections of the urinary tract and sexually transmitted diseases (STDs).

Etiologic and Predisposing Factors

One of the normal physiologic adaptations of pregnancy is a decreased immunologic response to infection. This change is thought to result from maternal physiologic acceptance of the placenta and fetus. Both are genetically and immunologically different tissues from the woman's own tissue. When infection occurs in pregnancy, the woman's entire immunologic defense response is less efficient and protective than when she is not pregnant (Gabbe et al., 1991).

Diagnosis

Techniques for diagnosing infection have improved dramatically in recent years. This is especially true for isolating viral agents. However, appropriate screening and diagnosis depends on careful identification of women likely to be at risk for infection. In many cases, the risks associated with some infections are severe enough that all women should be screened (see the accompanying display). In other cases, screening is chosen based on a careful assessment of the woman's medical and social history.

Treatment

Pregnancy alters the body's absorption and response to antibiotic therapy: gastric motility is slowed, blood volume is increased, and liver function is altered. Antibiotics cross the placenta, so the consequences of therapy for the fetus must be considered.

In some cases, specific antibiotic treatment is available and can be administered safely for some infections during pregnancy. Infections such as syphilis, gonorrhea, streptococcus B, and chlamydia fall into this category. However, viral infections that cause significant maternal, fetal, and neonatal sequelae such as herpes, hepatitis, and human immunodeficiency virus (HIV) cannot be treated at present. The following section addresses treatment modalities for specific types of infection during pregnancy.

Maternal, Fetal, and Neonatal Implications

Individual organisms vary greatly in their ability to cause maternal and fetal illness. Some organisms cause no maternal symptoms but pose fetal risk. Others can be transmitted across the placenta or only during fetal passage through the vagina. Teratogenic infections cause abnormal embryonic or fetal development. Most teratogenic infections are caused by viruses and are thus not responsive to antibiotic therapy.

Prenatal Screening for Infection

The nurse should be aware that women should be screened for the following infections early in prenatal care, and based on risk of exposure, may require testing again late in pregnancy.

Rubella
Streptococcus B
Herpes (if history of previous infection)
Hepatitis B
Tuberculosis
Chlamydia
Syphilis
Gonorrhea
Human immunodeficiency virus

Accurate screening is not possible for the following infections (see Table 16-4), but they have implications for fetal and neonatal well-being:

Cytomegalovirus
Parvovirus
Toxoplamosis

Implications for Nursing Care

Although there are specific implications for nursing care based on the particular infection involved, general implications also apply to the care of all pregnant women diagnosed with an infection. These general principles guiding the care of the pregnant woman with an infection are discussed below.

• • Assessment

A major responsibility of nurses in the prenatal period is obtaining an accurate health history. The pregnant woman is questioned in regard to infections before the pregnancy. The nurse assesses factors that put the pregnant woman at risk for infection during pregnancy. Based on risk factors and exposure, the nurse should ensure that women are appropriately screened for infections.

• • Nursing Diagnosis

The following nursing diagnoses may be applicable in the care of the pregnant woman with a systemic infection:

- Fear related to threat to fetal well-being
- Pain related to the inflammatory process
- Grieving related to personal losses associated with diagnosis of chronic, untreatable infection
- Decisional Conflict related to continuation of pregnancy after teratogenic infection exposure
- Noncompliance with prescribed antibiotic therapy related to side effects and cost

• • Planning and Implementation

The care of the pregnant woman with an infection focuses on providing the woman with information necessary to understand the significance of the infection for maternal and fetal well-being. The nurse also provides support to the woman and her family as they cope with those implications.

If the fetal effects of infection can be detected before fetal viability, the woman may be faced with a decision about whether the pregnancy should be continued. When the effects of infection cannot be known, the nurse should assist the woman and her family in coping with the uncertainty about fetal well-being. The nurse provides anticipatory guidance about potential health problems that may occur if the fetus is infected.

When infection represents a chronic condition for which there is no treatment, the need for psychosocial support to the pregnant woman and her family will be significant. The nurse may be responsible for explaining the nature of the infection. Self-care measures to prevent spread of the infection and to preserve optimal maternal and fetal well-being should be implemented. Planning for nursing care in the intrapartum and postpartum periods will include instructing the woman about special care that may be required for her and her neonate and providing anticipatory guidance. The nurse should explain that breastfeeding is generally unaffected by maternal infections and that separation from the neonate is usually not necessary.

Expected Outcomes

- The infected pregnant woman discusses the relative risks to herself and her fetus.
- The infected pregnant woman discusses self-care activities to relieve pain.
- The pregnant woman's partner provides support during counseling sessions.
- The infected pregnant woman decides whether pregnancy should be continued after receiving necessary information.
- The infected pregnant woman explains the rationale for prescribed medical and self-care activities.

• • Evaluation

The nurse is responsible for evaluating the pregnant woman's response to the diagnosis of infection as well as to her response to treatment. It is especially important for the nurse to be available to provide supportive care to those women diagnosed with an infection for which no treatment is available and which poses fetal risk. When the plan of care does not achieve expected outcomes, the nurse revises the plan and works collaboratively with others to ensure that optimal ongoing care is being provided.

The diagnosis of infection during pregnancy can be an intensely frightening experience for the woman and her family. It is an important nursing responsibility to evaluate how the woman and her family cope with the added stress and to provide supportive care as needed.

Systemic Infections in Pregnancy

Some infections are systemic in the sense that they can affect a major organ such as the lung or liver. Systemic infections have the capacity to produce organ system abnormalities in the fetus by transplacental transmission. The major categories of infection addressed in this section are hepatitis, tuberculosis, and teratogenic (formerly called TORCH) infections.

Hepatitis

The incidence of hepatitis has risen sharply over the last decade. Viral hepatitis is one of the most serious infections that can occur during pregnancy. There are four forms of hepatitis.

Hepatitis A is a relatively benign, self-limiting disease. It is transmitted person to person or from fecal–oral contamination. It occurs once in every 1000 pregnancies. Maternal illness is short, and serious complications are rare. Perinatal transmission does not occur.

Hepatitis B is a more serious form of hepatitis. The incidence of hepatitis B has increased markedly over the last decade. Acute infection occurs in 1 to 2 pregnancies per 1000 in the United States. Chronic infection is found in 5 to 15 pregnancies per 1000. Up to 75% of infections are asymptomatic; when symptoms occur, they include mild skin rash, low-grade fever, arthralgia, and hepatosplenomegaly. Transmission can occur from sexual contact although perinatal transmission is the major factor in the spread of this disease, largely through neonatal contact with maternal body fluids at delivery.

All women should be tested for hepatitis B as part of prenatal care because of the serious nature of this disease. Immunization is available and should be administered during pregnancy for women who test negative but are at high risk for exposure. Current recommendations for preventing hepatitis B in the United States include routine immunization of all neonates.

Hepatitis non-A, non-B (hepatitis C) accounts for approximately 10% to 20% of all cases of hepatitis in the United States. The C virus is detected on blood testing, and about 50% of those infected have chronic disease. Currently no immunization and no treatment are available. The fetus or neonate is rarely infected.

Hepatitis D is found only in individuals already infected with hepatitis B. Chronic infection occurs in over half of those infected and is likely to be severe. Neonatal infection is rare because immunization against hepatitis B also prevents hepatitis D infection (ACOG, 1992).

Etiologic and Predisposing Factors

These forms of hepatitis are caused by viruses, most of which are spread by fecal–oral, sexual, or body fluid routes. Risk factors for hepatitis infection include:

- Needle use
- Multiple sexual partners
- Exposure to blood products or needle sticks
- Work in an institution where oral–fecal contamination may occur (prisons, shelters, institutions for mentally retarded)

Diagnosis

Diagnosis of viral hepatitis is accomplished largely by detection of specific antibodies to the viruses in blood. The American College of Obstetricians and Gynecologists (ACOG, 1992) currently recommends routine screening of all pregnant women for hepatitis B. Testing for surface antigen is generally done at the first prenatal visit. A positive test for surface antigen may indicate chronic infection or past acute infection. Thus, an infection work-up for any pregnant woman with a positive surface antigen test for hepatitis B is indicated.

Treatment

There is no treatment available for viral hepatitis, except for supportive therapy during acute infection and for those chronically infected. Neonates born to women positive for hepatitis surface antigen should receive immunization against hepatitis B within 12 hours of birth to prevent infection.

Maternal, Fetal, and Neonatal Implications

Chronic hepatitis can be debilitating and can lead to permanent liver dysfunction. Women with chronic infection are more likely to acquire other opportunistic infections. Because perinatal transmission is preventable through immunization, maternal infection should have limited impact on neonatal well-being.

Implications for Nursing Care

Nursing care in the prenatal period focuses on ensuring that women are screened for hepatitis B. Pregnant women at risk for the infection are immunized during the prenatal period. An important nursing responsibility is preventing transmission through the scrupulous use of universal precautions for blood-borne infection. This is especially true in the intrapartum period when neonatal exposure is a major risk (see the Nursing Procedures on Universal Precautions in Chapters 20 and 31). The neonate should receive hepatitis B immunotherapy within 12 hours after delivery and the nurse should verify that pediatric follow-up with hepatitis B vaccine and boosters is planned.

Tuberculosis

After decades of declining incidence, tuberculosis has increased in recent years, primarily in urban areas. This infection, when untreated, can cause destruction of lung tissue. Disseminated infection and destruction of other target organs may occur if the disease progresses.

Etiologic and Predisposing Factors

This infection is caused by the tubercle bacillus; it is spread by airborne transmission. Infection is more likely in individuals with poor nutritional status living in crowded conditions and in poverty and is more prevalent among immigrants in the United States.

Diagnosis

Diagnosis is generally accomplished by chest radiography. A positive skin test for tuberculosis indicates the need for a chest x-ray. If lesions are noted on chest x-ray, active disease can be diagnosed by identifying tubercle bacilli in sputum.

Treatment

The drug of choice for treating tuberculosis is isoniazid. This medication must be taken orally over a period of 12 months or longer to ensure cure of active disease. Isoniazid is extremely toxic to the liver, and liver function studies should be done periodically during therapy. However, treatment is generally recommended and is considered safe during pregnancy.

Maternal, Fetal, and Neonatal Implications

All pregnant women should receive skin testing for tuberculosis using the PPD (purified protein derivative) or the Mantoux test unless they have a documented history of previous positive skin tests. Any pregnant woman with a positive skin test should have a chest x-ray with lead shielding in the first trimester. Medication for active disease should be started during pregnancy to prevent progression of the disease. Even if no lesions are noted, prophylactic drug therapy should be considered in the postpartum period after breastfeeding has ceased. Transplacental transmission is rare. However, infection of the neonate occurs 50% of the time if the mother has active disease because of airborne transmission (Gabbe et al., 1991).

Implications for Nursing Care

Prevention of tuberculosis depends on early identification and treatment of active disease. Thus, nurses working with childbearing populations in which tuberculosis may be prevalent should take active steps to ensure that women and their families are adequately screened for the disease. Women with active tuberculosis during pregnancy must be encouraged to comply with the treatment regimen. This prevents the possibility of spreading the disease to their neonate in the postpartum period.

Teratogenic Infections

Teratogenic (formerly called TORCH) infections are often discussed collectively. These infections have the ability to actively infect the fetus during pregnancy. The older name TORCH infections was derived from the first letter of each infectious condition: toxoplasmosis; other (syphilis, hepatitis, and HIV); rubella; cytomegalovirus; herpes.

However, a newer label of teratogenic infections has evolved because it describes the risk these infections pose during pregnancy. These infections may or may not be sexually transmitted. However, they all share the ability to infect the fetus. Infection of the fetus and neonate occurs by the virus crossing the placenta or by way of an ascending infection after rupture of the membranes and cervical dilatation.

When the organism crosses the placenta in early pregnancy, the fetus may develop major malformations. If the organism crosses the placenta in the latter half of pregnancy, the neonate may be born with active disease. The neonate has an immature immunologic system. Therefore, an ascending infection may become overwhelmingly systemic, causing encephalitis, meningitis, or both. If the neonate survives, the infant may suffer severe neurologic impairment.

The nurse should be aware of the role viruses play in contemporary health problems. They are more virulent than bacteria, more insidious, less responsive to treatment, and more devastating in their sequelae. These conditions are increasing in incidence and are often difficult to detect in the adult. Teratogenic infections may not be obvious in the neonate until weeks or months after birth. All of these conditions may be diagnosed by testing for a serum antibody titer level that indicates a past or current infectious process.

Table 16-4 describes etiologic factors; diagnosis and treatment; and maternal, fetal, and neonatal implications of teratogenic infections.

Infections of the Urinary Tract

Urinary tract infections (UTIs) are frequent complications of pregnancy and can have serious consequences. Asymptomatic bacteriuria (ASB) is a condition in which significant numbers of bacteria are found on urine culture (greater than 100,000 colonies/mL urine) in the absence of symptoms. Although this condition may not have deleterious consequences in the nonpregnant woman (see Chapter 6), it is more worrisome in pregnancy. Without treatment, 20% to 40% of pregnant women with ASB will go on to develop more

Table 16-4. Teratogenic Infections

Organism and Mode of Transmission	Diagnosis and Treatment	Maternal, Fetal, and Neonatal Implications	Nursing Implications
Rubella			
Virus transmitted via naso-pharyngeal secretions and trans-placentally	Titer of >1:32 indicates immunity from past exposure. Vaccine available but not safe in pregnancy. Communicable 1 wk before and 4 d after rash and mild illness.	If maternal infection in first trimester, 50% of fetuses infected, with resulting abortion, microcephaly, heart defects, cataracts, and deafness.	All women should receive serologic testing prenatally. Those without immunity should avoid exposure, and receive vaccine postpartum. Infected neonate must be isolated due to viral shedding.
Toxoplamosis			
Protozoan transmitted via cat feces and transplacentally	Serologic test required for diagnosis. No treatment known. Maternal illness may be asymptomatic or mild lymphadenopathy and malaise.	If infected in pregnancy, 60% of fetuses infected. Infected neonate may have intrauterine growth retardation, hydrocephalus, microcephaly, mental retardation, chorioretinitis, cerebral calcification.	Pregnant women should avoid exposure to cat feces; use careful handwashing.
Cytomegalovirus			
Member of herpesvirus family; transmitted by body fluids	Virus is ubiquitous, highly contagious in children. Serologic test available, but high rate of false-positive results. Infection is usually asymptomatic. No treatment or immunization available.	Half of woman are infected before pregnancy; 1% will transmit virus to fetus. Neonate may have subclinical to severe disease, including hepatosplenomegaly, pneumonitis, encephalitis, mental retardation. Approximately 10% of asymptomatic neonates develop hearing loss.	Women working with children highly susceptible; should consider limiting exposure in pregnancy. Infected neonate should be isolated due to viral shedding.
Varicella Zoster			
As shingles or chickenpox; member of herpes virus family; spread by droplet or transplacentally	Serologic tests show past exposure. Infectious 1 wk before macular eruption.	If infected between 8–20 wk, congenital anomalies such as limb reduction, cataracts, microcephaly. Neonate can develop severe infection with 10% mortality rate within 5 d of birth.	Women without immunity should receive varicella-zoster immune globulin (VZIG) within 4 d of exposure to prevent maternal complications, but offers no fetal protection. VZIG in exposed neonates may reduce complications. Isolate exposed newborn.
Parvovirus			
Transmitted by droplet or transplacentally	Serologic test for immunity; 30%–60% of adults test positive and are immune. No treatment available. Mild erythematous rash, fever, joint pain.	Rare reports of abortion; fetal hydrops may result from disrupted erythrocyte development; anemia and congestive heart failure. Maternal drop in hematocrit due to disruption in erythrocyte precursor development.	Women working with children may benefit from prenatal testing and limiting exposure in pregnancy.
Streptococcus B			
Mode of perinatal transmission unclear	Can be isolated by culture; present in cervical and vaginal secretions of 35% of women. Treatment with antibiotics prenatally not effective in preventing neonatal infection.	Most common cause of neonatal sepsis and meningitis. Transmission at delivery from infected woman in 1% of neonates.	With rupture of membranes and onset of labor, women with documented streptococcus B receive IV antibiotics to decrease neonatal infection.

From Gabbe, S., Niebyl, J., & Simpson, J. (1991). *Obstetrics: Normal and problem pregnancies.* New York: Churchill Livingstone; ACOG (1992). *Hepatitis in pregnancy* (No. 174). ACOG Technical Bulletin. Washington, DC: Author.

serious infection, including pyelonephritis (North, Speed, & Weiner, 1990).

Cystitis in the pregnant woman generally is associated with some combination of dysuria, frequency, urgency, suprapubic pain, increased nocturia, and occasionally, hematuria. A low-grade fever may be present.

Pyelonephritis in pregnancy is a more serious complication. Generally, onset of pyelonephritis is marked by sudden onset of chills and fever. Costovertebral angle pain, often on the right side, is a sign of pyelonephritis. Malaise, nausea, vomiting, and lack of appetite may be present. When pyelonephritis is accompanied by a lower UTI, the woman may complain of frequency, urgency, and dysuria. Pyelonephritis is most common in the latter part of pregnancy and often is the result of an unidentified and untreated lower UTI.

Etiologic and Predisposing Factors

The normal physiologic changes that accompany pregnancy place the woman at risk for urinary stasis and infection. These changes include:

- Slight enlargement of the kidneys
- Dilation of renal pelves and ureters
- Elongation of the ureters
- Changes in bladder position
- Changes in urine composition, such as glucosuria, which support bacterial growth

Diagnosis

Diagnosis of UTI is made on the basis of the history, clinical symptoms, and urine culture results. Typically, a single organism is responsible for asymptomatic bacteriuria. *Escherichia coli* is the most common infective organism. Urine cultures may also show the presence of *Klebsiella* and *Proteus* species.

Diagnosis of pyelonephritis is made on the basis of clinical symptoms, urinalysis, and urine culture. Urinalysis will usually show the presence of white blood cell casts. Multiple organisms are usually present in the urine in pyelonephritis. Blood cultures may be drawn to evaluate the possibility of sepsis.

Treatment

Pregnant women with asymptomatic bacteriuria can be safely treated with nitrofurantoin, ampicillin, cephalosporins, and short-acting sulfa drugs. Sulfa compounds are generally avoided near term because they interfere with protein binding of bilirubin in the fetus and may cause hyperbilirubinemia in the neonate. Treatment of lower UTIs should be followed by a repeat culture to verify that bacteria are no longer present in the urine.

Upper UTI or pyelonephritis is usually treated more aggressively. There are increased risks to the pregnant woman and the fetus. Usually, the woman is hospitalized, and intravenous fluids and antibiotics are administered. Bed rest is required, and pain medication is often prescribed.

Maternal, Fetal, and Neonatal Implications

Asymptomatic bacteriuria and cystitis, when promptly treated, generally do not result in problems for the pregnant woman or the fetus. Although less common, pyelonephritis is much more serious and can be life threatening. Maternal sepsis, premature labor, and intrauterine growth retardation can result from inadequately treated or untreated pyelonephritis in pregnancy.

Implications for Nursing Care

Infections of the urinary tract are common in pregnancy. The nurse has a particularly important responsibility to ensure that women are adequately screened. It is imperative that treatment is initiated promptly when infection is diagnosed. A careful initial assessment as well as ongoing assessments of the woman's urinary status are an important part of quality prenatal care.

• • Assessment

Because UTIs can occur in pregnancy without the usual clinical symptoms, the nurse should be certain that every pregnant woman is screened for bacteriuria during the course of prenatal care. This can be done reliably and inexpensively with a dipstick test. The nurse should inquire at each prenatal visit about the presence of any signs or symptoms of UTI.

• • Nursing Diagnosis

The following nursing diagnoses may be applicable in the care of the pregnant woman with a suspected or actual UTI:

- Fear related to diagnosis of infection and increased pregnancy risk
- Pain related to dysuria

• • Planning and Implementation

The nurse follows up on any reports of urinary symptoms to ensure that physical examination and a clean-catch urinalysis is completed immediately. The woman should be given a careful explanation of the importance of completing the prescribed course of antibiotics. The nurse teaches the pregnant woman about the signs of recurring infection and other warning signs during pregnancy (see Chapter 15).

The nurse instructs the woman on self-care techniques that will aid recovery from infection and prevent reinfection, such as:

- Maintaining adequate fluid intake of at least eight (8-oz) glasses of water a day
- Voiding frequently and when the urge to void occurs
- Wiping from front to back after bowel movements
- Voiding before and after intercourse
- Wearing cotton-lined underwear to keep perineal area dry
- Avoiding carbohydrate "binges" that contribute to glucosuria

Expected Outcomes

- The pregnant woman with symptoms of UTI seeks immediate care.

- The pregnant woman verbalizes symptoms of UTI and importance of early treatment.
- The pregnant woman with UTI states she has decreased the frequency of carbohydrate "binges" as a self-care technique to prevent glycosuria.

• • Evaluation

The nurse evaluates the woman's response to medical management once UTI is identified and treated. The nurse can assist the woman in self-care practices that will speed recovery and prevent recurrence. It is important for the nurse to evaluate the woman's urinary status on an ongoing basis because reinfection is common.

Sexually Transmitted Diseases

Sexually transmitted diseases were discussed in the context of women's health in Chapter 6. Refer to that chapter for detailed discussion of etiologic and predisposing factors and diagnostic procedures for these conditions.

The presence of STD in pregnancy can result in serious perinatal complications. The following section discusses STDs, presents medical treatment in pregnancy, and discusses implications for maternal, fetal, and neonatal well-being. Finally, implications for nursing care of the pregnant woman with an STD will be discussed.

Chlamydia

Chlamydial infections are the most common form of STD. More than half of all women have no clinical signs or symptoms, and rates among pregnant women range from 5% to 30% (Gabbe et al., 1991).

Etiologic and Predisposing Factors

Chlamydia shows an affinity for the squamocolumnar junction of the cervix. Adolescent women are at particular risk because of the prominence of this region of the cervix.

Diagnosis

Women with chlamydial infections are often asymptomatic. If symptoms are noted, they include mucopurulent vaginal discharge, postcoital bleeding, and diffuse low abdominal pain. Chlamydial infection is impossible to distinguish from gonorrhea on the basis of clinical signs. Further, chlamydial infection frequently coexists with gonorrhea, so concomitant testing for gonorrhea is standard. Diagnosis of chlamydia is made by cervical culture.

Treatment

Treatment for chlamydial infection during pregnancy is unchanged from that for the nonpregnant woman. Generally, treatment is a 10-day course of erythromycin, tetracycline, or doxycycline. The pregnant woman should be advised that reinfection is possible and that sexual partners should be screened and treated, as needed.

Maternal, Fetal, and Neonatal Implications

Chlamydial infection during pregnancy has been associated with premature rupture of membranes, preterm labor and birth, and low birth weight (Gabbe et al., 1991). The neonate can be infected during passage through the birth canal. Neonatal complications from untreated infection may include conjunctivitis, pneumonitis, asthma, and chronic otitis media.

Herpes Genitalis

Herpes genitalis (or herpes simplex virus or HSV) has become a major cause of STD. There is no treatment for HSV. Therefore, it has long-term implications for the pregnant woman who becomes infected. However, the more serious implications are for the neonate.

Etiologic and Predisposing Factors

The herpesvirus is spread through intimate, usually sexual contact. The virus enters the body through a mucosal surface such as the mouth, cervix, or conjunctiva or through small cracks in the skin. The infection is most common in European Americans between the ages of 15 and 35 years. Those with multiple sexual partners and those who do not use condoms are at significantly greater risk.

Diagnosis

Diagnosis is generally made on the basis of clinical symptoms. Testing to verify the diagnosis can be done using a Pap smear, enzyme-linked immunosorbent assays (ELISA), and cultures.

Treatment

There is no treatment for HSV infection. Acyclovir orally or in ointments to speed healing of lesions is not recommended during pregnancy because drug safety in pregnancy has not been established.

The following are recommendations for obstetric management of the pregnant woman with HSV infection to prevent neonatal infection:

- In any pregnant woman with suspicious lesions, the lesions should be cultured for HSV. Lesions in pregnant women with a history of HSV should be cultured weekly as delivery approaches, and the woman should be observed carefully for presence of vulvar lesions.
- If a woman with documented HSV infection has no visible lesions at onset of labor, vaginal delivery is acceptable. Presence of lesions requires cesarean delivery if labor begins or membranes rupture (ACOG, 1988).

Maternal, Fetal, and Neonatal Implications

Because pregnancy can act as an activator of HSV, pregnant women with active HSV lesions must be counseled about the use of safe sexual practices. Although complications of HSV infection, such as meningitis, encephalitis, arthritis, hepatitis, endometritis, and thrombocytopenia, have been noted in pregnant women, they are extremely rare.

Fetal and neonatal implications of maternal HSV infection are serious. Infection may occur in utero, by transplacental or ascending infection. Transplacental or ascending infections are rare, and no preventive measures currently exist. Exposure to vaginal lesions during delivery is more common.

Neonatal herpes is a serious complication that can result in disability or death and affects 1 in 7500 births (see Chapter 33). This infection can produce significant central nervous system damage, resulting in mental retardation and other brain abnormalities. Localized damage to the eye and skin are possible outcomes of neonatal herpes.

The neonate at greatest risk is one born during the primary episode of maternal genital infection although this occurs rarely. Infection of the neonate is more likely to occur during a secondary episode (see Chapter 6). Infection of the neonate usually occurs from exposure to a viral lesion in the vagina during delivery or from maternal contact in the immediate postpartum period (Jenkins & Kohl, 1992).

Condyloma Acuminata (Human Papilloma Virus)

Condyloma acuminata (genital warts) are caused by human papilloma virus (HPV) infection. Such infections are relatively common, with an incidence of 50/100,000 population.

Etiologic and Predisposing Factors

The virus is transmitted through sexual contact. Infectivity of this virus is high, with 50% to 70% infection rates found in sexual partners of infected individuals (Nettina & Kaufman, 1990). Individuals with multiple sexual partners and who engage in intercourse without condoms are at increased risk.

Diagnosis

Symptoms of HPV include the development of soft, gray, wartlike lesions in the genital area. Some women who report symptoms of recurrent vaginal infections unresponsive to treatment may have microscopic lesions. These lesions cannot be detected by clinical inspection (Tinkle, 1990).

Diagnosis may be made on clinical appearance alone or with the help of a Pap smear or biopsy, because it is important to differentiate condyloma from other lesions, some of which may be malignant. Careful cervical screening is necessary because of the association of HPV with precancerous changes in the cervix.

Treatment

Treatment of HPV focuses on reducing or removing the condyloma and preventing reinfection. Lesions may grow dramatically during pregnancy due to hormonal effects and immunosuppression. Cryotherapy or laser therapy may be used to remove the growths or significantly reduce their size. Sexual partners should be screened for infection and treated, as needed.

Maternal, Fetal, and Neonatal Implications

In pregnancy, condyloma acuminata may grow more rapidly and become extensive. Use of cytotoxic agents such as podophyllin or 5-fluorouracil are contraindicated because they have been associated with preterm labor and fetal death. The neonate may become infected during passage through the birth canal or may contract the infection in utero. Laryngeal papillomata may develop in some children born to women with HPV (Smith, Johnson, Cripe, Pignatari, & Turek, 1991).

Gonorrhea

Like syphilis, gonorrhea has become an endemic disease in minority populations in the United States. One million cases are reported in the United States annually. The prevalence of infection in pregnant women ranges from 0.5% to 7%, depending on the population studied (Csonka, 1990).

Etiologic and Predisposing Factors

Gonorrhea is transmitted by sexual contact. Risk factors for this infection include low socioeconomic status, urban residence, early onset of sexual activity, and multiple sexual partners.

Diagnosis

Definitive diagnosis of gonorrhea is made on the basis of cultures from the urethra, cervix, or rectum. Because gonorrhea is often asymptomatic in women, cervical cultures for this infection are routinely done as part of prenatal care.

Treatment

Treatment during pregnancy is similar to that for infected nonpregnant women. Treatment is likely to include a one-time administration of ceftriaxone intramuscularly and a 7-day course of erythromycin. Pregnant women should be advised of the need for abstinence or use of condoms until cure has been verified by repeat cervical culture. The woman's partners should be screened and treated, if necessary.

Maternal, Fetal, and Neonatal Implications

The most significant risk of untreated gonorrhea in women is the risk of progressive infection. Untreated infection can result in PID (see Chapter 6) and creates the potential for subsequent scarring of the fallopian tubes. Because ascending infection generally occurs during or after menstruation, infected pregnant women may be relatively protected from ascending infection. Further, if infection occurs after the third month of pregnancy, the cervical mucous plug appears to prevent ascending infection. However, gonococcal infection of the chorioamnion can occur and may lead to preterm labor, chorioamnionitis, and postpartum endometritis (Gabbe et al., 1991). Infection of the neonate can result in gonococcal ophthalmia neonatorum (see Chapter 33). Prophylactic administration of erythromycin or tetracycline ophthalmic preparations is required by law in most states.

Syphilis

Syphilis is reemerging as an endemic disease among minority heterosexual populations in the United States. For this reason, serologic testing of all pregnant women at the initial prenatal screening and again in the third trimester is recommended.

Etiologic and Predisposing Factors

Syphilis is caused by the spirochete *Treponema pallidum*. Between 1986 and 1990, the number of reported cases doubled to a total of 49,000, including 1747 cases of congenital syphilis in infants of infected mothers (Tillman, 1992).

Diagnosis

Diagnosis is made on the basis of blood tests, such as the VDRL (Venereal Disease Research Laboratories), RPR (rapid plasma reagin), or the FTA-ABS (fluorescent treponemal antibody absorption test). Screening for syphilis is a routine part of prenatal care. The VDRL and RPR are nonspecific tests for syphilis; false-positive results on these tests can be caused by pregnancy. The FTA-ABS is a more specific test for syphilis. For this reason, this test may be used to confirm a positive VDRL or RPR test.

Treatment

Treatment of syphilis during pregnancy is the same as for nonpregnant women, that is, with benzathine penicillin G. One month after treatment is completed, serology tests should be obtained in a series. Treatment is successful if maternal titers decrease over three tests.

Maternal, Fetal, and Neonatal Implications

Untreated syphilis puts the pregnant woman at risk for progression to the systemic form of the disease as described in Chapter 6. Infection during pregnancy places the fetus at risk for congenital syphilis. The risk of transmitting the infection depends on the stage of maternal disease. Risk of transmission to the fetus has been estimated at 50% in primary or secondary syphilis, declining to 10% in late syphilis.

Transmission to the fetus is blocked by a layer of chorion up until 16 to 18 weeks' gestation. However, this layer begins to atrophy after that point, thus making transmission possible.

If maternal infection is treated before 18 weeks, there are rarely any fetal effects. However, if treatment is delayed, fetal consequences are severe. In one of four cases, fetal death by midtrimester spontaneous abortion or stillbirth will occur once the fetus is infected. In utero fetal infection can also cause intrauterine growth retardation and preterm labor (Gabbe et al., 1991). The neonate with congenital syphilis presents with unexplained rhinitis, hepatosplenomegaly, and dermal rash (see Chapter 33).

Human Immunodeficiency Virus

Infection with HIV, which causes acquired immunodeficiency syndrome (AIDS), is a growing problem among pregnant women. In 1989, 1.5 in each 1000 women giving birth were HIV infected (ACOG, 1992). AIDS has become one of the leading causes of death in children, and over 80% of children with HIV acquire the infection in utero (Butler, 1991).

Relatively little is known about the progression of the disease in pregnant women. To date, no conclusive evidence indicates that pregnancy accelerates the course of the disease or that HIV affects pregnancy outcomes during early stages of the disease. Rather, available evidence suggests that outcomes of pregnancy in HIV-infected women and the subsequent progression of the disease are more directly related to how advanced maternal disease was at the time of pregnancy (Tinkle, Amaya, & Tamayo, 1992).

Etiologic and Predisposing Factors

The major mode of transmission of the HIV virus in women is unprotected heterosexual intercourse with infected men. Risk factors for HIV infection include unsafe sexual practices, needle sharing, and the presence of other STDs, which appears to allow a portal of entry for the virus through inflammation and lesions caused by the STD.

Diagnosis

The prenatal medical, social, and sexual history may provide clues to risk factors for HIV (history of intravenous drug use, sex with a bisexual man or intravenous drug user, history of prostitution, history of multiple sexual partners, and unprotected intercourse). Initial screening is possible with the use of ELISA tests. A positive test detects the antibody to HIV and indicates past or present infection. False-positive ELISA results can be a result of autoimmune disease, a history of multiple pregnancies, or multiple transfusions. False-negative ELISA results can result from blood testing after infection but before serum antibodies appear or late in the disease. When an ELISA test is positive, a Western blot test is administered to eliminate false-positive results.

Clinical signs of HIV infection in women include vaginal or esophageal moniliasis, HSV disease, and general physical debilitation and wasting (Hankins & Handley, 1992). Screening for hepatitis B, cytomegalovirus, and tuberculosis should be performed. These conditions are frequently found in HIV-infected women and require treatment.

Treatment

There is no cure at present for HIV and AIDS. Recent research indicates that zidovudine (AZT) is well tolerated by pregnant women, and there is no evidence of negative effects on perinatal outcomes (Sperling et al., 1992). AZT may delay the progression of symptoms, but the effect of AZT on the risk of perinatal transmission of the virus to the fetus is unknown. Side effects of AZT include anemia, thrombocytopenia, and granulocytopenia as a result of bone marrow suppression. Pregnant women with HIV may be given blood transfusions if hemoglobin levels fall below 11 g/dL. (Tinkle et al., 1992).

Other treatment to prevent opportunistic infections may be recommended. The most common of these infections is *Pneumocystis carinii* pneumonia (PCP). Currently available drugs that appear to be effective in preventing PCP include trimethoprim with sulfamethoxazole and aerosol pentamidine isethionate. Information on the fetal effects of these drugs is limited (Tinkle et al., 1992).

Maternal, Fetal, and Neonatal Implications

Some evidence indicates that pregnancy may hasten the progression of HIV and AIDS in women who are already symptomatic (Efantis & Sinclair, 1990). Other implications of infection for the pregnant woman include possible loss of employment and health insurance, denial of health care, social isolation, and anguish in regard to her own future and her fetus. Perinatal transmission of HIV from the pregnant woman to the fetus is reported to be 40%. The risk of transmission may increase in the presence of advanced maternal disease (Fletcher, 1990; Butler, 1991).

Because AZT readily crosses the placenta, there is the possibility of suppression of fetal bone marrow with resultant fetal anemia and intrauterine growth retardation. Because HIV-infected pregnant women are considered at high risk for poor pregnancy outcomes, fetal surveillance is critical. Careful monitoring of fetal growth and biophysical profiles are important tools in evaluating fetal status. After 32 weeks of gestation, weekly nonstress testing may be recommended. More invasive procedures, such as amniocentesis, should be carefully considered and discussed with the pregnant woman because they increase the risk of infecting a noninfected fetus with HIV (Efantis & Sinclair, 1990).

Implications for Nursing Care

The major goals of care for the HIV-infected women during the intrapartum and postpartum periods are preventing and identifying maternal, fetal, and neonatal complications, providing psychosocial support, and preventing nosocomial infection (see the Nursing Care Plan). Care for the asymptomatic women differs little from standard intrapartum and postpartum care. However, the woman with symptomatic HIV will require more sophisticated medical and nursing support to allow for safe delivery for the woman and the fetus.

Hemorrhage and infection are two major concerns. Women with HIV disease are often thrombocytopenic and anemic, and additional blood loss stresses an already stressed physiologic system. Infection is a significant concern because the woman's immune system is already compromised. Invasive procedures such as urinary catheterization, intravenous fluid administration, and vaginal examinations can all place the woman at increased risk for nosocomial infection.

Breastfeeding represents another source of HIV transmission, and women infected with HIV are not encouraged to breastfeed (Porcher, 1992). Diagnosis of HIV infection cannot be made reliably in the infant prior to 15 months because the presence of maternal antibodies can result in a positive antibody test in the infant.

Progression of HIV and AIDS appears to be more rapid in children. The main clinical features of AIDS in children are failure to thrive, high recurrent fever, persistent cough, chronic diarrhea, recurrent respiratory infections, hepatosplenomegaly, generalized lymphadenopathy, and oral candidiasis. Children with an early onset of opportunistic infection and severe encephalopathy may have a survival rate of less than 50% at 3 years of age (Blanche et al., 1990).

Until an effective treatment or cure is found for HIV and AIDS, prevention must be a major nursing priority. Education about risk factors for STDs of all types, including HIV and AIDS, is necessary before individuals become sexually active and must be targeted to the learning needs of specific identifiable groups. The accompanying Nursing Research display describes research on self-identification of risk status for HIV among a population of pregnant women.

Implications for Nursing Care

The diagnosis of an STD during pregnancy can be a particularly disturbing experience. The pregnant woman with an STD may have concerns about her relationship with her partner and about her own well-being and that of the fetus. The following section addresses general guidelines for nursing care of the pregnant woman with an STD.

• • Assessment

The nurse is responsible for conducting a thorough and sensitive health history and is in a position to identify pregnant women at risk for STDs. The nurse should be alert for signs and symptoms of STDS and should be certain that women are evaluated promptly if symptoms are present. Screening for some STDs is a standard part of prenatal care (see previous display on Prenatal Screening for Infection). The nurse should remember that, in many cases, pregnant women with STDs are asymptomatic and that only routine screening will identify infection in them. A pregnant woman should also be evaluated for the presence of STD if she requests screening or if she reports the following symptoms:

- Increased or malodorous vaginal discharge
- Vulvar itching
- Dysuria
- Dyspareunia
- Bleeding after sexual intercourse
- Presence of any sore or lesion in the genital area

• • Nursing Diagnosis

The following nursing diagnoses may be applicable in the care of a pregnant woman with a suspected or diagnosed STD:

- Fear related to increased risk to self and fetus
- Ineffective Individual Coping related to strain on sexual relationship as a result of STD exposure
- Situational Low Self-esteem related to shame and guilt regarding STD diagnosis
- High Risk for Recurrent STD Infection

• • Planning and Implementation

The nurse caring for a pregnant woman with an STD is responsible for verifying that appropriate treatment and follow-up are initiated, providing education to reduce risk of reinfection, and providing psychological support as needed.

Based on the nurse's assessment of the woman's knowledge about STDs, information about safe sexual practices and avoidance of STDs is reviewed with the pregnant woman. The nurse provides information about the disease, its transmission, treatment and follow-up plans, and the nature of risk (if any) to the woman and fetus.

The nurse should remind the woman that the full course of medical therapy should be carried out because disappearance of symptoms does not indicate that the infection has been eliminated. The woman should be encouraged to have her sexual partner screened and treated, if necessary. The importance of avoiding reinfection, both for her own health as well as for the fetus, should be stressed.

The nurse can provide psychological support by listening and responding to the woman's questions and concerns in a nonjudgmental and matter-of-fact way. If the woman is diagnosed with a condition that cannot be treated (herpes, HIV), the nurse should be prepared to maintain supportive

Nursing Care Plan

The Pregnant Woman With HIV Infection

PATIENT PROFILE

History

R.S. is a 26-year-old G3/P2 at 22 weeks' gestation. She is a divorced mother living in subsidized housing with her two children, ages 4 and 2. She states that her ex-husband is the biologic father in current pregnancy as well. She was diagnosed with HIV infection 2 months ago at prenatal intake with current pregnancy. Probable source of infection is ex-husband who is IV drug user for 10 years. R.S. has one symptom suggestive of HIV infection, a vaginal moniliasis identified at last visit and treated successfully. She continues to come in for regular prenatal care and social work assistance. R.S. reports feeling "so depressed about everything . . . I can't even think about not being around for my babies." R.S. is tremulous, quiet and appears to be tired.

Physical Assessment

R.S. demonstrates weight gain and uterine size appropriate for gestation. Reports no symptoms of vaginal moniliasis since treatment. No evidence of oral candidiasis noted.

COLLABORATIVE PROBLEMS/POTENTIAL COMPLICATIONS

- Recurrent monilial infection
- Maternal anemia, thrombocytopenia
- HIV wasting syndrome
- IUFD, fetal compromise

(See the accompanying Nursing Alert display.)

Assessment	*Nursing Diagnosis*	*Nursing Interventions*	*Rationale*
R.S. reports depression, difficulty sleeping; concern about future of children as her condition worsens.	Fear related to anticipated worsening of health status.	Acknowledge verbal and nonverbal expressions of grief and anger.	Conveys support, may help to decrease sense of isolation. Validates reality or R.S.'s situation.
	Anticipatory Grieving related to future loss of life.	Encourage expression of negative emotions.	
	Expected Outcome R.S. will demonstrate movement through grieving process.	Provide caring physical presence and prevent emotional isolation.	
		Encourage self-care activities and concrete plans for future.	Reinforces future planning as R.S. appears to be ready for these activities.
	R.S. will interact with others without marked and prolonged withdrawal.	Assess available support systems. Discuss with R.S. how to mobilize those supports as needed.	Mobilization of support systems will be necessary for care of self and children as disease worsens.
		Provide information as desired; correct misconceptions regarding prognosis but avoid destroying hope.	
R.S. asks about whether fetus can be tested for HIV "now"; questions her own decision to continue pregnancy. Expresses concerns about transmitting HIV to newborn.	Fear related to potential transmission of HIV to fetus.	Acknowledge legitimacy of fears.	Risk of prenatal transmission of HIV to fetus cannot be predicted, but transmission after delivery can be prevented.
	Decisional Conflict related to continuation of pregnancy with HIV infection.	Discuss facts regarding transplacental and postpartum transmission.	HIV-infected women must be provided caring and sensitive support as they make decisions regarding pregnancy. If such support is not provided, they may discontinue or delay needed health care.
	Expected Outcome R.S. will discuss her fears openly with nursing staff and expresses some relief of concerns after doing so.	Allow reexploration of decision.	
	R.S. will use nursing staff as support system in process of decision making about continuation of pregnancy.	Express willingness to support her decision and implement arrangements as needed.	

(*Continued*)

The Pregnant Woman With HIV Infection

(Continued)

Assessment	*Nursing Diagnosis*	*Nursing Interventions*	*Rationale*
R.S. is in asymptomatic stage of HIV. She is maintaining AZT regimen as prescribed (100 mg × 5 daily). She maintains regular prenatal care visits.	Health Seeking Behavior (preventive behavior) related to HIV/AIDS progression and pregnancy. ***Expected Outcome*** R.S. will remain free of infection. R.S. will maintain adequate weight gain during pregnancy.	Reinforce positive health behaviors. Advise R.S. about self-care in regard to prevention of infections. Assess carefully for signs of infection: cough, elevated temperature, lymphadenopathy.	Infections are major cause of deterioration and death in HIV-infected pregnant women.
		Assess for side-effects of AZT: anemia, thrombocytopenia, nausea and vomiting.	Medications for HIV may have side-effects that may affect maternal well-being during pregnancy.
R.S. states she is worried about whether the fetus will "grow."	Fear related to potential fetal compromise. ***Expected Outcome*** The fetus will show normal growth pattern and normal response to nonstress testing.	Reinforce positive behaviors.	Optimal nutritional status is especially important to ensure adequate maternal weight gain.
		Assess weight gain and dietary intake carefully.	Weight loss or failure to gain with more than adequate dietary intake may suggest HIV wasting syndrome in absence of other causes.
		Discuss plans for weekly nonstress testing in third trimester.	Careful fetal surveillance needed in third trimester to evaluate fetal growth and possible effects of maternal disease and medication.
R.S. states she is worried about who will care for her children during hospitalization for delivery.	Anxiety about future child care needs. ***Expected Outcome*** R.S. will state she feels less anxious knowing she will have child care while she is hospitalized.	Assist R.S. to plan for transportation and child care needs during third trimester. Advise social service of increasing transportation needs.	Concerns about child care are a major stressor for HIV-infected women, and suitable child care is often difficult for women to arrange without assistance.

EVALUATION

R.S. agrees to attend support group for HIV-infected women upon advice of nurse. Data collected from telephone follow-up initiated by nurse after first support meeting suggest that R.S. found the group helpful in regard to her concerns and worries about her family. R.S. continues to maintain regular prenatal visits, and remains free of signs/symptoms of opportunistic infection. Weight gain continues within normal limits by gestational age. At 28 weeks of gestation, weekly nonstress testing is begun to monitor fetal status. At 37 weeks, RS calls to report her membranes have ruptured. She arranges for friends from her support group to care for her children, and is admitted for evaluation. After 24 hours of observation, R.S. and her physician agree to begin induction of labor. After 17 hours of oxytocin induction, R.S. delivers a 2890 g (6 lb, 6 oz) male infant without complications. R.S. is discharged home at 3 days with her infant. The discharge planning nurse arranged for homemaker services for 1 week postpartum to allow R.S. to rest and recover. Perinatal nursing staff arrange for transfer of R.S.'s care to the HIV clinic after her 6-week checkup.

NURSING ALERT

SIGNS AND SYMPTOMS OF OPPORTUNISTIC INFECTION IN HIV-INFECTED PREGNANT WOMEN

The nurse should remember that pregnancy is associated with more rapid development of AIDS in women, and that women sometimes have subtle and nonspecific signs of worsening HIV infection. The pregnant HIV-infected woman is more susceptible to a range of infections, including *Candida* (vaginal and oral infection), toxoplasmosis, herpes simplex, hepatitis, and pneumocystis.

The pregnant woman with HIV should be counseled about avoiding exposure to all forms of infection. Consideration of the risks to her own health and that of others posed by sexual activity should be discussed. The woman with children may need assistance with child care arrangements (such as avoiding placing her children in group care, where exposure to infection is high). This will help to minimize risk of exposure. The nurse can stress the importance of handwashing, proper nutrition, and rest in preventing infection.

The HIV-infected pregnant woman should recognize the following signs of infection and seek immediate medical care:

- Unusual fatigue, loss of appetite
- Fever, cough, sore throat, night sweats
- Illness of unknown origin in children or other intimate contacts.

contact with the woman or refer her to other resources to assist her in coping with the implications of the diagnosis.

The nurse also works with the woman and other care providers to plan for labor and delivery if the woman's diagnosis requires it. Women diagnosed with HIV, herpes, and other viral STDs may require anticipatory guidance in regard to fetal evaluation, surveillance for viral lesions, and planned cesarean delivery if circumstances require.

Expected Outcomes

- The pregnant woman with an STD explains the nature of the diagnosis and its implications for her fetus, her own health, and her sexual partners.
- The pregnant woman with an STD states the importance of the treatment plan.
- The woman's sexual partner seeks screening and appropriate treatment.
- The woman discusses her problems with self-esteem.
- The pregnant woman with an STD of a chronic or long-term nature uses available services appropriately for ongoing care.

• • Evaluation

The nurse evaluates the pregnant woman's response to the proposed plan of care and modifies the plan as needed. The nurse should follow up to verify that treatment has been

Nursing Research

Self-Identification of Risk for HIV and AIDS in Pregnant Women

Women of childbearing age are increasingly recognized as a group at risk for HIV infection and AIDS. However, in many cases, educational programs about HIV infection and risk reduction target adult populations in general and are not specifically designed for women of childbearing age or for pregnant women. A survey was conducted by nurse researchers to determine the extent to which pregnant women receiving care at a military medical center were well-informed about their relative risk for HIV infection.

A questionnaire was administered to 700 pregnant women, asking questions that assessed knowledge, attitudes, beliefs, and self-identification of risk. Over 80% of the sample were military dependents, and the remainder were women who were active duty military. The average age of the respondents was 23 years, and the majority (49%) were European American.

The findings of the survey showed clearly that most women (58%) did not regard themselves as being at risk. However, 29% regarded themselves as being at some risk, yet only 8% in fact reported a specific risk factor for the disease. This suggested that some women had misinformation about specific risks for the disease and may be overestimating their own risk.

Over 90% of the women reported a desire for more information about HIV and its prevention. The survey also showed that women with less formal education and Hispanic women were most likely to have misinformation or inadequate information about HIV prevention.

The investigators suggested that a needs assessment approach may be useful in identifying clinical populations in particular need of focused HIV and AIDS health education efforts. This would enable nurses to use available resources efficiently to provide the information to those who need it most in a manner tailored to that group's specific needs. They conclude that health education is the most effective and economical weapon for combating the spread of AIDS among women during their childbearing years.

McNicol, L., Hadersbeck, R., Dickens, D., & Brown, J. (1991). AIDS and pregnancy: Survey of knowledge, attitudes, beliefs, and self-identification of risk. *Journal of Obstetric, Gynecologic, and Neonatal Nursing, 20*(1), 65–72.

successful, that the woman's sexual partners have been advised to seek screening and treatment, and that the woman is using self-care strategies to avoid reinfection.

A decreased immunologic response to infection is one of the normal physiologic adaptations to pregnancy. Thus, infections are a major source of perinatal morbidity and neonatal mortality. Careful identification must be made of women at risk for infection so that the pathogen can be isolated. Because antibiotics cross the placenta, consideration of the fetus must be made when prescribing therapy. Infections may be systemic (such as hepatitis, tuberculosis, teratogens), UTIs, or STDS (chlamydia, herpes, condyloma acuminata, gonorrhea, syphilis, HIV, and AIDS). Nurses are responsible for gathering a complete health history that will help identify women at risk for infection. Part of the nursing responsibility may be to teach the pregnant woman how to prevent infections; what the outcomes of infections may be to the woman, her fetus, and her neonate; and how to care for herself if the condition is chronic.

Perinatal Substance Use and Abuse

Chemical addiction and illegal drug use are significant perinatal problems. Both create significant risk to maternal and fetal well-being. The global use of illegal drugs has risen dramatically over the past 25 years, until it has reached epidemic proportions in some areas of the world. It is estimated that Americans consume 60% of the world's illicit drugs. The total number of women using both legal and illegal drugs during pregnancy is approximately 10% to 15%. The incidence is much higher among some groups. Several studies have discovered rates of substance abuse approaching 20% or higher in poor women living in decaying urban areas (Evans, 1991).

Chemical addiction is defined as a mental and physical state resulting from an interaction between the living organism and the drug. Addiction is characterized by a compulsion to take the drug to experience positive euphoric effects or to avoid the physical or emotional discomfort that occurs with abstinence (Buckley, 1990). Some experts define chemical addiction as a chronic disease with lifelong implications for treatment and prevention of recurrence. Nurses working in all areas of perinatal and child health encounter problems related to perinatal substance use and abuse.

The consequences of drug use pose both immediate emergencies and long-term and permanent disabilities. The physical, emotional, and economic costs of perinatal substance abuse are devastating. Medical costs related to perinatal cocaine use exceed $500 million dollars each year (Phibbs, Bateman, & Schwartz, 1991). The ability to provide appropriate care and services is often complicated by economic constraints and major legal and ethical considerations. Current inadequacies in the medical management of chemical addiction, particularly during pregnancy, compound the difficulties inherent in caring for women who abuse drugs during the perinatal period.

Etiologic and Predisposing Factors

The underlying causes for chemical addiction are only partly understood. Several theories have been proposed to explain an individual's predilection to the use and abuse of drugs. These include biologic, psychological, and environmental explanations. Currently, arguments in favor of a biopsychosocial model have gained ground. A genetic predisposition to drug use and chemical dependency may be expressed when the person experiences psychological stressors or environmental pressures.

Research has identified a genetic marker for alcoholism. Specific biologic characteristics of the drug used will also influence the likelihood of physical and psychological addiction. Nicotine and crack cocaine, for instance, are known to have strong physical addictive properties. In contrast, marijuana (cannabis) is more likely to result in psychological dependence.

The crack cocaine epidemic provides a model for the biopsychosocial theory of chemical dependency. The use of crack cocaine reached epidemic proportions during the 1980s in part because of its relatively low cost, wide availability, addictive properties, and the social climate of despair fueled by poverty. Initial lack of knowledge about the drug and its effects, combined with limited financial resources for research, education, and treatment, resulted in rapid spread of crack cocaine to all levels of society.

Diagnosis

The diagnosis of substance use and chemical addiction during the perinatal period is often based on presenting signs and symptoms. Although "hard core" addiction may be easily recognized by the health care provider, so-called recreational drug use, such as occasional smoking of marijuana or snorting cocaine, may be overlooked. The use of illicit substances commonly preferred by adolescents (amphetamines, marijuana, alcohol, and inhalants) is often missed in pregnant teenagers.

Many signs and symptoms of substance abuse are related to the specific action, common side effects, and adverse reactions of the drugs used. Life-style changes secondary to drug-seeking behavior, such as criminal activity and prostitution, are common. The woman's physical condition will deteriorate as a result of poor nutrition and hygiene, infection, adverse effects of the drug, and physical violence. Characteristics of "hard core" drug use are generally evident to health professionals. However, in the early stages of the disease, obvious signs of drug abuse or dependency may be absent. Subtle signs of drug use may be difficult to identify (see the accompanying display).

The woman may deny drug use despite strong indicators of chemical dependency. She may be unable to provide a reliable history of substance abuse. The diagnosis may be confirmed in some cases by toxicology screening tests. The most commonly used test involves maternal or neonatal urinalysis (urine toxicology screen). Advances in technology permit detection of drugs in samples of maternal and neonatal hair or meconium stool. Because hair growth is slow and meconium is produced by the second trimester, these methods provide long-term data on drug use.

The prevalence of perinatal substance abuse has led to

Signs and Symptoms of Chemical Addiction and Recreational Drug Use During Pregnancy

Chemical Addiction ("Hard Core") Use

Physical Signs

- Emaciated, poor weight gain
- Poor hygiene, strong body odor
- Skin infections, abscesses, cellulitis, skin parasites
- Track marks with intravenous injection
- Pinpoint pupils (with narcotic use)
- Rhinitis, sinusitis, polyps, and conjunctivitis (with cocaine freebasing and heavy marijuana use)
- Nasal septum perforation (with intranasal inhalation of cocaine)
- Poor dentition: carries, abscesses, missing teeth
- Cardiac murmurs
- Thrombosed veins with intravenous injection of drugs
- Hypertension and tachycardia (with cocaine and amphetamine use)
- Asthma, pneumonia (particularly with drug inhalation)
- Respiratory depression with narcotics
- Hepatomegaly secondary to hepatitis B
- Abruptio placentae, precipitous labor (with cocaine and amphetamines)
- Preterm labor and birth
- Fetal intrauterine growth retardation (IUGR) and intrauterine fetal death (IUFD)
- Sexually transmitted diseases, condyloma accuminata

Psychological Signs

- Psychosis, paranoia, panic attacks
- Rapid mood swings, agitation, irritability
- Depression
- Lethargy, disorientation, stupor, coma (with narcotic addiction)
- Abstinence syndrome (with narcotics and tranquilizers)

Behavioral Signs

- No prenatal care
- Frequent drop-in visits to labor and delivery
- Homeless or incarcerated
- Chain smoking, frequent requests to smoke, craving for cigarettes
- Seeking health care for battering
- Violence and abusive behavior directed against health care providers
- Inability to follow requests or directives
- Poor pain tolerance, repeated requests for pain medication without evidence of active labor
- Rapid, nonstop talking (common with cocaine and amphetamine use)

Recreational Substance Use

Physical Signs

- Underweight, poor weight gain during pregnancy
- Chronic rhinitis, sinusitis, polyps, dry mouth (marijuana use)
- Conjunctivitis, ptosis (marijuana use)
- Nasal septum excoriation or perforation (or history of septal repair—common with nasal snorting of cocaine)
- Hypertension, tachycardia (cocaine and amphetamines)

Psychological Signs

- Euphoria, lethargy, confusion
- Restlessness, agitation, panic attacks
- Depression

Behavioral Signs

- Reluctance to give urine specimen
- Seeking health care for battering
- Frequent accidents (falls, cuts, motor vehicle mishaps)
- Questions about effects of drugs on fetus or neonate
- Chronic bronchitis, "smoker's cough" (cigarettes and marijuana)

mandatory screening for drug use in some states. This occurs when a pregnant woman presents with common signs and symptoms of chemical dependency. In other cases, suspicion of drug use occurs after delivery of the neonate, when the neonate begins to exhibit signs and symptoms of narcotic withdrawal, called narcotic abstinence syndrome, or neurobehavioral aberrations. This serious condition is described in more detail in Chapter 33. It is characterized by extreme irritability and agitation, hypertonicity, feeding disorders, diarrhea, and dehydration. A sample of the neonate's urine, hair, or stool is then obtained for analysis. The ability to detect drugs in the urine, blood, hair, or meconium stool depends on the following factors:

- Timing and amount of last drug use
- Mode of excretion
- Half-life of the drug
- Sensitivity of equipment used to analyze specimen

Treatment

A significant approach to perinatal drug use and abuse must include prevention. However, in cases of clear abuse of alcohol or illegal drugs, treatment is a priority. Two forms of treatment for pregnant women who abuse drugs are available: residential treatment and drug therapy.

Residential Treatment. Treatment of substance abuse and addiction will depend in part on the type of drug used, maternal and fetal complications identified, and resources available in the community and hospital. Residential programs are the most effective modality for successful treatment of women addicted to cocaine or heroin. The woman (and her other children) may in some cases be removed from the community where poverty, violence, and easily available drugs combine to make abstinence and a healthy life-style nearly impossible.

While in residence the woman participates in group (or individual) therapy and classes on chemical addiction, child care, and infant and child development. Continued support from other residents, health care providers, psychologists, and social workers help the women refrain from drug use while they rebuild their lives. Referrals may be made for eventual relocation to a safer environment. Vocational training is encouraged. These strategies are essential to break the vicious cycle of poverty, lowered self-esteem, depression, and hopelessness that predisposes the woman to drug use.

Drug Therapy. Few drugs have been found to be useful in the treatment of chemical dependency. Pharmacologic treatment of severe withdrawal from alcohol, barbiturates, or tranquilizers may be necessary to prevent seizure activity or other adverse physiologic reactions to abstinence. Abrupt withdrawal (going "cold turkey") from any drug is not recommended because of the deleterious physiologic effects for the pregnant woman and fetus. Sudden withdrawal may result in fetal death. Gradual detoxification is often successful when the woman is dependent on nicotine, marijuana, barbiturates, or tranquilizers.

In the case of opiate addiction, treatment with methadone, a synthetic narcotic, is the therapy of choice. The goal of methadone maintenance treatment is to reach a dose of 20 mg/day or less by delivery (Buckley, 1990). In some case, slow detoxification from opiates and methadone may be accomplished before birth of the neonate. A contract is established between the woman and the agency dispensing the drug (usually a formal methadone maintenance program). The woman receives a daily dose of methadone to prevent acute narcotic withdrawal. To receive the drug and other benefits of the program, she must refrain from using narcotics or other illicit drugs.

One major advantage of the methadone maintenance program is that women do not have to engage in unhealthy drug-seeking behaviors to obtain heroin or other illicit substances. Profound life-style changes are possible when the woman participates in a methadone maintenance or detoxification program. The woman is expected to obtain routine prenatal care (often available through the program). She should participate in the residential or ambulatory treatment program, which usually includes individual or group therapy.

Maternal and neonatal outcomes can be greatly improved with appropriate treatment. Regular prenatal care, improved nutrition, treatment of medical and obstetric complications, and other changes in life-style and behavior can result in improved outcomes. The nurse has a key role in identifying pregnant women who are substance abusers and assisting them in obtaining appropriate treatment.

Maternal, Fetal, and Neonatal Implications

Maternal consequences of drug use are based on multiple factors, enumerated in the accompanying display.

Drug-specific maternal, fetal, and neonatal complications associated with substance use and chemical dependency are described in the following section. Neonatal conditions are discussed further in Chapter 33.

Smoking and Nicotine Use. Although the dangers of smoking are well publicized today, more than 20% of women continue to smoke during pregnancy. Nicotine is a stimulant and euphoriant. It may also cause a sensation of relaxation

Factors That Influence Maternal and Neonatal Outcomes When Substance Use and Chemical Addiction Complicate Pregnancy

Factors Influencing Maternal Outcomes

- Type, amount, and frequency of drug(s) used
- Period in gestation when drug used
- Life-style changes associated with drug-seeking behavior
- Presence of other medical or obstetric problems unrelated to drug use
- Preexisting problems related to drug use (ie, bacterial endocarditis)
- Educational level, intellectual abilities, mental status
- Motivation to change life-style
- Ability and desire to obtain regular prenatal care
- Family and community resources available to the woman
- Treatment modalities available for the specific chemical dependency
- Attitudes and knowledge of health care providers

Factors Influencing Neonatal Outcomes

- Type, amount, route, and frequency of drug(s) used
- Period in gestation when drug used
- Maternal health and nutritional status
- Maternal and fetal genetic status
- Environmental factors (pollutants, other chemical toxins)

when deep inhalation ("heavy dragging") is the mode of drug administration. Nicotine is one of the most addictive chemicals identified, causing both physiologic and psychological addiction. Nicotine is fat and water soluble and is rapidly distributed throughout the body.

The woman who smokes is at increased risk for upper respiratory tract infections, bronchitis, and asthma. Chronic smoking is associated with a higher incidence of cancer. Another serious consequence of smoking includes an increase in the rate of spontaneous abortion (as high as 24% versus 8% in the nonsmoking population).

The greatest risks posed by smoking during pregnancy are to the fetus. Heavy smokers denied cigarettes during hospitalization may experience symptoms of nicotine withdrawal, which is characterized by irritability, depression, alteration in sleep patterns, anxiety, and a pronounced physical and psychological craving for cigarettes. Little research has been conducted to document the effects of nicotine abstinence syndrome on the fetus. Neonates born to women who smoke are significantly more irritable (Buckley, 1990), perhaps due to nicotine withdrawal.

Smoking is estimated to be responsible for 25% of all perinatal morbidity and mortality. The most common effect of maternal smoking is reduced birth weight. The reduction may range from 40 to 430 g (1.4 to 15 oz), the average reduction being 200 g or 7 oz. This effect may be due to the high level of carboxyhemoglobin in the fetal circulation, which results from the transfer of carbon monoxide through the placenta. The amount of oxygen available to the fetus is decreased, causing hypoxia. The vasoconstrictive action of nicotine may further reduce the delivery of oxygen and nutrients to the fetus. The reduction in birth weight is directly related to the number of cigarettes smoked by the woman.

There does not appear to be a strong association between smoking and the risk of fetal malformations. However, several studies have found an increased incidence of cleft lip and palate. Smoking after age 35 is associated with a fivefold increase in intrauterine growth retardation (Wen et al., 1990) and a higher incidence of preterm labor and birth. An increased fetal death rate during labor and neonatal death rate have been noted in neonates of smoking women. Women who smoke 11 or more cigarettes per day increase their risk of having a stillborn neonate by greater than 50%.

The risk of sudden infant death syndrome (SIDS) is twice that of infants of nonsmoking mothers. Diseases of the respiratory system are also higher in infants of smokers, including respiratory infections and asthma. Studies suggest an increase in childhood cancer rates in infants and children who are reared in homes where parents smoke. Nicotine is secreted into breast milk and can be detected 7 to 8 hours after the last cigarette. Its concentration in the milk depends on the amount and depth of inhalation. The adverse of effects of long-term ingestion of nicotine during breast feeding have not been examined.

Alcohol. It is estimated that 65% of women consume alcohol during the first trimester, and 20% continue to drink regularly during the remainder of pregnancy (Serdula, Williamson, Kendrick, Anda, & Byers, 1991). Approximately 11% of women who continue to ingest alcohol have a drinking problem or are alcoholics. Alcohol contains ethanol and many other chemicals such as aldehydes that cause serious fetal anomalies, growth retardation, and death. The greatest risk of acute alcohol intoxication in women is injury or death secondary to automobile accidents. Severe alcoholics may experience acute withdrawal, including delirium tremens, if hospitalization prevents continued ingestion of the drug.

The effects of alcohol on fetal growth and development have been well documented. The constellation of physical, developmental and intellectual abnormalities are termed fetal alcohol syndrome (FAS). These problems are discussed in more detail in Chapter 33.

Precisely how alcohol causes FAS is not known. The fetal blood alcohol level remains much higher than the woman's blood level because the fetal liver is immature and unable to metabolize the drug. Risk to the fetus increases when the woman takes two or more drinks daily. Subtle facial anomalies are commonly present (Rostand et al., 1990). Ingestion of five or more drinks at a time, on a regular basis, increases the risks of structural brain anomalies and mental retardation in the neonate.

Because the precise level of alcohol required to cause fetal abnormalities is not known, all women should be counseled not to consume alcohol during pregnancy. Alcohol is found in breast milk after women drink. Cases of neonatal intoxication secondary to maternal alcohol consumption have been reported.

Marijuana. Marijuana contains over 400 known chemicals causing both therapeutic and adverse reactions. Clinical trials have demonstrated the benefits of marijuana in controlling nausea associated with chemotherapy. The psychoactive component of marijuana, tetrahydrocannabinol (THC), provides the "high" characteristic of the drug when it is inhaled as a cigarette or ingested in food. Cannabinoids are compounds also found in marijuana that cause increased heart rate, reddened conjunctiva, impaired memory, and psychomotor performance. These last two side effects may persist for 24 hours or longer and can delay reaction time required when operating an automobile or other complex machinery.

Marijuana is the most frequently used illicit chemical. It is estimated that 10% to 30% of woman may take the drug during pregnancy. The greatest risks to women who smoke marijuana are accidental injuries related to impaired coordination or injury and death secondary to motor vehicle accidents. The woman who smokes on a regular basis may suffer from chronic sinusitis, pharyngitis, polyps, and upper respiratory infections, which decrease the quality of health and well-being.

Many women who are heavy users of marijuana also smoke and ingest alcohol, thereby increasing the risk to the fetus of permanent injury. Marijuana has a potent inhibitory effect on reproductive hormones in adults. Although these effects appear to be reversible after discontinuation of the drug, individuals with impaired fertility (ie, women over age 40) or young adolescents should be particularly cautious about the use of marijuana.

Although THC reaches the fetus through placental transfer, no current evidence indicates that it is associated with congenital anomalies or fetal distress. Intrauterine growth retardation and preterm birth are more frequently observed and are dose dependent (Evans, 1991). It has been suggested that the neonate may suffer from subtle neurobehavioral disorders that are not currently fully understood or appreciated (Day & Richardson, 1991).

Tetrahydrocannabinol has been found in the breast milk of women who use marijuana, and cases of neonatal cannabis intoxication have been reported. Lactation can be affected by moderate to heavy marijuana use. The amount of milk produced is reduced as a result of a decrease in mammary gland enzymes necessary for growth of normal mammary tissue.

Opiates. Opiate addiction during the perinatal period remains a significant problem. It can cause life-threatening complications for the woman, fetus, and neonate. Opiate use imposes a tremendous burden on society because of the associated costs of medical care and the potential loss of life.

The rate of opiate dependence during pregnancy has remained relatively stable at 6% to 10%, depending on the population studied. Heroin and other opiates have strong physiologic and psychological addictive properties. They often produce significant alterations in life-style, which further threaten maternal and fetal well-being.

Heroin is the most dangerous opiate used illegally because it is sold on the street in uncertain concentrations and mixed with a variety of impure "cutting" agents. The combination can be lethal. Opiates can be taken by the oral, intranasal, pulmonary (smoking), intramuscular, or intravenous route.

Many maternal complications are related to opiate use. An immediate risk remains acute toxicity, respiratory depression, and death secondary to respiratory arrest. Sharing of contaminated syringes and needles results in the spread of HIV and hepatitis B virus. The physical, psychological, and economic consequences of opiate addiction have assumed even greater significance. Perinatal AIDS continues to grow in part due to opiate use. The woman with an opiate addiction often trades sexual services for drugs. This places her at greater risk for other STDs such as syphilis, gonorrhea, and herpesvirus. Other medical complications associated with narcotic addiction are listed in the accompanying display.

Fetal and neonatal consequences of maternal opiate addiction are devastating. The fetus is exposed to many other infections that can result in permanent injury, developmental disabilities, and mental retardation. Fetal death is common, and many fetuses do not survive the lethal exposure to drugs and intrauterine infection. Physical trauma to the fetus may occur if the woman is battered. Fetal distress is more common during labor. Many neonates are born prematurely and suffer from severe intrauterine growth retardation. The neonate may suffer from narcotic withdrawal or neonatal abstinence syndrome. In addition, the neonate may suffer from STDs and problems related to prematurity.

Cocaine and Amphetamines. The growing use of cocaine in the 1980s has had catastrophic results for maternal and neonatal well-being in the United States. Cocaine is one of the most powerfully addictive chemicals, possibly due to its affect on dopaminergic pathways (Farrar & Kearns, 1989).

Medical Problems Associated With Perinatal Opiate Addiction

Infection

Tetanus
Pneumonia
Tuberculosis
Bacterial endocarditis
Urinary tract infection
Sexually transmitted diseases and pelvic inflammatory disease
Cellulitis and abcesses

Cardiovascular Disease

Valvular disease secondary to endocarditis
Thrombophlebitis and thromboembolism
Hypertension

Pulmonary Disease

Asthma
Pulmonary edema
Chronic bronchitis

Psychological Disorders

Depression
Suicide

Other Problems

Diabetes mellitus
Anemia and nutritional deficiencies
Trauma, rape, and battery
Amputation due to severe infections secondary to intravenous drug injection

Perinatal cocaine use is estimated to be approximately 10% to 15% and much higher among indigent women living in urban areas. The use of cocaine has, in the past, been underestimated in middle-class women. Studies have reported the incidence of cocaine use at about 7% to 15% in this population (Chasnoff, Landress, & Barret, 1990).

Adverse effects of cocaine result from intense activation of the sympathetic nervous system. Pronounced vasoconstriction and resultant ischemia are responsible for many problems. Major complications include:

- Hypertension and cerebral vascular accidents
- Tachycardia, arrhythmias, and myocardial infarction
- Pulmonary edema
- Seizures
- Intestinal ischemia

Serious obstetric complications can threaten the life of the pregnant woman and fetus or neonate. Tumultuous labor often follows cocaine use and may result in abruptio placentae, hemorrhage, and preterm labor and birth. Fetal distress and death are common due to these complications. Studies examining the teratogenic effect of cocaine have yielded conflicting findings. Because polysubstance abuse is common in cocaine-addicted women, it is difficult to isolate the effect of the drug on fetal growth and development.

The neonate of a cocaine-addicted woman often suffers from severe intrauterine growth retardation and prematurity and may demonstrate evidence of infarcts in major organ systems secondary to vasoconstriction. Cerebral, myocardial, and intestinal infarcts have been reported. Because the woman often trades sexual services for drugs, the neonate is at increased risk for STDs and their sequellae. The risk of perinatal AIDS transmission is greater in this group of women, as is the rate of neonatal AIDS in their offspring. Several studies have reported a higher incidence of SIDS.

Neonates born to women who use cocaine do not suffer from the classic neonatal abstinence syndrome observed with narcotic-addicted mothers, unless of course, opiates are also taken during pregnancy. In many neonates, subtle neurobehavioral symptoms (increased startles, slightly increased or decreased tone, altered sleep patterns, or poor feeding) may be the only signs of maternal cocaine use (Peters & Theorell, 1991).

Many of the effects of amphetamines are similar to those observed with cocaine. Amphetamines activate the sympathetic nervous system, producing euphoria and side effects similar to those noted with cocaine use. There is a significant variation in the frequency and amount of amphetamine use throughout the United States. The greater incidence is found in the western United States (Evans, 1991).

Maternal, fetal, and neonatal complications are similar but are often less severe. Hypertension, increased uterine activity, and poor pregnancy weight gain often result in intrauterine growth retardation, abruptio placentae, and prematurity. Mild neurobehavioral aberrations have been documented in the neonate. Congenital anomalies and the classic neonatal abstinence syndrome are not associated with maternal amphetamine use and addiction.

Implications for Nursing Care

The nurse has a range of responsibilities in the care of the pregnant woman who abuses illegal drugs or alcohol. A major responsibility is the careful assessment of the woman's situation and planning for appropriate referral for care if the woman appears ready to make that decision.

• • Assessment

Treatment of substance abuse and chemical dependency begins with the initial prenatal assessment. All women should be screened for chemical use during pregnancy, beginning with questions about the use of nonprescription drugs, coffee, cigarettes, and alcohol. The assessment should progress to include questions about "recreational" drug use such as marijuana. Initial assessment concludes with queries about other drugs and problems with abstaining from drugs. It should be determined if the woman has had previous problems with chemical dependency. Assessment of maternal substance use should continue on an ongoing basis throughout pregnancy.

The nurse may be required to obtain a urine sample for toxicology screening. Several states have passed statutes that mandate drug testing when chemical dependency is suspected. In some cases mandatory reporting to social or child-protective services or law enforcement agencies is required when drugs are detected by the tests. Unfortunately, many of these laws target poor women. Middle-class women with health insurance who may also have significant problems related to drug use are often ignored. This raises issues highlighted in the Legal/Ethical Considerations display.

During the intrapartum period, the nurse should review the prenatal record to determine the woman's pattern of chemical use. If drug use is noted or if the woman reveals that she has had a chemical dependency problem during the pregnancy, the nurse should determine the time of last use and the amount and type of drug used. A supportive, nonjudgmental, matter-of-fact approach to the collection of information is essential to obtain accurate data.

• • Nursing Diagnosis

Appropriate nursing diagnoses are identified during the course of the initial and ongoing assessments during the prenatal and intrapartum period and may include the following:

- Altered Nutrition: Less than Body Requirements related to substance use
- High Risk for Infection related to drug-seeking and drug-use behaviors
- High Risk for Injury (trauma) related to drug-seeking behaviors
- High Risk for Self-directed Violence related to mental disorientation
- Fear related to side effects of drugs or complications of chemical dependency

• • Planning and Implementation

To provide effective care, the nurse must convey respect for and acceptance of the person (not the self-destructive behaviors). Many individuals with substance abuse problems have had negative experiences with nurses and physicians in the past. They may be distrustful of the nurse and demonstrate hostile or abusive behaviors initially. The nurse must be skilled in setting limits, expressing concern while remaining firm about inappropriate conduct, and remaining calm when the woman is unable to control her actions (Byrne & Lerner, 1992).

During the prenatal period, the nurse should praise the woman for health-seeking behaviors. It is important to develop a trusting relationship with the woman, offering positive feedback and reinforcement when appropriate. Referrals should be made to drug treatment programs or to members

Legal/Ethical Considerations

Mandatory Screening, Reporting, and Treatment of Chemical Dependence

The crack cocaine epidemic is unique among drug waves to hit the United States. Many young women of childbearing age are addicted to cocaine. It is estimated that as many as 350,000 neonates exposed to cocaine prenatally are born each year, many with significant physical and developmental problems. Some states have passed laws requiring health care professionals to participate in mandatory screening, reporting, and treatment initiatives.

In some cases, mandatory reporting does not result in treatment but the application of criminal penalties. By the early 1990s, there were more than 50 efforts to prosecute women for perinatal drug use (including alcohol). The charges have ranged from fetal abuse to murder. Unfortunately, almost all the women targeted have been indigent, with limited education or English language skills. The majority of these women are non-European American. The nurse has been drawn into this legal/ethical dilemma as the health care provider most often responsible for obtaining specimens for drug testing.

AWHONN (formerly NAACOG, the Organization for Obstetric, Gynecologic and Neonatal Nurses, 1990) and the American College of Obstetricians and Gynecologists (ACOG, 1990) have published position statements opposing enforced treatment and criminalization of chemical dependency. Punishing the woman for drug use may result in more women avoiding prenatal care. Mandatory reporting statutes change the basic nature of the physician– and nurse–client relationship; the health care provider is viewed as an informer and punisher. Furthermore, incarceration of the pregnant woman does not ensure fetal well-being. Women in jail are often exposed to unhealthy living conditions and receive inadequate diets and prenatal care.

In line with the position statement formulated by ACOG, nurses should oppose the passage of laws that require mandatory reporting of drug use to *law enforcement agencies* and the *criminalization* of perinatal chemical dependency. Efforts should be focused on the development of adequate treatment modalities and residential treatment programs for pregnant women. When obtaining specimens for toxicology screening, the nurse should verify that there is a physician's order or written protocol or policy governing the collection of specimens for drug screening. Even when state laws mandate screening, the woman should be informed by the nurse that the specimen will be tested and ask for verbal permission to conduct the test. If the woman objects to drug screening, the physician or midwife should be notified so that he or she can discuss this issue with the pregnant woman. The nurse should refrain from assuming the role of "enforcer," "informer," or "punisher."

ACOG Committee on Ethics. (1990). *Patient choice: Maternal-fetal conflict.* Committee Opinion No. 55. Washington, DC: Author.

Chavkin W. (1991). Mandatory treatment for drug use during pregnancy. *Journal of the American Medical Association, 266*(11), 1556.

NAACOG. (1990). *Substance abuse in women.* Position Statement. Washington, DC: Author.

of the health care team responsible for making arrangements for therapy.

When the woman presents with complications related to substance abuse or when the onset of labor occurs, the nurse must provide intensive nursing care. The primary goal of care is to maintain maternal and fetal physiologic stability. Plans should be made for adequate pain control during childbirth. The woman with a narcotic dependency problem has a high tolerance to narcotic analgesics and may have a low pain threshold. Collaboration with the obstetrician and an anesthesiologist (if available) is essential in providing appropriate and adequate pain relief. Regional epidural anesthesia may be indicated, decreasing the need for opiate administration.

The nurse should notify neonatal personnel well in advance of the impending birth when the woman with a chemical addiction arrives in the labor and delivery unit. If possible, neonatal staff should discuss the plan of care regarding the neonate in advance of the birth. If the woman's condition is stable and adequate pain relief has been accomplished, the neonatal staff can begin establishing a working relationship with the woman. The woman can begin to express her needs and concerns, and the health care team can answer her questions.

After birth of the neonate, the goal of postpartum interventions is to promote maternal-infant interactions. This process may be delayed by maternal and neonatal complications secondary to substance abuse. Maternal physiologic recovery may be protracted by poor nutrition, anemia, and infections. The neonate often requires special care due to asphyxia, prematurity, or infection. Sensitive, nonjudgmental care often eliminates barriers between the nurse and woman. This encourages the woman to ask questions and express her feelings and concerns more openly. Support of the parenting role may build maternal self-esteem. Efforts to motivate the woman to begin or continue with therapy and remain drug free are important to the woman's well-being and that of her family.

Expected Outcomes

- The woman demonstrating signs of substance abuse during pregnancy discusses suitable treatment alternatives.
- The woman who abuses drugs during pregnancy verbalizes the dangers of drug use for her own health and that of the fetus.
- The woman with a history of drug use during pregnancy requests medically appropriate and adequate pain relief for labor.

• • Evaluation

The physiologic and emotional status of the woman who is chemically dependent may change rapidly during the course of the pregnancy, birth, or postpartum periods. Fetal status is often in jeopardy. The nurse must perform frequent evaluations to assess the effectiveness of nursing care and medical therapy. If nursing interventions are successful, the woman will remain drug free or will continue with a methadone maintenance program (if addicted to narcotics). When deviations occur in expected outcomes, the nurse alters the plan of care to reflect the identification of new problems.

One of the greatest challenges facing the maternity nurse is caring for the woman who uses drugs or is chemically dependent. Acute and chronic health problems frequently arise, requiring expert nursing care. However, significant legal and ethical dilemmas may complicate the nurse's ability to provide this care. Positive outcomes are more likely to be achieved when the nurse approaches the woman and her family with respect and makes an effort to include them in planning care. Ongoing support and encouragement can be a strong motivator for the woman to continue care, remain drug free, and deliver a viable and healthy neonate.

Chemical addiction and illegal drug use cause significant problems in the perinatal period. The nurse has various responsibilities in the care of the pregnant woman who abuses chemical substances. All pregnant women should be screened for chemical use, including nonprescription drugs, coffee, cigarettes, and alcohol. Questions about recreational drugs should be asked. Positive outcomes are more likely to be achieved when the nurse approaches the family with respect. Significant legal and ethical dilemmas complicate such care. The nurse should counsel the woman in health-seeking behaviors. Referrals should be made for drug treatment. Special care must be provided for pain relief during labor and birth. Neonatal personnel should be notified in advance of the birth so that preparations may be made for a high-risk neonate.

Trauma in Pregnancy

The most frequent cause of death in women under age 35 is related to trauma. Trauma complicates 1 in 12 pregnancies (ACOG, 1991a).

Etiologic and Predisposing Factors

Trauma during pregnancy can result from motor vehicle accidents, domestic violence, falls, and burns. Factors predisposing women to traumatic injury vary. They include drivers under the influence of drugs, inconsistent or nonuse of seat belts, and increasing employment of pregnant women in physically demanding jobs.

The most frequent cause of trauma in women are motor vehicle accidents. Women typically wear seat belts more consistently than men, but use decreases with pregnancy. This pattern is a result of misperceptions about seat belt use and safety during pregnancy. The leading cause of fetal death is maternal death. No evidence indicates that seat belt use increases fetal loss or injury, but ample evidence shows that nonuse increases risk of maternal injury or death (ACOG, 1991b).

Diagnosis

The effect of trauma depends on the type and severity of insult, the extent to which normal uterine and fetal physiology is disrupted, and gestational age. For example, until 12 weeks of gestation, the uterus is a pelvic organ and is thus protected from direct impact by the bony pelvis. Later, when the uterus is an abdominal organ, there is increasing risk of impact.

Diagnostic procedures frequently include the use of radiographic studies. Such studies are generally thought unlikely to cause fetal abnormalities from radiation exposure after 20 weeks of gestation (Pearlman, Tintinalli, & Lorenz, 1990). In all cases, the risks of diagnostic procedures for the fetus must be weighed against the risk of maternal death if precise diagnosis is not accomplished.

Treatment

In general, treatment of trauma in the pregnant woman is specifically directed toward maintaining maternal and fetal physiologic stability. Medical decisions must balance both maternal and fetal well-being. These decisions must be discussed with the woman and her family and should be discussed by the entire treatment team to the extent possible.

Treatment may occur in an intensive care unit, with consultation from perinatal physicians and nurses. Some hospitals have specialized obstetric intensive care units, which are staffed with perinatal physicians and nurses specially trained to care for pregnant women who are victims of trauma.

In every case of trauma, medical and nursing actions must be considered in light of the effects on the pregnant woman, the fetus, and the family. For instance, if cardiopulmonary resuscitation is required, care must be taken to deflect the gravid uterus from chest compressions. Another example of necessary modification in standard intensive care practice may be relaxation of family visitation routines.

Maternal, Fetal, and Neonatal Implications

Implications of trauma for the pregnant woman and the fetus or neonate depend on the mechanism of injury, the gestational age of the fetus, and associated complications. These factors will determine the maternal and fetal response to treatment. Of most concern are injuries that compromise maternal hemodynamic and pulmonary function because deterioration in these systems is life threatening (Daddario & Johnson, 1992).

Trauma can result both from compression of the uterus as well as the kinetic force generated by sudden stops, such as in a fall or a motor vehicle accident. Fetal trauma from abdominal compression is infrequent, but uterine injury due to shearing forces on impact may lead to other problems. Injury to the pregnant woman may not be apparent in an initial examination. The most common obstetric consequence of trauma in pregnancy is abruptio placentae. This condition may occur as late as 5 days after the initial injury.

Trauma in pregnancy is not limited to abdominal insult. Maternal injuries to the head, neck, and chest can affect vital functions and compromise fetal status. Initial assessment focuses on maternal status in terms of cardiopulmonary function. Significant hemorrhage may be masked by the hypervolemic state of pregnancy. Thus, the pregnant woman's hemodynamic state may appear to be stable, yet the fetus is at extreme risk for hypoxic injury.

Implications for Nursing Care

Acute accidental trauma during pregnancy requires joint efforts of emergency room, intensive care, and obstetric personnel. Perinatal units in many hospitals are updating services to provide trauma care to pregnant women in an obstetric intensive care unit. Specialized units allow the woman to receive sophisticated hemodynamic monitoring and mechanical ventilation, if needed. In every case, care must be directed toward maintenance of maternal hemodynamic stability, adequate pulmonary function, fetal well-being, and maternal and family psychosocial well-being (May, 1992).

The nurse can play a critical role in ensuring that the psychological needs of the pregnant woman and her family are met. This is challenging because of the constraints of providing lifesaving and life-sustaining care simultaneously. Recognition of the multiple stressors facing the woman and her family will assist the nurse in providing sensitive, humane, and expert care.

Trauma complicates 1 in 12 pregnancies. The most frequent cause of trauma in women is motor vehicle accidents, although other trauma includes domestic violence, falls, and burns. The effect of trauma depends on the type and severity of the accident, the extent to which normal uterine and fetal physiology is disrupted, and the gestational age of the fetus. Treatment generally is toward maintaining maternal and fetal physiologic stability.

Chapter Summary

Complications in pregnancy cause the pregnant woman and her family stress, anxiety, and fear. The health care team expands in relation to the severity of complications. The nurse plays a pivotal role on the health care team by coordinating activities to achieve the care necessary for health maintenance throughout the pregnancy. The nurse plays an advocacy role, serving as the person consistently available to the family and knowledgeable about the care. In this way, nursing care can strongly influence the family's childbirth experience to promote health and optimal adaptation.

The nurse plays a similar role in the care of women whose pregnancies are complicated by medical conditions. The challenge to the health care team is to maintain the best balance possible between care of the medical condition and care of the pregnancy. It often requires the patient and her family to adjust their life-style to accommodate the self-care required. In the process, the woman undergoes physiologic changes in her health status and psychosocial changes in her identity, her family relationships, and possibly her entire social network. The nurse is challenged to address the full scope of individual and family needs in facilitating access to appropriate health care and community resources.

Study Questions

1. *A woman is 10 weeks pregnant and comes to the emergency room with brown vaginal spotting. She asks, "Does this means I am losing the baby?" How will you respond?*
2. *What is the major risk associated with placenta previa?*
3. *A woman complains of abdominal pain and shoulder pain. She was screened in the clinic 4 weeks ago and told she was pregnant. What is the nurse's assessment of the situation? What is the first nursing action?*
4. *What are three clinical findings that may indicate the presence of twins?*
5. *What is the rationale and mechanism of action of RhIgG prophylactic therapy?*
6. *What is the major physiologic complication associated with intrauterine fetal demise?*
7. *Why is iron supplementation not effective in the treatment of anemia as a result of hemoglobinopathy? Why is folic acid supplementation important?*
8. *What are the classic symptoms of a UTI?*
9. *What three STDs can be transmitted to the fetus?*
10. *What are common signs and symptoms of recreational and "hard core" substance abuse during pregnancy?*
11. *What health teaching points would the nurse use to help women avoid accidental trauma in pregnancy?*

References

ACOG (1992). *Hepatitis in pregnancy* (No. 174). ACOG Technical Bulletin. Washington, DC: Author.

ACOG (1991a). *Trauma during pregnancy* (No. 161). ACOG Technical Bulletin. Washington, DC: Author.

ACOG (1991b). *Automobile passenger restraints for children and pregnant women* (No. 151). ACOG Technical Bulletin. Washington DC: Author.

ACOG (1990). *Ectopic pregnancy* (No. 150). ACOG Technical Bulletin. Washington DC: Author.

ACOG (1989a). *Multiple gestation* (No. 131). ACOG Technical Bulletin. Washington DC: Author.

ACOG (1989b). *Diagnosis and management of postterm pregnancy* (No. 130). ACOG Technical Bulletin. Washington, DC: Author.

ACOG (1988). *Perinatal herpes simplex virus infections* (No. 122). ACOG Technical Bulletin. Washington, DC: Author.

Bachman, J. (1992). Postpartum ovarian vein thrombophlebitis: Etiology diagnosis, treatment and nursing implications. *Journal of Vascular Nursing, 10*(2), 13–18.

Blanche, S., Taudieu, M., Duliege, A., Rousiouz, C., LeDeist, F., Fukunaga, K., Caniglia, M., Jacomet, C., Messiah, A., & Griscelli, C. (1990). Longitudinal study of 94 symptomatic infants with perinatally acquired human immunodeficiency virus infection. *American Journal of Diseases in Children, 144*(11), 1210–1215.

Buckley, K. (1990). Substance abuse. In K. Buckley & N. Kulb (Eds). *High Risk Maternity Nursing Manual*. Baltimore: Williams & Wilkins.

Burrow, G., & Ferris, T. (1988). *Medical complications in pregnancy* (3rd ed.). Philadelphia: WB Saunders.

Butler, K. (1991). Transmission, diagnosis and treatment of HIV infection in children. *Journal of Intravenous Nursing, 14*(3), 13–24.

Byrne, M., & Lerner, H. (1992). Communicating with addicted women in labor. *American Journal of Maternal Child Nursing, 17*(1), 22–24.

Chasnoff, I., Landress, H., & Barret, M. (1990). The prevalence of illicit drug or alcohol use during pregnancy and discrepancies in mandatory reporting in Pinellas County, Florida. *New England Journal of Medicine, 322*(17), 1202–1205.

Csonka, G. (1990). *Sexually transmitted diseases: A textbook of genitourinary medicine*. New York: Baillere Tindall.

Daddario, J., & Johnson, G., (1992). Trauma in pregnancy. In L. Mandeville & N. Troiano (Eds.). *High risk intrapartum nursing*. Philadelphia: JB Lippincott.

Day, N., & Richardson, G. (1991). Prenatal marijuana use. *Clinics in Perinatology, 18*(1), 77–84.

Efantis, J., & Sinclair, B. (1990). Antepartum management of pregnant women with HIV infection. *NAACOG's Clinical Issues in Perinatal and Women's Health, 1*(1), 41–46.

Evans, A. (1991). Perinatal chemical use. In K. Niswander & A. Evans (Eds.). *Manual of obstetrics* (4th ed., p. 30). Boston: Little, Brown.

Farrar, H., & Kearns, G. (1989). Cocaine: Clinical pharmacology and toxicology. *Journal of Pediatrics, 115*(5), 665–672.

Fletcher, J. (1990). Human immunodeficiency virus and the fetus. *Journal of the American Board of Family Practice*, 3(3), 181–193.

Gabbe, S., Niebyl, J., & Simpson, J. (1991). *Obstetrics: Normal and problem pregnancies*. New York: Churchill Livingstone.

Golan, A., Barnan, J., & Vexler, R. (1989). Incompetent uterine cervix. *Obstetrical and Gynecological Survey, 44*(2), 96–107.

Hankins, C., & Handley, M. (1992). HIV disease and AIDS in women: Current knowledge and a research agenda. *Journal of Acquired Immune Deficiency Syndrome, 5*(10), 957–971.

Jenkins, M., & Kohl, S. (1992). New aspects of neonatal herpes. *Infectious Disease Clinics of North America, 6*(1), 57–64.

Mabie, P. (1992). Placenta previa. *Clinical Perinatology, 19*(2), 426–435.

May, K. (1992). Psychosocial implications of high-risk intrapartum care. In L. Mandeville & N. Troiano (Eds.). *High risk intrapartum nursing*. Philadelphia: JB Lippincott.

Nettina, S., & Kauffman, F. (1990). Diagnosis and management of sexually transmitted genital lesions. *Nurse Practitioner, 15*(1), 34–39.

North, D., Speed, J., & Weiner, W. (1990). Correlation of urinary tract infection with urinary screening at the first antepartum visit. *Journal of the Mississippi State Medical Association, 31*(10), 331–332.

Pearlman, M., Tintinalli, J., & Lorenz, R. (1990). Blunt trauma during pregnancy. *New England Journal of Medicine, 323*(23), 1609–1613.

Peters, H., & Theorell, C. (1991). Fetal and neonatal effects of maternal cocaine use. *Journal of Obstetric, Gynecologic, and Neonatal Nursing, 20*(2), 121–127.

Phibbs, C., Bateman, D., & Schwartz, R. The neonatal costs of maternal cocaine use. *Journal of the American Medical Association, 266*(11), 1521.

Porcher, R. (1992). HIV-infected pregnant women and their infants: Primary health care implications. *Nurse Practitioner, 17*(11), 49–50.

Rostand, A., Kaminski, M., Lelong, N., Dehaene, P., Delestret, I., Klein-Bertrand, C., Querleu, D., & Crepin, G. (1990). Alcohol use in pregnancy, craniofacial features, and fetal growth. *Journal of Epidemiology and Community Health, 44*, 302–307.

Serdula, M., Williamson, D., Kendrick, J., Anda, R., & Byers, T. (1991). Trends in alcohol consumption by pregnant women: 1985 through 1988. *Journal of the American Medical Association, 265*(7), 876–882.

Scott, J. (1990). Immunologic disorders in pregnancy. In D. Danforth & J. Scott (Eds.). *Danforth's Obstetrics and Gynecology*. Philadelphia: JB Lippincott.

Smith, E., Johnson, S., Cripe, T., Pignatari, S., & Turek, L. (1991). Perinatal vertical transmission of human papillomavirus and subsequent development of respiratory tract papillomatosis. *Annals of Otology, Rhinology, and Laryngology, 100*(6), 479–483.

Sperling, R., Stratton, P., O'Sullivan, M., Boyer, P., Watts, D., Lambert, J., Hammill, H., Livingstone, E., Gloeb, D., & Minkoff, H. (1992). A survey of zidovudine use in pregnant women with human immunodeficiency virus infection. *New England Journal of Medicine, 326*(13), 857–861.

Tillman, J. (1992). Syphilis: An old disease, a contemporary perinatal problem. *Journal of Obstetric, Gynecologic, and Neonatal Nursing, 21*(3), 209–214.

Tinkle, M. (1990). Genital human papillomavirus: A growing health concern. *Journal of Obstetric, Gynecologic and Neonatal Nursing, 19*(6), 501–507.

Tinkle, M., Amaya, M., & Tamayo, O. (1992). HIV disease and pregnancy. Part 1. Epidemiology, pathogenesis, and natural history. *Journal of Obstetric, Gynecologic and Neonatal Nursing, 21,*(2), 86–93.

Wen, S., Goldenberg, R., Cutter, G., Hoffman, H., Cliver, S., Davis, R., & DuBard, M. (1990). Smoking, maternal age, fetal growth, and gestational age at delivery. *American Journal of Obstetrics and Gynecology, 162*(1), 53–58.

Williams, M., & Wheby, M. (1992). Anemias in pregnancy. *Medical Clinics of North America, 76*(3), 631–647.

Suggested Readings

Helman, N. (1990). Sickle cell disease in pregnancy. *NAACOG's Clinical Issues in Perinatal and Women's Health Nursing, 1*(2), 194–201.

Hoegerman, G., & Schnoll, S. (1991). Narcotic use in pregnancy. *Clinics in Perinatology, 18*(1), 51.

Johnson, J., & Oakley, L. (1991). Managing minor trauma during pregnancy. *Journal of Obstetric, Gynecologic, and Neonatal Nursing, 20*(5), 379–384.

Knuppel, R., & Drukker, J. (1993). *High-risk pregnancy: A team approach* (2nd ed.). Philadelphia: WB Saunders.

Lynch, M., & McKeon, V. (1990). Cocaine use during pregnancy. *Journal of Obstetric, Gynecologic, and Neonatal Nursing, 19*(4), 285.

Sullivan, K. (1990). Maternal implications of cocaine use during pregnancy. *Journal of Perinatal and Neonatal Nursing, 3*(4), 12–16.

Summers, L. (1992). Understanding tuberculosis: Implications for pregnancy. *Journal of Perinatal and Neonatal Nursing, 6*(2), 12–24.

Wen, S., Goldenberg, R., Cutter, G., Hoffman, H., Cliver, S., Davis, R., & DuBard, M. (1990). Smoking, maternal age, fetal growth, and gestational age at delivery. *American Journal of Obstetrics and Gynecology, 162*(1), 53–58.

CHAPTER 17

Nutrition During Pregnancy

Learning Objectives

After studying the material in this chapter, the student will be able to:

- Identify steps to assess, maintain, and promote the nutritional status of pregnant women.
- Identify and relate nutritional risk factors during pregnancy.
- Use dietary guidelines in helping pregnant women meet their nutritional needs.
- Specify recommended daily intake of vitamins and minerals that are particularly important during pregnancy.
- Offer appropriate nutrition counseling to pregnant women based on assessment of economic, religious, and cultural factors.

Key Terms

body mass index
calorie
folic acid
iron cost
iron deficiency anemia
kilocalorie
megadose
nutritional requirement
pica (geophagia)
Recommended Dietary Allowances

Pregnancy is a unique period in the life cycle; at no other time is the well-being of one individual (the fetus) so directly dependent on the well-being of another (the mother). An important determinant of the woman's well-being and that of her fetus is her nutritional status.

Counseling and nutrition education are necessary to ensure normal fetal growth and development in underweight, undernourished, obese, and adolescent pregnant women. Nutritional care is also important for women who have good eating habits but need additional guidance during pregnancy. The nurse must appreciate the importance of nutrition and be knowledgeable about how the normal physiologic changes during pregnancy relate to nutritional needs.

This chapter presents basic information on the effects of maternal nutritional status on the course and outcome of pregnancy and describes daily nutritional requirements during pregnancy. Factors that affect women's dietary patterns during pregnancy are discussed, and nutritional risk factors are identified. Finally, the nursing process is used to plan quality care.

Basis of Nutritional Care During Pregnancy

The entire health team plays a role in carrying out nutritional care. The health team members must communicate through progress notes in the patient record and through case conferences. Documentation and communication help to ensure consistency in the nutritional advice given to the pregnant woman.

All health professionals involved in the delivery of prenatal nutrition services should be able to do the following:

- Evaluate current dietary practices.
- Counsel on nutrient needs and recommended diet during pregnancy and infancy.

- Refer, as necessary, to community resources, such as social services and food assistance programs.
- Monitor and interpret clinical data pertinent to nutritional assessment of the woman.
- Identify risk factors.
- Seek consultation and refer women considered to be at high nutritional risk.
- Provide information and advice on breastfeeding or alternative methods of infant feeding.
- Counsel on nutrient needs during lactation.

Much of this knowledge and many of these skills are necessary for the early identification, treatment, and referral of women with major nutritional problems. Health care professionals who provide direct nutritional services for women with nutritionally high-risk conditions or for parents of infants with nutritionally high-risk conditions require specialized knowledge.

To ensure optimal outcome, direct services to high-risk women and infants should be developed and delivered by the registered dietitian or nutritionist and approved by the provider responsible for quality care.

In addition to having the knowledge and skills identified for the uncomplicated pregnancy, the registered dietitian is uniquely trained to evaluate and manage the nutritional care of pregnant women with complex medical and surgical problems. These high-risk problems might include diabetes mellitus, chronic renal disease, cardiac problems, and chronic lung disease. Evaluation and management of nutritional care include screening for nutritional problems, monitoring and assessing nutritional status, developing and implementing complicated management plans, and providing instructional resources for special dietary modifications (California Department of Health Services, 1990). A registered dietitian is able to develop and ensure continuity of nutrition care plans. This includes coordination and referral to local agencies with food and nutrition resources, as well as providing follow-up services and monitoring and evaluating results of nutrition intervention.

Importance of Nutrition During Pregnancy

Good nutrition is a product of lifelong eating patterns; improved dietary habits during pregnancy cannot make up entirely for previous deficiencies. However, many pregnant women are highly motivated to change eating patterns for the good of their unborn children. Routine prenatal care allows for ongoing nutritional guidance, reinforcement, and support. For these reasons pregnancy is an excellent opportunity to assist women in choosing healthier diets for themselves and their families. If positive changes in eating habits become part of a life-style, they can contribute to improved family health for years to come. The nurse can have a significant impact on family health and well-being through nutritional care provided during pregnancy.

The importance of adequate maternal nutrition to the course and outcome of pregnancy can be well appreciated when indicators of fetal development and perinatal mortality and morbidity are examined. Adequate nutrition during pregnancy reduces the risk of some maternal complications, helps ensure that tissue growth proceeds normally, and increases the likelihood that the neonate will attain an optimal birth weight. Mothers with nutritional deficiencies before and during pregnancy are more likely to experience certain complications. These complications include pregnancy-induced hypertension and anemia and a higher perinatal morbidity and mortality caused by problems associated with low birth weight, malformations, and disturbances in cell development (Worthington-Roberts & Klerman, 1990)

Inadequate maternal nutrition has a significant effect on brain development in the fetus and newborn. The period of maximum brain growth in humans occurs late in fetal development. If the mother's nutrition is not adequate, the fetal brain will not develop fully, and the number of brain cells will be low. The infant can never replace brain cells that did not develop in utero, although some researchers argue that the quality of brain cells can be improved by a good diet in infancy (Institute of Medicine, 1990).

Numerous studies have reported a strong relationship between birth weight and maternal prepregnant weight and weight gain during pregnancy. This indicates the importance of nutritional guidance before pregnancy and early nutritional care during pregnancy. Some maternal factors have a direct impact on the nutritional status and birth weight of infants. For instance smoking interferes with metabolic processes in the body, resulting in low–birth-weight infants (Institute of Medicine, 1990).

Adolescent mothers are at higher risk of producing premature and low–birth-weight babies than women in their 20s. This may reflect the fact that many adolescent mothers come from socioeconomically disadvantaged families and have especially poor nutritional patterns before and during their pregnancies. However, when adequate maternal weight gain during pregnancy is achieved despite the presence of such risk factors, the chances that the infant will achieve optimal infant birth weight are increased.

The importance of nutrition during the childbearing years extends to the well-being of the infant in the first years of life. The infant's brain development can be arrested if it is malnourished in the early weeks of life. This may occur when impoverished families cannot afford infant formula and substitute other foods. However, infant malnutrition also can occur when the mother is too undernourished to produce sufficient amounts of high-quality breast milk.

Malnutrition among infants is a major contributor to infant mortality. Malnutrition in the very young does not usually kill outright, but rather lowers resistance to infections and parasitic diseases that would not be life-threatening to a well-nourished infant. The most comprehensive investigation of infant mortality conducted in the Western hemisphere was carried out by the Pan American Health Organization in the early 1970s. Examining data on 35,000 infant deaths in 15 regions of North and South America, it found that undernutrition was associated with 34% of these deaths in Latin American communities. Infant death was due to diarrhea, measles, pneumonia, or some other disease for which malnutrition set the stage. Another third of the deaths was caused by prematurity, which is often a product of undernutrition in the mother.

Physiologic Changes During Pregnancy Affecting Nutrition

The mother undergoes many complex physiologic adjustments during pregnancy. Some of these adjustments regulate maternal metabolism and promote optimal fetal growth and development. Others preserve maternal homeostasis and prepare the mother for labor, birth, and lactation. These physiologic changes affect the mother's appetite, digestion, absorption, and use of nutrients in many ways.

Hormonal Effects on Nutrition

During pregnancy the placenta assumes a major role in the production of hormones. Some hormones are produced only during pregnancy. They are human chorionic gonadotropin (HCG), human placental lactogen (also called human chorionic somatomammotropin), and human chorionic thyrotropin. Other hormones, such as progesterone and estrogen, are produced at higher levels during pregnancy and have direct effects on metabolism and nutrition.

Progesterone causes a relaxation of the smooth muscles, including the gastrointestinal tract. This relaxation of the gastrointestinal tract reduces motility in the gut, allowing more time for the nutrients to be absorbed. Other metabolic effects of progesterone are increased maternal fat deposition and increased renal sodium excretion. Estrogen has a hygroscopic, or water-retaining effect. As a result many pregnant women complain of excess fluid retention, which is regarded as normal. Nausea, which can have a significant impact on the mother's dietary intake, is believed to be caused in part by elevated HCG levels.

Metabolic Changes During Pregnancy

Some maternal physiologic adjustments have effects on overall metabolism and are the basis for the increased nutritional requirements and dietary allowances during pregnancy. These metabolic adjustments are described in detail in Chapter 11. They include the following:

- Increase in plasma volume
- Progressive increases in blood lipids
- Increase in red blood cells
- Increase in white blood cells
- Changes in renal function
- Increase in cardiac output

These metabolic adjustments require an overall increase in nutrient and food energy requirements. The next section discusses specific nutritional needs, providing the necessary background for nursing interventions related to nutritional care during pregnancy.

Nutrient Requirements During Pregnancy

During pregnancy the woman must meet not only her own nutritional needs, but also the needs of the growing fetus. There are additional demands from the growth of new fetal and maternal tissue. Although this growth process means increased nutritional requirements during pregnancy, some nutrients are of particular importance. The following summary of requirements for food energy, protein, vitamins, and minerals during pregnancy is based on nationally recognized Recommended Dietary Allowances (RDA) (National Research Council, 1990). This information is necessary for the nurse to advise pregnant women about adequate nutritional intake to meet the increased demands of pregnancy.

Energy

Additional calories are needed during pregnancy to support increased tissue synthesis by the pregnant woman and fetus. Additional metabolic cost is incurred by new tissue growth. Adequate intake of kilocalories (kcal) for energy is necessary for optimal protein use and tissue growth.

The total energy cost of pregnancy is 55,000 kcal (Institute of Medicine, 1990). This translates to an additional 300 kcal/d over nonpregnant needs during the second and third trimesters of pregnancy. Additional energy is probably not required during the first trimester of pregnancy because metabolic demands are not as high (National Research Council, 1990). Because caloric requirements are difficult to predict and vary widely among pregnant women, factors such as maternal age, activity, height, prepregnant weight, health, and stage of pregnancy must be considered. Differences in these parameters require that individual caloric needs be calculated for each individual to advise the pregnant woman accurately about dietary intake. One method of determining an individual woman's energy needs during pregnancy is shown in the accompanying display.

Determination of Energy Needs During Pregnancy

1. Determine nonpregnant body weight in kilograms (weight in pounds divided by 2.2).
2. Determine resting energy expenditure (REE) using the following values:
   28.5 kcal/kg for 11–14 years
   24.9 kcal/kg for 15–18 years
   23.3 kcal/kg for 19–24 years
   21.9 kcal/kg for 25–50 years
3. Multiply the REE by the activity factor, which is the following:
   1.3 for very light activity
   1.5 for light activity
   1.6 for moderate activity
   1.9 for heavy activity and
   2.2 for exceptionally heavy activity
4. Add 300 kcal for pregnancy during the second and third trimesters.

Adapted with permission from Recommended Dietary Allowances: 10th Edition. Copyright 1989 by the National Academy of Sciences. Courtesy of the National Academy Press, Washington, D.C.

Caloric expenditure is not distributed evenly throughout gestation. There is a slight increase during early pregnancy, with a sharp increase near the end of the first trimester. This level then remains constant until term. During the second trimester most of this extra caloric expenditure is devoted to maternal factors (blood expansion, uterine growth, breast tissue growth, and fat storage); during the last trimester the caloric expenditure is due primarily to the growth of the fetus and placenta.

Protein

Protein is needed in increased amounts during pregnancy to provide sufficient amino acids for fetal development, blood volume expansion, and growth of maternal breast and uterine tissues. The current RDA for protein intake is an additional 10 g of protein per day over the nonpregnant needs of adult women. It is important to remember that adequate protein intake without adequate calories should be avoided. If caloric intake is below the required amount, protein will be used for maternal energy needs rather than for its primary function of tissue building and maintenance. Steps in determination of protein needs during pregnancy are given in the accompanying display.

Determination of Protein Needs During Pregnancy

1. Determine the nonpregnant weight in kilograms (weight in pounds divided by 2.2).
2. Multiply by the following:
   1 g/kg for 11–14 years
   0.8 g/kg for 14–50 years
3. Add 10 g of protein for pregnancy.
4. Use this value or 60 g of protein per day, whichever is higher.

National Research Council. (1990). Recommended dietary allowances *(10th ed.). Washington, DC: National Academy Press.*

Carbohydrate and Fat

Carbohydrate and fat content of the diet should be adequate to meet energy needs. The proportion of carbohydrate in the diet of the pregnant woman is the same as for her nonpregnant counterpart. Carbohydrates should supply 55% to 60% of calories in the diet. Most of this intake should be in the form of complex carbohydrates, such as whole-grain cereal products, starchy vegetables, and legumes. The intake of simple sugars should be minimized.

Fat should not provide more than 30% of the energy in the diet. Saturated fat should be limited to no more than 10% of total calories. The remainder of the fat can be either polyunsaturated or monosaturated, though the latter is considered the preferred type of dietary fat.

Vitamins

Generally most vitamin requirements are increased during pregnancy (Tables 17-1 and 17-2). The accelerated energy and protein metabolism require increased amounts of vitamins for tissue synthesis and energy production.

In the past folic acid was routinely supplemented during pregnancy. This vitamin functions as a coenzyme in the synthesis of DNA and plays an integral role in red blood cell formation. The major dietary sources of folic acid are fruits, vegetables, and whole-grain cereals, which are readily available in the American diet. Therefore, routine supplementation of this vitamin is no longer advised.

Vitamin D is synthesized in the skin after exposure to the ultraviolet rays of the sun. It also is available in vitamin D fortified milk. Lack of this vitamin may be of concern for women who do not routinely consume milk. This concern is compounded in northern latitudes in the winter where the exposure to ultraviolet light is minimal. Women who, due to cultural beliefs, have little exposure to sunlight, may be at risk for vitamin D deficiency. Because vitamin D is necessary for the absorption and use of calcium, adequate intake is of considerable importance in pregnancy.

Minerals

Mineral requirements also are increased during pregnancy. This section discusses specific needs for iron, calcium, sodium, and zinc. Recommended dietary intake of these minerals during pregnancy is listed in Table 17-3.

Table 17-1. Recommended Intake of Fat-Soluble Vitamins

	Nonpregnant Intake				Pregnant Intake			
Age in Years	Vitamin A (μg RE)*	Vitamin D (μg)	Vitamin E (mg TE)†	Vitamin K (μg)	Vitamin A (μg RE)	Vitamin D (μg)	Vitamin E (mg TE)	Vitamin K (μg)
11–14	800	10	8	45	800	10	10	65
15–18	800	10	8	45	800	10	10	65
19–24	800	10	8	45	800	10	10	65
25–50	800	5	8	45	800	10	10	65

* RE = retinol equivalents.
800 = 4,000 IU (International units)
1000 = 5,000 IU (International units)
† TE = tocopherol equivalents
Adapted with permission from *Recommended Dietary Allowances: 10th Edition.* Copyright 1989 by the National Academy of Sciences. Courtesy of the National Academy Press, Washington, D.C.

Table 17-2. Recommended Intake of Water-Soluble Vitamins

	Age in Years			
Vitamin	11–14	15–18	19–24	25–50
Nonpregnant Intake				
Vitamin C (mg)	50	60	60	60
Thiamin (mg)	1.1	1.1	1.1	1.1
Riboflavin (mg)	1.3	1.3	1.3	1.3
Niacin (mg)	15	15	15	15
Vitamin B_6 (mg)	1.4	1.5	1.6	1.6
Folacin (μg)	150	180	180	180
Vitamin B_{12} (μg)	2	2	2	2
Pregnant Intake				
Vitamin C (mg)	70	70	70	70
Thiamin (mg)	1.5	1.5	1.5	1.5
Riboflavin (mg)	1.6	1.6	1.6	1.6
Niacin (mg)	17	17	17	17
Vitamin B_6 (mg)	2.2	2.2	2.2	2.2
Folacin (μg)	400	400	400	400
Vitamin B_{12} (μg)	2.2	2.2	2.2	2.2

Adapted with permission from *Recommended Dietary Allowances: 10th Edition.* Copyright 1989 by the National Academy of Sciences. Courtesy of the National Academy Press, Washington, D.C.

Iron

Pregnancy imposes substantial demands for iron, primarily because of the increased volume of the maternal blood supply and the growth of fetal and maternal tissues. Most iron in the body is in the form of hemoglobin, which is responsible for carrying oxygen to the body's cells, and the adequacy of the mother's iron store is reflected in the concentration of hemoglobin.

The "iron cost" of a full-term pregnancy with a single fetus has been calculated to be approximately 1000 mg. This means that approximately 3 mg absorbed iron is required daily during pregnancy. Both the fetus and the placenta effectively use iron and folate from the mother, even if she is grossly deficient. This iron drain reaches a peak after the 20th week of pregnancy. Iron balance also is influenced by the mode of delivery: a blood loss of 500 mL, which may occur with an operative delivery or excess maternal blood loss, represents more than 200 mg of iron lost from the system.

Although a portion of these needs could be met from the

Table 17-3. Recommended Intake of Minerals

	Age in Years			
Mineral	11–14	15–18	19–24	25–50
Nonpregnant Intake				
Calcium (mg)	1200	1200	1200	800
Phosphorus (mg)	1200	1200	1200	800
Magnesium (mg)	280	300	280	280
Iron (mg)	15	15	15	15
Zinc (mg)	12	12	12	12
Iodine (mg)	150	150	150	150
Pregnant Intake				
Calcium (mg)	1200	1200	1200	1200
Phosphorus (mg)	1200	1200	1200	1200
Magnesium (mg)	320	320	320	320
Iron (mg)*	30	30	30	30
Zinc (mg)	15	15	15	15
Iodine (mg)	175	175	175	175

*Supplemental iron is needed daily in addition to dietary sources.

Adapted with permission from *Recommended Dietary Allowances: 10th Edition.* Copyright 1989 by the National Academy of Sciences. Courtesy of the National Academy Press, Washington, D.C.

iron stores in the bone marrow, liver, and spleen, rarely are these sufficient to cover all the woman's needs without compromising her well-being. In men iron stores range from 500 to 1500 mg, but in women they tend to be much lower or even nonexistent. This is because women tend to have diets low in iron and because blood is lost regularly through menstruation.

Women with borderline iron stores will develop iron deficiency anemia if their iron intake is not supplemented during pregnancy. Even a woman whose nutritional status is excellent will complete a pregnancy with a deficit in available iron if her dietary intake is not supplemented.

Iron Deficiency Anemia. The most common nutritional disorder of pregnancy is iron deficiency anemia. Its symptoms include fatigue, anorexia, pallor, inability to concentrate, listlessness, and irritability. This condition causes a reduction in the capacity to do energy-requiring tasks. Iron deficiency imposes a limit on the body's ability to transport oxygen to the tissues.

The presence of iron deficiency anemia is confirmed by a hemoglobin of less than 11, along with other laboratory evidence of iron deficiency. Once the diagnosis is made, additional iron supplements may be prescribed. If this occurs, zinc and copper also will need to be supplemented because high doses of iron interfere with the use of these nutrients.

Nonpregnant women absorb only approximately 10% of the available iron in food. Thus, the dietary requirement of 15 mg/d for the nonpregnant woman produces an average of 1.5 mg/d for the body's use. During the second half of pregnancy the efficiency of iron absorption from food increases to approximately 25%. The mother's iron loss is lessened by the cessation of menstruation. However, even with these physiologic adjustments, the increased iron requirement during pregnancy cannot be met by the iron content in typical American diets. The average American's diet contains only approximately 6 mg iron per 1000 calories. Thus, it is recommended that 30 mg of ferrous iron (approximately 150 mg of ferrous sulfate, 300 mg of ferrous gluconate, or 100 mg of ferrous fumarate) be given in the form of a daily supplement during the second and third trimesters of pregnancy (Institute of Medicine, 1990).

Iron is best used when the supplements are taken on an empty stomach. However, this may cause gastrointestinal distress in some individuals. If this occurs, it is advisable to try a different form of iron supplement (ie, change from ferrous gluconate to ferrous sulfate). Some individuals will tolerate one form better than another.

Calcium and Phosphorus

During pregnancy extra calcium is required for fetal bone development. In the third trimester the fetus accumulates calcium at an average rate of 300 mg/d. If calcium intake is inadequate, fetal needs will be met by demineralization of the maternal skeleton. Pregnancy is accompanied by extensive adjustments in calcium metabolism; hormonal factors, phosphorus, and vitamin D positively affect maternal calcium retention. The recommended dietary requirement for calcium in pregnancy is 1200 mg/d.

The requirement for phosphorus is similar to that for calcium; however, phosphorus is so widely available in foods that a dietary deficiency is rare. Calcium and phosphorus exist in a balanced ratio in the blood. This ratio can be disturbed by the amounts of calcium and phosphorus in foods. The American diet is high in phosphorus. High levels are found in most animal protein foods, and even greater amounts are found in processed foods, meats, and soft drinks. With the exception of dairy products, foods that are high in phosphorus contain only small amounts of calcium. The pregnant woman needs 1200 mg of phosphorus per day.

Sodium

Much has been learned in recent years about the normal physiology of pregnancy. One result is that sodium or salt restrictions are no longer advocated for pregnant women. In years past sodium restriction was recommended for pregnant women to prevent edema; this was thought to reduce the risk of pregnancy-induced hypertension. However, it is now known that sodium metabolism is altered during pregnancy. In a normal pregnancy the glomerular filtration rate is increased by approximately 50%. Compensatory mechanisms come into play to maintain fluid and electrolyte balance. The increased fluid normally retained during pregnancy actually increases the body's need for sodium.

The typical American diet contains 4 g of sodium per day or more. Moderation in the use of salt and other sodium-rich foods is appropriate for everyone, not just pregnant women. Although no RDA has been established for sodium, 2 to 3 g of sodium per day is adequate to meet maternal needs during pregnancy.

Zinc

The role of zinc in the synthesis of DNA and RNA makes it a highly important element in reproduction. In humans the incidence of central nervous system malformations appears to be increased in areas where zinc deficiency is common. Marginal zinc deficiency has been documented in the United States. More recently, impaired taste acuity and subnormal growth in children have been associated with marginal zinc deficiency.

Marginal zinc deficiency may develop over a period of weeks. Therefore, it is important that zinc be supplied in the mother's diet daily. The RDA for zinc in pregnancy is 15 mg/d, an increase of 3 mg/d over the nonpregnant RDA. Animal proteins constitute the principal dietary sources of zinc. Meat, liver, eggs, and seafood (especially oysters) are the best sources of zinc. Milk, wheat germ, and legumes are good sources. Zinc intake is closely related to protein intake in the diet.

Multiple Vitamin and Mineral Supplements

With the exception of iron, which is recommended for all pregnant women, vitamin and mineral supplementation is not recommended unless the woman is at nutritional risk. Some health professionals routinely recommend vitamin and mineral supplementation during pregnancy as a form of "insurance" even when supplements are not strictly indicated. While this practice may not be harmful, megadoses of some vitamins and minerals can be deleterious to the health of the woman and the fetus. This is especially true of the fat-soluble vitamins, which are stored in the body and can reach toxic levels in tissue. Vitamin or mineral supplements used during pregnancy should not provide more than the RDA for pregnant women, except in the specific circumstances described in the accompanying display.

The pregnant woman undergoes many complex physiologic adjustments that affect appetite, digestion, absorption, and use of nutrients. Metabolic adjustments require an overall increase in requirements for nutrients and food energy. Additional calories are needed to support increased tissue synthesis by the pregnant woman and fetus. Protein is needed in increased amounts to provide sufficient amino acids for fetal development, blood volume expansion, and growth of maternal breast and uterine tissues. The accelerated energy and protein metabolism require increased amounts of vitamins for tissue synthesis and energy production. Pregnancy imposes substantial demands for iron, primarily because of the increased volume of the maternal blood supply and the growth of fetal and maternal tissues. Even a woman whose nutritional status is excellent will complete a pregnancy with a deficit in available iron if her dietary intake is not supplemented. With the exception of iron, which is recommended for all pregnant women, vitamin and mineral supplementation is not recommended unless the woman is at nutritional risk.

Vitamin Supplementation Recommendations for Women at Nutritional Risk

Pregnant women thought to be at nutritional risk are the following:

- Those with poor dietary intake
- Those carrying multiple fetuses
- Those who are heavy cigarette smokers or abuse alcohol and other drugs

Women at risk should take one between-meal supplement each day. This supplement should be taken during the second and third trimesters and should contain the following nutrients:

- Iron, 30 mg
- Zinc, 15 mg
- Copper, 2 mg
- Calcium, 250 mg
- Vitamin B_6 2 mg
- Folate, 300 μg
- Vitamin C, 50 mg
- Vitamin D, 5 μg

Other recommendations regarding vitamin and mineral supplementation during pregnancy including the following:

- Complete vegetarians and others who do not drink vitamin D fortified milk should take 10 μg of vitamin D per day.
- Women younger than age 25 whose dietary intake of calcium is less than 600 mg/d should take 600 mg of calcium at mealtime.
- Complete vegetarians should take 2 μg of vitamin B_{12} daily.
- Women taking more than 30 mg of iron supplementation per day also should take 2 mg of copper and 15 mg of zinc per day.

Reprinted with permission from *Nutrition During Pregnancy and Lactation: An Implementation Guide.* Copyright 1992 by the National Academy of Sciences. Courtesy of the National Academy Press, Washington, D.C.

Implications for Nursing Care

The nurse's role in nutritional care of the pregnant woman involves careful assessment of nutritional status, intervention based on identified needs, and ongoing evaluation of the woman's nutritional status as pregnancy progresses. The nurse working in the outpatient setting has an important responsibility in meeting the pregnant woman's needs for nutritional care, especially if the setting does not allow for routine contact with a registered dietitian. The pregnant woman's attitude and understanding will be affected by the nurse's own positive teaching strategies about nutrition. The nurse's enthusiasm, sensitivity, and awareness of the individual woman's needs contribute greatly to effective nutritional counseling. Knowledge of principles and goals in nutritional care is essential in providing quality nursing care.

• • Assessment

Cultural, socioeconomic, family, and developmental factors are influential in forming nutritional habits. The nurse collects pertinent information on these factors as part of his or her assessment of a pregnant woman's nutritional status.

Obtaining a General Nutritional Assessment

The nurse must rely on four types of data in the basic assessment of the pregnant woman's nutritional status: health history, physical examination, laboratory tests, and dietary history.

Health History

Assessment of the pregnant woman's nutritional status begins with a carefully taken health history, with special attention to obstetric history. These data help to identify nutritional problems that may be risk factors in the current pregnancy. For instance, multiple, closely spaced pregnancies or previous complications that may have lead to blood loss may put a woman at risk for iron deficiency anemia in a subsequent pregnancy. An excess weight gain with a previous pregnancy may not have been lost. The health history is especially important in identifying factors that put pregnant women at nutritional risk.

Physical Examination

The physical examination is an important aspect of nutritional assessment. Probably the most important part of the physical examination is assessment of the prepregnant and pregnant weight and height. The prepregnancy weight should be determined by history and often is used as a measure of nutritional status before conception. Height should be a measured value, not self-reported.

Once height and weight are obtained, a prepregnancy body mass index (BMI) is calculated. The BMI is a ratio of weight to height. To calculate the BMI weight is converted to kilograms by dividing the weight in pounds by 2.2, and height is converted from inches to meters by multiplying the height in inches by 0.0254. The formula for obtaining the BMI is weight (in kg) divided by height (in meters^2). Optimal weight gain recommended for pregnant women is based on this BMI.

Physical examination may identify signs of nutritional deficiencies. Many signs of nutrient deficiency develop in exposed parts of the body—hair, face, neck, eyes, lips, gums, teeth, arms, hands, and lower extremities. Indicators that may suggest specific nutrient deficiencies on the physical examination are shown in Table 17-4.

Laboratory Tests

The findings of many laboratory tests are altered by normal gestation. Reference to standards for pregnant women is necessary when interpreting test results. If the standards for nonpregnant individuals are used, test results can falsely suggest deficiency states. For instance blood levels of glucose, calcium, trace minerals, most amino acids, and nearly all water-soluble vitamins decline with pregnancy. Levels of other blood components, such as lipids and fat-soluble vitamins, rise during gestation. Normal laboratory values during pregnancy are listed in the appendix.

Dietary History

During the pregnant woman's first or second prenatal visit, the nurse obtains a dietary history. The woman should receive a complete explanation of the purpose of the dietary history. The explanation gives the nurse an excellent opportunity to emphasize the importance of good nutrition during pregnancy and to encourage the pregnant woman to eat well. The nurse's goal is to determine if the pregnant woman's dietary intake is adequate in the amounts and quality of nutrients for her own needs and for the growth and development of the fetus. The nurse screens for potential dietary problems, such as oversupplementation, ingestion of nonfood substances, or eating disorders. The latter is discussed in the Nursing Research display.

The dietary history is an indispensable part of the nutritional assessment. In a busy clinic, however, it may be done hurriedly or overlooked altogether. The nurse should remember that the accuracy of the information obtained depends on the pregnant woman's understanding of the reasons for the interview. The woman is encouraged to share this information with the nurse in detail.

The 24-Hour Diet Recall. A sample of the 24-hour diet recall is shown in the accompanying Assessment Tool. The nurse should first inquire about the pregnant woman's general pattern of daily activity and food intake. This is done by leading the woman through her usual routine from the time she gets up in the morning until she retires at night. The "24-hour diet recall" is then usually cross-checked with a food list to find out how food intake may vary throughout a typical week. The nurse asks about general food habits, overall frequency of food choices, allergies or food intolerance, cultural reasons for food choices, patterns of preparation, seasoning, size of portions, and general likes and dislikes, rather than confining her questions to any specific day's food intake. This will ensure that the nurse obtains information about long-standing dietary practices, as well as any short-term or recent changes. Use of the 24-hour diet recall in planning an adequate diet is discussed later in the chapter.

Table 17-4. Indicators of Nutrient Deficiency on Physical Examination

Physical Finding	Nutrient Deficit
Significant nondependent edema	Protein
Filiform papillary atrophy of the tongue	Iron/folate
Diffusely enlarged and visible thyroid gland (goiter)	Iodine
Follicular hyperkeratosis of upper arms	Vitamin A
Diffusely swollen red interdental papillae of gums in a clean mouth	Vitamin C
Angular fissures and cheilosis of lips	Riboflavin

Assessing Factors That Influence Dietary Patterns

Socioeconomic background, cultural associations, and developmental status and preferences for and emotional responses to food directly affect attitudes toward nutrition and nutritional habits. The nurse should recognize the importance of these factors and take them into account when assessing a pregnant woman's nutritional status.

Meaning of Food and Food Consumption

Food and food consumption acquire meanings that, for most people, go well beyond the basic need for food as sustenance. Eating patterns develop very early, and food habits are among the most difficult patterns of behavior to change. Food in early childhood is associated with security and love. Attitudes and responses to food develop in relation to family and cultural practices. Children may be rewarded, punished, consoled, or controlled with food. For adults, eating is part of social interaction and is culturally defined as part of celebration, mourning, friendship, recreation, and gift giving. Eating may become especially important at certain times in life for culturally or socially defined reasons. The saying that a pregnant woman is "eating for two" is one such example.

Nursing Research

Pregnancy and Lactation After Anorexia and Bulimia

Bulimia and anorexia may be deleterious to normal reproductive functioning and, if pregnancy occurs, to maternal and infant well-being. Incidence of these disorders may be as high as 20% of women in the United States, presenting a significant population at increased pregnancy risk.

This case study describes a 26-year-old woman who successfully conceived and carried a pregnancy to term, 10 years after the onset of anorexia and bulimia. At age 15 the patient experienced vomiting after meals, her weight dropped from 102 lb (46.3 kg) to 95 lb (43.1 kg), and she became amenorrheic. A diagnosis of anorexia nervosa was made; however, the patient denied that an eating disorder existed and consistently resisted treatment. By age 19 the patient weighed 47 pounds (21.3 kg). During the next year she began treatment but was informed that her amenorrhea and consequent infertility might be irreversible.

Menses returned at 95 lb (43.1 kg) or 93% of ideal body weight and a body mass index of 18.3, lower than the normal of 20.8. By age 25 her weight was 102 lb (46.3 kg), 8 lb less than her ideal body weight of 110 lb (49.9 kg). She conceived after 4 months of marriage and gained 43 lb (19.5 kg) during pregnancy.

The patient experienced no concerns about weight gain or body size during pregnancy and maintained a balanced dietary intake with few nutrient deficiences. She delivered a healthy full-term infant, and breastfed the infant exclusively for 5 months. At 1-month postpartum the patient weighted 115 lb (52.2 kg), and at 3 months her weight stabilized at 102 lb (46.3 kg).

When assessing a patient's ability to conceive, complete a pregnancy, and breastfeed following recovery from anorexia or bulimia, it is important to review the medical and nutritional history and support adequate weight gain and nutritional balance without placing undue emphasis on it. The nurse should be alert for negative comments related to body image or weight gain, and counseling should be advised if any signs of relapse are noted. Further research is recommended on pregnancy and breastfeeding outcomes in this population.

Bowles, B., & Williamson, B. (1990). Pregnancy and lactation following anorexia and bulimia. *Journal of Obstetric, Gynecologic, and Neonatal Nursing, 19*(3), 242–249.

Socioeconomic Status

Socioeconomic status has a direct and profound effect on nutritional habits. When finances are strained, the food budget often is made up of the money that remains after fixed and more pressing costs, such as rent, transportation, and medicine, are met. Low-income families often cannot afford high-quality foods and purchase less expensive foods low in nutritional value but high in calories. Low-income families also may copy patterns of food buying advertised in the media. Unfortunately, highly advertised items tend to be "prestige" food items that do not improve the overall nutritional value of the diet, such as coffee, soft drinks, and snack foods.

Employment patterns may directly affect nutritional status. As more women enter the work force, traditional food preparation patterns are giving way to the use of more "convenience" foods. Processed foods often are high in phosphorus, which can interfere with calcium use. Diets that contain a lot of processed convenience foods and "fast foods" tend to be higher in calories, fats, and sodium and lower in fiber than more traditional diets.

Cultural Influences

Food and food habits usually are prescribed culturally. Most cultures have a wealth of traditional dishes that use a variety of ingredients. This variety in traditional diets often leads to a well-balanced intake of essential nutrients. As people abandon traditional diets for more modern dietary patterns, they may end up with a less varied and less nutritious diet. This new dietary pattern may be high in sodium, fat, and calories.

Some ethnic groups have developed dietary patterns in response to food intolerances found in that group. One common type is lactose intolerance. The symptoms of lactose intolerance include abdominal distention, nausea and vomiting, diarrhea, and cramping after consumption of milk. In the United States lactose intolerance is common among African Americans, Asian Americans, Native Americans, and Mexican Americans. Milk consumption generally is low in the traditional diets of these groups. The enzyme lactase, which is available under the brand name Lactaid, may be added to milk to minimize the effects of lactose intolerance and allow the pregnant, lactase-deficient woman to consume adequate dairy products.

Although it is instructive to examine dietary patterns among cultural groups in the United States for overall nutritional adequacy, most people are exposed to multicultural food patterns. People may adhere to their traditional food patterns at main meals, yet reflect mainstream cultural patterns during other meals or snacks. This underscores the importance of examining what families actually do in terms of food selection and preparation, rather than relying only on assumptions about cultural dietary patterns.

Text continues on page 401

Assessment Tool

Dietary Intake
(RECORD DE COMIDA)

DO NOT WRITE IN THIS SPACE NO ESCRIBA EN ESTE ESPACIO
INTAKE SUMMARY

Name/Nombre	Age/Edad	Height/Altura	Weight/Peso

TIME HORA	PLACE LUGAR	AMOUNT CANTIDAD	FOODS EATEN ALIMENTOS CONSUMIDOS	Animal protein	Veg. protein	Milk products	Breads/cereals/grains	Vit. C. frt./veg.	Vit. A frt./veg.	Other fruits/veg.	Unsaturated fats

INFLUENCES ON DIET, COMMENTS, AND FOLLOW-UP	SUMMARY									
	Servings eaten									
	Servings needed									
	Difference									

Condition/diagnosis	Visit no.	Weeks gestation	Date	Interviewer

(continued)

Assessment Tool *(continued)*

Nutritional Assessment for Pregnant Women

Name: ______________________ I.D. #: __________ Date: __________

Please answer the following questions by checking the appropriate box "yes" or "no" or by filling in the blank. Answer only the questions that apply to you. All information is confidential.

For office use only

1. a. How many times have you been pregnant? ______________________
   b. If you have children, list their birth dates and birthweights below.

Birth date and birthweight	Birth date and birthweight
____________	____________
____________	____________
____________	____________

2. Do you now have or have you ever had any of the following?

Yes	No		Yes	No		Yes	No	
☐	☐	Abnormal pap smear	☐	☐	Liver disease/hepatitis	☐	☐	Premature infant
☐	☐	Allergy/asthma	☐	☐	Tuberculosis	☐	☐	Infant weighing less than 5½ lbs. (2,500 g)
☐	☐	Anemia	☐	☐	Venereal disease			
☐	☐	Cancer	☐	☐	Miscarriage	☐	☐	Infant weighing more than 8 lbs. 13 oz. (4,000 g)
☐	☐	Diabetes	☐	☐	Twins/triplets			
☐	☐	Heart disease	☐	☐	Cesarean delivery	☐	☐	Infant with medical problems
☐	☐	High blood pressure	☐	☐	Excessive bleeding during/after delivery			
☐	☐	Intestinal problems				☐	☐	Infant death
☐	☐	Kidney disease						
☐	☐	Other ______________						

3. Have you had any of the following during this pregnancy?

Yes	No		Yes	No		Yes	No	
☐	☐	Nausea	☐	☐	Diarrhea	☐	☐	Stress
☐	☐	Vomiting	☐	☐	Heartburn	☐	☐	Cold/flu
☐	☐	Constipation/ hemorrhoids	☐	☐	Leg cramps	☐	☐	Other illness ________

4. a. Before this pregnancy, what was your usual weight? ________ Pounds/kilos ☐ Don't know

   b. If you have been pregnant before, how much weight did you gain during your last pregnancy?

   ________ Pounds/kilos ________ Don't know

   c. How much weight do you expect to gain during this pregnancy?

   ________ Pounds/kilos ________ Don't know

5. a. How often do you exercise (besides housework, child care)? ______________

   b. What types of exercise do you do? ______________

6. During your pregnancy, have you wanted to eat any of the following?

Yes	No		Yes	No		Yes	No	
☐	☐	Ice/freezer frost	☐	☐	Laundry starch	☐	☐	Plaster
☐	☐	Cornstarch	☐	☐	Dirt or clay	☐	☐	Other: ________

7. Are there any foods that you avoid eating ☐ Yes ☐ No If yes, what: ____________

   ______________________ Why? ______________________

8. Are you now on any of these special diets?

Yes	No		Yes	No		Yes	No	
☐	☐	Diabetic	☐	☐	Low salt	☐	☐	High protein
☐	☐	Low fat	☐	☐	Weight loss	☐	☐	Other: ________

   If yes, who suggested the diet? ______________________

(continued)

Assessment Tool *(continued)*

Nutritional Assessment for Pregnant Women (continued)

For office use only

9. a. Are you a vegetarian? ☐ Yes ☐ No
   b. If yes, do you consume milk products (milk, cheese, yogurt) and/or eggs? ☐ Yes ☐ No

10. During this pregnancy, are you taking the following?

Yes	No		Yes	No		Yes	No	
☐	☐	Prenatal vitamin-mineral formula	☐	☐	Antihistamines/cold remedies	☐	☐	Birth control pills
☐	☐	Iron	☐	☐	Laxatives/antacids	☐	☐	Other prescription drugs
☐	☐	Other vitamins	☐	☐	Other nonprescription drugs	☐	☐	Marijuana/cocaine
☐	☐	Other minerals				☐	☐	Other drugs
☐	☐	Aspirin						

11. How many cups of the following liquids do you usually drink per day?

_______ Water _______ Sodas with sugar _______ Coffee

_______ Juice _______ Diet soda, diet punch _______ Tea

_______ Milk _______ Punch, Kool-Aid, Tang _______ Other: _______

12. a. How often do you drink beer, wine, hard liquor, or mixed drinks? ☐ Daily ☐ Weekly ☐ Monthly
    b. When you drink, how many drinks do you have? ☐ One ☐ Two ☐ Three ☐ More
    c. During this pregnancy, how many times have you had more than four drinks on any single occasion?
    ____

13. How many cigarettes do you smoke each day?
    ☐ Do not smoke ☐ Fewer than 10 cigarettes ☐ 11–20 cigarettes ☐ More than 20 cigarettes

14. What is the highest grade or year of regular school you have completed?
    ☐ Less than 6 years
    ☐ Elementary school (6 years)
    ☐ Junior high school (9 years)
    ☐ High school (12 years)
    ☐ Two-year college (14 years)
    ☐ Four-year college (16 years)
    ☐ Graduate school (17+ years)

15. Do you live: ☐ Alone ☐ With own family ☐ With other people

16. Check if you have the following: ☐ Stove ☐ Oven ☐ Refrigerator

17. a. Do you plan your own meals? ☐ Yes ☐ No
    b. Do you buy your own food? ☐ Yes ☐ No
    c. Do you prepare your own food? ☐ Yes ☐ No

18. How would you describe the type and amount of food in your household?
    ☐ Enough of the kind you want
    ☐ Enough, but not always the kind you want
    ☐ Sometimes not enough
    ☐ Often not enough

19. Are you receiving any of the following?
    ☐ Food stamps
    ☐ WIC
    ☐ Medi-Cal
    ☐ AFDC/welfare
    ☐ Donated food/meals
    ☐ Other: _______

20. a. How do you plan to feed your baby?
    ☐ Breastfeed ☐ Both breast and formula
    ☐ Formula-feed ☐ Other: _______
    b. Have you ever breastfed or tried to breastfeed before? ☐ Yes ☐ No
    c. If yes, how long did you breastfeed? _______
    d. Why did you stop breastfeding? _______

Reviewed by:

California Department of Health Services, Maternal and Child Health Branch. (1990). *Nutrition during pregnancy and the postpartum period: A manual for health care professionals.*

Mexican American Dietary Patterns. Mexican Americans make up a major cultural subgroup in the United States, particularly in the Southwest and West. Many Mexican Americans eat one "good" meal daily at noon. This meal is usually a hot meal that includes soup, beans, tortillas, and meat. Snacks may be taken throughout the day, especially if the main meal is delayed until the evening. Foods found in Mexican restaurants, such as tacos, enchiladas, and tamales, may not be a large part of a family's actual diet, especially if the mother is employed outside the home or if the family adopts the accelerated lifestyle common in the United States.

Milk is not typically consumed as a beverage in the Mexican American pregnant woman's diet, although it may be used occasionally in cooking. Vegetable and fruit consumption tends to be irregular. Well-liked vegetables include peppers, lettuce, tomatoes, and corn. Overcooking vegetables often results in a loss of much of their nutritional value. Fruits commonly eaten are apples and bananas. Chilies, which are frequently used, may be an adequate source of vitamin C, but the ascorbic acid content of this food often is destroyed in processing. Sweets are consumed frequently. Fats, usually lard and butter, are commonly used in preparation, often by frying. Major nutrients that may be lacking in the Mexican American diet are vitamin A, vitamin C, and calcium. Iron consumption may be adequate because pinto beans, which are high in iron, form a significant part of the diet (California Department of Health Services, 1989).

The pregnant Mexican American woman may be at nutritional risk for several reasons. First, she may not receive early prenatal care because of poverty, language and cultural barriers, or the belief that pregnancy is a normal state and does not require routine health care. For these reasons dietary deficiencies may not be detected until late in pregnancy. If she snacks frequently on fast foods, sweets, or soft drinks, she may be consuming adequate calories but insufficient protein. The strong orientation toward the family and the high value placed on children in Mexican American culture may provide the opportunity for nutrition education for other family members. Improvement of family health status may be a strong motivator for the pregnant woman to improve her dietary habits (California Department of Health Services, 1990).

Asian American Dietary Patterns. The largest Asian American populations in the United States are on the coasts, predominantly in larger cities. Asian American groups actually represent a variety of distinct and widely different ethnic groups, including Chinese, Japanese, and Southeast Asian. Among Asian people, food is an important aspect of the culture. For thousands of years the Chinese have used food and herbs to improve and promote health and to treat disease. Traditional beliefs among Chinese and some Southeast Asian people divide food into "hot" (Yang) foods, such as meat, eggs, and ginger, and "cold" (Yin) foods, such as winter melon, bananas, and fish. It is thought that these two groups should be balanced in each meal. Certain types of food may be prescribed or restricted on the basis of physical health in Asian American culture.

Asian American diets include many vegetables, such as cabbage, snow peas, mushrooms, bean sprouts, and sweet potatoes. Generally food is cooked quickly so that nutrient values are not lost. Food usually is purchased fresh and prepared the same day. White rice and noodles are the staples of the diet and may be eaten at every meal. Meat intake is moderate; fish and chicken are the main protein sources rather than meat. Fresh fruit is often used. Milk and dairy products are rarely used in traditional diets. Asian Americans may avoid milk products because of lactose intolerance. Sweets are not commonly used (California Department of Health Services, 1990).

Asian American diets often are very nutritious and contain adequate protein and nutrient levels. Calcium intake may be of concern because milk intake may be low. The pregnant Asian American woman who adheres to a more traditional diet often is in excellent nutritional status, except for calcium intake. Tofu (soybean curd) is an appropriate substitution; 1/2 cup of tofu contains the same amount of calcium as 1/2 cup of milk and the same amount of protein as two eggs. Asian Americans often regard the childbearing period as a very important time. Women may be motivated to make adjustments in their diets because of the value placed on childbearing (California Department of Health Services, 1990).

African American Dietary Patterns. Dietary patterns among African Americans vary widely according to region and socioeconomic status. Diets in middle-class or upwardly mobile African American families may be traditionally American and involve a high intake of red meats, starches, and snack foods. Poor families may spend food budgets on foods that are high in calories, fat, and carbohydrates. They may have extremely limited intakes of protein, fresh fruits, and vegetables. As income improves, families typically spend increasing amounts of the food budget on meat. African Americans may experience mild lactose intolerance and use little milk or dairy products in the diet. For many African Americans "soul food" has strong cultural associations. This diet is based on a diet common in rural regions. It relies heavily on foods available on subsistence farms, such as pork products, fried foods, gravies, field vegetables, and starches. Milk or dairy products are used very little (California Department of Health Services, 1990).

The pregnant African American woman may be at nutritional risk because of caloric imbalance in the diet. High intake of fats and carbohydrates, coupled with inadequate protein intake, contribute to obesity. These foods may cause too-rapid weight gain during pregnancy. The high incidence of pregnancy-induced hypertension among poor African American women may reflect dietary imbalance. Women living in extreme poverty are typically undernourished and at risk for inadequate weight gain during pregnancy.

Vegetarianism. Vegetarianism is widespread and diverse in the United States. This is due in part to the growth of "alternative life-styles" that may involve various forms of vegetarianism. An increased interest in fitness and health promotion and increasing numbers of ethnic minorities for whom vegetarianism is a cultural norm contribute to the number of pregnant women who may practice vegetarianism. Generally, those adhering to vegetarian patterns can be classified in two broad groups.

Traditional vegetarians are those whose cultural or religious affiliation prescribes their diet, such as Seventh Day Adventists or Hindi sects. Groups with long-standing customs usually evolve adequate diets through the consistent use of a wide variety of foods. "New" vegetarians are those who have adopted vegetarian dietary patterns recently for reasons that are personal or philosophic, rather than religious or cultural. Dietary intake varies more widely in this group and may be associated with the use of so-called health foods.

Within these two groups of vegetarians, there are dietary subdivisions. There are many forms of vegetarianism, some more beneficial during pregnancy than others. Vegans are those who consume no animal foods of any kind. Lactovegetarians consume milk and dairy products but exclude meat, poultry, fish and seafood, and eggs. Lacto-ovovegetarians include milk products and eggs in their diets. Partial vegetarians may exclude a specific type of animal food, usually meat, from their diet but may consume fish and poultry. Fruitarians are those who consume large amounts of fruit as a staple diet. Macrobiotics consume highly restricted vegan diets, with the goal of achieving a diet of 100% cereals; this diet may result in severe nutritional deficiencies.

In general, a well-planned lacto-ovovegetarian diet, consisting of a variety of largely unrefined plant foods supplemented with milk and eggs, meets all known nutrient needs. Such a diet can be planned to meet calorie, nutrient, and protein requirements during pregnancy. Iron and folic acid supplements are recommended, as with other prenatal diets. If a mother adheres to a vegan diet, consultation with a registered dietitian or nutritionist is advisable to ensure a safe calorie intake. Adequate protein intake using grains, seeds, nuts, and vegetables can be accomplished if the pregnant woman is knowledgeable about types and amounts of foods to consume during pregnancy.

Identifying Nutritional Risk Factors

Nutritional risk in pregnancy is identified by 18 factors. The recommended definition of maternal nutritional risk factors is listed in the accompanying display. The Assessment Tool provides parameters that must be examined to identify nutritional risk.

Adolescence

The pregnant adolescent is likely to be at nutritional risk for several reasons. First, because musculoskeletal growth can continue for several years after ovulation begins, the pregnant adolescent must meet her own nutrient needs for growth and maturation in addition to those of the fetus. The increased demands for protein, calories, and nutrients are reflected in the recommended daily requirements for adolescents (see Tables 17-1 through 17-3). Adolescents tend to have high activity levels, which pose additional nutritional demands. Dietary patterns may be less than optimal because of concerns about body weight, peer pressure, and heavy commercial marketing of snack foods directed at adolescents. (See Chapter 9 for additional discussion of nursing care for the pregnant adolescent.)

Caffeine and Alcohol Use

The nurse should screen for caffeine and alcohol use. Questions or concerns the mother may have can be answered at the time of the assessment. Because of reports in the media and a general increase in interest in the health effects of diet, many pregnant women are concerned about the possible effects of various substances on the fetus.

The nurse should recognize that conclusive research findings on the effects of substances on human pregnancy and birth are rare. Most preliminary work relies on animal research and retrospective studies of large numbers of pregnant women. With the exception of a direct link between excessive alcohol use and the risk of fetal alcohol syndrome (described below), scientific evidence of a direct link between use of certain substances and problems in pregnancy may be tenuous at best. However, women can be advised that because nearly all substances ingested by the mother affect her own health and potentially the health of her fetus, it is wise to cut down on or avoid caffeine and alcohol during her pregnancy.

Caffeine. In 1980 the Food and Drug Administration issued a recommendation that pregnant women avoid, or use sparingly, foods and drugs containing caffeine. In part this recommendation was based on animal research that suggested that caffeine was associated with decreased intrauterine growth, skeletal anomalies, and low birth weight. However, as with all animal research, the applicability of findings to humans is uncertain because of differences in mode and amount of the drug consumed and differences in human metabolism. Based on the evidence, caffeine appears to have little effect on pregnancy outcome. However, in view of a possible association between caffeine use and low birth weight and premature rupture of membranes, the nurse should encourage moderation in caffeine intake during pregnancy. Caffeine is found in many food and drug products, including coffee, tea, cola drinks, chocolate, and cough remedies.

Alcohol. In recent years ethanol has been shown to be teratogenic in humans. Fetal alcohol syndrome is characterized by craniofacial abnormalities, delayed motor development, low birth weight and smallness for dates, and mental retardation. It occurs in 1 in 4000 to 5000 births. There is evidence that women who drink large amounts of alcohol (five or more drinks per day) regularly place their unborn fetus at increased risk for fetal alcohol syndrome. The risk of congenital abnormalities and low birth weight is increased even among mothers who drink moderately (two to four drinks per day). The risk of fetal alcohol syndrome appears to increase proportionately with increases in average daily intake of alcohol. The effects of very low consumption of alcohol have not yet been determined. Fetal alcohol syndrome is discussed further in Chapter 33.

The nurse should routinely screen for level of alcohol use among pregnant mothers. Women should be advised of the potential risks to the fetus. Because safe intake levels have not been established, the safest practice is to abstain from all alcohol use during pregnancy. Women who are addicted to alcohol during pregnancy require specialized support and treatment for their condition.

Maternal Nutritional Risk Factors*

Anthropometric

Moderately Overweight

- Greater than 120% of desirable pregravid weight for height
- BMI of greater than 26 to 29

Very Overweight

- Greater than 135% of desirable pregravid weight for height
- BMI of greater than 29

Underweight

- Less than 90% of desirable pregravid weight for height
- BMI less than 19.8

Inadequate Weight Gain (During Pregnancy)

During trimesters 2 and 3:

- Less than 1 lb (0.5 kg) per month for very overweight women
- Less than 2 lb (1 kg) per month for all other women

Excessive Weight Gain (During Pregnancy)

- More than 6.5 lb (3 kg) per month

Biochemical (Laboratory)

Anemia

- Nonpregnant, 12–14 years old:
  Hb below 11.8 g/dL (or 118 g/L)
  Hct below 35.5% vol % (or 0.35)
- Nonpregnant, 15 years or older:
  Hb below 12.0 g/dL (or 120 g/L)
  Hct below 36.0 vol % (or 0.36)
- Pregnant, weeks 1–13:
  Hb below 11 (or 110 g/L)
  Hct below 33 (or 0.33)
- Pregnant, weeks 14–28:
  Hb below 10.5 (or 105 g/L)
  Hct below 32 (or 0.32)
- Pregnant, weeks 29+:
  Hb below 11 (or 110 g/L)
  Hct below 33 (or 0.33)

Hypovolemia (Inadequate Plasma Volume Expansion During Pregnancy)

- Between 24 and 34 weeks:
  Hb above 13.9 g/dL (or 139 g/L)
  Hct above 41.9 vol % (or 0.419)

Abnormal Glucose Levels

- 1-hour glucose loading test:
  Venous plasma glucose above 140 g/dL (7.8 mmol/L) 1 hour after 50-g oral glucose load
- 3-hour 100-g oral glucose tolerance test—two or more of the following venous plasma concentrations must be met or exceeded:
  Fasting, 105 mg/dL (5.8 mmol/L)
  1-hour, 190 mg/dL (10.6 mmol/L)
  2-hour, 165 mg/dL (9.2 mmol/L)
  3-hour, 145 mg/dL (8.1 mmol/L)

Clinical (Physical, Medical, Obstetric)

Previous Obstetric Complications

- Hyperemesis gravidarum
- Gestational diabetes
- Preeclampsia
- Anemia
- Preterm labor
- Inadequate weight gain
- Neonatal death (death within first 28 days after birth)
- Stillbirth (greater than 20 weeks' gestation)
- Fetal loss (less than 20 weeks' gestation)
- Premature delivery (less than 37 weeks' gestation)
- Low–birth-weight infant (less than 2500 g)
- Small-for-gestational-age infant
- High–birth-weight infant (more than 4000 g)
- Congenital anomaly
- Postpartum hemorrhage

Adolescence

- Less than 18 years at last menstrual period
- Less than reproductive biologic year 3 (biologic age = chronologic age minus menarcheal age)

High Parity

- Five or more previous deliveries at greater than 20 weeks' gestation

Short Interpregnancy Interval

- 12 months or less between delivery (or termination or pregnancy) and conception

Breastfeeding

- Breastfeeding during current pregnancy
- Inadequate milk supply

(Continued)

Maternal Nutritional Risk Factors* (Continued)

Current Medical or Obstetric Complications

- Diabetes (insulin-dependent, non–insulin-dependent, or gestational)
- Hypertension (chronic or associated with preeclampsia)
- Chronic renal disease
- Chronic liver disease
- Cancer
- Cardiopulmonary disease:
  - Functional heart disease (N.Y. Heart Assoc. class 2 or higher)
  - Organic disease (eg, tuberculosis, pneumonia)
  - Asthma requiring treatment
- Thyroid disease
- Gastrointestinal disease (including parasites, malabsorption more severe than lactase deficiency)
- Use of prescribed drugs known to affect or suspected of affecting the fetus (eg, Dilantin or phenobarbital for epilepsy)
- Multiple pregnancy
- Intrauterine growth retardation
- Severe infection (eg, pyelonephritis, hepatitis, toxoplasmosis, listeriosis, HIV positive)
- Venereal disease (positive VDRL, genital herpes, chlamydia, trichomoniasis)
- Anesthesia, surgery, or trauma shortly before or during the perinatal period
- Systemic evidence of nutritional deficiency

Socioeconomic

Low Income

- Eligible for local, state, or federal assistant programs

Substance Abuse

- Alcohol:
  - Average daily intake of more than 1 oz absolute alcohol (1 oz absolute alcohol = two mixed drinks of two cans beer or two 6-oz glasses wine)
  - Binge drinking
- Cigarettes:
  - More than 10 cigarettes per day
- Recreational or street drugs:
  - Use of narcotics, cocaine, hallucinogens, marijuana, amphetamines, or other recreational or street drugs
- Over-the-counter (OTC) medications and herbal remedies:
  - Chronic use of laxatives, antacids, or other OTC drugs known to affect nutritional status
  - Use of herbal remedies known or suspected to cause toxic side effects
- Vitamin and mineral supplements:
  - Excessive use of nutrient supplements (over toxicity limits):
    - Vitamin A >8000 IU daily
    - Vitamin D >400 IU daily
    - Vitamin C >2000 mg daily
    - Vitamin B_6 >100 mg daily
    - Iodine >11 mg daily
- Caffeine:
  - Excessive intake of caffeine (more than 300 mg/d). This amount of caffeine is found in approximately three cups coffee, four cups tea, or six cans of cola

Pica

- Eating of nonfood substances

Psychological Problems

- Depression influencing appetite or eating
- Current or past history of eating disorders (eg, anorexia nervosa, bulimia)
- Mental retardation
- Mental illness

Dietary

Poor Diet/Inappropriate Food Consumption

- Less than minimum recommended servings from each food group in the Daily Food Guide for Woman
- Excessive intake of fat, sugar, or salt

**Broader and more inclusive definitions for these risk factors are appropriate to determine eligibility for public health programs, such as WIC, because they identify individuals who may be predisposed to poor nutritional status and will benefit from nutritional education.*

California Department of Health Services. (1990). Nutrition during pregnancy and the postpartum period: A Manual for Health Care Professionals.

Pica

Pica or geophagia is defined as the craving for or eating of nonfood substances. Sometimes pregnant women consume dirt (geophagia), laundry starch, or other items that are not usually considered to be foods. Though it has been theorized that these nonfoods are being consumed to satisfy the need for a nutrient missing from the diet, this has not been substantiated. The main problem with eating dirt or clay is the potential for ingestion of bacteria or parasites. Some individuals "bake" dirt to minimize this risk. Another area of concern is that the intake of nonfoods will replace other foods in the diet, thus leading to inadequate nutrient

Assessment Tool

Nutritional Assessment for Pregnant Women

Source | Date
Identification

NUTRITIONAL RISK FACTORS

Very overweight	☐	Hypovolemia	☐	Medical/obstet. complications	☐
Underweight	☐	Prev. obstet. complications	☐	Low income	☐
Inadequate gain	☐	Adolescence	☐	Substance abuse	☐
Excessive gain	☐	High parity	☐	Pica	☐
Anemia	☐	Short interpreg. interval	☐	Psychological problems	☐

VISIT 1

Week gest. ________ Weight ________

BP________ Alb______ Ket________

Comment______ Glu______ Edema______

COMMENTS:

LABORATORY OBSERVATIONS

TEST	Values			
	Date	Date	Date	Date
Hemoglobin (g/dL)				
Hematocrit (%)				
MCV (μ^3 ir fL)				
Cervical cytology				
1-hour oral glucose load				

DIETARY ASSESSMENT

Daily average from ________ days:

Food Group	Minimum Amt./Serv.	Amt./Serv. Eaten	Sugg. Change
Animal protein	6 oz.		
Vegetable protein	1		
Milk products	3		
Breads/cereals/grains	7		
Vitamin C-rich frt./veg.	1		
Vitamin A-rich frt./veg.	1		
Other fruit/veg.	3		
Unsaturated fats	3		

Excessive: ☐ Fat ☐ Sugar ☐ Salt ☐ Caffeine

California Department of Health Services. (1990). *Nutrition during pregnancy and the postpartum period.*

intake. Finally, nonfood ingestion may interfere with nutrient absorption and may cause intestinal obstruction. It is important to identify pica in pregnant women, so the woman can be advised of the health risks. However, pica or geophagia may persist, despite warnings about harmful effects, because it is learned and is frequently cultural in origin.

Assessing Weight Gain

Adequate prenatal care must include repeated measurements of body weight (Fig. 17-1). Appropriate weight gain during pregnancy is essential to the continued good health of the mother and normal development of the fetus. Both prepregnant and pregnant weight are critical factors in the assessment of nutritional status. Prepregnant weight, fetal growth rate, and weight changes all reflect the woman's pattern of food use, particularly her caloric intake. The pregnant woman's weight at conception and her usual dietary practices and activity patterns must be evaluated before her optimal weight gain can be determined. The surest evidence of an adequate caloric intake is steady weight gain. Weight loss or failure to gain weight during pregnancy places mother and fetus at serious risk.

Recommendations for weight gain during pregnancy are based on the prepregnant BMI, and are shown in Table 17-5. A woman who is normal weight for height at conception should gain a total of 10 to 14 kg (25 to 35 lb) during the pregnancy. Women who are underweight at conception should gain more weight; those who were overweight should gain less. The weight gain should be at least 6 kg (15 lb) during the pregnancy. During the second and third trimesters, weight gain should occur at the rate of 0.4 kg (1 lb) per week for normal weight women, 0.5 kg (1.1 lb) per week for underweight women, and 0.3 kg (0.66 lb) per week for overweight women (Institute of Medicine, 1990).

Pregnant women are particularly susceptible to excess weight gain because of hormonal changes and increased appetite. Excess weight gain usually can be slowed if the woman is encouraged to satisfy her appetite with "high-quality" calories (eg, from cottage cheese, lean meats, fish, tofu, whole grains, fruits, and vegetables). The pregnant woman is counseled to avoid excess intake of fats and sugar.

Restriction of food intake to reduce weight gain poses a serious threat during pregnancy. Women with low weight gain during pregnancy, especially those already 10% or more below the recommended weight for height, are at increased risk of delivering a low–birth-weight neonate. If the mother's food intake is insufficient to provide for the fetus' need for energy, fetal growth and development will be impaired. The woman's body will not mobilize or "burn" maternal skeletal muscle to provide additional needed energy to the fetus. With the exception of iron, calcium, and folate, which the fetus claims from maternal stores, the fetus depends entirely on the mother's dietary intake to furnish nutrients and energy. For this reason restrictive dieting to limit weight gain during pregnancy is not recommended.

Table 17-5. Recommended Total Weight Gain Ranges for Pregnant Women,* by Prepregnancy Body Mass Index (BMI)†

Weight-for-Height Category	Recommended Total Gain kg	Recommended Total Gain lb
Low (BMI <19.8)	12.5–18	28–40
Normal (BMI 19.8 to 26.0)	11.5–16	25–35
High‡ (BMI >26.0 to 29.0)	7.0–11.5	15–25

*Young adolescents and African American women should strive for gains at the upper end of the recommended range. Short women (<157 cm, or 62 in) should strive for gains at the lower end of the range.

† BMI is calculated using metric units.

‡ The recommended target weight gain for obese women (BMI >29.0) is at least 6 kg (15 lb).

Reprinted with permission from *Nutrition During Pregnancy*. Copyright 1990 by the National Academy of Sciences. Courtesy of the National Academy Press, Washington, D.C.

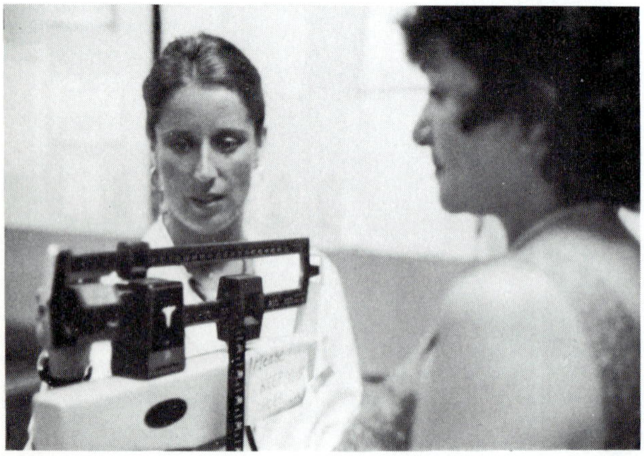

Figure 17-1.
Assessment of the pattern of weight gain during pregnancy is an important nursing responsibility. (Courtesy of the former Booth Maternity Center, Philadelphia.)

The Underweight Woman With Rapid Weight Gain

If the underweight woman tends to gain weight rapidly at the beginning of the first trimester, often as much as 0.4 kg (1 lb) per week, by 20 weeks of gestation she will have gained 7.2 to 8 kg (18 to 20 lb). It is important that this weight gain be recognized because it is different from the one that health professionals usually associate with pregnancy. If a nurse has only had experience with pregnant women who gain the standard recommended weight of 0.8 to 1.2 kg (2 to 3 lb), this nurse may be uncertain about how to manage the woman who shows rapid weight gain starting at the beginning of pregnancy.

The fetus will gain most of its weight in the last trimester. If the woman is advised to cut food intake at that point in an attempt to restrict her weight gain, the overall goal of producing a neonate of optimum birth weight may be jeopardized. The nurse should remember that the increased physiologic demand for food energy makes it difficult for most pregnant women to restrict caloric intake during the second and third trimesters of pregnancy because they are normally very hungry. The woman experiencing rapid weight gain in early pregnancy should be advised to satisfy her appetite with intake of high-quality foods in a regular pattern throughout the day. The woman should be advised to keep her caloric intake within the recommended limit, if possible, to allow an optimal weight gain later in pregnancy.

The Normal or Obese Woman With Excess Weight Gain

The nurse may encounter pregnant women who are at or above normal weight at the beginning of pregnancy but who exceed the usual recommended gain. If weight gain exceeds 3 kg (6.5 lb) per month, especially after the 20th week of gestation, the nurse's assessment is first directed at determining the cause of the weight gain. Nursing activities include the following:

- Verifying the prepregnancy weight
- Taking a 24-hour diet recall and calculating the woman's calorie and protein intake
- Ruling out excessive edema and hypertension
- Checking the woman's usual activity level, especially if her caloric intake does not appear to be excessive
- Encouraging the woman to increase her activity, primarily by walking

The nurse should keep in mind that nondietary factors can affect weight gain. For example the woman could be eating the recommended 2400 kcal/d, but she also might have increased blood pressure and excess fluid retention. This could account for a weight gain of 1.2 kg (3 lb) or more per week.

Certain conditions indicate the need to look more closely at the woman's diet. These conditions include the possibility of pregnancy-induced hypertension and excess fluid retention, weight gain as a result of multiple fetuses, or error in the measurement and recording of weights. If these factors are eliminated, a weight gain of greater than 3 kg (7.5 lb) per month indicates the need to look more closely at the patient's diet.

Assuming the caloric need is 2400 kcal and the actual intake is 3000 kcal, the nurse recommends nutritional intervention. The goal of this intervention for the woman who is gaining weight too rapidly in her pregnancy is not to decrease weight or to stop weight gain. The nurse should not advise the woman to significantly decrease calories or food intake. Attempts at weight reduction by dieting should be discouraged. If fat is catabolized or "burned," ketonemia and ketonuria result, and these in turn can be life-threatening to the fetus and can cause intellectual impairment in the offspring. Rather, the goal is to slow the rate of weight gain.

Two actions should be taken at this point. First, the weight goal for the pregnancy should be adjusted upward to account for the too-rapid gain to date. Second, the pregnant woman should be counseled to curb excessive calorie intake by reducing fat intake, controlling portion sizes, or both.

The Woman With Insufficient or Slow Weight Gain

The nurse may encounter pregnant women who demonstrate a consistently slow weight gain. This pattern may lead to insufficient total gain when calculated by weeks or trimesters. Weight gain during pregnancy is considered to be insufficient if the total gain is less than 10 kg (25 lb) in a normal weight woman, less than 6 kg (15 lb) for an obese woman, or if a satisfactory weight gain pattern has not been established by midpregnancy (20 to 24 weeks' gestation). However, a slow weight gain or actual weight loss in the first trimester should also be evaluated. The nurse's assessment is directed at determining the cause of the failure to gain weight. The nurse should do the following:

- Verify prepregnant weight and determine if weight loss during the first trimester is due to nausea or vomiting. If the mother is frequently nauseated, encourage her to eat dry toast or crackers in the morning before arising. She also should take small amounts of food frequently; the less she eats, the more her appetite will be depressed, and the more likely it is that nausea will persist. The nurse can encourage high-calorie, high-protein drinks, such as homemade milkshakes (milk, ice-cream, and fruit); drinking approximately 4 ounces every 2 hours often will ensure adequate protein and calories while stimulating the appetite.
- Check the woman's activity level, and compare it to her daily dietary intake. Activities that require much walking, child care, and strenuous exercise of any kind result in tremendous energy expenditures and may slow or stop weight gain.
- Check for food intolerances that might be causing frequent stomach upsets, diarrhea, or decreased appetite.
- Check environmental influences, such as hot weather, disruptions in family circumstances, or significant changes in routine. These influences may be related to cultural practices. For example a Hispanic woman living in a hot climate might drink rice water frequently to quench her thirst. Her reasoning might be that this is a healthy practice, because rice water is often given to babies. In fact, however, the carbohydrate level in rice water is sufficient to reduce her appetite for other food without providing enough nutrition to support adequate weight gain.
- Check economic status and ability to buy food. Poor women are at particular risk for protein and iron deficiency. The low-income mother should be encouraged to participate in community food programs. (See the section on counseling the low-income mother later in this chapter.)
- Assess the woman's emotional response to the pregnancy and to additional weight gain. If she is obese or disturbed about the pregnancy, she may be consciously or unconsciously limiting her weight gain. The nurse should reinforce that dieting during pregnancy is not recommended, because it deprives mother and fetus of nutrients needed for tissue growth. Weight loss often is accompanied by maternal ketosis, a direct threat to fetal well-being.

• • Nursing Diagnosis

Nursing diagnosis in nutritional care focuses on identifying the causes of nutritional risks to maternal and fetal health. Once risk factors are identified, nursing care to reduce nutritional risk can be planned and implemented. The following nursing diagnoses may be useful in nutritional care during pregnancy:

- Altered Nutrition: Less than Body Requirements related to nausea
- Altered Nutrition: More than Body Requirements related to increased appetite during pregnancy
- Constipation related to iron supplementation

• • Planning and Implementation

The process of planning and implementing nutritional care for the pregnant woman is based on an accurate assessment of nutritional status. The nurse uses a variety of resources to plan, implement, and evaluate individualized care for the pregnant woman. The first step in planning care is identifying dietary needs based on the nutritional assessment.

Planning an Adequate Diet

The 1990 Maternal and Child Health Daily Food Guide has been developed to ensure an intake of at least 90% of the RDA for pregnant and lactating women of average height (162 cm or 64 inches) and average weight (48 kg or 120 pounds prepregnant). Food groups are based on key nutrients within each group, so it is possible to substitute within a group. This Daily Food Guide is given in Table 17-6.

The recommended number of servings from each group represents a minimum number to maintain a healthy diet during pregnancy. If the guide is followed and recognizing that each food group has more nourishing and less nourishing choices within it, an intake of at least 90% of the recommended RDAs will be met. Therefore, this tool is the most practical and best available for the nurse to evaluate the adequacy of the pregnant woman's diet. After the 24-hour recall (see the Assessment Tool earlier in this chapter) has been completed, the food intake reported is compared with the Daily Pregnancy Food Group Guide (see Table 17-6).

Calories. Depending on the choice of foods within each group, the caloric intake can range from 1700 to 2900 calories for the pregnant woman. If the woman chooses only the lower calorie items in each group (those low in fat and sugar), she will need to eat more than the minimum number of servings to meet her caloric needs. Conversely, if her choices tend toward the high-fat, high-sugar foods, she should be encouraged to include some of the more nutrient-dense foods too.

Protein Foods. Each serving of protein food listed on the guide supplies approximately 6 g of protein. These foods also are good sources of vitamin B_6, iron, and zinc. Animal proteins provide vitamin B_{12}. Plant protein foods supply folate, magnesium, and fiber.

Milk Products. Each serving of this group supplies at least 250 mg of calcium. Milk is a good source of vitamin D, protein, phosphorus, riboflavin, vitamins A, B_6, and B_{12}. For some women this food group provides the primary source of protein in the diet. If the recommended number of servings from this group is not met, the calcium intake is likely to be inadequate.

Breads, Cereals, and Grains. This group is divided into two parts: whole grains and enriched products. Whole-grain products have much more fiber, vitamin B_6, folate, magnesium, and zinc than the enriched products. At least four servings each day should be of the whole-grain variety.

Fruits and Vegetables. Fruits and vegetables are divided into three groups: those high in vitamin C, those high in vitamin A, and other fruits and vegetables. All of these groups provide fiber, vitamins, and minerals. Those listed under vitamin C contain 30 mg of ascorbic acid, vitamin B_6, folate, and vitamin A. Those listed in the vitamin A group provide 2000 IU of vitamin A and are good sources of vitamin B_6, folate, and magnesium.

Cultural Patterns

The Daily Food Guide offers ideas for meeting the different cultural patterns of the pregnant woman. The sample menus shown in Figure 17-2 illustrate how cultural variations may be taken into account when a nutritionally adequate prenatal diet for an adult woman is being planned. All of these supply recommended daily allowances of calories, protein, vitamins A and C, and calcium. Iron intake for each plan is in an acceptable range (Mexican American, 21.9 mg; African American, 20.1 mg; Asian American, 15.3 mg; and vegetarian, 12 mg). Iron and folic acid supplementation would still be recommended during pregnancy. It is important to remember that these menus serve as guidelines and that each woman's preferences and food habits should be considered.

Expected Outcome

- The pregnant woman identifies appropriate dietary choices to best meet her caloric, protein, vitamin, and mineral needs during pregnancy.

Teaching for Effective Self-Care

Teaching the pregnant woman about nutrition is a high priority. The major emphasis in promoting optimal nutritional status during pregnancy is by providing information and encouragement (Fig. 17-3). The goal of this intervention is to help women make well-informed decisions about their diets.

In some settings the nurse may work closely with a dietitian to provide this care, while in other settings the nurse has primary responsibility for providing nutritional information and encouragement to mothers regarding their dietary patterns. The following sections provide some suggestions for the nurse as guidelines for teaching.

Parameters for effective nutrition teaching are the same as those for any kind of teaching provided by the nurse: sensitivity, rapport, and enthusiasm. Adequate time is scheduled, and appropriate teaching aids are used. Pictures of food in magazines may be useful in helping mothers estimate portion sizes, reinforcing information about food groups, and stimulating mothers to introduce more variety

Table 17-6. Daily Food Guide for Women

Food Group	One Serving Equals		Recommended Minimum Servings: Nonpregnant/Nonlactating 11–24 yrs.	Nonpregnant/Nonlactating 25+ yrs.	Pregnant/Lactating
Protein Foods Provide protein, iron, zinc, and B vitamins for growth of muscles, bone, blood, and nerves. Vegetable protein provides fiber to prevent constipation.	**Animal Protein** 1 oz cooked chicken or turkey 1 oz cooked lean beef, lamb, or pork 1 oz or 1/4 cup fish or other seafood 1 egg 2 fish sticks or hot dogs 2 slices luncheon meat	**Vegetable Protein** 1/2 cup cooked dry beans, lentils, or split peas 3 oz tofu 1 oz or 1/4 cup peanuts, pumpkin, or sunflower seeds 1 1/2 oz or 1/3 cup other nuts 2 tbsp peanut butter	5	5	7
			A half serving of vegetable protein daily		One serving of vegetable protein daily
Milk Products Provide protein and calcium to build strong bones, teeth, healthy nerves and muscles, and promote normal blood clotting.	8 oz milk 8 oz yogurt 1 cup milk shake 1 1/2 cups cream soup (made with milk) 1 1/2 oz or 1/3 cup grated cheese (like cheddar, monterey, mozzarella, or swiss)	1 1/2–2 slices presliced American cheese 4 tbsp parmesan cheese 2 cups cottage cheese 1 cup pudding 1 cup custard or flan 1 1/2 cups ice milk, ice cream, or frozen yogurt	3	2	3
Breads, Cereals, Grains Provide carbohydrates and B vitamins for energy and healthy nerves. Also provide iron for healthy blood. Whole grains provide fiber to prevent constipation.	1 slice bread 1 dinner roll 1/2 bun or bagel 1/2 English muffin or pita 1 small tortilla 3/4 cup dry cereal 1/2 cup granola 1/2 cup cooked cereal	1/2 cup rice 1/2 cup noodles or spaghetti 1/4 cup wheat germ 1 4-in pancake or waffle 1 small muffin 8 medium crackers 4 graham cracker squares 3 cups popcorn	7	6	7
			Four servings of whole-grain products daily		
Vitamin C-Rich Fruits and Vegetables Provide vitamin C to prevent infection and to promote healing and iron absorption. Also provide fiber to prevent constipation.	6 oz orange, grapefruit, or fruit juice enriched with vitamin C 6 oz tomato juice or vegetable juice cocktail 1 orange, kiwi, mango 1/2 grapefruit, cantaloupe 1/2 cup papaya 2 tangerines	1/2 cup strawberries 1/2 cup cooked or 1 cup raw cabbage 1/2 cup broccoli, Brussels sprouts, or cauliflower 1/2 cup snow peas, sweet peppers, or tomato puree 2 tomatoes	1	1	1
Vitamin A-Rich Fruits and Vegetables Provide beta-carotene and vitamin A to prevent infection and to promote wound healing and night vision. Also provide fiber to prevent constipation.	6 oz apricot nectar or vegetable juice cocktail 3 raw or 1/4 cup dried apricots 1/4 cantaloupe or mango 1 small or 1/2 cup sliced carrots 2 tomatoes	1/2 cup cooked or 1 cup raw spinach 1/2 cup cooked greens (beet, chard, collards, dandelion, kale, mustard) 1/2 cup pumpkin, sweet potato, winter squash, or yams	1	1	1
Other Fruits and Vegetables Provide carbohydrates for energy and fiber to prevent constipation.	6 oz fruit juice (if not listed above) 1 medium or 1/2 cup sliced fruit (apple, banana, peach, pear) 1/2 cup berries (other than strawberries) 1/2 cup cherries or grapes 1/2 cup pineapple 1/2 cup watermelon	1/4 cup dried fruit 1/2 cup sliced vegetable (asparagus, beets, green beans, celery, corn, eggplant, mushrooms, onion, peas, potato, summer squash, zucchini) 1/2 artichoke 1 cup lettuce	3	3	3
Unsaturated Fats Provide vitamin E to protect tissue.	1/8 med. avocado 1 tsp margarine 1 tsp mayonnaise 1 tsp vegetable oil	2 tsp salad dressing (mayonnaise-based) 1 tbsp salad dressing (oil-based)	3	3	3

California Department of Health Services, Maternal and Child Health Branch. (1990). *Nutrition during pregnancy and the postpartum period: A Manual for Health Care Professionals.*

SAMPLE MENUS TO MEET THE DAILY FOOD GUIDE FOR PREGNANCY

			Food Groups						
CHINESE AMERICAN	**JAPANESE AMERICAN**	**SOUTHEAST ASIAN AMERICAN**	**Protein**	**Milk**	**Grains**	**Vit. C**	**Vit. A**	**Other Frt./Veg.**	**Unsat. Fat**
Breakfast:									
1 egg, soft-boiled	1 egg, hard-&boiled	1 oz pork roast	1						
1 cup oatmeal, cooked	1 cup rice, steamed	1 cup noodles in broth			2				
1 cup lowfat milk	1 cup lowfat milk	½ cup evaporated milk		1					
Sugar*		(in decaf coffee)							
Lunch:									
Chicken & soup noodles:	*Soup & salad:*	*BBQ beef:*							
2 oz chicken, stir-fried	2 oz beef, stir-fried	2 oz beef strips, grilled	2						
1 tsp soy oil	1 tsp. safflower oil	1 tsp vegetable oil							1
Soy sauce, ginger*	Miso soup broth*	Lemon grass, garlic*							
1 cup noodles, boiled	1 cup buckwheat	1 cup rice noodles			2				
½ cup snow peas	noodles (soba)	6 oz orange juice				1			
½ cup bean sprouts,	½ cup broccoli	1 cup green leaf lettuce						1	
onions	1 cup head lettuce,	Fish sauce, hot							
Jasmine tea*	white radish	red pepper*							
	Seasoned rice vinegar*								
Dinner:									
Mongolian beef:	*Teriyaki salmon:*	*Stir-fry chicken:*							
3 oz beef, stir-fried	3 oz fresh salmon fillet,	3 oz chicken	3						
Garlic, soy sauce, green	broiled	Fish sauce*							
onions*	Shoyu marinade*	1 cup white rice, steamed			2				
1 cup white rice, steamed	1 cup white rice, steamed	½ cup bean sprouts						1	
½ cup onions, stir-fried	½ cup cucumber salad	Soup: ½ cup mustard					1		
½ cup bok choy, stir-fried	½ cup carrots, tempura	greens, 1 oz pork	1						
Soup: 3 oz tofu,	Soup: 3 oz tofu, 1 cup	Broth*							
chicken broth*	miso broth with onion*	2 tsp vegetable oil							
2 tsp vegetable oil	2 tsp vegetable oil	(for frying)							2
(for frying)	(in carrots)								
Snacks:									
1 cup lowfat milk	1 cup lowfat milk	1 cup lowfat milk		1					
1 medium apple	½ cup grapes	1 medium banana						1	
8 whole-wheat crackers	8 whole-wheat crackers	8 whole-wheat crackers			1				
		Totals:	7	2	7	1	1	3	3

Each menu contains at least the minimum number of servings for each food group in the Daily Food Guide for Pregnant Women, except the milk products group. Women who are able to drink milk or who will take lactose-reduced milk can include more milk products to meet their need for calcium. Additional calcium is supplied by broccoli, greens, and tofu.

None of these menus supplies the recommended minimum servings from whole grains, and the Southeast Asian American menu does not include the recommended one serving of vegetable protein, because the menus reflect usual cultural practices. Women should be encouraged to eat more whole grains and vegetable protein to obltain the recommended minimum number of servings.

* Indicates foods that provide extra calories only or are used for seasoning.

Figure 17-2.
Sample menus to meet the Daily Food Guide for pregnancy.

into their diet. Food group guides and nutrition information charts are ideal for reinforcing teaching and serving as references for the nurse and the pregnant woman.

Dietary patterns often are deeply ingrained habits and are difficult to change. The pregnant woman should be encouraged to make changes one step at a time.

Teaching Considerations

Because some aspects of nutrition are especially important during pregnancy, the nurse should take special care to provide information and practical guidance in these areas. However, the nurse must consider individual needs when developing appropriate teaching strategies.

Weight Gain. Many women do not welcome the increase in body weight and size that comes with pregnancy. However, they may accept it more readily if the nurse stresses that weight gain is the only way the fetus can be supplied with the nourishment it needs. It may be helpful to reinforce that some added body fat will be burned and that it provides necessary energy during lactation if the woman chooses to breastfeed.

SAMPLE MENUS TO MEET THE DAILY FOOD GUIDE FOR PREGNANCY

			Food Groups						
MEXICAN AMERICAN	**AFRICAN AMERICAN**	**LACTO-OVO-VEGETARIAN**	**Protein**	**Milk**	**Grains**	**Vit. C**	**Vit. A**	**Other Frt./Veg.**	**Unsat. Fat**
Breakfast:									
1 slice white toast	1 slice whole-grain toast	1 slice whole-wheat toast			1				
1 tsp margarine	1 tsp margarine	1 tsp margarine							1
½ cup oatmeal	½ cup grits	½ cup Wheatena			1				
1 cup lowfat milk	1 cup whole milk	1 cup nonfat milk		1					
Sugar*	Bacon*	Sugar*							
Lunch:									
Tostadas:	*Chiliburger:*	*Soup & Salad:*							
2 oz chicken breast	2 oz hamburger	1½ cups lentil soup	2						
½ cup refried beans	½ cup chili beans	1 egg hard-boiled	1						
2 corn tortillas	1 hamburger bun, white	(in salad)							
Fresh chili salsa:	Cole slaw:	2 whole-grain rolls			2				
½ tomato + ½ tbsp	½ cup cabbage	Salad:				½			
chili pepper	½ cup french fries	1 fresh tomato						1	
1 cup romaine lettuce	½ cup whole milk	1 cup romaine lettuce							1
¾ oz monterey	2 tsp salad dressing	½ cup nonfat milk		½					
jack cheese	(mayonnaise-type)	1 tbsp Italian dressing							
1 tsp corn oil (in beans)									
Dinner:									
Bistec ranchero:	*Pork chops:*	*Stuffed pita:*							
3 oz chuck steak	3 oz pork chop	½ cup kidney beans	}						
½ cup kidney beans	½ cup baked beans	6 oz tofu	}4						
		½ cup hummus							
½ cup red potatoes	½ cup mashed potato	½ cup mushrooms							
Fresh chili salsa:								1	
½ tomato + ½ tbsp	½ medium orange	¼ cup tomato puree				½			
chili pepper	2 whole-grain rolls	1 pita, whole-wheat			2				
2 corn tortillas	½ cup mustard greens	½ cup carrots, raw					1		
¼ fresh mango	1 tsp margarine (on rolls)	1 tsp olive oil							
1 tsp corn oil (for frying)		(in hummus)							1
Snacks:									
Licuado:		*Smoothee:*							
1 cup lowfat milk	1 cup fruit yogurt	4 oz nonfat milk + ½ cup		1					
1 banana + sugar,	½ cup grapes	yogurt							
vanilla*	8 whole-wheat crackers	1 banana + honey*						1	
¾ cup corn flakes	¾ oz American cheese	8 whole-wheat crackers			1				
½ cup lowfat milk		¾ cup frozen yogurt		½					
		Totals:	7	3	7	1	1	3	3

Each menu meets the minimum number of servings for all groups in the Daily Food Guide for Pregnant Women.

* Indicates foods that provide extra calories only or are used for seasoning.

California Department of Health Services. (1990). *Nutrition during pregnancy and the postpartum period: A manual for health care professionals.*

Protein Intake. The nurse stresses the importance of meeting the daily requirement of 60 g of protein. Protein can be described as providing "building blocks" for the woman's own tissues, as well as those of the fetus. For many women dairy products will be a major source of protein. If a woman does not drink milk, the nurse may point out that milk may be used in preparation of foods, such as soups, custards, and sauces. Cheese, yogurt, and ice cream are alternative sources.

The nurse should review food groups with the woman, reminding her that meat, poultry, fish, eggs, and legumes are good sources of protein. It may be helpful to encourage economic ways to boost protein intake, such as creating complementary proteins by combining a small amount of complete animal protein with an incomplete plant protein. Sample combinations include beans or pasta and cheese, eggs and whole-grain bread, and poultry or fish and rice. Women who practice vegetarianism often are quite knowledgeable about nutrition. However, they should still carefully assess their protein intake and, with the help of

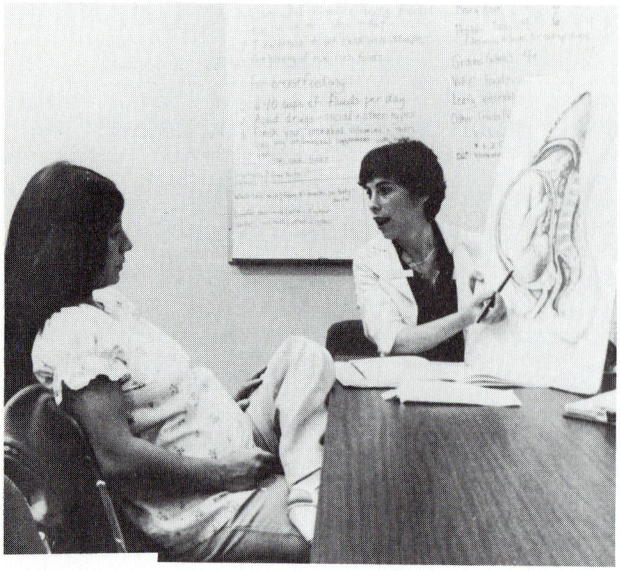

Figure 17-3.
Nutrition teaching should assist the pregnant woman to appreciate the direct connection between good nutrition and fetal well-being. (Photo by Michele Vignes.)

the nurse, use supplements, such as high-protein drinks if indicated.

Carbohydrate and Fat Intake. Carbohydrates and fats can be described as providing fuel for energy. The woman should be encouraged to choose natural sources, such as fruits and whole grains. She should avoid processed foods high in sugar, because natural sources provide other needed nutrients without concentrated calories. The nurse can stress that this change in habits, if sustained, can be very helpful in weight control after pregnancy as well. The nurse can point out that the typical American diet is high in fat and that the woman would be wise to choose low-fat or nonfat dairy products, to trim off fat from meats, and to substitute broiling or baking for frying.

Appetite Management. Women whose appetites are markedly increased during pregnancy may gain weight more rapidly than they would like because they feel hungry "all the time." The nurse should encourage women with this problem to take frequent small meals rather than one or two large meals a day. The woman should plan healthy, protein-containing snacks for herself, trying to eat small amounts before she becomes very hungry.

Iron Supplementation. Many women advised to take iron supplements are not in the habit of taking vitamins or any medication on a regular basis. They often complain that remembering to take their supplement is difficult. The nurse should encourage the woman to keep her supplement in a safe place where she will see them and to associate taking them with another daily activity, such as meals, brushing her teeth, or washing dishes. The constipation that may result from iron supplementation can be avoided by increasing the intake of fluid, high-fiber food, and increasing physical activities such as walking.

"Giving Up" versus "Cutting Down." Many women will be concerned about the effects of caffeine and alcohol in their diet but have difficulty giving up certain food habits. The nurse should explain that habits often are difficult to change. Cutting down gradually by setting realistic goals is often more effective than totally giving up favorite foods or beverages, feeling deprived, and then rebelling against the restriction. The nurse may suggest use of a food diary for a few days to help women who want to change habits but are experiencing difficulty. The woman simply keeps a log of what she eats, when, in what surroundings, and how she was feeling at the time. Keeping a food diary can allow a woman to "see" how her dietary intake is based on long-standing habits and what cues trigger her food habits. If a woman is motivated and keeps a food diary, this also allows for an excellent diet recall useful in assessing her progress.

Food Cravings. The nurse should reassure women that food cravings are not uncommon. As long as the rest of the woman's dietary intake is well balanced, there is probably little harm in indulging occasionally. Some cultures hold specific beliefs about food cravings, such as a particular craving "marking" the fetus physically. Although the nurse may gently provide accurate information and reassurance if a mother appears to be worried about a specific practice, this should be done without demeaning the mother's underlying cultural belief.

Breastfeeding versus Bottle Feeding. The decision to breastfeed an infant is a very personal one and should not be made hastily. The pregnant woman should be given information about lactation early in pregnancy and should be encouraged to make an informed decision about her infant feeding method. Many nurses and dietitians have strong opinions about the advantages of breastfeeding, and there are documented benefits for the infant in most cases (see Chapter 35 for an in-depth discussion of infant feeding). The nurse should be supportive in her interactions with pregnant women, providing education that encourages breastfeeding. However, the nurse also should provide support and assistance to women who choose to formula feed.

Expected Outcomes

- The pregnant woman identifies resources to help her improve her dietary habits and those of her family.
- The pregnant woman takes iron supplementation as recommended by her care provider.
- The pregnant woman uses high-fiber foods and increased fluid intake and exercise to avoid constipation.

Counseling Women at High Risk

Individual patients known to be at high nutritional risk, such as adolescents, impoverished women, or those with previously identified nutritional problems, will require additional time for individualized teaching and counseling. The nurse must anticipate the need for referral to community programs and be familiar with the services and programs available in the area. The nurse must plan time in routine prenatal visits for nutritional counseling and teaching. Providing effective and appropriate printed materials and teaching aids will enhance teaching effectiveness. When a dietitian is available for prenatal care, the nurse and dietitian should plan together how resources can be used most effectively to meet identified needs of the pregnant woman.

Low-income pregnant women are especially vulnerable to nutritional deficiency, particularly protein and iron deficiencies. Improving the quality of the diet on a restricted income requires specialized guidance about food buying, storage, and preparation. Referral to programs designed to ensure adequate provision of food to pregnant women and new mothers may be warranted. The nurse should ensure that the low-income mother is seen by a dietitian and social worker whenever possible and should encourage the mother to take advantage of these services. Local public health nurses are excellent sources of information for the nurse and the low-income mother.

The special supplemental feeding program for women, infants, and children (WIC) is a federally funded program designed to provide supplemental foods to infants and children younger than 5 years of age and to pregnant, lactating, or postpartum women. Individuals determined to be at nutritional risk by health care professionals can receive supplements of high-quality foods. This program requires that pregnant women receive nutritional counseling and routine health care. The eligibility criteria for the WIC program are as follows:

- Recurrent need for medical care
- Conformity with federal income guidelines
- Residence in a local agency's target area
- Determination by a health professional that "nutritional risk" is present

Expected Outcome

- The pregnant woman at nutritional risk demonstrates a weight gain during pregnancy appropriate to BMI.

• • Evaluation

The nurse uses physiologic and behavioral indicators to evaluate the effectiveness of nutritional care during pregnancy. Physiologic indicators of optimal nutritional care include:

- Adequate maternal weight gain during pregnancy
- Adequate maternal iron stores as reflected by hemoglobin and hematocrit levels before and after birth
- Optimal infant birth weight

Behavioral outcomes may not be as readily measurable but may be just as important to consider when evaluating the effectiveness of nursing interventions directed at nutritional needs. The nurse can assess the woman's satisfaction with her management of her own diet and with her level of nutritional knowledge.

The nurse's role in nutritional care of the pregnant woman involves careful assessment of nutritional status, intervention based on identified needs, and ongoing evaluation of the woman's nutritional status as pregnancy progresses. The health history is especially important in identifying factors that put pregnant women at nutritional risk. The prepregnancy weight should be determined and used as a measure of nutritional status before conception. Appropriate weight gain during pregnancy is essential to the continued good health of the mother and normal development of the fetus. The nurse should recognize the importance of and take into account socioeconomic background, cultural associations, and developmental status. Preferences for and emotional responses to food directly affect attitudes toward nutrition and nutritional habits. The major emphasis is placed on teaching and counseling. Individual patients known to be at high nutritional risk, such as adolescents, impoverished women, or those with previously identified nutritional problems, will require additional time for individualized teaching and counseling.

Chapter Summary

Adequate maternal nutrition is important in preventing perinatal morbidity and mortality and in achieving optimal fetal growth and development. Pregnancy causes significant changes in digestion and metabolism while increasing demands for specific nutrients, protein, and caloric intake. Maternal intake of iron and folic acid is especially important, and supplementation is commonly used to prevent iron deficiency anemia and to provide an adequate supply of these nutrients to the developing fetus.

The woman's cultural background, socioeconomic status, and developmental level directly influence her dietary patterns and her overall nutritional status. The nurse must understand the need for a comprehensive nutritional assessment, including a healthy history, physical examination, dietary history, and an ongoing assessment of maternal weight gain. This information provides the basis for planning prenatal nutritional care that meets the individual needs of the pregnant woman. Major nursing interventions include ongoing assessment of maternal nutritional status, teaching mothers effective self-care in relation to their dietary habits, and providing support and encouragement.

Study Questions

1. *How does the RDA for nonpregnant women and pregnant women differ?*
2. *What do US nutrition studies show about the adequacy of dietary intake of iron during pregnancy?*
3. *Why is the nutritional status of women before pregnancy important to pregnancy outcome?*
4. *What are the food groups and the number of servings from each group that should be included in the daily diet of a pregnant woman?*
5. *What are good sources for each of the following essential nutrients: calcium, iron, zinc, and vitamins C and D?*
6. *What should the nurse do when faced with a pregnant woman who uses megadoses of vitamin supplements?*
7. *Why are sodium and calorie restrictions not appropriate for most pregnant women?*

8. *What criteria should be used for the selection of prenatal vitamin and mineral supplements?*
9. *What important considerations are needed if you advise calcium supplements during pregnancy?*
10. *When should lactation information be given to the pregnant woman?*
11. *What are several teaching strategies that can be used when counseling pregnant women about nutritional needs?*

References

California Department of Health Services, Maternal and Child Health Branch. (1990). *Nutrition during pregnancy and the postpartum period: A manual for health care professionals*. Sacramento, CA: Author.

Institute of Medicine, National Academy of Sciences. (1990). *Nutrition during pregnancy*. Washington, DC: National Academy Press.

National Research Council, National Academy of Sciences. (1990). *Recommended dietary allowances* (10th ed.). Washington, DC: National Academy Press.

Worthington-Roberts, B., & Klerman, L. (1990). Maternal nutrition. In Merkatz, I., Thompson, J., Mullen, P., & Goldenberg, R. (Eds.): *New perspectives on prenatal care* (pp. 41–59) New York: Elsevier.

Suggested Readings

Alton, I. (1990). *Guidelines for nutritional care during pregnancy*. Chicago: Department of Health and Human Services, U.S. Public Health Service, Region 5.

Institute of Medicine, National Academy of Sciences. (1992). *Nutrition during pregnancy and lactation: An implementation guide*. Washington, DC: National Academy Press.

Worthington-Roberts, B. (1993) *Nutrition in pregnancy and lactation*. St. Louis: C.V. Mosby.

UNIT IV

Adaptation in the Intrapartum Period

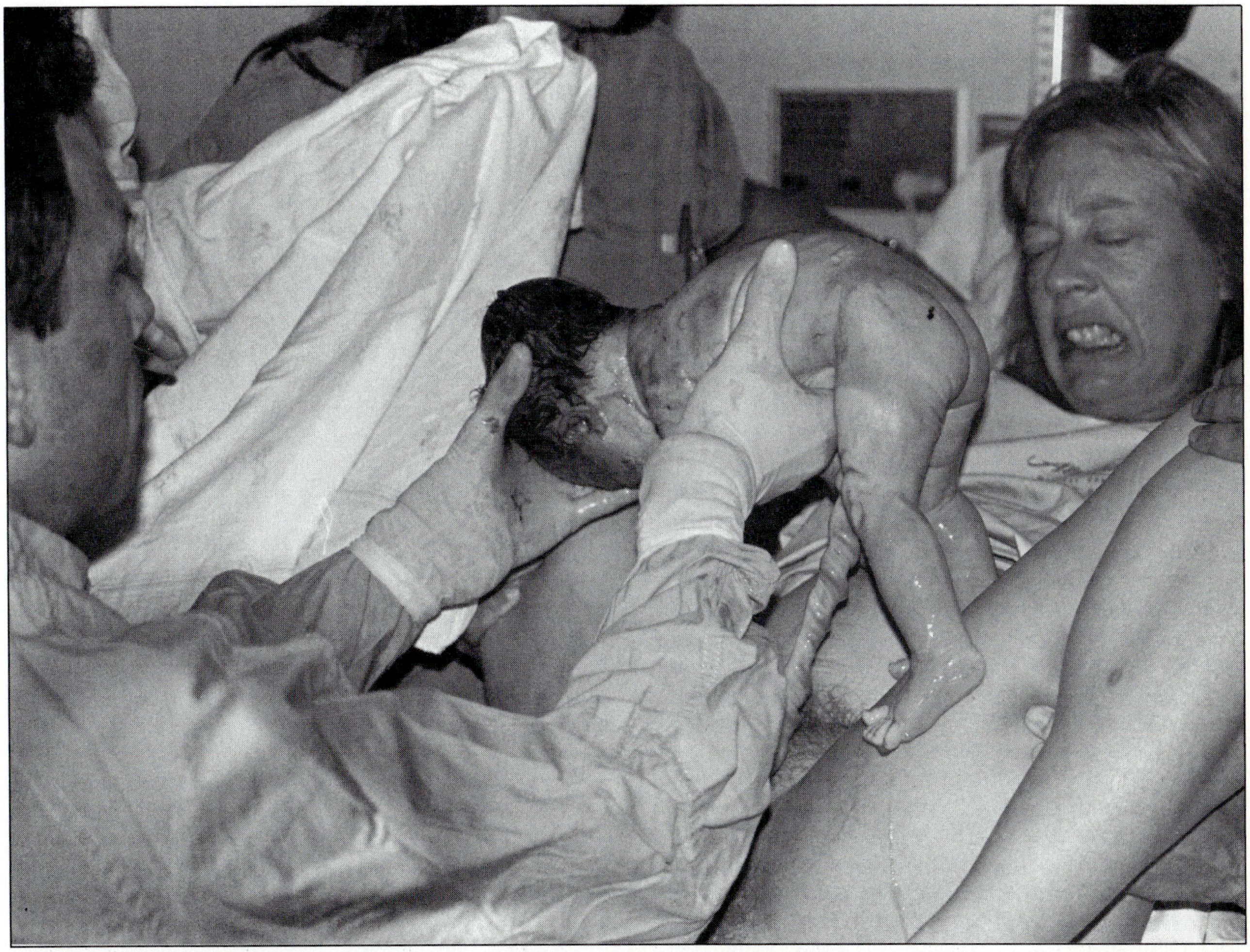

CHAPTER 18

Comprehensive Education for Childbirth

Learning Objectives

After studying the material in this chapter, the student will be able to:

- Describe the major trends and influences in childbirth education.
- Recognize ways in which the childbirth education movement has affected obstetric nursing care.
- Identify the documented benefits of childbirth education.
- List the organizations involved in childbirth education and certification of childbirth educators.
- Outline the basic components of childbirth education programs.
- Describe commonly used labor-coping techniques, and explain the underlying theory of their effectiveness.
- Explain the key points of appropriate nursing care of women using specific labor-coping techniques.
- Explain how the nurse can serve as an advocate for parents wishing to follow a birth plan.
- Discuss examples of programs designed for groups with particular needs for education during the childbearing year.
- Discuss nursing roles in childbirth education.

Key Terms

birth plan	progressive relaxation
conditioned response	psychoprophylaxis
effleurage	sensate focus
hyperventilation	signal or cleansing breath
preconception education	visualization

Most people are interested in how they can have a healthy pregnancy. No longer passive recipients of health care, consumers are actively choosing their caregivers and where and how they will give birth. Women with special needs also are seeking information. Couples are looking beyond the labor and birth to their transition to parenthood.

Because childbirth practices continue to change, the maternity nurse needs to be aware of past and current trends in preparation for childbirth. The nurse will encounter some women who have had formal preparation for childbirth. An understanding of the content of current childbirth education programs will enable the nurse to support families who are prepared. Knowledge of specific techniques and approaches for coping with labor will provide the nurse with the ability to support the unprepared woman and her family.

This chapter provides information about the content and changing nature of comprehensive childbirth education. With an understanding of the content of prepared childbirth classes, the nurse will be able to deliver safe and appropriate care to women and their families. Furthermore, with an understanding of the theoretical basis of childbirth education, the nurse will be able to better fulfill the role of advocate during childbirth as it continues to evolve.

Historic Trends in Childbirth Education

The history of childbirth and preparation for childbirth has influenced and continues to influence the experiences of childbearing families. The history of childbirth is discussed in Chapter 1. In the following section the historic trends affecting preparation for childbirth are presented. They are closely related.

Before the early part of the 20th century, birth was seen as a natural and inevitable event in the family's life. Women were prepared for childbirth and for their roles as mothers through life experiences. Many lacked fundamental understanding about reproduction and childbirth. Birth took place primarily in the home and frequently was regarded as something to be endured.

As birthing moved to the hospital setting, physicians became the primary caregivers and, under their direction, maternity nurses provided care for women during labor and the postpartum period.

Medicalization of Childbirth

As physician care of women during childbirth became the norm, so did the development and use of medical intervention and technologies to deal with the problems that physicians observed. Although changes in obstetric care were introduced with the intention of improving the health of women and their neonates, some practices clearly were not in the best interests of mothers, fathers, or newborns.

Anesthesia and forceps used for difficult births are examples of early medical interventions. As childbirth moved into the hospital, practices used in other areas of medicine, such as surgery, became part of routine management. Some practices, such as adherence to aseptic technique, were adopted with the intention of protecting women and their newborns. Hospital-acquired infections were a significant contributor to maternal and newborn mortality and morbidity, especially before the development of antibiotics. Other practices, however, were for the convenience of the staff, such as the use of the lithotomy position on a surgical table for birth. Routine perineal shaves and enemas in labor fit with the view of childbirth as a medical or surgical event, rather than a normal process. Birth in this context excluded the participation of family members and other support people who were not a part of the medically dominated team.

Standard obstetric practice gradually included the use of more analgesia. A drug regimen known as "twilight sleep," a combination of morphine and scopolamine, was an example. Women who received this regimen were unaware of their surroundings and had no memory of the birth. The use of morphine and opiate substitutes and general anesthesia for normal labor followed. Many of the anesthetic and analgesic agents caused respiratory depression in the neonate. Both mother and neonate required more intensive medical and nursing management.

The increased use of medical technology in normal childbirth had other undesirable effects on families. Fathers were barred from participation and even from any direct contact with the neonate. Frequently, they were only able to view their offspring through the nursery window. Participation and hospital visitation by other family members were practically unheard of (Wertz & Wertz, 1989).

Beginnings of the "Natural Childbirth" Movement

In response to the increasing medicalization of birth, a grass roots movement began that promoted the advantages of "natural childbirth." Dr. Grantly Dick-Read's book *Childbirth Without Fear*, published in the United States in 1944, gained popularity in Great Britain and North America. Dick-Read suggested that a cycle of "fear–tension–pain" resulted from women's lack of knowledge about childbirth. The author proposed that education would interrupt the cycle. The use of muscular relaxation and slow breathing was recommended to break the fear–pain–tension cycle. Women who had used these principles and had successful birth experiences, along with interested professionals, began to organize classes for other women.

The International Childbirth Education Association (ICEA) developed from this early childbirth education movement. Today the ICEA remains a major force in childbirth education and maternity services in general. It promotes "freedom of choice based on knowledge of alternatives" (ICEA, 1987).

Not long after the introduction of Dick-Read's methods the work of a French obstetrician became known through the publication of *Thank You, Dr. Lamaze* (Karmel, 1959). Lamaze proposed that through training, based on the Pavlovian conditioning concept, women could experience "childbirth without pain through the psychoprophylaxis method." It is based on the belief that the perception of pain could be greatly reduced or eliminated through conditioned responses to uterine contractions. This method soon gained popularity. Deep relaxation, concentration and focusing, and complex breathing patterns were the techniques used to decrease the perception of pain. A coalition of parents and professionals began organizing classes, and nationally recognized teacher-training programs followed. Their efforts led to the formation, in 1960, of the American Society for Psychoprophylaxis in Obstetrics (ASPO).

The next major force in the natural childbirth movement was an American obstetrician, Robert Bradley. His 1965 book, *Husband Coached Childbirth*, advocated the role of the spouse as the most effective person for supporting a woman during childbirth. Deep relaxation techniques and reduced responsiveness to external stimuli to promote comfort in labor were stressed.

The methods and techniques of these childbirth reformers continue to influence childbirth preparation today. Contemporary childbirth preparation classes may use an eclectic mixture of techniques. Further discussion appears in the section Preparation for Childbirth later in this chapter.

Struggles to Reform Childbirth

The views of the previously mentioned childbirth reformers met considerable resistance from the medical and nursing professions in the 1960s and 1970s. The struggle was so intense that in 1973 a bill was introduced in the U.S. House of Representatives (H.R. 1502). If this bill had passed, it would have made it mandatory for all hospitals receiving federal funds to permit the father to attend labor and delivery as long as he had the permission of the woman and the physician. Many nurses and physicians who joined parents in support of H.R. 1502 were ostracized, and in some cases, nurses lost their jobs.

Introducing change in childbirth has been (and continues to be) difficult. Most of the impetus for change has come from outside the health care system, from consumers and childbirth educators. There has been little organized support from medicine and nursing. The importance of the labor room nurse in the parents' experience was largely ignored by proponents of reform. Adversarial rather than collaborative relationships between parents who wanted some control over their birth experience and health professionals were a frequent result. This may have delayed the acceptance of family-centered care in many areas of North America. In some cases, conflict still hinders acceptance of reform.

The work of reforming childbirth continues. Recently, two French obstetricians, first Dr. Frederick Leboyer (1975) and then Dr. Michel Odent (1984), have focused on the birthing environment for women and neonates. In *Birth Without Violence* (1974) Leboyer advocated gentle handling of the neonate and a warm, dimly lit environment for birth. Warm water as a soothing element for the neonate after the stress of birth was proposed. In *Entering the World: The Demedicalization of Childbirth* (1984) Odent suggested that the environment in which labor and birth occurs affects the woman's ability to cope. Familiarity with the place of birth and privacy facilitate the birth process. Mobility and upright or squatting positions for labor and birth and water baths for pain relief were promoted. This movement supported less medical intervention for normal labor and birth.

The natural childbirth movement has been successful not only in promoting education and preparation for birth, but also in paving the way for the development of family-centered care and "alternative" birth practices (see Chapter 2). All of the childbirth reformers have shared goals of enabling women to cope with labor and birth and turning the trend against the medicalization of childbirth in general.

Education for Childbearing: A Social Trend

Education for childbearing increasingly has become a standard part of prenatal care in North America. The scope of prenatal education has broadened beyond simply teaching parents techniques for coping with labor. There is considerable agreement among major prenatal education organizations about the content areas that should be included. The basic components of prenatal education programs are listed in the accompanying display. In some hospitals most parents will have attended prenatal classes; however, childbirth education is still mostly a middle-class phenomenon. Programs may not be accessible to members of disadvantaged and minority groups. For a variety of reasons programs may inadequately address the needs of the participants.

Women who attend childbirth education classes are more likely to be primiparous, more affluent, and better

Basic Components of Prenatal Education Programs

The following are basic components of prenatal education programs, according to the *ICEA Position Paper on Planning Comprehensive Maternal and Newborn Services for the Childbearing Year* and NAACOG *Guidelines for Childbirth Education:*

- Human reproduction, including the anatomy, physiology, and psychology of labor, birth, and the postpartum period; signs of pregnancy; normal physical and psychological changes during pregnancy; health maintenance and care during pregnancy; fetal development; signs and stages of labor; postpartum health care
- Basic nutritional needs and their relationship to fetal development
- Self-help techniques and comfort measures for pregnancy, labor, birth, and the postpartum period, including posture, body mechanics, maintenance of muscle tone and physical fitness, control of tension and relaxation, breathing techniques, childbirth, and postpartum exercises
- Role and support techniques for the companion in labor and birth
- Social and psychological roles and relationships in the family; sexual roles
- Roles of health care providers in the management of labor, birth, and the postpartum period
- Options in labor and birth procedures and in the birth environment; rooming-in; early discharge; family visitation; home care follow-up
- Rights of the expectant family; responsibilities of the childbearing woman for self-care and decision-making
- High-risk birth, including indications and procedures for prenatal tests for fetal growth and well-being, electronic fetal monitoring, intravenous fluids, induction and augmentation, analgesia, anesthesia, episiotomy, forceps, and cesarean birth, as well as the risks and benefits associated with them and alternatives when appropriate; parents' participation in the care of a sick newborn
- Preparation for parenting, including the roles of family members, infant care, infant feeding (breast and bottle), child growth and development, child safety, well-baby care, immunizations, family planning, and the couple's sexual relationship; identification of community resource groups dealing with breastfeeding, parenting, cesarean family support, nutritional programs, and physical fitness
- Tour of maternity-newborn unit

Adapted from Young, D. (1982). Changing childbirth: Family birth in the hospital. *Rochester: Childbirth Graphics.*

educated. They are already highly motivated to learn what they can do to achieve a positive pregnancy outcome and experience. Furthermore, these women are more likely to have a positive self-esteem, favor nontraditional gender roles, plan to have their partner present at birth, and breast-feed than are nonattenders.

Education for the childbearing population has grown from the activities of small, scattered groups of largely self-taught childbirth educators to the formation of national organizations including ASPO/Lamaze and ICEA. These organizations have developed teacher-training and certification programs to ensure that childbirth educators have a sound knowledge base and specific competencies. Childbirth educators certified by these organizations may add the initials CCE (certified childbirth educator) or some similar designation after their names. Childbirth education is not regulated by law. Anyone may practice as a childbirth educator. Some professionals believe that regulation is desirable. Some also believe the view that only people with formal educational or professional qualifications (such as registered nurses or those with a degree in health education) should be allowed to practice as childbirth educators.

The nurse can become informed about local childbirth organizations and obtain information about the standards and competencies they require of their teachers. Nurses can work toward effective collaborative relationships with such groups in the community and can encourage parents to become informed about the qualifications of those teaching the classes they are contemplating attending.

Most communities now have childbirth educators in private practice and in hospital-based programs (Fig. 18-1). Community organizations, such as the Red Cross, and community colleges sponsor a wide range of classes for expectant and new parents. Libraries and book stores also offer a wide range of written material. There is a growing trend toward offering a greater variety of classes for childbearing families; these classes include preconception classes, early pregnancy classes, classes for siblings and grandparents, and programs designed for special groups, such as adolescents.

Changes are occurring in the way classes are organized. The usual format has been a series of evening sessions. Variations, such as weekend intensive courses, "prenatal-in-a-day" refresher courses, and weekend retreats, are some examples of nontraditional formats.

Organizations involved in childbirth education have a history of leadership in many aspects of maternity care. Education for the childbearing year is now a familiar concept. Individuals and groups involved in education for childbirth have had a profound influence on childbirth in North America.

Birth Plan

Many childbirth consumers are choosing to express their preferences for care during labor and the early postpartum period in the form of a birth plan. Such a plan represents a desire by women and their partners to have some control over the care they receive. Therefore, birth plans represent a shift from a passive recipient of care to an active participant.

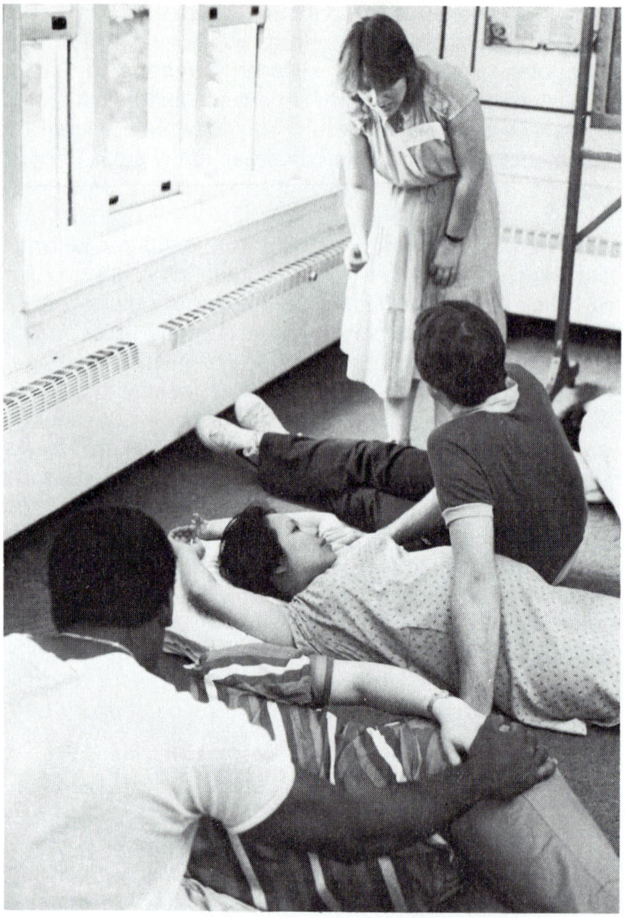

Figure 18-1.
A maternity nurse/childbirth educator provides individualized teaching for expectant parents in childbirth preparation classes. (Courtesy of the former Booth Maternity Center, Philadelphia.)

Not all caregivers are comfortable with this power shift. Some may feel threatened when consumers come with a written plan in hand.

Determination of a woman's preparation for childbirth, wishes, and preferences is an essential element in assessment of all women admitted to a birthing area. The maternity nurse, as the person providing the most direct care during labor, is in a position to act as an advocate for the fulfillment of the wishes of the woman and her family. This is true whether the wishes are presented verbally or are written. When hospital policies, practices, and routines make it difficult for nurses to provide the choices requested by consumers, the nurse is in a position to work within the system as a change agent. The nurse also must keep the requirement of informed consent in mind, remembering that women must give consent for any treatment or procedure.

For women, their partners, and childbirth educators the birth plan can be a useful educational tool. The process of discussing a birth plan in a group setting provides an opportunity to consider all possible approaches, interventions, and outcomes that might be encountered. Unexpected events, such as operative delivery, fetal distress, and even perinatal loss, may be raised. Couples have the opportunity to acknowledge the uncertainty inherent in childbirth. The birth plan also enables women and their partners to consider the important aspects of this experience. Who will be at the birth and what roles they will play can be thought through. Specific fears and preferences often surface in the process of discussing the birth plan. An effectively conducted discussion acknowledges the individuality of women and their partners as they contemplate labor and birth. Thus, the process reinforces the reality that there is no one right way to labor and give birth.

Critics of birth plans express the concern that one cannot plan for a birth and that birth plans create unrealistic expectations that in turn lead to dissatisfaction with the birth experience. This stereotypical view is not supported by the results of a study by Green, Coupland, and Kitzinger (1990). Their prospective study of 825 women in England suggested that high expectations are not bad for women but low expectations may be.

Birth plans often begin with an introductory statement about the woman's or couple's beliefs about childbirth. The plan includes a statement acknowledging that circumstances might arise in which interventions are required (Carty & Tier, 1989). The following topics might be addressed:

- Management of labor, including preferred coping strategies and techniques
- The birth environment, including who will be present and their roles
- Feelings about interventions and the decision-making process for interventions
- Immediate care of the neonate
- Wishes for family time to welcome the neonate
- Length of hospital stay
- Infant care and feeding and family involvement during the postpartum period
- Wishes in the event of unexpected outcomes, including perinatal loss

Nurses may encounter parents who have developed birth plans during prenatal care or on admission to the labor and delivery unit. Ideally, the parents would have discussed their birth plan with their physician or nurse midwife, and it would have been noted in the patient record. If not, the labor and delivery nurse should review the birth plan with parents on admission and take parental preferences into account when planning nursing care.

Childbirth practices have been influenced by trends in medical care and more recently by a trend toward more consumer choice about how birth is managed. Educating the woman and her family about childbirth and helping the woman plan for childbirth and communicate her concerns and desires to the health care team has become an important nursing priority.

Evaluation of Childbirth Education

Preparation for childbirth is widely believed to be of value. However, little scientific evidence exists to document these supposed benefits. Unfortunately, many studies have been poorly designed and thus their findings are unreliable. Reports indicated that consumers of childbirth education differ as a group from women who do not avail themselves of this service. Enkin (1990) and Shearer (1990) suggested that many researchers have been attempting to measure the wrong outcomes. They pointed out that obstetric outcomes were more dependent on other variables, such as the caregivers the woman encountered during pregnancy and childbirth, than on the childbirth preparation itself.

Childbirth education classes differ widely according to who teaches them and the underlying philosophy. Enkin, Kierse, and Chalmers (1989) suggested that classes offered by community-based childbirth education organizations differ from those sponsored by hospitals. The former frequently base their teaching on a philosophy of promoting choice, while hospital-based classes may serve to encourage parents to comply with the hospital's routine approaches and practices.

Overall, present research cannot substantiate most of the claimed benefits of prepared childbirth. Many aspects, and in particular new programs and approaches, have yet to be systematically evaluated.

Documented Effects of Prepared Childbirth

The singular, well-documented, positive effect of childbirth preparation is the use of less pain medication in labor by prepared women when compared with unprepared women. Thus, the techniques taught in childbirth education classes can, in general, be said to be helpful for women who wish to avoid or minimize their use of pain medication in labor. This does not mean that prepared women experience less pain.

Studies of labor pain indicate a wide range in women's experience of pain in labor, and they tell us that the average woman experiences a high level of pain (Enkin et al., 1989). Unlike the pioneers of prepared childbirth, such as Dick-Read and Lamaze, claims of painless childbirth as a result of preparation are no longer made. Rather, experts believe the learned relaxation and other strategies enable women to endure the pain of labor with less reliance on medication.

Unsupported Claims About Childbirth Education

The nurse must be aware that overenthusiastic proponents sometimes exaggerate the benefits of new and innovative developments in health care. Parents may hear that prepared childbirth will "make them better parents," "increase parent–infant attachment," or "improve the couple's relationship." Although couples may believe they experienced these benefits, no evidence indicates that preparation for childbirth has a long-term effect on couple or parent–infant relationships.

Many parents wish to become better informed about the processes of pregnancy, labor, and birth. Empowering women through knowledge of the choices they may have to make may enhance their self-esteem and decrease dissatisfaction with the birth experience (Enkin et al., 1989). These same authorities suggested that as the number of educated consumers increases, the health care system will be challenged to be more responsive to their needs.

As childbirth education has gained in popularity, it also have become the focus of debate regarding its effectiveness. Women and their families generally regard childbirth education as a valuable service, and many health professionals strongly support it. However, there is still no clear scientific evidence of measureable effects on birth outcomes. One problem may be that research to date has focused on measuring outcomes that are strongly affected by factors outside the influence of childbirth education techniques. More research is needed to determine the effects of childbirth education in a variety of populations.

Preparation for Childbirth

Theoretical Basis

Despite the lack of evidence for specific benefits of childbirth education, programs are proliferating. Knowledge from other disciplines continues to contribute to the theoretical basis for prepared childbirth practices. This knowledge will enable the maternity nurse to better support laboring women who use techniques they have learned in childbirth education classes. In this section, theories that support specific childbirth preparation techniques are outlined.

The major schools of prepared childbirth in North America evolved separately, and each used a different theory as its basis. Dick-Read (1959) stressed the importance of information to reduce fear of the unknown and thus minimize muscle tension. A cycle of fear–tension–pain described how fear of the unknown intensifies muscular tension, increasing the perception of pain.

The Lamaze method focuses on the idea that pain and uterine contractions are separate phenomena that have become linked in the human mind. The Lamaze method is directed toward reducing the negative preconceptions women have about labor. This is accomplished through education and the formation of new conditioned reflexes in response to uterine contractions. Selective breathing and active relaxation techniques are practiced until they can be repeated with ease. It has been suggested that pain impulses are blocked in the dorsal horn cells of the spinal cord. This occurs by creating varied tactile and pressure stimuli together with selective focusing on breathing and relaxation (the "gate control" theory). The effectiveness of these activities also has been linked to the body's ability to produce its own endorphins (Nichols & Humenick, 1988).

Shrock (1988) elaborated on the benefits of relaxation for decreasing the stress response in labor. Fear triggers a series of physiologic responses that, if prolonged, can adversely affect labor and birth. Relaxation has been shown to be an effective tool in reducing the stress response. Thus, combined with specific information that decreases the fear of the unknown, the laboring woman can respond more effectively, physiologically and psychologically, to the sensations of labor. In addition, relaxation of muscles not involved in the labor process avoid unnecessary energy drain and fatigue, which can lead to an increased perception of pain.

Virtually all childbirth preparation methods advocate having a prepared support person present during labor. This person provides psychological support and encourages the woman to use specific techniques. Providing simple comfort measures, being a familiar and continuous presence, and acting as a spokesperson are some of the functions of the labor support person. This role complements the role of the nurse who provides knowledgeable information on the progress of labor and the well-being of the woman and fetus.

Most often the support person is the woman's mate but may be a friend, her mother, or another relative. Some women choose to hire a labor support person. In this case more than one support person may be present.

Childbirth preparation and support in labor can be seen as a form of adaptation. The woman is able to draw on her knowledge and on a number of techniques and skills and the support of those involved with her as she faces and copes with the sensations of labor.

Goals and Practices

The nurse caring for childbearing women must be aware of the goals and practices of prepared childbirth. The following section outlines the goals and the content of contemporary childbirth education programs. Specific techniques are detailed. This knowledge will enhance the nurse's ability to care for all childbearing women.

Childbirth Education Goals and Content

In recent years the distinctions between the schools of prepared childbirth have faded. Many childbirth educators present an eclectic approach to labor techniques. There is general agreement about the goals of childbirth education, including:

- To provide the childbearing couple with the knowledge and skills they need to cope with the stress of pregnancy, labor, and birth
- To prepare the childbearing couple to become informed consumers of maternity care
- To assist the childbearing couple in achieving a safe, positive, and rewarding birth experience

The content most frequently associated with prepared childbirth classes is that which deals relaxation techniques and breathing techniques. These techniques are thought to promote a relaxed physical state in the woman and to allow her to cope with the changing sensations of labor. The following section presents a discussion of these techniques.

Relaxation Techniques

Relaxation is "a state of low arousal in which such bodily responses as muscle tension, heart rate, breathing rate, and metabolism diminish so as to bring these functions into equilibrium" (Shrock, 1988). The stress response, the opposite of relaxation, can interfere with any of the four major physiologic systems—muscular, vascular, hormonal, or neurotransmitter.

Relaxation techniques are designed to help the woman achieve a deep level of relaxation of muscles not directly involved in the work of labor. Uterine contractions use tremendous amounts of energy. Avoiding unnecessary muscular tension conserves energy and oxygen reserves needed for the work of labor. Few people are skilled at achieving and maintaining states of mental and physical relaxation, so specific techniques must be learned and practiced in preparation for birth (Fig. 18-2). Techniques for relaxation are most effective when they are selected according to which physiologic system is in disequilibrium.

Preparation for childbirth involves many types of relaxation techniques. Some of the most frequently taught are the following:

- *Progressive relaxation* is a technique in which muscle groups are systematically tensed and released in a patterned sequence to attain a state of deep physical relaxation.
- *Neuromuscular dissociation* is a technique in which one muscle group is consciously tensed and released, while deep relaxation is maintained elsewhere in the body.
- *Visualization* is a technique of consciously using calming and peaceful mental and visual images to maintain emotional equilibrium.

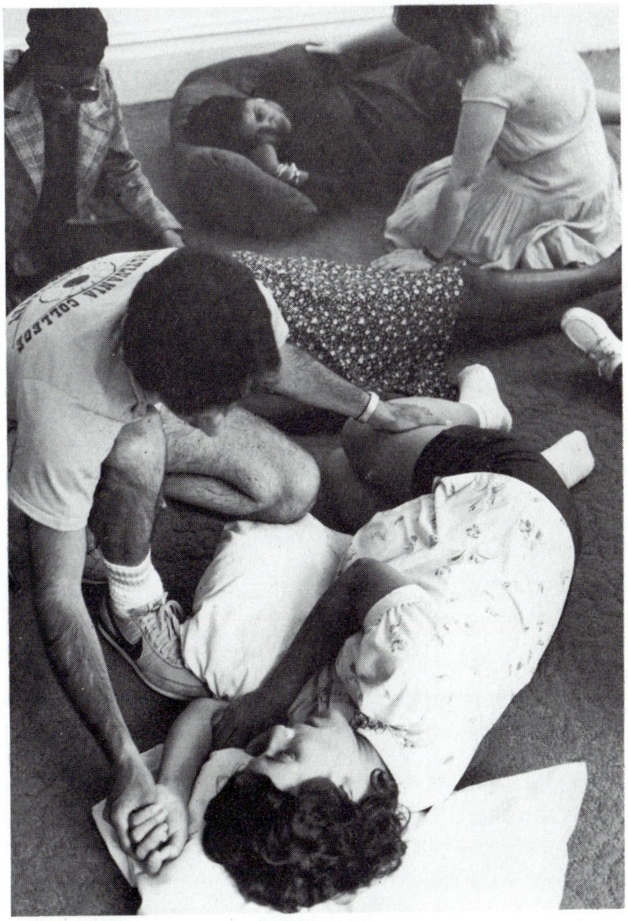

Figure 18-2.
The father or support person helps the mother learn to use relaxation techniques in preparation for childbirth. (Courtesy of the former Booth Maternity Center, Philadelphia.)

Several other techniques that can enhance relaxation are taught in many childbirth classes. The most common of these are the use of a sensate focus (or focal point), gentle massage, counterpressure to the back, and effleurage, a specialized form of massage. The nurse should be able to identify the particular techniques a woman and her support person have been taught and assist in their use. The nurse also should observe the woman's level of relaxation and comfort throughout her labor and be prepared to suggest and teach other techniques that might be useful.

Table 18-1 describes these and other types of relaxation techniques and approaches to teaching them. The nurse should be familiar with these to help laboring women and their partners to use relaxation as a coping technique during labor. This will enable the nurse to assist the woman in achieving and maintaining optimum relaxation and will help the support person to do the same. The nurse's familiarity and comfort with these techniques sometimes makes the difference between adequate and excellent supportive nursing care during labor.

Another important point is that relaxation training is probably one of the safest, most effective, and most underused interventions in nursing. Relaxation can be safely and effectively used in a variety of nursing situations, such as caring for a patient in pain or assisting a patient to relax and sleep.

Progressive Relaxation

Progressive relaxation exercises are not used during actual labor but are taught to enable the woman to achieve a relaxed state easily and release tension when it develops in a particular body part.

Neuromuscular Dissociation

Neuromuscular dissociation exercises are believed to be useful for simulating the experience of a uterine contraction while keeping other muscles relaxed.

Visualization

Visualization can be used during labor and can be an effective means of pain management. It may be used to induce a generalized response similar to that achieved by progressive relaxation. The goal may be to accomplish a specific physiologic response. During labor, visualizing the opening cervix may help to minimize unproductive tension. At the birth, picturing the fetus moving down the birth canal may mobilize the forces needed for delivery. Generalized relaxation responses may come from the suggestion to picture and recall the sensations associated with pleasant places the woman has been, to build an imagined picture after the verbal suggestions of her partner, or to visualize energy flowing into her body or the diminution of some symbol of pain. Imagery can be effectively used with an untrained woman if suggestions are simple and within the woman's frame of reference. The nurse's skill in assessing the woman's particular fears and in establishing trust will be particularly valuable. The accompanying display gives an

Table 18-1. Approaches to Teaching Relaxation Techniques

Name and Type	Description	Feedback
Progressive relaxation (modifies muscular responses)	Consists of systematically tensing and releasing muscles. Developed by E. Jacobson, modified by J. Wolpe into a 6-wk approach with home practice.	Primary feedback from awareness of participant, who focuses on sensation of tensing and relaxing each muscle. Either coach or electromyograph can provide further feedback.
Neuromuscular dissociation (modifies muscular responses)	Modifies progressive relaxation by asking the participant to tense some muscles and relax others simultaneously. Introduced in this country by E. Bing.	Feedback from coach who checks relaxation and tension. Introduced by Karmel and Bing. Not mentioned by Lamaze or Chabon.
Autogenic training (mental control modifies muscular and autonomic systems responses)	Uses suggestions, such as "my right arm is heavy" or "my left arm is warm." Effects include slowing heart and respiration, as well as cooling forehead. Developed by J. Schultz and W. Luther.	Primary feedback from awareness of participant. Biofeedback equipment, thermometers, and so forth also may be used.
Meditation (modifies vascular and neurotransmitter responses)	Is defined by H. Benson as dwelling on an object (repeating a sound or gazing at an object) while emptying the mind of all thoughts and distractions in a quiet atmosphere in a comfortable position. Used in transcendental meditation and yoga.	Self-monitoring by participant or feedback from coach on concentration on a focal point or breathing patterns.
Visual imagery	Includes techniques such as visualizing oneself on a warm beach or as a bag of cement or going down a staircase. Often precedes introduction of other kinds of relaxation. Also may be used to visualize and potentially affect specific body parts, as in cancer therapy. May be used in desensitization, in which one relaxes while visualizing a potentially threatening situation. Used in labor rehearsals.	
Touching/massage	Has always been a way for one person to calm another. There is evidence of actual transfer of energy through some forms of touching. In childbirth preparation touching is associated with muscular relaxation.	Feedback from coach, which includes informing the subject when muscle tension is felt. Advanced coaching needed. Coaches may need first to discern relaxation by moving a limb.
Biofeedback	Uses various devices: Electromyograph: measures neuromuscular tension. Thermometer: measures skin temperature at extremities. Galvanic skin reflex: records conductivity changes because of the action of sweat glands at the surface of the skin. Electroencephalograph: distinguishes alpha, beta, and theta waves in the brain.	Feedback from all of these machines in one or more of these forms: visualization of a meter, listening to a sound, or watching a set of flashing lights.

Adapted from Humernick, S. (1984). Teaching relaxation. *Childbirth Education 3*(4):48.

example of a simple visualization exercise for childbirth preparation.

Sensate Focus

Focused concentration on a particular sensory stimulus can be quite effective in achieving and maintaining a level of deep relaxation. Lamaze teachers typically instruct women to select an external focal point—an object, such as a small toy, a picture, or a vase of flowers—on which to focus their eyes during contractions. Other childbirth teachers, especially those using Bradley techniques, encourage women to close their eyes during a contraction and concentrate on the sound of their support person's voice, taped music, or a particular body sensation, such as the touch of the support person's hand. All of these examples operate on the same principle—the idea that deliberate attention to a sensate focus can alter and diminish the perception of pain. For this technique to be effective, consistency and avoidance of interruptions during contractions are important.

Gentle Massage and Counterpressure

Some methods of childbirth preparation encourage the use of gentle massage to enhance the relaxation and comfort of the woman in labor. Several massage techniques are

Visualization Exercise for Childbirth Preparation

Go to a quiet, tranquil place where you won't be disturbed. Lie down in a comfortable position with your body well supported with pillows. Close your eyes, inhale slowly as you breathe in fresh oxygen, then exhale completely while you release your body tension. As you continue to inhale oxygen and release tension, your breathing will become slower and more even.

Continue to rest and allow your mind to take you to a very special place where you feel comfortable, safe, and tranquil. Allow yourself to enter this favorite place. Take in the sights, sounds, and smells of this place, and allow those feelings to enter your body.

What sounds are you hearing? Pause and listen to all that you can. What scents are you smelling? Pause and enjoy the fragrances. What sights are you seeing? Pause and look around to enjoy all that you are seeing, the vibrant colors, the various shapes and sizes of all that you see.

Note the temperature in this special place, the warmth, the coolness, and allow your body to enjoy all the sensations while feeling comfortable, safe, and secure.

While in this special place, imagine your baby growing in your womb, being comfortable, safe, and secure.

Stay in this special place for a few minutes and enjoy all the good feelings of being there. . . . Now, bringing those good feelings with you, slowly come back to the here-and-now by counting backwards from 5 to 1. Five—move your feet and toes. Four—move your upper body. Three—open your eyes and take a good look around. Two—take a good stretch. One—sit up slowly as you come back to your present surrounding.

shown in Figure 18-3. Effleurage, a light, rhythmic, circular stroking of the abdomen with the fingertips, may be soothing to the woman and may complement the use of learned breathing techniques.

Gentle massage of the back and shoulders using talcum powder or lotion to reduce friction on the skin also can be comforting to the woman. This can be done in a variety of ways, allowing the woman to decide what is most effective for her. Massage of the legs should be done only lightly and *with caution;* there is a small increased risk of thrombosis in pregnant women. Vigorous massage might dislodge a blood clot, causing an embolism.

Firm counterpressure also may be offered as a counterirritant to sensations of internal pressure and pain, particularly in the lower back. Other areas where pressure can exert a calming effect are the pelvis, thighs, feet, shoulders, and hand. The effectiveness and comfort provided by gentle massage and counterpressure during labor must be reevaluated frequently. The amount of comfort the woman in labor derives from massage may change as her labor proceeds, and a touch that was relaxing early in labor may become intolerable later. For this reason the nurse and support person should observe the woman's nonverbal behavior closely, assess her comfort level regularly, and make adjustments as necessary. Figure 18-4 shows several ways a labor partner may apply counterpressure and other comfort measures to relieve back pain during labor.

Breathing Techniques

Most childbirth preparation methods teach some kind of learned breathing techniques for use in response to contractions during labor. Although specific techniques may vary, the underlying principles are the same. First, *deliberate, controlled, learned breathing patterns are directly linked to optimum relaxation*. Breathing techniques are not in themselves effective for pain management. They must be combined with relaxation techniques. In Lamaze, in particular, the *concentration* on performing complex breathing patterns alters the perception of pain and helps the women cope with the sensations of labor, rather than be overwhelmed by them. *Each breathing pattern is used according to need, not according to a particular stage of labor*. Thus, if one breathing pattern is not effective at a particular point in labor, then another one (usually a more complex pattern) may be used. Finally, *all commonly used breathing techniques must be done in a way that maintains adequate respiratory function without tiring the woman unnecessarily*. Practicing breathing techniques incorrectly can lead to hyperventilation, causing changes in blood chemistry.

The four major breathing techniques commonly used in childbirth preparation are slow paced breathing, modified paced breathing, patterned paced breathing, and expulsion breathing. All techniques can be individualized to promote optimum relaxation and oxygenation. In determining the pace and depth suitable for each woman the nurse should consider body position, the woman's usual respiratory rate, learned breathing techniques, and the progress of labor. Women and their support person(s) will use a variety of techniques, depending on the type of childbirth education they attended, their skill and confidence, and the effectiveness of the selected techniques in enabling the woman to cope with the labor. The nurse must be flexible and adjust care as much as possible to the couple's individual pattern during labor.

Slow Paced Breathing

The technique called slow paced breathing in the Lamaze method also is taught as slow abdominal breathing in other methods. It involves breathing at approximately half the normal breathing rate. It can be done through the nose, mouth, or both throughout the duration of a contraction. Slow paced breathing provides the best oxygenation, is calming, and is the least fatiguing of the breathing techniques. To counteract the tendency to habituate to this technique, thereby reducing its effectiveness in altering pain perception, the woman should be encouraged to vary its use

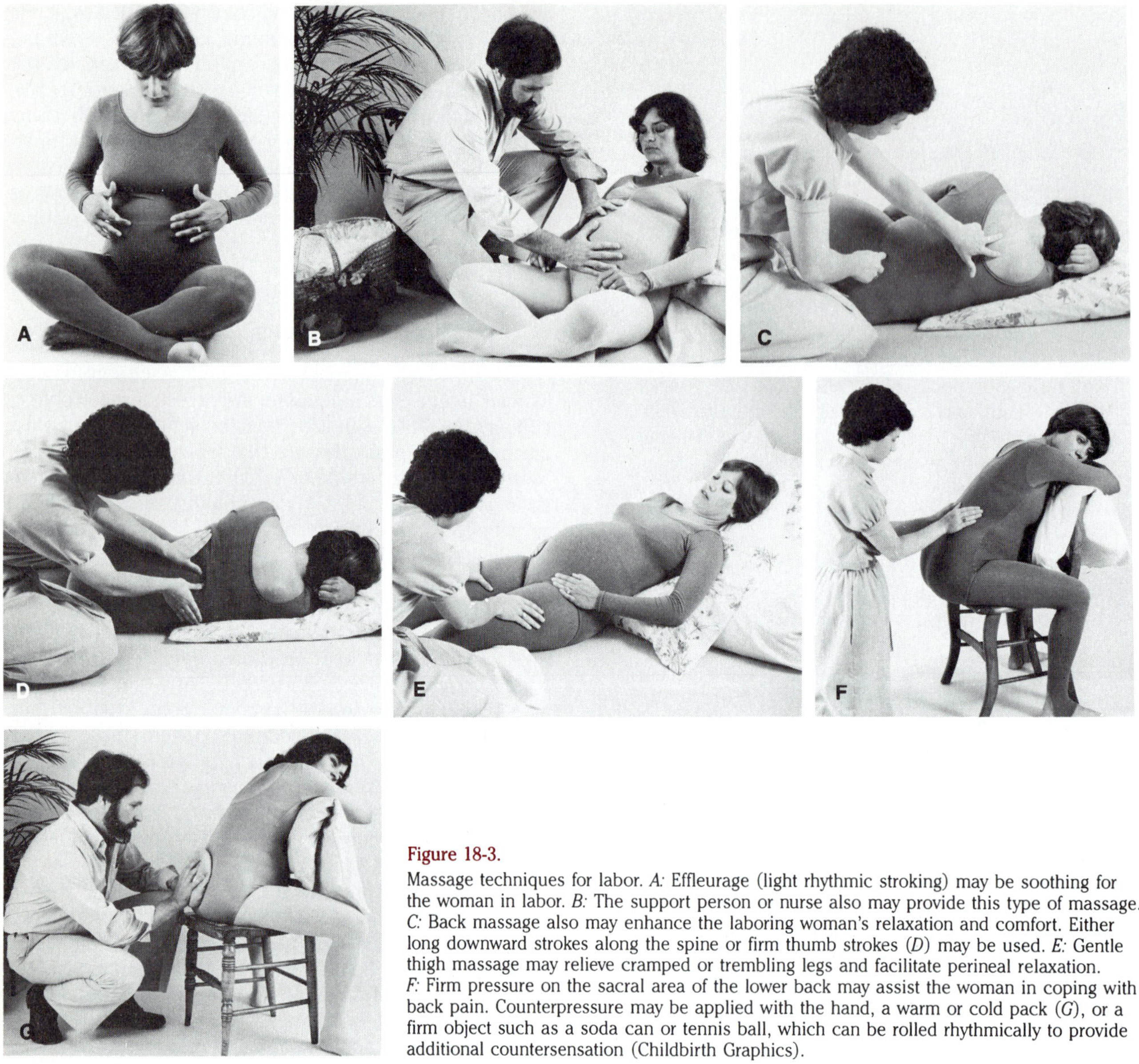

Figure 18-3.

Massage techniques for labor. *A:* Effleurage (light rhythmic stroking) may be soothing for the woman in labor. *B:* The support person or nurse also may provide this type of massage. *C:* Back massage also may enhance the laboring woman's relaxation and comfort. Either long downward strokes along the spine or firm thumb strokes (*D*) may be used. *E:* Gentle thigh massage may relieve cramped or trembling legs and facilitate perineal relaxation. *F:* Firm pressure on the sacral area of the lower back may assist the woman in coping with back pain. Counterpressure may be applied with the hand, a warm or cold pack (*G*), or a firm object such as a soda can or tennis ball, which can be rolled rhythmically to provide additional countersensation (Childbirth Graphics).

by incorporating a variety of other strategies. Some of these might be counting with each inhalation and exhalation, picturing the breath moving throughout the body, coordinating breathing with the support person's touch, walking or rocking in rhythm to the breath, or chanting a word or phrase with each exhalation. After delivery of the neonate, the woman may use slow paced breathing and relaxation techniques to deal with the discomforts of the early postpartum period. For instance, breathing techniques can be used to cope with uterine cramping or perineal pain, which may occur in the early postpartum period.

Modified Paced Breathing

Modified paced breathing is used when slow, rhythmic breathing is no longer effective, and a more alert state is needed. It begins with a cleansing breath (a deep inhalation through the nose and exhalation through the mouth) at the beginning of a contraction, shifts to breathing characterized by a slightly accelerated rate and increased use of the intercostal muscles, and ends with a cleansing breath. The rate should not exceed twice the woman's average respiratory rate. The primary considerations in determining rate are adequate oxygenation and the woman's comfort.

If this breathing technique alone is not effective, the strategies mentioned previously for use with slow paced breathing or effleurage may be added. Effleurage is done slowly but in rhythm with the breathing. Again, the concentration required for this complex combination helps alter the woman's perception of the pain associated with the contraction.

Preventing Hyperventilation. If respirations become deep and rapid as the pace of respiration increases, there is a risk of hyperventilation. Hyperventilation results in excessive carbon dioxide loss and respiratory alkalosis. Symptoms include lightheadedness and tingling of lips, face, hands, or

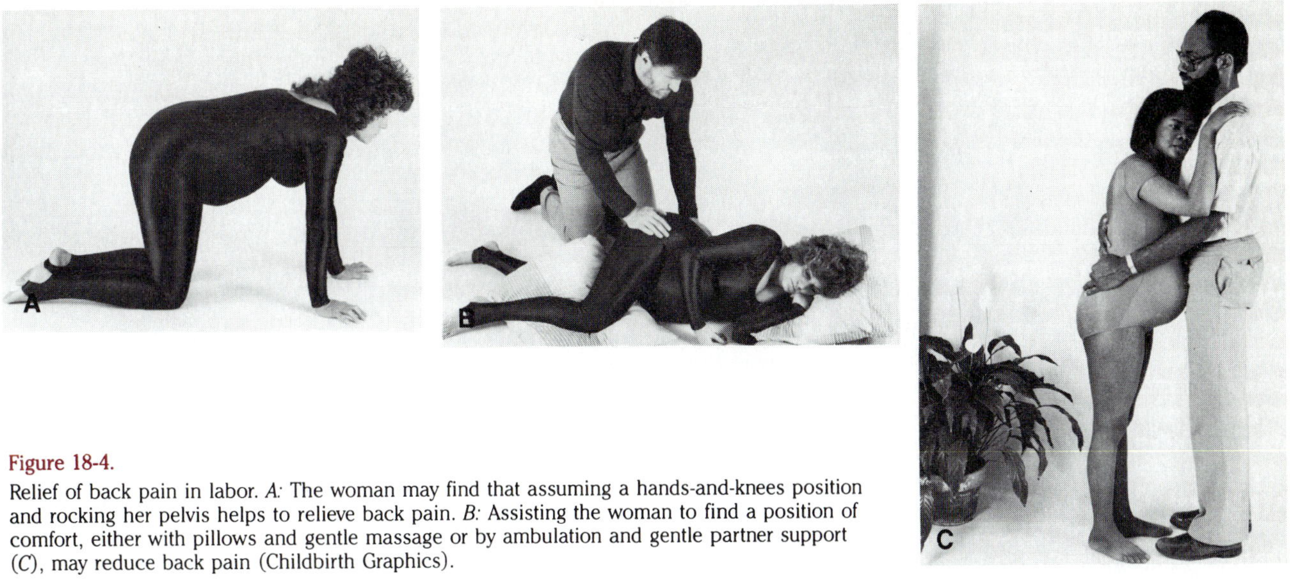

Figure 18-4.
Relief of back pain in labor. *A:* The woman may find that assuming a hands-and-knees position and rocking her pelvis helps to relieve back pain. *B:* Assisting the woman to find a position of comfort, either with pillows and gentle massage or by ambulation and gentle partner support (*C*), may reduce back pain (Childbirth Graphics).

feet. Hyperventilation can occur if the woman or support person is breathing too rapidly or begins to panic. If this occurs, the nurse should have the hyperventilating individual breathe into their cupped hands or a paper bag until the symptoms disappear. Measures to restore relaxation, such as verbal reassurance in a quiet, calm manner or a firm touch, should be taken. When the breathing pattern is resumed with the next contraction, respirations should be kept moderate to slow in rate. With careful assessment and action, such episodes usually are brief. However, prolonged hyperventilation eventually can cause loss of consciousness, severe maternal respiratory alkalosis, and a resulting decrease in uterine blood flow, which could put the fetus at risk.

Patterned Paced Breathing

During the last phase of cervical dilatation (7 to 10 cm) and the beginning of the second stage of labor, often called "transition," the woman may experience the sensations associated with labor most intensely. During this time she may require a rhythmic breathing pattern to assist her in working with her labor. Patterned paced breathing is a series of 1 to 6 breaths of the same quality as modified paced breathing but interspersed with a soft blow at regular intervals. The rhythmic quality and the need for concentration on a pattern make this technique effective for the most stressful periods of labor. If the woman begins to experience the urge to push before her cervix is completely dilated, she should be encouraged to use a series of soft blows to counteract the desire to push. This technique also can be used to avoid strong maternal pushing efforts, thus slowing the descent of the fetal head. This is sometimes necessary to avoid a too rapid delivery that might be difficult for the birth attendant to control.

Expulsion Breathing

The teaching of techniques for bearing-down efforts has more recently undergone a change (Nichols & Humenick, 1988). Women may be taught to push with a closed glottis (breath holding) or with an open glottis (exhaling). Conclusive evidence on the advantages and disadvantages of each technique is still lacking. Although pushing with a closed glottis, the traditional method, is taught and encouraged in many labor and delivery settings, there is some controversy about whether for an extended period of time it is the safest and most effective method for childbirth. It may cause an increase in intrathoracic pressure, which in turn causes a reduction in venous return to the heart and a decrease in cardiac output. This decreased cardiac output may cause reduced placental blood flow. Reduced placental perfusion is known to cause a decrease in available oxygen to the fetus, with resulting fetal hypoxia and acidosis. Proponents of open-glottis pushing assert that forced exhalation of air while pushing ("candle blowing" or groaning) does not inhibit venous return to the heart and causes the abdominal muscles to contract and press on the uterus, aiding in expulsion of the fetus. (See Chapter 21 for a more detailed discussion of bearing-down efforts during labor.)

The goals of childbirth education focus on providing information and techniques useful to the woman and her support person as she copes with labor and birth. Most childbirth educators use an eclectic mix of techniques, but relaxation and patterned breathing techniques are widely used. These techniques are designed to help the woman establish and maintain emotional and physical relaxation as she encounters the stresses of labor. These techniques can be used readily by the nurse to enhance the quality of the birth experience.

Preparation for the Childbearing Year

Education for childbearing families has grown beyond the original focus of preparing women for labor and birth. It has become part of a broader health promotion movement. Programs now exist for the period before conception on into the postpartum period. Traditional childbirth education classes have been criticized for continuing to meet the needs of only a segment of the population. However, more and more programs are being developed for groups with special needs, either for a particular emphasis or for approaches suited to the group's characteristic.

Community initiatives that aim to improve perinatal outcomes are being developed in some neighborhoods. These programs recognize support for expectant women and the promotion of prenatal care as important elements. Community-based childbearing women's support groups are an example of such initiatives. These groups provide more than education for childbirth. They also recognize the need to empower women within the context of their life circumstances. Helton (1990) in describing one such program identifies four elements as essential to the support group structure: a drop-in format; an agenda set by the women; some time devoted to labor, delivery, and parenting content; and the opportunity for women to share experiences and support each other.

To be effective such programs must consider the cultural makeup of the population. Important considerations in providing culturally appropriate educational programs include styles of verbal and nonverbal communication and forms of address. The educator must consider how decisions about health care and practices are made in the family's kinship network. Community programs that reach key family members may be necessary. Whenever possible, classes should be in the woman's primary language. When this is not possible, specific techniques, such as avoiding medical terminology, ample use of audiovisual materials, and speaking slowly, will help (Tripp-Reimer & Afifi, 1989).

Preconception and Early Pregnancy Education

Education for childbearing families should begin before pregnancy. The importance of the woman's health and life-style before pregnancy and in the first trimester is the impetus for such programs.

Preconception Education

Care in the period before conception is not a new concept, but a variety of factors make it more of a real possibility for women and couples today (Cefalo & Moos, 1988). Fundamental to preconception education is the ability to control reproduction with effective contraceptive methods. Combined with an increase in public knowledge about the influence of life-style, age, and health status on the outcome of pregnancy, planning for pregnancy motivates women to seek information to enable them to have the best possible pregnancy outcome. Medical advances in the management of chronic diseases and disabilities have opened the possibility of childbearing to women and couples who might previously have felt this was not an option.

Preconception care and counseling often are carried out on a one-to-one basis, particularly for women with health concerns, such as diabetes, previous pregnancy loss, and advanced maternal age. In some medical centers, preconception clinics offer this service. Cephalo and Moos (1988) described the goals of such a program as identifying individuals at risk, providing nonjudgmental and personalized education, and referral for in-depth assessment and teaching for those identified as at risk. Women may be referred for nutritional counseling, genetic counseling, or behavioral modification.

Programs for women and couples who may not have particular health risks are now becoming available in communities. These preconception classes have the overall goal of enabling women to "make informed decisions about conception, lifestyle and choices" in health care (Cephalo & Moos, 1988). Program content includes the following:

- Nutrition, weight, and exercise
- Effects on pregnancy of chemical substances (including alcohol, tobacco, caffeine, prescription, and illicit drugs)
- Environmental and occupational hazards
- Infectious diseases
- Prenatal diagnosis and testing
- General life-style and relationship concerns
- Health care during childbearing

Preconception education has the potential for improving outcomes for women and their neonates, but the effectiveness has yet to be studied. It may be important to reach beyond the women. St. Clair and Anderson (1989), in a study of 185 inner-city women, found that many received advice from their mothers, partners, sisters, and other relatives during pregnancy. Frequently, this advice differed from the advice of health care providers, and some of it, such as limiting weight gain, was potentially harmful.

Early Pregnancy Education

Early pregnancy classes, sometimes called "early bird" classes, address the concerns and interests of women in the first trimester. The overall goal is to encourage positive health behaviors for the woman's well-being and for fetal growth and development. Much of the content is the same as for the preconception period. Nutrition during pregnancy often is a particular focus. Content also includes reproduction, fetal development, maternal physiology, couple relationships, and sexuality in pregnancy.

Education for Transition to Parenthood

Although content about the early postpartum period, infant care, and transition to parenthood are included in most childbirth education series, parents often take in little of this information. Some parents report that they were not ready in the prenatal period to take in much detail about the postpartum period.

To meet the learning needs of new parents, programs are now being developed that are designed to enhance parents' feelings of competence and to offer a supportive group experience. These groups often are structured on a drop-in basis. Some offer a particular topic at each session and may be linked with other activities, such as postpartum fitness classes. Others are unstructured, with a group facilitator who encourages the parents to set the agenda and learn from each other. The opportunity to share the ups and downs of being a new parent is seen as beneficial and helps parents feel less isolated. Coping strategies for the realities of parenting and adjustment to parenting roles are frequent topics of discussion. The classes also offer the possibility of establishing ongoing relationships with other new parents.

Some childbirth education programs include a postpartum session with the class series. This may take the form of a structured class or may be primarily a social "reunion." There may be an opportunity to review birth experiences. Sexuality and family planning are content areas frequently addressed.

Women and their family members have many varied learning needs as they go through the childbearing cycle. Communities and institutions are responding to these needs. Educational programs for the childbearing population will undoubtedly continue to expand and evolve. The accompanying display lists groups with specialized learning needs. These needs may be addressed in specialized childbirth education classes.

Groups With Special Needs

High-Risk Women

When women become high risk and/or are hospitalized for prenatal complications, many of their hopes and plans are thwarted, including attending childbirth education classes. If already enrolled in hospital-based classes they may still be able to attend, but the classes may no longer address their concerns. The maternity nurse may be in a position to meet the learning needs of high-risk pregnant women, either individually or as a group. Alternatively, the nurse may facilitate the provision of special classes on the prenatal unit and encourage women and family members to participate. Avery and Olson (1987) described a course format designed for these women. The basic course content differs little from standard childbirth preparation classes. However, high-risk women will want a more in-depth understanding of the interventions they are more likely to encounter. Specifics of the care of high-risk neonates need to be discussed, including breastfeeding in such situations.

Relaxation techniques and strategies for coping with pain in labor are relevant regardless of the planned method of delivery. Such techniques are useful to decrease anxiety in general, to cope with discomfort during diagnostic tests, and to deal with postoperative pain management if cesarean delivery is required.

Ideally, classes provide an opportunity for group discussion and are held at times when partners or other support people can attend (Avery & Olson, 1987). When class attendance is not possible (eg, the woman is on strict bed rest) the maternity nurse should make an individual assessment of learning needs and use available resources, such as audio and video tapes and printed material that the woman can understand. Teaching is directed at meeting the individual's learning needs.

Groups with Specialized Learning Needs

- Adolescents
- Grandparents
- HIV-positive women who are pregnant
- Hospitalized high-risk pregnant women
- Immigrant women
- Multiparas who want to review childbirth preparation content
- Siblings
- Single women who are pregnant
- Couples with multiple gestation
- Women planning a vaginal birth after cesarean
- Women who have conceived after infertility treatment
- Lesbian women who are pregnant

Adolescents

Traditional childbirth education classes have little appeal for adolescents. Not only do they feel uncomfortable in a group of older, mostly married couples, but the class structure usually is unappealing. However, many professionals see specialized childbirth education programs to offer the possibility of improving outcomes for adolescent women and their neonates.

Programs for adolescents need to recognize the developmental challenges (described in detail in Chapter 9) facing the young pregnant woman. One study suggested that specialized classes can have a positive impact on obstetric complications for this group (Slager-Earnest, Hoffman, & Beckman, 1987). In this study, emphasis was placed on the biopsychosocial tasks facing the pregnant teenager. Smoke and Grace (1988) outlined content for a class series that is not significantly different from that of traditional childbirth education classes. The authors emphasized the need for the content to be at an appropriate age level. Their classes provided structured content and informal time for group discussion and interaction.

Other Family Members

With the trend toward family-centered maternity care, childbirth educators have become interested in other members of the family. Thus, special classes have been developed for grandparents and siblings. The accompanying display describes classes for expectant grandparents.

Classes for siblings take two forms: those that focus on helping the sibling adapt to a newborn in the family and those for children who are to be included in the actual birth. Spadt, Martin, and Thomas (1990) described experiential classes for siblings-to-be. They recommend an action-ori-

Family Considerations

Expectant Grandparents Classes

Classes for parents of childbearing couples are a recent phenomenon. In the past grandparents were the experts, but their role has been largely supplanted by health professionals. Childbirth practices and the teaching about newborn care and feeding are radically different from the practices many grandparents were advised to follow when they were new parents. These differences can lead to conflict between the generations. Conflict undermines the support grandparents can provide and may cause rifts between family members. Thus, the primary goal of classes for grandparents is to bridge the generation gap.

Many new parents want the support and practical help their parents can provide, particularly in the early postpartum period. By providing new grandparents with information about changes in childbirth practices and newborn care, especially breastfeeding, conflicts may be avoided.

Classes for grandparents emphasize positive ways to support new parents and enhance family role adaptation. Positive aspects of the grandparents' role, such as family historian, are explored. Finally, participants in these classes gain an appreciation of their children as parents with their own beliefs and practices.

Maloni, J. A., McIndoe, J. E., & Rubenstein, G. (1987). Expectant grandparent classes. Journal of Obstetric, Gynecologic, and Neonatal Nursing, 16*(1), 26–29.*

ented approach that helps prepare children for the arrival of their sister or brother through activities that include creating anatomic drawings, pushing a doll through a pelvis, and actually handling a newborn.

Some organizations offer classes for parents and children that prepare children to be present during the birth of a sibling. These classes focus specifically on the birth experience. In *Birth—Through Children's Eyes*, Anderson and Simkin (1981) listed the essential content:

- Understanding basic anatomy and physiology
- Sounds of labor and wetness of birth
- Intensity, hard work, and pain of labor
- Episiotomy or tear and repair
- The placenta
- What new babies are like

These authors believe that when children are properly prepared, family integration and attachment are strengthened. Coloring books, birthing dolls, and films are useful tools to help children prepare for the birth of a sibling.

Preparation for childbirth includes health education, which ideally should start in the preconception period. Women can be encouraged to make behavioral changes to increase health and well-being, thus promoting a healthier pregnancy later. Some groups may have specialized learning needs, such as pregnant adolescents or women with high-risk pregnancies. Family members, such as fathers, siblings, and grandparents, also may have unmet learning needs. Education for the early days and weeks of the transition to parenthood should be an important nursing priority.

Implications for Nursing Care

Individual nurses have played important roles in the evolution of childbirth education in the United States. Many of the first practicing childbirth educators were nurses who became involved in childbirth education through their professional work or their own experiences in childbearing. Proba-

Nursing Research

Perceptions of the Nurse's Role in Labor and Birth

A study was conducted to examine the role of the labor and delivery room nurse as perceived by expectant mothers trained in the Lamaze method, mothers without Lamaze training, and labor and delivery nurses themselves. The authors hypothesized that the Lamaze-trained women would perceive the nurses' role to be more important in terms of physical support, whereas the non–Lamaze-trained women would perceive the nurse's role to be more important in terms of emotional support, and their expectations of the nurse would be met more easily. However, none of these hypotheses were supported; that is, expectations of the nurse's role in labor and delivery were generally consistent between trained and untrained women and the nurses themselves.

The authors suggest that this study underscores the importance of both emotional and physical support for the laboring woman. Care must be individualized, based on the woman's expectations and perceptions; however, it is unwise to make assumptions about the importance of one aspect of nursing support over another, based only on the woman's level of childbirth preparation.

Collins, B. (1986). The role of the nurse in labor and delivery as perceived by nurses and patients. *Journal of Obstetric, Gynecologic, and Neonatal Nursing, 15*(5), 412–419.

bly the most important nursing role is the effective and compassionate nursing support of couples during labor in the hospital setting. This is when nurses make a unique contribution to the quality of the childbirth experience. The nurse plays a key role in helping parents put into practice what they have learned in prenatal education or in teaching useful techniques to assist unprepared couples in labor and birth. The nurse should never underestimate the effect of attitudes, skills, and knowledge implemented in caring for childbearing families.

The nurse's role in caring for women or couples using prepared childbirth techniques is the same as any other labor situation, except that the woman is a better informed and prepared patient. Nursing care during labor and birth is discussed in detail in Unit IV. However, some aspects of care should be emphasized when the nurse is caring for a woman or a couple using prepared childbirth techniques. These can be broken down into several areas: supporting the support person, providing comfort and reassurance, maintaining relaxation and concentration, and giving information.

• • Assessment

The nurse in the labor and delivery setting initially must assess what, if any, formal childbirth education the woman has had and what her expectations are in regard to particular coping techniques. In some cases these plans already may have been articulated in a written birth plan. This information is gathered and recorded as part of the nursing history. The nurse must assess the woman's responses to the sensations of labor, as well as the effectiveness of any particular technique in helping her cope with the stress of labor. The process of assessment of the laboring woman is detailed in Chapters 20 and 21.

• • Nursing Diagnosis

The nurse assesses the woman's responses to labor, as well as those of the father or support person on an ongoing basis throughout labor and formulates working nursing diagnoses that help to direct nursing care. Some nursing diagnoses that may be addressed in independently providing labor support for the woman and her support person include:

- Anxiety related to expectations of "coaching performance" in labor
- Pain related to uterine contractions
- Fatigue related to physical exertion of labor
- Knowledge Deficit related to coping techniques for labor
- Fear related to maternal expressions of pain and maternal panic

• • Planning and Implementation

The process of integrating "prepared childbirth techniques" into nursing care is discussed in Chapters 20 and 21. Some key interventions related to the nursing diagnoses listed in the previous section are highlighted in those chapters.

Supporting the Support Person(s)

The nurse must be present to monitor progress, assess the well-being of the woman and the fetus, and support the woman and her support person(s). Support includes providing the woman's support person with specific information about the progress of labor (Fig. 18-5).

The father is the person most often accompanying the laboring woman. He provides emotional support and encouragement for his mate. It is not his responsibility to make judgments about the progress of labor or make decisions on the woman's behalf, no matter how well prepared he may be. Furthermore, he may not be able to provide effective emotional and physical support continuously throughout the labor. The father who acts as a support person during labor is in a situation that may be extremely stressful and sometimes frightening. As he watches his partner struggle with the difficult, painful work of labor, he may feel as if he is helpless to assist her in a meaningful way. Even when labor is going well, he is intensely concerned about the safety and well-being of his partner and the fetus. If the nurse is not working with him closely and supporting his efforts, he is likely to feel anxious and alone. The woman will probably pick up his emotional discomfort, and this cannot help but increase her feelings of vulnerability and fear.

The nurse can assist by giving frequent and appropriate reassurance and feedback about the support person's effectiveness. The nurse should talk to *both* the woman and the support person, not just one or the other. Many prepared couples have discussed their hopes and expectations in advance so that the support person can "speak for" the woman in labor. The nurse should take note of the support

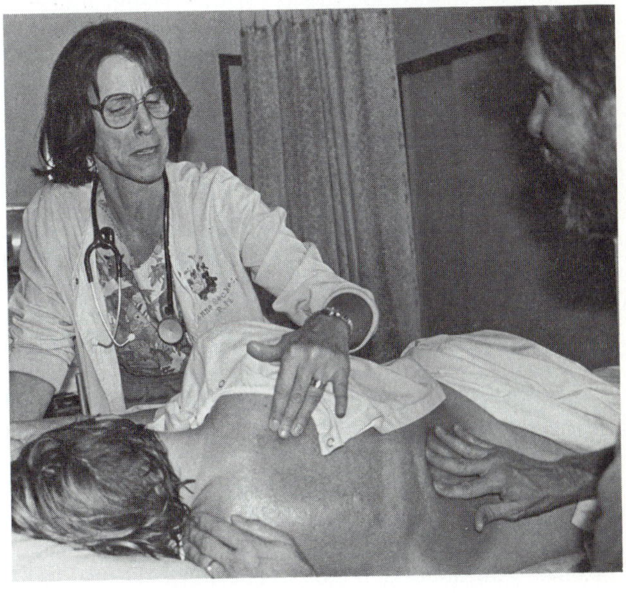

Figure 18-5.
The nurse should assess the support person's adaptation to the labor situation and assist him in his efforts to help his partner. (Photo by Kathy Sloane. Courtesy of Alta Bates Medical Center.)

Family Considerations

The "Father" Versus the "Coach"

The nurse should be especially careful not to "typecast" the father as the "coach" during labor and birth for several reasons. First, the coach concept tends to focus attention on the father's role during a relatively brief period on the childbearing cycle—labor and delivery—and detracts attention from other important aspects of father involvement in pregnancy, the growing bond between fetus–newborn and the father, and the emotional preparation necessary for fatherhood. Second, the concept of "father as coach" reinforces stereotypical and sexist gender roles, while it holds both parents to unreasonable expectations. At best, the concept of "coach" reinforces the image of the father as just a prop and deemphasizes him as a unique individual in the process of sharing a challenging life experience with his partner. At worst, it implies that the father should provide direction and should assume responsibility if things go badly during labor and birth, while it discourages the woman's reliance on her own self-knowledge and ability during childbirth.

Nurses should encourage expectant couples to "fire" the coach, and help fathers find their own place in the experience of birth by the following:

- Substituting the label "support person" for "coach" and not using "father" and "support person" synonymously. The father may provide labor support, but that is not all he does.
- Changing arbitrary institutional policies that restrict women to one labor-support person, and then encouraging parents to consider arranging for additional labor support, regardless of whether the father intends to provide labor support.
- Reminding fathers that nursing personnel are responsible for providing support and professional care during labor and he does not have to "do it all."

May, K. (1988). The father's role: Is it time to fire the coach? Childbirth Educator, *2, 30–35.*

person's view of the situation and assess the condition of the woman in labor directly; comments or actions that might be seen as discounting the support person's opinion should be avoided.

The nurse should observe whether the support person is comfortable and suggest breaks, reassuring the woman and the support person that someone will be available to stay with her. It is important that the nurse recognize the cumulative effects of stress and fatigue on the support person. Late in labor the support person's emotional and physical energy may be at a low point, and he or she will need additional encouragement and relief.

If the woman is to be transferred to another room for the birth, the nurse should prepare the support person well in advance to avoid an unsettling last-minute rush. The support person should be told specifically what preparation, such as scrubbing or special attire, is required. The nurse should give clear instructions to the support person about the type of "coaching" needed during the actual delivery and should frequently observe the support person's level of comfort during this time.

Maximizing the support person's effectiveness by providing assistance and encouragement not only benefits the woman in labor, but also helps to make the birth experience positive. If the father is the support person and he feels as if he has been effective in that role, this may indirectly affect his feelings about his spouse and neonate and his future role as a father.

Providing Comfort and Reassurance

A major aspect of caring for couples using prepared childbirth techniques is providing for their comfort and reassuring them that they are managing well and making progress. The presence of a caring nurse, even if no words are spoken, is reassuring. While taking into account a couple's need for privacy and uninterrupted periods, the nurse should avoid leaving couples alone for very long during labor, even if they seem to be managing well.

Comfort measures for the woman—ice chips, a cold cloth for her face, propping her with pillows in a comfortable position, back or leg rubs with talcum powder, balm for chapped lips, or a warm shower—may be particularly helpful. The support person may not remember to suggest such measures or may not be aware of them. The nurse can model this behavior for the support person and seek his or her opinion about what the woman may find comforting.

Sometimes prepared childbirth techniques and other comfort measures are not effective. If the woman is clearly struggling and in a great deal of pain and she is still more than 2 hours from expected delivery, the nurse should discuss appropriate analgesia with the woman and her support person. Comments like "you don't need to go all the way" imply failure and should be avoided. Instead, the nurse may point out that other techniques have not helped and explain that the woman's emotional and physical comfort is important for a safe birth. The nurse should assist the woman and her support person in making their own decision about the use of analgesia, within the limits of safety for the woman and fetus. Parents should be reminded that the desired outcome is a healthy newborn and a healthy and happy mother and father, and in some cases analgesia and other types of medical intervention will help achieve that goal.

Maintaining Relaxation and Concentration

The nurse also can intervene to assist the woman and her support person to establish and maintain high levels of relaxation and concentration throughout the labor process. One way is to make the environment conducive to the work of labor. The nurse should promote a calm and relaxed atmosphere by keeping the activity level and distractions in the labor room to a minimum. Distractions, such as unnecessary conversation late in labor, will drain energy the woman needs. The nurse should encourage rest and sleep between contractions. As labor intensifies, the nurse and support person should keep directions and questions short and relevant. Voices should be low and comforting. Lowering, rather than raising the voice and whispering directly into the woman's ear during the most intense parts of labor may be the most effective way of regaining control during periods of panic. The support person should sit down or get at the woman's eye level when supporting her through a contraction.

Giving Information

Couples who have attended childbirth education classes generally are knowledgeable about the progress of labor and will expect to be kept informed. The nurse should give the woman and her support person frequent information about the progress of labor, including the degree of dilatation and effacement and descent of the fetal head. If electronic fetal monitoring is used, the nurse should explain the significance of tracings; it is especially important to explain some of the common "nonemergencies" that may arise with monitoring equipment, such as the need to shift the tocodynamometer and the appearance of artifacts on the tracing, and to give hints on how to position electric cords. This should be done early in labor so that couples are not unnecessarily worried about these common problems.

Supporting the "Unprepared" Woman

The nurse should not assume that all pregnant women want to take prepared childbirth classes or want to use prepared childbirth techniques in their labor. Cultural and family backgrounds strongly affect a woman's expectations about labor and birth. Women from some ethnic groups (Hispanic and some Middle Eastern groups, for example) choose not to attend childbirth classes because it is not customary or acceptable for men to accompany their wives in labor. Some women will moan or scream throughout their labor because this is a culturally acceptable practice for them. Others may find the idea of a labor and birth without anesthesia horrifying and regard the traditional hospital birth with general anesthesia as modern and desirable. In these situations the nurse must explain the risks of unnecessary medication and assist these women in making safe decisions for themselves and their newborn. However, the labor and delivery suite is not the place to try to change women's expectations about birth, nor is it appropriate to impose the nurse's value judgments about a "good" labor on these patients.

On occasion the nurse provides care for women and family members who have not taken any kind of prepared childbirth classes and who are not well informed about what to expect in labor and birth. If the nurse has a working knowledge of labor-coping techniques, it may be possible to teach some of these techniques on the spot if the woman seems to be interested in learning ways to cope with her labor. Visualization may be particularly effective if the nurse can encourage pleasant imagery with suggestions appropriate to the woman's frame of reference. An "unprepared" support person can be taught to give effective comfort measures, some as simple as hand-holding and loving, reassuring talk.

• • Evaluation

Evaluating the effectiveness of care directed toward supporting prepared childbirth techniques is probably most often done by collecting information about the family's satisfaction with their birth experience. Most often, couples who have made specific plans for childbirth preparation are likely to regard their birth experience more positively if these plans are taken into account to the extent made possible by the health care team.

Of course most parents recognize that obstetric problems may require medical interventions, which make their birth plan impossible. However, the nurse plays a critical role in explaining how plans can be modified within the demands of a given labor situation and in assuring that parental wishes are respected to the maximum possible extent. Indeed, the difference between a satisfying and an unsatisfying birth experience for some well-prepared and goal-oriented couples may be the nurse who genuinely listened to their desires and helped the parents actualize as much of their birth plan as possible. Thus, it is essential the nurse be well versed in the types of childbirth preparation available to patients and be prepared to individualize intrapartum nursing care on that basis.

Chapter Summary

Preparation for childbirth evolved in response to consumer concerns about the increasing medical control and technologic management of normal labor and birth. Early proponents developed techniques intended to reduce pain perception and increase relaxation during labor and birth. Their goal was to reduce the need for analgesia, anesthesia, and other types of medical intervention in childbirth. Childbirth education attained early popularity among middle-class groups. Specialized educational services have been developed to meet the needs of disadvantaged and other high-risk groups, but more work is needed in this area.

Most types of childbirth education include factual information about the process of labor and birth, specific techniques for achieving and maintaining relaxation, and coping techniques to use in response to the sensations of labor. The nurse must be knowledgeable about the range of techniques taught in childbirth classes to act as a resource for parents seeking prenatal education and to provide effective and supportive care to women in labor and their families. Groups such as adolescents, single women, and women experiencing high-risk pregnancies may have specialized learning needs that should be addressed through innovative approaches to childbirth education. Education for the early days and weeks of the transition to parenthood should continue to be an important nursing priority. Nurses have played an important role in the development of innovative programs of parent education. High-quality and creative parent education during the childbearing year must continue to be a priority of nurses involved in maternity care.

Study Questions

1. *What are the major components of childbirth education programs?*
2. *How effective is childbirth education?*
3. *Can you name two national childbirth education organizations and describe the role of these organizations in establishing standards for childbirth education?*
4. *Considering the content of childbirth education, what preparation do you think is necessary for competent practice as a childbirth educator?*
5. *What groups of women whose needs have not been met in the past have been addressed by childbirth education programs? What programs fill some of the gaps in childbirth education programs?*
6. *What labor-coping techniques are used? What is the rationale for their use?*
7. *What are some supportive actions the nurse can use when caring for couples during childbirth?*

References

Anderson, S. V., & Simkin, P. (1981). *Birth—Through children's eyes*. Seattle, WA: Pennypress.

Avery, P., & Olson, I. M. (1987). Expanding the scope of childbirth education to meet the needs of hospitalized, high-risk clients. *Journal of Obstetric, Gynecologic, and Neonatal Nursing, 16*(6), 418–421.

Bradley, R. (1965). *Husband-coached childbirth*. New York: Harper & Row.

Carty, E. M., & Tier, D. T. (1989). Birth planning: A reality-based script for building confidence. *Journal of Nurse-Midwifery, 34*(3), 111–114.

Cefalo, R. C., & Moos, M. K. (1988). *Preconceptional health promotion: A practical guide*. Rockville, MD: Aspen.

Dick-Read, G. (1959). *Childbirth without fear*. New York: Harper & Row.

Enkin, M. W. (1990). Commentary: Are the correct outcomes of prenatal education being measured? *Birth, 17*(2), 90–91.

Enkin, M., Keirse, M. J. N. C., & Chalmers, I. (1989). *A guide to effective care in pregnancy and childbirth*. Oxford: Oxford University Press.

Green, J. M., Coupland, V. A., & Kitzinger, J. V. (1990). Expectations, experiences and psychological outcomes of childbirth: A prospective study of 825 women. *Birth, 17*(1), 15–23.

Helton, A. S. (1990). A buddy system to improve prenatal care. *MCN: American Journal of Maternal Child Nursing, 15*, 234–237.

ICEA. (1987). *ICEA position paper: The role of the childbirth educator and the scope of childbirth education*. Minneapolis: Author.

Karmel, M. (1959). *Thank you, Dr. Lamaze*. Garden City, NY: Doubleday.

Leboyer, F. (1974). *Birth without violence*. New York: Knopf.

Nichols, F. H., & Humenick, S. S. (Eds.). (1988). *Childbirth education: Practice, research, and theory*. Philadelphia: W.B. Saunders.

Odent, M. (1984). *Entering the world: The de-medicalization of childbirth*. New York: Marion Boyars.

Shearer, M. H. (1990). Effects of prenatal education depend on the attitudes and practices of obstetric caregivers. *Birth, 17*(2), 73–74.

Shrock, P. (1988). The basis of relaxation. In F. H. Nichols & S. S. Humenick (Eds.), *Childbirth education: Practice, research, and theory* (pp. 118–132). Philadelphia: W.B. Saunders.

Slager-Earnest, S. E., Hoffman, S. J., & Beckman, C. J. A. (1987). Effects of a specialized prenatal adolescent program on maternal and infant outcomes. *Journal of Obstetric, Gynecologic, and Neonatal Nursing, 16*(6), 422–429.

Smoke, J., & Grace, M.C. (1988). Effectiveness of prenatal care and education for pregnant adolescents. *Journal of Nurse-Midwifery, 33*(4), 178–184.

Spadt, S. K., Martin, K. R., & Thomas, A. M. (1990). Experiential classes for siblings-to-be. *MCN: American Journal of Maternal Child Nursing, 15*, 184–186.

St. Clair, P. A., & Anderson, N. A. (1989). Social network advice during pregnancy: Myths, misinformation and sound counsel. *Birth, 16*(3), 103–107.

Tripp-Reimer, T., & Afifi, L. A. (1989). Cross-cultural perspectives on patient teaching. *Nursing Clinics of North America, 24*(3), 613–619.

Wertz, D., & Wertz, R. (1989). *Lying in: A history of childbirth in America* (2nd ed.). New Haven: Yale University Press.

Suggested Readings

Eakin, P. (1986). *The American way of birth*. Philadelphia: Temple University Press.

Leavitt, J. (1986) *Brought to bed: Childbirth in America, 1750–1950*. New York: Oxford University Press.

Simkin, P., & Enkin, M. (1989). Antenatal classes. In I. Chalmers, M. Enkin, & M. Keirse (Eds.), *Effective care in pregnancy and childbirth* (pp. 318–334). Oxford: Oxford University Press.

CHAPTER 19

The Process of Labor and Birth

MATERNAL AND FETAL ADAPTATIONS

Learning Objectives

After studying the material in this chapter, the student will be able to:

- Describe the dynamic relationship between the bony pelvis, the fetus, and the pelvic and perineal muscles and ligaments during the process of labor and birth.
- Define and describe the stages of labor.
- Describe the cardinal movements of the fetus during labor and birth.
- Explain the possible causes of onset of labor.
- Describe the processes of cervical effacement and dilatation and their significance for progress in labor.
- Discuss maternal psychophysiologic responses during labor and birth.
- List the signs of labor and distinguish between false and true labor.
- Outline maternal physiologic and behavioral adaptations during labor and birth.
- Outline fetal physiologic and behavioral adaptations during labor and birth.

Key Terms

bregma	lie
cephalic	linea terminalis
cephalopelvic disproportion	mentum
contraction	molding
crowning	occiput
dilatation	position
dilatation and curettage	presentation
effacement	sinciput
engagement	station
fontanelle	true pelvis
labor	vertex

The process of labor and birth is a fairly predictable sequence of events that usually occurs in a harmonious fashion and results in a healthy mother and neonate. Many individual and environmental factors affect this process, causing each labor and birth experience to be unique. The course of labor can be prolonged or accelerated, painful or gentle. Labor may require aggressive medical and nursing management or only supportive care.

Nursing care during childbirth can change dramatically in minutes as the woman moves through the stages of labor. To accurately assess the woman's progress through labor and to anticipate and meet her needs, the nurse must have a thorough understanding of the anatomic and physiologic changes that occur during labor and birth. The nurse's understanding of this process will allow for the provision of appropriate and effective care. Factors that influence the labor and birth process are listed in the accompanying display.

This chapter reviews these anatomic and physiologic changes and discusses behavioral changes in the woman and the fetus. Chapters 20 to 26 discuss nursing care for women and their families or partners in normal, moderate-risk, and high-risk labor and birth.

Forces of Labor: Passage, Passenger, Powers, and Psyche

Four factors, commonly known as the "four Ps," are of critical importance in the process of childbirth. They are the *passage, passenger, powers, and psyche*. In normal labor the pelvic anatomy (passage) must be spacious enough to accomodate the fetus. The fetus (passenger) must be in an advantageous position and small enough to fit through the passage. Uterine contractions (powers) must be rhythmic, coordinated, and efficient enough to dilate and efface the cervix, and maternal emotional resources (psyche) must be adequate to accomplish the delivery of the fetus. All of these

Factors Influencing Progress in Labor and Birth

Maternal Age

Maternal age may affect the progress of normal labor and birth. The very young woman (younger than 16 years) may have an immature, small pelvis, increasing the risk of cephalopelvic disproportion. She is at increased risk for preeclampsia. The older woman (older than 35 years) is more likely to have twins, breech, or occipitoposterior presentations, and a longer second stage of labor.

Maternal Weight

Overweight women are at risk for delays or arrests in latent or active phases of labor and for soft-tissue dystocia, the slowing of the second stage, as a result of excessive weight.

Birth Interval

When the interval since the last birth is less than 1 year, the woman is at risk for a more rapid labor and a smaller infant.

Birth Weight and Gestational Age

Preterm and small fetuses are usually born after a fast labor, whereas large fetuses are generally associated with longer labors, especially a longer second stage of labor. Gestational age of less than 37 weeks is associated with a higher rate of malpresentation, which can affect the progress of labor. Gestational age of more than 42-weeks is associated with macrosomia, or large body size in the fetus, and a higher risk of birth complications.

Fetal Position

Labor progresses most effectively when the fetus is in a well-flexed vertex position.

Status of Amniotic Sac

Early rupture of the amniotic sac may interfere with the progress of labor because the synthesis in the chorion of prostaglandins, substances that cause uterine contraction, is impaired. There is no evidence that rupture of the amniotic sac shortens labor and some evidence that the fetus may be at higher risk for acidosis when membranes are ruptured before the second stage of labor.

Site of Placental Implantation

High or fundal implantation of the placenta has been shown to be associated with prolonged labor, possibly because of interference with myometrial contractility in the area.

Maternal Position During Labor

The woman's position during labor has been shown to affect uterine activity. Standing or upright positions have been found to be most efficient in dilating the cervix and have been associated with lower incidence of umbilical cord compression and increased maternal comfort.

The lateral recumbent position appears to result in less efficient uterine contractions than the upright position. The supine position is associated with more frequent but less efficient contractions.

Psychological Factors

Maternal psychological status has direct effects on the progress of labor. Stress and anxiety stimulate the release of stress hormones called catecholamines, which are known to inhibit uterine activity. Childbirth preparation has been shown to be helpful in reducing stress and anxiety associated with labor and birth and may contribute to a more favorable labor progress and outcome.

Medications

The use of narcotic analgesia has been shown to slow down the active phase of labor. Magnesium sulfate, used in the treatment of preeclampsia, has been shown to diminish the frequency and intensity of uterine contractions and reduce the resting tone of the uterus. There is some controversy about whether regional anesthesia, such as epidural anethesia, slows the progress of labor and contributes to increased need for oxytocin augmentation and cesarean delivery.

factors interact dynamically with the environment to accomplish spontaneous delivery in most cases.

An alteration in any component, such as a decrease in the effectiveness of uterine contractions or an increase in the size of the fetus, may delay the process of labor. Active intervention, such as the use of uterine stimulants or forceps, may be required to accomplish delivery when problems such as these occur. In many cases the nurse can prevent alterations in the labor process. This is accomplished by providing the woman with guidance about position and activity during labor that facilitate the physiologic progress. Specific aspects of nursing support and guidance that facilitate normal labor and birth are discussed in Chapters 20 and 21.

Passage: The Pelvis

The passage is determined by maternal pelvic anatomy—the bony pelvis and the muscles of the pelvic floor and perineum. (See Chapter 4 for the muscular and bony anatomy of the pelvis and Chapter 13 for the classification and assessment of pelvic types.) Specific pelvic landmarks and measurements are important when considering the complementary relationship between the bony pelvis and the fetus.

Pelvic Planes and Measurements

The pelvis consists of four bones: two innominate bones (formed by the ilium, ischium, and pubis), the sacrum, and the coccyx. The configuration of these bones is of considerable importance when measuring the capacity of the pelvis.

Planes

For obstetric purposes the pelvis is described as having three planes: the inlet, the midpelvis, and the outlet, as shown in Figure 19-1.

Pelvic Inlet. The pelvic inlet is bounded by the sacrum posteriorly, the linea terminalis laterally, and the symphysis pubis anteriorly. The linea terminalis separates the true pelvis from the false pelvis. The fetus must pass through the true pelvis to be born vaginally. Four diameters of the pelvic inlet are important for measurement purposes: the anteroposterior, the transverse, and the two oblique diameters. The anteroposterior diameter is designated the *obstetric conjugate* (Fig. 19-2) and represents the most important inlet diameter in most cases. The obstetric conjugate is the most significant inlet diameter because it represents the *shortest* distance between the promontory of the sacrum and the symphysis pubis. The fetal presenting part must first pass successfully through this diameter before further descent and eventual vaginal delivery can occur. The obstetric conjugate usually measures 10 cm or more, but if considerably shortened, the fetal presenting part may never pass through the inlet.

Because the obstetric conjugate cannot be measured directly by vaginal examination, the physician or midwife can only estimate its length. The distance from the lower margin of the symphysis pubis to the promontory of the sacrum, known as the *diagonal conjugate*, can be measured with the examining fingers (Fig. 19-3*A*). A vaginal examination is performed. The physician or midwife advances the hand posteriorly until the fingertips touch the sacral promontory. While maintaining contact with the sacrum, the hand is slightly elevated until it makes contact with the lower border of the symphysis pubis. The hand is then removed, and the distance from the tip of the finger to the point where the symphysis pubis made contact with the hand is measured in centimeters. By subtracting 1.5 to 2 cm from the diagonal conjugate, the obstetric conjugate is estimated (see Fig. 19-3*B*).

Midpelvis. The plane of the midpelvis is bounded anteriorly by the bottom of the symphysis pubis and at the sides by the ischial spines. The midpelvis has great obstetric

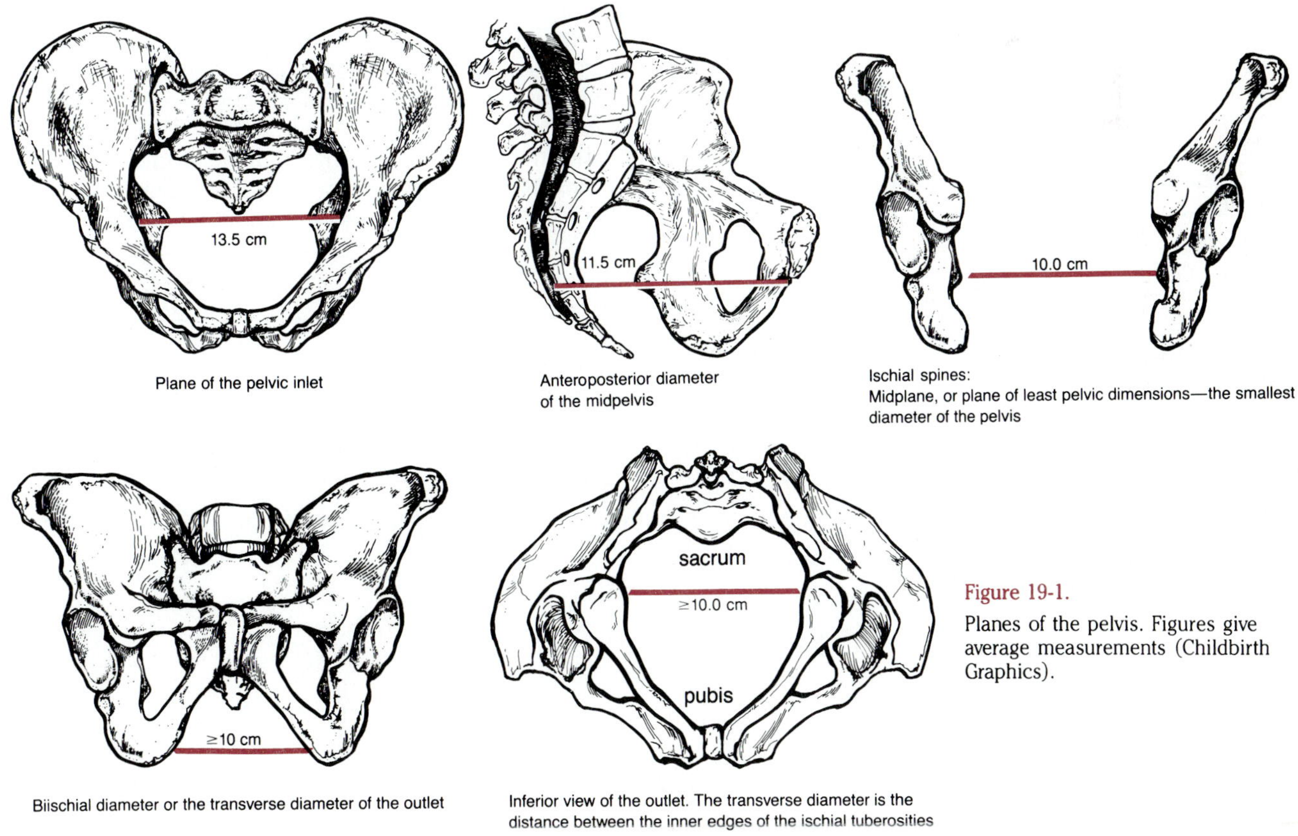

Figure 19-1.
Planes of the pelvis. Figures give average measurements (Childbirth Graphics).

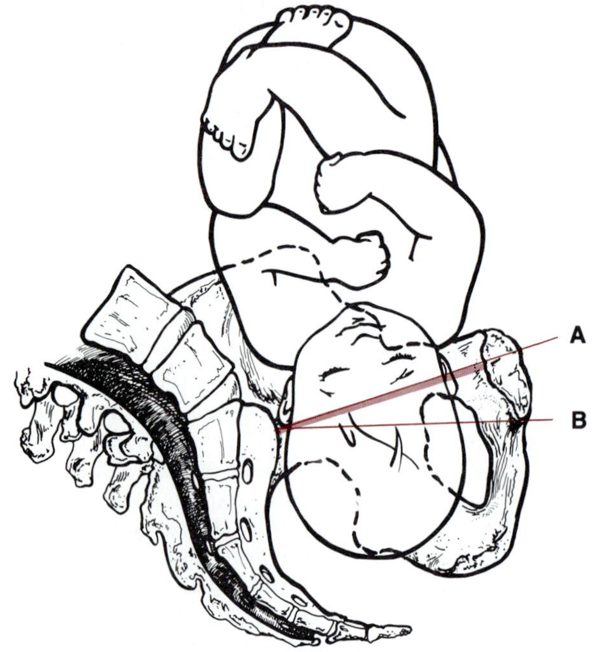

Figure 19-2.

A: Obstetric conjugate. This obstetrically important diameter is the shortest anteroposterior distance between the sacral promontory and symphysis pubis. *B:* Diagonal conjugate. Because the obstetric conjugate cannot be measured directly, its length is estimated by measuring the diagonal conjugate, which is the distance between the sacral promontory and the lower border of the symphysis pubis (Childbirth Graphics).

significance because it normally contains the *narrowest* portion of the pelvis. The smallest diameter of the pelvis is the transverse diameter between the two ischial spines (*interspinous diameter*), usually measuring approximately 10 cm. When the transverse diameter of the midpelvis is narrowed (less than 10 cm), fetal descent and further progress in labor may occur. The shortest anteroposterior diameter at the ischial spines usually measures 11.5 cm and is of less obstetric importance.

Pelvic Outlet. The pelvic outlet consists of a line drawn between the two ischial tuberosities (*biischial diameter*). This line, the transverse diameter of the outlet, usually measures 10 cm or more. In some cases the coccyx is immobile or the sacrococcygeal joint juts sharply inward. When this occurs the anteroposterior diameter of the pelvic outlet is narrowed and may delay or arrest further descent and birth of the fetus.

Pelvic Shape and Capacity

When assessing pelvic capacity, other important landmarks and measurements are considered. The curve and length of the sacrum determine the posterior capacity of the pelvis in all three planes. The sacrum may be concave, flat, or convex; the latter two characteristics decrease pelvic capacity. The characteristics of the ischial spines also are important when assessing pelvic capacity for childbirth. Sharp, encroaching spines greatly decrease the transverse diameter of the midpelvis. The pubic arch, or subpubic angle, should be wide and rounded at 90 degrees or more to allow the fetal head to pivot under it. A narrow or acute pubic angle will force the fetal head down onto the perineum and may cause major perineal tears or require an operative delivery.

The physician or nurse midwife will draw conclusions about the capacity of a woman's pelvis for normal childbirth from clinical evaluation of the pelvis and estimates of fetal weight and position. (See Chapter 20 for a detailed review of the pelvic examination.) The labor nurse also is usually expected to evaluate the shape and capacity of the pelvis during labor. A diagnosis of *cephalopelvic disproportion* (CPD) indicates that the combination of fetal size, fetal position, and pelvic architecture is not favorable for a vaginal delivery. This usually leads to a decision for a cesarean delivery. Unless gross pelvic inadequacies are found, the diagnosis of CPD is not safely made on the basis of clinical evaluation alone for several reasons. First, clinical evaluation of pelvic size and architecture by vaginal examination depends on the skill and experience of the examiner and may be open to subjective error. Second, fetal size is sometimes difficult to estimate accurately without the support of so-

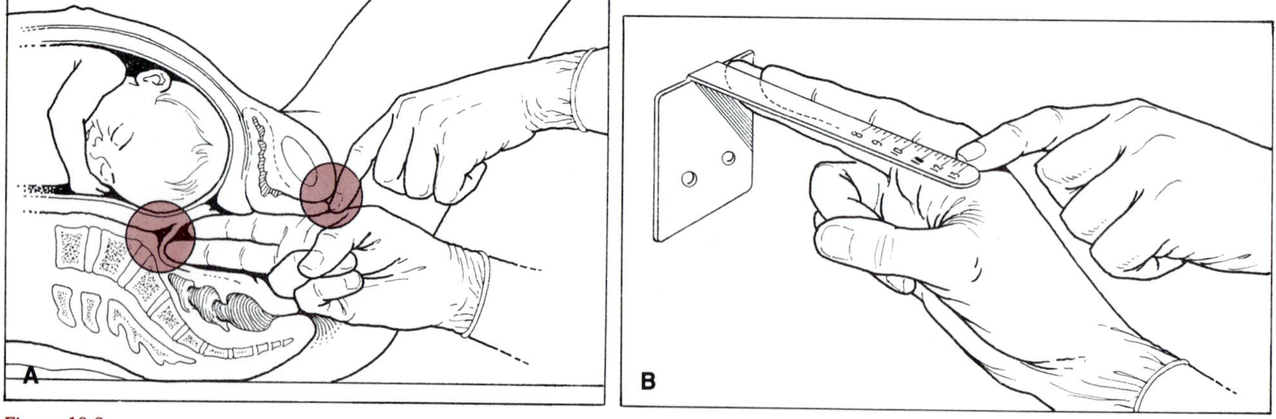

Figure 19-3.

Measurement of the diagonal conjugate. *A:* A vaginal examination is performed to measure the diagonal conjugate. The examiner touches the sacral promintory P, then marks the hand where it touches the symphysis pubis P. *B:* The distance between the two points is measured by subtracing 1.5 to 2 cm from this measurement. The obstetric conjugate is measured.

nography. Finally, a fetus that is well positioned or flexed may be able to negotiate passage through a tight pelvis, while another fetus of the same size but in a less favorable position may not.

Pelvimetry Techniques

Pelvic and fetal size may be measured using a variety of technologies. The physician or midwife who suspects CPD may order specific diagnostic tests to clarify the exact nature of the problem. Recent advances in ultrasonography and the development of computed tomography (CT) scanning have increased the accuracy of pelvimetry.

X-Ray Pelvimetry. X-ray pelvimetry is sometimes used to gain information about the shape and inclination of the pelvis, its length and diameters, and the relationship and fit of the fetus to the pelvis. However, the value of pelvimetry is controversial. The pelvic capacity and position of the fetus are only two of the many factors that determine obstetric outcome, and the prognosis for a successful vaginal delivery cannot be established on the basis of x-ray pelvimetry alone.

Computed Tomography Pelvimetry. Because traditional x-ray pelvimetry has been shown to have limited usefulness in predicting the progress of labor, a new technique, CT pelvimetry, is being used in selected settings to evaluate the adequacy of the maternal pelvis. A very low dose of radiation (22 mrad) is absorbed in comparison to conventional x-ray pelvimetry (885 mrad). Its usefulness in assessing pelvic dimensions in breech presentations and in estimating shoulder widths in macrosomic fetuses also is being evaluated (Cunningham, MacDonald, & Gant, 1989).

Ultrasonography. The use of diagnostic ultrasound also has been suggested to assist the physician or midwife in the evaluation cephalopelvic dimensions. Morgan and Thurnau (1988) have devised a technique for predicting the likelihood of CPD known as the *fetal-pelvic index*. This estimate is calculated through a combined measurement of maternal pelvic dimensions obtained by x-ray pelvimetry and fetal head and abdominal diameters estimated by linear array ultrasonography. Current research suggests that the fetal-pelvic index may be useful in predicting CPD in nulliparous women at high risk for this problem (Morgan & Thurnau, 1992).

Passenger: The Fetus

The fetus as passenger must undergo a series of predictable and synchronized maneuvers to descend through the maternal pelvis. The anatomy and placement of the fetal head in the bony pelvis and the movements of the fetus through the pelvis play an important part in the progress of normal labor.

Fetal Head

In normal labor and birth the head, or cranium, is viewed as the most important part of the fetus. The head is most often the presenting part; is not compressible, as is the softer tissue of the rest of the body; and, along with the shoulders, represents the largest part of the term infant.

Fetal Cranial Anatomy

The fetal cranium is composed of the occipital bone, two parietal bones, two temporal bones, and two frontal bones (Fig. 19-4*A*). At birth these bones are only partially ossified and are joined by tough, membranous connective tissue. This allows some movement and overlapping of the bones under pressure. This adaptation in the size and shape of the the fetal head as it passes through the maternal pelvis during labor is called *molding*.

The membranous spaces between the bony plates of the cranium are called sutures. Where these sutures intersect there are wide, membranous spaces called fontanelles. The characteristic arrangement of sutures and fontanelles provides a useful way of determining the position of the fetal head in relation to the maternal pelvis. In a vaginal examination during labor the examiner can feel the sutures and fontanelles through the dilated cervix.

The sagittal suture is the most readily felt. It runs in an anteroposterior direction between the two parietal bones, connecting the anterior and posterior fontanelles. The frontal suture is the anterior continuation of the sagittal suture between the two frontal bones. The coronal sutures, extending in a transverse direction from the anterior fontanelle, lie between the parietal and frontal bones. At the back of the head, the lambdoid sutures extend in a transverse direction from the posterior fontanelle, dividing the occipital bone from the parietals.

Other important landmarks of the fetal skull are shown in Figure 19-4*B*. These areas of the cranium are as follows:

- Occiput: back of the head formed by the occipital bone
- Vertex: top of the head between the two fontanelles
- Bregma: front of the head formed by the frontal bone
- Mentum: chin
- Sinciput: brow
- Glabella: elevated area between the orbital ridges
- Nasion: root of the nose
- Parietal eminences or bosses: widest areas on each side of the parietal bones

Diameters of the Fetal Skull

The diameters of the fetal skull are the distances between reference points in the cranium (Fig. 19-5). In general the fetus descends through the maternal pelvis by movements that present the *smallest* diameter of the fetal skull known as the *suboccipitobregmatic diameter*. The suboccipitobregmatic diameter extends from the lower edge of the occipital bone (near the neck) to the bregma, or forehead. This is the *anteroposterior diameter* of the fetal skull that presents to the maternal pelvis when the fetal neck is well flexed. The suboccipitobregmatic diameter averages 9.5 cm at term. The reader is reminded that the smallest transverse diameter of the midplane (interspinous diameter) is usually 10 cm or greater. When the fetal neck is well flexed and the suboccipitobregmatic diameter (9.5 cm) presents, there is generally enough room to pass through this important midpelvic diameter.

In obstetrics the *biparietal diameter* is the most significant fetal skull diameter (Fig. 19-6). It is the distance between the parietal bosses and represents the *largest* transverse diameter of the fetal head, averaging 9.25 cm at term. This diameter can be measured by ultrasonic measurements

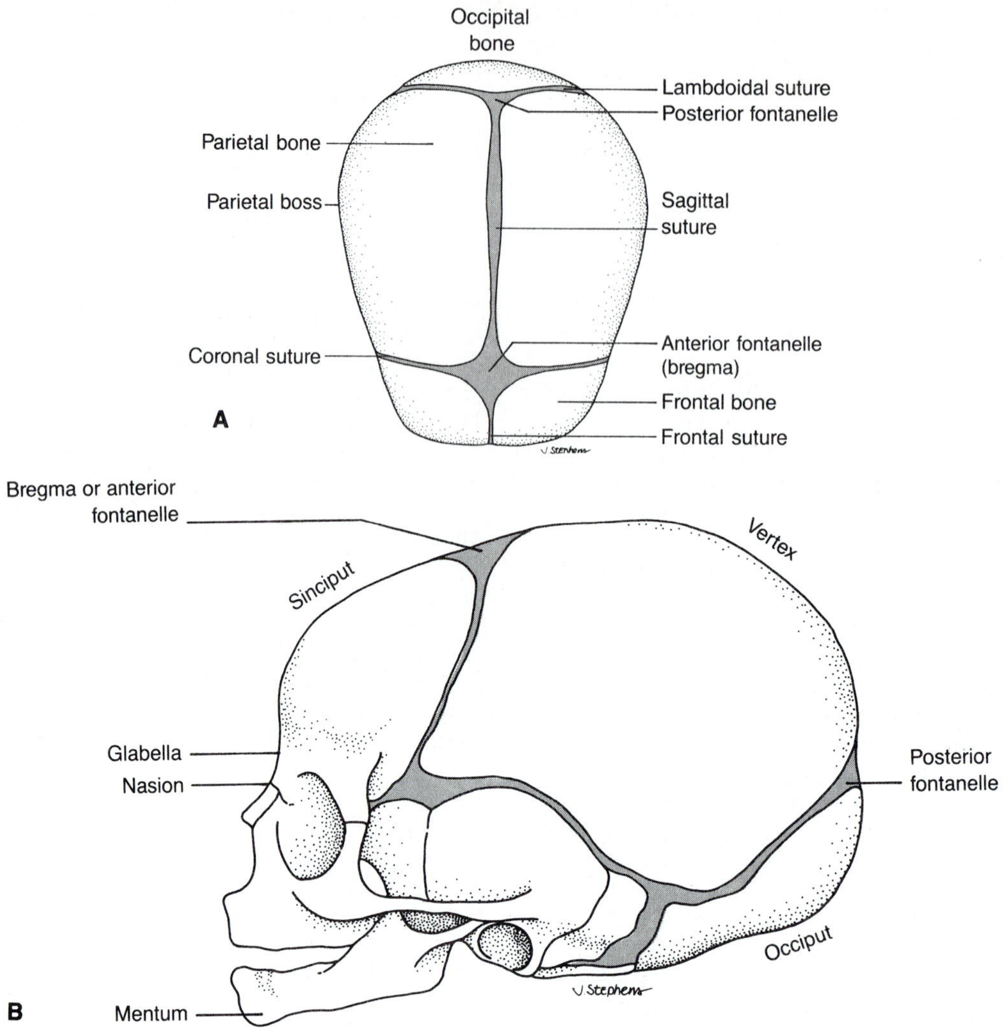

Figure 19-4.
The fetal cranium. *A:* Superior view. *B:* Lateral view (Childbirth Graphics).

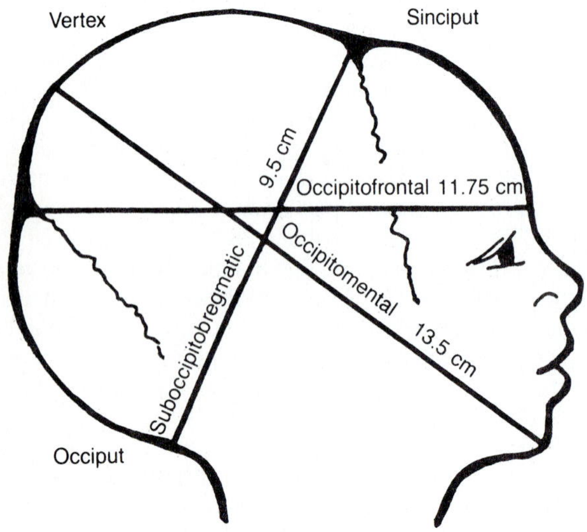

Figure 19-5.
Diameters of the fetal skull (Childbirth Graphics).

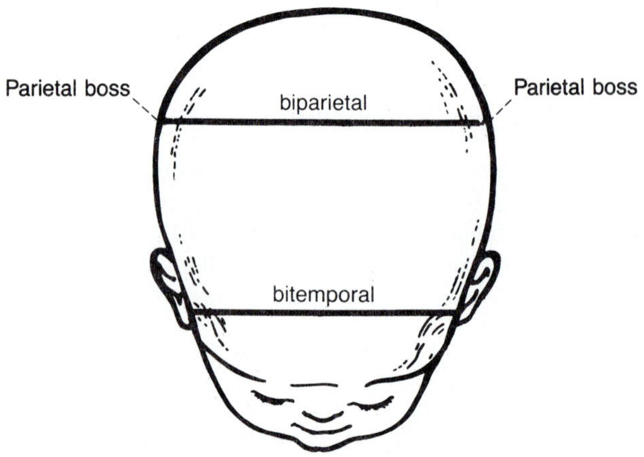

Figure 19-6.
The biparietal diameter of the fetal skull represents the largest transverse diameter of the fetal head. It averages 9.25 cm at term.

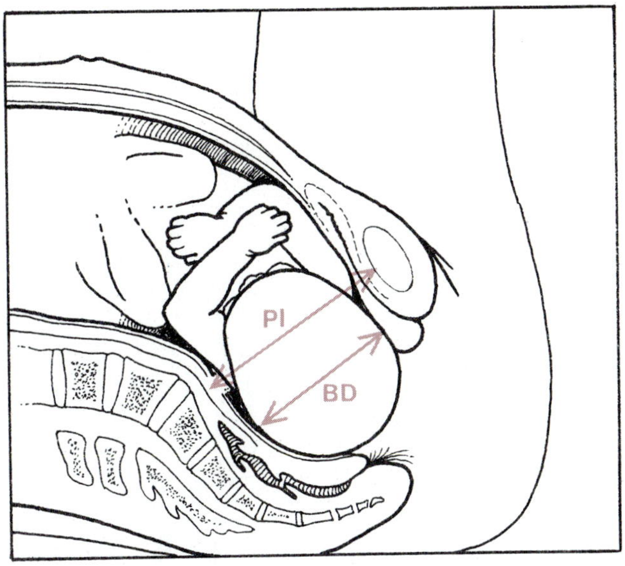

Figure 19-7.
When the biparietal diameter of the fetal skull has passed through the pelvic inlet, engagement has occurred.

of fetal head size. When this widest transverse diameter of the fetal head passes through the pelvic inlet, the fetal head is *engaged*. This is confirmatory evidence that the pelvic inlet is adequate in size to accommodate the fetal head. Engagement may be ascertained by vaginal examination (Fig. 19-7).

When the fetal neck is not well flexed or is partially or completely extended, larger anteroposterior diameters of the fetal skull will present to the maternal pelvis (see Fig. 19-5). When larger diameters present, the fetal head may be prevented from passing through the pelvis, necessitating a cesarean birth. The *occipitofrontal diameter* extends from the external occipital protuberance (back of the head) to the glabella. This diameter presents to the maternal pelvis when the fetal head is neither well flexed nor well extended but straight. The fetus is sometimes said to be in a "military attitude." The *verticomental diameter* extends from the vertex to the mentum and presents in the pelvis as a brow presentation with partial extension of the head. The *submentobregmatic diameter* presents with complete extension of the head, as in face presentations.

Attitude

Attitude refers to the relationship of fetal parts to each other. The fetus usually assumes a flexed position, in part to accommodate the shape of the uterine cavity. The back is flexed, the chin is placed on the chest, the arms are folded across the chest, and the thighs are drawn up against the abdomen with the knees flexed. The attitude of the head determines the part of the head and the diameter of the skull that presents. If the fetal head is flexed, the *occiput* presents first, and the posterior fontanelle is palpable when a vaginal examination is performed. If the head is extended, the *brow* will present; if the head is hyperextended, the *chin* (*mentum*) will present. If the head is neither flexed nor extended (ie, the fetus is in the military attitude), the bregma will present (*sinciput*), and the anterior fontanelle will be palpable when a vaginal examination is performed (Fig. 19-8).

Synclitism and Asynclitism

Synclitism and asynclitism refer to the position of the fetal head in relation to the anteroposterior diameter of the maternal pelvis (Fig. 19-9). *Synclitism* refers to the position of the fetal head when the sagittal suture (which runs from front to back along the top of the head) is halfway between the sacral promontory and the symphysis pubis, so the planes of the maternal pelvis and the fetal skull are parallel. *Asynclitism* refers to the position of the fetal head when the sagittal suture is closer to the sacral promontory (posterior asynclitism) or the symphysis pubis (anterior asynclitism). These positions occur normally as the fetal head shifts to accommodate the irregular shape of the pelvic cavity. Exaggerated or prolonged asynclitism, however, usually reflects CPD.

Fetal Shoulder Diameter and Chest Circumference

In most cases the head presents the largest diameter of the fetal body during labor. When the fetus is unusually large (macrosomic), the diameter of the shoulders (bisacromial diameter) may be larger than the head. The chest circum-

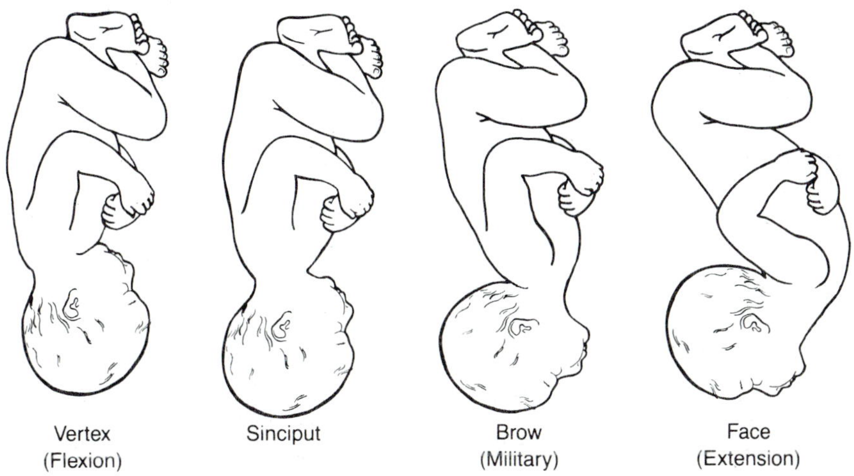

Figure 19-8.
Fetal attitude (Childbirth Graphics).

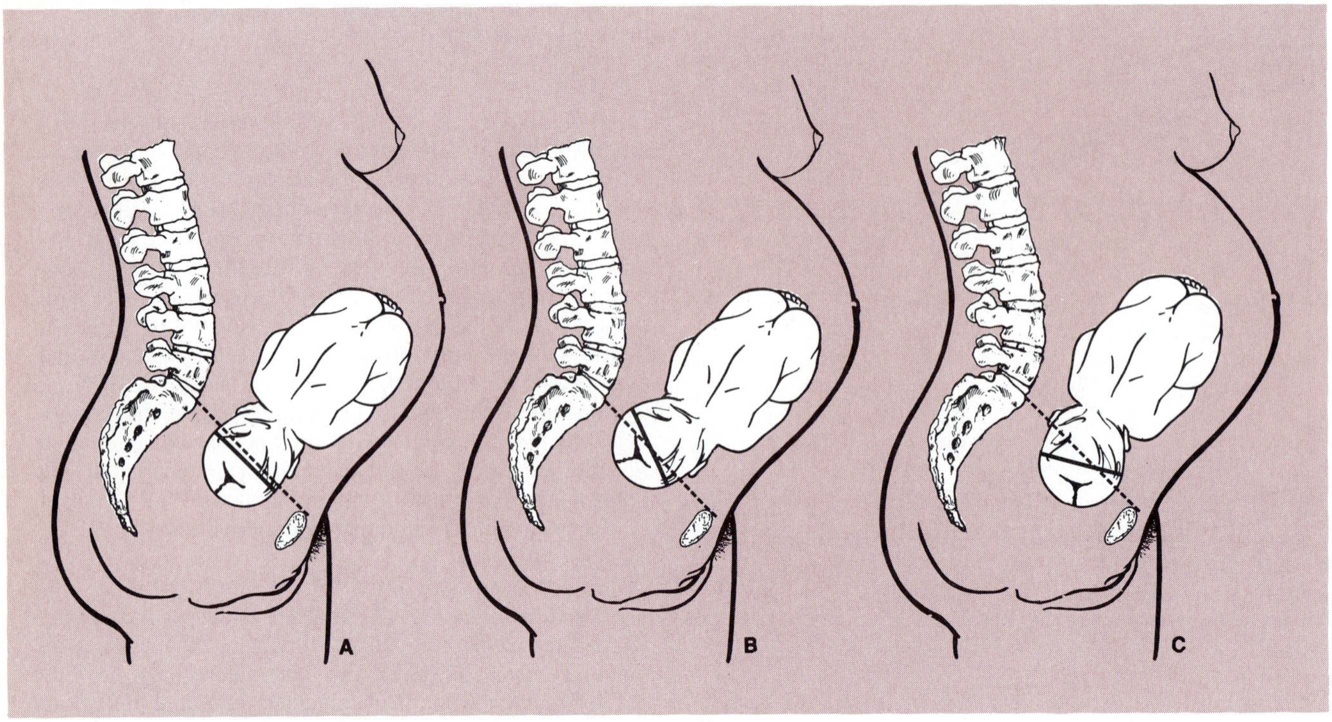

Figure 19-9.

A: Synclitism. Position of the fetal head when the sagittal suture is halfway between the sacral promontory and the symphysis pubis. *B:* Posterior asynclitism. Position of the fetal head when the sagittal suture is closer to the sacral promontory. *C:* Anterior asynclitism. Position of the fetal head when the sagittal suture is closer to the symphysis pubis (Childbirth Graphics).

ference also may be larger than normal. This is more common when the fetal weight exceeds 4000 g and may result in slowing fetal descent and increasing the risk of CPD. Research is ongoing to measure accurately chest circumference and bisacromial (shoulder) diameter and estimate the fetal weight. The reader is referred to Chapter 26 for a complete discussion of intrapartum complications related to fetal macrosomia.

Fetopelvic Relationships

Another set of terms is used to describe the relationship of the fetal body to the maternal pelvis. These terms are useful in describing the positioning of the fetus in the pelvis and the level of its descent through the pelvis.

Station

The term *station* refers to the level of the presenting part of the fetus, usually the head, in relation to the ischial spines in the midpelvis, as shown in Figure 19-10. When the biparietal diameter has passed through the pelvic inlet (engagement), the presenting part can be palpated at the level of the ischial spines during a vaginal examination. When the presenting part is felt at the level of the ischial spines, it is said to be at 0 station. Levels above the ischial spines are referred to as minus stations; stations of −4 to −1 indicate centimeters above the ischial spines. Levels below the ischial spines are plus stations; stations of +1 to +4 indicate centimeters below the level of the spines.

Fetal Lie

The term fetal *lie* refers to the relationship of the long axis of the fetus to the long axis of the woman, as shown in Figure 19-11. A longitudinal lie, with the fetal and maternal spines parallel, is normal and occurs most often. In a transverse lie the fetus is in a horizontal position relative to the maternal spine; in an oblique lie the fetus is at a slight angle off a true transverse lie. Transverse and oblique lies will prevent the fetus from entering the bony pelvis. They eliminate the possibility of a vaginal delivery, unless they convert to a longitudinal lie at the beginning of labor.

Presentation

The term *presentation* refers to the part of the fetus that enters, or presents to, the maternal pelvis. The major variations in fetal presentation are shown in Figure 19-12. The most common is cephalic or *vertex* presentation, which occurs in 95% of labors. *Breech*, or buttock, presentations occur in approximately 4% of labors. Breech presentations can be further divided into three types:

- Frank breech is the most common type, characterized by flexion of the fetal thighs and extension of the knees; the feet rest alongside the fetal head.
- Complete breech is characterized by flexion of the fetal thighs and knees; the fetus appears to be in a "squatting" position.
- Footling or incomplete breech is characterized by extension of the fetal knees and thighs; one or both feet may present in the pelvis and as descent occurs, through the cervix.

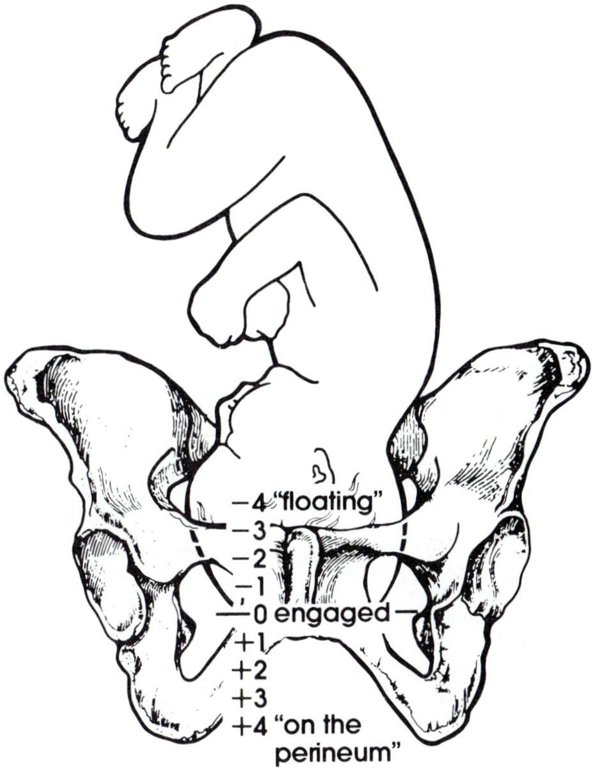

Figure 19-10.
Stations of the fetal head (Childbirth Graphics).

Breech presentations are shown in Figure 19-13.

Less common types of presentations are *shoulder* and *face* presentations. *Compound presentation* involves the prolapse of an extremity alongside the presenting part. The prolapse of a hand or arm alongside the head is more often seen; a hand also may present with a breech presentation.

Depending on the estimated size of the fetus and the progress of labor, some breech presentations can be successfully delivered vaginally. However, many cases of breech presentation and virtually all shoulder and face presentations require cesarean delivery.

Position

Position refers to the relationship of a particular reference point on the fetal presenting part to the maternal pelvis. In vertex presentations the reference point on the head may be the occiput, the brow, or the chin, depending on whether the head is flexed or extended. In breech presentations the reference point is the fetal sacrum, and in shoulder presentations it is the fetal scapula.

In describing fetal position the maternal pelvis is divided into four segments: right and left anterior and right and left posterior. These segments of the pelvis are labeled according to the woman's perspective: the *left* or *right* side of the maternal pelvis or the *anterior* or *posterior* part of the maternal pelvis.

The first step in determining the fetal position is to verify the fetal presentation by vaginal examination (eg, occiput, chin, sacrum, shoulder). Then the examiner determines whether the presenting part is facing the right or left side of the woman's pelvis. Finally, the examiner determines if the presenting part faces the posterior (back) or anterior (front) segment of the woman's pelvis. Figure 19-14*A* demonstrates a fetus in the right occipitoanterior position, and Figure 19-14*B* represents a fetus in the left occipitoposterior position. In some cases the fetal presenting part is oriented neither posteriorly nor anteriorly but faces directly opposite the woman's right or left hip. This is described as a transverse orientation. Figure 19-14*C* illustrates a fetus in the right occipitotransverse position.

Fetal position is described using a formal set of abbreviations. Each position is denoted by 3 letters of the alphabet (see the display of standard abbreviations). The orientation of the fetal presenting part is indicated by the abbreviations R for right, L for left, A for anterior, P for posterior, and T for transverse. The fetal presenting part is designated as O for occiput, M for mentum or chin, and S for sacrum. Thus, when

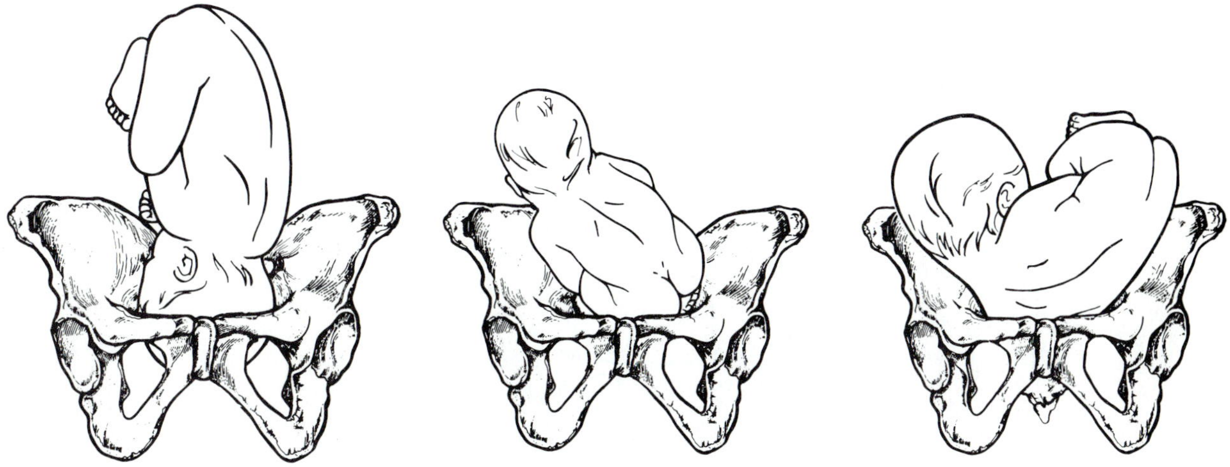

Figure 19-11.
Fetal Lie. Longitudinal lie occurs most often (Childbirth Graphics).

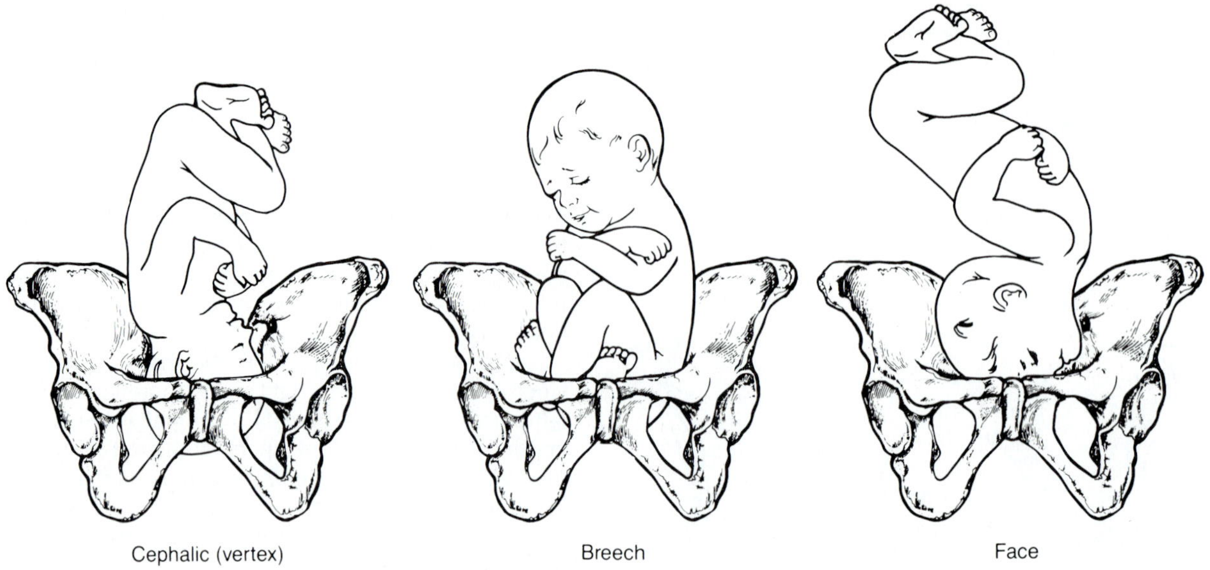

Figure 19-12.
Fetal presentations. Cephalic (vertex) presentation is most common (Childbirth Graphics).

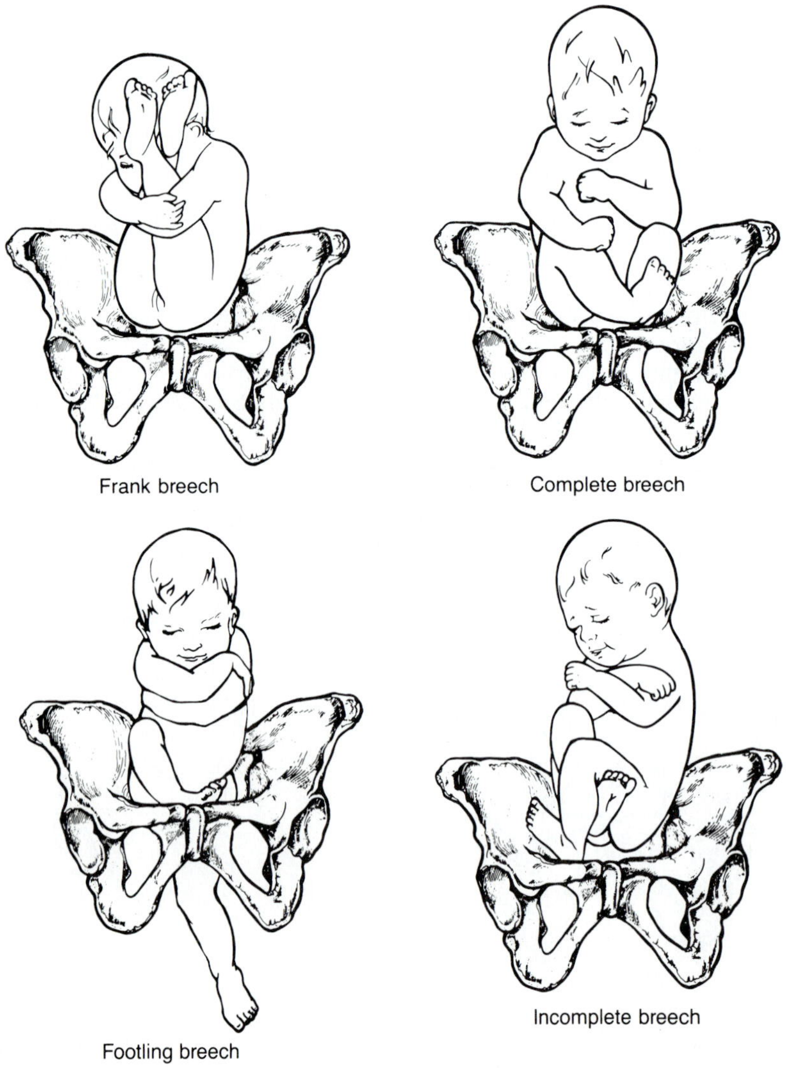

Figure 19-13.
Types of breech presentations (Childbirth Graphics).

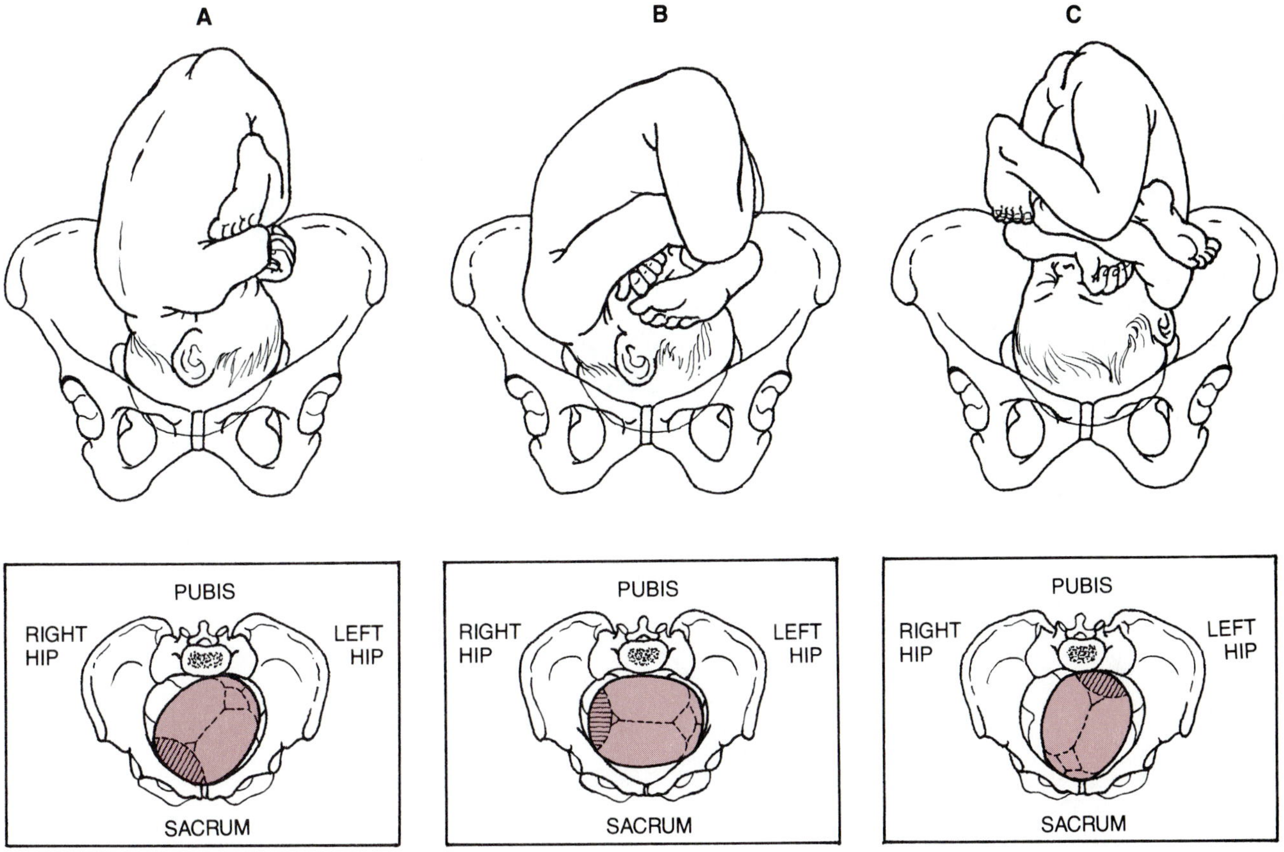

Figure 19-14.

Fetal positions. *A:* Infant in the right occipitoanterior position. The occiput (in red) faces the right, anterior segment of the woman's pelvis. *B:* Left occipitoposterior. The occiput (in red) faces the left, posterior segment of the woman's pelvis. *C:* Right occipitotransverse. The fetal occiput faces the woman's right hip.

the fetus is in the right occipitoanterior position, this is designated as ROA. See Figure 19-15 for further examples of fetal position.

Occipitoposterior Position. When the fetus is in the occipitoposterior position labor usually progresses more slowly than normal, with accentuated maternal back pain. When the woman experiences this persistent backache due to the occipitoposterior position, it is sometimes referred to as "back labor." Most fetuses in the occipitoposterior position during labor spontaneously rotate anteriorly, and birth proceeds normally. Certain maternal positions, such as kneeling on all fours or lying on the side opposite to the one on which the fetal occiput is detected, may allow gravity to rotate the fetal spine and occiput toward the anterior position. Approximately 10% of fetuses in occipitoposterior positions do not rotate, and the infant is born in a face up or infant face to maternal symphysis pubis position. Alternatively, the birth attendant may attempt to rotate the infant to an anterior position manually or with forceps to facilitate delivery.

Cardinal Movements

The cardinal movements of the fetus during labor have been described since the 18th century. These movements or

Standard Abbreviations Describing Fetal Position

Side of Maternal Pelvis

L—left
R—right
T—transverse

Presenting Part

O—occiput
S—sacrum
Sc—scapula
M—mentum

Part of Maternal Pelvis

A—anterior
P—posterior

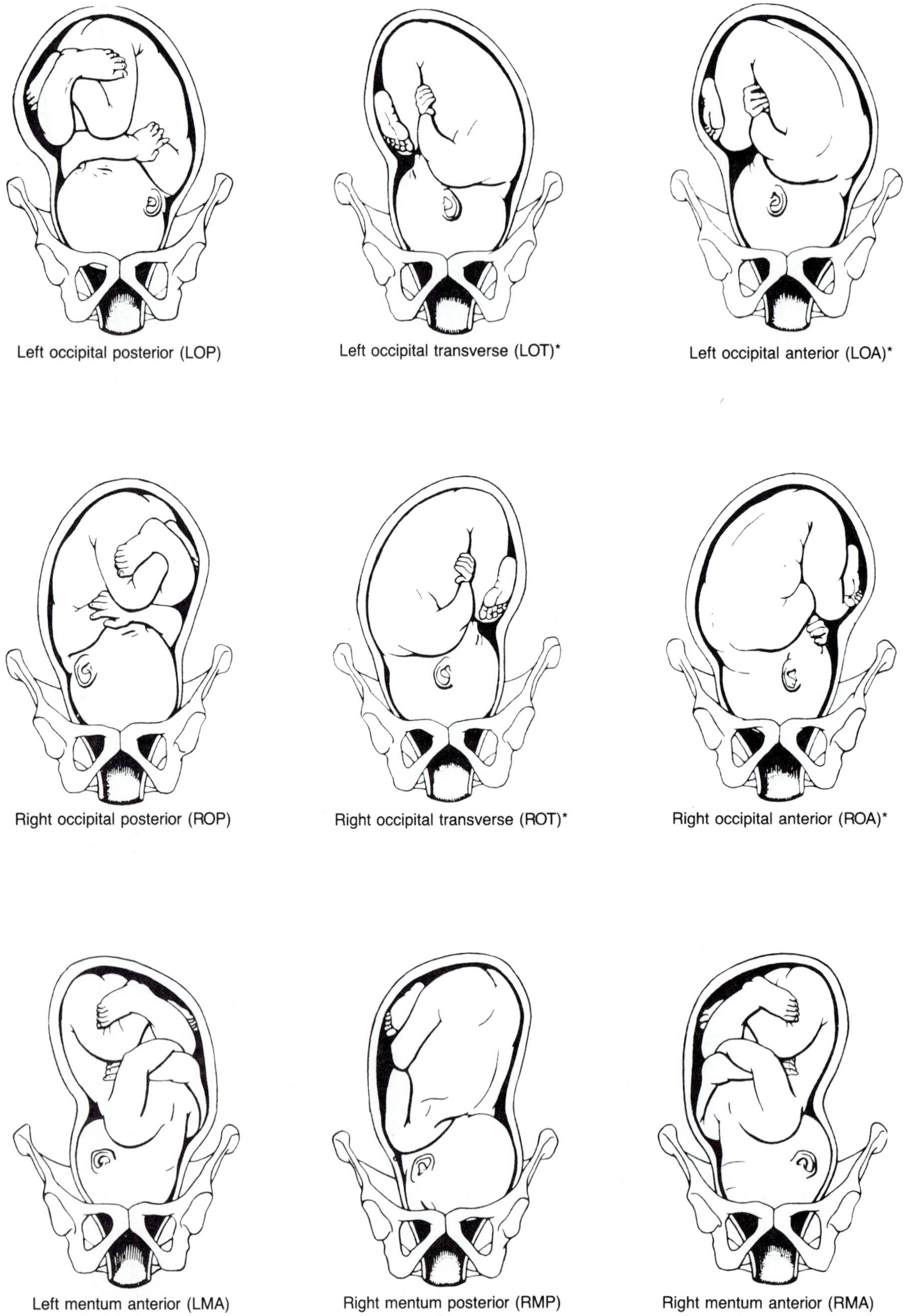

Figure 19-15.
Fetal positions. *LOT, LOA, ROT, and ROA are the most frequently occurring fetal positions (Childbirth Graphics).

mechanisms are a series of passive adjustments of position as the fetus descends through the pelvis during labor (Fig. 19-16). These movements flow smoothly and often overlap as labor progresses; failure to achieve one or more of these adjustments usually indicates a need for some form of obstetric intervention.

Descent. Descent, or the downward movement of the fetus, continues throughout normal labor. Descent is brought about by four mechanisms: (1) pressure of the amniotic fluid; (2) pressure of contractions, specifically pressure of the uterine fundus on the fetal breech; (3) bearing-down efforts of the woman during the second stage of labor; and (4) extension and straightening of the fetal body. An upright maternal position in labor allows gravity to aid in the descent of the fetus.

Flexion. Flexion is the natural attitude of the fetus because of the shape of the uterine cavity and, during labor, because of the resistance of the pelvic floor to fetal descent. Flexion also is aided by thickening of the uterine fundus, which decreases the available space; the fetus is forced to flex into a compact, ovoid shape. Flexion of the fetal head is important because, as mentioned previously, it causes the smallest fetal head diameter (suboccipitobregmatic diameter) to present to the maternal pelvis. Flexion begins at the pelvic inlet and continues until the head reaches the pelvic floor.

Internal Rotation. The fetal head usually enters the pelvis in a transverse or oblique position. Internal rotation involves a 45- to 90-degree rotation of the fetal head to the occipitoanterior or occipitoposterior position (see Fig. 19-16*A*). This must occur for the head to pass through the narrowest transverse diameter of the maternal pelvis, which is the midpelvic transverse (interspinous) diameter. In most cases the head rotates to an occipitoanterior position because of the shape of the bony pelvis and the downward and forward slope of the pelvic musculature. Internal rotation must occur for completion of labor, except during the birth of a very small infant. Internal rotation usually occurs during the second stage of labor. However, in multiparous women it may occur earlier in labor and is sometimes accomplished in one contraction.

Extension. Flexion of the head usually continues until crowning so that the smallest diameter of the fetal head presents and distends the perineum (see Fig. 19-16*C*). Extension of the fetal head is then caused by the continued downward pressure of uterine contractions and the resistance of the pelvic floor to continued descent of the fetus (see Fig. 19-16*B*). As the base of the occiput passes under the symphysis pubis, it causes the head to extend (see Fig. 19-16*D*). As the head extends the brow, face, and chin move past the sacrum and coccyx and are born over the perineum. At this point the infant's head is in an occipitoanterior position. Extension is said to be complete when the entire head is born.

Restitution. Normally, the head is born in a direct occipitoanterior position, with the face oriented toward the maternal sacrum. The shoulders remain in the oblique or transverse position; thus, the infant's neck is slightly twisted at birth (see Fig. 19-16*E*). After the head is born it rotates toward the right or left ischial tuberosity. The direction of rotation depends on the original position of the head before delivery. For instance if the head was directed toward the right ischial tuberosity, the occiput rotates to the right. Once the head rotates to the oblique or transverse position, it returns to its normal relationship with the shoulders. This is known as restitution.

External Rotation. Once restitution of the fetal head occurs, the fetal body rotates so that the shoulders are in the anteroposterior diameter of the maternal pelvis (see Fig. 19-16*F*). One shoulder rests behind the symphysis pubis, and the other is oriented posteriorly toward the sacrum.

Expulsion. Once the shoulders have rotated to the anteroposterior diameter of the maternal pelvis, the anterior shoulder is born under the symphysis pubis, and the posterior shoulder slides out over the perineum (see Fig. 19-16*G*). The head and shoulders are delivered, and the rest of the infant's body is expelled through the woman's bearing-down efforts.

Powers: The Uterus in Labor

A major force contributing to the process of labor and birth is the power of uterine contractions. The appropriately timed and coordinated onset of labor, uterine contractility patterns, and progressive cervical effacement and dilatation must occur to bring about fetal descent and birth.

Theories on Causes of Initiation of Labor

A complex interaction of maternal, fetal, and placental–decidual factors is responsible for initiating labor; however, the exact mechanism by which labor is initiated is still not well understood. Many theories have been proposed to explain the onset of labor, but none can stand alone as the complete explanation. Additional research will undoubtedly provide answers in the future. The following explanations are among those currently being investigated.

Uterine Stretch Theory. The uterine stretch theory proposes that labor begins when the uterus is stretched to a certain point. Stretching of uterine muscle also stimulates the production of the prostaglandins, endogenous hormones, and powerful uterine stimulants. This theory partially explains the early onset of labor in multiple gestations and cases of polyhydramnios (an excess amount of amniotic fluid) but does not help to explain what causes preterm labor.

Pressure Theory. The pressure theory of labor initiation proposes that the descent of the presenting part stimulates pressure receptors in the lower uterine segment. This in turn causes increased secretion of oxytocin by the maternal posterior pituitary gland. Oxytocin stimulates the myometrium to contract and start labor.

Text continues on page 451

Internal Rotation

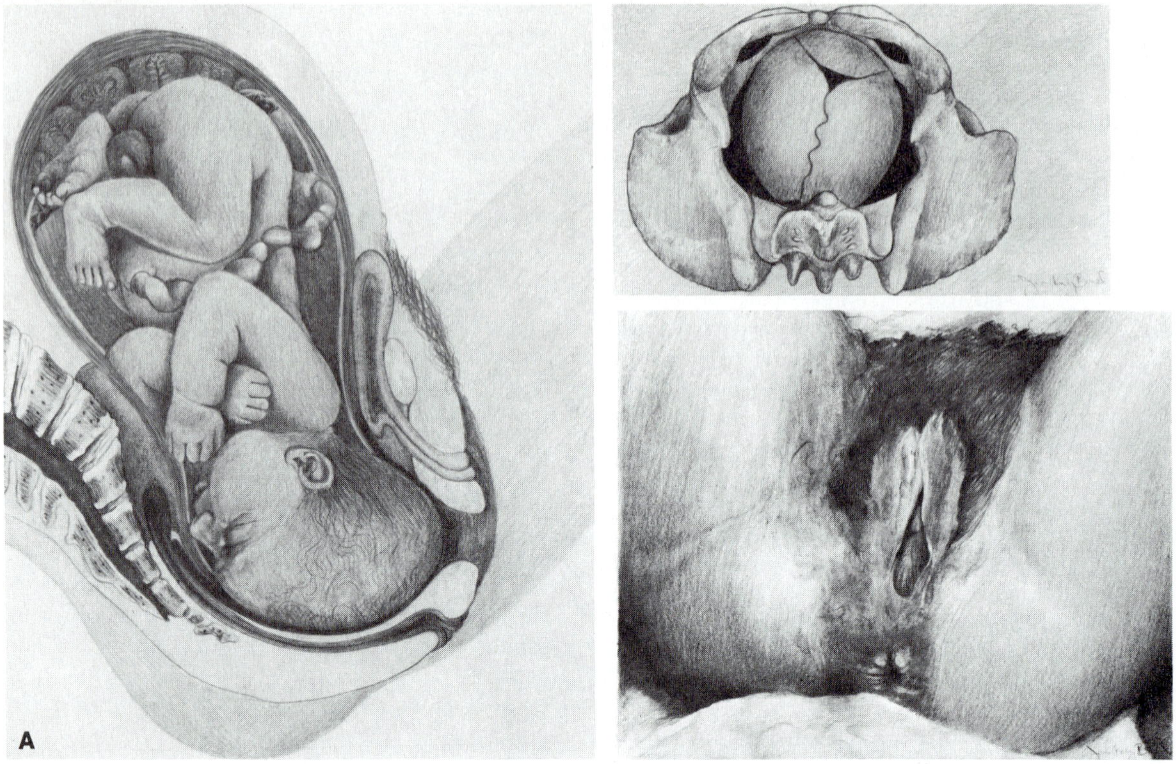

Figure 19-16.

A: Internal rotation. Internal rotation occurs as the fetal head enters the bony pelvis in a transverse position and rotates to an anteroposterior position because of pressure from the encroaching ischial spines. The bispinous diameter is too small to admit a normal-size head in a transverse position.

Extension Beginning

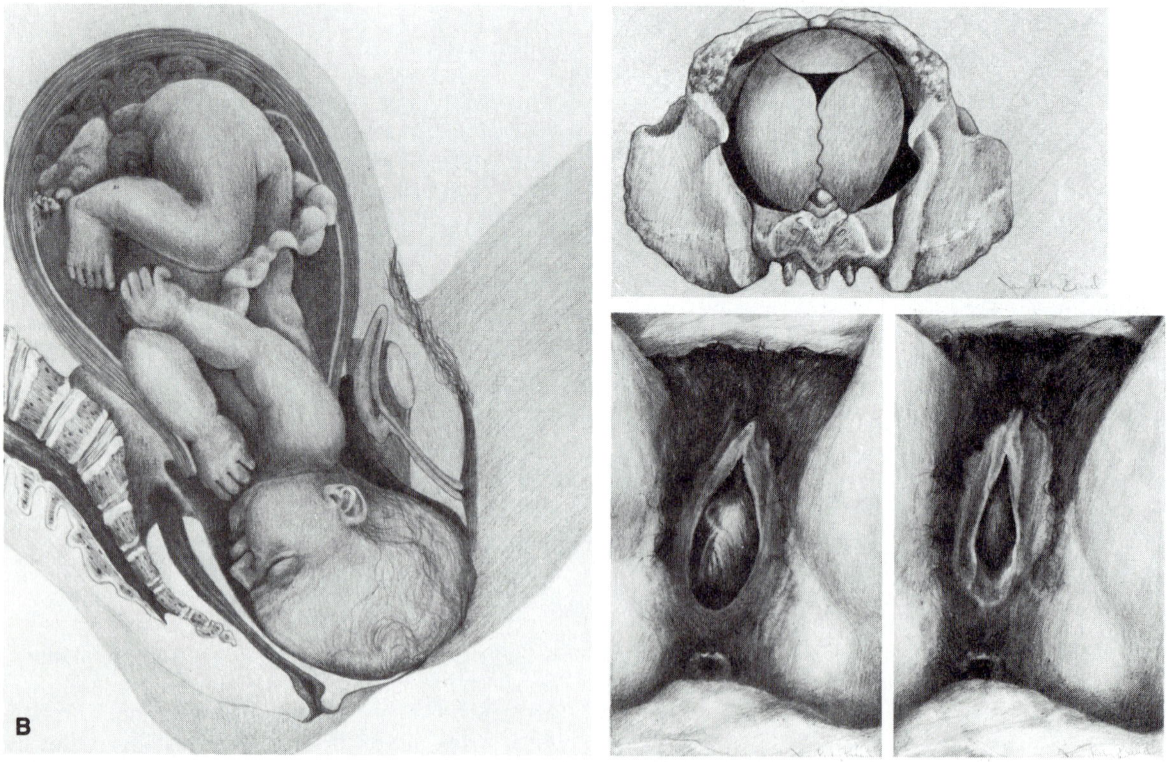

Figure 19-16 (*continued*).

B: Extension beginning. Extension occurs when the head reaches the pelvic floor and is deflected anteriorly away from the sacrum. The distention of the perineum becomes apparent. The head can be seen to advance with contractions and bearing down efforts and to retreat between contractions.

Crowning

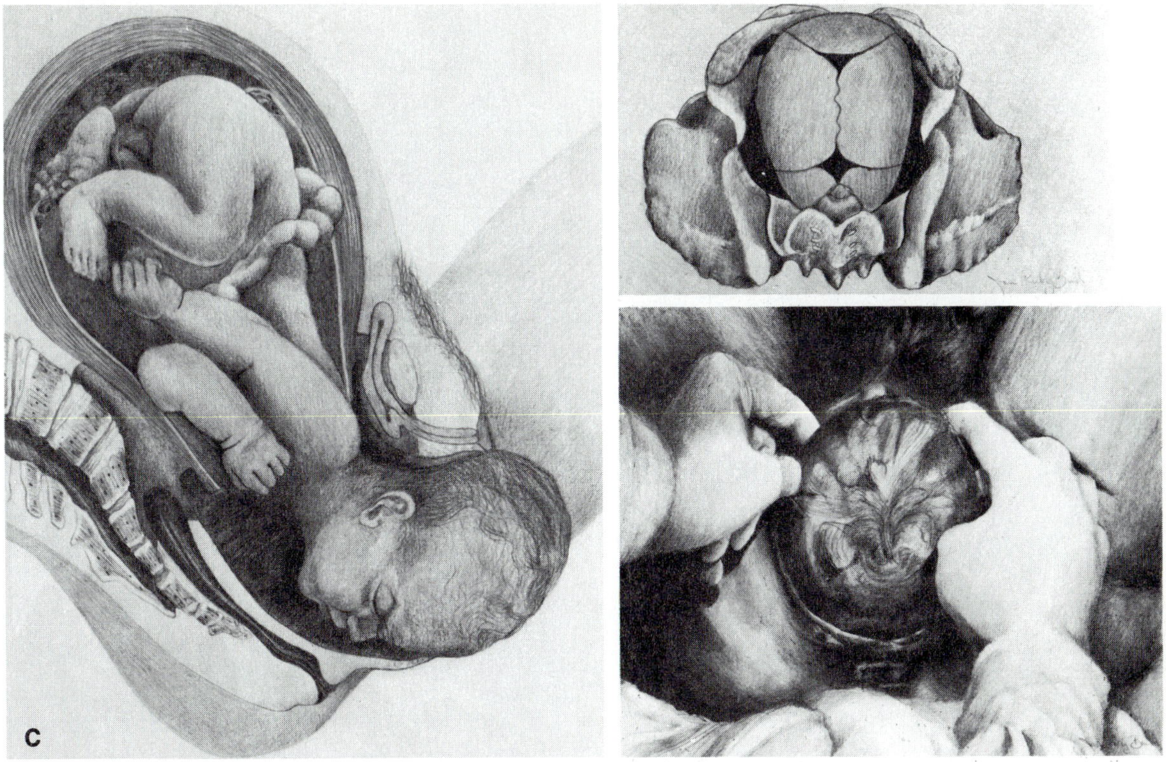

Figure 19-16 (*continued*).

C: Crowning occurs when the head distends the perineum maximally so that the head is fully encircled.

Extension Complete

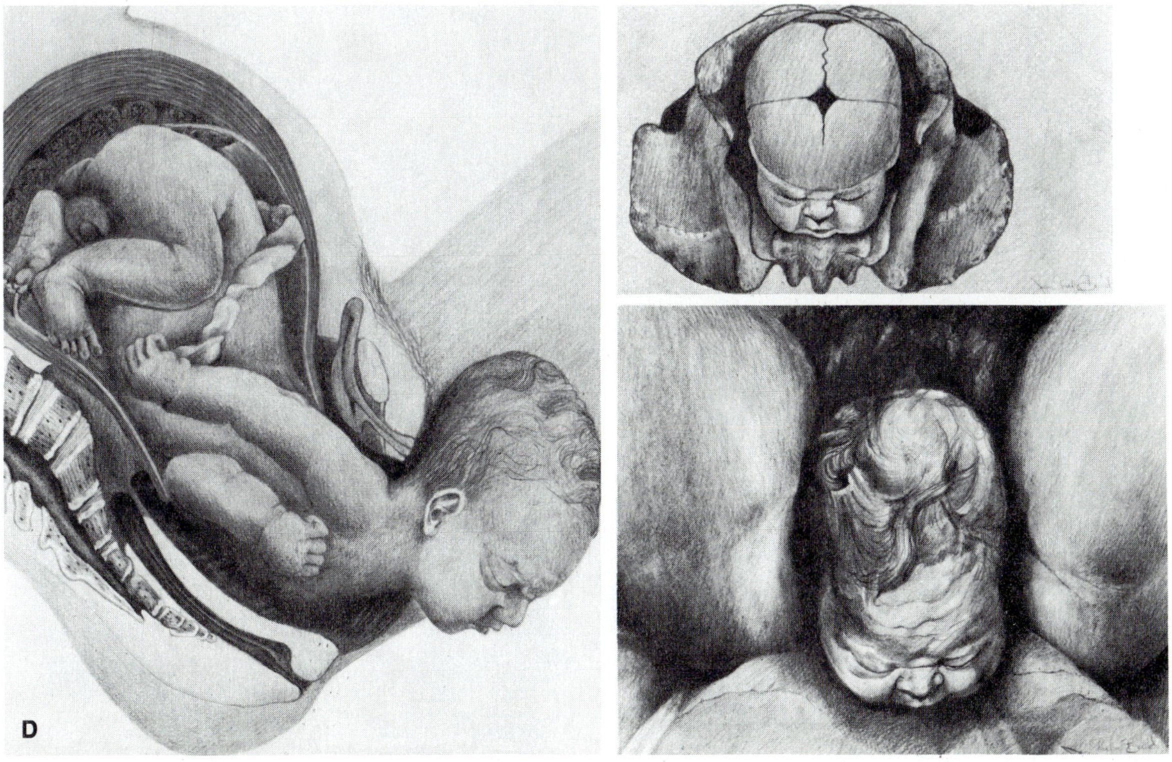

Figure 19-16 (*continued*).

D: Extension complete. As the head emerges the symphysis exerts pressure on the neck. The continued downward pressure from contractions forces the baby's head to pivot under the symphysis.

External Rotation (Restitution)

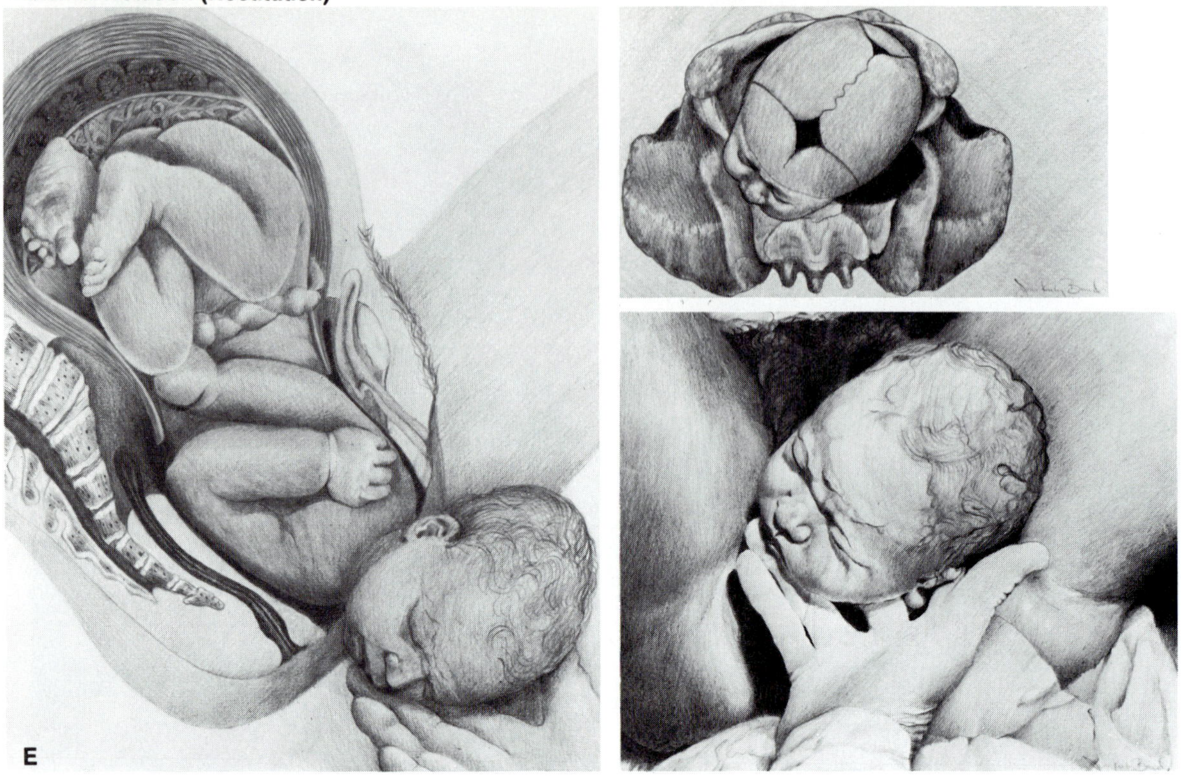

Figure 19-16 (*continued*).
E: External rotation (restitution). Restitution occurs when the head rotates back to the oblique position in which it entered the pelvis, thus realigning the head, neck, and shoulders.

External Rotation (Shoulder Rotation)

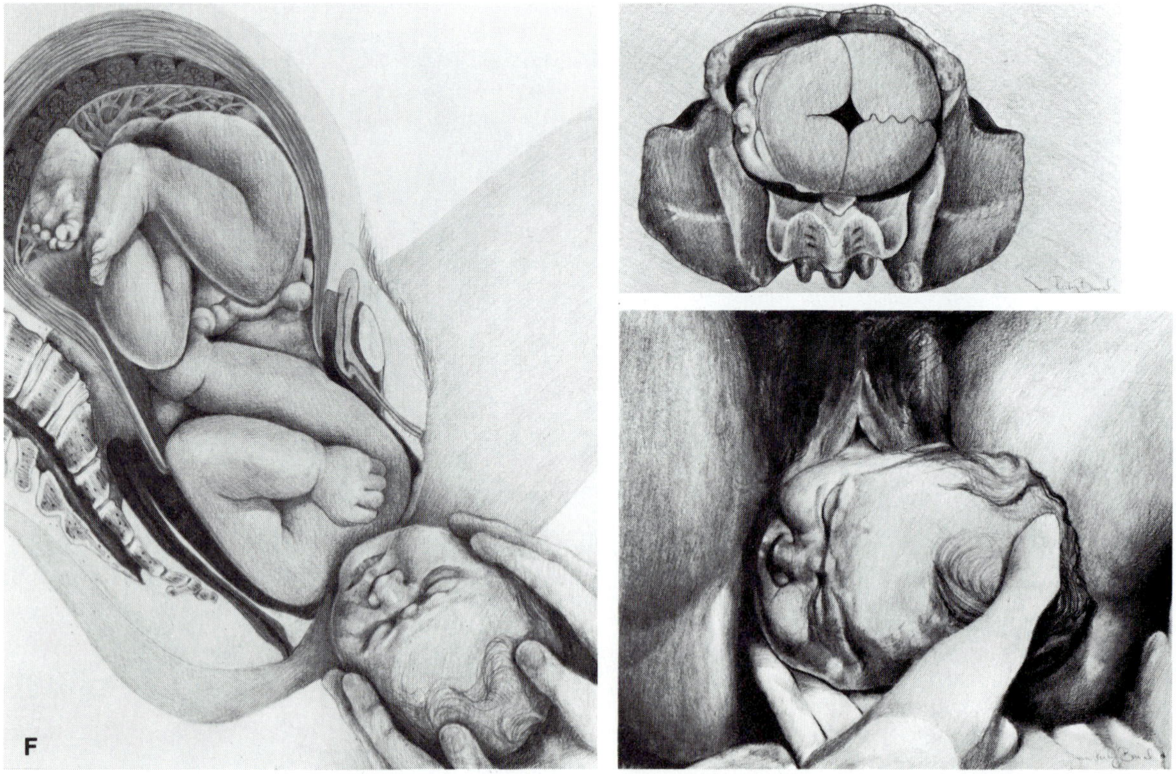

Figure 19-16 (*continued*).
F: External rotation (shoulder rotation). The fetal body rotates so that the shoulders are now in an anteroposterior position; the anterior shoulder is born under the symphysis, and the posterior shoulder slides over the perineum.

Expulsion

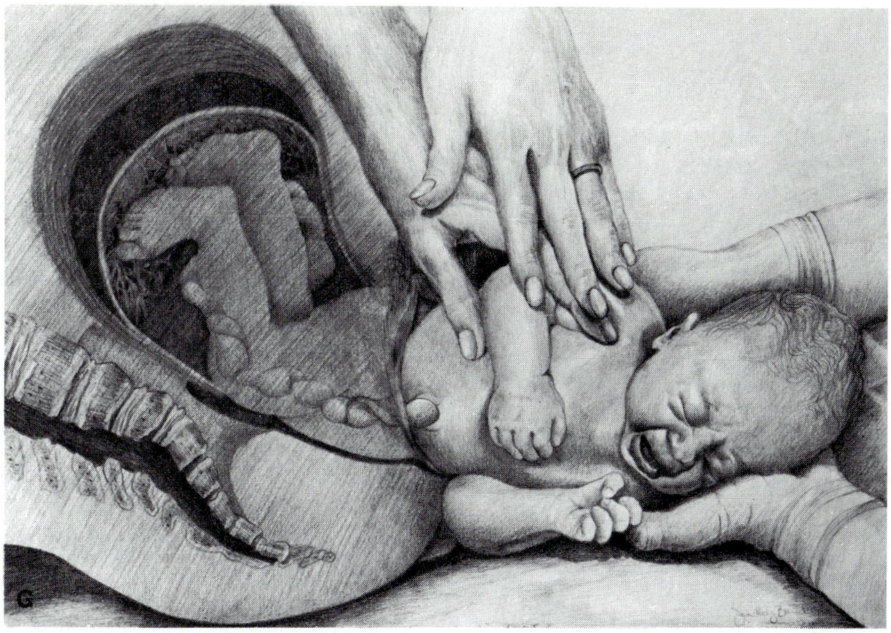

Figure 19-16 (*continued*).
G: Expulsion. Expulsion occurs as the rest of the body is born; because the head and shoulders are the largest part of the neonate, the rest of the body is delivered easily.

Hormonal Initiation Theory. Several hormones (oxytocin and prostaglandins) are potent uterine muscle stimulators. While blood levels of oxytocin do not appear to rise until late in active labor, oxytocin receptors in the uterine muscle are increased near the end of gestation. Furthermore, oxytocin promotes the release of *prostaglandin* F_2 *alpha* from the uterine endometrial decidua. During labor there also is a dramatic rise in *prostaglandin* E_2 in amniotic fluid. Most recent studies suggest that oxytocin and prostaglandin do not maintain a primary role in the onset of labor but that their release is triggered by earlier and unknown biochemical and physical changes in the woman and or fetus.

During pregnancy the proper balance between concentrations of estrogen and progesterone allows pregnancy to continue. Research has demonstrated that as *progesterone* levels decrease, prostaglandin formation increases. However, no evidence exists to demonstrate a progesterone decrease before the onset of human labor. Maturation of fetal adrenal glands and the release of *fetal cortisol* also has been suggested as a contributor to the onset of labor. It does not appear, however, that fetal adrenal development is a fundamental component of the initiation of labor; it may provide one trigger in the cascade of events that results in parturition (Cunningham, MacDonald, & Gant, 1989).

Uterine Decidua Activation Theory. One of the most recent theories implicates the release of bioactive agents from the uterine decidua into amniotic fluid. A complex biochemical cascade is proposed, which results in the onset of labor. Markers of this process found in amniotic fluid include *platelet-activating factor* (*PAF*) and *interleukin-1B*. PAF appears to increase calcium concentrations in uterine myometrial cells, resulting in uterine contractions (Zhu, Word, & Johnston, 1992). PAF also stimulates the production of prostaglandin E_2 by the fetal membranes, indirectly increasing uterine activity (Morris, Kahn, Sullivan, & Elder, 1992).

There is a tenfold increase in arachidonic acid concentrations in amniotic fluid during labor. Arachidonic acid is a precursor of prostaglandins, a very powerful uterine stimulant. Interleukin-1B appears to stimulate arachidonic acid release and prostaglandin formation.

Uterine Contractions

Although much is still to be learned about the mechanisms that trigger labor, the mechanisms of labor itself are better understood. The actual work of labor is accomplished through uterine contractions, which, over a period of hours, thin and open the cervix and facilitate descent of the fetus. Uterine contractions are augmented by the "power" of bearing-down efforts of the woman in the second stage of labor.

A contraction is a periodic, rhythmic shortening or tightening of the uterine musculature in response to a stimulus. Each contraction has three phases: the increment, the period during which the intensity of the contraction increases; the acme, the strongest point of the contraction; and the decrement, the period of decreasing intensity. The intervals between contractions are characterized by a relaxation of the muscle to its normal resting tone or tonus. During normal labor contractions occur 2 to 20 minutes apart, last 15 to 90 seconds, and are of varying intensity depending on the stage of labor. A typical pattern of uterine contraction is shown in Figure 19-17.

Contractions serve several purposes in labor: They efface and dilate the cervix; they facilitate the descent and

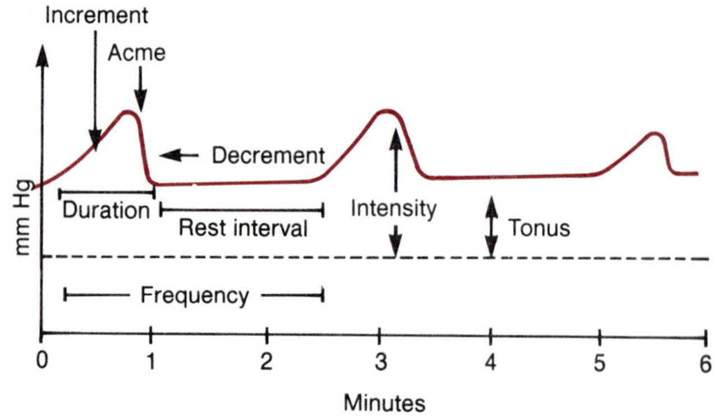

Figure 19-17.
Characteristic pattern of uterine contraction.

rotation of the fetus; they cause the separation and expulsion of the placenta after birth; and after the expulsion of the placenta, they maintain hemostasis of the uterus by compressing blood vessels. Normal uterine contractions are involuntary, rhythmic, and intermittent. Intervals between contractions allow the uterine muscle to rest and receive uninterrupted blood circulation.

If contractions are too frequent (with intervals of less than 30 seconds between contractions) or prolonged (lasting more than 90 seconds), medical evaluation of the woman is necessary. Strong, constant uterine contractions may result in rupture of the uterine muscle. Furthermore, vasoconstriction occurs during the contraction because of the pressure of the contracting tissue, dramatically reducing oxygen exchange with the fetus. The interval between contractions allows the flow of oxygenated blood into the intervillous spaces to resume. If intervals between contractions are too short (less than 30 to 40 seconds), the fetus is at risk for hypoxia.

Contractions increase in intensity, frequency, and duration throughout labor because of the mechanical stretching of the cervix. This phenomenon is known as Ferguson's reflex; contractions stimulate stretch and pressure receptors in the cervix. These receptors act to stimulate increased oxytocin secretion, which in turn stimulates the uterus to contract more vigorously.

The uterine contraction has been described as having three major characteristics. First, contractions normally start in a pacemaker near the uterotubal junction of the fundus at the top of the uterus and radiate downward toward the cervix. This characteristic is called fundal dominance. Second, the contraction diminishes in intensity as it moves away from the pacemaker, so that contraction of the upper segment of the uterus is stronger than contraction of the lower segment. Third, the duration of the contraction diminishes as it moves away from the pacemaker. Thus, contraction of the upper segment is longer than that of the lower segment. All three of these characteristics must be present to ensure efficient uterine functioning and normal progress in labor. For reasons not completely understood, contractions sometimes start in another area of the uterine muscle and spread in an uncoordinated fashion through the uterus rather than in this orderly fundus-to-cervix pattern. Contractions of this sort are not efficient and will not contribute to the work of thinning and opening the cervix in labor.

Changes in the Uterus During Labor

The process of labor requires the uterus to change dramatically in shape. These changes reflect two different processes: the development of the upper and lower uterine segments and cervical dilatation and effacement. Both processes facilitate the descent and eventual delivery of the fetus.

Development of the Uterine Segments

As labor contractions proceed the uterus differentiates into two distinct portions or segments. The upper segment is the more active fundal region; it becomes thicker and its muscle fibers become shorter as labor advances. The upper uterine segment contracts, retracts, and forces the fetus to descend and eventually be expelled from the uterus. The upper uterus never totally relaxes during labor, and the muscle becomes fixed at its shorter length to maintain the downward pressure it attains with each contraction. As a result of this contraction and retraction, the upper uterine segment becomes thicker through the first and second stages of labor. The upper segment thickens the most after the third stage of labor.

The lower segment is much less active. Its muscle fibers relax and stretch, and during labor the lower segment becomes a thin-walled passage for the fetus. The differentiation between the two segments becomes quite marked during labor. The boundary between them is called the physiologic retraction ring.

Cervical Effacement and Dilatation

The second major change that occurs in the uterus during labor is the process of cervical effacement and dilatation (Fig. 19-18). Effacement is the softening, thinning, and shortening of the cervical canal. According to traditional teaching, the length of the cervix at term was thought to be approximately 2 cm. With recent advances in ultrasonography the average length of the cervix has been estimated to be 3 to 4 cm by the third trimester of pregnancy (Holcomb & Smeltzer, 1991). As labor progresses the cervix is shortened and thinned until it is completely assimilated into the lower uterine segment. This change results from the contractions of the uterus and the pressure of the presenting part and the amniotic sac.

Effacement usually is evaluated during labor in terms of percentages: 0% indicates no effacement, and 100% indicates complete effacement. With the advent of ultrasonographic measurement of the cervix in cases of preterm labor, cervical effacement is described in terms of cervical length (2 cm [or greater], 1.5 cm, 1 cm, and 0.5 cm). Frequently, especially in multiparas, the cervix will be 50% or more effaced by Braxton Hicks contractions before labor begins. After labor begins effacement and dilatation will occur simultaneously in a multigravida, whereas in the primigravida effacement is usually advanced before dilatation of the os begins.

Dilatation, sometimes known as dilation, is the opening

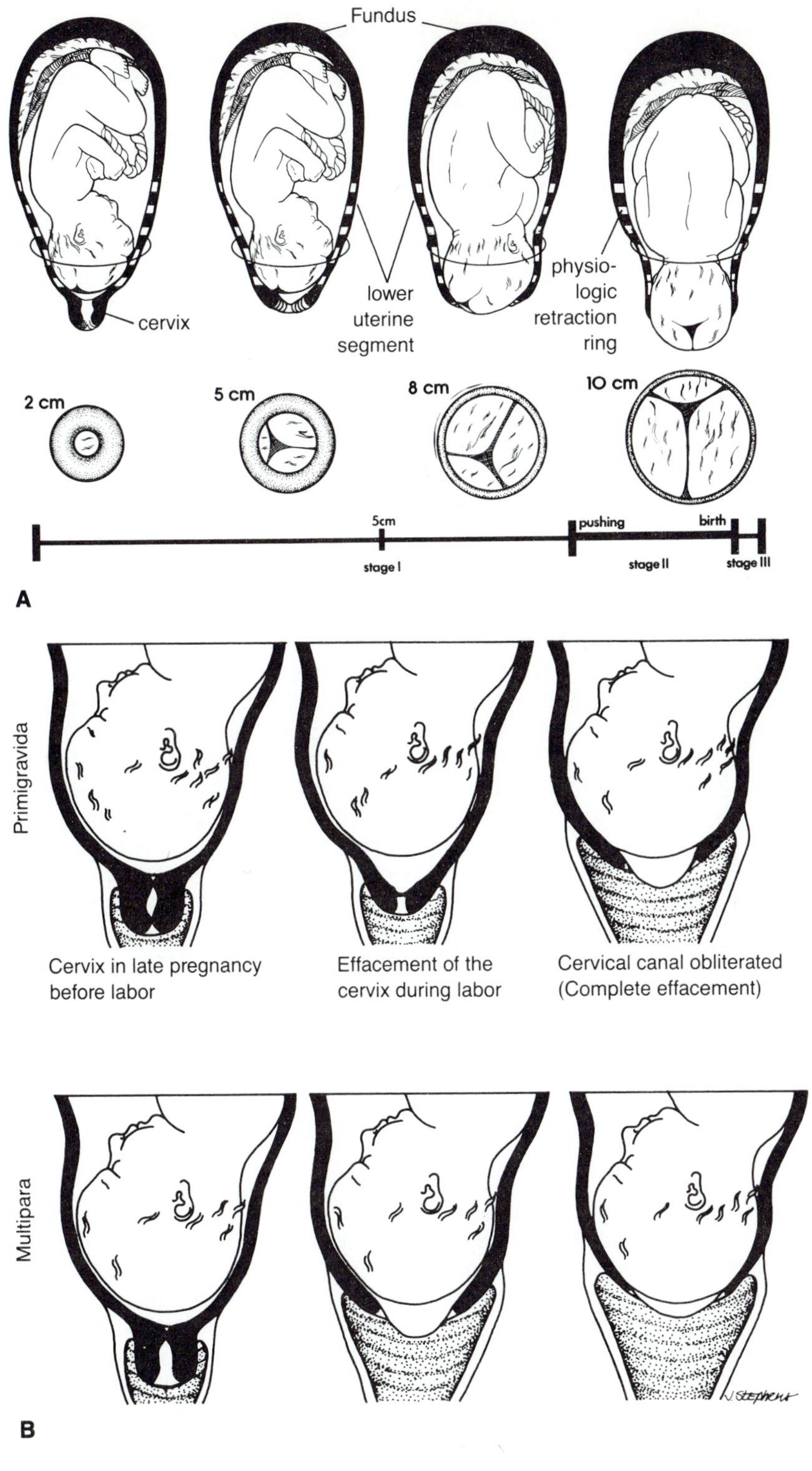

Figure 19-18.
A: Cervical effacement and dilatation. *B:* Comparison of cervical effacement and dilatation in the primigravida and multipara (Childbirth Graphics).

and enlargement of the external cervical os from a few millimeters during pregnancy to 10 cm at complete dilatation in labor. Dilatation is caused by the retraction of the cervix into the lower uterine segment as a result of labor contractions and the pressure of the amniotic sac.

Assessment of cervical effacement and dilatation during labor is accomplished by direct fingertip palpation of the cervix during vaginal examination (Fig. 19-19). Practice is necessary to develop consistency and accuracy in the assessment of cervical effacement and dilatation. Even experienced clinicians may report some small differences in assessments of the cervix in the same woman.

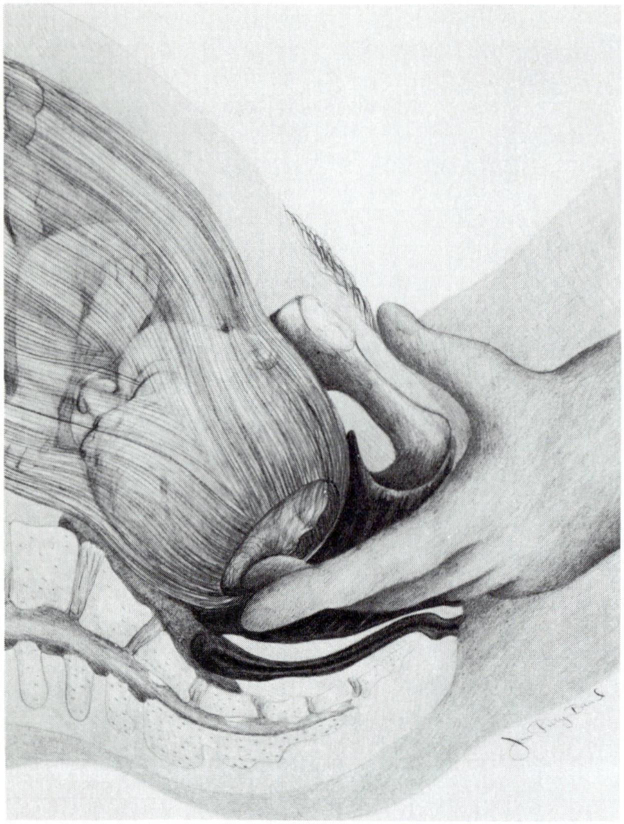

Figure 19-19.
Cervical dilatation. The degree of cervical effacement and dilatation is determined by manual examination. The examiner's first and second fingers are placed in the vagina, and the cervix is located. The fingers are swept over the cervical margin from one side to the other to determine its approximate dilatation in centimeters and to estimate its effacement. When the cervix is fully dilated, its diameter is approximately 10 cm. At the same time, the level of the presenting fetal part in the birth canal (station) is identified (Childbirth Graphics).

Psyche: The Woman's State of Mind

The woman's state of mind also is a critical aspect in the process of labor and birth. Her perception of the process of birth is influenced by several factors, including self-confidence, patterns of coping with uncertainty and stress, attitudes and expectations about labor and birth, and her response to pain, anxiety, and other alterations in functioning that occur during labor.

A knowledgeable and sensitive nurse can support the woman in making the most positive adaptation to labor possible, given the unique characteristics and course of each labor and birth. Chapters 20 and 21 address in more detail some specific nursing actions to facilitate healthy psychosocial and physiologic adaptation to labor and birth. A few key areas important to an overall understanding of the impact of the psyche on labor and birth are highlighted in this chapter.

Negative Attitudes About Childbirth

Some women see childbirth as a challenge to be met or as a brief experience to be endured and forgotten. Other women have much more negative attitudes about childbirth or are extremely fearful of it. These attitudes often affect the progress of labor and birth.

Childbirth as a Threat to Safety

Negative attitudes toward childbirth may arise from the threat it poses to physical safety—to the woman and her fetus. These fears are based to some degree on fact, because childbirth entails an element of physical risk that cannot always be anticipated or reduced. Fears are likely to be intensified by "horror stories" shared and sometimes embellished by other women. If the woman is a primigravida, she fears the unknown. If she has had children before, she may fear a repetition of previous negative experiences or if earlier births were easy, worry that this one will be difficult. Such attitudes may be hard to change for two reasons: (1) These fears are in part based in reality, and (2) friends, family members, and the woman's partner are likely to respond to the dangerous aspect of childbirth and unintentionally reinforce the woman's own fears.

Childbirth as a Threat to Self-Image

Childbirth also can be seen as a significant threat to the woman's self-image. Birth requires giving up control of one's body and one's behavior to a certain degree, which can be quite disturbing to some women. Childbirth also represents a real threat to a woman's body image. In addition she may view childbirth as the symbol of motherhood, and if she has negative feelings about what motherhood entails, such as loss of physical beauty or sexual attractiveness, increasing dependency on others, or loss of occupational potential, she is likely to be less positive about birth itself. A woman also may have unrealistic expectations about herself in relation to childbirth and childrearing and may see herself as having something to prove to herself or others. Such expectations may contribute to negative attitudes toward childbirth.

The "Medicalization" of Childbirth

Childbirth in Western society is viewed as an illness state requiring medical intervention, including hospitalization, medical management, the use of technology, and sometimes surgery to accomplish delivery. At times this trend contributes to a view of the childbearing woman as dependent, passive, and even childlike, with no real role in decision making. More women today reject this passive role, but the view that childbirth is a medical condition requiring treatment, instead of a normal physiologic process, is still prevalent. Labor and birth usually take place in the hospital setting, where the woman and her support person are relatively isolated. This restricts the amount of "second-hand" knowledge women gain about childbirth by viewing other women—family and friends—giving birth. It also may reduce the amount of emotional support the laboring woman may have from friends, family, and experienced women.

Although these negative attitudes may have some impact on the woman's psychosocial adaptation to labor, they usually can be assessed and addressed to some extent through effective nursing care. Attending childbirth preparation classes and receiving anticipatory guidance during pregnancy from a maternity nurse may go a long way toward reducing their effects in labor. As noted previously, however, each labor is unique and in some ways unpredictable. Thus, the woman's psychosocial adaptation to labor will depend in large part on her perception of events as they unfold. One of the most important factors affecting her adaptation is her response to labor pain.

Pain in Labor and Birth

Most women anticipate and do experience some pain in childbirth. Labor pain is sometimes described as the most intense pain a person may experience, and the pain of labor is often the aspect of childbirth most worrisome to expectant parents. There is a physiologic basis for pain in labor, although the intensity of the pain experienced varies a great deal from one woman to another. Although pain is usually associated with pathology, in the case of childbirth it is due to normal physiologic processes.

Factors Affecting Perception of Pain in Labor

A woman's responses to pain in labor are influenced to a great extent by her own history of pain, her cultural background, her psychological and physical state, and her interpretation of the pain-producing situation. The intensity of reported labor pain increases as labor progresses, peaks during the transition phase, declines during the second stage, and then increases during the last moments when the newborn's head and body are born. The perception of pain is influenced by the woman's confidence in her ability to cope with labor (see the accompanying Nursing Research display on maternal confidence). Research also indicates that continuous emotional support by a woman experienced in normal labor and birth reduces the woman's need for analgesia during labor (Kennell, Klaus, McGrath, Robertson, & Hinkley, 1991).

All of these factors—threats to personal safety and self-image, the medicalization of childbirth, and the meaning of pain—may arouse anxiety in the woman and alter the normal course of labor and birth. Excessive anxiety can alter the woman's perception of labor, intensifying her response to pain and fatigue. In a landmark study Lederman et al. (1978) discovered that high levels of anxiety during labor are related to the secretion of catecholamines, which in turn may inhibit uterine activity and increase the risk of intrapartum complications. Later research has supported these findings (Lederman et al., 1985). There is some evidence that preparation for childbirth may reduce anxiety during labor by minimizing the fear of the unknown and allowing the woman to interpret the sensations of labor more accurately.

Four major factors influence the process of labor and delivery by determining its length and the ability of the woman to deliver her neonate vaginally. They are the passage, passenger, powers, and psyche. Dysfunction in any factor may delay the progress or normal process of labor. The nurse plays a central role in the assessment of labor by evaluating these critical variables. In most

Nursing Research

Maternal Confidence in Coping With Labor

A woman's confidence in her ability to cope with labor can significantly influence her perceptions of pain. Maternal confidence has been defined as "self-efficacy," the individual's assessment of her capability to cope with the multiple stressors encountered during labor and birth. The woman's belief that she can "make it" through childbirth is based on four major factors:

- Past success coping with childbirth
- Observing another woman cope successfully with childbirth
- Confidence-building discussions with significant others and health care providers
- Physiologic arousal mechanisms to anticipated or actual sensations of labor and birth that reinforce level of confidence.

A second major component of maternal confidence involves the woman's assessment that a particular behavior will result in a given outcome. For example "I believe that relaxing my body during a contraction will reduce my level of pain."

Because each labor is unique, however, it is not easy to predict the woman's actual ability to cope with childbirth. The labor nurse can support the woman's self-confidence by building and reinforcing the woman's sense of competence. Providing positive feedback, manipulating the environment in ways that enhance feelings of control, and encouraging behaviors that result in successful coping are suggested. Continued research is recommended to delineate all dimensions of self-efficacy and identify nursing interventions that enhance maternal confidence to cope in labor.

Lowe, N. (1991). Maternal confidence in coping with labor. *Journal of Obstetric, Gynecologic, and Neonatal Nursing, 20*(6), 457.

cases labor progresses in a predictable fashion. When an abnormality is noted in the pelvic structure, fetal size or position, force of uterine contractions, or the woman's emotional status, the nurse must notify the midwife or physician immediately.

Stages of Labor

Labor is divided into four stages during which cervical effacement, dilatation, and the cardinal movements of the fetus occur.

The First Stage

The first stage of labor begins with the onset of regular contractions and ends with complete dilatation of the cervix (10 cm). The first stage is further divided into three phases: the latent phase, the active phase, and transition (Table 19-1).

Latent Phase

The latent phase begins with the initiation of true labor contractions and is completed when the cervix is dilated 3 to 4 cm. It is the longest of the three phases, and in primigravidas it is the period during which the cervix effaces. Uterine contractions during the latent phase usually are mild. The uterus is easily indented with the fingertips when it is palpated through a contraction, and the contraction exerts a pressure of only 20 to 30 mm Hg. Contractions often last only 15 to 30 seconds and are relatively infrequent (occurring as infrequently as every 10 to 20 minutes). Many women complete the latent phase at home in the comfort of familiar surroundings. They are able to ambulate without difficulty, at times even through contractions.

Active Phase

The active phase of labor, also called the dilatation phase, begins at 4 cm dilatation and ends at approximately 7 cm. Contractions become longer (45 to 60 seconds), stronger (exerting up to 50 mm Hg pressure or greater), and occur more frequently (as often as every 3 to 5 minutes). The uterus feels firm when palpated during a contraction. It may be more difficult for the woman to continue walking during contractions, and the nurse will note an obvious change in the woman's behavior, which is described later in this chapter. Mild cramping sensations and a low, dull backache may give way to perceptions of mild-to-moderate discomfort or pain during contractions. By 7 cm dilatation many women wish to sit or recline for periods of time and may find ambulation difficult or impossible at the acme of the contraction.

In traditional medical descriptions of labor the active phase begins at 4 cm dilatation and ends when the woman's cervix is completely dilated. It is subdivided into three periods: (1) the acceleration phase (4 to 5 cm), (2) the phase of maximum slope (5 to 9 cm), and (3) the deceleration phase (9 to 10 cm). This division of the active phase is useful in the diagnosis of abnormal labor patterns characterized by delayed dilatation or fetal descent.

Transition Phase

The transition phase is the interval between 8 and 10 cm cervical dilatation. During this phase the cervix dilates most rapidly. Uterine contractions continue to increase in frequency (every 2 to 3 minutes), intensity, and duration (60 to 90 seconds). There is often an increase in bloody show. The uterus is very firm or hard when palpated during strong contractions. The woman may experience moderate-to-severe discomfort or pain in the latter half of this phase. The laboring woman may experience intense sensations of discomfort or pain and an urge to bear down as she begins to feel the pressure of the fetal presenting part deep in the pelvis.

Nausea, vomiting, increased irritability, and even a sense of panic may occur as she is bombarded with multiple, intense stimuli. The culmination of the transition phase of labor is often characterized by a slight slowing in the rate of cervical dilatation. A noticeable change in the woman's responses to labor may be noted as she approaches complete dilatation. She may feel more relaxed and perceive less pain or discomfort, or the intensity, frequency, and duration of contractions may peak along with an irresistable urge to push.

The Second Stage

The second stage of labor, or the stage of expulsion, begins with complete dilatation of the cervix and ends with the birth of the neonate (see Table 19-1). Uterine contractions often decrease in intensity, frequency, and duration for a short period of time. The woman may immediately feel an urge to push, or it may take time for fetal descent to stimulate stretch receptors in the lower pelvis. Therefore, it may be appropriate in some instances to allow the woman a short period of rest, especially after a tumultuous first stage, before initiating bearing-down efforts.

Intraabdominal pressure is now combined with uterine contractions to expel the fetus. The perineum begins to bulge and flatten out as the presenting part emerges (see Fig. 19-16*B*). Protrusion of the rectal mucous membrane through the anus also may occur. The labia majora and minora begin to separate as the head emerges. With each contraction, a larger portion of the presenting part is visible at the introitus and is referred to as crowning. The woman may experience intense rectal pressure and a sensation of stretching, tearing, or burning of the perineum as the head is born. With the birth of the head, there is a sudden sense of relief, as well as diminution in pressure and pain. The shoulders and body are then expelled.

Rupture of Membranes

The membranes may rupture at any time before or during the first stage of labor, but occasionally they remain intact until the cervix is completely dilated. The birth attendant will usually artificially rupture the membranes if they have not ruptured during the course of the second stage of labor. This is done to visualize the color of the amniotic fluid. If meconium (fetal intestinal contents) has been expelled in utero, a special suction technique is required at birth to prevent aspiration of meconium by the neonate as it takes its

Table 19-1. Stages and Phases of Normal Labor and Related Physical Characteristics

Stage	Phase	Dilatation	Contractions: Frequency	Contractions: Intensity	Contractions: Duration	Physical Characteristics
First Stage (0–10 cm)	Latent	0–4 cm	Q. 10–20 min but may occur more often: 5–10 min.	Mild	15–30 sec	Mild "menstrual-like" cramps Low, dull backache Sensation of uterine tightening Expulsion of mucous Light bloody show Diarrhea Possible rupture of membranes Ambulation without difficulty
	Active	4–10 cm				Mild-to-moderate discomfort or pain with uterine contractions
	Acceleration	4–5 cm	Q. 3–5 min	Moderate	30–45 sec	Increased bloody show Possible rupture of membranes Persistent backache with occipitoposterior position Ambulation without difficulty
	Maximum slope	5–9 cm	Q. 2–3 min	Moderate to intense	60–90 sec	Moderate-to-severe discomfort or pain with uterine contractions Increased bloody show Increasing rectal pressure Intermittent urge to push Nausea, vomiting, hiccuping, leg cramps, diaphoresis Involuntary shaking Periods of amnesia Possible rupture of membranes Ambulation difficult or impossible with uterine contractions
	Transition	8–10 cm				Increased bloody show Increasing urge to push Increasing rectal pressure Possible rupture of membranes
	Deceleration	9–10 cm	As frequent as Q. 1–2 min	Moderate to intense	45–90 sec	Moderate to severe discomfort or pain with uterine contractions
Second Stage (10 cm to birth of infant)			(May initially decrease in frequency, intensity, and duration). As frequent as 1–2 min			Strong urge to push with descent of presenting part Increasing rectal and perineal pressure Desire in some women to assume squatting position Bulging of perineum Prolapse of rectal mucosa Emergence of fetal presenting part—"crowning" Possible rupture of membranes
Third Stage (Birth of infant to birth of placenta)			(Initial cessation of contractions)	Moderate		Sensation of burning, stretching, or tearing as head is born Perineal anesthesia due to extreme stretching of perineum Mild-to-moderate uterine cramping with reinitiation of uterine contractions Feeling of fullness in vagina as placenta is expelled
Fourth Stage (1–4 h postbirth)			(Continuous contraction of uterus to prevent bleeding from spiral arteries)			Perineal tenderness Intermittent mild-to-moderate menstruallike cramps Involuntary shivering in some women (neurogenic response to intensity of labor)

first breath. (See Chapter 21 for a further description of suctioning.)

The Third Stage

The third stage of labor, or the placental stage, begins with the birth of the infant and ends with delivery of the placenta (see Table 19-1). Contractions may cease for several minutes after the neonate is born, and with their resumption (usually within 5 minutes) the placenta is delivered in two phases: the separation phase and the expulsion phase.

The Separation Phase

With the birth of the neonate, the uterus contracts, becomes smaller and firmer, and often appears to stand up in the maternal abdomen. Within minutes after the infant has been expelled, the uterus becomes a thick muscular sac. The walls of the uterine cavity collapse, eliminating the large cavity that was recently occupied. This sudden decrease in uterine size results in a decreased area for placental attachment and causes the decidua and fetal membranes to fold. The placenta is forced to accommodate to the decreased surface area by buckling off the wall of the uterus in the decidua spongiosa layer. The blood vessels in this central area begin to bleed, and a hematoma forms between the placenta and the remaining decidua. As this retroplacental hematoma enlarges, it forces additional cleavage of the placenta from the uterine wall, as shown in Figure 19-20. Visible maternal bleeding is usually minimal during this process, but there may be a gush or spurt of blood from the vagina, signaling placental separation.

It is believed that separation of the placenta usually begins in the central area within minutes of delivery. The peripheral areas are more firmly attached. Part of the decidua comes off with the placenta, and a varying amount remains attached to the myometrium to be shed during the next several weeks. The fetal membranes are peeled off the uterine wall by contraction of the myometrium and traction of the separated placenta.

The placenta may be expelled from the uterus and vagina by increased abdominal pressure due to maternal pushing efforts. Other methods of assistance may be needed if the woman is in a recumbent position. If she is in an upright position, gravity will aid expulsion. A commonly used method of assistance in placental delivery involves applying a hand over the uterine fundus and using the uterus as a piston to expel the placenta while applying very gentle cord traction at the same time (Fig. 19-21).

After the placenta separates from the uterine wall, the uterus contracts to ligate the blood vessels that are disrupted by the placental detachment process. Uterine musculature is arranged in three layers: the outer layer, which arches over the fundus and extends into the various uterine ligaments; the inner layer, which consists of sphincterlike fibers that surround the openings into the uterus, the fallopian tubes, and internal os of the cervix; and the substantial middle layer, which forms a dense crisscrossing network of muscle fibers in which the many blood vessels of the uterus are interlaced.

As a result of this structure the contraction of the middle-layer muscle fibers results in hemostasis of the uterine blood vessels at the placental site. Immediately after placental

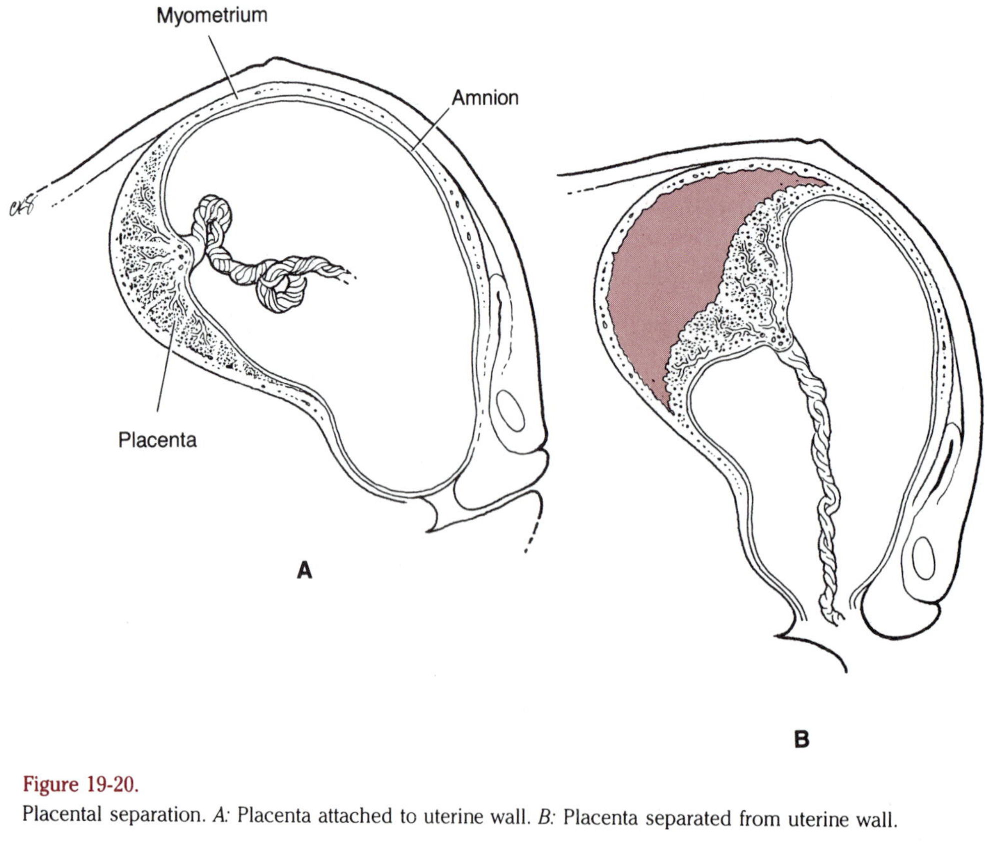

Figure 19-20.
Placental separation. *A:* Placenta attached to uterine wall. *B:* Placenta separated from uterine wall.

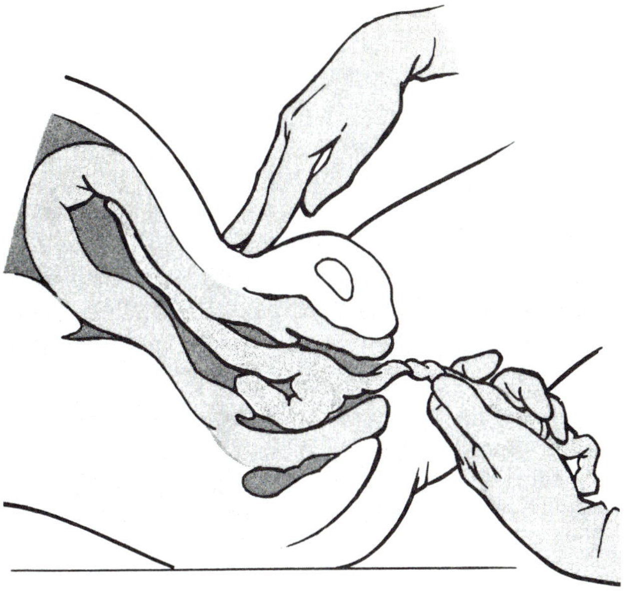

Figure 19-21.
Placental delivery. Note that attendant applies gentle traction to the umbilical cord.

delivery, the uterine muscle should feel firm and the fundus should be apparent at or below the umbilicus.

Normally, the third stage of labor lasts from a few minutes to 30 minutes. The incidence of complications increases after 30 minutes. The classic signs of placental separation are the following:

- A gush of blood from the vagina
- A change in the size, shape, and consistency of the uterus
- Lengthening of the umbilical cord from the vagina
- Maternal report of a contraction

Expulsion

There are two mechanisms by which the placenta can be expelled from the uterus. The more common of these is called the Schultze mechanism. In the *Schultze mechanism* the central region of the placenta separates first. As bleeding from torn vessels continues, a retroplacental hematoma is formed, and this further eases the placenta off the uterine wall. The central portion is followed by the peripheral portions. The hematoma and any free bleeding are contained in the trailing membranes as they are inverted behind the placenta. The shiny fetal surface of the placenta appears first at the introitus.

In the *Duncan mechanism* separation of the placenta occurs first at the periphery. Blood collects between the placenta and the uterine wall and may spurt or gush from the vagina when separation occurs. The placenta descends sideways in this case, and the dull, irregular maternal surface appears first at the introitus. Placental separation by the Duncan mechanism carries a slightly increased risk of retained placental fragments in the uterus after delivery because of incomplete separation. Because of the quality of the presenting surface in the two mechanisms, they often are remembered as shiny Schultze and dirty Duncan.

The Fourth Stage

The first several hours after delivery of the placenta are frequently referred to as the fourth stage of labor. This is a period of dramatic physiologic and psychologic changes in which the woman makes the first adaptations to the nonpregnant state. The physiologic and psychologic characteristics of this stage and appropriate nursing care of the woman during this early postpartum period are described in detail in Chapter 21.

The normal course of labor is divided into four stages, during which the cervix dilates and effaces and the fetus accomplishes the cardinal movements of birth. The nurse is responsible for examining the cervix periodically during labor to determine the stage. The skilled labor nurse can often identify movement from one stage of labor to the next by monitoring the woman's physical and emotional reactions. As the woman moves through the first stage and its phases, the nurse informs the woman and her birth attendant (midwife or physician) of her progress. The major goals of nursing care are to support the normal physiologic processes of childbirth and to monitor maternal and fetal responses to this process.

Duration of Labor

The length of time required to complete the work of childbirth varies according to a number of factors—fetal size and position, strength and pattern of uterine contractions, maternal position and activity, and maternal age and parity, to name a few. However, certain patterns in the duration of each stage and in the course of labor help to indicate whether a woman's labor is progressing normally.

Perhaps the most comprehensive study of the duration and progress of normal labor and birth was undertaken by Emmanuel Friedman, an obstetrician. He studied a large number of births and examined how long individual stages and the entire course of labor lasted under normal conditions in cases with good outcomes (Friedman, 1978). The results of his study on the length of stages of labor among primigravidas and multigravidas are shown in Table 19-2. The upper ranges represent the longest time that labor continued and still concluded normally. The characteristically shorter labor of the multigravida can be seen in this table. These results are used widely as guidelines for judging whether the progress of a particular woman's labor is within normal limits. However, these findings may have limitations and must be used cautiously.

The Friedman Curve

These guidelines have been translated into a graphic representation of the progress of labor (Fig. 19-22). The so-called Friedman curve frequently is used in labor assessment and may appear in hospital settings in preprinted labor progress records on which the woman's progress is charted. The nurse should recognize that these guidelines must not be used in isolation but must always be used with other clinical data, such as fetal heart rate and maternal status, to

Table 19-2. Lengths of Phases in Normal Labor

	Primigravidas		Multiparas	
Phase	Average	Upper Normal	Average	Upper Normal
First stage	13.3 h	28.5 h	7.5 h	20.0 h
Latent phase	8.6 h	20.0 h	5.3 h	14.0 h
Active phase	5.8 h	12.0 h	2.5 h	6.0 h
Transition phase*				
Second stage	57 min	150 min	18 min	50 min
Rate of cervical dilatation in active phase	Less than 1.2 cm/h is abnormal		Less than 1.5 cm/h is abnormal	

* Transition is not seen as a separate phase of labor in the medical model.

determine whether more active management of labor is needed.

Further, there is some evidence that the Friedman curve may not always accurately represent the upper safe limits of time in labor. Research on the length of the second stage of labor suggests that it may safely extend to 3 hours or longer for a primigravida and 2 hours or more for the multipara, as long as the woman and the fetus appear to be doing well. The original guidelines developed by Friedman may not accurately reflect patterns of normal labor in unmedicated and ambulating or upright women or women who receive epidural anesthesia during labor (Piper, Bolling, & Newton, 1991). Chapter 24 discusses the effect of epidural anesthesia on the duration of labor. As research continues, these guidelines may be revised further.

The duration of labor is usually predictable for both the primigravida and the multipara. Variations occur secondary to physiologic dysfunction, emotional distress, and iatrogenic factors such as the administration of medication. When labor is abnormally short or long, it may pose risks for the woman and her fetus. The nurse retains primary responsibility in most settings for monitoring and documenting the duration of labor. Major goals of nursing care during labor are to evaluate the progress of labor in relation to time, and to distract the woman in labor from focusing on the passage of time.

Signs and Symptoms of Labor

Before the onset of labor, certain phenomena may alert the woman to approaching labor.

Approaching Labor

Braxton Hicks Contractions. Although Braxton Hicks contractions occur throughout pregnancy, these tightenings of the uterine musculature become more noticeable in the last 4 to 6 weeks. Multigravidas often experience more discomfort from them than primigravidas. Braxton Hicks contractions usually are painless, irregular in frequency and intensity, and may be unusually long in duration. They are noted as a tightening or pulling sensation low in the abdomen over the pubic bone. These contractions may be helpful in developing the neuromuscular pathways needed for the coordinated contractions of labor. They also may assist in

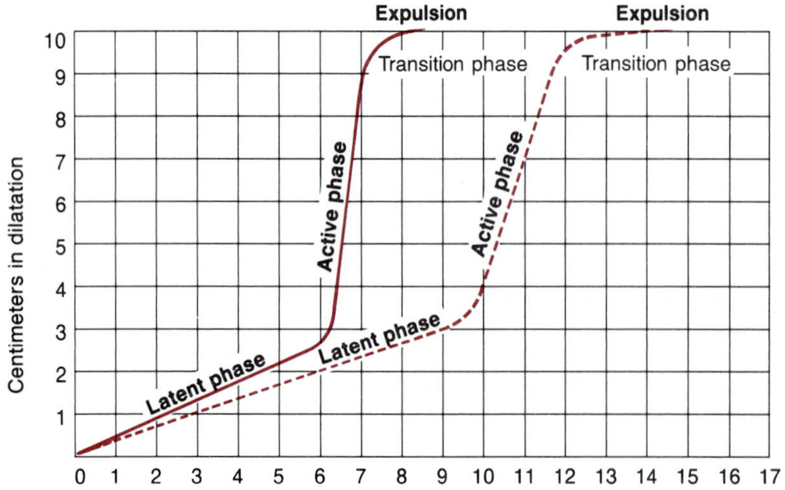

Figure 19-22.
Graphic analysis of labor using Friedman's curve. The mean labor duration for primigravidas is shown by the dotted line, and the mean for multigravidas is shown by the solid line.

early changes of the cervix before labor begins. A series of Braxton Hicks contractions may be referred to as false labor.

Lightening. Lightening refers to the settling or engagement of the presenting part in the maternal pelvis. It usually occurs 2 to 3 weeks before the onset of labor in primigravidas and may not occur in multigravidas until labor begins. Although it is often described as a subjective sensation felt by the woman, lightening may be evident as a decrease in prenatal fundal height near 37 or 38 weeks of gestation. The woman is usually aware of this settling of the fetus in the lower uterine segment, which is often described in lay terms as the "baby dropping." She feels increased movement low in the uterus, may experience less difficulty breathing, and observes that her uterus protrudes more. In addition, bladder capacity is further decreased and urination may be frequent. Leg cramps, pedal edema, and pelvic pressure also may increase.

Cervical and Vaginal Changes. Cervical changes, often referred to as "ripening," include softening, effacement (shortening and thinning), and sometimes dilatation. Uterine contractions late in pregnancy begin to pull the cervix upward as the lower uterine segment is formed. This results in the loosening of fibrous connective tissue of the cervix. The cervix becomes softer, shorter, more pliable, and thinner in preparation for dilatation. It also may move from a posterior to an anterior location in the vagina. There may be an increase in vaginal discharge due to pelvic congestion in early labor.

Persistent Backache. Relaxin, the placental hormone responsible for relaxation of pelvic ligaments, has maximally affected the sacroiliacs and other pelvic joints by late pregnancy. As a result strain on the muscles of the lower back is increased. Postural changes associated with pregnancy may add to this problem.

Weight Loss and Gastrointestinal Upset. As estrogen and progesterone levels change in late pregnancy, electrolyte shifts result in loss of body water. Weight loss of 1 to 3 pounds can occur. Many women also experience diarrhea 1 or 2 days before labor begins; the cause of this is unknown.

Nesting Behavior. Women commonly experience a sudden burst of energy and increased physical activity in the final days before labor begins. The woman can feel compelled to "have everything ready" for the arrival of the newborn. There is speculation that hormonal changes may contribute to this phenomenon; however, no research findings confirm this hypothesis.

Signs of True Labor

Uterine Contractions. True labor contractions usually occur at regular intervals. The contractions get closer, increase in duration and intensity, and bring about progressive change in the cervix and descent of the fetus. Women describe true labor contractions as starting in the back and radiating to the front. A change in activity, such as walking, may increase the intensity of true labor contractions.

Spontaneous Rupture of Membranes. Rupture of the membranes may occur as a leak or a gush of amniotic fluid. This fluid usually is clear and odorless, although in some cases it may be greenish because of meconium staining or fetal passage of intestinal contents in utero, a sign of possible fetal distress. Labor contractions usually start within 8 to 12 hours of spontaneous rupture; if labor does not ensue, more active obstetric management to stimulate labor may be advised because of the increasing risk that infection will ascend into the uterus and threaten the fetus.

Bloody Show. Bloody show, or blood-tinged vaginal secretions, may occur at the onset of labor or several days beforehand. It is caused by rupture of minute capillaries in the cervix as it softens, dilates, and effaces in preparation for labor.

The onset of labor is a time of excitement and uncertainty. Early signs of labor are often subtle, and both the woman and the nurse may be unsure of their significance. The woman should be educated about the signs of labor during the prenatal period so she is prepared for its onset. The skilled labor nurse must evaluate the presenting signs and determine their significance. When labor progresses normally, early or prodromal signs will correlate with cervical effacement and dilatation. When presenting signs of labor resolve or do not result in cervical change, the nurse must implement strategies that provide the woman with physical and emotional support until true labor ensues.

Maternal and Fetal Adaptations

Maternal Physiologic Adaptations

In addition to the adaptations that occur in the reproductive system, there are also normal alterations in other body systems, which indicate a healthy adaptation to the process of labor and birth.

Neurologic Adaptations

Neurologic adaptations have not been extensively studied. As noted previously, certain behavioral responses may occur just before the onset of labor, such as nesting behavior and energy spurts, which may reflect central nervous system adaptations. The neurochemical basis for these alterations in activity is poorly understood. Sleep disturbances also have been noted and have been attributed to frequent fetal movement, Braxton Hicks contractions, the need to urinate frequently, and the woman's inability to assume a comfortable resting position in late gestation. Hormonal changes in pregnancy may alter circadian rhythms and thus the percentage of time spent in REM sleep, further contributing to sleep disturbances.

Beta-endorphin levels (potent endogenous opiates) increase during pregnancy, giving rise to speculation regarding their impact on pain perception during labor. More research is needed before the role of beta-endorphins in the mediation of labor pain is understood (see the accompanying Nursing Research display).

Nursing Research

The Role of Beta-Endorphins in the Modulation of Pain During Labor

A major goal of nursing care during childbirth is the management of discomfort and pain. Beta-endorphins, powerful endogenous opiates, induce varying degrees of analgesia when produced by specialized cells in the central and peripheral nervous system. During pregnancy beta-endorphin levels are elevated. Efforts have been made to identify the role of endogenous opiates in the modulation of pain associated with childbirth. Cahill recently examined the relationship between self-reported perceptions of pain during labor and plasma beta-endorphin levels. While levels of beta-endorphins were significantly higher in pregnant women than in nonpregnant controls, subjects reported increased pain as labor progressed. Although plasma levels of beta-endorphins rose slightly during labor, they did not keep pace with the perceived level of pain. An interesting finding was that reported pain levels were higher *between* than during contractions. It is possible that endogenous opiates do modulate perception of painful stimuli but do not ameliorate generalized sensations of discomfort experienced between contractions. Further research is indicated before recommendations regarding nursing care or childbirth preparation classes can be made.

Cahill C. (1989). Beta-endorphin levels during pregnancy and labor: A role in pain modulation? *Nursing Research, 38*(4), 200.

Cardiovascular Adaptations

Cardiac Output. The woman's cardiac output steadily rises during labor, with a 15% to 20% increase during contractions. This occurs because catecholamine release due to pain and anxiety results in transient tachycardia. Furthermore, approximately 300 to 500 mL of blood is redistributed from the placental vascular bed and the uterus to the systemic circulation (Blackburn & Loper, 1992). Cardiac output decreases when the woman is in the supine position and increases during labor when she is placed in the lateral decubitus position. Cardiac output may increase as much as 40% to 50% in the second stage of labor, with expulsive efforts and peaks in the third stage at 80% above prelabor levels. This is caused by the loss of the uteroplacental vascular bed and the release of pressure on the vena cava.

Blood Pressure. Arterial blood pressure increases during labor. The woman's systolic pressure may increase an average of 15 mm Hg, and the diastolic pressure may increase 5 to 10 mm Hg. Higher levels may indicate pathology (see Chapter 27). During contractions the blood pressure may rise temporarily higher with pain sensations, anxiety, and catecholamine release, as well as by compression of the distal aorta and common iliac arteries. This is considered a normal physiologic response to contractions.

Heart Rate. The woman's pulse rate increases with time to 100 bpm or slightly higher by the second stage of labor, with sensations of pain, anxiety, increased activity, and catecholamine release. During the peak of contractions, a reflex bradycardia may occur, which results from the increase in cardiac output and blood pressure. Between contractions the pulse rate returns to the resting rate, which averages 80 to 90 bpm.

Stroke Volume and Blood Volume. There also is a progressive increase in stroke volume during labor, which peaks at delivery. There is no change in blood volume during normal labor; however, during delivery the woman may lose up to 500 mL of blood. The hypervolemia of pregnancy allows the woman to adapt to the rapid blood loss. Other cardiovascular responses that also aid in the successful adaptation include elimination of the large uteroplacental vascular bed and fluid shifts from the extravascular compartment back to the circulatory system.

Hematologic Adaptations

Blood coagulation time decreases slightly during labor, but plasma fibrinogen levels increase. There is a progressive leukocytosis (an average increase to 15,000 mm^3) by the end of the first stage. With heavy exertion the white cell count may rise to 25,000 to 35,000 mm.

Pulmonary Adaptations

The woman's respiratory rate increases during labor. This is due to anxiety, pain, physical exertion, and the increased demand for oxygen secondary to the rise in metabolic rate and the work of labor. Oxygen consumption also increases. Recent research indicates that many healthy women in labor experience drops in oxygen saturation without negative sequelae (Minnich, Brown, Clark, Miller, & Thompson, 1990). The frequency and severity of desaturation episodes increase in women who receive narcotics and with hyperventilation-induced hypocarbia. The risk of desaturation also is increased in obese women.

Some women may hyperventilate during the peak of contractions, but persistent hyperventilation is abnormal. Hyperventilation-induced hypocarbia (low $Paco_2$ levels) is common. The $Paco_2$ level normally declines throughout the first stage of labor. Arterial carbon dioxide levels as low as 17 mm Hg (normal range in pregnancy is 31.3 to 34.3 mm Hg) have been recorded in women with painful labors who are hyperventilating. During the second stage of labor $Paco_2$ levels may rise when breath holding accompanies bearing-down efforts. Significant changes in $Paco_2$ levels are potentially hazardous to the woman and fetus during labor. Extremely low $Paco_2$ levels may reduce placental perfusion. Elevated $Paco_2$ levels result in a shift in the oxygen-hemoglobin dissociation curve and impairs the release of oxygen from the maternal hemoglobin molecule to the fetus. If underlying maternal or fetal pathology preexists, aberrations in $PaCO_2$ may further compromise the fetus (Blackburn & Loper, 1992). Nursing efforts should be aimed at reducing inappropriate breathing patterns that result in "hyperventilation syndrome" (nausea, vomiting, and paresthesias) or breath holding during bearing-down efforts. (See Chapter 21 for a detailed discussion of nursing actions that reduce $PaCO_2$ abnormalities and acid–base shifts).

Biochemical Adaptations

While the maternal pH usually remains within normal limits (7.35 to 7.45), during labor acidosis can occur with pain, anxiety, physical exertion, strong contractions, ketosis, and drug administration. A rise in blood lactate and a fall in pH often are noted in the transition phase of labor when pain sensations and uterine contractions may be intense. During the second stage of labor $PaCO_2$ levels may rise if the woman holds her breath while bearing down. This results in respiratory acidosis. Respiratory alkalosis also is common and may occur with hyperventilation.

Renal Adaptations

Increased fluid losses and changes in electrolyte balance during labor result from several significant factors. Polyuria is common with increased cardiac output and a resultant rise in the glomerular filtration rate. Diaphoresis and hyperventilation contribute to insensible water loss. Reduced oral intake of fluids due to nausea, pain sensations, and the administration of analgesia or anesthesia further alter fluid and electrolyte balance. The hypervolemia of pregnancy protects the woman to some extent, but dehydration, ketonuria, and electrolyte aberrations are observed with prolonged labor, persistent nausea and vomiting, and maternal exhaustion.

Slight proteinuria (trace) is noted in as many as one third to one half of women secondary to an increased metabolic rate and muscle breakdown during the work of labor. Greater levels of proteinuria indicate pathology (see Chapter 27).

Inability to void and bladder distention often are observed in the laboring woman. A relaxed bladder muscle tone occurs when progesterone levels in pregnancy predispose the woman to distention. Compression of the urethra and bladder by the uterus and fetus may make it impossible for her to void. Distention may cause a reflex diminution in the forces of labor and can lead to trauma of the bladder mucosa during the birth of the infant.

Gastrointestinal Adaptations

Gastrointestinal motility and absorption decrease during labor, as do gastric secretions. The presence of pain and anxiety can further reduce gastrointestinal function. Thus, gastric emptying time is prolonged, and undigested food may remain in the stomach throughout labor. Nausea and vomiting are not uncommon, especially in the transition phase. Liquids are absorbed rapidly, however, and the woman experiencing an uncomplicated labor and birth is encouraged to ingest clear fluids, high in glucose, to meet energy requirements. Diarrhea also may be observed in some women, particularly as a sign of impending labor.

Metabolic Adaptations

The increased metabolic activity that occurs during labor causes an increased pulse rate, respiratory rate, body temperature, and insensible fluid loss. The slight elevation in body temperature should not exceed 0.5°C to 1°C (0.5°F to 1°F) and any increase should be observed closely, because it may indicate maternal dehydration, infection, or chorioamnionitis.

Aerobic and anaerobic carbohydrate metabolism increase during labor secondary to muscle activity and catecholamine release. Blood sugar levels decrease during labor, and the woman may require fluids with glucose supplementation during prolonged labor or with persistent nausea and vomiting.

Immunologic Adaptations

Alterations in immune activity occur in the woman during pregnancy. The stress of birth appears to further stimulate immunologic adaptations. Increased levels of interleukin-1, an immunoregulatory hormone that mediates the acute phase response to infection is increased in the amniotic fluid of women in labor. Polymorphonuclear leukocyte function is decreased. Nurse researchers have identified a significant association between anxiety levels and decreased immunoglobulin (Ig) A concentrations during labor. Lower IgA levels were associated with a greater incidence of postpartum complications and neonatal illnesses (Annie & Groer, 1991).

Maternal Behavioral Adaptations

A woman's responses to the pain and physical demands of labor produce systematic changes in behavior and require alterations in her psychological functioning as labor progresses. Many experienced labor nurses can judge with great accuracy how far cervical change has progressed in an unmedicated laboring woman by observing the woman's behavior and interaction with the environment. Excitement and anticipation are typical in early labor, and the woman interacts easily with her partner, other support people, and staff. Conversations or other activities readily distract the woman from attending to her labor, and only the recurring contractions refocus her attention on the process that has begun.

However, as labor becomes well established, the physical sensations become more compelling. As she reaches the midway point of cervical dilatation, the woman must work to cope with contractions. Interactions with others are limited to the work at hand, and only between contractions can her attention be directed away from the sensations she is experiencing. Observers have described this as a process of ego constriction: The woman's attention gradually narrows from her normal engagement with the outside world to the world of her labor room.

The nurse may observe a gradual loss of modesty as the work of labor becomes paramount in the woman's mind. A woman who in early labor was concerned about keeping her body covered may not even notice when she is uncovered during active phase. As labor reaches a peak during transition, she may actively remove coverings. The woman in active hard labor gradually becomes less and less able to focus on matters not directly related to her own comfort and safety. As she approaches complete dilatation, the sensations associated with contractions may be almost overwhelming. The woman's attention is totally self-focused. She may fall asleep or close her eyes between contractions and interact little with others, except to respond to directions or ask for help.

Once dilatation is complete, the sensations associated with labor compel the woman to bear down, and this work of pushing demands her full concentration. However, as she makes progress and delivery becomes imminent, attention expands to include the soon-to-be-born infant. She may watch the crowning and the birth with growing excitement and react with joy at the first sight of the infant. The woman often will then "reconnect" with her support person, especially if it is the father; she may look to see his response or share tears of joy and laughter with him. Rapidly, the mother's psychologic space expands to include newborn and father.

This process of behavioral adaptation to labor is influenced by many factors. Obviously, if regional anesthesia is used during labor, changes in the woman's behavior may be far less dramatic. If complications arise, the woman is forced not only to cope with labor, but also to adjust to a rapidly changing "risk" situation. She may become acutely attuned to interactions around her, looking for information and reassurance. Anxiety, sensory alterations, and the supportive presence of others also affect the woman's psychological adaptation to labor.

Fetal Physiologic Adaptations

In addition to the positional and attitudinal adaptations that occur in the fetus during labor and birth, the following adjustments are made.

Neurologic Adaptations

An intact brain and autonomic nervous system function to regulate fetal heart rate, cardiac output, and blood pressure. The parasympathetic nervous system (cardiodecelerator system) and its primary nerve—the vagus nerve—increase in dominance during gestation, and the fetal heart rate gradually slows. During labor, when the vagus nerve is stimulated, for example by compression of the fetal head during contractions, the heart rate will temporarily slow until pressure on the head ceases.

The sympathetic nervous system (cardioaccelerator system) has nerve fibers that are widely distributed in heart muscle. When stimulated by the mild hypoxia the fetus experiences during contractions, the heart rate is increased. The parasympathetic and sympathetic nervous systems interplay to control the fetal heart rate and the variability in the heart rate pattern. The balance between these systems is altered by changes in the intrauterine environment, fetal activity, external stimuli, and changes in maternal or fetal Po_2 or Pco_2 concentrations (Murray, 1988).

Cardiovascular Adaptations

Heart Rate. During labor, the fetal heart rate normally ranges between 120 and 160 bpm. In some term or post-term fetuses, the baseline heart rate ranges between 100 and 120 bpm as a result of neurologic maturity (Murray, 1988). With uterine contractions the increase in uterine tension reduces the flow of oxygenated maternal blood to the intervillous spaces. At approximately 50 mm Hg pressure, blood flow ceases, and the fetus must rely on oxygen reserves in the intervillous spaces. If these reserves are exhausted, fetal hypoxemia and tissue hypoxia will occur. Mild hypoxia causes an increase in fetal heart rate, and with moderate to severe hypoxia the fetal heart rate will slow.

Blood Pressure. Baroreceptors at the junction of the internal and external carotid arteries and chemoreceptors in the aortic arch, carotid bodies, and brain control fetal blood pressure and heart rate. If fetal blood pressure increases, baroreceptors cause a reflex decrease in cardiac output and blood pressure. This may occur with sudden compression of the fetal umbilical cord. Umbilical arteries are compressed, preventing outflow of fetal blood and increasing systemic blood pressure. Baroreceptors then slow the fetal heart rate and lower the blood pressure.

Chemoreceptors located in the brain are stimulated by adverse changes in fetal pH, Po_2, and Pco_2 and cause an initial increase in fetal heart rate and blood pressure. This initial rise in pressure is a protective mechanism that improves blood flow to the brain. With moderate to severe hypoxia, blood is selectively shunted to essential fetal organs (brain, heart, and adrenal glands) and away from the gastrointestinal tract, skeletal muscles, and skin. If blood shunting is prolonged and marked, it can result in permanent compromise of the renal and gastrointestinal system.

Hematologic Adaptations

Oxygen use by the fetus is very high during labor. The fetal Po_2 is approximately 30 to 35 mm Hg in the carotid artery. Although this is an extremely low oxygen tension, the fetus is able to meet its metabolic demands for oxygen in other ways. During uterine contractions a fall in cerebral blood flow is noted in the healthy fetus without a fall in oxygen saturation (Peebles et al., 1992). Hemoglobin levels are very high (15 to 20 g/dL). Fetal hemoglobin has a greater affinity for oxygen and a greater oxygen-carrying capacity than in the adult.

Pulmonary Adaptations

The placenta functions as the organ of respiration during intrauterine life. With the onset of labor, small amounts of fetal lung fluid are expelled from fetal airways during passage through the birth canal. This allows for an easier inflow of air when the neonate takes its first breath after birth. Ultrasonic examination of the fetus during labor confirms the continuation of rhythmic fetal breathing movements, which began early in the gestational period.

Gastrointestinal Adaptations

The healthy fetus may pass meconium (intestinal contents) during labor without adverse outcomes. Meconium also may be swallowed and reabsorbed. However, many studies have reported lower Apgar scores, lower pH values, and higher perinatal morbidity and mortality rates among neonates who pass meconium in utero (Katz & Bowes, 1992). In instances of moderate to severe intrauterine hypoxia, compensatory mechanisms shunt blood from the fetal gastrointestinal tract, and this may result in necrosis of intestinal tissue postnatally.

Renal Adaptations

The fetal kidneys produce urine, and the fetus may urinate in utero during labor without adverse sequelae. In instances of moderate to severe intrauterine hypoxia, compensatory mechanisms shunt blood from the fetal renal system, and this may result in postnatal renal dysfunction or failure.

Biochemical Adaptations

Normal fetal pH ranges between 7.25 and 7.35 during labor. Fluctuations in fetal pH occur with uterine activity. Fetal blood pH decreases during contractions by as much as 0.05 pH units. Between contractions excess carbon dioxide and acid metabolites are transported to the intervillous spaces and across the placental membrane. Carbon dioxide diffuses across the placental membrane at a much faster rate than lactic acid (at least 20 to 30 minutes), so the fetus can remain acidotic for some time after a hypoxic episode (Murray, 1988).

Fetal pH also is influenced by maternal pH. Maternal starvation, increased muscle activity, and catecholamine release will falsely decrease the fetal pH in the absence of hypoxia. Correction of the maternal condition will, in these cases, reverse the lowered fetal pH.

Hormonal Adaptations

Studies indicate that concentrations of catecholamines (epinephrine and norepinephrine) rise during labor as a result of the normal stressors associated with birth. These include pressure changes, decrease in fetal pH, and alterations in oxygen and carbon dioxide pressures. The production of catecholamines is beneficial, acting directly on the fetal heart and cardiovascular system to increase blood pressure, heart rate, and the force of myocardial contractility. They also increase the newborn's metabolic rate at birth and accelerate the breakdown of stored nutrients into available forms of energy for all organ systems (Cooper & Goldbenburg, 1990).

Fetal Behavioral Adaptations

Only recently have researchers begun to explore behavioral states in the human fetus during birth. Using ultrasound technology, investigators have identified awake states in the fetus characterized by mouthing movements (opening or closing of the jaw), eyelid closure and opening, and general body movements (rotation, flexion, and extension of extremities). The fetus also exhibits periods of quiet and active sleep, even with increasing intensity of labor and rupture of membranes. Habituation, the decreasing response to a repetitive stimuli, is also present in healthy term neonates and is an indicator of neurologic integrity (Goldkrand & Litvack, 1991).

The woman and the fetus undergo major physical and behavioral adaptations during the four stages of labor. During the first stage of labor the woman experiences an increasing intensity in physical and psychological sensations as the cervix dilates and the fetus begins its descent through the birth canal. During the second stage the physical work of labor reaches its peak as the woman must literally push the newborn into the world. The fetus also experiences drastic changes in pressure, position, and posture, which require complex physiologic adaptations. While the third stage is characterized by relief and elation for the new mother as the placenta is delivered, the neonate is faced with its greatest challenge as it makes the transition to extrauterine life. During the fourth stage maternal physiologic stability is achieved, but the psychological adaptation to parenthood is just beginning.

Chapter Summary

The essential components of childbirth can be summarized as the "four Ps:" passage, passenger, powers, and psyche. Each of these components involves a complex set of maternal and fetal adjustments. The passage, or maternal pelvis, must be adequate in size and shape to accommodate the descent and delivery of the fetus. The passenger, or fetus, must negotiate passage through the pelvis by fitting the smallest parts of its body to the narrow diameters of the pelvis. This is accomplished through a series of position changes known as the cardinal movements of labor. The powers, or uterine contractions, must be coordinated and of sufficient strength and quality to dilate and efface the cervix. This is achieved in concert with maternal expulsive efforts, which push the fetus down and eventually cause birth. The psyche, or maternal adaptation, must allow the woman to cope with the pain and physical demands of labor so that she can maintain physiologic and emotional balance and can actively push the fetus out during the second stage of labor.

Study Questions

1. *What are the three pelvic planes?*
2. *What are five maternal factors affecting birth outcome?*
3. *What are the definitions of the following terms: fetal lie, presentation, station, position, attitude, and synclitism?*
4. *What are the cardinal movements of labor? Why does each movement occur?*
5. *What are three current theories regarding the initiation of labor?*

6. *What actions are taken during the process of cervical effacement and dilatation?*
7. *What are the major stages and phases of labor? What are major defining characteristics of each?*
8. *What are the major maternal physiologic and behavioral adaptations that occur during labor and birth?*
9. *What are the major fetal physiologic and behavioral adaptations that occur during labor and birth?*
10. *What is the typical labor pattern of a primigravida compared with that of a multigravida?*
11. *What factors are known to influence a woman's perception of labor and her satisfaction with the birth experience?*

References

Annie, C., & Groer, M. (1991). Childbirth stress. *Journal of Obstetric, Gynecologic, and Neonatal Nursing*, *20*(5), 391–393.

Blackburn, S., & Loper, D. (1992). *Maternal, fetal, and neonatal physiology*. Philadelphia: W.B. Saunders.

Cooper, R., & Goldenberg, R. (1990). Catecholamine secretion in fetal adaptation to stress. *Journal of Obstetric, Gynecologic, and Neonatal Nursing, 19*(3), 223.

Cunningham, G., MacDonald, P., & Gant, N. (1989). *Williams obstetrics* (18th ed.). Norwalk, Ct: Appleton & Lange.

Friedman, E. (1978). *Labor: Clinical evaluation and management* (2nd ed.). New York: Appleton-Century-Croft.

Goldkrand, J., & Litvack, B. (1991). Demonstration of fetal habituation and patterns of fetal heart rate response to vibroacoustic stimulation in normal and high-risk pregnancies. *Journal of Perinatology*, *11*(1), 25–28.

Holcomb, W., & Smeltzer, J. (1991). Cervical effacement: Variation in belief among clinicians. *Obstetrics and Gynecology*, *78*(1), 43.

Katz, V., & Bowes, W. (1992). Meconium aspiration syndrome: Reflections on a murky subject. *American Journal of Obstetrics and Gynecology*, *166*(1), 171.

Kennell, J., Klaus, M., McGrath, S., Robertson, S., & Hinkley, C. (1991). Continuous emotional support during labor in a US hospital. *Journal of the American Medical Association*, *262*(17), 2197.

Lederman, R., Lederman, E., Work, B., et al. (1985). Anxiety and epinephrine in multiparous women in labor: Relationship to duration of labor and fetal heart rate pattern. *American Journal of Obstetrics and Gynecology*, *153*, 870.

Lederman, R., Lederman, E., Work, B., et al. (1978). The relationship of maternal anxiety, plasma catecholamines, and plasma cortisol to progress in labor. *American Journal of Obstetrics and Gynecology*, *132*, 495.

Minnich, M., Brown, M., Clark, R., Miller, F., & Thompson, D. (1990). Oxygen desaturation in women in labor. *Journal of Reproductive Medicine*, *35*(7), 693.

Morgan, M., & Thurnau, G. (1992). Efficacy of the fetal-pelvic index in nulliparous women at high risk for fetal-pelvic disproportion. *American Journal of Obstetrics and Gynecology*, *166*(3), 810.

Morgan, M., & Thurnau, G. (1988). Efficacy of the fetal-pelvic index for delivery of neonates weighing 4000 grams or greater: A preliminary report. *American Journal of Obstetrics and Gynecology*, *158*(5), 1133.

Morris, C., Khan, H., Sullivan, H., & Elder, M. (1992). Effects of platelet-activating factor on prostaglandin E2 production by intact fetal membranes. *American Journal of Obstetrics and Gynecology*, *166*(4), 1228.

Murray, M. (1988). *Antepartal and intrapartal fetal monitoring*. Washington, D.C.: NAACOG.

Piper, J., Bolling, D., & Newton, E. (1991). The second stage of labor: Factors influencing duration. *American Journal of Obstetrics and Gynecology*, *165*(4), 976.

Peebles, D., Edwards, D., Wyatt, J., et al. (1992). Changes in human fetal cerebral hemoglobin concentration and oxygenation during labor measured by near-infrared spectroscopy. *American Journal of Obstetrics and Gynecology*, *166*(5), 1369.

Zhu, Y., Word, A., & Johnston, J. (1992). The presence of platelet-activating factor binding sites in human myometrium and the role in uterine contraction. *American Journal of Obstetrics and Gynecology*, *166*(4), 1222.

Suggested Readings

Benzaquen, S., Gagnon, R., Hunse, C., & Foreman, J. (1990). The intrauterine sound environment of the human fetus during labor. *American Journal of Obstetrics and Gynecology*, *163*(2), 484.

Eganhous, D. (1991). A comparative study of variables differentiating false labor from early labor. *Jounral of Perinatology*, *11*(3), 249.

Mattison, D., Angtuaco, T., Miller, F. et al. (1989). Magnetic resonance imaging in maternal and fetal medicine. *Journal of Perinatology*, *9*(4), 311.

Romero, R., Brody, D., Oyarzun, E., Mazor, M., Wu, Y., Hobbins, J., & Durrum, S. (1989). Interleukin-1: A signal for the onset of parturition. *American Journal of Obstetrics and Gynecology*, *160*(5), 1117.

Van Loon, A., Mantingh, A., Thijn, C., et al. (1990). Pelvimetry by magnetic resonance imaging in breech presentation. *American Journal of Obstetrics and Gynecology*, *163*(4), 1256.

Winn, H., Rauk, P., & Petrie, R. (1992). Use of the fetal chest in estimating fetal weight. *American Journal of Obstetrics and Gynecology*, *176*(2), 448.

CHAPTER 20

Nursing Care in Normal Labor

FIRST STAGE

Learning Objectives

After studying the material in this chapter, the student will be able to:

- Discuss the application of the nursing process in caring for a woman in active labor and her family.
- Identify the signs of labor.
- Distinguish between false and true labor.
- Outline the differences between physiologic and active management of labor.
- Explain the technique of timing and palpating uterine contractions.
- Describe nonpharmacologic strategies for pain relief during labor.
- Outline the standard of nursing care for assessment of the woman in the latent, active, and transition phases labor.
- Describe the advantages and disadvantages of electronic fetal monitoring.

Key Terms

active management of labor
active phase of labor
bloody show
caput (succedaneum)
effleurage
electronic fetal monitoring
intrapartum
latent phase of labor
molding
prodromal labor
transition phase of labor

One of the most rewarding roles for the maternity nurse is participation in the birth of a neonate. Although childbirth requires little obstetric intervention for most women identified as "low risk," the presence of a professional nurse is essential. The nurse provides comfort, monitors the status of the woman and fetus, and implements physical and emotional support. In healthy, low-risk women, physiologic management of labor is appropriate. The primary goal of physiologic labor management is a healthy woman and fetus during the labor process. Physiologic management of labor is based on the following principles:

- Most childbearing women are healthy and at low risk.
- In most cases labor is a normal physiologic process.
- The healthy fetus benefits from minimal obstetric intervention.
- For most normal labors medication and other obstetric interventions are usually unnecessary, unless preferred by the woman.
- Women are generally more comfortable and less stressed when care emphasizes physiologic management.
- If deviations from the normal course of labor appear, more active management is needed.
- Active management of labor features interventions to promote and improve the body's own mechanisms.

For the last 50 years, obstetrics has been moving toward a more active management style, and many women do not object to the judicious use of analgesia, anesthesia, and interventions such as electronic fetal monitoring (EFM). However, some consumers and health care professionals question this approach and the need for intervention in normal labor and birth. They maintain that active interventions generally can be reserved for situations in which health problems or abnormal labor progress may increase risks to the woman or fetus.

Nursing care of families during labor focuses on maintaining normal physiologic and emotional status of all family members—woman, fetus and newborn, and father or signifi-

May: MATERNAL AND NEONATAL NURSING, 3rd. ed. © 1994 J.B. Lippincott Company.

cant others—as they move through the rapid changes of the intrapartum period. When the woman and her birth attendant desire more active management of the process, the nurse assists with implementation of appropriate interventions. The labor nurse individualizes care to meet the family's needs and desires within the physician's or nurse midwife's framework of obstetric management.

Appropriate nursing care during the process of labor is essential to ensure the well-being and security of the childbearing family. Labor and birth, as a progression of normal physiologic and psychological events, require expert nursing assessment skills and timely problem identification, intervention, and evaluation on a continuous basis. This chapter focuses on nursing care during the first stage of labor. Chapter 21 addresses nursing care from the second stage through delivery and immediate postpartum recovery. (Note: Throughout this chapter we use the terms "support person[s]," "family," "father," or "partner" to reflect the great diversity in family constellations and support systems available to women during childbirth.)

Environmental Considerations During Labor and Birth

When planning and implementing effective care, it is critically important to understand how the environment influences the process of labor and birth. Most hospitals in North America have developed birthing units that create a homelike environment for the childbearing family. The birthing unit may be a freestanding facility or a department within the hospital itself. A family-centered philosophy of childbirth has driven the development of these centers. The goal of care is to facilitate the process of birth and the transition to parenthood in a comfortable and safe setting (Fig. 20-1).

A labor lounge often is available for families to use during the early stages of labor. A television set, videotape recorder, reading materials, and games are often available as diversionary aids. Wireless telemetry is available in some units, allowing the nurse to monitor the fetal heart rate (FHR) while the woman ambulates. Women may be encouraged to ambulate to optimize the forces of labor and to use the shower or a whirlpool bath to promote comfort and relaxation. Emergency equipment, monitors, and supplies needed for delivery are usually concealed behind partitions or screens, enhancing the homelike nature of the setting. The nurse focuses on physiologic management of labor.

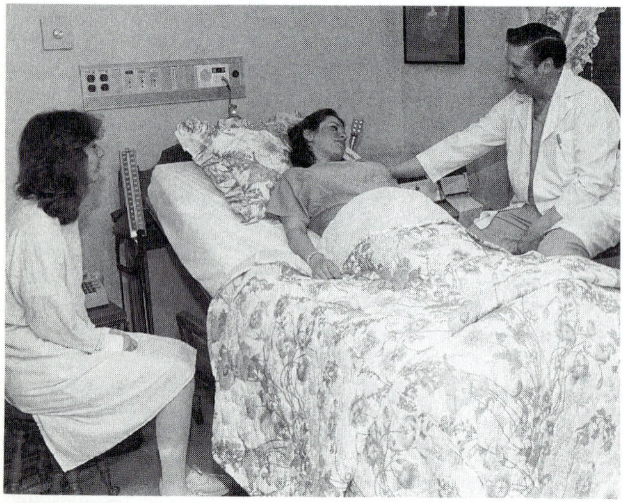

Figure 20-1.
Birthing unit.

If complications arise during the birthing process, the woman usually is transferred to a traditional labor and delivery unit where advanced monitoring and intensive nursing and medical care can be implemented. The woman may be confined to bed and the number of people present for the birth may be limited. The woman and her family may experience disappointment and anxiety that can adversely affect the progress of labor. Feelings of loss of control can arise. The nurse must be skillful in manipulating the environment to reduce unnecessary stimuli, promote comfort, and foster a family-centered birth experience in this potentially stressful setting.

The Onset of Labor

• • Assessment

The woman is normally instructed to contact her nurse midwife or physician if she believes that labor has begun or the membranes have ruptured. In some settings, particularly public hospitals, she may come directly to the labor or birthing unit, and the nurse is responsible for making a preliminary determination of whether the woman is in labor. Determining the onset of labor and providing appropriate information and guidance to the woman require an accurate assessment of the woman's physical and emotional status. These triage activities are critical for efficient functioning of the unit and provision of safe and effective care. Legal and ethical aspects are discussed in the accompanying display.

In some settings the nurse in labor and delivery units may be called on to answer questions regarding signs and symptoms of impending labor or other concerns by telephone. When providing information or advice by telephone, the nurse must use a systematic documentation form to record the patient contact and teaching. Formal documentation provides a method for organizing information obtained from the woman, describing her questions or complaints, and listing any advice or recommendations made by the nurse. Additionally, the labor and delivery unit should implement a mechanism for notifying the nurse midwife or physician when their patients call the nursing staff.

Distinguishing Between True and False Labor

The strength of contractions experienced during prodromal labor can be quite intense at times, without resulting in cervical dilatation. The phenomenon is often referred to as false labor. It is not uncommon for women experiencing prodromal signs of labor (backache; mild, irregular contractions; expulsion of mucous plug) to come to the birthing unit.

Legal Ethical Considerations

Triage Function of the Labor Nurse

The triage role of the nurse has been well developed in emergency room and disaster nursing, but it is a relatively new concept in maternity nursing. The current malpractice crisis and the growing accountability of nurses for their actions in emergency situations have encouraged refinement of this role for the labor nurse. The functions of the triage nurse include the following:

- Obtaining an accurate identification of the problem
- Determining the nature of care needed
- Deciding on the urgency of the condition
- Assigning the order in which patients will be seen
- Assigning or informing the appropriate nursing and medical personnel
- Decreasing patient waiting time
- Minimizing congestion in waiting areas

Nurses assuming the triage role should be experienced clinicians with advanced skills in labor and delivery care and strong problem-solving and organizational capabilities. The triage nurse must be prepared to make rapid decisions under stressful conditions based on sound professional judgment. Every labor and delivery unit should have a formal description of the triage role and a policy defining conditions under which triage functions are initiated.

Angelini, D., Zannieri, C., Silva, V., Fein, E., & Ward, P. (1990). Toward a concept of triage for labor and delivery: Staff perceptions and role utilization. Journal of Perinatal Neonatal Nursing, 4(3), 1–11.

The labor nurse is often called on to help make the initial determination about the onset of labor. Helping the woman distinguish between true and false labor can reduce anxiety, enhance feelings of competence, and reduce unnecessary visits to the birthing unit or hospital. Distinguishing characteristics of true and false labor are shown in Table 20-1.

• • Nursing Diagnosis

Although nursing diagnosis and planning usually do not begin until the woman is admitted, the following diagnoses may be useful when caring for women in false or the early latent phase of labor who seek telephone advice or come to the birthing unit for evaluation:

- Altered Health Maintenance related to labor and birth
- Fear/Anxiety related to impending labor and birth
- Pain related to prodromal labor sensations
- Sleep Pattern Disturbance related to prodromal labor sensations
- Fatigue related to discomfort and reduced quality of sleep

• • Planning and Implementation

Regardless of the setting chosen for birth, many women spend the first hours after the onset of true labor at home. If the nurse has telephone contact with the woman, nursing interventions in very early labor are primarily aimed at meeting the woman's need for information, promoting effective self-care and comfort measures, and providing emotional support.

Providing Information and Promoting Self-Care

Teaching considerations are given in the accompanying display. The healthy, low-risk woman may be advised to remain at home until her contractions occur every 5 minutes with regularity. The nurse should review comfort measures, relaxation techniques, and signs of true labor with her. Ambulation, use of a rocking chair, and a warm shower are excellent activities to reduce discomfort and enhance relaxation. The woman should be encouraged to continue taking clear liquids, and some physicians or midwives may permit eating lightly (low fat, high carbohydrate foods), until she comes to the birthing unit or hospital. Even if the woman already has information about directions to the hospital, the location of the unit, and what to bring to the hospital, review-

Table 20-1. Distinguishing Between True and False Labor

True Labor	False Labor
Uterine Contractions	
Show regular pattern	Show irregular pattern
Usually become closer together, stronger and longer	Usually vary
Increase in intensity with walking	May stop with walking or position change
Are usually felt in lower back, radiating to lower abdomen	Are usually felt in back, upper fundus
Are not stopped by relaxation techniques, such as hot bath, heating pad, alcoholic drink, or sedation	Will eventually stop with relaxation techniques
Cervix	
Softens, effaces, and dilates	May soften; no significant change in dilatation or effacement
Fetus	
Starts descent into pelvis	No noticeable change in position

Teaching Considerations

Early Labor

The nurse can use the following points in teaching women in early labor:

- Rest, relax, and conserve energy.
- Keep your mind occupied with something enjoyable.
- Try comfort measures, such as a warm bath, walking, or massage.
- Empty your bladder frequently and eat lightly (unless otherwise directed by your birth attendant).
- Keep taking clear fluids, such as water, juice, or soothing teas.
- Time your contractions, and don't use labor-coping techniques (such as breathing techniques) until you really need them to help you stay comfortable.

ing these quickly may alleviate worry and increase the woman's confidence about upcoming events.

A woman is advised to come to the birthing unit immediately if she reports strong, regular contractions; rupture of membranes; or abnormal signs and symptoms, such as profuse vaginal bleeding. If telephone consultation reveals that a woman has not received prenatal care, early admission also is strongly recommended. Health care providers will need ample time to complete the assessment process and laboratory tests and prepare the woman and her family for labor and birth. (See the display entitled "Providing Nursing Care When the Woman in Labor Has Not Received Prenatal Care.")

If a woman enters the labor and delivery unit and it is determined that she is not in labor, the nurse may direct her to return home after consulting with the nurse midwife or physician. When a diagnosis of false labor is made, the woman may express disappointment, embarrassment, or discouragement. The nurse should reassure the woman that this situation is not uncommon. A review of the characteristics of true labor and techniques to promote comfort and rest may alleviate any distress or uncertainty the woman feels at this time, as well as reduce the number of prelabor visits made by the woman (see the Nursing Research display).

Research conducted by Eganhouse (1991) found that women experiencing false labor report significant levels of anxiety, depression, and discomfort and have a greater incidence of abnormal labor requiring obstetric interventions. The nurse plays an important role in providing physical and emotional support and appropriate teaching when false labor is diagnosed.

Expected Outcomes

- The woman and her support person distinguish between true and false labor as evidenced by coming to the hospital or birthing center when a regular labor pattern is established.
- The woman uses effective comfort and relaxation techniques at home until a regular labor pattern is established.

Providing Nursing Care When the Woman in Labor Has Not Received Prenatal Care

A woman may enter labor and delivery without prenatal care. Often she is frightened, lacks basic information about the birth process, and may feel intense guilt regarding the lack of prenatal care. She also may have life-style problems that compromise maternal, fetal, and newborn well-being. These could be nutritional deficiencies and anemia, sexually transmitted diseases, domestic violence, or substance abuse.

Medical and obstetric problems that develop during pregnancy have not been treated, and the woman may require intensive intrapartum nursing and medical care. Fetal distress and neonatal asphyxia are more common. The situation may be complicated by language barriers, inadequate social support, and anxieties about financial considerations.

Often the labor nurse is the first health care professional the woman encounters as she enters the hospital to give birth. Although the nurse may feel frustrated or disapprove, the nurse is in a unique position to offer support and information and to reinforce health care-seeking behavior. Special aspects of nursing care for this group of women should include the following:

- A nonjudgmental approach (verbalizing disapproval may heighten the woman's anxiety, fear, guilt, or anger).
- Positive reinforcement (offering negative feedback may deter the woman from seeking care in the future).
- Culturally sensitive care (respecting childbirth practices that are influenced by culture will strengthen trust in health care providers).

Reproduced from Perez-Woods, R. (1990). Barriers to the use of prenatal care: Critical analysis of the literature 1966–1987. Journal of Perinatology, 10*(4), 420* with permission from Mosby-Year Book, Inc.

Nursing Research

Recognizing the Onset of Labor

The woman and her partner or coach may spend many hours in the birthing unit before the diagnosis of "false labor" is made. The woman expends physical and psychological energy needed for true labor. The nurse plays a critical role in reducing preadmission visits. Bonovich designed a low-cost, time-efficient intervention that significantly reduced the number of prelabor visits to a large community hospital. Nurses in the prenatal clinic made a careful assessment of the woman's knowledge base, reinforced correct information, and completed teaching regarding the signs and symptoms of true labor when knowledge deficits were identified. All nurses working in childbirth education classes, prenatal services, and birthing units can effectively reduce prelabor visits and the concomitant stress experienced by the expectant woman by implementing a systematic patient education protocol.

Bonovich, L. (1990). Recognizing the onset of labor. *Journal of Obstetric, Gynecologic, and Neonatal Nursing, 19*(2), 141–145.

Providing Emotional Support

The nurse should provide anticipatory guidance and include the support person(s) in communications. If the partner is going to be an active participant in the labor, the nurse assesses how well he or she is adapting to early labor and the level of support he or she is giving his partner. It also may be useful to review guidelines about family or support-person participation in labor and birth, if they are not already familiar with that information. The nurse identifies the nature of the woman's support system during early latent phase labor to plan appropriate care. It is essential that the nurse maintain an open, nonjudgmental, and supportive approach toward individuals the woman has selected to share in the birth experience.

Expected Outcome

- The support person verbalizes understanding of his or her part in the labor and birth process.

• • Evaluation

The nurse evaluates the effectiveness of nursing interventions that are aimed at preparing the woman for eventual admission to the birthing unit. With appropriate guidance and support, the healthy, low-risk woman will remain at home until the latent phase labor is well established. She will consume adequate fluids and calories and use a variety of self-care techniques to remain comfortable and relaxed. When the decision is made to come to labor and delivery, she will have sufficient energy reserves to meet the physical and emotional challenges of childbirth.

The period surrounding the onset of labor is often accompanied by feelings of heightened anticipation, anxiety, and uncertainty. For the primigravida prodromal signs of labor, including backache, pelvic pressure, and Braxton Hicks contractions, may be mistaken for true labor. The woman may telephone or come to the birthing unit before labor has been well established, seeking reassurance and information about her condition. The nurse plays a central role in providing guidance, encouragement, and support. The goals of nursing care at this time are to review signs of true labor and reinforce self-care activities that promote rest and comfort.

The Latent Phase of Labor

Admission to the Labor and Delivery Unit

Most women arrive on the birthing unit near the end of the latent phase of labor (0 to 4 cm dilatation). The physician, nurse midwife, or labor nurse will decide when admission is appropriate, based on the findings of the vaginal examination. Key components of this assessment focus on the cervical dilatation and effacement, the status of amniotic membranes, and the pattern of uterine contractions. An important nursing responsibility is to orient the woman and her support person or family to the unit and promote relaxation. Gentle touch should be used as indicated to communicate nonverbal caring. The accompanying Nursing Procedure outlines nursing care and rationales.

• • Assessment

Assessing Cervical Effacement and Dilatation and Determining Fetal Position, Descent, and Presentation

In most birthing units the nurse performs the first and subsequent vaginal examinations to assess the extent of cervical effacement and dilatation and descent of the fetal presenting part. Once contraindications to performing a vaginal examination have been eliminated, such as vaginal bleeding or premature rupture of the membranes, the nurse proceeds with the assessment. The nurse explains the procedure to the woman, suggests appropriate relaxation techniques to reduce discomfort, and then positions her for the examination. (The vaginal examination procedure is outlined in the accompanying Nursing Procedure.) The cervical os is located, and the nurse then estimates the degree of dilatation and effacement. The ischial spines are used as landmarks to determine descent of the fetus through the pelvis. With adequate descent of the fetal head, the nurse

NURSING PROCEDURE
Supporting the Woman and Support Person During Admission

Purpose: To reduce the level of anxiety that may accompany the admission procedure.

NURSING ACTION	*RATIONALE*
1. Introduce yourself to the woman and her support person(s).	To convey respect and let them know who will be completing the admission procedure.
2. Communicate your role as a supportive, nurturing, and knowledgeable nurse verbally and nonverbally.	To make the woman and her support person aware of the professional nurse's role during the labor and birth.
3. Orient the woman and her support person(s) to her surroundings, including how the labor bed works, location of bathroom, call light, towels, tissues, emesis basin, water, ice, and other items useful during labor.	To increase the woman's level of comfort about her surroundings.
4. Show approval, consideration, and regard for the woman and support person(s).	To provide positive affirmation and enhance the woman's sense of self-esteem.
5. Keep woman and support person(s) informed of progress after pelvic examinations.	To reduce anxiety related to procedures. To enhance the woman's sense of involvement in childbirth.
6. Act as liaison between woman and the physician, midwife, or nurse.	To facilitate communication between the woman and all members of the health care team.

also may be able to ascertain the position of the presenting part.

Assessing the Status of Amniotic Membranes

Another important nursing assessment is to determine whether amniotic membranes are intact or ruptured. If the nurse ascertains that the woman has already experienced persistent leaking or a gush of fluid, she should inquire about its color and odor, if any. If membranes have ruptured, the nurse should note the time of rupture and the color, amount, and odor of amniotic fluid. Normally amniotic fluid is clear or pale amber and has a slight fleshy odor. Any unpleasant odor or thick consistency of fluid suggests infection (amnionitis). Greenish fluid suggests recent fetal passage of meconium. Yellowish fluid may suggest meconium passage more than 36 hours before rupture of membranes or possibly fetal hemolytic disease. Wine-colored amniotic fluid indicates the presence of blood and may signal premature separation of the placenta, known as a placental abruption.

Women often are unsure whether they have experienced rupture of membranes or urinary incontinence caused by the pressure of the uterus on the bladder, a symptom not uncommon in late pregnancy. The labor nurse performs several tests to help establish membrane status. *Nitrazine* paper, which is sensitive to pH, will turn deep blue when applied to moist vaginal tissue or a perineal pad if membranes are ruptured. The blue color indicates the slight alkalinity of amniotic fluid. With urine and vaginal fluid, which are slightly acidic, the yellow color of the strip remains unchanged.

Ferning is the characteristic frondlike pattern of crystallization in amniotic fluid when it dries. It may be observed by placing a specimen of vaginal fluid on a microscopic slide, allowing it to dry, and then observing it under magnification. Urine and vaginal discharge will not show this pattern.

Pooling of fluid in the vagina can be observed on sterile speculum examination. The woman may be asked to bear down or cough, which will force amniotic fluid through the cervix and into the vagina if membranes are ruptured.

None of these tests is an absolute indicator of ruptured membranes. When the status of the membranes is uncertain, however, they are helpful determinants. If membranes are ruptured, subsequent vaginal examinations to determine the progress of labor should be kept to a minimum to reduce the risk of infection.

Evaluating the Uterine Contraction Pattern

An essential part of the nurse's initial and ongoing assessment in labor is an evaluation of the pattern of uterine contractions. To palpate contractions, the nurse places the

NURSING PROCEDURE
Using HIV Precautions in Labor and Delivery

The Centers for Disease Control (CDC) reports that health care workers have acquired human immunodeficiency syndrome (AIDS) viral (HIV) infection after their unprotected mucous membranes or broken skin were exposed to the body fluids of AIDS patients. The labor and delivery nurse is employed in an environment with a high risk of exposure to body fluids, including blood, amniotic fluid, urine, and feces. Emergency situations and sudden changes in patient status occur frequently, and the practitioner has limited time to don barriers such as gloves, impermeable cover gowns, goggles, or face shields to prevent direct contact with body fluids. *Universal blood and body fluid precautions should be used in the care of all patients, but the labor and delivery nurse should take added precautions based on the nature of the setting.*

Purpose: To prevent exposure to HIV while caring for the woman during childbirth

NURSING ACTION	***RATIONALE***
1. Wear clear glass or prescription lens eye wear at all times in labor and delivery.	To prevent unexpected splashes with body fluids (ie, sudden rupture of membranes, snapping of an umbilical cord during birth).
2. Carry a pair of unsterile gloves in a pocket at all times.	To have protective hand covering in case of precipitous birth or sudden hemorrhage.
3. Wear unsterile gloves whenever assisting birth attendants with vaginal exams, insertion of internal fetal monitor probes, or amniotomies.	To prevent exposure caused by fluid splashes or contamination of linens.
4. Place impermeable barrier gowns in each labor room.	To prevent contamination during precipitous delivery or sudden hemorrhage.
5. Stock knee-high boots for birth attendants and scrub nurses to wear.	To prevent contamination of the lower legs during birth.
6. Stock face shields in areas where birth occurs.	To prevent exposure during surgical or other procedures that generate splashes.
7. Institute a policy for placing all used sharps (i.e., suture needles and local anesthesia infusion needles) in one specified location on the delivery table.	To prevent housekeeping personnel or nurses from accidentally receiving puncture wounds.
8. Place sharps containers at every bedside.	To eliminate need for nursing staff and other personnel to carry open, contaminated needles long distances before disposal. To discourage nursing staff from deferring disposal of contaminated needles because a disposal container is not readily available.
9. Do not recap needles.	To prevent accidental skin puncture during the recapping effort.

pads of her fingertips on the woman's abdomen over the uterine fundus. Sometimes the nurse will feel tension or tightening of the uterus with the fingertips before the woman senses the contraction's onset. The nurse's assessment must include intensity, duration, and frequency.

The intensity of the contraction normally will increase, reach a peak, and then slowly diminish. Intensity is described as mild, moderate, or strong. With mild contractions the fingertips can indent the abdomen easily (similar to feeling the fleshy cheeks of the face). With moderate contractions the fingertips can indent the fundus only slightly (similar to feeling the chin). With strong contractions the fingertips cannot indent the abdomen (similar to feeling the forehead). See Figure 20-2 for a nurse assessing uterine contractions.

Intensity of uterine contractions may be described and documented in several ways:

- Mild, +1, soft
- Moderate, +2, firm
- Strong, +3, hard

If internal uterine monitoring is initiated, the strength of uterine contractions can be measured in millimeters of mercury. (The reader is referred to Chapter 22 for further discussion of intrauterine pressure monitoring and electronic monitoring.)

Duration is estimated from the beginning or onset of one contraction to the end of the contraction and is measured in seconds. *Frequency* is measured from the beginning of one contraction to the beginning of the next contraction.

NURSING PROCEDURE

Performing a Vaginal Examination to Assess Progress in Labor

Purpose: Vaginal examinations are performed to assess progress in labor by noting changes in cervical softening, dilatation, and effacement, as well as fetal descent.

NURSING ACTION	***RATIONALE***
1. Examinations are done only when necessary and only with aseptic technique.	To decrease the risk of infection.
2. Vaginal examinations are contraindicated if vaginal bleeding is present until placenta previa is ruled out.	To prevent hemorrhage caused by dislodgement of a low-lying or complete placenta previa.
Technique	
1. Place the woman comfortably in a supine position with legs flexed and separated. A pillow should be used to support the woman's head.	To promote relaxation during the examination.
2. Place a small pillow or rolled towel under the woman's right hip.	To prevent the heavy uterus from pressing on the vena cava and causing supine hypotension.
3. Explain that the vaginal examination will allow an assessment of progress in labor and, while it may be uncomfortable, should not cause pain.	To reduce anxiety regarding the procedure. To reduce knowledge deficits related to the procedure.
4. Put on a sterile glove. (Some facilities may require use of an antiseptic solution.)	To prevent infection.
5. Lubricate the gloved examining hand.	To reduce friction and tissue trauma related to the procedure.
6. Use sterile water as a lubricant if rupture of membranes has yet to be determined.	To prevent alteration in Nitrazine paper test for rupture of membranes. (Some antiseptic solutions affect Nitrazine paper, making it impossible to determine if membranes are ruptured using this diagnostic methods.)
7. Introduce the index and middle fingers into the vagina with slight downward pressure. Pause briefly. Then advance the fingers and rotate the hand so that the thumb rests outside and above the symphysis pubis.	To position the hand in the appropriate plane for examination of the cervix. The examiner pauses briefly after entering the vagina to allow the woman to become accustomed to the sensation.
8. After inserting one hand in the vagina, place the other hand on the mother's abdomen to allow slight downward pressure on the fundus.	To apply the presenting part more directly to the cervix, which may help determine fetal position by palpation of the fetal presenting part.
9. Advance the examining hand so that the cervix can be felt. This pressure may be uncomfortable, especially during a contraction. Encourage the woman to use relaxation techniques, and reassure her during the examination.	To decrease discomfort associated with the examination. To promote relaxation of skeletal muscles so that the hand may be advanced more easily.

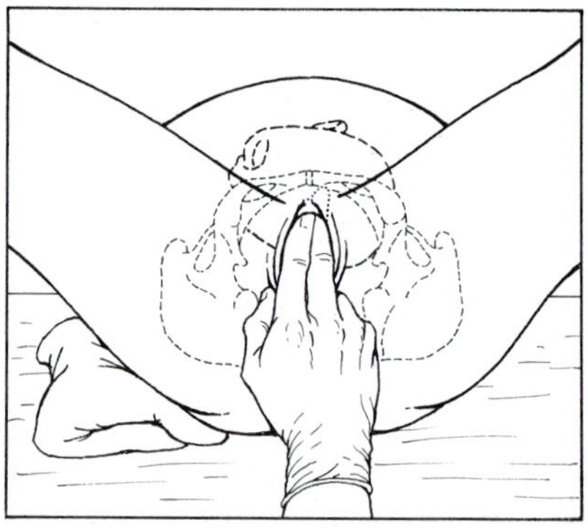

Step 7

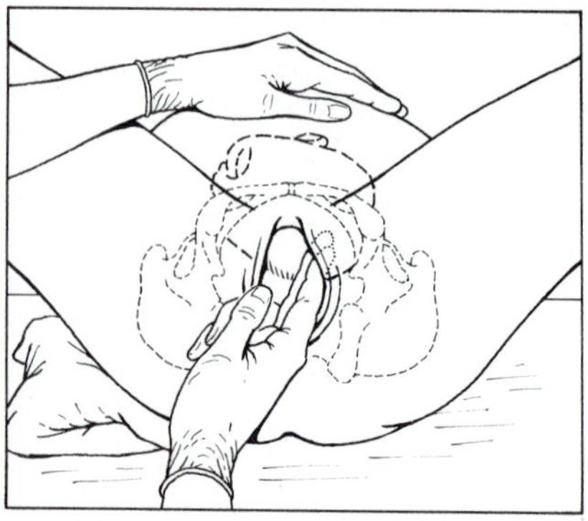

Step 7

(Continued)

NURSING PROCEDURE
Performing a Vaginal Examination to Assess Progress in Labor (Continued)

NURSING ACTION	*RATIONALE*
10. Make the following assessments: • Status of membranes (intact/ruptured/bulging) • Status of cervix (dilatation/effacement/consistency/position) • Fetal presentation (head/breech/shoulder) • Fetal position (left/right/anterior/posterior) • Fetal station (floating/ballotable/engaged)	To determine stage of labor and relationship of fetus to maternal pelvis.
11. Remove the examining hand gently, and explain the findings to the woman and her partner.	To keep them informed. To enhance woman's sense of participation in the labor and birth experience.
12. Dry the perineal area, and place clean absorbent pads under the buttocks. Help the woman to a comfortable position.	To promote comfort.

Obtaining the Admission History and Performing the Physical Examination

When a woman is admitted to the labor unit, a complete history and physical assessment are needed. A labor admission is recorded, and a labor and delivery assessment is begun. The nurse reviews the woman's history, which should contain the following items:

- Identifying information, such as name, age, gravidity, parity (including the number of full-term births, preterm births, and spontaneous and therapeutic abortions), last menstrual period, and estimated date of delivery
- History of current pregnancy, including prenatal care, laboratory work, special tests (amniocentesis, sonography); details of any complications or problems and their treatment; a complete review of the prenatal record, if available
- History of past pregnancies, including number, previous complications, size of infant(s), birth intervals, length of labor, and condition of children (eg, normal, term, or premature; congenital defects; early death [sudden infant death syndrome])
- Medical and family history (obtained from the prenatal chart), including drug allergies, other allergies, previous

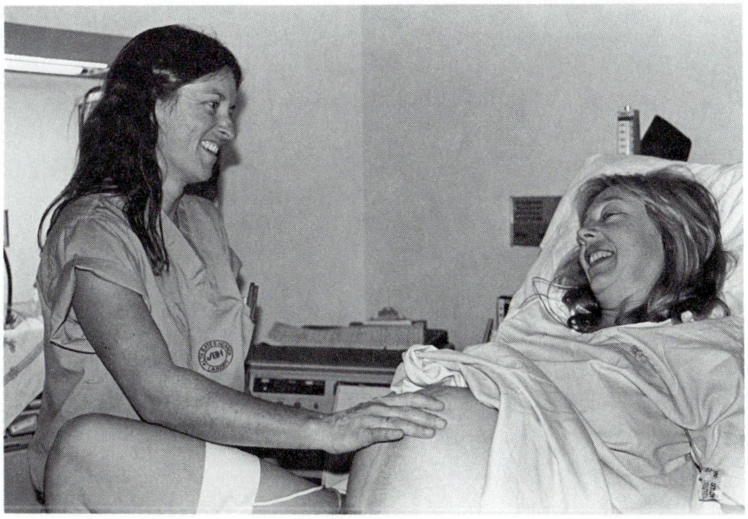

Figure 20-2.
The labor nurse assesses the intensity of the woman's contraction by palpation and observes the woman's response to the first stage of labor. (Photo by Kathy Sloane. Courtesy of Alta Bates Medical Center.)

Assessment Tool

Labor Admission Record

AGE	GRAVIDA	PARA	EDC	WEEKS FROM LMP
DATE LMP / /	LIVE BIRTHS: Living	Dead	OTHER TERMINATIONS: < 20 Wk	≥ 20 Wk
BLOOD TYPE	ANTIBODY SCREEN	SEROLOGY	RUBELLA	
TIME OF ADMISSION	DATE	TEAM		

FEEDING: ○ BREAST ○ BOTTLE Admitted to Alt. Birth Room: ○ YES ○ NO

EARLY DISCHARGE: ○ YES ○ NO

UNIT NUMBER

PT. NAME

BIRTHDATE

LOCATION DATE

PRIVATE PEDIATRICIAN ALLERGIES:

Previous Pregnancy Problems: Date Last Live Birth (Mo./Yr.) [/] Date Last Termination (Mo./Yr.) [/]

Present Pregnancy Problems:

History of Labor: Onset: ________ Character of Contractions ________ Comment: ________

Weight Gain [ ] kg Prenatal Care: ○ Regular ○ Teen ○ HiRisk ○ Private ○ Other

Month First Prenatal Visit [ ] (1st, 2nd, etc.) Total Number Visits [ ]

Comment: ________

Phys. Exam: Weight [ ] kg Height [ ] cm Blood Pressure [ ] T [ ] °C R [ ] P [ ]

○ Normal Head & Neck ○ Abnormal: ________ (Describe)

○ Normal Heart & Lungs ○ Abnormal: ________ (Describe)

○ Normal Breasts ○ Abnormal: ________ (Describe)

Abdomen: Presentation [ ] Position [ ]

FHT [ ] EFW [ ] g

○ Normal Extremities ○ Abnormal: ________ (Describe)

○ Normal Reflexes ○ Abnormal: ________ (Describe)

Vaginal: Dilatation [ ] cm Station [ ] Effacement [ ] cm

Pelvimetry: ________

Membranes: ○ Intact ○ Ruptured ○ Spontaneous ○ Artificial Date/Time [/ /]

Fluid: ○ Clear ○ Light meconium ○ Thick meconium

Laboratory: Hct [ ] % Urine Protein [ ] Sugar [ ]

Other: ________

Diagnosis: ________

Proposed Management: ________

________ M.D. __ __ __ __

________ Clinical Clerk

________ M.D. __ __ __ __

Assessment Tool

Labor and Delivery Nursing Assessment

I. ADMISSION DATA:
A. Medication taken during pregnancy: ______
B. Date and time of last dose: ______
C. Contact with communicable disease: (Circle one) Rubella – Measles
Hepatitis – Mumps – Herpes – Gonorrhea – Other
D. BP range during pregnancy: ______
E. Date and time of last meal: ______
F. Valuables: Yes No G. Disposition of valuables: sent home – held in safe – to postpartum
H. Fatigue level: Rested – Tired – Exhausted
I. Anxiety level: Alert – Excited – Maintains control – Fearful – Anxious – Out of control
J. Support person present: ______

II. ADMISSION ASSESSMENT: ______

Nurse's Signature: ______ Date: ______ Time: ______

III. DELIVERY AND PARENTAL–INFANT INTERACTION DATA:
A. Behavior of infant (Circle appropriate response):
1. Crying: None – Periodic – Almost continuous
2. Affect: Difficult to arouse – Dozes – Eyes open – Very alert
B. Verbal responses of mother (Circle those that apply):
1. Calls baby by name
2. Comments on beauty of baby and/or on realistic defects
3. Talks about baby
4. Asks husband or nurse if baby is all right
5. Voices unhappiness over sex of baby
6. Answers in monosyllables
7. Complains of difficult labor and delivery
8. Doesn't talk about baby
9. Requests baby be taken to nursery
10. Calls baby "it"
11. Uses unhappy or scolding inflection
C. Nonverbal responses of mother (Circle those that apply):
1. Looks, reaches out to baby
2. Hugs, kisses baby
3. Smiles at baby
4. Positive eye contact with partner
5. Holds hand of partner
6. Breast feeds baby
7. Sleepy, not drug-induced
8. Tenses face, arms
9. Turns head from baby
10. Unresponsive to partner/nurse
11. Doesn't touch baby
12. Doesn't look at baby
13. Pushes baby away
14. Cries unhappily

IV. ASSESSMENT OF PARENT RESPONSE TO BABY: ______

Did this family meet their expectations of labor and delivery? ______
If no, why not? ______

Signature ______ Date/Time ______
Nurse

blood transfusions, and major medical problems (should be reconfirmed with the woman)
- Assessment of attendance at childbirth preparation classes

The nurse is responsible for conducting a complete systems assessment of the woman. This is performed regardless of the type of birthing facility she has chosen and whether or not the birth attendant also is present to evaluate her status. Nursing diagnoses can be made only after the following systems review is completed by the nurse:

- Assessment of vital signs, including temperature, pulse, and respirations
- Assessment of blood pressure in a sitting position and left lateral position
- Gross examination and systems review

The last entry includes the following:

- *Neurologic system*: deep tendon reflexes and evidence of clonus, headache or visual disturbances, syncope or convulsions, numbness or tingling in extremities or around mouth
- *Cardiovascular system*: heart rate and rhythm, skin color and capillary fill time in nailbeds, edema (presence, extent, and location), and varicosities
- *Hematologic system*: pallor, petechiae or ecchymosis, and bleeding from mucous membranes or venipuncture sites
- *Respiratory system*: respiratory rate and pattern; breath sounds; dyspnea, shortness of breath, or cough; hiccups; and odor of breath (fruity or alcohol)
- *Gastrointestinal system*: nausea, vomiting, or diarrhea; epigastric distress; and time of last meal and fluid intake
- *Urinary system*: urine-specific gravity and pH; leukocytes, glucose, protein, or blood in urine on urine dipstick; costovertebral tenderness; and urinary frequency or dysuria
- *Musculoskeletal system*: deformities, fractures, or chronic back pain
- *Genital*: bloody show or mucous discharge, active vaginal bleeding, leakage or gush of fluid from vagina (color, odor, and amount), lesions of external genitalia (signs of sexually transmitted disease, such as vesicles, rash, or condyloma), redness or edema of external genitalia (signs of vaginitis), vulvar varicosities, and scars (prior episiotomy, lacerations, or female circumcision)
- *Skin and mucous membranes*: skin turgor; rashes, lesions, lacerations, or ecchymosis; track marks (substance abuse); nasal discharge or nosebleeds; scars (previous surgery); jaundice; moistness of mucous membranes; and use of dentures, eyeglasses, contact lenses, or hearing aids

In addition the nurse should weigh the woman to determine if there has been a sudden weight gain or loss.

The present labor history is obtained, including onset of contractions, bloody show, rupture of membranes, fetal movement, and frequency, duration, and intensity of contractions.

Finally, a thorough abdominal and pelvic examination is essential. In many settings this assessment is a nursing responsibility. An abdominal examination should include the following:

- General observation of the abdomen for scars, contour, and size
- Abdominal palpation for fetal presentation, lie, position, estimated size, and station (fetal head floating or fixed)
- Fundal measurement (to be compared with weeks of gestation and used in assessment of fetal size)
- Assessment of pattern, strength, and duration of contractions
- Assessment of pelvic capacity, including reevaluation of diagonal conjugate, bluntness or prominence of ischial spines, mobility of the coccyx, and angle of the pubic arch
- Auscultation, Doppler, or external electronic monitoring of FHR
- Observation of any fetal movement

A pelvic examination should include assessment of the following:

- Cervical effacement and dilatation
- Position of the cervix (anterior, posterior, or midposition)
- Fetal station
- Presenting part and position, if possible
- Presence of molding or caput
- Status of amniotic membranes
- Pelvic capacity
- Status of perineum

The comprehensiveness of this nursing assessment is modified if the woman presents in very active labor or delivery is imminent; however, it is imperative that as much information as possible be elicited to provide her with appropriate nursing care.

Obtaining and Reviewing Laboratory Tests

The woman's prenatal laboratory tests should be evaluated, especially the hematocrit (which may reflect anemia), blood type, and Rh test (which will determine the need for Rh immunoglobulin administration in the immediate postpartum period). On admission to the labor unit, a hematocrit value is repeated, and a urinalysis for protein, glucose, and ketones is performed. A blood sample is collected for typing and crossmatching in case transfusion becomes necessary, and a complete blood count (CBC) is obtained to establish a baseline for later assessment. The nurse should review findings of prenatal laboratory studies and note any pending studies as part of the initial assessment. The nurse reviews the information provided by the history, physical examination, and laboratory tests to assess the woman's level of obstetric risk.

Identifying Birth Plans and Preferences

As part of the comprehensive nursing assessment, the nurse should determine the woman's desires and expectations regarding the childbirth experience. Many women have discussed their options and alternatives with the midwife or physician during the prenatal period (see Chapter 13). A "birth plan" form may be completed before labor and attached to the prenatal record or brought to the birthing unit at the time of admission. The nurse should review this form with the woman and her support person and incorporate their preferences into the plan of care. If the assessment reveals abnormal findings or significant problems, the birth attendant and nurse should discuss how they will alter the birth plan.

Determining Maternal and Fetal Risk Status

Each maternity unit has explicit risk criteria, which are used to determine the type of obstetric and nursing care

Birthing Room Risk Criteria

Factors Precluding Admission to the Birthing Room

Social Factors

- Less than three prenatal visits
- Maternal age: primipara over 35 years of age; multipara over 40 years of age*
- Maternal substance abuse

Preexisting Maternal Disease

- Chronic hypertension
- Moderate or severe renal disease
- Heart disease, Class II–IV
- History of pregnancy-induced hypertension with seizures
- Diabetes
- Anemia (hemoglobin level less than 9.5 g/100 mL)
- Tuberculosis
- Chronic or acute pulmonary problem
- Psychiatric disease requiring major tranquilizer

Previous Obstetric History

- Previous stillbirth of unknown etiology
- Previous cesarean birth
- Postpartum hemorrhage
- Rh sensitivity
- Multiparity greater than 5†
- Previous infant with respiratory distress syndrome at same gestation

Factors in Present Pregnancy

- Pregnancy-induced hypertension
- Insulin-dependent diabetes
- Gestational age less than 37 weeks or more than 42 weeks
- Multiple pregnancy
- Abnormal presentation
- Third-trimester bleeding or known placenta previa
- Prolonged rupture of membranes (over 24 hours)
- Evidence of intrauterine growth retardation
- Contracted pelvis on any plane
- Excessive weight gain (>40 lb) and fetal macrosomia
- Pelvic diseases, such as adnexal mass, uterine malformation, herpes, pelvic tumors, polyhydramnios
- Treatment with reserpine, lithium, or magnesium
- Induction of labor
- Spinal or general anesthesia
- Any other acute or chronic medical or psychiatric illness that would increase risk to mother or infant

Factors Developing After Admission That Require Transfer to Labor and Delivery Unit‡

- Hemoglobin level less than 9.5 g/100 mL
- Temperature over 100.4°F (38°C)
- Significant variation in maternal blood pressure from previous recordings
- Meconium-stained amniotic fluid
- Abnormal fetal heart rate pattern
- Prolonged true labor (over 24 hours)
- Prolonged second-stage of labor (over 2 hours for primagravida; over 1 hour for multigravida)
- Arrest of labor in active phase
- Significant vaginal bleeding
- Development of any factor that requires continuous electronic fetal monitoring
- Any labor pattern or maternal–fetal complication that the physician, nurse midwife, or nurse believes requires more sophisticated diagnosis or treatment than is available in the birthing room

**Relative contraindication: patient may use the birthing room after a period of fetal monitoring in active labor.*
†May use the birthing room with an IV during labor.
‡Should the problem resolve, the woman may be moved back to the birth room.

given to the woman and her family. An example of criteria used in determining whether a delivery may take place in a birthing room is shown in the accompanying display, Birthing Room Risk Criteria. Admission to the hospital or birthing center during active labor is a stressful event for most women and their partners. As part of the admission procedure, the nurse should focus on stress reduction for the laboring woman and her support person(s). Earlier studies have established that excessive stress and anxiety are harmful for the woman and fetus (Lederman, Lederman, Work, & McCann, 1979; Lederman & Lederman, 1985). The nurse can play a key role in stress reduction while beginning to care for a woman in labor by providing support, minimizing noxious environmental stimuli, and teaching or reinforcing relaxation techniques.

Notifying the Birth Attendant

Once the nurse has completed the initial assessment of the woman in labor, the birth attendant is notified of findings. In many instances the physician or nurse midwife is not present in the birthing unit, and a telephone report is made. Critical elements of the report are presented in the accompanying display. The physician or nurse midwife depends on the labor nurse to provide an accurate and complete report to make appropriate decisions about care.

Report to Attending Physician or Nurse Midwife

When the patient has been admitted and assessed by the nurse, the attending physician or nurse midwife should be notified. A report should be given in an orderly manner to facilitate care. The following order of report is suggested:

Identifying Data

- Name
- Age
- Gravida, para
- LMP and EDC
- Weeks of gestation by dates and by examination

Assessment

- Chief complaint or problem (eg, normal labor, active phase)
- Significant prenatal history
- Significant medical or obstetric problems
- Significant laboratory data
- Current vital signs and urinalysis
- Other symptoms—edema, hyperreflexia, costovertebral angle tenderness
- Results of abdominal evaluation—height of fundus, fetal lie, presentation, position, estimated fetal weight, FHR, other significant findings
- Results of pelvic examination—station, effacement, dilatation, status of fetal membranes, fetal position, other significant findings
- Maternal and family responses to labor—emotional status and comfort level as evidenced by self-report and observed behavior
- Significant aspects of birth plan

Performing Ongoing Assessments During the Latent Phase

Maternal Physiologic Status

The nurse must be totally cognizant of adaptations that occur during labor and birth and their resultant impact on maternal vital signs. Standards of nursing practice require evaluation of maternal status at specific time intervals. Table 20-2 lists recommendations for the assessment of vital signs during the three phases of the first stage of labor.

If at any time aberrations in vital signs are noted, the birth attendant must be notified, and the woman must be evaluated more frequently. The following changes in maternal vital signs are indications of potential complications:

Blood pressure: Greater than 140/90 or 10 to 15 mm Hg elevation over prepregnancy levels may signal developing preeclampsia. Lower than 90/50 mm Hg may indicate complications associated with epidural anesthesia or hemorrhage.

Pulse rate: Greater than 120 bpm may indicate an elevated maternal pulse due to anxiety, pain, or excitement, but persistent tachycardia above 120 bpm is abnormal.

Respiratory rate: Greater than 24 breaths per minute at rest or between contractions may indicate cardiovascular or pulmonary disease.

Temperature: An elevation in temperature (greater than 37.5°C [99.6°F]), pulse, or respiration may signal maternal dehydration, developing infection, or hemorrhage.

An elevated pulse rate often is the first sign of maternal hemorrhage and precedes any drop in blood pressure after rapid blood loss.

Progress in Labor

Progress in cervical dilatation, effacement, and fetal descent should be charted in the medical record, as well as on a labor graph (see the labor graph later in the chapter). Vaginal examination should be performed on admission, when any change in labor pattern occurs, and when the woman reports an urge to push. (The nursing procedure for a vaginal examination is provided earlier in this chapter.) Other parameters of progress in labor that should be evaluated and documented at regular intervals include the presence of bloody show; rupture of membranes; color, amount, and unusual odor of amniotic fluid; nature of contraction pattern; and alterations in behavioral states. Table 20-2 summarizes these signs and recommended standards for frequency of nursing assessment.

Fetal Physiologic Status: Heart Rate

Although current research suggests that EFM of the low-risk woman provides no beneficial effects over intermittent auscultation, it is now strongly recommended that the fetus be evaluated initially for 15 to 20 minutes with an external EFM when the woman is admitted to the birthing unit. Electronic fetal surveillance yields more precise information regarding variability in the FHR pattern over time and may identify positive signs of adaptation (accelerations in the heart rate) and nonreassuring signs in fetal status with the onset of labor.

Once a 15- to 20-minute recording is obtained, formal policy normally guides the nurse in the appropriate method of ongoing FHR assessment. Whether continuous EFM or intermittent auscultation of the FHR is performed, both the baseline FHR and the response to contractions should be evaluated and documented at regular intervals throughout labor, according to the Association of Women's Health, Obstetric, and Neonatal Nursing (AWHONN) (formerly NAACOG) guidelines (1990). A list of times to reevaluate FHR is given in the accompanying display.

If the woman and fetus are determined to be low risk, the FHR pattern is assessed and documented:

- Every hour in latent phase
- Every 30 minutes during the active and transition phases
- Every 15 minutes during the second stage of labor

If the FHR is outside the normal range or problems are identified that place the woman or fetus in a high-risk category, assessment and documentation should be performed:

Table 20-2. Standards of Care for Assessment of Maternal Vital Signs and Maternal Progress During the First Stage of Labor

	Latent Phase (0–4 cm)	Active Phase (5–7 cm)	Transition Phase (8–10 cm)
Blood Pressure	60 min	60 min	60 min
Pulse and Respirations*	60 min	60 min	60 min
Temperature†	4 h	4 h	4 h
Contraction Pattern	30–60 min	30 min	15 min‡
Bloody Show	60 min	30 min	15 min‡
Amniotic Fluid	60 min	30 min	15 min‡
Behavior Pattern	60 min	30 min	15 min‡

*An increase in pulse or respiratory rate may be the first indication of maternal infection.

†When membranes rupture, the temperature is assessed every 2 hours.

‡Although the women should be evaluated *at least* every 15 minutes, the nurse's continuous presence at the bedside may be indicated because rapid alterations in maternal status occur in the transition period.

- Every 30 minutes in latent phase
- Every 15 minutes during active and transition phases
- Every 5 minutes during second stage

The baseline FHR should remain between 120 and 160 bpm. Baseline FHR is determined between contractions. If intermittent auscultation is performed, the FHR is counted for 1 full minute between contractions.

Screening for periodic changes also is essential and performed by observing the EFM strip for accelerations or decelerations in the FHR. If auscultation is selected as the method for fetal assessment, periodic changes are identified by listening to the FHR throughout a contraction and for 30 seconds afterward for evidence of acceleration or slowing of the FHR.

Assessment of FHR variability, an important indicator of fetal well-being, can be obtained only by EFM. Further discussion of FHR characteristics, including short-term and long-term variability, is provided in detail in Chapter 22. Indications for EFM and nursing actions are given in the accompanying Nursing Procedure.

The nurse should exercise clinical judgment about the mode of fetal monitoring when maternal or fetal abnormalities occur (NAACOG, 1990). Auscultation may be replaced by continuous external monitoring for at least a 15- to 20-minute interval to determine the nature of any variation detected on auscultation. Appropriate nursing interventions also are implemented to correct nonreassuring FHR patterns.

Equipment Used for Intermittent FHR Assessment. The *Doppler unit* (*Doptone*) is a portable electronic instrument that is used like a stethoscope. The unit emits ultrasound (high-frequency sound) waves that, when reflected off a moving object, in this case the fetal heart, produce echoes. The unit processes these echoes and transmits audible "clicks" to the listener at the rate the fetal heart is beating. The advantages of the Doppler unit are that (1) it is effective when FHR is difficult to hear with a fetoscope or when the nurse has difficulty locating the FHR with an external EFM; (2) it will usually detect the FHR regardless of maternal position; (3) it may reduce the stress and anxiety experienced by some women when continuous electronic monitoring is used; and (4) it allows for freedom in ambulation. The disadvantages of the fetoscope and Doppler units are that (1) the nurse is unable to evaluate FHR variability, an important indicator of fetal well-being; (2) abnormalities in FHR patterns that occur between auscultation are missed; (3) some women dislike the interruptions that occur when the nurse must perform frequent intermittent auscultation; and (4) it requires a one-to-one nurse–patient ratio when every 15-minute assessment is indicated (NAACOG, 1992), which may not be possible in a busy obstetric unit.

Reevaluation of the Fetal Heart Rate

When intermittent FHR auscultation has been selected as the method of evaluation, the nurse must reassess the FHR prior to and after the following interventions or activities:

Reassess Before:

- Initiation of labor-enhancing procedures (ie, rupture of membranes)
- Administration of analgesia or anesthesia
- Administration of other medications
- Ambulation

Reassess After:

- Recognition of abnormal uterine activity
- Alteration in infusion rate of oxytocin
- At the peak effect time of medications
- Rupture of membranes
- Urinary catheterization
- Vaginal examinations
- Expulsion of enema
- Period of ambulation

NAACOG. (1990). OGN Nursing Resource. Fetal heart rate auscultation. *Washington, DC: Author.*

NURSING PROCEDURE
Monitoring Electronic Fetal Heart Rate

Purpose: To identify abnormal fetal heart rate patterns. The following FHR patterns detected by auscultation indicate further, more precise assessment is required:

Baseline Fetal Heart Rate
- Tachycardia: FHR of 160 beats per minute or faster for 10 minutes or more.
- Bradycardia: FHR below 120 beats per minute for 10 minutes or more.

Periodic Changes
- Acceleration: Transitory (usually less than 10 minutes) increase above the FHR baseline.
- Acceleration is not associated with fetal distress, but when it occurs consistently and uniformly with uterine contractions, it may be a forerunner of fetal compromise.
- Deceleration: Transitory (less than 10 minutes) decrease the FHR baseline. Deceleration that occurs with the onset of contractions and in which FHR returns to baseline rate by the end of the uterine contraction (early deceleration) is not of clinical concern. All other deceleration patterns require further assessment.

If any of these FHR variations are detected, do the following:

NURSING ACTION	***RATIONALE***
1. Initiate continuous external electronic monitoring of FHR.	To collect additional data regarding fetal status, including long-term variability and periodic changes that may not be identified by intermittent auscultation.
2. Place the mother in a left, sidelying position.	To eliminate possible maternal supine hypotension or positional cord compression.
3. Turn to the right side if no change occurs or deceleration worsens.	To determine if fetal cord compression can be corrected by placing the woman in other positions.
4. Alert the physician or nurse midwife to the nature of the FHR variation and response to position change.	To obtain appropriate assistance from the primary health provider.
5. Administer 100% oxygen.	To improve fetal oxygenation.
6. Administer oxygen by tight face mask at 8 to 12 L/min.	To provide maximum oxygen concentration. The use of nasal prongs for the administration of oxygen is insufficient when signs of hypoxia occur. A maximum oxygen concentration of only 45% can be delivered at the highest recommended flow rate of 6 L/min. Mouth breathing will further reduce the oxygen concentration when nasal prongs are used.
7. Initiate an intravenous infusion if nonreassuring pattern persists.	To improve maternal circulation and provide access for medications.
8. Explain actions to woman. Explain that more evaluation, and possibly treatment, may be needed.	To reduce the woman's level of anxiety and to reduce knowledge deficits related to treatment.

The external electronic fetal monitor is an instrument that allows for intermittent or continuous monitoring of FHR and the duration and frequency of uterine contractions through sensors strapped to the woman's abdomen. It may be used for intermittent auscultation or continuous FHR evaluation. External EFM uses an ultrasound transducer to monitor the FHR in the same way as the portable Doppler unit. The EFM usually displays a digital readout of the FHR and produces amplified sound and a continuous graphic display of the FHR pattern. In addition the monitor also has a tokodynamometer (tocodynamometer), which, when positioned on the uterine fundus, records the frequency and duration of uterine contractions.

EFM has the following advantages (adapted from Murray [1988]):

- Reliably identifies healthy fetuses
- Permits evaluation of FHR variability
- Improves outcome for low–birth-weight infants
- Identifies more acidotic fetuses than intermittent auscultation
- Allows woman or coach to see contractions and assist woman with breathing
- May reassure woman to hear heartbeat
- Avoids need to interrupt woman to auscultate FHR during contractions

- Provides permanent record of FHR patterns and nursing and medical interventions

EFM has the following disadvantages (adapted from Murray [1988]):

- Reduces maternal mobility in labor
- May increase maternal discomfort (monitor belts or decreased position options)
- May interfere with effleurage (monitor belts and abdominal elastic binder)
- May cause anxiety in woman and labor support person
- May lead to unnecessary obstetric interventions and higher cesarean rate when used by clinicians inexperienced with interpretation
- Has limited value between 20 and 30 weeks of gestation
- May cause nurse to spend more time observing monitor than woman

The *fetoscope* is a modified stethoscope with a headpiece that allows FHR to be heard more clearly by using bone conduction and air conduction of sound. Although it is an inexpensive and noninvasive method, it is rarely used today in traditional hospital settings. The instrument is most effectively used to auscultate during and immediately after a uterine contraction. Only gross abnormalities can be detected, however, and if the woman is obese, effectiveness is reduced. The fetoscope can be used during labor with the woman in a sidelying or semisitting position.

Nursing Research

Women's Expectation of the Labor and Delivery Nurse

The expectations of women regarding the roles and responsibilities of the labor nurse vary significantly. Mackey and Lock discovered that, while many women expressed a need for close and frequent contact with an expert labor nurse, others desired limited nurse involvement during labor. Women who desired limited contact were well prepared for childbirth with their husbands, saw themselves as able to manage the labor process, and viewed themselves as the primary decision makers in establishing goals and planning care. All participants in the study expected nurses to perform assessments and monitor and keep them informed of the progress of labor. They also wanted the nurse to answer questions and provide salient information about labor and birth. The desire and need for the provision of support and comfort measures was expressed most frequently by women who desired close and extended contact with the nurse. These findings should sensitize nurses to the possibility that childbearing women will have varying needs and expectations about their care. The nurse should identify and respect the woman's expectations and clarify for her essential aspects of nursing care.

Mackey, M., & Lock, S. (1989). Women's expectations of the labor and delivery nurse. *Journal of Obstetric, Gynecologic, and Neonatal Nursing, 18*(6), 505–512.

Assessing Behavioral Adaptation

Maternal Responses

The nurse's assessment of the emotional status and behavioral adaptation of the woman and her partner or support person(s) completes the data base that will guide nursing care planning. The labor nurse notes psychosocial factors likely to affect how the parents will respond to labor, including the following:

- Mood or affect
- Signs of anxiety
- Attention span
- Body language
- Energy level

As the labor nurse completes admission procedures and the initial assessment, he or she asks questions regarding the woman's feelings and concerns about being in labor and observes nonverbal cues that indicate her emotional status. The nurse should observe the woman's responses to admission procedures, her partner or support person, and the uterine contractions. Is she excited and eager for information? Does she understand what is said and appear well prepared for labor? Does she appear fearful, uncomfortable, and confused by conversations and activities around her? Does she have a birth plan? The nurse should ask the woman how she has been feeling for the last 24 hours before admission: Has she been sleeping well or poorly? Has she been unusually active? Does she feel tired now? When did she last eat? Does she feel as though things are "under control" at home? These factors help the nurse assess the nature of psychological adaptations to early labor and to plan for support strategies as labor progresses.

Social, cultural, and demographic factors to be assessed are the following:

- Age, educational level, and socioeconomic level
- Overall response to pregnancy
- Previous experience with childbearing
- Cultural background
- Type of health care provider (certified nurse midwife or physician)
- Extent and type of health insurance
- Extent of prenatal care
- Family constellation and support system
- Extent and type of preparation for birth and parenthood

Considerations in the maternal support system include the following:

- Family constellation (single parent, nuclear, extended, blended family)

- Marital or partner status
- Nature of relationship (traditional or lesbian couple)
- Extent of father involvement
- Presence of siblings at birth
- Designated labor coach
- Individuals selected to participate in birth

The nurse should observe the woman's interaction with her support person(s) and try to identify how she is likely to use that support. The presence of a caring person during labor and birth, especially the father, has a positive effect on the length of labor and the woman's perception of childbirth. The person's supportive presence, rather than training or skill in labor coaching techniques, seems to be the important factor. In several studies women have reported that they were more comfortable, less fearful, and perceived their childbirth experience more positively when their partners or other support persons were present (Hofmeyr et al., 1991; Mackey & Lock, 1989; and Birch, 1986).

One way the nurse can determine the nature of the support relationship is to ask how the couple prepared for childbirth and what they desire from the nurse in terms of support and coaching during labor. Does the woman rely on her partner to assist with labor coping techniques (such as breathing or relaxation) or for reassurance and emotional support? Does she desire her partner, family, or friends to be present for "the experience" but expect the nurse to assist with coaching? How the woman seeks out and uses support systems during labor is an important aspect of the nurse's assessment, because the most effective nursing interventions will be tailored to fit that pattern.

For instance if the woman relies on her support person(s) for emotional sustenance and reassuring presence, the nurse can help by facilitating close contact. The nurse may want to concentrate her activities on coaching efforts and provision of physical comfort. If a designated labor coach is present to assist the woman, the nurse can "coach the coach." The nurse provides positive feedback to that person, offers frequent snack and bathroom breaks, and assists with additional coping techniques when requests for help or nonverbal cues suggest the need for intervention.

Paternal and Support Person Responses

Nurse researchers have examined the unique responses and roles of the father during labor. The nurse plays a critical role in the expectant father's actions and perceptions during childbirth and can strongly influence the quality and nature of the experience.

Whether the support person is the father, family member, or friend, the nurse should assess his or her responses to early labor and to the admission procedures. Does the individual appear confident or unusually anxious? Does he or she appear to understand conversations and activities surrounding the admission? Are there spontaneous efforts to physically or emotionally support the laboring woman?

A critical aspect of the nursing assessment is to determine the role the support person plans to perform during labor and birth. Although an increasing number of fathers attend the birth of the infant, the type and nature of support varies widely and is influenced by socioeconomic status, cultural and ethnic background, education, and previous experience with childbirth. In a qualitative study by Chapman (1992) three distinct expectant father labor roles were identified: "coach," "teammate," and "witness." The nurse should respect the decision made by the couple regarding the expectant father or support person role.

Nursing Research

Expectant Fathers' Experience During Labor and Birth

Nurses have been instrumental in reducing barriers to father and family presence in the birthing unit. Currently there is strong support and encouragement for father presence and participation in the birth of the infant. Little research, however, has been conducted to determine the concerns, needs, and roles of father during childbirth. Chapman conducted a qualitative study in which expectant fathers were observed during childbirth and later interviewed about their experiences. The men functioned in three roles: coach, teammate, or witness. Coaches colabored with their mates, directing them in breathing, relaxation, and pushing efforts. Men who viewed themselves as teammates provided a wide range of physical and emotional comfort and support. Witnesses were primarily observers of the birth process. The woman in labor and the nurse strongly influenced the expectant father's development and redefinition of his role. The labor nurse should attempt to identify the expectant father's role as early as possible in labor and encourage and respect the man's efforts to intensify or withdraw from involvement as the labor progresses.

Chapman, L. (1991). Searching: Expectant fathers' experiences during labor and birth. *Journal of Perinatal and Neonatal Nursing, 4*(4), 21–29.

• • Nursing Diagnosis

Based on a systematic assessment the nurse identifies nursing diagnoses that will direct ongoing care during the latent phase of first-stage labor. The following nursing diagnoses indicate needs of families admitted in the latent phase of labor. They may be addressed independently and priorities based on the nursing diagnoses assigned.

- Anxiety related to unfamiliar surroundings, pain, or lack of knowledge about the process of labor
- Pain related to uterine contractions
- Fatigue related to prolonged labor
- Ineffective Individual Coping related to prolonged labor
- High Risk for Infection related to premature rupture of membranes

- Altered Systemic Tissue Perfusion (vena cava syndrome) related to maternal position during labor

• • Planning and Implementation

After establishing appropriate nursing diagnoses, the labor nurse collaborates with the woman and her birth attendant to plan care for the woman in labor. Written or verbal orders are given to guide the nurse in provision of care. Preprinted standing orders for labor and delivery frequently are used by physicians or midwives to expedite the admission process. An example of standing orders is provided. Specific procedures, such as the type of fetal monitoring to be performed, are determined. An admission "prep" may be ordered at this time. See the accompanying display regarding routine preps. The nurse discusses the plan of care with the woman before implementing any procedure and allows time for questions from the woman and her support person.

Providing Emotional Support

By the last few weeks of gestation, most women are eager for the birth of the infant and the concomitant release from minor and more disabling discomforts of pregnancy. As the first signs of labor begin, however, the woman may become anxious because of perceived threats to herself and the fetus. Perceptions of pain may heighten the anxiety, and knowledge deficits add another dimension to the woman's fears. Nursing interventions are aimed at minimizing anxiety. A warm, supportive, and empathetic demeanor can put the woman and her partner at ease. All procedures should be explained before implementation. Admission procedures and orientation to the unit or birthing room should be accomplished without haste in the latent phase of labor to minimize the risk of sensory overload. The family should be encouraged to voice concerns and to ask questions as they arise. The woman is made to feel at home in her new surroundings and free to have her support system with her. Indigent patients or those from other cultures may require special nursing attention as they enter the hospital environment (see the accompanying Legal and Ethical Considerations display).

Expected Outcome

- The woman in labor demonstrates a decrease in anxiety as evidenced by verbalization of her understanding of interventions and her satisfaction with the emotional support provided by the nurse.

Promoting Rest and Comfort

Although uterine contractions are generally mild during the latent phase of labor, each woman's perceptions of discomfort is different. The body area most affected by pain sensations also varies. Many strategies may be used to alleviate discomfort, and a major responsibility of the labor and delivery nurse is promoting comfort and using nonpharmacologic techniques to minimize pain. The nurse should encourage ambulation and rest in an upright position (at least a 30-degree elevation). Suggesting a refreshing shower or bath and recommending massage by the labor coach can help the woman in the early stage of labor to reduce sensations of restlessness, discomfort, and anxiety. It may be helpful for the woman to listen to soothing music. Television viewing may be an effective distraction strategy for others. Breathing techniques can be used but should not be started too early or maternal exhaustion might occur later. The woman should be encouraged to take light nourishment or clear liquids and to empty her bladder at least every 1 to 2 hours. Normalizing the experience for the woman is the key to promoting comfort. For a discussion of pharmacologic measures, see Chapter 24.

Expected Outcomes

- The woman in labor uses strategies such as ambulation, effective breathing and relaxation, and comfortable positioning to adjust to her level of discomfort or pain.
- The woman in labor uses effective relaxation strategies to reduce fatigue, maintains adequate fluid and caloric intake to meet energy needs, and verbalizes her understanding of interventions used to promote sleep or encourage active labor.

Providing Support in Prolonged Latent Phase of Labor

Careful monitoring and active nursing management may be required for some women whose latent phase of labor does not follow normal patterns. The most common problems of this type are prolonged latent phase, or prodromal labor, and premature rupture of membranes (PROM). Patients experiencing these problems are likely to be admitted to the labor unit for observation and obstetric intervention.

The latent phase of labor is prolonged if it exceeds 20 hours for the primigravida or 14 hours for the multipara. The unripe cervix is the most common cause, especially in primigravidas, because time and continued uterine activity are required for cervical softening, thinning, and effacement. When this is accomplished, the woman's labor will often proceed normally. Other causes for a prolonged, latent phase of labor include abnormal fetal position, cephalopelvic disproportion, dysfunctional labor, and administration of sedation or analgesia early in labor.

Although a prolonged latent phase is not harmful to the fetus, it can cause sleep deprivation, maternal exhaustion, and increased anxiety. Nursing support should include reassurance, encouragement, and information about the nature of the problem. The nurse should suggest comfort measures, such as warm showers, ambulation, rest, and diversion. Special care must be taken to maintain energy levels and adequate hydration with juices and other clear liquids. An intravenous line may be initiated to maintain fluid balance and prevent ketosis.

The nurse should consult with the nurse midwife or physician when active management of labor is indicated and collaborate in a new plan of care when a prolonged latent phase of labor is diagnosed. Ambulation or possibly nipple stimulation may be encouraged to increase secretion of oxytocin, which enhances uterine activity (Stein, Bardeguez, Verma, & Tegani, 1990). Mild sedatives or narcotics may be used in some cases to promote sleep and avoid maternal exhaustion. (See Chapter 23 on modifying labor pattern.)

Assessment Tool

Standing Orders Form

INSTRUCTIONS
(Doctors write in black ink, nurses in red. Nurse checks orders with the time as she notes them. Doctors and nurses sign their notes. When an order is discontinued, doctor writes "Discontinue, etc." giving date and naming order.

Authorization is given for dispensing by non-proprietary name unless drug order is initiated by the physician opposite the name of the drug.

DATE	TIME

STANDING ORDER—LABOR AND DELIVERY

Admit to Labor and Delivery

Diagnosis:

Allergies:

Activity:

Diet: Clear Liquids

Vital Signs: Maternal—Temperature every 4 hours. (Every 2 hours if R.O.M.)

BP, P+R every 2–4 hours in early labor, and every 1 hour in active stage.

Obtain initial fetal heart rate/uterine contraction tracing for 20 minutes.

Monitoring:

Fetal Heart Rate:

Uterine Activity:

Labs: Urine—Dipstick for glucose/protein/ketones

Blood—Hold clot for blood bank and purple top. Spin hct.

Notify Anesthesia of patient's admission.

Additional Orders:

SIGNATURE ______ M.D. ___

______ Checked By ______ R.N. Time: ______

Expected Outcomes

- The woman verbalizes a reduction in fatigue with the implementation of measures that promote rest and comfort
- The woman demonstrates signs of progress in labor with the implementation of active management techniques.

Preventing Infection Related to Prolonged Rupture of Membranes

Rupture of the membranes 1 hour or more before the onset of labor is defined as PROM. This occurs in 10% to 12% of all pregnancies. The cause of premature rupture in term pregnancies is unknown. Spontaneous labor occurs within 48 hours in 50% to 70% of women with PROM. Premature rupture increases perinatal morbidity and mortality slightly, with an increased risk of infection to woman and infant. Other risks are involved, and they are discussed in Chapter 27.

The optimal obstetric management of premature rupture in term pregnancies is controversial. Some physicians and nurse midwives watch closely for signs of ascending infection or fetal distress but wait several days to see if labor begins spontaneously. Others wait only 6 to 12 hours before initiating steps to induce labor.

Nursing intervention varies to some degree. Nursing support should include monitoring fetal status, decreasing risk of infection, and providing support for the woman and her family. Fetal status may be assessed by frequent or continuous fetal heart monitoring (see Chapter 22). Infection prevention includes limiting vaginal examinations to reduce the risk of introducing contaminants and close monitoring for signs of maternal infection, such as maternal tachycardia, tachypnea or fever, and fetal tachycardia. Vital signs and temperature are recorded every 1 to 2 hours, and maternal CBC is taken every 24 hours. In some situations prophylactic antibiotics may be ordered as well.

Active nursing management includes interventions aimed at promoting labor, as described previously for the prolonged latent phase. In addition the nurse may be responsible for administering and monitoring oxytocin (Pitocin) by intravenous drip to induce labor. (See Chapter 23 for nursing care during induction and augmentation of labor.)

Expected Outcomes

- The woman demonstrates her understanding of the danger of infection as evidenced by her use of appro-

Routine "Preps" for Labor and Birth

The routine use of a perineal prep and an enema in early labor is controversial and is declining in most areas. Some clinicians believe that shaving the perineum facilitates postdelivery repair and improves perineal hygiene in the postpartum period. The routine administration of an enema in early labor is believed by some to stimulate labor and avoids the possibility of expelling bowel contents with consequent embarrassment to the woman during bearing down efforts in the second stage of labor.

Other care providers point out that shaving the perineum may increase the risk of infection and does not aid in postdelivery repair. Further, an enema is likely to be uncomfortable and embarrassing to the woman in labor and does not ensure that bowel contents will be totally absent by the second stage of labor. Many patients also question the need for perineal shaving and an enema in early labor. The nurse should determine the woman's wishes, verify the attending physician's or midwife's directions, and identify contraindications for routine perineal prep and enema before proceeding.

Rapid labor progress with imminent delivery is a contraindication for a routine prep and enema, because monitoring maternal and fetal status and preparation for delivery are nursing priorities in these circumstances. A history or presence of vaginal bleeding contraindicates the administration of an enema, because these signs suggest a placental problem, such as placenta previa or placental abruption; in both cases stimulation of labor must be avoided. Administration of an enema also is contraindicated in the absence of labor and a well-engaged presenting part, because peristalsis and straining caused by the enema may contribute to premature rupture of membranes and umbilical cord prolapse

Legal/Ethical Considerations

Nursing Care of the Homeless or Indigent Childbearing Family

The birth experience for homeless families and those with severely limited resources often occurs in public hospitals. These facilities frequently are affiliated with teaching institutions (medical and nursing schools), and patients may be asked to participate in research or permit assessment and care by students. Privacy is limited.

The nurse, in this setting, must be particularly vigilant in the role of patient advocate. When women in labor are asked for their permission to perform procedures or to conduct research, it must be determined that language barriers or limited education do not prevent informed consent. Every effort must be made to respect the woman's rights, and the nurse must be resourceful in manipulating the environment to provide the best childbirth experience possible.

priate perineal hygiene techniques to reduce the risk of infection.
- The woman remains free of signs and symptoms of infection secondary to PROM.

• • Evaluation

During the latent phase of labor the nurse determines the effectiveness of nursing activities that are focused on maintaining maternal and fetal physiologic integrity and psychosocial well-being. A major goal of care is conservation of maternal energy reserves for the ensuing active phase of labor. The woman should verbalize satisfaction with interventions aimed at promoting comfort and rest, and ingest adequate fluid and calories. She also should remain free of significant complications. The support person or partner will demonstrate comfort with the support role and gain increasing confidence with coaching and assistance with implementing comfort measures for the woman.

A woman in the latent phase of labor often expresses feelings of excitement and relief. The long-anticipated birth of the neonate has now arrived. The discomfort created by uterine activity and cervical dilatation is not yet intense, and most women can maintain self-care activities that promote comfort and rest. The major goals of nursing care are to reinforce these self-care activities and review relaxation and pain control techniques appropriate for this phase of labor. Efforts are made to normalize this phase of the first stage of labor by encouraging continued mobility and diversional activities.

The Active Phase of Labor

The active phase of labor (5 to 7 cm dilatation) is distinguished by a marked change in the pace and intensity of the labor process. The major characteristics of this phase are increased uterine activity and descent of the fetus into the bony pelvis. Nursing care is focused on monitoring maternal physiologic and behavioral adaptations, as well as fetal adjustments during this time of rapid change. Goals of care include assuming self-care activities for the woman as she moves through active labor, providing appropriate emotional support and comfort measures, and monitoring for fetal well-being and normal labor progression.

• • Assessment

Nursing assessment continues throughout labor. If the woman is admitted in active labor, the initial assessment is especially important. The nurse's initial assessment of the physical and emotional status of the woman and of the father or support person lays the foundation for nursing care. In active labor the nurse modifies the patient evaluation. The minimal components of the assessment include an evaluation of cervical dilatation and effacement, membrane status, contraction pattern, fetal and maternal physiologic status, and a brief review of the prenatal history. A physical examination is conducted and may be abbreviated if labor is intense and rapid. The nurse also obtains essential laboratory tests (CBC, blood type, and hold clot). Psychosocial and emotional status are briefly assessed. After completing the initial assessment, the nurse begins the process of assessing the maternal, fetal, and family responses to labor. This ongoing assessment focuses on the following major areas:

- Maternal physiologic status
- Progress of labor
- Status of membranes and amniotic fluid
- Fetal physiologic status
- Behavioral adaptations

Performing Ongoing Assessments

Maternal Physiologic Status

Maternal vital signs should be assessed throughout labor. Table 20-2 summarizes the standards for assessment of maternal vital signs in active labor. Care should be taken to obtain vital signs between contractions as uterine activity, controlled breathing patterns, and pain can significantly alter maternal blood pressure, pulse, and respiratory rate.

The nurse also must monitor fluid balance. With the increase in uterine activity and level of discomfort that frequently accompany the active phase of labor, the woman may reduce her oral intake. Dehydration and ketosis can occur and will decrease energy levels and adversely affect the fetus. If an intravenous line is inserted, the amount of intravenous fluids administered must be closely monitored. Likewise, pain and fatigue may interfere with the woman's attention to bladder function. Measuring output and performing periodic dipstick evaluations of urine to determine specific gravity and detect ketonuria is an essential aspect of nursing care. Frequent palpation of the bladder for distention is an integral component of assessment, particularly when analgesia or regional anesthesia are administered, because they may further reduce the urge to void.

Progress of Labor

If epidural anesthesia is not used, an experienced nurse will be able to estimate the extent of cervical change and progress in labor by observing the woman's behavioral cues. The accompanying display lists behavioral cues to the phases of labor.

During the active phase of labor, vaginal examinations are performed periodically to evaluate progress in cervical effacement and dilatation, determine station and position of the fetal presenting part, and establish the status of membranes. The degree of fetal head molding and the development of caput succedaneum (scalp edema) also are noted and documented if they occur. The frequency of vaginal examinations depends on the woman's condition, and status of membranes, contraction pattern, behavioral cues, and fetal physiologic status. It is important to monitor closely cervical dilatation and effacement when epidural or regional anesthesia, which reduce sensations of labor, is administered.

If membranes have ruptured, pelvic examinations should be restricted in number to reduce the risk of infection. In this circumstance vaginal examinations are done to verify

Behavioral Cues to the Phases of Labor

Latent Phase

Anticipation
Excitement
Animation, happiness
Relief that labor has started
Some fear and anxiety
Relaxation

Active Phase

Seriousness, growing apprehension
Sense of purpose
Introspection
Fear of being alone, desire for companionship
Change from relaxation to tension
Internal conflict of confidence versus fear
Ill-defined doubts and fears

Transition Phase

Acute sensitivity and irritability
Difficulty in controlling behaviors
Uninhibited behaviors
Fatigue, sleepiness
Amnesia
Horror of being left alone but little desire for interaction
Discouragement and fright
Frustration
Pronounced introspection
Many physical symptoms, including leg cramps, shaking and chills, perspiration, hiccuping, belching, flatulence, nausea and vomiting, heavy bloody show, pulling and stretching sensations low in the pelvis, and severe backache.

significant changes in cervical dilatation as suggested by changes in the woman's behavioral patterns or affect and to confirm complete dilatation before the woman is guided in pushing efforts. An examination also is in order when nonreassuring FHR patterns develop or with fetal bradycardia. The nurse always reevaluates cervical status before pain medication is administered, because sudden progress in labor may be the cause of the increased pain level. The purposes and technique of the vaginal examination during labor are outlined in the nursing procedure in the latent phase of labor.

The progress of labor, as noted by periodic vaginal examinations, is recorded on a labor graph, such as the one shown in the accompanying Assessment Tool. Such graphs can then be compared to Friedman curves for normal labor, which are discussed in Chapter 26.

The pattern and intensity of uterine contractions also are noted; the nurse palpates the intensity of contractions at the fundus and assesses the woman's response to uterine activity. Most women experience an increase in the frequency, intensity and duration of contractions as labor progresses. In some cases the contractions occur so frequently that placental perfusion is reduced and fetal oxygenation compromised. The nurse must palpate the uterus to determine if the uterine muscle is adequately relaxed between contractions.

Placental perfusion is decreased during uterine contraction. Healthy fetuses can tolerate this over the course of labor in the following circumstances:

- If the uterus relaxes well between contractions for long enough (more than 30 seconds) to allow normal perfusion between contractions.
- If contractions are not unusually long (ie, last less than 90 seconds).

Abnormally long, strong contractions, termed tetanic contractions, may follow oxytocin administration to stimulate or augment labor and placental abruption. If uterine contractions last more than 90 seconds or there is 30 seconds or less between contractions, do the following:

- Stop oxytocin administration.
- Change woman to left lateral position.
- Administer oxygen by tight face mask at 8 to 12 L/min.
- Assess FHR pattern.
- Notify physician or nurse midwife.

Other important data, such as quality of contractions and contraction patterns, maternal vital signs, FHR, administration of medications or intravenous fluids, and intake and output, often are charted using a nursing flow chart such as the one shown in the Assessment Tool.

Fetal Physiologic Status

Fetal well-being is evaluated throughout labor. Presentation, position, and station of the presenting part; baseline FHR; and heart rate patterns are critical components of the nursing assessment. Fetal presentation, position, and station are evaluated during maternal pelvic examinations. The presence of fetal head molding and caput helps the nurse assess progress of the fetus through the maternal pelvis.

The FHR is heard most clearly over the upper aspect of the fetal back. To evaluate the FHR the nurse uses Leopold's maneuvers to locate the fetal back and then places the ultrasonic device or fetoscope on the maternal abdomen over this area. This point is called the point of maximum intensity. Because the point of maximum intensity changes as the fetus descends and rotates, the nurse may need to alter the orientation of the ultrasound device, Doppler, or fetoscope on the maternal abdomen to maximize the pickup of the FHR.

When FHR is not being recorded continuously with the EFM, the ultrasonic device or fetoscope is used. It should be placed over the point of maximum FHR intensity. The nurse listens to the FHR for a full minute between contractions to determine the baseline in beats per minute. The nurse then listens to the FHR during the next contraction and for at least

Assessment Tool

Labor Graph

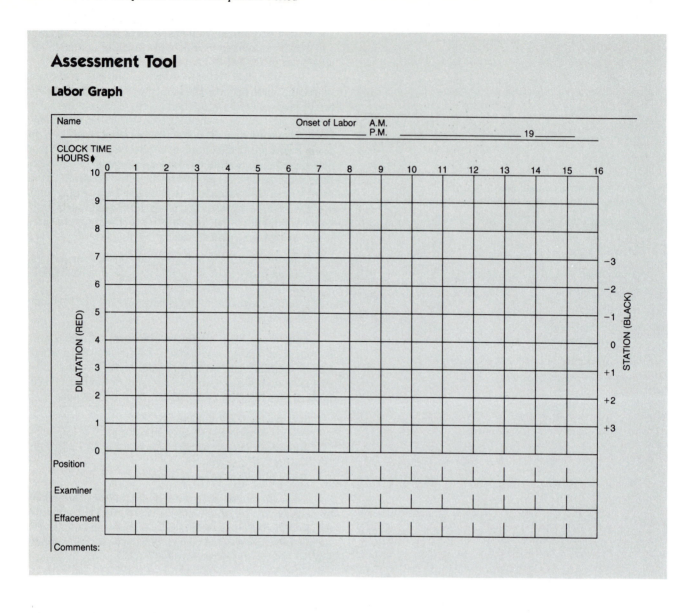

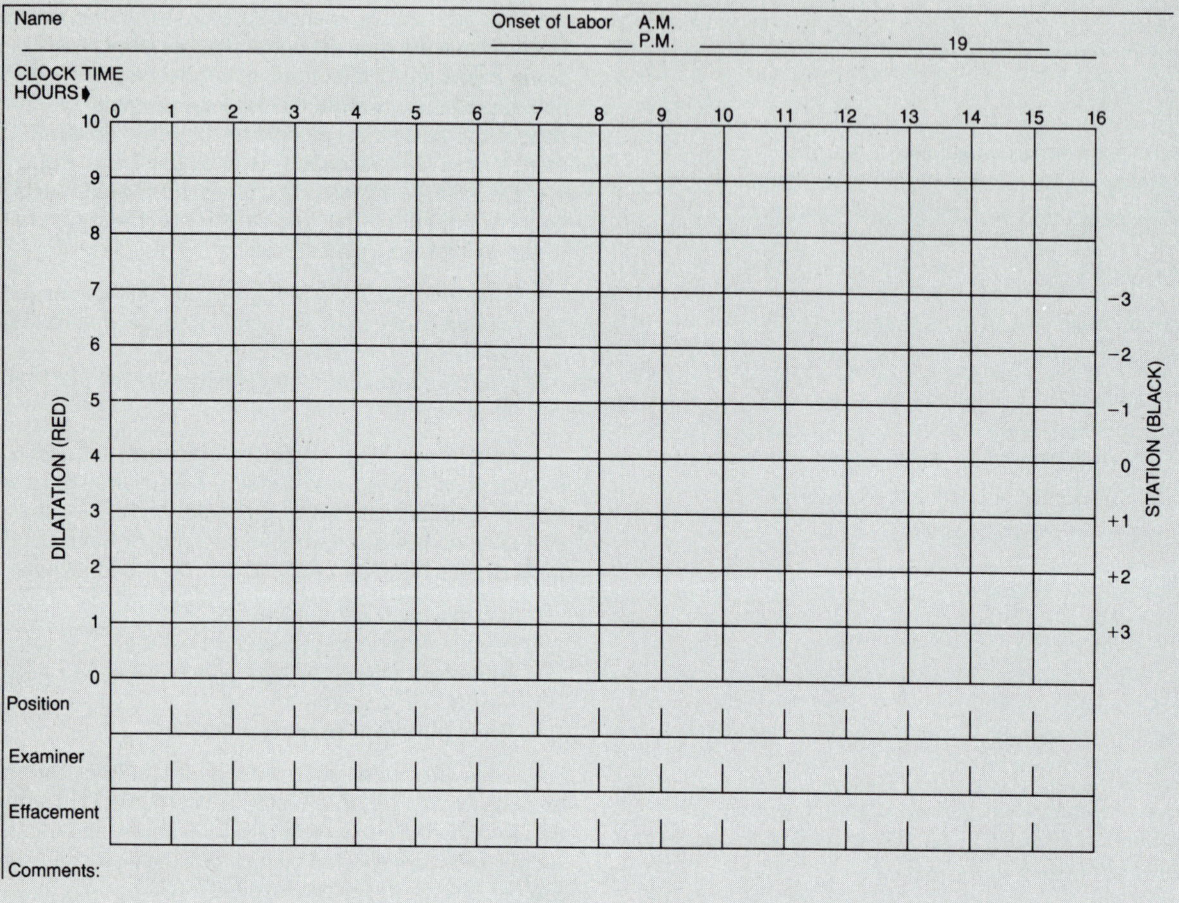

30 seconds after the contraction. Any irregularity or decelerations should be documented, and an external EFM should be applied for 20 minutes to evaluate the FHR pattern further. The nurse should palpate the uterus while listening to determine if the FHR changes in relation to the contraction. If the FHR slows, continuous external electronic monitoring may be indicated to assist in determining the precise nature of the FHR changes (see Chapter 22).

Whether intermittent auscultation or continuous EFM is selected for evaluation of the FHR, the nurse must follow guidelines for FHR evaluation established by AWHONN and discussed in the display that appears earlier in this chapter.

Status of Membranes

Once the membranes rupture, an ongoing assessment of the amniotic fluid characteristics is essential. The color and amount of fluid are noted every time linen or plastic linen protectors are changed and documented at least every 30 minutes to 1 hour. Changes in odor or consistency are immediately noted and reported to the midwife or physician. If meconium staining occurs at any time during labor, the FHR should be reevaluated immediately. When EFM is available the nurse may apply the monitor for 20 minutes to evaluate the FHR and variability and to determine the presence and nature of decelerations. The certified nurse midwife or physician is notified of the nurse's findings.

Assessing Behavioral Adaptation

The nurse also must assess the woman's and her partner's psychosocial responses to active labor on an ongoing basis. The following areas are important parts of the nurse's assessment of both partners as they adapt to the demands of active labor:

- Body posture and movement
- Interaction with partner and staff
- Perceptual status
- Energy or fatigue level
- Responses to disturbing stimuli
- Expressions of discomfort or pain

Each is discussed in more detail in the following sections.

Assessment Tool

Obstetric Flow Chart

DATE		6 AM PM	7	8	9	10	11	DATE 12	1	2	3	4	5	6
39	240													240
	230 ∨													230
38	SYSTOLIC 220													220
	210													210
37	200													200
	190													190
36	∧ 180													180
	DIASTOLIC 170													170
35	160													160
	150													150
34	140													140
	130													130
	120													120
	110													110
	100													100
	90													90
	80													80
	70													70
	60													60
	50													50
	40													40
	30													30
	20													20
	10													10
	0													0
CVP														
DTR/CLONUS														
LABS														
NOTES														
INITIAL														
FHR														
FHRV (NI, ↓, ⍉)														
PERIODIC CHANGES OF FHR														
FSS														
EFM, IFM, ASCUL														
CONTRACTIONS freq x dur x quality														
Montevideo u														
MEMBRANES I=Intact; SROM / AROM (color, date, time, no. hours, odor)														
MEDICATIONS 1														
2														
3														
4														
5														
6														
7														
8														
ALLERGIES														

T° = C
· = ORAL
X = RECTAL
o = Axillary

PULSE
● = RADIAL
x = APICAL

(continued)

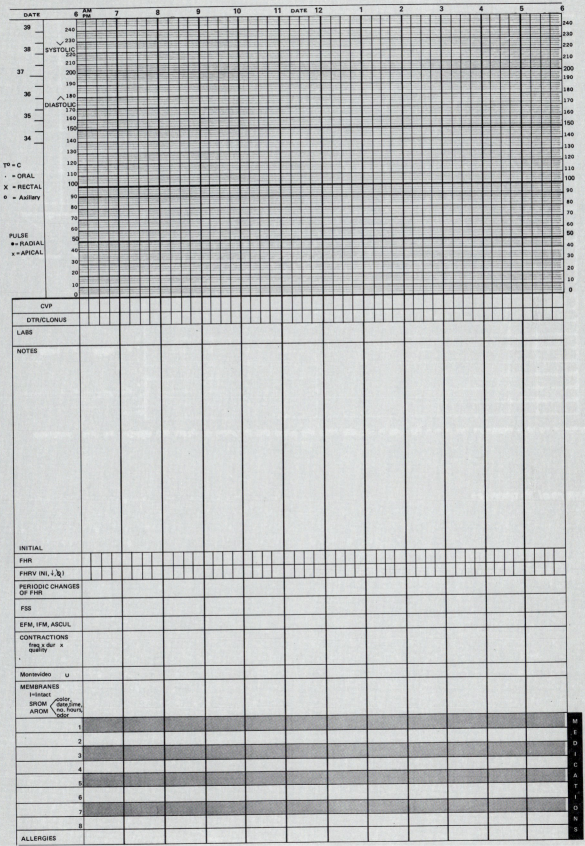

Assessment Tool (continued)

HOURLY INTAKE	I.V.												
	PO												
	OTHER												
HOURLY OUTPUT	URINE												
	OTHER												
UA	PROT												
	SG												
	GLUCOSE												
	KETONE												
	HEME												
	OTHER												

START TIME	BOTTLE NO.	PARENTERAL SOLUTION & ADDITIVES	TIME CHECKED	AMOUNT ABSORBED	LEFT IN BOTTLE	BLOOD	

INTAKE	A I.V. P	PO
	BLOOD	OTHER
	12° TOTAL	
OUTPUT	URINE	EBL
	EMESIS	OTHER
	12° TOTAL	
WEIGHT		

This section of the labor assessment tool permits the nurse to calculate intake and output and document significant data regarding the urine composition.

Maternal Responses

The woman's responses to labor involve physiologic and psychological adaptation to stress. The nurse should observe her body movements and posture for cues of growing fatigue, tension, or pain. If the woman is using relaxation techniques, growing muscular tension should be noted as a sign of increasing stress. However, the nurse should not assume that certain body movements signal an increase in pain. Cultural patterns play a significant part in a woman's behavior in labor; thrashing and crying out may be expected and do not necessarily indicate a need for immediate nursing intervention. Likewise, quiet, stoic behavior does not always indicate that the woman is experiencing little discomfort. The nurse should ask the woman frequently about her discomfort and make use of what the woman says and of observations of the woman's behavior. The woman's interactions with her partner and staff also give important cues to the progress of labor (Fig. 20-3).

The woman's attention and energy normally become inwardly focused as labor progresses, and interaction will become more difficult. This process requires the support person and staff to use more direct methods of interaction and direct, short instructions for communication. The woman's inward focus also will diminish her perceptions of the external environment. She may not hear or fully appreciate information or directives given by the nurse or labor coach. The woman may gradually lose concern about bodily modesty; she may remove clothing and bedding as she focuses intensely on coping with labor. However, the woman's perceptual acuity may increase if she becomes anxious. She may respond dramatically to small bits of information, such as an overheard conversation or a slight change in an attendant's facial expression.

The woman's energy and fatigue level will shift as labor progresses. This will be most noticeable in the later part of active labor. She will gradually avoid unnecessary activity and will rest or even sleep between contractions. She may respond to disturbing stimuli with greater irritability, however, for example, by pushing helping hands away, not permitting painful vaginal examinations or other procedures, or attempting to remove monitor or intravenous lines. The laboring woman's expressions of discomfort and pain are a major focus of the nurse's assessment. The nurse should observe for increasing restlessness and muscular tension. These signs may indicate that pain is increasing and that more effective comfort measures are needed. Another reason that the nurse should be alert for these signs is that they may signal rapid cervical change and faster progress toward delivery. The woman's responses to labor also reflect how well the actual experience fits with her expectations. For

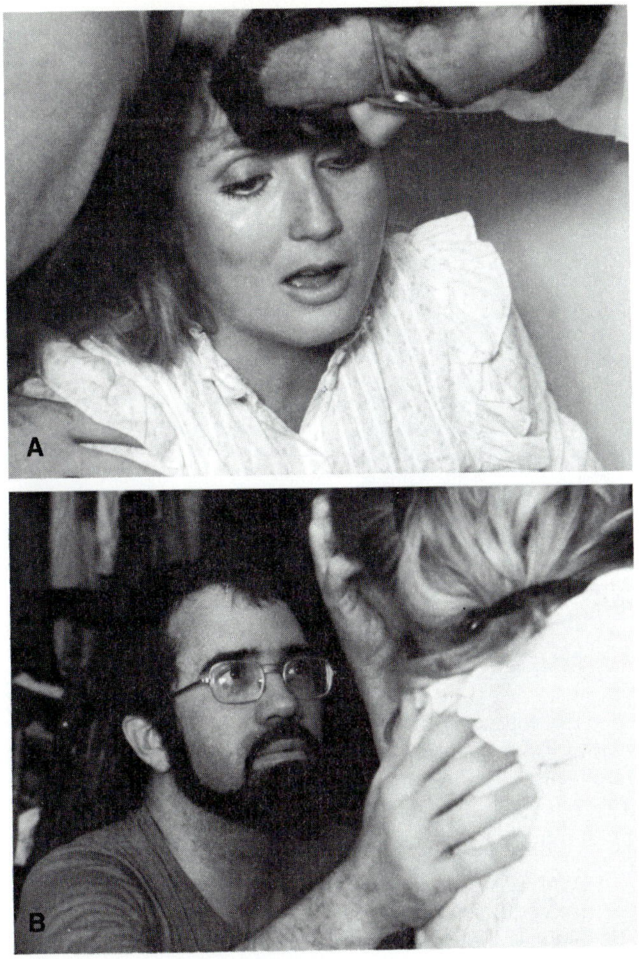

Figure 20-3.
The labor nurse should assess how well the mother responds to her partner's support (*A*) and how well the father is able to interpret his mate's needs as labor progresses (*B*). (Photo by BABES, Inc.)

instance, if she expected breathing techniques to reduce her pain and they seem to have little effect, she is likely to become increasingly anxious and uncomfortable. If she expected labor to progress quickly and it does not, or if unexpected problems arise, she is likely to become discouraged and doubt her ability to make it. This emotional state will decrease her ability to tolerate the demands of labor until she gathers additional energy and support to help her cope.

Paternal and Support Person Responses

The behavior of the father and other support people during labor shows more variability because their responses are based not only on physiologic changes, but also on the type of involvement that has been established. The nurse should keep in mind that virtually all support people and family members are to some extent fearful and concerned about the well-being of the woman and her fetus. No matter how involved they are in the labor process or how well prepared they appear for labor coaching, most individuals feel uncomfortable and unsure of themselves in this situation. They may become unsettled or anxious by some aspects of the birth process. Commonplace events on a labor unit may be mystifying or frightening to them. Nursing care should be directed toward reducing the support person's fears by providing information and emotional and practical support.

The nurse should observe body posture and nonverbal cues. The partner may stay very close to the laboring woman, actively supporting her through contractions, or may stay on the periphery, observing. A change in the posture or position may signal increasing fatigue or fear and should be further evaluated. The nurse also should observe the actively involved partner or family member for signs of muscle fatigue and the strain of bending over or physically supporting the laboring woman. Relief should be provided as necessary.

The partner's interactions with the woman and nursing staff will depend in large part on the type of involvement desired by that individual and the woman in labor. An actively involved partner may need occasional assistance in interpreting the woman's needs. Sometimes the person will need to be shown how to touch or comfort the woman in a different way. The nurse should provide guidance in a positive and supportive manner so that the partner's confidence is not undermined. Responses to labor are not always predictable. Trial and error may be needed to find the best way to comfort the woman.

The support person's perceptions and energy and fatigue level will change as labor progresses. The nurse should suggest frequent breaks for bathroom use, rest, and food and provide relief as needed. Especially during a long or painful labor, the partner is likely to become somewhat discouraged and unable to follow or understand events as they occur. Offering reassurance and pointing out tangible signs of progress may help.

The nurse should be especially alert to family member responses to potentially distressing stimuli. Anxiety-producing stimuli include the woman's appearance (grimacing, gradual loss of bodily modesty, bloody vaginal discharge) and vocalizations (moans, cries, use of expletives, and grunting with pushing efforts). Vaginal examinations, painful procedures, and dramatic perineal changes late in labor also may cause anxiety. Whenever possible, the nurse prepares the woman and her support person(s) for procedures and expected sensations before they occur and observes for signs of increasing emotional distress or discomfort. If family members are disturbed by these sights, they can be encouraged to take short breaks. The nurse also can suggest that the support person move toward the head of the labor bed to comfort the woman, thus limiting their view of some sights that may be disturbing (Fig. 20-4).

Sibling Responses

Settings in which older siblings are present typically have protocols designed to ensure a positive birth experience for all concerned. Such protocols nearly always require that each child have a support person whose responsibility it is to attend to the child's needs and monitor his or her responses to labor. In addition the protocol identifies the circumstances in which siblings will be excluded from attending labor and birth. The nurse's responsibility is limited to monitoring the sibling's and parent's responses (see the accompanying Family Considerations display). When the presence of the child is stressful for the parents or if the child

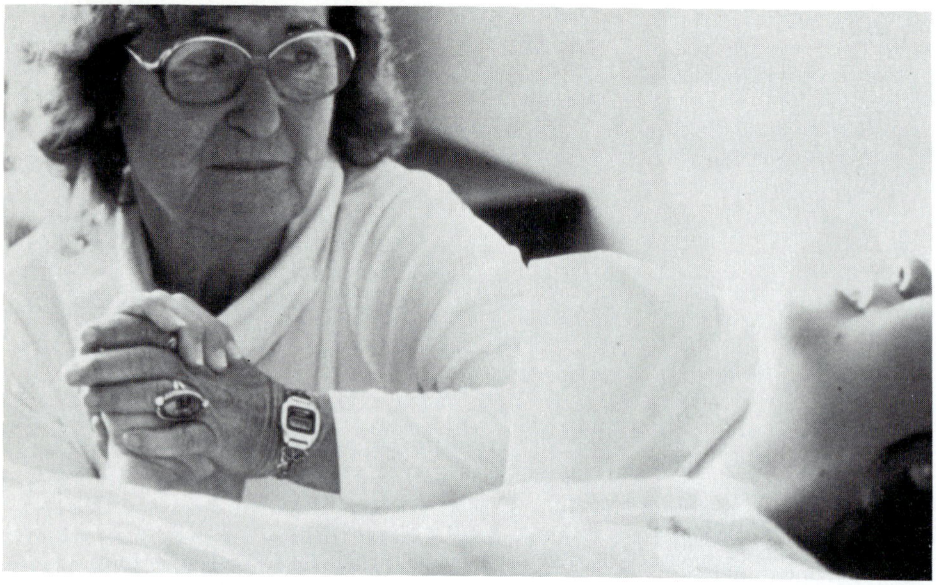

Figure 20-4.
It is helpful for the support person to be at the head of the bed to give encouragement. (Photo by Kathy Sloane.)

appears upset, the nurse should discuss her observations with the parents and support person. It may be advisable to limit the presence of the children during labor if their attention span is limited and the sights and sounds are disturbing to them. They may be invited into the room shortly before the birth.

Family Considerations

Presence of Siblings at the Birth of the Infant

Many facilities have instituted programs to prepare children for the birthing experience. It is often required that an adult, other than the labor coach or partner, be present to supervise the child. The nurse must, however, also assess the sibling's reaction and be prepared to provide comfort and guidance at any time. Behavioral responses will vary with the age of the child. The clinician must be alert to subtle cues of discomfort, mild anxiety, or distress and be prepared to direct the support person if he or she is unable to deal effectively with an upset child. Research suggests positive outcomes for the family when a properly prepared sibling participates in the birth experience. However, further study is indicated to distinguish benefits among different age groups and to identify the risks of permitting siblings to be present during childbirth.

Daniels, M. B. (1988). The birth experience for the sibling. Description and evaluation of a program. J Nurse-Midwifery, *28(5), 21–26.*

Nursing Diagnosis

The following nursing diagnoses may be useful when caring for women and their families in the normal physiologic and behavioral problems of the active phase of labor. These nursing diagnoses may be addressed independently by the nurse and priorities established based on them.

- Altered Nutrition: Less than Body Requirements related to insufficient intake during labor
- Fluid Volume Deficit related to decreased oral intake, nausea, or vomiting
- Altered Urinary Elimination related to pressure of the presenting part or epidural anesthesia
- Anxiety related to perceived threat to self or fetus from impending birth
- Ineffective Individual Coping related to fatigue and discomfort of labor
- Pain related to contractions or nausea and vomiting
- Impaired Physical Mobility related to discomfort, pain, or interventions
- Sensory-Perceptual Alterations related to pain, fatigue, or analgesia
- Self-Care Deficit: Hygiene related to energy depletion and pain in labor

Complications requiring collaboration with other team members may arise during the active phase. Such potential complications include fetal distress, labor dystocia, and maternal hyperventilation. All are discussed at the end of this chapter.

Planning and Implementation

The nurse's assessment and diagnoses may indicate successful physiologic management of active labor. More active nursing management is required when deviations from normal progress arise.

Promoting Nutrition and Hydration

Normal, healthy women may be permitted to eat lightly in early labor and should stop eating in active labor. Low-residue, simple, energy-packed foods, such as toast with honey, crackers, Jello, broth, or frozen juice bars are recommended for early labor. Soothing decaffeinated teas with honey, water, fruit juice, or ginger ale also can be taken. Restricting oral intake and using intravenous infusions during normal labor is not always necessary or justified.

Once the active phase of labor ensues or if the woman requests or requires narcotic analgesics or an epidural anesthesia in the latent phase of labor, she will usually be restricted to clear oral liquids or will remain NPO until the birth of the infant. An intravenous line also will be initiated for administration of fluids and drugs. Many facilities restrict the intake of food or fluids when active management of labor is elected, such as in oxytocin augmentation of labor. Restriction reduces the risks of vomiting and aspiration if a cesarean birth is required or if adverse reactions to the interventions occur. An intravenous infusion is initiated to meet fluid needs in this case. The nurse must be aware of physician and nurse midwife preferences and orders, as well as established hospital policies regarding oral intake during labor and should advise women of these policies. If labor does not proceed as expected, if complications arise, or if the woman is unwilling to take oral fluids or vomits frequently, intravenous hydration is indicated.

When intravenous fluids are ordered during labor, the nurse's responsibility includes administration and monitoring. Physiologic solutions, such as 5% dextrose in Ringer's lactate or plain Ringer's lactate, often are ordered and administered at 100 to 150 mL/h. The nurse should guard against the rapid infusion of dextrose. When rapid hydration is indicated, a physiologic solution such as Ringer's lactate should be infused. Glucose-containing solutions can then be added and administered at a controlled rate of less than 150 mL/h when indicated to meet energy requirement.

Fluid overload must be prevented, especially when oxytocin is administered (due to antidiuretic effect). Careful recording of intake and output is an essential aspect of nursing care.

Expected Outcomes

- The woman in labor maintains an adequate caloric intake to meet energy needs.
- The woman in labor maintains adequate fluid intake to prevent dehydration.

Promoting Bladder Elimination

As the fetal head descends through the birth canal during labor, sensations of pain and pressure may decrease the woman's sensitivity to bladder filling and stretching. Direct pressure of the fetal head on the bladder neck or stretching of the urinary meatus may make it difficult or impossible to urinate. A full bladder can impede fetal descent, is uncomfortable for the woman, and may become a predisposing cause of postpartum hemorrhage. The woman is encouraged to void at least every 2 hours. Nursing measures to aid micturation, such as running water, providing privacy, and pouring warm water over the perineum, are used. Catheterization may become necessary if efforts to keep the bladder empty fail. The possibility of urinary tract infection after catheterization in labor is great, so strict aseptic technique should be used (see the Nursing Procedure on catheterizing the bladder during labor).

Expected Outcome

- At least every 2 hours, the woman in active labor voluntarily voids a minimum of 100 mL/h which is free of ketones, and she maintains urine-specific gravity below 1.020.

Providing Emotional Support and Promoting Effective Coping

One of the strongest childbirth recollections for many women, particularly those who expect frequent, supportive contact with the nurse during labor, is the quality of nursing care. Most women never forget the professional nursing support (or lack of support) provided. A major nursing responsibility is providing the woman in labor and her partner with reassurance and encouragement as labor progresses. The woman becomes increasingly uncomfortable and fatigued as active labor progresses. Interaction with others becomes more difficult for her, because she is preoccupied with coping with contractions. Gradually, she will be less able to tolerate distractions and interruptions and may begin to doubt her ability to cope with labor. She finds it difficult to relax and needs constant reminders and encouragement. Touch, facial expression, and tone of voice are all critical aspects of the nurse's therapeutic role (see the Nursing Research display).

An enthusiastic, reaffirming approach by the nurse may best reinforce the positive feelings of excited happy women in early labor. ("You're doing a great job. We're ready for the birthday party!") If the woman verbalizes fearfulness or is tense or tearful, empathy and understanding are conveyed by the nurse through gentle touch, a soothing tone of voice, and frequent contact. ("Take a deep slow breath in. Hold it. Now let it out and relax all the muscles in your chest. Beautiful!") During the transition phase of labor, inner sensations may overwhelm the woman. Establishing close eye contact, speaking quietly into her ear, and providing brief, clear directives ("Pant! Blow! Perfect!") can be most effective in helping the woman focus her energies and maintain control.

The nurse periodically notes the woman's changing behavior and tailors interventions to her changing needs. The nurse should reiterate progress in labor, provide positive reinforcement, offer expert advice when asked, and communicate empathy for the woman and her family.

Time is often seen as an enemy during labor. The longer labor lasts, the more worried the woman and professionals become. The nurse should avoid focusing on the passage of time. Families often are unaware of the amount of time spent in labor, unless the staff reminds them and directs attention to time as a limiting factor. When no serious complications arise, time during labor can be viewed as an ally. With enough passage of time, many problems are solved in labor without intervention. The nurse's attention should more appropriately be focused on assessing the woman and family and on meeting other needs for comfort, relaxation, and safety.

NURSING PROCEDURE
Catheterizing the Bladder During Labor

Catheterization of the bladder during active labor may require special techniques to prevent infection and trauma, as well as maternal supine hypotension.

Purpose: To empty the bladder when the woman is unable to void as a result of direct pressure of the fetal presenting part on the bladder neck or urinary meatus.

NURSING ACTION	RATIONALE
1. Perform a pelvic examination	To determine the station of the fetal head.
2. Have a second nurse or physician stand by if the presenting part is low.	To assist with the procedure. If the presenting part is low, it may obstruct the flow of urine when the catheter is advanced.
3. After explaining the procedure, place the patient in a supine position, with a pillow or pad under the right hip.	To prevent supine hypotension.
4. Cleanse the vulva.	To remove blood, mucus, and amniotic fluid. This allows for better visualization of the meatus and prevents the gloved hand that retracts the labia from slipping during the procedure.
5. Apply sterile gloves.	To prevent infection.
6. Lubricate the catheter (usually a 14 French).	To prevent tissue trauma when the catheter is passed.
7. Prep the labia minora and meatal opening with a bacteriocidal agent.	To prevent infection.
8. Insert the catheter between contractions.	To reduce maternal discomfort. To reduce the possibility of the fetal presenting part impeding the passage of the catheter. During contractions the presenting part may be pushed downward, making it more difficult to advance the catheter.
9. Do not use force if unable to advance the catheter. Have the assistant place a hand above the symphysis pubis and apply gentle upward pressure on the presenting part while the catheter is advanced.	To prevent tissue trauma. To move the fetal presenting part off of the meatus so the catheter can be advanced.
10. If the catheter still advances with difficulty, attempt to direct it slightly downward toward the sacrum.	To angle the catheter downward so that it advances below the presenting part and into the bladder.
11. In rare circumstances the assistant may need to put on a sterile glove, place the hand in the vagina, and apply direct upward pressure to the presenting part.	To remove pressure from the bladder neck or meatus so the catheter can be advanced and the bladder emptied.

Expected Outcomes

- The woman in active labor verbalizes feelings related to her current emotional state.
- The woman in active labor uses effective coping strategies to enhance feelings of control and well-being.
- The woman in labor makes appropriate decisions with the input of support person(s) and the health care team to change problem situations.

Promoting Comfort

Many nursing support measures facilitate comfort and relaxation throughout labor. Patients will vary in their need for and response to these measures. Careful and thorough nursing assessment and evaluation are needed to meet the individualized needs of each woman and each labor.

Massage

Various forms of massage, including effleurage (light stroking of the abdomen), kneading, and counterpressure, often are soothing to the woman. This tactile stimulation helps with relaxation and pain relief. Effleurage often is used on the lower abdomen, over the lower half of the uterus. It also can be used on the legs or face. Kneading is particularly useful for reducing tension in the neck, shoulders, and back. (Occasionally, this is helpful for the support person(s) as well!) Massage of the feet can be relaxing for some women. Counterpressure is frequently used over the sacrum or the

Nursing Research

The Meaning of Touch During Childbirth

The act of touching is an integral, essential strategy in maternity nursing. Weaver discovered that most nurse-initiated touch was reported to involve intuition—an unconscious, automatic, intuitive action. Examples of therapeutic touch include massage, effleurage, selected pressure (ie, sacral), stroking, hand holding, and even hugging or embracing women in special circumstances. Touch was viewed as a potentially powerful modality for giving and receiving messages. While touching was strongly influenced by intuition, the use of touch can be a learned competency for nurses.

Weaver, D. (1990). Nurses' views on the meaning of touch in obstetrical nursing practice. *Journal of Obstetric, Gynecologic, and Neonatal Nursing, 19*(2), 157–160.

inner thighs (see section on massage techniques in Chapter 18).

Baths and Showers

Baths and showers to promote comfort and relaxation have been underused. Unfortunately, many labor and delivery units do not have bathtubs. Sometimes the staff views labor in the bathroom as undesirable, either because it is inconvenient or because the bathroom is shared with other patients. Ideally, for each woman in labor there should be a private bathroom, including tub and shower. If this is not possible, flexible rules should be established for the use of the bath or shower, including the presence of a support person. The advantages of hydrotherapy include relaxation and pain relief, distraction, and maintenance of the upright position. In a normal labor these advantages would seem to outweigh any inconveniences incurred by the staff.

A single long warm bath or shower may be helpful to the woman. During a long or very painful labor, several 1- to 2-hour sessions may be helpful and assist with general cleanliness. Little is known about the possible risk of ascending infection when bathing with ruptured membranes. Therefore, the woman should use the tub only when membranes are intact. Showers may be taken regardless of membrane status (Waldenstrom & Axel-Nilsson, 1992).

Cold Packs and Heating Pads

Cold packs and aquathermic heating pads can be used to promote relaxation and pain relief, as well as maternal comfort. Cold packs can be made from an ice bag or rubber glove filled with ice. A silica gel cold pack also can be used. Cold packs are particularly helpful over the sacral area. They can be used with counterpressure or alternated with counterpressure when backache is severe. Cool, moist cloths on the forehead, back of the neck, or upper chest can be soothing and refreshing to the perspiring woman.

Heat may be used over the sacral area; it can be soothing when placed on the lower abdomen. Heat applications and massage can be alternated. Care must be taken not to harm the woman's skin with excessive heat, because sensation will diminish after repeated applications of heat or cold. In the past hot compresses made from hot water bottles, or a towel soaked in hot water and wrapped in plastic were used when women desired heat applications. Malpractice suits have been initiated by women who have been burned when these "unapproved" heating pads and compresses have been used. Nurses who choose to use heat as a therapeutic modality should use only hospital-approved aquathermic heating pads.

Relaxation and Visualization

Some women will have practiced relaxation exercises prenatally. They will have spent time consciously focusing on the muscles of the body in a relaxed state and on rhythmic breathing to facilitate relaxation. The nurse should encourage the use of these relaxation and breathing methods and assist the support person in using the techniques. Simple relaxation methods can be taught on the spot to those who have not previously learned them.

The nurse can ask the woman to relax specific muscle groups, such as the legs, neck, face, and perineum. Relaxed rhythmic breathing can be encouraged to help "breathe out the tension" with each exhalation. Relaxation allows the woman to focus her mind on her body, thus experiencing the labor as a psychophysical experience. She neither controls the experience nor totally yields to it. The process of labor and birth is very much affected by the degree of integration between the mind and the body. Sammons (1984) conducted a pioneering study to explore the effects of music during labor. Findings suggest that music may enhance relaxation for some women.

Visualization, or mental picturing of the biophysical events of labor and birth, also can encourage women to work with, rather than resist, the normal progression of labor and birth. The nurse may suggest the use of visualization to strengthen the mind–body connection during labor. The nurse can enlist such images as contractions opening the cervix for the newborn (rather than being just painful); breathing bringing in healthy, cleansing oxygen to the fetus and getting rid of waste products and tension; and the newborn sliding down the birth canal.

The nurse should communicate in a calm, soothing voice and reduce noxious environmental stimuli that detract from relaxation and visualization. The nurse also should explain these techniques to the father or support person, who may be able to help the woman visualize calm, favorite scenes or who may have special knowledge about things the woman finds calming. (See Chapter 18 for further discussion and sample visualization exercise and Chapter 24 for managing maternal pain.)

Expected Outcome

- The woman in labor uses a variety of techniques to enhance comfort and reduce pain, as evidenced by her verbalization of a reduction in discomfort or pain.

NURSING PROCEDURE
Providing Nursing Care When the Umbilical Cord Prolapses

The umbilical cord can become prolapsed at any time in active labor if the presenting part is not well applied to the cervix. However, cord prolapse is most likely to occur at the time of rupture of membranes or shortly thereafter and in presentations other than vertex.

Purpose: To reduce pressure of the fetal presenting part on the umbilical cord until emergency cesarean delivery can be performed.

NURSING ACTION	***RATIONALE***
1. Auscultate FHR immediately after rupture of membranes and with next contraction.	To identify abrupt, persistent deceleration in the fetal heart rate suggesting cord compression.
2. If cord prolapse is suspected, perform sterile vaginal examination.	To determine if cord has prolapsed through the cervix or into the vagina.
3. If cord is palpable in the vagina, call for help, and apply two fingers against presenting part with cord in between fingers. Press presenting part up into pelvis.	To relieve pressure on cord, which disrupts blood flow to the fetus.
4. While maintaining upward pressure on presenting part, instruct others to assist mother to a knee–chest position with hips elevated as high as possible.	To allow gravity to pull presenting part off prolapsed cord.
5. Instruct others to administer oxygen by mask at 8 to 12 L/min.	To improve fetal oxygenation.

Encouraging Ambulation and Position Changes

Most women should be encouraged to ambulate during labor. Walking increases the level of comfort and promotes *less* frequent, *more* efficient contractions. The upright position allows gravity to support the process of labor. It encourages descent of the fetus into the true pelvis and accelerates dilatation and effacement by direct application of the presenting part to the cervix. Arrested labors may be augmented by walking (Liu, 1989). The slight movements of the joints during walking may facilitate rotation and descent of the fetus. Walking reduces discomfort, including pain from contractions and backache. A laboring woman will be most able, willing, and interested in walking if she is unencumbered by machinery and if she is awake and aware, not drowsy from medication. Telemetric EFM may soon be more widely available so that ambulation and continuous monitoring can be done simultaneously.

In some obstetric units, women are encouraged to stay in bed once they are admitted in labor because of concern about cord prolapse during ambulation. This is a highly unlikely event, even when membranes are ruptured. If membranes rupture during ambulation, the woman should be examined immediately for the presence of prolapsed cord and the FHR should be auscultated (see the Nursing Procedure, Providing Nursing Care When the Umbilical Cord Prolapses).

To evaluate the possible risk of cord prolapse, the woman can be examined vaginally in a standing position to assess how well the fetal head is applied to the cervix. If the head is not well applied or the fetal presentation is breech, risk of cord prolapse is increased. When the head is not well applied and ambulation is not advisable, raising the head of the bed to a 30-degree angle will facilitate fetal descent and the process of labor.

Position changes during labor can be used to enhance maternal comfort or to correct or prevent problems in labor. Position change is a simple, harmless tool the nurse or the woman herself can use. Research indicates that women prefer a mixture of positions, including sitting and standing or walking for most of the first stage and lying down only late in labor (Read, Miller, & Pauh, 1983). Maternal positioning can be used to prevent or correct malpositions of the fetus. An all-fours or sidelying position combined with the pelvic rock motion may be used to turn an occiput posterior fetus to a more favorable position. Prolonged backlying or semisitting and even prolonged sidelying may impede rotation and progress in labor. Frequent position changes appear to be effective in facilitating fetal rotation and descent. Some of the commonly used positions for labor are described and illustrated in the accompanying display.

Position changes are sometimes helpful in alleviating mild fetal distress if the distress is due to supine hypotension syndrome or cord compression. If evidence of umbilical cord compression occurs, trial and error methods must be

Physiologic Positions for Labor and Birth and Their Advantages

Standing

- Takes advantage of gravity during and between contractions
- Produces less painful and more productive contractions
- Aligns fetus with angle of pelvis
- May speed labor
- May increase urge to push in second stage
- Can be used with electronic fetal monitor

Standing and Leaning Forward

- Takes advantage of gravity during and between contractions
- Often produces less painful and more productive contractions
- Aligns fetus with angle of pelvis
- May speed labor
- Relieves backache
- May be more restful than standing
- Can be used with electronic fetal monitor

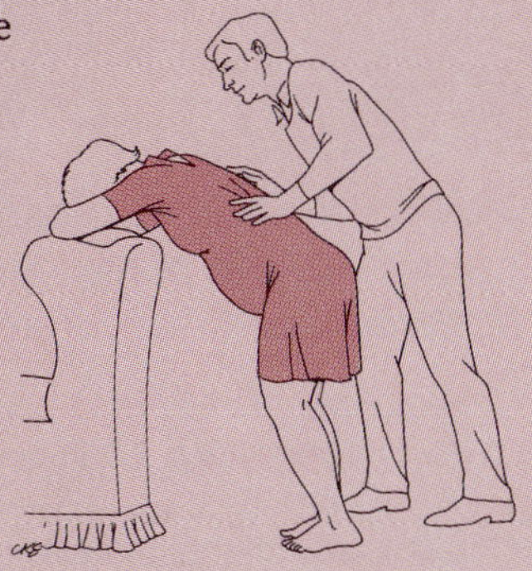

Walking

- Takes advantage of gravity during and between contractions
- Often produces less painful and more productive contractions
- Aligns fetus with angle of pelvis
- May speed labor
- Relieves backache
- Encourages descent through pelvic mobility

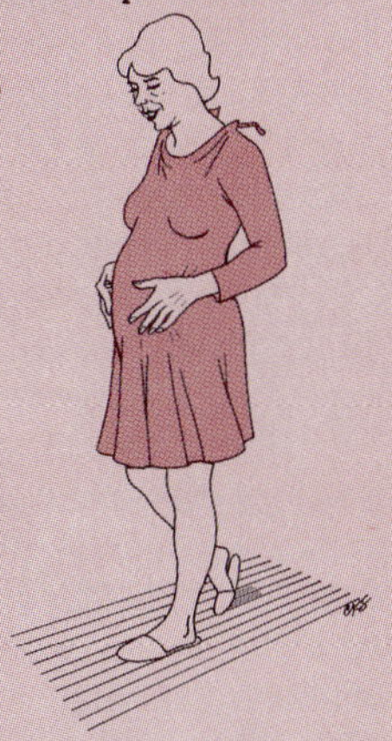

Sitting Upright

- Provides good resting position
- Provides some gravity advantage
- Can be used with electronic fetal monitor

Semisitting

- Provides good resting position
- Provides some gravity advantage
- Can be used with electronic fetal monitor
- Makes vaginal examinations possible
- Provides ease in getting onto bed or delivery table

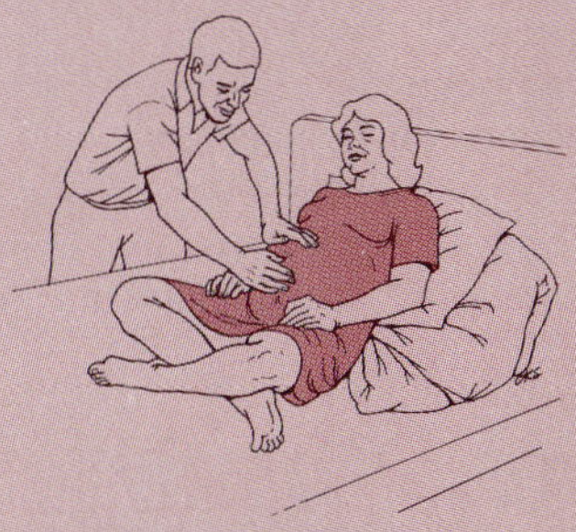

Sitting, Leaning Forward with Support

- Provides good resting position
- Has some gravity advantage
- Can be used with electronic fetal monitor
- Relieves backache
- Provides good position for back rub

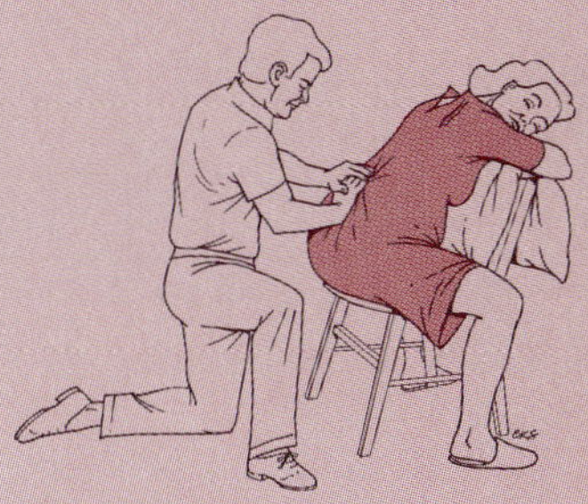

Hands and Knees

- Helps relieve backache
- Assists rotation of baby in occiput posterior position
- Allows for pelvic rocking and body movements
- Allows for vaginal examinations
- Takes pressure off hemorrhoids

Kneeling, Leaning Forward with Support

- Helps relieve backache
- Assists rotation of baby in occiput posterior position
- Allows for pelvic rocking
- Uses less strain on wrists and hands than hands and knees position

(Continued)

Physiologic Positions for Labor and Birth and Their Advantages (Continued)

Sidelying

- Provides excellent resting position
- Is convenient for many interventions
- Helps lower elevated blood pressure
- Provides safety if pain medications have been used
- May promote progress of labor when alternated with walking
- Provides neutral gravity
- Slows a very rapid second stage of labor
- Takes pressure off hemorrhoids
- Facilitates relaxation between pushing efforts
- Allows posterior sacral movement in second stage
- Can be used with electonic fetal monitor

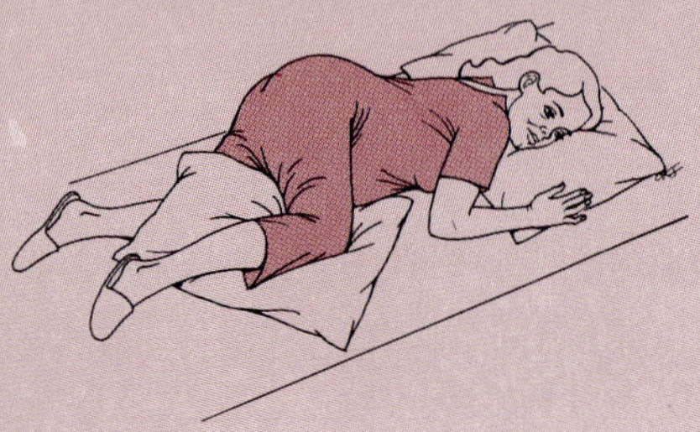

Sitting on Toilet or Commode

- May help perineum for effective bearing down
- Takes advantage of gravity

Squatting

- May be comfortable and relieve backache
- Takes advantage of gravity
- Widens pelvic outlet to its maximum
- Requires less bearing-down effort
- May enhance rotation and descent in a difficult birth
- Is relaxing if mother does not feel an urge to push
- Allows freedom to shift weight for comfort

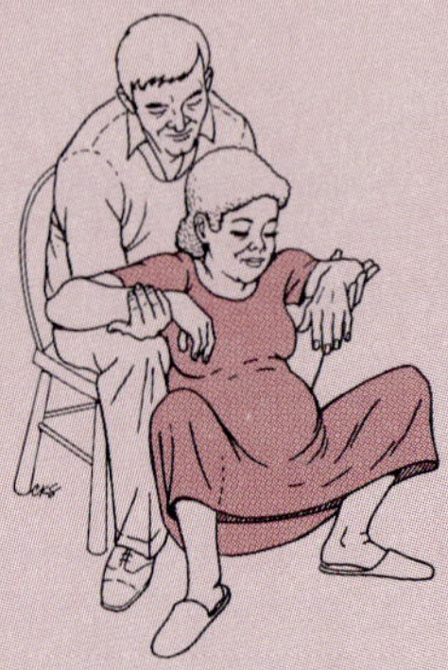

Supported Squat (mother leaning with back against support person who holds her under the arms and takes all her weight)

- Maximizes diameters of bony pelvis
- Permits relaxation while avoiding stretching of pelvis muscles
- Takes advantage of gravity

used by monitoring FHR in various positions to determine which to avoid and which to encourage in each woman.

When backache, often called back labor, occurs, it is usually caused by pressure of the presenting part on the sacrum, which refers pain to the lower back. It is particularly acute with a posterior presentation. Positioning can facilitate rotation and promote maternal comfort and relaxation. Other measures can be used as well, including counterpressure, heating pads or cold packs, and showers. (See Chapter 18 for relief measures for back labor.)

Expected Outcome

- The woman in active labor ambulates in the area and voices her increased comfort as evidenced by less frequent, more effective contractions.

Minimizing Sensory Overload

Some degree of sensory overload can be expected during labor. The unfamiliar physical environment of the birth setting alone may contribute to this disruption of senses. Uterine contractions, unusual secretions, rupture of membranes, nausea and vomiting, and pelvic pressure may range from mild and easily tolerable to overwhelming. Routine care, such as vaginal examinations, use of monitoring devices, laboratory tests, room changes, and personnel changes, introduce additional sensory input. Unusual situations that demand quick staff responses, such as instances of fetal distress or other developments requiring emergency procedures, can contribute to the sensory overload experienced by the woman in labor.

During the active phase of labor the nurse can minimize sensory overload by approaching the woman in labor in an unhurried, gentle manner. All procedures should be explained before they are implemented, and time should be provided for the woman to prepare herself for pelvic examinations and other necessary interventions. The environment should be conducive to rest and relaxation. Bright overhead lights can be dimmed, and natural light or small table lamps used whenever possible to reduce visual stimuli. The nurse should speak in a low, calm voice, and efforts should be made to reduce noise and unnecessary conversations immediately outside the woman's room. If an EFM is used, the audio output for the fetal heart beat should be reduced.

If a support person or coach is not present, the woman

in labor will benefit by the nurse's frequent or continuous presence. One of the most frightening experiences for the woman in active or the transition stage of labor is to be left alone. If the woman has neither family nor friends present, the nurse becomes her link to reality. She translates the intense sensations and often overwhelming stimuli into an understandable experience and reassures the woman that she will not be alone during the birth of her newborn.

Expected Outcome

- The woman in active labor verbalizes feeling relaxed and supported.

Supporting Appropriate Self-Care

Supportive care becomes increasingly important as labor progresses and the woman becomes less able to meet her own needs effectively. The nurse can assist the woman in maintaining a sense of control by encouraging her to perform easy self-care measures, such as effleurage, mouth care, and oral intake of fluids.

The nurse also can encourage the partner or support person to assume some care measures for the woman. These activities provide a sense of purpose and reward when it is evident that they help the woman. The support person may be especially helpful in assisting the woman with maintaining the room environment the way she prefers it (door open or shut, lights dimmed or bright, music or quiet). Other comfort measures they can assist with include massage, heating pad, or cold packs on the lower back; sips of fluid or ice chips; and comforting physical contact. The support person also may help the woman into a warm shower or bath and provide reassuring physical contact and assistance. One area in which the woman and her partner can exercise effective self-care is in promoting progress in labor. Ambulation and upright positions may encourage progress. If the progress of labor continues to be slow, the partner may assist the woman with breast or nipple stimulation to promote cervical ripening and labor (Fig. 20-5) (Stein et al., 1990). The nurse can explain this option and assist the couple by providing privacy. In some cases this technique may help to avoid the need for other measures to stimulate labor, such as artificial rupture of the membranes or oxytocin augmentation of labor. These interventions, although useful for many laboring women, have potential risks. (See Chapter 23 for further discussion.)

As the woman's energy resources are depleted, the nurse assumes a larger share of the care needs. The nurse provide perineal care after vaginal examinations, with rupture of the membranes, and when bloody show is evident. A sponge bath may be very refreshing at the end of the transition period, before the woman begins the expulsive stage of labor. Cool cloths to the forehead may be welcome. Attention to mouth care is important, because breathing efforts and decreased oral intake dry the mucous membranes.

Expected Outcomes

- The woman in the active phase of labor (or her support person) implements specific self-care measures.
- The woman in the active phase of labor verbalizes satisfaction with care and hygiene measures performed by others.

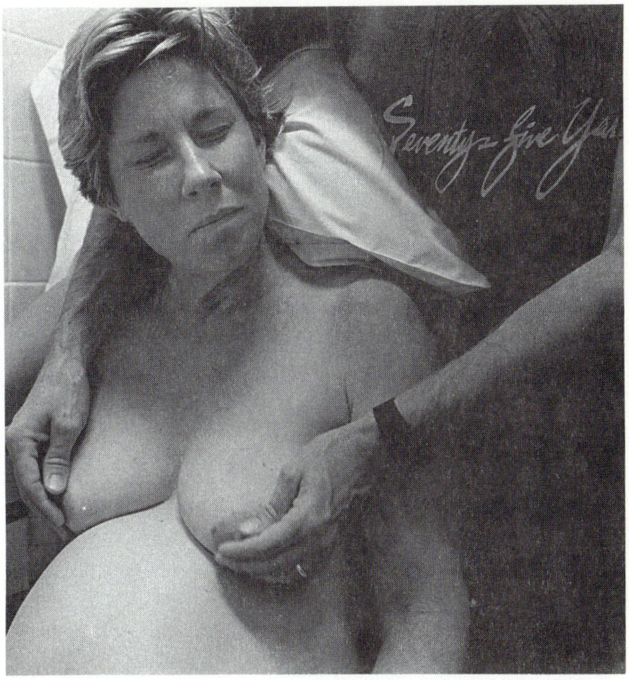

Figure 20-5.
Breast or nipple stimulation promotes cervical ripening and labor. The partner may assist with stimulation. (Photo by Kathy Sloane, Courtesy of Alta Bates Medical Center.)

• • Evaluation

As the level of physical sensation escalates in the active phase of labor, the nurse evaluates the woman's responses to interventions aimed at promoting physiologic and emotional stability. Maternal vital signs and characteristics of the FHR will remain within normal limits, and progress in cervical dilatation, effacement, and fetal descent should be noted. The woman will demonstrate effective alterations in breathing patterns and relaxation geared to cope with the growing intensity of the labor process, and her partner will remain comfortable and competent in his or her support role. Although the woman may verbalize anxiety as labor progresses, she should demonstrate effective coping strategies with appropriate nursing support and encouragement.

As the progress of labor accelerates, the woman will require increased physical and emotional support and encouragement from the nurse. Regardless of how active the role of the support person is in coaching the woman, the nurse plays a critical role in assessment and care during the active phase of labor. Close monitoring of physiologic and behavioral adaptations is essential as the stressors of labor are intensified. The nurse often assumes responsibility for self-care activities as the woman focuses on the physical sensations of labor. The primary goals of nursing care during the active phase of labor include assistance with comfort measures and pain control efforts, assumption of self-care activities, and continued encouragement of the support person.

The Transition Phase of Labor

The transition phase marks the end of the first stage of labor. It begins when the cervix reaches 8 cm dilatation and ends with complete dilatation (10 cm). Skilled and intensive nursing care is required at this time. Because of the overwhelming sensations that many women experience and the rapid progress to complete dilatation, especially in multigravidas, the woman is often unable to cope effectively without constant attention and support. The support person or partner also may require additional attention from the nurse during this dramatic period of labor.

• • Assessment

Characteristic responses may suggest to the nurse that the first stage of labor is ending. As the nurse performs ongoing assessments, specific behavioral cues will alert her to impending birth. The transition phase often is described as the most intense phase because of the heightened physical and emotional sensations. The woman may exhibit marked apprehension, restlessness, and irritability. As the cervix continues to dilate, often at a rapid pace, the woman's attention is focused only on her situation, and she may have difficulty responding to others. Many women do not wish to be touched or comforted but cannot cope with labor alone. The woman may appear confused and unable to understand directions. She may feel overwhelmed by the contractions and have little strength to cope with the demands of labor. She may experience panic and beg to be "put to sleep" or ask for the staff to "get the baby out."

Objective signs of transition phase include diaphoresis, in particular, a fine sheen of perspiration forming on the upper lip and across the bridge of the nose and cheek bones. The woman may feel nauseated, and vomiting is common. A sudden urge to push may occur. Some women may bear down involuntarily or state, "I have to have a bowel movement!" This sensation is a result of the rapid descent of the fetus through the pelvis and pressure of the presenting part on the woman's rectum. Table 20-2 summarizes the standards of care during the transition phase.

• • Nursing Diagnosis

Several significant nursing diagnoses are commonly noted during the transition phase of labor, and they highlight the intensity of this period:

- Ineffective Individual Coping related to the sensations experienced during transition phase
- Pain related to uterine contractions, rapid cervical dilatation, and pressure of the fetal presenting part
- Sensory-Perceptual Alterations related to rapid body changes experienced during transition phase
- Fear related to sensations experienced during transition phase and impending birth
- Ineffective Breathing Pattern related to physiologic demands and apprehension

• • Planning and Implementation

Transition marks an especially demanding phase in the care of the laboring woman and her family. If progress appears to be normal, the nurse begins to plan for imminent delivery—especially for the multipara, who will likely move through this phase in 15 to 20 minutes or less. (Table 20-3 lists nursing support measures.) The labor nurse should not leave the woman alone at this time and may need other staff assistance for preparations. The father or support person will need to be prepared for the birth. If special clothing is needed, the father should be shown where to change, what clothes are needed, and how they are to be worn. The physician or nurse midwife should be called if not already present. If the birth is to occur in the labor bed, any equipment likely to be needed at birth is collected.

Controlling the Urge to Push

As noted, a common variation in normal labor during the transition phase, which may require active nursing management, is the premature urge to push before the cervix is completely dilated. Traditional obstetric practice encourages attendants to prevent the woman from pushing until the cervix is completely dilated. The dangers to the woman and the fetus of pushing against an undilated cervix are not well documented. They are believed to include increased fetal head compression, cervical laceration, cervical edema, a subsequent prolonged labor, and maternal exhaustion as a result of prolonged ineffective pushing.

The urge to push is a reflex action stimulated by descent of the presenting part. The stretch and pressure receptors of the lower uterine segment and vagina are activated as the fetus descends. The obstetric conditions usually accompanying a premature urge to push are advanced labor, cervical dilatation of at least 8 cm, rapid fetal descent, and moderate to strong uterine contractions. The accompanying Nursing Care Plan discusses pain associated with an uncomplicated labor.

Nursing interventions focus on assisting the woman to avoid pushing or bearing down until the cervix is completely dilated. The nurse must explain to the woman why bearing down should be delayed and encourage her to "blow the contractions away" by blowing out short breaths of air through pursed lips during the urge to push with contractions. The nurse can increase the effectiveness of this technique by maintaining close eye contact with the woman and breathing with her. She should be helped to a gravity-neutral position, such as the sidelying position, to decrease the intensity of downward pelvic pressure. The nurse also may suggest that the woman visualize the last rim of the cervix being retracted over the neonate's head with a strong contraction; this may help her to focus her attention and resist the urge to push.

Because the urge to push may signal rapid movement into the second stage of labor the nurse also should be alert for signs of progress in labor. For this reason the nurse should perform a vaginal examination when the woman experiences a sudden urge to push. If rapid progress is noted, she should never be left alone. The skilled labor nurse

Table 20-3. Nursing Support Measures During Transition

Common Physiologic Characteristics	Nursing Interventions
Shaking, chills	Hold extremities; use warm blankets
Perspiration, feeling hot	Use fan; wipe with cool cloth; give ice chips
Restlessness, irritability, increased apprehension	Give encouragement; work on relaxation techniques; avoid behaviors irritating to woman; increase verbal cues for relaxation
Inability to focus; confusion	Give firm but kind instruction; repeat instruction and show understanding; breathe with woman; use eye contact
Increased pain, especially sacral	Apply sacral counterpressure
Inability to cope	Give reassurance; maintain physical presence; focus on shortness of phase
	Give overwhelming support: "baby is almost here"; take one contraction at a time; provide other comfort measures
Exhaustion	Facilitate rest and sleep between contractions; alert woman to beginning of contraction
Hiccuping, burping, flatulence	Woman is often embarrassed; reassure that this is normal.
Nausea and vomiting	Reassure that this is normal and will be over soon; use comfort measures, such as cold cloth to mouth or throat; position with head elevated or turn on left side
Urge to push	Check for complete dilatation; if not complete, try sidelying position and "blowing contractions away."
Carpopedal spasm	Extend woman's leg and flex foot; check for warmth of extremities; provide blanket as needed

takes seriously the woman's prediction of impending birth, particularly if the woman is a multipara. Verbalizations by the woman such as "my baby is coming" may herald a precipitous delivery. Full dilatation and birth can occur in several contractions for the multiparous woman in active labor. (See the Nursing Procedure for nursing responsibilities during a precipitous birth.)

Expected Outcome

- The woman demonstrates correct techniques to resist the premature urge to push.

Promoting Comfort

When maternal and fetal status and the progress of labor are normal, nursing care is directed toward providing comfort and emotional support (see Table 20-3). The nurse should assist the woman during transition by providing whatever physical comfort measures are possible and by providing encouragement and a calm presence. If the woman is using relaxation and breathing techniques, the nurse can help the support person keep the woman focused on these activities.

During this time sacral counterpressure, cool cloths on the forehead, and ice chips may be especially welcome. An emesis basin should be kept on hand; if the woman experiences nausea, deep breaths and moving her to a sitting or semisitting position may help.

Expected Outcome

- The woman verbalizes an acceptable decrease in discomfort or pain after implementation of specific techniques to reduce pain or pressure.

Managing Sensory Overload

For many women the potential for sensory overload is greatest during the transition period. The nurse's presence is absolutely essential to support her and her partner through this period of overwhelming sensory stimuli. Profound changes in behavior that frighten the partner may occur. Previously successful coaching techniques may fail to help the gravida because of the intensity of the experience.

It may be necessary to speak directly into the woman's ear or maintain close eye contact to prevent her from feeling overwhelmed by her contractions. The nurse should give firm, precise directions when needed and keep unnecessary conversation to a minimum to allow the woman to concentrate on coping with each contraction. The woman should be encouraged to rest and sleep, if possible, between contractions. Interruptions should be minimized to allow for quiet, undisturbed rest.

The nurse should explain to the partner or support person that the woman's irritable or angry behavior is a normal response to this part of labor. The woman may find certain kinds of contact very irritating, such as touch or

Text continues on page 507

Nursing Care Plan

The Woman Experiencing Pain Associated With Uncomplicated Labor and Birth

PATIENT PROFILE

History

NP is a 18-year-old G1/PO at $41^{2}/_{7}$ weeks' gestation. She is a single woman whose mother will remain with her during labor and birth. She tells the nurse that she did not attend childbirth preparation classes. "My mom has lots of experience, and she's going to help me. I want to do this without drugs. I'm really nervous about taking drugs for me and the baby. That's why I held out so long before coming in." A vaginal examination reveals that her cervix is 6 cm dilated and 75% effaced. The fetus is at a +1 station and in an occiput posterior position. Her membranes are intact.

Physical Assessment

During the admission process NP is tremulous. She states, "I'm scared stiff about this. I didn't think it would really happen, and now the contractions are so close and strong. My teeth are chattering!" When a contraction begins, NP begins to hold her breath. At the acme of the contraction she begins to scream and hyperventilate.

NP is unable to follow the nurse's directions for a more effective breathing pattern during the contraction. "I can't help it. The pain is horrible, and my back is killing me!" During the next several contractions NP is also noted to push intermittently. She tells the nurse, "I feel so much pressure sometimes, I can't help bearing down. Will pushing help me get this over sooner?"

COLLABORATIVE PROBLEMS/POTENTIAL COMPLICATIONS

- Cervical edema or trauma with premature pushing
- Hyperventilation syndrome

(See the Nursing Alert display and the Managed Care Path following the Care Plan.)

Assessment	*Nursing Diagnosis*	*Nursing Interventions*	*Rationale*
NP is an 18-year-old G1/PO and has not attended childbirth classes. NP states, "I'm really nervous about taking drugs. I'm scared stiff about this. My teeth are chattering." NP is tremulous, screams or hyperventilates with contractions, and is unable to follow directives. NP's mother will remain with her during labor and birth.	Anxiety related to unfamiliar situation of labor and fear of drugs, labor, and pain sensations *Expected Outcome* NP will verbalize a decrease in anxiety. NP will demonstrate a decrease in anxiety as evidenced by a cessation of tremulousness and ability to perform effective relaxation and breathing techniques.	Provide NP with brief, simple explanations of current status, cause of painful sensations, and how to cope with contractions.	Anxiety will reduce NP's ability to hear and understand explanations and directions. Having a basic understanding of her status and expected progress will promote NP's feelings of control and reduce anxiety. Helping NP to cope more effectively with her contractions will enhance her sense of competency and reduce her level of fear.
		Remain continuously with NP. Provide consistent coaching with each contraction, and demonstrate correct techniques.	Staying with NP and providing consistent physical and emotional support will lessen fears and may increase NP's ability to cope with anxiety.
		Listen to expressions of anxiety. Establish rapport with NP and her mother.	Listening to NP, establishing rapport, and giving positive feedback will convey genuine concern and caring, helping to reduce fear.

(*Continued*)

The Woman Experiencing Pain Associated With Uncomplicated Labor and Birth

(Continued)

Assessment	*Nursing Diagnosis*	*Nursing Interventions*	*Rationale*
		Give positive reinforcement and praise.	
		Use reassuring touch.	
		Explain all procedures briefly before performing.	
		Reassure NP that her anxiety and fears are normal but can be reduced by relaxation and breathing techniques.	Understanding that her fears are normal may reduce anxiety. Routine care may be misinterpreted as unusual or a cause for alarm, thus increasing anxiety.
		Provide guided imagery between contractions for relaxation, pain control, and anxiety reduction.	Refocusing attention to imagery may lessen preoccupation with anticipated pain and lessen fear.
		Encourage NP's mother to participate in support. Guide her in correct coaching techniques. Offer her support and encouragement.	Having the support of her mother may further reduce NP's level of anxiety. NP's mother may be most effective in reducing her level of anxiety.
NP is 6 cm dilated and has not attended childbirth classes. NP states, "I want to do this without drugs." Fetus is at +1 station and in an occiput posterior position.	Acute pain related to contractions, cervical dilatation, fetal descent, and occiput posterior position	Ask NP where she feels pain most intense.	Guidance in techniques to reduce pain will depend on the location, nature, and intensity of pain.
NP screams and holds breath and intermittently pushes with contractions.	***Expected Outcome*** NP will verbalize a decrease in pain sensation.	Provide brief, simple explanations of procedures and progress of labor.	Pain and anxiety will reduce NP's ability to hear and process information.
NP states, "The pain is horrible, and my back is killing me."	NP will demonstrate a decrease in pain sensation as evidenced by muscle relaxation between and during contraction, use of effective breathing patterns, and cessation of screaming.	Provide explanation and demonstration of effective breathing and relaxation techniques. Briefly explain why premature pushing is contraindicated.	Teaching effective breathing patterns is important as breath holding may decrease level of oxygen causing lactic acid accumulation and increased pain with uterine muscle contraction.
	NP will perform effective breathing and relaxation techniques.	Demonstrate "pant–blow" technique when NP has urge to push.	Actual demonstration of effective pain control strategies may increase NP's ability to perform correctly.
	NP will verbalize a decrease in pain sensation during contractions.		Premature pushing may delay progress of labor and increase level of pain and fatigue.

(Continued)

The Woman Experiencing Pain Associated With Uncomplicated Labor and Birth

(*Continued*)

Assessment	Nursing Diagnosis	Nursing Interventions	Rationale
		Reposition NP in sidelying or hands and knees position.	Sidelying position may decrease urge to push and facilitate rotation of fetus to occiput anterior position. Hands and knees position, application of sacral pressure, heating pad to lower back, and pelvic rocking may reduce sensation of back pain associated with occiput posterior position.
		Apply firm back pressure during and between contractions. Apply heating pad to lower back. Demonstrate pelvic rocking technique. Encourage voiding every 1 to 2 hours.	Alleviating secondary sources of pain, such as full bladder, fixed position, and muscle tenseness, will reduce sensations of pain.
		Encourage position change every 20 to 30 minutes.	Position changes reduce stiffness, tension, and pressure soreness.
		Promote general comfort by providing ice chips, fluids, clean dry linens, pillows, and comfortable room temperature and lighting.	General comfort affects the woman's overall perception of pain and tolerance of labor.
		Encourage mother to support techniques as taught to NP.	NP's mother may be most effective in guiding and encouraging her efforts at pain control, thus reducing painful sensations.
		If pain becomes intense and efforts to control pain are unsuccessful, discuss pharmacologic pain relief techniques with NP.	Intense, unrelieved pain may have physical and psychological adverse effects on NP.
NP is 6 cm dilated with fetus at +1 station. NP is intermittently pushing with contractions.	High Risk for Injury related to premature pushing ***Expected Outcome*** NP will stop pushing before she is completely dilated.	Briefly explain why premature pushing is contraindicated.	NP may be more motivated to resist urge to push if she understands reasons to delay bearing-down efforts.
		Demonstrate "pant–blow" technique when NP has urge to push.	Actual demonstration of "pant–blow" technique may improve NP's success with performing technique.

(*Continued*)

The Woman Experiencing Pain Associated With Uncomplicated Labor and Birth

(Continued)

Assessment	*Nursing Diagnosis*	*Nursing Interventions*	*Rationale*
		Reposition NP in sidelying or hands and knees position.	Placing NP in a gravity neutral position may decrease sensations of pressure and urge to push.
		Use guided imagery techniques to reduce urge to push.	Guided imagery may enhance the effectiveness of "pant–blow" technique and distract NP from urge to push.
		Remain with woman constantly and reinforce "pant–blow" technique with each urge to push.	Constant reinforcement and praise will encourage NP in her efforts to resist pushing.
		Offer positive reinforcement and praise.	
EVALUATION	With 30 minutes of coaching and support, NP stopped trembling and was able to follow directions and perform breathing and relaxation techniques. NP also verbalized a decrease in anxiety level and pain sensation. The intense pain persisted in her back until she was 9 cm dilated. The fetus then rotated to an occiput anterior position. As a result she did not need analgesia during labor. NP was successful in resisting the premature urge to push for most contractions until she reached 10 cm dilatation. No cervical edema or trauma was noted.		

conversation. The nurse can explain this and help to reduce these irritating stimuli as much as possible. The nurse also may need to interpret the woman's needs to other staff, based on the observations and knowledge acquired from working with the woman throughout her labor.

Expected Outcome

- The woman verbalizes a decrease in sensations of sensory overload after implementation of techniques that reduce unnecessary stimuli.

Providing Emotional Support

The woman and her support person are more likely to need reassurance and calm guidance at this point in labor than at any other time. The nurse should encourage them and commend them frequently on their efforts. Information about labor progress should be given freely when it is likely to be encouraging. The woman can be reminded that the neonate will soon be born and that she needs to cope with labor only a little while longer, if that can be said with reasonable certainty. The partner or support person may be particularly distressed over the woman's obvious discomfort and pain and may need additional encouragement and reassurance. To help the partner adjust more easily to the faster pace of activity, the nurse should anticipate questions and concerns and explain what the partner can expect in the next few minutes.

Expected Outcome

- The woman in transition experiences less anxiety and fear, as evidenced by her verbalization of feelings and of satisfaction with the emotional support provided by significant others and the health care team.

Preventing Hyperventilation

Because of the intense physiologic demands and her apprehension, the woman is prone to hyperventilation during this time, especially if she is using shallow, patterned breathing in an effort to cope with her contractions. Hyperventilation results from breathing too rapidly or too deeply, causing an excess amount of carbon dioxide to be blown off and leading to respiratory alkalosis. Symptoms of hyperven-

NURSING ALERT

NURSING RESPONSIBILITIES DURING PAINFUL LABOR

Uncontrolled, intense pain or pressure sensations during labor can result in several significant complications that may compromise the woman or her fetus. Hyperventilation may result in hypocarbia and altered acid–base balance, which can adversely affect fetal well-being. Premature pushing before the cervix completely dilates can cause cervical edema, which may retard the progress of labor. It also may result in cervical tears and bleeding.

The nurse must intervene promptly to prevent these complications.

- Briefly describe why hyperventilation or premature pushing is inadvisable
- Provide actual demonstration of techniques to eliminate the behavior
- Use eye contact, physical touch, and firm commands directed close to the woman's ear to reinforce desired behavior pattern
- Have woman breathe into a paper bag to correct hypocarbia if hyperventilation is the problem
- Have woman assume gravity-neutral position when premature pushing persists
- Perform vaginal examination to determine if rapid progress or fetal descent is the cause of hyperventilation or premature pushing
- Notify midwife or physician if problem hyperventilation persists

If the woman is unable to stop hyperventilating or pushing, analgesia or anesthesia may be indicated. Close consultation with the birth attendant and the anesthesiologist is essential to prevent complications when intense, unremitting pain or pressure persists.

tilation include numbness and tingling in the lips, fingers, or toes; dizziness; light-headedness; and confusion. The support person also may hyperventilate, either from excitement or from attempting to assist the woman to control her breathing. Treatment for hyperventilation consists of rebreathing exhaled carbon dioxide either from cupped hands around the mouth or from a paper bag.

Expected Outcome

- The woman in transition and her partner use effective techniques to prevent hyperventilation.

Monitoring for Potential Complications

Potential Complication: Fetal Compromise

The nurse must maintain a close watch on fetal status during the transition phase of labor. If intermittent auscultation of the FHR is performed, the heart rate should be monitored at the end of each contraction. Because contractions may be longer and more frequent with little resting time in between, placental oxygenation is decreased and fetal hypoxia is possible. Variable decelerations indicating umbilical cord compression often are evident if EFM is used and are usually benign. If the nurse auscultates decelerations in the FHR at this time, however, it is advisable to apply an external electronic monitor for continuous evaluation of the heart rate.

MANAGED CARE PATH

Labor/Delivery/Recovery—Vaginal Delivery

Expected Length of Stay: 12 hours

	Labor	Delivery	Recovery
Key Goals	Obtains pain relief option Adequate progress/labor	Vaginal delivery of infant Hemodynamically stable	Discharge to postpartum in 1–2 h Hemodynamically stable Ambulate with assist
Consults	Anesthesia		Parent education prn
Tests/Labs	EFM, dipstick urine, type and screen, complete blood count	Direct Coombs on cord blood if Apgar <7	
Meds	Pain med, pitocin aug prn	Pitocin after placenta	Pain med prn
Treatment	Mini prep prn Enema prn Assess VS per routine IV fluid, I&O	Assess VS per routine	Assess VS per routine D/C IV, I&O prn Ice to perineum
Teaching	EFM, unit routine, pain relief		Self care, perineal care, unit routine, pain relief
Equipment	EFM belts, infusion pump, bedpan, IV start kit, Chuks, maternity kit		
Diet	Clear liquid, NPO with ice chips after epidural		Diet as tolerated
Activity	Up ad lib, bedrest with pain med, epidural		Up with assist
D/C Plan	Coordinate with postpartum and nursery		Social work, parent ed prn

Adapted from collaborative paths developed by the Department of Nursing Service, Vanderbilt University Medical Center, Nashville, TN.

NURSING PROCEDURE
Participating in a Precipitous Birth

Purpose: To facilitate safe delivery of the infant and prevent maternal perineal lacerations.

NURSING ACTION	*RATIONALE*
1. Call for assistance.	To obtain supplies needed for delivery and additional help to support the woman and the infant. Fetal asphyxia can occur as a result of tumultuous contractions that prevent adequate placental perfusion and fetal oxygenation.
2. Instruct the woman in simple, direct terms to begin a pant–blow pattern.	To reduce the risk of an expulsive birth, which may result in perineal lacerations. Commands to "stop pushing" may be ineffective if not coupled with specific directions to "pant–blow."
3. Maintain a calm, reassuring demeanor, while providing the woman with brief, precise directives and support.	To reduce anxiety. The sudden and rapid birth of an infant can be an extremely frightening experience for the laboring woman and her partner.
4. Apply gloves quickly. Clean, nonsterile gloves may be used if sterile gloves are not immediately available.	To prevent exposure to body fluids. The precipitous birth of an infant can occur in 15 to 30 seconds, but even in extreme emergencies the nurse *must* observe universal body substance precautions.
5. Place the palm of the hand firmly against the perineum and emerging fetal head.	To support the perineum and decrease the expulsive forces that can lacerate the perineum and rectum.
6. If time permits, turn the woman to a sidelying or Sims' position	This position may decrease the urge to push and may reduce the risk of perineal or rectal lacerations.
7. When the head is born, quickly suction the infant's mouth and nares.	To clear the airway and prevent aspiration of blood, amniotic fluid, and mucus.
8. Quickly check for presence of a nuchal cord (umbilical cord around neck), and if present do the following: • Attempt to gently slip the coil of cord down and over the fetal head. • If gentle efforts to slip the cord over the fetal head fail, apply two clamps to the umbilical cord and cut between the clamps.	To prevent birth asphyxia or tearing of the umbilical cord. When a nuchal cord is present, continued expulsion of the fetus will tighten the cord around the infant's head, or the cord may rip.
9. Efforts should be made to suction the mouth and nares immediately after delivery of the infant if it has not been done before this time.	To prevent aspiration of blood, amniotic fluid, or mucus. In a precipitous birth the head and body may be born very rapidly in one expulsive motion before the airway can be cleared.
10. Clamp the umbilical cord (as noted in action 8) approximately 4 to 5 cm from the fetal abdomen. Leave 4 to 5 cm of umbilical cord.	To permit a plastic clamp to be applied to infant's umbilical cord stump.
11. Provide positive feedback about the woman's efforts and information about the condition of the infant.	To reduce anxiety and enhance maternal self-esteem.

• • Evaluation

The evaluation process during transition requires rapid reappraisal of the maternal and fetal condition, progress of labor, and effectiveness of nursing interventions. Although intense physical and emotional reactions are common, with appropriate nursing support the woman will demonstrate the ability to understand brief explanations and follow simple directions. The woman will be able to maintain an effective pant–blow pattern if the urge to push occurs, and expulsive efforts will be suppressed or minimized until the second stage of labor. The woman's partner will remain effective and comfortable in the support role with guidance and encouragement from the nurse.

The dramatic changes observed during the transition phase of labor herald the impending birth of the neonate. The woman is often overwhelmed by the intense physical sensations experienced at this time and requires constant coaching and support. The partner or support person may need additional guidance and encouragement at this time from the nurse. The primary aims of nursing care during the transition phase of labor include monitoring maternal and fetal physiologic status, progress of dilatation, and fetal descent and coaching the woman in appropriate breathing and relaxation techniques to prevent premature expulsive effort. Close collaboration with the birth attendant is essential to coordinate efforts for the birth of the newborn.

Chapter Summary

The first stage of labor is a period of concentrated nursing attention to the changing needs of the woman, the fetus, or the support person. The nurse must systematically assess and diagnose needs as they change through the latent, active, and transition phases of labor. Furthermore, the nurse must implement care and evaluate its effectiveness in meeting the woman's needs in the context of ongoing changes in response to labor. As the intensity of labor increases during the transition phase, the nurse begins to prepare for the second stage of labor and the dramatic event of birth.

Study Questions

1. *How would you help a woman distinguish between true and false labor during a telephone conversation?*
2. *What information should you give to a woman calling the labor unit who suspects that her membranes have ruptured? Why is this information important?*
3. *How would you instruct the partner supporting a woman in early labor to distinguish between mild, moderate, and strong contractions?*
4. *Which signs and symptoms most commonly characterize the transition phase of labor? What subjective comments by the woman would alert the nurse to the onset of transition phase?*
5. *Why might oral intake be limited or contraindicated during labor? What implications does maintenance of NPO status during labor have for nursing care?*
6. *Why are rapid infusions of intravenous glucose solutions contraindicated during labor?*
7. *How would you assist the woman experiencing a precipitous birth who is not attended by a physician or midwife?*

References

Birch, E. (1986). The experience of touch received during labor. *Journal of Nurse-Midwifery*, *31*(6), 270.

Chapman, L. (1992). Expectant fathers' roles during labor and birth. *Journal of Obstetric, Gynecologic, and Neonatal Nursing*, *21*(2), 114–120.

Eganhouse, D. (1991). A comparative study of variables differentiating false labor from early labor. *Journal of Perinatology*, *11*(3), 249.

Hofmeyr, G. J., Nikodem, V. C., Wolman, W. L., Chalmers, B. E., & Kramer, T. (1991). Companionship to modify the clinical birth environment: Effects on progress and perceptions of labour, and breastfeeding. *British Journal of Obstetrics and Gynecology*, *98*, 756.

Lederman, R., & Lederman, E. (1985). Anxiety and epinephrine in multiparous women in labor: Relationship to duration of labor and fetal heart rate pattern. *Obstetrics and Gynecology*, *153*, 870.

Lederman, R., Lederman, E., Work, B., & McCann, D. (1979). Relationship of psychologic factors in pregnancy to progress in labor. *Nursing Research*, *28*, 94.

Liu, Y. (1989). The effects of the upright position during childbirth. *Image*, *21*(1), 14.

Mackey, M., & Lock, S. (1989). Women's expectations of the labor and delivery nurse. *Journal of Obstetric, Gynecologic, and Neonatal Nursing*, *18*(6), 505.

Murray, M. (1988). *Antepartal and intrapartal fetal monitoring*. Washington, DC: NAACOG.

NAACOG. (1990). *OGN Nursing Practice Resource. Fetal heart rate auscultation*. Washington, DC: Author.

NAACOG. (1992). *Nursing responsibilities in implementing intrapartum fetal heart rate monitoring*. Washington, DC: Author.

Read, J. A., Miller, F. C., & Pauh, R. H. (1981). Randomized clinical trial of ambulation vs. oxytocin for labor enhancement: A preliminary report. *American Journal of Obstetrics and Gynecology*, *139*, 669.

Sammons, L. N. (1984). The use of music by women during childbirth. *Journal of Nurse-Midwifery*, *29*(4), 266–270.

Stein, A., Bardeguez, A., Verma, U., & Tegani, N. (1990). Nipple stimulation for labor augmentation. *Journal of Reproductive Medicine*, *35*(7), 710.

Waldenstrom, V., & Axel-Nilsson, C. (1992). Warm tub bath after spontaneous rupture of the membranes. *Birth*, *19*(2), 57–63.

Suggested Readings

Beaton, J. (1990). Dimensions of nurse and patient roles in labor. *Health Care for Women International*, *11*, 393.

Church, L. (1989). Water birth: One birthing center's observations. *Journal of Nurse-Midwifery*, *34*, 165.

Daniels, K. (1989). Waterbirth: The newest form of safe, gentle, joyous birth. *Journal of Nurse Midwifery*, *34*, 198.

Douglas, M. (1988). The case against a more liberal food and fluid policy in labor. *Birth*, *15*(2), 93–94.

Gerlach, C., & Schmid, M. (1988). Second skill educational development of personnel for a single-room maternity care system. *Journal of Obstetric, Gynecologic, and Neonatal Nursing*, *17*, 388.

Martin, J. (1990). *Intrapartum management*. Baltimore: Williams & Wilkins.

McKay, S., & Mahan, C. (1988). Modifying the stomach contents of laboring women: Why and how. *Success and Risks*, *15*(4), 213.

McNiven, P., Hodnett, E., & O'Brien-Pallas, L. (1992). Supporting women in labor: A work sampling study of the activities of labor and delivery nurses. *Birth*, (*19*)1, 3–7.

Phillips, C. R. (1988). Single-room maternity care for maximum cost-efficiency. *Perinatology-Neonatology*, *Mar/Apr*, 22–31.

CHAPTER 21

Nursing Care in Normal Birth

SECOND STAGE OF LABOR THROUGH RECOVERY

Learning Objectives

After studying the material in this chapter, the student will be able to:

- Discuss the application of the nursing process in caring for a woman and her family during the second stage of labor through recovery.
- Describe the types, indications, risks, and benefits of an episiotomy.
- Assess the placenta, cord, and fetal membranes for normalcy and completeness.
- Perform an assessment of the woman in the immediate postpartum period.
- Perform an immediate assessment of the neonate at delivery.
- Explain the procedure and rationale for fundal massage in the postpartum period.
- Identify maternal and neonatal needs during the first hour after birth.
- Discuss family needs and identify advantages of family-centered birth care.

Key Terms

Apgar score	cotyledon
atony	crowning
bearing down	episiotomy
birth attendant	introitus

The physiologic and behavioral changes of the first stage of labor become increasingly dramatic in the second stage, as the process of fetal descent becomes dominant. Nursing care centers on enhancing the body's own mechanisms for expulsion of the fetus and monitoring maternal and fetal status to detect deviations from normal. The nurse continues to assess maternal, fetal, and family well-being and identifies nursing diagnoses and collaborative problems that direct care. The plan of care is continually revised in light of changing needs as labor progresses. In addition the nurse collaborates with the birth attendant in preparation for and management of the actual delivery of the neonate. Finally, the nurse assists the family during the immediate postpartum recovery period.

Care of the Family During Early Second Stage of Labor

The second stage of labor begins with complete dilatation of the cervix and ends with birth. This stage can last from several minutes to several hours or more. During this stage the fetus descends through the maternal pelvis and the vaginal canal. This descent is caused by continuing uterine contractions and by the pushing or bearing-down efforts of the woman. The labor nurse provides one-to-one care at this time and is responsible for support and active nursing management.

• • Assessment

Nursing assessments in the second stage of labor focus on monitoring maternal and fetal physiologic status, evaluating the effectiveness of bearing-down efforts, and assessing the emotional state of the woman and her support person. Ongoing evaluation of the woman's energy level, fluid balance, and caloric intake (often intravenous glucose) is an essential aspect of nursing assessment if the second stage extends beyond 2 hours.

Monitoring Maternal and Fetal Physiologic Status

The woman's blood pressure, pulse, and respirations are monitored every 5 to 30 minutes throughout the second stage, depending on her condition and risk status. The temperature is taken every 2 hours once the membranes have ruptured. The nurse assesses the woman's energy level. Some women experience a "physiologic lull" during which contractions temporarily diminish in intensity and frequency before the urge to bear down is felt. As the second stage progresses effects of fatigue and increased physical activity become apparent. Flushing, increased perspiration, muscle weakness, and tremors may be observed. It is not unusual for women to become somnolent, awakening only with contractions.

The nurse continues to evaluate fluid balance and the adequacy of caloric intake for energy expenditure while pushing. Dehydration can occur if expulsive efforts exceed 2 hours and oral intake is reduced. Urine output is measured and the urine tested for the presence of ketones. The bladder also should be assessed for signs of distention, especially if intravenous fluids have been administered during labor. Furthermore, pressure of the fetal presenting part on the woman's bladder may result in decreased sensation and urge to void, even when the bladder is full.

Fetal heart rate (FHR) should be assessed by auscultation or electronic fetal monitor (EFM) and recorded according to AWHONN (formerly NAACOG; 1992) guidelines:

- Every 15 minutes in low-risk women
- Every 5 minutes in high-risk women

Marked changes may be noted in the FHR due to contractions and maternal bearing-down efforts and should be monitored closely. It is common to see early decelerations, which are periodic changes in the FHR pattern indicative of head compression. In the second stage of labor the FHR is usually best heard over the midline in the lower abdomen as fetal descent progresses (Fig. 21-1).

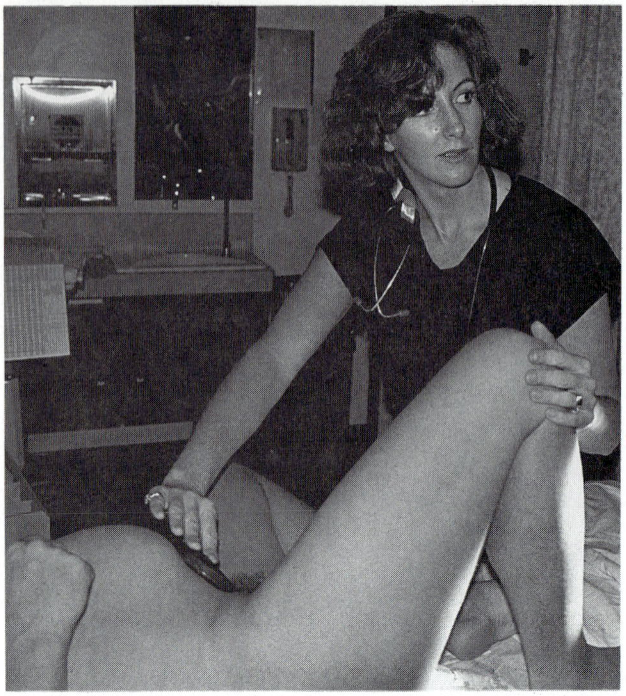

Figure 21-1.
Intermittent fetal heart rate monitoring with a Doppler ultrasound device in low-risk labor. (Photo by Kathy Sloane. Courtesy of Alta Bates Medical Center.)

Evaluating the Progress of Labor: Bearing-Down Efforts

The nurse should observe the woman's bearing-down efforts and assist her in positioning and pushing efforts that will result in labor progress. Effective expulsive efforts will result in steady descent of the fetal head and in the final phase of the second stage, flattening, then distention and bulging of the perineum (Fig. 21-2). Once the head is visible at the introitus, the nurse should observe that the head advances with bearing-down efforts and retreats slightly between contractions. However, the head should make steady, noticeable progress toward the perineum.

Identifying Behavioral Adaptations

Despite the physical demands of labor, the woman may be able to cope more easily with contractions when she begins to push. The end is now in sight, and some women experience a burst of energy as they move toward the goal of birth. They may vocalize during pushing efforts, involuntarily urinate or defecate, and when encouraged, assume positions that facilitate pushing, such as squatting or kneeling. Other women may become visibly fearful, fighting the strong urge to bear down, or refusing to push. They may cry out, "I can't do this!" or verbalize embarrassment if they become incontinent. This "holding back" or inability to "let go" also is common. The nurse must attempt to identify the reasons for the woman's hesitation to push, while encouraging her to "work with" her body's sensations.

The woman and her partner are extremely vulnerable at this time and may become fearful and discouraged if progress is slow; this is especially true if the labor is being managed with an eye toward a time limitation for the second stage (traditionally 1 hour for multiparas and 2 hours for nulliparas). These time limits have been relaxed recently, especially in women receiving epidural anesthesia, who may have a diminished reflex urge to bear down and who require more time to push effectively. If maternal and fetal physiologic status is stable, the second stage may be allowed to progress at a slower pace and may last 3 or more hours. The nurse can assist by providing encouragement and keeping the woman and support person informed of any progress and by active nursing management to facilitate the progress of labor.

Assessing Maternal Comfort

The woman experiences multiple foci of discomfort and pain during the second stage of labor. Pain caused by vaginal and perineal distention becomes prominent as the fetus descends into the birth canal. Persistent, intense back pain

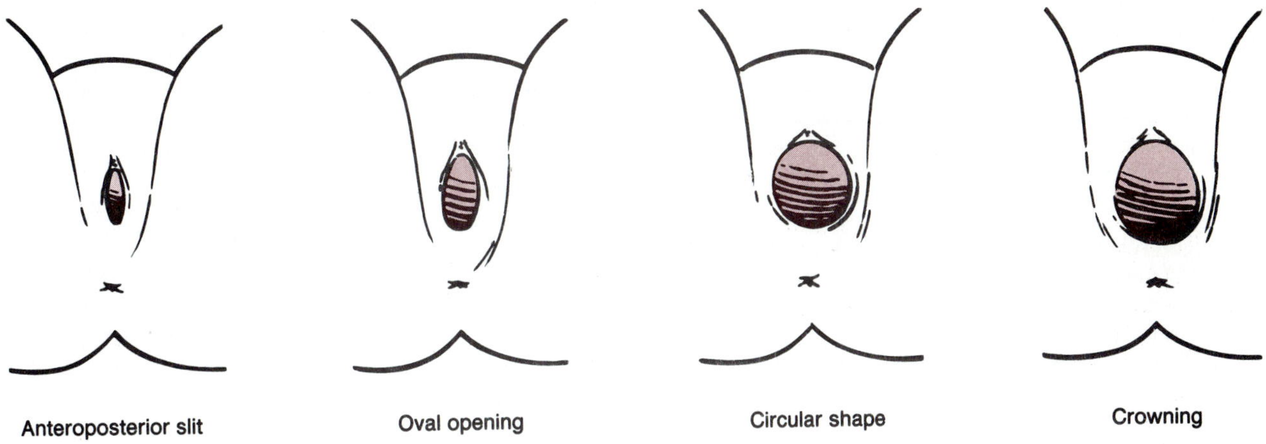

Figure 21-2.
Perineal changes in the second stage of labor.

also can occur, especially with an occipitoposterior presentation of the fetal head. The woman may experience painful leg cramps and general muscular achiness after long hours of labor. Fatigue adds to the general sense of discomfort during the expulsive stage of labor. As birth of the presenting part occurs, women often report an intense burning or tearing sensation.

The nurse continues her surveillance of the woman's comfort level and the location, nature, and extent of discomfort or pain. This may require questioning the woman gently. She may be unable to express herself well by the onset of the second stage because of sensory-perceptual alterations, fatigue, and pain. Body cues can alert the nurse to the location of pain. For example the woman may reach for her lower back with each contraction. The nurse also should assess the general comfort of the partner. Hours of coaching, including physical support of the woman and massage, may exhaust the support person after a long labor.

Nursing Research

Holding Back: Maternal Readiness to Give Birth

Holding back may occur when the woman is ambivalent about becoming a parent, fearful of the overwhelming feelings surrounding birth, or distressed by the noises she makes or incontinence that often occurs. Many women need time to gather emotional and physical strength before committing themselves to birth.

The labor nurse must recognize problems related to "letting go" and assist the woman as she works through her feelings. Behavioral and verbal cues that should alert the nurse include the following:

- Verbal protestations: "I can't do this!" "Not yet!" "I'm not ready!"
- Ineffectual "half-hearted" pushing efforts with correct coaching
- Rectum retracts during pushing efforts rather than bulges
- Obvious efforts to restrain any vocalizations during pushing
- Concern about the possibility of incontinence or distress with incontinence

Strategies that support emotional adaptations during the second stage include the following:

- Explore with the woman any negative comments regarding pushing.
- Encourage woman to stop pushing and renew her energies.
- Provide time alone for the woman and partner to exchange thoughts and feelings.
- Reassure woman that she is physically and emotionally able to "make it."
- Assist the woman who has strong fears of incontenence to the bathroom. Place bedpan under toilet seat, and have her begin pushing efforts.
- Reassure woman that making noises is perfectly normal.
- Have the woman begin with gentle pushing efforts to become familiar with the sensations.

McKay, S., & Barrows, T. (1991). Holding back: Maternal readiness to give birth. MCN: *American Journal of Maternal Child Nursing, 16*(5), 251.

• • Nursing Diagnosis

Based on data obtained from these assessments, the nurse formulates applicable nursing diagnoses. The following are nursing diagnoses reflecting possible problems that may arise during the second stage of labor and that may be addressed independently.

- Fatigue related to bearing-down efforts
- Pain related to fetal descent, pressure sensations, and perineal stretching
- Fear related to impending birth
- Ineffective Coping related to fatigue, sleep deprivation, and fears of impending birth
- Fluid Volume Deficit related to decreased oral intake and work of labor

Complications also may arise during the second stage of labor. They are related to bearing-down efforts and include alterations in maternal tissue perfusion, fetal compromise, and perineal injury. The nurse is responsible for monitoring for potential complications.

• • Planning and Implementation

Nursing interventions during the second stage of labor focus on supporting pushing, promoting comfort, providing support, and monitoring for potential complications.

Supporting Pushing Efforts

The role of the nurse in support of bearing-down efforts is critical. The nurse serves as the primary coach or collaborates with the woman's partner (Fig. 21-3). Some women do not begin to bear down until the presenting part descends far enough to stimulate nerves in the pelvic region that produce the urge to push. Epidural anesthesia also may interfere with the urge to push. Unless complications occur that require timely delivery of the infant, the woman who does not feel a desire to push at the onset of the second stage can be encouraged to rest or take a refreshing shower (Cosner & deJong, 1993).

Once sensations of pressure stimulate pushing efforts, the nurse should help the woman into a comfortable position. A variety of effective positions can be assumed to facilitate effective expulsive efforts. Many women assume a semisitting position (elevation of upper body at least 30 degrees) with legs well flexed at the hips. The woman's hands are positioned behind the knees or she can grasp special handles attached to the birthing bed or hold on to the bedrails. The woman also may choose to push in a squatting or kneeling position.

The nurse must assess the appropriateness of the woman's position and the efficacy of efforts to expel the fetus. Figure 21-4 illustrates a variety of commonly used positions for pushing in second-stage labor. If the woman is uncomfortable with a particular position or efforts appear ineffective in bringing down the presenting part, the nurse should not hesitate to try a different approach. Whatever position is selected, the woman should use the diaphragm and abdominal muscles to help in bearing down. Keeping other muscle groups as relaxed as possible will decrease fatigue. Nursing research indicates that allowing the woman to set the timing and pace of pushing efforts results in a shorter second stage than an approach that directs the woman to begin pushing vigorously as soon as she is completely dilated (Liu, 1989).

Traditional Methods of Pushing

Research has questioned the exclusive use of the lithotomy and other recumbent positions for pushing in the second stage of labor (Roberts, 1989). These positions cause maternal supine hypotension (due to aortal compression by the heavy uterus), which may result in fetal distress. Furthermore, the traditional methods of pushing or bearing down during the second stage have used the Valsalva maneuver. When the woman uses this type of bearing-down effort, she closes the glottis and pushes throughout a contraction, holding her breath as long as possible to build up intrathoracic pressure to assist in expelling the fetus. Hemodynamic changes result. Blood is driven from the pulmonary circulation into the left chambers of the heart, causing the woman's blood pressure to rise. However, as breath holding continues, the blood pressure begins to fall steadily. The longer the breath is held, the lower the blood pressure may drop.

Subsequent breath holding has a cumulative effect as well. Effects on the woman include exhaustion, cardiovascular strain due to blood pressure changes, and possible tissue damage with the birth. Fetal effects may be even more pronounced. During a Valsalva maneuver of 6 seconds or more, the woman's oxygenation is impaired and placental blood flow decreases. This may result in decreased fetal blood pH, decreased Po_2, increased Pco_2, and an increased incidence of FHR abnormalities. Prolonged bearing-down efforts may result in fetal hypoxia and acidosis and in lower Apgar scores for the newborn.

The valsalva maneuver also has been found to stimulate the sympathetic nervous system and thus increase catecholamine release. This response may decrease uterine activity, adversely affecting progress in labor.

Open-Glottis Pushing

An alternative style of pushing has been proposed for use in the second stage. Called "open-glottis" or "gentle" pushing, this style encourages the woman to push in short, 6- to 7-second periods and only when she has the urge to do so (not continuously through each contraction). She should push while exhaling slightly, which ensures an open glottis. When the woman in labor exhales while pushing, cardiovascular changes are not as pronounced. High intrathoracic pressure is not maintained, and there is minimal rise and fall in the woman's blood pressure. Open-glottis pushing has other benefits as well. It allows for relaxation of the perineum and gentle delivery of the neonate's head. It also is a pushing style women naturally adopt when they have not been trained to push in the traditional manner.

In open-glottis pushing the urge to push comes and goes, occurring in "surges" three to five times during each contraction. The nurse may feel the surges by palpating the fundus. Increased tension in the uterus is felt for 5 to 7 seconds. If the woman is encouraged to behave spontaneously, her behavior will include short, 5- to 7-second breath holds during these surges, with time for several

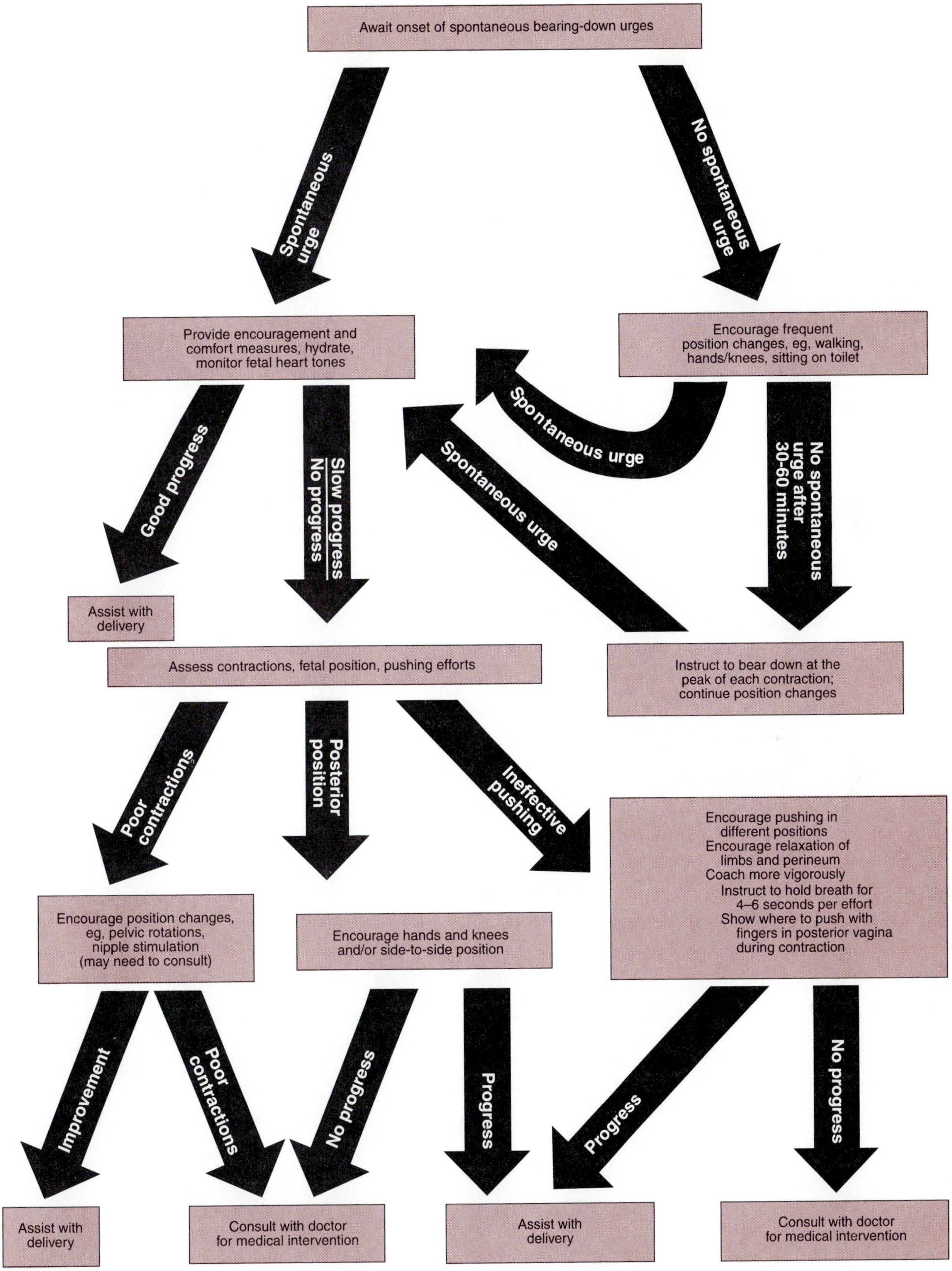

Figure 21-3.
Flow sheet for management of the second stage of labor. (From Cosner, K., & deJong, E. [1993]. Physiologic second stage labor. *American Journal of Maternal Child Nursing, 18*(1), 38–43.)

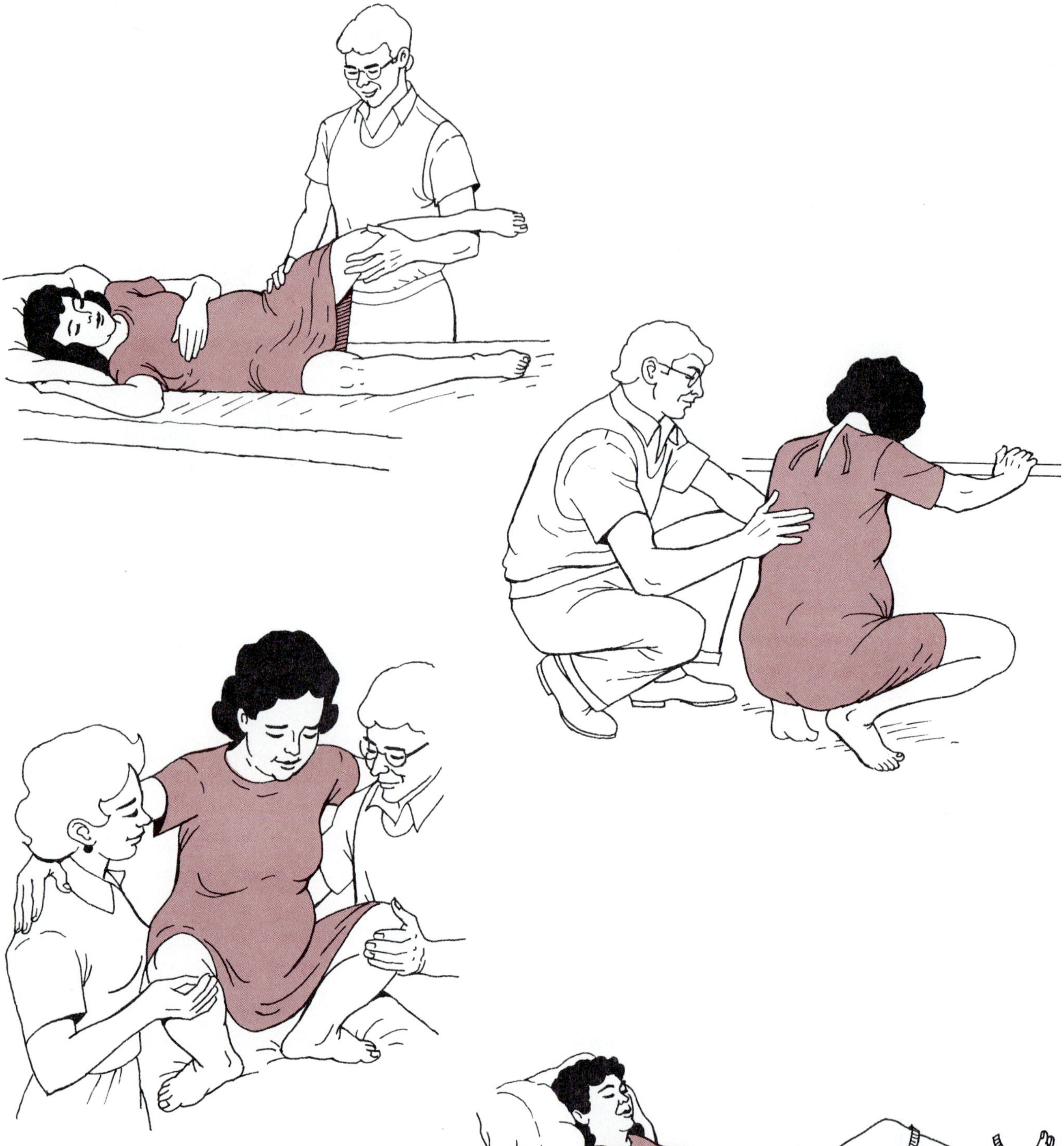

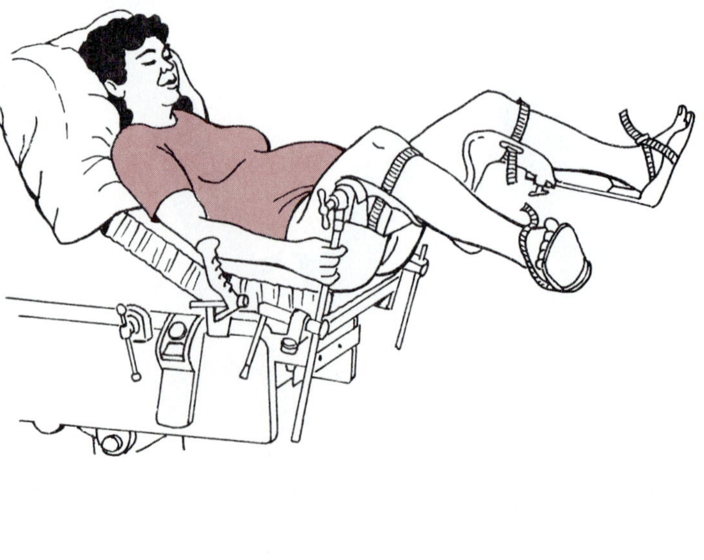

Figure 21-4.

Some commonly used positions for pushing in the second stage of labor. Most of these positions take advantage of gravity to aid bearing-down efforts. Laboring women will naturally assume many of these positions for bearing down if position choices are not restricted.

breaths in between. Grunting or other expiratory sounds may be heard.

Restraint in Pushing

In some instances uterine contractions are so intense and descent of the fetal head so rapid that expulsive efforts must be restrained to prevent perineal lacerations. In this case the woman must be coached to pant or pant-blow through the contractions. Assuming a sidelying position also may help to decrease the urge to push.

The woman's position can be varied during the second stage for the following reasons:

- Promote comfort
- Enhance or slow fetal descent
- Rotate a malpositioned fetus
- Avoid exacerbation of hemorrhoids
- Increase bearing-down sensations
- Protect the perineum from lacerations or episiotomy
- Intervene when fetal distress occurs due to umbilical cord compression or supine hypotension

Expected Outcomes

- The woman in labor uses effective breathing and expulsive techniques.
- The woman in labor assumes positions that facilitate expulsive efforts, maintain placental perfusion, and prevent or alleviate umbilical cord compression.

Promoting Comfort

The nurse encourages the woman to relax the perineum and to visualize the perineum thinning out to accommodate the fetus. Providing a mirror and helping her see the fetal head as it becomes visible or touch the fetal head may help her to do this. The woman should be reminded to relax as much as possible between contractions, and to keep her face, neck, and mouth as relaxed as possible during bearing-down efforts. Warm compresses to the perineum, perineal massage, or "ironing the perineum" (massaging and flattening the perineum between a finger inserted over the lower inner aspect of the vagina and the thumb) may help to promote perineal relaxation and tissue flexibility.

Shortly before birth, the woman may become unable to concentrate. The nurse can assist her by giving repeated and direct instructions on bearing-down efforts and by giving encouragement. Backache caused by fetal descent or an occiput posterior position may be alleviated in several ways. Pelvic rocking and counterpressure on the lower back may ameliorate the discomfort (see Chapter 18). Position changes should be frequent (at least every 15 minutes). The positions selected should promote physiologic bearing-down efforts. Squatting or hands-and-knees positions may be especially comfortable during the second stage. However, the nurse must be aware that the woman will require careful physical support in these positions.

The nurse should continue such comfort measures as supplying cool compresses and ice chips, because the woman typically becomes quite warm from the exertion of the second stage of labor. Mouth dryness is especially common because of mouth breathing with bearing-down efforts and because of dehydration. Sucking on large, hard, candy lollipops (not small candies, which may be kept in the mouth and might be aspirated) or frozen juice bars may be especially welcome and provide a source of food energy.

Expected Outcomes

- The woman in labor verbalizes her understanding of the interventions used to promote comfort.
- The woman verbalizes a decrease in her discomfort or pain.
- The woman demonstrates visible signs of relaxation between expulsive efforts.

Providing Emotional Support

The nurse should observe the interaction between the woman and her partner and be prepared to model encouragement and support techniques (Fig. 21-5). Support persons may have a tendency to become either overenthusiastic or too nondirective in their coaching efforts during the second stage. The nurse should explain what is needed and demonstrate it to the partner, reassuring the support person that he or she is doing well. The woman and partner should be well informed of progress during this phase, and the nurse should provide encouragement if progress appears slow. Slow progress can be especially demoralizing, and nursing support of the parents' confidence and spirits can be very helpful.

Expected Outcome

- The woman in labor and her support person verbalize a decrease in anxiety.

Monitoring for Complications

Complications in the second stage of labor primarily are related to the efforts of bearing down. The nurse must remain in constant attendance as the woman begins pushing. Perineal injury may result with sudden emergence of the fetal head. Position changes that reduce the effect of gravity, firm support of the perineum, and coaching the woman to begin a pant-blow pattern may reduce or prevent perineal trauma.

FHR decelerations and bradycardia can occur due to increased abdominal and intrauterine pressures, rapid changes in fetal position, and fetal head and umbilical cord compression. Closed-glottis pushing and the supine lithotomy position can result in further reductions in fetal oxygenation. While most fetuses demonstrate FHR decelerations in the second stage of labor, persistent bradycardia between 60 and 80 bpm signals severe acidosis and warrants active management (Roberts, 1989). Position changes, the administration of oxygen, temporary cessation of pushing efforts, and stimulation of the fetal scalp may alleviate the problem. If birth is not imminent and the bradycardia persists, timely obstetric intervention is indicated, such as performing an episiotomy to facilitate delivery.

• • Evaluation

The nurse performs ongoing evaluations during the early second stage of labor. If nursing interventions directed toward support of expulsive efforts and promotion of comfort

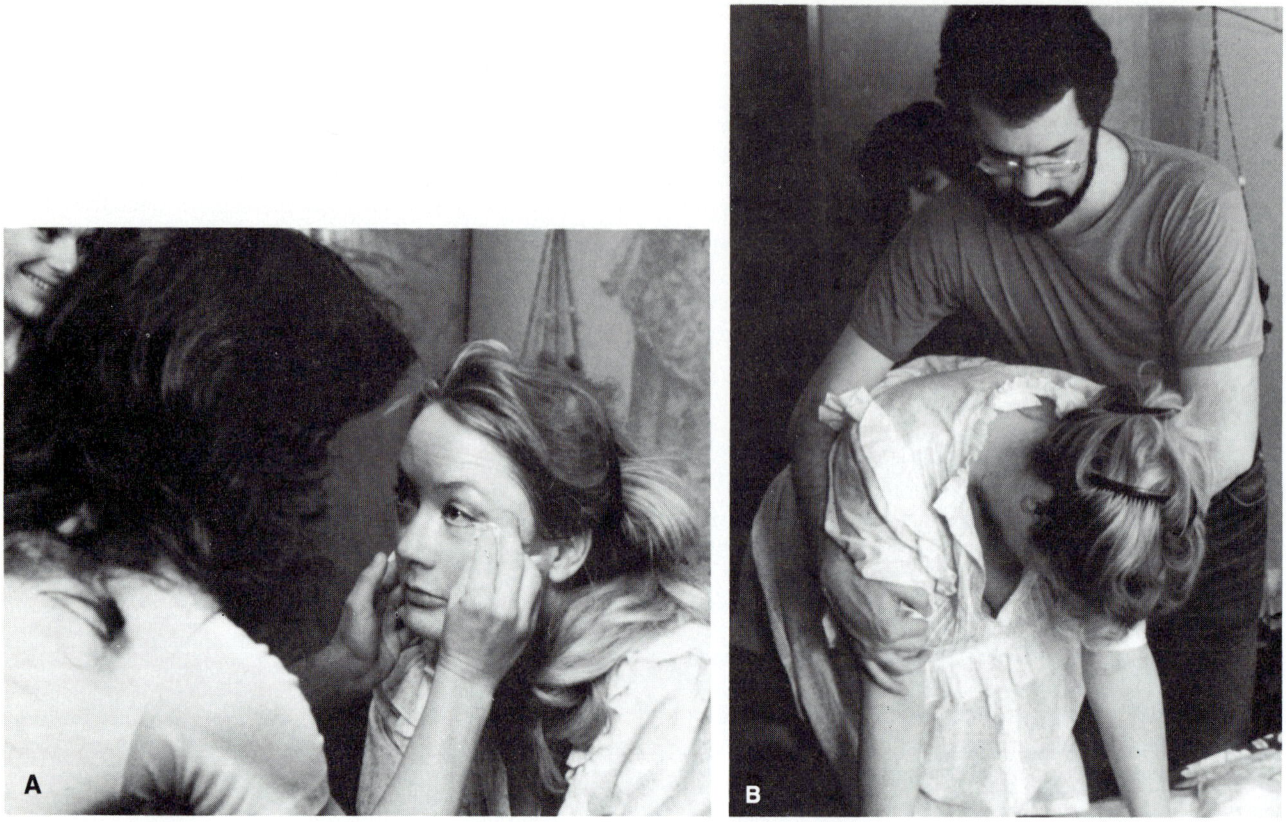

Figure 21-5.
A: The labor nurse provides comfort and encouragement to the laboring woman. *B:* The woman's partner supports here in active labor. This woman has chosen to labor in a hands-and-knees position. (Photo by BABES, Inc.)

are successful, the woman will demonstrate effective pushing techniques that result in steady descent of the fetus, and she will rest comfortably between contractions. The woman will maintain physiologic stability, and the FHR will remain within normal limits, although common variations frequently observed during second-stage expulsive efforts (for example, early decelerations with head compression) may be noted. The support person or partner will be able to continue in the support role and provide encouragement as the woman approaches the time of delivery.

The early second stage of labor often is characterized by a decrease in the intensity and pace of labor. This physiologic "lull" provides the woman with an opportunity to recoup her physical and emotional resources required for the bearing-down efforts demanded during the second stage. Particularly in primigravid women, time is usually available for resting, emptying the bladder, and changing positions to promote comfort. The goals of nursing care include encouraging rest, preparing women for bearing-down efforts (teaching and position change), and reassuring and revitalizing the support person for this period of labor. In multiparous women the early second stage may last several seconds to several hours and requires adjustments in the nurse's plan of care.

Care of the Family During Late Second Stage of Labor

• • Assessment

As birth of the infant approaches, the nurse is engaged in a variety of tasks that require great organizational skills. The nurse must move very quickly at times to prepare for the impending birth and to provide the woman with ongoing support and guidance and the birth attendant with necessary equipment and supplies.

Continuous appraisal of maternal and fetal status must be integrated with these essential nursing tasks. The perceptions of the woman, her support person, and family will be strongly influenced by the demeanor of the nurse during this potentially hectic period just preceding the birth of the newborn. A calm, reassuring approach will reassure the woman and facilitate an optimum birth experience.

Monitoring Maternal and Fetal Physiologic Status

The nurse continues to monitor the woman's vital signs (blood pressure, pulse, and respirations) and FHR at 5- to 15-minute intervals during the final moments before birth, depending on the maternal and fetal condition. If abnormalities are noted, the FHR should be auscultated after each contraction, or continuous EFM may be used. If EFM is used and the woman is transferred to a delivery room for the birth, it is imperative that the monitor be reapplied when she is positioned on the delivery table and that the fetus be continuously monitored until birth.

Assessing Emotional Responses and Coping Mechanisms

The impending birth of the infant may cause dramatic emotional responses in the woman and her partner or support person. The woman may cry out as the perineum is stretched and the head begins to emerge. It is quite common for the woman to ask that the infant be taken out immediately by forceps or cesarean delivery, or she may verbalize her inability to perform the last few pushes needed to deliver the infant—"I can't do it! Help me!" or "Take it out! I'm ripping apart!" The support person may become frightened or feel faint at this time. The nurse should assess the woman's and partner's responses at this time and offer immediate guidance and support.

• • Nursing Diagnosis

Several nursing diagnoses may be appropriate as the fetal head begins to crown, and birth is imminent:

- High Risk for Infection related to traumatized tissues and environmental factors
- Anxiety related to increased activity in the labor room
- Ineffective Individual Coping related to the physical sensations or emotional significance of impending birth
- Pain related to stretching of the perineum
- Powerlessness related to the activity and environment of the delivery room
- Fear related to impending birth

• • Planning and Implementation

The nurse prepares the woman for delivery by maintaining asepsis in equipment and supplies, summoning personnel needed for delivery, positioning the woman, and supporting the woman in her final expulsive efforts.

Maintaining Aseptic Technique and Providing Sterile Supplies

If the woman is positioned on the delivery table, a perineal scrub is often performed, and the area is draped. A delivery pack of sterile supplies will be opened and laid out for the physician or nurse midwife. This pack contains the instruments used for an episiotomy, for suctioning the neonate, and for clamping and cutting the umbilical cord. Sterile technique is observed in the conventional hospital delivery room or operating room to prevent nosocomial infections. Caps, masks, shoe covers or protective leggings, and sterile gowns and gloves are required for personnel. The support person is given a cap, mask, shoe covers, and gown.

In a labor room or birthing room delivery, a small sterile field may be created by putting a sterile drape under the woman's buttocks just before delivery. The sterile supplies and instruments are usually placed on a cart next to the birthing bed. A perineal scrub is optional and may be limited to cleansing of the perineum and anal area. Before the AIDS epidemic, guidelines for asepsis were somewhat relaxed in the birthing room. Clean cover gowns and sterile gloves usually were worn by the birth attendant. Today, the Centers for Disease Control guidelines and the Department of Labor, Occupational Safety, and Health Administration (OSHA) guidelines for universal body substance precautions (1991) mandate observance of universal precautions by the nursing and medical staff at all times. Splash-resistant gowns, gloves, and face masks that incorporate eye shields or goggles must be worn by all personnel directly involved in the birth. Support persons who will come in direct contact with body secretions also should wear appropriate barrier attire.

Expected Outcome

- The woman and support person verbalize an understanding of the universal precautions used by nursing and medical staff during the birth of the infant.

Providing Equipment and Summoning Personnel Needed for Delivery

A large quantity of equipment is not necessary for a spontaneous vaginal birth. Essential equipment, usually provided in a standard delivery pack, includes the following items:

- Sterile gown and gloves for the birth attendant
- Sterile drapes
- Gauze sponges for drying the neonate's face
- Bulb syringe for suctioning the neonate
- Two clamps for the umbilical cord
- Two scissors: one for the cord and one for the episiotomy, if needed
- A large basin for the placenta
- Gauze sponges and ring forceps for inspection of the vagina and perineum

In addition an infant linen pack contains infant blankets, sterile towels for handling the neonate, and a cap. All equipment and linens should be handled with aseptic technique and should be readily available to the birth attendant. An additional light source should be available in case it is needed. A radiant warmer for use during the initial assessment of the neonate and access to resuscitation equipment are important. The nurse should verify that this equipment is present and in working order before delivery (Fig. 21-6).

A birth attendant and a labor nurse should be present. When neonatal complications are anticipated, a pediatrician and a nursery nurse are essential and should be called in advance. If additional staff are called, the labor nurse should provide them with a brief summary of the labor and introduce them to the parents.

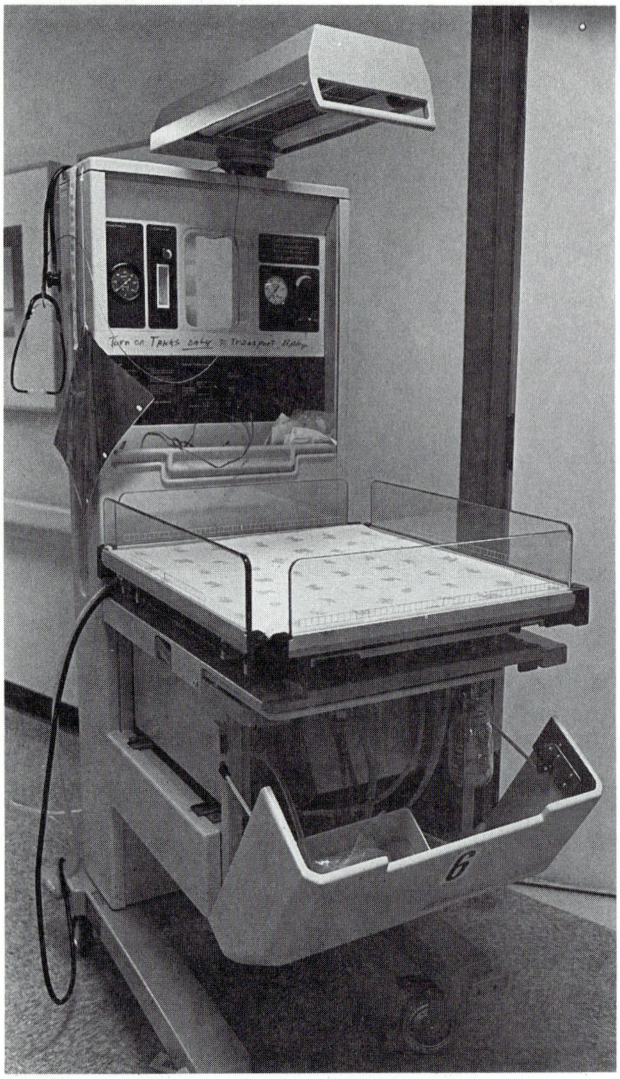

Figure 21-6.
A radiant heat crib used in the conventional delivery room setting. (Photo by Kathy Sloane.)

Expected Outcome

- The woman and support person verbalize an understanding of the equipment used and the personnel present for the birth of the infant.

Transferring the Woman to the Delivery Room

In many settings today labor and birth can occur in the same room, thus eliminating the inconvenience and discomfort of transferring the woman during the final stages of expulsion. If for any reason the birth is to take place in the delivery room, the primigravida is usually transferred by gurney or in the labor bed when the perineum is bulging. The multipara often is transferred at 8 to 9 cm of cervical dilatation, because birth can occur rapidly with complete dilatation of the cervix. If EFM has been used, it is reapplied in the delivery room. To the extent possible the nurse should leave ample time for a calm transfer, allowing the woman to move between contractions. Efforts must be made to maintain the woman's privacy and comfort during the move.

Expected Outcome

- The woman participates in the decision-making process regarding the setting for birth and verbalizes satisfaction with the environment.

Positioning the Woman for Delivery

The Lithotomy Position

Throughout history women have preferred the upright position for childbirth. However, in the last 50 years most women in the United States have given birth in the lithotomy, modified lithotomy, or recumbent position. Many reasons have been suggested for these positions, including increased use of analgesics and anesthesia, operative delivery, continuous EFM, episiotomy, and the more active management of delivery by the attendant.

This practice has come into question. The lithotomy position for birth has been linked to increased perineal lacerations and the woman's discomfort caused by stretching the leg muscles, torsion on the hip joints, and pressure on the coccyx. Thus, the lithotomy position does not facilitate physiologic labor and birth and can be a disadvantage to the woman and fetus. However, the lithotomy position is the position of choice when operative procedures are needed to complete the delivery. The technique is described in the accompanying Nursing Procedure.

Alternate Positions for Birth

Any delivery position used should allow the bearing-down efforts of the woman to be aided by gravity, promote fetal descent and rotation, and avoid supine hypotension. Descent and rotation are best aided by a position that provides for mobility of the pelvis into a pelvic tilt so that the sacral promontory is pulled away from the uterus, creating larger pelvic diameters in all planes. Radiographic studies have shown an increase of 0.5 to 2 cm in pelvic diameters when the woman is in a squatting position or on her hands and knees. Figure 21-7 illustrates physiologic positions for delivery. The left sidelying (Sims) position also may be used for birth and may be particularly beneficial for women with hypertension during pregnancy.

No one position is ideal for the second stage of labor and birth. Each position must be evaluated according to the particular circumstances. Modern delivery tables allow a variety of positions for delivery that promote the woman's comfort and give the birth attendant a clear view and good access to the perineum. The woman's body should be supported so she can curl forward and pull on handles with bearing-down efforts yet relax between contractions. Ongoing research has revealed positive and negative aspects of birth in a squatting or sitting position and with the use of the birthing chair (see the accompanying Nursing Research display). Birthing beds and birthing chairs that permit conversion to the traditional lithotomy position are being used increasingly in labor and delivery units today. In many set-

NURSING PROCEDURE
Supporting the Woman in the Lithotomy Position for Birth

The lithotomy position is used during specific procedures, including forceps delivery, vacuum extraction, and in some cases the repair of the episiotomy or lacerations.

Purpose: To promote comfort, and prevent injury while the woman is maintained in the lithotomy position.

NURSING ACTION	RATIONALE
1. Place a rolled towel or cushion under the woman's right hip.	To displace the uterus to the left to alleviate the effects of the supine hypotension syndrome.
2. Pad the stirrups.	To prevent pressure points that may injure tissue or constrict circulation in the legs.
3. Raise both legs simultaneously when placing them in the stirrups.	To prevent torsion, stretching, or injury to the sacroiliac joint or the ligaments, tendons, or muscles in the legs.
4. Readjust the stirrups so that the legs are aligned symetrically in relation to each other.	To prevent torsion, stretching, or injury to the sacroiliac joint or the ligaments, tendons, or muscles in the legs.
5. Dorsiflex the woman's feet if she experiences leg cramps.	To reduce contraction of the muscle through gentle stretching.
6. Minimize the length of time this position is used.	To reduce muscle soreness related to prolonged positioning in the lithotomy position.
7. Remove both of the woman's legs together from the stirrups.	To avoid injury to the sacroiliac joints, or the muscles, ligaments or tendons in the legs.

tings the traditional delivery table is often reserved for high-risk births (Fig. 21-8). Regardless of the equipment used, positioning the woman properly on the delivery table or bed is an important nursing responsibility.

If a conventional delivery table is to be used, the woman should be positioned in a semisitting position with the head of the table elevated 30 to 60 degrees or with pillows and partner assistance used to support the woman's back and head as shown in Figure 21-9. The bottom of the delivery table should remain extended until the birth attendant is present.

If stirrups are to be used, the woman's legs should be moved into position simultaneously. Both stirrups should be adjusted for the woman's comfort. The nurse should check that excessive pressure is not placed on the calf or popliteal area because this may predispose the woman to thrombophlebitis in the postpartum period. The nurse should never leave a woman unattended once she is positioned for delivery and should respect the woman's modesty by covering her as much as possible while preserving an easy view of the perineum.

Expected Outcome

- The woman verbalizes comfort with the position selected or required for birth.

Supporting the Woman During Final Expulsive Efforts

As the woman pushes the fetal head will advance, receding between bearing-down efforts until the vaginal opening completely encircles the head. This event is known as "crowning." The nurse prepares the woman and her support person for their first contact with the newborn. This can be done by providing a mirror so the woman can see the fetal head or guiding her hand to touch the fetal head if she desires to do so. The woman may express an inability to push past the pain or intense burning sensation experienced as the largest diameter of the fetal head stretches the perineum. The nurse must provide continuous physical and emotional support during these final moments before birth and reinforce any directions the birth attendant gives the woman at this time.

If the amniotic sac is still intact at this point, the birth attendant will rupture it to prevent the neonate from aspirating amniotic fluid with its first respiratory effort. If it appears that the vaginal opening will lacerate before the head is delivered, the birth attendant may administer local anesthesia, either through infiltration of the perineum or by pudendal block, and perform an episiotomy.

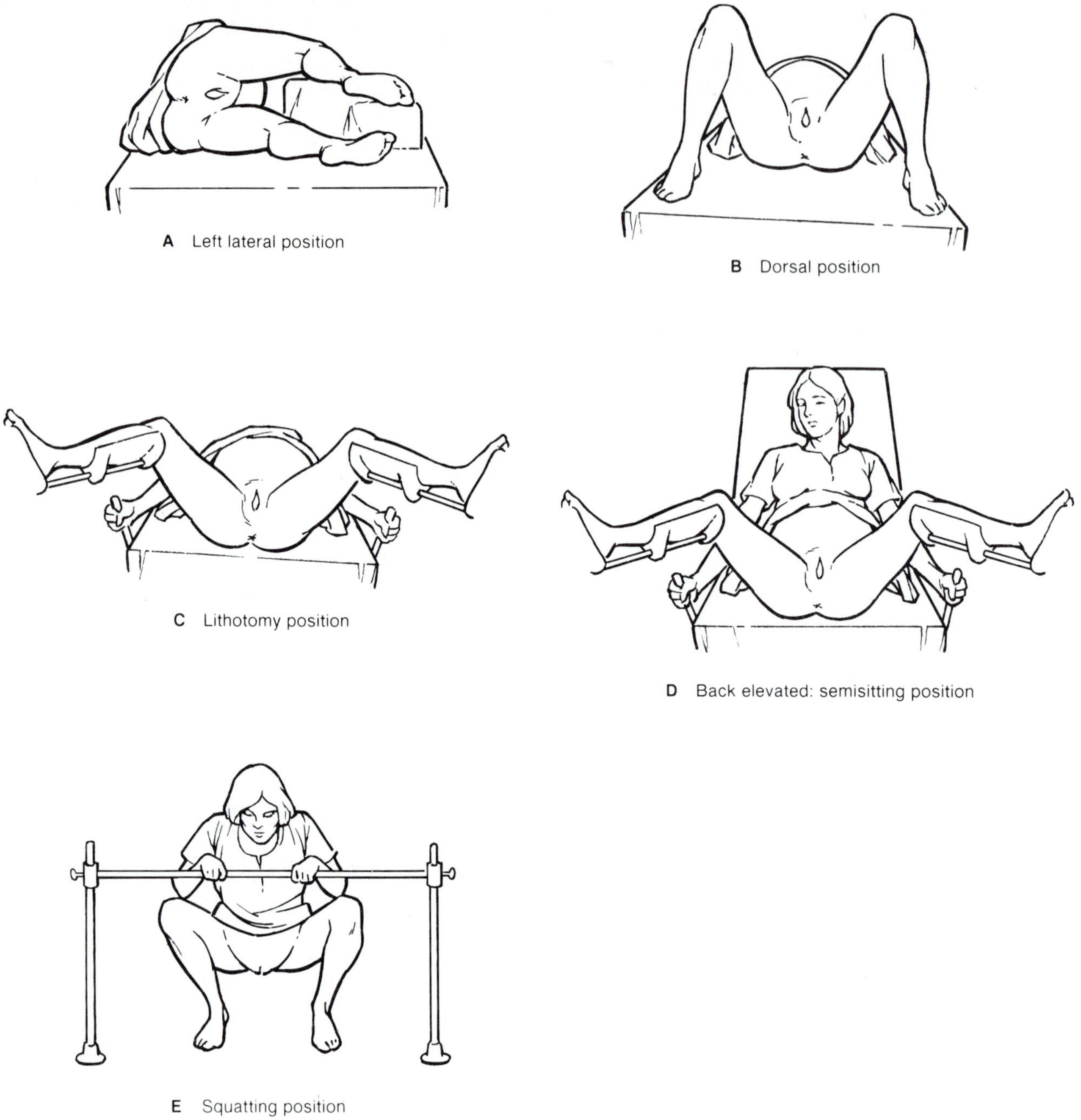

Figure 21-7.
Positions for delivery. *A:* Left lateral position. *B:* Dorsal position (with slight left tilt). *C:* Lithotomy position (with slight left tilt). *D:* Back elevated and semisitting position. *E:* Squatting position.

Expected Outcome

- The woman maintains an effective, physiologically safe, and comfortable position during birth of the newborn.

Preparing the Woman for Episiotomy

If the physician or midwife elects to perform an episiotomy, the nurse reinforces information and support to the woman as preparations are made. The nurse supplies the birth attendant with necessary equipment.

An episiotomy is an incision made from the lower aspect of the vaginal opening into the perineum during the second stage to enlarge the opening to accommodate the fetal head; this is done to prevent tearing the underlying muscle and fascia as the head is born. Episiotomy is the second most common surgical procedure performed. More than 65% of vaginal deliveries in the United States include episiotomy. Among primigravidas the incidence reaches 80% to 90% depending on the facility and whether the birth attendant is a physician or midwife.

Nursing Research

The Effects of the Birthing Chair or Stool on Maternal Outcomes in Labor and Delivery

Researchers have reported mixed findings concerning the use of the birth chair or stool, Crowley and associates (1991) found a reduction in episiotomy rates but no beneficial effects on the incidence of perineal trauma. Several studies have demonstrated a shortened second stage of labor for multiparas using the chair. Other investigators have found no differences. The effect of the birthing chair on blood loss, perineal swelling, and lacerations also is unclear. Waldenstrom and Gottval (1991) found a greater mean estimated blood loss and cases of postpartum hemorrhage in women using a birthing chair or stool, while Gardosi, Hutson, and Lynch (1989) found fewer perineal tears. Women using a birth chair have scored higher on comfort scales and reported lower perceptions of pain during the second stage when using the chair.

Some clinical researchers suggest that the chair should be pivoted to a horizontal position after birth of the infant or significant blood loss can occur with placental separation and from the episiotomy site. Further study is indicated. Practitioners may continued to use the birthing chair, but they should observe the perineum closely during second-stage expulsive efforts for signs of edema. They also may consider changing the position of the chair to the horizontal plane immediately after birth if an episiotomy was performed or significant bleeding occurs.

Crowley, P., Elbourne, D., et al. (1991). Delivery in an obstetric birth chair: A randomized controlled trial. *British Journal of Obstetrics and Gynaecology, 98,* 667.

Gardosi, J., Hutson, N. & Lynch, C. (1989). Randomised, controlled trial of squatting in the second stage of labour. *Lancet, 2,* 74.

Waldenstrom, U., & Gottval, K. (1991). A randomized trial of birthing stool or conventional semirecumbent position for second-stage labor. *Birth, 18*(1), 5.

Shannahan, M., & Cottrell, B. (1991). The effects of birth chair delivery on maternal perceptions. *Journal of Obstetric, Gynecologic, and Neonatal Nursing, 18*(4), 323.

The routine use of episiotomy is controversial. Nurse midwifery practice has historically relied on nonsurgical methods of protecting the perineum during the second stage, including perineal massage and the use of alternative positions to enhance perineal stretching while minimizing pressure on the tissue. Physicians may perform episiotomy more often because they have not had extensive experience in delivering over an intact perineum. Scientific studies to date have not demonstrated benefits of episiotomy in well-controlled clinical trials, and the risks of episiotomy are not insignificant (Thorp & Bowes, 1989). Maternal and fetal benefits and risks in episiotomy are discussed in the following display.

Types of Episiotomy

The two major types of episiotomy are the median and the mediolateral, shown in Figure 21-10. Both usually are performed under local anesthesia by the physician or nurse midwife, as shown in Figure 21-11. In some cases the perineum is naturally numbed by stretching and the pressure of the fetal head, and the episiotomy can be performed without anesthesia, if necessary. Infiltration of the perineum with lidocaine produces perineal anesthesia for the episiotomy and for its repair. Injection of lidocaine, using long needle guides, into the vaginal walls near the ischial spines blocks pain impulses through the pudendal nerve and provides anesthesia of the lower two thirds of the vagina and the perineum. This technique, known as pudendal block, also provides short-duration anesthesia for delivery and perineal repair. It is safe and effective and has little effect on the fetus. Pudendal block may temporarily blunt the woman's urge to bear down in the second stage.

The *median episiotomy* incision is the type most commonly used in the United States. It is reported to be easier to repair, less painful, less disfiguring, and associated with less blood loss and more rapid healing than the mediolateral incision. A disadvantage of the median incision is a higher incidence of extension (tearing beyond the incision) through the anal sphincter into the rectum.

The *mediolateral episiotomy* incision is used frequently in Europe and other parts of the world. Its advantages are that it provides more room for obstetric maneuvers and has less tendency to extend into the rectum than the median episiotomy. However, its disadvantages are regarded as significant and account for the rarity of its use in the United States. They include increased difficulty in repairing the incision, longer wound healing time, increased blood loss, greater distortion in perineal configuration, and consequent sexual dysfunction, including persistent dyspareunia.

The decision concerning the necessity of an episiotomy must be made by the birth attendant with as much participation as possible by the woman. No woman can be guaranteed that episiotomy will not be necessary, because many unexpected events may occur during labor and birth. The nurse can play an important role in minimizing the need for episiotomy during the intrapartum period.

Expected Outcomes

- The woman gives informed consent for an episiotomy.
- The woman verbalizes satisfaction with the decision to use an episiotomy.

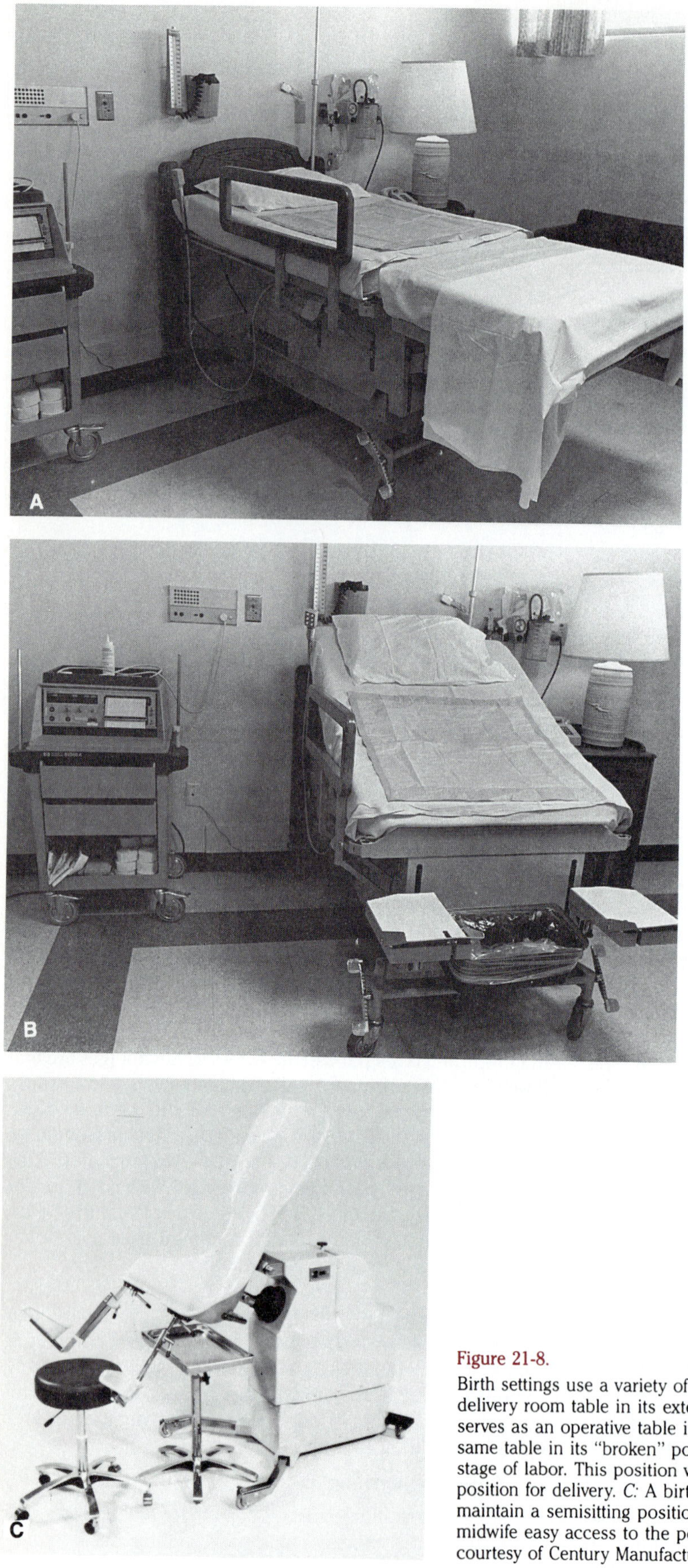

Figure 21-8.

Birth settings use a variety of beds and equipment. *A:* A standard delivery room table in its extended or flat position. The table also serves as an operative table if cesarean delivery is needed. *B:* The same table in its "broken" position, ready for use in the second stage of labor. This position will support the woman in a semisitting position for delivery. *C:* A birthing chair that enables the woman to maintain a semisitting position while still allowing the physician or midwife easy access to the perineum. (*A* and *B* by Kathy Sloane, *C* courtesy of Century Manufacturing Co, Inc.)

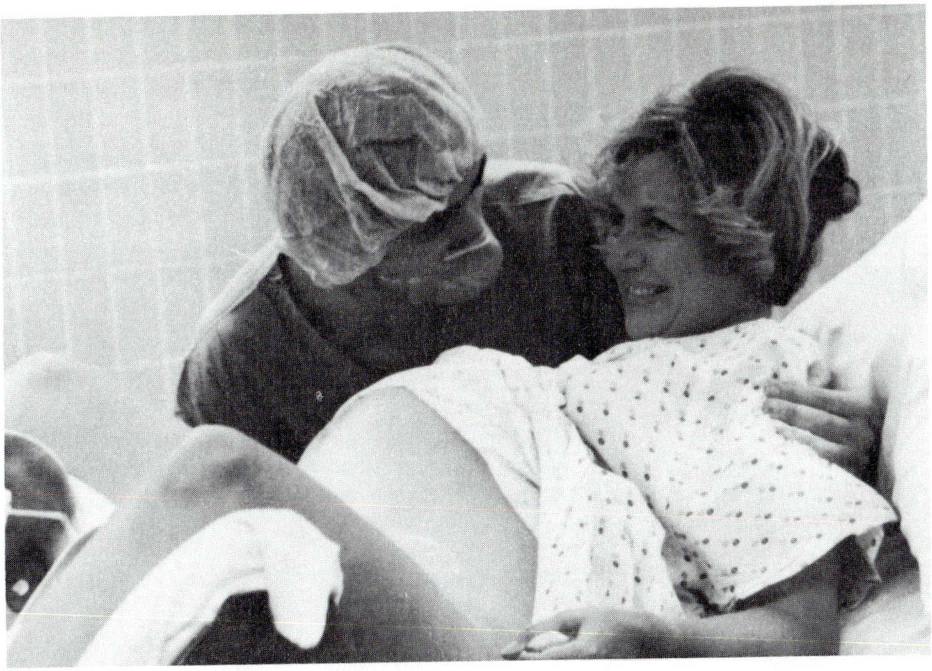

Figure 21-9.
Bearing-down efforts in a conventional delivery room. The woman is supported in a semirecumbent position by pillows and by the support person. Her legs are supported by well-padded stirrups; handholds are in place to assist pushing efforts. (Photo by BABES, Inc.)

Helping the Woman Maintain an Intact Perineum

When the woman wishes to avoid episiotomy and the birth attendant is cooperative, the nurse may use the following techniques to maximize the chances that the perineum will remain intact.

- Apply warm compresses to the perineum during the second stage of labor to promote relaxation, increased circulation, and increased pliability of the perineal tissues.
- Encourage gentle pushing during the second stage to allow for gradual distention of the perineal tissue.
- Encourage the woman to avoid bearing-down efforts when crowning occurs.

Benefits and Risks of Episiotomy

Benefits of Episiotomy

The following list reflects general beliefs that are based on observations in clinical practice and are not necessarily documented by clinical research.

Maternal Benefits

- May maintain pelvic floor integrity
- May lower incidence of serious lacerations with delivery of large infant
- Heals more rapidly than a laceration

Fetal Benefits

- Shortens second stage, which may be important with compromised fetus
- May prevent fetal brain damage by reducing pressure on fetal head from pelvic floor; may be important with premature fetus

Obstetric Benefits

- Facilitates obstetric maneuvers, such as forceps delivery and vacuum extraction
- Facilitates delivery of malpresenting or large infants
- Shortens second stage

Risks of Episiotomy

The following risks have been documented in clinical research and practice.

- Increased risk of third-degree and fourth-degree perineal lacerations
- Severe postepisiotomy pain is estimated to occur in 60% of women
- Risk of infection is increased
- Pain and edema may inhibit urination and defecation after delivery
- Risk of significant blood loss is increased
- Risk of persistent dyspareunia, which may last 6 months or more, is increased

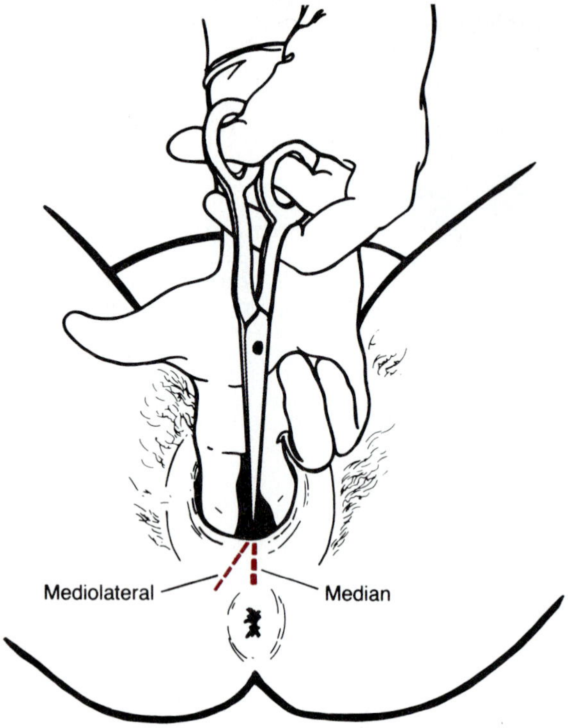

Figure 21-10.
Episiotomy types.

- Use a lubricant to massage the perineum during the second stage.
- Apply an ice pack on the clitoral or periurethral area during crowning to reduce the burning and stinging that accompany stretching of the vagina and to enhance perineal relaxation.
- Use positions for delivery that avoid overstretching the perineum, such as the sidelying or semisitting positions. When stirrups are used, position to avoid hyperextension of the legs and extreme perineal stretching.

Some conditions necessitate the use of episiotomy, and the birth attendant is in the best position to determine the best course of action for the health of the mother and newborn. The nurse can encourage women to avoid unnecessary episiotomy by using these techniques but should discourage women from focusing on this intervention to the detriment of the rest of the birth experience.

Expected Outcomes

- The woman verbalizes an understanding of the techniques used to reduce perineal trauma.
- The woman follows specific instructions regarding positioning and bearing-down efforts so that perineal trauma is minimized or eliminated.

• • Evaluation

The nurse continues to make rapid evaluations of the maternal and fetal responses to final expulsive efforts and impending birth. Successful adaptations are reflected in continuous emergence and crowning of the fetal presenting part. The woman and her support person are able to follow directions in terms of positioning and ongoing expulsive efforts. Although some variation in the woman's vital signs can be expected in the last few minutes of the second stage, the woman's condition will remain stable in the final moments before birth. Pressures exerted on the fetal head also may result in temporary fluctuations in the FHR, but short- and long-term variability will remain within normal limits.

The final moments before birth require the utmost attention and concentration on the part of the woman. The

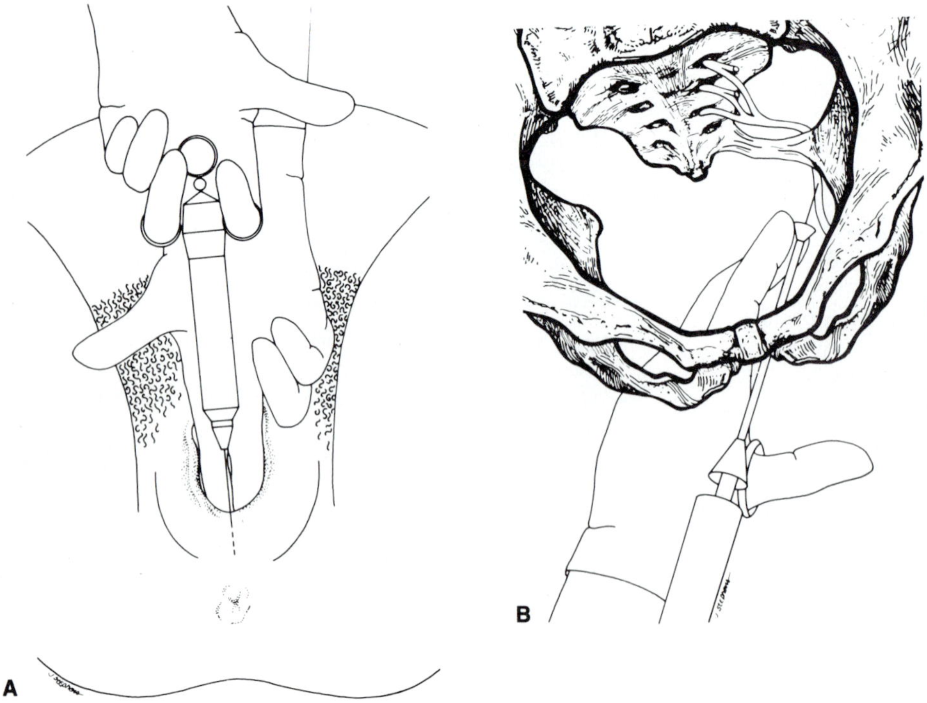

Figure 21-11.
Local anesthesia for episiotomy. *A:* Local infiltration of the perineum. *B:* Pudendal block (Childbirth Graphics).

nurse must use a variety of communication techniques that aid the woman in directing her energies on the final expulsive efforts. The nurse must be skilled in aseptic and surgical techniques and able to respond rapidly to the needs of the woman and the birth attendant. Goals of nursing care at this phase include preparing the supplies needed for birth, assisting the physician or midwife, and providing physical and emotional support to the woman at the time when her energy levels are often low or depleted.

Birth of the Neonate

The birth of the neonate is the culmination of the pregnancy; for most families it is the highlight of the labor process. While the woman and her support person are generally focused on the newborn, the nurse must simultaneously remain alert to the needs of the woman, neonate, support person, and birth attendant. The immediate physiologic needs of the woman and neonate will take precedence, but once the nurse confirms that the condition of both is stable, a major goal is to promote a family-centered experience.

• • Assessment

As the head is born the nurse must remain vigilant to the development of complications, including the presence of a tight nuchal cord (cord looped around the fetal neck) or impaction of the fetal shoulders (shoulder dystocia). The nurse must work closely with the birth attendant to identify the need for rapid interventions to prevent problems related to these conditions or the untoward sequelae of other complications. If the birth proceeds in an uneventful manner, the nurse can focus on behavioral responses of the woman and family members. Attention should be paid to the support person's responses. While it is uncommon for partners or support persons to faint during the birth, the nurse should observe their reactions and attend to any physical indicators of impending syncope.

• • Nursing Diagnosis

The birth is a rapid event, and the experienced nurse responds automatically to the process. However, several pertinent nursing diagnoses may emerge during the actual birth:

- High Risk for Injury (maternal) related to precipitous birth
- Ineffective Airway Clearance related to aspiration of fluids
- High Risk for Injury (fetal) related to precipitous birth

• • Planning and Implementation

The nurse must accomplish multiple tasks almost simultaneously during and immediately after the birth of the newborn. The following section describes the process of delivery and the roles of the birth attendant and nurse during this period.

Assisting With the Delivery of the Fetal Head

The birth attendant applies gentle pressure on the advancing head to control the delivery and prevent too-rapid expulsion. The other hand supports the perineum and prepares to receive the head as it emerges. The woman is instructed to pant or breathe through her contractions and to bear down only when asked to do so. The nurse may demonstrate this technique to guide the woman or should explain that this assists in controlling the birth and reduces the risk of a too-rapid delivery. The head is usually delivered between contractions.

Expected Outcome

- The woman follows the birth attendant's directives during the expulsion of the fetal head.

Suctioning of the Airway

Once the head is delivered the birth attendant suctions the neonate's mouth and then the nose with a bulb syringe. Because suctioning of the nares can create involuntary gasping, the mouth is always suctioned *first* to prevent aspiration of fluids in the oral cavity. The nurse often is required to provide equipment for suctioning or to assist in the procedure when mechanical suctioning is indicated. Suctioning with a mechanical suction device attached to a 10 French catheter is performed to clear the nasopharynx when the fetus has passed meconium before birth. The mouth and nares are still suctioned with a bulb syringe. The catheter is inserted into the mouth, pharynx, and then the nose to remove as much viscous, meconium- stained fluid as possible before the neonate's body is delivered.

Expected Outcome

- The newborn demonstrates normal breathing after the airway is cleared of fluids.

Delivering the Shoulders and Body

The birth attendant checks for the presence of a nuchal cord. This is done by inserting two fingers along the back of the neonate's neck. A nuchal cord (a loop of umbilical cord around the neonate's neck) is found in approximately 25% of deliveries and usually causes no difficulty. The loose loop is pulled out and slipped over the newborn's head to allow for delivery (Fig. 21-12); the attendant should then feel for a second loop and remove it in the same way. If the loop is too tight to be pulled over the head, it is double-clamped and cut between the clamps. The nurse guides the woman in resisting the urge to bear down until the birth attendant directs her to do so.

The birth attendant then holds the head in both hands and applies gentle downward pressure to ease the anterior shoulder under the symphysis. The woman is then asked to push gently to deliver the anterior shoulder; gentle upward pressure is then applied to deliver the posterior shoulder. The rest of the newborn slips out easily once the shoulders are delivered. The birth attendant suctions the mouth and nares again and observes for the onset of respirations and the change in color from cyanotic to pink, evaluates the muscle

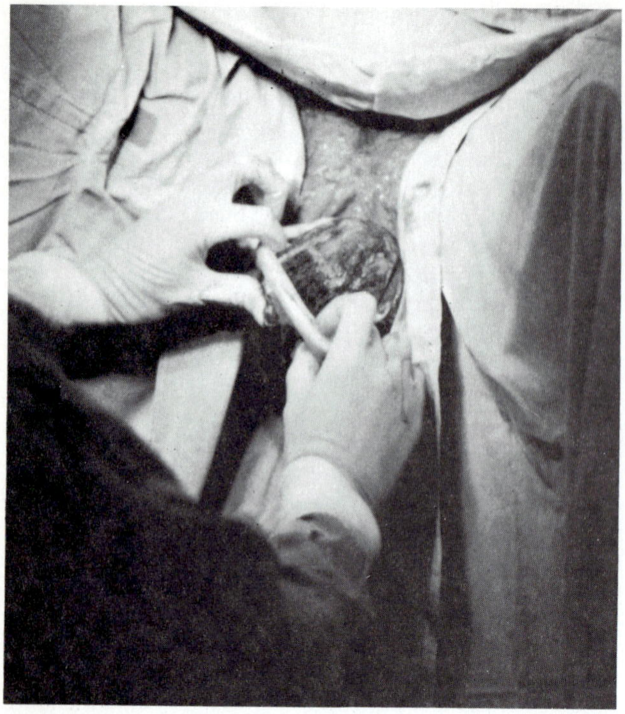

Figure 21-12.

The birth attendant finds the nuchal cord and slips the loop over the neonate's head. Notice the sterile draping in a delivery room setting. (Photo by BABES, Inc.)

tone, and makes an initial decision regarding the infant's condition. Two sterile clamps are placed on the cord 2 to 4 in from the umbilicus, and the cord is cut between the clamps with sterile scissors. Some birth attendants permit the father to cut the cord under close supervision, as seen in Figure 21-13.

The nurse should note the time of delivery for recording purposes and begin the timing for evaluation of the 1- and 5-minute Apgar scores. When an uncomplicated birth is anticipated, the nurse will place baby blankets on the women's abdomen. If the newborn is healthy and no signs of distress are evident at delivery, the birth attendant will place the newborn in the blanket on the mother's abdomen. The nurse can assist the mother to dry the neonate as the first abbreviated initial newborn assessment is performed. The 1- and 5-minute Apgar scores are then normally assigned by the nurse as he or she supports initial parent–newborn interaction. (See discussion of Apgar scoring and Table 21-1 later in this chapter.)

Other nursing responsibilities include preparation and application of the identification bracelets. The identification bracelets are matching identity bands that are usually placed on the infant's wrist and ankle and the mother's wrist. In some facilities with a central nursery, the father of the newborn also may receive a matching identification wrist band so that he may transport the neonate to and from the nursery. These bands are checked to confirm the identity of the newborn each time the neonate is taken to the mother and when procedures such as circumcision are performed. (The accompanying Nursing Procedure describes the procedure for identification.)

Expected Outcomes

- The woman demonstrates the ability to follow directions during the delivery of the neonate's body.
- The woman verbalizes satisfaction with her role in the birth of the neonate.
- The woman and support person identify the importance of identification techniques.

Obtaining Blood Samples

While awaiting placental separation the birth attendant will obtain a sample of blood from the umbilical cord. This sample is passed to the nurse or another physician who is responsible for placing the blood in the appropriate collection receptacles and labeling the specimens. Laboratory tests are completed later for neonatal blood type and Rh factor and a Venereal Disease Research Laboratories screen for syphilis. Many facilities also obtain umbilical cord blood samples at this time to evaluate the biochemical status of the neonate. A 4- to 6-inch length of cord is cut, clamped, and handed to the delivery room nurse, who then may obtain venous and arterial blood samples for analysis (see the Nursing Procedure, Obtaining Umbilical Cord Blood Samples for Biochemical Analysis).

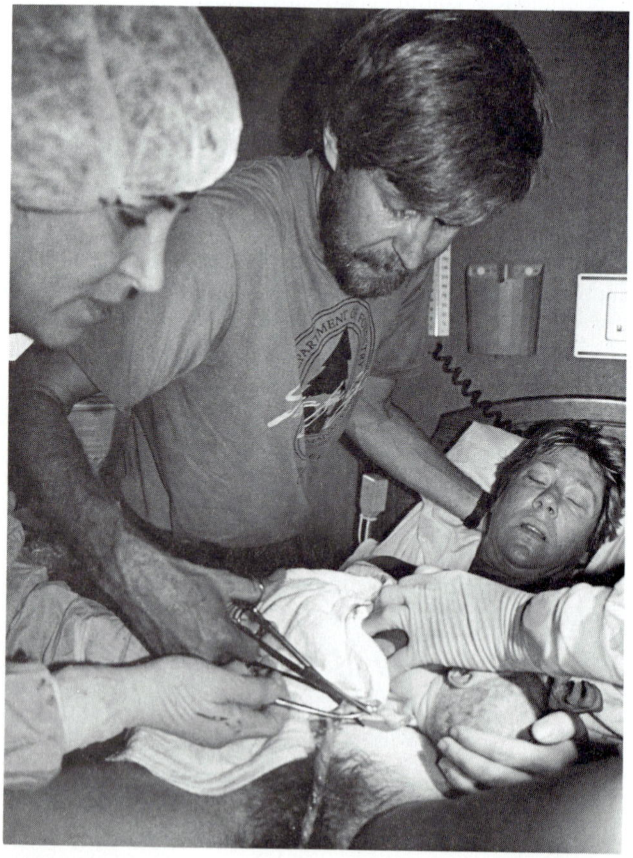

Figure 21-13.

This father is permitted to cut the cord after the birth attendant has clamped it. (Photo by Kathy Sloane. Courtesy of Alta Bates Medical Center.)

NURSING PROCEDURE
Identifying the Neonate

Purpose: To establish accurate identification of the neonate before mother and infant are separated.

NURSING ACTION	*RATIONALE*
1. Apply matching identification bands showing woman's first and last name and patient record number on both mother and infant.	To prevent accidental mismatching of parent and infant.
2. Place two bands on the infant (one wrist and one ankle). Place matching band on mother's wrist. In many units a band is also placed on the wrist of the father or partner.	To permit mother *or* partner to take infant from nursery or accompany the infant to procedures.
3. Place bands on infant snugly, but verify that circulatory compromise has not occurred.	To prevent identification band from slipping off. Infant weight loss (5% to 10% of birth weight) is common in the first days of life.
4. (If hospital policy requires fingerprinting or footprinting.) Take care to clean and dry skin surfaces before taking the prints.	Moisture, blood, mucus, or vernix can reduce clarity of print.
5. When taking an infant to its mother, address the woman by name, and verify that her band and infant's bands match.	To prevent accidental mismatching of parent and infant.

Expected Outcome

- The woman verbalizes an understanding of the procedures and techniques used to maintain the health of the newborn.

• • Evaluation

The nurse performs ongoing evaluations of the woman and fetus during delivery. Successful completion of the cardinal movements of labor are indicated by a smooth, uncomplicated delivery of the neonate's head, shoulders, and body. The woman will be able to follow the directions of the birth attendant to push or restrain from pushing as required to facilitate the delivery. The FHR may demonstrate wide variations in rate, rhythm, and periodic changes in the several moments before birth; however, the heart rate will be greater than 100 bpm at delivery, the neonate will breathe spontaneously, and he or she will receive an Apgar score of 7 or greater at 1 and 5 minutes. The woman and her partner will verbalize satisfaction with the birth and their roles in the process.

During the process of birth the nurse remains at the woman's side, offering final words of encouragement and remaining ready to assist the birth attendant as the infant is born. The nurse, in most cases, must attend to the immediate needs of the woman and neonate. This challenge requires that the nurse be skilled in neonatal assessment, Apgar scoring, and newborn resuscitation, as well as immediate support of normal adaptations and management of emergencies in the postpartum woman. Goals of care at this time include offering physical support and precise instructions to the woman to facilitate the birth of the neonate and assisting the birth attendant as indicated.

Care of the Family During the Third Stage of Labor

The third stage of labor is defined as the period from delivery of the neonate through separation and expulsion of the placenta. This period usually is one of dramatic release and high emotion for the new mother and her partner as they greet the neonate. Nursing responsibilities during this relatively short time are many and pressing, such as ongoing assessment of maternal and neonatal status, completion of delivery records, obtaining and labeling laboratory samples, and facilitating early parent–neonate interaction. The nurse must anticipate the woman's needs during this period. This includes monitoring for signs of excessive postpartum bleeding and obtaining any additional instruments or supplies needed by the birth attendant.

NURSING PROCEDURE

Obtaining Umbilical Cord Blood Samples for Biochemical Analysis

Clinical research indicates that umbilical cord blood analysis provides a more objective measurement of newborn acid–base status than the Apgar score. The ability to diagnose and treat significant metabolic acidemia in the infant is improved with knowledge of the infant's biochemical status.

Purpose: To obtain blood samples from one umbilical artery and and the umbilical vein for pH and blood gas analysis.

NURSING ACTION	RATIONALE
1. Flush two 1-mL syringes with 25-g needles with heparin, or obtain two syringes that have preinjected dry heparin.	To prevent clotting of the blood samples.
2. Set aside two rubber syringe stoppers to cap syringes after sample is obtained, or obtain special syringes that have built in safety cap.	To avoid recapping the syringe with contaminated needle. Recapping is one of the most common needle stick accidents to occur in the clinical setting.
3. Obtain 3- to 6-inch segment of umbilical cord clamped at both ends from birth attendant.	To ensure that a large enough segment is available from which to draw blood samples.
4. Dry cord segment and identify artery and vein.	To prevent cord from slipping when drawing blood samples.
5. Draw arterial blood sample first.	If umbilical cord blood is drawn first, artery may be more difficult to visualize and puncture.
6. Draw at least 0.6 mL of blood.	To provide sufficient amount of blood for pH and gas analysis.
7. Expell any air from syringe.	To prevent mixing of ambient oxygen with gas in blood sample.
8. Repeat procedure to obtain venous sample of blood.	
9. Remove needles and discard them. Seal syringe with rubber caps.	Sample must be airtight to prevent mixing of ambient oxygen with gas in blood sample.
10. Send to appropriate laboratory for biochemical analysis within 45 minutes.	Accurate analysis must be performed within 60 minutes of obtaining sample. Studies indicate that if iced, the heparinized syringe is good for up to 3 hours.

ACOG. (1991). Utility of umbilical cord blood acid–base assessment. Committee on Obstetrics: Maternal and Fetal Medicine. Opinion Number 91.

Delivery of the Placenta

The birth attendant observes for signs of placental separation (slight gush of blood from the vagina, lengthening of cord, rising of rounded uterine fundus palpable through the abdomen). When these signs are observed the woman is asked to push slightly with a contraction to deliver the placenta. The placenta is received into a basin for later examination. The birth attendant or nurse will then massage the uterus through the abdomen until it is well contracted, and bleeding from the site of placental detachment is controlled.

Examination of the Reproductive Tract

Once the uterus is contracted the vagina and perineum are routinely examined after delivery for lacerations or extension of an episiotomy. The cervix may not be inspected routinely because of the woman's discomfort, but if cervical bleeding is suspected, inspection will be necessary. It may be done under pudendal block or, less frequently, under light inhalation anesthesia. The nurse assists with the examination by providing the birth attendant with needed supplies, positioning the woman, and assisting with control or relief of discomfort or pain. Slow breathing and relaxation exercises may be sufficient for brief examinations, or the woman may require anesthesia or analgesia.

The perineum, the vagina, occasionally the cervix, or rarely the body of the uterus may be lacerated during delivery. Cervical or uterine lacerations usually occur in association with difficult deliveries or operative procedures for delivery. Factors associated with lacerations of the perineum and vagina include the following:

- Rapid, precipitous, uncontrolled delivery
- Malpresentations, such as occipitoposterior or face presentation
- Use of perineal anesthesia
- Friable or tense maternal tissue

- Operative delivery
- Inadequate length of episiotomy incision

Lacerations are classified according to the tissues involved, as follows:

- First degree: involving the skin or vaginal mucosa but not extending into the muscular layers
- Second degree: extending from the skin and vaginal mucosa into the muscles of the perineum
- Third degree: extending from the skin, vaginal mucosa, and muscle into the anal sphincter
- Fourth degree: extending through the rectal mucosa into the lumen of the rectum

Other genital lacerations that may result from vaginal delivery include periurethral tears, which occur near the urethral meatus, and periclitoral tears, which occur near the clitoris. Lacerations may bleed profusely, depending on their location and degree. They are generally repaired in the same way as an episiotomy.

Repair of the Episiotomy and Lacerations of the Perineum and Vaginal Tract

The birth attendant often will begin repair of the episiotomy or lacerations while awaiting the birth of the placenta. If the woman has not received regional anesthesia for delivery, the perineal and vaginal tissues will be infiltrated with a local anesthetic by the birth attendant. Suturing of the incision or edges of the lacerations continues after the placenta is expelled until the repair is completed. The nurse provides sutures and other equipment as requested by the birth attendant.

• • Assessment

Nursing priorities during this period focus on the assessment of maternal and neonatal physiologic status, support of uterine contraction, prevention of hemorrhage, and evaluation of early family responses to the newborn.

Monitoring Maternal Physiologic Status

Maternal physiologic status during the third stage of labor is determined primarily by monitoring the woman's vital signs and blood loss. The woman's blood pressure, pulse, and respirations should be monitored before and immediately after signs of placental separation are noted and every 15 minutes for the first hour after delivery of the placenta. If uterine bleeding is excessive, an increasing pulse rate may be the first sign of hypovolemic shock. Although the increase in blood volume provides some protection for blood loss at the time of delivery, hypotension and hypovolemic shock can develop quickly in the woman when the volume lost exceeds 500 mL.

Assessing Neonatal Physiologic Status

The nurse also is responsible for most aspects of the initial assessment of the normal newborn. Apgar scores are recorded officially at 1 and 5 minutes after birth. However, initial assessments of the newborn's condition and necessary steps to support respiration and cardiac function begin immediately after birth. The nurse is generally responsible for designating the Apgar score after the birth of a normal newborn, because the birth attendant's attention is focused on the woman's adaptations and well-being. The Apgar scoring system is used to assess heart rate, respiratory effort, muscle tone, reflex irritability, and color. The optimum score is 10, with 2 points being given for each criterion, as shown in Table 21-1. The nurse also examines the neonate for evidence of trauma or the presence of congenital anomalies.

The neonate's heart rate can be assessed by palpating the umbilical artery pulsations with a hand under the blankets or by auscultating if needed or desired. Respiratory effort, reflex irritability, muscle tone, and color can be evaluated as well. If the assessment is difficult to perform or if a change in the status of the neonate occurs, the nurse should reposition the neonate. The neonate also may be placed under a radiant warmer immediately after birth to facilitate the assessment or the performance of other necessary procedures.

Table 21-1. Apgar Scoring

	Score*		
Sign	0	1	2
Heart rate	Absent	Slow (below 100)	Over 100
Respiratory rate	Absent	Slow, irregular	Good, crying
Muscle tone	Flaccid	Some flexion of extremities	Active motion
Reflex irritability†	No response	Grimace	Cry
Color	Blue, pale	Body pink, extremities blue	Completely pink

*This method is used for evaluating the immediate postnatal adjustment of the neonate. The total score of the five signs is 8 to 10 when the initial adjustment is good. Newborns with lower scores require special attention. Scores under 4 indicate that the neonate is seriously depressed.

†Tested by inserting the tip of a catheter into the nostril.

Courtesy of Virginia Apgar, M.D., and Smith, Kline & French Laboratories, Philadelphia

Identifying Family Responses to the Neonate

The nurse observes and notes the parent's first responses to the newborn. These responses often give clues to the extent to which parents have attached to their neonate prenatally and provide information that helps direct ongoing family-centered care. Parents often are overjoyed with the arrival and immediately ask about the neonate's gender and health and call the neonate by name (Fig. 21-14). First-time parents often express wonder and pleasure at the newborn's appearance.

However, behavioral responses vary widely and depend on many factors, including the following:

- Maternal fatigue level
- Administration of analgesia or anesthesia
- Level of discomfort or pain
- Maternal parity
- Cultural background

The nurse must be cautious about drawing conclusions regarding the nature of the parent–newborn acquaintance process based on initial maternal responses. Many birthing units use an assessment tool that documents the woman's behavioral responses in the immediate postpartum period. The data collected should be viewed only as a beginning evaluation of parent–newborn attachment, and this nursing assessment must be placed within the context of the factors listed previously.

If family responses to the newborn do not seem to fit the expected norm, additional observation and interaction with the parents will be needed before a conclusive nursing diagnosis can be made. Responses that reflect some difficulty in prenatal attachment or signal that the parent–newborn relationship may be at risk include an unwillingness to hold or look at the newborn, expressions of displeasure about the appearance or sex, and blaming the newborn for a difficult labor and birth. If these responses continue into the postpartum period, the parent–newborn relationship may be at risk.

• • Nursing Diagnosis

The following nursing diagnoses reflect possible problems that may arise during the third stage of labor for the woman and her neonate and may be addressed independently by the nurse. Priorities in care may be established based on these diagnoses. Nursing diagnoses concerning the mother may include the following:

- High Risk for Infection related to trauma to the birth canal
- High Risk for Injury related to uterine prolapse
- High Risk for Fluid Volume Deficit related to hemorrhage

Nursing diagnoses to be considered for the neonate include the following:

- Ineffective Airway Clearance (neonate) related to aspiration of fluid during birth
- Hypothermia (newborn) related to immature thermoregulation
- High Risk for Altered Parenting related to difficulty in prenatal attachment

Complications requiring collaboration with other health care team members may arise during the third stage of labor.

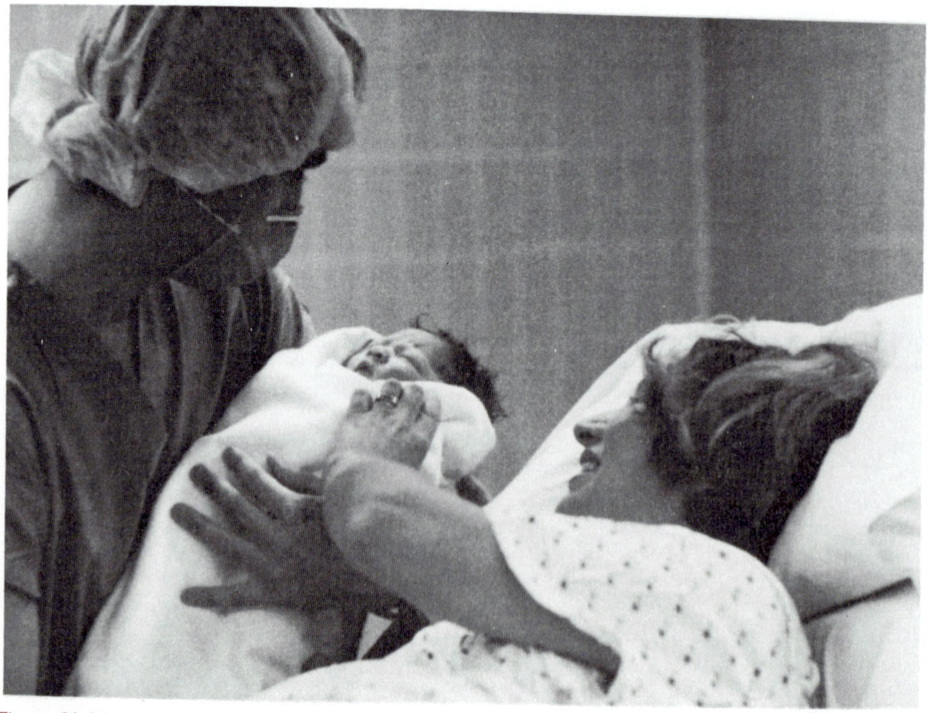

Figure 21-14.
The happy couple greet their newborn. (Photo by BABES, Inc.)

In addition to routine nursing care, the nurse is responsible for monitoring for potential complications. Such complications include postpartum hemorrhage (maternal), need for perineal repair, and cord or placental abnormalities.

• • Planning and Implementation

Nursing interventions during the third stage of labor center on supporting maternal and neonatal physiologic status, promoting the neonate's transition to extrauterine life, and fostering early interaction and breastfeeding. The nurse also remains alert to the needs of the birth attendant and provides any required assistance or supplies to repair the episiotomy or lacerations.

Promoting Maternal Physiologic Adaptation

The nurse watches for signs of placental separation and may need to alert the woman to assist placental delivery with bearing-down efforts. The nurse is ready to perform uterine massage, administer uterine tonics, and if blood loss exceeds 500 mL, initiate an intravenous line (see discussion of postpartum hemorrhage in following sections). The woman also may experience a sudden shaking chill, a benign response to birth, and will require a warm blanket.

Expected Outcomes

- The postpartum woman expels the entire placenta without complications within 30 minutes of delivery.
- The woman maintains normal blood pressure, pulse, and respiratory rate.
- The woman remains afebrile during the third stage of labor.

Massaging the Uterine Fundus

Massage of the uterine fundus in the immediate postpartum period stimulates the myometrium to contract and promotes hemostasis and the expulsion of clots. The nurse uses two hands for fundal massage: One hand anchors the lower uterine segment just above the symphysis, while the other gently massages the fundal area as shown in Figure 21-15. Fundal massage must be done gently, with adequate support of the lower segment, because the uterine suspensory ligaments are relaxed after delivery and offer little resistance. Aggressive massage may result in partial or complete uterine prolapse, a serious obstetric complication. Further, fundal massage should be done only when the fundus is not firm, because overstimulation of the myometrium can contribute to muscle fatigue and a tendency toward relaxation.

The nurse should explain to the woman why the fundal massage is necessary and that she may experience discomfort or cramping due to contraction of the uterine muscle. For further discussion see Chapter 26.

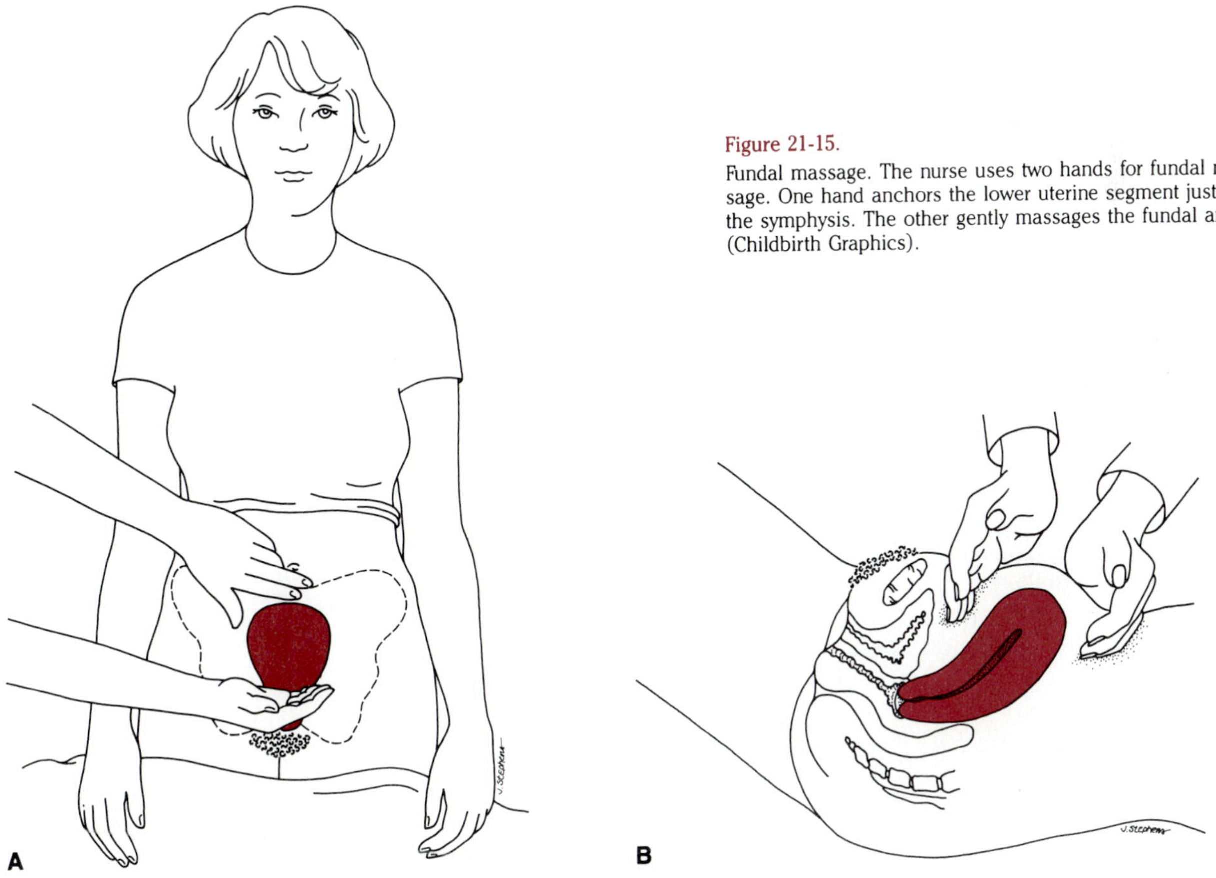

Figure 21-15.
Fundal massage. The nurse uses two hands for fundal massage. One hand anchors the lower uterine segment just above the symphysis. The other gently massages the fundal area (Childbirth Graphics).

Expected Outcomes

- The postpartum woman expresses minimal discomfort with fundal massage.
- The woman's uterus contracts in a firm tone.
- The woman maintains normal maternal vital signs.

Examining the Placenta, Membranes, and Umbilical Cord

The nurse or birth attendant examines the placenta and membranes to determine their completeness and to check for any abnormality. A thorough evaluation of the placenta may clarify the cause of an adverse maternal or neonatal outcome. A technique for examining the placenta and membranes follows.

1. With the placenta maternal side down, grasp the membranes and approximate the edges to determine if they are complete.
2. Inspect the fetal side.
   a. Check the location of the insertion of the cord (central, marginal, or velamentous).
   b. Trace blood vessels to the periphery to detect any torn vessels, which might indicate a succenturiate or extra lobe of the placenta.
3. Inspect the maternal surface.
   a. Check the placental cotyledons to determine if they are all present and intact.
   b. Observe for areas of abruption, infarction, or calcification.
4. Inspect the umbilical cord.
   a. Check the number of blood vessels (two arteries and one vein).
   b. Check the length of the cord (appropriate, long, or short).
   c. Check for the presence of a true knot, varicosities, or other abnormalities.

The nurse should chart the examination of the placenta and document the weight, noting any abnormalities. If the birth attendant requests microscopic and gross examination of the placenta by a pathologist, the nurse is responsible for proper labeling and storage of the organ according to facility guidelines. Placental abnormalities are discussed in greater detail in Chapter 26.

Expected Outcome

- The postpartum woman passes a complete placenta.

Measuring Maternal Blood Loss

Although the birth attendant is usually responsible for estimating the woman's blood loss, the nurse most frequently makes direct measurements from the placenta basin or other collection containers and by estimating the amount of blood on drapes, towels, sponges, and the floor. On the average, a 300- to 400-mL blood loss can be expected during vaginal delivery with an episiotomy. Most of the bleeding comes from the placental site. In addition, blood loss can result from any cervical, vaginal, or perineal tears or episiotomy.

The nurse must know the amount of blood lost during delivery to plan appropriate care in the immediate postpartum period. The extent of bleeding provides an indication of the woman's relative risk for hypovolemic shock in the immediate postpartum period and the need for monitoring hemoglobin and hematocrit levels during the postpartum recovery (see the accompanying display, Guidelines for Estimating Blood Loss).

Guidelines for Estimating Blood Loss

Nursing studies indicate that many nurses are unable to reliably and consistently estimate blood loss. The nurse's accuracy is influenced by the method used to assess blood loss (peripad count, milliliter measurement, visual estimate of fluid volume, weight measurement of linens, sponges, drapes, and clots). Traditional descriptions of blood or lochia flow as "scant," "small," "moderate," or "large" are inadequate and have proven to be unreliable in studies to date. Research findings support the need for objective measurements of blood loss. Nurses should receive a standardized orientation to the measurement and estimation of blood loss. Specific suggestions to assist nurses follow:

- Use a commercial under-the-buttocks drape that incorporates a milliliter collection chamber so that blood flowing from the vagina is caught and can be measured.
- Determine the amount of blood required to saturate the unit-specific peripads used in the facility (ie, Curity brand pads saturated by 80 mL of blood).
- Weigh blood clots, drapes, sponges, and linens saturated with blood and report in grams. In infants 1 mL of blood = 1 g. Although the correlation in adults is only approximate, it provides an objective measurement for the birth attendant.
- Draw a hemoglobin (Hgb) and/or hematocrit (Hct). The loss of 500 mL of blood decreases Hgb by 1.0 to 1.5 g and Hct by 3% to 4%

Luegenbiehl, D., Brophy, G., Artigue, G. Phillips, K., & Flak, R. (1990). Standardized assessment of blood loss. MCN: American Journal of Maternal Child Nursing, 15*(4), 241.*

Expected Outcome

- The postpartum woman exhibits blood loss within the normal range.

Assisting with Perineal Repair

The episiotomy or perineal lacerations are repaired by the birth attendant after the placenta is delivered and when the woman's condition permits. First-degree lacerations that are small (less than 1 cm) and not bleeding often are not repaired, because they will heal well without suturing. Other lacerations are sutured to ensure approximation of the wound edges and to reduce formation of scar tissue.

Perineal repair requires adequate anesthesia, usually through pudendal nerve block or local infiltration of the perineum. Sutures and new sterile gloves are supplied by the nurse. The birth attendant also may request new sterile drapes. The woman's vulva, perineum, and vagina are examined for lacerations and possible extension of the episiotomy into the rectum. The birth attendant applies direct pressure to bleeding sites using sterile pads; the vaginal incision will tend to bleed most. The nurse or birth attendant should explain the procedure to the woman and assess the adequacy of perineal anesthesia as suturing is begun. The vaginal mucosa is sutured first, beginning at the apex and working toward the perineum. Then the perineal muscle layers, the subcutaneous layers, and finally the skin edges are approximated and sutured.

During administration of anesthesia and repair of the perineum, it may be advisable to have the father or support person hold the infant. Repositioning of the woman and some degree of pain may make it difficult for the new mother to safely hold the infant or maintain her former level of attention and interaction with the neonate.

Expected Outcome

- The woman verbalizes no or very little discomfort with repair of the episiotomy or lacerations and other procedures performed during the third stage of labor.

Monitoring for Complications

Potential Complication: Postpartum Hemorrhage

Brisk bleeding after delivery is usually caused by relaxation of the uterus (uterine atony). Fundal massage, administration of oxytocics, and nipple stimulation may help to promote uterine tone and hemostasis.

The nurse must be alert for signs of impending postpartum hemorrhage. If fundal massage and nipple stimulation are not sufficient to keep the uterus well contracted, the nurse must notify the birth attendant, who may order administration of oxytocics. If bleeding is brisk and the uterus is firm, the placenta should be examined thoroughly for evidence of missing fragments or membranes that may be retained inside the uterus. Retained placental fragments or membranes will prevent the myometrium from completely contracting. Placental fragments may be retained if uterine force is insufficient to expel the entire placenta, attempts to remove the placenta manually do not result in total removal of all placental tissue, or defects exist in the decidua. Retained placental fragments must be removed manually by the physician under sterile conditions, or bleeding will continue and infection can occur. Once this is done, the uterus usually contracts firmly to maintain hemostasis.

If the fundus is firm but a steady, pulsating stream or a constant trickle of blood continues to ooze from the vagina, cervical, vaginal, or perineal tears should be suspected. An unligated vessel in an episiotomy also can bleed profusely. The repair must be done promptly to prevent further blood loss.

Administration of Uterine Tonics. Uterine tonics include oxytocics, ergot agents, and prostaglandins. The nurse administers these as directed.

Some birth attendants advocate the administration of *oxytocics* (Pitocin, Syntocin) immediately after delivery to promote uterine contractility and ensure hemostasis. Oxytocics may be given intramuscularly or added to intravenous fluids as the placenta is delivered. The usual dose is 10 to 20 IU given intramuscularly or 10 to 40 IU added to 1 L of IV fluid and infused at 10 to 40 mU/min. This medication generally is available in ampules containing 10 IU/mL. Oxytocin is usually not given in an intravenous bolus because doing so can induce hypotension and tachycardia. Intramuscular injection usually causes a transient burning sensation at the injection site.

Ergot agents include Ergotrate (ergonovine), a natural ergot preparation, and methylergonovine (Methergine), a synthetic ergot. They may be given intramuscularly to stimulate a sustained tetanic-type contraction to control postpartum hemorrhage. The usual dose is 0.2 mg given intramuscularly or orally. A single dose is usually sufficient to achieve hemostasis, but it can be repeated in 2 to 4 hours if needed. These drugs are never administered intravenously or before delivery because they are powerful vasoconstrictors. Ergotrate is slightly more likely to cause elevation in blood pressure in normotensive women than methylergonovine. Sudden hypertensive crisis and cerebral vascular accident may result with intravenous administration. These drugs also are contraindicated for women with hypertensive disease and for women who have received regional anesthesia because they are at risk for vasomotor instability. Either drug can be used safely in combination with oxytocin.

Prostaglandins also may be used. The Food and Drug Administration has recently approved the 15-methyl derivative of prostaglandin F2 alpha (Prostin/15M) for treatment of postpartum hemorrhage due to uterine atony. If the administration of oxytocin or Methergine is ineffective in stimulating uterine contraction, 250 μg (0.25 mg) of Prostin/15M can be administered intramuscularly and can be repeated as necessary at 15- to 90-minute intervals. This drug also is noted to result in sudden acute hypertension in some women and should be avoided in patients with preexisting hypertension.

If pharmacologic efforts to contract the uterus fail, the birth attendant can perform a bimanual compression and massage of the uterus. See Chapter 26 for a further discussion of uterine atony.

Expected Outcome

- The woman verbalizes an understanding of the purpose for the administration of uterine tonics.

Documenting Intrapartum Events, Procedures, and Care

A major nursing responsibility during the third stage of labor is accurate documentation of intrapartum procedures and care. Important details of this documentation include the following:

- Time of delivery of neonate and placenta
- 1- and 5-minute Apgar scores
- Results of umbilical cord blood gas analysis (if obtained)
- Any immediate neonatal care required
- Extent and repair of perineal lacerations or episiotomy
- Estimated maternal blood loss
- Medications administered before, during, and after delivery
- Placement of identification bands on mother and neonate
- Maternal vital signs
- Names of personnel attending the birth and responding to requests for assistance

Most institutions have standard forms for documenting intrapartum care; an example is shown in the accompanying assessment tool.

Supporting Neonatal Physiologic Adjustment

Immediately after birth the newborn should be dried and the head covered while it is on the mother's abdomen. Infant skin to maternal skin contact is an excellent method for prevention of heat loss and hypothermia. Mucus should be suctioned from the nares and mouth with a bulb syringe as needed during this period and the respiratory effort and color observed carefully. If the nurse has concerns about the newborn's status, the neonate should be moved to a radiant warmer within sight of the parents, so careful observation is possible and heat loss can be prevented. If the newborn's status is good, a more complete neonatal assessment usually is deferred until after the third stage of labor is completed.

A critical aspect of nursing care to support neonatal adaptation is correct positioning of the neonate. Correct positioning of the normal, healthy neonate immediately after birth is essential to accomplish the following:

- Facilitate drainage of secretions
- Maintain a patent airway
- Permit frequent assessment by the nursing staff
- Ensure safety and prevent injury

Any number of positions would meet these criteria, depending on the status of the neonate. One commonly used position is placement of the neonate so that his or her abdomen is in contact with the mother's abdomen. The neonate usually clutches the mother's body, and the woman or her partner can easily place a hand to secure the newborn. The neonate's head can be turned to the side easily to facilitate drainage of secretions. Warm blankets should be used to cover the neonate, or a radiant warmer can be directed over the area. While it is important to facilitate early maternal–newborn attachment, if the woman experiences significant pain, blood loss, or other problems, it may be inadvisable for her to hold the newborn. The support person or father may be enlisted in this case to hold the newborn, or the nurse may place the newborn on a bed under a radiant warmer unit.

Expected Outcomes

- The newborn breathes spontaneously.
- The newborn maintains a respiratory rate of 30 to 60 breaths per minute.
- The newborn maintains a patent airway.

Supporting Neonatal Thermoregulation

At birth the neonate's body temperature drops 2°C to 3°C (3.5°F to 5.3°F) because it is no longer protected by the uterus, and its body heat is conducted to cold objects that touch the newborn's skin. Body heat is lost through the evaporation of moisture from wet skin, radiation to a cool environment, or convection to cool air. The heat loss causes an increased need for oxygenation. In addition the newborn responds by vasoconstricting and increasing heat production through nonshivering thermogenesis, using stored brown fat. Hypothermia and resulting cold stress can become life-threatening if severe or prolonged as heart and respiratory rates decrease. (See Chapter 30 for an in-depth discussion of neonatal thermoregulation.) Body heat can be maintained in the normal newborn by observing the following procedures:

- Providing a warm, draft-free environment for birth
- Avoiding placing the newborn in contact with cold instruments, hands, blankets, or other equipment
- Drying the newborn thoroughly immediately after delivery
- Using radiant heat or skin-to-skin contact and covering the newborn with warm blankets
- Placing a cotton cap on the newborn to prevent evaporative heat loss from wet hair

Expected Outcome

- The newborn maintains a body temperature as measured by axillary body temperature between 36.4°C and 37.2°C (97.5°F to 99.0°F) in the first hour.

Promoting Parent–Newborn Interaction

If the newborn is placed on the mother's abdomen immediately after delivery, the nurse can encourage the parents to touch the newborn and to assist with drying and wrapping. If early breastfeeding is desired, the nurse should assist the woman into a comfortable position and help her with initial efforts to breastfeed. The nurse may want to stress that the newborn may be more interested in looking at the parents' faces than in breastfeeding in the first moments after birth. The parents will progressively explore their neonate, often unaware of other events around them.

The nurse also can encourage the father or partner to hold the newborn in the first minutes after birth. The nurse should assess the partner's physical and emotional state before encouraging immediate interaction. Some individ-

Assessment Tool

Delivery, Third Stage, and Newborn Record

LABOR

SEROLOGY TYPE Rh

○ SPONTANEOUS ○ NONE
○ AUGMENTED ○ MEDICAL AGENT ______
○ INDUCED ○ SURGICAL

○ NORMAL ○ FAILURE OF DESCENT
○ PROLONGED LATENT ○ TRANSVERSE ARREST
○ ACTIVE PHASE ARREST ○ PERSISTENT OP
○ SLOW SLOPE ACTIVITY ○ PROLONGED 2ND STAGE
○ NONE

LABOR ONSET: DATE TIME END OF 1ST STAGE: DATE TIME

MONITORING: ○ INTERNAL ○ EXTERNAL ○ BOTH ○ NONE

FETAL SCALP SAMPLING: ○ NO ○ YES NUMBER [ ] 1st STAGE HRS.-MIN.

ANESTHESIA ○ GENERAL ○ EPIDURAL ○ SADDLE-BACK ○ LOCAL/PUDENDAL ○ PARACERVICAL ANESTHESIA TIME HRS.

MEDICATION DURING LAST HOUR OF LABOR:

DELIVERY POSITION AT DELIVERY: STATION: DATE TIME

VAGINAL ○ VERTEX: ○ SPONTANEOUS (○ ASSISTED ○ UNASSISTED) 2nd STAGE HRS.-MIN.
○ VACUUM EXTRACTOR (○ LOW ○ MID*)
○ FORCEPS (○ LOW ○ MID*) ○ *ROTATE FROM TO METHOD ○ Manual ○ Forceps ○ Vacuum
○ BREECH:* ○ SPONTANEOUS (○ MAN. ASSIS. ○ EXTRACT ○ FORCEPS)

EPISIOTOMY ○ MEDIAN ○ MEDIOLATERAL ○ NONE

LACERATIONS:

ALTERNATIVE BIRTH PROGRAM: LABOR: ○ NO ○ YES DELIVERY ○ NO ○ YES POST PARTUM ○ NO ○ YES

LOCATION OF DELIVERY: ○ DR ○ LABOR ROOM ○ ABC ○ OR ○ Other ______

SECOND STAGE COMPLICATIONS:

CESAREAN DELIVERY ○ LOW TRANSVERSE ○ LOW VERTICAL ○ STERILIZATION OPERATING TIME HRS.
○ CLASSICAL ○ HYSTERECTOMY ○ OTHER ______

THIRD STAGE PLACENTA: ○ EXPRESSED ○ SPONTANEOUS ○ REMOVED DATE TIME

UTERUS EXPLORED: ○ NO ○ YES COMMENT: ______

EBL [ ] ML PLAC. WT. [ ] gm CORD VESSELS [ ] 3rd STAGE MIN.

THIRD STAGE COMPLICATIONS: ______ TOTAL LABOR HRS.-MIN.

MEDICATIONS:

INFANT ○ FEMALE ○ MALE WEIGHT [ ] gms SUSTAINED RESPIRATION ○ < 90 SEC. ○ > 90 SEC.

RESPIRATION SPONTANEOUS: ○ YES ○ NO RESUSCITATED: ○ O_2 ○ MASK ○ INTUBATION ○ OTHER ______
NASOGASTRIC TUBE PASSED: ○ LEFT ○ RIGHT

GASTRIC ASPIRATE: [ ] cc ROM: [ ] HRS.

APGAR SCORE						
TIME	HEART RATE	RESP. EFF.	MUSCLE TONE	REFLEX	COLOR	TOTAL
1 MIN.						
5 MIN.						

AMNIOTIC FLUID: ○ NOT DONE ○ CLEAR ○ MECONIUM: INTUBATED: ○ YES ○ NO ○ CLOUDY
______ ASPIRATE [ ] cc

BABY TO: ○ ICN ○ REGULAR NURSERY

CORD BLOOD ○ YES ○ NO

ANESTHESIOLOGISTS
______ MD __ __ __ __
______ MD __ __ __ __
NURSE: ______ RN

OBSTETRICIANS
______ MD __ __ __ __
______ MD __ __ __ __
______ MD __ __ __ __
D/C/A

○ NEWBORN ABNORMALITIES: ______

(ORIGINAL—OB RECORD; COPY—NEWBORN RECORD; PINK—LOG)

691-01 5/81

MEDICAL RECORD COPY

uals, especially first-time fathers, may be very excited and shaken after birth, and may feel unprepared to handle the newborn immediately. The nurse may ask the partner to take a seat at the woman's side before handing over the well-wrapped newborn.

Expected Outcomes

- Parents and newborn have an opportunity for face-to-face interaction.
- Parents have an opportunity to explore the newborn's face and body.

• • Evaluation

Ongoing evaluation of maternal and neonatal adaptations during the third stage of labor is an essential aspect of the nursing process. The woman's vital signs should remain stable and the uterine fundus firm so that vaginal bleeding is minimized. The neonate makes effective adjustments to the extrauterine environment. Cardiovascular and pulmonary systems function within normal limits during this transition period, and vital signs remain stable. The woman and her neonate can begin the acquaintance and bonding process, which is facilitated by close physical contact and breastfeeding.

For most women the moment of birth represents the culmination of a process begun 40 weeks earlier and marks the creation of a new family unit. The physical and emotional tension that mounts in the final minutes of the second stage of labor gives way as the birth occurs. Many women experience a sudden surge of energy as their attention is drawn to the neonate. The fatigue and pain are temporarily forgotten as the new mother receives the newborn. The goal of nursing care during this very special time is to support the physiologic adaptations of the mother and newborn and facilitate the beginning parent–newborn acquaintance process.

Care of the Family During the Fourth Stage of Labor

Technically the immediate postpartum recovery period is not part of labor, but sometimes it is called the fourth stage of labor because of its great importance. The first hour after the third stage has been completed is critical to maternal and neonatal recovery and important in the establishment of early family interaction and breastfeeding.

Many facilities that use conventional delivery rooms have a separate postpartum recovery room where women and their families are moved after the third stage of labor is completed. In other facilities the mother and newborn may recover in the delivery room for the first hour or two and then are transported to the postpartum unit. Settings with single-unit maternity systems allow the mother and newborn to recover and remain in their room until discharge. Regardless of how immediate postpartum recovery care is arranged, close nursing observation is absolutely essential to ensure optimal maternal and neonatal adaptation and to promote optimal family interaction in the first hour after birth.

• • Assessment

An essential aspect of postdelivery care is careful assessment of maternal and neonatal status and of family responses to the newborn. These assessments are performed frequently through the first hours after birth. Ideally, the nurse who accompanied the family during labor and birth also should provide this one-to-one recovery care.

Monitoring Maternal Physiologic Status

The nurse should complete a systematic assessment of the mother's physiologic status. Frequent assessments are necessary because changes in the woman's status that can result in life-threatening complications—most notably excessive bleeding and postpartum hemorrhage—can occur very rapidly. Often the initial assessment is conducted while the birth attendant repairs the episiotomy or lacerations.

The nurse monitors the following:

- Blood pressure, pulse, and respirations
- Position and tone of the uterus
- Amount and quality of vaginal bleeding
- Condition of the perineum
- Condition of the bladder

As noted in the previous section assessments are conducted every 15 minutes for the first hour. Continued observations will occur at 30-minute to 1-hour intervals until the woman is transferred to the postpartum unit or her condition stabilizes.

The woman's temperature also should be taken at least once during this time to check for elevation associated with dehydration or developing infection. Usually an elevation in temperature within 24 hours of delivery is due to dehydration and physical exertion and will respond to fluid replacement. However, if the temperature rises above 38°C (100.4°F) in association with prolonged rupture of membranes, infection should be suspected.

Assessing Uterine Tone and Position

The nurse palpates the uterus to assess tone. Usually uterine tone and the amount of vaginal bleeding are correlated. If the uterus is firmly contracted, vaginal bleeding will be slight. If the uterus is large and soft ("boggy"), flow will be moderate to heavy, and clots also may be expelled when the fundus is gently massaged. The nurse also should note the height and position of the uterus. The fundus should remain at or slightly below the level of the umbilicus in the midline. Enlargement may indicate that the uterus is filling with blood and clots and that a postpartum hemorrhage is imminent. Elevation and deviation of the fundus to one side, usually the right, often indicates that the uterus is being displaced by a full bladder. A full bladder will inhibit uterine contraction and may predispose the woman to postpartum hemorrhage. Steps must be taken promptly to alleviate bladder distention.

Monitoring Vaginal Bleeding

The nurse should observe the character and amount of vaginal bleeding while fundal massage is being performed. If the fundus is firm, the flow usually will be a slow, intermittent trickle composed of blood and decidual tissue known as lochia. Lochia will be bright red immediately after delivery (rubra lochia) and contain a few small clots. A continuous trickle of blood suggests a laceration of the cervix or vagina. Saturation of one perineal pad in less than 15 minutes (two pads in 30 minutes) or a rapid pooling of blood under the buttocks is considered excessive and requires immediate attention. If tissue is passed with the lochia, it should be saved for examination by the birth attendant. It may indicate the presence of retained placental tissue or fetal membranes.

Evaluating the Perineal Condition

The perineum is assessed frequently for increasing edema, asymmetric edema, bruising, gaping, and bleeding from perineal repair. The nurse should ask the woman if she is experiencing a great deal of perineal pain. Occasionally, a hematoma will form as a result of a broken blood vessel bleeding into the connective tissue underlying skin or mucosa of the vagina and perineum. A hematoma will feel fluctuant and is likely to be extremely painful when touched. The following symptoms of hematoma formation must be reported to the birth attendant promptly:

- Increasing, severe perineal pain
- Asymmetric perineal swelling
- Ecchymosis of the overlying skin or mucosa
- Increased tautness of skin or mucosa
- Complaint of rectal pressure

Monitoring Neonatal Physiologic Status

The labor and delivery nurse is usually responsible for ongoing assessment of the normal newborn in the first hour after delivery. Many labor and delivery units now provide family-centered recovery care, in which the newborn is screened for abnormalities in the delivery room and, if normal, stays with parents for the first hours after delivery. Other settings request that the newborn be taken away briefly for evaluation in the admission nursery and returned as soon as possible to the parents; still others request that the newborn spend some time in the admission nursery for observation.

The nurse should be sensitive to parents' wishes in this matter and attempt to maintain early parent–newborn contact within the limits of safe practice in that particular setting (Fig. 21-16). If the newborn is to remain with the mother and partner, the nurse must perform regular and systematic assessments of the newborn's physiologic status. The nurse must be alert for potential neonatal problems that necessitate close observation or admission to the nursery.

Nursing responsibilities in the initial neonatal assessment are discussed in detail in Chapter 31.

Assessing Family Responses to the Newborn

Usually the woman and partner are very joyful during this time and respond to their newborn with wonder, excitement, and delight. This early response can contribute to increased feelings of attraction and connectedness to the newborn and may lay the groundwork for and facilitate parent–newborn attachment. Behaviors thought to signify the beginning of positive parent–newborn interaction include the following:

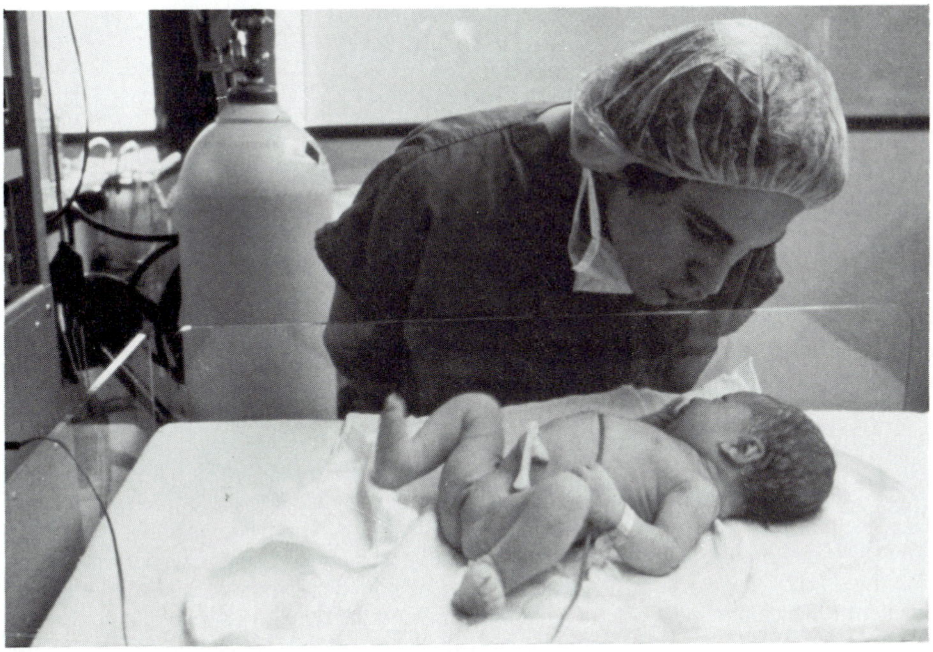

Figure 21-16.
This neonate was slightly hypothermic after delivery and was transferred to the admission nursery and put under a radiant heater. The father accompanies the neonate and has an excellent opportunity to explore and interact with his new daughter.

- Progression from tentative touch with fingertips to more confident touch and enfolding of the neonate
- Active reaching for the neonate rather than passive receiving
- Active attempts to make and hold eye contact with the newborn in the same vertical plane, known as en face positioning
- Expressions of approval or satisfaction with the neonate's sex, weight, condition, appearance, and size

The nurse should observe the nature of the parents' first responses, because they are the basis for the unfolding future relationship with the newborn. Close contact with the newborn in the first hours after birth is very important to many parents. The opportunity to be with the newborn in the first alert phase, which lasts 1 or 2 hours after birth, is precious and should be protected. The nurse will observe that most parents are overwhelmingly positive about their newborns and are eager for close contact and interaction.

However, some parents will seem less eager for interaction or will express concerns or disappointment about the newborn's appearance or sex. This reaction may be the result of a long, painful labor; of unmet expectations for the birth or the newborn; of physical pain and fatigue; of an unwanted pregnancy; or of cultural differences. The nurse should be careful not to assess such interactions as being atypical or worrisome too quickly; close observation and sensitive listening to and acknowledgment of parents' feelings and concerns and communication of observations to postpartum nursing staff are in order.

• • Nursing Diagnosis

Nursing diagnoses during the immediate postpartum recovery period guide the nurse in setting priorities for care in the first hours after birth. More immediate plans for transferring the family to the postpartum unit are made if necessary. Communication with the postpartum staff, who will be providing care throughout the rest of the hospital stay, will lead to a smooth transition of care.

The following are nursing diagnoses that may be useful in the care of families during the immediate postpartum period. Possible maternal nursing diagnoses follow:

- High Risk for Injury related to poor uterus tone and hemorrhage
- Altered Urinary Elimination related to childbirth or regional anesthesia
- Fluid Volume Deficit related to decreased oral intake, exertion, uterine atony, or lacerations
- Pain related to perineal trauma, uterine cramping, and postpartum chill
- Fatigue related to the process of labor and birth

Nursing diagnoses pertaining the neonate are the following:

- Ineffective Airway Clearance related to mucous secretions and developmental immaturity
- Ineffective Thermoregulation related to developmental immaturity
- Family Coping: Potential for Growth related to knowledge deficit concerning normal parent–newborn interactions after birth
- Ineffective Breastfeeding related to maternal anxiety, knowledge deficit, or immature neonatal sucking reflex

Complications of the immediate postpartum period include possible postpartum maternal hemorrhage and complications of the newborn, such as respiratory problems, hypothermia, and hypoglycemia. Part of the nurse's responsibilities during the fourth stage of labor is monitoring for possible complications.

• • Planning and Implementation

The period immediately after delivery often is the most rewarding time for the nurse working with a family during childbirth. The woman and her partner have completed the difficult work of labor and birth and now have the opportunity to become acquainted with their newborn. Nursing care for the woman and her family is directed at supporting maternal and neonatal physiologic status, providing for comfort needs, supporting family interaction, and monitoring for possible complications of the mother and newborn. Priorities for care are based on assessment data and nursing diagnoses.

Promoting Uterine Tone

The nurse assumes primary responsibility for promoting contraction of the uterine muscle, thus preventing excessive bleeding or postpartum hemorrhage. This is accomplished through fundal massage, administering uterine tonics, and teaching the woman to perform self-massage of the fundus. In some cultures the woman applies an abdominal binder in the immediate postpartum period to promote contraction of the myometrium. The nurse should respect this practice because there is no medical contraindication to it.

Expected Outcome

- The woman's uterus maintains its tone during the immediate postpartum period.

Promoting Hydration and Urinary Elimination

If the woman's condition is stable and alert, she should be offered clear liquids; if these are tolerated well, a normal or high-residue diet may be instituted. Both parents may be quite hungry at this point and may welcome a meal.

The woman should be encouraged to empty her bladder as soon as she is able to do so after delivery, whether or not she has the urge to urinate. Because of perineal anesthesia and postdelivery edema, she may not feel the urge to void even when the bladder is distended. Normal postdelivery diuresis and administration of intravenous fluids predispose the woman to bladder distention during this period. If bladder distention results in displacement of the uterus and increased bleeding and the woman is unable to void in the immediate postdelivery period, a standing order is frequently approved for bladder catheterization.

Expected Outcome

- The woman demonstrates complete emptying of bladder by voiding voluntarily within 6 hours after birth or when her bladder becomes full.

Promoting Comfort

Perineal edema and ecchymosis commonly occur secondary to birth trauma. Ice packs may be applied to the perineum for the first 24 hours postpartum to reduce pain, swelling, and resulting difficulty with voiding. Chemical ice packs are available, but a latex glove filled with crushed ice and covered with a cloth is just as effective. The nurse should explain the purpose of the ice pack. In some cultures cold is avoided for successful recovery from birth. In this case use of an ice pack may be objectionable, but the woman's initial concerns may be overcome by the nurse's sensitivity to cultural beliefs and careful teaching regarding the benefits of cold in the reduction of swelling.

If an episiotomy was performed or vaginal lacerations occurred, the woman may begin to experience perineal pain as the effects of the local anesthetic begin to wear off. If the woman has hemorrhoids, they also may contribute to sensations of pain. The application of a covered ice pack to the perineum during the first 24 hours may reduce pain sensations, but some women may require analgesia such as plain acetaminophen or a combination of acetaminophen and codeine. The nurse also can demonstrate techniques for sitting and getting out of bed that reduce tension on the episiotomy site.

Fundal massage is likely to be uncomfortable for the woman. The nurse can increase the mother's comfort by telling her why it is important and encouraging her to take some responsibility for this aspect of her care. The nurse then instructs the woman how to perform self-fundal massage. The nurse also reminds her to use relaxation techniques to ease this discomfort. Multiparas in particular may experience strong cramps because the uterine musculature is somewhat more relaxed. Many women experience temporary cramping with the initiation of breastfeeding. Ibuprofen (Motrin) may be ordered to relieve uterine discomfort.

Other nursing actions that contribute to the general comfort of the new mother include a sponge bath or shower and gentle perineal hygiene. Many units provide women with individualized "peri-bottles;" these are soft plastic squeeze bottles that can be filled with warm water that is gently squirted over the perineum for cleansing and to reduce stinging at the episiotomy site when the woman voids.

The new mother may experience shaking and chills in the first hour after delivery. The cause is unknown, but it may be related to an elevated core body temperature with relatively cool skin and extremities, or it may reflect a generalized immune response to fetal cells that entered the maternal circulation at the time of placental separation. See Chapter 28 for further discussion of the postpartum shivering phenomenon. The nurse should reassure parents that this is a normal phenomenon, cover the woman with a warmed blanket or two, and offer warm nonstimulating liquids, such as herbal tea or soup.

Expected Outcome

- The woman practices self-care comfort and pain-relief techniques resulting in decreasing levels of pain and increased maternal mobility.

Promoting Rest

The need for rest and sleep varies greatly in the immediate postdelivery period and depends on the following factors:

- Length of labor
- Complications experienced during labor and birth
- Administration of analgesia and anesthesia
- Degree of sleep deprivation experienced before the onset of labor
- Cultural background

Many women experience a burst of energy after the birth. The new mother may be energized, excited, and talkative. She may be ravenously hungry or very thirsty. Interaction with the newborn and attempts to breastfeed may be foremost in the woman's mind. Other women experience fatigue or somnolence after delivery. They may be strongly encouraged by family members or guided by cultural prescriptives to rest or sleep. The partner or other family member may assume primary responsibility for the neonate at this time. The nurse should be guided by knowledge of the labor and delivery history, the mother's behavioral cues, and stated preferences. It may be appropriate to reduce environmental stimuli and encourage family members and support people to withdraw temporarily so the mother can rest. The current trend for early discharge (24 hours or less in a growing number of facilities) also may predispose the woman to take every opportunity to rest before she returns home to the responsibilities of child care and daily life.

Expected Outcome

- The woman verbalizes satisfaction with the degree of sleep or rest experienced in the immediate postpartum period.

Promoting Neonatal Physiologic Adaptation

As long as the neonate's physiologic status is within normal limits, nursing support remains centered on preventing excessive heat loss and promoting effective airway clearance. The neonate is vulnerable to excessive heat loss in the first 1 to 2 hours after delivery. The nurse should ensure that the neonate is well dried and well covered at all times. A hat should be used to prevent heat loss from the head. The neonate also may need assistance in keeping the upper airway clear of mucus. The presence of excessive mucus is signaled by bubbling from the mouth, sneezing, or noisy respiration. The nares and mouth should be bulb suctioned as needed. (Thermoregulation and airway maintenance are discussed further in Unit 5.)

Expected Outcomes

- The newborn maintains a respiratory rate between 30 and 60 breaths per minute.

- The newborn maintains an axillary body temperature between 36.4°C and 37.2°C (97.5°F to 99.0°F) in the first 2 hours after delivery.

Promoting Parent–Newborn Interaction

An important nursing responsibility in the immediate postpartum recovery period is supporting family interaction and parent education. This phase of labor provides an excellent opportunity for parent–newborn interaction for several reasons:

- The newborn is likely to be in a quiet alert state for 1 or 2 hours, will gaze at faces, and will initiate breastfeeding with assistance (Fig. 21-17).
- Early contact with the alert newborn provides the parents with cues about its temperament and its needs, which helps them interact with the newborn as an individual.
- The woman and partner often are excited and eager to interact with the newborn as the reward for their hard work in labor; fatigue and discomfort may not be significant enough to interfere with this interaction.
- Parents may feel a special closeness with each other and with the newborn during this time, and interaction takes on a special significance.

The nurse can help in many ways to support family interaction during this special time. Promoting the comfort of both parents and helping them to become settled for a time will allow them to enjoy this interaction. Assessing the woman's physical comfort, providing food or fluids as appropriate, and providing extra blankets, a clean gown, or clean bedding may be helpful.

The nurse's regular assessments of the newborn's status provide an opportunity for teaching parents about their newborn. Although the nurse should take care not to overwhelm them with information, tips about important aspects of care—such as keeping the newborn warm, checking for excessive mucus, and using the bulb syringe—and information about the newborn's ability to see, hear, and orient to sounds may be new for first-time parents and will be especially welcome.

Assistance with early breastfeeding is often especially appreciated during this period. The newborn typically will not nurse long and may be more interested in gazing at faces. However, the mother–newborn contact will assist in maintaining uterine tone and hemostasis and may facilitate early initiation of lactation. The nurse should ensure that the woman is comfortably positioned and can support the newborn at the breast without fatigue or strain. This is easily accomplished by positioning the newborn on the breast and supporting its weight and the mother's arm on pillows.

The nurse should assess how much contact the father or partner wants with the newborn and facilitate father–newborn interaction as appropriate. Most women will ask their partner if he or she wants to hold the neonate, and many do not hesitate to do so. However, some individuals tend to hold back, either because they believe it is "more important" for the mother to hold the newborn or because they are uncertain about how to hold a newborn. The nurse should provide a comfortable chair, check that the neonate is well wrapped to prevent heat loss and provide ease in handling the neonate, and then hand the newborn to the partner. Reassurance, encouragement, and pointing out how the newborn orients toward and seeks out the partner's voice may provide powerful reinforcement to a person who is feeling unsure about his role.

Once these things are done, the nurse can ensure that the family has some private time without interruptions. This may require the nurse to reorganize the timing of periodic

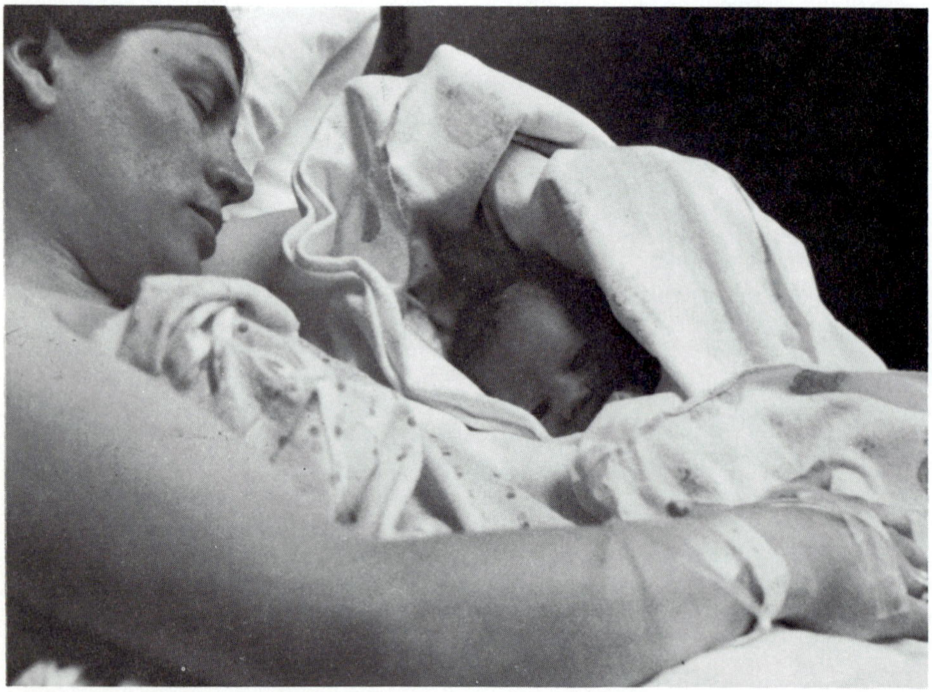

Figure 21-17.
Well wrapped and resting with his mother, the neonate is contentedly sucking on his hand in a quiet alert state. (Photo by BABES, Inc.)

NURSING PROCEDURE

Providing Nursing Care When Postpartum Hemorrhage Occurs

Immediate nursing action is required if any of the following conditions are noted in the first 1 to 2 hours after delivery:

- Two perineal pads are soaked within 30 minutes (excessive bleeding).
- The woman complains of light-headedness, nausea, or visual disturbances (possible impending hypovolemic shock).
- The woman is anxious, skin color is pale or ashen, and skin is clammy and cool (impending hypovolemic shock).
- Pulse and respirations are elevated, and blood pressure is unchanged or slightly lowered (impending hypovolemic shock).

Purpose: To maintain and support cardiovascular functioning and prevent uncompensated shock.

NURSING ACTION	***RATIONALE***
1. Summon help immediately by emergency call light; have care provider notified.	To obtain necessary supplies, equipment, and personnel required to support cardiovascular system.
2. Check uterine tone, massage fundus gently if not firm, and assess effect on bleeding or passage of clots.	Uterine atony will result in postpartum hemorrhage. Retained clots may result in relaxation of the uterus and postpartum hemorrhage.
3. Increase IV infusion, if present, or start IV infusion with a large-gauge angiocath (16 or 18 gauge).	To maintain IV access for the administration of blood products and IV fluids. To maintain adequate intravascular fluid volume for tissue perfusion.
4. Start oxygen at 8 to 12 L/min by mask.	To increase oxygenation of tissue.
5. Elevate the woman's legs, and lower head of bed.	To facilitate blood return to heart and increase brain perfusion.
6. Insert Foley catheter, and attach drainage bag.	To monitor urine output, which provides an indirect assessment of renal perfusion and the adequacy of fluid replacement.

assessments of maternal and infant status or of the administration of medications. However, this privacy can be very special to the family. The family should be assured that the nurse is nearby if needed, and the nurse should indicate when he or she will return. Whenever possible, the nurse should defer routine newborn care (eg, the administration of eye medication) until the second or third hour to allow the newborn to remain with the parents in a quiet, alert state.

Both parents are likely to experience great excitement and will interact with the newborn for a period. This is followed by growing awareness of their fatigue. At this point, the woman and her support person should be encouraged to rest. Once made comfortable, the woman will probably sleep intermittently. The nurse should help her find a comfortable position for rest and for breastfeeding. Pillows can be positioned to support the newborn. The partner should be encouraged to rest or sleep and offered a comfortable place with the new family if possible.

Expected Outcomes

- Parents demonstrate beginning attachment behaviors as evidenced by holding, smiling at, talking to, and seeking eye contact with their newborn.
- Parents demonstrate an understanding of neonatal characteristics as evidenced by positive verbalization of feelings about their newborn.

Monitoring for Complications

Potential Complication: Maternal Postpartum Hemorrhage

Maternal physiologic adaptations during the immediate postpartum period are dramatic and require nursing support if recovery is to be prompt. Of major importance is nursing intervention to ensure hemostasis and prevent excessive blood loss (see the accompanying Nursing Procedure).

Nursing actions to prevent excessive postpartum bleeding include close monitoring of uterine tone and the woman's blood pressure, administration of oxytocics, and maintenance of uterine tone by fundal massage. These are discussed earlier in this chapter and are discussed further in Unit 5.

Potential Complication: Neonatal Respiratory Distress, Hypothermia, or Hypoglycemia

The nurse continues to monitor for these major complications of the newborn. Airway clearance and thermoregulation are discussed in this chapter and are expanded in Unit 5. Prevention of hypoglycemia also is discussed in Unit 5. In the healthy neonate early initiation of breastfeeding also will aid in the prevention of hypoglycemia.

• • Evaluation

The nurse monitors the woman and newborn for indications of adaptation in the immediate postpartum period. Physiologic stability, including normal vital signs, maintenance of uterine tone, restoration of fluid balance and bladder function, provides evidence of successful postpartum adjustments in the new mother. Smooth neonatal transitions to extrauterine life and the establishment of early breastfeeding indicate that desired outcomes have been achieved for the neonate. Appraisal of parent–newborn interactions is an integral component of the evaluation process and provides additional data for the planning of ongoing nursing care and discharge teaching for the new family.

The fourth stage of labor is a period of vulnerability for the new family. The nurse plays a crucial role in supporting individual physiologic adjustments and family adaptations (see Chapter 28). Assessment of maternal and neonatal vital signs and physiologic functioning is essential. Complications that can occur during this period, such as uterine atony or neonatal hypothermia or hypoglycemia, are rare in healthy women and neonates but can result in significant compromise. The nurse plans and implements family-centered care that is individualized to meet the needs of the new family. Revisions in the nursing care plan are based on ongoing evaluation of the woman, her neonate, and the family.

Continuity of Nursing Care

Depending on the setting, the mother and newborn will be transferred to the postpartum unit after 1 or 2 hours. The nurse is responsible for the communication of important information about maternal, newborn, and family status at that time. All nursing care should have been recorded and a verbal report made to the nursing staff responsible for postpartum care. If the newborn is to be admitted to the nursery at this time, a report on the newborn's status also is necessary.

If the nurse is not going to have regular contact with the family during the postpartum period, he or she may want to "check in" on the family on an informal basis. The nurse who provides sensitive and expert care during labor and birth often becomes an important person to the mother and partner, if only temporarily. Visits from their labor nurse are seen as an expression of caring, and they give the new mother and partner an opportunity to relive their labor experiences and to fill in areas where their recall may not be clear.

Chapter Summary

The nurse plays a major role in supporting the woman and her family during the second stage of labor and in protecting maternal, fetal, and family well-being as they adapt to the normal physiologic and psychological stresses of birth. The needs of the woman and her family change throughout the course of second stage labor; nursing care must be continually adjusted to these changing needs. An important aspect of nursing care is attention to the appropriate use of technology and obstetric interventions. Nursing care for women at low risk for complications should provide physical and psychological support, monitor well-being so that variations from normal status can be identified and treated early, and provide family-centered care that promotes comfort and a positive, healthy beginning for the new family.

Study Questions

1. *The woman you are caring for is just fully dilated, but she tells you "I don't feel like pushing." What nursing interventions would you initiate in response to this comment?*
2. *How does "open glottis" pushing in the second stage of labor compare with traditional methods that use the Valsalva maneuver?*
3. *Which maternal positions and comfort measures may be helpful to a woman who is experiencing a slow second stage of labor?*
4. *What steps should you take in response to a woman who exclaims "My baby is coming!"? Give your rationale.*
5. *Which nursing actions are most effective in keeping the newborn warm immediately after birth?*
6. *You assess a woman in the 15 minutes after delivery and determine that she has saturated 2 peripads. What are the possible causes? What are appropriate nursing interventions? Give your rationale.*
7. *Why may some women desire limited interaction with the newborn after birth?*

References

Cosner, K., & deJong, E. (1993). Physiologic second stage labor. *American Journal of Maternal Child Nursing, 18*(1), 38–43.

Liu, Y. (1989). The effects of the upright position during childbirth. *Image, 21*(1), 14.

NAACOG. (1992). *Nursing responsibilities in implementing intrapartum fetal heart rate monitoring. Position Statement.* Washington, DC: Author.

CHAPTER 22

Monitoring the At-Risk Fetus

Learning Objectives

After studying the material in this chapter, the student will be able to:

- Identify indications for use of electronic fetal monitoring during labor.
- Describe advantages and disadvantages of internal and external fetal monitoring.
- Identify the key elements of fetal heart rate patterns and their normal range.
- Discuss the nurse's role in the application of electronic fetal monitoring and interpretation of its data.
- Describe the advantages and disadvantages of fetal scalp sampling and fetal scalp stimulation.
- Explain the kind of information obtained from fetal scalp sampling and scalp stimulation.
- Describe the new technologies and the kinds of information obtained.

Key Terms

baseline fetal heart rate
Doppler velocimetry
fetal distress
fetal stress
intrauterine pressure catheter
long-term variability
short-term variability
sinusoidal pattern
spiral electrode
tokodynamometer

Some women are known to be at risk for intrapartum complications because of preexisting conditions. Others will encounter unanticipated problems in the intrapartum period after an uneventful pregnancy. Both groups of women require *active obstetric management*, which includes the use of a variety of diagnostic tests and techniques designed to lower maternal–fetal risk in the intrapartum period.

When risk is increased, maternal care tends to become focused more on the medical management of the woman and fetus and less on the emotional needs of the woman. Family-centered care practices may be deemphasized or omitted because it is assumed that such practices would be unsafe or impractical. There is no clear evidence to support that assumption. Moderate- or high-risk women and their families benefit as much from family-centered maternity care as low-risk families (Loos & Julius, 1989).

Current maternity care includes a range of technologies and procedures designed to reduce intrapartum risk to the woman and fetus. Each procedure entails specific nursing responsibilities that must be carried out to provide safe and sensitive intrapartum care. However, the nurse must be prepared to care for women and their families so that the level of risk is reduced *and* emotional needs are met. The Organization for Obstetric, Gynecologic, and Neonatal Nurses (AWHONN) has formulated a statement on practice (1991) that emphasizes that the technology available to the nurse cannot take the place of hands-on individualized nursing care. This tenet is a central element of family-centered nursing.

Chapters 22, 23, and 24 highlight procedures intended to reduce maternal and fetal risk in the intrapartum period. Depending on the course of labor and the nature of the problem, several of these procedures may be implemented in the course of the woman's intrapartum care. In general risk-reducing procedures in intrapartum care can be grouped into three major categories:

- Procedures aimed at closer monitoring of fetal status
- Procedures aimed at safe and more effective management of maternal pain
- Procedures that involve modifying the pattern of labor and mode of delivery

This chapter focuses on monitoring the at-risk fetus. The chapters that follow discuss management of maternal pain and procedures that modify the pattern of labor and mode of delivery. Decisions to implement these procedures are made by the physician in consultation with the nurse midwife, the labor nurse, and the family. Discussions about risk reduction procedures must always take into account the relative benefits and risks of more active obstetric management.

Assessment of Fetal Status

The primary aim of fetal monitoring during the intrapartum period is the early identification of fetal distress to prevent asphyxia and permanent damage to the growing fetus. Although general imprecise terms have been used to describe the response of the fetus to a variety of stressors, in light of the current medicolegal climate, efforts have been made to delineate their meaning (Parer & Livingston, 1990).

Fetal stress is a term for the nonspecific biologic responses in the fetus elicited by adverse external influences. Fetal stress is a common feature of normal labor. The fetus is well equipped to withstand stress, and this ability is enhanced by catecholamine secretion (Copper & Goldenberg, 1990). It is generally believed that the intrauterine stress experienced during labor improves extrauterine adaptations that must occur in the first hours of postnatal life (Eskes, Ingemarsson, Pardi, Nijhuis, & Ruth, 1991).

Fetal distress generally is viewed as a state of physiologic decompensation or compromise in the fetus, caused by a lack of oxygen and nutrients required for normal physiologic functioning. Methods used to diagnose fetal distress during labor and delivery generally include biochemical tests (pH analysis of capillary or umbilical blood samples), electronic fetal monitoring (EFM), and most recently Doppler blood flow pattern analysis. Theoretically, the point at which distress results in permanent injury is unknown, but it is thought to depend on fetal reserves of oxygen and glucose, as well as the developmental state of the organ systems. Recent research indicates great "plasticity" in neurologic tissues of the fetus and neonate; this permits essentially normal growth and development, even after significant insult (Rowe, 1990).

Fetal asphyxia is a condition resulting from the absence of exchange of respiratory gases (oxygen and carbon dioxide) and may result in permanent organ damage. More precise terms, such as metabolic and respiratory acidemia, hypoxia, and hypercarbia, have been suggested to describe the specific nature and degree of fetal stress, distress, and asphyxia (ACOG, 1991). The extent of acidemia, hypoxia and hypercarbia may be measured during labor and immediately after birth and offer objective data regarding the condition of the fetus and neonate.

Fetal distress may be chronic or acute. If untreated, it can lead to fetal and neonatal morbidity and mortality. Even when it is treated promptly, intrauterine fetal distress can result in long-term problems, such as preterm birth, growth retardation, cerebral palsy, seizure disorders, and mental retardation. Researchers are attempting to define the degree of acidemia, hypoxia, and hypercarbia that causes fetal distress and permanent hypoxic damage (Portman, Carter, Gaylord, Murphy, Thieme, & Merenstein, 1990; Fee, Malee, Deddish, Minogue, & Socol, 1990).

When the fetus has been chronically comprised, the additional stress of labor compounds fetal risk. The extent to which repetitive uterine contractions contribute to fetal distress depends on the extent of previous fetal compromise and the quality of uterine activity. Diagnostic procedures of fetal well-being are discussed in Chapter 14.

Chronic Distress

Chronic fetal distress occurs when the physiologic exchange of nutrients, oxygen, and metabolites from the woman to her fetus is disrupted over time. This often is a result of systemic maternal problems. The disruption in oxygen and nutrients often is reflected in reduced blood flow to the placenta, abnormalities in placental structure, deficiency in placental functioning, and decreasing amniotic fluid volume. Maternal factors that can result in chronic fetal distress include the following:

- Vascular abnormalities associated with chronic maternal hypertension, pregnancy-induced hypertension (PIH) or eclampsia, or diabetes
- Inadequate systemic perfusion due to maternal cardiac or pulmonary disease
- Placental aging in post-term pregnancy
- Substance abuse
- Chronic intrauterine infection or sexually transmitted diseases

Fetal problems also can result in chronic fetal distress. The most frequent fetal causes of chronic distress are the following:

- Multiple gestation in which fetoplacental circulation is distributed unequally
- Congenital anomalies
- Infection, such as toxoplasmosis or cytomegalovirus
- Rh disease (erythroblastosis fetalis)

Chronic fetal distress is commonly diagnosed when uterine growth is less than adequate. The McDonald's measurements of fundal height will indicate a slowing of fetal growth. Clinical suspicions may be confirmed by the use of sonography (measurement of femur length or abdominal circumference). Ultrasonography has led to the development of other technologies to assist the health care provider in the diagnosis of intrauterine growth retardation (IUGR) and chronic fetal distress. These are discussed at the end of this chapter.

Acute Distress

Acute fetal distress can occur during the intrapartum period and is suggested by the presence of nonreassuring or ominous fetal heart rate (FHR) patterns, meconium-stained amniotic fluid, or abnormal blood gas and pH values (discussed later in this chapter). The major way to assess fetal risk during the intrapartum period is intensive monitoring of fetal physiologic status. This is primarily accomplished through continuous EFM and fetal blood sampling.

Technologic advances permit diagnosis of fetal well-being during the antenatal and intrapartum periods. The maternity nurse often functions in expanded roles and performs diagnostic tests of fetal physiologic status. The nurse who cares for the woman during the intrapartum period must have a comprehensive knowledge of these tests to plan and implement appropriate nursing care. During the intrapartum period, the nurse also may conduct additional diagnostic tests, such as the oxytocin challenge (contraction stress test), and must be skilled in all aspects of the procedure. Malpractice litigation in maternal–newborn nursing frequently surrounds issues of fetal well-being and the diagnosis of chronic or acute fetal distress. The maternity nurse must have a thorough understanding of fetal distress and the implications for nursing care when fetal distress is suspected. The following sections describe the use of EFM in the diagnosis of fetal distress and the role of the nurse in supporting fetal well-being when distress occurs.

Electronic Fetal Monitoring

The EFM is a device that provides a graphic display and a digital readout of the FHR (Fig. 22-1*A*). Uterine activity also can be measured and displayed. Data obtained from the fetal monitor usually are transcribed on a continuous strip of graph paper that runs at a speed of 3 cm/min (Fig. 22-1*B*). EFM data can be transmitted to a bank of video screens centrally located in the nurses' station for continuous assess-

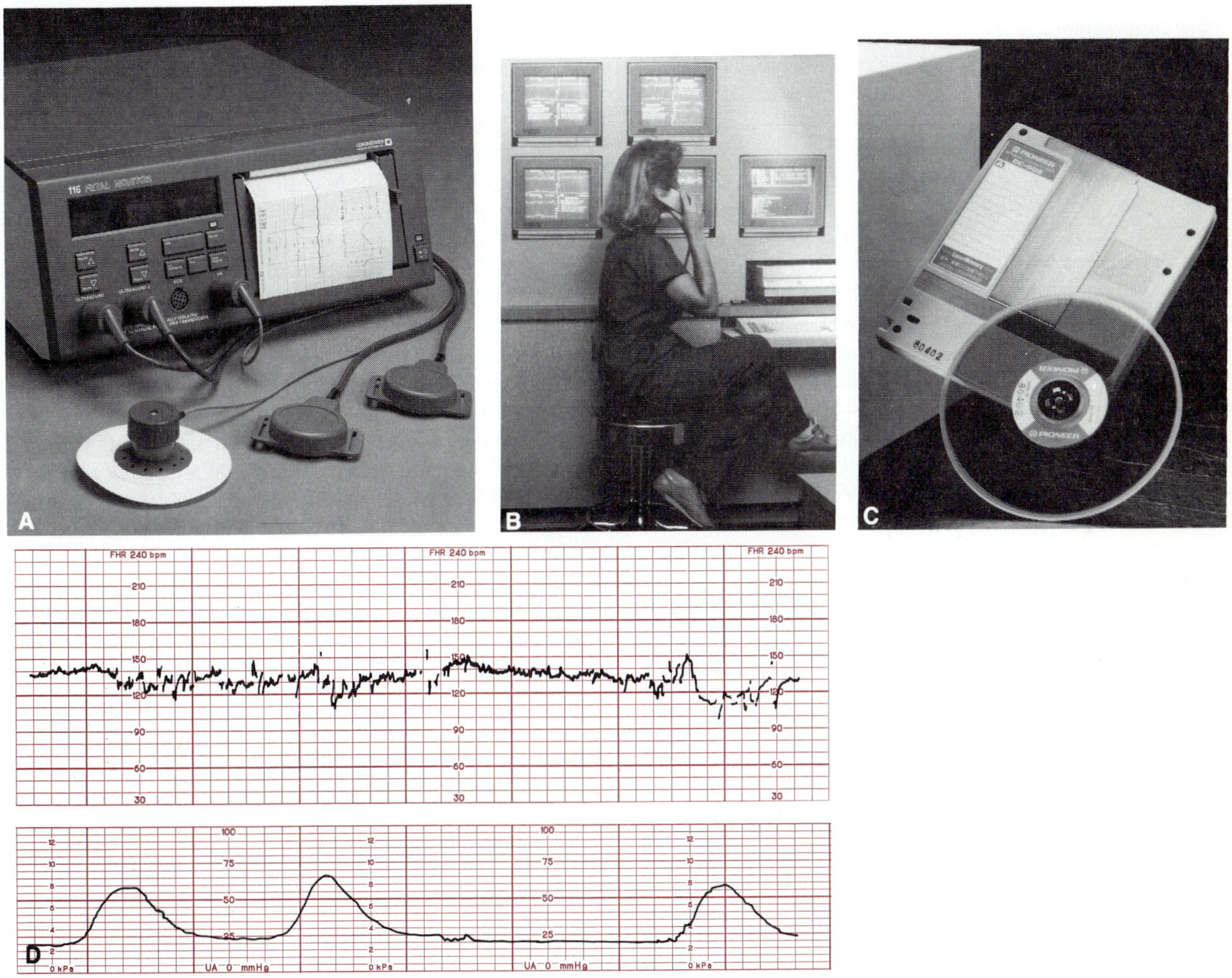

Figure 22-1.

Traditional EFM versus new EFM recording and retrieval systems. *A:* The traditional monitor machine displays a digital readout of the FHR, as well as a continuous graphic tracing of the FHR pattern and contraction pattern on specially marked paper. *B:* A much newer system is the central monitor. It consists of a bank of video screens, which allows the nurse to assess the fetal heart rate when out of the patient's room. *C:* Used in conjunction with the central monitor, the laser disk system permits computerized recording and storage of fetal heart rate data. (*A* courtesy of Corometrics Medical Systems Inc., Wallingford, CN; *C* and *D* courtesy of Peritronics Medical Inc., Brea, CA.) *D:* A monitor tracing from a traditional monitor machine shows the FHR pattern (top line) in beats per minute. The lower line shows the uterine contraction pattern in mm Hg. This allows observation of changes in FHR patterns in response to uterine activity.

ment when health providers are not at the bedside (Fig. 22-1*C*). Recent advances also permit electronic recording and storage of EFM data on optical laser disks (Fig. 22-1*D*). Many of these systems do not use graph paper or produce the EFM "strip." If the nurse wants to review FHR patterns or uterine activity, the information is retrieved using a computer system that permits electronic display of the data on a video screen.

Electronic monitoring can be accomplished by *external* (noninvasive) or *internal* methods. With internal monitoring an electrode is attached to the presenting fetal part and a pressure-sensing catheter is introduced into the uterus. This is performed after the membranes have ruptured. Nursing staff may routinely initiate external EFM; however, internal EFM is generally initiated by a physician or nurse midwife. Labor nurses also may apply the internal fetal monitor lead after they have completed a training course or acquired formal certification.

Routine continuous use of EFM is not recommended for low-risk women in normal labor. There is little disagreement about its value in the high-risk patient, particularly when indicators of fetal stress appear, but research has yielded conflicting results. Shy et al. (1990) discovered a higher incidence of cerebral palsy in preterm infants who had been monitored by EFM during labor. The time from diagnosis of an abnormal FHR pattern to delivery was prolonged in the EFM group compared with the nurse-monitored group evaluated by intermittent auscultation. The investigators suggested that the delay in delivery occurred because the obstetricians were reassured by specific characteristics of the FHR pattern and felt safe waiting until further evidence of distress occurred. Further research is needed to delineate the appropriate uses and value of EFM in high-risk patients.

Perhaps the greatest disadvantage of over-reliance on continuous EFM is the increased incidence of unnecessary obstetric intervention. Studies conducted in the 1980s indicated a twofold to threefold increase in the cesarean birth rate without an improvement in perinatal outcomes among women who received continuous EFM compared with women assessed by intermittent FHR auscultation (Placek, Keppel, Taffel, & Liss, 1984; McCusker, Harris, & Hosmer, 1988). Recent studies indicate the rate of cesarean birth remains more than 20% and clearly continues to be influenced by technology such as EFM (McCloskey, Petitti, & Hobel, 1992; Albers & Savitz, 1991).

External (Indirect) Monitoring

External EFM relies on ultrasound detection of the FHR, rather than a direct electrocardiogram display, such as that generated by internal monitoring. External EFM usually is used early in labor and may be used on an intermittent or continuous basis. The external monitoring is accomplished by two devices secured by belts or an elastic binder to the maternal abdomen and connected to a monitor, as shown in Figure 22-2.

The first of these devices is an *ultrasound transducer*, which detects fetal heart sounds. This device is placed, using a water-soluble conducting gel, on the maternal abdomen at the point of maximum intensity of the fetal heart tones and secured with the abdominal belt or elastic binder (see Fig. 22-2*B*). Ultrasound waves generated in this device bounce back from organs within the fetus. Information about internal movements (eg, movements of chambers of the fetal heart or of blood in fetal vessels) is then displayed on the monitor by a digital readout, by oscilloscope, and by graphic tracing. This transmission also may reflect movement of blood through a *maternal* vessel, so abnormally low readings may reflect the maternal pulse rather than the FHR. The nurse must count the maternal pulse rate while evaluating the FHR in this case to rule out true fetal bradycardia.

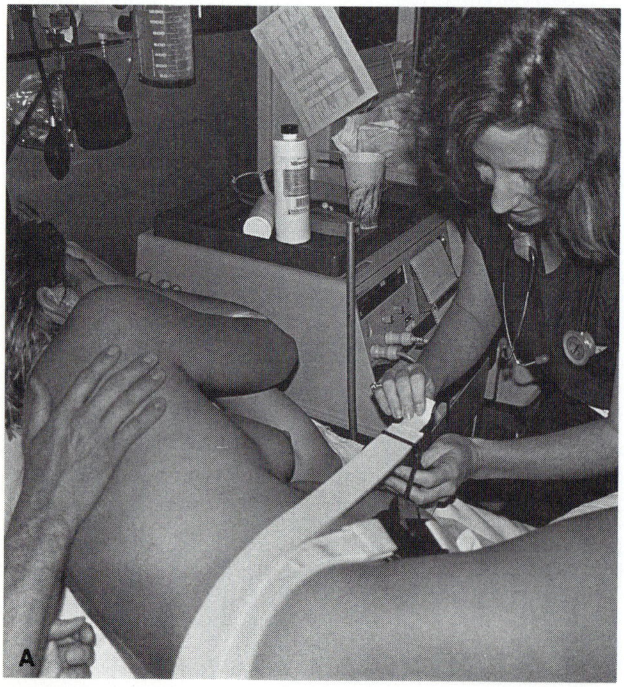

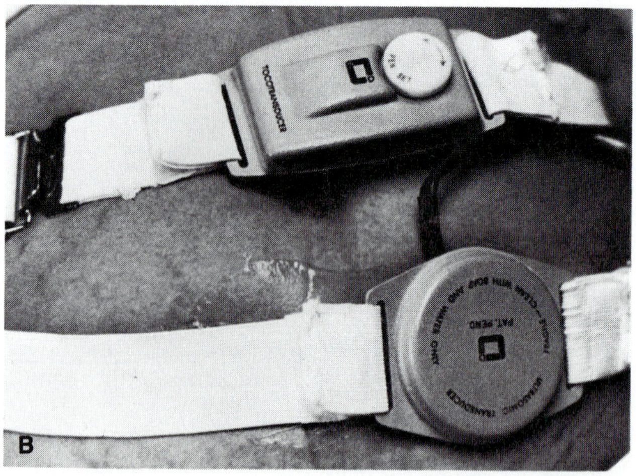

Figure 22-2.
External (indirect) electronic fetal monitoring in place. *A:* The nurse secures the two devices attached to belts to the woman's abdomen. *B:* The ultrasound transducer (bottom) detects fetal heart sounds. The tocotransducer (top) records the pressure of uterine contractions. (*A* by Kathy Sloane, Courtesy of Alta Bates Medical Center; *B* courtesy of BABES, Inc.)

The other device used for external EFM is a *tocotransducer* (tokodynamometer), a pressure-sensing instrument that records the relative strength of uterine contractions (see Fig. 22-2*B*). As the uterus contracts pressure is exerted against the tocotransducer and recorded on a graphic display or tracing, as shown in Figure 22-1*A*. This wavelike pattern can be used to record frequency and duration of uterine contractions. Intensity cannot be accurately recorded, because the height of the "wave" depends on the tightness of the belt securing the device to the abdomen and the woman's activity level. If belts are used, they should be secured tightly enough so that the monitor displays an increase in pressure just before or as the woman feels the contraction. This degree of tightness may be annoying to the woman. In many cases the elastic abdominal binder works as well as belts for recording contraction patterns. However, when belts must be used the woman should be told why they are needed, and they must be removed intermittently for temporary relief of the woman's discomfort. When precise measurement of contraction strength is needed, internal intrauterine pressure monitoring is indicated. However, internal (direct) monitoring cannot be initiated until the membranes have ruptured.

Indications and Contraindications

Indications include the following:

- Necessity of a baseline FHR for evidence of long-term variability
- Variations in FHR detected by auscultation
- Meconium-stained amniotic fluid
- Induction of labor
- Oxytocin augmentation of labor
- High risk for uteroplacental insufficiency or fetal compromise with hypertension, bleeding, preterm or postterm pregnancies, IUGR, abnormal fetal presentation, previous stillbirth, diabetes, sickle-cell disease, hemolytic disease of the fetus, or oligohydramnios

No absolute contraindications exist.

Advantages and Disadvantages

External EFM is most beneficial as an adjunct to repeated nursing assessments of fetal status and labor pattern by auscultation and palpation. Its advantages are that it can be initiated by nursing personnel, it is noninvasive and can be used when membranes are intact and the cervix is undilated, it provides useful information about fetal response to labor, and it may be reassuring and helpful to the woman as she copes with her labor.

Its disadvantages include its tendency to limit the woman's activity level and position changes. The relative lack of accuracy in recording FHR and uterine contraction strength also limits the usefulness of external EFM. Ultrasound transmission may record artifact sounds, including maternal bowel or cardiac sounds, and may be affected by fetal or maternal movement. Belts must be frequently repositioned, and external EFM does not give an accurate measurement of uterine contraction strength, even when the belts are applied carefully. Accuracy of external EFM is further limited by obesity, polyhydramnios, or a very active fetus.

Implications for Nursing Care

The externally monitored laboring woman should be encouraged to find a comfortable position and if ambulation is not contraindicated, to move around the room within the limits of the wire lengths that are attached to the monitor. Both the ultrasound transducer and the tocotransducer will require frequent checking and repositioning if the woman is mobile. However, the advantages of ambulation and frequent position changes, described in Chapter 20, outweigh any inconvenience this may cause. This should be explained to the woman and her support person because some women will limit their movement to avoid "bothering" the nurse to reposition the belts.

While preparing and placing the external monitoring devices, the nurse should instruct the woman and her partner about the function of each device and how it should be positioned. The nurse also should explain what information the monitor provides, how that information can be used to time uterine contractions, and how the volume of the monitor may be adjusted to hear the fetal heart pattern. The nurse should point out that attending to the monitor is helpful for some women but distracting for others. The nurse should explain that position changes, fetal movement, electronic interference, maternal sounds, ambulation, and occasional disconnection of leads will affect the readout data. Therefore, the woman and her partner should not be automatically alarmed by such a change but should alert the nurse.

Internal (Direct) Monitoring

Internal EFM and intrauterine pressure monitoring provide the most precise assessment of FHR and uterine contractility pattern. The FHR is directly monitored by recording electric impulses through an electrode attached to the presenting fetal part. Strength of uterine contractions is monitored through a pressure-sensing catheter placed inside the uterus (Fig. 22-3). Because of its invasiveness, internal EFM is used most often when accuracy of information about fetal response to labor or uterine contractility is essential. This type of monitoring is possible only after the membranes are ruptured.

Internal monitoring requires access to the fetus and the uterine cavity. The cervix must be dilated to at least 1 cm, and membranes must be ruptured artificially if spontaneous rupture has not occurred. In addition it is very difficult to attach the fetal electrode if the presenting part is not engaged and easily accessible through the cervix. The internal monitoring devices (ie, the fetal scalp electrode and the uterine pressure catheter) are applied under aseptic conditions in the following manner.

The Internal Spiral Electrode

The vulva may be cleansed with an antiseptic agent and a sterile vaginal examination performed to verify the nature of the presenting part (head, buttocks, foot), its position, and its station. A spiral electrode is inserted through a hollow guide into the vagina, through the cervix until the fetal presenting part is reached. The electrode is gently twisted so that its pointed tip punctures and slips beneath the fetal

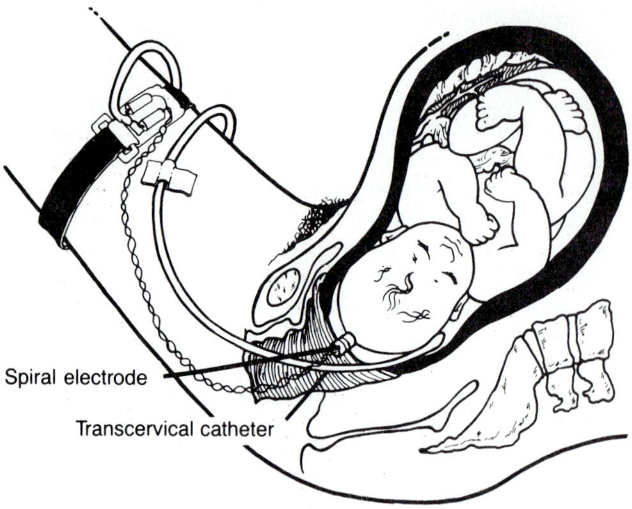

Figure 22-3.
Internal (direct) electronic fetal monitoring (Childbirth Graphics).

scalp and is secured in place. Extreme care is taken to avoid placing the electrode in such vulnerable body parts as the fontanelles, eyes, or genitals.

When the electrode is in place, the guide tube is removed, and the leads that are attached to the presenting part extend through the vagina to the outside. The ends of the scalp electrode are attached to a plate that is secured to the woman's thigh. This plate is connected to a cord leading to the fetal monitor.

The Intrauterine Pressure Catheter

Accurate measurement of uterine contraction strength is possible by inserting an intrauterine pressure catheter. Two types of catheter are available. A hollow, fluid-filled, plastic catheter was the first to be developed. Once the membranes are ruptured, it is threaded through a guide into the uterus and advanced until a mark on the catheter reaches the introitus. The catheter that extends from the vagina is connected to a strain gauge and then to the monitor. Recently a precalibrated, solid pressure catheter was developed. A computer chip located in the tip measures intrauterine pressure. No fluid is used, and once the catheter is calibrated and inserted, no further calibration can be done. Both catheters generate a similar uterine pressure tracing.

When intrauterine pressure is exerted on the fluid-filled catheter tip during contractions, it is transmitted through the channel of water in the catheter, across the transducer diaphragm, to the strain gauge. This mechanical energy is then converted to electric energy, amplified, and recorded on the monitor paper. When the solid catheter is used, pressure is transmitted electronically to the monitor rather than by mechanical energy generated by changes in water pressure.

When the fluid-filled catheter is used, sterile water *without* preservatives must be used. Saline can corrode the stainless steel diaphragm, and preservatives have been linked to morbidity and mortality in very low–birth-weight fetuses (Carlton, 1990). For accurate readings of intrauterine pressure, the strain gauge should be positioned at approximately the same level as the catheter tip. The transducer must be calibrated to atmospheric pressure after catheter insertion and every time the woman changes position. Occasionally the catheter tip becomes clogged with blood or meconium and must be flushed to ensure accurate measurements. The intrauterine pressure catheter measures the resting tonus of the uterus, as well as the frequency, duration, and strength of contractions, and it records this on a tracing calibrated to reflect pressure in mm Hg. This uterine pressure tracing is recorded simultaneously with the FHR. Accuracy of the measurement of uterine contraction strength can be checked by palpating a contraction and comparing this with the monitor tracing. An increase of 25 mm Hg over the resting tonus should correspond to a mild contraction, 50 mm Hg to a moderate contraction, and 70 mm Hg or more to a strong contraction. Patency of the catheter can be checked by asking the woman to cough or apply fundal pressure and by observing the tracing for a corresponding rise in intrauterine pressure.

Many birth attendants now use intrauterine pressure monitoring only when assessment of intensity and frequency of uterine contractions is particularly important—for example during administration of intravenous (IV) oxytocin.

Indications and Contraindications

Internal EFM provides the most accurate information about fetal response to labor and uterine contraction patterns, but because of its invasiveness, it is used less frequently than external EFM. Indications for internal EFM are the following:

- Variations in FHR detected by auscultation
- Meconium-stained amniotic fluid
- Induction of labor
- Oxytocin augmentation of labor
- High risk of uteroplacental insufficiency or fetal compromise
- Need for precise determination of FHR pattern, as when abnormality is suspected on the basis of external monitoring
- Failure to progress in labor with suspected uterine dystocia
- Possible vaginal delivery after previous cesarean birth

Contraindications include the following:

- Closed cervix
- Presenting part high in the pelvis
- Presenting part that cannot be identified with accuracy
- Presenting part such that application of the electrode would be the fetal face, fontanelles, or scrotum
- Maternal positive human immunodeficiency virus (HIV) status

Advantages and Disadvantages

Because of its invasiveness and potential risks, the disadvantages of internal EFM outweigh its advantages for routine use. However, when accurate information about a potentially compromised fetus is essential, internal EFM provides information about fetal status, allowing a margin of safety otherwise not possible.

An advantage of internal EFM is its ability to provide beat-by-beat assessment of the FHR. It also provides information on uterine contractility when palpation is difficult (because of obesity or presence of fibroids) or when assessment of uterine contractility must be continuous, such as during vaginal delivery after previous cesarean birth or during oxytocin infusion. Maternal or fetal position changes do not affect continuous recording of contractions when internal EFM is used.

Several disadvantages of internal EFM have been described. Before it can be used, the membranes must have ruptured. The fetus must have descended through the pelvis to a point where the examiner can reach the presenting part to attach the EFM electrode. The cervix also must be dilated to at least 1 cm before the electrode can be passed through the cervix. Skilled personnel are needed to apply the equipment and maintain it while in operation. Internal EFM is contraindicated with face presentation to prevent accidental insertion of the spinal electrode in the fetus's eye, and when the woman is HIV positive to reduce the risk of perinatal HIV transmission.

Several fetal and maternal complications can occur with EFM. Fetal scalp abscess or laceration of the scalp or other body part may result from insertion of the spiral electrode. In rare cases osteomyelitis, sepsis, and death have been reported after using the spiral electrode (Leatherman, Pachman, & Lawler, 1992). There also can be trauma to the fetal head because of lack of the amniotic fluid cushion to protect its head.

There is a risk of infection to the woman and of perforation of the uterus by the intrauterine catheter when it is used to measure uterine activity. Furthermore, the woman's stress level can be increased by early amniotomy. As noted previously the woman's movement is restricted, and the incidence of cesarean birth is increased. Finally, there can be a loss of attention to the laboring woman when health care providers and the support person focus on the monitor.

Implications for Nursing Care

The nurse should carefully explain to the woman and her partner why internal EFM is desirable and what the procedure involves, answering any questions they may have. Many will have initial reservations about the procedure and justifiably so, because it is not risk-free. However, when maternal or fetal conditions make internal monitoring desirable, women will usually permit the procedure when they receive an explanation of risks and benefits. The nurse must be aware that close attention to the monitor and its readings may result in decreased attention and concern for the woman's emotional well-being and comfort. The support person also should be alerted to the tendency of fixating on the machine instead of the woman who requires ongoing support and attention.

Nursing care should include encouraging the woman to change position frequently, using the fetus' heartbeat and uterine contraction patterns to assist with relaxation techniques. The anxiety level of the woman and support person can be decreased by explaining that variations in the recording of information on the graphic readout may be artifacts of movement or electric feedback (Fig. 22-4).

Some women welcome EFM because it reassures them and helps them to anticipate contractions. However, the irritation caused by the enforced immobility, loss of control, and loss of privacy may be exacerbated if the monitor receives the attention the woman desperately needs. Nurses should be particularly sensitive to the needs of women with EFM and remember that clinical skills in palpation of contractions and auscultation of FHR are crucial to verify EFM findings when caring for laboring women.

Ambulatory Telemetry

A recent innovation in internal EFM is ambulatory telemetry. A radio transmitter attached to a standard scalp electrode and intrauterine pressure catheter transmits information about the FHR and uterine contractions from an ambulating woman in labor to a central display screen and printer. Although not yet in common use, this telemetry system appears to promote maternal mobility, convenience, and comfort while maintaining the advantages of internal EFM.

Facsimile Telecopier Transmission of FHR

Many high-risk perinatal centers now offer long-distance consultation regarding FHR and uterine activity patterns to rural community hospitals. Using facsimile units, 24-hour transmission of FHR data to major referral centers is now possible. Low-cost facsimile units allow transmission of long

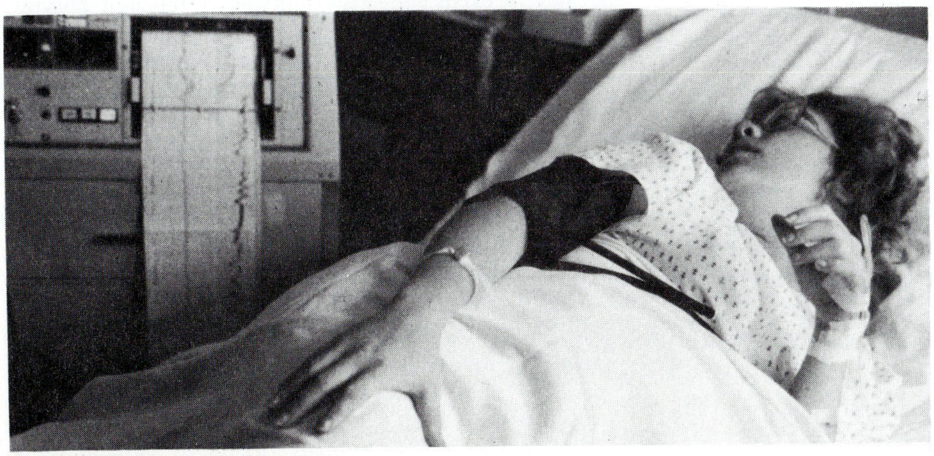

Figure 22-4.
The nurse must be sensitive to the woman's response to electronic fetal monitoring during labor and intervene to provide more information or support as needed.

documents (such as the fetal monitor strip) and permit perinatologists to offer medical consultation and advice to physicians and midwives providing care in low-risk settings far removed from medical centers. Early reports suggest improvement in patient care and a reduction in medicolegal liability (Clark, DeVore, Sabey, & Jolley, 1989).

In all labor and delivery settings the nurse maintains primary responsibility for implementing external fetal monitoring. In some settings the nurse may initiate internal EFM and is guided by unit protocols when implementing this method. Whether external or internal EFM is used, the nurse must have a comprehensive knowledge of both techniques. This is essential to assemble and safely use the equipment and to explain the risks, benefits, and purposes of EFM to the woman and her support person. With advances in technology, the nurse also is responsible for acquiring knowledge about computerized fetal monitoring, telemetry systems, and facsimile transmission of EFM data as they are introduced into the work setting.

Interpretation of Fetal Heart Rate Patterns

During each uterine contraction there is a transient reduction in maternal blood flow through the placenta. Under normal circumstances placental function and perfusion provide a "fetal reserve" of oxygen and nutrients, ensuring that stress to the fetus during labor is minimal. Labor has been described as a stress test for the fetus when certain conditions exist, including the following:

- Placental abnormality
- Maternal disease, such as diabetes, PIH (which produces early placental aging), or decreased perfusion
- Maternal hypotension
- Supine hypotensive syndrome
- Fetal disease, such as erythroblastosis fetalis
- Cord compression
- Analgesics or anesthesia

Intermittent auscultation of the FHR by fetoscope or Doppler during labor, especially if restricted only to the interval between contractions, is not effective for detecting subtle changes in the FHR pattern. As discussed, use of continuous EFM is indicated for high-risk fetal labors and when suspicious fluctuations of FHR are detected by fetoscope. Continuous monitoring provides an accurate reading of fetal response to the stress of uterine contractions. Many settings now use intermittent external EFM for low-risk women in labor (for example, one 20-minute readout strip on admission and every 1 to 2 hours thereafter) to complement auscultation by Doppler or fetoscope.

Assessment and interpretation of FHR patterns is a major nursing responsibility in intrapartum care. Interpretation of FHR patterns involves evaluation of baseline FHR and, more important, periodic FHR changes that appear in response to uterine contraction. The nurse must be able to recognize normal (reassuring) patterns and those that suggest fetal distress (nonreassuring and ominous patterns) (see the Nursing Procedure, Nursing Responsibilities When Abnormalities in FHR Are Noted).

Assessment of Baseline Fetal Heart Rate

Baseline FHR is determined by the range of the FHR in a 10-minute period in the absence of or between contractions. The normal baseline FHR is 120 to 160 bpm. This rate is influenced by the integrity of the autonomic nervous system of the fetus and also may be affected by such factors as prematurity, fetal hypoxia, medications, or maternal fever. If the FHR increases or decreases and remains at this new level for a 10-minute period during labor, this is referred to as a *baseline change*, and a new baseline is established.

Many electronic monitors display double counts or half counts of FHRs that are at the extreme ends of the recording range. If the FHR is 70 bpm or slower, the monitor may double the rate and display it as 140 bpm, while an FHR of 180 bpm or faster may be displayed as 90 bpm. This underscores an extremely important point: The nurse should never rely exclusively on monitor data for assessment of the maternal–fetal status. EFM *always* must be complemented by periodic auscultation of FHR and palpation of uterine contractions.

Fetal Bradycardia

Bradycardia exists when the baseline FHR is below 120 bpm for 10 minutes or more. Bradycardia is described in degrees from moderate to marked. Moderate bradycardia is said to exist if the FHR is between 100 and 119 bpm. This rate is not caused by fetal distress but is a benign change thought to be caused by a vagal response to head compression during labor. Vagal response, due to stimulation of the vagus or tenth cranial nerve, is characterized by parasympathetic nervous system activity, notably slowing of the heart. Marked bradycardia is said to exist if the FHR is less than 100 bpm. This rate is associated with progressive fetal acidosis due to hypoxia and is considered ominous, especially if accompanied by periodic FHR changes. Causes of fetal bradycardia are listed in Table 22-1.

Fetal Tachycardia

Tachycardia is said to exist if the baseline FHR is more than 160 bpm for longer than 10 minutes. Tachycardia is described as moderate or marked. Moderate tachycardia is said to exist if the FHR is between 161 and 180 bpm. This rate is associated with mild or progressive hypoxia. Marked tachycardia exists if the FHR is more than 180 bpm. This rate is considered an ominous sign when associated with periodic FHR changes or minimal baseline variability. Fetal tachycardia may be caused by the factors listed in Table 22-1.

Baseline Variability

Variability in the FHR is a sign of interaction between the fetal sympathetic and parasympathetic nervous systems. Normal FHR variability consists of two aspects: cyclic variations of 6 to 10 bpm amplitude around the baseline heart rate in 3 to 10 cycles per minute, also called *long-term variability*, and *beat-to-beat variability*. The latter is continuous beat-by-beat fluctuation in the heart rate of 2 to 3 bpm from the baseline. Variability creates a "waviness" or "jitteriness" that can be observed in the graphic FHR tracing. Because of the subtle nature of these changes, short-term variability can *only* be assessed by *internal* continuous EFM. External EFM

NURSING PROCEDURE

Nursing Responsibilities When Abnormalities in FHR Are Noted

Purpose: To attempt correction of nonreassuring FHR patterns and support fetal physiologic stability.

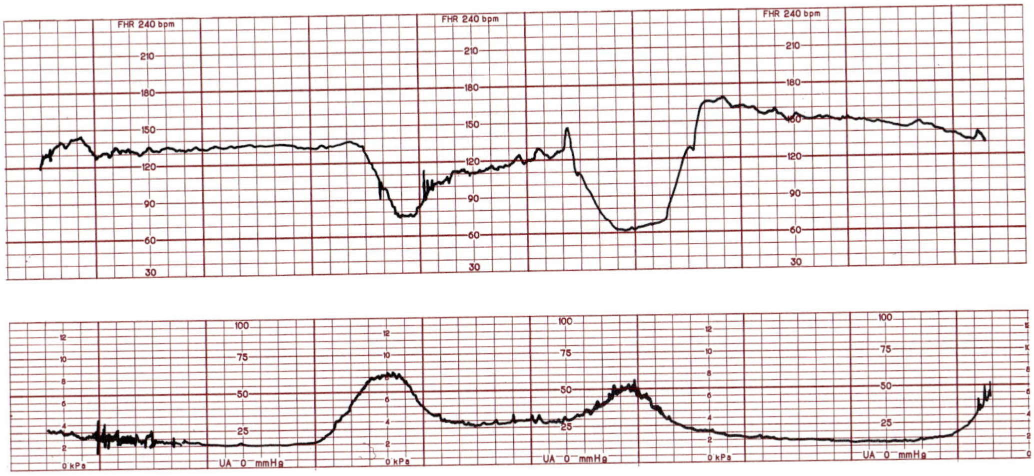

NURSING ACTION	***RATIONALE***
1. Observe EFM recording strip or perform intermittent auscultation of FHR according to standards of care, orders, and condition of woman.	To identify abnormality in timely manner. To initiate appropriate corrective actions based on the nature of abnormality.
2. Check that monitor belts and lines are properly secured and connected.	To obtain a technically accurate reading.
3. Explain purpose of FHR monitoring, equipment being used, and meanings of findings of readout data (with EFM).	To provide reassurance to woman and partner.
4. If performing EFM, confirm abnormality with portable Doppler, fetoscope, or ultrasound machine.	Electrical noise and limitations of equipment may result in unreliable data at times, such as doubling of very slow FHR (less than 120 bpm) or halving of very high FHR (more than 160 bpm).
5. Alert physician or nurse midwife about abnormal FHR promptly.	To obtain essential medical assistance in a timely manner.
6. Turn the woman to left lateral position.	To decrease supine hypotension and improve uteroplacental perfusion.
7. If EFM demonstrates variable decelerations, continue to change woman's position until pattern improves.	To reduce or eliminate cord compression; the woman's position may need to be altered several times before improvement is noted.
8. If IV is in place, increase infusion rate of mainline IV. If no IV line, initiate with large-gauge angiocath (16 to 18 gauge).	To increase uteroplacental perfusion.
9. Administer oxygen by face mask at 8 to 12 L/min.	To increase maternal blood oxygen level and the amount of oxygen available to the fetus.
10. If variable decelerations are severe, or prolonged decelerations are unimproved by nursing actions, perform vaginal examination.	To determine if decelerations are due to rapid progress of labor or if prolapse of umbilical cord is the cause.
11. If cord is prolapsed, move woman to knee–chest position.	To relieve pressure on umbilical cord.
12. Place bed in Trendelenberg position, and prepare for emergency cesarean delivery.	To deliver infant promptly to prevent asphyxia and possible permanent neurologic injury.
13. If oxytocin is infusing, stop administration	To decrease uterine activity and promote placental perfusion.
14. Be prepared to administer a tocolytic.	To reduce uterine activity and improve uterine blood flow.

Table 22-1. Causes of Baseline Changes in Fetal Heart Rate

Fetal Bradycardia	Fetal Tachycardia	Reduction in Fetal Heart Rate Variability
Fetal hypoxia Maternal drugs (anesthetics, oxytocics) Maternal hypotension Prolonged cord compression Congenital fetal cardiac lesion	Prematurity Mild hypoxia resulting in increased cardiac rate to compensate for oxygen debt Tocolytic agents given to the woman to treat preterm labor Maternal fever, which increases maternal metabolic levels and increases fetal oxygen needs Maternal anemia or hyperthyroidism Administration of phenothiazines or other atropinelike drugs, which interrupt vagal response in fetus Fetal activity Fetal infection Arrhythmia	Deep fetal sleep (should persist only 20–30 min) Prematurity Congenital anomalies Parasympathetic blocking agents (phenothiazines, atropine) Maternal analgesics Fetal hypoxia

produces an average FHR and does provide information about long-term variability. Beat-to-beat variability is described as present, decreased, or absent. Long-term variability is described in the degrees shown in Figure 22-5.

FHR variability has become one of the most important indicators in the clinical assessment of fetal well-being. Marked variability follows catecholamine release or sympathoadrenal activity in response to mild fetal hypoxia. It is most often observed in association with excessive uterine activity, especially during the second stage of labor. Reducing uterine activity or temporarily reducing pushing efforts will improve placental gas exchange and may improve this pattern (Chez, Harvey, & Murray, 1990). Decreasing variability is an indicator of developing fetal distress, and persistent minimal or absent variability is considered an ominous pattern suggesting profound fetal compromise. Some possible causes of reduction in FHR variability are listed in Table 22-1.

Sinusoidal Fetal Heart Rate Pattern

The sinusoidal FHR pattern is an unusual pattern that shows uniform wavelike long-term variability of 5 to 15 bpm every 3 to 5 minutes, minimal or absent beat-to-beat variability, and absence of specific responses to uterine contractions. The clinical significance of this pattern is controversial. It has been attributed to severe fetal distress, severe fetal anemia, and maternal medication during labor; however, its causes and implications for fetal well-being are still unclear.

Assessment of Periodic Changes in Fetal Heart Rate

Periodic FHR changes are fluctuations from the baseline rate that are associated with uterine contractions. An increase in the baseline associated with a contraction is called an *acceleration*, and a decrease is called a *deceleration*. These periodic FHR changes (Fig. 22-6) are thought to be related to mechanical and physiologic effects of uterine activity on the fetus.

Accelerations

An acceleration is an abrupt increase in the FHR that usually lasts less than 10 minutes and is associated with fetal movement. Accelerations are a result of an increase in beta-adrenergic sympathetic nervous system activity and are a reassuring indication of an intact nervous system. They may occur at any time during labor. Repetitive, uniform accelerations with each contraction may occur as an initial response to mild hypoxia that accompanies umbilical vein compression.

Decelerations

A deceleration is an abrupt decrease in the FHR that usually lasts less than 10 minutes and may be associated with hypoxemia and fetal distress. Decelerations are classified according to their timing in relation to uterine contraction and their shape or waveform as *early, late*, or *variable*. These three major types of decelerations; their causes, characteristics, and clinical significance; and the appropriate nursing interventions are summarized in Table 22-2.

Dysrhythmias

Dysrhythmias are irregularities in the fetal heart rhythm. They may be caused by a disturbance in the myocardial cells' ability to form and discharge electric impulses, resulting in ectopic or premature beats, tachycardia, or bradycardia. Disturbances in conductivity of impulses also occur, leading to heart block. Drugs, acidosis, hypoxia, electrolyte imbalances, and cardiac anomalies may precipitate altered rhythms. Many dysrhythmias are benign and require no treatment. It is important to listen to the FHR with a fetoscope before applying the external EFM to detect dysrhythmias and to differentiate them from artifact on the monitor printout.

Implications for Nursing Care

EFM has dramatically affected nursing responsibilities in the care of laboring women and their families, especially those who are regarded as being at increased risk in the intrapartum period. The nurse must be knowledgeable about

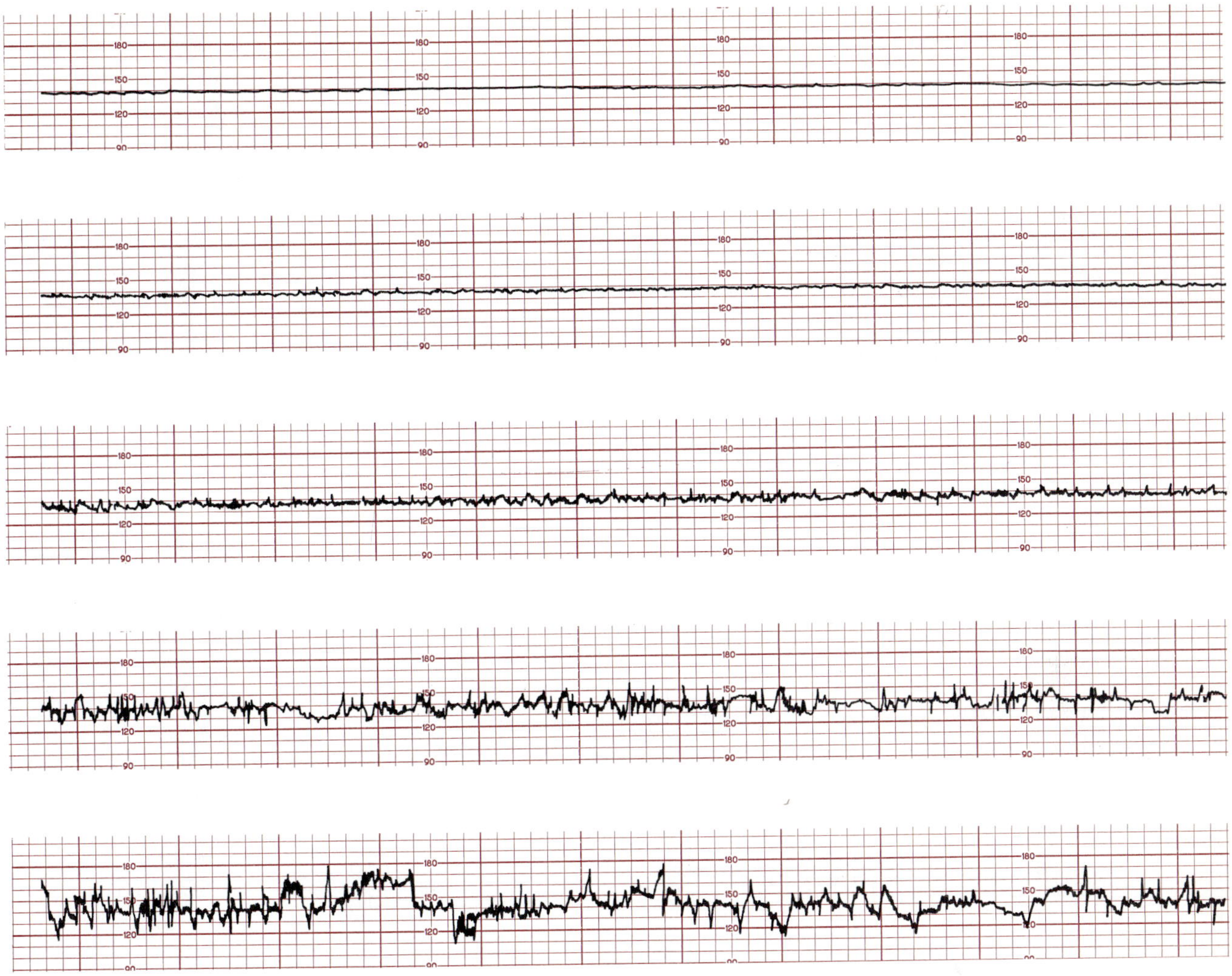

Figure 22-5.
Degrees and tracings illustrating long-time variability.

the appropriate use of intermittent and continuous EFM. He or she must be able to recognize and interpret patterns of FHR change, report them accurately, and initiate measures to enhance fetal well-being as needed (NAACOG, 1992). In addition the nurse must be able to rely on learned assessment skills rather than relying exclusively on monitors. Sensitive and safe nursing care must be provided to the woman and her family despite the potential intrusion of technology.

Evaluating Findings on Electronic Fetal Monitor Tracings

The nurse must have a systematic approach to evaluating findings on EFM tracings. When assessing FHR patterns, the nurse should first consider the *validity* of the recorded data. Are patterns clear, or does the tracing contain many artifacts and a great deal of "noise"? Are all leads connected? Does the recorded FHR correspond with that noted on auscultation? If it does not, the EFM may be picking up the maternal pulse or may be halving or doubling the actual FHR. Is the monitor recording the onset and end of uterine contractions simultaneously with the woman's sensation and her own palpation? If it does not, it is impossible to distinguish between early and late decelerations, a critically important difference. If recordings of uterine contractions are faulty, the intrauterine pressure catheter may have become dislodged, or the monitor may need to be adjusted or recalibrated. Events that may have affected the FHR or uterine contraction pattern and other information that aids interpretation must be noted directly on the tracing strip. The following types of information are typically recorded on the tracing strip:

- Findings of vaginal examination (station, cervical change, fetal position)
- Spontaneous or artificial rupture of membranes
- Maternal vital signs and position changes
- Administration of oxygen, medications, or IV fluids
- Changes in maternal status, such as emesis or bearing-down efforts
- Changing from external to internal monitoring equipment
- Evaluation of the fetal monitor strip by the birth attendant

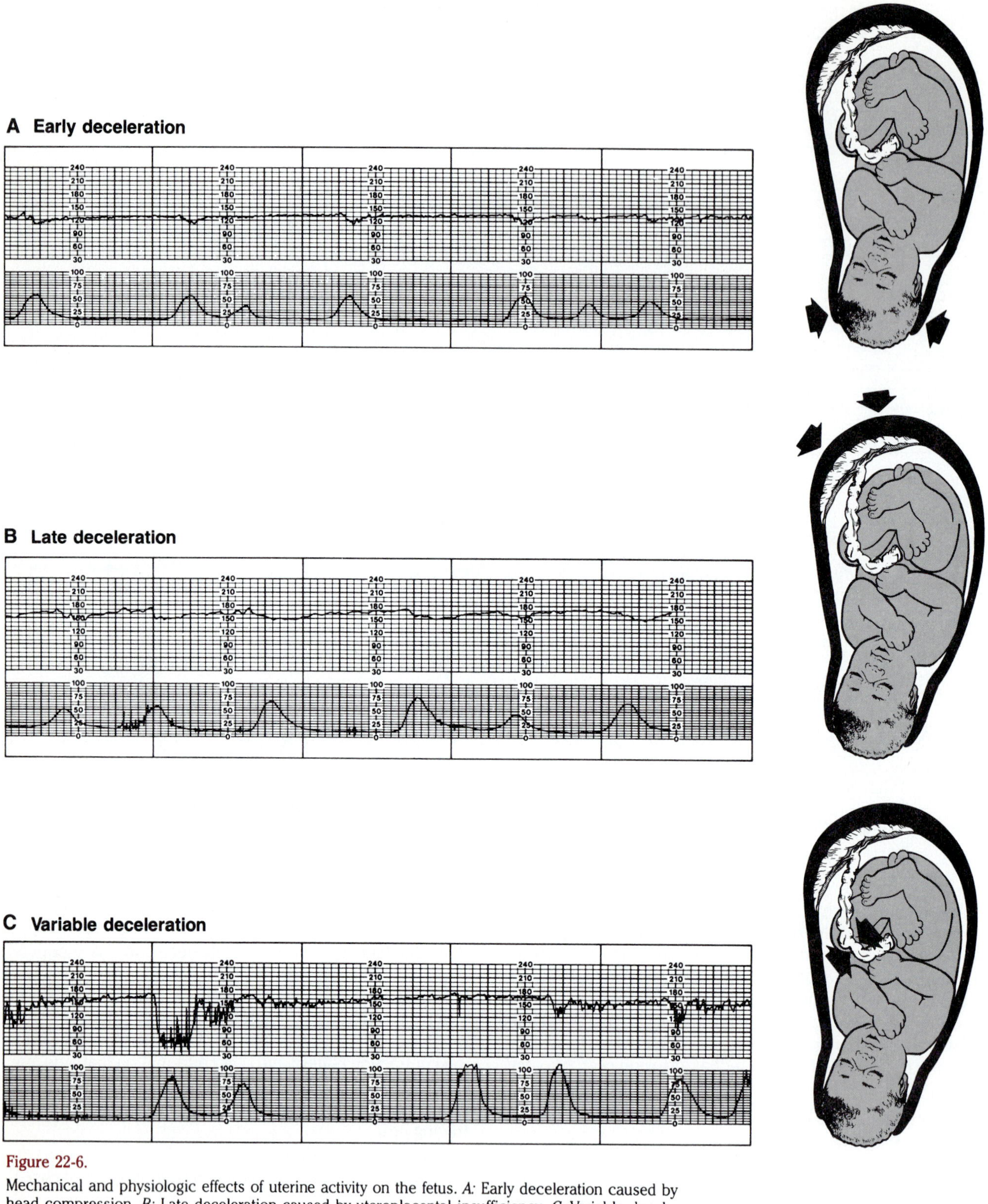

Figure 22-6.

Mechanical and physiologic effects of uterine activity on the fetus. *A:* Early deceleration caused by head compression. *B:* Late deceleration caused by uteroplacental insufficiency. *C:* Variable deceleration caused by umbilical cord compression. (All fetal art from Childbirth Graphics.)

Table 22-2. Patterns of Deceleration Observed on EFM and Appropriate Nursing Care

Type	Cause	Characteristics	Clinical Significance	Nursing Interventions
Early deceleration	Vagal stimulation from head compression	Onset of deceleration at onset of contraction Ends before contraction ends Uniform wave shape reflects shape of contraction Lowest point within normal limits at peak of contraction	Usually innocuous, reassuring pattern May be prevented by avoiding early rupture of membranes	Observe FHR closely to distinguish this from other ominous patterns.
Late deceleration	Uteroplacental insufficiency due to decrease blood flow during uterine contraction subsequent to: Hypotension (induced by supine position or anesthesia) Pregnancy-induced hypertension Tetanic or hypertonic contraction Abruptio placentae Postmaturity	Onset of deceleration at the peak of contraction Ends after contraction ends Uniform wave shape reflects shape of contraction Lowest point near end of contraction Tends to occur with every contraction Depth of deceleration does not reflect degree of fetal insult; variability and baseline also must be evaluated	Ominous sign indicating fetal distress Possible need for cesarean delivery Possible need for fetal scalp pH Severe fetal acidosis if baseline variability is lost	Change the woman's position to left side, right side, or Trendelenburg to alleviate pattern. Administer O_2 by mask at 8–12 L/min. Discontinue oxytocin. Increase intravenous fluids if hypotension is due to regional anesthesia. Notify physician. Prepare to give tocolytic to reduce uterine activity. Prepare for prompt delivery.
Variable deceleration	Umbilical cord compression against fetal bony part, short or knotted cord, possible prolapse	Deceleration unrelated to contractions Wave forms differ in shape from contraction and from each other Decelerations usually markedly altered by woman's position change or external manipulation of fetus	Possible severe fetal compromise if decelerations worsen, are prolonged, or are repetitive Possible need for fetal scalp pH Possible diminishing fetal reserve if bradycardia is prolonged following deceleration	Change woman to side-lying position. Initiate external manipulation of fetus. Place woman in knee-chest position if deceleration is uncorrected by change to sidelying position. Administer O_2 by face mask at 8–12 L/min. Perform vaginal exam ratio to rule out cord prolapse. Prepare to give tocolytic to reduce uterine activity. Prepare for intra-amniotic saline infusion.

- Adjusting or repositioning monitor leads or any recalibration

If the data are judged to be valid, the nurse then evaluates the tracing for baseline and periodic changes and assesses the quality of the uterine contraction pattern. Data on the tracing are compared with data collected through auscultation, palpation, and observation. Any deviations from normal patterns should be carefully examined and described, and the FHR pattern should be interpreted tentatively.

Discriminating Between Reassuring and Nonreassuring Fetal Heart Rate Patterns

Once the FHR pattern is interpreted tentatively, the nurse must be able to determine whether it is a reassuring or a nonreassuring FHR pattern. Examples of both types are listed in the accompanying display. Reassuring patterns are associated with fetal well-being and positive outcomes. Nonreassuring or "warning" patterns suggest decreasing fetal capacity to cope with the stress of labor and may signal frank

Fetal Heart Rate Patterns

Reassuring Patterns

Reassuring patterns are those with normal baseline FHR and average variability with

- Mild variable decelerations (less than 30 seconds in duration, with rapid return to baseline)
- Early decelerations (concurrent "mirror image" decrease with contraction)
- Accelerations without other changes

Nonreassuring Patterns (Warning Signs)

- Moderate tachycardia (more than 160 bpm)
- Decrease in baseline variability
- Progressive increase or decrease in baseline FHR
- Intermittent late decelerations with good variability

Ominous Patterns

- Persistent late decelerations, especially with decreasing variability
- Variable decelerations with loss of variability, tachycardia, or late return to baseline
- Rebound accelerations "overshoot" baseline FHR following each variable deceleration and absent variability
- True sinusoidal pattern with absent variability
- Absence of variability
- Severe bradycardia

Schifrin, B. (1990). Exercises in fetal monitoring. *St. Louis: Mosby Year Book.*

fetal distress. Ominous FHR patterns are known to be associated with rapidly developing fetal distress and markedly increased fetal risk.

The nurse must identify the nature of the change and report nonreassuring or ominous findings to the physician or nurse midwife (AAP/ACOG, 1988). Usually further careful evaluation of maternal and fetal status is then undertaken before decisions about management are made. However, the nurse should be prepared for additional obstetric interventions, such as fetal blood sampling or cesarean delivery.

Because nonreassuring patterns reflect decreasing fetal physiologic reserve to cope with uterine contractions, nursing interventions are directed at maximizing uteroplacental perfusion, providing support and reassurance to the woman, and preparing for additional obstetric intervention as necessary. The nurse must notify the physician or nurse midwife immediately and take the following actions to maximize uteroplacental perfusion:

- Position the woman on the left or right side to reduce the possibility of cord compression and supine hypotension.
- Discontinue oxytocin infusion; prepare for possible administration of tocolytics to reduce uterine activity and improve uteroplacental perfusion.
- Administer oxygen by face mask at 8 to 12 L/min to increase fetal oxygenation (see the accompanying Nursing Procedure).
- Start IV fluids, or increase rate of administration.
- Reassure and support the woman to decrease detrimental effects of catecholamine release on uterine blood flow.
- Prepare for possible intrauterine amnioinfusion to reduce umbilical cord compression.

Reassuring and supporting the woman and her partner are primary nursing responsibilities. The nurse should explain the need for the actions outlined previously and encourage the woman and her support person to ask questions. The nurse should stay with the family, offering encouragement and acknowledging their concerns; use of gentle touch can be very reassuring and quieting to the mother. Providing a calm atmosphere and an explanation of the situation and allowing parents to remain together as much as possible will help them cope with this unwanted turn of events.

If, after further evaluation of fetal status, the FHR is still considered ominous, the physician may decide that prompt delivery is needed. Birth is usually accomplished by cesarean delivery; occasionally forceps or vacuum extraction is used if the course of labor is well advanced, and delivery is anticipated shortly. Nursing responsibilities in these situations are discussed later in Chapter 23.

Computerized Fetal Heart Rate Analysis

Because visual interpretation of FHR patterns is unreliable, even by experienced clinicians, programs for computerized FHR analysis have been developed. Research findings indicate many advantages to computerized FHR analysis (Dawes, Moulden, & Redman, 1991). Interpretation is rapid and reliable and allows for correlation of FHR patterns with other objective data about fetal status (ie, meconium staining, scalp blood samples). New programs also provide information regarding trends in the FHR, such as increasing or decreasing variability or subtle shifts in the baseline rate. Quantitative analysis allows even novice clinicians to describe FHR patterns unambiguously. An increasing number of nurses and physicians will undoubtedly use these programs as an adjunct to FHR evaluation in the near future.

In all labor and delivery settings the nurse maintains primary responsibility for implementing external fetal monitoring. In some settings the nurse may initiate internal EFM guided by unit protocols. The nurse must have a comprehensive knowledge of external and internal EFM to assemble and safely use the equipment and explain the risks, benefits, and purposes of EFM to the woman and her support person. The nurse is responsible for assessing FHR patterns. Extensive knowledge and expertise are required to evaluate accurately the FHR and uterine contraction patterns derived from EFM data. The nurse must be able to differentiate technically poor EFM

NURSING PROCEDURE

Administering Oxygen With Nonreassuring or Ominous Fetal Heart Rate Patterns

Purpose: To attempt improvement in fetal oxygen concentrations if indicators of fetal compromise become evident by FHR assessment.

NURSING ACTION	***RATIONALE***
1. Administer 100% oxygen.	To maximize maternal PaO_2 level, which will increase oxygen available to fetus.
2. Use tight face mask. Do not use nasal cannula.	To ensure the delivery of a high concentration of oxygen. Many women in labor breathe through their mouths during contractions, and inspiration of room air (20.9% O_2) will decrease oxygen concentrations to 40% or less when nasal cannula used.
3. Administer at rates of at least 8 to 12 L/min.	High flow of oxygen will ensure maximum delivery of oxygen to woman.
4. Note for improvement in FHR within 1 to 6 minutes.	If maternal, placental, and fetal circulation is not severely compromised, fetal oxygen levels should improve in 1 to 6 minutes.

tracings or readout data from abnormal FHR patterns. Of critical importance is the ability to recognize nonreassuring or ominous FHR patterns and to implement corrective actions. The nurse collaborates with the midwife or physician when these abnormal patterns are identified and provides the woman with information and emotional support until the problem is resolved.

Fetal Blood Sampling

Fetal hypoxia and the resulting acidosis may be signaled by abnormal FHR patterns. However, at times FHR patterns are inconclusive, and the physician or midwife may need additional information to decide whether emergency delivery, usually by cesarean, is needed. If hypoxia is prolonged, the fetus becomes increasingly acidotic and the blood pH decreases. If acidosis is pronounced and uncorrected, fetal well-being is seriously threatened.

Information about fetal blood chemistry can be obtained by fetal blood sampling. A sample can be drawn from the presenting part (usually the scalp) and analyzed to determine pH, oxygen, and carbon dioxide levels. This information can then be used to corroborate or clarify FHR information. To obtain a fetal blood sample, a cone-shaped endoscope is inserted into the vagina through the cervix and is pressed against the presenting part, as shown in Figure 22-7. The scalp is swabbed clean and pricked with a small blade that permits a 2-mm deep incision. Fetal blood is collected in a heparinized capillary tube and sent immediately to the clinical laboratory for determination of pH and blood gas levels. For this reason fetal blood sampling is done largely in centers where findings can be interpreted within 10 to 15 minutes. Having to wait longer for results renders the findings of little value.

The fetal scalp blood pH values usually fall between those of the umbilical artery and vein (Porto & Nageotte, 1991) and are listed below:

Normal pH (7.25 to 7.35): No intervention needed; continue to monitor.

Borderline pH (7.2 to 7.25): Evaluate second sample in 15 to 30 minutes to check for downward trend; continue to monitor.

Acidotic pH (7.2 or less on two consecutive measurements): Severely acidotic fetus; immediate forceps or cesarean delivery is necessary.

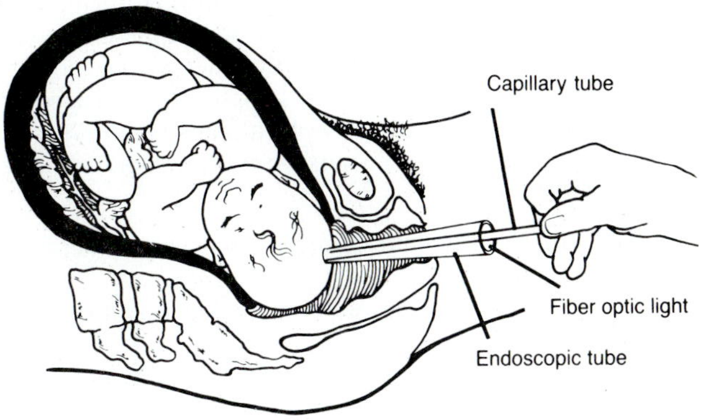

Figure 22-7.
Fetal blood sampling to verify fetal status and assess heart rate pattern as seen on the electronic fetal monitor.

Indications and Contraindications

Fetal scalp sampling requires access to the fetal presenting part through ruptured membranes and a cervix that is 2 to 3 cm dilated. Access to immediate laboratory analysis and ability to initiate emergency delivery also are necessary. Sampling is done when FHR patterns are inconclusive and potentially worrisome and when additional information about fetal status will make a difference in a decision to delay or expedite delivery. Thus, fetal blood sampling is contraindicated in the following situations (Chez, Harvey, & Murray, 1990):

- Obstetric emergencies, such as cord prolapse or vaginal bleeding, or when FHR patterns are ominous
- If the woman is a known carrier of hemophilia and the fetal gender is unknown
- If the woman is HIV seropositive
- If the woman has an active genital infection (ie, herpes, human immunodeficiency virus, group B streptococcus, or gonorrhea)

Advantages and Disadvantages

A major advantage of fetal blood sampling is that it gives direct information about fetal physiologic status that may be used to avoid unnecessary obstetric interventions, such as emergency cesarean delivery. Fetal blood sampling can confirm and clarify inconclusive FHR findings; however, the procedure also has its disadvantages. Fetal blood sampling requires considerable skill and is a difficult procedure even under optimal conditions. Furthermore, high-quality and immediately accessible laboratory support is necessary to yield accurate findings that can be used to manage obstetric care. Fetal blood sampling only provides intermittent data, and findings can be influenced by examiner skill and maternal physiologic status (pronounced maternal metabolic acidosis may result in fetal acidosis). Scalp samples may not accurately reflect pH and blood gas levels in the fetal central circulation, especially if the head is severely molded with marked scalp swelling (caput succedaneum). Finally, the incision site makes the fetus vulnerable to hemorrhage and subsequent infection.

Implications for Nursing Care

The nurse must be prepared for problems arising during labor that call for immediate recognition and decisive action (see the accompanying Nursing Care Plan). Problems arising suddenly during labor that cause suspicion about fetal status, especially nonreassuring FHR patterns, may indicate a need for immediate fetal blood sampling. The procedure demands prompt action and may be alarming to the woman and her support person. The nurse's primary responsibilities are the following:

- Describe the procedure, and reinforce information given by the physician.
- Provide emotional support to the woman and her support person.
- Gather the necessary equipment and alert laboratory personnel who will analyze the blood sample.
- Assist the woman into the lithotomy position.
- Assist with the procedure using strict aseptic technique.
- Provide ongoing information to the woman about what is happening and what she can do to help expedite the procedure.

While awaiting the pH results, the nurse optimizes maternal and fetal status by placing the woman on her left side and providing oxygen. If oxytocin has been infusing, it may be discontinued by physician's order to decrease uterine activity and increase uterine blood flow.

When scalp blood analysis indicates that the fetal pH is less than 7.20, the nurse will prepare for vaginal delivery by forceps or vacuum extraction or for cesarean birth. The method chosen for delivery will depend on the stage of cervical dilatation and the status of the fetus. The nurse reinforces information provided by the physician about the results and prepares the woman and her support person for delivery of the infant. Nursery personnel who normally attend the birth of high-risk neonates are alerted and are informed of the fetal scalp blood analysis results.

When FHR data are inconclusive, the physician may obtain a fetal scalp sample of capillary blood to determine fetal acid–base status. The nurse prepares the woman for this procedure by providing explanations, answering questions, and offering support and encouragement. The nurse also assists the woman with position changes and provides the physician with essential equipment required for the test. Because the risk of infection is increased with invasive procedures, the nurse plays a crucial role in maintaining strict asepsis during the procedure. The need for fetal scalp sampling reduces the woman's control over the process of labor. However, the nurse can enhance feelings of control and satisfaction with the birth experience by closely involving her in all plans and decisions.

Fetal Scalp Stimulation

If nonreassuring FHR patterns persist and a practitioner is not immediately available to perform fetal scalp sampling, a new technique has been suggested to assist in evaluation of fetal well-being. Brisk digital stimulation of the fetal scalp through the dilated cervix is accomplished by the examiner's gloved fingers. Immediate FHR accelerations in response to stimulation indicate a well-oxygenated brain and fetal reserve and have been associated with a scalp pH of greater than 7.20 (Porto & Nageotte, 1991). Accelerations are defined as an increase in the FHR baseline of at least 15 bpm for at least 15 seconds.

Another technique involves gentle traction on the fetal scalp electrode. Fetal movement and FHR accelerations were noted to occur within 15 seconds after this method of stimulation in healthy fetuses (Zimmer & Vadasz, 1989). This method requires that the membranes be ruptured and a scalp electrode be in place before it can be used.

Fetal scalp stimulation is easy to learn, requires no special technology, can be performed by the nurse, and may reduce the number of scalp sampling procedures performed. It also provides the clinician with objective data regarding fetal well-being. While the membranes do not need to be ruptured to attempt scalp stimulation, the fetus

Nursing Care Plan

The Woman in Labor With a Fetus in Distress

PATIENT PROFILE

History

M.L. is a 33-year-old G1/P0 at $40\frac{3}{7}$ weeks' gestation. She is admitted to labor in active phase labor with intact membranes. The EFM reveals an FHR in the 130 bpm range with 6 to 10 bpm LTV.

One hour after admission M.L. experiences spontaneous rupture of membranes. A small amount of thick, particulate meconium is noted. The baseline FHR is now in the 160 bpm range with 3 to 5 bpm LTV. Contractions occur every 3 minutes, last 60 seconds, and are strong. Variable decelerations are noted with each contraction. The FHR drops abruptly to 90 bpm for 60 seconds with prompt return to the baseline after the contraction. A vaginal examination finds that the cervix is 7 cm dilated and 100% effaced. The fetus is at −1 station. The physician orders an amnioinfusion.

Physical Assessment

Twenty minutes after initiation of the amnioinfusion, the nurse notes contractions every 2 minutes, which last 80 seconds and are strong. M.L. is resting on her left side when a contraction begins. The FHR abruptly drops to 60 bpm for 80 seconds with slow return to the baseline 60 seconds after the contraction ends. The same pattern occurs with the next contraction. The LTV is noted to be 0 to 2 bpm now. Turning M.L. to her right side does not improve the FHR pattern. M.L. asks the nurse, "What's happening to my baby? Why is the heart rate so slow?"

COLLABORATIVE PROBLEMS/POTENTIAL COMPLICATIONS

- Umbilical cord compression
- Uteroplacental insufficiency
- Fetal hypoxia and acidosis
- Meconium aspiration

(See the Nursing Alert display following the Care Plan.)

Assessment	*Nursing Diagnosis*	*Nursing Interventions*	*Rationale*
FHR in 160 bpm range. Decreased LTV (3 to 5 bpm range). Variable decelerations to 60 bpm lasting with 80 seconds with slow return to FHR baseline. Presence of thick particulate meconium.	Altered Tissue Perfusion related to umbilical cord compression *Expected Outcome* The fetus' heart rate baseline will return to normal range of 120 to 160 bpm with 6 to 10 bpm LTV. M.L. will use hands-and-knees position to relieve the variable deceleration pattern. M.L. will return to a sidelying position.	Assist M.L. to a hands-and-knees position, or place in Trendelenberg if turning from left side to right side does not improve FHR.	Position change often will correct FHR pattern by relieving cord compression. Severe variable decelerations can result in fetal acidosis, loss of baseline LTV, and fetal compromise.
		Administer O_2 at 8 to 12 L/min by mask.	Increasing maternal blood oxygenation increases O_2 available to fetus.
		Increase or initiate intravenous line and infuse rapidly.	Increasing IV fluids may improve placental perfusion, permitting more effective delivery orf oxygen to fetus.
		Perform vaginal examination.	Sudden severe variable decelerations may indicate rapid progress in labor, sudden fetal descent, or prolapsed cord.
		Call for help.	Additional staff will be required to support M.L. and implement corrective actions.

(*Continued*)

The Woman in Labor With a Fetus in Distress

(Continued)

Assessment	***Nursing Diagnosis***	***Nursing Interventions***	***Rationale***
		Notify physician.	Physician's presence is required to evaluate M.L. and perform further diagnostic tests.
		Prepare for internal fetal electrode placement or fetal scalp sampling.	Information about STV can be obtained only by internal EFM. Fetal scalp pH will clarify degree of fetal acidosis.
		Be prepared to administer tocolytic.	Tocolytic may decrease severity of variable decelerations by reducing uterine activity.
		Continue amnioinfusion.	Amnioinfusion may relieve cord compression.
Amnioinfusion is continued. Multiple vaginal examinations are performed.	High Risk for Maternal or Fetal Infection related to amnioinfusion and other invasives procedures	Maintain surgical asepsis in preparing equipment for invasive diagnostic tests and vaginal examinations.	Reducing number of vaginal examinations and performing perineal care reduces the risk of infection.
	Expected Outcome M.L will remain free of signs and symptoms of infection.	Minimize the number of vaginal examinations.	Increasing maternal blood oxygenation increases O_2 available to fetus.
	The fetus will remains free of signs and symptoms of infection.	Perform perineal care after M.L. voids, after vaginal examinations, and after diagnostic procedures.	
	M.L.'s vital signs and white blood count will remain within normal limits.	Monitor M.L.'s temperature, pulse, and respirations every 2 hours after rupture of membranes.	Maternal pulse and respirations are sensitive indicators of infection.
		Monitor FHR for evidence of tachycardia.	Fetal tachycardia occurs with chorioamnionitis and maternal fever.
		Assess amniotic fluid for evidence of prurulence or foul-smelling odor.	Purulent, foul-smelling amniotic fluid is commonly observed with chorioamnionitis.
		Palpate uterus for evidence of tenderness.	
		Monitor white blood count.	
M.L. asks, "What's happening to my baby? Why is the heart rate so slow?"	Fear related to changes in FHR and management of decelerations ***Expected Outcome*** M.L. will experience a decrease in the level of fear as evidenced by adaptive coping behavior.	Explain in brief, simple terms the nature of the problem and the reason for interventions or requests for position changes.	Fear or severe anxiety will reduce comprehension level and ability to respond to directives for position change. Women in labor are sensitive to caregiver reactions.
	M.L. will verbalize a decrease in level of fear	Notify M.L. promptly when improvement in FHR pattern is noted.	Providing woman with brief, simple explanations may reduce fear or anxiety level and support coping behaviors.

(Continued)

The Woman in Labor With a Fetus in Distress
(Continued)

Assessment	Nursing Diagnosis	Nursing Interventions	Rationale
			Fear results in catecholamine release, which causes vasoconstriction. This may reduce placental perfusion.

EVALUATION

When M.L. was assisted to a hands-and-knees position, the variable deceleration pattern was relieved. After 45 minutes of amnioinfusion, M.L. was able to return to a sidelying position. Intermittent mild variable decelerations were noted. The baseline FHR returned to 140 bpm and remained within normal limits. Amniotic fluid was not foul smelling. M.L. was able to follow directions and requests for position changes. M.L. continued to state concerns about her fetus.

must be in a vertex presentation and the presenting part low enough to be reached by the examiner's fingers.

Implications for Nursing Care

Once the correct technique for fetal scalp stimulation is learned, it may be used in the following situations described by Chez, Harvey, and Murray (1990) to increase the nurse's data base:

- Persistent late decelerations with normal short-term variability
- Persistent deep, variable decelerations with decreasing variability
- Sinusoidal FHR baseline
- Fetal bradycardia or tachycardia with decreasing variability
- Any nonreassuring pattern that cannot be resolved with standard interventions
- Inability to assess short-term variability (after administration of analgesia)
- FHR arrhythmia

The nurse communicates the findings of the fetal scalp stimulation technique to the midwife or the physician. The absence of accelerations in the FHR as a response to stimulation indicates the need for timely medical evaluation. Fetal scalp blood sampling or operative delivery may be anticipated by the nurse in this circumstance.

NURSING ALERT

INTRAUTERINE AMNIOINFUSION

When oligohydramnios is diagnosed or if membranes rupture prematurely, the fetus is at increased risk of umbilical cord compression during fetal movement and during contractions. Intrauterine amnioinfusion is being used in selected medical centers to increase intrauterine fluid volume and decrease pressure on the fetal umbilical cord. When severe variable decelerations persist after maternal position changes and oxygen administration have been implemented, amnioinfusion may be attempted.

Amnioinfusion is now also recommended when thick particulate meconium is noted in the amniotic fluid. Research indicates that amnioinfusion in the presence of meconium passage and oligohydramnios decreases the incidence of postnatal meconium aspiration syndrome (Macri, Schrimmer, Leung, Greenspoon, & Paul, 1992). Positive outcomes may be a result of reduced umbilical cord compression and mechanical flushing of meconium from the uterine cavity. A hollow intrauterine pressure catheter is inserted into the uterus, and warmed sterile saline is infused at 60 to 100 mL/h after an initial loading dose of 600 mL/h for the first hour. Continuous fetal monitoring is required. Potential complications of the procedure include overdistention of the uterus and increased uterine resting tonus. The infusion is therefore stopped every 30 minutes to record resting tone between contractions. Frequent linen protector changes (Chux pads) will be required to maintain patient comfort.

Macri, C., Schrimmer, D., Leung, A, Greenspoon, J., & Paul, R. (1992). Prophylactic amnioinfusion improves outcome of pregnancy complicated by thick meconium and oligohydramnios. American Journal of Obstetrics and Gynecology, 167*(1), 117.*

Advances in Technology

Recently, new diagnostic tools have been developed to assess fetal well-being during the intrapartum period. Many are still in the experimental stages of development or available

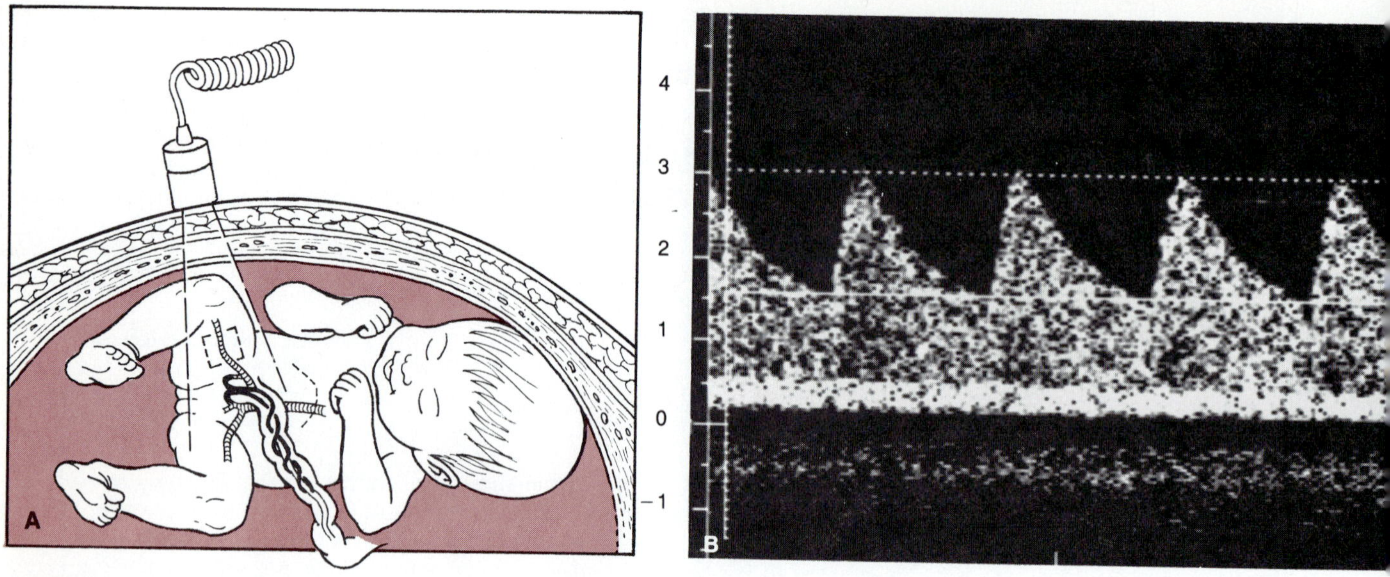

Figure 22-8.

Doppler velocimetry. *A:* Measurement of velocity of blood flow in the fetal aorta and umbilical artery is made by Doppler ultrasonography. *B:* Normal blood flow in the fetal umbilical artery.

only in selected medical centers. However, with the rapid advances in technology they may be expected to be used in a wide variety of clinical settings in the near future.

Doppler velocimetry (Fig. 22-8) is a noninvasive technique that permits measurement of blood flow velocity in the fetal aorta and umbilical artery using continuous-wave Doppler ultrasonography in labor (James, Parker, & Smoleniec, 1992; Marsal, 1991). A significant association was found between a decease in blood flow and fetal distress and neonatal depression, including low Apgar scores, the need for intubation, and abnormal blood pH studies. Doppler velocimetry is available currently in selected medical centers but is expected to be more widely available in the near future.

Cordocentesis or *percutaneous umbilical cord blood sampling* is the transabdominal needle aspiration of umbilical cord blood. The procedure allows the analysis of fetal blood gas and acid–base parameters. Furthermore, a complete blood profile, including complete blood count, liver enzymes, and immunoglobulin levels, can be obtained in an attempt to establish the exact cause of IUGR, chronic fetal distress, and chromosomal anomalies (Hickok, Mills, & Western Collaborative Perinatal Group, 1992). Although the procedure is available only in selected medical centers, it should become more widely available in the near future.

A method for continuous *fetal tissue pH measurement* is being refined and may eliminate the need for more invasive fetal scalp sampling in the near future. Studies indicate that a fiberoptic probe applied to the fetal scalp permits early warning of fetal hypoxia and distress (Nickelsen & Weber, 1991). Finally, efforts are underway to adapt pulse oximetry for fetal monitoring during the intrapartum period. Early studies indicate that trends in oxygen saturation can be used to confirm fetal well-being and reduce the need for fetal scalp sampling (Gardosi, Schram, & Symonds, 1991).

Chapter Summary

The nurse providing care for families during labor must be knowledgeable about procedures used for monitoring fetal status. EFM, fetal scalp stimulation, and fetal blood sampling enable the clinician to identify the degree of fetal distress and to institute treatment before fetal compromise becomes severe. Nursing responsibilities include recognizing women in labor who are likely to benefit from these procedures and safely implementing warranted technology. Interpretation of FHR patterns and data from fetal blood sampling has become an essential element of high-risk intrapartum care and requires the nurse to have up-to-date skills to maintain safe standards of practice.

Study Questions

1. *What nursing actions should be taken when FHR variability decreases or disappears?*
2. *What nursing actions are appropriate when severe variable decelerations occur?*
3. *What are the causes and significance of a late deceleration?*
4. *What would you tell a woman who refused EFM when meconium-stained fluid was the indication?*
5. *Which FHR deceleration patterns suggest fetal distress? Why?*
6. *What FHR patterns are considered reassuring, nonreassuring, and ominous? Why?*
7. *What is the purpose of fetal scalp sampling? What are normal and abnormal findings?*
8. *What is the purpose of fetal scalp stimulation? What*

fetal response would be considered reassuring when initiating scalp stimualtion?

9. *What information should be written directly on the fetal monitor strip?*

References

Albers, L., & Savitz, D. (1991). Hospital setting for birth and use of medical procedures in low-risk women. *Journal of Nurse-Midwifery*, *36*(6), 327.

American College of Obstetricians and Gynecologists. (1991). Utility of umbilical cord blood acid-base assessment. *ACOG Committee Opinion*, Number 91.

American Academy of Pediatrics and American College of Obstetricians and Gynecologists. (1988). *Guidelines for perinatal care* (2nd ed.). Washington, DC: Author.

Carlton, L. (1990). Basic intrapartum fetal monitoring. In E. J. Martin (Ed.). *Intrapartum management modules*. Baltimore: Williams & Wilkins.

Chez, B. F., Harvey, C., & Murray, M. (1990). Critical concepts in fetal heart rate monitoring. Baltimore: Williams & Wilkins.

Clark, S., DeVore, G., Sabey, P., & Jolley, K. (1989). Fetal heart rate transmission with the facsimile telecopier in rural areas. *American Journal of Obstetrics and Gynecology*, *160*(5), 1040.

Copper, R., & Goldenberg, R. (1990). Catecholamine secretion in fetal adaptation to stress. *Journal of Obstetric, Gynecologic, and Neonatal Nursing*, *19*(3), 223.

Dawes, G., Moulden, M., & Redman, C. (1991). The advantages of computerized fetal heart rate analysis. *Journal of Perinatology*, *19*, 39.

Eskes, T., Ingemarsson, I., Pardi, G., Nijhuis, J., & Ruth, V. (1991). Consensus statements round table "Fetal and Neonatal Distress." *Journal of Perinatal Medicine*, *19*(Suppl. 1), 126.

Fee, S., Malee, K., Deddish, R., Minogue, J., & Socol, M. (1990). Severe acidosis and subsequent neurologic status. *American Journal of Obstetrics and Gynecology*, *162*(3), 802.

Gardosi, J., Schram, C., & Symonds, M. (1991). Adaptation of pulse oximetry for fetal monitoring during labour. *Lancet*, *337*, 1265.

Goodlin, R. (1980). Low risk obstetric care for low risk mothers. *Lancet*, *10*(5), 1017.

Hickok, D., Mills, M., & Western Collaborative Perinatal Group. (1992). Percutaneous umbilical blood sampling: Results from a multicenter collaborative registry. *American Journal of Obstetrics and Gynecology*, *166*(6), 1614.

James, D., Parker, M., & Smoleniec, J. (1992). Comprehensive fetal assessment with three ultrasonographic characteristics. *American Journal of Obstetrics and Gynecology*, *166*(5), 1486.

Leatherman, J., Pachman, M., & Lawler, F. (1992). Infection of fetal scalp electrode monitoring sites. *American Family Physician*, *45*(2), 579.

Loos, C., & Julius, L. (1989). The client's view of hospitalization during pregnancy. *Journal of Obstetric, Gynecologic, and Neonatal Nursing*, *18*(1), 52.

Marsal, K. (1991). Doppler ultrasound examination as a clinical diagnostic test in obstetrics. *Journal of Perinatal Medicine*, *19*(Suppl. 1), 299.

McCloskey, L., Petitti, D., & Hobel, C. (1992). Variations in the use of cesarean delivery for dystocia. *Medical Care*, *30*(2), 126.

McCusker, J., Harris, D., & Hosmer, D. (1988). Association of electronic fetal monitoring during labor with cesarean section rate and with neonatal morbidity and mortality. *American Journal of Public Health*, *78*(9), 1170.

Morrow, R., & Ritchie, K. (1989). Doppler ultrasound fetal velocimetry and its role in obstetrics. *Clinics in Perinatology*, *16*(3), 771.

NAACOG. (1992). *Nursing responsibilities in implementing intrapartum heart rate monitoring: Position statement*. Washington, DC: author.

NAACOG Committee on Practice. (1991). *Appropriate use of technology in nursing care*. Washington, DC: Author.

Nickelsen, C., & Weber, T. (1991). The current status of intrapartum continuous fetal tissue pH measurements. *Journal of Perinatal Medicine*, *19*, 87.

Parer, J., & Livingston, E. (1990). What is fetal distress? *American Journal of Obstetrics and Gynecology*, *162*(6), 1421.

Placek, P., Keppel, K., Taffel, S., & Liss, T. (1984). Electronic fetal monitoring in relation to cesarean section delivery, for live births and stillbirths in the US, 1980. *Public Health Reports*, *99*(2), 173.

Portman, R., Carter, B., Gaylord, M., Murphy, G., Thieme, R., & Merenstein, G. (1990). Predicting neonatal morbidity after perinatal asphyxia: A scoring system. *American Journal of Obstetrics and Gynecology*, *162*(1), 174.

Porto, M., & Nageotte, M. (1991) Fetal heart rate monitoring. In K. Niswander & A. Evans (Eds.). *Manual of obstetrics* (4th ed.). Boston: Little, Brown & Co.

Rowe, M. (1990). Asphyxiated infants: Pathophysiologic consequences, parenting, and nursing management. *Neonatal Network*, *9*(4), 7.

Schifrin, B. (1990). Polemics in perinatology: The electronic fetal monitoring guidelines. *Journal of Perinatology*, *10*(2), 188–192.

Shy, K., Luthy, D., Forrest, B., Whitfield, M., Larson, E., Van Belle, G., Hughes, J., Wilson, J., & Stenchever, M. (1990). Effects of electronic fetal heart rate monitoring, as compared with periodic auscultation, on the neurologic development of premature infants. *New England Journal of Medicine*, *322*(9), 588.

Suggested Readings

Egley, C., Bowes, W., & Wagner, D. (1991). Sinusoidal fetal heart rate pattern during labor. *American Journal of Perinatology*, *8*(3), 197.

Lowery, C., Henson, B., Wan, J., & Brumfield, C. (1990). A comparison between umbilical artery velocimetry and standard antepartum surveillance in hospitalized high-risk patients. *American Journal of Obstetrics and Gynecology*, *167*(3), 710.

Mandeville, L., & Troiano, N. (1992). *High-Risk intrapartum nursing*. Philadelphia: J.B. Lippincott.

Mantel, R., Geijn, H., Ververs, I., & Copray, F. (1991). Automated analysis of near-term antepartum fetal heart rate in relation to fetal behavioral states: The Sonicaid System 8000. *American Journal of Obstetrics and Gynecology*, *165*(1), 57.

Murray, M. (1988). *Antepartal and intrapartal fetal monitoring*. Washington, DC: NAACOG.

NAACOG. (1988). Nursing responsibilities in implementing intrapartum fetal heart rate monitoring. Washington, DC: Author.

Piquard, F., Hsiung, R., Mettauer, M., Schaefer, A., Haberey, P., & Dellenbach, P. (1988). The validity of fetal heart rate monitoring during the second stage of labor. *Obstetrics and Gynecology*, *72*(5), 746.

Schifrin, B. (1990). Exercises in fetal monitoring. St. Louis: Mosby Year Book.

Sherwen, L., & Hoffman, N. (1990). Stress factors related to antenatal testing during high-risk pregnancy. *Journal of Perinatology*, *10*(2), 195.

Youchah, J., Chazotte, C., & Cohen, W. (1989). Heart rate patterns and fetal sepsis. *American Journal of Perinatology*, *6*(3), 356.

CHAPTER 23

Modifying Labor Patterns and Mode of Delivery

Learning Objectives

After studying the material in this chapter, the student will be able to:

- Distinguish between induction and augmentation of labor and identify the common modes of each.
- Discuss nursing responsibilities during and after amniotomy.
- List major precautions to be considered when infusing oxytocin.
- Identify indications for and precautions taken during forceps applications.
- State the indications for cesarean birth.
- Discuss nursing responsibilities in caring for the woman and her family before, during, and after cesarean birth.
- Describe the importance of emotional and family-centered support for the woman experiencing cesarean birth.
- Identify contraindications and necessary precautions for a trial of labor and vaginal birth after cesarean delivery.
- Explain nursing responsibilities when uterine hyperstimulation is identified during augmentation or induction of labor.

Key Terms

amniotomy	macrosomia
augmentation of labor	malpresentation
Bishop score	meconium
cervical ripening	oxytocin
cord prolapse	prostaglandin E_2 gel
forceps	stripping membranes
induction of labor	tetanic contraction
intrauterine fetal resuscitation	tocolysis
laminaria	version

Some women require interventions to modify a less than optimal labor pattern or a difficult labor. When this occurs, nursing care is focused on explaining the procedures, clarifying questions the woman or family may have, maintaining maternal and fetal physiologic status, and providing emotional and physical support. The nurse must be knowledgeable about obstetric procedures and the indications and contraindications for these procedures and must be able to identify both reassuring and worrisome maternal and fetal responses to them. To allow for the safest, most satisfying birth experience possible, the nurse must be able to balance a technologic approach to care with intensive emotional support.

Modifying the Labor Pattern

Maternal–fetal risk in the intrapartum period can be reduced by modifying the pattern of labor, accomplished through induction of labor, augmentation of labor, or by temporarily reducing uterine activity.

Induction of Labor

Induction of labor is the deliberate initiation of uterine contractions before they start spontaneously. Induction of labor is a long-standing practice in obstetrics, but it is not without its critics. Induction of labor entails some maternal and fetal risk, and expert medical and nursing care is required to ensure optimal maternal and fetal outcomes. However, induction of labor can also be a lifesaving measure when obstetric or medical indications for the procedure exist and when the procedure is carried out safely.

Indications and Contraindications

A specific obstetric or medical problem must be present for an induction to be termed *medically* indicated. Some of the more common obstetric indications for the induction of labor are listed in the accompanying display.

Indications and Contraindications to Induction of Labor

Indications

- Pregnancy-induced hypertension: This condition may progressively worsen unless resolved by delivery of the fetus.
- Maternal diabetes, classes B-R: Induction and delivery of the fetus 2 to 3 weeks before the expected date of delivery may be indicated to prevent fetal demise from placental insufficiency, especially if the diabetes is not well controlled during pregnancy.
- Premature rupture of membranes: Induction may be indicated to prevent uterine infection when membranes have been ruptured 24 hours or more.
- Rh isoimmunization: A rising Rh antibody titer in later pregnancy may indicate maternal sensitization and the need for prompt delivery to prevent erythroblastosis fetalis.
- Postmaturity (more than 42 weeks of gestation): Placental insufficiency and fetal compromise may result from prolonged pregnancy.
- Suspected fetal jeopardy: Fetal compromise as evidenced by biophysical and biochemical indicators may require prompt delivery.
- Intrauterine fetal demise: If fetal death has been diagnosed but labor does not ensue, induction may be indicated to reduce maternal risk of disseminated intravascular coagulation and unwarranted emotional distress.
- Chorioamnionitis
- Logistic factors: History of rapid labor and distance from hospital may place a woman at risk for precipitous delivery in an uncontrolled environment.

Contraindications

Maternal

- Previous uterine scar or trauma (classical cesarean incision)
- Abnormalities of the uterus, vagina, or pelvis
- Placental abnormalities (previa or suspected abruption)
- Active herpesvirus type II in genital tract
- Grand multiparity
- Overdistention of uterus (from multiple gestation, polyhydramnios)
- Invasive cervical carcinoma

Fetal

- Abnormal fetal lie (transverse, breech)
- Low birth weight or preterm fetus
- Fetal distress shown by electronic fetal monitoring
- Positive (abnormal) contraction stress test

When no medical condition indicates the need to initiate labor, an induction is called *elective* and is performed for the convenience of the physician or woman. Elective inductions are discouraged in some centers because of the increased maternal risk of uterine hyperstimulation and operative delivery and the danger of fetal distress. A recent study by Macer and associates (1992) found a 50% cesarean birth rate when an induction procedure was implemented in nulliparous women with a Bishop score of 5 or less. (Bishop scores are presented in Table 23-1.) Clearly the risks associated with elective or medical induction must be carefully weighed against the need for the procedure.

Contraindications to induction of labor exist when there are medical reasons to avoid or delay onset of labor or to avoid vaginal delivery. Contraindications to induction of labor can be classified as maternal or fetal in nature and are listed in the display.

Advantages and Disadvantages

In addition to resolving the obstetric or medical condition for which induction is indicated, labor induction offers other advantages in the care of the woman at increased intrapartum risk. Because the induction is often prescheduled, there is an opportunity for physical and emotional preparation for labor and birth. There is a decreased anesthetic risk, since the woman can be kept NPO and well hydrated to maintain intravascular volume. Planning the time of birth also allows for physician attendance and suitable nursing staff levels.

Disadvantages to induction of labor also exist. There is an increased risk of preterm birth and prematurity in the neonate if the expected date of delivery is miscalculated and the induction procedure is attempted before 37 weeks of gestation. Induction carries the risk of fetal distress caused by uterine hyperstimulation and the concomitant reduction of uterine and placental blood flow. Additionally, neonates have an increased incidence of hyperbilirubinemia when their mothers receive oxytocin during labor (American Society of Hospital Pharmacists, 1990).

Risks faced by the woman include uterine rupture, amniotic fluid embolus, precipitate labor and birth, cervical lacerations, and postpartum hemorrhage. The woman may experience water intoxication secondary to antidiuretic hormone release when a prolonged induction at high infusion rates (approximately 40 mU/min) occurs (Musacchio, 1990). A failed induction produces emotional and physical stress and is costly in staff time and actual expense to the woman. Finally, the use of analgesia and anesthesia may be increased if the onset of labor occurs rapidly and uterine contractions are frequent and intense. In evaluating outcomes of elective induction, Macer and associates (1992) found that 83% of women in the elective induction group

Table 23-1. Bishop Score for Assessing Readiness for Induction

	Assigned Value			
Factor	0	1	2	3
Cervical dilatation	0	1–2 cm	3–4 cm	5 cm or more
Cervical effacement	0%–30%	40%–50%	60%–70%	80% or more
Fetal station	−3	−2	−1, 0	+1, +2
Cervical consistency	Firm	Medium	Soft	
Cervical position	Posterior	Midposition	Anterior	

Adapted from Bishop, E. H. (1964). Pelvic scoring for elective induction. *Obstetrics and Gynecology, 24,* 266.

received epidural anesthesia, compared with 55% in the spontaneous labor group.

Implications for Nursing Care

The nurse must demonstrate independent judgment in the initiation of the induction process. This requires an assessment of maternal and fetal status and a review of the prenatal record for evidence of indications and contraindications to the specific procedure selected by the physician or nurse midwife (NAACOG, 1988). Before induction of labor is considered, the physiologic readiness of both the woman and fetus for delivery must also be evaluated.

Fetal maturity must be established before induction is attempted; otherwise, there is a possibility of delivering a preterm neonate, with all the associated risks and complications. The gestational age must be verified by establishing the date of the last menstrual period and reviewing the history of uterine growth and quickening. If there is a question about fetal maturity, other tests should be performed. Amniocentesis may be necessary to obtain an amniotic fluid sample to determine the lecithin/sphingomyelin (L/S) ratio and the presence of phosphatidylglycerol. These tests indicate fetal lung maturity required for pulmonary function in the newborn. In addition, ultrasound evaluation may be needed to estimate fetal size and gestational age (see Chapter 14).

Current fetal well-being must be confirmed before initiating the induction process. A 20- to 30-minute fetal heart rate (FHR) readout should be obtained by electronic fetal monitoring (EFM) to confirm the baseline FHR, provide evidence of long-term variability, and document any periodic heart rate changes that occur. If a nonreassuring or ominous FHR pattern is evident, the physician or nurse midwife should be consulted before the induction process is initiated. Identification of fetal contraindications to labor induction would also necessitate a consultation with the primary provider.

Maternal well-being should also be determined and documented before induction. Baseline vital signs should be obtained and recorded. Evidence of vaginal bleeding requires immediate notification of the physician or nurse midwife. The tokodynamometer should be applied to record uterine activity. Occasionally, the woman scheduled for an induction will present with uterine contractions requiring further evaluation before the induction procedure is initiated. Essential laboratory specimens should be obtained, and the nurse should verify that a clot for blood typing and crossmatching (if indicated) has been received by the blood bank. If the nurse identifies any factors that contraindicate the procedure, the nurse midwife and physician are consulted before the induction proceeds.

Maternal readiness for induction also includes evidence of cervical "ripeness." Changes normally occur in late pregnancy that prepare or "ripen" the cervix for labor. These changes include the development of a soft consistency, some degree of effacement or shortening, and a movement to the anterior or centered position relative to the axis of the vagina. The potential for a successful induction depends in great part on the status of the cervix. One of several assessment tools developed to determine the degree of cervical ripeness and used to predict the success of labor induction is the Bishop score. It is described in the next section. Although the physician or nurse midwife normally calculates the numerical value, the nurse should have knowledge of the score and the implications for success of the process based on the Bishop score.

Another factor that must be considered when readiness for induction is being assessed includes the woman's knowledge about the procedure. A well-informed woman can make more intelligent decisions about obstetric interventions. Informed consent should be obtained by the physician or nurse midwife before initiation of the induction. A review of the indications, relative risks, and probability of success of the procedure should be discussed in detail. The nurse then provides any additional information about the procedure the woman may request and reinforces and clarifies explanations given by the physician or nurse midwife. The ultimate choice rests with the woman, and her decision should be respected by the nursing and medical staff.

Ripening of the Cervix

The induction process is more likely to succeed when the cervix is "ripe." The Bishop score (see Table 23-1) is the most frequently used method for determining the probability of a successful induction. This score assesses cervical dilatation, effacement, consistency, and position as well as fetal station. Each factor is assigned a score from 0 to 3, and a total score is calculated. The higher the total score, the higher the likelihood of a successful induction. Scores of 6 or more suggest a high probability (95%) of successful induction. If induction is being considered and the cervix is not favorable for induction, ripening may be attempted through the use of cervical effacers and dilators.

Prostaglandin E_2 Gel

Prostaglandin E_2 (PGE_2) is a hormone produced by the cervix and placental trophoblastic tissue. PGE_2 causes effacement and softening of the cervix and also appears to stimulate uterine myometrium, thereby causing contractions. If an induction is planned using intravenous (IV) oxytocin, PGE_2 gel is first applied on the cervix or into the cervical os to begin the process of effacement and softening. Application of up to 5 mg of a prostaglandin suppository into the vaginal vault or 0.5 mg gel into the cervix once, or after several applications at 4- to 6-hour intervals, will produce cervical change within 48 hours.

Indications and Contraindications

PGE_2 suppositories or cervical gel is indicated for cervical ripening when the Bishop score is less than 5. Contraindications to the drug include a history of sensitivity or allergic response to the administration of PGE_2 drugs, often manifested by shortness of breath and hypotension. The presence of frequent uterine contractions also precludes the use of the drug because uterine hyperstimulation may result. Other contraindications include those listed in the display under contraindications to induction of labor.

Although PGE_2 gel or suppositories are now administered in many medical centers for cervical ripening, they are not yet formally approved for other than experimental use in the United States. Further evaluations of the drug's safety and effectiveness will be needed before Food and Drug Administration (FDA) approval is given; therefore, informed consent must be obtained before the drug is administered.

Advantages and Disadvantages

A major benefit of PGE_2 appears to be a reduction in the need for oxytocin infusion with its potential side effects and complications. Two recent studies indicate that with the administration of serial doses of PGE_2 gel (two to three instillations every 2 to 4 hours), labor occurred in 40% of women with intact membranes (Elliott, Clewell, & Radin, 1992) and 67% of women with ruptured membranes (Bigrigg, Rees, & Read, 1991) before the oxytocin induction was initiated. The cesarean birth rate is also reduced when PGE_2 gel is used before oxytocin induction in women with low Bishop scores. In another study the duration of labor after initiation of the induction was shortened when PGE_2 was administered before infusion of oxytocin (Rayburn, 1989).

In clinical trials, side-effects of PGE_2 gel appear to occur rarely. Many women report mild uterine contractions or backache shortly after administration. Shivering, backache, vomiting, and diarrhea, and shortness of breath (allergic response) have been reported, however, as well as uterine hypertonus, tachysystole, and even uterine rupture (Maymon, Shyulman, Pomeranz, Holtzinger, Haimovich, & Behary, 1991; Egarter, Husslein, & Rayburn, 1990). In nulliparous women, two to three applications of the drug are often required to achieve adequate cervical ripening (Milliez, Jannet, Touboul, Mahfoudh, & Paniel, 1991), which may extend the total length of hospital stay. A recent clinical study (Elliott et al., 1992), however, suggests that PGE_2 gel may be safely administered in an antenatal testing setting where oxygen, EFM, and medical assistance are readily available. After a 2-hour observation period, the woman may be able to return home for the night and return in the morning for initiation of the oxytocin induction.

Implications for Nursing Care

The woman is placed in bed and vital signs as well as a baseline fetal monitor strip (20 to 30 minutes in length) are obtained before administration of the gel. The tokodynamometer should also be applied to detect uterine activity. If uterine contractions are evident, the physician or nurse midwife should be notified. Administration of prostaglandin gel may be delayed or deferred when contractions are frequent or a true labor pattern has been established.

The woman may be placed on a bedpan to elevate the hips and facilitate placement of the gel. The nurse assists during the procedure by guiding the woman with relaxation techniques effective during pelvic examinations. Continuous fetal monitoring is required for at least 1 hour after administration. Many facilities place the woman in a modified Trendelenberg position for 1 or 2 hours to prevent leakage of the gel from the vagina. If underlying high-risk conditions exist, the woman may remain on the monitor until delivery.

The nurse should be particularly alert for signs of uterine hyperstimulation and fetal distress in the first hour after gel administration. If oxytocin is to be initiated, it should not be administered until 4 hours after the last application to avoid uterine hyperstimulation (ACOG, 1991a). The procedure as well as maternal and fetal responses to administration of prostaglandin should be documented in the patient record.

Stripping of Amniotic Membranes

Stripping of the membranes involves the digital separation of the amniotic membranes from the wall of the lower uterine segment near the cervix. It remains a common method of cervical ripening and labor induction. This is done manually during vaginal examination and is thought to initiate labor by stimulating an autonomic neural reflex that releases endogenous oxytocin and prostaglandins. McColgin and associates (1990) studied the effects of membrane stripping and found it a safe method for stimulating labor in nulliparous women with low Bishop scores; the method also reduced the incidence of postterm pregnancy.

The procedure presents several significant risks including premature rupture of the membranes, bleeding from an undiagnosed placenta previa, and infection. Because stripping the membranes poses risk and discomfort, the procedure should be discussed with the woman before it is performed, and informed consent should be obtained. Ultrasonography should be performed before stripping of membranes to exclude the presence of placenta previa or abnormal fetal presentation or lie.

Stripping of the membranes may occur before admission to the labor and delivery unit. If the procedure is done after admission, the nurse should first ascertain that placenta previa or abnormal fetal presentation or lie has been ruled out by ultrasonography. The nurse is responsible for assisting the physician or nurse midwife, evaluating the maternal and fetal status, and supporting the woman.

Continuous FHR monitoring should be obtained for 20 to 30 minutes before the procedure to establish the baseline

FHR parameters. The EFM should also remain in place during the procedure. The nurse guides the woman in relaxation techniques, which are effective during pelvic examinations, and observes for evidence of rupture of membranes or vaginal bleeding. The procedure and maternal and fetal responses to stripping of the membranes should be documented in the patient record.

Laminaria Tents

Until recently, cervical dilators were used to prepare the cervix for induction of labor. Laminaria tents are stems of round, smooth seaweed that have been dried and sterilized and that readily absorb water. After being placed into the cervical canal, moisture is absorbed by the stem and causes the tent to swell. This causes the cervix to become softened and slightly dilated. They are rarely used today. Synthetic cervical dilators (Dilapan) are more commonly used instead of seaweed laminaria in the preparation of the cervix for first and second trimester abortions.

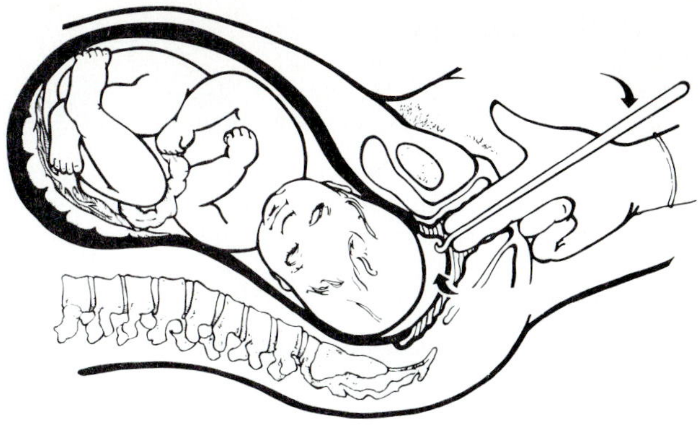

Figure 23-1.
Amniotomy (artificial rupture of the membranes) (Childbirth Graphics).

Stimulation of Uterine Contractions

Amniotomy

Amniotomy is the artificial rupture of the membranes (AROM), performed by inserting a sterile instrument, usually an Amnihook, into the vaginal canal during vaginal examination and puncturing the amniotic sac, as shown in Figure 23-1. This method of labor induction is thought to be effective because it promotes descent of the presenting part, and mechanical irritation from the presenting part on the parous cervix initiates uterine contractions. Furthermore, rupture of membranes is believed to release arachidonic acid, a precursor of prostaglandins, which also enhance uterine activity (Mandeville & Troiano, 1992). Labor usually commences within 12 hours.

The amount of amniotic fluid lost after amniotomy varies and depends on the amount of fluid contained in the amniotic sac. Descent of the fetal head against the cervix before amniotomy prevents rapid fluid loss and prolapse of the fetal umbilical cord. After amniotomy, small amounts of fluid may continue to leak slowly from the vagina throughout labor. Fluid should be clear or cloudy and odorless. Meconium will turn the fluid green, and thick yellowish-brown fluid (particulate meconium) indicates that the fetus has passed bowel contents for some length of time preceding the onset of labor. Occasionally placental abruption will be suspected when an AROM reveals blood-stained fluid. Foul-smelling fluid may indicate infection within the uterus (chorioamnionitis).

Indications and Contraindications

Indications for the use of amniotomy in induction include contraindications to the use of oxytocin infusion, desire for direct fetal monitoring, and desire to observe color of amniotic fluid.

Contraindications to amniotomy include high or unengaged presenting part (-2 stations or above), unknown presenting part of abnormal presentation such as transverse lie or breech, uncertain estimated date of conception (EDC), placenta previa, and herpesvirus type II present in vaginal tract.

Advantages and Disadvantages

One advantage of amniotomy is that the use of mechanical means to rupture the membranes avoids the systemic effects of PGE_2 and oxytocin. Amniotomy is also necessary for internal EFM and essential when close monitoring of fetal status is necessary. When fetal hypoxia and acidosis, uterine hyperstimulation, or other high-risk factors are suspected, the benefits of direct fetal monitoring outweigh the risks. For instance, an early amniotomy may reveal meconium-stained fluid, thus allowing timely interventions to avert more serious problems. Finally, when continuous fetal monitoring is indicated and a continuous, technically adequate FHR tracing cannot be obtained by external monitoring, amniotomy may be performed so that an internal fetal scalp electrode can be placed on the presenting part.

Amniotomy is not without risk to the woman and fetus. It has been associated with increased risk for infection, fetal head compression, and umbilical cord prolapse. Amniotomy also removes the protective cushion of the amniotic sac over the fetal head, exposes the presenting part to increased pressure as it is forced against the pelvis and maternal tissues, and causes distortion of the fetal skull. A recent study by Barrett and associates (1992) found a higher incidence of FHR abnormalities (early, late, and variable decelerations) after artificial rupture of the membranes. When performed during labor, amniotomy may shorten the length of labor, although studies in this area have been conflicting (Fraser, Sauve, Parboosingh, Sokol, & Persaud, 1991). In fact, no evidence exists to confirm that shorter labors are beneficial to the woman or fetus, and some authors suggest it may even be harmful to the fetus by increasing the risk of acidosis and head trauma.

Implications for Nursing Care

The nurse must be aware of the woman's status and of any obstetric or medical contraindications for amniotomy that may be present. The current medicolegal climate has implicated nurses in malpractice suits arising from claims of negligence surrounding amniotomy. Before the procedure,

NURSING PROCEDURE
Assisting With Amniotomy in Labor

Purpose: The presence of the nurse is essential during an amniotomy procedure to prepare and support the woman, provide essential equipment, and assist the physician or midwife. The nurse must also be ready to initiate emergency nursing measures if prolapse of the umbilical cord occurs with rupture of membranes.

NURSING ACTION	***RATIONALE***
1. Evaluate the woman's current status and discuss the rationale for amniotomy with the physician or midwife.	The nurse is responsible for identifying indications and contraindications to amniotomy to prevent complications related to the procedure.
2. Explain procedure to the woman, telling her she will experience no more discomfort than with a vaginal examination and that she will feel "warm and wet" from the amniotic fluid as it drains from the vagina.	To reduce anxiety and enhance the woman's ability to relax during the procedure and cooperate with the amniotomy
3. Assemble the required equipment, which includes an Amnihook, sterile gloves, lubricant, linens, Doppler device or EFM to evaluate the FHR.	To promote efficient use of time and appropriate monitoring of the fetus during and after the procedure
4. Help the woman to assume the correct position on her back, with her knees flexed and dropped apart. The woman may be placed on a bedpan.	To facilitate the vaginal examination To elevate the hips, facilitate the vaginal examination, and catch the amniotic fluid draining from the vagina
5. Displace the uterus to the left.	To prevent supine hypotension
6. Monitor the FHR just before and during the procedure.	To identify complications such as prolapsed umbilical cord
7. Assist the midwife or physician when requested, by applying fundal or suprapubic pressure.	To keep the fetal head well applied to the cervix, which reduces risk of umbilical cord prolapse
8. (After the amniotomy) perform and document the following: • Time of amniotomy • FHR pattern • Color, amount consistency, and odor of the amniotic fluid • Cervical status and fetal station	To communicate with other health care providers and complete a permanent record of medical and nursing care, progress of labor, and the maternal–fetal responses
9. Explain to the woman the results of the procedure and what is to be expected (onset of or increase in uterine contractions, and leakage of fluid).	To reduce anxiety
10. Change bed linens and give hygiene.	To promote comfort
11. Monitor the woman's temperature every 2 hours.	To assess for evidence of uterine infection (chorioamnionitis)

the nurse should assess the woman's condition. The station of the fetal presenting part should be verified and its application to the cervix confirmed to reduce the risk of fetal umbilical cord prolapse (ACOG, 1991a). When evidence suggests that the merit or safety of an amniotomy is in question, such as unengaged fetal head and bulging membranes, the nurse should discuss the findings and rationale with the physician or nurse midwife attending the woman. The availability of nursing, surgical, and anesthesia personnel as well as an operating room should be ascertained before the procedure is performed, should an emergency operative delivery be necessitated by a prolapsed umbilical cord. Circumstances can change in a short time, especially when an induction has been previously planned and time has lapsed since the last assessment of the woman.

The nurse is responsible for preparing the woman for amniotomy and assisting the physician or nurse midwife during the procedure. Steps in this process are detailed in the accompanying Nursing Procedure.

Labor usually begins within 12 hours of amniotomy. If labor has not been established by this time, IV oxytocin is normally initiated.

Intravenous Oxytocin Infusion

Endogenous oxytocin, a natural hormone, is released from the posterior lobe of the pituitary gland. When it is released, it binds to receptors in the uterine myometrium and stimulates contraction of the uterus. As pregnancy nears term, the uterus becomes sensitive to minute amounts of oxytocin. Synthetic oxytocics, such as Pitocin, when given intravenously, will also act on the uterine muscle, stimulating contraction.

Oxytocin has pronounced maternal cardiovascular and renal effects. Cardiac output and stroke volume are increased, and in some cases, a significant rise in baseline maternal blood pressure can be noted. If oxytocin is given in an IV bolus, profound hypotension and tachycardia may result. Urinary output decreases significantly because of the drug's antidiuretic effect and can result in water retention. Additionally, neonatal hyperbilirubinemia and jaundice can occur in the neonate of mothers who received oxytocin infusions for the induction of labor. The risk depends on both the dose of oxytocin administered and the gestational age of the fetus.

Oxytocin is the most efficient and frequently used drug for induction of labor; it is also used to augment labor already in progress (see Augmentation of Labor in the next section of this chapter). Because it is a powerful drug, the woman must be carefully assessed before and throughout oxytocin administration.

Indications and Contraindications

Indications for use of oxytocin to induce labor include all of the general indications listed earlier. Indications for oxytocin use include the following:

- Pregnancy-induced hypertension (PIH)
- Maternal diabetes, classes B to R, especially if diabetes is not well controlled during pregnancy
- Premature rupture of membranes
- Rh isoimmunization
- Postmaturity (more than 42 weeks of gestation): placental insufficiency and fetal compromise may result from prolonged pregnancy
- Evidence of fetal jeopardy (oligohydramnios)
- Intrauterine fetal demise

Contraindications to oxytocin include:

- Cephalopelvic disproportion (CPD)
- Abnormal fetal presentation (transverse, breech)
- Placental abnormalities (placenta previa, suspected abruption)
- Documented fetal distress
- Prematurity (unless maternal or fetal condition warrants delivery)
- Predisposition to uterine rupture (previous classical cesarean scar or history of uterine trauma, infection)

The FDA has banned the use of oxytocin for elective inductions and recommends it only for medically indicated inductions (Food and Drug Administration, 1978).

Advantages and Disadvantages

Advantages of oxytocin use for induction of labor include its efficiency and effectiveness in initiating and stimulating labor, its lack of direct action on the fetus, and its predictability of action.

Disadvantages of oxytocin use include the risk of abnormally strong or tetanic uterine contractions. Uterine overstimulation may result in fetal distress and, in rare cases, uterine rupture. Use of oxytocin has also been associated with increased incidence of cesarean births and the use of epidural anesthesia (Macer et al., 1992) and may result in preterm birth when the gestational age of the fetus has not been clearly established before induction of labor. Safe oxytocin induction requires the capability for internal (direct) EFM and intrauterine pressure monitoring. A physician who has privileges to perform cesarean deliveries must be readily available in the facility, and one-to-one expert nursing care is required.

Implications for Nursing Care

In most settings, the nurse is the primary care provider during the oxytocin infusion, and must be aware of all the data relating to the woman and fetus. Although the woman will previously have been screened by the physician or nurse midwife, the nurse has an independent duty to identify contraindications to the use of the drug. Any concerns regarding the procedure must be clarified before initiating the infusion.

The nurse then performs a complete assessment of the woman and fetus and obtains baseline vital signs and FHR pattern. In most facilities a 20- to 30-minute external EFM strip (or video terminal readout in the case of a computerized optical disk recording), is obtained to establish the FHR baseline, long-term variability, and periodic FHR changes. The woman's understanding of the induction process should also be ascertained at this time and her questions answered before beginning the procedure.

Initiating the Drip. Oxytocin is always administered intravenously when used for induction or stimulation of labor. Most hospitals have detailed policies and procedures concerning the preparation of the solution, as well as the amount and rate of oxytocin infusion. Before initiating an infusion, the policy should be reviewed. Use of an infusion pump is *required* because it offers precise control of the medication dose. An IV piggyback setup is used. The main IV line is started with a large-bore needle (usually 16- or 18-gauge) and connected to 1000 mL of a physiologic electrolyte solution such as Ringer's lactate. In a second liter of solution, 10 units (10,000 mU) of oxytocin is added. The piggyback line delivering the medication is connected at the most proximal location to the vein. This arrangement allows immediate discontinuation of the oxytocin when necessary, with no residual oxytocin solution remaining in the main IV infusion line.

The current standard of care requires a physician to be immediately available at all times during an oxytocin infusion to intervene in a timely manner if complications arise. The nurse is responsible for notifying the physician before starting the infusion. Since nursing supervision is mandatory and the woman must be monitored closely, adequate staffing should be ensured before the infusion is begun. The Association of Women's Health, Obstetric, and Neonatal Nursing (AWHONN) guidelines (NAACOG, 1988) recommend a 1:2 nurse–patient ratio, but a 1:1 nurse–patient ratio may be indicated in high-risk patients with complex problems and needs. Continuous EFM and tokodynamometer monitoring of uterine activity is indicated to appropriately assess the effects of the drug. Internal EFM and uterine monitoring may be implemented when the nurse is unable to obtain a technically adequate tracing with external monitoring or precise measurement of uterine activity is required.

Dosage Amounts. Recent evidence suggests that the current dosages of oxytocin administered during induction or augmentation of labor may be too high. According to AWHONN guidelines (NAACOG, 1988), the oxytocin infusion is started at 0.5 to 1.0 mU/min, using a standard infusion guide to calculate flow rate, as shown in Table 23-2.

This amount is gradually increased by 1 to 2 mU at every 30- to 60-minute interval until an optimal uterine response is achieved: contractions at a frequency of every 2 to 3 minutes, with duration of 45 to 90 seconds and moderate to strong (60 to 70 mm Hg) intensity with at least a 30- to 45-second rest period between contractions. More recently published ACOG guidelines (1991a) suggest a 40- to 60-minute interval for increase in oxytocin. This recommendation reflects current knowledge gained from research studies, which indicate that a 40- to 60-minute interval is required to reach a steady-state concentration of oxytocin in plasma after initiation of or change in the infusion rate (Seitchik & Castillo, 1983). Some controversy still exists, however, about the optimum dose and interval between increases in the oxytocin infusion rate. Hauth (1986) found an increase of 1 mU/min as often as every 15 minutes a safe and effective induction protocol. Ultimately, the nurse's decision to increase or decrease the rate of oxytocin infusion must be based on uterine and fetal responses to the drug.

Ongoing Assessments. To fully assess uterine activity during the induction process, the nurse must observe the contraction pattern obtained by tokodynamometry and printed on the EFM graph paper or visually displayed on a video terminal if a computer system is used (see Fig. 22-1).

The uterus is also manually palpated by the nurse both during and after contractions. It is critical that the nurse palpate the fundus between contractions because oxytocin can elevate the resting tone of the uterine muscle. As the resting tone rises above 15 to 20 mm Hg, uterine and placental perfusion is decreased, which can compromise fetal oxygenation. If an internal pressure catheter has not been inserted into the uterus, the nurse can identify an elevation in resting tone by palpating a continued degree of firmness in the uterine fundus between contractions. This condition should be reported to the nurse midwife or physician immediately. Palpation of the uterus is also essential to identify the development of a pathologic retraction ring, a complication that can arise when oxytocin infusion continues in the presence of an obstructed labor (see Chapter 26 for further discussion of this complication).

Sensitivity of the uterine muscle to oxytocin cannot be predicted with accuracy. Additional administration of the medication will continue to affect the myometrium after optimal uterine contraction has begun. Hyperstimulation of the uterus may result in tachysystole (frequent contractions), tetanic contractions, which are prolonged over 90 seconds, or an elevated resting tone. Tumultuous labor, or intense, rapid labor, may also result. Hyperstimulation may result in the following sequelae:

- Fetal distress due to impaired uteroplacental perfusion
- Abruption of the placenta
- Amniotic fluid embolism
- Lacerations of the cervix
- Uterine rupture
- Neonatal trauma

To accurately measure the effects of oxytocin on the uterine muscle, an intrauterine pressure catheter (IUPC) may be advanced through the cervix into the uterine cavity. The IUPC provides a direct measurement of the pressure generated by contraction of the uterine muscle in millimeters of mercury. (See Chapter 22 for a description of IUPC placement).

If signs of uterine hypertonicity are observed, the nurse should discontinue the oxytocin infusion immediately and notify the physician or nurse midwife (see the accompanying Nursing Care Plan). A tocolytic drug, usually 0.125 to 0.25 mg terbutaline, may be administered subcutaneously or intravenously to decrease uterine activity. Maternal plasma concentration of oxytocin falls rapidly after the infusion is discontinued, since the circulating half-life is 3 to 4 minutes. After reevaluation of the woman's status, the physician or nurse midwife may elect to restart the oxytocin at a lower dose or rate of infusion, stop the procedure, select another method of induction, or after obtaining informed consent, perform a cesarean delivery.

After optimal uterine activity is established, the nurse will need to assess the woman's progress in labor, her response to the process, and her comfort level. The nurse should be alert to individual and family needs for support and avoid the tendency to become focused too much on the procedure at hand. Oxytocin administration may be associated with increased pain and fatigue for the woman. The nurse should evaluate the need for analgesia or regional anesthesia, avoiding administration too early (which may prolong labor) and too late (which in the case of narcotic

Text continues on page 580

Table 23-2. Oxytocin Administration Flow Rate Guide*

Dosage in mU/min	Flow Rate mL/hr
0.5	3
1.0	6
2.0	12
3.0	18
4.0	24
5.0	30
6.0	36
7.0	42
8.0	48
9.0	54
10.0	60
12.0	72
14.0	84
16.0	96
18.0	108
20.0†	120

* This guide is for use in administration of oxytocin using IV pump that delivers 20 gtt/mL. Infusion solution is 10 units oxytocin in 1000 mL IV fluid (or 5 units in 500 mL).

† If desired contraction pattern is not achieved with dosage of 20.0 mU/min, consult with physician and obtain order for increased dosage, if appropriate.

Marshall C. (1985). The art of induction/augmentation of labor. *Journal of Obstetric, Gynecologic, and Neonatal Nursing, 14*(1), 22.

Nursing Care Plan

The Woman Receiving Oxytocin Therapy for Induction or Augmentation of Labor

PATIENT PROFILE

History

J.R. is a 22-year-old G3/PO at $42\,^{2}/_{7}$ weeks' gestation. Beginning in the 41st week of gestation she is evaluated in the antenatal testing center to identify signs of fetal compromise secondary to postmaturity. At 42 weeks her nonstress test is nonreactive and the amniotic fluid index is 2.5. J.R. is scheduled for an induction of labor. Four hours after cervical installation of prostaglandin gel, an oxytocin infusion is started.

At the end of the second day of induction J.R.'s labor is progressing slowly. She is 5 cm and 80% effaced. The fetus is at 0 station. The membranes are intact. J.R. is receiving oxytocin at an infusion rate of 16 mU/min (96 mL/hr of IV fluid). Maternal vital signs and the FHR have been normal. J.R. has been permitted to drink clear fluids in labor. She has consumed 1500 mL of liquids in the past 8 hours and her urine output was 450 mL during that time period. She has received no analgesia or anesthesia.

Physical Assessment

The nurse is beginning a physical assessment. J.R. rolls to the supine position with her knees drawn up. She is holding her abdomen and moaning. She says, "Oh God! Help me nurse! I'm in so much pain. This contraction is unbearable, and it seems to be going on forever." The nurse notes on the EFM that the uterine contraction is still intense after 120 seconds. The FHR drops to 60 bpm.

COLLABORATIVE PROBLEMS/ POTENTIAL COMPLICATIONS

Maternal
- Tetanic contractions
- Uterine rupture
- Soft-tissue trauma due to tumultuous labor
- Water intoxication
- Hypertension
- Hypotension
- Hypersensitivity/allergic reactions
- Precipitous labor and/or birth
- Postpartum uterine atony

(See the Nursing Alert display following the Care Plan.)

Fetal
- Hypoxia
- Fetal distress

Neonatal
- Hyperbilirubinemia

Assessment	*Nursing Diagnosis*	*Nursing Interventions*	*Rationale*
Uterine contraction lasting 120 seconds. J.R. is receiving an oxytocin infusion at 16 mU/min.	High Risk for Maternal Injury related to uterine hyperstimulation *Expected Outcome* The woman's uterus will subside in activity.	Stop the oxytocin infusion	Serum half-life of oxytocin is 2 to 3 minutes, thus stopping infusion will decrease uterine activity rapidly. Continued excessive uterine activity may result in uterine rupture or soft-tissue injury.
	The woman will verbalize relief from intense contraction	Call for assistance	Additional help will be needed to obtain medical assistance, evaluate woman, and provide therapy and drugs should tetanic contractions persist.

(*Continued*)

The Woman Receiving Oxytocin Therapy for Induction or Augmentation of Labor

(*Continued*)

Assessment	Nursing Diagnosis	Nursing Interventions	Rationale
		Prepare to administer tocolytic such as terbutaline. Palpate uterine fundus and or observe electronic monitor for evidence of uterine relaxation.	A uterine tocolytic may be ordered to reduce uterine activity if stopping the infusion does not result in rapid decrease in contraction frequency and duration.
		Remain with J.R. continuously. Do not restart oxytocin infusion until maternal and fetal status stabilize.	The woman should never be left unattended during an oxytocin infusion because of the danger of maternal injury or fetal distress.
Fetal heart rate is 60 bpm	High Risk for Fetal Injury related to uterine hyperstimulation Altered Tissue Perfusion related to uteroplacental insufficiency ***Expected Outcome*** The FHR will return to normal baseline.	Stop oxytocin infusion. Turn J.R. to her left side. Increase mainline IV infusion rate.	Stopping infusion, repositioning J.R., and increasing the mainline IV infusion will improve placental perfusion.
		Administer oxygen to J.R. at 8 to 12 L/min by tight face mask.	Administering oxygen will increase maternal oxygen supply available to fetus.
		Perform vaginal examination.	Sudden fetal distress may be the result of rapid progress in labor, descent of fetus, or prolapsed umbilical cord.
		Call for additional help.	Additional assistance will be needed to support J.R., provide therapy.
		Notify physician.	Physician or midwife must be notified of all significant changes in maternal–fetal status.
		Be prepared to administer tocolytic.	Administering tocolytic will reduce uterine activity and improve placental perfusion.
J.R. receiving 16 mU/min of oxytocin (high dose). IV intake of 96 mL/hr. Oral intake of 1500 mL in past 8 hours and urine output of 450 mL in past 8 hours	(Possible) Fluid Volume Excess related to water-retaining effects of oxytocin ***Expected Outcome*** Woman maintains fluid balance during course of oxytocin infusion.	Monitor intake and output. Decrease total IV infusion of mainline IV.	Oxytocin in high doses (above 16 mU/min) may exert an antidiuretic effect, resulting in water retention and decreased urine output.
		Follow unit policies for consulting with physician or midwife when high doses (16 mU/min or higher) are infused.	Nurse must notify physician or midwife when high levels of oxytocin are infused because of increased risk of water intoxication and need to reevaluate progress of labor.

(*Continued*)

The Woman Receiving Oxytocin Therapy for Induction or Augmentation of Labor
(Continued)

Assessment	***Nursing Diagnosis***	***Nursing Interventions***	***Rationale***
		Monitor J.R. for evidence of bounding pulse, peripheral edema, sacral edema, shortness of breath, increasing blood pressure, signs of lethargy, confusion, or altered mentation.	In addition to development of edema, water retention can result in hypertension, pulmonary or cerebral edema.
		Restrict fluid intake if signs of fluid retention are present.	
Tetanic contraction. Drop in FHR to 60 bpm. "Oh god. Help me nurse. I'm in so much pain."	Fear related to complication of oxytocin infusion Pain related to tetanic contraction	Provide J.R. with a brief explanation of problem and reason for implementation of corrective actions to reduce uterine activity and improve FHR.	Acute fear will reduce J.R.'s ability to receive and process information about her condition and the fetal status.
	Expected Outcome J.R. will follow simple directives. J.R. will verbalize a decrease in anxiety as her condition and status of fetus stabilize.	Answer questions with short, simple responses. Provide ongoing information as condition improves or if further interventions are necessary.	Offering ongoing information and answering questions may reduce level of acute anxiety, which may be experienced with complication.
		Provide brief directions for breathing pattern, which may be temporarily helpful to control pain until tetanic contraction stops.	Offering suggestions about short-term pain control technique may reduce pain and accompanying anxiety.
		Discuss nonpharmacologic and/or pharmacologic pain control methods when condition stabilizes.	When condition stabilizes, J.R. may wish to discuss additional pain control methods if contractions remain strong and regular.

EVALUATION

J.R. performed rapid shallow chest breathing until tetanic contraction ended. Within 60 seconds of stopping oxytocin infusion, the contraction ended, and contraction frequency was spaced out to every 2 minutes thereafter. The FHR returned to a baseline in 140 bpm range within 60 seconds of stopping oxytocin infusion and coincided with end of tetanic contraction. Vaginal examination of J.R. found the cervix dilated 6 cm and 100% effaced. The fetus was at +1 station and no prolapsed cord.

After J.R. understood the problem, her level of fear was reduced and she cooperated with efforts to correct the problem. After maternal and fetal status stabilized, J.R. requested intramuscular or IV narcotic analgesia for relief of pain.

NURSING ALERT

MONITORING FOR COMPLICATIONS WHEN THE NURSE MANAGES AN OXYTOCIN INFUSION

The nurse monitors for complications related to oxytocin administration during the induction or augmentation of labor. Complications fall into four major categories.

Uterine Hyperstimulation

The nurse monitors uterine activity by palpation and electronic monitoring. When internal pressure monitoring is implemented by the midwife or physician, the nurse is responsible for assembling, calibrating, and trouble-shooting the equipment. The nurse must be skillful in calculating Montevideo units and adjusting the oxytocin infusion rate based on measurement of uterine activity. All labor nurses must be prepared to initiate emergency supportive care when uterine hyperstimulation is identified (see Nursing Care Plan).

Blood Pressure Changes

The blood pressure is measured before each increase in the oxytocin infusion rate, or more often depending on the woman's condition and responses to the drug. Hypotension or hypertension may occur and require immediate nursing actions to prevent maternal or fetal injury.

Water Retention

Intake and output are monitored closely to identify signs of water retention. Ongoing assessment of peripheral and sacral edema as well as pulmonary and cerebral edema are essential. The nurse observes for alterations in cardiovascular status such as hypertension and bounding pulses, which may indicate water retention.

Allergic Reactions

The nurse determines if previous adverse reactions suggestive of allergy or hypersensitivity have occurred before beginning the infusion. The woman is monitored for signs and symptoms indicative of allergic reaction including shortness of breath, hypotension, uticaria, generalized anxiety, or altered mentation. The nurse must be prepared to initiate supportive care (airway maintenance, oxygen, and IV therapy) and administer emergency drugs such as epinephrine.

analgesics, may produce neonatal depression at delivery). In addition, the woman may make rapid progress in cervical change and fetal descent during oxytocin administration; vaginal examination is indicated when the contraction pattern suggests an effective contraction pattern or if there is an increase in maternal pain. If the woman is a multigravida, she may require more frequent vaginal examinations because labor often progresses more rapidly.

In addition to monitoring uterine activity, the FHR pattern is assessed and documented every 15 to 30 minutes. If a nonreassuring FHR pattern develops, the nurse must implement actions to correct the problem (see the accompanying Nursing Procedure, Correcting Nonreasurring Electronic Fetal Monitoring Patterns). The woman's blood pressure, pulse, and respirations are also reevaluated every 30 minutes or more frequently. Intake and output should be measured because of the drug's potential antidiuretic effect. Prolonged infusion of oxytocin may result in water intoxication, with symptoms of shortness of breath, rales on chest auscultation, alterations in mentation, and convulsions.

Discontinuing the Infusion. When labor is not established within 8 to 12 hours, the oxytocin infusion should be discontinued to permit rest and to prevent fluid imbalance problems associated with prolonged oxytocin administration. The main IV line may be maintained for access, or a saline or heparin lock inserted to permit greater comfort during the night. The oxytocin infusion is restarted the following day after the woman has had an opportunity to shower and complete other aspects of personal hygiene. Serial attempts to induce labor with oxytocin infusions are not uncommon, and the woman should be prepared for the process. Anxiety, disappointment, and a sense of failure are more acute when the woman is not forewarned that the induction procedure can span several days. If serial induction fails, cesarean delivery may be indicated.

Although the woman and her support person may verbalize disappointment regarding the need for labor induction, the childbirth experience can still be satisfying. When the nurse uses a family-centered approach to the active management of labor, the focus shifts from the technology and drugs necessary for the process to the woman and her support person. The nurse can also encourage active participation of the woman and family in the childbirth experience, thus reducing negative perceptions of the induction procedure.

Augmentation of Labor

Augmentation or stimulation of labor refers to the process of promoting more effective uterine contractions when labor has already begun but is dysfunctional or has stopped completely. The most commonly used methods of labor augmentation are also methods for induction of labor, namely, amniotomy and IV oxytocin infusion. In addition, breast (nipple) stimulation is used to stimulate uterine activity. Other physiologic techniques, such as ambulation and position change, are discussed in Chapter 20.

When uterine activity is insufficient to produce progressive cervical dilatation, *amniotomy* or AROM may be performed. Amniotomy is thought to release arachidonic acid, a precursor of prostaglandins, which enhance uterine activity. AROM also promotes descent of the presenting part, thus applying pressure on the cervix, which further stimulates contractions.

Labor may also be augmented by IV infusion of *oxytocin*. For augmentation of labor, the maximum infusion rate required to produce effective contractions is generally lower than that required to initiate labor.

Breast stimulation has been suggested as an alternative method in an effort to reduce invasive techniques for the augmentation of labor. Nipple stimulation is known to cause endogenous oxytocin release from the posterior pituitary gland, resulting in uterine contractions. Manual nipple rolling and the application of moist, warm wash cloths to the breast have been used to stimulate oxytocin release. A study by Stein and associates (1990) also evaluated the effectiveness of an electric breast pump; they found it a safe and

NURSING PROCEDURE

Correcting Nonreassuring Electronic Fetal Monitoring Patterns

Purpose: The nurse is responsible for monitoring maternal and fetal responses to the infusion of oxytocin. When nonreassuring or ominous FHR patterns are identified, or excessive uterine activity occurs, the nurse acts in a timely manner to correct the underlying problem(s).

NURSING ACTION	RATIONALE
1. Stop the oxytocin infusion.	To reduce uterine activity and improve uteroplacental perfusion
2. Call for immediate assistance.	Additional help will facilitate implementation of corrective actions
3. Turn the woman to the left side-lying position.	To improve uteroplacental blood flow and fetal oxygenation
4. Increase the mainline infusion rate.	To improve uteroplacental blood flow and fetal oxygenation
5. Administer oxygen at 8 to 12 L/min by tight face mask.	To improve fetal oxygenation
6. Perform a vaginal examination.	To determine cervical dilatation and to rule out complications such as prolapsed umbilical cord
7. Be prepared to administer a tocolytic (terbutaline 0.125 to 0.25 mg) subcutaneously or intravenously by physician or midwife order.	To reduce uterine activity and improve uteroplacental blood flow
8. Provide the woman with a brief explanation of the problem and the reasons for corrective actions.	To reduce anxiety and enhance the woman's ability to cooperate with directions for position change and oxygen administration
9. Notify the midwife or physician in a timely manner.	To communicate significant data To obtain appropriate physician or midwife directives

effective alternative to IV oxytocin infusion for the augmentation of labor.

Indications and Contraindications

Augmentation or stimulation of more effective uterine activity is indicated when hypotonic contractions occur, resulting in delayed progress in labor (dilatation and or fetal descent). Factors that often contribute to ineffective uterine activity include analgesia, regional anesthesia, chorioamnionitis, and overdistention of the uterus. Contraindications to augmentation of labor include fetal distress, strong evidence of CPD such as the development of a pathologic retraction ring, maternal hemorrhage, or exhaustion.

Advantages and Disadvantages

Several potential benefits of successful labor augmentation include reduction in the incidence of infection secondary to prolonged labor and a decrease in the cesarean birth rate due to failure in cervical dilatation and fetal descent. Early detection and treatment of hypoactive uterine contractions can reduce maternal fatigue and anxiety and the need for other procedures such as forceps application or vacuum extraction at the time of birth. When successful, amniotomy eliminates the discomfort and systemic effects produced by oxytocin infusions. Benefits of breast stimulation may include avoidance of pain related to an IV insertion, elimination of the risk of maternal hypertension and water intoxication secondary to an IV oxytocin infusion, increased patient control during the labor process, and early milk production for the breastfeeding client.

Enhancement of uterine activity by amniotomy, oxytocin infusion, or release of endogenous oxytocin through breast (nipple) stimulation is not without risk. Infection, fetal umbilical cord prolapse, and amniotic fluid embolus can occur with AROM. The infusion of exogenous oxytocin is associated with uterine hyperstimulation and has the potential to cause fetal distress, uterine rupture, cervical lacerations, and precipitous labor and delivery. Possible adverse effects that may limit the usefulness of breast stimulation are uterine hyperstimulation, fetal distress, nipple soreness, and milk production and engorgement in bottle-feeding clients. Some women find breast stimulation embarrassing.

NURSING PROCEDURE

Supporting the Woman Using Manual Breast Stimulation for Labor Initiation or Augmentation

Purpose: To provide the woman with instruction and support during manual breast (nipple) stimulation for the augmentation of labor and to evaluate maternal and fetal responses to the procedure.

NURSING ACTION	RATIONALE
1. Monitor FHR and contraction pattern data for 10 minutes before beginning procedure.	To obtain baseline data and to identify any contraindications (fetal distress or uterine hyperactivity) to the procedure
2. Instruct woman to roll or tug one nipple under her clothing for a 10-minute period or until the first contraction occurs.	To prevent uterine hyperstimulation, which may occur if both breasts are stimulated simultaneously
3. On contraction, instruct woman to stop stimulation immediately.	To prevent uterine hyperstimulation To permit evaluation of intensity and duration of contraction
4. Evaluate FHR pattern.	To determine fetal response to uterine contraction(s)
5. If FHR response and contraction quality are within normal limits, instruct woman to resume nipple rolling for another 10 minutes or until next contraction occurs.	The stimulation of adequate contractions may take some time and requires continued nipple stimulation.
6. Observe closely for uterine hyperstimulation and adverse FHR response.	Breast stimulation does not permit control of endogenous oxytocin release and may result in uterine hyperstimulation and fetal distress.
7. Instruct woman to discontinue breast stimulation if exaggerated uterine activity or adverse fetal response occurs.	

If no positive changes in labor pattern result, discontinue procedure.

Implications for Nursing Care

When an amniotomy is to be performed to augment labor, the nurse must assess the patient's condition and status of the labor and delivery unit to determine the advisability of the procedure. When the physician or nurse midwife and the nurse are in agreement with the plan of care, the steps are taken to prepare the woman and assemble the necessary equipment. A complete description of the nurse's role in amniotomy is presented in the display presented in the previous section of this chapter.

If oxytocin is used to stimulate more effective uterine activity, guidelines for preparation and administration of the drug and nursing care are identical to those used in induction. As noted, the infusion rate required to effect progressive dilatation is usually lower than that required for induction of labor. The oxytocin infusion may be initiated after several hours of inadequate progress, and the woman may already experience complications related to a prolonged labor including fatigue, dehydration, increased pain sensations, and infection. In addition, once the diagnosis of labor dystocia is made, based on the hypoactive labor pattern, the woman's level of anxiety and feelings of inadequacy or failure may be heightened. The nurse monitors the woman closely for evidence of complications and provides appropriate physical and emotional support to reduce the woman's fears and feelings of discouragement.

If breast stimulation is ordered, the nurse must carefully instruct the woman in the appropriate technique, closely monitor uterine and fetal responses to the procedure, and be prepared to administer tocolytics, as ordered, if uterine hyperstimulation occurs. The procedures for manual breast stimulation and breast pump stimulation are given in the two accompanying Nursing Procedures.

Reduction of Uterine Activity

Another technique to modify the labor pattern involves the temporary reduction in uterine activity or tocolysis. Terbutaline, a tocolytic drug, is used in some cases of fetal

NURSING PROCEDURE

Supporting the Woman Using Breast Pump Stimulation for Labor Augmentation

Purpose: To provide the woman with appropriate instruction and support during breast stimulation for the augmentation of labor when a breast pump is used and to evaluate maternal and fetal responses to breast stimulation.

NURSING ACTION	***RATIONALE***
1. Obtain an electric breast pump and instruct woman to apply moderate suction on her right breast for 10 minutes.	Use moderate pressure level and limit to 10-minute time interval to prevent breast tissue trauma or uterine hyperstimulation.
2. Repeat procedure on left breast until first contraction occurs.	More than 10 minutes may be required to stimulate contractions.
3. When contraction occurs, discontinue pumping for 10 minutes.	To prevent uterine hyperstimulation and fetal distress
4. Observe FHR and contraction pattern.	To identify adverse fetal response
5. Repeat the above cycle five times, evaluating closely for uterine hyperstimulation and fetal distress until contraction pattern is established.	To prevent excessive pressure to breast To permit immediate discontinuation of procedure if adverse response occurs

If no positive changes in labor pattern result, discontinue procedure.

distress when uterine activity is contributing to fetal hypoxia. This procedure, often referred to as *intrauterine fetal resuscitation*, is attempted to improve uterine perfusion and fetal oxygenation, which is sometimes compromised during contractions and with fetal umbilical cord compression. The recommended protocol is the administration of a single bolus of terbutaline (0.125 to 0.25 mg) intravenously over a 1-minute period (Burke et al., 1989; Shekarloo, Bauer, Cook, & Freese, 1989).

The nurse plays a central role in the augmentation or induction of labor. Because of the risks inherent in the procedures used by the nurse midwife or physician for stimulation of labor, the nurse has an independent duty to evaluate the appropriateness of the method(s) selected. The nurse must assess maternal–fetal well-being and clarify any questions that arise regarding the advisability of the procedure. This must be done before assisting the nurse midwife or physician or before administering an oxytocin infusion. If complications arise, the nurse provides immediate supportive care and must be prepared to assist the physician or nurse midwife with diagnostic procedures during an emergency delivery.

Modifying the Mode of Delivery

Obstetric interventions may be implemented to reduce maternal or fetal risk in selected circumstances. Common obstetric interventions that modify the mode of delivery include version, forceps application, vacuum extraction, cesarean birth, and trial of labor and vaginal birth after previous cesarean (VBAC).

Version of the Fetus

Version is the manipulation of the fetus to obtain a more favorable position for delivery. External cephalic version refers to manipulation of the fetus through the woman's abdominal wall, usually to convert a breech presentation to vertex or a persistent transverse lie into a longitudinal presentation. With the advent of ultrasonography, this procedure has become more common and is usually done at around 37 weeks of gestation; however, it can also be done in early labor. Successful versions, with the use of ultrasonography, tocolytics to relax the uterus, and EFM, can be accomplished in 60% to 77% of women with abnormal presentations (Donald & Barton, 1990).

Indications and Contraindications

External version may be attempted if a breech or transverse presentation is diagnosed and the following conditions exist:

- Ultrasound evaluation has been done to localize the placenta and rule out multiple gestation.
- The presenting part is not engaged in the pelvis.
- The maternal abdominal wall is thin, permitting accurate palpation of fetal position.
- The uterus is not irritable (prone to contraction with manipulation).

- There is enough amniotic fluid to allow easy movement of the fetus.
- Manipulation can be done without anesthesia, to avoid application of undue force.

Contraindications include the absence of any of these indications. External version may stimulate uterine activity and puts mechanical stress on the uterus, membranes, and placenta. Thus, the other contraindications are previous uterine trauma or surgery, any condition that would prohibit a vaginal delivery, or evidence of third trimester bleeding or a low-lying placenta.

Advantages and Disadvantages

Recent research findings suggest that external version, when done under optimal conditions, can reduce the risks associated with malpresentation and eliminate the need for a cesarean delivery. External version may be attempted after IV administration of a tocolytic agent to enhance uterine relaxation; however, several studies indicate success without the use of these agents. Even if conversion of a malpresentation is successful using this procedure, the fetus may later spontaneously return to the previous position. Risks associated with external cephalic version include placental dislodgment with bleeding, umbilical cord compression, and fetal bradycardia. Use of ultrasonography and EFM with external version has greatly reduced the incidence of these problems.

Implications for Nursing Care

After version, nursing responsibilities focus on close monitoring of maternal–fetal status for signs of hemorrhage or fetal compromise. Maternal blood pressure should be monitored every 5 minutes throughout the procedure, and continuous FHR monitoring should be in place. The procedure should be discontinued if abnormalities in the FHR appear. Assessment of maternal blood pressure and FHR should be continued during the first 30 minutes after the procedure. If external version is performed during the intrapartum period, the woman should be monitored closely for signs of postpartum uterine atony and developing hemorrhage secondary to uterine trauma.

Internal podalic version or direct manual manipulation of the fetus inside the uterus may be done to convert malpresentation of a second twin, after the birth of the first infant. Internal version poses significant risk to the fetus, however, and is usually done only in high-risk perinatal centers with the use of ultrasonography and EFM. It may be performed in other settings during extreme emergencies such as profound fetal distress with a prolapsed cord or the need for immediate delivery of a second twin when cesarean delivery cannot be accomplished in a timely manner. Nursing responsibilities when an internal podalic version is attempted include:

- Obtaining additional medical and nursing assistance (anesthesiologist and pediatric support staff)
- Providing the woman with a brief explanation of procedure
- Providing the woman with emotional support
- Monitoring the fetus with external EFM
- Monitoring maternal responses to the procedure

Forceps Application

Obstetric forceps are curved metal tongs used to facilitate the birth of the infant's head by providing traction and rotation, as shown in Figure 23-2. Blades of the forceps are specially shaped to fit the fetal head and the maternal pelvis. Both the blades and the shanks of the forceps are curved to provide the best traction angle for various situations. The incidence of forceps applications will vary according to the facility, the type of analgesia and anesthesia used for labor, customary maternal position for labor and delivery, and the skill and experience of the birth attendant.

Traction is needed when the woman is unable to push the infant out of the vagina spontaneously due to a tight fetopelvic fit, diminished urge to push, or decreased effectiveness of bearing-down efforts as a result of anesthesia, analgesia, fatigue, or improper positioning. In addition, traction may be needed to achieve a rapid delivery if maternal status is compromised or if fetal distress is detected late in the second stage. Preterm infants may be delivered using forceps to shorten the second stage and protect their vulnerable heads from the prolonged pressure of labor. Rotation of the infant by forceps may be done if the fetus presents in a persistent transverse or posterior position and maternal position changes have not been successful in achieving spontaneous rotation (see the display, Types of Obstetric Forceps).

Three types of forceps applications are acceptable (ACOG, 1991b). *Outlet forceps applications* are done when the fetal head is visible at the vaginal introitus without separating the labia. The forceps are used to guide and control the delivery of the head. In *low forceps applications*, the leading point of the fetal skull is at or greater than +2 station, but not yet visible at the introitus. The fetal head may need to be rotated more than 45 degrees to accomplish an anterior vertex delivery. *Midforceps applications* are those in which the fetal head is above a +2 station, but is at least at the level of the ischial spines and engaged. Midforceps deliveries are difficult, and current obstetric management may be replacing midforceps applications with cesarean delivery.

A former type of forceps application, high, is no longer used because of the high risk of severe maternal and fetal

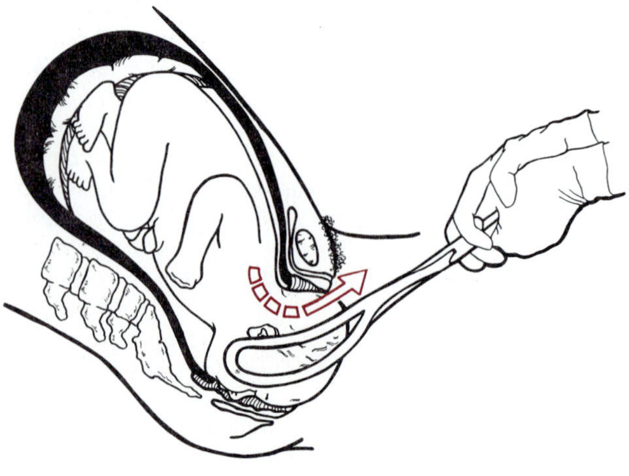

Figure 23-2.
Forceps delivery (Childbirth Graphics).

Types of Obstetric Forceps

Obstetric forceps are designed to facilitate delivery of the fetal head. They have blades that are either solid or fenestrated (with an opening), shanks, and handles. The blades are curved to fit the fetal head and the curve of the maternal pelvis. They are designed for specific obstetric purposes; the most commonly used types are described below.

Simpson forceps (similar to DeLee forceps) are used for low or outlet forceps applications. Note the shanks are well separated near the handle to allow an episiotomy incision to be made after the forceps have been applied.

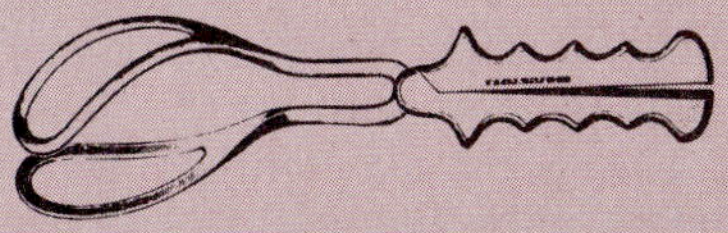

Tucker-McLean forceps are used for low forceps applications and with preterm infants. The solid blades allow easier application and removal, and lessen the potential for soft-tissue or head trauma.

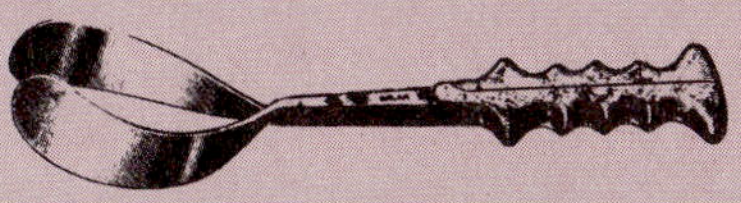

Piper forceps are specifically designed for delivery of the after-coming head in breech deliveries. The shanks are curved down, so that the blades can be higher than the handles when applied to the fetal skull. This allows for easier traction in a breech delivery.

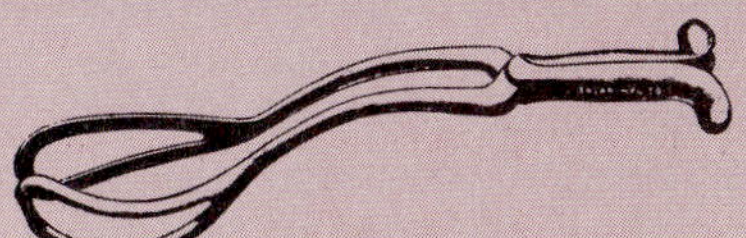

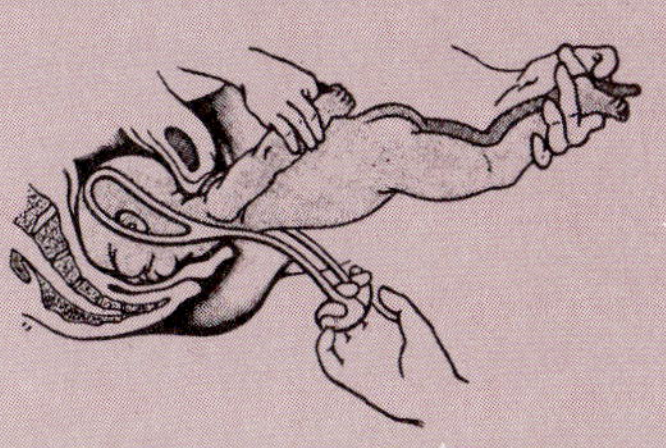

injury. This practice has been replaced by cesarean delivery (ACOG, 1991b). A failed forceps delivery is one in which an approved application was attempted but delivery could not be achieved. Cesarean birth is then indicated.

Indications and Contraindications

Indications for forceps application include those conditions that require a shortened second stage of labor: when the woman or fetus is in jeopardy or when assistance with maternal bearing-down is needed (certain cardiac or cerebrovascular diseases). Prolonged second stage of labor is a relative indication. ACOG guidelines (1991b) recommend evaluation of the need for forceps application in the following situations:

- Nulliparous woman when the second stage of labor exceeds 3 hours with an epidural anesthetic or 2 hours without a regional anesthetic.
- Multiparous woman when the second stage of labor exceeds 2 hours with an epidural anesthetic or 1 hour without regional anesthesia.

The following conditions must exist for a safe forceps delivery:

- Rupture of membranes
- Complete dilatation of the cervix
- Knowledge of fetal position: fetal head must be engaged
- Diagnosed vertex, breech, or face (mentum anterior) presentation
- Absence of CPD, sacral or pelvic outlet abnormalities
- Adequate regional or general anesthesia
- Empty maternal bladder to avoid trauma
- Ability to perform emergency cesarean delivery if problems occur

Without these conditions forceps delivery is unsafe, and cesarean birth is indicated.

Advantages and Disadvantages

Advantages of forceps applications include possible avoidance of cesarean delivery when vaginal birth can be safely achieved with mechanical assistance, protection of the preterm fetus's vulnerable head during the second stage of labor, and avoidance of maternal exhaustion from prolonged pushing during the second stage of labor. Disadvantages of forceps applications center on trauma to maternal tissue and the fetal head during delivery. Lacerations of the vagina and cervix may occur, but the most common injury results from extension of an episiotomy into the rectum. Rupture of the uterus can occur, and there is an increased risk of uterine atony and excessive bleeding after a forceps-assisted birth. Because of the invasive nature of the procedure, a higher incidence of infection occurs. Although less commonly observed, fracture of the coccyx and bladder trauma have been reported. Finally, there is the potential for trauma and bruising of neonate's head and neurologic damage secondary to skull fracture and intracranial hemorrhage.

Implications for Nursing Care

The decision for a forceps delivery is made by the physician or the nurse midwife. The nurse must be prepared to locate the appropriate type of forceps when requested. Forceps are placed one at a time on either side of the fetal head, while frequent checks are made to ensure proper positioning and to avoid trauma to the fetal head or maternal tissues. An episiotomy may be made after forceps are placed. Delivery of the infant is achieved by gentle traction on the forceps handles until full crowning of the fetal head is evident, after which they are removed. When crowning has taken place, the woman then can usually provide the final push to deliver the head and rest of the body.

The nurse must support the woman if she is awake,

Legal/Ethical Considerations

Nursing Responsibility During Forceps-Assisted Delivery

The courts have now ruled that the nurse has an independent duty to evaluate the physician's or midwife's decision to use forceps. In a recent lawsuit, the nurse was found negligent for failing to obtain additional medical assistance when the physician attempted a midforceps delivery of a fetus that had not engaged in the pelvis. Medical and nursing experts testified that, based on the nurse's knowledge of this particular labor, the nurse had an independent duty to seek additional medical consultation before providing the physician with the requested forceps.

Schifrin, B., & Hamilton, T. (1991). Abnormal labor curve with inappropriate use of forceps. Journal of Perinatology, XI *(1), 63.*

explaining what is being done and how she can assist in the prompt delivery of her infant. The woman's comfort level should be observed closely; forceps applications will involve sensations of pressure, but adequate regional anesthesia can be established so that pain can be controlled. Inhalation anesthesia may also be used to achieve adequate maternal relaxation for some forceps applications.

Because of the increased risk of maternal and fetal injury, claims of malpractice are more likely to occur with the application of forceps. The nurse should assess the FHR continuously by external EFM during the forceps application and traction. Fetal bradycardia may be observed as a result of head compression and should be transient. Midforceps applications are more dangerous to the fetus, and pediatric assistance should be available because intensive neonatal support may be necessary. The neonate delivered with forceps should be carefully examined for cerebral trauma or nerve damage (see Chapter 31). The nurse must be alert for possible risks associated with forceps deliveries. The woman should be observed carefully for excessive bleeding, severe perineal bruising and pain, difficulty in voiding, and cervical or vaginal lacerations.

Vacuum Extraction

Vacuum extraction is accomplished by use of a specialized vacuum extractor, which has a caplike suction device that can be applied to the fetal head to facilitate extraction, as shown in Figure 23-3. Once the suction cup is applied, it is connected with sterile tubing to the suction machine. Suction is initiated at 0.2 kg/cm^2, and gradually increased in equal increments to a maximum of 0.8 kg/cm^2. The negative pressure that is achieved pulls the fetal scalp tissue into the suction cup. Fluid accumulates in the subcutaneous tissue of the scalp and it becomes edematous, forming a caput, which fits snugly into the cavity of the vacuum cup. This allows traction forces to be applied to the head. Once the appropriate level of negative pressure is reached, the physician applies traction during uterine contractions until descent of the fetal head can be achieved. The suction device should be kept in place no longer than 20 to 30 minutes, and slippage or "pull off" should be avoided because it can cause trauma to the fetal scalp or maternal tissue. Caution should be taken to avoid placing the suction device over a previous scalp electrode or blood sampling site, if possible.

Indications and Contraindications

Indications for use of vacuum extraction are similar to those for forceps application. If the woman is unable to push the infant out of the vagina spontaneously due to a diminished urge to push or decreased effectiveness of bearing-down efforts secondary to anesthesia, analgesia, or fatigue, vacuum extraction may be used to shorten the second stage of labor. Contraindications include profound fetal or maternal distress requiring rapid delivery, evidence of CPD, or face or breech presentation.

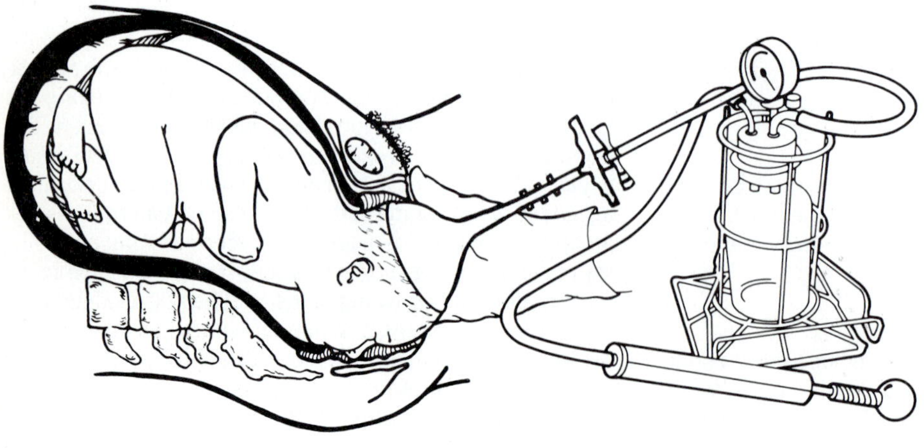

Figure 23-3.
Vacuum extractor with suction cup applied to scalp (Childbirth Graphics).

Advantages and Disadvantages

Vacuum extraction has several advantages over forceps applications. There is usually less trauma to the woman's bladder and vaginal tissue and a decreased risk of perineal tearing. Attachment of a vacuum extractor cup is easier than application of forceps when the presenting part fits snugly in the birth canal. Pressure on the fetal head is less intense than when forceps are used, and head trauma is less commonly observed.

Disadvantages include the fact that vacuum extraction cannot assist in an emergency where rapid delivery is needed and rotation of the presenting part cannot usually be accomplished; sometimes, however, spontaneous rotation occurs when traction is applied. Other disadvantages include the risk of fetal scalp bruising, blistering, avulsion, and other cerebral trauma from excessive suction or prolonged use (greater than 30 minutes). There is an increased incidence of cephalhematoma (localized bleeding beneath the periostomy of the neonatal skull) when vacuum extraction is used.

Implications for Nursing Care

Nursing responsibilities during vacuum extraction include assembling equipment, informing the woman and support person about the procedure, continued monitoring of maternal and fetal status, and assisting the birth attendant with the procedure. The FHR should be auscultated and documented at least every 5 minutes if continuous EFM is not used, and the nurse should be prepared for forceps application and neonatal resuscitation if prompt delivery is necessary.

During vacuum extraction, the nurse may need to help the physician by connecting the sterile tubing to the suction machine and starting the suction. The nurse may need to release the suction quickly if the cap slips off to avoid trauma to maternal tissue. When delivery is achieved, the neonate must be assessed at birth and observed throughout the immediate postpartum period for signs of cerebral trauma secondary to vacuum extraction. A caput succedaneum (localized swelling of the neonate's scalp) at the suction cap site is considered normal and will resolve within 24 hours.

Cesarean Birth

Cesarean birth is an operative procedure in which the fetus is delivered through a surgical incision in the woman's abdominal wall and uterus, as shown in Figure 23-4. The term cesarean comes from the Latin root, *caedere*, to cut. Previously called C-section, and considered major surgery, the preferred term for the procedure is now cesarean birth or cesarean delivery. This terminology deemphasizes the operative procedure and stresses the birth experience. Such deliveries may be planned (elective) or arise from an unanticipated problem (emergency).

Cesarean birth is the most common surgical procedure performed in the United States (with the exception of cervical biopsy). Currently the incidence of cesarean birth is approximately 25% of all births in the United States, up from the 4% rate of the late 1960s (Tighe & Sweezy, 1990). More than 900,000 cesarean deliveries are performed each year (Taffel, Placek, & Kosary, 1992). This increase may be due in part to the widespread use of EFM and the resulting concern for fetal well-being during labor, the increased safety of anesthesia and operative care, and the increasing numbers of moderate-risk and high-risk pregnancies being carried to term. In addition, cesarean delivery is performed in more than 80% of cases when breech presentation is diagnosed (Taffel, Placek, Moien, & Kosary, 1991), and is recommended by some experts when the estimated fetal weight is greater than 4500 g (9 lb, 14 oz) to avoid complications associated with shoulder dystocia (O'Leary & Leonetti, 1990).

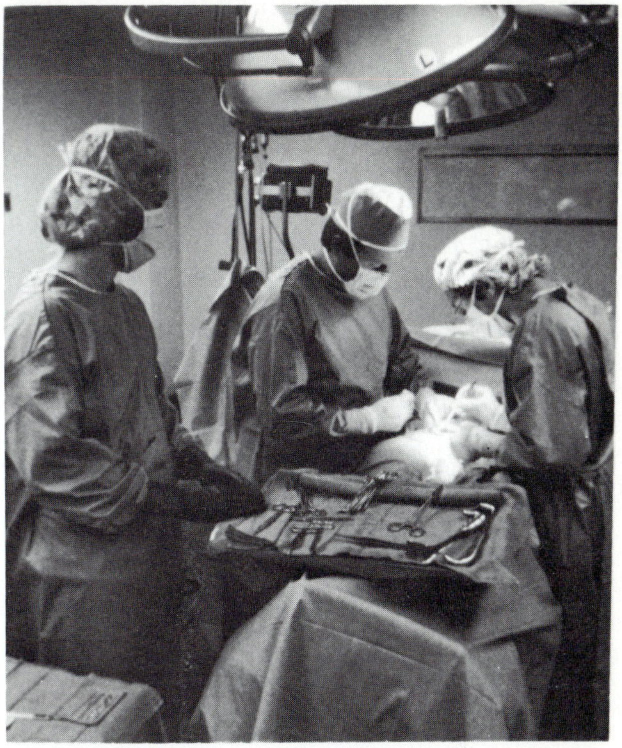

Figure 23-4.
Cesarean birth, once a measure of last resort, is now relatively safe and, in many cases, a lifesaving procedure. Nevertheless, it is major surgery and is not without risk for both the woman and the neonate. (Photo by BABES, Inc.)

Critics of the cesarean birth rate note that repeat cesarean deliveries contribute significantly to the total increase (Cunningham et al., 1989). In fact, repeat cesareans account for approximately 35% of all surgical births (Taffel et al., 1991). Current practice also reflects the nature of the obstetrician's education: a physician who receives obstetric training in a setting where medical and obstetric conditions are treated by surgical intervention has little opportunity to learn other, equally safe techniques for vaginal delivery. Individual physician practice style was, in fact, the only apparent determinant of cesarean rates in several studies conducted to identify reasons for cesarean birth (DeMott & Sandmire, 1990; Goyert, Bottoms, Treadwell, & Nehra, 1989). Finally, fears of malpractice suits may influence the decision to perform a cesarean delivery in a significant number of cases (Cunningham et al., 1989).

Types of Cesarean Birth

There are two major types of cesarean deliveries: low-segment and classical. The most commonly used is the low-segment procedure. In the low-segment delivery, the skin incision is made horizontally. This is called a Pfannenstiel incision or, more popularly, the "bikini cut" (Fig. 23-5). The cut is made transversely on the skin at the level of the mon pubis, and a horizontal incision is made in the lower segment of the uterus. Because the skin incision is low, it is later hidden by pubic hair; thus the name "bikini cut."

A major advantage of the low-segment incision is that there is less chance of rupture from the uterine scar in future pregnancies. The risk of rupture is decreased because the tissue of the lower uterine segment is less contractile than the body of the uterus. Blood loss is minimal because the lower uterine segment is thinner than the body of the uterus. There are fewer postdelivery complications with the low-segment incision, and it is easy to repair. Studies indicate that the woman also experiences less postoperative abdominal distention. Its major drawback is that the procedure takes longer to perform and thus is not practical in an emergency. Because of the anatomic features of the area, there is limited ability to stretch the incision and limited space in which to work. This limitation can be alleviated by use of a low-segment *vertical* incision in the uterus, which has the advantages of the low-segment transverse incision but which can be extended into a classical midline incision, if more room is needed to deliver the neonate.

In a classical cesarean delivery, a vertical midline incision is made in the skin and also into the wall of the body of the uterus (see Fig. 23-5). This incision is preferable when there are abdominal adhesions from previous surgery and when the fetus is in a transverse lie, because it permits easier access to the fetus for delivery. This type of cesarean is also commonly used in an emergency delivery because more rapid access to the fetus is possible; however, blood loss is increased because large vessels in the myometrium are cut. Furthermore, the uterine musculature is weakened by a midline incision, and there is a greater chance of rupture of the uterine scar in subsequent pregnancies and labor.

On rare occasions, a cesarean hysterectomy may have to be performed. In this case, the uterus is removed after delivery of the fetus. This is radical surgery reserved for frank

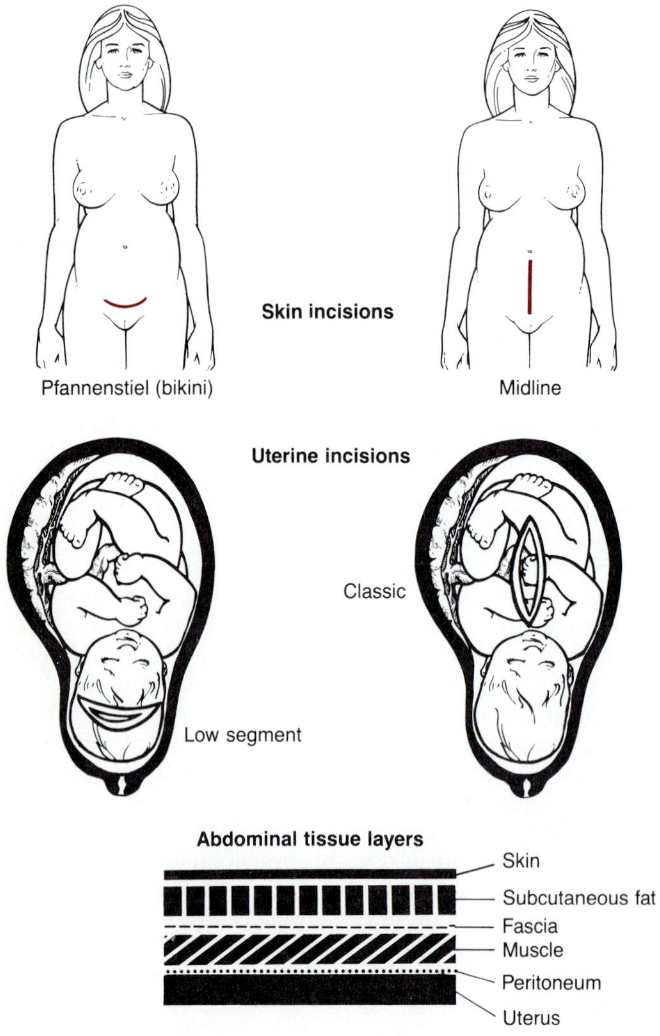

Figure 23-5.
Cesarean birth incisions (Childbirth Graphics).

obstetric emergencies, including uncontrolled uterine hemorrhage, placenta accreta (abnormal placental adherence to the uterine wall; see Chapter 26), uterine rupture, or fulminating uterine infection. The term *primary cesarean* refers to the woman's first cesarean delivery. The term *elective repeat cesarean* refers to a subsequent cesarean that is performed in the absence of a specific medical or obstetric indication for operative delivery. In the past, a previous cesarean delivery was considered a relative contraindication for subsequent vaginal delivery, even if the cause of the previous cesarean was nonrepeating (such as cord prolapse or breech presentation). Concern that the uterine scar would rupture during the stress of labor was the rationale for repeat elective cesarean delivery. Uterine rupture was thought to be a frank obstetric emergency with high maternal and fetal risk. As discussed later in this chapter, however, the risk of uterine rupture seems to have been overestimated; trial of labor and VBAC is increasingly regarded as a safe and appropriate mode of obstetric management for selected women.

Anesthesia for Cesarean Birth

The selection of anesthesia for cesarean birth depends on maternal status and medical history, fetal status, urgency of delivery, and site of the operative procedure. Regional anesthesia (either spinal or epidural block) as well as general anesthesia are commonly used for cesarean delivery (see Managing Pain During the Intrapartum Period, Chapter 23). In many settings, general anesthesia is used only in emergency situations when there is insufficient time for administration of regional anesthesia. Family-centered care is facilitated by use of regional anesthesia because the woman is alert during the birth and in many cases the father or support person may be present (Fig. 23-6).

Indications and Contraindications

The primary goal of a cesarean delivery is the preservation of the life and well-being of both the woman and fetus. A variety of conditions are considered relative indicators for a cesarean birth, whereas others are considered absolute. A discussion of each follows.

Cephalopelvic disproportion (*CPD*) is the most common reason given for cesarean birth and indicates a spatial inadequacy of the maternal pelvis in relation to the fetal head. This problem impedes the fetus from passing through the pelvic canal. A maternal history of a contracted pelvis or severe pelvic trauma, or a diagnosis of extreme fetal macrosomia with an estimated birth weight of greater than 4500 g (9 lb, 14 oz) suggests the likelihood of CPD and the need for a cesarean birth.

Malpresentation of the fetus exists when the fetus is in a transverse (sideways) or breech (buttocks or feet first) position. Vaginal delivery is potentially dangerous for the woman and fetus when these fetal positions exist. Although vaginal delivery of a fetus in the breech position may be uncomplicated, when the fetal head becomes obstructed at the vaginal opening, the problem is serious. For this reason, some obstetricians feel that in most circumstances breech presentations should be delivered surgically to protect the neonate's well-being. With the development of computed tomography pelvimetry and the ability to more accurately assess the woman's pelvic dimensions, evidence is growing that breech vaginal birth is a safe alternative to cesarean

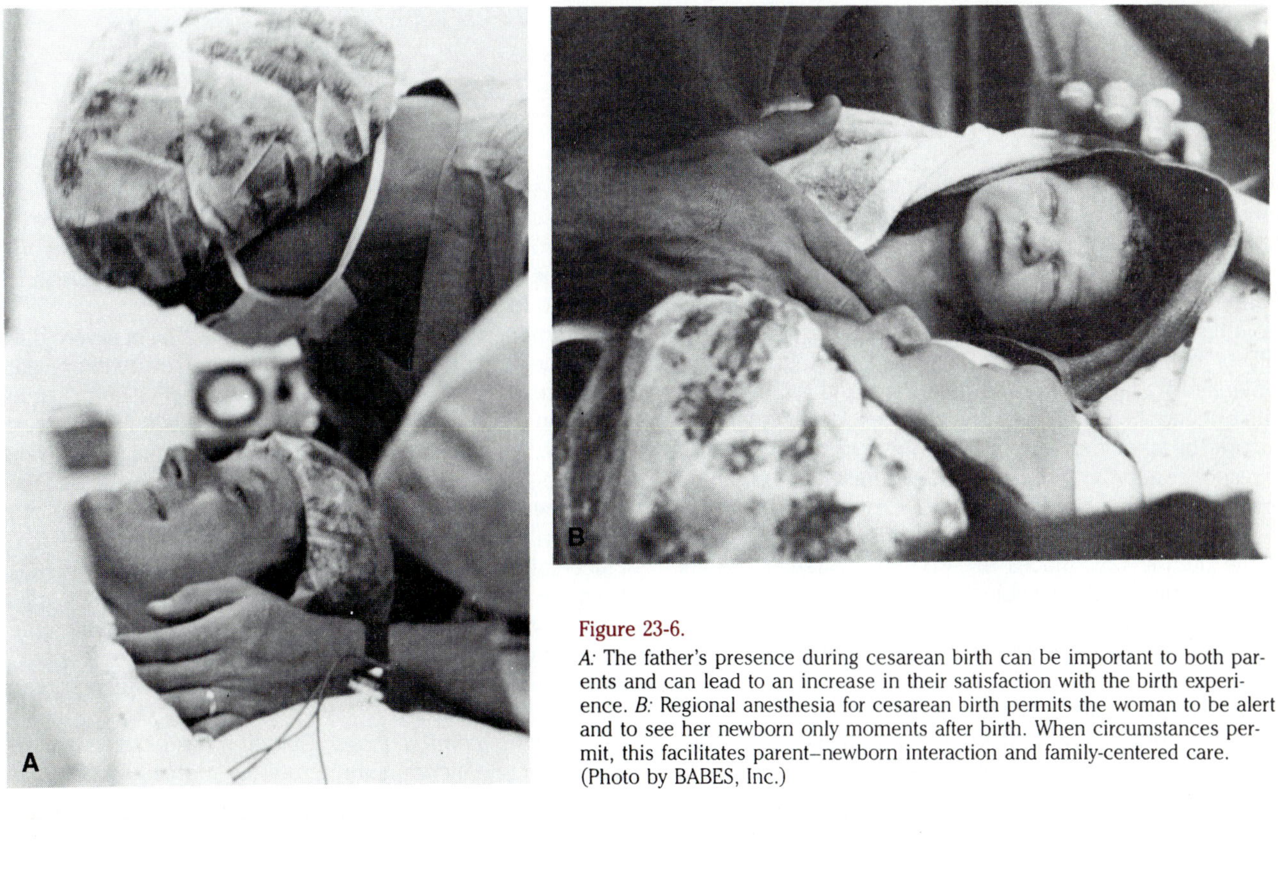

Figure 23-6.

A: The father's presence during cesarean birth can be important to both parents and can lead to an increase in their satisfaction with the birth experience. *B:* Regional anesthesia for cesarean birth permits the woman to be alert and to see her newborn only moments after birth. When circumstances permit, this facilitates parent–newborn interaction and family-centered care. (Photo by BABES, Inc.)

Legal/Ethical Considerations

Enforced Cesarean Birth

In the past decade, approximately two dozen courts have been asked to order enforced cesarean deliveries. One case in particular in 1987 received wide media coverage. A judge ordered a cesarean delivery for a 27-year-old woman suffering from terminal cancer who was 26 weeks pregnant. The surgery was performed against the express wish of the patient and her family and in violation of the ethical principle of autonomy (the right of each person to choose or refuse recommended medical treatment). The infant died of complications of prematurity several hours after birth; the mother died 2 days later—her death possibly hastened by the surgical procedure. In response to the current movement to treat pregnant women differently from other autonomous human beings. The Committee of Ethics of the American College of Obstetricians and Gynecologists drafted an opinion "Patient Choice: Maternal–Fetal Conflict." Major elements of the opinion are:

- The maternal–fetal relationship remains a unique one, requiring a balance of maternal health, autonomy, and fetal needs.
- Every reasonable effort should be made to protect the fetus, but the pregnant woman's autonomy should be respected.
- Consultation with the institution's ethics committee should be sought to aid the pregnant woman and obstetrician in making decisions.
- The use of courts to resolve conflicts is almost never warranted.
- The use of judicial authority to implement treatments to protect the fetus violates the pregnant woman's autonomy.

The nurse is often the first health professional to become aware of an impending conflict. Efforts must be made to open lines of communication between the woman, family, physician, and all other members of the health care team, who will participate in specific procedures. (These procedures are most often performed on poor, nonwhite women and on those whose first language is not English.)

When ethical principles are violated, nurses may be guided by the ACOG opinion statement as well as the American Nurses Association Code of Ethics. According to the Code, the nurse may morally refuse to participate in care on the grounds of patient advocacy or moral objection to a specific type of intervention. ANA also supports the nurse's participation in the institutional ethical review process, which is essential when maternal–fetal conflicts arise.

ACOG. (1987). Patient choice: Maternal-fetal conflict *(No. 55). ACOG Committee on Ethics Opinion.*
ANA. (1988). Ethnics in nursing: Position statements and guidelines. *Kansas City, Mo; ANA Committee on Ethics.*
Johnson, S. (1992). Ethical dilemma: A patient refuses a life-saving cesarean. American Journal of Maternal Child Nursing, *17(3), 121–125.*

when careful screening and monitoring are used. The practitioner must also be skilled in performing vaginal breech deliveries.

Labor dystocia describes inefficient or uncoordinated uterine contractions, inability of the cervix to dilate, and prolonged labor. Labor dystocia may also be associated with CPD or fetal malpresentation. Failure of labor to progress is evidenced by lack of cervical dilatation and fetal descent with documented adequate uterine forces. Unsuccessful induction of labor may occur when the cervix is unripe or unresponsive to oxytocin. In these circumstances cesarean delivery may also be required.

Previous "classical" cesarean incision through the body of the uterine wall places the woman at greater risk for uterine rupture when subjected to the stress of labor. Planned cesarean births are frequently advised. This trend may decrease as more physicians peform the low uterine segment incision.

Soft-tissue dystocia refers to the inability of the fetus to descend through the woman's pelvis or vagina due to excessive maternal or fetal adipose tissue or the presence of tumors such as uterine fibroids. Soft-tissue dystocia may also be caused by previous surgery or injury to the tissue of the reproductive tract, which causes cervical rigidity, stenosis of the vagina, or scars in the genital tract. A cesarean is required in this case.

Complications of pregnancy, such as PIH or severe diabetes mellitus may necessitate cesarean delivery to prevent severe maternal or fetal compromise. An active herpesvirus infection of the genital tract indicates the need for cesarean delivery. When herpes lesions in the birth canal are actively shedding virus at the time of delivery, as many as 50% of the infants will become infected. Neonatal herpes infection can result in neurologic injury, long-term disability, or death. Placental insufficiency and oligohydramnios, which results from the aging of the placenta in postterm pregnancy, may also suggest the need for an operative delivery. When prenatal testing of the postterm fetus reveals it to be in jeopardy and induction of labor is not feasible or successful, cesarean delivery is performed.

Maternal complications, including cardiac disease, hypertension, Rh incompatibility, uterine anomaly, or previous vaginal repair, may also be relative indications for cesarean delivery. Other *high-risk obstetric factors* are absolute contraindicators for a vaginal birth and signal the need for cesarean delivery. These factors include complete placenta previa, severe placental abruption and hemorrhage, umbilical cord prolapse, unrelieved fetal distress, conjoined twins, and persistent transverse lie.

Relative contraindications for cesarean delivery include the presence of a dead fetus or an immature fetus that could not survive outside the uterine environment. In these situations, the maternal risk of operative delivery is not justified.

Advantages and Disadvantages

Advantages of cesarean birth include the ability to deliver a fetus rapidly when fetal or maternal well-being is threatened or when this threat would be increased by continuing labor. The incidence of intraventricular hemorrhage may be lowered in preterm infants delivered by cesarean by reducing the pressure exerted on the fetal head during labor and birth (Philip & Allan, 1991). Operative birth may reduce the incidence of trauma and neonatal asphyxia associated with shoulder dystocia when the estimated fetal weight exceeds 4500 g (9 lb, 14 oz) and a diagnosis of severe fetal macrosomia is made. Although cesarean birth is generally thought to improve maternal and neonatal outcomes, current studies do not universally support this assumption. DeMott and Sandmire (1990) and Goyert et al., (1989) found that higher cesarean rates did not result in better neonatal outcomes. In fact a recent study by Belizan and associates (1991) indicates that infants born by elective cesarean delivery may experience greater morbidity such as prematurity and transient tachypnea and longer hospital stays. Otamiri and colleagues (1991) discovered lower noradrenaline levels, poorer muscle tone, and reduced arousability in the early neonatal period when infants are delivered surgically.

For the woman, the fact that cesarean birth is major abdominal surgery is the greatest disadvantage of this mode of delivery. Maternal mortality and morbidity are increased over that of vaginal birth. Surgical complications, such as hemorrhage, anesthetic reactions, embolization, injury to pelvic or abdominal organs, and infection, may result. Hospital costs and length of stay are increased. Maternal–infant interactions may be delayed or disrupted by postoperative pain, fatigue, or drowsiness secondary to narcotics administration. The initiation of breastfeeding may also be impeded, and if the woman is employed, the extended period required for recuperation may delay return to work.

Disruption in the woman's support network is another negative aspect of cesarean birth. Fathers and support persons are often excluded from the delivery room if a cesarean is required, despite growing evidence that their presence increases the woman's emotional comfort and may contribute to easier postnatal adaptation. Opponents to the presence of the father or support person in the surgical suite may be concerned about an increased infection rate, or fear that the sights and sounds of the surgery will be overwhelming, or that malpractice litigation will become more likely if complications arise and the person is a witness to the care rendered. Others argue that if the cesarean is done under general anesthesia, the father or support person cannot support the woman emotionally and therefore has no role in the delivery room. In fact, the opposite appears to be true; infection rates and malpractice cases have not increased in centers allowing the father or support person to attend cesarean birth (see Fig. 23-6). The birth can still be experienced as a special event. Many support persons desire the opportunity to stay with the woman, even if a general anesthetic is administered, to "welcome the infant" and take pictures to share with her later when she is awake (May & Sollid, 1984).

Finally, cesarean birth has been shown to have negative emotional consequences for some women. Certainly an unplanned cesarean delivery may be perceived as loss of the anticipated vaginal birth, and some women experience emotional upset when surgery is indicated. Other possible negative emotional reactions to cesarean birth identified by nurse researchers and other scientists include anger, depression, fear of dying, long-term grief, lowered self-esteem, distorted body image, sense of powerlessness, psychosomatic symptoms, distorted time perceptions, feelings of being unable to breathe, lack of confidence in ability to recover, feelings of indifference about the infant, and repression of some aspects of the experience (Schimmel, 1991).

These feelings, with the longer postcesarean recovery period, may predispose the woman to difficulty during her early adjustment to motherhood.

Implications for Nursing Care

In many facilities the labor nurse is responsible for preparing the woman for cesarean delivery, but the procedure itself takes place in the operating room. In other settings cesarean deliveries are done in the labor and delivery unit, and the labor nurse assists with all phases of the birth. Nursing responsibilities combine aspects of surgical and maternity care.

The nurse may function in one of two roles during the cesarean birth. The *circulating nurse* provides the surgeons and anesthesiologist with essential supplies and equipment, and if the woman is awake, continues to offer emotional support and encouragement. The preparation of the support person is usually the responsibility of the circulating nurse. The *surgical nurse* assists the surgeon by providing sterile instruments, sutures, and other supplies during the procedure, and has a central role in maintaining surgical asepsis. In many facilities, assessments of the FHR remain the responsibility of the labor nurse until the abdomen is scrubbed and draped or may be transferred to nursing personnel in the operating room who are trained to interpret fetal monitor data. Once the procedure begins, the anesthesiologist assumes responsibility for assessing the woman's vital signs and responses to the surgery and anesthetics.

Preparing the Family in Elective, Unanticipated, and Emergency Conditions. Some aspects of nursing care vary depending on whether the procedure is elective, unanticipated, or done under emergency conditions.

If the procedure is elective, the couple can be prepared through prenatal cesarean childbirth classes. Films, videotapes, books, and other teaching aids are available to these women and their partners or support persons. Childbirth educators play a key role in preparing families for an elective cesarean birth (see the accompanying Nursing Research display).

If the need for cesarean delivery was not anticipated before admission to labor and delivery, the labor nurse will help prepare the woman and her support person for the surgical birth. Although obtaining informed consent is a responsibility of the nurse midwife or physician, the nurse plays a critical role in clarifying and reinforcing information provided by the primary health care provider. The nurse also describes essential aspects of the procedure, and if time permits, discusses immediate postpartum events and care. At times the need to perform a cesarean delivery is communicated as urgent, when in fact the woman has time to consider the information and make an informed decision. In nonemergency situations, the woman should be given time alone with her support person to consider the need for cesarean birth, alternative approaches, and probable consequences of those approaches before giving consent. If a woman feels she has been consulted and has some control over what happens to her, she is more likely to respond favorably and perceive the birth experience more positively. The nurse should allow time for the woman to express concerns and encourage her to ask any questions she may have.

Because the woman's response will be strongly influenced by her educational level and cultural background, the nurse should take these factors into consideration when preparing her for an operative delivery (see accompanying display).

Under emergency conditions the nurse must support the woman and her support person during rapidly changing events. In many instances the cesarean birth is accomplished in 10 to 15 minutes. In these circumstances the nurse will have many pressing tasks to complete in preparation for the procedure; however, providing brief, clear explanations and emotional support to the woman remains an essential element of nursing care. When the need for delivery is urgent, cesarean birth constitutes a traumatic event. The woman's anxieties about an operative birth will be intensified by the emergency, and she or the support person may verbalize fears about bodily harm or death. The support person or father of the infant is often not permitted into the operating room during an emergency and can feel overwhelmed and abandoned. Efforts should be made to assign another staff member to remain with the support person until the infant is delivered and more information can be provided.

Nursing Research

The Effects of Culture, Educational Level, and Socioeconomic Status on Perceptions of Cesarean Birth

A major criticism of many research findings in the past is their limited generalizability because the majority of subjects were middle class whites. More recent studies have attempted to discover the experience of cesarean birth among women of different ages, ethnic backgrounds, and educational levels.

A study conducted among low-income, Mexican-born women giving birth in the United States found the majority satisfied with their delivery and perceived the cesarean birth as "normal." Eleven percent believed there was an advantage to cesarean birth. Studies of adolescents, and other Hispanic groups, and low-income African-American women, revealed positive feelings about the operative birth. A predominant theme was relief that labor was behind them and that the baby was healthy. Many attributed positive neonatal outcomes to the cesarean birth.

Nurses must attempt to understand the sociocultural context of cesarean delivery. Although many women may verbalize negative feelings about the surgical birth, not all will perceive the experience as unsatisfactory. The initial transition to parenthood may be easier for women who are satisfied with the cesarean birth experience and have a positive attitude regarding this mode of delivery.

Cummins, L., Scrimshaw, S., & Engle, P. (1988). Views of cesarean birth among primiparous women of Mexican origin in Los Angeles. *Birth, 15*(3), 164.

Giving Emotional Support. The nurse should always try to appreciate the effect that an at-risk labor and cesarean delivery may have on the emotional state of the woman and her partner. When possible, they should be given time alone to gather their strength and take in information and events. Anxiety, tension, and fear are appropriate responses, and they may be expressed through anger, withdrawal, crying, and agitation. The nurse should assess how the woman and her support person are coping with their apprehension and offer support as needed.

The nurse should also facilitate a family-centered approach to the cesarean delivery. If the woman desires it, the father or support person should be permitted to attend the birth. The nurse should explain the partner's role during the birth. If the support person cannot or chooses not to be present, the nurse should keep them together as long as possible to promote maternal comfort and emotional support. Many women are especially afraid of the administration of regional anesthetic. If the anesthesiologist approves, the partner's presence during that procedure may be helpful and reassuring to the woman. When the support person is present for the cesarean birth, the nurse obtains suitable operating room attire and ensures that the partner knows where to go once dressed for the delivery.

The support person is typically seated at the woman's head during cesarean delivery. From this position he or she can touch and converse with the woman, and the anesthesiologist or circulating nurse can provide explanations and any needed assistance. Both the woman's and partner's view of the surgical field is blocked by a screen. If the support person is to be present at a delivery performed under general anesthesia, he or she is usually seated off to the side of the room where the birth can be observed.

The partner present at the cesarean delivery is often the first one to hold the neonate after it is stabilized. If the support person cannot or chooses not to be present, he or she can be encouraged to stay nearby and perhaps observe through the delivery room window if there are staff who can remain near and provide reassurance and information. The partner can also be encouraged to carry the newborn to the nursery. It is a nursing responsibility to keep the support person well informed about the status of mother and newborn before, during, and immediately after the operative procedure. Nursing research suggests that the presence of the father during a cesarean birth will later enhance caretaking activities.

Providing Preoperative Teaching. The labor nurse should explain the sequence of events leading up to the delivery and what can be expected during postanesthesia recovery. As physical preparations are made, the nurse describes each procedure, why it is needed, and what sensations the woman may feel. If the father or support person is present, the nurse provides anticipatory guidance so support can be given the woman during these preparations. The nurse reinforces information given by the anesthesiologist or nurse anesthetist regarding the analgesia and anesthesia that will be administered during and after the birth. If regional anesthesia is used, the woman will be awake during the procedure and requires ongoing explanations. She should be told that she may feel some abdominal pressure and pulling during the delivery. Specific procedures, such as the use of an electrocoagulation machine to ligate blood vessels (the machine makes a characteristic noise and emits an odor) or the routine sponge count, should be described so that she is not surprised and worried.

If circumstances permit, the nurse should also describe postanesthesia recovery routines and when the woman and her newborn are likely to be transferred to the postpartum unit. The woman should understand that she will have some pain from the incision and that analgesia will be offered as needed. Preoperative teaching about the importance of early ambulation, coughing, and deep breathing in the postoperative period can be done at this time. The nurse should explain that although these activities will cause discomfort at first, they are essential to reduce the risk of postoperative complications, such as respiratory infection and thromboembolism, and will shorten her recovery time. The woman should be able to demonstrate the following skills before the delivery:

- Coughing and deep breathing techniques
- Use of incentive spirometer
- Splinting and supporting of incision
- Proper positioning when resting, sitting, and standing
- Using traction bar to rise to a sitting position and moving up to the head of the bed

Prepping the Woman Preoperatively. The activities described here are typically performed by the nurse assuming the role of "circulator" in the surgical delivery room.

- Ensure that the woman's identification bracelet is correct. Prepare the infant's identification bracelets.
- Help the father or support person with preparations to attend the delivery.
- Obtain or determine that preoperative laboratory tests, including complete blood count, electrolytes, clotting studies, and type and crossmatch, have been drawn and that the results are available.
- Shave the abdominal area beginning just below the breasts and including the mons pubis.
- Insert an indwelling urinary catheter to dependent drainage to prevent bladder distention during delivery. This procedure may be delayed until anesthesia has been administered to reduce the discomfort associated with bladder catheterization.
- Insert an IV line or assess the patency of an existing line to ensure an open route for administration of medications, fluids, and blood. The bore of the needle must be large enough (18 or 16 gauge) for the administration of blood replacement.
- Maintain NPO status. The nurse may, however, administer a nonparticulate antacid 15 minutes before induction of anesthesia. In the event of vomiting and aspiration of stomach contents during surgery, the gastric acids will have been neutralized, which helps to prevent aspiration pneumonitis.
- Assist the woman with transfer to the operative delivery table. Supine hypotensive syndrome can occur as a result of the woman lying on her back. The operating table is tilted slightly to one side to relieve pressure of the uterus on the vena cava and maintain optimal circulation to the placenta.
- Assist the anesthesiologist when anesthesia is administered.
- Ascertain that the woman's arms are properly aligned and secured to arm boards. Ascertain that the legs are properly aligned and restrained.
- Scrub the abdomen with antiseptic solution.
- Notify other members of the health care team that the delivery is imminent: pediatrician, intensive care nursery staff, and anesthesia staff.
- Monitor the FHR until the woman's abdomen is scrubbed and draped. If internal EFM is performed, the FHR may be monitored until the uterine incision is made. The circulating nurse then disconnects the fetal scalp lead.
- Verify that the suction and cautery machines are functioning correctly.
- Assist with gowning and gloving of the physicians.
- Perform an initial sponge count with the scrub nurse and physician.

Providing Intraoperative Nursing Support. An important function of the nurse is the timing and documentation of events both before and during the procedure. This includes the time of the initial incision, the exact time of delivery of the infant, and the time at which the procedure is completed. The nurse stands by to give support to the woman and her partner during the birth, and assists the surgical team by providing additional equipment and supplies. See the accompanying display for further discussion of the nurse's legal/ethical responsibilities during an operative birth.

The delivery room or circulating nurse may also be needed by the pediatrician to assist with care of the neonate. Help may be required with suctioning of the infant, administering oxygen when necessary, clamping the umbilical cord, evaluating the newborn, administering intramuscular vitamin K and erythromycin opthalmic ointment, and applying identification bracelets on the infant's arm and leg. If the newborn is compromised, cardiopulmonary support and resuscitation efforts are begun. The nurse assists, as needed, and provides information and support to the parents. When the neonate has been assessed and is stabilized, it is given to the woman or her partner to hold. Nursing support of the family at this time may help to alleviate some of the feeling they may have of being deprived of a family-centered birth.

After delivery of the infant, the placenta will be delivered manually. The anesthesiologist is responsible for administering IV oxytocin to the woman, as ordered, at delivery of the placenta and antibiotics or other drugs required at this time. The nurse is often responsible for obtaining umbilical cord blood samples for pH and blood gas analysis as well as other laboratory tests. The placenta is weighed and may be sent to pathology for examination. A final sponge count is made and recorded. A dressing is applied to the incision and the woman is assisted onto the gurney and transferred to the recovery unit.

Giving Immediate Postcesarean Care. Immediate postcesarean care of the woman and her family is similar in many ways to nursing care after a vaginal birth (see the Nursing Care Plan earlier in the chapter). If possible, the family should be kept together in the recovery area and time should be made for interaction and closeness. Intravenous fluids will be continued for 24 to 48 hours, so accurate intake and output records must be maintained. Blood-tinged urine from an indwelling catheter suggests surgical trauma to the bladder and should be reported to the physician. Dietary intake is generally limited to clear liquids until bowel sounds are heard and then advanced as tolerated to a regular diet.

If the woman received a regional anesthetic, her postoperative care must include assistance with positioning until she has adequate sensation in her legs for movement in bed. The nurse must assess return of sensation and level of anesthesia every 15 minutes until sensation has completely returned. If a general anesthetic is used, the woman is usually sent to a postanesthesia care unit until her condition is stabilized, and then she is transferred to the postpartum unit.

As soon as the woman is fully awake, she should be permitted to see her partner and her newborn, if possible. When possible the father or support person should be encouraged to bring the newborn to the mother and give her information about the infant to promote the sense of a shared experience. Nursing care for this woman also must include special attention to coughing and deep breathing in the immediate postoperative period to prevent congestion and risk of infection. It is especially important for the nurse to spend time in the postpartum period with the woman who delivers by cesarean birth to allow her to talk over her birth experience, to express any feelings of loss or inadequacy, and to be reassured that she did the best she could under difficult circumstances. The woman and support person may

Legal/Ethical Considerations

Nursing Responsibilities During a Cesarean Birth

In many birthing units, the labor or circulating nurse maintains responsibility for the woman's well-being during the cesarean procedure. When malpractice litigation arises as a result of injury sustained during surgery, the nurse is often involved in claims of negligence. Several types of injury are common during cesarean procedures and are attributed to breaches in the standard of nursing care:

1. Skin burns resulting from improper placement of electrocautery pads placed under the patient when electrocoagulation equipment is used
2. Brachial nerve injuries caused by improper alignment and torsion of the arm when it is placed on the delivery table arm board
3. Leg injuries or falls from the delivery table due to failure to secure or improper restraint of the lower limbs

In addition, nurses are often implicated in malpractice claims when laparotomy sponges or instruments are left in the woman's abdomen due to an incorrect sponge or instrument count. Failure to ensure the woman's safety and establish a correct count of instruments, needles, or lap sponges remain major allegations in nursing malpractice cases. The nurse must take special care to protect the woman from musculoskeletal and skin injuries, particularly after the administration of analgesic and anesthetic agents, which reduce sensory-motor function and level of consciousness. The nurse must also focus full attention on procedures required to verify that all instruments, needles, and sponges are accounted for before the cesarean incision is closed.

Tammelleo, A. (1992). Can doctors rely on nurses' sponge counts? Regan Report on Nursing Law, 32 *(11), 2.*
ANA. (1988). Liability prevention and you. *Kansas City, Mo: Author.*

have a need to "relive" the experience by telling it to others in detail. The woman may also have gaps in her memory of events; these should be filled in as much as possible by the support person or the nurse to facilitate integration of the birth experience. The nurse should encourage as positive a view of the experience as possible and help the family focus on the newborn. If the neonate's condition is uncertain, the family will need additional nursing attention and support in the early postpartum period.

Trial of Labor and Vaginal Birth After Cesarean Delivery

At one time women who had had previous cesarean births were routinely advised to have repeat cesareans, even if the cause of the previous cesarean did not recur. Fear of uterine rupture during a subsequent labor prevented physicians from considering trial of labor and VBAC as a safe mode of delivery, since the uterine musculature was believed to be significantly weakened. More recent research suggests that the risks of VBAC may have been overestimated, however, and the trend toward trial of labor appears to be increasing. Reasons for the increase in the number of VBACs include consumer pressure to avoid operative delivery, cost increases, and maternal and neonatal risks of an operative procedure.

The ACOG has established guidelines for VBAC. They have rejected the concept of "routine repeat cesarean birth" and recommend that women with previous cesarean births with low transverse incisions should be counseled and encouraged to attempt labor (ACOG, 1988).

Indications and Contraindications

The ACOG indications for VBAC center on the woman's desire to avoid a repeat cesarean, and on factors that suggest that maternal–fetal risk can be managed, including the following:

- Low-segment uterine incision with previous cesarean
- Availability of emergency surgical facilities
- Physician readily available during labor

Contraindications (ACOG, 1988) include any of the usual contraindications for vaginal delivery as well as those listed here:

- Any contraindications for vaginal delivery
- Previous classical (vertical) uterine incision
- Strong likelihood of CPD
- Strong likelihood of fetal macrosomia (greater than 4000 g [8 lb, 13 oz])

Advantages and Disadvantages

Advantages of VBAC include the fact that it reduces maternal and neonatal risk associated with an operative procedure. VBAC significantly reduces financial costs and length of hospital stay. For women and their partners who view a vaginal delivery as highly desirable, this option may increase satisfaction with the outcome. Disadvantages include the small risk of uterine rupture and the need for an emergency cesarean and the need for more intensive monitoring during labor. Some woman whose previous labor was unusually long and painful may be very anxious during the trial of labor, requiring continuous support and coaching. Women who are strongly invested in a vaginal birth may focus too much on this goal and are greatly disappointed if the trial of labor fails.

Implications for Nursing Care

Nursing management and care of the woman undergoing trial of labor and VBAC are similar to those for other at-risk patients in labor. Close monitoring of uterine contraction patterns and fetal status is necessary. The FHR and uterine contraction patterns must assessed and documented every 15 minutes in the first stage and every 5 minutes in the second stage of labor (Shearer, 1992). Most facilities require the use of continuous electronic monitoring (Flamm, 1992). The woman may have an IV infusion started in the event complications arise. The nurse must be alert to signs that labor is not progressing normally (arrest of progress, fetal distress, signs of uncoordinated uterine activity). Signs that suggest uterine scar weakening or rupture include maternal report of a "tearing" sensation, abrupt cessation of labor, and developing signs of maternal hypovolemic shock and fetal distress. If observed, these signs must be reported immediately, and and the nurse must be prepared for the likelihood of an emergency cesarean delivery.

Growing experience with VBAC has resulted in a relaxation of many restrictions imposed on the woman attempting a trial of labor. The ACOG (1988) recommends that normal activity be encouraged during latent phase labor, especially ambulation. Oxytocin infusions for induction or augmentation of labor have been administered safely and effectively, and regional anesthesia such as epidurals can be used for pain relief (Flamm, Goings, & Fuelberth, 1987). Recent studies have also demonstrated that forceps application or vacuum extraction can be used safely (Flamm, Lim, & Jones, 1988).

When complications arise that require the nurse midwife or physician to modify the normal mode of vaginal delivery, the nurse plays an important role in the procedure. The nurse assists the birth attendant by assembling necessary equipment and supplies and notifying additional staff members in a timely manner. The nurse also reinforces essential information about the procedure and answers additional questions the woman and her support person may have regarding the delivery. Although anesthesiology personnel often assume primary responsibility for monitoring the woman's physiologic status, physical and emotional support of the woman and assessment of fetal well-being remain nursing duties. The woman's perceptions of events are strongly influenced by the quality of nursing care provided during active management of labor and birth. The goal of nursing care at this time is to facilitate a family-centered birth experience, regardless of the mode of delivery.

Chapter Summary

When the woman or fetus is seen to be at increased intrapartum risk, various interventions can be used to reduce that risk. The nurse plays an important role in identifying women who are at increased risk as they begin the labor process as well as those who develop problems in the intrapartum period.

Modern obstetrics offers a range of techniques designed to reduce the risks, including intensively monitoring fetal status, managing maternal pain, modifying labor patterns, and modifying the mode of delivery. Each of these modes of risk reduction includes a number of obstetric interventions that can help ensure a positive birth outcome for many women and their newborns. Each obstetric intervention increases the need for expert nursing support in the intrapartum period.

The nurse strives to balance an increasingly technologic approach to labor care with an increasingly caring and human emphasis, for women at increased risk in labor and birth need this type of care, perhaps even more than normal, low-risk women. To achieve this balance, the nurse must be able to integrate technology and intensive intervention into care so that it supplements the professional hands-on assessment of the woman's status rather than substituting for it. The nurse must be capable of providing family-centered support for these women and their families despite the increased level of medical and nursing intervention required in their care. In this way, nursing makes a significant contribution to the safety and well-being of the woman and her fetus/newborn and to the emotional well-being of the family as a whole.

Study Questions

1. *Why is an amniotomy not recommended by some health professionals as a method for stimulating labor?*
2. *What is the appropriate nursing care for the woman who receives intravaginal prostaglandin gel for "cervical ripening?"*
3. *What are the nurse's responsibilities in the administration of oxytocin for the induction or augmentation of labor?*
4. *Under what conditions are forceps used during delivery?*
5. *What are the nurse's responsibilities during forceps application?*
6. *What is the purpose of the vacuum extraction delivery?*
7. *What are five common indications for cesarean delivery?*
8. *What preoperative preparation, teaching, and emotional support would the nurse offer a woman before cesarean delivery?*
9. *You are caring for a woman in labor who delivered her last child by cesarean section. What are the special aspects of your care based on her obstetric history?*
10. *What should be included in the nursing care of the woman who has given birth by cesarean delivery?*
11. *How can the nurse promote family-centered care in the event of an unscheduled cesarean delivery that requires administration of a general anesthetic?*

References

ACOG. (1991a). *Induction and augmentation of labor* (No. 157). ACOG Technical Bulletin.

ACOG. (1991b). *Operative vaginal delivery* (No. 152). ACOG Technical Bulletin.

ACOG. (1988). *Guidelines for vaginal delivery after a previous cesarean birth* (No. 64). ACOG Opinion.

American Society of Hospital Pharmacists. (1990). *American Hospital Formulary Society Drug Information*. Bethesda, MD: Author.

Barrett, J., Savage, J., Phillips, K., & Lilford, R. (1992). Randomized trial rof amniotomy in labour versus the intention to leave membranes intact until the second stage. (1992). *British Journal of Obstetrics and Gynaecology, 99*, 5.

Belizan, J., Quaranta, P., Paquez, E., & Villar, J. (1991). Caesarean section and fear of litigation. *Lancet, 338*, 1462.

Bigrigg, A., Rees, A., & Read, M. (1991). Induction of labour in the presence of ruptured membranes with prostaglandin E2 gel. *Clinical Experiments in Obstetrics and Gynecology, XVIII*(3), 197.

Burke, M., Porreco, R., Day, D., Watson, J., Haverkamp, A., Orleans, M., & Luckey, D. (1989). Intrauterine resuscitation with tocolysis. *Journal of Perinatology, IX*(3), 296.

Cunningham, G., MacDonald, P. & Gant, N. (1989). *William's obstetrics* (18th ed.). Norwalk, CT: Appleton & Lange.

DeMott, R., & Sandmire, H. (1990). The physician factor as a determinant of cesarean birth rates. *American Journal of Obstetrics and Gynecology, 162*(6), 1593.

Donald, W., & Barton, J. Ultrasonography and external cephalic version. *American Journal of Obstetrics and Gynecology, 162*(6), 1542.

Egarter, C., Husslein, P., & Rayburn, W. (1990). Uterine hyperstimulation after low-dose prostaglandin E2 therapy. Tocolytic treatment in 181 cases. *American Journal of Obstetrics and Gynecology, 163*, 794.

Elliott, J., Clewell, W., & Radin, T. (1992). Intracervical prostaglandin E2 gel. Safety for outpatient cervical ripening before induction of labor. *Journal of Reproductive Medicine, 37*(8), 713.

Flamm, B. (1992). Should the electronic fetal monitor always be used for women in labor who are having a vaginal birth after a previous cesarean section? *Birth, 19*(1), 31.

Flamm, B., Goings, J., & Fuelberth, N. (1987). Oxytocin during labor after previous cesarean section: Results of a multicenter study. *Obstetrics and Gynecology, 79*(5), 709.

Flamm, B., Lim, O., & Jones, C. (1988). Vaginal birth after cesarean section—results of a multicenter study. *American Journal of Obstetrics and Gynecology, 158*, 1079.

Food and Drug Administration. (1978). *New restrictions on oxytocin use*. Washington DC: FDA Drug Bulletin.

Fraser, W., Sauve, R., Parboosingh, T., Sokol, R., & Persaud, D. (1991). A randomized controlled trial of early amniotomy. *British Journal of Obstetrics and Gynaecology, 98*, 84.

Glazer, G., & Hulme, A. (1987). Prostaglandin gel for cervical ripening. *American Journal of Maternal Child Nursing, 12*, 28–31.

Goyert, G., Bottoms, S., Treadwell, M., & Nehra, P. (1989). The physician factor in cesarean birth rates. *New England Journal of Medicine, 320*(11), 706.

Hauth, J., Hankins, G., Gilstrap, L., Strickland, D., & Vance P. (1986). Uterine contraction pressures with oxytocin induction/augmentation. *Obstetrics and Gynecology, 68*, 305–309.

Macer, J., Macer, C., & Chan, L. (1992). Elective induction versus spontaneous labor: A retrospective study of complications and outcome. *American Journal of Obstetrics and Gynecology, 166*(6), 1690.

Mandeville, L., & Troiano, N. (1992). *High-risk intrapartum nursing*. Philadelphia: JB Lippincott.

May, K., & Sollid, D. (1984). Unanticipated cesarean birth: From the father's perspective. *Birth, 11*(2), 87.

Maymon, R., Shyulman, A., Pomeranz, M., Holtzinger, M., Haimovich, L., & Behary, C. (1991). Uterine rupture at term pregnancy with the use of intracervical prostaglandin E2 gel for induction of labor. *American Journal of Obstetrics and Gynecology*, *165*(2), 368.

McColgin, S., Hamptom, H., McCaul, J., Howard, P., Andrew, M., & Morrison, J. (1990). Stripping membranes at term: Can it safely reduce the incidence of post-term pregnancies? *Obstetrics and Gynecology*, *76*(4), 678.

Milliez, J., Jannet, D., Touboul, C., Mahfoudh, M., & Paniel, B. (1991). Maturation of the uterine cervix by repeated intracervical instillation of prostaglandin E2. *American Journal of Obstetrics and Gynecology*, *165*(3), 523.

Musacchio, M. (1990). *Oxytocins for augmentation and induction of labor*. New York: March of Dimes.

NAACOG. (1998). *The nurse's role in the induction/augmentation of labor*. OGN Nursing Practice Resource. Washington, DC: Author.

O'Leary, J., & Leonetti, H. (1990). Shoulder dystocia: Prevention and treatment. *American Journal of Obstetrics and Gynecology*, *162*(1), 5.

Otamiri, G., Berg, G., Ledin, T., Leijon, I., & Lagercrantz, H. (1991). Delayed neurological adaptation in infants delivered by elective cesarean section and the relation to catecholamine levels. *Early Human Development*, *26*, 51.

Philip, A., & Allan, W. (1991). Does cesarean section protect against intraventricular hemorrhage in preterm infants? *Journal of Perinatology*, *XI*(1), 3.

Rayburn, W. (1989). Prostaglandin E2 gel for cervical ripening and induction of labor: A critical analysis. *American Journal of Obstetrics and Gynecology*, *160*(3), 529.

Schimmel, L. (1991). Cesareans and care. In P. Chinn (Ed.). *Anthology on caring* (pp.). New York: National League for Nursing Press.

Seitchik, J., & Castillo, M. (1983). Oxytocin augmentation of dysfunctional labor. *American Journal of Obstetrics and Gynecology*, *145*(7), 777.

Shearer, E. (1992). Should the electronic fetal monitor always be used for women in labor who are having a vaginal birth after a previous cesarean section? *Birth*, *19*(1), 33.

Shekarloo, A., Bauer, C., Cook, V., & Freese, U. (1989). Terbutaline (intravenous bolus) for the treatment of acute intrapartum fetal distress. *American Journal of Obstetrics and Gynecology*, *60*(3), 615.

Stein, J., Bardequez, A., Verma, U., & Tegani, N. (1990). Nipple stimulation for labor augmentation. *Journal of Reproductive Medicine*, *35*(7), 710.

Taffel, S., Placek, P., & Kosary, C. (1992). U.S. cesarean section rates 1990: An update. *Birth*, *19*(1), 21.

Taffel, S., Placek, P., Moien, M., & Kosary, C. (1991). 1989 U.S. cesarean section rate steadies-VBAC rate rises to nearly one in five. *Birth*, *18*(2), 73.

Tighe, D., & Sweezy, S. (1990). The perioperative experience of cesarean birth: Preparation, considerations, and complications. *Journal of Perinatal Neonatal Nursing*, *3*(3), 14.

Suggested Readings

Afriat, C. (1990). Vaginal birth after cesarean section: A review of the literature. *Journal of Perinatal Neonatal Nursing*, *3*(3), 1.

Brodsky, P., & Pelzar, E. (1991). Rationale for the revision of oxytocin administration protocols. *Journal of Obstetric, Gynecologic, and Neonatal Nursing*, *20*, 440.

Commiskey, K., & Dawood, M. (1990). Induction of labor with pulsatile oxytocin. *American Journal of Obstetrics and Gynecology*, *163*, 1868.

Committee on Obstetrics. (1991). Fetal maturity assessment prior to elective repeat cesarean delivery. Number. Committee Opinion Number 98. Washington DC: ACOG.

Fawcett, J. (1990). Preparation for caesarean childbirth: Derivation of a nursing intervention from the Roy Adaptation Model. *Journal of Advanced Nursing*, *15*, 1418.

Fortier, J. C. (1988). The relationship of vaginal and cesarean births to father–infant attachment. *Journal of Obstetric, Gynecologic, and Neonatal Nursing*, *17*, 128–134.

Musacchio, M. (1989). *Oxytocics for augmentation and induction of labor*. White Plains, NY: March of Dimes Birth Defects Foundation.

Seitchik, J., Amico, J., & Castillo, M. (1985). Oxytocin augmentation of dysfunctional labor. V. *American Journal of Obstetrics and Gynecology*, *151*, 757.

Ward, C. (1991). Analysis of 500 obstetric and gynecologic malpractice claims: Causes and prevention. *American Journal of Obstetrics and Gynecology*, *165*(2), 298.

CHAPTER 24

Managing Pain During the Intrapartum and Postpartum Periods

Learning Objectives

After studying the material in this chapter, the student should be able to:

- Discuss the causes of pain in childbirth.
- Outline the adverse effects of pain on maternal and fetal well-being.
- Explain the behavioral cues of pain in the woman during labor and birth.
- Describe common verbal indicators of pain during childbirth.
- Identify the most common types of obstetric analgesia and anesthesia.
- List advantages and disadvantages of obstetric analgesia and anesthesia.
- Describe nursing responsibilities during the administration of analgesia or anesthesia.
- List major complications of obstetric analgesia and anesthesia.

Key Terms

analgesia
anesthesia
general anesthesia
local anesthesia
regional anesthesia

Most women approaching their expected date of delivery are concerned about the degree and duration of discomfort or pain they will have to endure. Each woman experiences the physical sensations of labor differently. For some, uterine contractions, the process of cervical dilatation, and fetal descent will create feelings of "discomfort" that range from mild to intense. Other women will describe labor and birth in terms of "pain." "Pressure" is a word often used by women to describe the predominant sensation accompanying childbirth. Even the multigravida will have concerns about the discomfort and pain of childbirth, because each labor is different, and no one can predict what subsequent labor experiences will be like in terms of pain (see the Nursing Research display, Differences in Perceptions of Pain in Primigravidas and Multigravidas).

Labor nurses differ philosophically in how to describe the sensations evoked by labor and childbirth. Many nurses have been educated to avoid the use of the word "pain" in relation to contractions. They have been taught that labor need not be painful when women are adequately prepared. Furthermore, it is suggested that using the word "pain" when speaking with the laboring woman may negatively influence her perceptions of sensations that are due more to pressure or stretching than pain. Other nurses believe that some degree of pain is experienced by most women during labor and birth, even though the pain varies widely in nature, extent, and location. These nurses believe that it is important to address the issue of pain, to question the woman about the nature and degree of pain, and to educate her about pharmacologic options in managing it.

Conversely, many new mothers and health professionals assume that pain is a common and expected problem in the postpartum period. Callahan-Faut and Paice (1990) identify two "myths" regarding pain that are prevalent among nurses who care for the women after birth:

- Myth 1: New mothers accept pain after delivery as unavoidable, just as they accept it during labor and delivery.

Nursing Research

Differences in Perceptions of Pain in Primigravidas and Multigravidas

Pain has been described as a multidimensional, subjective experience of discomfort composed of both sensory and affective components. Although few investigators have explored the differences in the experience of pain between primigravidas and multigravidas, nurse researchers have begun to systematically describe the dimensions of pain during labor in these two groups of women.

Johansson and associates (1988) found that the sensory component of pain was more severe than the affective dimension in *both* primigravidas and multigravidas during labor. Primigravidas reported more intense sensory pain during the first stage of labor and more affective pain in all stages of childbirth, even though they received more analgesia. Primigravidas also reported significantly higher sensory and affective pain in the study of labor pain by Brown and associates (1989). The authors noted that nonpharmacologic methods for pain relief may be useful for reducing the affective component of pain but that analgesia was more effective for lowering sensory pain intensity.

While formulating an individualized care plan for pain control, clinicians should bear in mind that primigravidas may in general experience greater pain and require more intensive emotional and pharmacologic support during labor and birth.

Brown, S., Campbell, D., & Kurtz, A. (1989). Characteristics of labor pain at two stages of cervical dilation. *Pain, 38,* 289.

Johansson, F. G., Fridh, G., Norvell, K. T. (1988). Progression of labor pain in primiparas and multiparas. *Nursing Research, 37*(2), 86–89.

- Myth 2: If mothers and infants are exposed to the dangers of analgesic therapy, appropriate maternal–infant bonding may not occur.

Although minor discomforts are common in the immediate postpartum period, unrelieved pain that interferes with rest and sleep and the ability to perform activities of daily living requires prompt alleviation. Unrelieved pain can, in fact, interfere with the maternal–infant acquaintance process and bonding. Women most likely to suffer from pain in the postpartum period are those who require operative interventions such as cesarean birth or the use of forceps or vacuum extraction at delivery.

This chapter reviews the causes of discomfort or pain experienced during childbirth and during the postpartum period and discusses pharmacologic methods used to control these sensations. Nursing responsibilities in reducing discomfort and pain and in the administration of obstetric analgesia and anesthesia are outlined in detail. Because nonpharmacologic techniques for pain control, such as breathing techniques, have been discussed in Chapters 18, 20, and 21, the emphasis in this section will be on pharmacologic modes of pain relief.

Pain and Discomfort During the Intrapartum and Postpartum Period

Many women have been told that childbirth is the most painful experience they will ever have, and they fully expect to suffer through labor and birth. Others have had previous labors in which their pain was not manageable by prepared childbirth techniques; such women approach labor worrying that they will not be able to tolerate that level of pain again. Other women may be shocked by a painful, difficult labor when their previous labors were more easily tolerated and will require pharmacologic pain relief. Still others will develop problems in the intrapartum period that require active obstetric intervention that may cause pain or that cannot be accomplished without anesthesia.

For most women, the actual birth leads to a pronounced reduction in sensations of pain, stretching, and pressure. The excitement accompanying birth also leads to a reduction in perceptions of pain. Complications or obstetric interventions can, however, result in tissue edema, perineal trauma (lacerations, hematomas, and bruising), an episiotomy, or cesarean incision. In some situations, sensations of pain can be intense and, unlike the pain associated with contractions, are continuous. The woman may be stoically resigned to this pain or refuse to take analgesics if she is breastfeeding, for fear that the drugs may harm the neonate. Others may be shocked and disappointed by the degree of pain and require maximum doses of analgesia to function.

Origins of Painful Stimuli

The sensations of discomfort, pain, and pressure that arise during vaginal birth originate primarily in the lower genital tract. Pain during labor may be related to a variety of physiologic factors including:

- Uterine hypoxia
- Stretching of the uterine ligaments
- Distention of the lower uterine segment
- Pressure on the nerve ganglia around the uterus and vagina
- Cervical stretching during dilatation
- Pressure on the bladder and urethra

Pain in first stage of labor is caused mainly by cervical stretching. These pain impulses are transmitted by sensory pathways that accompany the sympathetic nerves and pass through the spinal nerve to enter the spinal cord. Pain during this stage is usually felt in the lower abdomen and the skin over the lower lumbar spine and upper sacrum. With intense pain, sensations may also be felt above and below these areas, that is, in the upper thighs and the umbilical region.

Pain in the second stage of labor is caused primarily by the distention of the vagina and the perineum resulting from fetal descent. Pain impulses from these areas are transmitted by the sensory fibers of the pudendal nerves, which enter the posterior roots of the second, third, and fourth sacral nerves, as shown in Figure 24-1.

Many women will experience some discomfort from perineal edema, hemorrhoids, or muscle soreness in the immediate postpartum period. After several days, breast engorgement may also cause temporary discomfort. Varying sensations of pain are often present when obstetric interventions are implemented or complications arise that result in trauma or surgery, including:

- Vaginal, perineal, periurethral, or cervical lacerations
- Episiotomy
- Hematomas (vaginal or abdominal)
- Cesarean incision
- Fracture of the coccyx
- Hemorrhoids
- Backache secondary to spinal or epidural anesthesia
- Retained gas and abdominal distention postoperatively
- Spinal headache
- Infection (endometritis, episiotomy site)

Pain can be caused by edema, tension of incisions sites, inflammation, and pressure. Some women will describe the pain experienced during the postpartum period as more intense than the pain sensations felt during labor.

Effects of Pain

Physiologic Effects

Extreme distress from pain in childbirth itself can constitute a risk factor affecting both maternal and fetal status. When the woman experiences severe pain, significant physiologic changes can occur (Fig. 24-2), including an increase in cardiac output and blood pressure. Marked pain causes oxygen consumption to increase markedly; when hyperventilation is present, hypocarbia (excessive CO_2 loss) can re-

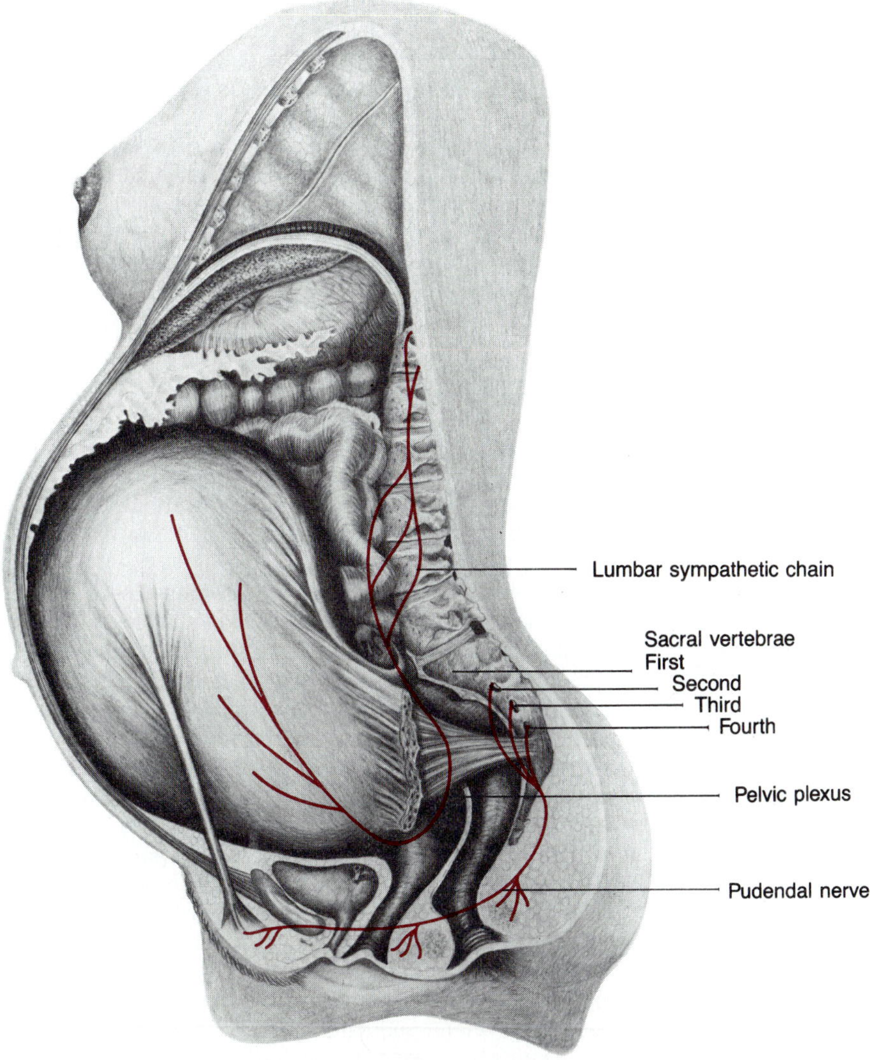

Figure 24-1.

Pain pathways during labor. The pain of vaginal delivery primarily originates in the lower genital tract, and painful stimuli from this region are transmitted through the pudendal nerve. Peripheral branches of this nerve provide sensory stimulation to the perineum and anus and to parts of the vulva and clitoris. Sensory fibers of the pudendal nerve originate from the ventral branches of the second, third, and fourth sacral nerves (Maternity Center Association, New York).

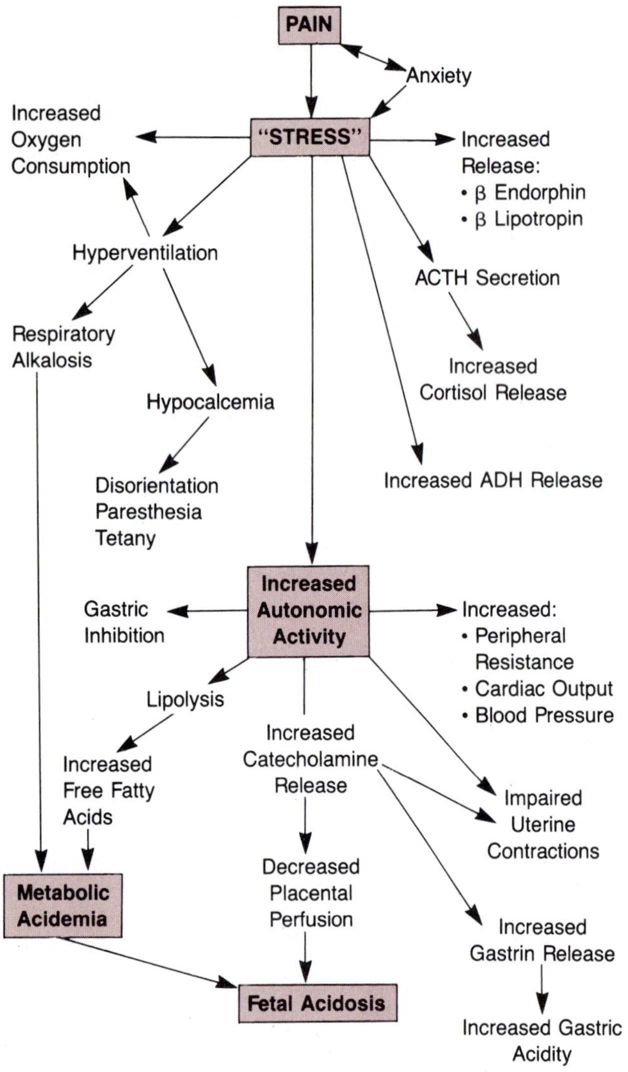

Figure 24-2.

Physiologic changes secondary to pain in labor. (From Brownridge, P., & Cohen, S. [1988]. In M. J. Cousins & P. O. Bridenbaugh [Eds.]. Neural Blockade, 2nd ed. Philadelphia: JB Lippincott.)

sult in decreased uterine and cerebral blood flow. Stress can result in increased secretion of epinephrine, which may in turn cause vasoconstriction and fetal hypoxia. Distress from pain exacerbates apprehension and muscular tension. This muscular tension increases the metabolic demands on the woman, contributing to acidosis, which may also affect fetal metabolic balance. Finally, muscular tension may result in reflex tightening of the pelvic floor, thus impeding descent and delivery of the fetus.

Postpartum pain can interfere with rest, which results in sleep deprivation and marked fatigue. Moderate to severe pain may interfere with breastfeeding by inhibiting the let-down reflex. Unrelieved pain after cesarean birth may prevent the woman from turning, coughing, deep breathing, and ambulating. This can lead to serious postoperative complications including pneumonia, thrombus formation, and delayed return in bowel and bladder function. Research clearly indicates that severe pain can also delay tissue healing.

Psychological Effects

The sensation of acute pain may also have immediate and long-term psychological effects. A woman who has previously been able to perform breathing and relaxation exercises during contractions and is suddenly unable to do so may become discouraged, frightened, or even panicky. She may experience a loss of self-esteem and confidence in her ability to maintain control of her physical and emotional responses. If the psychological need to remain in control is a strong aspect of the woman's personality, the loss of control can be devastating. Research indicates that fear of pain and helplessness can result in high levels of distress even in the early or latent phase of labor (Wuitchik, Hesson, & Bakal, 1990).

Pain during and after birth can have deleterious effects on the postpartum experience. Acute pain that lasts many hours leads to fatigue and distortions in perceptions of time, physical boundaries, and even reality. The woman may be unable to remember parts of her labor experience or the memories may be grossly distorted. After birth of the neonate, the woman may express anger toward her infant, viewing the newborn as the cause of the extreme distress experienced during childbirth. The fear of recurring pain in subsequent labors may diminish sexual responsiveness and create hesitancy to become pregnant again.

Unrelieved postpartum pain can interfere with the maternal–infant acquaintance process and the woman's ability to interact with other family members. She may become depressed, and feelings of failure or low self-esteem may surface. If nurses are unresponsive to the woman's verbalizations of pain or do not provide adequate analgesia to relieve pain, feelings of anger may also occur. The woman may doubt the validity of her feelings and the sensations of pain, further exacerbating feelings of low self-esteem.

Pain Management

Both *analgesia* (the absence or decreased awareness of pain without loss of consciousness) and *anesthesia* (the partial or complete loss of sensation with or without loss of consciousness) may be used to reduce pain during the intrapartum and postpartum periods.

Several major pharmacologic methods of pain relief are commonly used for childbirth. *Parenteral analgesics*, including narcotics combined with ataractics, and less frequently sedatives, are used to provide quick, effective, and easily administered pain relief during labor. They are given intravenously, intramuscularly, or subcutaneously. A new method of analgesia, *intrathecal analgesia*, is also being used in selected centers during labor and will be discussed in the next section of the chapter. *Conduction anesthesia*, which includes pudendal, epidural, and spinal anesthesia, uses anesthetic agents to provide pain relief by blocking sensory nerve impulses from a specific area of the body. *Inhalation anesthesia* may also be used in intrapartum care to provide brief periods of relief or to allow rapid induction of deep anesthesia for emergency operative procedures; it is also used when conduction anesthesia is not possible.

During the postpartum period, parenteral and oral analgesics are used to control pain. *Intravenous (IV) analgesia* may be provided through a relatively new method known as patient-controlled analgesia (PCA). It is usually reserved for the relief of pain after cesarean birth. *Intramuscular (IM) analgesia* is also administered, particularly when pain is intense or when the woman is NPO. If the woman is permitted oral intake, *oral analgesics* are often given to reduce mild to moderately intense postpartum pain. *Morphine (Duramorph)* can be injected into an *epidural* catheter to provide postoperative analgesia after cesarean birth.

Promotion of comfort and control of pain are important roles for the nurse during labor, birth, and the postpartum period. Research clearly indicates that pain management has been inadequate in many instances and results in negative outcome for the woman and her fetus (United States Department of Health and Human Services, 1992). The nurse administers many types of analgesics and other drugs useful in managing pain and must closely monitor maternal and fetal responses when analgesia and anesthesia are given. To effectively assist the woman with control of pain during childbirth and the postpartum period, the nurse implements the nursing process. This systematic approach to pain management begins with admission of the woman to the labor or birthing unit. The nurse assesses the woman's level of pain or discomfort, identifies immediate needs, and makes appropriate nursing diagnoses throughout the course of the hospital or birthing unit stay. Planning and implementation of nursing care to control pain are made in close collaboration with the woman. Evaluation of maternal–fetal responses to pain management is an essential component in the nursing process and will guide the nurse in revision of the care plan.

• • Assessment

Assessment of an individual woman's response to labor and the need for physical comfort, analgesia, or anesthesia requires sensitivity, experience, and a knowledge of research findings. The nurse must be knowledgeable about how various physiologic and psychological factors exacerbate pain. These factors include the quality of contractions, fatigue, anxiety, perceptions of childbirth, and readiness for and parenthood (see Chapter 20 and 21 for further discussion of pain and responses to pain during labor.)

Assessment begins with admission to the labor unit and may in part help to distinguish between true and false labor (see Chapter 20). The nurse must ascertain the nature, degree, and location of discomfort or pain. Determining the location of pain may alert the nurse to fetal presentation and position, stage of labor, and the presence of complications. For instance, low, persistent backache is associated with occiput posterior position, intense rectal pressure may herald the onset of the second stage of labor, and intense abdominal tenderness may indicate intrauterine infection or abruptio placentae.

In the postpartum period, ongoing assessment of the woman's level of discomfort or pain is also conducted. The nature of pain may suggest the development of specific problems. Constant rectal pressure in the first hours after birth may indicate the development of a vaginal hematoma. Uterine tenderness and low backache are common findings with uterine infection and subinvolution. Pain related to breastfeeding can occur with improper positioning of the infant on the breast and guides the nurse in the development of a teaching plan.

Assessing the Nature and Location of Pain

The nurse asks the woman to describe the pain; where it is most intense, whether it radiates, and if it is persistent or intermittent in nature. Other questions such as those that follow can help the nurse to identify the nature of discomfort and manage the woman's pain. Has the woman attempted to relieve the pain? What measures has she taken and have her attempts been successful? When did the pain begin? When did it change in intensity? The nurse should also discuss the woman's preparations, if any, for relief of discomfort and pain in labor. Did she attend childbirth preparation classes? What are her plans and desires for pain control and relief during labor? What is her knowledge base regarding breastfeeding and the use of analgesics? If she is a multipara, what has she experienced in previous pregnancies and what pain control methods were used? Finally, were these measures successful, and were any complications related to their use?

Verbal Reports of Pain

A persistent problem in assessment of discomfort and pain during labor is that pain itself is not observable. The nurse must rely on observations of behavior or the woman's own reports of pain. Many women will use terms synonymous with pain to describe labor sensations; others use terms that more accurately characterize pressure or tension. These descriptors help guide the nurse in pain management strategies. Table 24-1 lists common verbal descriptors of pain.

The intensity of pain, however, is *not* always congruent with the woman's verbal estimates of the degree of pain. Some women in early labor having very mild contractions may describe the sensations as "very painful," whereas

Table 24-1. Verbal Descriptors of Pain During Labor and Birth

Sensory	Affective
First Stage of Labor	
Cramping, pulling, aching, heavy, sharp, stabbing, cutting, intermittent, localized, global	Exciting, intense, tiring/exhausting, scary/frightening, bearable/unbearable, distressing, horrible, agonizing, indescribable, overwhelming, engulfing
Second Stage of Labor	
Painful pressure, burning, ripping, tearing, piercing, explosive, rending, localized	Exhausting, overwhelming, out-of-body feeling, inner focused/tunnel vision, exciting, horrible, excruciating, terrifying, less intense

others use the term "crampy" to explain the feelings experienced in the latent phase. Nurse researchers are using a variety of instruments to measure pain levels and explore the dimensions of pain during childbirth. These findings may help the labor nurse plan care for the woman in labor (Brown, Campbell, & Kurtz, 1989).

Nonverbal Cues of Pain

The nurse must be extremely sensitive to nonverbal cues of discomfort and pain during childbirth. This is particularly important if a language barrier exists between the woman and the health care provider. Restlessness, rapid breathing, diaphoresis, facial grimacing, and tensing of muscles are common nonverbal indicators of pain. Behavioral cues may also indicate the stage of labor. If a woman is able to smile or continue walking through contractions and suddenly stops walking and focuses on her breathing technique, it may herald the transition to a more active phase of labor. Conversely, knowing the woman's stage of labor may provide the nurse with some appreciation of the expected degree of pain. However, anxiety and fear may enhance sensations of mild discomfort, and abnormal labor or obstetric complications may produce intense pain even in the latent phase of labor.

Assessing Psychological Dimensions of Pain

To promote comfort and reduce pain, the nurse explores the woman's expectations about pain during labor, birth, and the postpartum period. Psychological factors play a central role in the perceptions of and response to pain. Some women will stoically accept intense pain without providing the nurse with physical or verbal cues to its presence. Other women may display an intense degree of discomfort when the first sensations of pain are perceived.

Nursing research suggests that a woman's confidence in her ability to cope with the pain during childbirth strongly influences her perceptions of discomfort (Lowe, 1991) and the course of labor and delivery. Extreme fear can actually slow the progress of cervical dilatation and prevent the woman from pushing effectively during the second stage of labor (McKay & Brown, 1991). Alterations in self-esteem may occur when the normally stoic woman or one with a strong need for control cries out in pain during labor or requests an anesthetic when she had planned for a "natural birth." Other women who anticipate early pharmacologic pain relief and do not receive it may experience profound disappointment in the birth experience.

Identifying Social and Cultural Influences on Pain Expression

Cultural beliefs and practices strongly influence the woman's perceptions and expressions of pain and her desire for analgesia or anesthesia. In some cultures women are cautioned against any expressions of pain during labor or after birth because they may alert "evil spirits" to the presence of a "defenseless" newborn. In other ethnic groups, loud vocalizations are expected and may be encouraged as a normal part of the childbirth experience. The attendance of another woman (doula) who has experienced childbirth to guide and support the primigravida is viewed as crucial in some societies. Recent research clearly demonstrates a strong relationship between the presence of a doula during labor and a decrease in the use of epidural anesthesia even among American women (Kennell, Klaus, McGrath, Robertson, & Hinkley, 1991). Many cultures prescribe specific herbs or other remedies to reduce postpartum discomfort or pain, and these women may not ask for pharmacologic agents.

Identifying Plans for Pain Management

The labor nurse must determine the woman's preference for pain relief during childbirth. Some women will come well-prepared with breathing and relaxation techniques, whereas others rely entirely on the nurse for guidance in strategies to control discomfort and pain. Many women have plans for specific types of analgesia and anesthesia. With the growing use of epidurals during labor, it is not uncommon for women to request this specific type of regional anesthesia when they are admitted to the labor unit. The nurse must be aware of the woman's preferences and convey this information to the birth attendant and anesthesiologist or nurse anesthetist.

The nurse determines the woman's preferences for pain relief during the postpartum period. Some women who experience only mild discomfort and are breastfeeding will avoid narcotics or other analgesics. Others desire guidance regarding the safety and efficacy of various agents. Women who are interested in assuming self-care activities as soon as possible may prefer help with comfort measures they can continue to practice at home. If pain persists through the time of discharge and the woman is still taking medication for pain, the nurse should ascertain that the woman has a prescription for the analgesic before she leaves the hospital or birthing unit.

Assessing Maternal and Fetal Responses to Analgesia and Anesthesia

Once analgesia or anesthesia has been administered, the nurse is responsible for assessing maternal and fetal responses to the pain control medications. Close monitoring of maternal vital signs, the labor pattern, and fetal heart rate (FHR) patterns in labor is essential because adverse reactions and complications can occur with the use of analgesics and anesthetics. With the growing use of both intrathecal analgesia and epidural anesthesia during labor, the responsibilities of the nurse in assessing and monitoring maternal and fetal well-being have increased. Nursing implications for these pain control methods as well as other types of medications and anesthetics are presented in the next section of this chapter.

• • Nursing Diagnosis

Based on the assessment, the nurse identifies the woman's specific needs and problems related to pain management. Nursing diagnoses commonly used in the plan of care include:

- Anxiety related to pain or anticipation of pain during childbirth
- Ineffective Breathing Patterns related to analgesia or anesthesia
- Impaired Verbal Communication related to pain
- Ineffective Individual Coping related to pain or anticipation of pain
- Decisional Conflict related to the use of analgesia or anesthesia during childbirth or the postpartum period
- Fear related to pain or the administration of analgesia or anesthesia
- High Risk for Injury related to the use of analgesia or anesthesia
- Knowledge Deficit related to pain control techniques or analgesia and anesthesia
- Pain related to the process of childbirth, obstetric interventions, or birth trauma
- Self-Esteem Disturbance related to need for analgesia or anesthesia
- Sensory–Perceptual Alterations related to pain, analgesia, or anesthesia
- Altered Urinary Elimination related to analgesia or anesthesia

• • Planning and Implementation

Planning and implementing nonpharmacologic nursing measures (described in Chapter 20) to relieve pain is a major nursing responsibility. The nurse must work closely with the woman and her support person to promote comfort and control pain sensations during labor. The nurse must also be familiar with commonly used methods of relaxation and pain relief taught in childbirth education classes. It is crucial to support the woman's efforts to "stay on top," "flow with," "go with," or "avoid fighting" the sensations with which she is bombarded during labor, using specific techniques. However, coping strategies may fail to control or relieve pain and require the skilled labor nurse to suggest pharmacologic pain relief methods.

The nurse should caution the woman about embracing the goal of "natural childbirth" as the most important element during childbirth. She should not have to suffer through an intensely painful labor experience or refuse medication that may actually improve labor progress to achieve this goal. On the other hand, a woman experiencing a difficult time during transition may respond positively to intensive support and encouragement. With support, she may be able to cope *without* analgesia for the short period of time needed to achieve complete dilatation of the cervix. The nurse's goal is to support the woman who wishes to avoid medication during labor. However, the woman should feel comfortable asking for pharmacologic pain relief if she needs it.

If comfort measures and relaxation techniques are not successful in helping the woman cope with pain, the nurse or the birth attendant will discuss the possibility of pharmacologic pain relief. It is essential that the woman be informed of the benefits, disadvantages, and risks of the method and agent selected for pain relief. Discussing this when the woman is experiencing intense pain, often compounded by fatigue and anxiety, is inadvisable. Ideally, the discussion about pain relief techniques should occur *before* the onset of labor. If the woman has not received prenatal care, the nurse should explore the woman's preferences for pain relief as soon as possible after admission and discuss available pain control methods well in advance of their need.

During the postpartum period the nurse should spend time evaluating the woman's understanding of the reasons for her pain, the benefits and risks of analgesia, and her usual coping methods when she experiences pain. Nonpharmacologic techniques can be implemented when the woman is opposed to analgesia and pain is mild to moderate in intensity. When pain is severe, the nurse must consult with the primary provider. Attempts must be made to discover why the woman is opposed to pain medication. Conversely, if the woman is requesting frequent administration of analgesia and complaints of pain are incongruent with her condition, a careful reassessment must be conducted to rule out complications. Regardless of the origins of pain (physiologic or psychological), the pain is real and should be viewed as real (Callahan-Faut & Paice, 1990).

The nurse has specific responsibilities when analgesia or anesthesia is used. In most facilities, analgesics are administered by the nurse who is responsible for preparing the drug and reviewing the woman's record to identify contraindications to its use. The nurse is responsible for the ongoing assessment and monitoring of maternal–fetal status during labor and the postpartum woman's condition after birth when analgesia and anesthesia are used. If an operative delivery is performed, the anesthesiologist is usually responsible for evaluating the woman's response to the agent during surgery. But if a morphine epidural is given postoperatively, the nurse is responsible for ongoing evaluation of the woman for the first 24 hours.

• • Evaluation

The nurse must determine if the analgesic or anesthetic administered is effective in managing pain. The woman is observed for evidence of reduced pain sensation and should verbalize a decrease in the level or intensity of pain sensations. Maternal vital signs and the FHR pattern should remain within normal limits, and the woman should remain free of adverse reactions to the drug(s). An important aspect of evaluation is to determine the effect of pain relief methods on the woman's ability to push during the second stage of labor. Decreased attention to pressure sensations or complete loss of sensory and motor function in the lower extremities may make it difficult for the woman to bear down. If new problems are identified during this evaluation process, the nursing care plan is modified. In the postpartum period, pain control should be adequate to permit self-care and infant care activities, including breastfeeding.

The nurse engages in an ongoing assessment of the woman's level of comfort and perceptions of pain to identify the need for pharmacologic pain relief. Decisions about the woman's comfort needs are based on verbalizations of pain, observation of behavioral cues, and maternal–fetal status. Planning and implementation of appropriate nursing interventions to control pain are based on expert knowledge regarding comfort measures and pain relief techniques available. The woman should be an active participant in the planning process. Evaluation of maternal and fetal responses to the administration of analgesia or anesthesia will guide the nurse in implementing further pain control techniques.

To assist the woman in pain management during labor and birth, the nurse must have a comprehensive knowledge regarding the causes of pain during parturition. Effective control of pain is essential because of the deleterious effects of severe, unremitting pain on both maternal and fetal well-being. Because pain is influenced by anatomic, physiologic, psychological, and social factors, the nurse must perform a comprehensive assessment of each woman as she begins the process of labor. The use of both nonpharmacologic and pharmacologic methods of pain control is based on identification of these four major factors. The nurse uses the nursing process to plan ongoing pain control strategies, and this problem-solving approach is described in the following section.

Obstetric Analgesia During Childbirth

Obstetric analgesia includes the use of analgesics, sedatives, ataractics, and tranquilizers (Table 24-2).

Parenteral Analgesics

Analgesics are natural or synthetic narcotic drugs that provide highly effective pain relief as well as some sedation, decrease in anxiety, euphoria, and antispasmodic action. Analgesics commonly used in labor include meperidine hydrochloride (Demerol), fentanyl (Sublimaze), and morphine sulfate. Morphine is most often used to induce sleep in women experiencing a prolonged latent phase of labor without progress (prolonged prodromal labor).

As systemic drugs, administered by the intravascular, IM, or subcutaneous (SC) route, analgesics readily cross the placental barrier. Because fetal liver and renal functions are immature, drugs are metabolized slowly. Thus, fetal blood levels remain higher for longer periods than do maternal blood levels. If an electronic fetal monitor (EFM) is used, a temporary decrease in FHR variability is often observed secondary to central nervous system (CNS) depression of the fetus. Research also indicates that a transient decrease in fetal blood oxygen levels may occur after IV administration. Therefore, narcotics should be avoided when fetal distress is evident (Baxi, Petrie, & James, 1988).

Depressive effects on the neonate are greatest when delivery occurs in the first 2 to 3 hours after administration. For this reason, administration of these agents within 3 hours of anticipated delivery is not recommended. The administration of narcotics in labor can have subtle effects on neonatal behavioral functioning in the first 24 hours of life, even if a narcotic antagonist is administered to the infant at birth. These effects, which include decreased alertness and responsiveness to stimulation and decreased consolability, may persist for several days. Many women who receive narcotics in the latent phase of labor experience a decrease in uterine activity that impedes progress in labor; thus, the woman should be encouraged to use nonpharmacologic measures to reduce pain until active labor is well-established. When administered in the active phase of labor, the woman receives the benefits of analgesia, without a slowing of cervical dilation.

Intrathecal Analgesics

A new technique, the intrathecal administration of analgesics, has been developed recently to manage pain during labor. In selected centers, narcotics such as meperidine (Demerol) and fentanyl (Sublimaze) are injected into the subarachnoid space to provide pain relief. This method is discussed in detail later in the Obstetric Anesthesia section.

Sedative-Hypnotics

Sedative-hypnotics do not relieve pain but induce relaxation and sleep. They may be used to potentiate the effects of analgesics or to promote rest and sleep when the woman is extremely apprehensive or becoming exhausted in the latent phase of labor. Among drugs in this class, barbiturates are most commonly used in intrapartum care, including secobarbital sodium (Seconal), pentobarbital sodium (Nembutal), and phenobarbital (Luminal). These drugs may be administered orally or intramuscularly. Thiopental sodium (Pentothal), an ultrashort-acting drug administered intravenously, is used for rapid induction of anesthesia for operative procedures.

Barbiturates cause sedation and relaxation. Side-effects may include restlessness (especially when used alone in the presence of moderate to severe pain), hypotension, vertigo, lethargy, and nausea and vomiting. Sedative-hypnotics (with the exception of IV thiopental) should not be used during active labor because of rapid transfer across the placenta, long-lasting effects in the newborn, and the lack of an antagonist to reverse these effects. Effects in the neonate include CNS depression, prolonged drowsiness, and delayed establishment of feeding (poor sucking reflex and lower sucking pressure, resulting in decreased intake).

Ataractics

Ataractics (or tranquilizers) are a class of drugs that do not by themselves relieve pain, but they decrease apprehension and anxiety and reduce the nausea sometimes produced by analgesics. They potentiate the action of sedatives and analgesics, thereby reducing the dosage needed to produce desired effects. Two groups of ataractics are commonly used during the intrapartum period: phenothiazines, including promazine (Sparine), promethazine (Phenergan), and propiomazine hydrochloride (Largon); and benzodiazepines, including hydroxyzine (Vistaril, Atarax).

Ataractics may cause maternal hypotension with resultant decreased fetoplacental circulation, drowsiness, and

Table 24-2. Drugs Used for Analgesia in Labor

Drug	Dosage/Route	Maternal Side-Effects	Fetal/Neonatal Side-Effects	Nursing Implications
Analgesics				
Morphine sulfate	8–15 mg IM or 1–2 mg IV; peak effect in 30–60 min after IM and 15–20 min after IV administration; duration 4–6 h	CNS depression, especially respiratory; nausea/vomiting; possible decrease in uterine activity	Transient decrease in FHR variability Neonatal CNS depression; peak effect 30 min to 1 h after IV administration and 2 h after IM administration	More commonly used to induce sleep in prodromal labor. Not commonly used in labor. Do *not* administer if maternal respiratory rate is below 12/min or other signs of CNS depression are present. Avoid administration 1–3 h (depending on route) before delivery. Administer IV drug slowly over 3–5 min. Prepare to administer narcotic antagonist (Narcan, 0.01 mg/kg) to neonate if depression is evident.
Meperidine hydrochloride (Demerol)	50–100 mg IM or 25–50 mg IV; peak effect in 40–60 min after IM and 5–10 min after IV administration; duration 3–4 h	CNS depression, especially respiratory; nausea/vomiting; hypotension; drowsiness; blurred vision; after initial decrease in contractility, a mild oxytocic effect with possible uterine hyperstimulation	Transient decrease in FHR variability CNS depression; hypotonia; lethargy up to 72 h after birth	Most commonly used narcotic drug for labor. Administered in active phase of labor, preferably at least 2 h before delivery to minimize CNS depression in newborn. Administer IV drug slowly over 3–5 min. Prepare to administer narcotic antagonist to neonate if depression evident (Narcan, 0.01 mg/kg).
Fentanyl (Sublimaze)	50–100 μg IM or 25–50 μg IV; peak effect in 20–30 min after IM and 3–5 min after IV administration; duration 30 min to 1 h IV and 1–2 h IM	CNS depression, especially respiratory; apnea; hypotension; nausea/vomiting; hypotension; skeletal and thoracic muscle rigidity	Transient decrease in FHR variability CNS depression	Short-acting drug appropriate for late active phase of labor in primigravidas. Have oxygen and suction equipment available as respiratory depression effects last longer than analgesic effects. Administer IV drug slowly over 3–5 min to reduce muscle rigidity. Prepare to administer narcotic antagonist to woman or neonate if depression evident.
Nalbuphine (Nubain)	0.2 mg/kg IM or 0.1–0.2 mg/kg IV; peak effect in 30 min after IV and 1 h after IM administration; duration 3–6 h	CNS sedation especially dizziness (vertigo) and respiratory depression; hypotension; nausea/vomiting; blurred vision; dry mouth; diaphoresis; mild antagonist effect may precipitate withdrawal in narcotic-dependent women	Transient decrease in FHR variability Respiratory depression	Do not administer to narcotic-dependent woman. Prepare to give Narcan (0.01 mg/kg) to neonate if signs of CNS depression evident. Administer IV drug slowly over 3–5 min.

(*continued*)

Table 24-2. Drugs Used for Analgesia in Labor (*continued*)

Drug	Dosage/Route	Maternal Side-Effects	Fetal/Neonatal Side-Effects	Nursing Implications
Barbiturates				
Sodium secobarbital (Seconal) Sodium pentobarbital (Nembutal) Sodium phenobarbital (Luminal)	100 mg IM or orally; peak effect in 30 min after PO and 10 min after IM administration; duration 1–4 h	Reduced tension, release of inhibitions; lethargy, hypotension, decreased sensory perception; restlessness in presence of pain or as idiosyncratic reaction in some women	CNS depression; neonatal hypotonia; delay in establishment of feeding. Used to induce sedation during latent phase labor. *Note:* There is no available antagonist; avoid use in active labor.	Used to induce sedation in prolonged latent phase of labor. *Note:* There is no available antagonist; avoid use in active labor—will cause marked restlessness if administered to woman in pain.
Ataractics				
Promazine (Sparine)	25–50 mg IM or IV; peak effect in 30 min after IM or IV administration; duration unknown	Potentiates narcotic effects; antiemetic. Use with analgesic; may produce pseudohypnotic effect	Potentiates CNS depression	Monitor closely; institute standard safety measures for medicated women (side rails, bed rest, frequent checking).
Promethazine (Phenergan)	25–50 mg IM or IV; peak effects are unknown; duration up to 2–8 h	As for promazine	As for promazine	As for promazine; administer IM dose deep into well-developed muscle
Hydroxyzine (Vistaril)	25–50 mg IM; peak effects in 2–4 h after administration; duration 4–6 h	As for promazine; pain at IM site	As for promazine	As for promazine Spasmodic eye or neck movements suggest extrapyramidal effect of phenothiazine; alert care provider. Do not use deltoid muscle. Administer IM deep into well-developed muscle, preferably with Z-track technique. Do *not* administer IV as may cause hemolysis.

vertigo. Drugs in the phenothiazine group can cause adverse reactions in the woman that mimic symptoms of meningitis, including spasmodic eye movements, neck stiffness and spasm, and arching of the neck and back. Ataractics cross the placenta readily, and metabolites can be found in the neonate's system for at least 7 days. Effects on the fetus may include tachycardia and loss of normal beat-to-beat variability on EFM. Effects extending into the neonatal period may include hypotonia, hypothermia, and generalized drowsiness, including reluctance to feed in the first days of life.

Amnesics

Amnesics are drugs that induce loss of memory. Scopolamine, a drug with sedative and tranquilizing effects, is also referred to as an amnesic because it produces near-total or complete loss of memory of events during its peak action. This drug was commonly used during the intrapartum period in the past. It is not used in contemporary practice because of several undesirable effects including marked delirium, hallucinations, and agitation of women in labor.

Indications and Contraindications

The decision to administer analgesics, sedatives, or tranquilizers should be a collaborative decision involving the woman in labor and the nurse or birth attendant. At times the woman in labor will specifically request analgesia. In other situations, the nurse may take the initiative and suggest that analgesia is indicated. The nurse is often given a standing order for analgesia and is expected to evaluate the woman's responses to labor and determine if and when it should be implemented. The nurse must conduct an ongoing assessment of the woman's success in controlling pain. If sudden changes in the woman's behavioral and verbal responses suggest an increased pain level, the nurse should perform a vaginal examination to evaluate the progress of labor. Any decision regarding the use of an analgesic is predicated on this vaginal examination. If birth is anticipated within several hours, the risk of neonatal narcosis may preclude the use of analgesia.

The risks and benefits of using pharmacologic agents must be weighed carefully. Factors to consider before administration of any analgesic include:

- Maternal plans and desires
- Maternal and fetal status
- Expected time frame for delivery
- Presence of complications that preclude narcotics

If the woman is opposed to and has refused the use of analgesics in the presence of severe pain, the nurse must remain in close attendance to assess maternal and fetal physiologic responses. As noted, pain can have adverse effects on the woman and fetus. The birth attendant should be informed of the woman's status and included in further discussions regarding pain relief options. If systemic analgesia is refused because of the placental transfer of the agent to the fetus, the woman may be less opposed to regional or conduction anesthesia. Occasionally the woman's partner or support person objects to the administration of analgesia or anesthesia even when the woman has requested it. The nurse must intervene quickly to reconcile the couple's expectations and needs (see the Legal/Ethical Considerations display).

Even when the woman desires pharmacologic pain relief during labor and pain is intense, several significant factors can preclude the use of parenteral analgesia. These factors include:

- History of adverse or idiosyncratic reactions to analgesics
- Allergy to the drug of choice
- Maternal hemorrhage
- Maternal hypotension
- Fetal distress
- Impending birth of the infant
- Objections to the use of analgesia by the woman

When these problems are evident, the nurse must consult closely with the birth attendant and anesthesiologist to determine the safest method of pain management.

Advantages and Disadvantages

Parenteral analgesia provides a rapid method for pain relief, particularly if the IV route is used for administration of the drug. If fatigue is a significant component of pain, analgesia may permit rest between contractions. With a prolonged latent phase, sedatives or narcotics may induce sleep and stop the abnormal labor pattern. The judicious use of analgesia may allow women to regain control when they are unable to perform breathing or relaxation techniques. This can restore their self-confidence and sense of competence to make it through labor and birth. Newer synthetic, short-acting drugs, such as fentanyl, may be given closer to the time of delivery. If the progress of labor is rapid and birth occurs before anticipated, the short half-life of the drug reduces the risk of neonatal depression. Finally, because sensation is not lost with analgesics, the woman has better control over the process of pushing during the second stage of labor.

Although the woman may realize significant benefits with the administration of analgesics during labor, there are distinct disadvantages to their use. As noted, maternal and neonatal respiratory depression can occur with the use of analgesia and may require the administration of narcotic antagonists or resuscitative efforts to restore breathing. Because of this risk, the use of analgesia may be inadvisable during a painful, but rapid labor, when birth appears imminent. Other significant side-effects may occur that jeopardize the well-being of the woman or fetus, including maternal hypotension and allergic reactions to the drugs used. Common side-effects such as nausea and vomiting can occur,

Legal/Ethical Considerations

When the Partner or Support Person Objects to Analgesia or Anesthesia

Occasionally the responses of the support person have a negative impact on the woman and require timely interventions by the nurse to reestablish a helping relationship. The partner or support person who objects to the administration of analgesia (or anesthesia), after the woman expressly requests it, creates a conflict that can interfere with the normal course of labor. It also poses an ethical dilemma for the labor nurse.

The nurse is guided by ethical principles to recognize and respect the woman's choice of support person during labor. When objections are voiced by that person about an intervention, the nurse must attempt to identify the reasons. Some partners may feel they have failed in the role of coach if the woman needs medication. Others may believe that the woman should "tough it out," and their role is to see that she does so. Before the onset of labor, a woman may ask her partner to intervene if she asks for pain relief—"If I break down, don't listen to me!" Concerns about the maternal and neonatal effects of analgesia or anesthesia may motivate opposition to the use of drugs.

If the woman persists in her request for pain relief and the nursing assessment indicates it is appropriate, the partner's wishes or demands may not be satisfied. The nurse may attempt to alleviate fears about the new role of the support person once the woman is medicated. However, when unresolved conflict occurs, the birth attendant should be notified immediately. A discussion between the primary provider and the couple may resolve the problem. Ultimately the woman's choices must be respected in this matter.

ANA Committee on Ethics. (1988). Ethics in nursing: Position statements and guidelines. *Kansas City, Mo: Author.*

and uterine activity may be temporarily decreased, prolonging the first stage of labor.

The use of analgesia reduces awareness and may result in "gaps" in the woman's memory about labor. She may be disappointed in the quality of the childbirth experience as a result of "losing time." If analgesia is given shortly before birth, the woman may be unable to interact with the neonate or breastfeed effectively because of sedation. Finally, immaturity in neonatal organ systems delays metabolism and excretion of analgesic drugs and sedatives and can result in temporary, subtle neurobehavioral aberrations in the neonate.

Implications for Nursing Care

When narcotic analgesics, tranquilizers, or sedatives are administered in labor, the nurse must monitor maternal and fetal physiologic functioning closely. The accompanying Nursing Care Plan outlines the appropriate care for the woman receiving intrapartum analgesia. The nurse assesses the woman at frequent intervals (at least every 15 minutes for the first 2 hours) to evaluate the effectiveness of the drug and to identify idiosyncratic or allergic reactions, side-effects, or other adverse maternal or fetal responses. Hypotension can occur, particularly after IV administration of analgesics. The blood pressure should be measured before administration of the drug and again when peak action of the drug is expected.

Respiratory depression is also a significant side-effect. Narcotic antagonists, such as nalorphine (Nalline), or naloxone (Narcan) must be on hand to counteract narcotic-induced respiratory depression. Narcotic antagonists may be administered to the woman intramuscularly 5 to 15 minutes before delivery or to the neonate immediately after birth to reduce narcotic-induced neonatal depression. Neonatal Narcan is given intramuscularly or intravenously by injection of a dilute solution of the medication into the umbilical artery. Extreme caution should be taken when the woman is known or suspected to be physically dependent on opioids. In such cases, an abrupt and complete reversal of narcotic effects may precipitate acute withdrawal syndrome in the woman.

If the woman continues to experience the same level or greater intensity of pain after peak action of the analgesic is reached, she should be reexamined to determine if further cervical dilatation has occurred. Rapid progress in dilatation and fetal descent often occurs when analgesia is given in active labor. The nurse should be alert for signs of the second stage of labor because the woman may be sedated and unaware of the impending birth.

The FHR is assessed after administration of analgesics. Once the woman in labor receives the analgesic, it is advisable to apply an external FHM and tokodynamometer (if intermittent auscultation has been previously used). This permits ongoing assessment of fetal status without disturb-

Table 24-3. Time Sequence for Nursing Support and Administration of Analgesics/Anesthetics During Labor

Latent Phase (1–3 cm dilatation)	Active Phase (4–7 cm dilatation)	Transition (8–10 cm dilatation)	Second Stage (pushing)	Birth
Provide nursing support and promote self-care, using the following: Breathing techniques Back massage Effleurage/stroking Application of heat or cold Position changes, ambulation Praise, encouragement Anticipatory teaching	Provide nursing support and promote self-care, using the following: Breathing techniques Back massage Effleurage/stroking Application of heat or cold Position changes, ambulation Praise, encouragement Anticipatory teaching	Provide nursing support and promote self-care, using the following: Breathing techniques Back massage Effleurage/stroking Application of heat or cold Position changes, ambulation Praise, encouragement Anticipatory teaching	Provide nursing support and promote self-care, using the following: Breathing techniques Back massage Effleurage/stroking Application of heat or cold Position changes, ambulation Praise, encouragement Anticipatory teaching	
	Caution woman against hyperventilation Encourage woman to change breathing techniques.	Instruct woman to blow out if she feels urge to push. Do not leave woman alone.	Assist woman with pushing technique. Assist with positioning if spinal or epidural anesthetic has been given.	
Sedatives (Seconal, Nembutal, Dalmane) or morphine may be provided to induce sleep with prolonged latent phase of labor.	Analgesics may be provided (Demerol, Fentanyl, Nubain).	Analgesic administration may be repeated if >2 h before expected delivery.	Local or pudendal anesthesia may be provided.	Narcotic antagonist may be provided.
	Epidural anesthesia may be provided.	Epidural anesthesia may be provided. Spinal anesthesia may be provided; Check for bladder distention.	Epidural anesthesia may be provided.	Epidural anesthesia may be provided.

ing the woman every 15 minutes to auscultate the FHR. Even when small doses of analgesics are given, the fatigued woman may sleep until the contraction reaches its acme. She may wake up confused and be unable to use the relaxation and breathing pattern used earlier. Using the FHM allows the labor coach to alert the woman as each contraction begins so that she is not startled or overwhelmed.

After receiving analgesics for relief of pain during labor or sedatives, many women experience transient mental impairment, vertigo, and somnolence. Safety measures must be implemented to prevent injury (side rails), and the patient should be instructed to remain in bed unless attended by the nurse. Nausea and vomiting are common side-effects; therefore, the woman should be placed on her side before administration of the drug, and an emesis basin should be provided.

Because the nurse recognizes that no medication provides completely safe and effective analgesia, the choice of analgesia in labor must always be made in regard to possible adverse effects on the woman, the progress of labor, and the fetus. However, when used wisely, parenteral analgesia can be safe and beneficial to the woman and presents little risk to the healthy fetus and newborn. Table 24-3 outlines nursing support with analgesic use during the labor stages and birth. The following nursing implications relate to the administration of *any* of these medications to the woman in labor.

- Because nausea and vomiting are common in labor and are also side-effects of the drugs, they are typically given intramuscularly and intravenously (see accompanying display).
- Dosages are kept to the smallest effective dose so that duration of effect can be better predicted and deleterious effects minimized.
- Routine precautions for administration of these medications should be taken: verifying drug, dosage, route, and patient name and checking for maternal allergies.
- Positive suggestion will potentiate the effects of analgesics administered to laboring women.
- Safety precautions are initiated to prevent injuries such as falls, nerve injuries due to improper injection technique, and aspiration of vomitus.

The nurse provides a wide variety of analgesics during the first stage of labor to reduce painful stimuli. Additional agents are often combined with analgesics to enhance their effectiveness, reduce side-effects, or promote sedation. Because nurses are generally responsible for the preparation and administration of analgesics, they must have a comprehensive knowledge regarding these agents, including the normal dosages, indications and contraindications for use, drug precautions, and effective antidotes to adverse reactions. Once analgesics are administered, the nurse monitors maternal and fetal well-being and continues to provide nonpharmacologic comfort measures to enhance their effectiveness.

Techniques for Administration of Intramuscular and Intravenous Drugs During Labor

Intramuscular Injection

Research indicates that drug absorption from the gluteus muscle is decreased in late pregnancy as a result of impaired venous return and edema in the lower extremities (Lazebnik, Kuhnert, Carr, Brashear, Syracuse, & Mann, 1989). In some women drug concentrations did not reach therapeutic levels. When the IM route is indicated, the nurse should consider the following:

- The needle should be long enough to ensure that the medication is placed in the muscle rather than subcutaneous fat.
- The deltoid muscle should be considered as an alternative site when 0.5 to 1.0 mL of drug is to be administered.

Intravenous Injection

- Follow guidelines regarding dilution of drug. Many drugs must be diluted before IV administration.
- Administer at a slow rate (1 mL/min or slower) to avoid too-rapid physiologic responses to drug, such as hypotension or muscular rigidity.
- Administer during a contraction to prevent bolus of drug passing through the placenta to the fetus. Placental circulation is decreased during a contraction.

Lazebnik, N., Kuhnert, B., Carr, P., Brashear, W., Syracuse, C., & Mann, L. (1989). Intravenous, deltoid, or gluteus administration of meperidine during labor? American Journal of Obstetrics and Gynecology, *160(5), 1184.*

Obstetric Anesthesia in Labor

Situations where systemic analgesics are contraindicated or more active obstetric management of labor is indicated may require the use of obstetric anesthesia. Recent advances in technology and ongoing research have resulted in new techniques for achieving obstetric anesthesia. This section presents commonly used methods of anesthetic pain relief, including regional and general anesthesia. Perineal and pudendal block, which are commonly used in low-risk labors, are discussed in Chapter 21. The major types of anesthesia are described, the relative risks and benefits are discussed, as well as specific nursing responsibilities in caring for patients requiring obstetric anesthesia.

Regional Anesthesia

Regional anesthesia refers to techniques that provide pain relief to a specific region of the body by directly affecting nerve impulse transmission. This class of anesthetic techniques, sometimes called *conduction anesthesia*, includes *subarachnoid* or *spinal*, *epidural*, *paracervical*, and *pudendal* anesthesia. In all cases, these methods produce analgesia and anesthesia through the injection of an anesthetic agent into a location where it can stabilize the cell membrane of nervous tissue. This prevents transmission of sensory impulses. Each method is characterized by a different injection site, which in turn enables different patterns of anesthesia, as discussed later in this section. Figure 24-3 shows pertinent spinal anatomy and the infiltration sites for regional anesthesia.

Agents Used in Regional Anesthesia

Several local anesthetic agents are used in regional anesthesia, based on the type of infiltration and the level of anesthesia desired. There are two major classes of these drugs: *ester-linked anesthetics*, such as procaine (Novocaine), chloroprocaine (Nesacaine), and tetracaine (Pontocaine); and *amide-linked anesthetics,* such as lidocaine (Xylocaine), mepivacaine (Carbocaine), and bupivacaine (Marcaine). These groups are metabolized differently in the body and vary in their duration of action and particularly in their effects on the fetus.

Ester-linked agents are metabolized by plasma cholinesterase in maternal serum, are relatively short acting, and do not readily cross into fetal circulation. These agents may require repeated dosages to achieve satisfactory anesthesia. Amide-linked agents, which are metabolized by liver enzymes, are longer acting and are favored for use in obstetrics for this reason. However, these agents cross the placenta readily and are not easily metabolized by the immature fetal liver, so fetal effects are prolonged.

The practice of administering *narcotics* into the subarachnoid or epidural space to provide pain relief during labor is growing. Opiate receptors are present in the dorsal horn of the spinal cord. Narcotics such as *morphine* (Du-

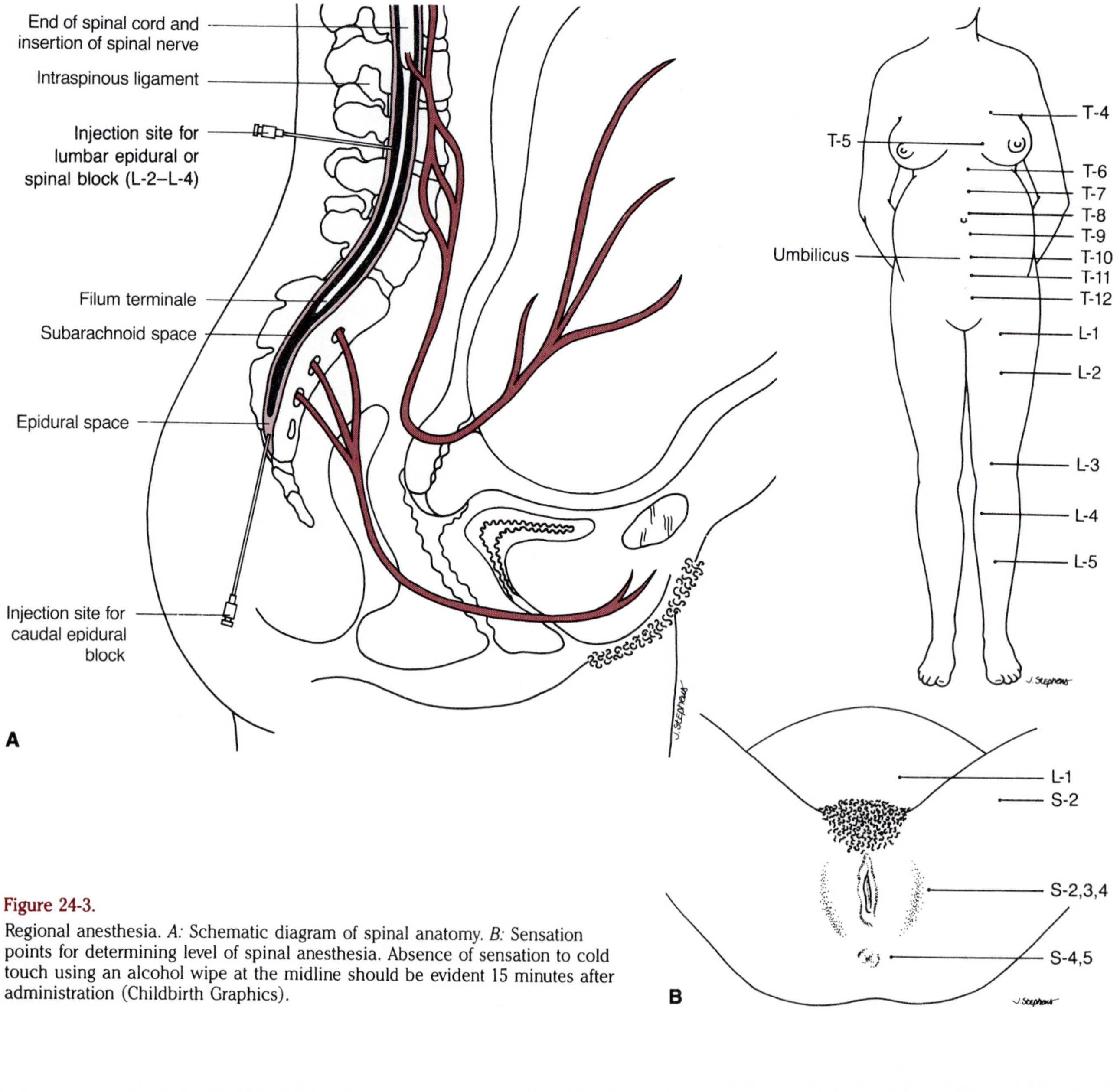

Figure 24-3.

Regional anesthesia. *A:* Schematic diagram of spinal anatomy. *B:* Sensation points for determining level of spinal anesthesia. Absence of sensation to cold touch using an alcohol wipe at the midline should be evident 15 minutes after administration (Childbirth Graphics).

ramorph), *meperidine* (Demerol), and *fentanyl* (Sublimaze) diffuse from the epidural or subarachnoid space to these receptor sites, inducing analgesia. The drugs used are also absorbed into the intravascular compartment and are detectable in both maternal serum and neonatal umbilical cord blood samples.

Intraspinal (intrathecal) and epidural narcotics appear to provide good to excellent pain relief during labor and birth. The choice of drug will be based in part on the desired onset and duration of action. Some narcotics, such as fentanyl and meperidine permit rapid analgesia due to their lipophilic properties. Peak blood levels are achieved in 10 to 15 minutes, but duration of analgesia is relatively short, ranging from 1 to 4 hours for women in labor. Other drugs, such as morphine, with low lipid solubility, reach peak blood levels in 30 to 60 minutes, but provide pain relief for up to 24 hours (Wild & Coyne, 1992). For this reason, fentanyl and meperidine are more commonly used during labor when fast-acting, shorter duration of effect is required. Morphine is more commonly administered at the time of cesarean birth to provide prolonged pain relief during the first 24 hours postoperatively. A detailed discussion of both intrathecal and epidural narcotics analgesia follows in the chapter.

Indications and Contraindications

Regional anesthetics may be indicated when parenteral analgesics have failed to relieve moderate to severe intrapartum pain. Some women do not wish to experience the CNS effects of narcotics such as sedation, euphoria, or altered sense of time. They wish to be active participants in the labor and birth experience, but they also desire a reduction in pain sensation. At times, active management of labor is indicated due to prolonged or arrested labor or other problems, which require potentially painful obstetric interventions. The woman and birth attendant may prefer a method, such as continuous epidural or subarachnoid anesthesia, which provides loss of sensation. Finally, when operative delivery appears likely, regional anesthesia is usually preferred to general anesthesia because it poses fewer risks to maternal, fetal, and neonatal well-being.

There are several contraindications to regional anesthesia. One of the most serious is a known allergy to the amide- or ester-linked anesthetics or narcotics commonly used in regional anesthesia. Women with significant back injuries or those who have undergone spinal surgery are usually not candidates for this method. The presence of hemorrhage and shock, bleeding disorders such as disseminated intravascular coagulation, or other coagulopathies would also preclude regional anesthesia. A suspicion or diagnosis of meningitis, spinal abscess, or generalized septicemia would also be a contraindication to this method. Morbid obesity may present technical difficulties that make the procedure more difficult, but it is not an absolute contraindication. In fact, if regional anesthesia can be achieved in the obese woman, it is preferable to general anesthesia.

Advantages and Disadvantages

The use of regional anesthesia for labor and birth has gained popularity in recent years. A major advantage is that the dangers of general anesthesia, particularly vomiting and aspiration of gastric contents, can be avoided. Additionally, the woman can be alert during the process of labor and birth. Other advantages include:

- Pain relief is complete in the area affected by the regional block.
- Anesthetic agents can be administered continuously through use of a catheter placed into the subarachnoid or epidural space.
- Fetal CNS and respiratory depression is avoided with spinal and epidural blocks.
- Newer subarachnoid narcotics provide analgesia without motor block, permitting the woman to push more effectively in the second stage of labor.

Disadvantages of regional anesthesia include:

- Administration requires specialized skill and cannot be done by nursing personnel.
- Anesthetic failures (no effect or only partial effect) can occur.
- Administration of epidural anesthesia too early in labor can reduce uterine contractility and progress of labor and may require oxytocin augmentation.
- An IV line is required for the administration of fluids to support normal blood pressure levels because hypotension is a common side-effect.
- Loss of bladder sensation may require insertion of a urinary drainage catheter to prevent bladder distention.
- Bearing-down efforts may be less effective, prolonging the second stage of labor.
- Forceps applications may be necessary because these blocks reduce the reflex urge to bear down.
- Administration of epidural anesthesia has been linked to an increased incidence of cesarean delivery.

Adverse Reactions to Regional Anesthesia

Another disadvantage of regional anesthesia is the possibility of significant adverse maternal reactions. Although they are rare, these adverse reactions demand prompt nursing intervention. The most frequent adverse maternal reactions to regional anesthesia are *maternal hypotension* and *acute systemic toxicity* to the drug itself. A rare but alarming problem is respiratory paralysis resulting from a *total spinal block*. Another less common side-effect is *infection* (meningitis or epidural abscess). Less alarming responses, but still distressing to the woman, are *postlumbar puncture headache* and *backache*, and *partial or total anesthetic failure*. These reactions and appropriate nursing actions are discussed here.

Maternal Hypotension. Maternal hypotension may follow administration of any regional anesthetic although it is more common after spinal or epidural block. The hypotension is caused by the sympathetic blocking action of the drug, with the resulting loss of peripheral vascular resistance, and may also be compounded by compression of the vena cava if the woman is supine. The nurse should monitor maternal blood pressure and pulse every 2 to 3 minutes for 20 minutes after injection of the anesthetic, and every 10 to 15 minutes thereafter. An electronic blood pressure monitor can be used to facilitate frequent blood pressure assessment. Nursing actions to prevent maternal hypotension include:

- Administration of an IV fluid bolus of 1000 mL of a physiologic solution (see the display, Prehydration Precautions)
- Maintaining adequate maternal hydration with IV fluid
- Avoiding compression of the vena cava by using the sidelying position

Early signs of developing hypotension include sudden nausea or vomiting or a change in maternal affect. The woman may verbalize "feeling funny." Tachypnea is a common sign. Any decrease in systolic pressure should be considered a possible early sign. The nurse should take the following steps if maternal blood pressure decreases:

- Increase flow rate of IV fluid.
- Place the woman in left sidelying position to relieve pressure on the vena cava and elevate legs to promote venous return.
- Administer oxygen at 8 to 12 L/min by face mask.
- Have another staff member notify the physician immediately.
- Remain with the woman and provide reassurance.
- Be prepared to administer Ephedrine, an α–β-adrenergic agonist that causes peripheral vasoconstriction.
- Observe FHR pattern for changes.

Inadvertent Total Spinal Block. Respiratory paralysis can result from spinal block at T-4 or above. This may occur after accidental penetration and injection of the dura with an epidural dose of anesthetic agent. Signs of respiratory paralysis include rapidly developing apnea and hypotension. If uncorrected, cardiac arrest will result. The nurse should note the woman's respiratory status carefully after the block has been administered. If hypotension develops accompanied by respiratory distress and apnea, the physician is alerted immediately and the nurse initiates emergency steps to maintain maternal cardiopulmonary status. Treatment includes implementing nursing actions described earlier for correcting hypotension. Respiratory effort must be supported, and endotracheal intubation and assisted ventilation may be necessary until the effects of the block have worn off.

Prehydration Precautions

Women receiving epidural or spinal blocks during childbirth are normally prehydrated with 500 to 1000 mL of IV fluid before the procedure to prevent hypotension. Hypotension is a common side-effect of conduction anesthetics, secondary to sympathetic blockade and concomitant vasodilation of the lower extremities. Recent research suggests that the rapid infusion of 5% dextrose in water can have a deleterious effect on fetal acid–base balance. Fetal hyperglycemia, metabolic acidosis, and neonatal hypoglycemia have been associated with a glucose solution bolus. The use of a balanced physiologic solution, such as Ringer's lactate or Plasma-lyte, is recommended for prehydration before administration of conduction anesthesia and for rapid IV infusion in cases of maternal hypotension and dehydration.

Philipson, E. H., Kalhan, S. C., Riha, M. M., & Pimentel, R. (1987). Effects of maternal glucose infusion on fetal acid–base status in human pregnancy. American Journal of Obstetrics and Gynecology, 157, *866–873.*

Allergic or Toxic Reaction. Both allergic and toxic reactions may occur in response to anesthetic agents. Allergic reactions include urticaria, laryngeal edema, and bronchospasm; this type of reaction is treated by IV injection of an antihistamine, usually diphenhydramine. Toxic reactions may also occur when high circulating levels of the drug are introduced, either by inadvertent intravascular injection or by rapid absorption. Although these reactions are *rare*, the nurse must note early signs and notify the physician immediately. The following are signs of drug toxicity, presented in the order of increasing severity.

- Lightheadedness, vertigo
- Slurred speech, metallic taste in the mouth, loud ringing in ears
- Numbness of tongue and mouth
- Muscle twitching
- Loss of consciousness
- Sudden cardiovascular collapse
- Generalized convulsions

These signs would also be present if the anesthetic agent is inadvertently injected into the maternal blood stream during initial placement of the needle or catheter.

Treatment of toxic reactions includes administration of oxygen and IV or IM injection of drugs to counteract convulsions. Administration of a short-acting barbiturate may be ordered to prevent convulsions. If convulsions are present, IV or IM injection of 40 to 60 mg succinylcholine will be ordered; this controls muscular spasm and allows endotracheal intubation for a patent airway. Once this has been accomplished, assisted ventilation will be initiated, and IV fluids and vasopressors will be administered rapidly to support cardiovascular function (Nicholson & Ridolfo, 1989).

Toxic reactions may also occur in the neonate and are characterized by alterations in CNS functioning, seizures, bradycardia, hypotonia, and apnea. Treatment of neonatal anesthetic toxicity includes inducing prompt diuresis with IV fluids, supporting respiratory and metabolic status, and using barbiturates or diazepam to control seizure activity.

Infection. Strict adherence to aseptic technique will minimize the risk of local or systemic infection. Regional anesthesia is contraindicated in generalized septicemia. Controversy exists regarding the use of regional anesthesia in patients with herpes simplex virus type 2, due to the possibility of disseminating shedding of the virus from the skin into the ganglia.

Headache. The most common complication associated with epidural anesthesia is headache after accidental lumbar puncture. The leakage of cerebrospinal fluid (CSF) from the hole created by the puncture in the dura results in a frontal or occipital headache that is aggravated by standing. The woman may also complain of nausea, vomiting, vertigo, and acute sensitivity to light and sound. Bed rest, increased fluid intake, and the use of an abdominal binder and mild analgesic may be successful in reducing or alleviating the headache. If headaches are severe and persistent, a saline injection or epidural blood patch may be performed. Either 40 to 60 mL sterile saline or 10 to 20 mL of the patient's blood is injected into the epidural space through a catheter, in an attempt to seal the leak. Although considered a less serious side-effect, severe headache with nausea, vomiting, photophobia, and acute sensitivity to noise may greatly reduce the quality of the postpartum experience. The woman may find it impossible to breastfeed or assume infant care activities. It may prolong the hospitalization period and delay the maternal–infant attachment process.

Partial or Total Anesthetic Failure. Occasionally regional anesthesia will be only partially established or will fail to provide adequate pain relief. There are various causes for this. Malabsorption of the agent may occur because of decreased vascularity in the injection area, dehydration, and poor maternal physical condition. Spinal abnormalities or inaccurate placement of the injection may result in anesthetic failure. In many cases a partial block can be increased by injecting additional medication. The catheter may need to be removed and another catheter inserted, which requires the woman to undergo the entire procedure a second time. In other cases maternal pain relief remains inadequate, and other methods, such as systemic or general anesthesia, may be necessary.

Implications for Nursing Care

Women receiving regional anesthesia for labor and birth are at slightly increased risk by virtue of the procedure itself and the potential complications described in the preceding section. Nursing care for patients before, during, and after administration of regional anesthesia is extremely important to ensure the safety of the woman and the fetus. The following general functions are of primary concern to the nurse caring for women receiving any type of regional anesthetic.

- Reinforce information provided by the birth attendant and anesthesiologist about the procedure.
- Insert an IV line (if not already done) and administer a preanesthetic fluid bolus as ordered to prevent hypotension.
- Encourage the woman to empty her bladder immediately before the procedure begins.
- Attach blood pressure, pulse, and fetal monitoring equipment.
- Position the woman for the procedure and direct the support person in the appropriate role and position during the procedure.
- Provide support and reassurance for the woman and her partner.
- Monitor maternal and fetal physiologic responses to the anesthesia.
- Observe closely for adverse reactions.

Once the procedure is completed, nursing care is focused on the following activities.

- Position the woman to maintain optimum uterine blood flow.
- Ensure patient safety by raising bed side rails and placing the call button within reach or applying a leg strap if the woman has been placed on the delivery table.
- Monitor maternal and fetal physiologic status.
- Monitor uterine activity for changes resulting from the anesthetic.
- Monitor for maternal urinary retention resulting from decreased bladder sensation.
- Catheterize the bladder if the woman is unable to void and has a distended bladder.
- Assess maternal comfort level.
- Evaluate the level of anesthesia and monitor for return of sensation.
- Initiate emergency measures in the event of adverse maternal or fetal responses.

These nursing responsibilities apply to care of patients receiving *any* type of regional anesthesia. The following section discusses each method in more detail and outlines specific nursing care.

Epidural (Lumbar and Caudal) Anesthesia

Epidural anesthesia can provide excellent anesthesia throughout the active phase and second stage of labor. It can be administered at any point in labor but is customarily administered at 4 to 6 cm of cervical dilatation. In some situations, dry catheters may be placed in early labor, and anesthetic agents are added later when pain relief is required. This is recommended when cesarean birth is likely, to avoid the risks inherent (failed intubation, vomiting, and aspiration) in the emergency induction of general anesthesia (ACOG, 1992).

Anesthesia is achieved by injecting the anesthetic agent into the epidural space outside the dura. The injection may be in the lumbar region at L-2 to L-4 or in the caudal region through the sacral hiatus at S-4. Epidural block typically produces blockade from T-10 to S-5, providing complete anesthesia from umbilicus to midthigh. It can be extended upward for cesarean delivery by administering larger doses of anesthetic.

Continuous epidural anesthesia has become the most common type of epidural block. The end of the plastic epidural catheter is attached to a continuous infusion pump and the anesthetic agent is delivered to the woman through the catheter at a set rate. If a continuous infusion of anesthetic is not implemented, the epidural catheter must be refilled or "topped up" each time the anesthetic is metabolized and pain sensation returns. A double-catheter approach using both a lumbar and a sacral catheter also can provide flexible and highly effective anesthesia throughout active labor and delivery.

Lumbar epidural blocks are administered with the woman in a sitting or sidelying position. Flexion of the back is not desirable because it reduces the peridural space and stretches the dura, making it more susceptible to puncture.

NURSING PROCEDURE

Aiding the Woman During the Epidural Block Procedure

NURSING ACTION	***RATIONALE***
1. Check that oxygen and suction equipment is available and properly functioning.	To be prepared for adverse reactions that require airway maintenance and oxygen
2. Administer 500 to 1000 mL prehydration bolus of IV fluid as ordered.	To reduce the risk of hypotension that occurs with epidural anesthesia
3. Verify that blood pressure monitor (or sphygmomanometer) and fetal monitor are functioning properly.	To obtain appropriate data on maternal–fetal status during the procedure
4. Position the woman on her left side with shoulders aligned and legs slightly flexed.	To facilitate optimum uterine blood flow during the procedure
5. When anesthesiologist is ready to begin procedure, have woman bring knees to abdomen, chin to chest, and round out back.	To increase the opening of the lumbar interspaces so that the epidural needle can be more easily advanced into the epidural space
6. Place the woman in a sitting position for the procedure if requested by the anesthesiologist.	To increase the opening of the lumbar interspaces when the side-lying position is not successful.
7. Verify patency of the IV line.	To facilitate rapid infusion of IV fluids should hypotension or other adverse reactions occur during the procedure
8. Assist woman to maintain appropriate position during procedure. Offer reassurance and support during the procedure.	It may be difficult for the woman to maintain the position, especially during contractions.
9. Monitor the affect and condition of the support person during the procedure.	Support person may feel uncomfortable or have physical reactions to the procedure.
Anesthesiologist Activities	
1. Scrub lower back with antiseptic solution and drapes area.	To maintain asepsis and prevent infection
2. Inject local anesthetic intradermally at the proposed insertion site.	To anesthetize the area into which the epidural needle will be placed
3. Introduce beveled epidural needle into interspace between L-2 to L-4.	To place catheter at level of spine required for anesthesia of uterus and cervix
4. Advance needle into the interspinous ligament. Attach air-filled syringe to hub of needle and begin slowly advancing needle to the ligamentum flavum. Attempt to inject air by gently "pumping" plunger of syringe. Resistance will be felt until peridural space reached.	To identify when epidural space is reached. When the epidural space is reached, air can be injected from the syringe into the space.
5. Advance needle another millimeter into the epidural space.	To facilitate correct placement of epidural catheter
6. Aspirate for CSF or blood.	To verify that epidural needle has not accidentally been inserted into the subarachnoid space

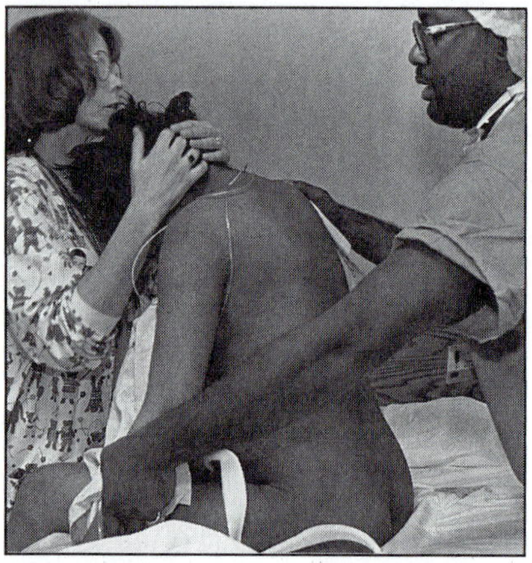

Step 6. Sitting position for epidural block. (Photo by Kathy Sloane.)

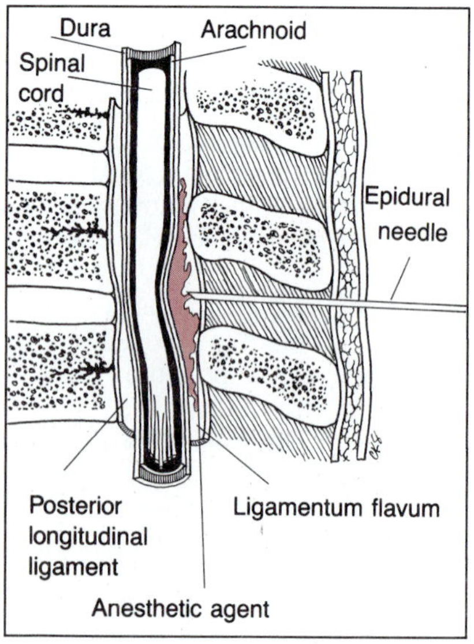

Step 4. Epidural injection.

(Continued)

NURSING PROCEDURE

Aiding the Woman During the Epidural Block Procedure (*Continued*)

NURSING ACTION	***RATIONALE***
7. If CSF or blood is aspirated, the needle is withdrawn and insertion is attempted at another site.	To prevent accidental injection of epidural anesthetic into the subarachnoid space, which would result in "inadvertent spinal" with significant adverse affects
8. Inject test dose of anesthetic agent. Ask woman if she is feeling any untoward effects such as vertigo, shortness of breath, ringing of ears etc.	To identify early signs of adverse effects or complications related to epidural anesthesia
9. Monitor for signs of inadvertent spinal anesthesia (onset of anesthesia after the test dose) or intravascular injection (circumoral tingling, vertigo, tinnitus) for 3 to 5 minutes.	To identify early signs of inadvertent spinal, so that corrective actions can be taken
10. Remove syringe and thread epidural catheter through needle into epidural space.	To permit injection of anesthetic agent into the catheter
11. Remove needle and administer appropriate amount of anesthetic.	To induce anesthesia
12. Tape catheter in place, allowing for additional injections by the anesthetist or physician as needed *or*	
13. Attach catheter to syringe filled with anesthetic and placed in continuous infusion pump and set appropriate infusion rate.	

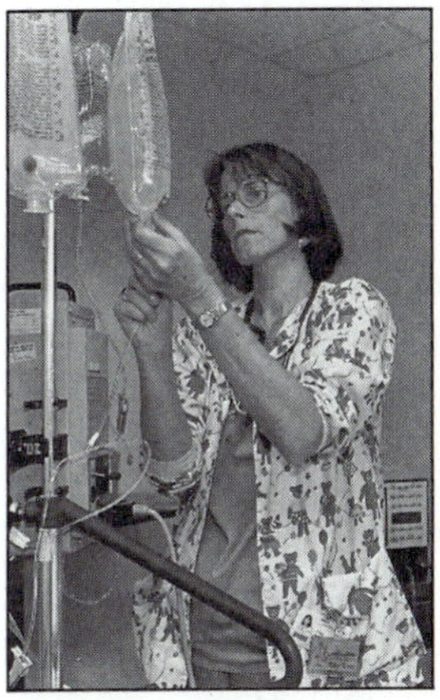

Step 13. Continuous epidural block.

Injection is made in an interspace between L-2 and L-4. First the syringe is aspirated to verify that the needle is correctly placed. Incorrect needle placement resulting in puncture of a vessel will yield blood; aspiration of CSF indicates the dura has been punctured. In either case, the needle is withdrawn and another injection is attempted. The procedure for lumbar and caudal epidural block is outlined in the accompanying Nursing Procedure.

If aspiration for blood and CSF is negative, a *test dose* of anesthetic is injected. The test dose usually consists of 3 mL of local anesthetic and may include epinephrine (15 to 20 μg). If accidental intravascular injection occurs, an increase in heart rate or blood pressure (or both) will be observed due to the effect of epinephrine. If epinephrine is *not* used, an intravascular injection of a small dose of local anesthesia will cause numbness or tingling of the tongue or circumoral area, lightheadedness, tinnitus, or a metallic taste. If the dura is inadvertently punctured, the test dose will produce a transient spinal anesthesia with loss of sensation and motor function in the lower limbs.

When the woman experiences warmth and tingling of the legs with the test dose without paralysis, sensory impairment, or signs of intravascular injection, the needle has been properly positioned in the epidural space and injection of the full dose can proceed. If continuous administration is desired, a catheter is inserted into the epidural space and attached to a continuous infusion pump.

Caudal epidural anesthesia is administered infrequently today. The fourth sacral vertebra has a U-shaped opening protected by a thin fibrous membrane; this opening is called the sacral hiatus and is the route through which a needle can be advanced into the lowest part of the epidural space. There is less risk of puncturing the dura with a caudal insertion than with a lumbar insertion. However, correct placement of the needle in the sacral hiatus is essential because incorrect placement may result in puncture of the maternal rectum or of the fetal head, a potentially lethal accident. For this reason, caudal blocks should not be attempted when the presenting part is on the pelvic floor.

Early signs of a successful caudal block include rapid perineal anesthesia and loss of anal sphincter reflex and numbness and tingling of toes and warmth and dryness of feet.

Indications and Contraindications

An epidural may be indicated when parenteral analgesics have failed to relieve pain. Women who want to be active participants in the labor and birth experience and avoid the sedative effects of parenteral analgesia may desire an epidural anesthetic. If active management of labor is indicated because of intrapartum complications, an epidural may be useful in reducing or eliminating the pain associated with painful obstetric interventions. When operative delivery appears a strong likelihood or an elective cesarean birth is planned, epidural anesthesia is usually preferred to general anesthesia because it poses fewer maternal–fetal risks.

Contraindications to epidural anesthesia are identical to those listed for regional anesthesia.

Advantages and Disadvantages

There are many advantages to the use of epidural anesthesia. It provides excellent pain relief in the first, second, and even third stage of labor (for repair of episiotomy or lacerations). It can also provide anesthesia for cesarean delivery and permits the woman to remain awake and alert for the birth. There is evidence that this method may improve maternal and fetal status when pregnancy-induced hypertension occurs by improving uterine blood flow and reducing blood pressure levels. Research suggests little or no identifiable effect on the fetus. In some cases, fetal status may even improve after epidural block because of increased uterine blood flow.

Several distinct disadvantages are evident with the use of epidural anesthesia. The time from administration of the anesthetic to the onset of pain relief is often 10 to 15 minutes. When the woman is experiencing intense pain, this delay may seem extremely long. If emergency cesarean birth or a rapid forceps or vacuum-assisted delivery is indicated, epidural anesthesia cannot be administered because of this delay in anesthetic effect.

The administration of epidural anesthesia restricts the woman to bed and makes spontaneous movement difficult due to partial or complete loss of motor function in the legs. Loss of sensation can result in bladder distention and the need for catheterization. Epidural anesthesia requires initiation of an IV line with its attendant discomfort and further restriction of movement, and oral intake is usually withheld once epidural anesthesia is administered.

The normal labor pattern may be disrupted and require use of oxytocin to stimulate uterine activity. The second stage of labor is also prolonged because pushing efforts may be less effective. Studies indicate an increase in vacuum extraction, forceps delivery, and cesarean birth rate.

Potential risks of maternal hypotension, toxic response to the anesthetic, and other complications of regional anesthesia require intensive nursing care and frequent blood pressure assessments. Many women complain of the discomfort caused by frequent automatic blood pressure measurements. These potential risks also require the use of electronic fetal and uterine monitoring.

Implications for Nursing Care

Nursing responsibilities in providing care for a woman receiving an epidural block center on adequately prehydrating the woman with IV solutions to prevent hypotension, assisting her into position for insertion of the catheter, closely monitoring maternal and fetal physiologic status, and providing emotional and physical comfort and support during and after the procedure. The woman is given information about the epidural by the anesthesiologist and must give informed consent. However, the nurse may need to answer additional questions and explain what the woman and her partner may expect. A Nursing Care Plan for the woman receiving epidural anesthesia during labor accompanies this section.

The nurse monitors both FHR and uterine activity and alerts the anesthesiologist to onset of contractions so that the block can be administered between contractions. This strategy may reduce the absorption of anesthetic systemically, as extradural venous distention occurs with contractions. Continuous fetal monitoring by EFM or Doppler is essential to evaluate fetal response to the epidural block. To facilitate frequent assessment of maternal vital signs, the nurse may use an electronic blood pressure monitor that automatically takes the blood pressure and pulse at preset intervals.

The nurse notes the woman's comfort level, evaluates level of anesthesia using an alcohol wipe, evaluates mental status (confusion, lethargy, or lightheadedness may indicate hypotension), and checks for signs of adverse reaction to the anesthetic as discussed earlier in the chapter. Care must be

Legal/Ethical Considerations

Fetal Monitoring During Administration of Regional Anesthesia

If the decision is made to administer an epidural or spinal anesthetic during childbirth, the nurse has specific responsibilities regarding fetal monitoring during the procedure. Recent changes in standards of practice have occurred as the result of litigation. Currently, the *nurse* assumes primary responsibility for assessing the fetal response during administration of anesthesia. An EFM of Doppler must be used *continuously* during the procedure.

Frequently, the external tokodynamometer belt must be removed during epidural or spinal administration. If the nurse is unable to continuously assess uterine activity, oxytocin infusions should be discontinued during the procedure. The nurse should manually palpate the uterus or ask the woman to inform her of each contraction to time their frequency and duration. The anesthesiologist should be notified immediately if fetal bradycardia or prolonged decelerations occur. The procedure should be stopped and measures should be instituted to oxygenate the fetus, improve uteroplacental perfusion, and reduce uterine activity. The birth attendant should examine the woman to rule out prolapsed cord or imminent birth.

Nursing Care Plan

The Woman Receiving Epidural Anesthesia During Labor

PATIENT PROFILE

History

R.A. is a 42-year-old G1/PO at 40 weeks' gestation. She has had a prolonged latent phase of labor (14 h). When the cervix is 5 cm dilated and 50% effaced, R.A. requests an epidural anesthesia. Her vital signs have been stable: 37°C (98.6°F), BP 110/60, p 88, RR 20; 1000 mL Ringer's lactate is infused intravenously as a preepidural bolus. The anesthesiologist then administers the epidural and begins a continuous infusion of 0.25% bupivacaine by pump.

Physical Assessment

One hour after administration of the epidural, the nurse is conducting an assessment. R.A. verbalizes complete pain relief. The nurse notes a large palpable bladder, and R.A. is unable to void when placed on a bedpan. "I just don't feel like my bladder is full. Everything is so numb down there, and I can't move my legs at all!" While R.A. is sitting on the bedpan, the electronic blood pressure monitor alarm is triggered. The nurse notes the following: BP 86/42, P 90. The FHR drops to 90 bpm and long-term variability is diminished. R.A. says, "I feel nauseated."

COLLABORATIVE PROBLEMS/POTENTIAL COMPLICATIONS

- Hypotension
- Allergic reaction/anaphylaxis
- Cardiovascular collapse secondary to accidental intravascular injection
- Respiratory arrest
- Postlumbar headache
- Infection at injection site
- Inadvertent spinal block

(See the Nursing Alert display following the Care Plan.)

Assessment	*Nursing Diagnosis*	*Nursing Interventions*	*Rationale*
R.A. is receiving epidural anesthesia R.A. is sitting in upright position on bedpan BP 86/42 P 90 R.A. says, "I feel nauseated."	Decreased Cardiac Output related to hypotension secondary to epidural anesthesia ***Expected Outcome*** R.A.'s blood pressure will stabilize within normal limits as evidenced by: Systolic BP >90 and <140 mm Hg Diastolic BP >50 and <90 mm Hg Mean arterial pressure >70 and <105 mm Hg	Call for help.	Additional help will be required to reposition R.A., administer fluids, and drugs in a timely manner.
		Have anesthesiologist notified.	The anesthesiologist must be notified when complications arise and may order additional therapy.
		Increase mainline IV infusion.	Rapid IV infusion will increase intravascular volume and elevate blood pressure. Epidural induced hypotension is due to relaxation of arteries below level of block. Ephedrine causes vasoconstriction, thus elevating blood pressure.
		Remove R.A. from bedpan. Lower head of bed.	Lowering head of bed will increase blood flow to brain.
		Place R.A. on left side and elevate her legs.	Turning R.A. to left will eliminate risk of supine hypotension. Raising legs will increase blood flow to brain.

(*Continued*)

The Woman Receiving Epidural Anesthesia During Labor
(Continued)

Assessment	***Nursing Diagnosis***	***Nursing Interventions***	***Rationale***
		Administer ephedrine 5–10 mg IV as ordered. Recycle electronic blood pressure monitor or take blood pressure q 1–2 min until stable.	More frequent monitoring will be required until blood pressure is stabilized.
		Monitor R.A. for alterations in mentation or complaints of nausea or vomiting.	Falling blood pressure will result in decreased tissue perfusion to brain and can result in altered mentation, nausea, or vomiting.
R.A. received 1000 mL IV fluid R.A. has no urge to void R.A. has epidural anesthesia	Altered Urinary Elimination related to decrease in sensation and motor function secondary to epidural anesthesia ***Expected Outcome*** R.A.'s bladder will not remain distended.	Monitor intake and output. Monitor R.A. for evidence of bladder distention.	Preepidural IV bolus and continued IV intake can result in bladder distention.
		If R.A. unable to void on bedpan, obtain order to catheterize her bladder or to insert Foley catheter to a drainage bag.	Even with anesthesia some women may be able to void when placed on bedpan. Epidural anesthesia may block normal sensations of urge to void or motor function required to urinate. Full bladder may impede fetal descent or may be traumatized during birth. If woman is not expected to give birth shortly, repeated catheterizations may result in urethral trauma and infection. Inserting a Foley catheter permits continuous urine drainage until delivery.
R.A. states, I just can't move my legs at all!" R.A. has epidural anesthesia	High Risk for Injury related to decreased sensation and motor function secondary to epidural anesthesia ***Expected Outcome*** R.A. will state she is pain free in legs and pelvis after the epidural was discontinued.	Place side rail up. Maintain legs in proper alignment. Use pillows to pad legs and prevent pressure points. Turn R.A. every 1–2 h. Obtain additional assistance when moving R.A. or transferring her from bed to delivery table.	Epidural anesthesia results in sensory and motor block, which eliminates perceptions of pressure, heat or pain or ability to move legs. Improper alignment can result in injury to muscles, tendons, or ligaments in legs or hips. Unrelieved pressure can result in decreased blood flow in legs and increases the risk of thromboembolic disorders.
		Do not use heating pad or warm packs on back, abdo-	Epidural will eliminate sensations of heat. Burns may oc-

(Continued)

The Woman Receiving Epidural Anesthesia During Labor

(Continued)

Assessment	Nursing Diagnosis	Nursing Interventions	Rationale
		men, or perineum after initiation of epidural.	cur if heat is applied to anesthetized areas.
		If legs placed in stirrups, pad the stirrups first and ascertain that legs are placed in proper alignment.	Improper alignment of legs while in stirrups can result in injury to muscle ligaments or tendons in legs or pelvis.
HR dropped to 90 bpm when R.A.'s pressure dropped to 86/42 HR long-term variability is diminished	High Risk for Fetal Injury related to epidural anesthesia ***Expected Outcome*** The FHR will remain within normal limits during administration of anesthesia as evidenced by: FHR baseline between 120–160 bpm. FHR long-term variability 6–10 bpm. No evidence of late decelerations.	Increase IV infusion rate. Turn R.A. to her left side	Increasing IV infusion and turning R.A. to her left side will improve uteroplacental perfusion and also increase R.A.'s blood pressure, which improves uteroplacental perfusion.
		Administer oxygen at 8–12 L/min by face mask.	Increasing R.A.'s blood oxygen level will increase the amount of oxygen available to fetus.
		Maintain continuous electronic fetal monitoring when epidural initiated Notify obstetrician of drop in FHR.	Continous EFM is indicated when anesthesia is administered during labor. It also permits immediate identification of fetal problems related to epidural anesthesia.

EVALUATION R.A.'s blood pressure was stabilized between 100/50 and 110/60. A Foley catheter was placed because R.A. had no urge to void; 800 mL clear amber urine was obtained. The Foley catheter was removed just before the birth. R.A. did not experience injury during labor and did not complain of pain or soreness in her legs and pelvis after the epidural was discontinued. The fetus was not injured because of the epidural anesthesia.

taken in positioning the woman to avoid injury to the lower extremities because sensory and motor function is diminished or lost. The left lateral position with the head of the bed slightly elevated will promote uteroplacental perfusion and patient comfort.

Bladder distention is a common problem during labor when epidural anesthesia is administered because the block eliminates bladder sensation to some extent. The problem is exacerbated by the administration of large volumes of IV fluids to prevent hypotension. The nurse must monitor intake and output carefully and observe and palpate for bladder distention at least every 30 minutes. The woman can be placed on a bedpan (walking is impossible with an epidural block due to loss of motor function), and some women will be able to void. If the woman is unable to empty her bladder, the birth attendant may decide to place a urinary drainage catheter in the bladder. This negates the need for repeated catheterization of the bladder when birth is not anticipated for some time.

Comfort measures such as position changes, frequent replacement of linen protectors as they become soiled, and perineal care are important. Because of the possibility of adverse effects with epidural anesthesia, the patient is usually given either nothing by mouth or clear liquids only once the epidural block is administered. Oral hygiene should be offered as needed to promote comfort and prevent dryness of the mucous membranes. Nausea or vomiting may occur with sudden hypotension, so an emesis basin should be placed within the woman's reach.

Because the woman will no longer feel uterine contractions, the nurse must evaluate their frequency, intensity, and duration by palpation and should apply the tokodynamometer to assist in this assessment. The woman will need assistance to push effectively during the second stage of labor

NURSING ALERT

NURSING RESPONSIBILITIES DURING ADMINISTRATION OF EPIDURAL ANESTHESIA

The nurse has primary responsibility for assessing and maintaining maternal and fetal physiologic stability during and after initiation of epidural anesthesia. Major complications can result in rapid, life-threatening decompensation. Before the anesthesiologist begins the procedure the nurse must:

- Administer 1000 mL prehydration bolus of IV fluid; have additional IV fluids at bedside (2 L Ringer's lactate).
- Ascertain that bedside oxygen and suction equipment is functioning.
- Ensure that emergency drugs including epinephrine, ephedrine, and benadryl are readily available.
- Attach an electronic blood pressure monitor or blood pressure cuff.
- Obtain portable FHR Doppler in case EFM is not possible during the procedure.

During the procedure, the nurse must maintain continuous FHR monitoring or frequent Doppler monitoring (q 5 min or more frequently) until EFM can be reinstituted. If IV oxytocin is being administered and the nurse is unable to monitor uterine activity during the procedure, the infusion should be stopped until the tokodynamometer can be reapplied. After the anesthetic is administered, the nurse remains continuously with the woman until vital signs are stable, assessing for evidence of:

- Hypotension
- Allergy or anaphylaxis
- Toxic reactions
- Total spinal block

The nurse must be skilled in resuscitation should adverse reactions occur. Ongoing nursing assessments of maternal vital signs and FHR must be conducted at least every 10 to 15 minutes.

In most settings the nurse is also responsible for periodic evaluation of anesthetic levels and should be skilled in this procedure.

because, as noted, sensation from the lower body is diminished or eliminated. She will need frequent feedback about the effectiveness of bearing-down efforts. The second stage is often somewhat longer than the traditionally defined 2 hours for primigravidas and 1 hour for multiparas, and the couple may need reassurance that this is to be expected.

Because of the loss of both sensation and motor function, safety remains a primary concern throughout labor, birth, and the recovery period. If the woman is moved to a delivery room, a roller may be needed to transfer her from the labor bed to delivery table. Once transfer is accomplished, the delivery table is mechanically tilted to the left to prevent supine hypotension. Care must be taken to protect her lower legs from sliding off the delivery table until they are secured in the stirrups. Proper alignment and padding of the legs is essential as lack of sensation makes it impossible for the woman to detect strain or pulling of ligaments or muscles. After birth, both legs should be carefully removed from the stirrups at the same time to prevent injury to ligaments or muscles. After birth of the neonate, the nurse must make certain that ambulation is not attempted until full motor and sensory function of the lower extremities is regained (see accompanying Legal/Ethical Considerations display).

Epidural Narcotics

A relatively new method of pain relief involves the injection of narcotics into the epidural space. Research indicates that epidural narcotics alone do not provide adequate analgesia for childbirth. However, when 75 to 80 μg of fentanyl (Sublimaze) is combined with a local anesthetic (bupivacaine), more rapid, complete pain relief of longer duration is experienced than when bupivacaine is administered alone. Fentanyl, a potent, short-acting narcotic, is currently the pre-

Legal/Ethical Considerations

Nursing Responsibilities in the Delivery Room After Administration of Regional Anesthesia

In many cases the woman receives an epidural or spinal anesthetic in the delivery room just prior to birth of the infant. Nursing malpractice cases frequently result from inadequate supervision of the woman during the interval between administration of anesthesia and birth. The nurse must take specific steps to ensure the safety and well-being of both woman and fetus until vaginal or cesarean birth.

- Continuous EFM and assessment of uterine activity is required.
- The uterus is displaced to prevent compression of the vena cava.
- Extreme caution must be exercised to prevent nerve and tissue damage resulting from pressure on or torsion of the legs.
- Care must be taken to restrain the lower limbs to prevent them from falling off the narrow delivery table.
- Care must be taken to prevent patient falls from the narrow delivery table, especially if it is tilted to facilitate uterine displacement.

The woman should *never* be left unattended in the delivery room. Her legs should be positioned in correct anatomic alignment, and stirrups should be padded. Leg restraints should not constrict blood flow. The fetal monitor should not be removed until birth of the neonate in the case of vaginal delivery or until abdominal prep is begun in the case of cesarean birth. If a urinary catheter is attached to a drainage bag, the nurse must verify that the tubing is not kinked and is patent during the delivery.

ferred drug for labor (Viscomi, Hood, Melone, & Eisenach, 1990).

The usefulness of epidural narcotics during and after cesarean birth has also been evaluated (Belzarena, 1992). The addition of fentanyl to the epidural anesthetic during cesarean birth reduces the pain, nausea, and vomiting frequently observed during uterine manipulation. A single dose of morphine (5 mg Duramorph) injected into the epidural catheter immediately after birth of the neonate results in up to 24 hours of analgesia (Nicholson, 1990). The need for additional parenteral pain relief may be reduced, allowing the mother greater mobility and alertness for ambulation and interaction with the neonate (Preston et al., 1988).

Indications and Contraindications

The addition of fentanyl to the epidural anesthetic is indicated when rapid induction of anesthesia is required. Women in the late active phase of labor or who are experiencing moderate to severe pain desire more rapid pain relief. The addition of fentanyl to the anesthetic may accomplish this goal. If the woman continues to perceive pain even with an adequate level of anesthesia (determined by a pinprick or alcohol swab test of the skin), she may benefit from the addition of fentanyl to the epidural local anesthetic.

There are very few contraindications to the use of epidural fentanyl. A known allergy to the drug would preclude its use. Maternal respiratory depression would be another factor. Several early studies examining the effects of fentanyl on FHR patterns discovered a temporary decrease in long-term variability. More recent studies have failed to duplicate these findings (Viscomi et al., 1990).

Advantages and Disadvantages

As noted, the addition of fentanyl to the epidural anesthetic can reduce the delay in onset of pain relief and results in a longer duration of epidural effect. The use of fentanyl may improve the woman's ability to push more effectively in the second stage of labor. This is possible because the degree of motor block experienced with epidural anesthesia can be decreased by adding fentanyl to a more *dilute* concentration of the epidural anesthetic. This can be accomplished without reducing pain relief.

Maternal and fetal cardiovascular, neurologic, and respiratory disturbances are rare with the use of epidural narcotics; however, delayed maternal respiratory depression and apnea have been reported. Nausea, vomiting, itching (particularly the mouth, face and eyes), and urinary retention are common side-effects. Some women may also experience euphoria or sedation as the drug reaches the opiate receptors in the dorsal horn of the spinal column. No significant effects on fetal distress, neonatal Apgar scores, umbilical cord pH values, neurobehavioral integrity, or state control have been demonstrated (Thorp et al., 1991).

Implications for Nursing Care

Nursing care of the woman who receives an epidural narcotic during labor requires careful monitoring of respiratory status. Respiratory depression is most likely to occur within the first hour after administration of the narcotic when peak blood levels are reached, and again 6 to 12 hours later when the opioids in the CSF reach the respiratory centers in the brain. The quality and rate of respiration are assessed every 10 to 15 minutes for the first hour and every 30 to 60 minutes for the remainder of labor. Naloxone should be available for reversal of respiratory depression. (A full discussion of the treatment of side-effects common with the administration of epidural narcotics follows later in the chapter.) Table 24-4 delineates nursing care during the use of an epidural analgesic.

Spinal (Subarachnoid) Anesthesia

Spinal anesthesia involves introduction of an anesthetic agent into CSF in the subarachnoid space through a spinal needle (Fig. 24-4). Spinal block can be used to provide anesthesia for vaginal delivery or for cesarean delivery by varying the level of sensation loss. Spinal block is usually effective for 1 to 2 hours and so is used primarily at the end of the first stage of labor and for delivery.

The *level of anesthesia* achieved with a spinal is described both as it relates to the specific location in the spinal column at which impulses are blocked and as it relates to the corresponding loss of sensation. A *saddle block* is achieved by blockade from level S-1 to S-4, with loss of sensation in the perineum, lower pelvis, and inner thighs; uterine contractions will still be felt, and pain with delivery will not be completely eliminated. A *low spinal block* for vaginal delivery requires blockage up to level T-10, with loss of sensation from the umbilicus to the toes. There is loss of sensation of uterine contractions and complete pain relief for delivery. A spinal block for cesarean delivery requires blockage up to the level of T-6, producing complete anesthesia from the nipple line to the toes.

The level of anesthesia is determined by altering the amount of medication injected and by changing the woman's position after injection. Because the anesthetic agent is hyperbaric (heavier than the CSF), changing the tilt of the delivery table or the woman's position will influence the level of anesthesia achieved. The injection is usually done at L-2 to L-5, preferably L-3 to L-4, for any spinal block, as shown in Figure 24-3. The block is usually administered with the woman in a sitting or sidelying position with the head slightly elevated. The woman is asked to place her chin on her chest and arch her back forward to widen the intervertebral space (see the accompanying Nursing Procedure, Aiding the Woman During the Spinal Block Procedure).

Injection during bearing-down efforts, coughing, straining, or vomiting must be avoided because these actions compress the subarachnoid space and force the anesthetic agent to a higher level than desired. If a saddle block or low spinal block for vaginal delivery is desired, the woman is generally kept in a sitting position for 5 minutes to allow time for the anesthetic to become bound to neural tissue. If a higher block for cesarean delivery is needed, more medication is injected, and the woman may be asked to move to a supine position immediately after injection. After 5 minutes, maternal position or actions will have little effect on the level of anesthesia produced. When the woman is placed in a supine position, the delivery table must be tilted to the left to prevent supine hypotension.

Table 24-4. Nursing Care of the Patient Receiving Epidural Analgesics

Assessment	Intervention
Inadequate pain relief	Notify anesthesiologist. Check for proper functioning of infusion pump. Check for kinks in epidural catheter. Evaluate anesthesia level. Perform vaginal exam to assess progress of labor. Do not administer parenteral narcotics until woman reevaluated by anesthesiologist and specifically ordered.
Localized pain (right or left side)	Turn woman to same side as pain if localized to redistribute medication.
Pruritus	Monitor for uticaria. Provide cool, moist cloth for skin. Administer antihistamine or naloxone as ordered.
Nausea or vomiting	Evaluate frequent causes of nausea and or vomiting: Hypotension Progress of labor Psychological factors Administer antiemetics as ordered. Provide mouth care.
Urinary retention	Monitor intake and output. Palpate for bladder distention. Administer naloxone as ordered. Ambulate early (when motor function returns after delivery).
Respiratory depression	Monitor and record respiratory rate: Every 10–15 min for first hour Every 30–60 min for duration of labor and for 24 h after morphine epidural If respiratory rate <12–14/min: Administer naloxone as ordered Administer oxygen 10–12 L/min by mask Monitor oxygen saturation with pulse oximeter Elevate head of bed to 30 degrees Notify anesthesiologist

Adapted from Nicholson, C. (1990). Nursing considerations for the parturient who has received epidural narcotics during labor and delivery. *Journal of Perinatal and Neonatal Nursing, 4*(1), 24. Reprinted with permission of Aspen Publishers, Inc., © 1990.

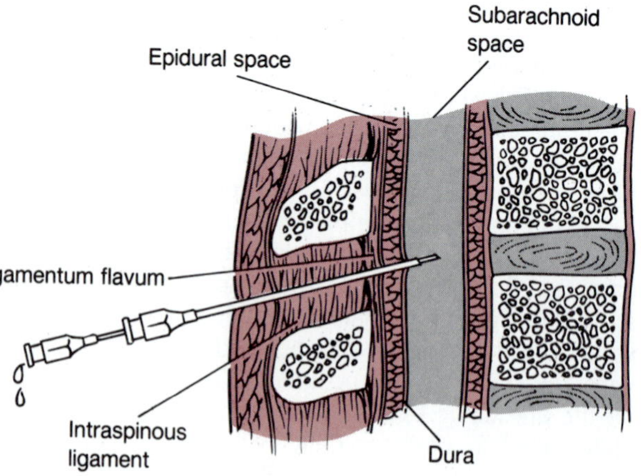

Figure 24-4.
Spinal injection is accomplished through a double-needle technique, in which a larger needle is introduced up to the ligamentum flavum, and a smaller needle is used for the injection into the subarachnoid space to minimize the puncture size.

Indications and Contraindications

Spinal anesthesia is indicated when complete sensory block is required. It is an excellent method for operative procedures such as forceps delivery, vacuum extraction, or cesarean birth. Induction of anesthesia is relatively rapid, but it would not be useful for emergencies.

Contraindications for spinal block include maternal hypotension or any factors that predispose to it (suspected hemorrhage, hypovolemia), neurologic disease, coagulation disorders or anticoagulation therapy, infection at the proposed injection site, or acute fetal distress. Spinal block will produce a rapid and dramatic fall in blood pressure as well as uterine and placental blood flow in women with hypertension. Thus, maternal hypertension may be considered a relative contraindication because of its deleterious effects on placental perfusion and fetal well-being.

Advantages and Disadvantages

Spinal anesthesia provides rapid and complete anesthesia for delivery and fourth stage of labor. There is little or no

NURSING PROCEDURE

Aiding the Woman During the Spinal Block Procedure

NURSING ACTION	*RATIONALE*
1. Administer the prehydration IV bolus.	To prevent hypotension and verifies that the infusion remains patient
2. Verify that blood pressure monitor (or sphygmomanometer) and fetal monitor are functioning properly.	To obtain appropriate data on maternal–fetal status during the procedure
3. Position the woman on her side with shoulders aligned and legs slightly flexed.	To facilitate optimum uterine blood flow during the procedure
4. When anesthesiologist is ready to begin procedure, have woman bring knees to abdomen, chin to chest, and round out back.	To increase the opening of the lumbar interspaces so that the epidural needle can be more easily advanced into the epidural space
5. Place the woman in a sitting position for the procedure if requested by the anesthesiologist.	To increase the opening of the lumbar interspaces when the sidelying position is not successful
6. Verify patency of the IV line.	To facilitate rapid infusion of IV fluids should hypotension or other adverse reactions occur during the procedure
7. Assist woman to maintain appropriate position during procedure. Offer reassurance and support during the procedure.	It may be difficult for the woman to maintain the position, especially during contractions; woman may be anxious about procedure.
8. After procedure, assist the woman into the desired position (supine with left tilt for cesarean birth, sitting for vaginal delivery for 3 to 5 minutes, then into a lithotomy position with left tilt).	To maintain adequate uterine perfusion
9. Continue to monitor FHR pattern.	To identify adverse response to anesthesia or to labor
10. Position legs for cesarean delivery and prevent them from sliding off of the delivery table by restraining them *or* place in stirrups and determine that legs are in proper alignment.	To prevent injury or circulatory compromise.
Anesthesiologist Activities	
1. Lower back is scrubbed with an antiseptic solution and draped.	To maintain asepsis and prevent infection
2. A skin wheal is raised between L-2 and L-5 (L-3 to L-4 preferred) interspace by intradermal injection of local anesthetic.	To facilitate proper injection of the spinal anesthetic
3. A 20- or 21-gauge needle is introduced into the wheal and advanced into the interspinous ligament, the ligamentum flavum, and the epidural space.	
4. A smaller gauge needle (25 or 26 gauge) is then inserted into the larger needle and advanced through the dura into the subarachnoid space. An attempt is then made to aspirate CSF.	The presence of CSF in the needle hub verifies that placement is correct.
5. Appropriate amount of anesthetic is injected slowly, and both needles are removed.	To provide anesthesia
6. Begin to monitor blood pressure, respiration, and pulse every 1 to 2 minutes for the first 10 minutes after administration.	To identify hypotension and signs of toxic reaction or respiratory difficulty, which signals possible respiratory paralysis.

direct effect on the fetus if maternal blood pressure is maintained.

Disadvantages of spinal block center on complications that may arise, including maternal hypotension and related fetal compromise; disruption of the normal pattern of labor with decreased effectiveness of bearing-down efforts; possible total or "high" spinal block, which interferes with respiration; postspinal headache; and increased risk of urinary retention in the immediate postpartum period. Each of these is discussed in detail. (The reader is referred to the earlier discussion of the adverse reactions to regional anesthesia.)

Implications for Nursing Care

Nursing responsibilities in providing care for a woman receiving a spinal block center on assisting the woman during administration of the block, closely monitoring maternal physiologic status, and promoting comfort and safety. The woman must receive an explanation about the procedure and give consent; usually this is performed by the anesthesiologist. However, the nurse may need to answer additional questions and explain what the woman and her partner should expect.

The nurse assists the woman into position for administration, explains the need to avoid movement, and supports her physically. The nurse also alerts the physician to onset of contractions so that the block can be administered between contractions. The nurse should recognize that spinal procedures are frightening to most patients and should provide emotional support and comforting touch during this time.

Once the woman has remained in the position necessary to establish desired anesthetic level for 5 minutes, the anesthesiologist or nurse anesthetist normally begins monitoring maternal blood pressure and vital signs. The nurse is responsible for assessing the woman's mental state and comfort level. Care must be taken in positioning the woman for delivery to avoid injury to the lower extremities, since self-protective pain sensation will be lost. The nurse is also responsible for continuous fetal monitoring until the birth of the neonate.

Intraspinal (Intrathecal) Narcotic Analgesia and Anesthesia

Another new technique being evaluated is the injection of *intraspinal* narcotics into the subarachnoid space to induce analgesia during labor. Meperidine (Demerol) has been used because of its combined analgesic *and* anesthetic properties. In recent studies (Swayze et al., 1991; Johnson et al., 1990), women who received meperidine during labor reported satisfactory to excellent pain relief. Onset of pain relief was rapid (approximately 4 minutes) and lasted over an hour. Motor block is rare, and women are able to push effectively in the second stage of labor. Side-effects of this new method are similar to those observed with epidural narcotics and include altered respiratory patterns, nausea, pruritus, and sedation. Further research will determine the usefulness of this method for the woman during labor and birth.

Paracervical Block

Paracervical block relieves uterine pain and thus is used to relieve pain of the first stage of labor only. The woman is placed in the lithotomy position, and the anesthetic agent (usually procaine or tetracaine) is injected into the lateral vaginal fornices on either side of the cervix, as shown in Figure 24-5. A paracervical block is administered in active labor, typically at 5 to 6 cm dilatation in a primigravida and 4 to 5 cm in a multigravida. It can be administered only while the cervix is still palpable. Anesthetic effect is nearly immediate and lasts 45 to 60 minutes.

Indications and Contraindications

Although paracervical block is rarely used today, it may be indicated for relief of pain in the first stage of labor when parenteral analgesics and epidural anesthesia are contraindicated.

Contraindications to the procedure include known hypersensitivity or allergy to the local anesthetic. Because of the high incidence of fetal bradycardia, use of paracervical block is contraindicated with fetal distress or when the fetus

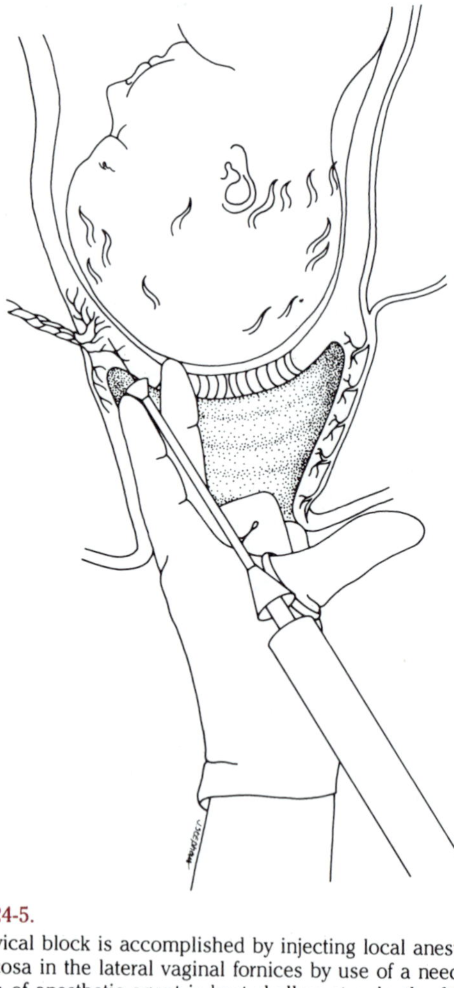

Figure 24-5.
Paracervical block is accomplished by injecting local anesthetic into the mucosa in the lateral vaginal fornices by use of a needle guide. Injection of anesthetic agent is kept shallow at a depth of 3 to 5 mm to avoid over-rapid absorption of the agent and accidental fetal injection (Childbirth Graphics).

is premature. It is also contraindicated when there is evidence of vaginal infection because of the risk of endometritis. (Insertion of a needle into the mucosa when infection is present may spread pathogens into underlying tissue and the uteroplacental circulation.)

Advantages and Disadvantages

The paracervical injection is a relatively simple procedure and provides good to excellent anesthesia for pain of uterine contractions and cervical dilatation. Maternal side-effects are rare; however, there is a small risk of maternal toxic reaction to the drug due to intravascular injection or rapid absorption after administration.

A major disadvantage of paracervical block is the fairly high incidence (25% to 85%) of fetal bradycardia after administration. This bradycardia is usually transient, appearing within 2 to 10 minutes after injection and lasting 10 to 30 minutes. There may also be loss of baseline variability and occasional late decelerations before the preblock FHR is reestablished. Finally, there is a small risk of injecting anesthetic directly into the fetus, which will result in toxicity and, possibly, fetal death. For these reasons few women receive paracervical blocks today.

Implications for Nursing Care

Nursing responsibilities in caring for a woman receiving a paracervical block include monitoring maternal and fetal physiologic response to the anesthetic and maintaining maternal physiologic functioning once anesthesia has been achieved. Continuous fetal monitoring is required, and the nurse must observe the FHR closely for evidence of bradycardia. If bradycardia is detected, the woman is kept in a side-lying position, and oxygen is administered. If FHR abnormalities persist longer than 30 minutes, the fetus should be considered potentially distressed, and the nurse should prepare for fetal blood sampling and emergency delivery.

General Anesthesia

General anesthesia, defined as pharmacologic intervention that results in progressive CNS depression with eventual loss of bodily sensation and consciousness, was routinely used in the 1950s and 1960s to manage maternal pain during labor and birth. However, this method of anesthesia is no longer widely used in normal intrapartum care because of the significant maternal and fetal risks it presents and because other modes of anesthesia now provide safer alternatives. However, general anesthesia is still appropriately used when emergency operative procedures including forceps delivery or cesarean birth are indicated.

The term *general anesthesia* is usually used in obstetrics to refer to inhalation anesthesia, or pain relief through administration of a gaseous agent mixed with oxygen and inhaled until loss of consciousness occurs. General anesthesia also includes the administration of IV anesthesia, usually a short-acting barbiturate, used in combination with inhalation anesthetics (see following section on combination or "balanced" anesthesia) to render the woman unconscious.

Agents used in general anesthesia include gas anesthetics and induction agents, usually IV drugs used to assist in the rapid induction of anesthesia. Some gas anesthetics can be self-administered by the patient with the use of an inhaler, a specialized mask that permits the woman to inhale the agent at the beginning of each contraction before pain is felt and to remove (or drop) the mask when anesthesia is sufficient. Inhaler masks should not be held in place for the woman by *anyone* but a skilled anesthetist or anesthesiologist because of the risk of rapid induction of deeper anesthesia and loss of consciousness. This method is rarely used in the United States.

Nitrous Oxide

Nitrous oxide produces analgesia and alteration of consciousness but not true anesthesia. It provides rapid, pleasant induction without interfering with maternal physiologic status at low dose concentrations (40% nitrous oxide, 60% oxygen). It can be administered by face mask or inhaler and should be given in combination with oxygen in concentrations no higher than 70% to avoid maternal hypoxia. Nitrous oxide has few side-effects and is often used both for analgesia in the second stage of labor and for induction of anesthesia in combination with other agents.

Methoxyflurane (Penthrane)

Methoxyflurane can be administered by inhaler for analgesia or in combination with other agents for anesthesia. It provides pleasant but somewhat slower induction and recovery than other gas agents. This agent also is associated with uterine relaxation and increased blood loss in the postpartum period, and for this reason use is typically restricted to low doses for relatively short periods.

Ketamine

Ketamine is an IV induction agent that produces analgesia, amnesia, and a sleeplike state with some CNS stimulation; it can be used as an induction agent for and in combination with inhalation anesthesia. Ketamine causes an increase in maternal blood pressure and pulse rate. It may cause unpleasant delirium and hallucinations and is rarely used in obstetrics.

Thiopental Sodium

Thiopental sodium (Pentothal) is an ultrashort-acting barbiturate that produces CNS depression and loss of consciousness within 30 seconds of administration. Its rapid action, its low potential for causing nausea and vomiting, and the prompt recovery time make it useful for induction in obstetric anesthesia. However, it does not produce anesthesia until doses are high enough to cause profound CNS depression; thus Pentothal is rarely used alone, being normally used with gas anesthetic agents.

Indications and Contraindications

Indications for general anesthesia for delivery are primarily conditions that require considerable uterine and pelvic relaxation (such as difficult forceps applications, breech deliveries, or the presence of tetanic contractions) with prompt effective maternal anesthesia. General anesthesia is often used in emergency vaginal deliveries and emergency cesarean deliveries for fetal distress. General anesthesia is regarded as the anesthetic of choice in the presence of maternal hemorrhage because regional anesthesia can compound maternal hypotension.

Contraindications to general anesthesia include situations where the fetus is already compromised and, because of the possible depressant effect on the fetus and newborn, where delivery cannot be anticipated within minutes of anesthetic administration.

Advantages and Disadvantages

Advantages of general anesthesia include the fact that it produces significant overall muscle relaxation, which is useful in difficult forceps extractions and in breech and cesarean deliveries. This property is also beneficial when the woman has severe preeclampsia or eclampsia because the muscle relaxation reduces the likelihood of convulsions. General anesthesia can also be rapidly administered and is ideal for emergency situations where delivery must be immediate and maternal pain relief is essential.

Disadvantages of general anesthesia for use in the intrapartum period include:

- Delivery must occur within 5 to 7 minutes after administration because inhalation anesthetics rapidly cross the placenta and will cause hypoxia and respiratory depression in the neonate.
- The risk of maternal aspiration of gastric contents with resulting life-threatening pulmonary complications is considerable.
- A skilled anesthetist or anesthesiologist is required for safe administration.
- Immediate postpartum recovery is more difficult, and there may be nausea and vomiting and increased risk of uterine atony and postpartum hemorrhage.
- The mother is not alert for the birth, and the partner is usually excluded from the delivery room.

Several of these points will be discussed in detail.

Respiratory Depression in the Fetus/Neonate. Most general anesthetics rapidly cross the placenta and enter fetal circulation within 2 minutes of administration. The degree of fetal CNS depression from anesthetic agents is proportional to the depth and duration of maternal anesthesia. If the fetus is already compromised by hypoxia or prematurity, the depressive effects of anesthesia are additive, and vigorous neonatal resuscitation may be needed at birth (see Chapter 32). The long-term effects of maternal anesthesia on neonatal status are not clearly understood. Effects of general anesthesia are similar to those of other medications but more pronounced; these include decreased response to stimuli, decreased rooting and sucking reflexes, hypotonia, and irritability.

Vomiting and Aspiration During General Anesthesia. Deaths related to anesthesia may account for as much as one half of maternal mortality; the most common cause of anesthesia-related death is pneumonia or chemical pneumonitis resulting from aspiration of gastric contents. General anesthesia reduces or eliminates the laryngeal and cough reflexes and often induces vomiting. Vomiting is especially likely during emergence from general anesthesia in circumstances where fundal pressure is applied to assist with the delivery.

In addition, the laboring woman is at increased risk for aspiration because gastric emptying time may be reduced during labor; she is likely to have particulate food matter in her stomach even hours after eating. Furthermore, the pH of gastric acid is lower in pregnancy and secretion of acid may be increased. Aspiration of particulate food matter typically leads to acute respiratory obstruction and aspiration pneumonia. Aspiration of even small amounts (less than 25 mL) of gastric acid is highly destructive to lung tissue and may lead to aspiration pneumonitis or Mendelson syndrome (adult respiratory distress syndrome).

Vomiting and aspiration during general anesthesia may be silent and unnoticed unless the patient is being monitored closely. Early signs of aspiration pneumonitis are restlessness and agitation, increased respiratory rate, tachycardia, cyanosis, and shock. Immediate treatment includes positioning the woman on her right side with head down at a 30-degree angle to facilitate airway clearance; endotracheal intubation with assisted ventilation and, possibly, a tracheostomy during the acute phase; systemic corticosteroids to limit the inflammatory reaction; and antibiotics to limit infection.

Measures to prevent aspiration during general anesthesia in the intrapartum period typically include:

- Administration of nonparticulate oral antacids (15 to 20 mL every 2 hours throughout labor and 30 to 50 mL within an hour before administration of general anesthesia)
- Maintenance of NPO status (with ice chips) for laboring women considered likely to require general anesthesia
- Smooth induction of anesthesia followed by prompt endotracheal intubation; intubation should be maintained until the woman is fully awake and has regained cough and laryngeal reflexes to protect her airway
- Application of cricoid pressure (downward pressure on the cricoid cartilage to compress the esophagus, preventing aspiration) during intubation and extubation and when vomiting has occurred

Increased Risk for Postpartum Hemorrhage. Another common problem related to general anesthesia in the intrapartum period is uterine atony and increased risk of postpartum hemorrhage. Most anesthetic gases used for general anesthesia produce profound uterine relaxation, preventing effective contractions and hemostasis. Treatment includes close monitoring of vaginal bleeding and continuous oxytocin infusion begun immediately after the delivery. This is done to maintain uterine tone until hemorrhage is no longer considered likely.

Implications for Nursing Care

Nursing responsibilities for care of the woman receiving general anesthesia for delivery include assisting the anesthetist as needed during the procedure. The nurse must be prepared to assist in emergencies such as acute respiratory obstruction. The nurse must be familiar with the location and use of emergency equipment and procedures needed for support of cardiopulmonary status. In the event of arrest, the nurse assists with cardiopulmonary resuscitation efforts. Nursing care during postanesthesia recovery is of special importance and, in most obstetric settings, the woman will be transferred to a postanesthesia unit. More intensive nursing care is required to avoid postanesthetic respiratory complications and to monitor for uterine atony and potential hemorrhage. Cardiopulmonary status is closely assessed until anesthetic effects have worn off. The reader is referred to a nursing text on surgical nursing for a more complete discussion of postoperative nursing care.

With recent advances in technology and the development of new methods of anesthesia, the nurse plays a central role in the safe use of anesthetic agents during labor and birth. The responsibility for supporting maternal and fetal well-being after anesthesia is initiated is based on a sound knowledge of the agents used, methods of administration, and potential complications. The nurse must recognize adverse reactions and must be prepared to initiate emergency supportive care when they arise. The goal of nursing care remains focused on a family-centered experience even after the administration of anesthesia. When general anesthesia is used, the partner or support person welcomes the neonate and becomes the link between mother and infant until she resumes consciousness.

Postpartum Analgesia

Most women who experience pain during the postpartum period experience mild or moderate pain, which is controlled by oral analgesics. If cesarean delivery is performed, parenteral narcotics or morphine epidural anesthesia is usually administered. A brief review of the most commonly used analgesics follows. For a detailed discussion of nonpharmacologic pain relief, the reader is referred to Chapter 28.

Nonsteroidal Antiinflammatory Drugs

Nonsteroidal antiinflammatory drugs (NSAIDs), the most widely used analgesics, include aspirin, acetaminophen, ibuprofen, and naproxen. In the postpartum period, inflammatory responses to lacerations, surgical incision, and trauma results in pain. NSAIDs indirectly inhibit the production of prostaglandins, which stimulate the inflammatory response. These drugs are available in oral, liquid, rectal, and in some cases, parenteral form. Common examples of NSAIDs used for mild to moderate postpartum pain include ibuprofen (Motrin), and acetaminophen (Tylenol). Ketorolac tromethamine (Toradol) is a parenteral NSAID. It may be administered to women who continue to experience postsurgical pain after administration of a morphine epidural, when concerns about respiratory depression preclude the use of narcotic analgesics.

Cross-sensitivity to aspirin should be assessed before administering ibuprofen or acetaminophen because allergic reactions may occur. Women who take NSAIDs may breastfeed. Side-effects are rare although prolonged use may result in gastric irritation. Women who are discharged with a prescription for NSAIDS should be warned about this potential side-effect.

Narcotics

Parenteral and oral narcotics are frequently administered during the postpartum period when NSAIDs are contraindicated or when pain is moderate to severe in intensity. Respiratory depression may occur, particularly when narcotics are administered by the parenteral route. Naloxone should be readily available to reverse respiratory depression. Sedation, a common side-effect of narcotics, may interfere with the woman's ability to assume self-care and infant care activities including breastfeeding. This disadvantage is observed more frequently in women after cesarean birth and is rare when oral doses are administered. Other side-effects include nausea and vomiting.

Some women may be hesitant to receive narcotics if they are breastfeeding. Others may be worried about narcotic dependence if repeated administration of the drug is necessary to control pain. The nurse must discuss the value of adequate pain control and the disadvantages of attempting self-care and infant care activities when significant pain and fatigue are experienced. The importance of receiving the next dose of narcotic analgesia *before* pain becomes severe should be stressed. Women who receive narcotics may breastfeed.

Patient-Controlled Analgesia

Patient-controlled analgesia (PCA) permits the self-administration of IV narcotics by the postpartum woman who has experienced a cesarean delivery. PCA permits the woman to control the amount and timing of drug administration. A solution of narcotic is drawn up into a syringe and placed into a computerized infusion pump. This pump has a "lock-out" device or security door that prevents unauthorized access to the prescribed opioid. Special tubing connects the syringe to the woman's IV line.

The infusion pump permits three types of infusion:

- Demand dosing, with preset limits established in the pump's computer for the frequency and total dose of medication that can be self-administered
- Continuous infusion of the narcotic analgesic
- Continuous infusion plus demand dosing of the narcotic analgesic

The woman pushes a button when she wishes to receive a dose of medication.

Research has demonstrated that this technique results in better pain control and greater patient satisfaction. Respiratory depression is rare. The patients receiving PCA infusions consumed more total narcotic in several studies than patients receiving intermittent IM injections, while experiencing less sedation. These findings support data suggesting that many patients may be reluctant to ask for more medication and fear the pain associated with IM injections (McIntosh & Rayburn, 1991). Patients also ambulated sooner and more frequently (Perez-Woods et al., 1991).

Disadvantages of this method include the possibility of respiratory depression. Cost has been noted to be a deterrent to the wider use of PCA. The infusion devices are expensive. Some women may be anxious initially about controlling the amount of narcotic received. However, with positive results (decreased pain, greater relaxation), most patients are satisfied or enthusiastic about the method.

Initial patient teaching about PCA and evaluation of the woman's use of the PCA pump are normally nursing responsibilities. Many facilities provide booklets that describe the method, its advantages, and its potential risks or problems. The nurse must continue to assess the woman's level of comfort and response to the narcotic. Monitoring of respiratory status is crucial, and naloxone should be readily available should respiratory depression occur.

Epidural Narcotics

Morphine (Duramorph) epidural is administered to provide postsurgical pain relief after cesarean birth. The analgesic effects last for up to 24 hours and permit earlier ambulation and assumption of self-care and infant care activities for most women who receive this method of pain control. Common side-effects are similar to those observed when intrathecal and epidural narcotics are administered during labor.

Respiratory status is monitored for 24 hours due to the longer duration of effect of this opiate. The respirations are assessed every 10 to 15 minutes in the first hour, then every 30 minutes for 3 to 6 hours, followed by evaluation every 30 to 60 minutes for the remainder of the first 24 hours. The anesthesiologist is notified immediately if respiratory depression becomes evident. Oxygen should be administered, and a pulse oximeter may be used to measure oxygen saturation levels. The head of the bed should be elevated 30 degrees to facilitate lung expansion and movement of the diaphragm. Protocols or anesthesia orders are often provided to guide the nurse in the treatment of adverse reactions. Narcotic antagonists, such as naloxone hydrochloride (Narcan), are administered to counteract respiratory depression. The drug can be administered intravenously (0.1-mg increments to a total of 0.4 mg). The nurse must be aware that the duration of action for naloxone is approximately 30 minutes, and respiratory depression may recur. The anesthesiologist may order a continuous infusion of naloxone if respiratory depression persists. The use of naloxone may unfortunately reduce the level of pain relief, and the woman may need parenteral analgesics. The anesthesiologist must be consulted before any additional narcotic analgesics are administered; however, parenteral NSAIDs may be given.

A small number of women experience moderate to severe itching after administration of epidural narcotics. Antipruritics (Benadryl) may be given to control discomfort from pruritus. Persistent nausea and vomiting may also occur and can be controlled with an antiemetic such as metoclopramide (Reglan) and droperidol (Inapsine). Compazine may also be administered, but should be used cautiously because it is a CNS depressant. Table 24-4 summarizes nursing care for the patient receiving epidural analgesics. The woman is also observed for other side-effects such as urinary retention and bladder distention. Naloxone has also been used to alleviate a persistent retention problem (see the Nursing Care Plan for the woman with a morphine epidural).

The advent of new methods of analgesia and anesthesia has increased the scope and responsibility of nursing practice in the postpartum period. These advances in pain control permit the woman who has experienced an operative delivery to assume self-care and infant care activities at an earlier stage in the postbirth period. They also reduce the risks of postoperative bed rest because the woman is generally able to ambulate earlier in the postpartum period. None of these methods is without side-effects and potential adverse reactions, however. The nurse must be knowledgeable about the method used and competent in providing relief from side-effects and emergency supportive care when complications arise.

Text continues on page 634

NURSING ALERT

NURSING RESPONSIBILITIES DURING ADMINISTRATION OF EPIDURAL MORPHINE

The nurse maintains primary responsibility for monitoring cardiovascular and respiratory status after the administration of epidural morphine. In most facilities, the nurse is guided by preestablished protocols in treatment of both minor and major complications of epidural narcotics. In other hospitals, the nurse must consult with the anesthesiologist before initiating treatment.

In either case, if respiratory depression or cardiovascular compromise is identified, the nurse must be prepared to initiate emergency cardiopulmonary support or resuscitation until the anesthesiologist arrives. The following nursing precautions should be taken:

- Monitor respiratory status with the frequency required by hospital protocol, physician order, and the woman's condition.
- Maintain a patent IV line for the administration of emergency drugs.
- Have a resuscitation bag and face mask at the woman's bedside or readily available, and ascertain that oxygen, bag and mask, and suction are functioning.
- Have naloxone and a 1-mL syringe available at the woman's bedside.
- Label woman's chart and place sign at bedside alerting all staff that a morphine epidural has been administered.
- Obtain order for incentive spirometer and begin deep-breathing exercises on admission to unit if not already begun in recovery room.
- Elevate head of bed at least 30 degrees to facilitate lung expansion.
- Notify anesthesiologist if downward trend in respiratory rate is noted before respiratory rate drops *below* 11 to 12 breaths/min.
- Apply pulse oximeter when downward trend is noted so that oxygen desaturation can be identified early.
- Be prepared to initiate artificial respiration if respiratory failure occurs.

Nursing Care Plan

The Postpartum Woman With a Morphine Epidural

PATIENT PROFILE

History

N.E. is a 22-year-old G1/P1 who has had a cesarean birth for failure to progress in labor. She received an epidural anesthetic during labor. After delivery of the infant, the anesthesiologist injected 5 mg Duramorph into the epidural space for postpartum pain control. Her baseline vital signs on admission to the postpartum unit are: T 37°C (98.6°F), BP 116/74, P 88, RR 22. N.E. verbalized complete pain relief at that time and had full return of sensation and motor function in her legs.

Physical Assessment

At 7 h postpartum the nurse performs an assessment and notes the following: The bed is flat, and N.E. is supine. During the assessment she begins to moan softly and places her hands over her abdominal dressing. N.E.'s vital signs are: T 36.8°C (98°F), BP 100/64, P 100, RR 11. She is alert and oriented. Her respirations are shallow. Breath sounds are diminished in the lower lobes bilaterally. Her abdomen is soft, nondistended. The incision dressing is dry. She has no bowel sounds. An emesis basin at the bedside has approximately 100 mL bile-stained fluid in it. N.E. has a Foley catheter, and the drainage bag has 450 mL clear amber urine. She is moving her lower extremities slowly. Her skin is pale pink, dry, and cool. Multiple scratch marks are present on her face, neck, and upper arms. N.E. states: "I feel horrible. I itch everywhere—like ants are crawling on me, and I'm in terrible pain. I thought this epidural was supposed to work for 24 hours! And I keep retching. I'm so nauseated. Can't you do something for me?"

COLLABORATIVE PROBLEMS/POTENTIAL COMPLICATIONS

- Respiratory depression/arrest
- Urinary retention
- Sedation/euphoria
- Pruritus
- Nausea/vomiting

(See the accompanying Nursing Alert display.)

Assessment	*Nursing Diagnosis*	*Nursing Interventions*	*Rationale*
N.E. has a morphine epidural anesthetic Respirations are 11/min Respirations shallow Breath sounds diminished in lower lobes N.E. is flat and in supine position N.E. is guarding abdomen due to pain	Ineffective Breathing Pattern related to epidural anesthesia *Expected Outcome* N.E. will maintain respiratory rate between 12 and 24/min. N.E. will demonstrate normal respiratory excursions with periodic inspiratory sighs. N.E.'s breath sounds will be clear and equal bilaterally in all lobes.	Notify anesthesiologist.	Anesthesiologist must be informed of complications related to epidural.
		Elevate head of bed 30 to 45 degrees.	Elevating head of bed will improve lung expansion.
		Administer 100% oxygen by mask (8–10 L/min) or nasal cannula (6 L/min).	Respiratory depression will result in decreased blood oxygen level.
		Administer naloxone per protocol or physician order: 0.2 mg IV (0.5 mL) and repeat q 2–3 min until respirations and respiratory effort are improved.	Naloxone is a narcotic antagonist and will reverse respiratory depression due to morphine. Naloxone has short half-life and may need to be readministered to maintain reversal of morphine-induced respiratory depression.

(*Continued*)

The Postpartum Woman With a Morphine Epidural

(Continued)

Assessment	Nursing Diagnosis	Nursing Interventions	Rationale
		Apply pulse oximeter.	Pulse oximeter will indicate oxygen saturation level and effectiveness of oxygen and naloxone administration.
		Initiate deep breathing exercises, preferably with use of incentive spirometer.	Deep breathing and ICS will increase lung expansion and improve gas exchange.
		Have anesthesia bag and mask at bedside. Ascertain that oxygen equipment and wall suction are functioning. Have naloxone and syringe at bedside.	Emergency equipment must be available to perform artificial ventilation should respiratory depression or arrest occur.
		Continue to monitor respiratory rate for 24 h according to protocol, doctor's order and N.E.'s condition. (Continuous until within normal limits q 10–15 min in subsequent hour; q 30 min for next 3 to 6 h; q 30–60 min for remaining 24 h.)	Continued assessment of respirations is essential until risk of drug-induced respiratory depression has passed (24 h).
N.E. has multiple scratch marks on face, neck N.E. has morphine epidural N.E. states, "I itch everywhere."	Altered Comfort (pruritus) related to morphine epidural ***Expected Outcome*** N.E. will verbalize a satisfactory decrease in sensations of itching within 45 min.	Administer antipruritics per protocol or physician's order: Naloxone 0.1 mg IV q 15 min PRN × 3 doses and then 0.1 mg q h if effective *or* Benadryl 25 to 50 mg IV or IM q 2 h *or* nalbuphine 10 mg SQ q 2 h. If no relief within 45 min, begin continous IV infusion of 1.6 mg (4 mL) naloxone in 1000 mL Ringer's lactate at 0.2 mg/h (125 mL/h of IV solution)	Pruritus is the most common side-effect of narcotic epidural anesthesia. Naloxone or nalbuphine, narcotic antagonists, appear to be most effective agents. Benadryl causes sedation, which may decrease awareness of itching sensation, but also may depress respiratory rate, respiratory effort, and interfere with maternal–neonatal interactions and breastfeeding.
		Apply cool wash cloths to skin until antipruritics begin to take effect.	Cool washcloths may decrease sensations of itching.
100 mL bile-stained emesis N.E. states, "I keep retching." N.E. has morphine epidural	Altered Comfort (nausea and vomiting) related to morphine epidural ***Expected Outcome*** N.E. will verbalize a satisfactory decrease in nausea and no further vomiting within 45 min of administration of antiemetic.	Administer antiemetics per protocol or physician order: Metoclopramide 10 mg IV q 2 h or droperidol 0.625 mg IV or IM q 4 h PRN for nausea.	Antiemetic may be required to control nausea due to morphine
		Provide mouth care.	Postsurgical patients are usually NPO for 24 h and will require month care.

(Continued)

The Postpartum Woman With a Morphine Epidural

(Continued)

Assessment	Nursing Diagnosis	Nursing Interventions	Rationale
		Decrease environmental stimuli until nausea and vomiting are controlled (light, noise, unpleasant odors, food odors).	Environmental stimuli may exacerbate nausea.
		Minimize activities that require woman to move and teach slow, deep-breathing exercises until nausea and vomiting are controlled.	Movement may increase nausea or precipitate vomiting.
N.E. has incision from cesarean delivery N.E. is moaning during nursing assessment N.E. is guarding abdomen N.E. states, "I'm having terrible pain."	Pain related to cesarean incision ***Expected Outcome*** N.E. will verbalize satisfactory pain relief within 45 min of receiving an analgesic.	Notify anesthesiologist. Administer analgesic per physician order: Ketorolac (Toradol) 30–60 mg IM × 1 followed by 30 mg q 6 h	Additional pain medication cannot be administered without evaluation of cardiovascular and respiratory status due increased risk of respiratory depression.
		If respiratory status stable: Morphine 1–2 mg IV q 1–2 h PRN or nalbuphine 5–10 mg IM q 2–3 h PRN or nalbuphine 1–2 mg IV q 1–2 h PRN.	Morphine is a respiratory depressant and may only be administered if respiratory rate is within normal limits (>18/min)
		Monitor pain level and administer analgesic based on respiratory status and level of pain sensation.	
		Implement additional nonpharmacologic pain relief methods to reduce pain sensations such as pillows for support, massage, use of imagery, and breathing techniques.	An NSAID may be drug of choice if respiratory rate is slow or if woman wishes to avoid sedation. Repeat doses of analgesics should be administered before pain sensations are intense because it will take longer for analgesia to reduce pain.
		Evaluate abdomen for evidence of distention, rigidity, increasing girth.	Uncontrolled pain will result in release of catecholamines, will increase fatigue, and may have an adverse effect on wound healing. Uncontrolled pain will also interfere with the woman's ability to perform self-care, interact with neonate, and breastfeed.

(Continued)

The Postpartum Woman With a Morphine Epidural
(Continued)

Assessment	Nursing Diagnosis	Nursing Interventions	Rationale
			Respiratory and cardiovascular status must be reevaluated before administering a drug that causes respiratory depression. Intense, unrelieved pain may be due abdominal distention secondary to intraabdominal bleeding.

EVALUATION

After administration of naloxone 0.2 mg IV × 2, N.E.'s respiratory rate rose to 18/min and remained in a range of 16 to 20/min. Respirations increased in depth. Periodic sighs were noted. Breath sounds were clear and equal bilaterally in all lobes by 18 h postpartum.

Because N.E. did not achieve a satisfactory decrease in sensations of itching after three doses of 0.1 mg naloxone IV, a continuous IV infusion of naloxone was infiltrated at 0.2 mg/h. Forty-five minutes after infusion, N.E. verbalized complete cessation of itching. Within 45 min of administration of 0.625 mg droperidol IV, N.E. verbalized total cessation of sensations of nausea. No further vomiting occurred.

N.E.'s incisional pain decreased within 50 min of Toradol administration. Additional doses were required at q 6-h intervals.

Chapter Summary

A major goal of nursing care during childbirth and the postpartum period is the provision of comfort and the control of pain. Uncontrolled pain has deleterious effects for both the woman and her fetus. When comfort measures fail to provide adequate pain control or when complications require immediate intervention such as cesarean birth, pharmacologic methods may be used. The nurse uses the nursing process to meet these objectives.

From admission through birth and the postpartum period, the nurse assesses the patient's level of discomfort, establishes appropriate nursing diagnoses, and plans effective strategies to manage pain. The safety and efficacy of analgesia and anesthesia depend in large part on the expertise of the clinician. The competent nurse must have comprehensive knowledge regarding the drugs and techniques commonly used in childbirth and the postpartum period.

Study Questions

1. *What are the major sources of discomfort and pain during labor, birth, and the postpartum period?*
2. *What are the physiologic and psychological effects of pain?*
3. *What are the nurse's primary responsibilities when administering analgesia during childbirth and the postpartum period?*
4. *Why is it inadvisable to administer analgesia during the transition stage of labor?*
5. *What are the advantages and disadvantages of PCA?*
6. *What are common forms of regional anesthesia?*
7. *What are the nurse's primary responsibilities when epidural or spinal block are administered?*
8. *What are the major advantages and disadvantages of regional anesthesia?*
9. *What are the common side-effects of epidural and intrathecal narcotics?*
10. *What are the nurse's responsibilities after administration of epidural narcotic?*
11. *What are the nurse's responsibilities in the first 24 hours postpartum after administration of a morphine epidural?*
12. *What are common adverse effects of epidural and spinal block?*
13. *What are the advantages and disadvantages of general anesthesia?*

References

ACOG Committee on Obstetrics. (1992). *Maternal and fetal medicine. Anesthesia for emergency deliveries* (No. 104). Washington DC: Author.

Baxi, L., Petrie, R., & James, S. (1988). Human fetal oxygenation ($tcPO_2$), heart rate variability and uterine activity following maternal administration of meperidine. *Journal of Perinatal Medicine*, *16*, 23.

Belzarena, S. (1992). Clinical effects of intrathecally administered fentanyl in patients undergoing cesarean section. *Anesthesia and Analgesia*, *74*, 653.

Brown, S., Campbell, D., & Kurtz, A. (1989). Characteristics of labor pain at two stages of cervical dilation. *Pain*, *38*, 289.

Callahan-Faut, M., & Paice, J. (1990). Postoperative pain control for the parturient. *Journal of Perinatal and Neonatal Nursing*, *4*(1), 27.

Johnson, M., Hurley, R., Gilbertson, L., et al. (1990). Continuous microcatheter spinal anesthesia with subarachnoid meperidine for labor and delivery. *Anesthesia and Analgesia*, *70*, 658.

Kennell, J., Klaus, M., McGrath, S., Robertson, S., & Hinkley, C. (1991). Continuous emotional support during labor in a US hospital. *Journal of the American Medical Association*, *262*(17), 2197.

Lowe, N. (1991). Maternal confidence in coping with labor. *Journal of Obstetric, Gynecologic, and Neonatal Nursing*, *20*(6), 457.

McIntosh, D., & Rayburn, W. (1991). Patient-controlled analgesia in obstetrics and gynecology. *Obstetrics and Gynecology*, *78*(6), 1129.

McKay, S., & Barrow, T. (1991). Holding back: Maternal readiness to give birth. *American Journal of Maternal Child Nursing*, *16*(5), 251.

NAACOG. (1991). Position statement on the role of the registered nurse in the management of analgesia by catheter techniques (epidural, intrathecal, intrapleural, or peripheral nerve catheters). Joint State of Nursing Organizations.

Nicholson, C., & Ridolfo, E. (1989). Avoiding the pitfalls of epidural anesthesia in obstetrics. *Journal of American Association of Nurse Anesthetists*, *57*(3), 220.

Perez-Woods, R., Gorhar, J., Skaredoff, M. et al. (1991). Pain control after cesarean birth. *Journal of Perinatology*, *XI*(2), 174.

Preston, P. G., Rosen, M. A., Hughes, S. C., Glosten, B., et al. (1988). Epidural anesthesia with fentanyl and lidocaine for cesarean section: Maternal effects and neonatal outcomes. *Anesthesiology*, *68*, 938–943.

Swayze, C., Walker, E., Skerman, J., et al. (1991). Efficacy of subarachnoid meperidine for labor analgesia. *Regional Anesthesia*, *16*, 309.

Thorp, J., Eckert, L., Ang, M. et al. (1991). Epidural analgesia and cesarean section for dystocia: Risk factors in nulliparas. *American Journal of Perinatology*, *8*(6), 402.

United States Department of Health and Human Services. (1992). *Acute pain management in adults: Operative procedures*. Rockville, MD: Author.

Viscomi, C., Hood, D., Melone, P., & Eisenach, J. (1990). Fetal heart rate variability after epidural fentanyl during labor. *Anesthesia and Analgesia*, *71*, 679.

Wild, L., & Coyne, C. (1992). Epidural analgesia. *American Journal of Nursing*, *92*(4), 26.

Wuitchik, M., Hesson, K., & Bakal, D. (1990). Perinatal predictors of pain and distress during labor. *Birth*, *17*(4), 186.

Suggested Readings

Blum, M. (1989). *Selected drugs used during labor and delivery: Effects on the fetus and neonate* (2nd ed.). Series 3. Intrapartum care. Module 1. White Plains, NY: The National Foundation/March of Dimes.

Daley, M. (1990). A comparison of epidural and intramuscular morphine in patients following C section. *Anesthesiology*, *72*, 289.

Geden, E. A., Beck, N. C., Anderson, J. S., Kennish, M. E., et al. (1986). Effects of cognitive and pharmacologic strategies on analogued labor pain. *Nursing Research*, *35*, 301–306.

Gribble, R., & Meier, P. (1990). Effects of epidural analgesia on the primary cesarean rate. *Obstetrics and Gynecology*, *78*, 231.

Henrikson, M., & Wild, L. (1988). A nursing process approach to epidural analgesia. *Journal of Obstetric, Gynecologic, and Neonatal Nursing*, *17*, 316.

Johnson, C., & Oriol, N. (1990). The role of epidural anesthesia in trial of labor. *Regional Anesthesia*, *15*, 304.

Kavee, E., & Ramanathan, S. (1991). The hypothermic action of epidural and subarachnoid morphine in parturients. *Regional Anesthesia*, *16*, 325.

Nicholson, C. (1990). Nursing considerations for the parturient who has received epidural narcotics during labor and delivery. *Journal of Perinatal Neonatal Nursing*, *4*(1), 14.

Types of Losses Arising in the Perinatal Period and Their Causes

Loss of "Real Versus Ideal" (Pregnancy)

- Maternal or fetal disease
- Need for hospitalization or transport to distant site
- Diagnosis of fetal anomalies
- Intrauterine fetal demise

Loss of "Normal" Labor Experience

- Development of complications
- Need for interventions (intravenous therapy, oxytocin infusion, oxygen)
- Need for external or internal fetal monitoring
- Fetal distress
- Need to remain in bed
- Need for analgesia or anesthesia

Loss of Emotional Control

- Screaming, crying
- Verbalization of anger, fear, discouragement
- Use of expletives

Loss of Physical Control

- Inability to push or inability to withstand involuntary urge to push
- Involuntary vocalizations, defecation, or urination during bearing-down efforts
- Inability to maintain breathing or relaxation techniques
- Vomiting
- Slapping or hitting coach, partner, medical or nursing staff, or physical objects
- Throwing objects

Loss of "Natural Birth" Experience

- Preterm birth
- Need for analgesia or anesthesia
- Need for episiotomy
- Need for forceps or vacuum extraction
- Need for cesarean delivery

Loss of Shared Experiences

- Absence of father, partner, or other significant family members or friends

Loss of Body Image

- Incompetent cervix
- Severe edema with preeclampsia
- Incision from cesarean birth

Loss of "Real Versus Ideal" (Neonate)

- Neonatal anomalies
- Birth injuries or asphyxia
- Preterm infant
- Need for transport to distant site
- Stillbirth/neonatal death

Loss of "Real Versus Ideal" (Postpartum Experience)

- Maternal trauma or disease
- Postpartum depression

Loss of Self-Image

- Maternal disease process
- Preterm labor or birth
- Fetal or neonatal death

Loss of "Real Versus Ideal" (Breastfeeding)

- Neonate unable to breastfeed due to prematurity, illness, or anomalies

Loss of Relationships

- Maternal hospitalization or transport to distant site
- Neonatal transport
- Fetal or neonatal death
- Partner withdraws during grief process
- With fetal or neonatal death, avoidance behaviors by family or friends

Loss of Life-style

- Disruption in work and daily living activities
- Alteration in sleep patterns
- Disruption in sexuality or intimacy with significant others

Loss of Life-style in Hospital

- Lack of privacy
- Inability to pursue leisure activities
- Lack of control over environment

overwhelming physical and emotional consequences of intrapartum death and bereavement. At other times perinatal complications result in relatively few or less significant deprivations. Sensitive nursing care and appropriate support often are all that are needed to help families weather temporary setbacks. When losses are identified, grieving occurs. The maternity nurse must be able to identify the grieving process and assist the woman and her family in the work of grieving.

The Grieving Process

When problems are diagnosed during the perinatal period, a grief response ensues in parents and close family members. Mourning occurs for the loss of the idealized pregnancy or childbirth experience or for the fantasized child if fetal or neonatal complications develop. The stages of grieving are essentially the same as those described by Kubler-Ross (1969).

Shock. The woman and her partner feel numb and are unable to comprehend the full import of the problem. They may withdraw, showing no evidence of discomfort or sadness to avoid the pain that will follow with full realization of the problem. This period may last from minutes to days.

Denial and Disbelief. The woman and her partner cannot believe that the stressful event is really happening to them. If the problem is not observable, they may deny that any problem exists. This phase also may be characterized by unrealistic optimism in the face of a very poor prognosis. Parents may say that the situation seems "unreal." The length of this period depends on the visibility of the disease or anomaly in the case of a neonate born with a congenital problem. It is more difficult to continue denying the problem when severe and obvious sequelae exist.

Anger. Once the woman and her partner permit themselves a full realization of the problem, feelings of anger surface. A healthy response is to displace the anger on staff members, family, or friends. An individual may verbalize feelings of anger or may react physically by throwing things or hitting people close by.

Sadness and Guilt. Painful feelings are now fully experienced. Physical symptoms of grief may be present, including tightness in the chest or epigastric distress. The woman or her partner may experience a feeling of emptiness. Self-recriminations and strong feelings of guilt also emerge: "What did I do to cause this to happen?" They will frequently review the entire course of pregnancy trying to pinpoint something he or she did to cause the problem.

Reorganization and Resolution. After a prolonged period (sometimes months to years) the feelings of sadness are blunted, the guilt feelings are resolved, and the individual is able to reorganize his or her life. If long-term disabilities remain, as in the case of a neonate with severe anomalies, the woman or her partner may regress to previous stages of grieving when new, related problems surface for the child.

Grief Work

Successful reorganization and resolution require an active effort to move through the stages of grief and have been described by Worden (1982) as the "work of grieving." The goals of grief work are to accept the loss, experience the pain of grief, adjust to the environment in which the loss has occurred, and reinvest the energy expended in grief to restore one's life (Worden, 1982).

Individual and Family Responses

Maternal Responses

Regardless of the nature of the problem or when it develops, the woman usually is anxious and in some situations may feel overwhelmed. If fetal well-being is jeopardized, her distress is heightened. Hospitalization during pregnancy or a prolonged stay due to complications occurring during birth or the postpartum period place additional stain on the woman. If the woman is already a mother, pragmatic considerations regarding child care may add to her emotional burden; concerns about disruption in employment and work responsibilities may be another source of anxiety. In the worst case fetal or neonatal death brings an abrupt ending to the pregnancy, which can be emotionally shattering.

Initially all of the woman's energies may be focused on dealing with the physical sensations associated with the problem, as well as the diagnostic tests and therapeutic interventions that are initiated. She may be tearful or withdrawn and unable to process a great deal of the information provided by health care professionals about her condition. Early signs of grief may be evident, including verbalizations of shock and disbelief. Physiologic signs of anxiety, including tremulousness, tachycardia, hyperventilation, nausea and vomiting, or cold, clammy extremities, may be evident. The nurse must be sensitive to these responses to plan and implement appropriate interventions that support physiologic functioning and reduce acute anxiety, which can be almost paralyzing at times.

Paternal or Partner Responses

The partner or father must come to grips with the vulnerability of the woman and fetus or newborn. Both parents are likely to feel that they are not prepared to deal with the complication. However, if the woman is completely incapacitated or unconscious, the spouse or partner must often assume responsibility for life-and-death decisions, as well as household duties and child care for siblings (Fig. 25-2). This can represent an overwhelming stressor for even the most competent adults. Financial concerns can represent an additional burden and source of anxiety.

Research has discovered an increased incidence of illness among men during the pregnancy and postpartum recovery of a spouse or partner (Ferketich & Mercer, 1989). There is also an increase in the report of pregnancy-related symptoms, known as the couvade syndrome, which includes nausea and vomiting, abdominal bloating, heartburn, backaches, leg cramps, and anxiety (Brown, 1988). Very few

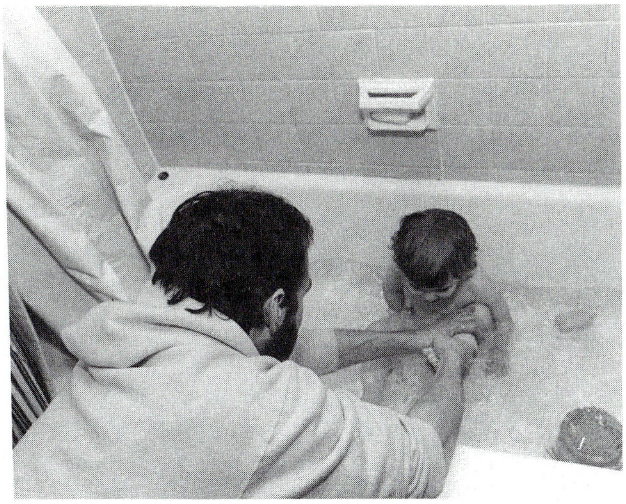

Figure 25-2.
Everyday routines of child care can feel like an overwhelming responsibility to the partner of a woman hospitalized for high-risk pregnancy.

investigators have examined the impact of high-risk pregnancy on the father's or partner's health. However, Conner and Denson (1990) suggest that some men may be at greater risk of physical or mental health problems when intrapartum problems arise. The responses of men may depend in part on their involvement in the pregnancy and when the complications arise.

Role expectations for men also may account for the responses of many partners to intrapartum complications. Research indicates that men's responses to loss closely conform to how they believe men should act, rather than how they need to act to confront the problem or resolve grief (Cordell & Thomas, 1990). Some men will appear stoic, very controlled, and hesitant to reveal their true level of distress. In addition the necessity of assuming the roles of "protector" and "provider" during a potential crisis may delay the work of grieving for many men.

Specific reactions to perinatal complications will vary greatly, however, and the nurse will observe many characteristic responses. Men should be permitted to express emotional distress openly and in an accepting and supportive environment when they are ready to do so. The nurse should also be prepared for many of the same physiologic responses observed in women.

Sibling Responses

Nurse researchers are beginning to explore the responses of siblings to intrapartum complications and loss. Children will react differently to the stress of unexpected problems or intrapartum death. Research findings indicate that children do mourn but do so differently from adults. They can continue with the business of play while dealing with the work of grief. Trouy and Larson (1987) note common grief reactions in children in response to the death of a sibling:

- Frightening thoughts about death that are difficult to express
- Attention-seeking misbehaviors
- Unexpressed guilt for having wished the sibling dead at some time
- Feelings of responsibility for the sibling's death
- Distancing behaviors from the grief of others; assuming an attitude of unconcern

Other common reactions include regression, somatic complaints, and sudden changes in eating and sleeping patterns. School-age children may have difficulty with lessons and fail to complete assignments. Because parents are their children's primary role models, grief reactions will be influenced strongly by the adult responses. Parents play a powerful role in facilitating or impeding the successful resolution of grief. Health care providers can provide parents with guidance in this area. Some nursing interventions are discussed in the nursing process section.

Assessment

The nursing assessment of the woman and her family includes identifying the stage of grief. Verbal and nonverbal cues will assist the nurse in this process. Characteristics of the early stages of the grieving process are listed in the accompanying Family Considerations display.

The nurse also attempts to identify adaptive and maladaptive responses and balancing factors that influence the ability to resolve the potential crisis (see Fig. 25-1). Physical reactions to stress may exacerbate the underlying physiologic problems experienced by the woman and complicate the assessment process.

The initial assessment often is conducted simultaneously with the implementation of emergency nursing and medical measures. The goal of this assessment is to pinpoint the most pressing individual and family needs and to reduce extreme levels of anxiety and distress. An in-depth and systematic assessment of family responses, strengths, and coping patterns often is deferred until physiologic stability is achieved in the woman and fetus or newborn. If the mother or neonate is transported to a perinatal center, other health care professionals, including social workers and psychiatric personnel, may be involved in the assessment process.

Nursing Diagnosis

Psychosocial problems usually will be identified when complications occur. The following are selected nursing diagnoses that reflect common difficulties for the individual or family:

- Knowledge Deficit related to the condition, procedures, and interventions
- Fear/Anxiety related to complications and procedures
- Impaired Verbal Communication related to anxiety or fear
- Family Coping: Potential for Growth related to constructive stress management, supportive social networks, or role changes

Family Considerations

Characteristics of the Early Stages of the Grieving Process

Shock

- Stunned silence
- Inability to verbalize
- Inability to follow simple explanations or directions
- Inability to give information
- Inability to understand what is said about neonate's condition
- Physical reactions—pallor, tremors, nausea or vomiting, feelings of faintness or actual syncope

Denial/Disbelief

- Withdrawal from neonate or other family members
- Physical abandonment of mother or neonate by father or partner
- Unrealistic optimism
- Expressions of feelings of unreality: "I can't believe this is happening."
- Refusal to speak about neonate's condition
- Refusal to see infant
- Refusal to participate in decisions about treatment of child

Anger

- Irritability
- Use of profanity
- Throwing objects
- Hitting others in the environment
- Verbal abuse of spouse, family members, or staff members
- Angry requests to be left alone
- Assignment of blame to staff or others
- Verbalizations of anger

Guilt

- Repeated reviews of course of pregnancy, labor, and delivery for causes of neonatal problems
- Repeated questions about possible causes of problem
- Verbalization of guilt: "It's my fault."
- Statements such as "If only I had not done . . . "
- Assignment of cause of problem to past actions, omissions, or "sins"
- Statements that the problem is "a punishment from God"

Sadness

- Loss of appetite
- Difficulty in sleeping
- Crying
- Restlessness
- Other somatic complaints
- Inability to focus attention
- Verbalization of sadness or depression
- Verbalization of sense of failure
- Verbalization of wanting to be left alone

- Ineffective Individual or Family Coping related to intrapartum loss, disruption in emotional bonds, inadequate social or psychological resources, or sensory overload
- Sleep Pattern Disturbance related to disease, treatment, or hospitalization
- Self-Care Deficit related to enforced immobility
- Situational Low Self-Esteem related to loss of body function, disease, loss, hospitalization, or surgery
- Anticipatory Grieving related to loss
- Decisional Conflict related to illness or hospitalization
- Spiritual Distress related to illness or loss
- Social Isolation related to hospitalization
- Powerlessness related to illness or hospitalization
- Hopelessness related to chronic illness or loss

• • Planning and Implementation

Planning and providing care to the at-risk family is a complex process. Although establishing physiologic stability is usually the foremost consideration, of critical importance is maintaining emotional equilibrium. Research indicates that the emotional distress associated with high-risk pregnancy can result in many deleterious physiologic effects for the woman and fetus; in the postpartum period psychological disequilibrium interferes with maternal and family adaptations and parenting activities.

Planning Appropriate Support

The woman, her partner, or other significant family members should be included in the immediate plan of care. If long-term hospitalization is anticipated for the woman or neonate, the nurse can discuss the expected course of therapy and answer questions about planned treatments and expected outcomes in conjunction with the physician. Routines for bathing, meals, rest, physical therapy, administration of medication, and diversional activities should be planned with the woman. Practical considerations should be discussed, including a review of visiting hours for family, siblings, and friends; pastoral support; and long-distance phone calls if the woman or neonate is transported far from home. Arrangements should be made for consultations with dietary, financial, and social services and when appropriate occupational therapy. A major goal of planning is to provide the woman and her partner with as much control as possible in a situation that often engenders feelings of lack of control.

Providing Family-Centered Nursing Care

The provision of family-centered maternity care is essential when complications arise during the intrapartum period; however, implementation of this approach often is difficult. If the woman or neonate is critically ill, initial care and treatment must be focused on physiologic functioning, limiting the ability of health professionals to address the emotional needs of the family. Long-term hospitalization or transportation often results in physical and emotional disruption of the family unit. The use of technology, such as monitors and incubators, also limits close physical contact between the neonate and family members. Some specific nursing interventions to provide family-centered care in the perinatal period are listed in the accompanying display.

Expected Outcomes

- The at-risk couple restates information given to them about problems, planned treatment, and procedures.
- The at-risk couple verbalizes comfort and appreciation for support.
- The at-risk couple uses coping techniques increasingly.

• • Evaluation

When perinatal complications result in the birth of a high-risk neonate or when fetal or neonatal death occurs, long-term follow-up is an essential aspect of nursing care. Most intrapartum units now have protocols for contact with families at specified intervals during the first year after the birth (or death) of the high-risk neonate.

Nurse researcher Kenner (1990) identified five areas of parental concern requiring ongoing evaluation and support: (1) informational needs, (2) grief counseling, (3) social support, (4) parent–newborn development, and (5) stress and coping problems.

Nurses in acute care and community health settings usually are involved in the ongoing evaluation and care of the family who has experienced an intrapartum problem. The neonatal nurse may make phone contact at 1 week, 1 month, 6 months, and 1 year after birth.

A new and rapidly growing area of practice involves home monitoring of the high-risk pregnant woman required to remain on bed rest for an extended time. Nurses who visit the home and evaluate the woman also are involved in the evaluation of family responses to perinatal complications. Goals of ongoing evaluation include identifying the need for further support or referrals and assisting in the resolution of the grief process. The following signs of pathologic grief are adapted from the Association of Women's Health, Obstetric, and Neonatal Nursing (formerly NAACOG, 1985):

- Unrelieved depression
- Delayed or postponed grief
- Overactivity without a sense of loss
- Extreme hostility against specific person
- Immediate attempts to become pregnant again
- Disruptions in relationships with family and friends
- Persistent loss of patterns of social interaction
- Initial diagnosis or exacerbation of psychosomatic disease
- Activities detrimental to personal, social, or economic survival

Although individual responses to the development of perinatal complications vary, most family members demonstrate a pattern of grieving that has fairly predictable stages. Whether anticipated or unexpected, each family member must cope with perceptions of loss. Behavioral and verbal clues assist the nurse in identifying the stage of the grieving process and initiating appropriate nursing interventions, which are described in the following section.

Periods in Which the Family is at Risk for Loss

The High-Risk Pregnancy

The diagnosis of high-risk pregnancy evokes varying degrees of anxiety and distress in the childbearing woman. When this diagnosis requires enforced bed rest at home or hospitalization, the family faces a potential crisis (Maloni & Kasper, 1991). Home bed rest often is recommended for preterm labor, incompetent cervix with cerclage placement, or placenta previa. Monahan and DeJoseph (1991) found that these women face many common stressors as a result of the following:

- Restriction in activity
- Uncertainty of pregnancy outcomes
- Reduced childbirth education options
- Reduced labor and birthing options
- Adverse effects of oral or subcutaneous tocolytics
- Disruption in career or work activities
- Disruption in patterns of sexuality and intimacy with partner
- Financial strains

Women who are hospitalized can be expected to experience many similar concerns and may verbalize greater levels of anxiety. Concerns often are initially focused on fears for self or the health of the fetus. The uncertainty regarding pregnancy outcomes can be unbearable at times. Side effects and adverse reactions to medications such as tocolytics and other treatments may exaggerate these fears and feelings of distress. (See Chapter 27 for a discussion of the medications and treatments used in preterm labor.) A common reaction is a sense of lowered self-esteem and competence regarding the ability to have a normal pregnancy and sustain and nourish the fetus.

If the maternal or fetal condition stabilizes, new worries surface about the change in family relations, loss of intimacy with one's partner, and the inability to continue employment. Feelings of depression are experienced frequently and

Nursing Interventions to Provide Family-Centered Care in the Intrapartum Period

General Strategies

- Advocate for open or flexible visiting hours, even in critical care units.
- Give primary nursing care to encourage development of close, trusting relationships between the family and nursing staff.
- Use nursing assessment instruments that incorporate psychosocial evaluation and data about the family unit.
- Develop a nursing care plan to ensure continuity and consistency of care.
- Urge frequent telephone contact with family members.
- Plan periodic family conferences with primary health care providers to evaluate and revise ongoing care.
- Involve family in the care provided as appropriate and when possible.
- Involve selected family members in high-risk birth experience.
- Support and promote breastfeeding when postnatal or postpartum complications occur.
- Encourage sibling visitation.
- Identify support groups for high-risk families.
- Develop long-term follow-up for high-risk families.

Interventions When Families Perceive Birth as a Loss of an Anticipated "Normal" Birth

- Use caring touch and reassurance generously.
- Give frequent explanations about necessary procedures and the woman's or neonate's status.
- Emphasize the unpredictability of some aspects of birth, and remind parents that they coped as best they could in a difficult situation, giving specific examples if possible.
- Allow parents to express their concerns or failed expectations, and acknowledge their feelings with statements such as "It's disappointing to have problems during your childbirth."
- Spend time with parents. Do not give the impression that you are "too busy" to listen.
- Make sure that the woman receives adequate analgesia and comfort care before seeing the baby.
- Tell the woman that she will begin to feel more like herself physically in a few days.
- Facilitate parent–newborn interaction by promoting frequent and *enjoyable* contact with their baby as the parents express readiness for it.

Interventions When Maternal Physical Health Is Jeopardized

- Organize care to give the woman physical and emotional support. (The woman will need to focus her energy on her own recovery.)
- Be sure that interaction with the neonate is enjoyable and tailored to the mother's physical and emotional status.
- Be alert for the possibility that the partner may interact with the neonate more often because of the mother's illness and may become more confident in his or her caretaking skills than the woman. (This may increase the mother's insecurity.)
- Provide for supportive mother–newborn interaction without devaluing the father's participation.
- Help the parents relive their experience by offering information and answering questions.

Interventions When Families' Perception is That of Loss of an Anticipated "Normal" Newborn

- Avoid global reassurances ("Everything will turn out for the best") or comments that fail to acknowledge the parents' feelings ("I know just how you feel").
- Stress that the neonate is getting good care.
- Give factual information to help parents reduce their stress. Reassure family that you are available.
- Avoid giving conflicting information. (Parents may be asking questions of many staff members and remembering only part of what they are told.)
- Verify your information before answering.
- Respect the parents' need for privacy.
- Avoid pushing parents into activities for which they are unready. (Refusals to see the infant or speak with physicians or other care providers may reflect a need to take things at a slower pace.)
- Allow parents to ventilate their feelings without staff responding defensively.
- Acknowledge parents' pain, disappointment, and feelings of helplessness.

Interventions to Help Siblings Cope With Loss and Grief

- Meet with parents before siblings are told, to offer them appropriate guidance.
- Provide parents with a safe, quiet environment in which to talk with their children.
- Advise parents to explain the problem in terms appropriate for the child's developmental level.
- Tell parents to assure children that they are not responsible for the problem.
- Let the children know that any questions and feelings are "ok."
- Advise family to transmit a sense of love and interest to the siblings so that not all attention is focused on the high-risk parent or neonate.
- Permit children to visit the sick parent or neonate, or, in some situations, to see the dead newborn (at least a picture of the newborn).
- Provide information to parents about support groups for parents or siblings.
- Discuss with parents the common reactions of children to intrapartum complications and loss.

appear strongly related to the quality of social support (Monahan & DeJoseph, 1991). Even levels of norepinephrine, one indicator of the stress response, are elevated in women who perceive less support from partners during a high-risk pregnancy (Kemp & Hatmaker, 1989).

In a study by Loos and Julius (1989), hospitalized high-risk women also expressed feelings of loneliness, boredom, and powerlessness. Loneliness and a sense of isolation are anticipated when women are separated from loved ones and friends and often are exacerbated by transportation to a distant perinatal high-risk center. At the same time, many women will feel a profound loss of privacy as they are subjected to many invasive procedures and as hospital personnel continually flow in and out of their room.

Loss of control and feelings of powerlessness are created by the hospital environment itself. Administration of medications and the need for repeated physical nursing assessments, physical examinations, and diagnostic evaluations all limit the ability of the woman to regulate her activities. Enforced bed rest further reduces her options. Uncertainty about the eventual outcomes also can produce a profound sense of frustration. In the best of settings in which family-centered maternity care is provided and individualized care is implemented, the woman must still learn to "let go" in many areas. This might include relinquishing personal control of housekeeping tasks, child care, and work responsibilities. Persistent struggles to maintain total control of the environment, therapy, and family relations indicate an ineffective coping pattern.

Implications for Nursing Care

When high-risk factors complicate the pregnancy experience for women, an interdisciplinary team approach is essential to support individual and family coping. Once physiologic stability is achieved, the woman's activities and physical surroundings should be normalized. Family visiting hours should be adapted to meet the needs of working partners or spouses or school-age children. Personal effects should be arranged to create a more humane and homelike environment. Providing structure to each day yet allowing the woman to determine the pace and timing of activities will reduce sensations of powerlessness and boredom. The sense of isolation also can be partially alleviated by expanding visiting hours and allowing hospitalized pregnant women with common problems to meet (via wheelchair or gurney if necessary) to share concerns and experiences.

Some degree of emotional distress may be present until the problem requiring home bed rest or hospitalization is resolved. The woman may exhibit marked swings in mood—elation as gestational age landmarks are reached or signs of fetal well-being are confirmed or depression when signs of deterioration occur in maternal or fetal condition. The nurse makes appropriate referrals for social services and psychiatric and pastoral counseling as needed. Plans should be made for childbirth education classes for the home-bound or hospitalized woman. Personalized instruction from a childbirth educator may be possible, or videotapes and books may be used. Telephone consultation or a visit from a labor and delivery nurse can be helpful when preparing the woman and reducing her level of anxiety regarding the anticipated birth. In some instances a tour of the delivery unit may be possible for the woman using a wheelchair or gurney if she is hospitalized in the facility where birth is planned.

Intrapartum Complications

The intrapartum period is one of heightened emotions and stress, even under normal conditions. When problems arise the woman and her partner will be more anxious and fearful. Furthermore, most women and their families have not dealt with intrapartum complications before and will feel as if all aspects of the situation are out of their control. When emergencies arise and the life of the mother and or fetus are threatened, a true family crisis may exist. The degree to which family members can adapt to and cope with this increased stress level will determine if they can resolve the crisis and how well they will function as a family in the intrapartum and immediate postpartum periods.

Intrapartum complications present the distinct threat of individual and family loss. Loss of the anticipated "normal" birth often is the greatest disappointment for many couples, but other losses can be experienced, as listed previously in this chapter. The contemporary emphasis on preparation for childbirth and family involvement in the birth event intensifies this natural anticipation for a "normal" birth and may deepen the disappointment when problems surface. The greater the perceived threat, the greater the stress under which the woman and her partner are operating. One particularly common event, cesarean delivery, is an excellent example. Even if maternal and neonatal outcomes are excellent, the woman may experience an emotional shock and later, anger or guilt at her "failure" to give birth "naturally." No matter how trivial these issues may seem to nursing and medical personnel, parents will have to resolve these losses through the grief process.

The woman's responses to intrapartum complications will be strongly influenced by the stage of labor, degree of pain and fatigue, and the administration of analgesics or anesthesia. Emotional reactions can be muted or exaggerated by these factors. Family members are likely to respond to complications with common tension-releasing behaviors, such as crying, pacing, or other repetitive physical activities. Characteristic ways of coping with intense emotional distress may be exhibited. These include denying the threat, seeking additional information to understand the problem, limiting the amount of information, or expressing feelings of guilt or anger.

The nature of changes in maternal and fetal status also will have an effect on how the woman and her family respond to intrapartum complications. Changes in maternal and fetal status can be sudden, dramatic, and clearly indicative of an emergency, or they may be gradual and subtle, apparent only to skilled professionals. When the threat to maternal and fetal status is obvious to the woman and her partner, such as hemorrhage or seizures, they may be better able to adjust to the situation and understand the need for prompt action; however, if signs are not obvious, the couple may be confused or object to active interventions.

Implications for Nursing Care

Although physiologic considerations take precedence, nursing care must still be directed at the psychosocial needs of the parents whose "normal" childbirth was not possible. The nurse should recognize that the intensity of the emotional reaction often is proportional to the gap between expectations and the real birth experience. Platitudes such as "the important thing is that you and your newborn are fine" or "thank goodness we have the technology to deal with these complications" should be avoided. Instead the nurse should acknowledge the sense of loss, answer any questions the couple may have, allow them to express their feelings, and listen empathetically. A nonjudgmental approach permits the woman and her family to respond authentically and express their true feelings. This allows the nurse to identify family strengths and coping patterns and plan and implement appropriate family-centered care.

An important nursing responsibility is providing anticipatory guidance to the woman and her partner about what they can expect when intrapartum problems complicate childbirth. The nurse should collaborate in this effort with the physician or nurse midwife so that information given to the parents is accurate and consistent. Such information helps the couple adjust to rapidly changing events, usually reduces their anxiety, and allows them to prepare emotionally and physically. Except in emergency situations, it also helps to ensure informed consent to any planned therapy or treatments.

The nurse evaluates how much information is useful and helpful and when it should be given. In stressful situations most people can take in some information about present and immediate future events if it is presented simply and calmly. However, some people cope by avoiding information and decision making and rely instead on health professionals. The nurse also must assess partner and family responses to the situation. Is the partner able to provide needed emotional and physical support for the woman without experiencing undue strain or anxiety and without creating additional demands on staff attention that cannot be accommodated? If siblings are present for the birth and problems occur, the children's reactions must be evaluated. It may be necessary for the children's support person to remove them from the immediate environment.

A plan for emergencies should be in place well before the anticipated date of birth to facilitate this process. Nursing personnel may assist the family in expediting these contingency plans when significant problems occur.

Many high-risk situations lend themselves to creative implementation of family-centered maternity nursing. Permitting the woman to have the partner, family member, or close friend at her side during labor and birth, whether a vaginal or cesarean delivery, can significantly reduce her level of anxiety and stress. This can be beneficial to maternal and fetal physiologic status. Integrating family-centered practices into high-risk intrapartum care also increases the likelihood that the family will perceive their birth experience positively. This in turn will promote favorable individual and family adaptations in the postpartum period.

Nursing Research

Predictors of Parental Attachment During the Early Postpartum Period

In the high-risk pregnant or postpartum woman, the parent–newborn attachment process may be altered by limited contact and the parents' physical and emotional condition. Research efforts suggest that skillful nursing care can support the attachment process.

Mercer and Ferketich (1990) examined the relationship between parent–newborn attachment scores and events during pregnancy, labor, and birth. A significant finding was that the earlier high-risk women held their newborns, the higher the attachment scores in the first week of life. The investigators suggest that a woman's concern for the neonate's welfare in a high-risk pregnancy may contribute to greater attachment. The parent's confidence in the parental role was also a major predictor of attachment.

It appears that the nature and quality of support provided by nurses, especially the implementation of family-centered maternity care, facilitates the maternal–newborn attachment process. Providing opportunities for early contact in high-risk women and enhancing parenting skills when readiness is observed in mother and father will foster the attachment process.

Mercer, R., & Ferketich, S. (1990). Predictors of parental attachment during early parenthood. *Journal of Advanced Nursing, 15,* 268.

Postpartum Complications

In some instances prenatal or intrapartum complications continue to pose problems for the woman after birth. In other cases trauma, postpartum hemorrhage, infection, or other unexpected difficulties complicate the postpartum period. If the neonate is healthy, the parents' concerns generally are focused on maternal well-being and disruptions in maternal–newborn bonding. However, some women will express anger at their newborn for having caused the complication. This by itself is not evidence of a disordered maternal–newborn attachment, but it is an expression of the grieving process. Further evaluation of maternal–newborn interactions is needed to determine the existence and extent of any problem once the mother has achieved physiologic stability and feels well enough to deal with the neonate. Other mothers initially may be tentative about holding or caring for their newborns because they feel they are too weak or unsteady to hold the newborn safely.

Feelings of loss are just as common in the postpartum period as in the prenatal period when problems arise. When the mother is deprived of the ability to interact fully with the newborn after birth and to feed and care for her infant, she may experience a profound sense of disappointment. The natural exhilaration and excitement after birth often is blunted or absent when the woman is ill, and grieving may occur when she is deprived of the anticipated period of joy, accomplishment, or even euphoria. If the complications are serious or life-threatening, significant gaps in memory may occur, and the woman may express feelings of unreality about the birth experience. She may have initial difficulty believing the neonate is hers. This is particularly true if the birth was accomplished under general anesthesia, or her awareness is diminished in the immediate postpartum period due to illness or the use of analgesics.

The father's or partner's responses are similar to those described previously. He or she may feel overwhelmed by worries about the woman and unable to give the neonate the loving care and attention planned before birth. This may give rise to feelings of anger or guilt. Financial concerns complicate this picture and may cause some partners to return to work early (if paternal leave was planned) to deal with unexpected hospital expenses. Some men may have difficulty expressing their true feelings because of their role expectations for men in general and husband–provider–father specifically. This may delay the ability to begin the work of grief and the resolution of a potential crisis.

Implications for Nursing Care

A primary nursing responsibility when postpartum complications occur is conservation of maternal energy to support a rapid return to physical and emotional health. This may require the nurse to assume greater responsibility for physical care and feeding of the infant or more intensive preparation of the partner to assume this role. The nurse should evaluate the family's plans for participation in infant care and in particular the father's or partner's desires and abilities. In some cases the partner's level of anxiety is greatly reduced by immersion in the parenting role; for others fear for the woman interferes with the ability to concentrate on the infant's needs. In some cultures another female family member will be expected to assume responsibility for the newborn.

While the mother remains ill and in the "taking-in" phase of the postpartum period, the nurse can provide her with brief periods of time with her infant, offering the opportunity to hold the newborn with adequate supervision and support. (See Chapter 28 for a complete discussion of the "taking in" phase of the postpartum period.) Questions about the neonate should be answered as they arise, and regular contact with nursery personnel should be established so that the mother receives periodic information about the neonate. If she has indicated a desire for this arrangement, rooming-in should be initiated for at least part of the day as soon as the mother's condition permits.

The woman may desire to talk about the labor and birth, filling in gaps or "missing pieces" in her memory about the event or clarifying unanswered questions. The labor and delivery nurses involved in the birth should be contacted to speak with her if she verbalizes an interest in discussing these "missing pieces." The nurse should reassure the woman or partner who expresses concern about interruptions in maternal–newborn bonding. The quality of the parent–newborn relationship develops with time and is not wholly dependent on contact during the first postnatal days.

Birth of a High-Risk Infant

One of the most obvious types of loss parents may experience occurs with the birth of a neonate who is premature, ill, injured, or has congenital anomalies. If the pregnancy was complicated, neonatal problems represent the parents' worst fears and create a long period of stress and uncertainty. When neonatal complications are unanticipated, the parents must deal with overwhelming shock and disruption, often on the heels of an exhausting and stressful birth experience. Parental adjustments in the subsequent days and weeks consume huge amounts of time and energy, inflict great emotional pain, and require drastic reorganization of their plans, goals, and physical, social, and financial circumstances.

The birth of a sick or high-risk neonate evokes a grief response in couples as they mourn the loss of the idealized child they fantasized about during pregnancy. Guilt is often a hallmark of the process; each parent may spend days reviewing every aspect of the pregnancy or birth in an attempt to identify something they might have done to cause the problem. While searching for answers, parents may question the nurse about specific behaviors or actions they engaged in that could have hurt the fetus. "I worked extra shifts in the beginning of the pregnancy to save up a little extra money for newborn things. Do you think that could have caused the infection?" "I sometimes smoked cigarettes when my wife was home. Is there any connection between smoking and cleft palate?" Even if no specific cause is found for the complication or anomaly, the woman may experience a profound sense of guilt and failure for being unable to produce a whole or healthy newborn.

When problems result in permanent impairment of the neonate, the sense of loss expands to include future events. The parents may mourn the fact that the newborn will be limited physically, mentally, or psychologically in some way by the intrinsic nature of the problem. Grief may never be totally resolved as new problems related to the condition surface throughout childhood. Uncertainty regarding the eventual outcome for the neonate may complicate the situation. Parents may hesitate to care for a very fragile newborn for fear of injuring him or her. They also may avoid or delay the attachment process with a neonate whose survival is uncertain. This is to reduce the pain associated with this loss (see the display, Barriers to Parent–Newborn Attachment in the Neonatal Intensive Care Unit). The couple will need extended time to adjust to the birth of a high-risk neonate. Physical separation through transportation to a distant medical center also lengthens the time it takes for adaptive responses to appear.

Implications for Nursing Care

An interdisciplinary team approach is used to care for the high-risk neonate; the primary nurse is often instrumental in coordinating its activities. Nursing care is planned in collaboration with other members of the health team, such as physicians, respiratory therapists, social workers, psychologists, physical therapists, financial counselors, and members of support groups and community agencies that help parents of sick infants (Brown, 1992).

The nurse is responsible for providing support and infor-

Barriers to Parent–Newborn Attachment in the Neonatal Intensive Care Unit

Physical

Distance

- Different floor or unit from postpartum unit
- Different hospital

Accommodations

- Lack of accommodations for parents near unit to permit 24-hour visiting when neonate's very ill or getting ready for discharge

Unit Space

- Inadequate space to comfortably accommodate a prolonged visit by parents

Mechanical

- Oxygen hoods that mask the neonate's face
- Ventilators that prevent or limit ability to hold neonate
- Phototherapy eye pads that prevent eye contact
- Incubators that enclose neonate
- Intravenous fluid lines that limit ability to hold neonate
- Thermal blankets or plastic heat shields that limit visibility of neonate and ability to touch

Psychological or Emotional Factors

- Lack of privacy
- Neonate's appearance and behaviors
- Parental feelings of guilt, inadequacy, or helplessness
- Nonsupportive employers (lack of parental leave)
- Parental belief system regarding sickness or anomalies

Nurse and Physician Factors

- Attitude of nursing and medical staff
- Too busy to interact with parents
- Belief that parents not competent to care for neonate
- Lack of notification when neonate's condition changes

From Griffin, T. (1990). Nurse barriers to parenting in the special care nursery. Journal of Perinatal and Neonatal Nursing, *4(2), 56.*

mation to the parents in the first few minutes after birth. The woman and her partner usually become aware that something is wrong almost immediately, either from the interactions of the staff in the first moments or more clearly from emergency measures that may be instituted. The labor nurse must first assist in initiating emergency care as needed, but once neonatal or other delivery room staff arrive, he or she should turn to the parents.

Preparing the Family for Viewing the Neonate. As soon as the neonate's condition permits, the parents should be given an opportunity for visual or physical contact to allow them to have a sense that the neonate is real. If there are visible defects, the nurse must make sure the parents are prepared for the neonate's appearance. This can be accomplished by describing the neonate's appearance in simple terms first, calling attention to normal features, and making sure that the father or support person is seated and with the mother before the neonate is brought to them. The nurse also must be aware of her own response to the newborn and should not exhibit distaste or pity by facial expression or verbal comments.

The maternity nurse should facilitate ongoing contact between the parents and the neonatal medical and nursing staff. Until both parents can see the neonate, an instant photograph may be helpful in preparing them for what they will see, as well as providing tangible evidence that the neonate exists. The mother still requires close nursing observation in the postpartum period, and this routine care provides the nurse with many opportunities to listen and give emotional support.

When the mother is stable and well enough to see the neonate, she should be prepared for the neonatal intensive care unit (NICU) environment. Family members can be overwhelmed initially by the NICU setting. Feelings can be so intense that they may feel physically ill at first. Comfortable chairs should be available; it is not unusual for the woman or family members to feel faint when first confronted with the many strange sights, sounds, and odors typically found in the NICU. The condition of the neonate also contributes to the sensations of fear, shock, and helplessness.

Ongoing nursing research has identified common parental reactions to the NICU and effective nursing interventions to reduce anxiety and promote parent–newborn interactions. Parents report that overall levels of stress in the NICU are low when the nursing staff takes time to orient them to the unfamiliar environment and to the complex methods of neonatal care (Perehudoff, 1990). Other nurse investigators have found that developing unstructured visiting hours, permitting extended family members to participate in care, and permitting sibling visitations greatly reduced parents' negative reactions to the NICU (Newman & McSweeney, 1990).

Promoting Family-Centered Care. Increasing awareness of the negative effect of the NICU environment on the parent–newborn relationship has led to the implementation of family-centered approaches to care in these "high-tech" settings. Initiating early parent participation in newborn care, providing positive feedback when they successfully accomplish tasks, and permitting the family to "room-in" 24 hours a day to prepare for discharge are elements of family-centered care. Nurses also must be flexible about issues of promptness and refrain from performing neonatal care tasks themselves if parents are late for a visit. When the nurse encourages frequent phone calls from parents, day or night, and consistently notifies them of changes in the neonate's condition or in therapy, they begin to believe that they are truly the most important people in the neonate's life.

Facilitating nurturant fathering behavior is important, particularly when the mother is ill and unable to interact with the newborn. Novak (1990), a nurse researcher, conducted a study to identify factors influencing fathers' nurturant behavior in the NICU. The following variables appear related to fathering behaviors:

- Sociocultural background
- Value placed on a nurturant fathering role
- Wife's support of nurturing behaviors in father
- Comfort level with the NICU environment
- Previous experience with infants
- Support of nursing staff

Novak found the role of the nurse to be central to father involvement. Empathetic guidance focused on the unique needs of each father without role assumptions had the greatest impact on father participation.

Grandparents and extended family members can support parents who are struggling with their concerns. Grandparents may experience an intense grieving process and may express a desire to help the parents and the newborn in any way possible. New nursing research suggests that in selected circumstances permitting grandparent involvement supports parental adaptation, assists in resolution of the potential crisis for both generations, and may be beneficial for the neonate. Rumpusheski (1990) suggests that when parents desire grandparent involvement, NICU staff should expand visitation privileges to them and to involve them in care of the infant in selected situations.

Preparing for Discharge. To respond effectively the parents must develop a realistic perception of the neonate's special problems and prognosis (see the Nursing Research display). Family members will need repeated explanations and reinforcement by the nursing and medical staff. Ongoing assessment includes the parents' response to the birth of the high-risk or sick neonate. The nursing staff must gather sufficient data to plan parent–newborn interactions and begin discharge teaching. The following information should be obtained as soon as possible:

- Mother's physical condition
- Current living conditions
- Distance from the hospital
- Family constellation
- Family support systems
- Parents' educational levels
- Family financial resources
- Religious background and beliefs
- Transportation available to family
- Availability of a telephone
- Work and home responsibilities
- Past experiences with high-risk neonates

Nursing Research

Discharge Teaching: Preparing the Family to Take the High-Risk Neonate Home

A growing body of nursing research confirms the importance of early discharge planning and complete preparation of parents to return home with the high-risk neonate. Furthermore, a landmark nursing study by Brooten (1986) indicates that early discharge of the high-risk neonate with home follow-up is safe, beneficial, and results in significant financial savings for the hospital and family.

Ideally, basic neonatal care skills should be taught by the primary nurse; however, parents of neonates requiring continuing care at home also may be instructed by specialists in neonatal cardiopulmonary resuscitation, as well as physical and respiratory therapists. The primary nurse or clinical nurse specialist plays an important role in coordinating this discharge teaching.

Information should be standardized, and instructions should be reinforced by materials printed in the family's primary language and that are geared to the parents' educational level. Systematic protocols should be developed to document all aspects of teaching and note satisfactory return demonstrations of neonatal care activities by parents. Parents and other care providers must have ample time to repeat complex tasks, such as the measuring and administering drugs, performing chest physiotherapy and suctioning, and caring for central venous lines.

Brooten, D., Kumar, S., & Brown, L. (1986). A randomized clinical trial of early hospital discharge and home follow-up of very low birth weight infants. *New England Journal of Medicine, 315*, 934.

Damato, E. (1991). Discharge planning from the neonatal intensive care unit. *Journal of Perinatal and Neonatal Nursing, 5*(1), 43.

Figure 25-3 lists adaptive and maladaptive parental responses after the birth of a high-risk neonate. Nurses must document their assessments of parental coping behavior and identify early indications of parenting disorders so that the health team can intervene as quickly as possible. Before determining whether a particular behavior is truly maladaptive, the nurse must have a working knowledge of these factors. For instance a mother who lives in a shelter for the homeless may not be able to visit the neonate after 4:00 PM because she must stand in line by that time each day to secure a bed for the night. A father or partner who works 12-

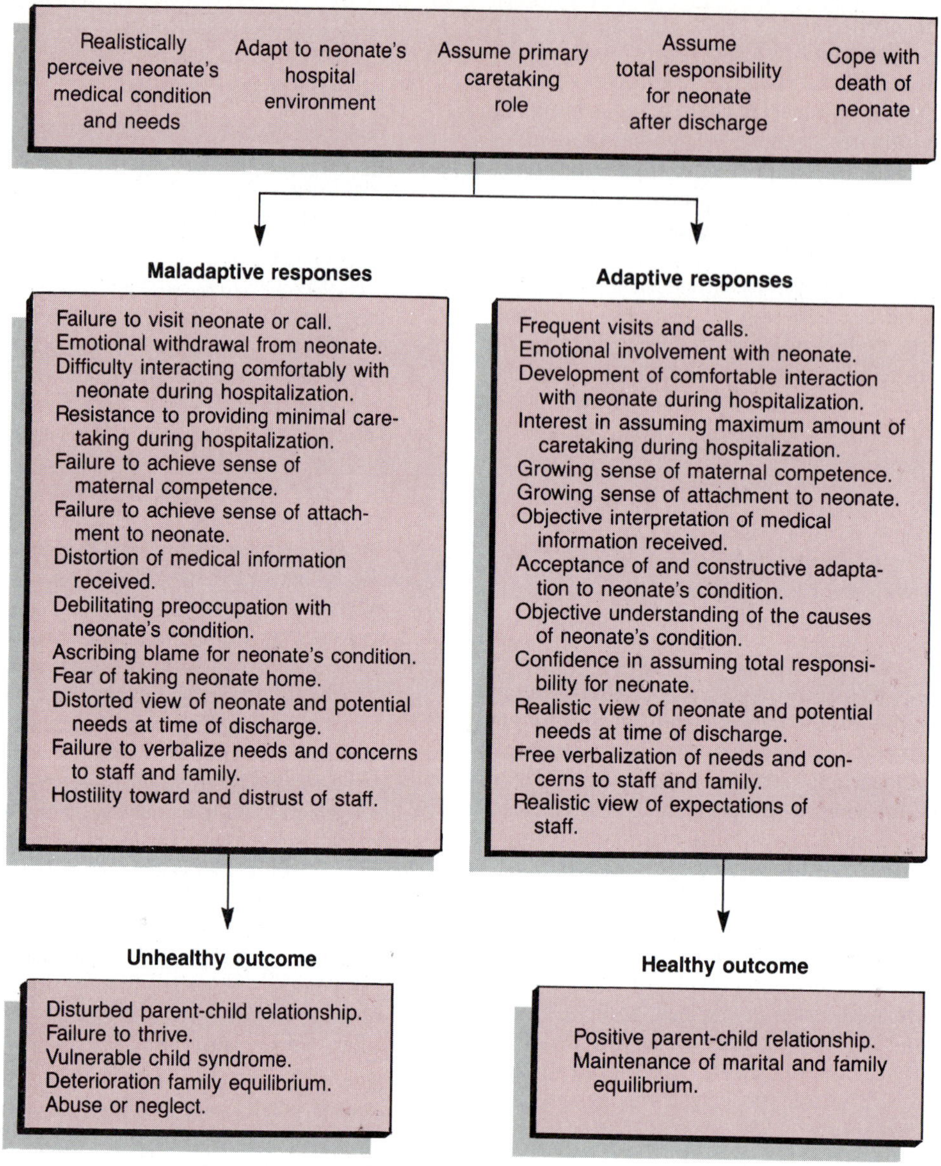

Figure 25-3.
Parents may show adaptive or maladaptive responses to the tasks of parenting a high-risk neonate. The nurse should assess the quality of parental adaptation so effective and appropriate intervention can be implemented. (From Grant, P. [1978]. Psychosocial needs of families of high-risk infants. *Family and Community Health, 11*, 93.)

or 14-hour days and has a long commute may not visit every day.

The goals of discharge teaching include the following:

- Maintaining the neonate's health
- Maximizing parental confidence and competence
- Decreasing the stress of the transition to home
- Minimizing the risks of illness and rehospitalization
- Reestablishing the family unit

As the time approaches for the neonate's discharge, the woman and her partner must be given ample opportunity to become skilled and comfortable with neonatal care activities, including the administration of any medications or provision of treatments. They are often taught resuscitation; this can be an anxiety-provoking activity. One of the most challenging tasks for parents is acquiring neonatal care skills, particularly when the neonate has permanent disabilities or is perceived as "fragile" in the eyes of the family. Parents can experience losses in self-esteem as they observe skilled nurses handle the most extraordinary care in a routine manner. Often parents perceive that the primary nurse is more attuned to the neonate's moods, temperament, and needs at any given time and despair of ever becoming competent enough to care for their neonate. The nurse should be aware of these common feelings and support the family's gradual assumption of care. Parents should be praised frequently for their efforts and progress in acquiring parenting skills, and the nurse should reinforce the fact that they are the most important people in the neonate's life.

Many units now provide live-in arrangements for parents; parents remain in the unit for several days before discharge to become familiar with the infant's schedule and special needs through a 24-hour cycle. Appropriate community referrals are made before discharge so that parents have ongoing support in the home. In addition the primary NICU nurse or a clinical nurse specialist involved in the acute phase of recovery may make periodic telephone calls to the family to answer questions and identify new problems.

Fetal or Neonatal Death

The most profound loss associated with childbearing is an intrapartum death—the loss of a fetus during pregnancy or childbirth—or neonatal death.

Intrauterine fetal demise (IUFD), with its attendant medical complications and psychological distress, is extremely traumatic to the woman and her family. The woman may expect the diagnosis of IUFD, or it may come as a sudden and unexpected shock. In the past it was assumed that the loss of a fetus did not result in the same intensity of grief as neonatal death because the woman did not have time to know her neonate. A growing body of research has refuted this assumption. Most women begin to form bonds with the fetus before birth, and the ability of ultrasound technology to visualize the fetus in all its stages of development may enhance the woman's appreciation of the fetus as a separate, living being (Layne, 1990).

Technologic advances have resulted in the short-term survival of many neonates. Other neonates may survive for weeks or months. The experience of *neonatal death* can be as devastating as the loss of a parent, spouse, or close friend. In third world countries very high infant mortality rates are often the norm, and death is often expected or accepted. In the American culture neonatal death usually comes as a shock to family and friends, particularly when the woman is healthy, has had prenatal care, and had anticipated no problems before the birth.

When intrauterine fetal death or neonatal loss occurs, the immediate responses range from stunned disbelief to violent reactions of anger, rage, or sorrow. Initially the woman's responses may be altered by her physical condition. She may not be aware of the loss for some time if she is critically ill or has received a general anesthetic for an emergency cesarean delivery. When the reality of the situation is fully appreciated, the nurse may expect to see behaviors that typify grief, including shock, disbelief, guilt, and anger. Searching behaviors to identify the reason for the loss often predominate the earlier period of grieving. Expressions of guilt, anger, or blame directed at medical or nursing staff also are common.

The grief experience of a woman who has suffered an IUFD differs from the bereavement that follows neonatal death. Phillips (1988) notes that because the woman has never experienced the neonate in the external world, the impact of the diagnosis may not be fully felt until birth. Many women do not totally accept the diagnosis until birth when they can hold and see the dead fetus. Therefore, it is not unusual for a woman to tell the nurse that she still feels fetal movement after fetal death has been confirmed. Furthermore, carrying a dead fetus can have a profoundly distressing effect on the woman; she appears pregnant, but something horrible is happening inside her body. The psychological devastation is exacerbated by physical threats to her well-being that result from the risks of the coagulation disorders that frequently accompany IUFD.

The labor and delivery experience often is acutely physically and psychologically painful for the woman with an IUFD. Labor may be induced, and the induction can be a long and painful process. The woman knows that the pain and effort experienced will not result in the birth of a viable neonate, and she may become profoundly depressed. It will add to her distress if nursing staff are uncomfortable with caring for her. Some family members may be too sad or frightened to remain with the woman during labor or to visit her after birth. The sense of unreality and isolation felt by the woman can be acute.

Paternal responses differ from the woman's reactions. In several recent nursing studies fathers experienced intense feelings of anger and responded in physical ways. Actions characteristic of rage included kicking or punching objects and tearing down curtains in the hospital environment (Cordell & Thomas, 1990). Crying out and verbalizing anger also were common responses. Flight reactions were observed in some men through increased alcohol use or leaving their spouses because of the grief connected with them (Kimble, 1991). Once the fathers released pent-up anger, they often switched to a detached mode of coping, becoming very restrained and focusing on instrumental tasks, such as preparing for the funeral and removing baby furniture and clothing before the woman returned home. Many men also express profound feelings of loss and guilt and may cry openly, especially if they believe that the nursing staff is supportive and accepting of this behavior (Lieberman & Huges, 1990).

Implications for Nursing Care

Providing care for families experiencing neonatal death is difficult because the nurse and physician must first come to grips with their own feelings of guilt, anger, and sadness. When professionals' ability to work with parents is compromised by their own response to the death, other staff should be brought in immediately to take over care of the family. The staff should be provided opportunities to discuss feelings and come to some resolution.

Ryan, Arsenault, and Sugarman (1991) recommend the use of an intrapartum loss checklist to ensure consistency and continuity of care. An example of such a checklist appears in the assessment tool. Use of a systematic checklist ensures that vital aspects of care are not omitted as the woman moves through the health care system and returns to the community after the birth of the infant. However, such protocols should not lead to a regimented or assembly line approach to perinatal loss. The nurse should be attuned to the individual needs of each family.

Confirming the Death. The confirmation of IUFD is most often made in the provider's office or a clinic, and nurses working in this setting must begin bereavement interventions that reflect current understanding of the grieving process.

If the woman has come to the office or clinic alone, she

Assessment Tool

Comprehensive Checklist for Perinatal Loss

Parents' names ______________________________

Address ______________________________

Phone ______________________________

Description of loss: ______________________________

Description of previous loss(es) ______________________________

L.M.P. ____________ E.D.C. ____________

Week of gestation ______________

Sex of baby (if known) ______________

Religious affiliation ______________

	Office Staff	E.R. Staff	Labor/Delivery	Postpartrum	Neonatal ICU	O.R. Staff	GYN/Post Op	Community Health	Date(s)
Received pregnancy confirmation									
Lab/amnio results	☐	☐	☐			☐			______
Sonogram photo	☐		☐			☐			______
Acknowledgment of loss/Impaired fertility	☐	☐	☐	☐	☐	☐	☐	☐	______
Bring up the subject									
Refer to the baby/expected child									
Call the baby by name									
Anticipatory guidance about normal grief									
Mother	☐	☐	☐	☐	☐	☐	☐	☐	______
Father	☐	☐	☐	☐	☐	☐	☐	☐	______
Family members	☐	☐	☐	☐	☐	☐	☐	☐	______
Postloss options given									
To go home/maternity floor/alternate floor	☐	☐	☐			☐			______
Father to remain with mother/private room			☐	☐			☐		______
Saw/touched/held baby or products of conception	☐	☐	☐		☐	☐	☐		______
If refused, later offers made			☐	☐	☐		☐		______
Family members included in offer	☐	☐	☐	☐	☐	☐	☐		______
Received mementos									
Footprints			☐	☐	☐				______
Bracelet			☐	☐	☐				______
Lock of hair			☐	☐	☐				______
Crib card			☐	☐	☐				______
Blanket			☐	☐	☐				______
Tape measure			☐	☐	☐				______
Certificate of life/remembrance	☐	☐	☐	☐	☐	☐	☐	☐	______
Photographs taken									
Given to parents			☐		☐				______
Filed with chart			☐		☐				______
Bathed/dressed baby			☐		☐				______
Postdeath options discussed	☐	☐	☐	☐	☐		☐		______
Need/desire for funeral director									
Type/location/timing of service									
Burial/cremation/hospital disposal									
Parent involvement									
Choosing burial outfit/mementos									
Announcements—public/personal									
Religious options									
Baby baptized	☐	☐	☐		☐	☐	☐		______
Clergy notified	☐	☐	☐	☐	☐	☐	☐	☐	______
Received information about									
Birth/death certificates	☐	☐		☐	☐		☐	☐	______
Autopsy option discussed	☐	☐	☐	☐	☐		☐		______
Marked chart/room with identifying symbol e.g., butterfly, rainbow, rose	☐	☐	☐	☐	☐	☐	☐	☐	______
Received literature/suggested readings	☐	☐	☐	☐	☐	☐	☐	☐	______
Hospital admitting office notified	☐	☐							______
SHARE/support group referral made	☐	☐	☐	☐	☐	☐	☐	☐	______

From Family Nursing Associates.

should not leave unescorted. If possible, a family member or close friend should be called to accompany her home or to the hospital. All records should reflect the diagnosis of IUFD, and the hospital should be called to update their copies of prenatal records. The woman should never be sent alone for diagnostic tests after a diagnosis of IUFD. She should not be abandoned.

In the case of an unexpected stillbirth or neonatal death, the woman and her partner should be informed together if possible. This should occur as soon as possible after the death occurs, so the parents may begin a normal mourning process. Information should be given in an unrushed, quiet manner.

Although privacy is important, withdrawal or avoidance behavior is inappropriate. The comforting presence of a professional is essential. The nurse also should reassure the family that they will not be left alone, but they should discuss their desires for privacy. Nursing care should be arranged to permit periods of uninterrupted quiet. The nurse offers to spend that time sitting with parents, talking about the experience, and answering their questions. Transferring the woman to another unit or arranging early discharge may further increase the woman's sense of isolation or may reinforce her feelings that she did something to cause the death. A sign on the door directs visitors to see the charge nurse; this directive makes sure visitors are aware of the death. The family responds with appreciation and is touched by genuine sorrow and caring by health professionals when IUFD or neonatal death occurs. The nurse should not hesitate to touch the woman, hold her hand, or embrace her when expressing distress at the outcome.

It is normal and common for family members to redirect overwhelming feelings of rage, anger, or guilt at health professionals. The staff should not react defensively. When family members vent their feelings, these feelings should be validated with simple comments such as, "I feel the same anger you do. This was horrible and senseless." Later, coherent discussions about the possible causes for fetal or neonatal death can be explored.

Facilitating the Grieving Process. Nurses and other health providers have long recommended specific interventions to support the grieving family. A recent study was conducted by Lemmer (1991) to explore parents' reactions to fetal or neonatal death. Nurses were singled out as health providers who most consistently demonstrated caring behaviors.

Nursing care in fetal demise is discussed in the nursing care plan. Other nursing interventions for loss are discussed earlier in the chapter. Nursing research (Lemmer, 1991; Welch, 1991) has identified specific interventions to facilitate the grieving process and support appropriate coping behaviors. They are summarized as follows:

- Acknowledge the loss, and avoid euphemisms.
- Express your feelings about the infant's death with consoling words.
- Touch parents in a caring fashion; words are not always necessary.
- Provide as much factual information about the neonate's death as is available.
- Describe the infant's appearance in factual and tender terms before bringing the newborn to the parents.
- Encourage the parents to see and hold the infant.
- Stay with the family as they examine the infant for the first time.
- Acknowledge the infant's death at first contact with the parents and daily thereafter; do not act as if the death has not occurred.
- Provide parents with physical tokens of the infant; wisp of hair, photograph, blanket, identification bracelet.
- Allow for sibling visitation if desired.
- Determine if the family wishes an autopsy.
- Encourage the parents to grieve openly.
- Spend extra time with the parents to review events surrounding the newborn's death.
- Encourage the parents to make arrangements for a spiritual or religious ritual to mark the neonate's death (baptism, funeral, memorial service).
- Suggest a "practice run" of the discharge process; help the family work through their feelings about going home without a newborn.
- Help parents prepare themselves for telling family and

Text continues on page 658

NURSING ALERT

THE WOMAN EXPERIENCING FETAL DEMISE

The woman who has experienced an intrauterine fetal demise (IUFD) may be at risk for several collaborative problems that require close nursing assessment. The majority of women with a diagnosis of IUFD experience spontaneous labor within 2 weeks of fetal death. When the dead fetus is retained for longer periods, disseminated intravascular coagulation (DIC) may develop. To prevent DIC, plans may be made for induction of labor if a significant delay in spontaneous labor occurs. If the induction of labor requires high doses of oxytocin infusion for several days, the woman also is at risk for water intoxication.

When the nurse cares for the woman at risk for DIC, she must be assessed frequently for the following signs of coagulopathy:

- Hematuria
- Ecchymosis
- Generalized petechiae
- Oozing at venipuncture sites
- Vaginal bleeding

The nurse also is responsible for monitoring serial "DIC screening tests" and coagulation studies for evidence of bleeding disorders. Of specific concern are the following abnormal findings:

- Fall in fibrinogen levels
- Rise in fibrin split products
- Delayed clotting time
- Thrombocytopenia

If evidence of DIC is present, the nurse must alert the physician or midwife in a timely manner and be prepared to institute therapy required to prevent massive hemorrhage. This may include the transfusion of whole blood, cryoprecipitate, fresh-frozen plasma, and platelets. Heparin may be administered in special cases to reverse the consumptive coagulopathy, preventing further depletion of clotting factors.

Nursing Care Plan

The Family Experiencing Fetal Demise

PATIENT PROFILE

History

F.D. is a healthy 25-year-old G1/P0 who works full time as a plumber. She and her husband have recently moved to the community and have no close friends or family nearby. At 37 weeks' gestation she is unable to feel fetal movement and calls her physician. An NST is scheduled for that morning, and when F.D. arrives for the test, the fetal heart rate cannot be found. A diagnosis of intrauterine fetal demise is confirmed by ultrasonography. A decision is made to admit F.D. to labor and delivery and induce labor. A blood specimen is obtained for coagulation studies. Ten hours later F.D. experiences a vaginal birth of a stillborn infant girl. There is a true knot in the umbilical cord. A minister who is present baptizes the baby. The baby is wrapped in a blanket and given to F.D. as she has requested.

Physical Assessment

The nurse remains at the bedside to support F.D. and her husband, monitor F.D.'s physiologic status, and assess the family's responses. F.D. says, "It can't be true. You look so perfect my Baby Annie." She looks at the nurse and says, "This all seems so unreal. I feel numb. Why can't I cry?"

F.D.'s husband touches the baby and then quickly leaves the room saying "I can't deal with this. I have to get out of here. I'll come back later."

After holding Baby Annie for about an hour, she asks the nurse to take the infant. Her husband has not returned. "I know she died because I worked too hard. I should have slowed down. Now I'll have to live with my mistake. That's why my husband left. He can't stand looking at me."

COLLABORATIVE PROBLEMS/POTENTIAL COMPLICATIONS

- Disseminated intravascular coagulopathy (DIC)
- Delayed delivery/failed induction of labor

(See the accompanying Nursing Alert display and Managed Care Path.)

Assessment	*Nursing Diagnosis*	*Nursing Interventions*	*Rationale*
Diagnosis of IUFD. F.D. states: "I can't believe it's true." "This seems unreal." "I feel numb. Why can't I cry.	Grieving related to fetal loss and still birth of infant ***Expected Outcome*** F.D. and her husband, after considering options, will make choices about how they wish to deal with the fetal death before, during and afterbirth.	Acknowledge fetal death.	Family often continues to hope that there has been an error in the diagnosis.
		Convey condolences and feelings about the loss.	Expressing condolences conveys empathy and sensitivity.
		Encourage family members to grieve openly.	Encouraging expressions of grief and accepting negative feelings support the "work of grieving."
		Accept expressions of grief, including anger directed at health providers.	
		Remain with woman, and provide physical and emotional support during process of labor.	The nurse's presence and physical support fosters trust and confidence.
		Explain and reinforce information about process of induction, labor, and birth.	Providing information as appropriate conveys respect and reinforces reality of event.
		Involve family, pastoral services, and social services.	Providing information as appropriate conveys respect and reinforces reality of event.

(Continued)

The Family Experiencing Fetal Demise

(Continued)

Assessment	Nursing Diagnosis	Nursing Interventions	Rationale
		After establishing relationship with family, inquire about preferences for: • Baptism or other religious ceremony at birth • Seeing, holding or touching infant at birth • Having picture or other physical mementos of infant	Involving other professionals in planning and implementing care facilitates grieving process. The nurse can only individualize care if the family's preferences are known. Theories of grieving suggest that holding and touching the infant permits "detachment" and facilitates grieving. Saving memorabilia acknowledges the reality of the infant and birth. If parents initially decline these items, they should be kept for at least 2 years so they can be retrieved later if family members change their minds.
		At birth confirm that the infant is dead. Assist with baptism or other religious ceremony as needed.	The family needs verification of the infant's death to continue with the process of grieving.
		Prepare infant for viewing: • Clean or bathe infant. • Wrap in warm blankets; put on stockinette cap. • Use cord clamp, not hemostat on umbilical cord. • Save cord with true knot so that F.D. can see this specific problem when she is ready to do so.	Viewing should occur as soon as possible after birth. The infant's physical appearance should be as normal as possible to emphasize the "humaness" of the baby. The family should be informed of any obvious problems that might explain the IUFD.
		During viewing of infant: • Allow family to unwrap and view entire infant. • Point out individual infant characteristics, such as color of hair, perfect fingers, toes, shape of mouth, and so forth.	The infant's uniqueness should be emphasized to make the family's memories of their baby real. Pointing out special attributes reinforces the infant's worth and value.
		• Ask family if they wish to be alone, but convey that you are very comfortable remaining with them.	Families may feel more comfortable expressing grief if done in private. The family may wish to say goodbye in private.

(*Continued*)

The Family Experiencing Fetal Demise

(Continued)

Assessment	Nursing Diagnosis	Nursing Interventions	Rationale
		• Do not limit the time for viewing. If significant family member arrives later, be prepared to obtain infant from morgue, and repeat the viewing process.	Nursing care must be individualized. The process of grieving and saying goodbye cannot be rushed.
		During labor or after birth, determine family's desire for: • Autopsy	The cause of most fetal deaths is unknown despite autopsy, but finding that the infant was normal may reassure the family of their ability to produce a "normal" infant. Finding a specific problem may allow parents to accept the death.
		• Funeral service/burial plans	Parents may desire a funeral service to assist in the grieving process or to fulfill religious ritual or requirements. Even very low–birth-weight or premature neonates may have a funeral and burial today.
		Provide information about support groups for families who have experienced fetal death.	Support groups may be very helpful in the "work of grieving," particularly when minimal social support is available.
		Inquire about woman's desires regarding early discharge or type of room she wishes (ie, postpartum room versus room on another unit).	The woman may feel more isolated if sent home immediately or if placed on a medical floor for recovery. Nurses on another unit may be unfamiliar with appropriate nursing support following IUFD or neonatal death. Providing choices promotes participation and feelings of control.
No family or close friends in the community (inadequate social support). Husband unable to remain with F.D. after birth of infant.	Altered Family Processes related to intrauterine fetal demise and still birth of infant ***Expected Outcome*** The family will begin adaptation process as evidenced by open discussion, reciprocal support, and ability to make decisions about disposition of fetal body.	Explore with woman and husband the possibility of family or friends coming to community to support woman. Enlist assistance of pastoral and social services.	Family may feel extremely isolated if family or friends are unavailable after an IUFD. Continued physical support by the nurse and follow-up care after discharge from the hospital may be essential to promote family adaptation

(Continued)

The Family Experiencing Fetal Demise

(Continued)

Assessment	Nursing Diagnosis	Nursing Interventions	Rationale
		Remain in room and maintain close physical presence unless woman or family request time alone.	
F.D. states, "I know she died because I worked too hard." "That's why my husband left. He can't stand looking at me."	Situational Low Self-Esteem related to feelings of guilt regarding fetal death ***Expected Outcome*** F.D. will demonstrate progressive reintegration of self-concept as evidenced by realistic statements about the cause of the infant's death.	Acknowledge woman's feelings of guilt, even if cause of death is not related to her behavior or a medical/obstetric problem (ie, diabetes or PIH).	Feelings of guilt are common and indicate that the woman is beginning the process of grieving. Attempting to correct woman's perceptions about the cause of death in the immediate postpartum period is not therapeutic and invalidates her feelings.
		Remain with woman, and plan to spend extra time with her until her husband returns. Validate woman's worth by demonstrating concern and respect for her.	Feelings of guilt for F.D. may be exacerbated by husband's behavior—leaving hospital.
		Initiate social service referral.	Ongoing assessment by health professionals is essential.
Husband unable to remain with wife after birth. Husband states, "I can't deal with this. I have to get out of here."	Ineffective Individual Coping related to fetal death and stillbirth of infant ***Expected Outcome*** Husband will begin process of adaptive coping as evidenced by return to hospital, ability to view infant, and ability to remain with wife.	Acknowledge husband's feelings, and accept inability to remain with wife.	Recognition of and nonjudgmental support of husband fosters trust and confidence in nursing staff.
		Make appropriate referral to pastoral, psychological, or social service for husband. Determine if another family member can travel to the hospital to provide support for F.D.'s husband. Provide information to husband when he returns about support groups formed to help parents who have experienced IUFD.	Husband will require additional professional counseling and support to begin the grieving process and develop adaptive coping mechanisms.

EVALUATION

Arrangements were made to place Baby Annie in a crib in a private area of the nursery. The labor nurse returned to F.D. and remained with her, encouraging her to express her feelings. F.D. was finally able to cry, and express her anger about the loss of her newborn. Approximately 30 minutes later F.D.'s husband returned to the delivery area and asked to see the neonate. The newborn was returned to the room, where both parents held her. They unwrapped her blankets, examined her body, and both wept. They requested that a priest be called to baptize the neonate.

The nurse made arrangements for immediate pastoral support. The parents remained in the room with the infant for 2 hours, at which time they requested that pictures be taken and a lock of the neonate's hair and her blanket be saved for them. By discharge to the postpartum unit, both parents were openly expressing their grief (verbalizations and crying), and had begun to make funeral arrangements.

MANAGED CARE PATH

Pregnancy Loss

Expected Length of Stay: 1 to 2 days

	Admission/Stabilization/Labor–Delivery	Maintenance/Postpartum
Key Goals	Counseling initiated Woman/family verbalizes understanding of situation	Counseling F/U plans Hemodynamically stable (postpartum)
Consults	Social work, pastoral services, genetics prn Anesthesia	Social work, pastoral care
Tests/Labs	Complete blood count (CBC), type and screen	CBC prn
Meds	Pain meds prn	Pain meds prn
Treatments	IV fluids, comfort measures	Comfort measures, parental grief materials
Teaching	Unit routine, medications, emotional response, pregnancy termination process, disposal of fetal remains	Grief follow-up, home care instructions
Equipment	IV pump/tubing, precip pack, emesis basin	
Diet	NPO to ice chips prn	Regular prn
Activity	Bed rest with bathroom priviledges	Up ad lib
D/C Plan	Social support, family, grief support	Social support, grief follow-up, transportation

Adapted from collaborative paths developed by the Department of Nursing Service, Vanderbilt University Medical Center, Nashville, TN.

friends and responding to others who do not know of the infant's death.

- Involve other family members or support people in preparations for going home.
- Discuss possible difficult times: dismantling the nursery, renewing their sexual relationship, seeing other infants.
- Provide referral to support services, such as parent support groups or counseling.
- Maintain postdischarge contact with parents through the first year.

There are several situations in which the family can experience a loss—in high-risk circumstances, during pregnancy, the intrapartum and postpartum periods, after the birth of a high-risk neonate, and with the death of a fetus or newborn. All of these are situations in which the nurse gives psychosocial care. An interdisciplinary team approach is also used in many of these situations. The most profound loss is intrapartum death; this type of loss is also difficult for the health care team.

Chapter Summary

The nurse is likely to be the health professional who has the most consistent contact with the family experiencing perinatal loss. Nursing care of the family must be based on a sound knowledge of the grieving process and crisis theory. The nurse is in a unique position to promote optimal health and adaptation after the stressful event of loss. This is accomplished through the use of the nursing process. A systematic assessment is conducted to identify individual and family strengths and weaknesses, coping behaviors, and the phase of the grieving process. Many nursing diagnoses are available to define the problems experienced by the woman and her family, and interventions are based on these diagnoses. Nursing care also must reflect current research findings about grief, loss, and death. Evaluation of family responses will guide the nurse in revising the plan of care. Clearly, the role of the professional nurse is central to resolution of the grief process and reintegration of the family unit.

Study Questions

1. *Why is the experience of perinatal loss considered a potential crisis?*
2. *What factors contribute to the resolution of crisis for the family experiencing perinatal loss?*
3. *What are the normal phases of the grieving process?*
4. *Why does a diagnosis of "high-risk pregnancy" represent a real or potential loss for the pregnant woman?*
5. *What are common emotional responses to the development of complications during the prenatal period?*
7. *How can the nurse support the woman and her family when prenatal complications occur?*
8. *What are the common emotional responses to the development of intrapartum complications? How can the nurse support the family experiencing life-threatening problems during labor and birth?*

9. *What signs might indicate maladaptive responses in the parents of a high-risk neonate?*
10. *What are specific nursing interventions the nurse can implement to support the parents of a high-risk neonate?*
11. *How do responses to IUFD and neonatal death differ for the mother?*
12. *What are common paternal or partner responses to IUFD or neonatal death? How do societal and cultural factors influence men's reactions to intrapartum loss?*
13. *Which nursing interventions at the time of birth have been found to facilitate the grieving process when a stillbirth or neonatal death occurs?*

References

Aguilera, D., & Messick, J. (1985). *Crisis intervention: Theory and methodology* (5th ed.). St. Louis: C.V. Mosby.

Aguilera, D. (1990). *Crisis intervention*. Philadelphia: C.V. Mosby.

Brown, M. (1988). A comparison of health responses in expectant mothers and fathers. *Western Journal of Nursing Research*, *10*, 527.

Brown, Y. (1992). The crisis of pregnancy loss: a team approach. *Birth*, *19*(2), 82.

Conner, G., & Denson, V. (1990). Expectant fathers' response to pregnancy: Review of literature and implications for research in high-risk pregnancy. *Journal of Perinatal and Neonatal Nursing*, *4*(2), 33.

Cordell, A., & Thomas, N. (1990). Fathers and grieving: Coping with infant death. *Journal of Perinatology*, *10*(1), 75.

Ferketich, S., & Mercer, R. (1989). Men's health status during pregnancy and early fatherhood. *Research in Nursing and Health*, *12*, 137.

Kenner, C. (1990). Caring for the NICU parent. *Journal of Perinatal and Neonatal Nursing*, *4*(3), 78.

Mercer, R., & Ferketich, S. (1990). Predictors of parental attachment during early parenthood. *Journal of Advanced Nursing*, *15*, 268.

Kemp, V., & Hatmaker, D. (1989). Stress and social support in high risk pregnancy. *Research in Nursing and Health*, *12*, 331.

Kimble, D. (1991). Neonatal death: A descriptive study of father's experiences. *Neonatal Network*, *9*(8), 45.

Kubler-Ross, E. (1969). *On death and dying*. New York: Macmillian Publishing.

Layne, L. (1990). Motherhood lost: Cultural dimensions of miscarriage and stillbirth in America. *Women & Health*, *16*(3/4), 69.

Lemmer, Sr., C. (1991). Parental perceptions of caring following perinatal bereavement. *Western Journal of Nursing Research*, *13*(4), 475.

Lieberman, J., & Hughes, C. (1990). How fathers perceive perinatal death. *American Journal of Maternal Child Nursing*, *15*(5), 320.

Loos, C., & Julius, L. (1989). The client's view of hospitalization during pregnancy. *Journal of Obstetric, Gynecologic, and Neonatal Nursing*, *18*(1), 52.

Maloni, J., & Kasper, C. (1991). Physical and psychosocial effects of antepartum hospital bedrest: A review of the literature. *Image*, *23*(3), 187.

Monahan, P., & DeJoseph, J. (1991). The woman with preterm labor at home: A descriptive analysis. *Journal of Perinatal and Neonatal Nursing*, *4*(4), 12.

NAACOG. (1985). *Grief related to perinatal death*. OGN Nursing Practice Resource. Washington, DC: Author.

Newman, C., & McSweeney, M. (1990). Descriptive study of sibling visitation in the NICU. *Neonatal Network*, *9*(4), 27.

Novak, J. (1990). Facilitating nurturant fathering behavior in the NICU. *Journal of Perinatal and Neonatal Nursing*, *4*(2), 68.

Perehudoff, B. (1990). Parents' perceptions of environmental stressors in the special care nursery. *Neonatal Network*, *9*(2), 39.

Phillips, C. (1988). Intrauterine fetal death: The maternal bereavement experience. *Journal of Perinatal and Neonatal Nursing*, *2*(2), 34.

Rumpusheski, V. (1990). Role of the extended family in parenting: A focus on grandparents of preterm infants. *Journal of Perinatal and Neonatal Nursing*, *4*(2), 43.

Ryan, P., Arsenault, D., & Sugarman, L. (1991). Facilitating care after perinatal loss. *Journal of Obstetric, Gynecologic, and Neonatal Nursing*, *21*(5), 385.

Trouy, M., & Larson, C. (1987). Sibling grief. *Neonatal Network*, *6*(2), 35.

Welch, I. (1991). Miscarriage, stillbirth, or newborn death. *Neonatal Network*, *9*(8), 53.

Worden, W. (1982). *Grief counseling and grief therapy*. New York: Springer-Verlag.

Suggested Readings

Blackburn, S., & Lowen, L. (1986). Impact of an infant's premature birth on the grandparents and parents. *Journal of Obstetric, Gynecologic, and Neonatal Nursing*, *15*(6), 173.

Brown, L., Gennaro, S., York, R., et al. (1991). VLBW infants: Association between visiting and telephoning and maternal and infant outcome measures. *Journal of Perinatal and Neonatal Nursing*, *4*(4), 39.

Corrine, L., Bailey, V., Valentin, M., et al. (1992). The unheard voices of women: spiritual interventions in maternal-child health. *MCN: American Journal of Maternal Child Nursing*, *17*(3), 141.

Driscoll, J. (1990). Maternal parenthood and the grief process. *Journal of Perinatal and Neonatal Nursing*, *4*(1), 1.

Kenner, C. (1990). Caring for the NICU parent. *Journal of Perinatal and Neonatal Nursing*, *4*(3), 78.

Kenner, C., & Lott, J. (1990). Parent transition after discharge from the NICU. *Neonatal Network*, *9*(2), 31.

Kimberlin, L., Kucera, V., Lawrence, P., Newkirk, A., & Stenske, J. (1989). The role of the neonatal intensive care nurse in the delivery room. *Clinics in Perinatology*, *16*(4), 1021.

Kolotylo, C., Parker, N., & Chapman, J. (1990). Mothers' perceptions of their neonates' in-hospital transfers from a neonatal intensive care unit. *Journal of Obstetric, Gynecologic, and Neonatal Nursing*, *20*(2), 146.

Kraft, L., & Wilson, C. (1988). Dilemmas in the care of impaired infants. *Neonatal Network*, *6*(5), 73.

Leon, I. (1992). Providing versus packaging support for bereaved parents after perinatal loss. *Birth*, *19*(2), 89.

Lieberman, J., & Hughes, C. (1990). How fathers perceive perinatal death. *MCN: American Journal of Maternal Child Nursing*, *15*(5), 320.

Novak, J. (1988). An ethical decision-making model for the neonatal intensive care unit. *Journal of Perinatal and Neonatal Nursing*, *1*(3), 57.

Penticuff, J. (1988). Neonatal intensive care: Parental prerogatives. *Journal of Perinatal and Neonatal Nursing*, *1*(3), 77.

Schmidt, R., & Levine, D. (1990). Early discharge of low birthweight infants as a hospital policy. *Journal of Perinatology*, *10*(4), 396.

Tolentino, M. (1990). The use of Oren's self-care model in the neonatal intensive care unit. *Journal of Obstetric, Gynecologic, and Neonatal Nursing*, *19*(6), 496.

Woldt, E. (1991). Breastfeeding support group in the NICU. *Neonatal Network*, *9*(5), 53.

CHAPTER 26

Intrapartum Complications

Learning Objectives

After studying the material in this chapter, the student will be able to:

- Compare and contrast the common causes, signs, and symptoms of placenta previa and abruptio placentae.
- Outline medical and nursing care for the woman when placenta previa or abruptio placentae complicates the intrapartum period.
- Compare and contrast the causes, signs, and symptoms of oligohydramnios and polyhydramnios.
- Outline the medical and nursing care when oligohydramnios or polyhydramnios complicates the intrapartum period.
- Identify risks of umbilical cord prolapse to the woman and fetus.
- Discuss the required emergency nursing interventions when umbilical cord prolapse occurs.
- Describe the four major causes of labor dystocia.
- Outline the medical and nursing care for the woman with labor dystocia due to the four causes.
- Compare and contrast the causes, signs, and symptoms of hypovolemic and septic shock.
- Outline nursing responsibilities in the treatment of hypovolemic shock.
- Discuss disseminated intravascular coagulopathy in terms of etiology, diagnosis, and medical and nursing care.
- Identify common causes, signs, and symptoms for uterine rupture.
- Outline nursing responsibilities in the care of the woman with uterine rupture.
- Identify common causes, signs, and symptoms for amniotic fluid embolus.
- Outline nursing responsibilities in the care of the woman with amniotic fluid embolus.

Key Terms

abruptio placentae
bicornuate uterus
chorioamnionitis
cor pulmonale
disseminated intravascular coagulopathy
dystocia
endotoxin
exsanguination
hypotonic labor
hypertonic labor
placenta previa
retraction ring
shock
vasa praevia
velamentous insertion

Labor and birth usually progress with few problems, and outcomes for the woman, neonate, and family generally are positive. However, when complications arise in the intrapartum period, they may develop rapidly and can have devastating effects on the well-being of the woman, fetus, or neonate.

The nurse must identify intrapartum problems and intervene in a timely manner to reduce or limit detrimental effects on the woman and fetus. Although many women with obstetric or medical complications may be transported to high-risk perinatal centers, all labor and delivery nurses must possess the knowledge and skills required to deal with obstetric emergencies. This chapter focuses on the major complications that occur during the intrapartum period and discusses appropriate medical and nursing management of the high-risk intrapartum woman.

Complications during the intrapartum period can be classified in a variety of ways. In this chapter they are divided into the following categories:

- Complications involving the placenta, membranes, and amniotic fluid
- Complications with the umbilical cord and fetus
- Complications in the progress of labor related to fetal descent
- Complications in the progress of labor related to uterine function
- Complications in the progress of labor related to pelvic structure

- Complications involving the reproductive tract
- Complications involving maternal physiologic systems

Specific obstetric complications are described, including etiologic or predisposing factors, maternal and fetal or neonatal implications, and treatment. Implications for nursing care are provided for each condition.

Specialization and Regionalization in Perinatal Care for High-Risk Families

Regionalized perinatal care was established in the late 1960s to provide access to specialized neonatal intensive care units. Facilities were classified according to the level of neonatal care that could be safely given, ranging from low-risk "primary" care to high-risk or "tertiary" level care. In the past complications in the intrapartum period were managed in the local facility, and the sick or compromised neonate was then transported to a tertiary center for care.

Advances in the understanding and treatment of maternal and fetal physiologic status have resulted in an increasing focus on intensive perinatal and intrapartum care. This has given rise to the practice of "maternal transport," or transfer of the woman who is at high risk during pregnancy or the intrapartum period to a center where a high level of perinatal and neonatal expertise is available. Maternal transport has been advantageous in such conditions as preterm labor and uncontrolled diabetes or when congenital anomalies requiring specialized prenatal mangement or surgery occur. Maternal transport is avoided if delivery is judged to be imminent to preclude the possibility of an out-of-hospital delivery; the woman can be moved to a specialized treatment center once her condition is stabilized. The accompanying display lists conditions that may indicate the need for maternal transport to a regional perinatal center.

Some critics question whether the advantages of maternal transport outweigh the hardships involved in removing the woman from her own community for delivery. Families often are separated for long periods (weeks or months), and the costs of specialized care often are prohibitive and continue to rise. However, effective treatment can forestall or prevent the birth of a preterm or physically compromised infant. It also can reduce the costs of neonatal intensive care and eliminate a prolonged hospital stay for the neonate.

Because of the inevitable connection between maternal status and fetal well-being, considerations for the fetus and newborn motivate the majority of maternal transports. Preterm labor is the most common, accounting for almost half of all transports. It is not unusual for a woman to have more than one indication for transport, such as diabetes, pregnancy-induced hypertension (PIH), and preterm labor. Transport teams frequently include a nurse with advanced training in the stabilization and care of high-risk women. Martin (1990) suggests that when the woman must be transported, the nurse can assist the woman, her support person, and other family members adjust to the process in the following ways.

Conditions That May Indicate the Need for Maternal Transport

- Preterm labor before 34 weeks
- Premature rupture of membranes before 34 weeks
- Multifetal gestation
- Severe intrauterine growth retardation
- Rh sensitization
- Severe pregnancy-induced hypertension
- Maternal substance abuse
- Fetal congenital anomalies
- Maternal diseases:
  - Cancer
  - Renal failure
  - Cardiac disease
  - Uncontrolled diabetes
  - Severe chronic hypertension
- Maternal trauma requiring intensive care or surgery beyond the capabilities of the referring hospital

- Ensure that the woman and family members understand the reasons for transport.
- Inform the woman and family about the regional hospital, including name, location, how family can get there.
- Provide name(s) of physician or nurse who will accompany the woman.
- Provide names of primary physician and nurse at center who will care for the woman and whom family may contact.
- Encourage the woman to express her concerns, fears, and questions.

The increasing specialization in perinatal services has implications for the delivery of nursing care in the intrapartum period. Many tertiary care settings have established intensive care intrapartum units. This has allowed the integration of family-centered practices into high-risk settings because staff are comfortable with individualizing care in a "high-tech" environment. Nurses in these settings have established a new standard of practice for the childbearing family experiencing complications. Nursing research findings have resulted in creative solutions to the problem of providing family-centered maternity care in an intensive care context (Harvey, 1992). Many nursing practices have overcome initial reservations and critcisms regarding perinatal regionalization as individual and family integrity is maintained under extremely stressful conditions. Martin (1990) suggests the following strategies to humanize the high-tech environment when the nurse admits a woman after transport to the regional perinatal center:

- Welcome the woman and her family with warmth and enthusiasm.
- Orient the woman to the unit when her condition permits this.

- Orient the family to the unit and the hospital.
- Provide information about overnight and long-term accommodations for family members that are available in the community.
- Facilitate telephone communication.
- Provide the family with privacy during the visits.
- Assist the family in contacting clergy, social services, a psychologist, or support groups.
- Maintain open visiting hours so family members can visit at any time.
- Encourage the woman to verbalize her fears, concerns, and questions.

Perinatal regionalization has made it possible to transport women with intrapartum complications when special treatment is required. Advances in perinatal care permit successful treatment of life-threatening problems. While this has improved physical outcomes for the woman and her neonate, transport disrupts family bonds and may produce psychological distress. The high-tech environment has the potential to dehumanize the birth experience. Maternity nurses must implement strategies that promote family-centered care. This approach will support the family unit while it adjusts to the intrapartum complication and the birth of the new family member.

Nursing Process

The nurse uses the nursing process to care for the woman with intrapartum complications. The nursing process provides the formal framework required to identify risk factors, diagnose patient problems, and implement effective care. It aids the nurse in setting goals and establishing expected outcomes.

• • Assessment

Providing intrapartum care for women and families experiencing complications is a complex process. First and foremost the nurse must identify factors that place the woman at risk for developing problems during labor and birth. Many potential problems can be anticipated by reviewing information in the woman's prenatal record. Preexisting diseases, such as diabetes or chronic hypertension, or problems such as maternal substance abuse will alert the nurse to the need for specialized intrapartum care.

While many risk factors may be identified in the prenatal period, others will only become evident on admission to the birthing unit or develop during labor and birth. The nurse plays a central role in promptly recognizing subtle and obvious abnormalities. When life-threatening complications occur, rapid appraisal of the woman's physiologic status is necessary to determine priority needs. The frequency of assessments is determined by the woman's condition, physician orders, and standards of care that guide nursing practice. Table 26-1 summarizes signs and symptoms that indicate the presence or development of intrapartum complications.

Once a problem has been identified and treatment implemented, the nurse also is responsible for ongoing assessment of maternal and fetal physiologic status and responses to treatment.

• • Nursing Diagnosis

When complications occur during the intrapartum period, the woman will present with a number of physiologic and psychological problems. Many nursing diagnoses are applicable, and they guide the nurse in establishing expected outcomes and planning care. The following are selected nursing diagnoses that reflect possible physiologic problems that may arise during the intrapartum period.

- Decreased Cardiac Output related to hemorrhage
- Pain related to invasive procedures
- Fluid Volume Deficit related to fever or vomiting
- Fluid Volume Excess related to disease processes (renal failure)
- Hyperthermia related to infection
- High Risk for Infection related to prolonged rupture of membranes, prolonged labor, or invasive procedures
- Sleep Pattern Disturbance related to pain, anxiety, and treatment
- Altered Tissue Perfusion related to hypotension

Nursing diagnoses related to psychosocial problems encountered when intrapartum complications arise are listed and discussed in Chapter 25. In addition to establishing appropriate nursing diagnoses, nurses must identify and manage specific physiologic complications (collaborative problems) that occur in high-risk women. Table 26-2 lists common collaborative problems encountered in high-risk women during the intrapartum period.

• • Planning and Implementation

Women who develop problems during the intrapartum period will require more intensive monitoring and intervention throughout the process of labor and birth. Therefore, these women will be cared for in conventional labor and delivery units or perinatal critical care units (as opposed to birthing rooms). Depending on the nature of the problem, the woman may be kept in the intrapartum unit, or she may be transferred to another facility where more intensive neonatal care is available. The challenge for nursing staff is to promote family-centered maternity care, reduce the stress of hospitalization as much as possible, and provide continuity and coordination of services.

The nurse must systematically approach the care of women with intrapartum complications. The following considerations should be addressed when problems arise.

- Which health care providers should be informed of this problem (perinatologist, neonatologist, or clinical nurse specialist)?
- What is the most appropriate setting for the woman (traditional labor and delivery unit or perinatal intensive care unit)?

Table 26-1. Signs and Symptoms Indicating Intrapartum Complications

Problem	Potential Complication
Central Nervous System	
Headache, visual disturbances	Pregnancy-induced hypertension
Hyperreflexia	Hemorrhage, shock
Decreasing consciousness, altered mentation	
Cardiovascular System	
Hypertension	Pregnancy-induced hypertension Eclampsia, chronic hypertension Cocaine-induced hypertensive crisis
Hypotension	Hemorrhage, shock
Tachycardia	Hemorrhage, shock, infection; cardiac disease
Chest pain	Cardiac disease
Marked edema	Cardiac disease Pregnancy-induced hypertension
Petechiae	HELLP syndrome, disseminated intravascular coagulopathy
Pulmonary System	
Shortness of breath	Pulmonary edema or emboli
Cough	Pulmonary edema or emboli
Tachypnea	Cardiac disease, infection, pulmonary edema or emboli
Gastrointestinal System	
Epigastric pain	Pregnancy-induced hypertension
Nausea and vomiting	Pregnancy-induced hypertension
Genitourinary System	
Proteinuria	Pregnancy-induced hypertension
Oliguria	Pregnancy-induced hypertension, shock
Vaginal bleeding	Placenta previa, abruptio placentae
Uterine tenderness	Chorioamnionitis, abruptio placentae

- Should this woman be transported to another facility for more intensive or specialized care?
- What are the unique risks that this problem poses for the woman or fetus and newborn?
- What type of maternal and fetal monitoring is necessary?
- What specialized equipment is required to provide care?
- Has or will the problem alter the course of labor and birth?
- Will it be necessary to modify (speed up, control, or slow down) the pattern of labor?
- How can maternal pain be safely managed?
- Will it be necessary to modify the mode of delivery to promote maternal and fetal or neonatal safety?
- How will the woman's educational level, prenatal preparation, and cultural background influence her understanding and response to the problem?
- What are the special legal and ethical dilemmas?

The time available for specifying nursing diagnoses and planning for nursing care is shortened when major intrapartum complications occur. Diagnosis, planning, and implementation of that plan of care may appear to be almost simultaneous as maternal and fetal status changes, and steps are taken to limit and reduce risk.

Common nursing interventions for high-risk intrapartum patients and their families tend to cluster in the following categories:

- Initiating emergency care to stabilize the woman or fetus
- Coordinating patient care services
- Implementing specific treatments and medications
- Monitoring and supporting maternal and fetal physiologic status
- Providing anticipatory guidance to the woman and her partner
- Promoting family-centered care

Initiating Emergency Care

The nurse often is the first health care professional to identify significant or life-threatening problems during the intrapartum period. All labor nurses must be skilled in managing obstetric and medical emergencies, even if the woman with complications eventually will be transported to another facility for intensive care. The nurse must be competent in the immediate management of hemorrhage, shock, hypertensive crisis, seizure activity, and acute fetal distress. Hospital policies and procedures guide the nurse when initiating emergency care, such as oxygen administration and intravenous (IV) lines, before the physician or midwife arrives.

Table 26-2. Common Collaborative Problems in High-Risk Intrapartum Patients

Medical Condition	Collaborative Problem
Cardiovascular System	
Pregnancy-induced hypertension	Hypertension Seizures Coma Pulmonary edema Renal failure edema Placental insufficiency Intrauterine growth retardation, fetal distress
Chronic hypertension	Renal failure Placental insufficiency, intrauterine growth retardation
Placenta previa/abruptio placentae	Hemorrhage and shock Disseminated intravascular coagulation Transfusion reactions Fetal distress
Cardiac disease	Congestive heart failure Pulmonary edema
Valvular disease	Pulmonary emboli
Marked vulvar varicosities	Hemorrhage
Respiratory System	
Adult respiratory distress syndrome	Hypoxemia
Genitourinary/Reproductive System	
Labor dystocia	Infection Birth trauma Fetal distress
Preterm labor	Infection Pulmonary edema Fetal distress
Previous cesarean birth	Ruptured uterus
Metabolic Functions	
Diabetes mellitus	Ketoacidosis Hypoglycemia Infections Nephropathy Hypertension Placental Insufficiency
Hyperthyroidism	Thyroid crisis "storm"
Miscellaneous	
Substance abuse	Infection Abruptio placentae Bacterial endocarditis Intrauterine growth retardation, fetal distress

Expected Outcome

- The woman with intrapartum complications and her fetus achieve physiologic stability.

Coordinating Patient Care Services

When intrapartum complications arise, health care professionals with specialized training are summoned to meet maternal, fetal, and neonatal needs. The nurse frequently is designated to coordinate patient care requirements. Once the midwife or physician is notified, other essential personnel are summoned. In most cases a perinatologist, neonatologist, or pediatrician is consulted to determine the special needs of the fetus or neonate. An anesthesiologist or nurse anesthestist is notified or alerted, because operative delivery may be anticipated or special pain management techniques indicated when complications arise. Depending on the nature of the problem, other services may be required to stabilize or treat the woman and her fetus or newborn. Timely notification of all essential health professionals is crucial to manage the problem and prevent further deterioration in the woman's condition.

Expected Outcome

- The woman and her family express verbal satisfaction with coordination of care.

Implementing Treatments and Administering Medications

The nurse is responsible for implementing a wide range of treatments and medication regimens when complications arise. With the creation of perinatal intensive care units, many nursing and medical functions and activities overlap. Nurses are educated to initiate specialized treatments, such as oxytocin induction and amnioinfusion. Agency policies, physician's orders, and practice guidelines developed by specialty organizations such as Association of Women's Health, Obstetric, and Neonatal Nursing (AWHONN, formerly NAACOG) guide the nurse in implementing care. While many aspects of care are task oriented, the nurse promotes a family-centered approach.

Expected Outcome

- The family verbalizes an understanding of the need for treatment and its regimen.

Monitoring and Supporting Maternal and Fetal Physiologic Status

Women at increased intrapartum risk require intensive monitoring and support of physiologic status. The nurse is responsible for regular and frequent monitoring of maternal vital signs and the progress of labor. Continuous external or internal electronic fetal monitoring (EFM) usually is established at the earliest opportunity. Other equipment, such as an electronic blood pressure monitor, pulse oximeter, or central venous or arterial monitor, often are used. The nurse must be familiar with procedures to support maternal and fetal physiologic status, including altering maternal position, changing IV infusion rates, and administering oxygen. (These are discussed in this chapter and in Chapters 23 and 27.)

Expected Outcome

- The laboring woman and her fetus maintain physiologic stability after implementation of appropriate treatment for intrapartum complications.

Providing Anticipatory Guidance

Research findings clearly indicate that catecholamines produced in anxiety-provoking conditions have a deleterious effect on maternal–fetal physiologic status. Even in extreme emergencies, the nurse must attempt to provide brief explanations to the woman and her support person regarding the nature of the problem and the interventions implemented to correct it. Under less stressful conditions, more detailed discussions and explanations will reduce anxiety levels and support individual and family functioning. Chapter 25 provides additional information regarding anticipatory guidance.

Expected Outcome

- The woman and her family exhibit an understanding of intrapartum problems, the plan of care, and procedures to be performed as indicated by their questions and restatement of information.

• • Evaluation

The appropriateness and adequacy of nursing care are based on the process of evaluation. When expected outcomes are met, the nurse continues with the established plan of care. If new intrapartum problems develop or desired outcomes and goals are not achieved, the nurse revises the care plan. When nursing actions are effective, the woman should achieve physiologic stability, progress through labor, and give birth to a viable, healthy neonate.

The nursing process provides the nurse with a systematic method of identifying intrapartum problems and planning appropriate care. The labor and delivery nurse reviews the woman's prenatal record to determine preexisting risk factors. Ongoing assessments of the woman's physiologic status are conducted so that early signs and symptoms of problems can be detected. Nursing diagnoses that reflect priority problems and needs are identified, and the plan of care is then formulated and implemented. Because many intrapartum complications pose a serious risk to maternal or fetal well-being, ongoing evaluation of responses to nursing care and medical therapy is essential. If expected outcomes are not achieved, revisions are made in the plan of care to achieve maternal and fetal physiologic stability.

Complications Involving the Placenta

Maternal and fetal status are so intertwined that classifying a problem as a maternal or fetal complication is an oversimplification of the situation. Placental problems, such as placenta previa and placental abruption, are life-threatening events for both patients (woman and fetus).

The placenta is the life support system of the fetus. Weighing approximately 450 g (1 lb) and measuring approximately 15 cm (6 inches) in diameter, it allows the exchange of oxygen, nutrients, carbon dioxide, and metabolic wastes. It also transports maternal antibodies, hormones, and other substances required for fetal growth and development. When placental functioning is disrupted during the intrapartum period, fetal hypoxia and distress occur.

Abnormalities often are evident in placental perfusion (diagnosed by Doppler velocimetry), in the site of attachment of the placenta in the uterus (localized by ultrasonography), or in tissue structure (identified by ultrasonography or postnatally by gross or microscopic examination of the placenta). When fetal death has occurred without apparent reason, the placenta may provide clues to the cause through evidence of infection, systemic vascular disease, or genetic abnormalities.

Placenta Previa

Placenta previa occurs when implantation of the trophoblast takes place in the lower uterine segment. The placenta grows to partially or completely cover the internal cervical os, as illustrated in Figure 26-1. The condition occurs in approximately 1 in 200 pregnancies (LoBue, 1991). Placenta previa may be classified as follows:

- *Low lying:* the placenta is implanted near the internal margin of the os.
- *Marginal:* the edge of the placenta borders on the os.
- *Partial:* a percentage of the placenta covers the cervical os.
- *Total:* the placenta completely covers and obstructs the os.

As the placenta increases in size and weight, pressure and stretching occur in the lower uterine segment and over the cervix, often stimulating uterine contractions and some degree of cervical dilatation and effacement. The placental tissue over the dilating os is torn from its implantation site and exposes open, bleeding blood vessels. Because this bleeding originates from the placenta, it cannot be stopped effectively until the infant and placenta are delivered.

The degree of placental placement over the internal cervical os determines the severity of the bleeding and onset of the initial episode. Women with central previa will have the first onset of bleeding by 28 to 30 weeks' gestation. The first episode of bleeding rarely is severe enough to be fatal to the woman or fetus.

Etiologic and Predisposing Factors

The precise cause of placenta previa is unknown. It is believed that when the vasculature in the uterine fundus is deficient, the placenta implants at a lower level where the blood supply is more conducive to placental growth. The following are among the factors known to place the woman at risk for placenta previa.

- Age greater than 35: placenta previa is three times greater at age 35 than age 25.
- Increasing parity: 80% of women experiencing placenta previa are multiparas.
- Presence of uterine scars.
- Prior placenta previa: the incidence among women who have already had a placenta previa is 12 times higher than in the general population.
- Development of a placenta with an abnormally large

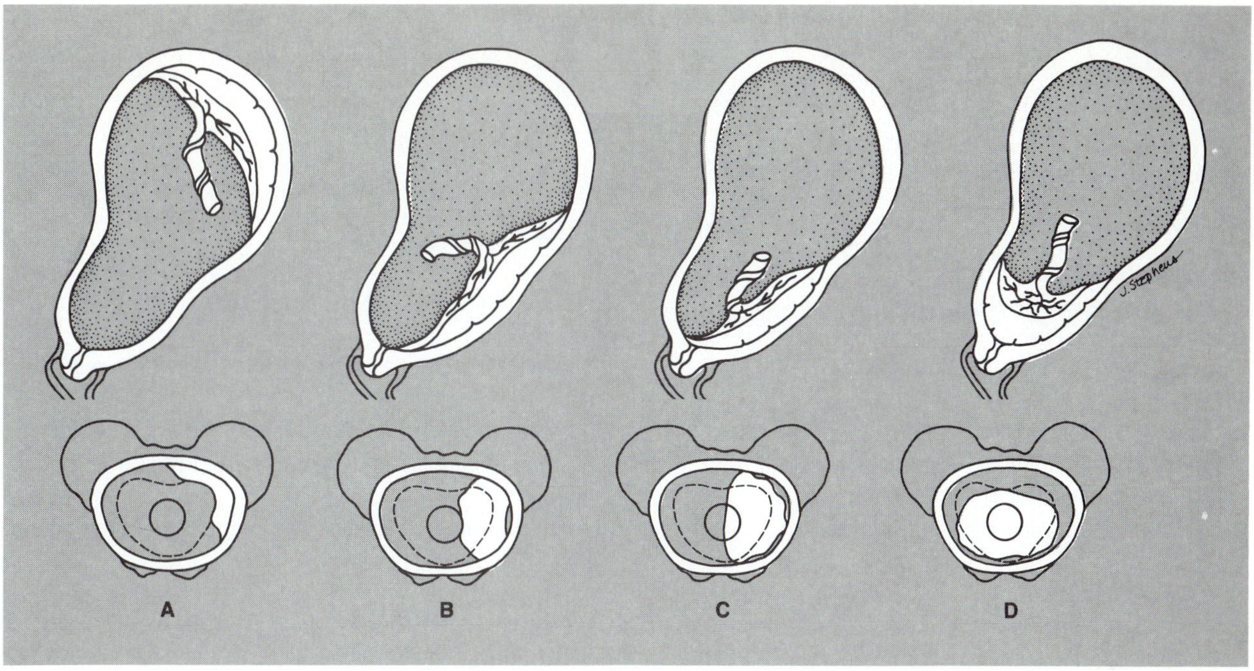

Figure 26-1.

Placental positions in normal pregnancy and with placenta previa. *A:* Normal position. *B:* Low implantation. *C:* Partial placenta previa. *D:* Total placenta previa (Childbirth Graphics).

surface area (multifetal pregnancy or Rh isoimmunization with erythroblastosis fetalis).

Other factors thought to be possible causes include late fertilization of the egg, in vitro fertilization, and delayed implantation.

Diagnosis

This condition often is revealed as painless, bright-red vaginal bleeding during the third trimester. However, due to stimulation of the lower uterine segment, some women present with signs and symptoms of preterm labor coincident with vaginal bleeding. If contractions are present, the uterus should relax between contractions. The existence of placenta previa may be discovered before bleeding occurs if ultrasonography has been performed for another indication, such as gestational age dating. When a woman presents in labor and delivery with vaginal bleeding, the diagnosis of placenta previa is confirmed by ultrasound localization of the placenta.

Manual or speculum examination of the cervix should *never* be performed on a woman who presents with vaginal bleeding until placenta previa has been ruled out. This is crucial because the speculum or examiner's finger may further stimulate cervical dilatation and dislodge the placenta, resulting in massive hemorrhage. When marginal placenta previa has been diagnosed by sonography, a sterile speculum examination of the cervix may be performed to evaluate the degree to which the cervical os is covered by placenta. The woman is transferred to a delivery room, and prepared for both vaginal and cesarean birth. Instruments, equipment, medical and nursing personnel, and crossmatched blood are immediately available to accomplish a cesarean delivery if profuse hemorrhage results from the examination. This is referred to as a double set-up procedure.

Maternal, Fetal, and Neonatal Implications

The first episode of bleeding in placenta previa rarely is serious for the woman. Maternal mortality is less than 1% (Kulb, 1990a). However, subsequent bleeding episodes may place the woman at risk for severe hemorrhage, embolism, and risks associated with emergency operative delivery. Up to 25% of women will experience hypovolemic shock with subsequent episodes of bleeding.

A major risk associated with this condition is preterm labor. If not recognized or controlled in a timely manner, hemorrhage and preterm birth may ensue. Other maternal risks are those associated with cesarean delivery, including exessive blood loss, infection, and aspiration pneumonia secondary to the administration of general anesthesia.

Women with placenta previa also are at increased risk for postpartum hemorrhage, because vessels in the lower uterine segment are not effectively compressed by contraction of the uterus. Significant postpartum bleeding can occur even when the fundus is very firm. If bleeding cannot be controlled with oxytocics or prostin 15 M, ligation of uterine vessels or hysterectomy may be necessary.

Hemorrhage requires early cesarean delivery regardless of fetal maturity. Prematurity accounts for 60% of the fetal deaths associated with placenta previa. Fetal death related to placenta previa also may result from intrauterine asphyxia or fetal hemorrhage, which may result from tearing of the placenta during cesarean delivery or from a vaginal examination that injures fetal vessels. The incidence of congenital

NURSING PROCEDURE
Administering Blood Products

Purpose: To replace serum or red blood cells, treat hypovolemic shock, or disseminated intravascular coagulopathy.

NURSING ACTION	***RATIONALE***
Preparation	
1. Insert large-gauge needle or angiocath (16 to 19 g in adults).	To prevent hemolysis of red blood cells (RBCs).
2. Attach blood tubing with inline filter (170 μm pore size).	To prevent hemolyzed cells and small clots from entering vein.
3. Use Y-type tubing system.	To permit simultaneous infusion of blood and IV fluids.
4. Prime blood tubing with 0.9 NaCl (normal saline). Use 0.9 NaCl *only* for flush of tubing.	To prevent clumping of or hemolysis of RBCs, which occurs with glucose solutions.
5. Obtain pretransfusion vital signs and record.	To have baseline parameters for comparison during and after transfusion.
Verification	
6. Obtain blood product from blood bank just prior to administration.	To prevent deterioration in blood product. Blood product cannot be returned to blood bank for reissue if kept at room temperature for longer than 30 minutes.
7. Check blood product against patient information with another registered nurse: • Verify ABO group and Rh type. • Match unit serial numbers on bag against original blood request slip. • Compare the name and ID number on the bag with the woman's ID bracelet. • Verify that blood product matches the original MD order.	To prevent accidental administration of wrong blood product to woman, which may result in life-threatening or fatal reaction.
• Check the expiration date on the blood bag. • Inspect the bag for evidence of leakage, discoloration, or bubbling.	To prevent administration of contaminated product or expired unit.
Administration	
8. Start infusion slowly: no faster than 30 mL in first 15 min while remaining with woman.	To allow identification of adverse reactions and timely intervention to reverse them.
9. Obtain vital signs after first 15 min and at least every hour thereafter.	
10. May use infusion pump approved for blood administration.	To prevent hemolysis of RBCs. Must use only approved pump.
11. Transfuse unit in 2 to 4 hours.	To avoid delayed infusion, which results in deterioration of blood product.
12. If rapid infusion indicated, use blood warming device.	To prevent too rapid infusion of cold blood, which causes hypothermia.
13. Change blood tubing after infusing 2 units of blood.	To prevent clogging of inline filter.

Adapted from National Blood Resource Education Program, Nursing Education Work Group. (1991). Choosing blood components and equipment. American Journal of Nursing, *91(6), 48–50.*

abnormalities is increased when placenta previa is present, for reasons not fully understood.

Treatment

Treatment of placenta previa during the intrapartum period centers on monitoring bleeding, preventing hemorrhage, and replacing blood when necessary to prevent shock (see the Nursing Procedure, Administering Blood Products). If bleeding has been controlled by bed rest and tocolytic therapy to prevent preterm labor, an elective cesarean birth can be planned when fetal maturity is assured. In some cases the woman may be permitted to return home on a regimen of complete bed rest. Ongoing assessment is provided by nurses skilled in home health care nursing (see next section on Implications for Nursing Care).

Once the gestational age is confirmed to be 36 weeks or greater, delivery can be safely planned. In many settings cesarean delivery is the method of choice. Some physicians may choose to proceed with vaginal delivery when the previa is partial at 30% or less. Labor may be induced with amniotomy to promote descent of the presenting part, which applies pressure to the bleeding site (tamponade) and may decrease blood loss. Careful Pitocin induction of labor is begun if the presenting part is low, the presentation normal, and the cervix favorable. If the woman presents with active bleeding that cannot be stopped through the use of bed rest and tocolytics, an emergency cesarean birth will be performed immediately regardless of gestational age.

Implications for Nursing Care

Nursing responsibilities center on prompt evaluation of maternal and fetal physiologic status and minimizing blood loss until delivery can be accomplished. A review of critical nursing responsibilities when third-trimester bleeding occurs is given in the accompanying Nursing Procedure. Emotional support is ongoing and occurs in conjunction with other nursing activities.

If the woman's condition stabilizes and she is permitted to return home, ongoing nursing assessments and care are arranged. The woman performs daily EFM and uterine monitoring at home using portable equipment. Data are transmitted by telephone to a regional perinatal center or a home health care agency. A nurse who is skilled in the interpretation of fetal heart rate (FHR) patterns and uterine activity will evaluate the strip and make recommendations based on the

NURSING PROCEDURE
Managing Third-Trimester Bleeding

Purpose: In the presence of third-trimester bleeding, the nurse never *performs a vaginal or rectal examination before placenta previa is ruled out. The following actions should be initiated by the nurse.*

NURSING ACTION	***RATIONALE***
1. Call for help. Have another staff person notify the physician or midwife.	To facilitate prompt initiation of supportive measures. To alert physician or midwife about the development of problems.
2. Initiate an intravenous line with a large-bore angiocath (16- or 18-g angiocath).	To provide access for administration of fluids, blood, and drugs.
3. If bleeding is profuse, insert *two* IV lines.	To provide additional route for rapid administration of blood and fluids.
4. Draw a blood sample and send to the laboratory for type, Rh factor, antibody screen, and crossmatching.	To ensure that blood is available and can be given promptly when required.
5. Draw additional samples for complete blood count and clotting studies.	To determine the extent of blood loss and depletion of clotting factors.
6. Administer oxygen at 8 to 12 L/min.	To improve maternal oxygenation and amount of oxygen available to fetus.
7. Place woman in Trendelenburg position, preferably on her left side.	To improve blood flow to brain. To prevent supine hypotension.
8. Initiate continuous external EFM and uterine monitoring.	To ascertain fetal status and uterine activity pattern.
9. Initiate frequent monitoring of maternal vital signs (Q 15 minutes or more frequently) until the woman's condition stabilizes.	To ascertain maternal status and detect early signs of change.
10. Initiate pulse oximetry monitoring.	To determine blood oxygen saturation levels.
11. Notify anesthesiologist, neonatologist (or pediatrician), nursery nurse manager, or charge nurse (of possible cesarean birth of compromised neonate).	To have additional staff available for emergency cesarean birth and support of the neonate at birth.
12. Measure all blood loss (peripad counts, weighing bed linen or linen protectors).	
13. Be prepared to insert Foley catheter.	To measure urine output and in preparation for cesarean birth.
14. Assemble supplies and equipment for cesarean birth.	To expedite prompt delivery of neonate.
15. Initiate preoperative checklist.	To ensure that all requirements for surgery have been met.

data. The nurse also reports the findings to the physician and collaborates on changes in the plan of care. Periodic visits are made by a perinatal nurse skilled in the in-home assessment and care of women with placenta previa.

Abruptio Placentae

Abruptio placentae is the premature separation of the normally situated placenta from its site of implantation after the 20th week of gestation. The incidence is estimated at 1 in every 100 pregnancies and appears to be increasing (Saftlas et al., 1991). As the placenta detaches, bleeding occurs in the space between the placenta and uterus, forming a retroplacental clot. As the clot grows, further placental separation occurs. Hemorrhage may be apparent (obvious vaginal bleeding) or concealed as shown in Figure 26-2. Placental abruption can be a slow process or occur rapidly. The severity of this complication depends on the degree of placental separation and amount of bleeding that results during the detachment process.

Abruptio placentae is classified on the basis of bleeding and symptoms (see the accompanying display). With cesarean delivery the uterus also may be observed to have large areas of hemorrhage in the musculature itself. This condition is known as Couvelaire uterus.

Etiologic and Predisposing Factors

The exact cause of abruptio placentae is unknown. It is suggested that defective placental vasculature causes arteriolar thrombosis, degeneration of the decidua, and disruption of the vessels. As noted, the incidence of abruption appears to be increasing. Recent research indicates that poverty, the inability to receive treatment for predisposing conditions such as hypertension, and the growing use of crack cocaine may be the primary reasons for this increase (Saftlas et al., 1991). The following factors have been implicated in the development of abruptio placentae.

- History of placental abruption (30 times greater than in general population)
- Increasing multiparity (six times greater than in general population)
- Poverty
- PIH
- Increasing maternal age
- Supine hypotensive syndrome
- Sudden uterine decompression (as in rupture of membranes with polyhydramnios)
- Short umbilical cord
- Trauma to the abdomen
- Cocaine and amphetamine use
- Cigarette smoking
- Excessive alcohol consumption

Diagnosis

The diagnosis of abruptio placentae generally is made from clinical signs and symptoms, which vary extensively depending on the degree of the placental separation and extent of bleeding. The classic presentation includes constant abdominal pain and uterine tenderness on palpation. Increased uterine tone (tetany) without relaxation between contractions is common. The uterus feels firm or "boardlike," and contractions may be difficult to palpate when the uterus is rigid. If external tokodynamometry is used in conjunction with EFM, a distinctive uterine pattern of very frequent, low amplitude contractions (tachysystole) may be noted. If vaginal bleeding is evident, the blood is noted to be dark or port-wine stained and does not clot (Dorman, 1989).

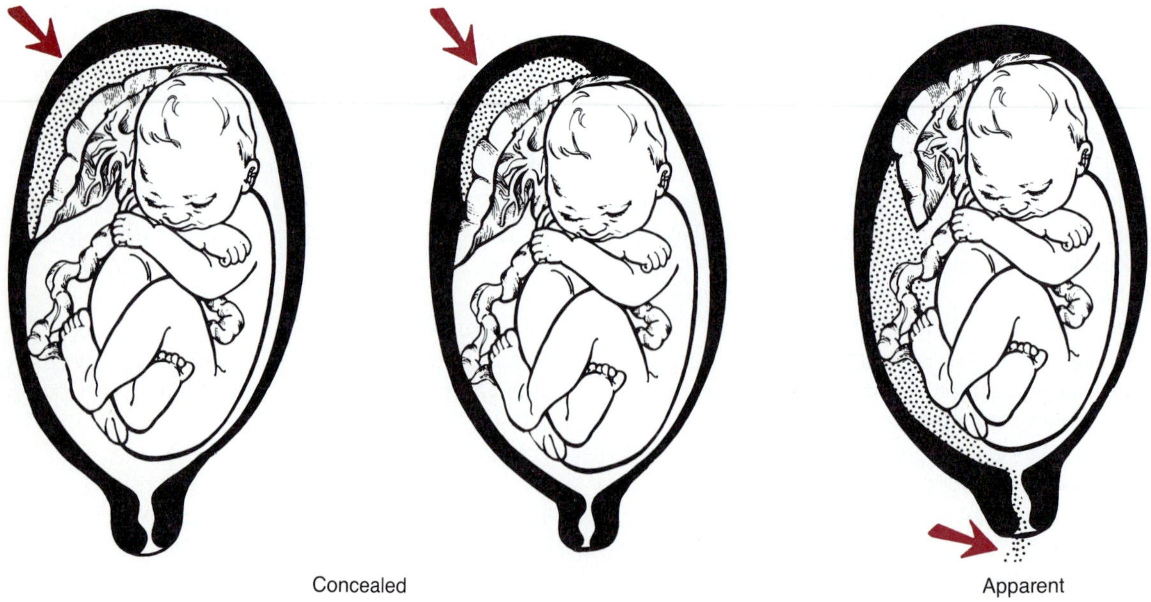

Figure 26-2.
Abruptio placentae. Hemorrhage may be concealed or apparent by vaginal bleeding (Childbirth Graphics).

Classification of Abruptio Placentae

Grade 0: Small retroplacental clot formed, or small rupture of a marginal sinus.

Bleeding is not significant (<100 mL) and may be concealed.

Woman is asymptomatic for pain, hypovolemic shock, and coagulopathy.

No fetal distress.

Grade 1: Small retroplacental clot may be formed; detachment of larger surface of placenta (<50% detachment).

Bleeding is slightly increased (>100 mL, <500 mL) but not significant; may be concealed.

Woman may experience mild uterine tenderness with slight degree of uterine tetany; no evidence of hypovolemic shock or coagulopathy.

No fetal distress.

Grade 2: Significant retroplacental clot formation may occur; detachment of large surface of placent (approaching 50%).

Bleeding is increased and closer to 500 mL; bleeding may be concealed; hypovolemia may occur.

Woman experiences significant uterine tenderness with increased uterine tone, and polysystole; mild, compensated shock often evident, and abnormal coagulation.

Fetal distress evident; fetal death may occur.

Grade 3: Significant retroplacental clot formation may occur; detachment greater than 50% (may be total).

Bleeding is greater than 500 mL; bleeding may be concealed; hypovolemia occurs.

Woman experiences extreme uterine tenderness; uterine tone is extreme (tetany) and reactive to palpation; polysystole evident; uncompensated shock; coagulopathy is common; maternal death possible.

Fetal distress and fetal death are common.

Adapted from LoBue, C. (1991). Third-trimester bleeding. In K. Niswander & A. Evans (Eds.), Manual of obstetrics. *Boston: Little, Brown and Co.*

Symptoms of shock will depend on the amount of blood lost. The severity of shock may not be consistent with the degree of vaginal bleeding noted, because a significant amount of bleeding may be concealed. Fetal distress may be evident but also will depend on the degree of blood loss.

Ultrasonography often is useful in confirming the diagnosis of abruptio placentae (Combs et al., 1992). The identification of retroplacental clots, placental thickening, and placental detachment is now possible with advances in sonographic technology.

Maternal, Fetal, and Neonatal Implications

Abruptio placentae is a serious problem resulting in maternal mortality and death. Maternal mortality is estimated to be between 0.5% and 5%. Major complications include hemorrhagic shock, disseminated intravascular coagulopathy (DIC), and ischemic necrosis of other organs, such as the brain, kidneys, or pituitary gland (Sheehan syndrome) secondary to shock. Couvelaire uterus, hemorrhage into the uterine myometrium, may prevent adequate contraction of the uterus after birth of the infant and placenta. This complication may require hysterectomy.

Women with placental abruption who are at greatest risk for serious complications are those with sudden, massive hemorrhage and complete placental detachment (often seen with women who inhale [freebase] crack cocaine). Women with slowly growing central clots who are undiagnosed until fetal demise and DIC occur also are at high risk for hemorrhage, organ necrosis, and death. When placental separation is minimal and prompt obstetric diagnosis and treatment are available, maternal mortality and morbidity are reduced.

Abruptio placentae is responsible for 15% to 25% of perinatal death (Combs et al., 1992). Among women presenting with signs of placental abruption, 20% will present with fetal demise, and another 20% will have fetuses experiencing fetal distress. Prospects for fetal survival are even worse when significant placental abruption occurs. Perinatal mortality associated with greater than 50% abruption ranges from 50% to 80%. In half of the cases of uncompensated maternal shock when blood transfusion is urgently needed, the fetus is likely to die. Of the neonates who do survive, many suffer increased morbidity from effects of hypoxia, birth trauma, and prematurity.

Treatment

Once the cause of third-trimester bleeding is determined to be abruptio placentae (after placenta previa has been ruled out), a vaginal examination may be performed to determine cervical status. The nature of treatment will depend on the degree of abruption and the severity of bleeding.

Mild Abruption (Grade 0). Women with grade 0 abruptions may be managed conservatively with tocolytics and bed rest when they are diagnosed before 37 weeks' gestation (Combs et al., 1992). The woman remains hospitalized. Continuous monitoring of fetal status and uterine activity and close evaluation of maternal status are implemented. The goal of treatment is to maintain the pregnancy until fetal maturity is achieved.

Moderate Abruption (Grade 1). When maternal and fetal conditions are stable and blood loss is not significant, oxytocin augmentation of labor may be instituted. This plan will depend on the fetal gestational age, cervical status, and the ability to perform an immediate emergency cesarean delivery if the degree of abruption and bleeding worsens. Vaginal delivery may then be attempted if the cervix continues to dilate, the fetus descends through the birth canal, and bleeding is not severe. Maternal and fetal status are constantly monitored, as well as the woman's hemoglobin, hematocrit, and clotting factors.

Moderate to Severe Abruption (Grade 2 or 3). Treatment consists of restoration and maintenance of maternal physiologic status. IV fluid and blood replacement are initiated to counteract hypovolemic shock. Central venous pressure monitoring may be instituted to assess accurately maternal hemodynamic status. DIC is treated with whole blood and platelet transfusions. Hypofibrinogenemia, if present, is treated with cryoprecipitate or fresh-frozen plasma. Arrangements are completed for immediate cesarean delivery.

Implications for Nursing Care

Nursing responsibilities in the care of a woman with suspected or diagnosed abruptio placentae center on the following:

- Early identification of clinical signs and symptoms or evidence of worsening abruption
- Initiation of measures to support maternal physiologic status (see Nursing Procedure on managing third-trimester bleeding earlier in this chapter)
- Monitoring maternal and fetal status
- Monitoring laboratory tests for evidence of DIC
- Preparing for and assisting with prompt delivery

The reader is referred to the Nursing Care Plan for the woman with abruptio placentae.

> ### *Placental Grading*
>
> Grade 0: Homogeneous immature placenta without calcification.
>
> Grade I: Echogenic densities begin to appear in the placenta.
>
> May be evident around 31 weeks' gestation.
>
> Rarely observed after 42 weeks.
>
> Grade II: Calcifications and indentations of the chorionic plate appear on the placenta.
>
> Become evident about 36 weeks' gestation.
>
> Grade III: Multiple indentations appear on placenta causing a "Swiss cheese" pattern.
>
> Becomes evident about 38 weeks' gestation.
>
> May become evident before 35 weeks' gestation in intrauterine growth retardation, maternal pregnancy-induced hypertension, or chronic hypertension.
>
> *Adapted from Murphy P. (1990). Assessment of fetal status. In K. Buckley & N. Kulb (Eds.),* High risk maternity nursing manual *(p. 44). Baltimore: Williams & Wilkins.*

Placental Infarction

Placental infarction occurs when the blood supply to an area of the placenta is blocked, and tissue necrosis results. This occurs during late pregnancy and indicates the normal placental aging process. Pathologic infarctions occur with maternal diseases that adversely affect her cardiovascular system.

Etiologic and Predisposing Factors

Pathologic infarctions are most often associated with vascular disease of the uteroplacental unit secondary to maternal hypertension. In the presence of PIH, nearly 33% of placentas will contain infarctions. The incidence increases to 60% in the presence of eclampsia. Infarctions are more common in women with severe type I diabetes.

Diagnosis

Advances in ultrasonography permit assessment of the placenta for evidence of aging, including the presence of infarctions. The technique, known as placental grading, provides a classification of changes in placental structure. The grading system is presented in the accompanying display. Pathologic infarctions may be suspected during pregnancy when intrauterine fetal growth retardation is diagnosed, or when placental perfusion is compromised during labor (late decelerations) in the woman with PIH.

After delivery of the placenta, the physician or midwife can confirm the diagnosis of infarction through visual inspection of the placenta. Infarctions occur most commonly on the maternal surface as circular areas ranging from dark red to yellow–white. They are seen frequently at the placental margin and may represent normal physiologic degenerative changes that occur with placental aging. They also may represent pathologic changes associated with the disease process. If neonatal asphyxia occurs, the placenta frequently is sent to pathology for a more complete gross and microscopic examination. The extent of placental infarction can be estimated more accurately.

Maternal, Fetal, and Neonatal Implications

Placental infarcts have no clinical effects on maternal status. Fetal circulation may not be immediately affected by placental infarction. Small marginal areas of infarction have no effect on fetal status. Blood will continue to flow through the ischemic villi for some time, but their capacity for metabolic exchange is limited. Affected areas eventually become fibrotic. However, if the circulation through the rest of the organ is sufficient, a fetus may survive when as much as 20% to 30% of the placenta is infarcted. If infarctions occur centrally and compromise the blood supply to the fetus, growth retardation or even death may result.

Treatment

Placental infarctions cannot be treated per se. However, early and comprehensive treatment of underlying maternal disease during pregnancy can decrease the severity and incidence of placental infarcts.

Implications for Nursing Care

During labor the nurse monitors the FHR for evidence of impaired uteroplacental perfusion. Although not a specific indicator of placental infarction, the presence of persistent late decelerations may suggest compromised placental per-

Text continues on page 676

Nursing Care Plan

The Woman With Abruptio Placentae

PATIENT PROFILE

History

A.P. is a 34-year-old G3/P2 at 30 weeks' gestation. She comes to labor and delivery because she is experiencing intense, frequent contractions and vaginal bleeding. She has had no prenatal care. She reveals to the nurse that she used "crack" cocaine several hours ago.

Physical Assessment

The nurse notes a moderate amount of dark red vaginal bleeding. There are no clots. The vital signs are B/P96/46; P 136; RR 26; T37.0°C (98.6°F). A.P. is conscious, restless, and moans continuously. Her skin is pale, cool, and clammy. Her nailbed CFT is 5 seconds.

A.P. is placed on an external EFM, and the following pattern is noted: FHR 170 BPM; 0–3 bpm LTV; persistent late decelerations. The uterine contractions are occurring every 1 to 1½ minutes, lasting 45 seconds (tachysystole). The uterus is very firm (boardlike) and does not relax between contractions.

A.P. clutches the nurse arm tightly and says, "I'm going to die, and my baby is going to die! Please help me. I don't want to die!" A.P. is visibly tremulous. She will not release the nurse's arm.

COLLABORATIVE PROBLEMS/POTENTIAL COMPLICATIONS

- Hypovolemic shock
- Disseminated intravascular coagulopathy
- Adult respiratory distress syndrome
- Sheehan's syndrome
- Renal tubular necrosis
- Fetal distress and intrauterine fetal death

Assessment	*Nursing Diagnosis*	*Nursing Interventions*	*Rationale*
B/P 96/46; P 136; RR 26 Moderate amount of dark red vaginal bleeding. Uterus firm (boardlike). Skin pale, cool and clammy. CFT × 5 seconds. A.P. is conscious and restless.	Decreased Cardiac Output related to hemorrhage Altered Tissue Perfusion related to hypotension. *Expected Outcome* A.P.'s vital signs will stabilize and remain within normal limits after initiation of therapy.	Call for help. Notify midwife or MD. Initiate an IV line with a 16–18 g angiocath. Insert a second line when help arrives.	Additional staff and physician presence are essential to treat shock and expedite delivery. Large-gauge angiocath is essential for rapid blood and fluid replacement.
		Use blood tubing for IV set up. Infuse physiologic IV solution rapidly.	Blood is essential to prevent irreversible tissue and organ damage. Blood tubing with filter is essential for blood administration. IV fluids are essential to restore circulating volume. Physiologic solution prevents hemolysis of RBCs and supports kidney function.
		Place A.P. on left side and in Trendelenburg position.	Turning on left side prevents supine hypotension. Trendelenburg improves return of blood to heart and brain.

(Continued)

The Woman With Abruptio Placentae

(*Continued*)

Assessment	***Nursing Diagnosis***	***Nursing Interventions***	***Rationale***
		Administer oxygen at 8–12 L/min by face mask.	Administration at this rate promotes optimum tissue oxygenation.
		Draw blood specimen for CBC, type and crossmatch, blood coagulation studies (PT/PTT, fibrinogen, fibrin split products).	Lab tests will assist in estimating blood loss and the development of DIC.
		Do not perform vaginal examination.	Vaginal exams are prohibited until placenta previa is ruled out.
		Insert in-dwelling Foley catheter.	Knowledge of kidney function will assist in determining the adequacy of fluid replacement.
		Monitor vital signs Q 5 min.	Vital signs are sensitive indicators of shock and response to therapy.
		Attach pulse oximeter and electronic blood pressure monitor if available.	Electronic monitor permits rapid appraisal of vital signs. Pulse oximeter provides data on oxygen saturation levels.
		Alert OR staff and prepare A.P. for emergency cesarean delivery.	If bleeding continues, the uterus must be emptied to prevent fetal death and continued uterine bleeding.
FHR is 170 bmp with 0–3 bpm LTV and repetitive late decelerations. A.P. took crack several hours ago. Contractions occurring Q $1^{1}/_{2}$ min and lasts 45 sec. Uterus is firm and does not relax between contractions.	Altered Fetal Tissue Perfusion related to hemorrhage and tachysystole contraction pattern ***Expected Outcome*** A.P. will deliver by cesarean surgery.	Place A.P. on left side and in Trendelenburg position.	To improve uteroplacental perfusion. To improve maternal cardiac output, which improves placental perfusion.
		Administer O2 8–12 L/min by mask.	Increasing maternal blood oxygen level will improve fetal and maternal tissue oxygenation.
		Give IV fluids and blood as ordered.	IV fluids and blood will stabilize maternal blood pressure and improve utero-placental blood flow.
		Be prepared to administer a tocolytic (if ordered and vital signs stabilize).	Tocolytics may decrease uterine tachysystole and improve fetal oxygenation. However with signs of shock, Beta-sympathomimetics, such as Terbutaline, are contraindicated.

(*Continued*)

The Woman With Abruptio Placentae

(Continued)

Assessment	*Nursing Diagnosis*	*Nursing Interventions*	*Rationale*
		Summon pediatric staff.	Pediatric or neonatal staff must be present at birth of preterm infant with evidence of fetal distress.
		Prepare A.P. for cesarean birth.	If bleeding and signs of shock continue, the infant must be delivered promptly or severe asphyxia or death will occur.
A.P. says, "I'm going to die, and my baby is going to die. Help me nurse. I don't want to die." A.P. clutches nurse's arm and will not release it. A.P. is visibly tremulous.	Fear related to bleeding episode, use of crack cocaine, gestational age, and impending cesarean birth ***Expected Outcome*** A.P. will verbalize a decrease in her level of fear. A.P. will demonstrate a decreased level of fear as evidenced by her ability to follow directions and cooperate in her care	Provide continuous support and encouragement. Reassure A.P. that someone will remain continuously with her. Reassure her that staff is doing all they can to help her and her baby. Offer brief, simple explanations regarding status and procedures.	Hemorrhage is extremely alarming and anxiety provoking for the woman. The woman should never be left alone because level of anxiety will escalate. Positive feedback about care may help to control the level of A.P.'s fear. Acute anxiety reduces the woman's ability to process or understand information and explanations.
		Inquire about A.P.'s support system and determine if she wishes to have someone with her.	The support of a family member or friend may reduce the level of anxiety.
		When possible, offer brief directions regarding relaxation and imagery as A.P. is prepared for emergency cesarean birth.	Providing A.P. with concrete directions regarding relaxation and imagery may enhance her coping skills.
		Maintain a calm demeanor.	Maintaining a calm demeanor will reassure A.P. that she has a competent nurse and that the situation is in control.

EVALUATION

A diagnosis of abruptio placentae was made, and it was decided that A.P. should deliver by cesarean birth. A.P. was able to decrease her fear enough to cooperate with the staff during preparation for the cesarean delivery. She continued to verbalize fears of dying until she received general anesthesia. A.P. held a nurse's hand and maintained eye contact with the nurse until she was unconscious. A.P. delivered a 1000-g baby girl 20 minutes after admission to the labor and delivery unit. The newborn's Apgar score was 2 at 1 minute (for a heart rate over 100 bpm) and 5 at 5 minutes. The newborn was intubated, received oxygen, and was taken to the neonatal intensive care unit. Ten units of packed cells were administered to A.P. A.P.'s vital signs stabilized and remained within normal limits.

fusion due to placental calcification, fibrin deposition, or infarction. This is particularly true when the pregnancy progresses beyond 42 weeks, or PIH has been diagnosed. The nurse must attempt to improve placental perfusion by changing the woman's position and initiating an IV line to increase maternal circulation. Persistent late decelerations must be reported to the physician or midwife.

The nurse frequently is responsible for examination of the placenta after delivery. When infarctions or other abnormalities are noted, the nurse should bring this to the birth attendant's attention. In most cases such findings have no clinical significance. However the American College of Obstetrics suggets that systematic pathologic examination of the placenta may be helpful in identifying possible placental abnormalities when adverse perinatal outcomes occur (Committee on Obstetrics, 1991).

Because of the vital role the placenta plays in fetal physiologic functioning, complications involving the placenta can result in fetal distress or death. The woman also is at risk for life-threatening hemorrhage when abnormal implantation or premature detachment occurs. The maternity nurse must be vigilant for signs of fetal distress or decompensation in the woman that may suggest placental problems. Prompt interventions are necessary to prevent decompensation, permanent disability, or death. Regardless of the setting, the maternity nurse must be prepared to initiate emergency measures to support the woman and fetus until medical help arrives when placental problems occur. The nurse also is responsible for examining the placenta after birth and identifying and reporting abnormalities.

Complications Involving the Membranes and Amniotic Fluid

Complications in the intrapartum period can arise from structural problems with amniotic membranes, infection of the membranes, or the volume of amniotic fluid. Premature rupture of membranes (PROM) or abnormalities in amniotic fluid volume will affect the fetus and alter the process of labor and birth. PROM is described in detail in Chapter 20.

Chorioamnionitis

Chorioamnionitis (sometimes referred to as amnionitis, intrapartum infection, or intraamniotic infection) involves infection of the chorion, amnion, amniotic fluid, and fetus. Although chorioamnionitis occurs most commonly after rupture of fetal membranes, it also may occur when membranes are intact.

Etiologic and Predisposing Factors

Infection of the fetal membranes is thought to occur by three routes (Fig. 26-3):

- Ascending infections from the vagina across intact or through ruptured membranes
- Transplacental infection from the maternal circulation to the amniotic sac
- Descending infection from the abdominal cavity through the fallopian tubes and into the uterus

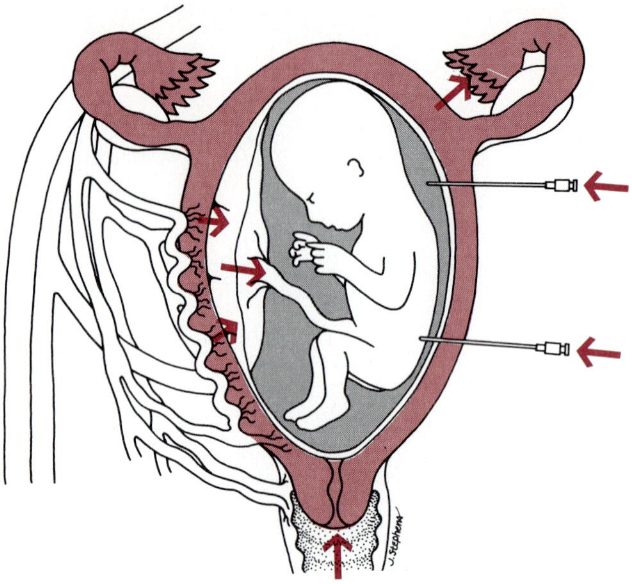

Figure 26-3.
Routes of intrauterine infection. Chorioamnionitis can result from contamination as a result of amniocentesis, ascending vaginal microorganisms, or maternal systemic infection through the placenta or the pelvic organs themselves (Childbirth Graphics).

During normal pregnancy the fetus and membranes usually are protected from infection ascending from the vagina by the mucous plug in the cervical canal, the intact amniotic membranes, and the normal antibacterial activity of the amniotic fluid. These protective mechanisms are lost with ruputure of the membranes. Infection begins when the membranes, exposed to the dilating cervix, become inflamed. The membranes become stretched and subject to decreased blood supply; they may become weakened and vulnerable to bacteria introduced during vaginal examinations and other invasive procedures. The risk of infection increases only slightly within the first 24 hours but exponentially thereafter. In rare cases ascending infections may spread from the vagina into the uterus across intact membranes. The causes and mechanisms for this form of ascending infection are not fully understood.

Other routes for the development of chorioamnionitis are less common. With maternal blood-borne infections, organisms migrate through the placenta into the amniotic sac. Listeriosis, or maternal listeremia, is a serious blood-borne infection that may cause an infection of the membranes and fetus, resulting in spontaneous abortion, preterm labor, and neonatal death. Descending infections are rare but may occur in women who begin pregnancy with chronic pelvic infections. Organisms travel through the fallopian tubes into the uterine cavity.

Ascending infections may be caused by bacteria, fungi, or viruses. Bacteria, protozoa, and parasitic organisms have been implicated in blood-borne infections. The organisms most commonly isolated as the cause of amnionitis are *Bacteroides* (25%), aerobic *Streptococcus* (13%), *group B Streptococcus* (12%), and *Escherichia coli* (10%). Genital mycoplasmas also may be found and may predispose the woman to preterm labor (Williams et al., 1991). Anaerobic bacteria should be suspected if foul-smelling amniotic fluid is present. When amniotic fluid is meconium stained, propagation of pathogenic organisms is greatly enhanced.

Sexual intercourse late in pregnancy has been implicated in the increased incidence and severity of amniotic infections in recent years. Some researchers suggest that sexual activity close to term may cause as much as a fourfold increase in fetal and maternal mortality.

Poor maternal nutrition also appears to be an important factor in chorioamnionitis. Malnourished pregnant women are at greater risk for contracting infection because their immune systems are less efficient. Other factors that predispose the laboring woman to chorioamnionitis include repeated vaginal examinations, internal fetal monitoring, presence of vaginitis or cervicitis, previous cervical cerclage, poverty, and substance abuse.

Diagnosis

Chorioamnionitis becomes clinically evident in 0.5% to 1% of pregnancies, although some researchers report incidences as high as 20% in women with PROM (Gibbs & Duff, 1991). Women developing chorioamnionitis usually have early symptoms that are nonspecific, including tachypnea, tachycardia (elevation of the pulse to more than 100 bpm), and temperature elevations of 38°C (100.4°F) or above. The FHR is a sensitive indicator of chorioamnionitis, and fetal tachycardia may precede all other signs of infection. Maternal symptoms worsen rapidly. Many women experience severe shaking chills, generalized malaise, and increasing uterine tenderness. The amniotic fluid may appear cloudy or purulent and maladorous. As organisms invade the uterine myometrium, uterine irritability and dysfunctional labor are common. Hypotonic contractions often occur, resulting in prolonged labor.

Diagnosis of chorioamnionitis often is made solely on the basis of the number and severity of maternal symptoms and the presence of fetal tachycardia. A rising white blood cell count also suggests infection. If membranes are intact, amniocentesis may be performed to provide a specimen of amniotic fluid. A variety of diagnostic tests of amniotic fluid have been developed to assist the physician or midwife. Culture and Gram stain of amniotic fluid may identify specific organisms. The presence of leukocyte esterase enzymes not normally found in amniotic fluid strongly suggests infection (Gibbs & Duff, 1991). A falling amniotic fluid glucose level is another indicator that may help confirm the diagnosis of chorioamnionitis. Glucose is consumed by organisms and white blood cells found in the amniotic fluid with infection. C-reactive protein, a nonspecific marker of the inflammatory process, has been proposed recently as a diagnostic indicator of infection (Williams et al., 1991). Further research is required before its usefulness is determined.

Definitive diagnosis of chorioamnionitis may be retrospective after delivery based on the following:

- Microscopic examination of the placenta confirming chorioamnionitis
- Isolation of organisms from cultures of maternal cervix, placenta, or blood
- Isolation of organisms from cultures of the umbilical cord, neonatal skin, blood, or spinal fluid
- Gram stain of fetal gastric contents for bacteria

Maternal, Fetal, and Neonatal Implications

The woman with chorioamnionitis often is very ill. She may have severe shaking chills, generalized muscle pain, high fever, and increased pain due to uterine tenderness and irritability. She is exposed to a greater number of invasive procedures, such as vaginal examinations and internal electronic fetal monitoring, which produce additional discomfort or pain. More frequent venipunctures also may be performed to monitor the white blood count. These physical sensations usually are made more unpleasant by the anxiety and fear generated by the development of complications. The woman generally requires analgesia or an epidural anesthesia to control pain sensations.

Chorioamnionitis influences the mode and outcome of delivery. Cesarean deliveries are up to three times as common when infection is present. This often is due to the adverse effect of infection on myometrial activity, resulting in hypotonic contractions and prolonged labor. The exact mechanism for hypotonic labor dystocia is not fully understood. The woman also is exposed to the increased risk associated with oxytocin augmentation when a hypotonic labor pattern occurs.

In addition the risk of a range of postpartum complications is increased, including septicemia, pelvic peritonitis, pelvic abscess formation, and septic thrombophlebitis. If the infection is unresponsive to antibiotic therapy, hysterectomy may be necessary to remove the source of the infection.

The neonate exposed to intrauterine infection is at high risk for sepsis (discussed further in Chapter 33). Infected amniotic fluid in the fetal lungs may result in pneumonia in the neonatal period. Introduction of infected fluid through the eustachian tube into the middle ear may cause otitis media and other septic complications.

Treatment

Some aspects of treatment of amnionitis remain controversial; however, there is agreement that treatment must include delivery of the infant, antibiotic therapy for the woman, and prophylactic antibiotic treatment of the neonate. Unresolved issues are related to the timing of antibiotic therapy. Several studies suggest a decreased incidence of neonatal sepsis when maternal therapy is initiated before birth (Gilstrap et al., 1988; Gibbs & Duff, 1991). However, treatment with antibiotics before birth makes identification of organisms in the neonate more difficult; maternal drugs cross the placenta and are present in the infant's bloodstream before blood cultures can be obtained at birth.

Research findings indicate that vaginal birth is preferred to cesarean delivery when chorioamnionitis occurs and labor progresses toward delivery. Operative delivery is criticized as unnecessarily risky for the woman, because preexisting infection increases the likelihood of difficulties in wound healing and other complications after surgery. Because labor dysfunction is common with chorioamnionitis, for reasons that are unclear, oxytocin frequently is required to augment uterine activity.

Implications for Nursing Care

Intrapartum nursing care of the woman with chorioamnionitis includes close observation of maternal and fetal status in relation to the stress of infection. Temperature, pulse, and respiration should be assessed every hour and the nature of amniotic fluid noted. Continuous EFM and uterine activity monitoring are indicated. Intake and output are monitored carefully because dehydration and ketosis are more common with infection. The nurse will initiate an IV line (if not already in place) to ensure adequate hydration and to permit administration of IV antibiotics. Oxytocin induction or augmentation may be ordered to promote uterine contractions and hasten delivery. Reduction of high body temperatures (38°C [100.4°F] or higher) is essential. The woman may require a cooling blanket or sponge baths, and acetominophen frequently is ordered when hyperthermia occurs.

When chorioamnionitis is diagnosed, the neonate must be regarded as at extremely high risk for infection. The nurse should make provisions for pediatric support staff to be present at delivery and if possible, to discuss with the woman proposed treatment of the infant after birth. On delivery cultures of the neonate's skin and gastric contents are taken, and prophylactic antibiotic therapy may be initiated. Signs of sepsis may be present in the neonate at birth or may develop later in the postnatal period. The neonate at risk for sepsis is monitored carefully in the first hours (see Chapter 33). Woman and neonate may require isolation care depending on the nature of the infection and hospital policy.

Imbalances of Amniotic Fluid Volume

Infection is not the only complication involving the intrauterine environment. Problems may arise if too much amniotic fluid accumulates, a condition known as hydramnios or polyhydramnios, or if too little fluid is present, a condition known as oligohydramnios. Amniotic fluid serves several functions, including the following:

- Protecting the fetus and umbilical cord from injury due to mechanical pressures
- Maintaining intrauterine temperature
- Allowing free movement and development of fetal limbs
- Facilitating fetal lung development
- Minimizing adherence of the amniotic membranes to the fetus

The volume of amniotic fluid increases as pregnancy progresses, peaking at approximately 980 mL at 34 weeks and then decreasing to approximately 830 mL at term and 550 mL by 41 to 42 weeks. Amniotic fluid is constantly being exchanged, at the rate of 3 to 4 L/h at term. The fetus plays an important role in maintaining amniotic fluid volume balance. Close to term, the fetus swallows between 400 and 500 mL amniotic fluid per day (approximately the amount of liquid consumed by the newborn infant) and micturates an equal volume, thus maintaining a steady volume. Interference with fetal intake or fetal output causes gross alterations in amniotic fluid volume.

Polyhydramnios

Polyhydramnios is the excessive accumulation of amniotic fluid in the amniotic sac. Amounts may reach levels of 2000 to 5000 mL or more. This accumulation may be gradual (chronic) or acute, occurring over a period of days to 2 weeks.

Etiologic and Predisposing Factors

Polyhydramnios is estimated to occur in 1.5% of all pregnancies. The etiology is unclear. An imbalance between fetal swallowing and micturition may be responsible in some cases. For instance polyhydramnios is much more common when the fetus has a tracheoesophageal fistula, a gastrointestinal anomaly that interferes with swallowing of amniotic fluid. However, support for this theory is not always conclusive, and in some cases a disruption in water transport in and out of the amniotic cavity may be responsible. The condition is associated with maternal diabetes, Rh-isommunization, anomalies of the gastrointestinal and central nervous systems, and multifetal pregnancy.

Diagnosis

The initial diagnosis of polyhydramnios may depend on the severity of the condition. As increasing amounts of fluid accumulate within the uterus, it becomes more difficult to palpate fetal position and to auscultate the FHR. The entire fetus also may be ballotable because of the large amount of fluid in which the body floats. The fundal height, when measured, may be larger than anticipated for gestational age. The woman may gain excessive weight or complain of an abnormally large abdomen. When palpated, the abdomen may feel tense, or a "fluid thrill" (a tremor detected on percussion of the abdomen) may be noted (Kulb, 1990b). The woman may experience more severe edema in the lower extremities and vulva due to the increasing size and weight of the uterus.

The development of ultrasonography has allowed the volume of amniotic fluid to be estimated. Polyhdramnios is defined as an amniotic fluid index in excess of 20 cm. The amniotic fluid index value is obtained by summing the largest vertical amniotic fluid pocket (in centimeters) found in each of the four uterine quadrants (Williams, 1991).

Maternal, Fetal, and Neonatal Implications

When polyhydramnios is severe, the woman experiences abdominal discomfort, dyspnea, edema, and varicosities of the vulva and lower extremities, as well as difficulty in mobility.

The uterine muscle becomes overstretched as amniotic fluid volume increases. This condition may contribute to preterm labor, intrapartum hypotonic labor, and increased risk of postpartum hemorrhage due to uterine atony. There is a small but significant risk of amniotic fluid embolus (see discussion of embolus later in chapter) at the time of birth. Diabetes mellitus also is associated with polyhydramnios, complicating the intrapartum course for this group of women (Phelan et al., 1990).

The woman is subjected to a variety of diagnostic tests to determine if fetal anomalies are present. Serial amniocentesis may be performed to remove excess amounts of amni-

NURSING PROCEDURE
Performing Needle Amniotomy

Purpose: To prevent a sudden, uncontrolled, spontaneous rupture of membranes during labor when polyhydramnious complicates the intrapartum period. To reduce the risk of umbilical cord prolapse with polyhydramnios or when the fetal head is not engaged, and artificial rupture of membranes (AROM) is indicated.

NURSING ACTION	***RATIONALE***
1. Verify that a maternal blood sample is held in the blood bank and has been typed and crossmatched.	To permit prompt administration of blood if cesarean birth is required or bleeding occurs.
2. Transport the woman to the delivery room and place on the delivery table.	To permit prompt cesarean delivery if prolapse of the cord occurs.
3. Tilt the delivery table to the left.	To prevent supine hypotension.
4. Place the woman in a slight Trendelenburg position.	To prevent a rapid gush of amniotic fluid from the sac when the membranes are punctured.
5. Assemble equipment required by the physician, including a 22-g spinal needle and sterile speculum.	Puncturing the membranes with a small needle permits a controlled release of fluid and reduces the risk of prolapsed cord.
6. Initiate an intravenous line with a large-gauge angiocath (16 to 18 g).	To permit rapid induction of labor if prolapse of the cord occurs.
7. Assemble staff and equipment required for an emergency cesarean delivery.	To facilitate prompt cesarean birth if prolapse of the cord occurs.
8. Attach external EFM and maintain continuous monitoring of FHR.	To identify occult prolapse of the umbilical cord and monitor fetal response to AROM.
9. Note the characteristics of the amniotic fluid as it drains from the vagina and document findings.	To identify the presence of meconium staining, blood, vernix, or a foul odor. To estimate the amount of fluid.
10. Continue to monitor maternal and fetal status, and return to the labor room if the condition of the woman and fetus remains stable.	To identify adverse responses to the needle amniotomy.

otic fluid before the onset of labor (Oi, 1991). Because the incidence of abnormal fetal presentation is increased and the woman may have an ineffective labor pattern, she may be at increased risk for cesarean delivery. With the increased risk of fetal anomalies associated with polyhydramnios comes an increased risk of fetal or neonatal death secondary to severe structural deformities. In the presence of polyhydramnios approximately 60% of surviving infants will be normal, and the remaining 40% will display some congenital abnormalities. The most commonly associated congenital problems include anencephaly, hydrocephaly, neural tube defects, and upper gastrointestinal abnormalities.

Another major risk to the fetus is acute hypoxia secondary to prolapse of the umbilical cord with rupture of the membranes. Prophylactic treatment to reduce this risk is described in the next section. An increased amniotic fluid volume also is associated with fetal macrosomia (secondary to maternal diabetes mellitus) and may result in trauma or asphyxia if shoulder dystocia occurs at the time of birth.

Treatment

Mild or moderate polyhydramnios may not cause significant distress to the woman, and no treatment may be needed. However, because of the increased risk of prolapsed umbilical cord with rupture of membranes during labor, the membranes may be "needled" to allow slow, controlled release of amniotic fluid before spontaneous rupture occurs. The procedure is performed in the delivery room in case sudden rupture of the membranes with resultant prolapse of the umbilical cord does occur (see the Nursing Procedure, Performing Needle Amniotomy). The membranes are punctured with a small needle to permit a slow release of fluid.

Implications for Nursing Care

Intrapartum nursing care for the woman with polyhydramnios focuses on providing comfort measures to relieve maternal respiratory distress. Ambulation may be contraindicated because of the risk of prolapsed umbilical cord with spontaneous rupture of the membranes. The majority of women must labor in a semi- or high-Fowler's position until rupture of membranes relieves pressure on the diaphragm and lower lungs. The nurse must always be alert for signs of cord prolapse when the membranes rupture. Continuous electronic monitoring of the FHR is indicated.

Because uterine distention often results in labor dystocia, the nurse closely monitors uterine activity and progress in cervical dilatation. An oxytocin infusion may be initiated to augment uterine contractions. The nurse continues to give information as labor progresses and offers anticipatory guidance regarding special procedures, such as needle amniotomy. If prenatal diagnosis of fetal anomalies has been made, the nurse must provide sensitive emotional support for the woman and her partner. Uterine tonics (oxytocin, methergine, and Prostin 15 M) are readied at the time of birth, because uterine atony and postpartum hemorrhage occur more frequently when polydramnios complicates labor.

Oligohydramnios

Oligohydramnios is a condition in which the volume of amniotic fluid is abnormally small.

Etiologic and Predisposing Factors

The precise causes of oligohydramnios are unknown. It can occur in postterm pregnancies and appears to be related to normal aging of the placenta (Trimmer et al., 1990). Oligohydramnios also is noted when there is chronic leakage of amniotic fluid and before term and with PROM after 38 weeks gestation. Conditions associated with or predisposing to oligohydramnios include the following:

- Placental insufficiency
- Intrauterine growth retardation (IUGR)
- Premature separation of the placenta
- PROM
- Twin-to-twin transfusion syndrome
- Fetal anomalies, especially renal abnormalities

Diagnosis

Oligohydramnios may be suspected when fundal height does not keep pace with the advancing pregnancy; the uterine fundus usually is small for gestational age, and the fetal outline may be easily felt through the abdominal wall. It can be strongly suspected when any of the conditions described in the previous section occur.

With advances in technology, the diagnosis of oligohydramnios is confirmed by obstetric ultrasonography. Oligohydramnios is defined as an amniotic fluid volume of 5 cm or less. This value is obtained by summing the largest vertical pocket of amniotic fluid found in the four uterine quadrants measured in centimeters. If the largest pocket of amniotic fluid is less than 1 cm by 1 cm by sonographic measurement, a diagnosis of oligohydramnios also is made.

Maternal, Fetal, and Neonatal Implications

There are no direct adverse effects of oligohydramnios on maternal well-being. In cases of oligohydramnios labor may be induced before term. Risks to the woman are related to invasive procedures. These procedures include internal EFM, oxytocin induction, and the initiation of amnioinfusion, a procedure used to relieve oligohydramnios. The woman also is exposed to the risks related to cesarean delivery. The incidence of cesarean delivery is increased with oligohydramnios because the fetus is predisposed to hypoxia due to umbilical cord compression, or decreased uteroplacental perfusion (Robson et al., 1992).

When little amniotic fluid is present, the intrauterine space decreases because the uterine walls are not distended by fluid. The fetus may assume a flexed and cramped attitude. When PROM and oligohydramnios occur before 38 weeks gestation, the fetus can suffer from skeletal deformities and pulmonary hypoplasia. Chronic cord compression may result in IUGR, fetal hypoxia, and meconium aspiration syndrome (Robson et al., 1992). At birth, surviving infants appear "starved" due to depletion of adipose tissue and are small for gestational age.

With advances in diagnostic technology, confirmation of oligohydramnios and IUGR is possible. It permits neonates to be delivered before term to prevent the negative consequences of intrauterine hypoxia or sudden death secondary to cord compression. However, the infant suffers from complications related to prematurity when it is delivered before term.

Renal abnormalities are implicated when oligohydramnios is present, because fetal urination in utero plays an important role in amniotic fluid balance. Many of these abnormalities are incompatible with life. Potter syndrome, a constellation of fetal abnormalities, including renal agenesis and pulmonary hypoplasia, also may be found in the presence of oligohydramnios.

Treatment

An amniotic fluid volume of 5 cm or less indicates the need for immediate delivery, regardless of gestational age. Some health care providers have attempted an IV bolus of fluid or have given the woman 2 L of water to improve the amniotic fluid volume (Kilpatrick et al., 1991), but results are variable. It is unclear how much fluid must be given to the woman to increase the amniotic fluid volume or how long the effect persists.

Timely delivery in the case of oligohydramnios is necessary to prevent sudden fetal death secondary to worsening chronic hypoxia or umbilical cord compression. The woman will be admitted to the labor and delivery unit and prepared for induction of labor.

Saline amnioinfusion may be initiated in an attempt to relieve umbilical cord compression if severe variable decelerations occur. A sterile solution of 0.9 normal saline is infused into the uterine cavity through a catheter passed into the vagina and through the cervical canal. Fluid is introduced at a continuous rate through an IV infusion pump. The goal is to relieve umbilical cord compression by increasing the amount of fluid in the uterus.

Amnioinfusion also has been used successfully to reduce the incidence of meconium aspiration syndrome, a complication frequently associated with oligohydramnios. Normal saline is infused into the uterus to dilute and flush the meconium out of the uterine cavity. Secondarily, further passage of meconium by the fetus may be prevented if it relieves umbilical cord compression, and concomitant fetal hypoxia. Studies indicate that dilution of meconium reduces the risk of aspiration, improves arterial umbilical cord pH, and reduces the need for mechanical ventilation of the infant after birth (Sadovsky et al., 1989).

Contraindications to amnioinfusion include the following:

- Suspected or diagnosed placental abruption
- Acute fetal distress
- Head engaged and tightly applied to cervix
- Inability to measure intrauterine pressures

Implications for Nursing Care

Intrapartum care of the woman with oligohydramnios requires intensive monitoring of fetal status. Continuous EFM is required to identify signs of acute hypoxic injury (late decelerations or severe variable decelerations). If amnioinfusion is ordered, the nurse is responsible for preparing the woman and initiating the procedure. Amnioinfusion has been implicated in the development of iatrogenic complications during the intrapartum period. Isolated cases of increased uterine activity and hypertonus, iatrogenic polyhydramnios, fetal distress, and even burns secondary to administration of hot saline have been reported with amnioinfusion. The nurse is responsible for safe administration of the saline infusion, monitoring maternal and fetal status during the procedure, and reporting problems to the birth attendant in a timely manner (see the Nursing Procedure, Assisting When Amnioinfusion Is Implemented).

The nurse prepares in advance for the possibility of emergency cesarean birth by doing the following:

- Reinforcing information provided by the physician or midwife
- Providing anticipatory guidance regarding planned or anticipated procedures
- Ensuring IV access for fluid boluses or emegency drugs
- Completing a preoperative checklist before initiation of induction or signs of distress occur
- Limiting intake to clear fluids, or maintaining NPO status
- Alerting surgical personnel and nursery staff to the possibility of operative birth

Fetal well-being is jeopardized when problems occur due to imbalances in amniotic fluid volume or in the integrity of fetal membranes. In some cases complications involving amniotic fluid may be due to preexisting congenital anomalies, increasing fetal risk. The maternity nurse plays a central role in the identification of problems, such as polyhydramnios, oligohydramnios, and chorioamnionitis. When infection of the fetal membranes occurs, maternal well-being also is threatened. The nurse must be skilled in the support of maternal and fetal physiologic functioning to ameliorate the negative affects of these complications. The woman often is exposed to invasive procedures to correct amniotic fluid imbalance. She will require supportive nursing care to cope with the physical and psychological impact of these intrapartum complications.

Complications Involving the Umbilical Cord

Abnormalities in the umbilical cord or cord prolapse compromise fetal oxygenation and may require emergency surgical delivery, which increases maternal risks. It is essential to provide sensitive emotional support to the woman and her partner, particularly if serious fetal anomalies have already been diagnosed.

Umbilical Cord Prolapse

Prolapse of the umbilical cord is a serious intrapartum complication, occurring in approximately 1 of 200 pregnancies. When a loop of umbilical cord is positioned alongside or in front of the presenting part, it may become compressed between the fetus and the woman's cervix or pelvis. If the fetal presenting part does not completely occlude the pelvic inlet, this loop may be carried down into the vagina by escaping amniotic fluid when membranes rupture. As the presenting part settles down into the pelvis, this prolapsed loop will be compressed, and fetoplacental perfusion will be compromised or cut off entirely.

Etiologic and Predisposing Factors

Many obstetric variables can cause cord prolapse. Any condition in which the fetal presenting part does not engage in the maternal pelvis may permit prolapse of the cord. The sudden release of pressure when the membranes rupture is a contributing factor. As fluid gushes out of the amniotic sac, it may carry the umbilical cord out of the birth canal in front of the presenting part. Common predisposing factors include the following:

- Abnormal fetal position: breech, shoulder, face, or brow
- Multifetal gestation
- Prematurity
- Polyhydramnios
- Fetopelvic disproportion
- Abnormally long umbilical cord
- Rupture of membranes before engagement of the presenting part

Cord prolapse also may be a result of obstetric intervention, such as amniotomy performed in the presence of a malposition or high presenting part, or obstetric maneuvers, such as manual rotation or flexion of the fetal head, which may disengage the presenting part and allow the cord to slip through and prolapse.

Diagnosis

The diagnosis of cord prolapse generally is made by vaginal examination. Sudden deceleration in the FHR, particularly after rupture of the membranes, often signifies prolapse of the cord. Three types of umbilical cord prolapse have been identified. The classification depends on the position of the cord in relation to the presenting part, as shown in Figure 26-4.

NURSING PROCEDURE

Assisting When Amnioinfusion Is Implemented

Purpose: Amnioinfusion may be ordered to achieve a variety of therapeutic goals, including the following:
- *To treat intrapartum variable decelerations due to cord compression*
- *To dilute and lavage meconium from the uterus*
- *To administer antibiotics when chorioamnionitis is diagnosed*

NURSING ACTION	RATIONALE
1. Assemble an intravenous infusion of 1000 mL of 0.9 normal saline.	To prevent fluid shifts in tissues caused by the infusion of hypotonic or hypertonic solutions, a physiologic saline solution is used.
2. If the solution is to be heated, a blood warming unit should be used and the solution is warmed to 37°C (98.6°F).	To prevent burns, saline should *never* be heated in a microwave oven or a blanket warmer because the temperature of the solution cannot be measured.
3. Warm fluid is indicated in preterm labor.	To prevent fetal hypothermia.
4. Attach infusion tubing to an infusion pump.	To precisely control the amount of fluid infused into the uterus.
5. If one intrauterine pressure catheter is to be inserted into the uterus, attach a stopcock to the site where the infusion tubing and the intrauterine catheter meet.	To permit temperature shut-off of the amnioinfusion so that intrauterine pressures can be measured periodically.

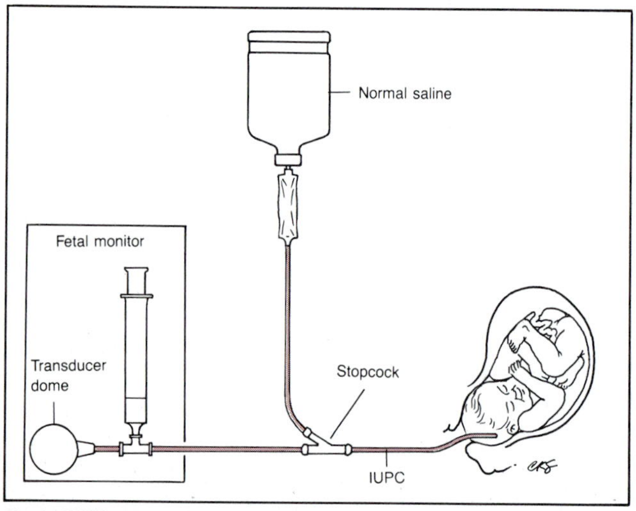

Single IUPC set-up. A stopcock must be used at the junction of the infusion tubing and IUPC so that intrauterine pressures can be measured intermittently. The infusion is turned off during measurement.

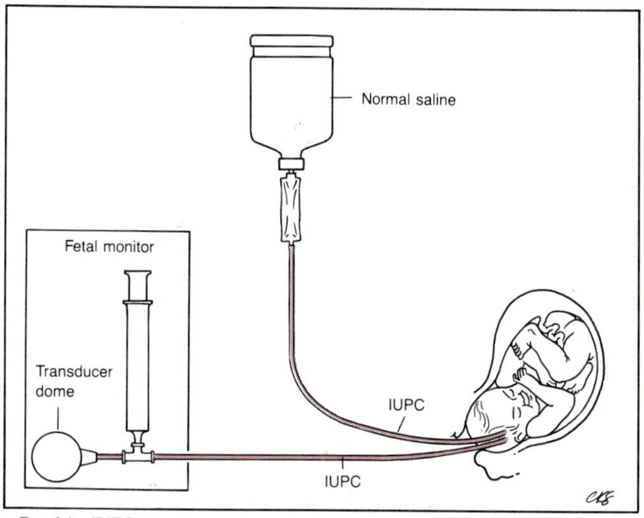

Double IUPC set-up when two IUPCs are used. The amnioinfusion does not have to be stopped while measurements are taken of intrauterine pressure.

NURSING ACTION	RATIONALE
6. Assist with the insertion of a second IUPC if the physician or midwife desire continuous measurement of intrauterine pressure.	To permit continuous measurement of intrauterine pressure during the amnioinfusion, a second intrauterine pressure catheter must be inserted into the uterus.
7. Administer a loading volume of 10 mL/min (600 mL/h) for 1 hour.	To rapidly increase the intrauterine fluid volume and reduce cord compression or lavage meconium from the uterus.
8. Initiate an infusion rate of 60 to 120 mL/h (1–2 mL/h) after infusion of the initial loading volume.	
9. Measure intrauterine pressures at least every 15 to 30 minutes.	To prevent fetal distress, because an elevated resting tone decreases placental perfusion, gas exchange, and fetal hypoxia.
10. Measure the amount of fluid leaking from the vagina by weighing bed linens or bed protectors.	To prevent iatrogenic polyhydramnios.

(*Continued*)

NURSING PROCEDURE

Assisting When Amnioinfusion Is Implemented (Continued)

NURSING ACTION	***RATIONALE***
11. Assist with ultrasonography.	Ultrasonography may be used to measure fluid pockets.
12. Maintain continuous EFM.	To monitor fetal responses to amnioinfusion.
13. Apply external tocodynamometer if only one IUPC is inserted.	To permit continuous monitoring of the frequency and duration of contractions.
14. If variable decelerations or persist after infusion of loading volume, notify the physician or midwife.	To permit physician or midwife to reevaluate the benefit of the procedure.
15. Change linen frequently.	To promote the woman's comfort.

Posner, M., Ballagh, S., & Paul, R. (1990). The effect of amnioinfusion on uterine pressure and activity: A preliminary report. American Journal of Obstetrics and Gynecology, 163*(3), 813.*

Haubrich, K. (1990). Amnioinfusion: A technique for the relief of variable decelerations. Journal of Obstetric, Gynecologic, and Neonatal Nursing, 19*(4), 299.*

- *Occult prolapse:* the cord lies alongside the presenting part; membranes are either intact or ruptured, but the cord cannot be palpated on vaginal examination.
- *Forelying prolapse:* the cord precedes the presenting part and is contained within intact membranes; the cord may be palpable through the membranes.
- *Complete prolapse:* membranes are ruptured, and the cord drops through the cervix into the vagina; the cord can be palpated on vaginal examination and may be visible at the introitus.

With advances in ultrasonography prenatal recognition of cord presentation is possible (Manning, 1989). When loops of umbilical cord are visualized between the fetal presenting part and the cervix, cord prolapse may be prevented (see treatment section).

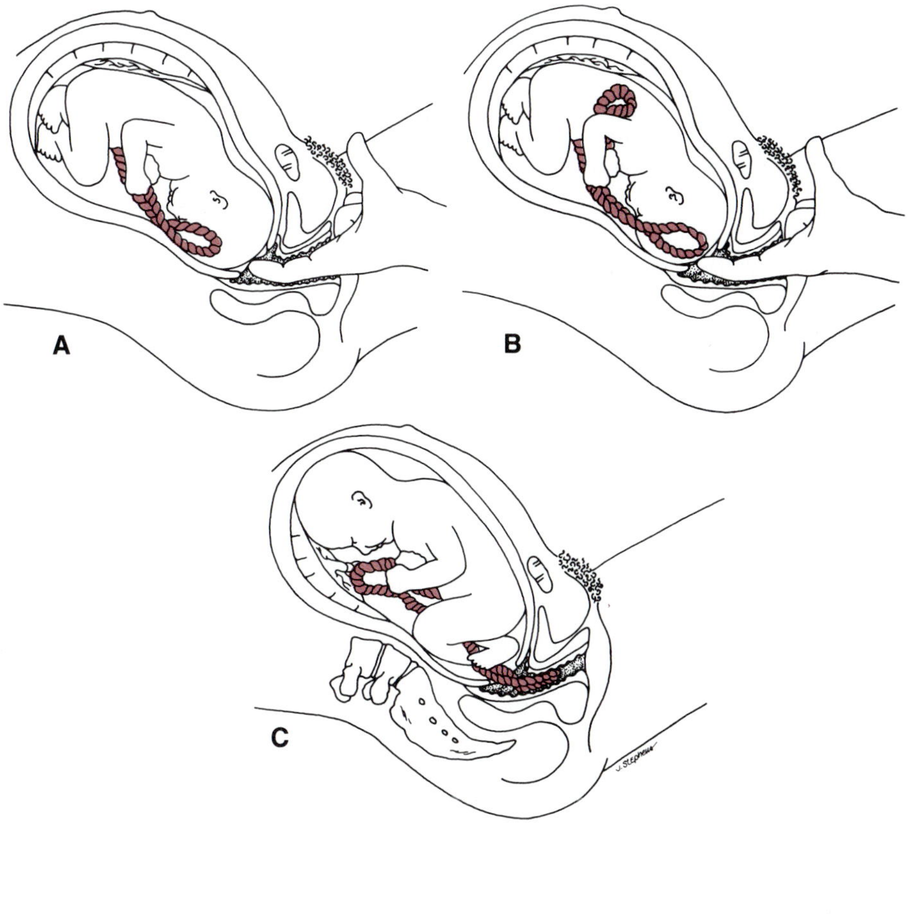

Figure 26-4.
Umbilical cord prolapse. *A:* Occult prolapse and compression of cord by fetal head. *B:* Forelying cord palpable in cervical os. *C:* Complete cord prolapse with breech presentation (Childbirth Graphics).

Maternal, Fetal, and Neonatal Implications

Cord prolapse in the intrapartum period produces an emergency situation in which swift action is needed to save the fetus. Immediate delivery will be attempted, either by cesarean or forceps application. The woman will be at increased risk for complications related to these emergency interventions, including trauma to the birth canal with rapid forceps extraction, uterine atony resulting from anesthesia, risk of excessive blood loss from operative delivery, and infection.

Perinatal morbidity and mortality are increased when cord prolapse occurs. The most critical factor in fetal survival is the interval between the actual prolapse and delivery. When delivery is accomplished within 15 to 30 minutes, fetal survival is approximately 70% to 75%; however, if delivery is delayed more than 1 hour, fetal loss may exceed 50%. Infants who survive may develop later complications related to prematurity, birth trauma, meconium aspiration, and hypoxia; the prognosis is especially guarded for premature infants when meconium staining is noted or when the cord pulse is weak.

Treatment

When prolapsed cord is diagnosed, rapid action is needed to preserve fetal well-being. The goals of obstetric management are the following:

- Alleviate as much pressure as possible on the umbilical cord.
- Deliver the infant as soon as possible.

Vaginal delivery with forceps application may be considered if the cervix is fully dilated, the presenting part is engaged and no malpresentation exists, and pelvic size is normal. If these criteria are not met, however, cesarean delivery is indicated to avoid the further risks of traumatic vaginal delivery. Clinical trials have recently been conducted to evaluate the effectiveness of manually reducing the umbilical cord (funic reduction) in selected situations. Barrett (1991) manually replaced the prolapsed umbilical cord in women at least 4 cm dilated while preparations were made for emergency cesarean birth. Continuous EFM was used, and gentle suprapubic pressure was applied to assist in elevation of the head. Seven of eight women went on to deliver vaginally. Infants had 5-minute Apgar scores of 7 or greater.

While preparations for delivery are being made, pressure on the prolapsed cord must be relieved. The fetal presenting part is elevated from the cord with direct manual pressure. A newer technique involves inserting a Foley catheter into the bladder and rapidly infusing 1000 mL of sterile saline (Koonings, Paul, & Campbell, 1990). This technique has in some cases elevated the fetal head and partially relieved cord compression. The woman may be placed in the Trendelenburg, knee-chest, or Sims' position to prevent further prolapse and to relieve pressure of the presenting part. Tocolytics also may be administered to reduced uterine activity.

Implications for Nursing Care

The nurse must identify women who may be at increased risk for cord prolapse and monitor fetal status carefully. If the birth attendant intends to rupture membranes before the head is engaged, the nurse should initiate a discussion about the plan and review the potential consequences of the intervention (see the Legal/Ethical Considerations display). When membranes rupture, the nurse should immediately auscultate or observe the FHR for 1 full minute after the rupture and also during the next uterine contraction to identify signs of acute fetal distress associated with cord compression. In addition vaginal examination should be performed to determine whether the presenting part is engaged and if the cord has prolapsed.

If the nurse identifies possible or actual cord prolapse, she must initiate the following emergency measures (see the Nursing Procedure about prolapsed umbilical cord in Chapter 20). Firm manual pressure should be applied to the presenting part to elevate it and relieve pressure from the cord. The nurse must take care not to further compress the cord. However, cord pulsations should be assessed constantly, because the pulse provides direct evidence of patency and fetal status. Under no circumstances should the hand be removed or the upward pressure released until delivery can be accomplished. Staff must be mobilized for the immediate birth of the infant, in most cases by cesarean delivery.

Oxygen and IV fluids will be administered to the woman to increase placental perfusion and reduce fetal hypoxia. Tocolytics may be administered to reduce uterine activity, which also improves placental perfusion and may improve fetal oxygenation. The nurse also should be prepared to insert a Foley catheter for possible saline infusion into the bladder. As the bladder is filled with saline, it may elevate the fetal presenting part, reducing pressure on the umbilical cord. If this effort fails to relieve cord compression, the bladder catheter will be needed for urine drainage during the cesarean delivery.

The nurse also is responsible for providing emotional support and reassurance to the woman and her partner. This situation is extremely frightening, and every effort should be made to provide information and assistance before, during, and after the delivery. The support person often is unable to attend the birth and remains behind in the woman's room. If possible, another staff person should be assigned to provide information as the infant is delivered.

Congenital Absence of the Umbilical Artery

Although umbilical cord prolapse is the most worrisome complication involving the cord, increased intrapartum risk to the fetus or neonate can result from structural abnormalities of the cord and unusual cord length. Normally, the umbilical cord contains two umbilical arteries and one vein. However, single umbilical arteries are observed in 0.08% to 1.9% of pregnancies.

Etiologic and Predisposing Factors

The etiology of this condition is unknown. The incidence is higher among white Americans than among African Americans and more common among infants of diabetic women. This condition also is associated with a higher

Legal/Ethical Considerations

When the Birth Attendant Artificially Ruptures Membranes

Current research confirms that some women may experience unnecessary emergency cesarean birth for prolapsed umbilical cord, because of inadvised artifical rupture of membranes by the birth attendant. This situation may result in the initiation of a lawsuit by the parents, particularly if adverse neonatal outcomes occur. Recently, nurses also have been implicated in these lawsuits, and allegations of negligence have been made when the nurse participates in artificial rupture of membranes, resulting in cord prolapse.

When the birth attendant indicates intention to artificially rupture the membranes, the nurse must independently assess the advisability of the procedure. The following points should be carefully considered before the nurse hands the birth attendant an amnihook and assists with the procedure:

- *Is the fetal head engaged?* The risk of prolapsed cord is greatly increased with artificial rupture of membranes (AROM) if the head is not engaged and the cervix is dilated.
- *If cord prolapse occurs, is a surgical suite available for immediate cesarean birth?* In several lawsuits all delivery rooms and surgical suites were occupied when the physician ruptured the membranes and cord prolapse occurred.
- *Has the woman been informed of the potential benefits and risks of AROM?* In several lawsuits women state that they had no idea that cord prolapse was a risk, or they would not have agreed to the procedure.
- *Is there an obstetric indication for AROM?* If there is an obstetric indication for AROM, the nurse can quickly discuss current unit conditions with the birth attendant that would influence the staff's ability to handle an emergency situation, such as cord prolapse.

Barrett, J. (1991). Funic reduction for the management of umbilical cord prolapse. American Journal of Obstetrics and Gynecology, 165*(3), 654.*

Mahlmeister, L. (1992). Professional accountability and legal liability for labor and delivery nurses. American Health Care Institute Workshop on Documentation, *January.*

incidence of other congenital anomalies. Of neonates with a single umbilical artery, 15% to 20% will have cardiovascular anomalies.

Diagnosis

Diagnosis may be made with ultrasonography in the prenatal period but often goes undetected until the time of delivery. When the umbilical cord is inspected, the absence of one artery will be noted.

Maternal, Fetal, and Neonatal Implications

There are no immediate maternal implications of this condition. The presence of a single umbilical artery may predispose the fetus or neonate to low birth weight. Anomalies may appear in any body system and are evident in as many as 25% to 50% of infants with single umbilical arteries. Other common congenital problems include renal anomalies, tracheoesophageal fistulas, and central nervous system lesions. The presence of a single umbilical artery also is associated with certain cytogenetic abnormalities, including infants with trisomy 13 and 18 (Saller et al., 1990).

Treatment

Treatment of the condition is not possible. If the diagnosis was made prenatally with the use of ultrasonography, appropriate pediatric support can be present at delivery to assess and care for the infant. Neonates with a single umbilical artery require careful screening for congenital anomalies and possible low birth weight.

Implications for Nursing Care

Nursing responsibilities include accurately identifying congenital absence of the umbilical artery on inspection of the umbilical cord at delivery. In collaboration with the physician the nurse may explain the problem to the parents, and provide them with information and support as further screening for congenital anomalies is undertaken. An interesting finding of recent research indicates that the absence of the normal helix or twist in the umbilical cord may be associated with the presence of only one umbilical artery (Lacro, Jones, & Benirschke, 1987).

Velamentous Insertion and Vasa Previa

The normal umbilical cord contains three blood vessels—two umbilical arteries and one umbilical vein—and is inserted into the central area of the fetal surface of the placenta.

Velamentous insertion is characterized by insertion of the umbilical cord on the fetal membranes. The three umbilical vessels traverse the membranes for some distance, protected only by the amnion, before entering the placental surface as shown in Figure 26-5. When velamentous insertion occurs in the portion of the fetal membranes presenting over the cervical os in front of the fetal presenting part, it is known as vasa previa.

Etiologic and Predisposing Factors

Normally, the embryonic body stalk, which will become the umbilical cord, aligns with the center of the trophoblastic cell mass of the developing placenta. Spontaneous rotation of the body stalk gives rise to eccentric insertions of the cord. The degree of rotation will influence how far the umbilical cord will be from the center of the placenta (eccentric, marginal, or true velamentous insertion) (Blackburn & Loper, 1992). These conditions are quite rare, occurring in less than 1% of all pregnancies. Velamentous insertion is more common with multifetal gestation and is associated with increased incidence of fetal anomalies.

Diagnosis

These conditions usually are not diagnosed before labor. It is possible to detect them by ultrasonography. Velamentous insertion usually is asymptomatic and may not be diagnosed until the placenta is examined after delivery. However, blood-stained amniotic fluid or small amounts of vaginal bleeding may suggest that fetal hemorrhage has occurred. Vasa previa may be diagnosed by vaginal examination. With assessment of the cervical os, the examiner may feel a vessel pulsating synchronously with the FHR in the membranes in front of the presenting part.

When amniotomy is accompanied by an excessive show of blood, the physician or nurse midwife may collect a small amount to be assessed for the presence of fetal cells using the Apt test. The purpose of this test is to differentiate between maternal and fetal blood. Blood is collected in a test tube to which water and potassium hydroxide are added; maternal hemoglobin will denature and turn brown but fetal hemoglobin will remain pink. Blood identified as fetal in origin is evidence of fetal hemorrhage, and emergency cesarean delivery is necessary.

Maternal, Fetal, and Neonatal Implications

As long as the unprotected vessels do not cross the site of amniotic sac rupture, velamentous insertion presents no hazards for the fetus, and most deliveries are without incident. When the condition is discovered, the neonate should be screened carefully for the presence of congenital anomalies. Vasa previa places the fetus at considerable risk; if tears in fetal vessels occur, risk of fetal demise due to exsanguination is 60% to 70%.

Treatment

Velamentous insertion requires no treatment unless evidence of fetal hemorrhage exists; emergency cesarean delivery is then indicated. Vasa previa presents an increased risk of fetal hemorrhage as labor progresses; the woman is kept on bed rest, and extremely close external monitoring of fetal heart tones is required. Cesarean delivery may be indicated if the physician believes the risk of hemorrhage is great. Any evidence of fetal bleeding or significant changes in FHR require emergency cesarean delivery.

Implications for Nursing Care

The nurse must recognize intrapartum signs of placental abnormality, such as pulsating vessels at the cervical os and blood-stained amniotic fluid, and alert the birth attendant at

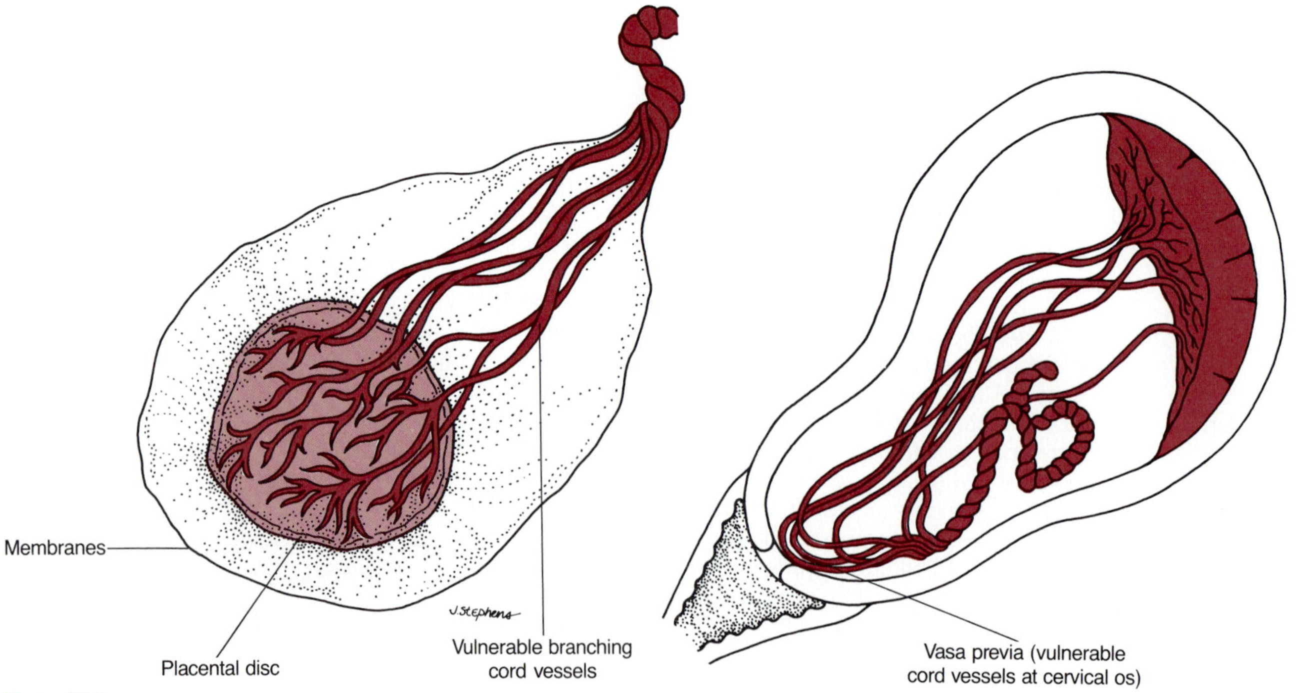

Figure 26-5.
Velamentous cord insertion and vasa previa (Childbirth Graphics).

once. Close monitoring of fetal heart tones is essential; any changes in FHR or incidents of vaginal bleeding must be evaluated immediately to rule out fetal hemorrhage. Stimulation or augmentation of labor is contraindicated for these women. The woman will be maintained on bed rest and will require an IV line to facilitate emergency obstetric management if needed. In collaboration with the birth attendant, the nurse should explain the situation to the woman and her partner and prepare them for the possibility of a cesarean delivery. Preparations for an emergency delivery—staff, including neonatal intensive care unit staff; supplies; and equipment—should be made in case one is needed.

Abnormal Umbilical Cord Length

The average length of the umbilical cord at term is 54 to 61 cm. In general larger infants have longer cords. However, there is considerable variation in individual cord lengths at term and at different points in gestation.

Etiologic and Predisposing Factors

It is believed that the length and spiral configuration of the cord is due to fetal movement (Benirschke, 1989). Fetal movement is greatest in the second and early third trimesters and indicates fetal well-being. Abnormally short cords may be related to genetic or neurologic abnormalities in the fetus that result in decreased movement and possibly poor intrauterine growth.

Diagnosis

Cord length is determined at delivery. An abnormally short cord is defined as less than 32 cm at term, approximately the minimum length necessary to permit a normal vertex delivery. Short cords, using this standard, may be observed in 1% of all deliveries. A cord in excess of 100 cm is considered abnormally long. Such long cords are found in 0.5% of all births.

Maternal, Fetal, and Neonatal Implications

Abnormal umbilical cord length may result in abruptio placentae due to excessive traction on a short cord as the fetus descends. This poses a serious health risk to the woman and fetus due to hemorrhage and shock. Although many neonates with short umbilical cords are delivered without ill effect, severe traction on the cord also may result in compromised blood flow and asphyxia at delivery. Although a rare complication, a short umbilical cord also may tear or completely rupture during second-stage labor, presenting the danger of fetal hemorrhage and hypoxia.

An abnormally long cord is susceptible to knotting or entanglement in utero, especially around the fetal neck, resulting in cord compression. When chronic mechanical stress (through knots or compression) impedes circulation in the cord, the fetus may be chronically denied adequate perfusion of oxygen, metabolites, and nutrients. This results in IUGR, a condition placing the neonate at risk for a variety of problems. Acute mechanical stress, such as compression from cord prolapse, a tight nuchal cord, or rupture during labor or birth, presents the danger of rapidly developing fetal hypoxia and death if not discovered promptly and treated. The risk of cord prolapse after rupture of the membranes is increased with an abnormally long umbilical cord.

Treatment

Unfortunately, no treatment exists to prevent the development of an excessively short or long umbilical cord. When signs of cord compression develop during labor, efforts are directed at improving the pattern, regardless of the cause. If position changes or amnioinfusion do not alleviate abnormal FHR patterns, the fetus is delivered by cesarean surgery.

Implications for Nursing Care

Nursing responsibilities in the intrapartum period center on identifying variable decelerations in FHR that are associated with cord compression and assisting the birth attendant as necessary in the event of a short or nuchal cord at time of delivery. In the event of cord problems the nurse must be prepared to initiate procedures to support the neonate who has experienced acute or chronic hypoxia (see Chapters 32 and 33).

Integrity of the fetal umbilical cord is essential for the transport of nutrition and the exchange of wastes and gases during the prenatal period. When complications threaten the integrity or function of the umbilical cord, the fetus is at risk for life-threatening problems. The woman often is at increased risk secondary to the invasive procedure used to correct the problem or to cesarean delivery. The nurse is responsible for assessing fetal status during labor and monitoring for evidence of cord compression or trauma. Regardless of the setting, the maternity nurse must initiate corrective measures to relieve umbilical cord compression until medical help arrives. After birth the nurse also is responsible for examining the umbilical cord and identifying abnormalities.

Complications Involving the Fetus

Congenital anomalies and fetal malpresentations or malpositions can result in fetal distress and deviations in the normal course of labor and birth for the woman. A variety of fetal problems may have particular significance in the intrapartum period, increasing maternal or fetal risk. A major concern is fetal distress, already discussed in Chapter 22. Other problems include fetal anomalies that influence the course of labor and birth; multifetal gestation, which poses additional risks to fetal well-being in the intrapartum period; and intrauterine fetal demise (IUFD), which affects not only the physiologic, but also the psychological process of labor and birth.

Multifetal Gestation

Prenatal care of women with multifetal gestation is discussed fully in Chapter 16. This section focuses on the intrapartum assessment of maternal and fetal well-being and management of the labor and birth process when multifetal gestation complicates the pregnancy.

Etiologic and Predisposing Factors

The etiology of spontaneous monozygotic twinning is unclear. The widespread use of ovulation-inducing drugs in the management of infertility has increased the number of multifetal pregnancies. The incidence among women given gonadotropins is estimated to be 20%. Of this group, 75% are twin gestations, and 25% are triplet or higher-number gestations. Among women treated with clomiphene, the incidence of multiple gestation is approximately 10%. These factors are discussed in detail in Chapter 16.

Diagnosis

Multifetal pregnancy often is suspected when the uterine size or fundal height is greater than dates. As the uses for obstetric ultrasonography grow, more women experience at least one sonogram during pregnancy. Multifetal gestation often is diagnosed during the prenatal period, either inadvertently during a sonographic examination or because the physician or midwife suspects a multifetal pregnancy and has ordered ultrasonography to confirm the diagnosis.

Maternal, Fetal, and Neonatal Implications

Although the woman with a multifetal pregnancy usually experiences a higher risk of morbidity than one with a singleton pregnancy, mortality is only slightly higher. Problems associated with multifetal gestation increase with three or more fetuses. Intrapartum complications frequently encountered when there is more than one fetus are listed in the accompanying display.

Labor frequently is complicated by a hypotonic uterine contraction pattern, because the myometrium is stretched due to uterine distention. The woman is exposed to the additional risks associated with induction or augmentation of labor or cesarean delivery. The incidence of postpartum hemorrhage is increased fivefold because of distention of the uterine muscle and subsequent atony. Infectious complications also are five times greater among women with multifetal pregnancy when compared with women with singleton deliveries. Fetal complications in the intrapartum period are numerous and are responsible for most perinatal deaths in multiple gestation. Complications associated with preterm delivery, especially when the fetuses weigh less than 2000 g (4 lb 6 oz), account for most of these losses. PROM with preterm labor resulting in delivery is a significant problem with multiple gestation; this occurs in 25% of twin pregnancies, 50% of triplet pregnancies, and 75% of quadruplet pregnancies (Benson, 1987).

The complexities of descent and delivery when more than one fetus is present also account for increased fetal risk. Fetuses may be in abnormal positions that disrupt circulation of one fetus, requiring immediate cesarean delivery. Cord prolapse is more common than with singleton pregnancies. Further, separation of the placenta sometimes occurs before delivery of the second twin, which may cause fetal distress, perinatal asphyxia, or death.

> ## *Intrapartum Complications Associated With Multifetal Pregnancy*
>
> - Preterm labor and birth
> - Pregnancy-induced hypertension
> - Placental accidents
>   - Abruptio placentae
>   - Placenta previa
> - Umbilical cord problems
>   - Entwinement
>   - Prolapse
>   - Vasa previa
> - Imbalances in amniotic fluid balance
>   - Polyhydramnios or oligohydramnios in twin-to-twin transfusion syndrome
> - Fetal distress due to intrauterine growth retardation

Treatment

Many intrapartum problems can be prevented, and fetal outcomes may be substantially improved with multifetal gestation when care is planned early. During the early intrapartum period the physician or midwife should discuss factors influencing the method of delivery, either vaginal or cesarean. To make decisions about the mode of birth, gestational age and fetal positions must be confirmed.

Factors Affecting Mode of Delivery. Vaginal delivery is not deemed appropriate when there are three or more fetuses. This is because there is an increased risk of cord entanglement or prolapse, malpresentations, and hemorrhage from the separating placenta during delivery. The following discussion regarding vaginal birth is therefore limited to women with twins. The ability of the woman to birth twins vaginally is based on a variety of factors including the following:

- Gestational age of the fetuses at delivery—some experts advocate cesarean delivery for twins with estimated weights of 1500 g (3 lb 5 oz) or less at birth to reduce the incidence of intraventricular hemorrhage.
- Presence of preexisting problems—if severe IUGR or oligohydramnios is evident in one twin due to twin-to-twin transfusion syndrome, cesarean delivery may be preferred to avoid birth asphyxia.
- Presentation of twins at birth—many experts advocate cesarean delivery if both twins are in a nonvertex presentation or if the second twin is in a nonvertex presentation.

If a vaginal delivery is planned, certain precautions must be taken. The delivery room must be prepared for immediate cesarean delivery, with any additional staff needed on hand, until the twins are successfully delivered. Anesthesia and analgesia must be carefully administered to avoid depression of the infants. Maternal discomfort may be managed by regional and local anesthesia. Continuous EFM is essential and must be maintained until delivery of the second twin. If the second twin is in a transverse lie and remains so after efforts at external version, cesarean delivery is then indicated.

Immediately after the first twin is delivered, the umbilical cord is clamped. A vaginal examination is performed to rule out cord prolapse and determine the presentation of the second twin. If the presentation is favorable and the second amniotic sac is still intact, it is gently pierced with a fine spinal needle to allow for slow descent of the second twin into the pelvis. This technique is used to prevent cord prolapse. A nurse must monitor the second twin's heart rate continuously throughout this procedure.

Unless some other threatening condition exists, there is no need for prompt delivery of the second twin. Labor may progress as long as the fetus and woman are stable (Jackson, 1989). A dilute solution of Pitocin may be started to stimulate effective contractions if uterine inertia occurs. When the second twin is delivered, the cord is clamped in such a way as to differentiate the umbilical cords for subsequent examination.

Cesarean delivery often occurs early in cases of three or more fetuses. This is because of preterm labor; maternal complications, such as uncontrolled diabetes or PIH; or decreasing fetal well-being. Although many twins may be successfully delivered vaginally, problems may arise that preclude a vaginal birth. Many complications involve abnormal position or presentation (Fig. 26-6), including:

- Transverse lie of first twin
- Transverse lie of second twin and unsuccessful attempt at external version after delivery of first twin
- Conjoined or interlocking twins
- Signs of fetal distress in either twin
- Prolapsed cord with rupture of membranes
- Evidence of placenta previa or abruptio placentae
- Uterine hypotonicity and failure to progress with oxytocin infusion

If a cesarean delivery is planned, the physician will make decisions regarding the type of anesthesia and abdominal and uterine wall incisions before surgery. The abdominal incision may be vertical to allow ample room for manipulation of abnormal presentations. The uterine incision may be low transverse unless fetal positions are difficult to verify, in which case a vertical incision may be used.

Implications for Nursing Care

As mentioned previously, multifetal gestation usually is diagnosed well before the woman is admitted to the labor and delivery unit. However, a missed diagnosis of twins may occur even at term. The nurse should evaluate the fundal height on her initial assessment and perform Leopold maneuvers to identify fetal extremities. If the fundal height measurement is large for gestational age or if many small parts are palpable, making it difficult to determine fetal position, the nurse should auscultate for two separate FHRs. The physician or midwife should be notified immediately of the nurse's suspicions of multifetal pregnancy.

Intrapartum care of the woman includes close evaluation of vital signs. PIH is a common complication, and ongoing assessments for signs of PIH, including edema, pro-

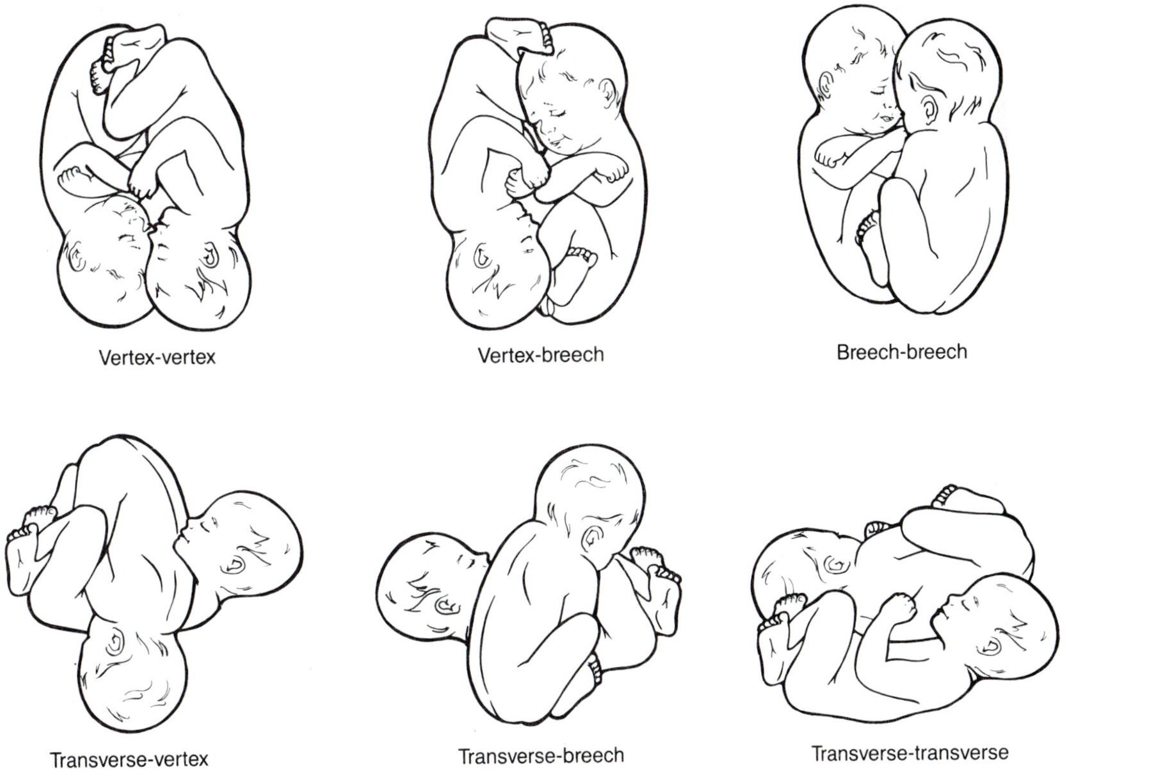

Figure 26-6.
Twin presentations.

teinuria, and hypertension, should be performed. The nurse should initiate external EFM for each fetus. Newer EFM machines permit simultaneous monitoring of both FHR patterns with one machine. Obtaining simultaneous FHR tracings when continuous EFM is initiated with twins often is difficult. Fetal position and movement may make it difficult to obtain a continuous reading. With three or more fetuses simultaneous monitoring may be impossible.

Furthermore, recent research indicates that synchronous FHR patterns occur when twins are very similar in size and weight or when there is a monochorionic or fused dichorionic placenta (Eganhous, 1992) (Fig. 26-7). The nurse may be unable to differentiate between a synchronous pattern that reflects two similar but independent heart rates and two recordings of the same twin's heart rate. Newer EFM monitors use paper with a single scale for monitoring both FHRs. The presence of a single FHR tracing may indicate that the same fetus is being monitored twice. If the nurse is unable to obtain the second FHR, the physician or midwife should be notified promptly. Ultrasonography may assist the nurse in locating the second twin's heart so that the ultrasound device can be more precisely situated. Once membranes have ruptured, it is possible to attached a fetal scalp electrode for direct or internal monitoring of the presenting twin.

Because uterine distension frequently results in labor dystocia, the nurse must carefully monitor the progress of labor and report any deviations to the birth attendant. An oxytocin infusion may be ordered to augment uterine activity. Most women with twins labor more comfortably in a semi- or high-Fowler's position; it reduces the dyspnea frequently experienced and decreases the risk of supine hypotension. It may be difficult to assume a comfortable position for any length of time, and position changes may be difficult due to the enlarged uterus. The use of an eggcrate mattress pad and pillows to support the back, abdomen, and extremities will reduce discomfort for many women.

The nurse usually is responsible for alerting the delivery team, including neonatal support staff, to prepare for small and possibly compromised infants. A neonatal team and a separate set of equipment and supplies should be available for each neonate. Preparations are made for an emergency cesarean delivery if needed, including having blood typed and crossmatched and a surgical team on hand. A nurse must monitor the FHR patterns of each twin continuously until delivery is accomplished.

The nurse is responsible for ensuring accurate identification of the infants, especially if they are born in rapid sequence. A second nurse is needed to receive the second twin while the first nurse cares for the first twin and the woman. Immediate postpartum care includes careful monitoring of maternal bleeding because of the increased risk of postpartum hemorrhage due to the overdistended uterus and large placental site. Oxytocin normally is administered to enhance uterine contractility and decrease maternal blood loss due to uterine atony. The woman and support person may be exhausted and overwhelmed by the interaction with two babies. The nurse should provide support and comfort measures, deferring extended contact with the babies until the parents are more comfortable. Parents also may need additional social support, and plans for public health or social work referral or contact with community support groups can be made at this time.

Three or More Fetuses

Problems associated with multifetal pregnancy increase with three or more fetuses. Although they are rare, the widespread use of ovulation-inducing drugs in the management of infertility has increased the number of multiple births. The incidence of multiple gestation among women given gonadotropins is estimated to be 20%. Of this group, 75% are twin gestations, and 25% are triplet or higher-number gestations. Among women treated with clomiphene, the incidence of multiple gestation is approximately 10%.

Cesarean delivery is preferred for these infants because of the increased risks of cord prolapse, hemorrhage from the separating placenta during delivery, malpresentations, and higher mortality risk to the last-delivered fetus. In cases of three or more fetuses, delivery often occurs early, because of preterm labor or diagnosed fetal distress.

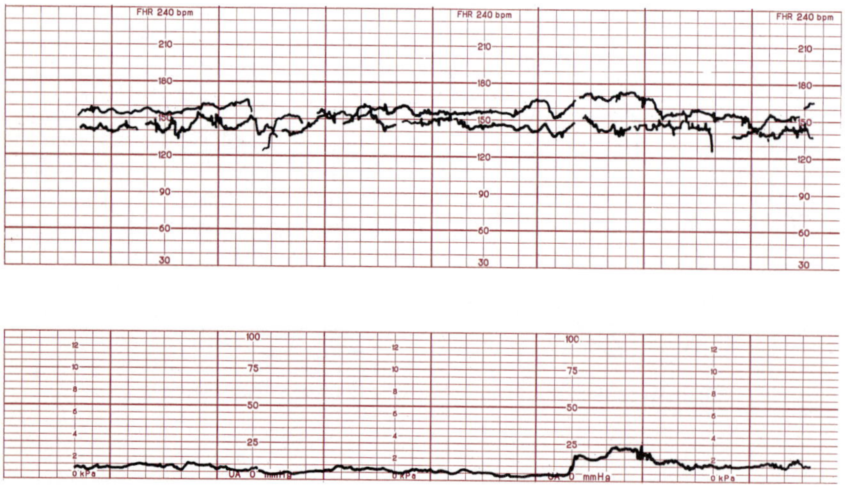

Figure 26-7.
Synchronous fetal heart rate tracings have similar frequency and timing of accelerations, baseline oscillations, and periodic changes.

Postterm Gestation and the Postmature Fetus

Postterm pregnancy is defined as a gestational period greater than 42 weeks. Approximately 6% to 12% of births occur after 42 weeks' gestation but fewer than 1% after 44 weeks. Placental aging, which occurs after 38 weeks' gestation, results in placental infarcts and the deposition of fibrin materials on the surface of the chorionic villi. These changes result in reduced provision of nutrients to the fetus and impaired gas exchange. The fetus is at risk for hypoxia, acidosis, and starvation with depletion of glycogen stores and fat deposits.

Etiologic and Predisposing Factors

The causes of postterm pregnancy are not clearly understood. A combination of the presence of inhibitory factors, such as progesterone, and absence of stimulatory factors, such as the release of oxytocin and prostaglandins, may operate to prolong the pregnancy. Maternal and fetal factors associated with postterm pregnancy are presented in the accompanying display.

Diagnosis

The diagnosis of prolonged pregnancy is possible when gestational age is well established by early pregnancy confirmation or with ultrasonographic dating (measurement of head and abdominal circumference, femur length, and biparietal diameter). Establishing a diagnosis of fetal postmaturity syndrome requires careful prenatal testing and evaluation of the fetus, including:

- Nonreactive nonstress test
- Sudden decrease in total volume of amniotic fluid
- Amniotic fluid volume index of 5 cm or less
- Decreasing biophysical profile score
- Evidence of placental aging, determined by ultrasound grading of the placenta

Maternal and Fetal Factors Associated With Postterm Pregnancy

- Multiparity
- History of postterm pregnancy
- Maternal age (<25 years and >35 years)
- Parity greater than gravida four
- Carriers of group B hemolytic *Streptococcus*
- Congenital anomalies
  - Anencephaly
  - Hydrocephaly
  - Adrenal hypoplasia
  - Osteogenesis imperfecta
- Occipitoposterior position*
- Short umbilical cord*

**Prevents stimulation of cervix and lower uterine segment by presenting part.*

Maternal, Fetal, and Neonatal Implications

The woman may be exposed to the risks of multiple obstetric interventions (oxytocin challenge test, amniotomy, amnioinfusion, and induction of labor) when postmaturity syndrome occurs, and efforts are made to deliver the fetus. Psychological distress is common. The woman frequently becomes frustrated and impatient when the pregnancy continues beyond the expected date of confinement, particularly when friends and relatives question her about when she is going to deliver. Feelings of inadequacy and failure may emerge. Fatigue and physical discomforts of late pregnancy are pronounced and may contribute to depression. Anxiety is aroused by concerns for the fetus, particularly when the health care team begins testing to determine fetal well-being.

The reduction of nutrients and oxygen in utero places the fetus at risk for hypoxia and asphyxia. The stress of labor can result in acute fetal distress. Other fetal risks include an increased incidence of umbilical cord compression and hypoxia secondary to oligohydramnios. As a result of intestinal and anal sphincter maturation, the postterm fetus may pass meconium in utero in response to hypoxia. With severe asphyxia the fetus gasps, drawing meconium into the airways and alveoli.

At birth the neonate suffers from meconium aspiration syndrome (discussed in Chapter 33). While amnioinfusion to dilute and flush thick meconium from the uterus and mechanical aspiration of meconium at birth has reduced perinatal morbidity and mortality, a small percentage of infants still succumb to this pulmonary insult. Permanent neurologic damage as a result of intrauterine asphyxia is another complication of postterm gestation.

As a result of prenatal testing, most fetuses suffering from IUGR secondary to placental aging are delivered before 42 weeks' gestation. Consequently, the greatest concern in postterm pregnancies is now fetal macrosomia (fetal weight above the 90th percentile for gestational age) and the attendant risks of shoulder dystocia and birth trauma. Intrapartum problems related to fetal macrosomia are discussed later in this chapter.

Treatment

Once postterm gestation is strongly suspected or confirmed, a series of tests is performed to assess fetal well-being, including biophysical profile, nonstress testing, amniocentesis to detect the presence of meconium, and recording fetal movement (kick counts). Many practitioners will schedule the woman for induction of labor after the 42nd week, even when signs of fetal well-being are present, particularly if the Bishop score indicates that the cervix is conducive to induction. Expectant management is acceptable with frequent ongoing assessment of fetal well-being, including weekly contraction stress testing.

Implications for Nursing Care

Whether the woman is scheduled for induction of labor or is experiencing spontaneous contractions, nursing care in postterm pregnancy focuses on optimizing uteroplacental perfusion and oxygenation of the fetus. Continuous EFM is indicated, and the woman is maintained in the left lateral recumbent position to improve placental perfusion. Oxygen is administered at 8 to 10 L/min by mask if a nonreassuring FHR pattern is identified. If oligohydramnios has been diagnosed, the nurse must observe the FHR for evidence of a cord compression pattern and attempt changes in the woman's position to correct the problem.

Amniotomy may be performed when possible to attach a fetal scalp electrode and to examine the amniotic fluid for the presence of meconium. The amniotic fluid is evaluated periodically for signs of meconium staining. Amnioinfusion may be implemented to correct severe variable decelerations or to dilute and flush thick meconium from the uterus. If fetal scalp sampling is performed, the nurse assists the physician and prepares and supports the woman through the procedure.

The nursery should be notified of the impending birth of a postmature infant. Pediatric staff or a health care professional skilled in intubation and mechanical aspiration of meconium should be present at the birth to care for the infant (see Chapter 32). The nurse should be prepared for sudden fetal decompensation and the need for an emergency cesarean birth, particularly when thick, particulate meconium is evident and administration of oxygen does not improve nonreassuring or ominous FHR patterns.

Because fetal macrosomia appears to be an increasing risk in postterm pregnancies, the nurse should be prepared to assist the birth attendant if shoulder dystocia occurs (discussed later in the chapter).

Fetal Abnormalities Affecting Labor and Birth

Unexpected fetal anomalies may cause difficult labor and delivery, trauma to the fetus, or even fetal—and rarely maternal—death. Most often these anomalies are associated with unusual body size or shape; fetal conditions that may cause dystocia include macrosomia, hydrocephalus, fetal tumors, and conjoined twins.

Macrosomia

Macrosomia is defined as a fetal weight above the 90th percentile for gestational age or a birth weight greater than 4000 g (8 lb 12.8 oz). This condition occurs in approximately 5% of all births and appears to be increasing.

Etiologic and Predisposing Factors

Macrosomia most often is associated with poorly controlled maternal diabetes and hyperglycemia. Other factors also can be responsible, including:

- Maternal birth weight greater than 4000 g (8 lb 12.8 oz)
- Body size of parents (constitutional factor)
- Maternal obesity
- Postdate pregnancy
- Fetal gigantism (Beckwith-Wiedemann syndrome)

Diagnosis

The diagnosis of fetal macrosomia is based on a strong clinical suspicion of excessive fetal size and ultrasound evaluation. The physician or midwife must take into consideration the following factors:

- Maternal weight and height
- Fundal height
- Presence of gestational diabetes
- Previous obstetric history of birthing a macrosomic infant
- Evaluation of the difference between fetal head and chest circumference

Unfortunately, diagnosis based on ultrasonographic measurement of fetal size (chest circumference and amount of adipose tissue) is imprecise and cannot be used as the sole diagnostic determinant of fetal size. During the intrapartum period, labor dystocia (including failure to progress or prolonged second stage labor) and failure of the fetal head to engage in the maternal pelvis strongly suggest fetal macrosomia.

Maternal, Fetal, and Neonatal Implications

When the maternal pelvis is sufficiently large, birth of a large infant presents no problem. However, when the maternal pelvis is of only average size, an oversized fetal head cannot accommodate to the pelvis. Cephalopelvic disproportion may cause distention of the myometrium, resulting in uterine inertia and requiring cesarean delivery. This condition also places the woman at increased risk for perineal trauma, uterine rupture, and postpartum hemorrhage. Serious risk to the fetus may result if the maternal pelvis is assumed to be adequate, fetal size is underestimated, and oxytocin augmentation is initiated to stimulate labor. Uterine contractions become regular and strong, forcing the fetal head against the unyielding bony pelvis. Cerebral trauma, neurologic damage, hypoxia, and asphyxia may result, with tragic long-term consequences even if cesarean delivery is ultimately performed. Shoulder dystocia is another significant risk with fetal macrosomia and can result in asphyxia and or birth trauma for the infant. The reader is referred to the discussion of shoulder dystocia presented later in the chapter.

Treatment

If maternal diabetes is diagnosed during pregnancy, strict plasma glucose control may reduce the incidence of fetal macrosomia. When the fetal weight is estimated to be greater than 4500 g (9 lb 4 oz), cesarean delivery is indicated (Nageotte, 1991). Instrument-assisted delivery (forceps or vacuum extraction) is to be avoided, particularly when fetal macrosomia is strongly suspected and labor has been prolonged. Maternal and fetal injuries can be severe and may result in permanent neurologic impairment of the neonate.

Implications for Nursing Care

The nurse is responsible for estimating fetal size on admission to the labor and delivery unit. The prenatal record is reviewed for maternal factors associated with fetal macrosomia, such as diabetes, excessive weight gain, or a history of birthing macrosomic fetuses. Fundal height should be measured, and performing Leopold maneuver will help the nurse make a gross determination of fetal size. The nurse notes if the fetal head is engaged and makes careful note of fetal descent during labor. The physician or midwife is notified in a timely manner if failure in fetal descent is noted. When there is strong suspicion of macrosomia, the nurse should discuss the findings with the physician or midwife and determine the medical plan.

Hydrocephalus

Hydrocephalus is a condition in which an excessive amount of cerebrospinal fluid accumulates within the fetal cranium, causing an abnormally large, softened fetal skull (see Chapter 34).

Etiologic and Predisposing Factors

The cause of hydrocephaly is unknown, but it may be genetically linked. Women who have had a previous hydrocephalic infant have a 2% to 5% risk of recurrence. The fetus of a diabetic woman also is at increased risk for the development of hydrocephalus.

Diagnosis

Hydrocephalus may be suspected when there has been rapid uterine growth in the last trimester, accompanied by hydramnios or failure of the fetal head to engage. Ultrasound assessment of the fetal cranium can allow for definitive diagnosis by measurement of the intraventricular width after the second trimester. When hydrocephalus is present, the fetal head may be palpable as a large symmetric mass over the pubis or in the fundus. Pelvic examination when the cervix is dilated may reveal abnormally widely separated fetal skull sutures; however, the softness of the skull may sometimes lead to an incorrect diagnosis of breech presentation.

Maternal, Fetal, and Neonatal Factors

The woman may have a difficult last trimester, with dyspnea, back and abdominal pain, and nausea and vomiting from the pressure the enlarged fetal head. The enlarged fetal head causes marked cephalopelvic disproportion (Fig. 26-8) and failure to progress in labor. If vaginal delivery is attempted as a result of failure to identify hydrocephaly, the woman is at risk for dystocia and uterine rupture.

Depending on the severity of the fluid accumulation, the damage to the fetal brain, and the availability of early obstetric intervention, the fetus may survive the intrapartum period. However, when the condition is not diagnosed before delivery, the risk of traumatic delivery markedly lowers the chances of fetal survival.

Treatment

Prenatal treatment for hydrocephalus is not widely available, but recent advances in fetal surgery permit surgical intervention in some cases. A ventriculoamniotic shunt has been developed that will allow for release of fluid from the fetal cranium, thus preventing brain damage from excessive pressure; this treatment, however, is still in its experimental stages (Manning, 1989).

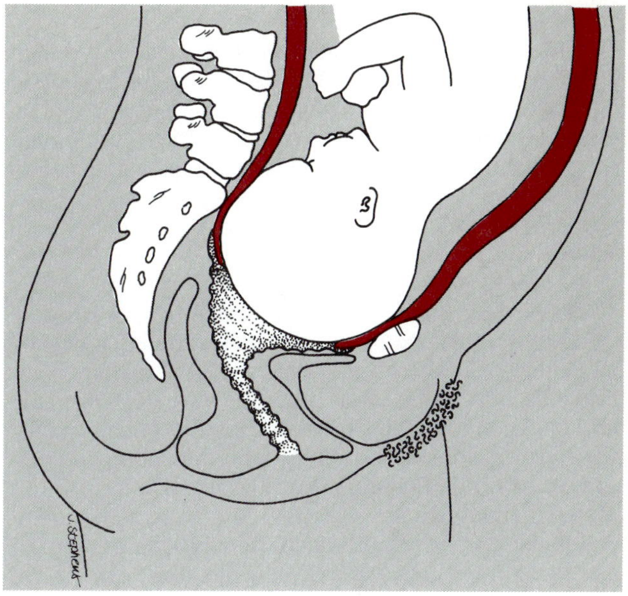

Figure 26-8.
Severe dystocia resulting from hydrocephalus. Note the disparity between the fetal head size and diameter of the pelvis between the symphysis and sacrum.

Implications for Nursing Care

In the majority of cases when the woman has received prenatal care, the diagnosis of hydrocephaly will be made before the intrapartum period. The woman will be scheduled for a cesarean birth. The nurse provides emotional support during the admission procedure and evaluates the woman's and partner's understanding of the problem. Preoperative teaching and preparation is completed by the nurse. The nursery staff is alerted so that they may be present at the neonate's birth. The reader is referred to Chapter 25 for a complete discussion of emotional support of the woman and her family when fetal/neonatal anomalies are diagnosed.

Anencephaly

Anencephaly is a condition in which the fetal cerebrum and cranium fail to develop. The appearance of the fetus is characteristic: The face is prominent with protruding eyes, and the cranial vault is absent. This condition is incompatible with life.

Etiologic and Predisposing Factors

The cause of anencephaly is unknown. Research findings suggest a polygenic or multifactorial etiology. Factors associated with this condition include the following:

- Amniotic band syndrome
- Polyhydramnios
- Maternal hyperthermia
- Maternal folate, zinc, and copper deficiency during pregnancy
- Twinning
- Geographic location (Eastern seaboard of United States, Western coast of Europe, and Ireland)

Diagnosis

The diagnosis of anencephaly can be made with a high degree of certainty. The maternal serum alpha-fetoprotein level is elevated in approximately 90% of cases and is elevated in amniotic fluid (Stumpf, 1990). Once the elevated maternal alpha-fetoprotein level is confirmed, sonography will be performed to identify the anomaly. Like other neural tube defects, anencephaly may be detected early with amniocentesis.

Maternal, Fetal, and Neonatal Implications

If the woman chooses to continue with the pregnancy once a diagnosis of anencephaly is made, intrapartum complications can cause serious problems. Anencephaly is the most common cause of polyhydramnios. The condition may cause extreme discomfort during labor secondary to pressure on the woman's lower extremities and diaphragm. The woman is exposed to the risks associated with polyhydramnios, including placental abruption, amniotic fluid embolus, and postpartum hemorrhage. Amniocentesis may be required to reduce dyspnea and abdominal pressure and increases the risk of maternal infection. Anencephalic pregnancies tend to be prolonged, especially if polyhydramnios is not present. Induction of labor often is difficult, because the overdistended uterus may not be responsive to oxytocin. Cesarean delivery may be required if induction of labor fails. The woman, aware of the prognosis for the neonate, often experiences extreme psychological distress.

Most anencephalic infants die within the first days after birth. Survival beyond 1 week is rare. However, survival for as long as 3 months has been reported (Stumpf, 1990). Early death of the neonate often involves varying degrees of withholding medical treatment that may prolong survival (IV fluids). In most cases cardiorespiratory arrest occurs before cessation of brain stem functions.

Implications for Nursing Care

The nurse is responsible for monitoring the woman's physiologic status for evidence of problems related to polyhydramnios when it complicates the diagnosis of anencephaly. Major goals of nursing care center on giving physical and emotional support to the woman and her partner, meeting comfort needs, and providing information sensitively. The nurse also must help the parents to acknowledge their loss so that grieving may begin.

Other Fetal Anomalies Affecting Delivery

Unusual tumors may cause enlargement of the fetal abdomen or neck, or strictures of the urethral valve may cause profound distention of the fetal bladder, causing enlargements that interfere with vaginal delivery. In addition conjoined (Siamese) twins may result in dystocia. These conditions may not be diagnosed until the intrapartum period when labor fails to progress. In other cases diagnosis may have been made prenatally.

These conditions generally are not amenable to treatment, and cesarean delivery often is chosen. In some cases fluid-filled tumors of the fetal abdomen may be reduced by insertion of a needle through the maternal abdomen to drain off fluid and reduce the size of the fetal abdomen. However, this procedure presents an obvious risk of trauma to the fetus.

When fetal problems complicate the intrapartum period, the focus of nursing care generally is on assessment of fetal well-being and support of fetal physiologic functioning. However, the woman also may be at increased risk due to mechanical problems (multifetal gestation or hydrocephalus) or invasive procedures required to assess fetal status or treat the underlying fetal problems. In many cases the woman is aware that significant fetal problems will be present at birth, even with the best of care. The nurse provides physical and emotional support to the woman while monitoring maternal and physiologic functioning. The nurse also prepares the family for special neonatal care and procedures that are anticipated after birth of the infant.

Complications Affecting the Process of Labor: Dystocia

Dystocia literally means difficult labor. Other synonyms include prolonged or abnormal labor and uterine inertia. Many factors contribute to the quality of labor; four factors, however, are of primary importance in determining whether progress is made:

- Fetal size, presentation, position, and ability of the fetal head to mold in the pelvis
- Ability of the uterus to contract efficiently
- Pelvic size and internal shape
- Structural abnormalities

Problems in any of these areas can cause dystocia. These factors may operate in combination, and labor outcome depends on the interaction of fetal, uterine, and pelvic factors in achieving fetal descent. The factors affecting fetal descent are summarized in the display and discussed in this section.

Fetal Factors Causing Dystocia

Fetal dystocia can result when the fetus has assumed an abnormal position or presentation, is unusually large (macrosomic), or has an anomaly that prevents descent into the bony pelvis. Malpresentations and malpositions, however, are more frequent causes of fetal dystocia. Malpresentations usually reduce the efficiency of labor. For instance the presenting part cannot adapt to the bony pelvis and exert pressure against the cervix; thus, it cannot aid in further dilatation and effacement. The quality and frequency of uterine contractions may decrease, prolonging labor. Malpresentations also may increase the likelihood of PROM. If labor continues when fetal descent is impossible, the integrity of the uterine muscle may be threatened.

Fetal position refers to the relationship of the fetal skull to the maternal pelvis. Fetal position may contribute to dystocia if the fetus is in a persistent occipitoposterior position. More frequently, however, fetal dystocia is related to such

Factors Complicating Fetal Descent: Dystocia

Fetal Factors

Unusually large fetus
Fetal anomaly
Malpresentations and malpositions

Uterine Factors

Pathologic retraction rings
Hypotonic labor
Hypertonic labor
Precipitous labor
Prolonged labor

Pelvic Factors

Inlet contracture
Midpelvis contracture
Outlet contracture

Soft-Tissue Factors

Structural abnormalities

malpresentations as breech, brow, face, and shoulder presentation and shoulder dystocia.

Occipitoposterior Position

In the occipitoposterior position the fetal occiput and small posterior fontanelle are located in the posterior segment of the maternal pelvis, and the brow and face are in the anterior segment.

Etiologic and Predisposing Factors

The occipitoposterior position occurs in 15% to 30% of labors. The exact incidence is unknown because most fetuses spontaneously rotate to an occipitoanterior position during labor. A right occipitoposterior position is five times more common than left. Factors related to occipitoposterior position include pelvic architecture in which posterior sagittal diameters are larger (android and anthropoid pelves) and cephalopelvic disproportion.

Diagnosis

The position is diagnosed through abdominal assessment and pelvic examination. During abdominal assessment the fetal back is not outlined well, while the fetal small parts are easily felt. The FHR may best be heard in the maternal flank, far from the midline. Occasionally, when the fetus is in occipitoposterior position, the contour of the maternal abdomen assumes an hourglass shape that can give the impression of a full bladder. Vaginal examination may reveal or verify the position. The fontanelles are at approximately the same level in the pelvis because of the typical military attitude assumed by the fetus in the occipitoposterior position. The anterior fontanelle is readily felt in the anterior segment of the maternal pelvis.

Maternal, Fetal, and Neonatal Implications

When the fetus is in occipitoposterior position, cervical dilatation and fetal descent often are slow. This is because the fetal head may not apply even pressure to the cervix. If the malposition is persistent, the fetal head does not completely flex to present a smaller diameter to the pelvic outlet. Labor may be significantly prolonged.

The woman may experience excessive backache (back labor) and coupling of uterine contractions. Typically, the membranes rupture in the latent phase, follwed by a prolonged active phase. Fatigue, dehydration, and frustration may occur, and she may become exhausted and anxious. Ketosis may develop with prolonged labor, maternal exhaustion, and dehydration. This poses a physiologic risk to the woman and fetus. If delivery occurs in a persistent occipitoposterior position, third- or fourth-degree perineal lacerations and periurethral lacerations occur. Several complications may occur when the fetus is in a persistent occipitoposterior position. If attempts at manual or forceps rotation of the occiput occur, the fetus is at risk for umbilical cord accidents (torsion or compression). The use of forceps may result in ecchymosis or lacerations of the face, facial nerve damage, and in rare cases intracranial injury.

Treatment

Many times the fetus in the occipitoposterior position rotates spontaneously during labor. Having the woman lie on the side of the occiput or in a knee-chest position may facilitate this. Occasionally, spontaneous delivery of the fetus in posterior position occurs. The birth attendant may attempt a manual rotation to the occipitoanterior position, followed by forceps delivery. In the case of a low midpelvic arrest with an anthropoid pelvis, an instrument rotation using Kielland's forceps also may be attempted. If manual and or instrument attempts fail, cesarean delivery is indicated.

Implications for Nursing Care

Once persistent occipitoposterior position has been diagnosed or is suspected, the nurse may initiate intervention to facilitate rotation and descent of the fetus (see the Nursing Research display). The nurse should encourage the woman to use positions for labor that facilitate fetal rotation, including squatting, knee-chest, hands-and-knees, standing and leaning forward, and sidelying on the side opposite the fetal back (which allows gravity to accomplish rotation to anterior position). With the woman in the hands-and-knees position, the nurse may try firm stroking of the maternal abdomen from the same side as the fetal back toward the midline; pelvic rocking movements may assist this technique.

Because dehydration and exhaustion can occur with prolonged labor, the nurse should monitor intake and output carefully, encourage adequate fluid and calorie intake, assess the urine for the presence of ketones, and measure its specific gravity. Frequent reassurance of the parturient is essential to prevent frustration and discouragement. The

Nursing Research

Positive Nursing Support When the Occipitoposterior (OP) Position Occurs

The woman who labors with the fetus in an OP position must endure many adverse effects, including the following:

- Backache
- Painful contractions that do not produce descent or dilatation
- Prolonged rupture of membranes with possible chorioamnionitis
- Third- or fourth-degree periurethral lacerations if delivery occurs in the OP position
- Increased risk of cesarean delivery for failure to progress

Biancuzzo (1991) conducted a retrospective chart review to determine the impact of nursing care on the outcome of labor for the woman with a fetus in the OP position. Significantly, labor nurses did not always perform Leopold maneuvers or vaginal examination to determine fetal position; active management to correct the OP position was not implemented or delayed for many hours. As a result labor was prolonged, and in some instances cesarean delivery was performed without attempting maternal position changes recommended to rotate the fetus.

When the OP position was diagnosed and nurses altered the maternal position, rotation of the fetal head occurred in as little as 40 minutes. The author suggests that the optimum time to facilitate rotation is during transition or the second stage of labor when the greater intensity of contractions speeds the rotation process.

Further research is definitely indicated to confirm these findings, identify the optimum time for changing maternal position, and strengthen recommendations for practice.

Biancuzzo, M. (1991). The patient observer: Does the hands-and-knees posture during labor help to rotate the occiput posterior position? *Birth, 18*(1), 40.

FHR should be monitored closely for deviations from the norm, particularly in second stage if attempts are made to manually rotate the fetal head or if forceps are applied.

Breech Presentation

Breech presentations are a common cause of dystocia and in many settings contribute significantly to the incidence of cesarean delivery. Dystocia is associated with breech presentation because the buttocks are soft and are not as effective as the head in dilating the cervix. With breech presentation, the body usually passes through the cervix before full dilatation. The head becomes entrapped because the cervix is not fully dilated, resulting in hypoxia and asphyxia. However, there are conditions under which vaginal breech delivery is acceptable (see the display, Vaginal versus Cesarean Delivery in Breech Presentations).

Etiologic and Predisposing Factors

Breech presentations are commonly found in the second trimester, but most usually spontaneously convert to the vertex presentation. Approximately 3% to 4% of singleton deliveries are breech presentations. The incidence is increased in multiple gestation and with fetal and uterine anomalies. Breech presentations also appear to correlate with fetal weight, decreasing as fetal weight increases. Breech presentations occur in approximately 20% of deliveries when fetal weight is 1000 g (2 lb 3 oz), decreasing to 12% at 1500 g (3 lb 5 oz), and less than 5% when fetal weight is 3000 g (6 lb 9 oz) or more. Breech presentations are classified in the accompanying display.

Diagnosis

Breech presentation usually is diagnosed prenatally by abdominal palpation in conjunction with bimanual examination. The vertex is palpable as a hard, round object in the fundus and is ballotable (ie, it can be moved independent of the rest of the body). The wider sacrum is palpated in the lower portion of the pelvis, and FHR is auscultated above the umbilicus. Internal examination when the presenting part is engaged may reveal the soft breech, legs, and feet or the absence of fontanelles. The genitalia of the fetus may be identifiable. When breech presentation is diagnosed, further assessment by ultrasound examination may be indicated to confirm fetal position and presentation, localize the placenta, assess fetal head and pelvic size, and identify possible fetal anomalies. Computed tomography (CT) pelvimetry also may be performed to evaluate pelvic measurements before a final decision is made regarding the mode of delivery (vaginal or cesarean).

Maternal, Fetal, and Neonatal Implications

Some increased maternal risk results from breech presentations, even if vaginal delivery eventually is successful. Because the fetal buttocks do not conform well to the lower uterine segment or to the bony pelvis, the membranes may rupture prematurely, producing increased risk of cord prolapse or infection. Labor may be prolonged and inefficient, because the breech is not as effective as the head in accomplishing cervical dilatation. Forceful delivery of the fetus through a tight pelvis with poor soft tissue dilatation before the descent of the head may cause lower uterine segment, cervical, vaginal, or perineal lacerations, especially if for-

Vaginal versus Cesarean Delivery in Breech Presentations

All the following criteria should be present for vaginal delivery:

- Frank or complete breech without hyperextension of the fetal head
- Fetal weight estimated at less than 3500 g
- Adequate pelvic size confirmed by computed tomography (CT) pelvimetry
- Gestational age of 36 to 42 weeks
- Birth attendant experienced in vaginal breech deliveries and pediatric support available in the event of neonatal problems

Cesarean delivery is preferable under the following circumstances:

- Absence of labor when fetal status requires delivery
- Premature fetus whose condition requires minimal stress in delivery
- Previous history of perinatal death or of a child with residual birth trauma
- Inadequate pelvis suggested by previous birth history or CT pelvimetry

ceps application is needed to hasten delivery of the head. Women who require cesarean delivery because of breech presentation are exposed to the additional risks associated with operative intervention.

Much of the increased fetal and neonatal morbidity and mortality associated with breech delivery come from related conditions, such as preterm birth, congenital malformations, PROM, or placental problems. Factors directly related to breech delivery include prolapse of the umbilical cord, entrapment of the fetal head, and trauma during vaginal delivery, primarily trauma to the after-coming head. This may result in central nervous system injuries, such as the following:

- Vertebral and medullary injury in infants with a hyperextended head
- Separation of the occipital bone and subdural hemorrhage resulting from pressure on the fetal cranium
- Erb palsy (facial nerve paralysis)
- Central nervous system damage resulting from hypoxia in delayed delivery

Other types of fetal trauma include muscle damage, bone fracture, and aspiration of amniotic fluid. The last is particularly troublesome, because amniotic fluid is more frequently stained with meconium in breech presentations, so the risk of meconium aspiration may be higher.

Classifications of Breech Presentations

Frank breech (65% of breech presentations): The fetal thighs are flexed at the hips, the legs are extended, and the feet are extended close to the face.

Incomplete or footling breech (25% of breech presentations): One or both thighs are not flexed, so one or both feet lie below the buttocks, and a knee or foot is actually the presenting part.

Complete breech (10% of breech presentations): The fetal thighs are flexed at the hips, and the knees are flexed.

Treatment

When breech presentation is diagnosed early in labor, the decision about the appropriate mode of delivery must be made. When time is needed to assess the fetus, its position, and the adequacy of the maternal pelvis during labor, a tocolytic agent may be administered to slow down or stop labor temporarily. Assessment of the fetus includes ultrasound examination to assess fetal weight, hyperextension of the fetal head, and type of presentation. The adequacy of the maternal pelvis also may be determined by CT pelvimetery. After these fetal and maternal factors have been considered, the decision for route of delivery is made, as shown in Figure 26-9. Research findings indicate that vaginal breech births can be accomplished successfully in selected women, using new sonographic and CT pelvimetry techniques, without an increase in fetal, maternal, or neonatal morbidity or mortality.

Implications for Nursing Care

Although most breech presentations are diagnosed prenatally, the nurse may sometimes discover an undiagnosed breech presentation in the course of the intrapartum assessment. The nurse should notify the birth attendant immediately, because this information may affect the plan of care, especially in settings where vaginal breech deliveries are rare, and cesarean delivery is the usual practice. In these cases the nurse should be prepared to answer the parents' questions and to provide support and reassurance as needed.

An IV line should be inserted in preparation for a possible cesarean delivery or in the case of a vaginal birth the administration of fluids or blood if maternal trauma occurs at delivery. The nurse should be prepared to administer tocolytics, such as subcutaneous terbutaline, to reduce uterine activity and allow time for ultrasonography or CT pelvimetry. Continuous electronic monitoring is indicated, particularly with meconium-stained amniotic fluid. Passage of meconium is common in breech presentation, but it does not preclude the possibility of fetal distress when staining of fluid occurs. Pediatric nursing and medical staff should be alerted and present for the delivery. Anesthesia personnel also should be informed, so they may be present at the birth.

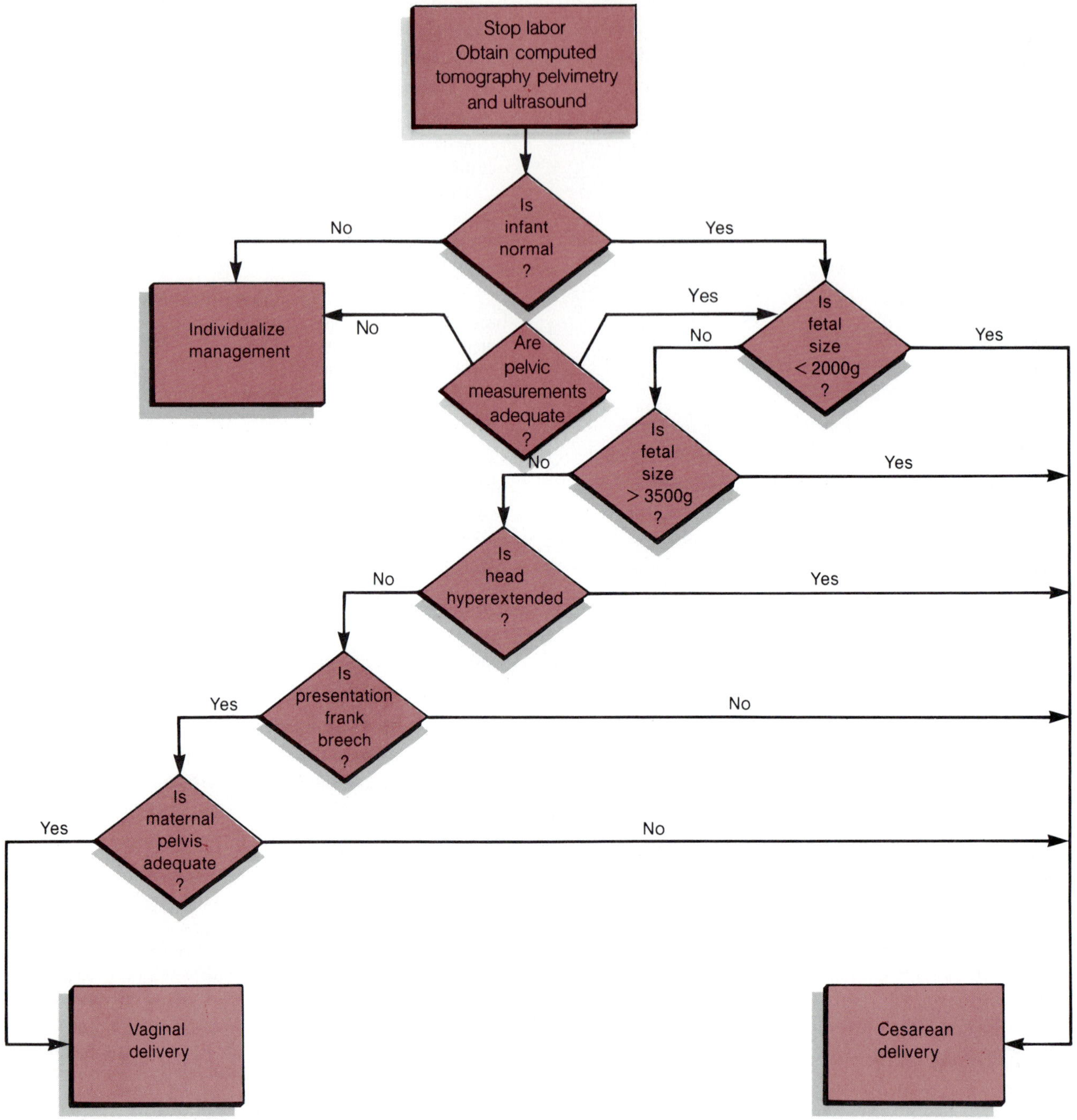

Figure 26-9.
Intrapartal management of breech presentations. (Adapted from Arias, F., Holcomb, W. [1984]. Abnormal fetal presentations and positions during labor. In F. Arias [Ed.], *High-Risk pregnancy and delivery* [pp. 324–325]. St. Louis: C.V. Mosby.)

Emergency resuscitation equipment should be checked before delivery, particularly when a vaginal birth is planned. If vaginal birth is attempted, the nurse should be prepared for prompt action if there are difficulties during the delivery of the head. The fetus should be monitored continuously for evidence of compromise, either from cord prolapse or from cord compression during the second stage. In some cases the nurse must be ready to assist with forceps application and occasionally with emergency measures, such as general anesthesia or cesarean birth, if complications threaten fetal well-being.

Brow Presentation

Brow presentation occurs when the fetus is in a head-down position with the head straight or slightly extended so that the brow and orbital ridges are the presenting part of the skull. This means that the largest skull diameter, the occipitomental, is presented to the pelvic inlet. Frequently, brow presentations convert to face or vertex presentations on descent into the bony pelvis.

Etiologic and Predisposing Factors

Brow presentations are thought to be caused by conditions that allow the fetal body to sag forward, resulting in straightening and extension of the neck. Brow presentations are more common in multiparous women or primiparas with small fetuses.

Diagnosis

Brow presentation is diagnosed when the fetal head is partially extended, and the fetal brow is palpable on vaginal examination.

Maternal, Fetal, and Neonatal Implications

If the maternal pelvis is adequate and conversion to a face or vertex presentation occurs, labor may proceed normally. Vaginal delivery with a persistent brow presentation usually results in perineal and vaginal lacerations.

Risks to the fetus in brow presentation are similar to those in face presentations: increased danger of trauma to the head, neck, and larynx and damage to the central nervous system. Trauma also may result from forceps application.

Treatment

Intervention is not needed in cases of brow presentation if the maternal pelvis is adequate and labor is progressing. In the presence of arrested labor or fetal distress, cesarean delivery is indicated.

Implications for Nursing Care

Nursing responsibilities in caring for a woman with a brow presentation include close monitoring of the progress of labor and fetal status throughout labor. Application of a fetal scalp electrode in contraindicated to prevent accidental insertion in the fetal eye. The nurse should explain the problem to the parents and assist them in coping with what may be a prolonged and difficult labor. The nurse also should be prepared for the possible need for forceps application and emergency cesarean delivery if fetal status is compromised. If the presentation converts to a face presentation during descent, the nurse should be prepared to explain to the parents the cause and expected duration of any facial swelling and bruising in the neonate and to provide reassurance as needed.

Face Presentation

Face presentation occurs when the fetus is in a head-down position but with the head hyperextended so that the face is the presenting part.

Etiologic and Predisposing Factors

Face presentation is rare, occurring in 0.2% of deliveries, and is more common among multiparous women. This is thought to be the result of brow presentations in which the fetal head has become hyperextended. Any factors that favor extension of the head while preventing its flexion may lead to a face presentation, such as the following:

- Small pelvis
- Large infant
- Congenital goiter or anencephaly (rare)
- Weakness of the maternal abdominal wall, which allows the fetal torso to sag forward, causing straightening of the neck
- Preterm labor

Diagnosis

Face presentation is diagnosed on vaginal examination. The facial features of the fetus can be palpated.

Maternal, Fetal, and Neonatal Implications

Vaginal delivery may occur in up to 80% of face presentations if the maternal pelvis is adequate and the chin (mentum) is anterior. In mentum posterior positions the chin often becomes arrested against the maternal sacrum. Because no further extension of the fetal head is possible, labor is arrested. Cesarean delivery often is indicated in this instance. However, if labor is progressing well and the fetus is in an anterior position, attempts to rotate the fetus manually to an occiput position should be avoided, and labor should be supported as long as progress continues. Labor may be prolonged, because the face is not as effective in dilating the cervix as the fetal head. Descent may be more painful, and the risk of trauma to the genital tract is increased.

When the maternal pelvis is adequate and the fetus is anterior, fetal distress is uncommon. Fetal membranes usually rupture early in labor, and the face becomes swollen, misshapen, and bruised from the pressure against the cervix and throughout descent. The neonate's facial appearance on delivery may be disturbing to the parents; however, swelling gradually resolves over several days. The molding of the fetal head may be pronounced, with the forehead and occiput protruding. Rarely, prolonged pressure on the infant's hyoid bone during labor may cause edema of the larynx. This may cause transient respiratory difficulty and requires close nursing observation throughout the first 24 hours of life.

Treatment

No treatment for face presentation is needed, unless arrest of progress or fetal distress occurs; in this event cesarean delivery is indicated.

Implications for Nursing Care

The nurse should closely monitor the progress of labor and fetal status and be prepared to offer support and provide information to the woman and her partner as they cope with what may be a difficult and prolonged labor. Application of a fetal electrode is contraindicated to prevent accidental placement of the device in a fetal eye. The nurse also should be prepared for the need for emergency delivery and resuscitation efforts if the infant is compromised. If vaginal delivery is successful or if a cesarean delivery is needed after considerable time in labor, the nurse should prepare the woman and support person for the infant's facial appearance. The attending pediatrician, should provide reassurance about the infant's normalcy and the expected resolution of facial swelling and bruising in 3 to 5 days.

Shoulder Presentation (Transverse Lie)

Shoulder presentation is rare and occurs in 0.3% of singleton births; it is more common among second twins and when fetal weight exceeds 4000 g (8 lb 12.8 oz). Shoulder presentation occurs when the fetus's long axis is perpendicular to the maternal axis in a transverse lie. Inspection of the maternal abdomen shows unusual wideness from side to side, decreased fundal height, and no discernible fetal parts in the fundus. The head and breech may be palpable on opposite sides of the abdomen. With rupture of membranes the fetal shoulder dips into the pelvis; an arm may prolapse into the vagina. Attempts to rotate the infant to a more favorable position are generally unsuccessful and may present significant risks of vaginal lacerations and lower uterine segment rupture.

Etiologic and Predisposing Factors

Factors that predispose to shoulder presentation include the following:

- Multiparity and lax abdominal musculature
- Preterm labor
- Conditions that inhibit normal engagement and descent, such as low-lying placenta, placenta previa, and inlet contracture
- Macrosomia

Diagnosis

Transverse lie that produces a shoulder presentation is suspected when Leopold maneuvers are performed. The diagnosis is confirmed by ultrasonography.

Maternal, Fetal, and Neonatal Implications

Labor can be dysfunctional, and pathologic retraction rings and even uterine rupture can result if the diagnosis of shoulder presentation is missed, and labor is permitted to progress. When transverse lie is persistent, vaginal delivery is impossible. There is an increased risk of cord prolapse with a transverse lie, as well as the risk of prolapse of the arm into the cervix and vagina.

Treatment

If the diagnosis of transverse lie is made before labor, external version can be performed to convert the presentation to a vertex or breech. Treatment for persistent shoulder presentation is cesarean delivery.

Nursing Implications

The nurse may suspect transverse lie and shoulder presentation from presenting risk factors for the condition. Leopold maneuvers are performed, and if the findings confirm suspicions of an abnormal lie, the midwife or physician should be promptly notified. Other responsibilities of the nurse include preparing the woman for external version if it will be attempted or for cesarean birth.

Shoulder Dystocia

Shoulder dystocia occurs during the second stage of labor when the fetal head is born, but the shoulders are too broad to rotate and to be delivered between the symphysis pubis and the sacrum. This may delay delivery of the body and poses significant risk of fetal asphyxia if the umbilical cord has been brought down and is compressed between the fetal body and the bony pelvis. The incidence of shoulder dystocia is increasing; this may reflect recommendations for increased maternal weight gain in pregnancy and a decrease in factors leading to IUGR and the birth of small-for-gestational age infants (O'Leary & Leonetti, 1990).

Etiologic and Predisposing Factors

The most common causes of shoulder dystocia are macrosomia and a tight or contracted pelvic outlet. Because of the many adverse effects of shoulder dystocia, efforts have been made to identify major risk factors associated with this complication. The risk factors associated with shoulder dystocia are listed in the accompanying display.

Diagnosis

The diagnosis of shoulder dystocia is made at birth after the fetal head has been delivered, and the shoulders fail to spontaneously traverse the pelvis. Prenatal and intrapartum signs listed in the accompanying display may provide earlier indicators to the likelihood of shoulder dys-

Risk Factors Associated with Shoulder Dystocia

Prepregnancy Factors

Maternal birth weight
Prior shoulder dystocia
Prior macrosomia
Preexisting maternal diabetes
Obesity
Multiparity
Advanced maternal age

Prepartum Risk Factors

Glucose intolerance of pregnancy
Excessive weight gain
Diagnosed or suspected fetal macrosomia
Abnormal pelvic size or shape
Postdatism

Intrapartum Risk Factors

Prolonged second stage
Protracted or arrest of descent
Pronounced fetal head molding
Need for midpelvic forceps delivery

Adapted from O'Leary, J., & Leonetti, H. (1990). Shoulder dystocia: Prevention and treatment. American Journal of Obstetrics and Gynecology, *162(1), 5.*

tocia. Another clue observed in the second stage of labor is the "turtle sign," so called because the head of the infant draws back into the perinuem with each pushing effort, much like the head of a turtle drawing back into its shell (Penney & Perlis, 1992).

Estimation of fetal weight by fundal height measurement and palpation of fetal parts also is important. However, estimates of weight are not highly reliable. Research also is being conducted to evaluate the effectiveness of ultrasound and CT scans to measure the fetal bisacromial (shoulder) diameter before delivery. It is too early to determine the usefulness of these measures.

Maternal, Fetal, and Neonatal Implications

If shoulder dystocia occurs, there is increased risk of vaginal or perineal trauma as the birth attendant attempts various maneuvers to facilitate delivery. Risk to the fetus is increased from asphyxia caused by prolonged cord compression, brachial plexus injury due to overstretching of the neck, and clavicle fractures sustained during emergency measures to complete delivery. This difficult second stage carries the possibility of cervical nerve damage in the neonate, and the newborn must be observed and assessed carefully for signs of neurologic damage.

Treatment

Shoulder dystocia can be prevented in many cases by careful assessment of the risk factors described in the accompanying display and selecting cesarean birth as the mode of delivery. When a fetus estimated to be large arrests in the midpelvis, vacuum or forceps extraction must be viewed as increasing the potential risk of shoulder dystocia and birth trauma and asphyxia.

When shoulder dystocia occurs the birth attendant may request assistance with manual attempts to extract the fetus. The nurse may be asked to assist in applying suprapubic pressure in an attempt to deliver the shoulder under the symphysis. In extreme cases when delivery cannot be accomplished, the physician may find it necessary to fracture the infant's clavicles or to perform an emergency cesarean birth. A protracted attempt at vaginal birth followed by cesarean delivery usually results in very poor neonatal outcomes.

Implications for Nursing Care

An important nursing responsibility is monitoring labor progress. If fetal descent is slow and difficult, especially when the fetus is estimated to be large, the nurse should be alert for any arrest of progress and notify the birth attendant. The nurse should review with the midwife or physician any prenatal or intrapartum factors that appear to increase the risk of shoulder dystocia. When shoulder dystocia occurs, the nurse must assist the birth attendant to facilitate delivery (see the accompanying Nursing Procedure). The neonate is assessed immediately for signs of asphyxia or trauma related to the delivery, especially fracture of the clavicle or brachial plexus injury. If the Apgar scores are low (below 7 at 5 minutes) umbilical cord blood should be obtained for gas and pH analysis to determine the degree of metabolic acidosis.

Uterine Factors Causing Dystocia

Uterine dystocia exists when contractions of the uterine muscle are not adequate to dilate the cervix and facilitate the descent of the fetus. Approximately 5% of all labors are complicated by uterine dystocia, most often among primiparas. Uterine dystocia is classified as primary, meaning that uterine contraction patterns appear to be abnormal from their onset, or secondary, meaning that a normal labor pattern has become abnormal.

As discussed in Chapter 19, normal uterine contractions begin in a pacemaker site, usually one of the two uterine cornua. From here electric impulses sweep down and across the uterus, stimulating a coordinated muscle contraction. As this wave moves away from the pacemaker, the duration and intensity of the contraction decrease so that the contraction is longer and stronger in the fundus than in the less contractile lower uterine segment. Thus, the fundus dominates uterine activity, which permits cervical dilatation and effacement and facilitates the descent of the fetus.

Pathologic Retraction Rings

One sign of dystocia, particularly in prolonged and obstructed labor, is the development of pathologic retraction rings in the uterus. A physiologic retraction ring is a ridge on the inner surface of the uterus marking the boundary between the contractile upper uterine segment and the passive, distensible lower segment. Physiologic retraction rings are normal findings and have little significance for maternal or infant status.

Pathologic retraction rings, also known as annular uterine strictures, are of two types: Bandl's rings and constriction rings (Table 26-3). The most common type, Bandl's ring, begins as a physiologic retraction ring. A constriction ring occurs when a ring-shaped portion of the uterine musculature becomes tetanic. A pathologic ring prevents fetal descent, and the fetus may become trapped; thus, a constriction ring is the cause rather than the result of arrested fetal descent.

Etiologic and Predisposing Factors

Pathologic retraction rings develop with prolonged, obstructed labor. Continuing uterine contractions without fetal descent (due to cepahlopelvic disproportion) result in overretraction of the upper uterine segment and overdistention of the lower segment. With each contraction the ring widens, and the lower uterine segment becomes thinner and more distended. Predisposing factors to the development of pathologic rings include fetal macrosomia, pelvic contactures, and oxytocin administration.

Diagnosis

Constriction rings can occur at any level, but the most common location is 7 to 8 cm above the level of the cervix. The ring may be palpable abdominally and causes severe abdominal pain but only when the abdominal wall is thin.

Maternal, Fetal, and Neonatal Implicatons

Formation of a pathologic ring is considered a sign of impending uterine rupture. The woman may feel pain in the

NURSING PROCEDURE
Assisting the Birth Attendant When Shoulder Dystocia Occurs

The incidence of fetal macrosomia and shoulder dystocia appears to be increasing. Lawsuits arising from adverse outcomes with shoulder dystocia also are increasing in number. The nurse may be implicated in allegations of negligence if steps taken to assist the birth attendant are delayed or inappropriate when shoulder dystocia is diagnosed.

Purpose: To facilitate birth and support the neonate after delivery.

NURSING ACTION	RATIONALE
1. Call for help.	To obtain additional nursing and medical help.
2. Call for pediatric or neonatal assistance.	To assist with resuscitation of the neonate if asphyxia occurs.
3. Call for anesthesia support.	Anesthesia may have to be administered to control pain or for emergency cesarean birth.
4. Note the the time that the head is delivered and the time that the shoulders and body of the neonate are delivered.	To determine the period of time required to deliver the shoulder. Risk of neonatal asphyxial injury increases as the time between delivery of head and delivery of shoulders lengthens.
5. Have the woman cease pushing efforts.	Further pushing efforts will not usually help and may further impact the anterior shoulder against the symphysis bone.
6. Implement the McRoberts maneuver (see art). The maneuver consists of placing the woman's legs in exaggerated flexion onto her abdomen.	To slightly alter the pelvic configuration and free the impacted anterior shoulder.
7. Apply suprapubic pressure (see art). On direction from the birth attendant, apply firm pressure directly posterior over the suprapubic area.	To attempt forcing of the anterior shoulder behind the pubic bone and under the symphysis.
8. Be prepared to place the woman in a hands-and-knees or lateral position.	To slightly alter the pelvic configuration and dislodge the impacted shoulder.

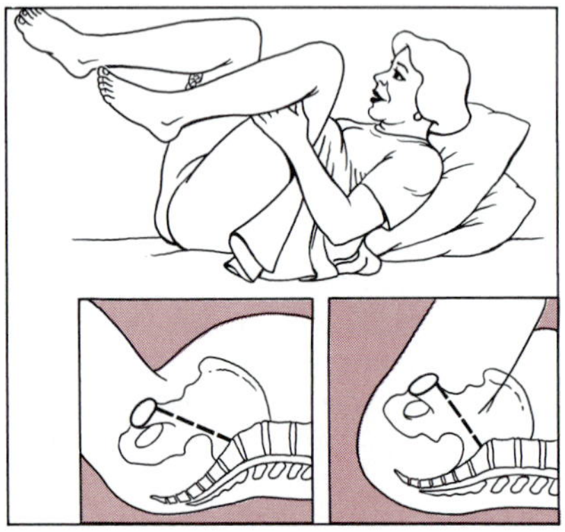

Step 6. McRoberts maneuver.

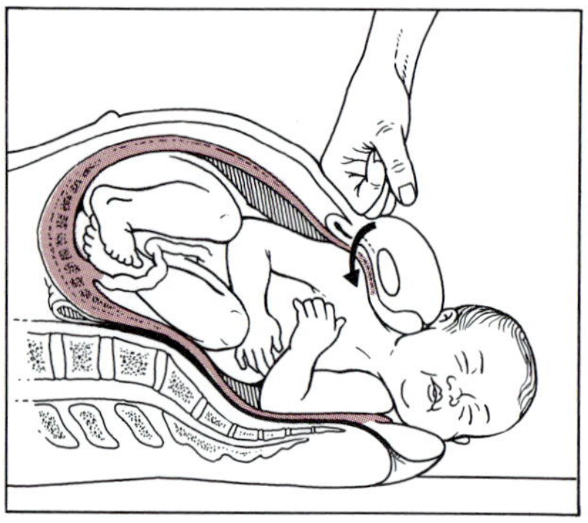

Step 7. Suprapubic pressure.

While efforts are being made to free the anterior shoulder and deliver the infant, other personnel should be assembling equipment for neonatal resuscitation and stabilization.

abdomen. However, if an epidural anesthesia is administered, sensations of pain may be absent. A Bandl's ring may actually impede labor further, because part of the fetus can become trapped above the ring. The woman often is in excruciating pain and experiences increasing anxiety as it becomes evident that the progress of labor is abnormal. Exhaustion and dehydration may occur if the underlying abnormality in the progress of labor is not identified, and delivery is not accomplished in a timely manner. If prompt treatment is not initiated, the woman also is at risk for uterine rupture and hemorrhage.

Because the pathologic ring is associated with prolonged, obstructed labor, fetal distress may occur. Continuing strong contractions impede uteroplacental perfusion and can cause fetal hypoxia, meconium passage, and asphyxia.

Treatment

Close monitoring of the progress of labor and fetal descent is essential to prevent the development of pathologic retraction rings. Analgesia or anesthesia may relax the constriction once it has developed. Vaginal delivery may be possible as long as fetal status is good and labor progresses well. However, in most cases when a pathologic retraction ring is identified, a tocolytic (terbutaline) is administered to reduce or stop uterine activity. Arrangments are then made for an immediate cesarean delivery. Maternal and fetal physi-

Table 26-3. Differential Diagnosis of Constriction Ring and Bandl's Ring

Constriction Ring	Bandl's Ring
Ring is localized area of spastic myometrium.	Ring is formed by excessive retraction of upper segment.
Ring may occur in any part of the uterus.	Ring is always at junction of upper and lower segments.
Muscle at the ring is thicker than above or below it.	Myometrium is much thicker above than below the ring.
Uterus below the ring is neither thin nor distended.	Wall below is thin and overdistended.
Uterus never ruptures.	If uncorrected, uterus may rupture.
Uterus above ring is relaxed and not tender.	Uterus above ring is hard.
Round ligaments are not tense.	Round ligaments are tense and stand out.
Ring may occur in any stage of labor.	Ring usually occurs late in the second stage.
Position of the ring does not change.	The ring gradually rises in the abdomen.
Presenting part is not driven down.	Presenting part is jammed into the pelvis.
Fetus may be wholly or mainly above the ring.	Part of the fetus must be below the ring.
Patient's general condition is good.	Patient's general condition is poor.
Uterine action is inefficient.	Uterine action is efficient or overefficient.
Polarity is abnormal.	Polarity is normal.
Ring results in obstructed labor.	Ring is caused by an obstruction.

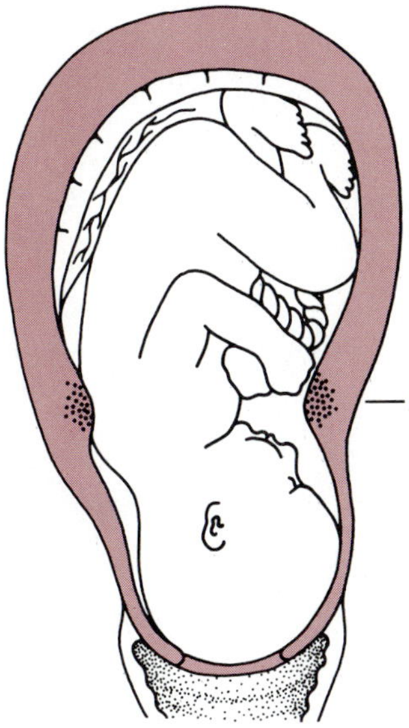

Constriction ring

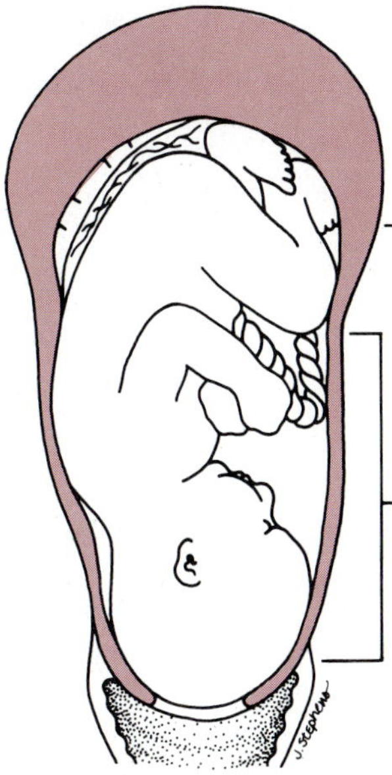

Pathologic retraction (Bandl's) ring

From Oxnorn, H. (1985). *Human labor and birth* (5th ed.). New York: Appleton-Century-Crofts.

ologic functioning are supported with IV fluids and oxygen until the delivery can be accomplished.

Implications for Nursing Care

The nurse monitors the progress of labor and fetal descent and in many cases is responsible for completing the labor graph. The midwife or physician must be notified promptly when abnormalities in progress are noted. If a retraction ring is palpated and oxytocin is being administered, the infusion is stopped immediately. The nurse should be prepared to administer tocolytics and may initate oxygen to improve fetal status if abnormal FHR patterns are evident. Continuous EFM is indicated until delivery.

The woman often complains of extreme pain when a pathologic retraction ring develops. The nurse may receive orders to administer analgesics or may assist in the administration of anesthesia. If a cesarean delivery is planned, the nurse prepares the woman for the procedure and provides guidance to the support person regarding his or her role during the birth.

Dysfunctional Labor Patterns

Uterine dystocia may be reflected in several different labor patterns: hypotonic labor, hypertonic labor, precipitous labor, and prolonged labor. These patterns also are referred to as dysfunctional labor patterns (Fig. 26-10).

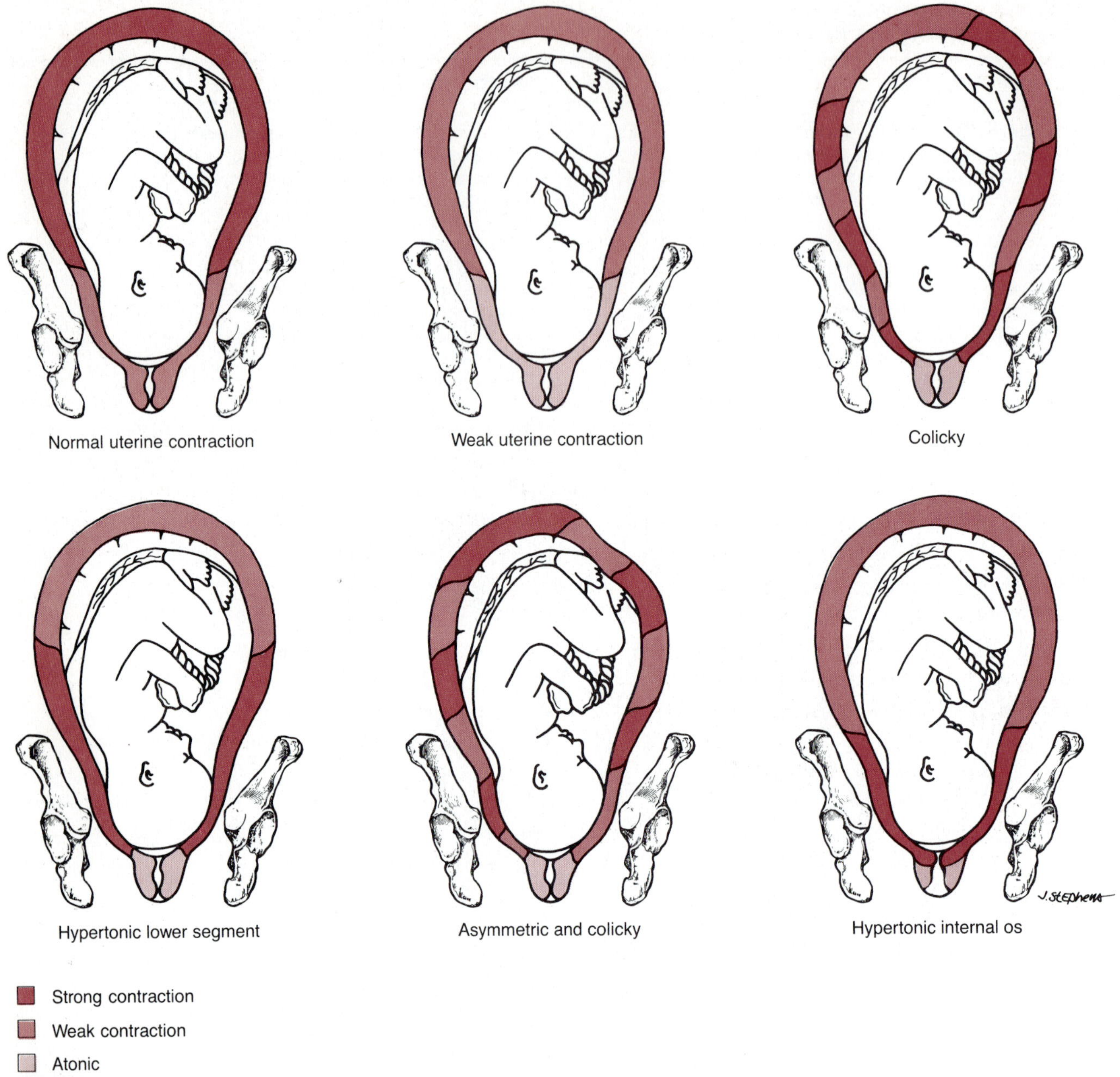

Figure 26-10.
Normal and dysfunctional uterine contraction (Childbirth Graphics).

Hypotonic Labor

Hypotonic labor is characterized by contractions that have a normal pressure gradient but are insufficiently intense or frequent to achieve cervical dilatation and fetal descent. This pattern may develop early in labor but also is observed in the active phase of labor.

Etiologic and Predisposing Factors

Hypotonic labor patterns may result from overstretching of the uterus, as in multifetal gestation or polyhydramnios. Administration of analgesia or epidural anesthesia has been implicated in this condition, particularly when given in early labor. Cephalopelvic disproportion and fetal malpresentation or malposition are predisposing factors, as is chorioamnionitis. Laboring in a supine position has been associated with prolonged labor due to less efficient contractions (Gillogley, 1991). Anxiety with the release of catecholamines also may result in hypotonic contractions (Smith, 1990).

Diagnosis

In hypotonic uterine dysfunction, contractions may exhibit a normal pattern early in labor, but then a pattern of infrequent contractions with poor intensity and low resting tone (less than 8 mm Hg on internal EFM) develops. Three patterns may be observed:

- Prolonged latent phase of labor
- Protracted or arrested active phase of labor
- Prolonged second stage of labor

Maternal, Fetal, and Neonatal Implications

Contractions are seldom painful in hypotonic labor. Labor of this kind, however, increases the risk of prolonged labor and PROM, with its attendant problems. There also is the possibility that the woman will become discouraged or frightened at the lack of noticeable progress and that her mental state will adversely affect her response to labor. She also is at increased risk for uterine atony and associated hemorrhage in the postpartum period.

If the fetus is otherwise in good condition, hypotonic labor usually does not cause adverse effects. However, fetal distress can be seen late in hypotonic labor, and subsequent neonatal sepsis may result; infection occurs secondary to prolonged labor.

Treatment

Appropriate treatment first requires that cephalopelvic disproportion, malpresentation, and obstruction due to pelvic or uterine abnormalities be ruled out. When these factors are absent, failure to progress can be assumed to be due to uterine dysfunction. Administration of IV oxytocin to augment labor usually is indicated. Thus, close monitoring of maternal and fetal status and subsequent progress in labor is essential.

Implications for Nursing Care

Nursing responsibilities in the care of a woman experiencing hypotonic labor center on close monitoring of labor progress and maternal–fetal status and promotion of effective labor through medical and nursing intervention (see the Legal/Ethical Considerations display). The nurse often is the first to identify hypotonic labor by careful analysis of labor progress and should call this to the attention of the birth attendant. The nurse also should evaluate whether maternal anxiety, sedation, or dehydration might play a role in hypotonic labor and whether comfort measures, ambulation, a change in position, or hydration and rest might facilitate effective uterine contractions. IV fluids may be ordered; the nurse must monitor intake and output and prevent bladder distention. Signs of infection should be monitored, especially if membranes are ruptured. Amniotomy may be used as a means of augmenting labor. If oxytocin administration is ordered, the nurse has a major responsibility in monitoring its effects, as discussed in Chapter 23.

Hypertonic Labor

Hypertonic labor is characterized by elevated uterine tone and an abnormal contraction pressure gradient. In such cases contractions usually are more frequent but are of only moderate intensity. Although contractions are of moderate intensity, they are not effective in dilating the cervix because fundal dominance is lacking. Hypertonic labor most often occurs in early labor and, if uncorrected, may develop into prolonged labor.

Etiologic and Predisposing Factors

Hypertonic labor occurs when fundal dominance of the contraction pattern is disrupted, often because two or more pacemakers are stimulating contractions. In most cases the

Legal/Ethical Considerations

The Role of the Labor Nurse in Determining Pelvic Shape and Capacity

In most birth settings the labor nurse is responsible for making an individual assessment of pelvic shape and size and estimating the general size of the fetus when the woman is admitted to the unit. This skill requires practice and experience but is crucial to anticipate potential problems. Specific findings that should alert the nurse to the possibility of cephalopelvic disproportion include the following:

- Fetal head unengaged during labor in the primigravid woman
- Excessively large (marcrosomic) infant
- Sharp, protruding ischial spines (narrow midpelvic transverse diameter)
- Flat or convex sacrum or immobile coccyx
- Narrow pubic arch (<90 degrees)
- Failure in fetal descent with strong uterine contractions
- Delay in the normal progress of cervical dilatation with strong uterine contractions

Expert witness testimony in medical malpractice cases has clearly established the central role of the nurse in the early identification of labor abnormalities and cephalopelvic disproportion. In most birth settings the labor nurse performs the initial pelvic examination and monitors the course of labor progress and fetal descent. The nurse is expected to update the labor graph with each vaginal examination and to notify the birth attendant in a timely manner when deviations in the normal progression of labor occur. Failure to alert the midwife or physician falls below the standard of care and makes the nurse vulnerable to allegations of negligence.

Schifrin, B., & Hamilton, T. (1991). Abnormal labor curve with inappropriate use of forceps. Journal of Perinatology, *XI(1), 63.*

cause of hypertonic labor is unknown, although cephalopelvic disproportion and fetal malposition are associated with the condition.

Diagnosis

The diagnosis is based on failure to progress in labor coupled with the observation of frequent, extremely painful contractions. When the uterus is palpated between contractions, the fundus does not completely relaxed (elevated resting tone). An internal uterine pressure catheter may be inserted to document the strength of contractions and the degree of resting tone.

Maternal, Fetal, and Neonatal Implications

The woman experiencing hypertonic labor quickly becomes exhausted and discouraged because she is making little progress and must cope with painful contractions far earlier in labor than is typical. The general resting tone of the uterus is increased, and the uterine muscle does not relax sufficiently between contractions to allow optimal perfusion of the muscle. Thus, the woman experiences increased pain with contractions due to the anoxic condition of the uterine muscle. In addition if this condition persists, her physiologic reserves will be depleted, leading to dehydration, acute fatigue, and increasing anxiety. Pain also can be intense, and the woman may need pharmacologic pain relief.

Hypertonicity of the uterus may decrease placental perfusion and place the fetus at risk for uteroplacental insufficiency and subsequent fetal distress. This may develop early and fairly rapidly, because fetal reserves are taxed by prolonged uterine contractions. Excessive pressure on the fetal head also contributes to excessive molding and to caput succedaneum and cephalohematoma formation.

Treatment

Treatment is aimed at stopping this discoordinate labor pattern and promoting more effective uterine contractions. This may be accomplished by encouraging relaxation and sleep through comfort measures and sedation. Morphine is the drug of choice to induce sedation. Often after a period of rest, the woman will awaken to a normal labor pattern. Rehydration by IV or oral fluids also may be beneficial. If this pattern persists into prolonged labor, the physician or midwife may elect amniotomy or oxytocin administration to establish more effective uterine contractions. If oxytocin is administered, close monitoring of intrauterine pressures (internal EFM) and FHR patterns is essential. Cesarean delivery is indicated if these treatment modalities fail to produce a normal labor pattern and progress in labor.

Implications for Nursing Care

With uterine hypertonicity, continuous monitoring of maternal and fetal status is especially important. FHR patterns should be carefully evaluated for signs of fetal distress. The nurse also must monitor uterine tone for tetanic contractions or development of a pathologic retraction ring (as discussed previously), because both conditions markedly increase the risk of uterine rupture. Because of the physiologic demands on the woman, adequate hydration is important; the nurse must closely monitor intake and output and observe for the presence of ketonuria, a reflection of inadequate energy and fluid balance.

The nurse also must face the challenge of finding effective comfort measures and assisting the woman and her partner in coping with this unanticipated and difficult labor experience. Pharmacologic pain relief often is indicated and may in fact be therapeutic because intense pain can be detrimental to fetal well-being with the release of catecholamines and other stress hormones.

Precipitous Labor

Precipitous labor lasts less than 3 hours before spontaneous delivery. It should be differentiated from precipitous delivery, a term applied to an unexpected and often unattended delivery.

Etiologic and Predisposing Factors

The most common cause for precipitous labor is abnormally low resistance of maternal tissue, which allows the fetus to pass easily through the pelvis and vagina. In some cases precipitous labor results from a pattern of abnormally strong and frequent uterine contractions, which may achieve an amplitude of 70 mm Hg or greater; in other cases this labor pattern is caused only by an unusually rapid sequence of uterine contractions of moderate intensity. Factors that predispose a woman to precipitous labor include the following:

- Multiparity
- Large pelvis
- Soft, pliable genital tissue
- Small fetus in normal vertex position
- Previous precipitous labor
- Cocaine abuse

Diagnosis

The diagnosis of precipitous labor is made retrospectively, although very rapid progress may alert the midwife or physician to the possibility of this condition. The woman may have very intense, frequent contractions. Progress in dilatation may occur in minutes rather than hours. When the labor graph is completed, and the total length of labor is 3 hours or less, the diagnosis is confirmed.

Maternal, Fetal, and Neonatal Implications

When the cervix is effaced and dilated and the maternal tissues are pliable, serious maternal complications rarely occur as a result of precipitous labor, despite past assertions that such dangers existed. However, maternal risk is substantially increased if precipitous labor occurs when the cervix is long and firm, contractions are vigorous, and maternal tissues are firm and resistant to stretching. These conditions place the woman at high risk for uterine rupture and lacerations of the genital tract; the risk of amniotic fluid embolism is increased as well. Postpartum maternal risk also is increased because vigorous uterine activity may predispose the woman to postpartum uterine atony and hemorrhage.

If there is minimal resistance to fetal descent and birth and if the fetus experiences adequate placental circulation despite the vigorous uterine activity, few fetal complications will result from precipitous labor. However, if the fetus is chronically stressed, its condition may further deteriorate during an abnormally brisk labor, because perfusion is reduced by uterine hypercontractility. If there is bony or soft tissue resistance to descent and delivery, trauma to the fetal head may occur. The risk of neonatal aspiration and hypothermia also is increased if the precipitous labor results in an unattended delivery where assistance is not readily available.

Treatment

If the woman has a history of precipitous labor and lives a considerable distance from the hospital, the midwife or physician may consider an elective induction of labor. This may prevent sudden, rapid labor outside of the birthing unit, with the woman unattended by her primary care provider or nurses. If a previous labor or birth occurred at home or on the way to the hospital, the benefits of elective induction of labor may outweigh its risks. If frequent, intense contractions result in fetal distress due to decreased uteroplacental perfusion, a tocolytic may be administered to reduce uterine activity.

Implications for Nursing Care

In the labor and delivery setting a woman may be admitted in advanced labor and exhibiting rapid progress toward delivery. The nurse must be prepared to evaluate the woman's labor status, alert the birth attendant and other staff as needed, and attend the delivery if necessary. The nurse immediately assesses the woman's labor pattern, stage of cervical dilatation and effacement, and fetal station and presentation. FHR should be auscultated at once and monitored for signs of apparent fetal distress. If time permits, electronic EFM is indicated to evalutate continuously the fetal response to a tumultuous labor.

Nurse-Attended Birth in the Hospital. The nurse may be required to attend the birth of an infant before the midwife or physician can arrive when precipitous labor occurs. The actions taken are described in Chapter 21 in the section discussing precipitous birth. When delivery is imminent the nurse should do the following:

- Reassure the woman that a competent nurse will remain continuously with her to assist with the birth.
- Instruct the woman in breathing techniques that facilitate relaxation and prevent forceful pushing efforts.
- Prepare sterile supplies and instruments.
- Have an additional nurse stand by, if possible, to support the parents during the birth and assist with assessing and stabilizing the infant.

Admission of the Woman Who Has Experienced an Out-of-Hospital Birth. Occasionally, the labor and delivery nurse may be required to care for a woman who has delivered before reaching the hospital. Birth may have occurred without medical and nursing assistance at home, in the car, or outside. The major goals of nursing care on admission to the unit include the following:

- Verifying or establishing effective respiratory effort in the infant
- Preventing neonatal hypothermia
- Assessing and maintaining uterine tone

The nurse must evaluate the woman for evidence of postpartum hemorrhage and should initiate an IV line if there is any indication of physiologic instability (hypotension, tachycardia, or frank bleeding). A pediatrician or nursery nurse also should be notified immediately to evaluate the infant; hypothermia, hypoglycemia, and polycythemia are common complications of an unattended precipitous birth. Giving birth without medical or nursing assistance may be a very traumatic experience for the woman and her support person, and sensitive emotional support is an essential aspect of nursing care.

Nurse-Attended Birth Out-of-Hospital. The nurse may find herself supporting a woman who unexpectedly delivers outside of the hospital or birthing center. Media accounts have profiled nurses assisting a woman during childbirth on aircrafts, in department stores, and other public places. Major objectives of care are as follows:

- Preventing maternal trauma
- Preventing transmission of infection
- Establishing the neonate's airway and maintaining respirations
- Minimizing maternal blood loss
- Preventing neonatal hypothermia
- Reasurring the woman and securing medical help

The woman should be coached in efforts that prevent expulsive pushing efforts. A Sims' or lateral position also may reduce tension on the perineum during birth. Encouraging the woman to "hold the legs together" is inappropriate. Using a clean cloth or paper barrier, the nurse may support the perineum as the head begins to crown.

Because of the risks of transmission of the human immunodeficiency virus and to prevent maternal infection, the nurse should avoid touching the vagina during the birth process. If possible, a piece of clothing or newspaper should be used as a barrier when supporting the perineum or handling the neonate at birth. Once the umbilical cord is dried, it can be tied with clean cloth ties and cut with a clean or boiled blade, new razor, or scissors if hospital care is unlikely for several hours. If hospital care can be obtained within several hours, the cord can be left intact to avoid the risk of infection from the cutting instrument. The placenta should be wrapped up and kept close to the newborn, avoiding traction on the cord. Clean cloths should be kept under the woman's buttocks, not against the perineum to catch lochial flow.

The nurse should place the newborn in a head-down position and can gently sweep the mouth with a clean cloth. Stroking the back or flicking the heels may stimulate the newborn who has not taken a first breath to initiate breathing efforts. If mouth-to-mouth resuscitation is indicated, the nurse should first take care to remove all secretions from the newborn's face to reduce the risk of infection transmission.

As soon as the infant is delivered, the nurse should observe for signs of placental separation (see Chapter 21). Traction should not be applied to the umbilical cord. Once the placenta has been delivered, the nurse should firmly massage the uterine fundus. The infant also should be placed on the breast to promote contraction of the uterine muscles.

Clean soft cloths can be used to dry the newborn. The newborn should be carefully dried, especially the head, because greatest heat loss will occur from that surface. A hat or head wrap should be fashioned from clean cloth and well secured. Hypothermia must be prevented by ensuring a consistent heat source for the newborn and woman. The newborn should be placed skin-to-skin against the mother in a position that allows for breastfeeding. The woman and newborn should be wrapped together in whatever clean materials are available, taking care not to obstruct the newborn's breathing. Once the pair are well wrapped, covers should be disturbed as little as possible, thus conserving body heat. Clean newspapers or plastic bags are good insulators and can be placed under and over the pair, followed by blankets, coats, or sleeping bags. If plastic is used, care should be taken not to cover the neonate's face. The nurse's own body can provide additional body heat to prevent neonatal hypothermia, if necessary.

The nurse should remain with the woman and newborn until help arrives and, if possible, should accompany the woman to a location where obstetric care can be provided. The nurse should then provide a report to the attending care provider about the circumstances of the birth to allow appropriate and continuous care for woman and newborn.

Prolonged Labor

Prolonged labor occurs in approximately 1% to 7% of laboring women. This complication, although relatively rare, can result in significant morbidity for the woman and the neonate.

Etiologic and Predisposing Factors

One of the major causes of prolonged labor is myometrial dysfunction. During the latent phase this may be caused by an unripe cervix (ie, one that is long, firm, and closed). Uterine contractions must work to overcome the passive resistance of the lower uterine segment and cervix. This process is impeded because the cervix must first be softened and thinned. During the active phase of labor, prolongation tends to be caused by factors that impede cervical dilatation through a lack of pressure by the presenting part, such as fetopelvic disproportion, fetal malposition, PROM, and excessive use of anesthesia or sedation, which decreases uterine motility. When these factors have been ruled out, prolonged labor, especially secondary arrest of dilatation, may be caused by myometrial fatigue and excessive maternal discomfort and anxiety.

Diagnosis

Prolonged labor is diagnosed by graphing cervical dilatation and fetal descent against time on the Friedman curve. Figure 26-11 illustrates an analysis of a primigravida experiencing an arrest disorder. In most cases the first stage is prolonged. The latent phase, active phase, or second stage of labor may also be longer than normal.

Prolonged Latent Phase of Labor. The latent phase normally lasts no longer than 20 hours in a primigravida and 14 hours in a multipara. A major challenge for the nurse or birth attendant in making a diagnosis of prolonged latent phase of labor is to distinguish between true and false labor.

Prolonged Active Phase of Labor. The active phase of labor normally lasts from 5.8 hours to 12 hours in the primigravida and 2.5 to 6 hours in the multigravida. The speed of cervical dilatation is the most important factor to consider in the active phase. Prolongation of the active phase of labor is further divided into two categories: primary dysfunctional or protracted labor and secondary arrest of dilatation.

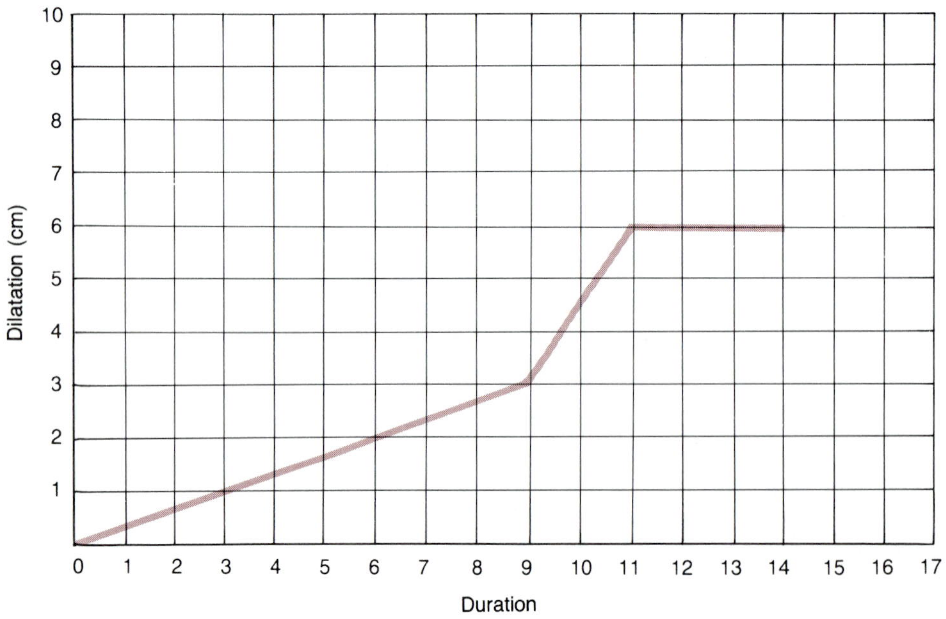

Figure 26-11.
Example of an arrest disorder in the labor of a primigravida as followed on the Friedman graph. The average normal labor duration for primigravidas is charted in Figure 19-22.

Primary dysfunctional labor occurs when there is steady progress but at a rate slower than normal; less than 1.2 cm/h in the nullipara and less than 1.5 cm/h in the multipara. Approximately 60% of women experiencing primary dysfunctional labor will deliver vaginally without assistance. The remainder may require augmentation of labor, forceps application, or cesarean delivery.

Secondary arrest of dilatation occurs when there is no cervical dilatation for 2 hours in the presence of adequate uterine forces.

Prolonged Second Stage of Labor. The second stage is considered prolonged when it exceeds 2 hours in the nullipara (3 hours with regional anesthesia) or 1 hour in the multipara (2 hours with regional anesthesia).

Maternal, Fetal, and Neonatal Implications

Exhaustion and severe emotional distress are common occurrences with dysfunctional labor. The woman and her partner are likely to become increasingly discouraged, especially if additional obstetric interventions, such as oxytocin induction, forceps application, or cesarean delivery, are performed. Infection is a common complication secondary to prolonged rupture of membranes, multiple vaginal examinations, or insertion of internal monitoring equipment. Prolonged labor also places the woman at increased risk for uterine atony and lacerations, resulting in hemorrhage and postpartum infection.

Risk of fetal morbidity and mortality increases as the length of labor increases. This risk comes primarily from the potential for fetal asphyxia as a result of reduced uteroplacental perfusion, infection, and cord prolapse when the presenting part has not engaged. Pressure on the fetal head from the bony pelvis or maternal tissue may cause soft tissue damage and occasionally cerebral trauma. Risk of head trauma also is posed by the possibility of forceps application, especially if fetal or maternal condition suddenly requires prompt delivery.

Treatment

Treatment depends largely on the type of prolonged labor and its cause. Management of prolonged latent phase of labor depends on the woman's status. If the woman is exhausted from sleep deprivation, she may be sedated and allowed to rest. In some cases labor will proceed normally when she awakens and contractions resume. If spontaneous labor does not occur, contractions can be stimulated; nipple stimulation, amniotomy, or oxytocin infusion may be initiated as discussed in Chapter 23. If dysfunctional labor continues after these measures, cesarean delivery is indicated.

If arrest of labor occurs during the active phase of labor, secondary arrest of labor, amniotomy, and an oxytocin infusion will be initiated. If no progress in cervical dilatation is noted after approximately 1 to 2 hours with adequate forces of labor, documented by intrauterine pressure monitoring, a cesarean birth is indicated.

Occasionally, prolonged second stage of labor will occur. If hypotonic or infrequent uterine contractions are diagnosed as the cause of prolonged second stage of labor, an oxytocin infusion is initiated. In some cases the administration of regional anesthesia often is an implicating factor in a prolonged second stage. If ineffective pushing efforts are a contributing cause, the birth attendant may elect to stop the continuous infusion of local anesthestic. Once regional anesthesia begins to wear off, the woman may exprience an urge to bear down; this may result in stronger bearing-down efforts.

Implications for Nursing Care

The nurse plays an indispensable role in the safe and humane care of women experiencing prolonged labor. Nursing responsibilities include close monitoring of maternal and fetal status for the adverse effects of protracted labor, including signs of fetal distress, infection, and an increasing risk of uterine rupture. The nurse administers and evaluates the effects of medications, such as analgesics, sedatives, and oxytocin. Providing comfort measures and emotional support to the woman and her partner is a major nursing function. Table 26-4 describes nursing interventions and rationale for these strategies in caring for women experiencing prolonged labor.

Pelvic Factors Causing Dystocia

In cases of pelvic dystocia the fetus is normal but labor and delivery are complicated because of problems in the size and shape of the bony pelvis. As discussed in Chapter 19, there are four types of pelves. The normal configuration, present in 50% of all women, is the gynecoid pelvis. When a normal fetus is present, dystocia in these women is rarely caused by pelvic factors. The major planes of the bony pelvis are the inlet, the midplane, and the outlet. When the diameter or shape of any of these planes is abnormal, the pelvis is said to be contracted. When more than one diameter is contracted, the risk of obstetric dystocia is significantly greater than when only one diameter is affected. Uterine contractions that would otherwise be effective are inadequate to produce fetal descent if the pelvis is too small or the head is too large (cephalopelvic disproportion).

Etiologic and Predisposing Factors

Pelvic dystocia is caused by contractures or abnormalities in the size or shape of the maternal pelvis. Variations in the shape of the pelvis result largely from genetic factors that dictate the size and configuration of the skeleton. Musculoskeletal deformities caused by rickets (due to vitamin D deficiency) or scoliosis also may lead to pelvic dystocia. Other factors, however, such as abnormal fetal size or presentation, may contribute to dystocia. A normal or average pelvis may be too small to permit the descent of a large or malpositioned fetus.

Diagnosis

The diameters of the pelvic planes can be precisely measured only by CT scan, ultrasonography, or x-ray pelvimetry. The fetal–pelvic index, a measurement of pelvic capacity and fetal head size, may be computed using a combination of x-ray pelvimetry, CT scan, and ultrasonography (Morgan & Thurnau, 1988). It may assist the primary provider in determining the likelihood of cephalopelvic dis-

Table 26-4. Nursing Interventions for Arrest of Labor

Causes of Arrest of Descent	Nursing Interventions	Rationale
Cephalopelvic Disproportion		
Maternal Factors		
Inadequate pelvic diameters	Facilitate maternal squatting position.	To increase pelvic diameters
Soft-tissue dystocia	Facilitate maternal upright position; hands and knees or supported squat. Remind patient to relax perineum.	To make use of gravity; relax perineal tissues
Excessive analgesia or anesthesia (especially regional)	Encourage more active bearing-down efforts. Allow medication to wear off	To offset decrease in urge to push caused by medication
	Use maternal upright positions, as tolerated.	To make use of gravity
Inadequate pushing	Briefly review physiology of second stage.	To offset possible lack of information
	Use maternal upright position.	To make use of gravity
	Hydrate and rest woman.	To avoid exhaustion and dehydration
	Encourage more active pushing.	
Fetal Factors		
Occipitoposterior or transverse arrest	Use upright positions; leaning forward, hands, and knees, or sidelying on the side opposite the back of the fetus.	To facilitate rotation to occipito anterior position
Deflexed head, brow, or face presentation	Use upright positions, especially squatting.	To make use of gravity to encourage flexion
Maternal Dehydration and Exhaustion		
	Rehydrate woman with oral or IV fluid.	To restore fluid, electrolyte, and glucose levels
	Encourage rest in sidelying position for 20 minutes.	
Inadequate Contractions		
Maternal stress	Reduce stress. Provide quiet, peaceful, supportive environment.	Maternal stress releases catecholamines that decrease uterine activity and blood flow.
Excessive analgesia or anesthesia	Avoid by using other comfort measures. Use nipple stimulation. Allow medication to wear off. Use upright positions, as tolerated.	Contractions are increased by oxytocin release with nipple stimulation.

proportion and dystocia. This diagnostic technique is relatively new and not universally available.

However, the maternal pelvis is clinically assessed prenatally by bimanual examination and may alert the midwife or physician to the potential for pelvic dystocia. Failure of the fetal head to engage and subsequent failure in fetal descent with intense, coordinated, and frequent contractions strongly suggest cephalopelvic disproportion. Severe fetal head molding, which may be determined during vaginal examinations, also indicates cephalopelvic disproportion.

Maternal, Fetal, and Neonatal Implications

Any pelvic contracture predisposes the woman to cephalopelvic disproportion or malposition and malpresentation of the fetus. The nature of the pelvic anomaly will determine outcomes and treatment for the woman, fetus, and neonate.

Inlet Contracture. The pelvic inlet, known also as the superior strait, is considered to be contracted when its anteroposterior diameter is 10 cm or less or when its transverse diameter is less than 12 cm. When the measurements of the inlet are smaller than normal, engagement of the presenting part may be difficult. This may result in malpresentations, particularly breech presentations, because the smaller breech may engage while descent of the fetal head is difficult or impossible.

Labor is likely to be prolonged and ineffective because the presenting part cannot descend and apply pressure to the cervix; cervical dilatation often is slow and incomplete. PROM is common, because the force of uterine activity is exerted on the membranes rather than on the fetal presenting part. If labor continues, the risk of pathologic retraction rings and uterine rupture increases.

Inlet contracture increases the risk of perinatal mortality, in part because of the higher percentage of malpositions and malpresentations. Because descent is impeded and the fetal presenting part does not occlude the cervix, the risk of cord prolapse with rupture of membranes is increased. If the fetal head is applied against the bony pelvis for long periods, there is greater danger of soft-tissue trauma, excessive molding, and skull fracture and intracranial hemorrhage.

Midpelvis Contracture. The midpelvis (midplane or plane of least dimensions) is at the level of the ischial spines. As the fetus enters the midplane, three important diameters must be negotiated successfully before it can descend to the pelvic outlet. Contractures are present if any of the following conditions exist:

- The interspinous or transverse diameter is less than 10.9 cm.
- The anteroposterior diameter measured from the inferior border of the symphysis pubis to the juncture of the sacral vertebra (S4-5) is less than 11.5 cm.
- The posterior sagittal diameter between the sacrum and the interspinous diameter is less than 4.5 cm.

Accurate measurement of these diameters requires CT pelvimetry. However, when large jutting ischial spines and a generally small pelvis are found on clinical examination, contracture of the midpelvis is probable.

Contractures of the midpelvis predispose to transverse arrest of the fetal head. If the contracture is marginal, uterine contractions may move the head past it without intervention. If this does not occur, however, cesarean delivery usually is indicated, because midforceps applications can result in significant trauma to maternal tissue and to the fetal skull. A midpelvis contracture may prevent anterior rotation of the fetal head, turning it into the hollow of the sacrum and impeding its downward progress. As with other contractures, if labor is prolonged, excessive pressure on the fetal head may result in soft tissue or skull trauma.

Outlet Contracture. The pelvic outlet is considered to be contracted when the interischial tuberous diameter is less than 8 cm. This condition commonly occurs in conjunction with other pelvic contractures.

If descent of the fetal head is protracted and forceps application is difficult, necrosis of maternal soft tissue may result, leading to the formation of fistulas in the vaginal walls. The risk of vaginal hematoma formation also may be increased.

Extreme molding and caput succedaneum formation may make it appear that the fetal head has descended lower into the birth canal than it actually has. This increases the chances that a forceps application will be difficult or unsuccessful.

Treatment

Treatment for a laboring woman with a suspected pelvic contracture includes close monitoring of labor progress and continuous monitoring of fetal status. Because the exact extent of pelvic contracture and its effect on fetal descent cannot always be accurately predicted, the birth attendant may suggest that the woman have a trial of labor with an oxytocin infusion. However, trial of labor is justified only if progressive dilatation, effacement, and fetal descent are occurring, and maternal and fetal status remains good. If trial of labor is unsuccessful and forceps application or vacuum extraction is considered unsafe, cesarean delivery is indicated.

Implications for Nursing Care

The nurse must be alert for indications of pelvic contractures. When caring for a nullipara, the nurse must recognize that the pelvis is "untested," and contractures may be present. A multiparous woman who is carrying a normal-sized fetus without evidence of malpresentation and who has had previous uncomplicated vaginal deliveries may be considered to be at less risk. Regardless of the woman's obstetric history, however, the nurse must look for any notations about pelvic adequacy on the prenatal chart and for signs of delayed engagement of the fetal presenting part, slow cervical dilatation and effacement, and a developing pattern of prolonged labor. The nurse often has primary responsibility for monitoring and documenting labor progress and therefore is responsible for alerting the physician or midwife to deviations that may suggest pelvic contractures and resulting cephalopelvic disproportion. (See the earlier Legal/Ethical Considerations display describing the nurse's responsibilities in measuring pelvic capacity.)

If a trial of labor is initiated, the nurse is responsible for administering and monitoring the oxytocin drip and for carefully observing maternal and fetal responses, as described in Chapter 22. The nurse also must pay special attention to the comfort and emotional needs of the woman and her partner, as they are experiencing a more difficult and frightening course of labor than they may have anticipated. The nurse must keep the parents informed about the progress of labor and the status of the fetus and be prepared to explain any obstetric interventions that may be needed if labor does not progress.

Soft-Tissue Factors and Structural Abnormalities Causing Dystocia

Intrapartum complications involving the reproductive tract can arise because of trauma to maternal tissue during delivery or because of preexisting structural abnormalities of the reproductive tract that affect uterine function or fetal descent through the birth canal. Structural abnormalities can occur in the vagina, cervix, and uterus, affecting the process of labor and birth.

The most common vaginal abnormality is the presence of vaginal septa. They usually are minor in significance and can be surgically removed so that vaginal birth may proceed normally.

Cervical abnormalities also may affect the course of labor and birth. Three general types of cervical abnormalities have been identified. The septate cervix consists of a ring of muscular tissue partitioned by a septum that either extends downward from the uterus or upward from the vagina or is contained completely within the cervix itself. A double cervix has two separate cervices in one uterus. A single hemicervix or half-cervix results from incomplete and asymmetric development in which only one müllerian duct matures.

Uterine abnormalities are manifested in a variety of forms, but four simplified types generally are recognized, as shown in Figure 26-12. The septate uterus appears normal from the exterior, but it contains a septum that extends partially or completely from the fundus to the cervix, dividing the uterine cavity into two separate compartments. The bicornuate uterus is roughly Y-shaped. The fundus is notched to various depths, and the woman may even appear to have a "double uterus"; however, there is only one cervix. A true double uterus results from a lack of midline fusion, and two complete uteri, each with its own cervix,

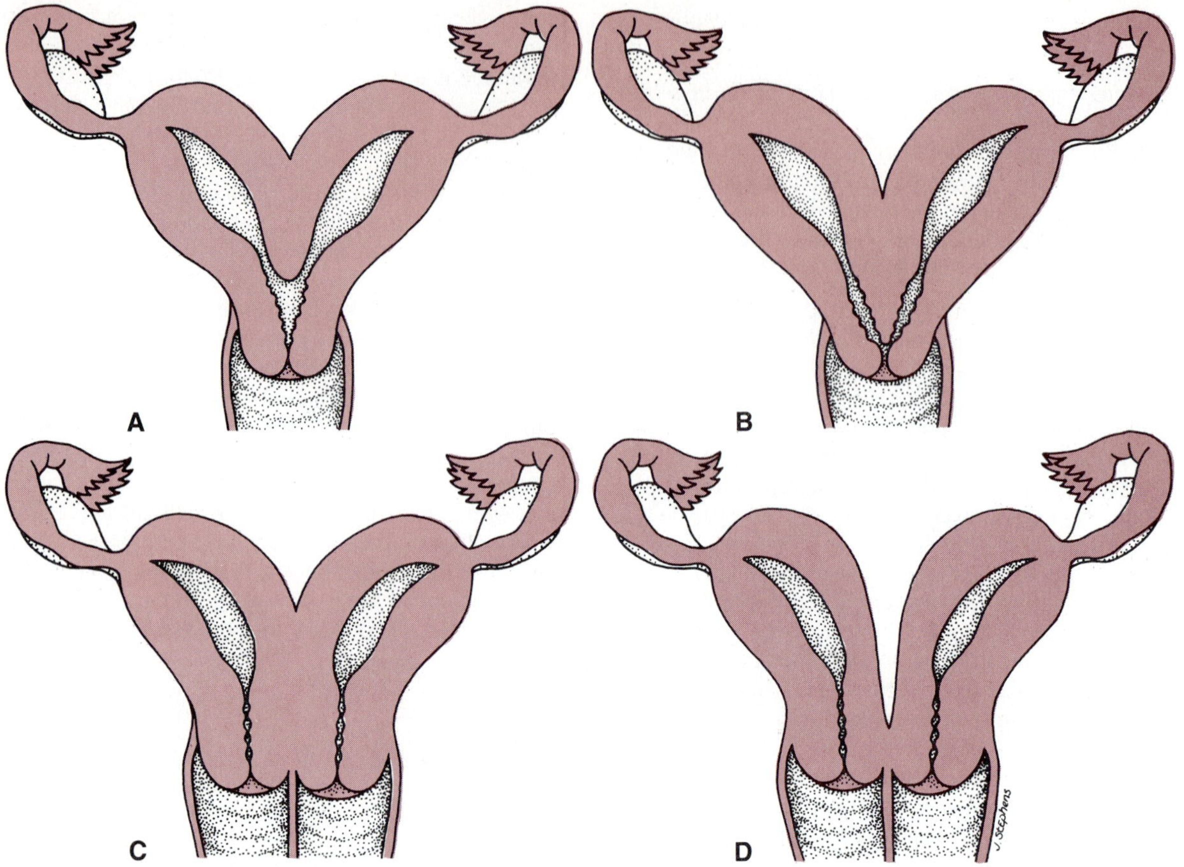

Figure 26-12.
Abnormal uterine types. *A:* Septate uterus. *B:* Bicornuate uterus. *C:* Double uterus. *D:* Uterus didelphys (Childbirth Graphics).

are formed. When both are fully formed, this anomaly may be referred to as uterus didelphys. Occasionally, one of the uteri will not fully form, remaining as a rudimentary organ without a cervix or uterine cavity. A single hemiuterus results when one müllerian duct fails to develop during embryonic growth, resulting in one uterine cavity and one oviduct.

Etiologic and Predisposing Factors

During fetal development the female reproductive tract is formed by the fusion of the two müllerian ducts. Anomalies arise primarily from the alteration of the fusion process. Failure of the ducts to fuse normally results in two partially or completely separated tracts. Failure of one duct to mature results in a one-sided tract. Incomplete fusion of one or both ducts causes faulty canalization and formation of a transverse vaginal septum or, more rarely, absence of the vagina. The cause of these disruptions in embryonic development usually is not known; however, some patterns of vaginal and cervical abnormalities have been identified in daughters born in the 1960s and 1970s to women who received diethylstilbestrol during pregnancy.

Diagnosis

Most vaginal and cervical abnormalities will be discovered prenatally when a vaginal examination is performed. Previously undiscovered uterine abnormalities may be detected after the onset of preterm labor or after the appearance of an abnormal pattern of uterine contraction in labor.

Maternal, Fetal, and Neonatal Implications

Malformations of the uterus may cause difficulty when pregnancy occurs. Depending on its configuration, the uterus may not be able to stretch sufficiently to accommodate the growing fetus and permit it to assume a normal position. The hemiuterus in particular presents a variety of problems because of its small size. Abortion, preterm labor, uterine dysfunction, and pathologic lie are more common. Uterine rupture also may be more common. Women with other uterine abnormalities may experience relatively few problems during labor and birth.

Cervical abnormalities affect labor and birth to varying degrees, depending on the ability of the cervix to dilate and efface to permit delivery. In many cases cesarean delivery is necessary; the septate cervix may function adequately to permit vaginal delivery, but vaginal birth is accompanied by an increased risk of cervical rupture and hemorrhage.

For women with minor reproductive tract abnormalities, chances for safe childbearing are good. When defects do not affect the maintenance of pregnancy and the normal development of the fetus, cesarean delivery may be selected to avoid the risk of dysfunction during labor. When uterine defects exist, perinatal loss is higher than among women without uterine abnormalities, in part reflecting a higher rate of spontaneous abortion. In addition the incidence of low birth weight due to problems in placental structure and function and of preterm labor is three times greater than in the normal population. The risk of uterine rupture during labor also is thought to be higher.

Treatment

If possible, the structural abnormalities are surgically treated before conception. Intrapartum management focuses on close monitoring of the labor pattern, uterine and cervical functioning, and fetal status. Vaginal septa usually do not present serious problems in terms of normal reproductive function. They are easily accessible and can be easily dilated or removed surgically, at which time labor and birth may proceed normally. Cesarean delivery will be performed if structural abnormalities impede normal progress or threaten fetal status.

Implications for Nursing Care

Nursing responsibilities in the intrapartum care of women with reproductive tract abnormalities include assessment and close monitoring of labor progress and maternal and fetal status and providing support and anticipatory guidance about likely outcomes of labor. Women with uterine abnormalities are more prone to preterm labor; the nurse must therefore carefully assess fetal gestational age by reviewing the woman's record for her last menstrual period, quickening date, and ultrasonography reports, when available, and by directly assessing the fundal height in centimeters. The nurse also must monitor the woman closely for signs of dystocia and impending uterine rupture. Nursing care for the woman with uterine complications, such as preterm labor, dystocia, and uterine rupture, is discussed earlier in this chapter. When vaginal delivery is being attempted, careful assessment of fetal descent and progress through the birth canal is especially important, as is close fetal monitoring.

Dystocia means difficult labor. It may result from fetal, uterine, or pelvic factors or abnormalities of the reproductive tract. Dystocia may impede the progress of labor and place the woman, fetus, and newborn at risk. When the progress of labor is prolonged, the nurse is responsible for notifying the midwife or physician immediately. Dystocia causes anxiety, pain, and fatigue for the woman. The nurse provides physical and emotional support while continuing to monitor progress and provide information.

Emergent Maternal Complications

Shock and DIC may develop during the intrapartum period. These maternal conditions involve several physiologic systems and pose a severe threat to the woman and fetus. These are true emergency situations, and although rare, they require immediate diagnosis and treatment to prevent maternal or fetal or neonatal death. The following sections discuss these conditions and a third intrapartum emergency, amniotic fluid embolism, which characteristically presents with both of these problems in the intrapartum patient.

Shock

Shock is the body's response to life-threatening physiologic conditions. A variety of mechanisms are used to protect the functioning of vital organs. However, the response itself can become a threat to survival and in extreme cases can be reversed only through aggressive therapy, often including cardiopulmonary resuscitation.

There are four types of shock: hypovolemic, septic, cardiogenic, and neurogenic. In pregnancy and especially in the intrapartum period, hypovolemic and septic shock are most common. The classification of shock associated with maternity care is summarized in the accompanying display and the following section discusses hypovolemic and septic shock.

Classification of Shock Associated With Maternity Care

Hypovolemic Shock

- Hemorrhagic shock associated with
  - Ectopic pregnancy
  - Placenta previa/abruptio placentae
  - Uterine rupture
  - Postpartum/postabortion hemorrhage
  - Obstetric surgery

Septic Shock

- Prenatal or postpartum infection
- Septic abortion
- Chorioamnionitis
- Pyelonephritis
- Postpartum systemic infection

Cardiogenic Shock

- Failure of left ventricular filling associated with
  - Cardiac tamponade associated with coagulation defects
  - Pulmonary embolism
  - Thrombophlebitis

Neurogenic Shock

- Chemical injury associated with aspiration of gastrointestinal contents
- Drug toxicity associated with spinal anesthesia
- Inversion of the uterus with vasomotor collapse
- Electrolyte imbalance associated with hyponatremia

Hypovolemic Shock

When large amounts of blood are lost, the body compensates by maintaining blood pressure to minimize the adverse effects of decreased perfusion on tissues. At first, increased respiratory efforts help to maintain venous flow to the heart. Generalized vasoconstriction resulting from catecholamine release from the adrenals ensures that blood pressure and blood flow to essential organs (such as brain, kidneys, heart muscle, and lungs) are temporarily maintained.

This compensatory mechanism is effective until 20% to 25% of circulating blood volume is lost; when this level is surpassed, shock becomes severe. Cardiac output may fall as much as 50%. The body's ability to supply oxygen is overcome, and the continued reduction in cell oxygenation results in an accumulation of lactic acid. Acidosis ensues, and vasodilation in arterioles results in pooling of blood. Perfusion of vital organs is compromised. Renal blood flow is reduced, and urinary output decreases. Massive electrolyte changes occur, and oxygenation of all tissues is compromised. Ultimately, if shock is not reversed, swelling of lung tissue leads to adult respiratory distress syndrome, profound metabolic acidosis, and death. Once adequate perfusion to the brain stops, brain damage and "brain death" occur within 5 minutes.

Septic Shock

The precipitating factor in septic shock usually is endotoxin from pathologic gram-negative organisms. The incidence of gram-negative sepsis among hospitalized patients has been increasing in recent years, and mortality averages 50% in documented cases. The early phase of septic shock may be referred to as "warm" and is characterized by normal or increased cardiac output and warm, dry skin. These symptoms may be easily overlooked, and by the time they appear oxygen consumption is already considerably reduced as a result of impaired cellular metabolism.

When septic shock is not recognized in this early phase and fluid replacement is not instituted, hypovolemic shock results, and the "cold" phase of septic shock begins. Severe cellular damage from the effects of endotoxins causes malfunction of the vascular system; blood pressure falls dramatically, causing markedly reduced tissue perfusion. At this point severe shock is present, with the associated problems of profound metabolic acidosis. Adult respiratory distress syndrome and death may result.

Etiologic and Predisposing Factors

The most common causes of hypovolemic shock in the intrapartum period are placental accidents, uterine rupture, uterine atony, and severe lacerations of the genital tract. Hypovolemic shock also may be triggered by hemorrhage associated with DIC. Obstetric patients who are at particular risk for septic shock are those with infections resulting from septic abortions, chorioamnionitis, pyelonephritis, and septic pelvic thrombophlebitis.

Diagnosis

Signs and symptoms of hypovolemic and septic shock appear in the accompanying display. The major goal of medical and nursing care is the early identification of signs and symptoms so that compensatory mechanisms can be supported and uncompensated shock averted.

Signs and Symptoms of Shock

Hypovolemic Shock

Signs

- Tachypnea (deep and rapid)
- Tachycardia
- Weak, thready pulse
- Hypotension
- Narrowed pulse pressure
- Increased capillary fill time (>4 sec)
- Oliguria (less than 20–30 mL/h)
- Urine sodium = 80 mEq/L
- Cool, clammy skin
- Pallor and peripheral cyanosis
- Hypothermia

Symptoms

- Anxiety, restlessness, disorientation
- Thirst, dry mouth
- Feeling chilled

Septic Shock

Signs

- Tachycardia
- Hyperdynamic pulse
- Tachypnea, respiratory alkalosis
- Hypotension
- Cerebral ischemia
- Polyuria, urine sodium 10 mEq/L
- Hyperthermia (in early septic shock)

Symptoms

- Palpitations
- Faintness, dizziness
- Anxiety, apprehension, disorientation, stupor

Maternal, Fetal, and Neonatal Implications

Hypovolemic or septic shock in the intrapartum period poses a direct threat to maternal survival. Symptoms can develop rapidly, producing the need for emergency interventions, including blood and fluid replacement, cesarean delivery, and cardiopulmonary resuscitation. The woman generally is aware of the seriousness of the situation as her condition deteriorates. She may be cognizant of her surroundings and events taking place, even if she cannot communicate verbally with staff. She may experience fear for her own survival and for her fetus if delivery has not been accomplished.

One consequence of severe hemorrhagic shock and DIC is postdelivery anterior pituitary necrosis, also known as

Sheehan's syndrome. This constellation of symptoms, reflecting partial or total loss of endocrine function, including thyroid, adrenocortical, and gonadal insufficiency, affects a small percentage of women who survive profound hemorrhagic shock and DIC. The exact cause of this syndrome is unknown. The symptoms, which include lactation failure, amenorrhea, breast atrophy, genital atrophy, and loss of pubic and axillary hair, suggest varying degrees of anterior pituitary damage and the resulting impaired secretion of its trophic hormones. Treatment, which includes hormonal replacement, is supportive, and the prognosis depends on the degree of damage sustained.

The fetus is directly threatened by maternal shock, primarily because uteroplacental perfusion is compromised. The fetal response is similar to the woman's. Hypoxemia and acidosis cause bradycardia, vasospasm, and shunting of blood to vital organs. As the maternal condition worsens and these compensatory mechanisms can no longer function, brain damage and fetal death occur.

Treatment

Treatment of maternal shock in the intrapartum period requires rapid response to the first signs of decompensation. The order of priorities in the management of shock is shown in the accompanying Nursing Procedure.

Intravenous Access and Provision of Blood and Fluids. The most immediate concern in shock is to gain access to the vascular system and maintain IV access for administration of blood and fluids. At least two IV lines are started with a 16- or 18-gauge angiocath to prevent hemolysis with blood transfusions. A lactated Ringer's solution is indicated for all types of hypovolemic shock and may be used as an emergency volume expander while blood is being typed and crossmatched. Rapid fluid replacement also is possible with 0.9 normal saline solution; however, hypernatremia, hypokalemia, and metabolic acidosis are major concerns when large volumes are infused. A central venous pressure line may be inserted to provide accurate measurement of venous return and adequacy of fulid replacement.

Blood transfusions are indicated with massive blood loss; whole blood, packed red blood cells, plasma, and 5% albumin are common components used in transfusions. Additional information about blood replacement is found in Table 26-5 and in the Nursing Procedure, Administering Blood Products. As a result of the acquired immunodeficiency syndrome epidemic, advances in blood collection and transfusion therapy may now permit certain women at high risk for hemorrhage during the intrapartum period to donate their own blood in advance of delivery (Penney, 1991). Research indicates that autologous blood transfusions are feasible and safe during pregnancy (see the Nursing Research display).

An indwelling urinary catheter is inserted to allow for accurate monitoring of urinary output; 50 mL/h or more indicates adequate renal perfusion. Output of less than 30 mL/h is not a reassuring sign, reflecting either worsening shock or inadequate fluid replacement.

Improvement of Oxygenation and Tissue Perfusion. The woman is placed in a sidelying or supine position with right hip elevated to improve venous return and increase uterine perfusion. Blood flow to the brain and other vital organs also is improved by the supine position. The legs may be elevated 20 to 30 degrees. A patent airway must be maintained, and oxygen is administered at 8 to 12 L/min by tight face mask.

Correction of the Underlying Problem. Medical management requires treatment of the underlying cause of shock in the obstetric patient. In the case of placenta previa, massive abruption, or uterine rupture, emergency cesarean delivery is indicated. Septic shock requires antimicrobial therapy; neurogenic shock due to an inverted uterus may in some instances require emergency hysterectomy.

Implications for Nursing Care

The role of the nurse in the identification and treatment of shock is critical to the long-term outcome for the woman and her fetus. Timely management is essential to prevent irreversible cellular damage and death. The appropriate steps in the immediate treatment of shock are described in the Nursing Procedure, Managing the Patient in Shock.

Identifying of Shock. A primary nursing responsibility is early detection of hemorrhage and signs of impending shock. Identifying risk factors that place the woman at risk for shock is an essential aspect of this process. Tachypnea or tachycardia may be the first signs, followed by hypotension. In septic shock warm, flushed skin; subtle alterations in mentation; and an increase in urine output may be the first indications of shock. (See the earlier display for a review of the signs and symptoms of hypovolemic and septic shock.)

Administering Blood and Fluids. The nurse must stay with the woman, alert other staff, and take quick action to intervene if, on the basis of these signs, impending shock is suspected. While waiting for assistance, the nurse should initiate an IV line with a large-gauge angiocath and begin infusion of fluids as described previously. The nurse's responsibilities in the administration of blood products are described in the Nursing Procedure, Administering Blood Products, which appears earlier in this chapter.

Monitoring and Supporting Maternal and Fetal Physiologic Status. The nurse positions the woman on her left side, begins oxygen administration, and prepares ventilation and suction equipment for use. The legs may be elevated 20 to 30 degrees.

Maternal pulse, respirations, and blood pressure must be checked and recorded every 2 to 5 minutes. The use of an electronic blood pressure monitor will facilitate this process. A pulse oximeter should be applied to evaluate blood oxygen saturation. Observations of skin color, temperature, and level of consciousness must be recorded as well. Continuous EFM is indicated to identify signs of developing fetal distress. Because shock may be complicated by DIC, bruising and signs of bleeding from puncture sites, nose, or gums indicate the need for immediate blood-clotting studies.

Fluid overload is a major complication of replacement

NURSING PROCEDURE
Managing the Patient in Shock

Purpose: To prevent uncompensated shock, exsanguination, and death.

NURSING ACTION	RATIONALE
Obtain Additional Assistance	
1. Call for help.	To obtain assistance with initiating the following steps and in notifying appropriate medical personnel.
Restore Circulating Volume	
1. Initiate an IV line with a large-gauge angiocath (16 or 18 g)	To permit rapid infusion of blood and fluids.
2. Insert a second line when help arrives.	
3. Attach extension tubing to the hub of the angiocath.	To permit multiple tubing changes as blood is transfused. Blood tubing must be change after every 2 to 3 units of blood are infused.
4. Use blood tubing when starting the intravenous line.	To permit blood replacement therapy and avoid a delay when blood arrives.
5. Administer lactated Ringer's solution or 0.9 normal saline rapidly until medical help and blood products arrive.	To provide a balanced salt (physiologic) solution and avoid hemolysis or swelling of red blood cells, which may occur with the rapid infusion of hypo- or hyperosmotic solutions.
6. Draw blood for type and crossmatching procedures and send to lab.	To permit prompt preparation of blood as it is ordered by the physician.
7. Assemble equipment for insertion of central venous or central arterial monitoring.	To permit more precise measurement of fluid replacement therapy.
Improve Tissue Perfusion and Oxygenation	
1. Maintain patent airway. Administer oxygen 10–12 L/min by tight face mask.	To improve oxygenation of tissues.
2. Place woman on left side in supine position.	To prevent supine hypotension syndrome.
3. Elevate legs 20 to 30 degrees.	To improve blood return to heart and brain.
4. Be prepared to assist with obtaining arterial blood for Ph and gas analysis.	To determine degree of shock and effectiveness of blood and fluid replacement therapy.
Administer Drug Therapy	
1. Avoid vasopressors, such as ephedrine, as a general rule.	May temporarily elevate blood pressure and mask severity of true blood loss.
2. Digitalize if in cardiac failure.	To improve cardiac function and tissue perfusion.
3. Administer Lasix as ordered if pulmonary edema develops.	To reduce fluid and lung and improve gas exchange.
4. Be prepared to administer other drugs, such as dopamine.	To improve cardiac output.
Evaluate Physiologic Status and Response to Treatment	
1. Apply appropriate monitoring equipment: pulse oximeter, cardiorespiratory monitor, electronic blood pressure monitor.	To permit rapid or continuous data regarding cardiopulmonary status.
2. Monitor central venous pressure or central arterial data.	To evaluate effectiveness of fluid and blood replacement therapy.
3. Evaluate color, capillary filltime, skin temperature.	To evaluate tissue perfusion
4. Assess breath sounds; observe for neck vein distention. Insert Foley catheter to drainage and measure output.	To identify signs of fluid overload and pulmonary edema.
5. Measure all blood loss (weigh linens or linen protectors).	To estimate total blood loss and to provide physician with information about blood loss.
Assist With Treatment of the Basic Problem	
1. Prepare woman for emergency surgery.	To correct source of hemorrhage (ie, placenta previa).

Nursing Research

Autologous Blood Transfusion During Pregnancy

In the past pregnant women were not permitted to donate homologous blood because of the unknown effects on the fetus. With the advent of electronic EFM and ultrasonography, it is possible to monitor fetal well-being during blood donation. Increasing concern for the transmission of transfusion-associated infectious diseases has led to research on the effects of autologous transfusions during pregnancy.

Possible indications for autologous transfusions include the following:

- Anticipated primary or repeat cesarean birth
- Placenta previa without antenatal hemorrhage or anemia
- History of large blood loss at previous delivery (ie, postpartum hemorrhage)
- History of transfusion at previous delivery
- Multiple gestation

Furthermore, some women who object to blood transfusion on religious grounds may be amenable to autologous transfusion.

Research indicates no adverse fetal effects during the donation on homologous blood, and the incidence of vasovagal reactions in the women was similar to non-pregnant donors. It appears that blood may be donated in the second or third trimester. One study found that women who donated blood during the final week before delivery were more likely to need transfusions. it is recommended that donation does not occur any later than 2 to 4 weeks prior to delivery to provide time for replacement of blood cell mass.

Andres, R., Piacquandio, & Resnik, R. (1990). A reappraisal of the need for autologous blood donation in the obstetric patient. *American Journal of Obstetrics and Gynecology, 163*(5), 1551.

Penny, D. (1991). Autologous blood use in obstetrics. *NAACOGs Clinical Issues in Perinatal and Women's Health Nursing, 2*(3), 344.

therapy. The nurse's role in the prevention and treatment of fluid overload includes the following actions:

- Carefully monitor fluid intake and urine output.
- Frequently monitor blood pressure; hypertension suggests overload.
- Observe for signs of pulmonary edema: rales, cough, shortness of breath, neck vein distension.
- Assess urine-specific gravity levels: decreasing value indicates hemodilution.
- Monitor central venous pressure; a significant rise indicates fluid overload (Fig. 26-13).

Providing Emotional Support. If the partner, other family member, or support person is present, the nurse should quickly explain the situation, assist him or her to a waiting area, and make an effort to obtain another staff member to keep the family informed and as comfortable as can be expected under the circumstances. The nurse also

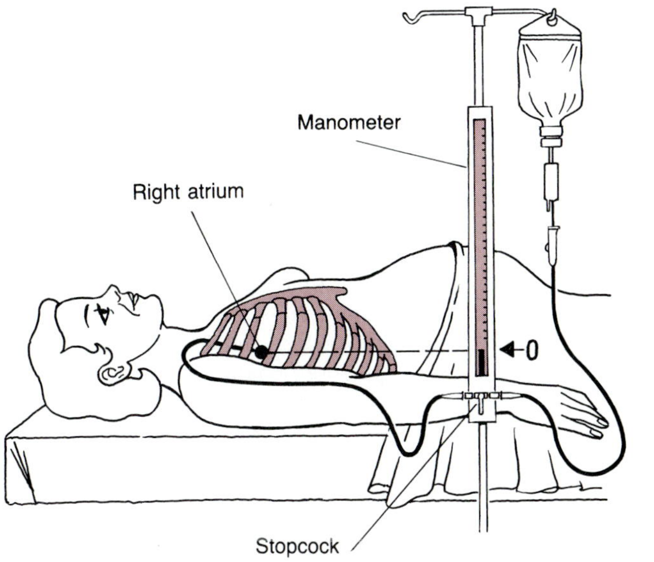

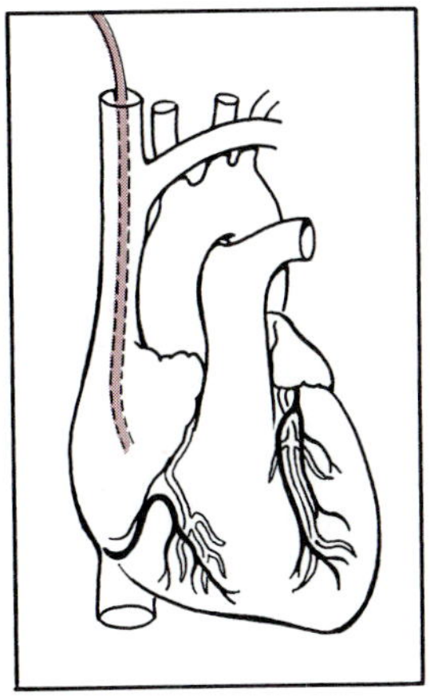

Figure 26-13.
Central venous pressure monitoring. A central venous catheter is inserted by a physician in the subclavian or internal jugular vein and threaded until the catheter tip rests in the superior vena cava or right atrium of the heart. The catheter is connected to a fluid-filled manometer, which permits measurements of central venous pressure (CVP). This procedure permits more precise monitoring of fluid replacement therapy.

must recognize that the woman may be cognizant of events although unable to communicate; an effort to explain procedures and provide reassurance should be made without disruption of emergency measures.

Disseminated Intravascular Coagulation

DIC may occur as a result of physiologic insult late in pregnancy or the intrapartum period. This condition is characterized by generation of increased prothrombin, platelets, and other coagulation factors that cause widespread formation of thrombi throughout the microvasculature. Eventually, the body's clotting factors are expended, and severe hemorrhage begins.

In normal pregnancy the levels of certain clotting factors are increased, which may help prevent exsanguination at birth. The most significant is a 50% increase in fibrinogen concentration over the nonpregnant state. This is believed to be related to the normally high levels of estrogen during pregnancy. Platelet count and prothrombin levels are not increased in normal pregnancy. However, conditions such as placental bleeding, IUFD, and sepsis predispose the pregnant woman to DIC. DIC may develop insidiously during pregnancy or suddenly.

Etiologic and Predisposing Factors

A pathologic event, such as IUFD or placental bleeding, activates normal clotting mechanisms and, if clotting factors are depleted, can initiate DIC. Such pathologic events may include the following:

- Septic shock
- Placental or profuse uterine bleeding
- Release of fetal thromboplastin after IUFD
- Amniotic fluid embolism
- Formation of thrombi in kidney, liver, or cerebral vessels secondary to preeclampsia and eclampsia

Diagnosis

Thrombocytopenia, decreasing fibrinogen, and prolonged prothrombin time are early signs of developing coagulopathy, and baseline laboratory studies should be obtained on women thought to be at risk for DIC. Maternal symptoms include bleeding from puncture sites and gums or other unusual bleeding, such as hematuria, and the presence of hemorrhagic areas in the skin (ecchymosis). Platelet count and fibrinogen levels decrease, while prothrombin and partial thromboplastin time increase. A tentative diagnosis of DIC can be made when coagulation studies are reported.

Maternal, Fetal, and Neonatal Implications

With diagnosis of DIC immediate intensive care is necessary. Often the woman is moved to an intensive care unit, with obstetric staff providing assistance in monitoring fetal status. The woman is extremely ill and will require extensive medical intervention to correct coagulopathy. She may be aware of the seriousness of the situation and is likely to be fearful for her own life and that of her fetus.

Fetal or neonatal risk is increased not by DIC, but by other maternal physiologic problems, such as sepsis, acidosis, and hypotension. The major risk facing the fetus or neonate is that of hypoxia. In catastrophic situations in which maternal status is deteriorating rapidly, emergency cesarean delivery may be necessary to save the life of the fetus.

Treatment

Treatment of DIC must include treatment of the causative factor, as well as replacement of maternal coagulation factors and support of physiologic functioning. The first 2 hours of care are critical to survival, and vital signs and renal output must be supported. Treatment of the cause usually involves delivery of the fetus, removal of the placenta, and stabilization of the maternal condition.

Except when amniotic fluid embolism is the cause, evacuation of the uterine contents often eliminates the cause of DIC. Vaginal delivery is preferable if maternal condition permits. Surgical procedures, such as episiotomy and cesarean delivery, place more stress on hemostatic mechanisms; however, many women are too ill for continued labor and vaginal delivery, and in such cases cesarean delivery is indicated.

Replacement of depleted coagulation factors usually is accomplished by whole blood infusion (donor fresh at 6 to 12 hours). Other blood components also may be used, as shown in Table 26-5.

Renal failure is a serious consequence of DIC; urinary output must be carefully monitored and output maintained at 30 to 50 mL/h. When blood components are rapidly available and used early, kidney function usually is adequately maintained.

Implications for Nursing Care

An important nursing responsibility is early detection of DIC in the intrapartum patient. The nurse should assess the woman's history for possible predisposing factors. If the woman is identified as at risk, emergency equipment for blood administration and blood components should be readily available. The reader is referred to the Nursing Procedure, Administering Blood Products, earlier in this chapter for further discussion of the nurse's responsibilities during blood transfusion.

The nurse must recognize signs of unusual bleeding and notify the physician immediately if bleeding occurs from IV puncture sites, gums, or nose or if there is unusual vaginal bleeding or hematuria. The nurse should alert other staff for assistance, stay with the woman, and apply direct pressure to bleeding puncture sites until bleeding stops. Vital signs and FHR must be monitored frequently. If the woman exhibits signs of anxiety or agitation, restraints or padded rails are needed to prevent bruising.

The nurse should expedite the process of obtaining laboratory studies and notifying the blood bank of the possible need for coagulation factors and other blood components. An IV line with large-bore needle for blood administration and an indwelling urinary catheter will be needed. The nurse should be prepared to assist with placement of a central venous pressure catheter in case one is needed. Oxygen administration by mask should be initiated and the woman placed in a left, sidelying position to prevent maternal hypotension and fetal hypoxia.

Table 26-5. Component Replacement

Replacement Component	Factors Present	Nursing Interventions
Fresh whole blood	All factors	Use immediately and complete transfusion within 2–3 hours. Perform careful pretransfusion check of blood type, RH factor, and patient identification. Make sure crossmatching is completed. Use blood tubing with inline filter. If infusing rapidly, use blood warmer. Observe closely for transfusion reactions (uticaria, fever, chills, shortness of breath). (See Nursing Procedure for blood transfusions.)
Fresh frozen plasma	All factors except platelets	Use within 30 minutes to minimize rapid deterioration of coagulation factors. Perform pretransfusion check of blood type, Rh factor, and patient identification. Verify that crossmatching was completed. Use blood tubing with inline filter. Observe for transfusion reactions (same as whole blood).
Platelets	Only platelets	Infuse as rapidly as possible. Infuse at room temperature. Perform pretransfusion patient identification check. Make sure donor plasma and recipient blood are typed for ABO incompatibility. Crossmatching is not necessary. Do not use standard, inline blood filter. Use nonwettable tubing kit provided with platelets. Observe for febrile reaction. Transfusion reaction rare because contains few red blood cells.
Cryoprecipitate	Fibrinogen, factor VIII, and factor XIII	Infuse as quickly as possible. Observe for febrile and allergic reactions.

The nurse also must recognize that the woman usually is fearful about the complication and its treatment. The nurse provides as much emotional support as possible, given the emergency situation; brief explanations of necessary procedures can be given without interrupting the flow of care. Other staff can be mobilized to stay with family members, keeping them informed and providing emotional support.

Uterine Rupture

Rupture of the uterus during labor is a potential obstetric catastrophe that threatens the woman and fetus. Although uterine rupture is rare in the United States, occurring in approximately 1 in 1500 deliveries, it is more common in underdeveloped countries where home deliveries are the norm and obstetric care is limited. Although better obstetric management has improved maternal and fetal outcomes after uterine rupture, it still accounts for 5% of all maternal deaths. When uterine rupture occurs, 50% of all instances result in fetal demise.

Rupture of the uterus can be complete or incomplete. Complete rupture extends through the entire uterine wall, and the uterine contents are extruded into the abdominal cavity (Fig. 26-14). Incomplete rupture extends through the

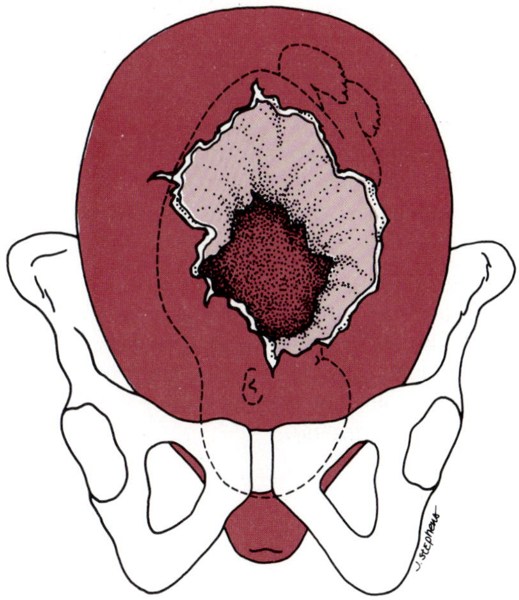

Figure 26-14.
Uterine rupture (Childbirth Graphics).

endometrium and myometrium, but the peritoneum surrounding the uterus remains intact. Uterine rupture often occurs in the thinned-out lower uterine segment. Incomplete tears may occur along previous uterine scars. Another term used synonymously with incomplete rupture is dehiscence, the bursting open of a surgical scar.

Etiologic and Predisposing Factors

The most common predisposing factor for traumatic uterine rupture is a preexisting scar, which results in a weakening or defect in the myometrium that does not stretch as well as surrounding tissue. Rupture is considered more likely from a vertical (classic) cesarean incision. Low transverse uterine incisions from previous cesarean deliveries are not as prone to rupture and thus do not preclude a subsequent normal labor (see Chapter 23 for a discussion of vaginal birth after a cesarean delivery).

Rupture of the pregnant uterus may be classified as traumatic or spontaneous; either type can occur in the presence or absence of a uterine scar. Traumatic uterine rupture usually is associated with a previous uterine scar and the application of excessive force to the labor, sometimes from imprudent obstetric interference. Causes of traumatic uterine rupture include the following:

- Trauma from instruments (such as use of a uterine sound or curet or tools used to induce abortion)
- Obstetric intervention: forceps delivery
- High vacuum extraction
- Excessive fundal pressure
- Tumultuous labor
- Violent bearing-down efforts
- Internal podalic version
- Forceps rotation
- Shoulder dystocia
- Induced uterine hypertonicity from oxytocin infusion
- Manual removal of the placenta (rare)

Spontaneous uterine rupture before the onset of labor is rare. During labor it is most likely to occur under the following conditions:

- Previous uterine surgery, such as low-segment cesarean section, myomectomy, salpingectomy, curettage, or manual removal of the placenta
- Grand multiparity combined with the use of oxytocic agents to stimulate labor
- Cephalopelvic disproportion, malpresentation, or hydrocephalus

Uterine rupture that occurs in the absence of a scar often is an obstetric emergency. Maternal death from hemorrhage and shock may occur. On the other hand uterine dehiscence or small ruptures actually may go undetected. Signs that reflect an abnormal thinning of the uterine wall may signal an impending uterine rupture.

Signs and Symptoms in Uterine Rupture

Signs and Symptoms of Impending Uterine Rupture

- Restlessness and anxiety
- Severe lower abdominal pain
- Lack of progress in cervical dilatation or fetal descent
- Presence of a palpable ridge of uterus above the symphysis pubis
- Presence of retraction ring (indentation across the lower abdominal wall) between upper and lower uterine segments
- Acute tenderness above the symphysis
- Tetanic contractions

Signs and Symptoms of Incomplete Uterine Rupture

- Tenderness or pain in the abdomen associated with increasing uterine irritability before the onset of labor
- Small amounts of vaginal bleeding
- Persistence and intensification of abdominal pain and tenderness between contractions
- Rebound tenderness of the abdomen
- Abdominal distention beyond that expected in normal pregnancy
- Appearance of a retraction ring across the lower abdomen
- Thinning and ballooning of the lower uterine segment, similar in appearance to a full bladder
- Lack of progress in cervical dilatation

Signs and Symptoms of Complete Uterine Rupture

- Intense, sharp, tearing pain in the lower abdomen
- Palpation of fetal parts outside the uterine wall
- Abrupt cessation of uterine contractions
- Ascent of presenting part on vaginal examination relative to previous position
- Gross hematuria from bladder damage
- Rapid onset of signs of fetal distress
- Loss of fetal heart rate (fetal death)
- Progressive signs of maternal hypovolemic shock

Diagnosis

Symptoms of rupture may appear immediately or may not appear until the postpartum period, when anesthesia or sedation has worn off. This reflects the fact that signs and symptoms of uterine rupture may vary from very mild to severe and acute (see the display, Signs and Symptoms of Uterine Rupture). Factors that determine when symptoms appear and their severity include the following:

- Site and extent of the rupture
- Degree of extrusion of the uterine contents
- Occurrence or absence of intraperitoneal spill of amniotic fluid and blood

Complete ruptures, those involving the lower uterine segment and the body of the uterus, and those in which extrusion is marked or there is intraperitoneal spill usually are associated with rapid onset of severe symptoms. However, symptoms of uterine rupture often are difficult to differentiate from those of other pathologic events. Women in labor may report an internal tearing sensation, which may or may not be painful, just before the actual rupture; this may be the most characteristic symptom of uterine rupture.

The most common symptom of uterine rupture is diffuse pain or pain localized to the umbilical and epigastric region, which may be referred to the shoulder (reflecting diaphragmatic irritation). Women who have experienced uterine rupture before the onset of labor may experience continuous or intermittent pain that may easily be confused with labor.

When diagnosis of uterine rupture is not clear on the basis of these clinical signs, other diagnostic tests may be used. X-ray films of the abdomen may show the fetus lying abnormally high and outside the uterus. Free fluid or air may be seen in the abdominal cavity. Ultrasonography may show the absence of the amniotic cavity within the uterus. Culdocentesis (aspiration of fluid through the posterior vaginal fornix) may reveal the presence of blood in the abdominal cavity.

Maternal, Fetal, and Neonatal Implications

Maternal risks associated with uterine rupture depend on the extent of the injury. Small tears may be asymptomatic; they may heal spontaneously and remain undetected until subsequent labor strains the scar, resulting in more serious damage. More severe ruptures present the risk of irreversible maternal hypovolemic shock or subsequent peritonitis. Maternal hypovolemia and fetal extrusion out of the uterus through the rupture with loss of placental circulation present major risks to the fetus. Anoxia is very common, and fetal or neonatal death occurs in 50% to 75% of all cases of complete rupture. Survival depends on prompt surgical delivery and immediate neonatal resuscitation.

Treatment

Vaginal delivery generally is not attempted if signs of possible uterine rupture are present, because vaginal delivery will present greater risks to the woman and fetus. If symptoms of uterine rupture are severe, emergency cesarean delivery will be performed to attempt immediate delivery of the fetus, establish hemostasis, and allow for surgical repair of the uterus. The type of surgical procedure required will vary according to the extent of uterine damage. A repair of the uterine tear may be attempted, or hysterectomy may be required. Hysterectomy may be lifesaving for the woman if bleeding cannot otherwise be controlled.

A central venous pressure catheter may be inserted by anesthesia personnel to permit assessment of blood loss and to monitor effects of fluid and blood replacement. A radial artery line also may be inserted so that blood samples may be obtained for gas and pH analysis.

Implications for Nursing Care

Nursing responsibilities begin with identification of maternal factors that may predispose a woman to uterine rupture and close monitoring of the labor pattern to identify uterine hypertonicity or signs of a weakening uterine muscle.

When uterine rupture occurs, the first nursing concern after calling for help is to correct maternal hypovolemic shock and prepare for an emergency cesarean birth. Time is of the essence; the priority is to control hemorrhage and prevent fetal death through rapid surgical intervention. The following procedures will be implemented in preparation for delivery:

- Insertion of an IV line for administration of fluids and blood
- Rapid infusion of a lactated Ringer's solution or 0.9 normal saline
- Administration of oxygen to prevent or reduce maternal and fetal hypoxia
- Insertion of an indwelling Foley catheter

The woman is transported to the delivery room or surgical suite, and if time permits, the abdomen may be shaved while general anesthesia is administered. Continuous monitoring of maternal vital signs and FHR is required until the obstetrician arrives to perform the delivery.

The nurse must respond in a calm, efficient manner and provide reassurance and support to the woman and her partner, explaining briefly what has happened and what can be anticipated. Once surgery has begun, the nurse should see that the partner and family members have staff support and are told when they will receive information about the woman and neonate.

Amniotic Fluid Embolism

Amniotic fluid embolism is a rare obstetric catastrophe and has been called the most unpredictable and unpreventable cause of maternal death. Its incidence has been reported as ranging from 1 in 8000 to 1 in 80,000 births. It is characterized in most cases by rapid and simultaneous onset of shock and DIC. Few women survive amniotic fluid embolism. In the past this diagnosis could not be confirmed until autopsy, and if the woman survived, the diagnosis was questioned; current diagnostic capabilities and advanced life support suggest that survival is possible (Esposito et al., 1990).

An amniotic fluid embolism occurs when a large amount of amniotic fluid gains access to the central maternal circulation (Fig. 26-15). Multiple emboli form in the pulmonary capillaries, resulting in rapid onset of respiratory distress and shock.

Etiologic and Predisposing Factors

Amniotic fluid embolism typically occurs in the intrapartum period. There is considerable speculation about the mechanism involved. One theory suggests that a leak of fluid may occur when a tear in the amnion and chorion allows fluid to enter the chorionic plate; under pressure from the contracting uterus, the fluid is forced into the maternal circulation. It also is postulated that amniotic fluid may enter the maternal circulation through a laceration in the cervix or uterus.

The following have been identified as predisposing factors for amniotic fluid embolism:

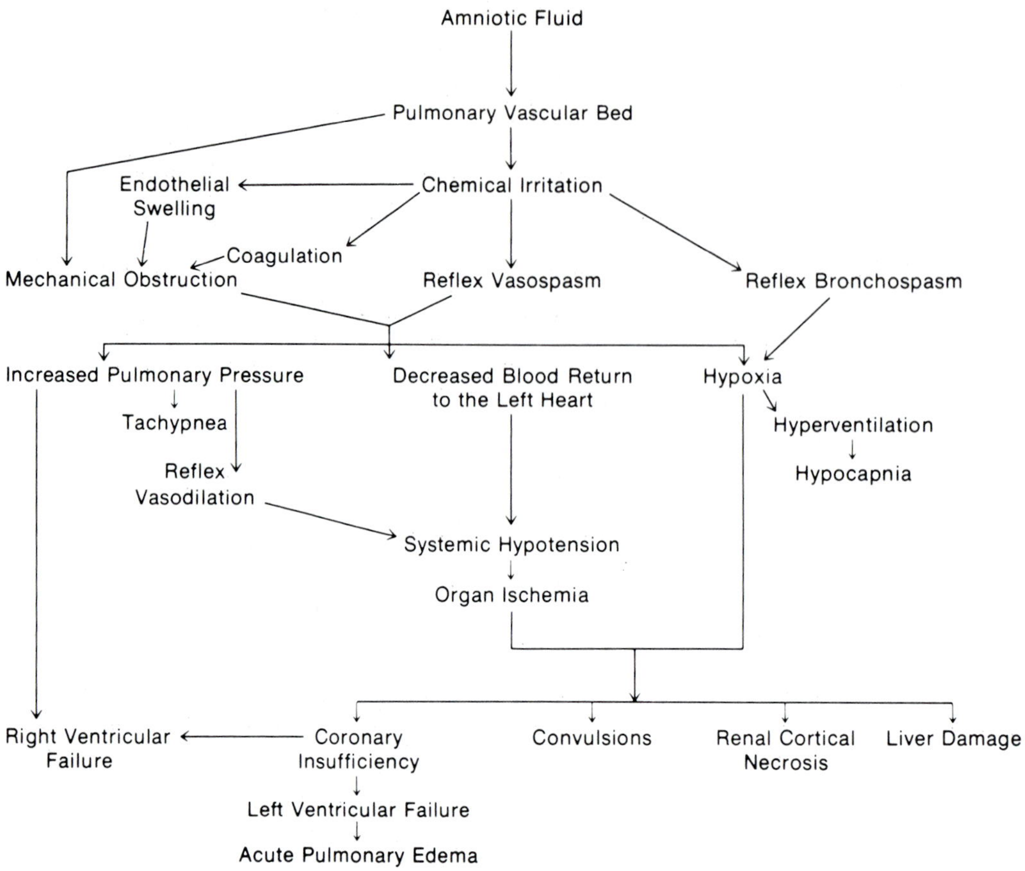

Figure 26-15.

Sequence of events leading to cardiopulmonary complications of amniotic fluid embolism. (Abouleish, E. [1977]. *Pain control in obstetrics.* Philadelphia: J.B. Lippincott.)

- High parity
- Advanced maternal age
- Short or tumultuous labor
- Polyhydramnios
- Oxytocin augmentation
- Intrauterine fetal death
- Abruptio placentae

The underlying pathology of this condition is not yet well understood. This is the only instance in which the agent that triggers defibrination and resulting DIC has been clearly identified. Amniotic fluid and mucus contain thromboplastinlike material that activates the coagulation cascade.

Events leading to cardiopulmonary collapse are initial pulmonary hypertension, cor pulmonale (acute right heart strain and failure), reduced left atrial pressure, reduced carbon dioxide, and systemic hypotension. The cause of the initial pulmonary hypertension is not fully understood. It may result from obstruction of the capillary bed by debris (fetal squamous epithelium, lanugo, mucus, and meconium) in the amniotic fluid; the presence of this material in pulmonary vessels at autopsy confirms the diagnosis of amniotic fluid embolism.

Diagnosis

Diagnosis is based on presenting signs and symptoms and the presence of predisposing factors. DIC is confirmed by laboratory tests, which demonstrate the following aberrations in coagulation:

- Prolonged thrombin time, prothrombin time, and partial thromboplastin time
- Decreased platelet count
- Elevated fibrin split products
- Decreased coagulation factors: factor V, VIII, and X

Signs and symptoms of amniotic fluid embolism are listed in the accompanying display.

Maternal, Fetal, and Neonatal Implications

Approximately 25% of women diagnosed with amniotic fluid embolism die within 1 hour of the onset of symptoms. Mortality for all cases is estimated to be more than 80%. The interval between onset of symptoms and death ranges from 1 to 32 hours. Coagulation failure occurs in up to 50% of patients within 1 hour of onset. Significant hemorrhage usually occurs. Among women surviving the initial crisis, uncontrollable uterine hemorrhage may begin within minutes or hours.

The fetus is at profound risk because of the rapid deterioration of maternal status, and immediate delivery is essential. FHR is continuously monitored until delivery can be accomplished. Forceps application and emergency vaginal delivery may be possible if labor has progressed sufficiently;

Signs and Symptoms of Amniotic Fluid Embolism

Premonitory Signs and Symptoms

Shaking chill and diaphoresis
Increasing restlessness and anxiety
Coughing with frothy pink sputum
Chest pain
Vomiting
Seizures

Cardinal symptoms

Rapidly developing dyspnea, tachypnea, and cyanosis
Shock out of proportion to blood loss
Hemorrhage
Coma

otherwise, emergency cesarean delivery is necessary. Neonatal support personnel are needed to attend to a neonate who may be severely compromised and to allow delivery room personnel to attend to the woman.

Treatment

Treatment is largely symptomatic. At the first signs of respiratory distress, oxygen is administered under positive pressure until endotracheal intubation can be accomplished. IV administration of blood components and heparin will be initiated. Close monitoring of cardiopulmonary status is essential; a central venous pressure line should be established to guard against the risk of fluid overload when blood components are being administered; this risk is especially great in the presence of right heart strain or failure. Respiratory and cardiac arrest is common, and cardiopulmonary resuscitation must be initiated immediately. Recent reports indicate that in some cases the woman's prognosis for survival may be improved with aggressive therapy. Treatment consists of placing the woman on cardiopulmonary bypass, and surgically removing the pulmonary thrombus (Esposito et al., 1990).

Management of the coagulopathy consists of the following therapy:

- Interruption of the coagulation cascade
- Deactivation of the fibrinolytic system
- Replacement of coagulation factors
- Replacement of blood and fluids

Implications for Nursing Care

Nursing responsibilities include prompt identification of early symptoms and initiation of emergency care. Initial nursing actions include administration of oxygen, alerting staff and obtaining assistance, and monitoring maternal vital signs. This situation often is handled by delivery room staff assisted by the cardiopulmonary resuscitation team because of the complex nature of this emergency. The nurse assists in the emergency procedures previously described.

If the partner or other support person is present, the nurse should make sure that they are escorted to a place where they can wait and that they are kept informed and supported while emergency care continues. If maternal or fetal death occurs, the nurse should immediately mobilize specialized support for family members, including the chaplain or another spiritual leader and other nursing staff whose attention can be directed solely to the family's needs during this catastrophic experience.

Because unanticipated problems can emerge at any time during the intrapartum period, the nurse must remain alert to the possibility of their development throughout the course of labor and birth. Regardless of the setting, all maternity nurses must be skilled in the provision of emergency care and support until medical personnel arrive. While maintaining maternal and fetal physiologic functioning is the primary goal of care, the nurse must provide emotional support and encouragement. The sudden onset of life-threatening problems can be extremely frightening for the woman and her partner. The presence of a sensitive, caring nurse can make the difference in how the experience is viewed and how well the family copes in the postpartum period.

Chapter Summary

Birth is unpredictable. Complications arise that can threaten maternal and fetal well-being and that require expert medical and nursing intervention to ensure positive outcomes. The nurse plays a crucial role in the care of families at risk for, or actually experiencing, complications in the intrapartum period. The nurse assesses maternal and fetal status, detects early signs of developing complications, observes signs of impending danger, and often offers the first emergency interventions to preserve maternal and fetal well-being. A systematic approach to care, reflected in the nursing process, is required to ensure that nursing actions are based on accurate data and that care is provided in an orderly fashion, even in emergencies. The constantly developing technology of perinatal care allows health care professionals greater precision and effectiveness in their treatment of complications associated with childbirth.

Study Questions

1. *What are the classic signs of placenta previa and abruptio placentae?*
2. *Why are vaginal examinations contraindicated when the woman first presents with complaints of vaginal bleeding in the third trimester?*
3. *How can the nurse determine if pathologic infarctions of the placenta are present during labor?*
4. *What signs in the FHR pattern would suggest umbilical cord compression?*

5. *How can the nurse identify a prolapsed umbilical cord?*
6. *What are the primary nursing responsibilities when prolapse of the umbilical cord occurs?*
7. *What characteristics of pelvic structure can be determined by the nurse during a vaginal examination?*
8. *What are the primary nursing responsibilities when caring for the woman with prolonged labor?*
9. *What are the major nursing responsibilities during labor and birth when caring for the woman experiencing a postterm gestation?*
10. *What are the primary nursing responsibilities when assisting a woman during an out-of-hospital birth?*
11. *What signs and symptoms would indicate to the nurse that the woman was experiencing hypovolemic shock or DIC?*
12. *What are the major nursing responsibilities during a blood transfusion?*
13. *What are the classic signs of uterine rupture?*
14. *What emergency support does the nurse provide when a uterine rupture is suspected?*

References

Andres, R., Piacquandio, A., & Resnik, R. (1990). A reappraisal of the need for autologous blood donation in the obstetric patient. *American Journal of Obstetrics and Gynecology*, *163*(5), 1551–1553.

Aumann, G. (1988). New chances, new choices: Problems with perinatal technology. *Journal of Perinatal and Neonatal Nursing*, *1*(3), 1.

Barrett, J. (1991). Funic reduction for the management of umbilical cord prolapse. *American Journal of Obstetrics and Gynecology*, *165*(3), 654.

Benirschke, K. (1989). Normal development. In R. Creasy & R. Resnik (Eds.), *Maternal-fetal medicine* (2nd ed.) (p. 116). Philadelphia: W.B. Saunders.

Benson, R. (1987). Multiple pregnancy. In R. Benson (Ed.), *Current obstetric and gynecologic diagnosis and treatment* (6th ed.) (p. 187). Los Altos, CA: Lange Medical Publications.

Blackburn, S., & Loper, D. (1992). Maternal, fetal, and neonatal physiology. Philadelphia: W.B. Saunders.

Combs, A., Nyberg, D., Mack, L., et al. (1992). Expectant management after sonographic diagnosis of placental abruption. *American Journal of Perinatology*, *9*(3), 170.

Committee on Obstetrics. (1991). *Maternal and fetal medicine. Placental pathology*. Committee Opinion Number 102. Washington, DC: American College of Obstetrics.

Dorman, K. (1989). Hemorrhagic emergencies in obstetrics. *Journal of Perinatal and Neonatal Nursing*, *3*(2), 23.

Eganhouse, D. (1992). Fetal monitoring of twins. *Journal of Obstetric, Gynecologic, and Neonatal Nursing*, *21*(1), 17.

Esposito, R., Grossi, E., Coppa, G., Giangola, G., Ferri, D., Angelides, E., & Andriakos, P. (1990). Successful treatment of postpartum shock caused by amniotic fluid embolism with cardiopulmonary bypass and pulmonary artery thromboembolectomy. *American Journal of Obstetrics and Gynecology*, *163*(2), 572.

Flannagan, T., Mulchahey, K., Korenbrot, C., et al. (1987). Management of term breech presentation. *American Journal of Obstetrics and Gynecology*, *156*(6), 1492.

Gibbs, R., & Duff, P. (1991). Progress in pathogenesis and management of clinical intraamniotic infection. *American Journal of Obstetrics and Gynecology*, *164*(5), 1317.

Gillogley, K. (1991). Abnormal labor and delivery. In K. Niswanter & A. Evans (Eds.), *Manual of obstetrics* (4th ed.) (p. 443). Boston: Little, Brown and Co.

Gilstrap, L., Leveno, K., Cox, S., et al. (1988). Intrapartum treatment of acute chorioamnionitis: Impact on neonatal sepsis. *American Journal of Obstetrics and Gynecology*, *159*(3), 579.

Harvey, M. (1992). Humanizing the intensive care unit experience. *NAACOG'S Clinical Issues in Perinatal and Women's Health*, *3*(3), 369.

Jackson, V. (1989). Delivery of the second twin. *Journal of Perinatal and Neonatal Nursing*, *3*(1), 22.

Kilpatrick, S., Safford, K., Pomeroy, T., et al. (1991). Maternal hydration increases amniotic fluid index. *Obstetrics and Gynecology*, *78*(6), 1098.

Kulb, N. (1990a). Abnormalities of the placenta and membranes. In K. Buckley & N. Kulb (Eds.), *High risk maternity nursing manual*. Baltimore: Williams & Wilkins.

Kulb, N. (1990b). Abnormalities of the amniotic fluid. In K. Buckley & N. Kulb (Eds.), *High risk maternity nursing manual*. Baltimore: Williams & Wilkins.

Lacro, R. V., Jones, K. L., & Benirschke, K. (1987). The umbilical cord twist: Origin, direction, and relevance. *American Journal of Obstetrics and Gynecology*, *157*, 833.

LoBue, C. (1991). Third trimester bleeding. In K. Niswander & A. Evans (Eds.), *Manual of obstetrics*. Boston: Little, Brown and Co.

Manning, F. (1989). General principles and application of ultrasound. In R. Creasy & R. Resnik (Eds.), *Maternal-fetal medicine* (2nd ed.) (p. 195). Philadelphia: W.B. Saunders.

Martin, E. (1990). Maternal transport. In E. Martin (Ed.), *Intrapartum mangement modules*.Baltimore: Williams & Wilkins.

Morgan, M., & Thumau, G. (1988). Efficacy of the fetal-pelvic index for delivery of neonates weighing 4000 grams or greater. *American Journal of Obstetrics and Gynecology*, *158*, 1133–1136.

Nageotte, M. (1991). Fetal growth abnormalities. In K. Niswander & A. Evans (Eds.), *Manual of obstetrics* (4th ed.) (p. 317). Boston: Little Brown and Co.

Oi, R. (1991). Diseases of the placenta. In K. Niswander (Ed.), *Manual of obstetrics* (p. 457). Boston: Little, Brown and Co.

O'Leary, J., & Leonetti, H. (1990). Shoulder dystocia: Prevention and treatment. *American Journal of Obstetrics and Gynecology*, *162*(1), 5.

Penney, D., & Perlis, D. (1992). Shoulder dystocia. *MCN: American Journal of Maternal Child Nursing*, *17*(1), 34.

Penney, D. (1991). Autologous blood use in obstetrics. *NAACOGs Clinical Issues in Perinatal and Women's Health Nursing*, *2*(3), 344.

Phelan, J., Park, Y., Ahn, M., et al. (1990). Polyhydramnios and perinatal outcome. *Journal of Perinatology*, *X*(4), 347.

Robson, S., Crawford, R., Spencer, J., et al. (1992). Intrapartum amniotic fluid index and its relationship to fetal distress. *American Journal of* Obstetrics and Gynecology, *166*(1), 78.

Sadovsky, Y., Amon, E., Bade, M., et al. (1989). Prophylactic amnioinfusion during labor complicated by meconium: A preliminary report. *American Journal of Obstetrics and Gynecology*, *161*(3), 613.

Saftlas, A., Olson, D., Atrash, H., et al. (1991). National trends in the incidence of abruptio placentae, 1979–1987. *Obstetrics and Gynecology*, *78*(6), 1081.

Saller, D., Keene, C., Sun, C., et al. (1990). The association of single umbilical artery with cytogenetically abnormal pregnancies. *American Journal of Obstetrics and Gynecology*, *163*(3), 922.

Smith, S. (1990). Dystocias of labor. In K. Buckley & N. Kulb (Eds.), *High risk maternity nursing manual* (p. 389). Baltimore: Williams & Wilkins.

Stumpf, D. (1990). The infant with anencephaly. *New England Journal of Medicine*, *322*(10), 669.

Williams, M., Mittendorf, R., Lieberman, E., et al. (1991). Cigarette smoking during pregnancy in relation to placenta previa. *American Journal of Obstetrics and Gynecology*, *165*(1), 28.1

Suggested Readings

Galvan, B., Van Mullem, C., & Broekhuizen, F. (1989). Using amnioinfusion for the relief of repetitive variable decelerations during labor. *Journal of Obstetric, Gynecologic, and Neonatal Nursing*, *18*(3), 222.

Haubrich, K. (1990). Amnioinfusion: A technique for the relief of variable deceleration. *Journal of Obstetric, Gynecologic, and Neonatal Nursing*, *19*(4), 299.

Koonings, P., Paul, R., & Campbell, K. (1990). Umbilical cord prolapse. *Journal of Reproductive Medicine*, *35*(7), 690.

Mashburn, J. (1988). Identification and management of shoulder dystocia. *Journal of Nurse-Midwifery*, *33*(5), 225.

Phelan, J., Park, W., Ahn, M., et al. (1990). Polyhydramnios and perinatal outcome. *Journal of Perinatology*, *X*(4), 347.

Querin, J., & Stahl, L. (1990). Two simple sensible steps for successful blood transfusions. *Nursing 90*, *20*(10), 68.

Saller, D., Nagey, D., Pupkin, M., et al. (1990). Tocolysis in the management of third trimester bleeding. *Journal of Perinatology*, *X*(2), 125.

Shenker, L., Reed, K., Anderson, C., et al. (1991). Significance of oligohydramnios complicating pregnancy. *American Journal of Obstetrics and Gynecology*, *164*(2), 1597.

Sherer, D., Cullen, J., Thompson, H., et al. (1990). Transient oligohydramnios in a severely hypovolemic gravid woman at 35 weeks gestation. *American Journal of Obstetrics and Gynecology*, *162*(3), 770.

Wingeier, R., & Griggs, R. (1990). Management of retained placenta using intraumbilical oxytocin injection. *Journal of Nurse-Midwifery*, *36*(4), 240.

CHAPTER 27

Perinatal High-Risk Challenges

Learning Objectives

After studying the material in this chapter, the student will be able to:

- List predisposing factors associated with preterm labor and birth.
- Compare and contrast tocolytics currently used in the treatment of preterm labor in terms of dosages, route of administration, side affects, adverse reactions, and nursing implications.
- Discuss fetal and neonatal complications related to preterm premature rupture of membranes.
- Outline the medical management and nursing care for the woman with preterm premature rupture of membranes.
- Discuss current theories regarding the etiology of pregnancy- induced hypertension.
- Outline the classic signs and symptoms of pregnancy-induced hypertension.
- Outline the medical management and nursing care of the woman with pregnancy-induced hypertension.
- Define eclampsia and describe the major nursing care when eclamptic seizures occur.
- Compare and contrast the etiology and clinical signs and symptoms of disseminated intravascular coagulopathy and HELLP syndrome.
- Describe pregnancy changes that predispose the woman to the development of carbohydrate intolerance and diabetes.
- Identify maternal, fetal, and neonatal risks when diabetes complicates pregnancy.
- Define diabetic ketoacidosis, its medical treatment, and appropriate nursing care.
- Describe signs and symptoms of hypoglycemia and the nurse's role in its treatment.
- Outline major aspects of nursing and medical management when cardiac disease complicates pregnancy.

Key Terms

disseminated intravascular coagulopathy
eclampsia
ketoacidosis
neuropathy
petechiae
plasma oncotic pressure
preeclampsia
pregnancy-induced hypertension
premature rupture of membranes
preterm labor
retinopathy
scotoma
tocolytic

Some women begin pregnancy with underlying medical problems that may compromise maternal, fetal, and neonatal well-being (see the accompanying display). Others develop significant obstetric complications that alter the subsequent course and outcome of the childbearing process. Unlike many of the relatively minor disorders that occur in pregnancy, these high-risk challenges do not resolve with prompt medical treatment. They require active, ongoing medical and nursing management throughout the gestational period, during childbirth, and in the immediate postpartum period. In many instances, the neonate also may require long-term care as a result of the woman's condition.

The woman with a major obstetric or medical problem during pregnancy usually experiences less than optimal adaptations in both physiologic and psychological function. She may be transported to a perinatal high-risk center (see Chapter 26) so that specialized medical treatment and expert nursing care can be provided. Close monitoring is required to ensure early detection of further compromise in maternal or fetal status. A perinatal team consisting of obstetricians, perinatologists, nurses, respiratory therapists, physical therapists, social workers, and other health care specialists is often required to plan and implement care for these women.

A medical or obstetric problem that complicates the course of pregnancy, birth, and postpartum recovery presents a challenge for the maternity nurse. Whether the

Conditions Influencing Maternal, Fetal, or Neonatal Status During the Childbearing Cycle

Preexisting Conditions

- Cardiac disease
- Chronic hypertension
- Thromboembolic disorders
- Pulmonary disease
- Diabetes mellitus
- Renal disease
- Hyperthyroidism
- Orthopedic deformities
- Pelvic fractures
- Neoplastic disease
- Substance abuse
- Sexually transmitted diseases
- Human immunodeficiency syndromes

Problems of Pregnancy

- Gestational diabetes
- Premature rupture of the membranes
- Preterm labor and delivery
- Pregnancy-induced hypertension

woman remains in her own community or is transported to a perinatal center, expert nursing care is required to maintain maternal and fetal physiologic well-being. Meeting the emotional needs of the woman and her family becomes crucially important when major threats to physiologic integrity occur.

This chapter describes major complications that occur during the perinatal period. They are responsible for a large percentage of perinatal morbidity and mortality. Perinatal high-risk medical or obstetric problems often require intensive medical and nursing care for an extended time during the prenatal period. They include both medical and obstetric problems including diabetes. The underlying pathophysiology of these high-risk conditions, as well as etiology, diagnosis, and medical and nursing management are described. Maternal, fetal, and neonatal implications of each complication are discussed. The reader is referred to Chapter 25 for an in-depth discussion of emotional consequences of perinatal complications and appropriate nursing care of families in crisis.

Obstetric Complications During the Perinatal Period

Preterm Labor

Labor that begins before the 38th week of gestation is defined as preterm labor (PTL). Premature labor and birth is the greatest single problem in contemporary obstetrics. In the United States, complications from preterm birth cause two thirds of all perinatal and neonatal morbidity and mortality not related to congenital defects (Graf & Perez-Woods, 1992). Thirty percent of all neonatal mortality is directly attributable to complications resulting from preterm delivery. Among those preterm newborns who survive, long-term physical, developmental, and intellectual handicaps are found, particularly when the neonate is born before 28 weeks of gestation.

Preterm labor occurs in approximately 7% of all births in the United States. However, the incidence is double that figure (approximately 15%) in African American women (Williams, 1991b). This higher occurrence is believed to be related to socioeconomic factors. Poverty is a strong predictor of premature labor and birth.

Etiologic and Predisposing Factors

The cause of PTL is not completely understood. In 20% to 40% of cases, medical and obstetric complications, such as diabetes or placenta previa, contribute to PTL and premature birth. A variety of behavioral factors and physical problems may place a woman at higher risk (see the accompanying display). Unfortunately, iatrogenic factors such as

Risk Factors Associated With Preterm Labor and Birth

Obstetric Factors

- Polyhydramnios
- Prenatal bleeding
- Multifetal gestation
- Prior preterm delivery
- Cervical incompetence
- Uterine or cervical anomalies
- Reproductive tract infection
- Poor pregnancy weight gain
- Abdominal surgery during pregnancy
- Previous second trimester abortion
- Cervical dilatation more than 2 cm by 32 weeks

Medical Factors

- Renal disease; pyelonephritis
- Chronic hypertension
- Diethylstilbestrol exposure in utero

Social and Behavioral Factors

- Race other than European American
- Age (under 19 or over 40 years)
- Inadequate prenatal care
- Low socioeconomic status
- Prepregnancy weight under 4.5 kg (100 lb)
- Domestic violence (battering)
- Smoking: alcohol intake; substance abuse
- Psychological stress

Table 27-1. Preterm Labor Risk Assessment Tool*

Score	Socioeconomic Conditions	Past History	Daily Habits	Current Pregnancy
1	2 children at home; low socioeconomic status	1 abortion; <1 y since last birth	Work outside home	Unusual fatigue
2	<20 y old >40 y old Single parent	2 abortions	More than 10 cigarettes/day	Albuminuria Hypertension Bacteriuria
3	Very low socioeconomic status Under 5 ft tall Under 100 lb	3 abortions	Heavy work; long tiring trip	Breech at 32 wk Weight loss of 5 lb Head engaged Febrile illness
4	Under 18 y old	Pyelonephritis		Metrorrhagia after 12 wk; Effacement; dilatation; uterine irritability
5		Second trimester abortion DES exposure		Uterine anomaly; placenta previa; polyhydramnios Uterine myoma
10		Preterm delivery; repeated second trimester abortion		Twins; abdominal surgery

*Although many nurses use preterm labor assessment tools, their accuracy in predicting preterm labor has not been established.

This risk assessment instrument is used at the initial prenatal visit and again at 26 to 28 weeks' gestation. (Creasy, R., & Merkatz, I. (1990). Prevention of preterm birth: Clinical opinion. *Obstetrics and Gynecology, 76*(1), 2–45.)

From Creasy, R., & Herron, M. (1981). Prevention of preterm birth. *Seminars in Perinatology, 5*, 297.

elective induction of labor or repeat cesarean delivery account for 10% to 15% of neonatal intensive care unit (NICU) admissions for prematurity (Graf & Perez-Woods, 1992).

Attempts have been made to develop a scoring system that will accurately identify women at risk for PTL. Pioneering research by Creasy and Herron (1981) led to the development of several instruments currently used in clinical practice to predict PTL (Table 27-1). The goal of risk assessment is early identification of vulnerable women and prevention of preterm birth. Ongoing research with special populations is needed to develop more precise risk assessment instruments.

Diagnosis

Signs and symptoms of PTL, listed in the accompanying display, are often subtle and difficult to differentiate from minor discomforts frequently experienced during pregnancy.

The diagnosis of PTL is based on the presence of uterine contractions and the finding of progressive cervical effacement or dilatation. A single cervical examination is not sufficient to establish the diagnosis of PTL. Fifteen percent of primigravidas and more than 10% of multigravidas may be at least 1 cm dilated before 38 weeks' gestation (Kulb, 1990a). A repeated cervical evaluation 30 to 60 minutes after the first assessment needs to be performed (preferably by the same examiner) to confirm cervical change. Factors to be assessed in the digital examination of the cervix include:

- Cervical effacement
- Cervical dilatation
- Consistency of cervix (soft, medium, firm)
- Position of cervix (posterior, midposition, anterior)
- Fetal station

Because specific organisms such as *Chlamydia trachomatis* have been implicated in the etiology of PTL, many experts recommend that a sterile speculum examination be performed *before* the initial digital examination of the cervix. The vagina should be assessed for evidence of amniotic fluid leakage, and cervical cultures for group B streptococcus, *C. trachomatis*, and *Neisseria gonorrhoeae* need to be obtained. When chorioamnionitis is strongly suspected as a

Signs and Symptoms of Preterm Labor

Signs

- Change in character of vaginal discharge
- Increased vaginal discharge
- Vaginal spotting or bleeding
- Rupture of membranes
- Diarrhea
- Fetus engaged before 32 weeks
- Urinary tract infection (pyelonephritis)

Symptoms

- Low backache
  - Pelvic pressure
  - Thigh pressure
- Sensation of uterine tightening
- Abdominal cramping
  - Intermittent urge to void occurs with regularity
  - Dysuria, urinary frequency, burning when woman urinates

cause of PTL, a Gram stain and culture of amniotic fluid obtained by amniocentesis may also be performed.

Maternal, Fetal, and Neonatal Implications

Maternal complications of PTL and premature birth are associated with current treatment modalities such as tocolytic therapy (to inhibit uterine activity), bed rest, or cesarean delivery. Cardiopulmonary complications of tocolytics may be life threatening (Grimes, Schulz, Hadi, & Albazzaz, 1989). Bed rest is commonly prescribed as a treatment for PTL. However, no research results have been published on the physiologic consequences of prolonged bed rest during pregnancy at this time. Problems associated with bed rest include an increased risk of thrombus formation, muscle wasting, calcium loss from bone, renal calculi, constipation, decreased appetite, and sensory deprivation. Postpartum recovery and ability to assume neonatal care is delayed when the woman has experienced prolonged bed rest.

More attention has been focused on the psychological and social consequences of bed rest. Monahan and DeJoseph (1991) found that prolonged bed rest resulted in feelings of anger, depression, boredom, and isolation in women experiencing PTL. If extended hospitalization occurs, separation from one's partner or other children and family members can result in further anxiety and emotional distress. Disruption in daily activities, household routines, infant and child care, and loss of income (if the woman was forced to quit her job) are potential stressors. Worry about fetal or neonatal well-being can precipitate a crisis (see Chapter 25 for a full discussion of the emotional impact of PTL).

Cesarean delivery may be recommended as the mode of delivery for very low–birth-weight, preterm neonates or those with sudden fetal distress. A classic incision may be performed because of the small size of the uterus. As a consequence, the woman will generally require elective repeat cesarean deliveries in future pregnancies. The woman is at increased risk for all of the complications associated with cesarean birth and the administration of anesthesia.

Preterm labor and birth pose life-threatening risks for the fetus and neonate. Mortality is greatest among preterm neonates born between 23 and 28 weeks' gestation. The major threat to survival is respiratory distress syndrome (RDS) resulting from pulmonary immaturity. Other threats are also due to immaturity of organ systems including patent ductus arteriosus, necrotizing enterocolitis, and intraventricular hemorrhage. A complete discussion of the problems related to prematurity is presented in Chapter 33.

Even when PTL is successfully suppressed, the fetus and neonate may experience adverse effects from tocolytic therapy. Neonatal cardiovascular toxicity (Thorkelsson & Loughead, 1991) and myocardial necrosis (Fletcher et al., 1991) have been reported secondary to long-term subcutaneous infusion of terbutaline. Pulmonary hypertension and premature closure of the ductus arteriosus have been documented with the use of indomethacin (Indocin) (Eronen et al., 1991). The long-term infusion of magnesium sulfate has resulted in neonatal bone abnormalities (Holcomb, Shackelford, & Petrie, 1991) and depressed calcium levels and hypotonia in the neonate (Hankins, Hammond, & Yeomans, 1991).

Treatment

Medical treatment of PTL encompasses a variety of therapies. Because the incidence of preterm delivery has not decreased significantly in the past 10 years, greater emphasis is placed on determining the benefit of commonly used modalities.

Bed Rest. For more than 30 years, bed rest has been extensively used to treat PTL, particularly in women with multifetal gestation and placenta previa. The rationale for bed rest includes reducing pressure of the fetal presenting part on the cervix when the fetal head is engaged, improving uterine blood flow, and promoting rest. Recent research does not support the supposed benefits of bed rest in all cases (Malone & Kasper, 1991). Further research is needed to determine the value of bed rest.

Hydration. Several studies indicate that uterine activity can be suppressed in some cases by hydrating the woman with signs or symptoms of PTL. The tocolytic effect of hydration is attributed to inhibition of the antidiuretic hormone. If hydration is not effective in stopping PTL, the subsequent administration of tocolytics (ritodrine or magnesium sulfate) or corticosteroids to accelerate fetal lung maturity may predispose the woman to pulmonary edema due to increased fluid volume (Armson et al., 1992). It is recommended that fluid hydration therapy be restricted to approximately 100 mL/h (total fluid), using a physiologic solution such as Ringer's lactate intravenously.

Tocolytic Therapy. In the event that PTL cannot be suppressed by use of bed rest and hydration, the woman may be hospitalized for more intensive treatment. Various types of drugs, known as tocolytics, have been used to arrest labor. The most common group of tocolytics include:

- Smooth muscle relaxants (magnesium sulfate)
- Beta-sympathomimetics (ritodrine and terbutaline)
- Calcium channel blockers (nifedipine)
- Prostaglandin synthetase inhibitors (indomethacin)

Each of these drugs may afford some degree of success. However, studies indicate that delivery is on an average delayed only 3 to 7 days (Kulb, 1990a). All tocolytics have side effects that must be closely monitored (Table 27-2). Certain groups of women, such as individuals with cardiac disease, may not be candidates for tocolytic therapy. Long-term use of these drugs requires ongoing research to determine the drug's safety.

The precise mechanism for the tocolytic effect of *magnesium sulfate* ($MgS0_4$) is not precisely understood. Magnesium interferes with the transport of intracellular and extracellular calcium, reducing its availability for coupling with actomyosin, thus decreasing muscle contractions and the conduction of nerve impulses (Neal & Bockman, 1990).

Magnesium sulfate is most often given intravenously. A loading dose is administered over 15 to 30 minutes followed by a maintenance infusion. A single dose of subcutaneous terbutaline (0.125 mg intravenously or 0.25 mg subcutaneously) may be prescribed as adjunct therapy. This may successfully suppress uterine activity until a therapeutic serum magnesium level is achieved. Magnesium sulfate is adminis-

Table 27-2. Drugs Used in Treatment of Preterm Labor

Drug	Dosage/Route/Action	Maternal Side Effects	Fetal Side Effects	Nursing Implications
$MgSO_4$	IV: 4 g loading dose in 50–100 mL 5% dextrose in water (infused slowly over 15–30 min) Follow with maintenance dose of 1–4 g/h to maintain uterine relaxation Standard solution is 20–40 g $MgSO_4$ in 1000 mL IV solution **Indication/Action** Neuromuscular sedative that decreases the amount of acetylcholine produced by motor nerves, effectively blocking neuromuscular transmission, thereby suppressing uterine activity	CNS depression, skeletal and smooth muscle relaxation, resulting in: drowsiness, lethargy, ptosis, blurred vision, slurred speech, muscular weakness and generalized hypotonia, respiratory depression or paralysis, loss of deep tendon reflexes Vasodilation, resulting in: flushing, feeling of warmth, hypotension and possible cardiovascular collapse Other side effects: nausea and increased thirst Pulmonary edema has been associated with $MgSO_4$ tocolysis. Exact etiology is unknown, but is often associated with IV hydration of the woman	Possible decrease in FHR variability in preterm fetus Possible bone abnormalities with prolonged maternal administration	Monitor maternal vital signs closely during loading dose. Monitor maternal vital signs, DTRs, urinary output every 30 min to 1 h until stable serum therapeutic level is achieved. (4–7.5 mEq/ liter) Then monitor vital signs, as ordered, when client is stable. Notify physician of Respirations <12/min Urinary output <25–30 ml/h Absent DTRs Signs of toxicity: increasing lethargy, hypotonia, hypotension, extreme thirst Limit intake to prevent pulmonary edema (usually 2000 to 3000 mL/24 h). Have resuscitation equipment at bedside. Have antidote, 10% calcium gluconate, at bedside. Provide for continuous EFM and toco monitoring. Prepare client for common side effects of drug. Obtain serum Mg levels, as ordered.
Ritodrine (Yutopar)	150 mg in 500 mL fluid yields concentration of 0.3 mg/mL IV: 0.05–0.1 mg/min increasing every 10 min to maximum of 0.35 mg/min or until adequate response obtained Oral: 10 mg every 2 h for 24 h (administered 30 min before IV infusion is discontinued), then decreased 5–10 mg every 4–6 h; not to exceed 120 mg/d **Indication/Action** Stimulates sympathetic beta-2 receptors; inhibits uterine contractility Metabolized by liver; 70%–90% excreted in urine in 10–12 h	ECG changes and cardiac arrhythmia; dose-related tachycardia; decreased blood pressure; increased pulse pressure; flushing; sweating; nausea and vomiting; tremors; headache Pulmonary edema (more frequent when used concurrently with corticosteroids and in cases of multiple gestation) Positional hypotension (may be exacerbated by anesthesia) Transient increases in serum insulin, glucose, and free fatty acids; decrease in serum potassium Risk of overdose (signaled by exaggeration of cardiac and other side effects) Maternal deaths reported (from pulmonary edema)	Drug crosses placenta; increased FHR; hypoglycemia (infrequently); cardiac arrhythmia (occasionally)	Closely observe blood pressure and maternal and fetal heart rates; maternal heart rate should not exceed 130 bpm. Check apical heart rate for arrhythmia. Observe closely for signs of pulmonary edema; monitor input and output; maintain fluid restrictions. Ritodrine therapy may unmask occult heart disease and must be used with caution in hypertensive, diabetic, and preeclamptic patients. Drug is contraindicated with active bleeding. Obtain maternal serum potassium, glucose, and ECG baselines before initiating IV therapy.

(*Continued*)

Table 27-2. Drugs Used in Treatment of Preterm Labor (*Continued*)

Drug	Dosage/Route/Action	Maternal Side Effects	Fetal Side Effects	Nursing Implications
Terbutaline (Brethine, Bricanyl): experimental—not currently approved by FDA for use as tocolytic, but used widely throughout US for tocolysis	IV: 5 mg/500 mL fluid Initiate at rate of 1 mg/min to maximum of 8 mg/min; continue 8–12 h; then subcutaneously 0.25 mg every 4 h for 24 h May be given orally or subcutaneously for home management: 2.5–5 mg PO every 4–6 h, or 0.25 mg continuous subcutaneous infusion **Indication/Action** Beta-adrenergic agent; suppresses uterine contractility Partially metabolized by liver; excreted through gastrointestinal tract and kidneys Similar to those of ritodrine; but less severe	Nervousness, restlessness, tremors, headache, insomnia, hypertension, tachycardia, palpitations, pulmonary edema (with IV tocolysis), nausea, vomiting, hypokalemia	Similar to ritodrine	See ritodrine
Nifedipine (Procardia)	Initial dose: Sublingual or PO: 10 mg; may repeat 10 mg dose at 15–20 min intervals for three more doses until contractions resolve Maintenance dose: 10 mg q 6h **Indication/Action** Inhibits transport of calcium via slow calcium channels resulting in relaxation of uterine muscle	Flushing, vertigo, headache, nervousness, nasal congestion, dyspnea, hypotension, syncope, tachycardia, myocardial infarction, nausea, heartburn, diarrhea, constipation, muscle cramps, fever	Tachycardia; possible fetal acidosis	Monitor blood pressure, pulse, and respirations just before administration, q 15–20 min during repeated initial doses. Monitor intake and output, breath sounds, weight gain for evidence of pulmonary edema Observe for tachycardia, chest pain, palpitations Monitor renal and hepatic function tests as obtained If administered sublingually, puncture capsule with sterile needle, and squeeze to deliver into buccal pouch
Indomethacin (Indocin)	Initial dose per rectum: 100 mg Maintenance dose PO: 25 mg q 6 h for a maximum of 48 h **Indication/Action** Inhibits prostaglandin synthesis thereby inhibiting stimulation of uterine muscle	Nausea, heartburn, gastrointestinal ulceration, decreased renal function	Closure of ductus arteriosus, oligohydramnios, neonatal pulmonary hypertension	Continuous EFM and uterine monitoring during therapy Observe woman for evidence of gastrointestinal side effects Cross-sensitivity with other nonsteroidal antiinflammatory agents including aspirin; observe closely for developing hypersensitivity Administer with meals or with food, or administer antacids to decrease gastrointestinal irritation

(*Continued*)

Table 27-2. Drugs Used in Treatment of Preterm Labor ***(Continued)***

Drug	Dosage/Route/Action	Maternal Side Effects	Fetal Side Effects	Nursing Implications
Betamethasone (Celestone)	IM: 12 mg every 24 h for two doses IM: 5 mg every 24 h for two doses **Indication/Action** Increases lung maturity in fetus expected to be delivered preterm Thought to bind with glucocorticoid receptors in alveolar cells to increase production of surfactant Peak effect 48 h after first dose; lasts 7 d	Increased white blood cell count; possibly decreased resistance to infection; increased risk of pulmonary edema if used concurrently with betamimetic therapy for preterm labor Possible production or exacerbation of maternal hypertension	Potential for fetal demise secondary to maternal hypertension or placental insufficiency No documented long-term effects	All listed compounds *except* hydrocortisone are suspensions for IM use only; IV use is contraindicated. Monitor mother closely for signs of infection; ruptured membranes may be a relative contraindication, since medication may mask signs of developing infection

CNS, central nervous system; DTR, deep tendon reflex; ECG, electrocardiogram; EFM, electronic fetal monitoring; FDA, Food and Drug Administration; FHR, fetal heart rate.

tered for 12 to 24 hours and then is slowly decreased. An oral tocolytic may be given, and the magnesium infusion is discontinued 30 minutes later.

Initial trials with oral magnesium have suggested the drug may be as effective as oral terbutaline. Oral magnesium was found to produce far fewer side effects and at one third the cost of the beta-adrenergic agent (Ridgway et al., 1990) Diarrhea and fatigue appear to be the main side effects of oral magnesium therapy (Ricci et al., 1991).

Beta-sympathomimetics are ritodrine and terbutaline, epinephrine derivatives that selectively stimulate beta-adrenergic receptors in the uterus. This results in smooth muscle relaxation. Initial therapy is administered intravenously. The infusion rate is increased approximately every 15 to 30 minutes until adequate tocolysis is achieved and contractions stop. The medication is usually continued for 12 to 24 hours. The infusion rate is then slowly decreased, and if significant uterine activity does not recur, the intravenous infusion is stopped 30 minutes after the first dose of an oral tocolytic is given. In some cases, continuous subcutaneous tocolytic infusion therapy is instituted when oral tocolytic therapy is inadequate (Allbert et al., 1992). The adverse effects of beta-adrenergic agents, particularly cardiopulmonary effects, limit their use, and ritodrine is used less often today than magnesium sulfate.

Indomethacin (Indocin) is the most common *prostaglandin synthetase inhibitor* used as a tocolytic. This agent suppresses cyclooxygenase, an essential enzyme in the production of prostaglandins, which are potent uterine tonics. The drug is administered by the oral or rectal route; the rectal route may be preferred initially due to rapid absorption of drugs from the rectal mucosa. Indocin may cause premature closure of the fetal ductus arteriosus and has been associated with the development of neonatal pulmonary hypertension and oligohydramnios (Besinger, Niebyl, Keyes, & Johnson, 1991); its use is limited. The drug is not administered after the 32nd week of gestation because of the fetal and neonatal side effects.

Calcium channel blockers are another type of tocolytic. A newer pharmacologic approach to suppress uterine activity is the calcium antagonist, nifedipine. The drug has a selective inhibitory effect on slow calcium channels, which prevents calcium from diffusing through the cell membrane. This action blocks contraction of the uterine muscle. Nifedipine is administered orally or sublingually. No serious maternal or fetal side effects have been documented with nifedipine; however, it is not approved for use as a tocolytic agent by the Food and Drug Administration (FDA).

Antibiotic Administration. When infection is believed to be a causative factor in the onset of PTL, antibiotics may be administered. The development of pyelonephritis, an infection in the kidney during pregnancy, is strongly associated with PTL. Prompt antibiotic therapy is essential to prevent sepsis and preterm birth. The prophylactic use of antibiotics when specific agents such as *Mycoplasma hominis*, *Ureaplasma ureolyticum*, and group B streptococci have been cultured from the cervix or vagina remains controversial. Treatment of *C. trachomatis* and *N. gonorrhoeae* infections is definitely indicated, not only to reduce the risk of PTL, but to prevent serious neonatal consequences.

Betamethasone Administration. If fetal lung *immaturity* is confirmed by the absence of phosphatidylglycerol (PG) and a lecithin/sphingomyelin (L/S) ratio of less than 2.0, the physician may elect to administer corticosteroids (betamethasone). Betamethasone is given to the woman to enhance the process of fetal lung maturity and reduce the risk of RDS. The fetus must be between 28 and 34 weeks' gestation with delivery delayed for 24 to 48 hours for the drug to achieve its therapeutic effect. The fetal side effects and long-term consequences of steroid treatment are not known; however, the risks of RDS of prematurity are considered to outweigh these possible problems.

Preterm Delivery. When PTL is advanced or unresponsive to tocolytic therapy, the health care team prepares for delivery of a preterm neonate. Several factors affect the management of a preterm delivery to optimize the birth of a healthy neonate. Important factors to be considered in determining the mode and timing of delivery include:

- Gestational age
- Estimated birth weight
- Estimated fetal lung maturity and the risk of RDS
- Status of the membranes (ruptured or intact)
- Presence of infection (chorioamnionitis)
- Evidence of fetal distress

Preterm labor resulting from chorioamnionitis does not warrant suppression of labor. Continuing the pregnancy increases the risk of sepsis and fetal death. Labor may be suppressed long enough to ensure safe maternal transport.

The delivery itself is managed to minimize risk to the vulnerable premature fetus. Use of analgesia is minimized to avoid compromising neonatal respiratory efforts. Regional epidural anesthesia may be used if maternal hemorrhage or hypovolemia does not contraindicate its use.

If possible, rupture of the membranes is delayed until cervical dilatation has reached 6 cm to afford additional protection for the soft skull of the preterm fetus. This also reduces the risk of cord prolapse. An episiotomy may be performed to avoid perineal pressure on the skull. Outlet forceps also may be used to retract maternal soft tissue and guide the head over the perineum. Delivery must be attended by a neonatal support team skilled in providing immediate care and resuscitation to the preterm neonate.

Emergency cesarean delivery is generally considered acceptable practice when fetal distress occurs. Surgical intervention at 23 to 26 weeks' gestation carries with it ethical concerns about fetal viability and the potential risks to the woman (see the Legal/Ethical Considerations display). Elective cesarean birth to prevent fetal head trauma and intraventricular hemorrhage remains controversial. Studies regarding the benefits of cesarean birth for delivery of the preterm neonate have yielded conflicting results.

Legal/Ethical Considerations

Aggressive Management of Preterm Labor Between 23 and 26 Weeks of Gestation

Central to the issue of preterm labor management is the tremendous uncertainty about the final outcome for the very preterm neonate. Infants of similar gestational ages and weights experience very different postnatal outcomes. Women who present in advanced stages of labor may have to make rational decisions regarding treatment options for the neonate in a short period of time. Nurses may be asked to implement care that they find morally or philosophically objectionable.

Parents must be included in the decision-making process. They should be encouraged to voice concerns, fears, and questions. The nurse is able to help parents view issues from various perspectives, providing information and assisting families as they cope with complex life-and-death decisions. Recognizing the importance of parental preference is more likely to lead to a decision acceptable to both parents and caregivers, regardless of the outcome.

Aumann, G. (1988). New chances, new choices: Problems with perinatal technology. Journal of Perinatal and Neonatal Nursing, 1*(3), 1.*

• • Assessment

The nurse screens the woman during each prenatal visit for signs and symptoms of PTL and complications that may cause PTL, such as pregnancy-induced hypertension (PIH) or pyelonephritis. The nurse may obtain urine and cervical cultures to identify organisms associated with PTL when they are indicated.

When the woman experiences PTL, assessment includes continuous monitoring of uterine activity using the tokodynamometer. In addition to questioning the woman about signs of PTL, the nurse must be skilled in palpating for contractions and identifying subtle contractions and irritability patterns (low amplitude, high frequency contractions) on the fetal monitor. Numerous problems complicate the early identification of uterine activity.

Because contractions may not always be evident, the woman must be observed closely for subtle signs and symptoms of PTL. Complaints of minor discomfort such as cramping or urinary frequency should be reported promptly to the physician or midwife. A vaginal examination should be performed to determine if progressive cervical effacement or dilatation is occurring. The nurse may perform this examination after consulting with the physician or midwife.

When uterine activity continues or recurs despite tocolytic therapy, the nurse must monitor the progress of labor closely. This is critical because labor and birth may occur much more rapidly than at term. If the woman's condition is stabilized, a prolonged period of bed rest may be prescribed to suppress uterine activity. The nurse performs periodic assessments to identify complications frequently encountered with bed rest.

When the woman receives intravenous tocolytics, intensive monitoring is required to document therapeutic effects as well as identify adverse reactions and life-threatening complications of the drug. Frequent assessment of maternal vital signs is essential and facilitated by the use of an electronic blood pressure monitor. Continuous electronic fetal monitoring (EFM) and tokodynamometer monitoring of contractions are also implemented. A complete record of intake and output is maintained along with daily weights to detect fluid retention. Breath sounds are auscultated every 4 to 8 hours to assess for pulmonary edema. When magnesium sulfate is administered, deep tendon reflexes (DTRs) are evaluated periodically. Serum magnesium determinations may be ordered. The nurse is responsible for monitoring the

Nursing Research

Self-Diagnosis of Preterm Labor

The incidence of preterm labor (PTL) and birth remains higher in the Unites States than in many other industrialized nations. A major goal of prenatal education is to teach women about the signs and symptoms of PTL, so that they will seek medical help promptly.

Patterson (1992) conducted a qualitative study to learn how women come to recognize PTL and what they do when they realize something is wrong. Participants in the study, both private and clinic patients, described four processes in dealing with PTL: self-treating, ignoring symptoms, positive thinking, and waiting. Seeking professional help was found to be the strategy of *last resort* when symptoms could no longer be ignored. Even when women were told by caregivers to come to the office or hospital for evaluation, some continued to delay seeking help.

Freda (1991) surveyed women in an inner-city clinic to determine their knowledge about preventing preterm birth. Fifty percent of the women did not know when PTl could occur, and 30% did not know that a neonate born prematurely could have health problems. The study found that 25% could not name one symptom of PTL or could not say what to do if they felt symptoms of PTL.

Further research is needed to determine if specific teaching strategies are more effective in alerting women to subtle signs of PTL. It is important to convey to the woman what to do when she recognizes PTL. Based on the finding of delay in seeking professional evaluation and help, the most important question for nurse researchers to answer is "What factors lead to a delay in seeking care?" In the interim, nurses need to emphasize the importance of prompt reporting of symptoms regardless of the hour or day of the week. When providing telephone advice, the nurse should clearly delineate the risks of delaying evaluation and treatment, encouraging the women to seek help and evaluation as quickly as possible.

Freda, M. C., Damus, K., & Merkatz, I. (1991). What do pregnant women know about preventing preterm birth? *Journal of Gynecologic, Obstetric, and Neonatal Nursing, 20*(2), 140.

Patterson, E., Douglas, A., Patterson, P. & Bradle, J. (1992). Symptoms of preterm labor and self-diagnostic confusion. *Nursing Research, 41*(6), 367.

findings to determine if therapeutic drug levels (4–7.5 mEq) have been achieved or exceeded. Renal function, electrolyte values, and glucose levels are reassessed periodically when beta-sympathomimetics are administered. The nurse needs to be aware of significant changes in these test results.

Home Uterine Monitoring

Another area of nursing assessment involves monitoring uterine activity and maternal and fetal status while the woman remains at home. Current advances in technology permit recording of uterine activity and fetal heart rate (FHR) using a portable EFM system. Data are then transferred by telephone modem to a center where they are evaluated. Nurses most often assess this information.

Perinatal nurses may also visit the home to assess maternal and fetal status. Home monitoring is cost effective in comparison to long-term hospitalization when PTL occurs.

Studies evaluating the benefits of home uterine monitoring have yielded conflicting results. Several clinical trials have demonstrated earlier detection and treatment of PTL (Mou et al., 1991), or a reduction in the incidence of preterm birth with home monitoring (Hill et al., 1990). Other investigators have reported no reduction in preterm birth as a result of home uterine monitoring alone (Grimes & Schulz, 1992). A positive outcome has been found for high-risk women who received prenatal education and daily telephone contact with nurses (Merkatz & Merkatz, 1991). The American College of Obstetricians and Gynecologists (ACOG) recommends further clinical trials to validate the benefits of home uterine activity monitoring before formulating an official position statement regarding its use (ACOG, 1992).

• • Nursing Diagnosis

A number of problems may be identified when the woman experiences PTL, particularly when tocolytic therapy is implemented. Nursing interventions are based on the following sample of diagnoses:

- Knowledge Deficit related to PTL and treatment
- Impaired Gas Exchange related to pulmonary edema
- Fluid Volume Excess related to beta-sympathomimetic or magnesium sulfate tocolysis
- Altered Nutrition: Less than Body Requirements related to bed rest or tocolytic therapy
- Constipation related to bed rest or tocolytic therapy
- Ineffective Breathing Pattern related to magnesium sulfate tocolysis
- Pain related to tocolysis or prolonged bed rest
- Altered Tissue Perfusion related to beta-sympathomimetic tocolysis

- Impaired Physical Mobility related to prolonged bed rest
- Anxiety related to diagnosis of PTL or impending preterm birth
- High Risk for Fetal Injury related to PTL and preterm birth

• • Planning and Implementation

Providing Information for Self-care

Nursing care of the woman at risk for PTL focuses on education. The goal of teaching is to promote self-monitoring and early recognition of PTL. Important aspects of self-care teaching are included in the Teaching Considerations display.

Expected Outcome

- The woman demonstrates effective self-monitoring activities, as evidenced by daily assessment of uterine activity and prompt reporting of signs and symptoms.

Teaching Considerations

Self-Care to Identify Preterm Labor

The nurse can use the following points in teaching the woman at risk for preterm labor.

The following signs and symptoms should be reported to the care provider *immediately:*

- Uterine contractions that may be felt as abdominal tightening, with or without pain
- Menstrual-like cramping, often rhythmic and felt just above the pelvic bone
- Pelvic pressure or fullness noted in pelvic area, back, or thigh
- Intestinal cramps with or without diarrhea
- An increase in vaginal discharge; the consistency may change from mucousy to watery

If you feel any of these warning signs perform the following steps:

1. Lie down on your left side; use a pillow to support your back.
2. Place your fingertips on your skin, on each side of your abdomen (above the level of your umbilicus), so that you can press inward and feel the differences between tightness and relaxation of the uterus. (If you feel tightening, you are having a contraction.)
3. Use your watch to time the frequency and length of the contractions.
4. If, after an hour, you have four or more contractions in that hour call your physician or midwife *immediately.*
5. Go to the labor and delivery unit immediately if you cannot reach your health care provider.
6. If you have a gush, or a continuous leakage of fluid from the vagina, or a pink or brownish discharge, call the midwife or physician *immediately.*

Providing Support for Tocolytic Administration

The nurse prepares the woman for special tests that may be ordered to determine maternal and fetal status during pregnancy. If the woman is placed on oral tocolytics or a subcutaneous terbutaline infusion pump, the nurse is responsible for explaining the purpose of therapy, describing common side effects, and teaching appropriate self-medication activities. The nurse supervises the woman until she demonstrates proficiency in tasks such as counting her pulse before self-administration of oral terbutaline or changing the site of the subcutaneous needle when an infusion pump is used. When intravenous tocolytic therapy is implemented, the nurse must provide intensive nursing care during the initial administration of the medication.

Rapid implementation of tocolytic therapy is often necessary. The nurse needs to be skilled in providing essential information while preparing to administer the ordered drug. A brief, simple explanation of common side effects is the nurse's responsibility. The woman may be anxious. She is often unprepared for unpleasant side effects and may experience greater fear and distress if she does not understand the treatment's side effects.

Basic nursing care of the woman who is treated for PTL with intravenous tocolytics is outlined in the Nursing Procedure display. If adverse reactions occur after the tocolytic infusion is initiated, the nurse acts to stabilize the woman and maintain physiologic integrity. The nurse stops the infusion, calls for assistance, and proceeds with supportive care.

Total fluid intake is restricted to 2400 to 2500 mL daily to reduce the risk of pulmonary edema. The woman is provided with supplies that permit frequent mouth care because thirst and dry mucous membranes can make her uncomfortable. Once the woman's status is stable and she is permitted to eat, a consultation with a registered dietitian may be necessary to determine her food preferences and appropriate dietary intake. Small frequent meals may be better tolerated than three large meals a day when the woman is restricted to bed and is in the Trendelenberg position. Fruits and vegetables with a high water content, such as watermelon or cucumbers, must be limited because they add to the total fluid intake. Support of the woman receiving magnesium sulfate is given in the Nursing Care Plan.

Once a maintenance dose of the tocolytic has been achieved and contractions cease, the nurse is responsible for weaning the woman from the intravenous drug according to a standardized protocol or physician's order. This is accomplished by slowly reducing the infusion rate, while monitoring uterine activity. If the woman remains stable, the infusion is reduced to a rate equal to the dose of an oral tocolytic. The infusion is stopped 30 minutes after administration of the first dose of the oral tocolytic.

NURSING PROCEDURE

Supporting the Woman Receiving Tocolytic Therapy

Purpose: To support maternal and fetal physiologic status during administration of tocolysis and to identify and treat adverse reaction to specific drugs.

NURSING ACTION	*RATIONALE*
1. Maintain strict bed rest in lateral decubitus position.	To prevent injury secondary to orthostatic hypotension and improve uteroplacental perfusion.
2. Place bed in Trendelenberg position.	To reduce pressure of fetal presenting part on cervix.
3. Apply external fetal monitor and tocotransducer.	To obtain baseline data on fetal heart rate pattern and uterine activity.
4. Obtain baseline vital signs.	To determine effect of tocolytic on maternal vital signs and status.
5. Obtain sterile urine specimen by catheterizing the bladder.	To rule out urinary tract infection as causative factor in preterm labor.
6. Obtain cervical and vaginal cultures as ordered.	To identify pathologic organisms implicated in preterm labor.
7. Obtain lab studies including CBC with differential, electrolytes, glucose, blood type and hold as ordered.	To obtain baseline value and identify significant changes that may occur due to infection or tocolysis.
8. Assist with or obtain ECG if ordered before initiation of tocolytic therapy.	To identify undiagnosed cardiac disease before initiating beta-sympathomimetics especially in women who have not received prenatal care or are poor historians regarding medical history.
9. Initiate an intravenous line and use a physiologic solution such as Ringer's lactate as the mainline.	To provide intravenous access should the tocolytic have to be stopped or emergency drugs be administered.
10. Restrict oral and IV fluid intake to 100 mL/h or less.	To prevent fluid overload, which could lead to pulmonary edema.
11. Explain common side effects of medication.	To prepare woman for unpleasant side effects that may frighten her.
12. Piggyback tocolytic to mainline and administer via an infusion pump.	To control drug administration and prevent accidental overdose.
13. Monitor blood pressure, pulse and respiration every 10 to 15 minutes during initial infusion, and until maintenance dose of tocolytic is achieved and maternal fetal vital signs are stable.	To determine the effect of tocolytic therapy on maternal vital signs. To identify adverse reactions to drug.
14. Auscultate heart rate and rhythm every 10 to 15 minutes during initial infusion and until maintenance dose is established, vital signs and maternal-fetal status are stable.	To identify adverse cardiac reaction to beta-sympathomimetic.
15. Instruct woman to notify nurse immediately if chest pain, pressure, or tightness, shortness of breath or cough develops.	To permit rapid treatment of serious cardiopulmonary complications of tocolytic therapy.

Expected Outcomes

- The woman verbalizes correct understanding of the purpose of tocolytic therapy and its side effects and adverse reactions.
- The woman's uterus and cervix respond positively to the therapy.
- The woman maintains an adequate intake of nutrients, as evidenced by appropriate weight gain.
- The woman's condition stabilizes so she can be discharged home.

Providing Comfort

Until the woman is discharged from the hospital, her basic comfort needs are met by the nurse. An eggcrate mattress pad is often placed on the bed. Extra pillows to support the woman's back or placed between her legs will enhance comfort. Sheepskin pads may be used to prevent excoriation of the woman's elbows, knees, or ankles. The nurse must provide frequent pericare until the woman is permitted bathroom privileges.

Text continues on page 740

Nursing Care Plan

The Woman With Preterm Labor Receiving Magnesium Sulfate

PATIENT PROFILE

History

P.L. is a 43-year-old G1/PO at 28 weeks' gestation with twins. She has been admitted to the prenatal unit for PTL. Her condition was stabilized in the labor unit, but she could not be weaned from intravenous magnesium sulfate. She is not a candidate for a continuous terbutaline pump due to an adverse reaction to beta-adrenergics. She is receiving 2.5 g $MgSO_4$/h. She is on a regimen of bed rest with bathroom privileges. She is on a regular diet and her total fluid intake is restricted to 2500 mL/24 h. The physician has ordered Colace 250 mg b.i.d., and iron therapy for anemia.

Physical Assessment

Three days after admission the nurse is performing an assessment and notes the following: T 37.0°C (98.6°F); B/P 100/68, P 80, RR 22; FHR in the 150 bpm range. Ongoing pattern of 1–3 contractions per hour (unchanged since admission); P.L. is lethargic, but awake and oriented; DTRS +1; regular heart rhythm; breath sounds clear and equal bilaterally; hypoactive bowel sounds, with last BM 48 h ago; abdomen soft, but distended with air; eating 50% of food on meal trays; maintaining the 2500-mL fluid restriction regimen; voiding approximately 2200 mL/24 h. Skin is warm, pink, and dry; excoriations on elbows, knees, and ankles.

P.L. denies urinary frequency or dysuria, backache, pelvic pressure, or cramping. She does not feel the 1–3 contractions she has each hour. She states, "I am so sleepy all the time, but I haven't had a decent night's sleep with all the interruptions. I know I should be eating more, but I hate the food here, and I don't have much of an appetite anyway. I'm terribly bloated. I usually have a bowel movement every day."

COLLABORATIVE PROBLEMS/POTENTIAL COMPLICATIONS

- Respiratory depression
- Pulmonary edema
- Paralytic ileus

(See the accompanying Nursing Alert display.)

Assessment	*Nursing Diagnosis*	*Nursing Interventions*	*Rationale*
P.L. is on bed rest and receives 2.5 g $MgSO_4$/h. She has hypoactive bowel sounds and has a soft abdomen distended with air. She is receiving iron therapy and Colace. Her fluid intake is restricted to 2500 mL/24 h. P.L. has had no bowel movement for 48 h and her usual bowel habit is every day.	Constipation related to bed rest, iron therapy, $MgSO_4$, and fluid restriction ***Expected Outcome*** P.L. will have a bowel movement within 6–12 h of taking a laxative. P.L. will verbalize some degree of relief of abdominal distention. P.L. will eat foods high in fiber.	Teach P.L. about foods that are high in fiber and encourage their intake.	High-fiber food may prevent constipation.
		Administer Colace as ordered.	Colace is a stool softener that reduces risk of constipation.
		Notify physician of alteration in bowel function.	Physician should be apprised of P.L.'s condition to assess her needs and order appropriate treatment of constipation.
		Administer laxative (ie, Milk of Magnesia) or antiflatulent as ordered.	Mild laxative may be required to relieve constipation.
		Eliminate gas-forming foods.	Combination of bed rest, $MgSO_4$, and ingestion of gas-forming food may cause significant abdominal distention. Antiflatulent may decrease discomfort associated with gas formation.
		Assess for bowel sounds and evidence of distention each shift. Monitor bowel habits daily.	Close monitoring is essential to prevent the development of constipation, which may increase uterine activity.

(*Continued*)

The Woman With Preterm Labor Receiving Magnesium Sulfate

(*Continued*)

Assessment	Nursing Diagnosis	Nursing Interventions	Rationale
P.L. is on bed rest and receives an IV $MgSO_4$ infusion. She does not like the foods offered for her meals. P.L. is eating only 50% of food on trays. P.L. states, "I know I should be eating more but I hate the food here."	Altered Nutrition, Less than Body Requirements related to tocolytic therapy, bed rest, and dissatisfaction with food served to her. ***Expected Outcome*** P.L. will select foods she prefers to eat. P.L. will consume sufficient calories in balanced proportions for her needs and fetal growth and development.	Make referral to registered dietitian or assist P.L. with selection of foods she prefers.	Selecting preferred foods may stimulate P.L.'s appetite. $MgSO_4$ and bed rest will depress P.L.'s appetite. Dietitian may suggest high-calorie foods when P.L.'s appetite is depressed.
		If possible, have family members bring in home-cooked meals, or favorite restaurant food.	P.L. may ingest more calories if she receives home-cooked meals that appeal to her.
		Offer frequent mouth care.	The appetite may be stimulated by mouth care.
		Serve meals when P.L. prefers to eat if microwave is available to heat food.	Encouraging P.L. to eat when hungry may result in her eating more foods.
		Weigh P.L. daily and monitor weight loss or gain.	Weight loss is contraindicated in pregnancy and can deprive the fetus of essential nutrients for growth and development.
P.L. in on bed rest and has excoriations on elbows, knees, and ankles.	Altered Skin Integrity related to bed rest and hospital linen. ***Expected Outcome*** P.L.'s skin will demonstrate healing of excoriations on elbows, knees, and ankles. P.L. will demonstrate no further skin breakdown.	Apply eggcrate mattress to P.L.'s bed. Use sheepskin pads over bony prominences or sheepskin pad over sheet.	Continuous pressure and friction will contribute to excoriation and breakdown of skin.
		Keep P.L.'s skin dry. Change wet or soiled linen promptly.	Moisture facilitates bacterial growth and breakdown of skin.
		Use soap sparingly. Use lotion to soften skin.	Soap destroys acid mantle of skin and dries skin, contributing to cracking and breakdown.
P.L. is on bed rest and states, "I'm so sleepy, but I haven't had a decent night's sleep with all the interruptions."	Sleep Pattern Disturbance related to bed rest, tocolytic therapy, nursing care activities, and hospitalization. ***Expected Outcome*** P.L. will verbalize satisfaction with the quality of rest and degree of sleep.	Coordinate nursing activities to minimize frequent interruptions.	Hospital routine and frequent interruptions by staff and visitors can prevent adequate periods of time for rest or sleep. Providing periods of uninterrupted rest will enhance quality of rest and may promote sleep.
		Decrease environmental stimuli (dim lights, reduce noise, turn off phone) during periods of rest. Place "Do not disturb" sign on door during periods of rest. Offer massage to enhance rest. Place eggcrate mattress on bed and provide extra pillows for comfort.	Physical discomforts associated with prolonged bed rest, sleeping in strange bed, and limitation in movement due to IV therapy, will interfere with quality of rest.

(*Continued*)

The Woman With Preterm Labor Receiving Magnesium Sulfate
(Continued)

Assessment	Nursing Diagnosis	Nursing Interventions	Rationale
		Suggest P.L.'s family bring in radio, tape cassette or CD player, or device to provide white noise, if feasible.	Listening to restful music or using "white noise" machine has been found to reduce the person's awareness of usual environmental sounds and may promote rest.

EVALUATION P.L had a bowel movement 8 h after receiving Milk of Magnesia. She verbalized some relief of abdominal distention. Adjustments were made in types of food and timing of meals to meet P.L.'s preferences. P.L. consumed 75% to 80% of food on each tray and two daily snacks provided by diet kitchen. P.L.'s husband brought special foods for the dinner meal when he visited after work. After she was placed on an eggcrate mattress and sheepskin pads were applied, P.L. verbalized increased comfort. Her skin excoriations healed within 3 days. P.L. limited the number of phone calls and visitors and listened to her favorite cassettes. She was pleased with the improved quality of her rest and sleep.

NURSING ALERT

NURSING RESPONSIBILITIES WHEN CARING FOR THE WOMAN RECEIVING INTRAVENOUS TOCOLYTICS

The woman receiving intravenous tocolytics (magnesium sulfate or ritodrine) is at increased risk for developing life-threatening cardiopulmonary complications. Myocardial decompensation, respiratory depression, and pulmonary edema are usually the most serious problems that may arise. The nurse must be alert for signs and symptoms of adverse reactions and be prepared to implement emergency supportive care. Before initiating intravenous tocolytic therapy, the nurse should verify that oxygen and suction equipment are readily available and functioning. Emergency drugs required to reverse the effects of tocolytics (ie, calcium gluconate for magnesium sulfate toxicity) and other adverse responses also should be easily accessible. Close monitoring of the woman is essential to identify early signs of drug toxicity, allergic reactions, or severe side effects. In case of adverse reactions to tocolytic agents, the nurse must be prepared to stop the infusion and implement supportive care such as oxygen administration. The nurse must also initiate cardiopulmonary resuscitation should the woman experience cardiac or respiratory arrest.

The woman's emotional needs should not be neglected. The nurse encourages frequent visits from the partner and other family members. A referral to occupational therapy may be initiated early. Creative strategies that reduce isolation can be devised, such as permitting the woman to leave the unit in a wheelchair or on a gurney for a short time when her condition is stable. Some prenatal units have developed support groups for women who require extended hospitalization. Women may be placed in wheelchairs or on gurneys and transported to a room where small groups can meet periodically to share their feelings and concerns. The neonatal nursing staff should initiate contact with the woman and answer her questions regarding special care should birth occur prematurely.

Expected Outcomes

- The woman verbalizes satisfaction with the implemented comfort measures.
- The woman verbalizes satisfaction with family contact and diversional activities.

Preparing the Woman for Preterm Birth

If preterm birth appears inevitable, the nurse prepares the woman for the delivery and anticipated events in the immediate postpartum period. Neonatal personnel must be notified of the impending birth in a timely manner so they are present at the delivery. The nurse assists the physician with the delivery, provides needed supplies, and keeps the woman informed about the fetal condition and procedures being performed. Lynam and Miller (1992) found that women experiencing PTL had a strong desire for frequent information about the fetal status and that this need was often not appreciated by the labor nurse.

Expected Outcome

- The woman verbalizes satisfaction with her level of participation in the birth and the information provided by the nurse.

MANAGED CARE PATH

Preterm Labor

Expected Length of Stay: 1–10 days

	Admission/Stabilization/ Labor–Delivery	Maintenance/Postpartum
Key Goals	No cervical change, fetus stable Hemodynamically stable, no s/s infection or pulmonary edema (L & D) Pain relief option, adequate progression of labor vaginal delivery of infant	No cervical change, fetus stable No s/s infection (PP) discharge to PP 1–2 hours after delivery (PP) Up with assistance
Consults	Anesthesia, NICU. Social work prn	Social work, parent ed., dietary prn
Tests/Labs	CBC with diff., UA, C&S, cervical culture, T&S, SMA 6, biophysical profile (BPP). Amnio prn. (L & D) EFM, dipstick UA, T&S, CBC with diff direct Coombs, Rh on umb. blood, cord gas if Apgar <7	WBC, amniocentesis prn
Meds	Tocolytic, antibiotic, steroid prn. Stool softener, pain med, sedative prn. (L & D) Pain med, antibiotic, pitocin augmentation and after placenta prn	Tocolytic, antibiotic, steroid prn. Stool softener, pain med, sedative prn
Treatments	Assess per protocol (EFM, DTR, pulse oximetry) Foley, IV, I&O, urine cultures prn (L & D) as above	Assess per protocol (EFM, UCs) IV fluids prn (PP) D/C IV, I&O prn
Teaching	Plan of care (EFM, meds, BPP, VS, meds) Palpation of UCs Prep for L & D prn	S & S labor, PROM, vag. bleeding Limitations (sexual/physical activity) Prep for L/D
Equipment	Foley, IV kit, infusion pump, speculum, bedpan	Heplock with flush for IV prn
Diet	NPO to clear liq	Regular with snacks ×2
Activity	Bedrest or bedrest with BRP. (L & D) Up ad lib with assist	BR with BRP, wheelchair prn. (PP) up ad lib
D/C Plan	Social support, family, housing	Eval. for d/c., home care, transport needs.

Adapted from collaborative paths developed by the Department of Nursing Service, Vanderbilt University Medical Center, Nashville, TN.

Evaluation

For effective management of PTL, the high-risk woman will recognize early signs of PTL and report them promptly to the physician or midwife. She will be actively engaged in self-care activities recommended by the health team to prevent PTL, including self-administration of tocolytics. Ideally, the pregnancy will be extended, and a healthy neonate will be born at term. If problems arise that result in recurring PTL, the nurse adapts the plan of care to meet the changing needs of the woman and her fetus.

Preterm Premature Rupture of Membranes

When rupture of the membranes occurs prior to 37 weeks' gestation, it is described as *preterm premature rupture of membranes (PPROM)*. This condition is distinct from premature rupture of membranes (PROM) after 37 weeks of gestation in terms of complications, medical management, and nursing care. Women experiencing PROM at term usually begin labor within 24 hours in 80% to 90% of cases. With

PPROM, 20% to 40% of women may not begin labor (latency period) for 7 days or longer (Williams, 1991a). In some cases of PPROM, small ruptures in the membranes appear to reseal, permitting continuance of pregnancy to term (Johnson, Egerman, & Moorhead, 1990).

Etiologic and Predisposing Factors

The precise cause of PPROM is unknown. Infections of the reproductive tract have been implicated in PPROM including beta-hemolytic streptococci, *C. trachomatis*, and *Listeria* species. Specific predisposing factors include the following:

- Previous preterm birth
- Cigarette smoking
- Fetal anomalies
- Coitus
- Amnionitis
- Vaginal colonization with group B streptococci
- Prenatal vaginal bleeding in more than one trimester
- Increased intrauterine volume (polyhydramnios and multiple gestation)

Diagnosis

Early and accurate evaluation of membrane status is essential if PPROM is suspected. This is accomplished through sterile speculum examination and nitrazine and fern testing (see Chapter 20). Digital examination of the cervix is contraindicated. The risk of preterm delivery and maternal and neonatal infection is increased significantly when digital examinations are performed after PPROM (Lewis et al., 1992).

When PPROM is suspected but the woman does not present with gross leakage of fluid or pooling of fluid in the vagina, other tools may be used to confirm the diagnosis. Ultrasonography can be used to measure amniotic fluid volume (AFV), which is reduced with PPROM. If all other tests are inconclusive, an amniocentesis may be performed to instill indigo carmine or Evans blue dyes (FDA class C) into the amniotic fluid. The nurse then observes the patient for leakage of blue-colored fluid from the vagina. Methylene blue (class D if instilled into amniotic fluid) is no longer recommended for this procedure because of the potentially toxic effects on maternal and fetal tissues (Williams, 1991a).

Maternal, Fetal, and Neonatal Implications

There is an increased risk of intrauterine infection known as chorioamnionitis if labor does not begin within 12 to 24 hours after PPROM. Individual risk factors such as smoking, poverty and poor nutritional status also predispose the woman to infection. Postpartum endometritis (infection of the endometrial lining of the uterus) subsequent to PPROM also is common. Women with PPROM are at two to three times greater risk for abruptio placentae (premature separation of the placenta). The leading cause of fetal death associated with PPROM is infection.

The greatest risks for the neonate are respiratory distress of prematurity and infection when PPROM is followed by PTL and delivery. A neonatal mortality rate of 29% has been reported with PPROM before 34 weeks' gestation. Mortality rises to 37% in neonates when PPROM occurs *before* 26 weeks' gestation (Major & Kitzmiller, 1990). However, perinatal survival has improved dramatically with technologic advances in the care of preterm neonates. Sixty-eight percent of the surviving neonates born before 26 weeks in the study by Major and Kitzmiller (1990) had normal neurologic and physical development at 1 year of age. PPROM before 20 weeks' gestation results in postbirth problems, such as pulmonary hypoplasia, which are generally fatal to the neonate (see Chapter 33).

Treatment

Treatment of PPROM is strongly influenced by the gestational age, as summarized in Table 27-3.

Once rupture of membranes is confirmed, initial management includes the following steps:

- Verification of gestational age
- Determination of fetal pulmonary maturity
- Identification of pathologic bacterial infections
- Detection of fetal anomalies and compromise

Active Management. Active management of PPROM may include:

- Tocolytic therapy to prolong the pregnancy after PPROM
- Antibiotic therapy to treat specific infections identified on culture of the cervix, vagina, or amniotic fluid or to prevent infection
- Steroid administration to accelerate lung maturation
- Amnioinfusion (see Chapter 26) to reduce fetal skeletal compression deformities or pulmonary hypoplasia with prolonged PPROM

Controversy surrounds the use of *tocolytic drugs* that inhibit uterine activity when PPROM occurs. PTL may be initiated by asymptomatic intrauterine infection, in which case prompt delivery of the fetus is indicated. Once infection

Table 27-3. Medical Management of Preterm Premature Rupture of Membranes Based on Gestational Age of the Fetus

Fetal Gestational Age	Medical Management
34–36 wk	The risk of infection is generally greater than the risk of respiratory distress of prematurity. If labor does not begin spontaneously, oxytocin induction is usually planned
28–33 wk	Amniocentesis may be performed to determine fetal gestational age and to identify evidence of infection If no signs of infection or labor, observation and bed rest If signs of infection develop, delivery is planned by the vaginal route or by cesarean delivery if signs of fetal distress occur
Under 28 wk	80% of fetuses deliver within 1 wk. Hydration by IV route to increase the amniotic fluid volume or by amnioinfusion has been attempted experimentally, with limited success, to prevent compression anomalies

is ruled out (ie, by cultures and normal leukocyte count), tocolysis may be implemented for one of two reasons:

- To prolong the latency period for several days to allow fetal lung maturation
- To prolong the latency period for several weeks to lessen the neonatal problems related to extreme prematurity and low birth weight

Antibiotic therapy is recommended by some experts when beta-hemolytic streptococci or *C. trachomatis* is identified in cervical cultures. Chlamydia is associated with neonatal conjunctivitis and pneumonia. Beta-streptococcal infection is associated with significant morbidity and mortality in the neonate (Williams, 1991a). Prophylactic administration of antibiotics has been evaluated as a preventive measure against maternal, fetal, and neonatal infection. (Johnston, Ramos, Vaughn, Todd, & Benrubi, 1990; McGregor, French, & Seo, 1991).

Corticosteroids such as betamethasone have been used to promote fetal lung maturity; conflicting research findings continue to cast doubts on their value. The use of steroids is not without risk. Fluid retention secondary to steroid use may increase the risk of pulmonary edema in the woman when underlying infection complicates PPROM or tocolytics are administered.

Saline amnioinfusions have been used experimentally to avoid the unfavorable effects of oligohydramnios on umbilical cord circulation and pulmonary development. Imanaka and coworkers (1989) initiated a continuous amnioinfusion of a saline solution containing antibiotics, with an indwelling cervical catheter. Amniotic fluid volume was increased and pregnancy was extended by an average of 8 days. This procedure will require extensive evaluation before it can be recommended in the active management of PPROM.

Many aspects of active management, particularly before 23 to 24 weeks' gestation, remain controversial. The boundaries of perinatal medicine are expanding; the value of implementing extraordinary treatment at 20 to 22 weeks' gestation remains questionable and raises significant ethical dilemmas.

Conservative Management. Expectant or conservative management of PPROM involves careful observation; invasive interventions are withheld unless signs of chorioamnionitis or fetal distress are seen. When PPROM occurs, the risks associated with maintaining *or* terminating the pregnancy are considerable; conservative management may be preferred by the woman and her partner. Conservative management in this case would include bed rest, frequent assessment of maternal vital signs for infection, and monitoring fetal well-being (biophysical profile and nonstress testing; see Chapter 22).

• • Assessment

Nursing responsibilities in the care of women experiencing PPROM center on minimizing the risk of infection and promoting optimal maternal and fetal status. The goals are to prolong pregnancy and to achieve a safe delivery of the neonate without risk to the woman or fetus.

After PPROM, the woman's temperature and pulse and respiratory rates are monitored every 2 to 4 hours. Elevations in respirations and pulse rate often precede a rise in temperature. Intermittent or continuous external FHR monitoring is initiated. The FHR is another sensitive indicator of chorioamnionitis. Fetal tachycardia often occurs before an elevation in the woman's temperature is noted. The woman is observed for other signs and symptoms of chorioamnionitis including:

- Shaking chills and fever
- Uterine tenderness
- Uterine irritability (frequent, low amplitude contractions)
- Malodorous amniotic fluid
- Purulent vaginal discharge
- Rising white blood cell count

The FHR is intermittently evaluated and continuous or intermittent tokodynamometry is initiated with the EFM. The nurse assesses for evidence of uterine activity. When PPROM occurs before 26 to 28 weeks, subtle contractions may be difficult to detect on the electronic monitor or by palpation. The woman should be evaluated for other signs of uterine activity including cramping, low backache, and pelvic pressure.

Ongoing assessments of the woman's physical and psychological reactions to PPROM and its treatment are conducted. If antibiotic therapy is initiated to prevent infection or amnioinfusion is implemented to reduce cord compression, the nurse monitors maternal and fetal responses. The nurse is responsible for initiating treatments such as oxytocin induction of labor and administration of betamethasone or antibiotics. The nurse should verify that the woman understands why these treatments are being implemented and what the risks and benefits are for each procedure.

• • Nursing Diagnosis

A variety of nursing diagnoses related to physiologic problems may be identified on assessment of the woman with PPROM, including:

- Anxiety related to tests and procedures
- High Risk for Maternal/Fetal/Neonatal Infection related to PPROM
- High Risk for Fetal Injury related to oligohydramnios
- Decreased Fetal Cardiac Output and Tissue Perfusion related to umbilical cord compression
- Fluid Volume Excess (maternal pulmonary edema) related to administration of steroids (betamethasone)
- Pain related to diagnostic procedures or initiation of therapy

• • Planning and Implementation

During the initial evaluation of the woman, the nurse assists with diagnostic tests and prepares the woman for necessary procedures. Although obtaining informed consent is the responsibility of the physician or midwife, the nurse often answers questions and clarifies areas of concern for the woman and her partner. If complicated treatment decisions must be made, the nurse should verify that the woman has had as much time as possible to discuss her options with her family and health care providers.

The nurse takes steps to minimize infection while caring for the woman who has suspected or diagnosed PPROM. Vaginal examinations are avoided or kept to a minimum. Surgical asepsis should be maintained during the performance of invasive procedures such as amniocentesis. The woman with PPROM is frequently maintained on strict bed rest. Pericare should be provided after use of the bedpan and with the daily bed bath. The importance of wiping the perineum from front to back should be reinforced to reduce the risk of ascending vaginal infection.

Expected Outcomes

- The woman verbalizes understanding of her condition, fetal prognosis, and treatment options.
- The woman verbalizes satisfaction with the decision-making process in the treatment of PPROM.
- The woman verbalizes understanding of the procedures performed to treat PPROM before they are implemented.
- The woman and fetus remain free of signs and symptoms of chorioamnionitis.

• • Evaluation

The nursing process mandates ongoing evaluation of maternal and fetal responses to PPROM and its treatment. If expected outcomes are achieved, the woman and her fetus will remain free of infection, and delivery will be delayed until fetal pulmonary maturity is achieved. The woman will be an active participant in the decision-making process regarding management of her condition. Given the opportunity, she will verbalize satisfaction with the process. The fetus will demonstrate evidence of well-being while in utero, and when delivery occurs, will achieve physiologic stability after birth. If the stated goals of care are not realized, the nurse revises the nursing care plan to reflect new priorities.

Pregnancy-Induced Hypertension

Hypertension is considered the most significant medical complication of pregnancy and remains the second leading cause of maternal death in the United States. It is estimated that hypertension complicates approximately 10% of pregnancies. This constitutes a major challenge for the maternity nurse. Hypertension is a generic term referring to a variety of conditions that include an elevation in blood pressure during the prenatal, intrapartum, or postpartum period. To clarify the differences among hypertensive diseases during pregnancy, the ACOG developed a clinical classification, as presented in the accompanying display.

Pregnancy-induced hypertension is a hypertensive disorder unique to pregnancy. PIH is further differentiated into two serious diseases: preeclampsia and eclampsia. *Preeclampsia* is a slowly progressive, multisystem disease that occurs primarily after the 20th week of gestation, but most frequently near term. If it occurs in the first trimester, it is associated with hydatidiform mole or Rh isoimmunization and hydrops fetalis. *Eclampsia* is an extension of PIH and represents a worsening of the condition. It is characterized by the development of grand mal seizures.

A major pathologic feature of both preeclampsia and eclampsia is a marked increase in *peripheral vascular resistance due to vasospasm*. This vascular change is responsible for the blood pressure elevations commonly observed. However, hypertension is *not* the major pathologic problem in PIH, except when blood pressure levels are extremely high (above 160/110). Life-threatening cerebral, renal, and hepatic changes characteristic of PIH pose greater risks for the woman.

Classification of Hypertensive Disorders of Pregnancy With Diagnostic Criteria

Pregnancy-Induced Hypertension (PIH)

Preeclampsia: Hypertension with proteinuria, edema, or both developing after the 20th week of gestation

Mild: B/P of 140/90 or greater; *or* an increase of 30 mm Hg in the systolic or 15 mm Hg in the diastolic over baseline

Severe: B/P of 160/110 or greater; proteinuria of 5 g/24 h; cerebral disturbances, pulmonary edema, or HELLP syndrome

Eclampsia: Extension of preeclampsia with tonic–clonic seizures

Chronic Hypertension

Hypertension (140/90 mm Hg) before pregnancy; or discovery of hypertension before the 20th week of gestation; or continuation of hypertension indefinitely after pregnancy

Chronic Hypertension With Superimposed PIH

Preexisting chronic hypertension complicated by PIH

Superimposed preeclampsia

Superimposed eclampsia

Late or Transient Hypertension

Transient elevations of blood pressure during labor or in the early postpartum period, returning to baseline within 10 days of delivery

From The American College of Obstetricians and Gynecologists. (1986). Management of preeclampsia. *ACOG Technical Bulletin #91. Washington, DC: ACOG. © 1986.*

Etiologic and Predisposing Factors

Despite decades of research, the pathogenesis of PIH is still not completely understood. PIH was formerly termed *toxemia* because it was theorized that some unknown toxin was responsible for the pathologic processes. Research suggests that a yet-to-be-identified toxic substance may be implicated in the etiology (Taylor et al., 1991). A growing consensus attributes the development of preeclampsia to *maternal vascular endothelial cell injury*, possibly as a result of a circulating toxin (Khong, Sawyer, & Heryet, 1992). Damage to this single layer of cells lining the inner lumen of both arteries and veins is suggested as the underlying cause of subsequent pathologic changes associated with PIH. The underlying cause of maternal endothelial cell damage remains a mystery. One theory proposes that impaired vascular invasion of the uterine lining by trophoblasts is responsible for initial endothelial damage. There is some indication that an autoimmune response may be responsible in some cases. Easterling and Benedetti (1989) suggest that an abnormally elevated cardiac output in early pregnancy creates excessive pressure in arterioles, causing damage to endothelial cells. See Figure 27-1 for more information on the pathophysiology of preeclampsia.

Pathophysiology of PIH

Pregnancy-induced hypertension is a *multisystem disease*, with classic signs and symptoms resulting from damage in many organs. The nurse caring for the woman with preeclampsia or eclampsia must have a comprehensive knowledge of these changes to identify danger signals and plan appropriate care.

Alterations in Central Nervous System (CNS) Function. Newer technologies, such as computed tomography scanning and magnetic resonance imaging have helped to delineate changes in the maternal brain induced by PIH. Hypertension and damage to the endothelial cells in the brain results in cerebral hemorrhage, edema, and thrombosis. The most common cause of death in PIH is cerebral hemorrhage, which occurs in approximately 60% of women who die after eclamptic seizures (Ferris, 1988). Headache, visual disturbances including blurred or double vision and scotoma, hyperreflexia, clonus, altered consciousness, and seizures are consequences of brain pathology.

Alteration in Cardiovascular Function. Maternal cardiac function may be greatly altered, particularly with severe PIH. Research indicates that pregnancy complicated by PIH results in an elevation of cardiac output in the early stages of the disease. As vasoconstriction and hypertension worsen, a dramatic change in hemodynamics occurs (Easterling & Benedetti, 1989). *Preload*, the filling volume of either ventricle before systole, is decreased due to hemoconcentration and the lowered circulating blood volume. *Afterload*, the amount of vascular resistance the left ventricle must contract against during systole, is elevated. This is due to vasospasm, vasoconstriction, and the dramatic increase in systemic vascular resistance. The combination of these two factors (low preload and high afterload) may lead to cardiac decompensation, compromised coronary perfusion, and hypoperfusion of major organ systems including the brain and kidney.

Alterations in the Hematologic System. Thrombocytopenia, a decrease in platelets, is the most common hematologic abnormality in PIH. It is attributed to platelet deposition at the site of endothelial damage and decreased lifespan of the cell. The development of overt thrombocytopenia, a platelet count less than 100,000/μL, is an ominous sign of worsening PIH and the possible development of disseminated intravascular coagulopathy (DIC).

Alterations in the Pulmonary System. Clinically, women with PIH are noted to develop pulmonary edema. It is suggested that decreased plasma oncotic pressure and increased permeability in the vascular endothelial lining permit movement of fluid into the pulmonary interstitial space. These changes result in pulmonary edema.

Alterations in the Renal System. Damage to the vascular endothelium in the kidneys results in the development of a characteristic lesion—*glomerular capillary endotheliosis*. Glomerular cells swell and capillary loops are variably dilated and contracted. Vasoconstriction causes a 60% to 80% decrease in renal perfusion and glomerular filtration in PIH (Ferris, 1988). There is a corresponding elevation in serum creatinine and uric acid levels and a reduction in creatinine clearance.

Proteinuria develops with endothelial damage and is usually a late sign in the course of PIH. Some women will develop proteinuria before overt hypertension occurs. Hematuria may be present due to red blood cell destruction. With severe PIH, oliguria and renal failure may occur.

Alterations in the Hepatic System. Significant lesions may develop in the liver. Periportal hemorrhage and necrosis of liver cells occur. Later, hepatic infarctions may develop. Bleeding from hemorrhagic lesions may extend beneath the liver capsule to form a subcapsular hematoma. In some instances the capsule will rupture, requiring immediate surgical intervention to prevent maternal and fetal death. Severe PIH will result in alteration in tests of hepatic function, including elevations in serum aspartate aminotransferase (AST) and alanine aminotransferase (ALT). The nausea, vomiting, right upper quadrant abdominal pain, and epigastric pain often experienced with severe PIH are attributed to hepatic injury.

Risk Factors for the Development of PIH

Risk factors for the development of PIH have been delineated and include:

- Parity: First pregnancy or first pregnancy with current partner
- Age: Women under age 21 who are nulliparas and women over age 35 who are multiparous
- Family prevalence of the PIH
- Preexisting diabetes or renal disease
- Preexisting chronic hypertension
- Multifetal pregnancy
- Hydatidiform mole
- Hydrops fetalis

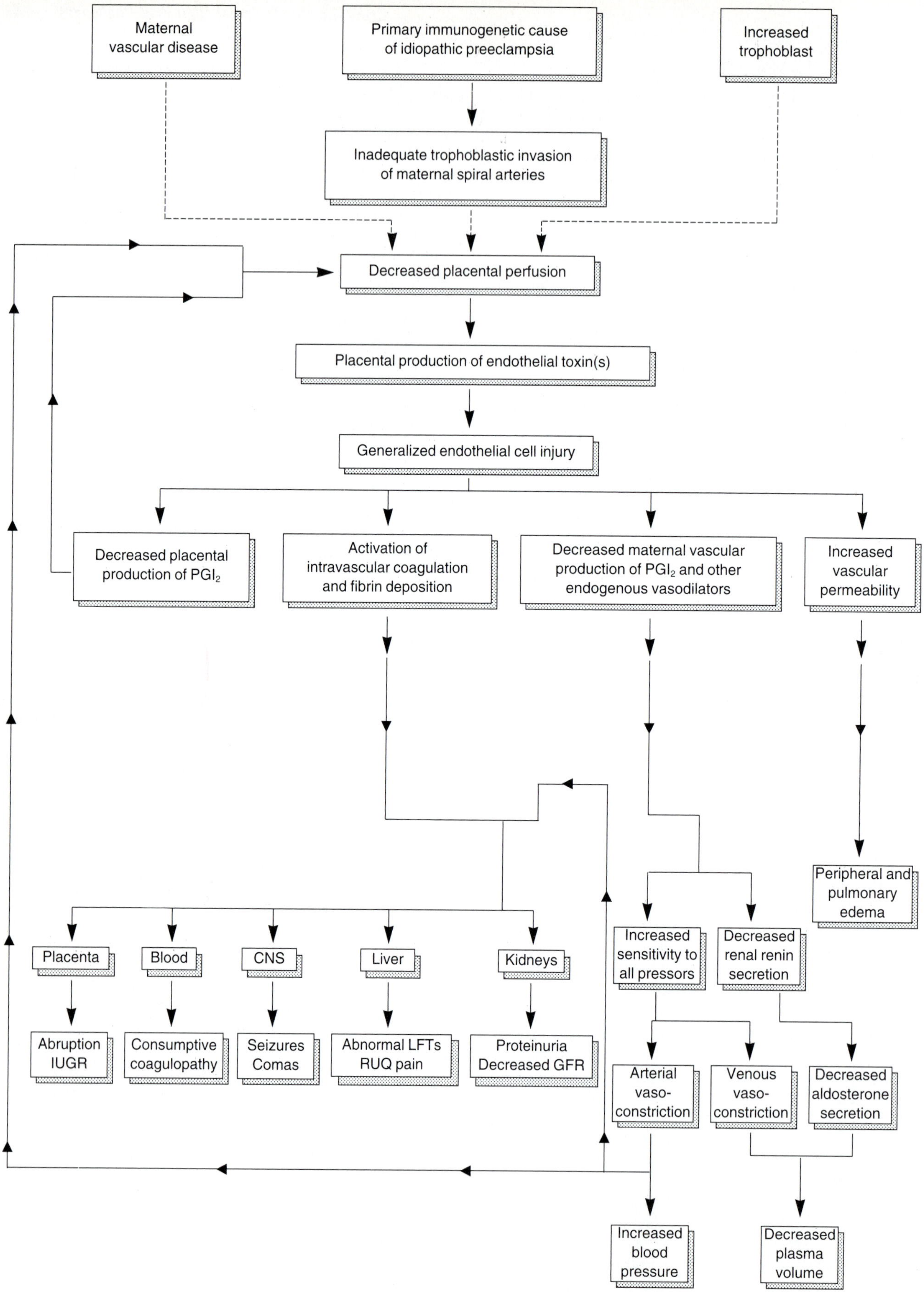

Figure 27-1.

Proposed model illustrating the pathophysiology of preeclampsia. (From Friedman, S., Taylor, R., & Roberts, J. [1991]. Pathophysiology of preeclampsia. *Clinics in Perinatology, 18*[4], 661–678.)

Signs and Symptoms Related to Organ System Involvement in Pregnancy-Induced Hypertention

Central Nervous System

- Headache
- Tinnitus
- Altered mentation
  - Lethargy
  - Somnolence
  - Coma
- Hyperreflexia
- Seizures

Visual Sensory System

- Visual disturbances
  - Scotoma
  - Diplopia
  - Blurred vision
  - Spots or flashes of light in visual field
  - Blindness
- Retinal changes (on fundoscopic exam)
  - Segmental arteriolar narrowing
  - Wet, glistening appearance due to edema
  - Retinal detachment

Cardiovascular System

- Hypertension
- Edema
  - Generalized
  - Hand and face
- Cardiac failure
  - Jugular venous distention

Pulmonary System

- Pulmonary edema
  - Dyspnea
  - Basilar rales

Gastrointestinal System

- Nausea and vomiting
- Hematemesis

Hepatic System

- Right upper quadrant pain
- Epigastric pain
- Hepatic enlargement

Genitourinary System

- Decreased urine output
  - Olguria
  - Anuria
- Hematuria
- Proteinuria

In a recent study, employment during pregnancy more than doubled the risk for preeclampsia, regardless of the work setting (Eskenazi, Fenster, & Sidney, 1991).

Diagnosis

Signs and Symptoms of PIH. The classic triad of symptoms resulting from pathologic changes associated with PIH are:

- *Hypertension*: Defined as a blood pressure of 140/90, or an increase in systolic pressure of 30 mm Hg, or a diastolic pressure of 15 mm Hg above nonpregnant levels.
- *Edema*: Defined as clinically evident swelling or a sudden, rapid weight gain of 1 lb (0.5 kg) a week in second trimester or 216 (0.9 kg) a week in third trimester or greater; nondependent edema of the hands and face is significant.
- *Proteinuria*: Defined as the excretion of 500 mg of protein in 24 hours or a reading of 1 + or greater on a urine dipstick analysis.

The diagnosis of preeclampsia may be more difficult when the classic triad of symptoms is not evident. Research indicates that some women may develop significant organ system injury before the development of overt hypertension. The diagnosis may be delayed when the *relative* rise in the blood pressure is overlooked. This is particularly true when a woman's prepregnancy blood pressure is normally low (90/50 to 100/60 range).

Other signs and symptoms of PIH, which relate to organ system injury, include those listed in the accompanying display. Laboratory findings are extremely useful in the early diagnosis of PIH and are listed in Table 27-4.

Pregnancy-induced hypertension may range from *mild* to *severe*. The progression of the disease is usually slow. Changes in prostaglandin levels and coagulation factors may precede the development of classic signs and symptoms by months. In rare cases, the progression of PIH may be rapid, with mild PIH progressing to its severe form or eclampsia in a matter of days or even hours.

Signs and Symptoms of Eclampsia. Eclampsia, a serious obstetric emergency, represents a worsening of pre-

Table 27-4. Laboratory Findings With Pregnancy-Induced Hypertension

Laboratory Test	Significance
Complete Blood Count	
Hematocrit	Hemoconcentration with subsequent rise in hematocrit is common Hematocrit >40% is significant
Blood smear	To detect schistocytes, fragmented erythrocytes, which occur with hemolysis in HELLP syndrome
Red blood cell count	
Renal Function Tests	
Serum uric acid	≥5.5 mg/100 mL is a strong biochemical indicator Levels > 6.0 mg/100 mL indicate severe PIH
Creatinine	≥1.0 mg/dL Because of the physiologic changes in renal function during normal pregnancy, an elevated creatinine level in preeclampsia is often in a range that would be considered normal for nonpregnant women 2.0–3.0 mg/dL indicates severe PIH
Blood urea nitrogen	8–10 mg/100 mL indicates PIH 10 mg/–16 mg/100 mL indicates severe PIH
Creatinine clearance	<150 mL/min
Coagulation Tests	
Platelets	Usually reduced because of aggregation and decreased life span. <100,000 uL indicates severe PIH or HELLP syndrome
Prothrombin time (PT)	Usually normal levels May increase (>16 s) with severe PIH complicated by abruptio placentae or DIC
Partial thromboplastin time (PTT)	Usually normal levels May increase (>38 s) with severe PIH complicated by abruptio placentae of DIC
Fibrinogen	Usually normal levels <285 mg/dL is significant for coagulopathy
Fibrin degradation products	8–10 μg/mL is abnormal ≥16 μg/mL has been observed with severe PIH Frequently elevated due to localized coagulopathy at site of endothelial cell damage
Liver Function Tests	
Serum alanine aminotransferase (ALT)	Usually normal levels, but may be elevated with liver damage secondary to severe PIH Reference value (0–35 U/L)
Serum aspartate aminotransferase (AST)	Usually normal levels, but may be elevated with liver damage secondary to liver damage Reference value (0–35 U/L)

existent preeclampsia. The cardinal sign of eclampsia is *tonoclonic seizures*. Signs and symptoms signaling an impending convulsion include:

- Epigastric or upper right quadrant pain
- Increasing hyperreflexia
- Development or worsening of clonus

Hypertensive crisis and coma may occur with eclampsia. Other signs that characterize eclampsia are shown in the accompanying display.

Hyperreflexia is an exaggeration of normal, involuntary deep tendon reflexes and indicates increased CNS irritability. It may be caused by the cerebral edema and ischemia, which occur with PIH. The Nursing Procedure display reviews the procedure for evaluating DTRs and ankle clonus.

Clonus refers to a rapid, alternating contraction and relaxation, of a muscle group. The development of clonus is an indicator of increasing CNS irritability. Ankle clonus, a rhythmic jerking contraction of the foot, may be observed when the foot is rapidly dorsiflexed by the nurse.

Convulsions and hypertensive crises associated with eclampsia may appear before, during, or after labor or in the early postpartum period. It is estimated that approximately one third of women who develop eclampsia do so in the postpartum period. The risk of convulsions is greatest in the first 24 hours postpartum.

During an eclamptic convulsion, the maternal pulse rate increases dramatically, and blood pressure may reach 200 mm Hg systolic with hyperpyrexia of 39°C (103°F) to 40°C (104°F). A typical convulsion may last for 15 to 20 seconds

Signs and Symptoms of Eclampsia

Symptoms of Impending Eclampsia

- Severe headache
- Visual disturbances
- Epigastric pain
- Vomiting
- Increasing clonus

Signs Characterizing Eclampsia

- Increasing hyperreflexia
- Seizures*
- Worsening hypertension (>160/110)
- Proteinuria: 5 g/24 h
- Oliguria: 500 mL/24 h or less
- Hyperreflexia (4+ DTR or sustained clonus)
- Pulmonary edema
- Congestive heart failure

**Eclampsia is defined as the extension of pre-eclampsia with* seizure activity.

and begins with facial twitching and rolling of the eyes. The muscles of the entire body quickly become rigidly contracted; the face is distorted; the eyes protrude; the arms are flexed; and the hands are clenched. Fixation of the diaphragm occurs and respiration ceases.

After 20 seconds of this tonic contraction, clonic contractions begin with violent opening and closing of the eyes and jaws and contraction and relaxation of the extremities. The woman will thrash about and will need protection to avoid injury. She may bite her tongue at this time. When the seizure ends, the patient will take a long, labored breath. Gradually more normal respiration will resume. Coma ensues, and consciousness is gradually regained over a number of hours. Once they begin, convulsions usually recur unless treatment is initiated.

Diagnosis of HELLP Syndrome. A serious complication of PIH affecting approximately 8.5% of women is known as *HELLP syndrome*. *HELLP* is an acronym for the major pathologic findings of this disorder:

- **H**: Hemolysis of red blood cells
- **EL**: Elevated liver enzymes
- **LP**: Low platelet count (less than 100,000)

Women with HELLP syndrome generally present with symptoms of a viral-like illness, including malaise, nausea, and vomiting. Epigastric or right upper quadrant pain is a common complaint. The woman may seek medical care for other nonspecific symptoms of illness such as edema, jaundice, hematuria, flank or shoulder pain, or diffuse abdominal pain. Hypertension is absent in 20% of cases and is mild in another 30% of women with the disease (Sibai, 1991). Proteinuria is uncommon or a late finding. As a result, the diagnosis of HELLP syndrome may be missed initially. Laboratory studies are used to make a differential diagnosis.

The identification of *microangiopathic hemolytic anemia*, based on altered red blood cell morphology, is strongly diagnostic of the disorder. Examination of a peripheral blood smear most often reveals *schistocytes*, small irregularly shaped red blood cells, and *echinocytes* (burr cells), contracted erythrocytes with spiny projections. Elevated liver enzymes (ALT and AST) occur as a result of focal necrosis and hemorrhage in the liver. Thrombocytopenia (less than 100,000 μL) is indicative of coagulopathy.

Symptoms of HELLP often have a gradual onset and appear from as early as the 17th week of gestation to the first postpartum week. Recent studies indicate that the disease peaks in intensity 24 to 48 hours *after* delivery, followed by rapid recovery if appropriate treatment is initiated (Martin et al., 1991). Hypertension is absent or mild in approximately 50% of women with HELLP syndrome.

Maternal, Fetal, and Neonatal Implications

The major maternal and fetal complications of PIH are those associated with eclampsia and its associated seizures or hypertensive crisis, HELLP syndrome, and DIC. Death from mild PIH itself is relatively rare, whereas maternal mortality among women with eclampsia is estimated to be 10% to 15%. The most frequent cause of maternal death associated with eclampsia is cerebral hemorrhage. Other causes of maternal mortality include congestive heart failure (CHF), hemorrhage and shock secondary to abruptio placentae, hepatic rupture, HELLP syndrome, or DIC.

For women who survive PIH, the majority experience a complete resolution of the multisystem disease process within 6 weeks to 2 months postpartum. Blood pressure levels may return to normal within 1 to 2 days of delivery. Some women may experience mild elevations in pressure for 6 to 8 weeks after delivery. Recent research indicates that recurrent PIH is more likely in subsequent pregnancies. Women who develop severe PIH in the second trimester have the greatest risk of recurrent severe PIH with the next pregnancy (Sibai, Mercer, & Sarinoglu, 1991).

The major risk to the fetus is placental insufficiency and ischemia related to vasoconstriction. The fetus often suffers from intrauterine growth retardation. Prematurity is more common due to maternal complications that necessitate early delivery. Abruptio placentae may occur, resulting in acute fetal distress or death. Fetal mortality has been reported to range from 10% to 30% (Kulb, 1990b).

The neonate is at risk for all of the complications related to chronic hypoxia, intrauterine growth retardation, birth asphyxia, and prematurity. If the woman has received large doses of magnesium sulfate during labor, the neonate may experience temporary CNS depression due to hypermagnesemia.

Treatment

Prevention. As a greater understanding of the etiology of PIH is achieved, the potential for prevention appears likely. One preventive strategy that is receiving attention is the use of low-dose aspirin therapy. In several studies, administration of 60 to 100 mg of aspirin daily has resulted in the

NURSING PROCEDURE

Assessing Deep Tendon Reflexes and Clonus

Purpose: To identify signs of increased CNS irritability.

NURSING ACTION	***RATIONALE***
1. Place the limb to be tested in a relaxed, semiflexed position.	To elicit the DTR, the tendon must be in a relaxed state. Voluntary muscle contraction by the woman, may inhibit or prevent elicitation of DTRs.
2. Palpate for the tendon to be stretched and place your thumb on the skin directly over the tendon.	To identify the correct tendon To maintain contact with the tendon
3. Tap your thumb briskly with the pointed end of the reflex hammer and note the reflex contraction of the muscle and flexion of the limb.	To stretch the tendon and elicit contraction of the muscle which is attached to the tendon
4. *Estimate the strength of the reflex contraction of the muscle.	To determine the degree of CNS irritability or depression
5. Compare reflex responses on left and right sides. Note and record any asymmetry.	Asymmetry may indicate CNS injury such as focal ischemia or cerebral hemorrhage.
Biceps Reflex	
1. Palpate for the tendon of the biceps brachii muscle in the bend of the elbow and place your thumb over it.	To identify the correct tendon
2. Follow steps 3 through 5.	
3. Observe for flexion of the forearm.	If the tendon of the biceps reflex has been correctly elicited, and CNS depression is not present, the forearm will be flexed.
Quadriceps Reflex	
1. Support the leg under the knee with one arm and palpate the patellar tendon just below the patella.	To identify the correct tendon
2. Follow steps 3 through 5.	
3. Observe for the reflex extension of the lower leg.	If the quadriceps reflex is correctly elicited, and CNS depression is not present, the lower leg will extend.
Presence of Clonus Irritability and Ankle Clonus	
1. If DTRs are increased, assess for ankle clonus. Position the patient so the knee is slightly flexed.	To determine the degree of CNS excitability
2. Support the leg under the knee with one arm. With the other hand, grasp the foot, dorsiflex it quickly, and maintain this position.	To elicit the clonic contraction
3. Observe for the rhythmic, repetitive jerks or beats of clonus and chart the number of beats.	If present, clonus indicates increased CNS excitability and worsening PIH.

** The strength of the DTR is measured using a numerical scale of 0 to 4+:*
0 No response
+1 Low normal or somewhat diminished reflex response
+2 Normal or average reflex response
+3 Above average briskness in reflex response
+4 Very brisk, hyperactive reflex response; often associated with clonus, a series of convulsive ankle movements that occur when the foot is dorsiflexed

reduction of PIH in women at high risk for developing the disease (Wallenburg et al., 1991; and Schiff et al., 1989). There were no adverse effects on maternal or fetal status.

Aspirin must be used with caution and is not recommended for the general population of pregnant women at this time. The drug should be reserved for use after the first trimester because studies indicate that aspirin has teratogenic effects. Aspirin also inhibits platelet aggregation and may contribute to maternal and fetal coagulation disorders (Repke, 1991). It is therefore recommended that administration of the drug be stopped 5 to 10 days before anticipated delivery.

Promising research is being conducted on the use of calcium supplementation in the prevention of chronic hypertension and PIH. Several recent studies have demonstrated a significant reduction in the incidence of PIH and preterm delivery when 1.5 g elemental calcium (calcium carbonate) was administered orally (Repke et al., 1989; Repke & Villar, 1989).

Treatment in Mild PIH. When a diagnosis of mild preeclampsia is made, the woman may be hospitalized for an initial evaluation of maternal and fetal status. Bed rest, with the woman in the left lateral decubitus position, is often prescribed; bathroom privileges are allowed. Serial blood pressures are taken to assess the degree of hypertension. A 24-hour urine specimen is collected for evaluation of proteinuria and creatinine clearance. Laboratory studies to determine renal and hepatic function, hematocrit and coagulation status, and the presence of anemia or thrombocytopenia are performed. Fetal assessment is conducted including nonstress testing, biophysical profile, growth parameters, and fetal maturity determination. (See Chapter 14 for a complete discussion of the fetus at risk.)

If maternal and fetal status remains stable, the woman may be discharged home on a regimen of bed rest with bathroom privileges. Generally, a regular diet that does not restrict salt or fluid intake is recommended. Frequent assessments of blood pressure (every 4 hours) and daily weight and fetal movement count can be performed by the woman herself. The woman is instructed to report signs of worsening PIH immediately. A referral may be made for a perinatal home health nurse to periodically evaluate the woman's blood pressure, DTRs, urine protein, weight, and extent of edema. The woman is seen every 2 to 3 days for laboratory evaluation of urine protein, hematocrit, platelet count, liver function tests, and fetal well-being (Sibai, 1991). The goal of care is to safely extend the pregnancy until fetal maturity permits delivery.

In some cases, due to the social situation or living conditions, it may be necessary to continue hospitalization of the woman with mild PIH until delivery of the neonate. Sibai (1991) noted that for some women, hospitalization is preferred and is cost effective because it prolongs gestation and prevents the birth of a sick or premature neonate. Research findings have not supported the use of antihypertensive drugs or sedatives for mild PIH. Diuretics have no place in the treatment of PIH unless pulmonary edema or CHF develops. These drugs worsen maternal hemoconcentration, which characterizes PIH, and reduce uteroplacental blood flow. If at any time the maternal or fetal condition deteriorates, regardless of gestational age, delivery should be planned by induction of labor or cesarean birth.

Treatment in Severe PIH. The woman with severe PIH or eclampsia is admitted to a traditional labor and delivery unit or perinatal intensive care unit supplied with equipment and drugs used in the management of labor, obstetric emergencies, and eclampsia. The goal of care is to prevent further deterioration in maternal and fetal status. If severe PIH develops before 34 weeks' gestation and fetal distress occurs or the woman's life is in jeopardy, delivery is indicated.

The woman is kept on strict bed rest to reduce the risk of injury should seizures occur and to improve uterine blood flow. She should be maintained in a lateral recumbent position. To optimize the intrauterine environment, oxygen is administered at 8 to 12 L/min by tight face mask when PIH is moderate or severe, or when nonreassuring or ominous FHR patterns are noted.

A major goal of treatment is to prevent seizures and the serious sequelae of convulsions (maternal injury or cerebral hemorrhage and fetal hypoxia). Administration of magnesium sulfate by an intravenous infusion may prevent seizures. It permits stabilization of the woman's neurologic status while plans are made for delivery of the neonate. Table 27-5 lists appropriate drugs with dosage and administration.

Magnesium sulfate has minor side effects. Most women are able to tolerate the minor effects; however, major adverse effects may cause maternal CNS depression and death. The drug must be administered by an intravenous pump. Constant attendance by a perinatal nurse is essential during the magnesium infusion.

Serious complications and adverse reactions are related to toxicity. Signs and symptoms of toxicity, related to the serum magnesium level, are diminished DTRs, respiratory depression, hypotension and cardiac conduction, and depression. Antihypertensive drugs are indicated only in cases of severe hypertension (diastolic pressure above 100 to 110 mm Hg) when the risk of cerebrovascular accident is high. The goal is to stabilize the diastolic blood pressure between 90 and 100 mm Hg. Lowering the diastolic pressure too rapidly, and below 90 mm Hg, may significantly reduce uteroplacental perfusion and can compromise fetal status. Hydralazine is usually the drug of choice and may be given to counteract the generalized vasospasm associated with eclampsia. It also enhances renal blood flow. Labetalol, a combined alpha- and beta-adrenergic blocker, has been found effective in the treatment of acute hypertensive crisis associated with PIH.

Another important aspect of the management of severe PIH is to improve intravascular fluid volume without creating fluid overload. Hypovolemia and hemoconcentration are characteristic of PIH and the woman will require intravenous fluid replacement. Administration of a lactated Ringer's solution at a carefully controlled rate of 75 mL to 125 mL/h is recommended (Silver, 1991). Pulmonary edema is a common complication of aggressive intravenous fluid therapy. A central venous pressure (CVP) line or pulmonary artery catheter (Swan-Ganz catheter) may be necessary to accurately measure circulatory volume and to prevent circulatory overload. Lasix may be administered if pulmonary edema occurs.

Acute renal failure is a rare complication of PIH, but pathologic changes in the kidney secondary to PIH often result in oliguria (less than 30 mL/h). Women with underlying kidney disease or those who suffer abruptio placentae and hemorrhage are at increased risk for renal failure and anuria. An indwelling Foley catheter should be inserted and a drainage bag should be used, which permits precise measurement of output (urometer bag).

Delivery of the Neonate. Induction of labor is the recommended course of obstetric management when PIH is moderate or severe. In cases of severe PIH or eclampsia, the woman must be delivered regardless of the gestational age of the fetus. Most women respond favorably to oxytocin induc-

Table 27-5. Drugs That May Be Indicated in Control of Severe Pregnancy-Induced Hypertension/Eclampsia

Drug	Dosage	Indication	Nursing Implications
Magnesium sulfate	Loading dose: 4–6 g of a 10% solution IV Maintenance dose: 1–2 g/h	For prevention of seizures in PIH	Infuse slowly via infusion pump over 15–30 min diluted in 50–100 mL of 5% D/W Add 40 g $MgSO_4$ to 1000 mL in Ringer's lactate Piggyback to mainline and administer via infusion pump Assess urine output, deep tendon reflexes and respiration q 1h. Stop infusion if urine output is <20–30 mL/h, respirations <12/min, DTRs disappear, or serum magnesium level is <7.5 mEq/L, and notify physician immediately. Have antidote (calcium gluconate) at bedside.
Hydralazine (Apresoline)	5–10 mg IV	Diastolic B/P ≥110 mm Hg	Inject at 15–20 min intervals. Administer slowly at a rate of 10 mg over 1 min. Administer until diastolic B/P stable between 90–100 mm Hg. Check B/P q 5 min until stabilized.
Diazepam (Valium)	5–10 mg IV	Control of seizures	Inject undiluted. Administer slowly at a rate of 5 mg over 1 min. May be repeated at intervals of 5–10 min up to a dose of 30 mg in 1 hour. Observe for respiratory depression or apnea.
Diazoxide (Hyperstat)	30 mg or 1 mg/kg	Hypertensive crisis	Reserved for hypertension resistant to hydralazine. Must be given in smaller dose than recommended for nonpregnant patients. May cause precipitous drop in BIP. Must monitor B/P q 1–2 min until stable; q 5 min for 30 min and than q 15 min thereafter.
Furosemide (Lasix)	20–40 mg IV	For treatment of pulmonary edema	Inject 20 mg over 1 min. Monitor urine output. Indwelling catheter may be ordered for precise measurement of urine output.

tion, even before term. Uterine irritability is common in severe PIH, and many women may present with signs of early labor. If the condition of the woman or fetus deteriorates rapidly, or induction fails, cesarean birth is indicated. Reversal of symptoms occurs shortly after delivery for most women, but the risks of seizures and other complications remains high for 24 to 48 hours.

• • Assessment in Mild PIH

Nursing care of the woman with PIH will depend on the severity of the disease and the development of complications. Women with mild PIH are often followed in an ambulatory care setting, although they may be hospitalized. A perinatal nurse may evaluate the woman who is at home on a modified bed rest regimen.

During the first prenatal visit, the nurse identifies risk factors for the development of PIH. The nurse assesses every woman for signs and symptoms of PIH beginning at the 20th week of gestation. A critical component of this assessment is taking accurate blood pressure readings. The woman is screened during each prenatal visit for other signs of PIH including edema, rapid weight gain, proteinuria, and subjective symptoms (headaches, visual disturbances, and epigastric pain).

When a diagnosis of mild PIH is made, ongoing assessments and laboratory tests are performed to identify the severity of the disease. The nurse also performs assessments of fetal status including measuring the FHR during each prenatal visit and conducting other tests of fetal well-being as they are ordered (ie, nonstress test, biophysical profile, and oxytocin challenge test).

• • Nursing Diagnosis in Mild PIH

After the nurse completes the assessment process, nursing diagnoses are identified that reflect the following common problems for the woman with mild PIH:

- High Risk for Fluid Volume Excess related to pathophysiologic changes of PIH
- Altered Tissue Perfusion related to vasospasm and thrombosis
- Knowledge Deficit related to signs and symptoms of PIH
- Anxiety related to the diagnosis of mild PIH
- Diversional Activity Deficit related to bed rest

• • Planning and Implementation in Mild PIH

The nurse plans and implements nursing care in close collaboration with the midwife or physician, as well as the woman herself. The success of treatment often depends on the woman's understanding of the disease, the importance of bed rest, and self-monitoring for symptoms. Patient education is an important component of nursing care. The following are important areas to be covered when teaching the woman about PIH and its management:

- Signs and symptoms of worsening PIH
- Importance of modified bed rest
- Self-monitoring of blood pressure
- Laboratory studies (purpose and frequency)
- Assessment of fetal well-being

If the woman with mild PIH is hospitalized, nursing care is focused on encouraging bed rest in the lateral decubitus position and supporting adequate nutritional and fluid intake. The nurse implements strategies to relieve the discomforts associated with bed rest and increasing edema. Although rest is important, the woman's family and close friends should be encouraged to visit to help reduce the woman's sense of isolation and boredom associated with prolonged hospitalization. A referral may be made to occupational therapy so that the woman can be provided with appropriate diversional activities.

Expected Outcomes

- The woman demonstrates appropriate self-care activities that promote maternal and fetal well-being.
- The woman lists the danger signals of worsening PIH.
- The woman verbalizes a decrease in discomfort related to bed rest or edema.

• • Evaluation in Mild PIH

The nurse evaluates the success of nursing care and self-care activities in preventing extension of the disease process. If the woman maintains a modified bed rest regimen and performs other self-care activities that promote maternal and fetal well-being, her blood pressure will be reduced or remain stable. Other signs of worsening PIH will not develop, and the delivery will be delayed until fetal maturity is achieved. If signs of severe PIH and physiologic decompensation develop, the nurse modifies the plan of care to meet the needs of the woman and her fetus.

• • Assessment in Severe PIH

If the woman develops severe PIH, she will be hospitalized immediately. The nurse plays a central role in the assessment and support of maternal and fetal physiologic status. Even if the woman is eventually transported to a perinatal regional center, life-threatening complications such as HELLP syndrome, DIC, or abruptio placentae must be dealt with immediately.

The woman with severe PIH and her fetus require continuous and intensive monitoring. Blood pressure, pulse, respirations, level of consciousness, and DTRs are assessed *every 15 to 30 minutes* or more frequently depending on her condition. Use of an electronic blood pressure monitor is recommended and will facilitate the process. If pulmonary status is unstable, a pulse oximeter is also applied to monitor oxygen saturation levels. In some cases, an arterial line will be placed to permit central blood pressure monitoring and provide access for blood gas analysis. The nurse is responsible for calibration of this equipment and interpreting the data.

Meticulous measurement of all intake is required to determine fluid needs and prevent pulmonary edema. Urine output is monitored and a bladder catheter may be inserted to facilitate evaluation of urine output when kidney function is compromised. The urine is tested for proteinuria periodically. If oliguria develops, a urometer collection bag should be used to permit accurate measurement of very small volumes of urine. The degree of pitting edema is also periodically evaluated. Edema will develop first in dependent areas such as the sacral or hip area. Breath sounds are auscultated every 30 to 60 minutes for evidence of rales because circulatory overload and pulmonary edema are greater risks with severe PIH or eclampsia. The nurse monitors for signs and symptoms of worsening preeclampsia or impending seizure activity:

- Blood pressure of 160/110 or greater
- Severe headache
- Visual disturbances
- Sudden nausea and vomiting
- Epigastric distress or acute upper right quadrant pain
- Worsening hyperreflexia or the development of clonus
- Altered mentation or complaints of altered sensory function

The woman is observed for petechiae, ecchymosis, or oozing at venipuncture sites. These skin and mucous membrane changes are indicators of DIC. Evaluation of laboratory findings is another aspect of nursing assessment. Table 27-4 describes the biochemical tests most frequently evaluated in the intrapartum management of preeclampsia. The nurse monitors serum magnesium levels as they are reported and notifies the physician if the level exceeds 7.5 mEq/L.

Continuous fetal monitoring is initiated immediately on admission, and an electronic fetal scalp electrode is applied as soon as feasible. Fetal scalp sampling may be performed during the course of labor to evaluate fetal pH and blood gas status. The nurse assesses the electronic monitor data for evidence of fetal distress including loss of FHR variability, repetitive late decelerations, or sudden bradycardia.

Ongoing assessments continue through delivery and for the first 24 to 48 hours after birth of the neonate. Pathophysiologic changes do not immediately resolve after birth. After delivery, uterine tone is closely monitored. This is essential because there is a greater risk of uterine atony due to the relaxant effect of magnesium sulfate on smooth muscle. Bladder function must also be assessed frequently because mobilization of extravascular fluid and diuresis can result in the production of more than 2000 to 3000 mL of urine per day in the first 24 to 48 hours. Once the Foley catheter is removed, the bladder is assessed hourly for distention, and the woman should be assisted to void frequently.

• • Nursing Diagnosis in Severe PIH

Based on assessment data, the nurse identifies appropriate nursing diagnoses for the woman with severe PIH, including:

- High Risk for Injury related to seizure activity

- Impaired Gas Exchange related to pulmonary edema
- Ineffective Airway Clearance related to seizure activity
- Fluid Volume Excess related to renal injury
- Decreased Cardiac Output related to decreased preload or antihypertensive therapy
- Altered Maternal and Fetal Tissue Perfusion related to generalized vasospasm and thrombosis
- Pain related to headache or epigastric pain
- Fear related to development of severe PIH

• • Planning and Implementation in Severe PIH

Ensuring Patient Safety

Safety precautions are implemented on admission to the intrapartum unit to prevent injury during seizures. Strict bed rest is observed, and side rails are used and may be padded, if seizures appear likely or occur. Suction and oxygen equipment and a nasopharyngeal airway are placed at the bedside. The woman is kept NPO to prevent aspiration of vomitus or secretions after seizure activity. The room is kept dimly lit and quiet, and stimulation (including procedures) is minimized because CNS irritability may trigger seizures. Visitors may be permitted on a limited basis; however, the nurse must explain to them the need for a calm, quiet environment.

If assessment indicates that the woman's condition is deteriorating or if seizures occur, the nurse must remain with her at all times, but call for immediate help. The midwife or physician is notified, and anesthesia personnel may be summoned to assist with airway management (see the Nursing Care Plan).

If seizures occur, the nurse's first concern is maintaining a patent airway and protecting the woman from injury. The patient should be turned on her side to decrease the risk of aspiration should vomiting occur. Past nursing practice for eclamptic patients included attempts to insert a padded tongue blade ("bite stick") or plastic oral airway at the first sign of seizure activity to prevent tongue biting. Current emergency management of seizures does not include the use of tongue blades or oral airways.

A nasopharyngeal airway (nasal trumpet) should be kept at the bedside and may be inserted by medical or nursing staff after a seizure. The nasal airway must be well lubricated with water-soluble lubricant before insertion. Right and left nasal airways can be distinguished by the pharyngeal end opening, which should face the midline. Once in place, connection tubing can be used for suctioning or for oxygen administration. Oxygen should be administered at 8 to 12 L/min by mask during the convulsion to maximize fetal oxygenation.

Because delivery does not immediately reverse the pathophysiologic effects of PIH, it is necessary to continue assessment and nursing care of the woman during the immediate postpartum period. Intravenous magnesium sulfate is continued for 24 to 48 hours postpartum and is accompanied by monitoring of vital signs, urinary output, and DTRs. The goal of therapy in the postpartum period is to prevent eclamptic seizures and subsequent injury and neurologic damage to the new mother.

Expected Outcome

- The woman maintains normal respiratory function during administration of magnesium sulfate after a seizure.

Monitoring the Woman During Fluid and Drug Administration

The nurse implements physician directives for essential fluids and drugs used in the treatment of PIH (see Table 27-5). Because of the unstable circulatory status observed in severe PIH, intravenous fluids should be administered by infusion pump to prevent accidental volume overload.

Magnesium sulfate is prepared and administered intravenously, and the nurse observes the woman for side effects as well as signs of toxicity. The magnesium infusion is continued through delivery of the neonate and as noted, for 24 to 48 hours postpartum, until the blood pressure stabilizes and the risk of seizures is significantly reduced. When magnesium sulfate is administered, calcium gluconate, the antidote for magnesium overdose, should be kept at the bedside (see Table 27-5).

NURSING ALERT

NURSING CARE OF THE WOMAN WITH SEVERE PREGNANCY-INDUCED HYPERTENSION

The woman with severe PIH is at risk for the development of multiple life-threatening complications, including cerebrovascular accidents, congestive heart failure, pulmonary edema, and disseminated intravascular coagulopathy. In addition, she is at high risk for seizures. The nurse is responsible for close monitoring of maternal–fetal status and support of physiologic adaptations. In many cases, the nurse is guided by printed protocols that permit the implementation of care as the woman's condition changes or when medical assistance is not immediately available.

When the woman develops severe PIH, the nurse initiates the following protective and supportive actions:

- Initiate seizure precautions.
  Place side rails up and pad with linen or blankets.
  Have suction and airway equipment at bedside.
  Have emergency drugs to control seizures at bedside.
  Reduce environmental stimuli.
- Maintain the woman in the left lateral position.
- Implement frequent blood pressure monitoring (q 15 min or more frequently).
- Implement continuous EFM and uterine monitoring.
- Initiate oxygen at 8 to 12 L/min by face mask and attach a pulse oximeter.
- Insert Foley catheter to drainage bag for hourly urine output measurement.
- Initiate an intravenous line if not yet implemented.

The nurse remains in continuous attendance, providing both physical and emotional support of the woman. The goals of care are to identify early signs of complications, obtain medical help in a timely manner, institute supportive care, and protect the woman from injury should seizures occur.

Text continues on page 758

Nursing Care Plan

The Woman With Severe Pregnancy-Induced Hypertension

PATIENT PROFILE

History

H.N. is a 21-year-old G1/PO at 36 weeks' gestation. She has been admitted to labor with a diagnosis of PIH. Her admission assessment reveals the following data: B/P 148/96, P 82, RR 22; +2 generalized edema; +2 proteinuria on dipstick of a urine specimen obtained by catheterization; +3 DTRs; no clonus. H.N. complains of a mild headache without visual changes (no blurring or scotoma). She is placed on bed rest in the left lateral recumbent position. An oxytocin infusion is started for induction of labor. A 4-g loading dose of magnesium sulfate is given intravenously by infusion pump to prevent seizures. Twenty minutes later, a maintenance dose of $MgSO_4$ is started at 1 g/h intravenously. An indwelling urinary catheter is inserted to measure urine output.

Physical Assessment

Four hours after admission H.N. is examined and her cervix is 2 cm dilated and 50% effaced. On assessment, the nurse notes the following: B/P 168/116, P 100, RR 28; +4 DTRs; 1 beat of clonus; a total of 40 mL of urine output in past 2 h. Faint rales bilaterally in lower lobes of lungs.

H.N. complains of a severe headache and sudden, constant right upper quadrant pain. She states, "I see sparks of light in my eyes." The physician orders hydralazine 10 mg slow IV push for H.N.'s blood pressure. As the nurse prepares to administer the drug, H.N. has an eclamptic seizure. The FHR drops to 80 bpm with the seizure.

COLLABORATIVE PROBLEMS/POTENTIAL COMPLICATIONS

- Cerebral vascular accident
- Renal failure
- Disseminated intravascular coagulopathy
- Congestive heart failure
- Pulmonary edema

(See the accompanying Nursing Alert display.)

Assessment	*Nursing Diagnosis*	*Nursing Interventions*	*Rationale*
H.N. has diagnosis of PIH B/P 168/116 +4 DTRs/1 beat clonus H.N. complains of headache, visual disturbances, and right upper quadrant pain. H.N. receiving $MgSO_4$ 1 g/h.	High Risk for Injury related seizure activity. ***Expected Outcome*** H.N. will not experience physical trauma or organ system injury related to seizure activity.	Call for assistance	Additional staff will be needed to protect H.N. and provide care.
		Protect H.N.'s head and limbs from striking headboard or side rails. Protect IV site.	During clonic phase of seizure H.N. may strike head or limbs or fall from bed if not supported. IV may be dislodged during seizure; IV access will be needed for administration of emergency drugs.
		Be prepared to administer Valium to control seizures.	Valium is a CNS depressant and drug of choice for controlling seizures.
		When seizure stops, turn H.N. to left side.	Placing H.N. on side will permit drainage of secretions from mouth and will improve uteroplacental perfusion.
		Open airway (suction secretions from mouth and nares).	Secretions can collect in mouth during seizure, obstructing airway; secretions may be aspirated if not removed from airway.

(*Continued*)

The Woman With Severe Pregnancy-Induced Hypertension

(*Continued*)

Assessment	*Nursing Diagnosis*	*Nursing Interventions*	*Rationale*
		Administer oxygen 8–12 L/min by face mask.	Respiratory arrest and hypoxemia occur during seizure. Increasing maternal oxygen level may increase amount of oxygen available to fetus.
		Apply pulse oximeter.	Pulse oximetry will provide data on level of blood oxygen saturation and effectiveness of therapy.
		If no spontaneous respirations initiate artificial ventiliation.	Respiratory arrest is rare, but may occur after seizure.
		After H.N.'s condition stabilizes, continue to monitor vital signs q 15 min or more frequently.	Eclamptic seizure may worsen H.N.'s condition. Continued rise in blood pressure may occur.
		Monitor H.N. for evidence of increasing DTRs, clonus, or complaints of headache, visual disturbances, RUQ or epigatric pain.	Seizure activity may recur, and the nurse must continue to monitor H.N. for evidence of impending seizure or worsening PIH.
		Minimize environmental stimuli; remain continuously at bedside; pad side rails.	Decreasing external stimuli may reduce CNS irritability and risk of seizure.
H.N. has severe PIH. Respirations 28/min. Urine output of 40 mL in past 2 h. Faint rales in lower lobes of lungs bilaterally. H.N. has eclamptic seizure.	Ineffective Breathing Pattern related to seizure. Impaired Gas Exchange related to pulmonary edema ***Expected Outcome*** H.N. will maintain normal respiratory function, as evidenced by spontaneous respirations between 12 and 24 breaths/min.	Insert indwelling bladder catheter and attach "urometer" drainage bag for precise measurement of urine. Monitor and record intake and output q 1 h.	With severe PIH, renal failure may occur; continuous monitoring or urine output is essential to detect decreasing renal function and fluid retention.
		Notify physician if urine output less than 40–50 mL/h.	Physician must be apprised of deterioration in H.N.'s status to reevaluate and order appropriate tests and treatment. Urine output of less than 40 mL/h may signal impending renal function deterioration.
		Maintain fluid restrictions as ordered.	Intake must be restricted when renal function decreases to prevent fluid overload and pulmonary edema.
		Assess for evidence and degree of edema.	Edema is evidence of capillary fluid leak and pathologic change associated with PIH.
		Auscultate breath sounds q 1 h.	Rales will occur with pulmonary edema.
		Administer oxygen at 8–12 L/min and apply pulse oximeter if altered respiratory function occurs.	Oxygen administration will improve maternal blood oxygen level when pulmonary edema occurs.

(*Continued*)

The Woman With Severe Pregnancy-Induced Hypertension

(Continued)

Assessment	Nursing Diagnosis	Nursing Interventions	Rationale
			Pulse oximetry will provide data on level of blood oxygen saturation and effectiveness of therapy.
		Be prepared to administer furosemide (Lasix) IV as ordered.	In some cases, diuretics may be given to promote urine production (contraindicated in frank renal failure).
		Be prepared to assist with initiation of central venous or (arterial) hemodynamic monitoring.	With severe PIH, invasive arterial or venous monitoring will provide data about fluid overload and effectiveness of therapy.
H.N. has severe PIH. B/P 168/116. H.N. has an eclamptic seizure. FHR drops to 80 bpm during seizure.	Altered Placental Tissue Perfusion related to vasospasm ***Expected Outcome*** H.N. maintained her placental perfusion.	Maintain H.N. in left lateral decubitus position.	Uterine perfusion is optimum in left lateral decubitus position.
		Administer oxygen 8–12 L/min continuously.	Increasing maternal blood oxygen increases oxygen available to fetus.
		Maintain continuous EFM.	Continuous EFM is required to permit immediate detection of fetal distress.
		Observe the FHR for evidence of late decelerations, absent long-term variability, or bradycardia.	Decreased placental perfusion results in late deceleration pattern; with severe reduction in oxygen delivery, bradycardia will occur.
		Administer hydralazine IV push as ordered to maintain diastolic B/P between 90 and 100 mm Hg.	Hydralazine is a vasodilator that may improve uterine blood flow; lowering the diastolic B/P below 90 mm Hg, however, may decrease uteroplacental perfusion.
		Be prepared for emergency cesarean delivery if bradycardia does not resolve when seizure stops.	Acute fetal hypoxemia occurs during seizure, but may result in decompensation. If FHR does not return to baseline, immediate delivery is indicated.
		Notify neonatal team of maternal seizure and fetal bradycardia.	Neonatal staff must be notified of significant changes in fetus and must be present for birth of neonate to provide support or resuscitation.

EVALUATION

H.N.'s seizure activity ceased after 15 mg Valium was administered by IV push. No physical trauma was experienced, and no further seizures occurred before delivery. Hemodynamic monitoring was initiated, a radial artery catheter was inserted. Lasix 20 mg IV push was given. Urine output increased to 40–60 mL/h. H.N. maintained normal respiratory function, and breath sounds were clear and equal bilaterally. Pulmonary edema was resolved. H.N.'s FHR rose to 90–100 bpm range for 2 minutes after seizure and then returned to FHR baseline of 150 bpm over next 2 minutes. No late decelerations or bradycardia were noted. LTV remained in the 3–5 bpm range until delivery.

MANAGED CARE PATH

Pregnancy-Induced Hypertension

Expected Length of Stay: 3–4 days

	Admission/Stabilization/ Labor–Delivery	Maintenance/Postpartum
Key Goals	Hemodynamically stable, no s/s/ pulmonary edema No seizure activity, fetus stable Pain relief obtained (L & D)	Hemodynamically stable Stable PIH assessment, fetus stable No s/s pulmonary edema (postpartum) Tolerates po intake (postpartum)
Consults	Anesthesia NICU, social work prn	Dietary Social work, perinatal ed prn
Tests/Labs	CBC, T&S, SGOT, LDH 24hr urine protein, urine dipstick, Doppler flow	PIH tests prn Doppler flow prn
Meds	$MgSO_4$, steroids, antihypertensives prn Pain med, $MgSO_4$ prn (L & D)	PNV, stool softener, sedatives, steroids, antihypertensives, Heplock with flush, antacids prn
Treatments	Assess: weight (daily), Foley, EFM, I&O Pitocin after placenta delivered (L & D) Direct Coombs, type, Rh on umb.cord blood, placenta to pathology	Assess: weight, EFM, I&O. urine protein, pulse oximeter prn (postpartum)
Teaching	EFM, unit routine, medications, plan of care antepartum testing, s/s PIH	S & S PIH, unit routine, medications, birth plan, self-care, and discharge (postpartum)
Equipment	Foley cath w/meter, infusion pump/ tubing	Infusion pump prn
Diet	NPO. Ice chips prn	Regular. Clear liq to reg (postpartum)
Activity	Bed rest	Bathroom privileges, wheelchair
D/C Plan	Social support	Social support, transportation, housing F/u appointments made

Adapted from collaborative paths developed by the Department of Nursing Service, Vanderbilt University Medical Center, Nashville, TN.

In addition to administering drugs commonly used in the treatment of severe PIH, the nurse will be responsible for the infusion of oxytocin if induction of labor is indicated. Chapter 23 discusses specific nursing actions when oxytocin is ordered.

At the time of delivery, oxytocin should be immediately available and is often necessary to prevent uterine atony secondary to the relaxant effects of magnesium sulfate. Methergine and Prostin/15M (Carboprost) are contraindicated when hypertension occurs. The nurse is often responsible for administering oxytocin prophylactically after delivery of the placenta. Use of other agents is often reserved for cases of uterine atony and postpartum hemorrhage that do not respond to intravenous oxytocin administration.

Expected Outcome

- The woman maintains adequate fluid balance, as evidenced by urine output greater than 30 mL/h.

Providing Physical Comfort and Emotional Support

A major nursing responsibility is providing physical comfort and emotional support during this period of physiologic instability and uncertainty. The woman must maintain a left, lateral recumbent position as much as possible, which can become uncomfortable. An eggcrate mattress pad may reduce discomfort, as will a periodic gentle massage of the left side. Pharmacologic pain relief is indicated early in labor to avoid the deleterious physiologic effects of pain. Regional anesthesia (epidural) may be given, and the nurse assists with this procedure.

The woman may benefit from quiet visits from her partner or other family members. Some patients rest more easily when family members are present. The nurse must also remember the strain on family members during this time; efforts should be made to reassure them, to allow for close interaction and mutual support, and to create as normal a birth environment as possible.

Expected Outcomes

- The woman verbalizes satisfaction with the techniques used to enhance comfort.
- The woman verbalizes satisfaction with the emotional support provided by her partner, family, friends, and the nurse.

• • Evaluation in Severe PIH

Rapid changes in the plan of nursing care are often required on evaluation of expected outcomes when the woman has severe PIH. Even when prompt treatment and intensive nursing care are implemented, the maternal or fetal condition may deteriorate. The nurse must perform frequent evaluations to modify the plan of care and implement emergency supportive measures. When nursing actions are effective, the woman and fetus will maintain physiologic stability, and delivery will occur before significant deterioration occurs in maternal or fetal status. Resolution of PIH will occur rapidly within the first 24 to 48 hours postpartum, and the woman and her neonate will not suffer permanent physiologic or emotional impairment.

Significant obstetric complications alter the course and outcome of pregnancy. Among obstetric complications are preterm labor (PTL), preterm premature rupture of membranes (PPROM), and pregnancy-induced hypertension (PIH). Although new pharmacologic agents have been developed to treat PTL, the incidence of preterm birth remains essentially unchanged. Research indicates that, in some cases, the nurse is more effective in preventing PTL than sophisticated technology or the development of new pharmacologic agents. PPROM poses serious risks for both the woman and her fetus. Technology has improved the survival of even very premature, low–birth-weight neonates, so that active management of PPROM is often advocated to gain time for fetal pulmonary maturation. Although PIH remains the most significant obstetric complication, advances in medical and nursing science have improved maternal and fetal outcomes. The nurse has a central role in the early identification and treatment of these disorders.

Medical Complications of the Perinatal Period

Diabetes Mellitus

Diabetes mellitus is a chronic familial disease characterized by inadequate insulin production or use. Insulin is needed to transport glucose across the cell membrane. When transport does not occur, hyperglycemia results. As the plasma glucose level rises, it exceeds the renal threshold, resulting in glucosuria. Fats and proteins are catabolized to meet energy needs. When fats are oxidized, ketonemia and ketonuria develop. Long-term systemic effects of diabetes result in vasculopathy, nephropathy, and neuropathy. During pregnancy, diabetes may compromise maternal and fetal well-being and presents a major challenge for the perinatal health team.

The National Diabetes Data Group has classified diabetes according to insulin dependency and etiologic factors (see the accompanying display on diabetes classification).

The pregnant woman may have preexisting diabetes (type I or type II) or may develop gestational diabetes mellitus (GDM or type III) during the course of pregnancy. In either case, the woman, fetus, and neonate are at increased risk of morbidity or morality. The greatest complications develop for women with preexisting diabetes or in cases where delayed diagnosis of GDM occurs (Cousins et al., 1991). Perinatal outcomes will depend primarily on the degree of control of plasma glucose levels. Fetal growth and development will be affected by the severity of the woman's disease for 3 to 6 months *preceding* pregnancy and at the time of conception (Evans & Benbarka, 1991).

Etiologic and Predisposing Factors

It is estimated that 2% to 3% of all women will develop GDM (type III) during pregnancy. Most of these women do not have a prior history of carbohydrate intolerance. Women with preexisting diabetes (type I or type II) will experience a worsening of the disease during pregnancy. Aberrations in carbohydrate metabolism are caused by hormonal changes that occur during the gestational period.

Hormonal influences can best be appreciated if they are divided into the first and second half of pregnancy. The first 20 weeks of pregnancy are characterized by *insulin sensitivity*. Increases in estrogen and progesterone induce metabolic alterations causing:

- Pancreatic beta cell hyperplasia and increased insulin production
- Increased glycogen synthesis
- Increased tissue glucose use
- Increased tissue glycogen storage
- Decreased liver synthesis of glucose

As a result of these changes, the action of insulin is facilitated. Maternal fasting plasma glucose levels are *decreased*, and significant hypoglycemia can occur, particularly in type I diabetic women. Insulin requirements often drop. Hypoglycemia can be exacerbated by the nausea and vomiting that frequently occur in the first trimester of pregnancy.

During the second half of pregnancy, observed changes in carbohydrate metabolism suggest *insulin resistance*. Diminished tissue responsiveness to insulin is thought to be due to a variety of hormones secreted by the placenta, including human placental lactogen (HPL), progesterone, estrogen, and pituitary prolactin. HPL and other placental hormones including prolactin and progesterone also stimulate lipolysis and spare glucose for fetal growth and development. Plasma glucose levels begin to rise and maternal hyperglycemia occurs. Insulin requirements may rise dramatically for the insulin-dependent diabetic woman (Fig. 27-2).

Predisposing risks and factors associated with type III GDM are: obesity, glucosuria, over age 30, hypertension, polyhydramnios, family history of diabetes, previous birth of

National Diabetes Data Group Classification of Diabetes

Type I: Insulin-Dependent Diabetes

Usual onset in childhood or young adulthood

Lack of insulin production by pancreatic beta cells

Prone to ketoacidosis

Type II: Non–Insulin-Dependent Diabetes

Usual onset after age 30

70%–80% of people with disease are obese

Have adequate insulin, but delay release or abnormal reaction in peripheral tissues

Type III: Gestational Diabetes Mellitus (GDM)

Onset during pregnancy

May be controlled by diet or may require insulin

Usually resolves after pregnancy

Type IV: Secondary Diabetes

Develops secondary to a disease process

macrosomic neonate, previous history of GDM, and previous fetal death of unknown etiology.

Diagnosis

Type I and II Diabetes. The four classic signs and symptoms of diabetes are polyphagia (increased appetite), polydipsia (increased thirst), polyuria (increased urine volume), and loss of weight and muscle strength. These characteristics are caused by aberrations in carbohydrate metabolism, which should be controlled in type I or type II diabetic women *before* pregnancy.

Diagnostic tests focus on determining the plamsa glucose level, ongoing insulin needs, and the severity of complications related to the disorder in women with preexisting diabetes. Laboratory tests also are performed to determine the percentage of *glycosylated hemoglobin*.

With prolonged maternal hyperglycemia, a percentage of the total hemoglobin will remain saturated with glucose for the remaining life of the cell. Glycosylated hemoglobin (Hgb A_{1c}) reflects the overall plasma glucose status of the woman during a 4- to 6-week period *before* the test. The incidence of fetal malformations is increased when glycosylated hemoglobin levels are greater than 7% to 9% of the total hemoglobin (Lucas, Leveno, & Williams, 1989). The risk of anomalies is elevated when Hgb A_{1c} levels are elevated 6 to 12 months before conception and during the first trimeter (Hollingsworth & Moore, 1989). Elevated Hgb A_{1c} levels are also positively associated with fetal macrosomia and large-for-gestational age at birth (Howard, 1992).

When possible, a *preconceptual* assessment of the woman's diabetic status should be performed to determine the extent of hyperglycemia. This information allows the health team to counsel the woman about maternal and fetal risks and achieve optimum plasma glucose control. The woman also is screened for evidence of cardiovascular and renal disease, as well as ophthalmologic and neurologic problems common in diabetes.

It is common for women with preexisting but undetected type II diabetes to be diagnosed during pregnancy (Evans & Benbarka, 1991). The common signs of type II diabetes that alert the midwife or physician to the possibility of the disease include polydipsia, polyuria, and polyphagia. The woman may complain of blurred vision, lethargy, or an increased number of vaginal infections. Dipstick glucose readings exceeding +2 may be noted. Most women with preexisting type II diabetes are obese. The diagnosis is confirmed by a 50-g oral glucose test (see the next section on GDM). The glycosylated hemoglobin level is often elevated.

Type III—Gestational Diabetes. The American Diabetes Association (ADA, 1987) has recommended universal screening of *all* women for glucose intolerance during pregnancy. Screening is accomplished by determining the plasma glucose level 1 hour after oral administration of a 50-g glucose drink. Because carbohydrate intolerance occurs in the second half of pregnancy, screening is recommended between 24 and 28 weeks' gestation. Women who have identified risk factors for the development of GDM should be screened at the first prenatal visit. If this initial screening is negative, and the woman develops signs and symptoms of diabetes later, such as fetal macrosomia, excessive weight gain, or glucosuria, she should be rescreened.

The 50-g glucose test for GDM screening currently requires no prior fasting. Test values in excess of 140 mg/dL for plasma glucose are an indication for further testing with the 3-hour oral glucose tolerance test (OGTT). Recently, a test value of 130 mg/dL has been recommended as a more sensitive indicator of carbohydrate intolerance in pregnancy (Cousins et al., 1991).

Three-Hour Glucose Tolerance Test. If the 1-hour test is abnormal, a 3-hour glucose tolerance test is performed. A 100-g glucose drink is administered orally. The woman is given specific instructions to ensure accuracy of the test. A high-carbohydrate diet (150 g) is eaten for 3 days before the test. Eating or smoking is not permitted after midnight the day of the test. The woman may have water before the test, but caffeinated beverages should be avoided because they increase plasma glucose levels. Strenuous exercise should be avoided 30 minutes before taking the glucose solution.

A blood specimen is drawn to determine the fasting plasma glucose level just before the woman drinks the 100-g glucose. Repeat blood specimens are drawn at 1, 2, and 3 hours after ingestion of the glucose. If two of the following plasma glucose levels are exceeded, the woman is diagnosed as having GDM:

- Fasting: 105 mg/dL
- 1 hour: 190 mg/dL

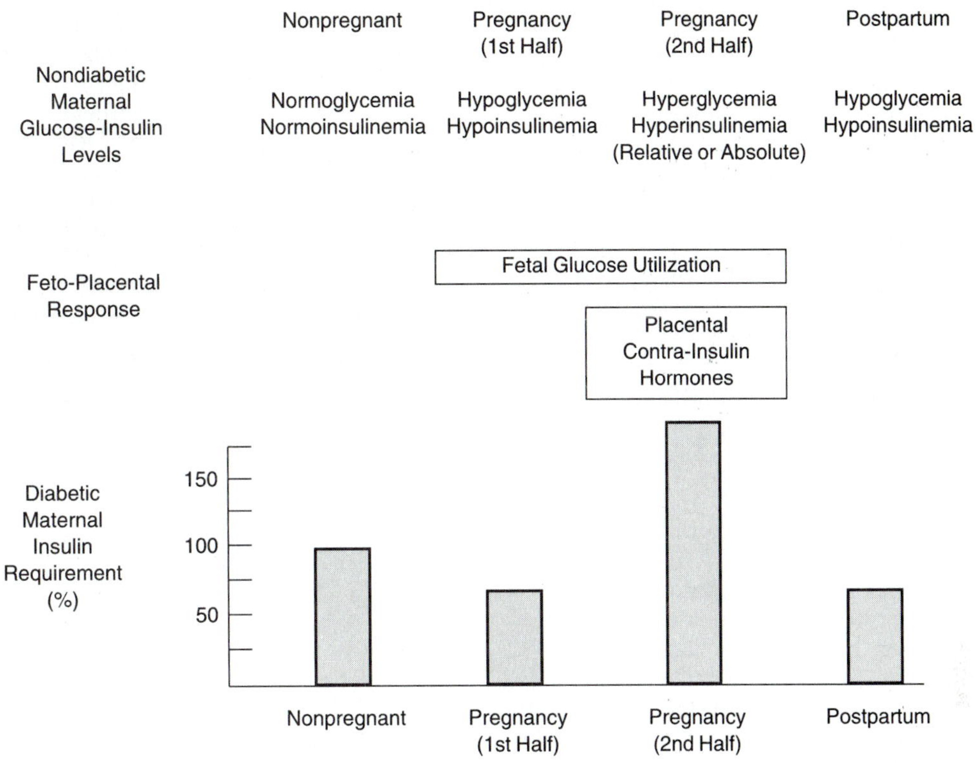

Figure 27-2.

Influence of pregnancy on glucose and insulin levels in nondiabetic subjects and on insulin requirements in diabetic subjects. The pregnancy insulin dose is shown as 100%. The insulin requirement may decline in the first half of pregnancy and after the birth and is increased in the second half of pregnancy. (From Coustan, D., & Felig, P. [1988]. *Medical complications during pregnancy*. pp. 34–64. Philadelphia: W.B. Saunders.)

- 2 hours: 165 mg/dL
- 3 hours: 145 mg/dL

Maternal, Fetal, and Neonatal Implications

Before the advent of insulin, women with type I diabetes were frequently infertile. In women who were able to conceive, one third died during pregnancy, and few neonates survived. The use of insulin therapy has resulted in improved fertility among diabetic women. Maternal health has shown significant improvement. Nevertheless, maternal, fetal, and neonatal complications are still seen today.

The woman with GDM who maintains consistent glycemic control develops the fewest problems during pregnancy and the intrapartum period. However, recent research confirms that even with tight glycemic control, women with diet-controlled GDM have an increased incidence of sudden fetal death and give birth to macrosomic neonates more frequently than pregnant women with normal carbohydrate tolerance (Girz, Divon, & Merkatz, 1992).

Infection. Infections are more common in all diabetic women, particularly urinary tract and vaginal infections. Asymptomatic bacteriuria is three times more common, regardless of diabetic classification. Pyelonephritis is a significant complication predisposing the woman to preterm labor and birth. *Candida* vaginitis is most frequently found in the diabetic woman. It often recurs, requiring repeated therapy throughout pregnancy.

Hypertensive Disorders. The incidence of chronic hypertension and PIH is increased in type I and II diabetes, probably due to underlying renal disease. However, essential hypertension and PIH occur more frequently even in women with GDM who have no renal problems, particularly when the diagnosis of GDM is made before 24 weeks' gestation (Berkowitz et al., 1992). Diabetic nephropathy and retinopathy can accelerate with pregnancy, particularly with the development of hypertension (Rosenn et al., 1992). Fetal intrauterine growth retardation is more common with chronic hypertension and PIH.

Hypoglycemia. Hypoglycemia is a serious complication of type I or type II diabetes. It rarely occurs in GDM unless the woman is receiving insulin to control hyperglycemia. Mild hypoglycemia is usually observed when the plasma glucose level falls *below* 50 mg/dL. Signs and symptoms of profound hypoglycemia usually occur when the plasma glucose level is 40 mg/dL or lower (Plovie, 1991). Signs and symptoms of hypoglycemia include hunger, nausea, headache, sweating, tremulousness, weakness and fatigue, blurred or tunnel vision, numbness around lips and tongue, altered mentation or disorientation, stupor, loss of consciousness, coma, and seizures.

Hypoglycemic (insulin) shock usually occurs in the insulin-treated diabetic patient when the plasma glucose level is less than 30 to 40 mg/dL. The person will generally lose consciousness and requires immediate emergency care or will suffer irreversible brain damage or death. The fetus will generally survive mild to moderate episodes of maternal hypoglycemia because fetal supplies of glucose are sufficient to meet its metabolic needs. Severe hypoglycemia that compromises maternal cardiac function may result in decreased uteroplacental function and result in fetal distress.

Diabetic Ketoacidosis. Diabetic ketoacidosis (DKA) is a life-threatening complication for the woman and her fetus during pregnancy. It is a multisystem disorder that results from extreme hyperglycemia (plasma levels above 350 mg/dL) and ketonemia (plasma ketone levels above 5 mmol/L) and acidosis. Signs and symptoms of DKA are:

- Severe dehydration
- Rapid respirations (Kussmaul respirations)
- Alterations in mentation
- Fluid and electrolyte imbalances
- Loss of intracellular potassium

Diabetic ketoacidosis is often precipitated by an underlying stressor such as infection or extreme stress. The type I pregnant diabetic is more predisposed to develop DKA and at a lower threshold of hyperglycemia due to the "diabetogenic" effect that occurs during the second half of gestation (Harvey, 1992). Maternal mortality is due to profound hypovolemic shock secondary to dehydration or electrolyte imbalance with associated cardiac arrhythmias. Fetal mortality may be as high as 50% to 80%. It is thought that fetal death is secondary to decreasing placental perfusion and hypoxia. Ketonemia may play a secondary role in fetal loss.

Congenital Anomalies. The fetus of the diabetic woman is also at risk for neural tube, cardiac, and gastrointestinal anomalies. The rate of abnormalities is three to four times the incidence in the general population. This is thought to result from maternal metabolic aberrations (glucose, protein, and fat metabolism) in early pregnancy. The highest rate of fetal abnormalities is among women with glycosylated hemoglobin levels greater than 9.5% (Lucas, et al., 1989). Fetal anomalies are currently the most common cause of fetal and neonatal death when diabetes complicates pregnancy (Samson, 1992).

Fetal Macrosomia. Macrosomia is defined as a weight that is above the 90th percentile for the gestational age of the fetus. Fetal macrosomia remains the most common complication of diabetes for the fetus, even with uncomplicated GDM. It is thought to occur because of maternal hyperglycemia. Maternal glucose diffuses through the placenta, stimulating fetal hyperinsulinemia. This, in turn, causes a massive transport of glucose into fetal cells.

Birth trauma is more common with macrosomic neonates, resulting in facial palsy, fracture of the humerus and clavicle, bruising, and cephalhematoma (see Chapter 33 for a discussion of these neonatal problems).

Intrapartum Complications. The intrapartum period is often complicated for the diabetic woman because she is at increased risk for hypertension and PIH. When fetal macrosomia has been diagnosed, the woman may experience prolonged labor due to cephalopelvic disproportion. Polyhydramnios, PTL, hypotonic contractions, prolapsed umbilical cord, and amniotic fluid embolism are added risks. Uterine atony and postpartum hemorrhage are secondary problems that may occur with fetal macrosomia and polyhydramnios.

During the intrapartum period, fetal well-being may be further jeopardized by hypoxia because of the decrease in uteroplacental perfusion secondary to contractions. The risk of intrauterine fetal demise (IUFD) is decreasing as a result of strict glycemic control and careful prenatal monitoring of fetal status.

Neonatal Morbidity and Mortality. The neonate of the diabetic woman suffers from increased morbidity and mortality. RDS is five times more common in full-term neonates. Fetal hyperinsulinemia is thought to play a role in the delayed development of pulmonary maturity. The neonate is also at increased risk for hyperbilirubinemia, neuromuscular irritability, and hypoglycemia during the neonatal period. Care of the neonate of a diabetic woman is discussed in Chapter 33.

Treatment

Preconceptual Care and Counseling. When the woman has preexisting type I or type II diabetes, management of the disease should begin 3 to 6 months *before* pregnancy. The objective is to achieve normal plasma glucose levels (euglycemia) and thereby reduce the incidence of congenital malformations among infants of diabetic mothers (IDM). Goals during this time are directed toward:

- Achieving strict plasma glucose control
- Reducing glycosylated hemoglobin levels to 7% or less
- Assessing for vasculopathy, neuropathy, nephropathy, and retinopathy
- Providing or referring for genetic counseling
- Enhancing the woman's knowledge of diabetes during pregnancy

Prenatal Management. White (1978) developed a classification system (Table 27-6) to guide the physician in the management of the pregnant woman with diabetes and to predict perinatal outcomes. It is based on the duration of the disease, age of onset, and degree of vascular complications.

The major areas of medical management and care of the pregnant woman with diabetes are described in the following section. Although the physician determines medical therapy, the nurse is instrumental in implementing specific aspects of the medical plan.

Strict control of the woman's plasma glucose levels is necessary and may be accomplished through diet, regulated physical activity, insulin use when necessary, monitoring of *capillary* blood glucose (CBG) levels, and adjusting insulin and activity when special circumstances arise.

Total caloric intake during pregnancy is approximately 30 to 35 calories/kg per day, which results in 1800 to 2400 calories for each 24-hour period. This is provided as four to six meals daily, including snacks. Calories are distributed in the following manner:

Table 27-6. White Classification of Diabetes in Pregnancy With Implications

Class	Characteristics	Implications
A_1	Glucose intolerance diagnosed during pregnancy	Treatment with diet is adequate to maintain euglycemia Least risk of complications
A_2	Glucose intolerance diagnosed during pregnancy	Treatment requires administration of insulin in addition to diet More likelihood of fetal macrosomatia
B	Onset after age 20; duration less than 10 y No vascular disease	Some endogenous insulin secretion Characterized by insulin resistance Insulin treatment *before* pregnancy Increased risk of PIH, hypertension, fetal anomalies, and macrosomatia
C	Onset between age 10 and 20 No vascular disease	Insulin treatment *before* pregnancy Increased risk of PIH, hypertension, fetal anomalies, and macrosomatia
D	Onset before age 10; duration more than 20 y Retinopathy	Fetal growth retardation is possible Retinopathy may accelerate during pregnancy and then regress Increased risk of PIH, hypertension, fetal anomalies, or intrauterine growth retardation possible
F	Diabetic nephropathy with proteinuria	Anemia, hypertension, PIH, preterm labor common; anomalies and intrauterine growth retardation common
H	Coronary artery disease	Grave maternal and fetal risk for death

- Complex carbohydrates: 55% to 60%
- Protein: 20%
- Fat: < 30%

The care of the pregnant woman with diabetes requires the professional services of a registered dietitian or diabetes educator for assessment, diet prescription, and teaching. In the United States, most diabetes educators are registered nurses, many with expertise in the care of the pregnant diabetic patient.

Physical activity has a major impact on plasma glucose levels. Significant changes in daily activity can adversely affect glycemic control. A regular, consistent level of physical activity and exercise is required (Evans & Benbarka, 1991). The woman should plan physical activity in close collaboration with the physician and a diabetes educator skilled in counseling about exercise (Plovie, 1991).

The woman's need for insulin is usually based on finger stick CBG monitoring, an indirect measure of plasma glucose levels. The following pattern of surveillance is recommended:

- Fasting level in morning before breakfast
- Preprandial (premeal) values 30 to 45 minutes before breakfast, lunch, dinner, and evening snack
- One hour postprandial (postmeal) level

The goal of medical management is to maintain plasma glucose levels in the range described here (Evans & Benbarka (1991):

- Before meals and snacks: 60 to 80 mg/dL
- One hour postprandial: < 120 mg/dL
- Between 2 AM and 6 AM: 60 to 80 mg/dL

Insulin is prescribed if nutritional therapy is insufficient to control the blood glucose level or the woman has preexisting diabetes requiring insulin therapy before pregnancy. When the plasma glucose level exceeds the recommended range (60 to 120 mg/dL), insulin therapy is initiated. The most common therapy consists of a combination of short-acting (regular Humulin) and intermediate (NPH, or Lente) insulin. The standard regimen is a prebreakfast and predinner dose of combined regular and NPH insulin.

Supplemental regular insulin is added on a "sliding scale" if the glucose level is higher than the desired range. An increase in the dose of insulin is anticipated in the second half of pregnancy. For instance, if the preprandial glucose level is between 140 and 160 mg/dL, 3 U regular insulin is added to the usual dose. If the preprandial level is between 160 and 180 mg/dL, 4 U is added, and so forth.

If the woman's plasma glucose levels cannot be adequately controlled by intermittent injections of insulin, an insulin pump may be ordered for continuous infusion of the drug. Insulin pumps are approximately the size of a pocket calculator. All pumps infuse regular insulin through a catheter attached to a 26- to 27-gauge needle inserted by the woman into the subcutaneous tissue. The needle and site are changed every 2 to 3 days. The pumps are set to deliver a basal infusion rate. Boluses can be preset into the pump's computer for intermittent delivery. For some women, the pump is more effective because it mimics normal pancreatic insulin release.

The physician must make periodic adjustments in the woman's insulin dose and activity level. Insulin requirements generally decrease during the first trimester. Illness including influenza, the common cold, or morning sickness will require prompt adjustments in activity and insulin to protect the health of the woman and her fetus. Some women, particularly those with type I diabetes, will experience the *Somogyi effect*, which is a hypoglycemic episode between 2 AM and 4 AM. A reduction in the evening NPH dose of insulin or an increase in the evening snack calories will correct this problem. As the pregnancy progresses, synthesis of placental ("diabetogenic") hormones will increase insulin requirements.

Ongoing evaluation of the woman is performed to identify the development or worsening of renal disease, chronic hypertension, neuropathies, or ophthalmologic problems. Tests are conducted periodically to determine if underlying problems, such as retinopathy, are accelerating. The woman is screened at each visit for evidence of PIH, polyhydramnios, PTL, or infection.

Antihypertensive drugs may be administered if blood pressure levels rise to unacceptably high levels. Tocolytics may be given to suppress PTL. Magnesium sulfate is the drug of choice for PTL because beta-sympathomimetics such as ritodrine may exacerbate the diabetic state. Antibiotic therapy is initiated if urinary tract infection occurs or asymptomatic bacteriuria is identified because the diabetic woman is at increased risk for pyelonephritis.

Fetal surveillance is important throughout the gestational period. Observations include evaluation for congenital anomalies, macrosomia, appropriate fetal growth, and fetal lung maturity (L/S ratio). Prenatal assessment may include nonstress or contraction stress testing and biophysical profile. Testing generally begins at 32 weeks' gestation or earlier if the woman exhibits poor plasma glucose control. (See Chapter 14 for a complete discussion of fetal assessment.)

If induction of labor or a cesarean delivery is planned, confirmation of fetal pulmonary maturity is determined by amniocentesis. Delayed fetal pulmonary maturity and neonatal RDS are common problems when pregnancy is complicated by diabetes (Evans & Benbarka, 1991). Whereas 99% of normal fetuses have achieved pulmonary maturity by 37 weeks, the fetus of a diabetic woman does not, on average, achieve maturity until after 38.5 weeks.

Intrapartum Management. When the plasma blood glucose level has been well controlled and no complications arise, the diabetic woman may anticipate a vaginal delivery, with close monitoring of maternal and fetal status throughout labor. If labor does not begin spontaneously by 40 weeks' gestation, an oxytocin induction is usually scheduled (Hollingsworth & Moore, 1989). Oxytocin induction of labor or cesarean delivery may be planned before 40 weeks' gestation if fetal or maternal well-being is jeopardized and delivery is indicated (see the accompanying display).

The night before induction of labor, the woman eats her dinner and then receives the usual evening dose of insulin. Food is withheld after midnight. Once in labor and delivery, a mainline intravenous infusion of 5% dextrose in lactated Ringer's is initiated at 125 mL/h. This delivers approximately 6 g carbohydrate an hour (Palmer & Inturrisi, 1992). Plasma glucose or finger stick capillary glucose levels are then monitored hourly.

Regular insulin, 25 U, is added to 250 mL normal saline (1 u/10 mL). The solution is piggybacked to the intravenous mainline and is infused using an insulin administration protocol to maintain plasma glucose levels between 60 and 120 mg/dL (Table 27-7). The insulin infusion rate is determined by the plasma glucose level. If the plasma glucose level rises above 130 mg/dL, the mainline infusion of 5% dextrose in Ringer's lactate is discontinued. This protocol not only reduces the risk of maternal hyperglycemia during labor, but also the incidence of neonatal hyperinsulinism and hypoglycemia (Plovie, 1991).

The non–insulin-dependent woman with GDM may be permitted to eat light meals during early labor. Once active labor begins, food is usually withheld. An insulin infusion is implemented if the plasma glucose level rises above 130 mg/dL.

Postpartum Management. The continuous insulin infusion is usually stopped after delivery because insulin

Delivery of the Infant of a Diabetic Mother

Indications for Induction of Labor

- Pregnancy of 40 weeks or more gestation
- Severe pregnancy-induced hypertension
- Fetal macrosomia, with or without polyhydramnios
- Decreasing fetal well-being as noted by biophysical profile and or nonstress test

Indications for Cesarean Delivery

- Cephalopelvic disproportion
- Fetal macrosomia, (>4500 g)
- Previous cesarean birth with classic incision
- Worsening complications associated with diabetes
- Malpresentation, especially breech, in a macrosomic fetus

Table 27-7. Guidelines for the Intrapartum Administration of Insulin

Plasma Glucose Level (mg/dL)	Insulin Dose (U/h)
<70	No Insulin
71–90	0.5
91–110	1.0
111–130	2.0
131–150	3.0
151–170	4.0
171–190	5.0
>190	Notify physician

Adapted from Palmer, D., & Inturrisi, M. (1992). Insulin infusion therapy in the intrapartum period. *Journal of Perinatal and Neonatal Nursing, 6*(2), 25–36, with permission of Aspen Publishers, Inc., © 1992.

requirements decrease rapidly with the birth of the placenta. The goal of treatment for all women (type I, II, and III) is to maintain the fasting plasma glucose level under 100 mg/dL and the 2-hour postprandial level below 150 mg/dL. Plasma glucose levels are monitored by fasting and preprandial finger stick glucose tests, performed 30 minutes before meals. Insulin is administered by the subcutaneous route when the glucose level exceeds these limits.

The insulin-dependent woman who has had a vaginal birth may be permitted to eat a calorie-controlled diabetic diet. If the woman has had a cesarean delivery and is NPO, an intravenous infusion of 5% dextrose in Ringer's lactate is administered at 125 mL/h to meet energy needs until she may eat. The woman with GDM often has normal glucose levels in the immediate postpartum period.

Breastfeeding is encouraged, and extra fluids are added to the woman's diet to meet the demands of lactation. Women who breastfeed often experience episodes of hypoglycemia 30 to 45 minutes after nursing the infant. This can be prevented by drinking a glass of milk before breastfeeding (Hollingsworth & Moore, 1989).

• • Assessment

If the woman with preexisting diabetes has received preconceptual counseling, she is often prepared for the changes in medical regimen and self-care because of her disease. The newly diagnosed pregnant diabetic woman may have more difficulty adjusting to the diagnosis. The success of this adjustment rests largely with the woman's ability to integrate the requirements of self-care and the medical therapy into her usual daily activities. The nurse plays a key role in promoting effective coping behaviors and uses the nursing process to facilitate successful adaptations.

The diabetic clinical nurse specialist or nurse diabetes educator is often part of the health care team involved in determining the prepregnancy status of the diabetic woman and the most likely risks for her and her fetus after conception. Of particular importance is the ongoing assessment of plasma glucose and glycosylated hemoglobin levels. Strict control of the plasma glucose level is essential *3 to 6 months before* conception to minimize the risk of fetal anomalies.

During the prenatal period, the nurse assesses the woman to determine the likelihood of effective self-care including:

- Knowledge of diabetes and its treatment
- Knowledge of dietary adjustments
- Adherence to dietary restrictions
- Accuracy and consistency of self-glucose monitoring
- Techniques for measurement and self-administration of insulin
- Preventing, recognizing, and treating insulin reactions
- Emotional status and coping mechanisms

Although a diabetes educator (most often a nurse) is often the health team member who teaches dietary adjustments and insulin requirements, the nurse is responsible for the ongoing assessment of the woman's compliance with the diet, glucose monitoring, and insulin administration. The nurse should be familiar with the specific division of kilocalories for the required 24-hour intake, insulin requirements and administration, and recommended glucose levels. When the woman is unable to comply with the plan of care, the nurse must attempt to identify obstacles to effective self-care activities and communicate her findings to the physician and diabetes educator.

The woman is screened at each visit for evidence of complications associated with diabetes including PTL, PIH, and infection. The nurse obtains vital signs and the woman's weight. The urine is tested for evidence of protein, glucose, and ketones. The nurse asks the woman about her general health and the development of complications. The woman's plasma glucose values obtained at home through self-monitoring are reviewed. Abnormal findings are brought to the physician's or diabetic nurse educator's attention. The nurse reviews the woman's record for previous test results including assessments of fetal well-being. If the woman is screened periodically for diabetic retinopathy or neuropathy, the nurse should be aware of the findings.

On admission to the labor and delivery unit, the nurse reviews the woman's prenatal history to determine the following:

- Degree of glycemic control
- Development of medical or obstetric complications
- Fetal gestational age
- Findings of fetal assessment tests
- L/S ratio and presence of PG
- Diagnosis of congenital anomalies
- Suspicion or anticipation of fetal macrosomatia
- Medical plan for mode of labor and delivery

During the intrapartum period, the nurse assumes responsibility for glucose monitoring. The woman may perform her own finger sticks and glucose evaluations during the early phases of labor. The woman is monitored closely for evidence of hypoglycemia, particularly when an intravenous insulin infusion is initiated. The FHR is assessed by EFM for evidence of decreased uteroplacental perfusion. The woman is observed closely for the development of PIH, which may occur during labor or the early postpartum period.

After birth of the neonate, insulin resistance and insulin requirements decline dramatically. The nurse observes the woman for signs and symptoms of hypoglycemia. This is particularly important if the woman is breastfeeding because it is not uncommon for the plasma glucose level to decrease during the breastfeeding session. The insulin-dependent woman's plasma glucose levels should be monitored hourly for the first 4 to 6 hours and then every 2 hours until stable (Plovie, 1991).

• • Nursing Diagnosis

On assessment of the pregnant diabetic woman, the following nursing diagnoses may be identified:

- Knowledge Deficit related to diabetes, self-monitoring, or diet
- Fear related to diagnosis of diabetes or impact on maternal or fetal well-being

- Altered Nutrition: More than Body Requirements related to dietary intake
- High Risk for Infection related to diabetes
- Altered Nutrition: Less than Body Requirements related to insulin administration
- High Risk for Injury related to hypoglycemia or hyperglycemia
- Altered Tissue Perfusion related to diabetic ketoacidosis
- Fluid Volume Deficit related to diabetic ketoacidosis
- Pain related to multiple finger sticks and venipuncture
- Anxiety related to concerns about future pregnancies
- Altered Uteroplacental Tissue Perfusion related to diabetic vasculopathies

• • Planning and Implementation

Planning and implementing care for the pregnant woman with diabetes must be a team effort. The nurse is often responsible for coordinating all services involved in the woman's care.

Providing Information for Self-Care

Teaching is a central focus of nursing interventions throughout the childbearing cycle. Essential components of teaching are listed in the accompanying display.

The woman with a diagnosis of preexisting diabetes (type I or II) or GDM (type III) is referred to a diabetes educator. The woman will need to learn (or review) self-monitoring of glucose levels. Self-monitoring is possible with the development of a glucose reflectance meter device. A drop of capillary blood obtained by finger stick is placed on a glucose oxidase strip. After a specified period of time, the excess blood is removed from the strip and then placed in the reflectance meter for measurement of the CBG level. The goal of education is to prepare her to perform glucose self-monitoring and to self-administer insulin.

Expected Outcomes

- The woman verbalizes an accurate understanding of diabetes, insulin therapy, glucose self-monitoring, and medical treatment.
- The woman demonstrates correct self-monitoring of glucose and insulin administration techniques.

Supporting the Diabetic Woman in the Prenatal Period

An important aspect of prenatal nursing care includes scheduling and preparing the woman for laboratory studies and fetal assessment. If the woman is admitted to the hospital for evaluation or stabilization of plasma glucose levels, the nurse provides supportive care. The goal is to maintain physiologic integrity and promote comfort. In the first trimester, nausea and vomiting may result in episodes of hypoglycemia. The nurse assists the woman in self-evaluation of glucose levels and adjustments in insulin doses to prevent hypoglycemia. Profound hypoglycemia is a medical emergency and requires prompt nursing action to prevent permanent neurologic damage or death. The following Nursing Care Plan illustrates such a case. Nursing and medical management of hypoglycemia is outlined in the Nursing Procedure display, Supporting the Woman With Maternal Hypoglycemia.

If DKA occurs, the nurse implements emergency measures to stabilize the woman's physiologic functions. The nurse must be knowledgeable regarding pathophysiology of DKA. Standardized protocols often guide the nurse in the provision of care (see the Nursing Procedure describing emergency treatment of DKA).

Expected Outcomes

- The woman exhibits plasma glucose levels within the recommended range of 60 to 120 mg/dL.
- The woman verbalizes comfort after she is stabilized.

Providing Insulin Support in the Intrapartum Period

Intensive nursing care is required for the insulin-dependent woman during labor and birth. Precise orders are required for adjusting the woman's insulin infusion according to blood glucose determinations. The nurse is responsible for assembling all necessary equipment for care of the diabetic woman in labor and delivery and preparing the insulin solution. Insulin binds to glass and plastic; therefore, 50 mL of the insulin-intravenous solution mixture should be run through the intravenous tubing to coat it and ensure delivery of accurate insulin dosage in the subsequent administration.

The continuous insulin infusion is piggybacked to the primary intravenous line. The insulin must be administered using an infusion pump. Because many diabetics suffer from PIH or are scheduled for induction of labor, oxytocin and magnesium sulfate may be administered concurrently with insulin. These two drugs are compatible with the insulin infusion.

Expected Outcome

- The woman maintains plasma glucose levels within the recommended range of 60 to 120 mg/dL during labor and birth.

Monitoring for Hypoglycemia in the Intrapartum Period

The nurse should have glucagon, 500 mL of 10% dextrose and 50 mL of injectable dextrose 50% available to treat maternal hypoglycemia. Close monitoring for signs and symptoms of hypoglycemia is essential. If hypoglycemia occurs, the insulin infusion should be stopped immediately.

Expected Outcome

- The woman's blood level stabilizes in the recommended range after appropriate treatment of hypoglycemia.

Meeting Comfort Needs

Meeting the comfort needs of a diabetic woman is difficult. The woman is most often confined to bed, and free movement is hindered by multiple intravenous infusions and electronic fetal and uterine monitoring. Frequent position

Essential Aspects of the Teaching Care Plan for the Pregnant Diabetic Woman

Preconceptual Counseling and Teaching

- Importance of low glycosylated hemoglobin level
- Risk of congenital anomalies
- Risk of accelerating retinopathy, neuropathy, or kidney disease
- Complications associated with diabetes in pregnancy (ie, PIH)
- Anticipated changes in self-care and life-style

Prenatal Counseling and Teaching

Diet

- Need for regular intake at established times
- Specific dietary requirements (calories and percentage of carbohydrates, protein, and fats)
- Use of American Diabetes Association exchange list in meal planning
- Desired weight gain during pregnancy
- Contraindication to sugar substitutes and diet beverages during pregnancy

Insulin

- Dose, route, timing
- Storage of drug
- Physiologic effects of drug
- Technique for drawing up and self-administering drug
- Recommendations regarding rotating injections within a chosen area
- Differences in absorption of insulin by area of injection
- Relationship between intake, activity, and insulin dose
- Use and maintenance of insulin pump (if ordered)
- Use of sliding scale insulin administration
- Signs and symptoms of hypoglycemia

Activity

- Importance of consistency in exercise
- Type of exercise recommended during pregnancy
- Timing of exercise in relation to insulin injections
- Selection of site for insulin injection that will not be exercised
- Importance of checking insulin before and after exercise
- Need to carry carbohydrate snack during exercise

Self-Monitoring Glucose

- Importance of glucose monitoring
- Timing of glucose monitoring
- Use of home glucose monitoring system
- Correct technique for obtaining capillary blood sample by finger stick
- Correct application of blood sample to glucose oxidase strip
- Recording glucose values
- Reporting abnormal values
- Treating hypoglycemia
- Testing for urine ketone levels

Complications

- Recognizing early signs of diabetic ketoacidosis
- Recognizing and treating hypoglycemia
- Recognizing and reporting symptoms of urinary tract infections
- Recognizing and reporting signs of PIH
- Reporting illness (ie, flu or colds)
- Reporting decreased fetal movement

Plan for Fetal Assessments

- Purpose and timing of:
  Ultrasonography
  Amniocentesis
  Nonstress test
  Contraction stress test

Intrapartum Counseling and Teaching

Plan for Delivery

- Mode and timing
- Anticipated medical and nursing care in labor
- Analgesia and anesthesia
- Glucose monitoring
- Insulin administration

Postpartum Counseling and Teaching

- Need for ongoing glucose monitoring
- Insulin requirements (in any)
- Breastfeeding
- Contraception

changes and the use of pillows or an eggcrate mattress pad can enhance comfort.

Analgesia and anesthesia may be administered as labor progresses. Plans for pain control should be discussed before the onset of labor. When the woman has severe renal or cardiovascular complications secondary to diabetes, the anesthesiologist should be consulted well before labor occurs. This ensures that adequate assessment and appropriate decisions can be made regarding analgesia and anesthesia.

The woman is subjected to multiple finger sticks or venipuncture procedures for plasma glucose monitoring.

Text continues on page 771

Nursing Care Plan

The Woman With Diabetes Mellitus During Pregnancy

PATIENT PROFILE

History

D.M. is a 17-year-old G2/PO at 32 weeks' gestation. She is single and this was an unplanned pregnancy. She plans to keep her baby and says she is "excited about being a mother." She is recently diagnosed type III gestational diabetic, who has been noncompliant with her prescribed diet and glucose self-monitoring regimen. She weighs 192 lb and has gained a total of 48 lb during the pregnancy. She is admitted for glycemic control and treatment of a recurrent urinary tract infection. She is also found to have a *Candida* vaginitis.

D.M. is placed on insulin therapy: IOU Regular Humulin insulin and 3 U NPH insulin b.i.d. (prebreakfast and predinner). She says, "I don't mean to cheat on my diet, but when I'm out with my friends its hard to do this food group stuff. And you forget to check your sugar every single time. How am I supposed to give myself insulin too? Why do I need insulin anyway?" She is learning how to draw up the prescribed dose of insulin, but is refusing to practice injection techniques. "I hate needles so much I won't even get my ears pierced. I can't do it!"

Physical Assessment

Two hours after breakfast, on the 2nd hospital day the nurse enters D.M.'s room and notes the following: D.M. is standing in the bathroom and is pale, diaphoretic, and tremulous. She stays, "I feel weird, like I'm gonna pass out." She reveals to the nurse that she flushed most of her breakfast down the toilet. "I guess I should have eaten more, but I'm so fat now I hate myself. And I hate breakfast."

COLLABORATIVE PROBLEMS/POTENTIAL COMPLICATIONS

- Hypoglycemia/hyperglycemia
- PIH
- Infection
- Fetal macrosomia

(See the accompanying Nursing Alert display.)

Assessment	*Nursing Diagnosis*	*Nursing Interventions*	*Rationale*
D.M. is an insulin-dependent type III gestational diabetic.	Altered Nutrition: Less than Body Requirements related to inadequate intake and insulin administration.	Call for help and assist D.M. back to bed.	Additional staff are needed to support and monitor D.M. and provide needed supplies.
She is noncompliant with the diabetic self-care regimen.	High Risk for Injury related to hypoglycemia.	If D.M. remains conscious give her 12–14 oz of milk or juice to drink followed by a protein snack.	D.M. requires rapidly digestible source of glucose to counteract hypoglycemia.
She received 10 U of regular and 3 U of NPH insulin prebreakfast.	***Expected Outcome***	If decreased consciousness or unconsciousness occurs, give glucagon, 1 U (1 mg) IV, IM, or SC, or give 50% glucose IV if glucagon not available, as ordered.	Glucagon stimulates hepatic production of glucose.
D.M. flushed most of her breakfast down the toilet.	D.M.'s glucose level will stabilize between 60 and 120 mg/dL.		IV glucose may also be given but is more likely to result in hyperglycemia.
She is pale, diaphoretic and tremulous.	D.M. will verbalize resolution of symptoms of hypoglycemia.		
D.M. states, "I feel so weird, I think I'm gonna pass out."		Draw blood specimen as quickly as possible and repeat 20 minutes after snack or glucagon.	To document degree of hypoglycemia and effectiveness of therapy.

(*Continued*)

The Woman With Diabetes Mellitus During Pregnancy

(Continued)

Assessment	*Nursing Diagnosis*	*Nursing Interventions*	*Rationale*
		Remain with D.M. continuously. Note and record vital signs and level of consciousness every 5 to 10 minutes. If no improvement or deterioration in D.M.'s condition repeat glucagon in 5 to 10 minutes.	Plasma levels may continue to drop and D.M. may lose consciousness, requiring additional glucagon or glucose.
		Notify physician of D.M.'s condition and problem with compliance.	Physician must be apprised of D.M.'s condition to plan therapy.
D.M. has type III diabetes. D.M. is noncompliant with treatment regimen. She has a recurrent urinary tract infection and *Candida* vaginitis.	Infection related to diabetes and hyperglycemia. ***Expected Outcome*** D.M. will demonstrate self-care activities which will reduce risk of infection.	Administer antibiotics and antifungal drugs as ordered. Teach D.M. about causes of increased risk of infection with diabetes and pregnancy.	Drug therapy is required to eliminate pathogenic organisms. Treatment of urinary tract infection may prevent pyelonephritis.
		Instruct D.M. in self-care activities that reduce risk of vaginal candidiasis and urinary tract infections: • Wear cotton underwear • Wear loose-fitting slacks • Wear nylons with cotton crotch • Wipe front to back when cleaning perineum • Avoid douching and perineal hygiene products with perfume • Maintain plasma glucose level between 60 and 120 mg/dL • Drink at least 6–8 glasses of water per day. • Urinate after sexual intercourse. • Drink cranberry juice. • Avoid caffeine-containing products.	Self-care activities that promote health will reduce risk of recurrent infection. *Candida* organisms thrive in warm, dark, moist environment. Use of cotton underwear and nylons with cotton crotch wick moisture from skin. Loose underclothing improves circulation of air. Wiping front to back prevents contamination of vagina and urethra with pathogenic organisms. Douching and perfumes destroy normal flora. Tissue hyperglycemia is an excellent medium for the growth of pathogenic organisms. Drinking adequate fluids prevents urine stasis and growth of pathogenic bacteria. Cranberry juice changes pH of urine and inhibits growth of pathogenic organisms. Caffeine is a bladder mucosa irritant.
D.M. is 17-year-old gestational diabetic.	Altered Health Maintenance. Instrumental Self-Care Deficit related to developmental maturity level and values.	Use open-ended questions when discussing D.M.'s condition with her.	Open-ended questions permit exploration of feelings/questions.

(Continued)

The Woman With Diabetes Mellitus During Pregnancy

(Continued)

Assessment	Nursing Diagnosis	Nursing Interventions	Rationale
D.M. does not follow prescribed self-care and self-monitoring regimen. D.M. states, "How am I supposed to give myself insulin? I hate needles." D.M. is resistant to learning self-injection techniques. D.M.'s pregnancy was unplanned.	***Expected Outcome*** D.M. will identify healthy alternatives to present coping behaviors. D.M. will demonstrate more effective coping mechanisms. D.M.'s support system will reinforce health-promoting behaviors.	Identify D.M.'s feelings, major fears, and concerns about her disease and the pregnancy.	Nursing interventions may be more appropriately planned when the woman's major concerns are identified.
		Identify D.M.'s support system and enlist their aid in reinforcing health-promoting behaviors.	Supportive peers and family can reinforce positive, health-promoting behaviors.
		Determine if a diabetes support group is available for pregnant women/adolescents.	A peer support group tailored to the developmental level of the adolescent will be more effective in promoting change.
D.M. is a recently diagnosed diabetic. She asks, "Why do I need insulin?" D.M. is 17-years-old. D.M. plans to keep her baby.	Knowledge Deficit related to self-administration of insulin. Knowledge Deficit related to the effects of her condition on her fetus. ***Expected Outcome*** D.M. will verbalize a correct understanding of effects of poor glycemic control on maternal, fetal, and neonatal status. D.M. will attend diabetes education classes in the hospital.	Determine D.M.'s understanding of her disease process and the effects of poor glycemic control on fetal growth, development, and well-being.	Correct understanding of her disease process may improve compliance with plan of care and insulin administration.
		Initiate referral for formal diabetes education if available in the hospital or community.	Ongoing education may enhance D.M.'s confidence in her ability to perform self-care.
		Teach D.M. about the effects of poor glycemic control on fetal and neonatal status and her physical health.	Knowledge of adverse effects of poor glycemic control on fetal and neonatal well-being may be a powerful motivator for change.
		Make community referral for follow-up by nurse.	Ongoing assessment and reinforcement of self-care is essential to support D.M. and promote healthy behaviors.

EVALUATION

D.M.'s symptoms resolved with a 14-oz glass of orange juice. The first plasma glucose level drawn immediately after D.M. reported symptoms was 53 mg/dL; 20 minutes after treatment it was 120 mg/dL. The father of D.M.'s fetus and his 17-year-old sister were D.M.'s major support system; they verbalized a commitment to encouraging her to comply with the plan of care. They attended the training sessions with D.M. in which she learned self-administration of insulin and supported her in her learning. D.M. attended two diabetes education classes while she was in the hospital. By discharge she demonstrated self-care activities and compliance with insulin administration.

NURSING ALERT

NURSING RESPONSIBILITIES WHEN CARING FOR THE WOMAN WITH DIABETES MELLITUS DURING PREGNANCY

The insulin-dependent pregnant woman with diabetes is vulnerable to both hypoglycemic shock and episodes of diabetic ketoacidosis (DKA). The nurse must be prepared to respond promptly should the woman demonstrate sudden deterioration in physiologic stability because of extreme abnormalities in the plasma glucose level. Emergency equipment should be readily available, and the nurse should verify that it is functioning properly. Frequently administered drugs and intravenous fluids, such as insulin and glucagon, also should be easily accessible. The nurse must be alert for subtle signs and symptoms of hypoglycemia and prodromal indicators of DKA.

The nurse is responsible for implementing emergency supportive care until medical help arrives. Essential aspects of care include initiating an intravenous line, maintaining a patent airway, promoting respiratory function, and administering oxygen. Glucagon may be required in cases of hypoglycemia or insulin when DKA occurs, and these drugs should be administered promptly. In some settings the nurse may be guided by physician orders or standardized protocols, so that emergency measures can be instituted before the physician arrives.

During the course of normal labor, hourly capillary glucose evaluation results in several dozen skin punctures. The woman's fingers may become sore, and the usually minor discomfort of a finger stick can become acutely painful. The peripheral aspects of the finger are less sensitive than the ball of the finger and are the preferred areas for puncture. The thumb and fourth finger have a better vascular supply and are preferred sites for obtaining a specimen (Palmer & Inturrisi, 1992). If the woman prefers, other body areas can be used for blood sampling, such as the heel of the foot or the earlobe.

Expected Outcome

- The woman verbalizes satisfaction with comfort measures implemented to reduce pain.

Notifying Neonatal Staff of Impending Birth

At the time of delivery, neonatal staff should be present to evaluate and support the neonate because macrosomia remains a common problem for neonates of diabetic women. The nurse should be prepared to assist the birth attendant if impaction of the fetal shoulders occurs during vaginal delivery (see Chapter 26 for a discussion of shoulder dystocia). Neonatal asphyxia and birth trauma are common complications resulting from shoulder dystocia.

Neonates of diabetic women are at high risk for many problems secondary to maternal metabolic aberrations including hypoglycemia, hypocalcemia, and RDS. Congenital anomalies may also present a problem. The neonate is usually placed in an observation or special care unit until its condition stabilizes. Further discussion of the needs of a neonate of a diabetic woman occurs in Chapter 33.

Expected Outcome

- The neonate maintains physiologic stability, including normal plasma glucose levels, in the postbirth period.

Supporting the Family in the Postpartum Period

The nurse usually discontinues the intravenous insulin infusion after birth of the neonate and placenta. Administration of subcutaneous doses of insulin may be required if the fasting plasma glucose level exceeds 100 mg/dL or 150 mg/dL 2 hours after a meal. The woman is supported in her efforts to resume self-care activities including monitoring of CBG levels.

If the woman plans to breastfeed the neonate, the nurse alerts the woman to the possibility of hypoglycemia during breastfeeding sessions. The nurse provides additional milk or a snack before the woman breastfeeds the neonate as ordered by the physician. If the neonate must remain in the nursery for observation or treatment of complications related to maternal diabetes, the nurse provides information about the neonate's condition (see Chapter 33 for a complete discussion of neonatal problems related to maternal diabetes). The woman is escorted to the nursery as soon as possible, so that she can begin the maternal-newborn acquaintance process.

Discussion of family planning options is an essential aspect of discharge teaching for all women. The presence of diabetes mellitus must be considered when discussing contraception. Oral and injectable contraception may be contraindicated when diabetes is poorly controlled and is absolutely contraindicated in women with cardiovascular disease secondary to diabetes.

Expected Outcomes

- The woman resumes CBG self-monitoring and insulin self-administration as indicated by her condition.
- The postpartum woman maintains a fasting plasma glucose level below 100 mg/dL and a 2-hour postprandial plasma glucose level under 150 mg/dL.
- The woman verbalizes an understanding of her contraceptive options.

• • Evaluation

Ongoing evaluation of maternal and fetal status is essential to determine adequacy of nursing and medical care. If nursing interventions are effective, expected outcomes will be achieved. The woman will maintain her plasma glucose levels within the recommended range and will remain free of complications of diabetes including hypoglycemic episodes or DKA. Medical and obstetric problems will be minimized, and the woman will maintain physiologic stability during pregnancy and the intrapartum and postpartum periods. Fetal growth and development will proceed in a normal fashion, and the woman will give birth to a viable and healthy infant.

NURSING PROCEDURE
Supporting the Woman With Maternal Hypoglycemia

Purpose: To raise plasma glucose levels and prevent neurologic injury secondary to profound hypoglycemia.

NURSING ACTION	***RATIONALE***
1. Be particularly alert for signs and symptoms during peak action of insulin: • 2 to 4 hours after regular Humulin • 2 to 15 hours after NPH or Humulin N with illness, or vomiting (morning sickness)	To promote early recognition and treatment of hypoglycemia
2. If the woman is conscious and exhibits mild symptoms of hypoglycemia, (40–60 mg/dL) give 20 g carbohydrate (14 oz of whole milk or 12 oz of apple or orange juice).	To provide a solution that will raise the plasma glucose level but will not result in rebound hypoglycemia
3. Perform a finger stick glucose test as quickly as possible, while the woman is drinking the milk or juice.	To determine the plasma glucose level
4. Draw a venous sample if ordered.	To verify the accuracy of the reflectance meter reading
5. If the woman remains stable and conscious, wait 20 minutes, and repeat finger stick glucose test.	To determine the effectiveness of treatment and to prevent overtreatment and hyperglycemia
6. If the woman is vomiting, *or* disoriented, *or* unconscious—indicators of severe hypoglycemia—(less than 40 mg/dL), call for help.	Additional staff is needed to support woman and provide emergency drugs and supplies.
7. Give glucagon 0.5 to 1 U (0.5–1 mg) IV, IM, or SC.	Glucagon is preferred over rapid infusion of glucose because its action is physiologic and is less likely to result in hyperglycemia.
8. If glucagon is given, turn woman's head to side and have suction available.	To prevent aspiration because vomiting may occur after administration of glucagon
9. If woman does not respond to administration of glucagon, give second dose in 5 to 20 minutes.	Additional glucagon may be required with profound hypoglycemia.
10. If glucagon not available, may give 50 mL of 50% glucose IV as ordered or by protocol.	

Cardiac Disease

Cardiac disease is a rare but serious problem complicating pregnancy and the postpartum period. It occurs in approximately 1% of pregnancies and may jeopardize both maternal and fetal well-being (Troiano, 1992). The nurse must have a sound understanding of the normal cardiovascular adaptations of the childbearing cycle and how they may affect the woman with underlying cardiac dysfunction. The nurse must also be knowledgeable about the most common cardiac problems encountered during the childbearing cycle.

Etiologic and Predisposing Factors

Normal cardiac function is altered during pregnancy and may worsen preexisting cardiac disease. The most significant physiologic changes are:

- Increase in cardiac output by 40%
- Increase in plasma volume by 40% to 50%
- Rise in stroke volume by 30% to 40%
- Decrease in vascular resistance

Rheumatic heart disease (RHD) accounts for 65% to 80% of all cardiac disease. The incidence of RHD is decreas-

NURSING PROCEDURE
Managing Diabetic Ketoacidosis in the Pregnant Woman in an Emergency

Purpose: To prevent reduce maternal hyperglycemia, ketonemia, maternal death, fetal distress, or intrauterine fetal demise secondary to diabetic ketoacidosis.

NURSING ACTION	RATIONALE
1. Start IV infusion of isotonic (0.9%) saline at a rate of 500 mL/h.	To correct hypovolemia and electrolyte imbalance and acidosis
2. Administer insulin loading dose (10–20 U regular insulin) via infusion pump.	To correct hyperglycemia, ketonemia, and acidosis
3. Administer maintenance IV insulin infusion (5–10 U/h) after loading dose completed.	
4. Obtain blood and urine samples as ordered by physician.	To determine further need for insulin therapy
5. Administer oxygen at 8 to 12 L/min by face mask. Be prepared to assist with insertion of arterial line or mechanical ventilation.	To correct hypoxia, and improve fetal oxygenation To permit evaluation of blood pH $Pa{O_2}$ and $Pa{CO_2}$ levels To provide ventilatory support if the woman is unconscious
6. Maintain woman in lateral decubitus position and have suction equipment available.	To prevent supine hypotension To prevent aspiration should the woman vomit
7. Be prepared to assist with insertion of nasogastric tube.	To prevent vomiting and aspiration of gastric contents
8. Insert indwelling Foley catheter.	To permit measurement of urine volume and evaluate adequacy of therapy
9. Maintain strict intake and output.	
10. Implement cardiorespiratory monitoring.	To identify cardiac arrhythmias secondary to electrolyte imbalance
11. Implement electronic blood pressure monitoring.	To permit rapid assessment of vital signs
12. Implement electronic fetal monitoring if fetal gestational age is 20 weeks or greater.	To determine FHR and status
13. Perform rapid physical assessment.	To detect shock and other physiologic complications secondary to DKA
14. Monitor plasma glucose levels as indicated by woman's condition and response to treatment.	To determine ongoing therapy

ing due to a reduction in acute rheumatic fever and subsequent injury to the heart valves. RHD most commonly causes mitral valve stenosis, pulmonary vascular congestion, and dyspnea.

Congenital heart disease (CHD) is the next largest category of cardiac disease observed during pregnancy. Anomalies that may be encountered include intracardiac septal defects, coarctation of the aorta, and tetralogy of Fallot. CHD is growing because advances in treatment permit female infants with congenital anomalies of the heart to survive and reach childbearing age. Many women with CHD have had corrective heart surgery before pregnancy. Both genetic and environmental factors have been identified in the etiology of CHD.

Mitral valve prolapse is encountered in many pregnant women and in most cases is a benign syndrome. The changes in vascular resistance and blood volume characteristic of pregnancy may result in overt symptoms of cardiac disease including arrhythmias, chest pain, and peripheral emboli.

Coronary artery disease and *myocardial infarction* remain rare causes of morbidity and mortality during the childbearing cycle. The trend toward delayed childbearing (see Chapter 10) may lead to an increase in these cardiac problems during pregnancy. This is particularly true for women over the age of 40.

Diagnosis

In some cases women begin pregnancy with recognized cardiac disease. Diagnosis in other women is not made until signs and symptoms of cardiac decompensation develop. Signs and symptoms of cardiac dysfunction are listed in the accompanying display.

Several diagnostic modalities can be used to confirm the diagnosis of cardiac disease including chest radiography, electrocardiography (ECG), and echocardiography.

Maternal, Fetal, and Neonatal Implications

Maternal morbidity and mortality will depend on the type and severity of cardiac disease and the availability of appropriate medical and nursing care during the childbearing cycle. A classification system has been developed to estimate the risk of mortality (see the accompanying display). As symptoms of cardiac disease increase, the woman's ability to complete activities of daily living will be limited. With acute cardiac decompensation, the woman may be confined to bed or hospitalized.

This risk of cardiac decompensation is greatest immediately after the delivery of the placenta. Shifts in fluid balance occurring during this time are responsible for increasing cardiac workload. Eighty percent of maternal deaths occur during this critical time period. The probability of postpartum decompensation is greatest when the woman has class III or class IV cardiac disease.

Two cardiac problems pose severe threats to the woman's life, and pregnancy is not recommended (Blackburn & Loper, 1992). *Pulmonary hypertension* (Eisenmenger syndrome) carries a 50% maternal mortality rate. The pregnant woman can die at any time during the childbearing cycle, but she is most vulnerable at the time of birth and during the first postpartum week due to the profound hemodynamic changes that occur. *Marfan syndrome* results from a weakness of connective tissues, including the vascular system. Death is commonly caused by dissection and rupture of the aorta after blood volume and cardiac output increase in the second half of pregnancy.

Fetal morbidity and mortality also depend on the severity of maternal cardiac disease and the availability of medical and nursing services. When maternal cardiac decompensation occurs, fetal mortality may reach 50% due to reduced uteroplacental perfusion and profound hypoxia. When genetic factors are implicated in the development of maternal cardiac disease, the fetus is evaluated for the presence of inherited heart abnormalities. Recent advances in ultrasonography make early diagnosis of fetal heart anomalies possible, and arrangements can be made for immediate postnatal support of the neonate.

Mortality Risk Associated With Cardiac Disease During Pregnancy

Group I: Mortality Less Than 1%

Atrial septal defect
Ventricular septal defect
Patent ductus arteriosus
Pulmonic and tricuspid disease
Corrected tetrology of Fallot
Biosynthetic valve prosthesis

Group II: Mortality 5% to 15%

Aortic stenosis
Mechanical valve prosthesis
Previous myocardial infarction
Uncorrected tetralogy of Fallot
Marfan syndrome with normal aorta
Mitral stenosis, NYHA class III or IV
Mitral stenosis with atrial fibrillation
Coarctation of the aorta (uncomplicated)

Group III: Mortality 25% to 50%

Pulmonary hypertension
Coarctation of the aorta, complicated
Marfan syndrome with aortic involvement

From Clark, S. L. (1991). Structural cardiac disease in pregnancy. In S. L. Clark, G. Hankins, D. Cotton, & J. Phelan (Eds.). Critical care obstetrics *(2nd ed.). Boston: Blackwell Scientific Publishers.*

Signs and Symptoms of Cardiac Disease During Pregnancy

- Chest pain
- Severe dyspnea
- Diastolic murmur
- Large, harsh systolic murmur
- Pulmonary rales
- Peripheral cyanosis
- Clubbing of fingers
- Distended neck veins
- Postural syncope (fainting)
- Coughing and hemoptysis
- Resting tachycardia or tachypnea
- Increased cardiac size (cardiomegaly)
- Dysrhythmias (except sinus tachycardia and paroxysmal tachycardia)

New York Heart Association Functional Classification (Modified)

Class I

No limitation of physical activity

Class II

No symptoms at rest

Minor limitation of physical activity (fatigue, palpitations, minor dyspnea, etc.)

Class III

No symptoms at rest

Marked limitation of physical activity due to symptoms of cardiac disease

Class IV

Symptoms at rest

Discomfort increased with any physical activity

From Malkasian, G., Noller, K., Aaro, L., et al. (1981). Miscellaneous medical complications. In Iffy, L., Kaminetzky, H.A. (Eds.). Principles and practice of obstetrics and perinatology, *Volume 2. New York: John Wiley & Sons.*

Treatment

Medical management of the pregnant woman with a cardiac condition is guided by the New York Heart Association classification, shown in the accompanying display. It is based on the type of symptoms the woman experiences and the degree of disruption in activities of daily living.

Management of Class I and II Heart Disease. The management of the pregnant woman in class I or II is centered on early recognition of cardiac decompensation and prevention of problems that exacerbate cardiac disease. The goal of treatment is to reduce cardiac workload by:

- Ensuring adequate rest
- Limiting strenuous activity
- Implementing a low-salt diet
- Avoiding anemia
- Avoiding excessive weight gain
- Aggressively treating infections

The balance between rest and activity is determined after the woman's symptoms are assessed. An evaluation of the living situation will aid in determining how activity must be altered. For example, the woman who has to climb stairs to enter the home may be hindered from leaving the house as often as desired unless adjustments in living arrangements can be made.

The benefits of rest include avoiding cardiac exertion and improving uteroplacental perfusion. The woman should be instructed to rest in the left lateral recumbent position and obtain a minimum of 8 to 10 hours of sleep per day. An effort should be made to take frequent rest periods during waking hours. Absolute bed rest will be required when cardiac decompensation is a potential or real problem.

The degree of salt restriction in the diet depends on the severity of the condition. Fluid and salt restriction is essential to prevent fluid overload, cardiac decompensation, and pulmonary edema. Anemia is avoided through sound nutrition, with an emphasis on foods high in iron and the prescription of supplemental iron.

Because infection of any kind may exacerbate cardiac disease, the woman is counseled to avoid people with known infections. The woman should receive pneumococcal and influenza vaccines. Prophylactic antibiotics are administered to women with valve disease or prosthetic valves if invasive procedures such as dental work or surgery are performed. This is done to prevent the development of bacterial endocarditis. Although controversial, some experts recommend initiation of ampicillin therapy during labor when valve disease exists, to reduce the risk of endocarditis.

Prenatal monitoring of the fetal status is initiated at 32 weeks or earlier depending on the woman's condition. A vaginal delivery may be planned if the maternal and fetal condition is stable. Adequate analgesia and anesthesia are essential to reduce pain and anxiety, which can stress the heart. Epidural anesthesia is often used.

If the woman remains free of all signs and symptoms of cardiac decompensation, she may be permitted to push during the second stage of labor. If any signs of cardiac decompensation occur, such as a pulse rate over 100 bpm, or a respiratory rate of 24/min, pushing efforts are stopped and forceps assisted delivery or cesarean delivery is performed (Kulb, 1990b).

During the postpartum period the woman with class I or II disease may resume activities of daily living as soon as desired. Breastfeeding should be encouraged.

Management of Class III or IV Heart Disease. Management for the woman with class III or IV cardiac problems is directed at avoiding congestive failure and pulmonary edema. These complications result from the cardiac decompensation. Treatment includes strict bed rest, administration of oxygen and medications, and planning for delivery. Table 27-8 list drugs commonly used to treat cardiac disease in pregnancy.

Close monitoring of maternal and fetal status is essential. A cardiologist with expertise in the care of pregnant women with heart disease should be consulted. Early delivery may be indicated to save the life of the woman.

• • Assessment

Ideally, women with diagnosed cardiac disease will have access to preconceptual counseling regarding the risks and potential complications of pregnancy. When pregnancy

Table 27-8. Common Maintenance Drugs for the Cardiac Patient

Drug	Dosage and Route	Therapeutic/Adverse Effects	Nursing Implications
Digoxin (cardiac glycoside)	0.5–1 mg/d PO, IM, or IV digitalizing dose; 0.125–0.5 mg/d, PO, IM, or IV maintenance dose	Increases the force of cardiac contraction and refractory period Decreases conductivity May cause headache, blurred vision, yellow vision, arrhythmias, bradycardia, nausea, vomiting, anorexia, fatigue Depletes potassium when given with thiazides Ingestion with high-fiber meals may reduce absorption No adverse effects reported on fetus	Take apical pulse for a full minute before administration. Withhold dose if pulse <60. Withhold dose and notify physician if pulse is <60/min. Monitor ECG periodically throughout therapy for arrhythmias. Withhold drug if GI disturbances are noted. Monitor laboratory findings for hypokalemia. Provide/encourage intake of foods high in potassium.
Hydrodiuril (thiazide diuretic)	50–100 mg/d PO	Promotes excretion of water, sodium, and chloride Used as an adjunct in treating edema in congestive heart failure May cause lethargy, weakness, hypotension, hyperglycemia, nausea, vomiting, anorexia, hyperuricemia, muscle cramps, photosensitivity Causes excretion of potassium, bicarbonate, and other ions	Weigh patient daily. Monitor intake and output. Observe for signs of electrolyte imbalance. Review laboratory studies of renal function and electrolytes, especially hypokalemia and hyponatremia. Provide/encourage intake of foods high in potassium. Caution patient to make position changes slowly to prevent orthostatic hypotension. Advise patient to use sunscreen and protective clothing when in the sun to prevent photosensitivity reactions.
Heparin (anticoagulant)*	10,000 U followed by 5000–10,000 U q 4–6 h IV or SC *or* 10,000–20,000 U followed by 8000–10,000 U t.i.d. IV or SC	Interferes with most aspects of clotting mechanism Prolongs clotting time but does not affect bleeding time Increases risk of hemorrhage Is highly acidic, so incompatible with most antibiotics Does not cross the placenta	Assess patient for signs of bleeding (bleeding gums, nose; unusual bruising, tarry stools, hematuria). Monitor daily coagulation studies. If SC injection, rotate injection sites. Check sites for hemorrhage and avoid massage. Type and crossmatch patient on admission.
Quinidine (antiarrhythmic)	0.2–0.3 g t.i.d. or q.i.d., PO, IM, or IV	Depresses cardiac excitability, conduction velocity, and contractability Has an anticholinergic action Effect is reduced if hypokalemia is present May cause tinnitus, headache, vertigo, blurred vision, photophobia, hypotension, nausea, diarrhea, anorexia, bitter taste No adverse effects reported on fetus	Monitor ECG periodically for arrhythmias. Monitor serum electrolytes frequently. Administer PO dose with 8 oz of water on empty stomach 1–2 h after meals.
Beta-adrenergic blockers (ie, Inderal)	Generally contraindicated during pregnancy because it may reduce uterine blood flow and cause intrauterine growth retardation, may cause premature closing of fetal ductus arteriosus; may cause bradycardia, hypotension, and hypoglycemia in the neonate.		
Calcium channel blockers (Nifedipine) See Table 27-2			
Vasodilators (hydralazine) See Table 27-5			

*Oral anticoagulants have been known to cause hemorrhage in the fetus and therefore they are contraindicated in pregnancy.

is contraindicated, the woman should be offered appropriate contraceptive counseling.

Assessing the Woman in the Prenatal Period

Ongoing assessment of the woman's cardiac status begins in the prenatal period. The nurse reviews signs and symptoms of cardiac decompensation at each prenatal visit and reports problems to the physician promptly. The nurse evaluates the woman's understanding of her disease, diet, and sodium restrictions. It is important to determine the woman's ability to comply with the medical regimen of rest and activity based on her cardiac classification and condition.

Referrals may be made to a community or home health nursing service. This allows for assessment of the home environment to determine any special circumstances that may have an impact on treatment or the woman's ability to accomplish self-care. Family members' understanding of the disease is encouraged by a supportive nurse who understands the full impact of the disease on normal family functioning.

If the woman is hospitalized for cardiac decompensation, frequent monitoring of maternal and fetal status is imperative. Assessment of vital signs and the FHR is preformed every 15 minutes or more frequently until the woman's condition is stabilized. A pulse oximeter should be applied to determine the percentage of blood oxygen saturation. If a cardiac monitor or invasive hemodynamic monitoring is implemented (ie, a Swan-Ganz catheter), nurses skilled in the use of this equipment and interpretation of data should assume responsibility for patient assessment. Intake and output are monitored, and daily weights are obtained as ordered.

Close monitoring of fluid balance is essential to prevent CHF. The nurse observes the woman for signs and symptoms of fluid volume overload and CHF including tachycardia, rising blood pressure, bounding pulses, distended neck veins, generalized edema, pulmonary rales, and dyspnea. The nurse also assesses the woman's response to drug therapy.

Assessing the Woman in the Intrapartum Period

The period during labor and birth is a critical time for potential cardiac decompensation. Intensive monitoring of maternal and fetal status is necessary. Electronic blood pressure, cardiac monitoring, pulse oximetry, and continuous EFM are indicated and permit frequent maternal and fetal assessments. Close monitoring of intake and output is essential. Assessment of physiologic responses to pain and the exertional effort of pushing during the second stage of labor must be performed.

Assessing the Woman in the Postpartum Period

The risk of cardiac decompensation remains high in the immediate postpartum period because of the dramatic fluid shifts that occur at this time. Close assessment of maternal vital signs, oxygen saturation levels, and fluid balance is essential. The woman may be transferred to a cardiac care unit that permits hemodynamic monitoring, until physiologic stability is achieved. On admission to the postpartum unit, the nurse evaluates the woman's level of fatigue and cardiac responses to the assumption of self-care, neonatal care activities, and breastfeeding.

• • Nursing Diagnosis

The following nursing diagnoses may be applicable to problems arising secondary to cardiac disease:

- Activity Intolerance related to cardiac disease
- Constipation related to bed rest
- Decreased Cardiac Output related to cardiac disease
- Altered Tissue Perfusion related to cardiac decompensation
- Fatigue related to cardiac disease
- Fluid Volume Excess related to cardiac decompensation
- Knowledge Deficit related to disease, therapy, or activity limitations
- Impaired Gas Exchange related to pulmonary edema

• • Planning and Implementation

Supporting the Woman in the Prenatal Period

During the prenatal period, nursing care is focused on patient education to recognize and prevent deterioration in the woman's condition. Essential components of the teaching plan include information about:

- The nature of the cardiac disease and its treatment
- Rest and activity
- Diet and sodium restrictions
- Avoidance of anemia
- Avoidance of infection
- Danger signs and symptoms
- Self-administration of drugs

Women should rest in the left lateral recumbent position to facilitate vascular flow. This promotes diuresis and improves uteroplacental perfusion. When sitting, the woman should elevate her feet above the level of her heart to prevent circulatory stasis in the lower extremities and dependent edema. If the woman is hospitalized for cardiac decompensation, essential aspects of nursing care include:

- Providing oxygenation
- Maintaining fluid restrictions (as ordered)
- Suggesting appropriate guidelines for rest and activity
- Providing skin care
- Promoting good nutrition
- Preventing constipation
- Administering medications and intravenous fluids
- Providing emotional support

Meticulous control of intravenous fluids is critically important to prevent fluid overload. All intravenous fluids should be administered by an infusion pump.

Expected Outcomes

- The woman verbalizes understanding of her disease and the anticipated medical management.
- The woman reports danger signs and symptoms to the nurse or physician in a timely manner.
- The woman demonstrates correct techniques required for self-administration of medications.

Preparing the Woman for Birth

The work of labor and birth and the profound fluid changes that occur in the immediate postpartum period can result in cardiac decompensation. During the intrapartum period, the nurse assumes many self-care activities for the woman in an effort to minimize the maternal cardiac workload. The nurse collaborates with the woman and her physician in planning the timing of analgesia and anesthesia and to determine if bearing down efforts will be permitted during the second stage of labor. If the woman develops an involuntary urge to push and bearing down should be avoided, the nurse will need to demonstrate techniques that may be effective to resist the pushing urge (see Chapter 21) and notifies the physician immediately. After delivery, the nurse assists the woman with breastfeeding and the gradual assumption of neonatal care activities.

Expected Outcomes

- The woman participates in planning for the actual labor.
- The woman demonstrates understanding of techniques to use so she can resist the urge to push.

Supporting the Woman in the Postpartum Period

Once physiologic stability is achieved, the nurse assists the woman to assume self-care and neonatal care activities. If cardiac disease requires the new mother to limit physical activity and increase periods of rest, the nurse assists her to plan for these requirements. The partner and other family members should be included in the discussion of how household activities will be adjusted so that the woman can follow the prescribed medical regimen.

The nurse may initiate a referral for community or home health nursing services before the woman is discharged. This is particularly important when significant cardiac disease persists in the postpartum period. Contraceptive counseling is an essential aspect of discharge teaching. Oral contraceptives and intrauterine devices are generally contraindicated when the woman has cardiac disease (see Chapter 7 for a complete discussion of family planning).

Expected Outcomes

- The woman gives birth to a viable, healthy neonate while maintaining stable cardiac function.
- The woman assumes self-care and neonatal care activities permitted by her cardiac status.

• • Evaluation

The effectiveness of nursing and medical care are determined through ongoing evaluation of the woman's condition and response to treatment. The woman should demonstrate appropriate self-monitoring and self-care activities and maintain a stable cardiac function. If complications arise during any phase of the childbearing cycle related to the woman's cardiac disease, the nurse makes appropriate changes in the plan of care. An important aspect of evaluation is to determine the woman's emotional response to her cardiac condition, medical treatment, restricted activity, and prognosis. The success of therapy will in large part depend on the woman's psychological status. Prompt alterations in the nursing care plan are essential when the woman demonstrates emotional disturbances.

Two major medical complications that represent a serious threat to maternal and fetal well-being in the perinatal period are diabetes mellitus and cardiac disease. Advances in the medical management of diabetes during pregnancy have improved outcomes for the woman and her neonate, but comprehensive nursing care is essential to achieve these positive outcomes. Likewise, in cardiac disease, skilled nursing care is required to prevent or recognize complications. Because the greatest maternal risks often occur in the immediate postpartum period, the nurse must remain vigilant for signs of cardiac decompensation after the birth of the neonate. The goal of care in medical complications is to provide a family-centered experience while monitoring and supporting maternal status throughout the childbearing cycle.

Chapter Summary

Although significant advances have been made in perinatal care during the 20th century, nurses are faced with many challenges in the provision of maternity care. Although maternal mortality and morbidity have steadily declined throughout the 20th century, the infant mortality rate has not dropped as rapidly. During the perinatal period, nurses still must deal with significant problems that threaten the well-being of the woman, fetus, and her neonate. A family-centered philosophy is used to plan and implement care when significant obstetric or medical complications arise. The primary goal is to provide humane, sensitive nursing care while maintaining maternal and fetal physiologic functioning.

Study Questions

1. *What are the primary nursing responsibilities when stabilizing the woman admitted with a diagnosis of preterm labor?*
2. *What are the major fetal and neonatal risks associated with preterm labor and tocolytic therapy?*
3. *What are the nurse's responsibilities when the woman experiences an adverse reaction to beta-sympathomimetic or magnesium sulfate tocolytic therapy?*
4. *What are the major maternal and fetal risks associ-*

ated with premature rupture of membranes?

5. *What can the nurse do to reduce the risk of infection related to PPROM?*
6. *What are the primary nursing responsibilities when the woman is hospitalized for severe PIH?*
7. *What are the primary nursing responsibilities when the nurse administers magnesium sulfate to prevent seizures?*
8. *What nursing interventions are required when an eclamptic seizure occurs.*
9. *What are the primary nursing responsibilities when the diabetic woman exhibits signs or symptoms of hypoglycemia?*
10. *What is the primary focus of nursing care in the prenatal care of the woman with diabetes?*
11. *What are the major nursing responsibilities when caring for the diabetic woman during the intrapartum period?*
12. *What are the signs and symptoms of cardiac decompensation?*

References

ACOG Committee on Obstetrics: Maternal and Fetal Medicine. (1992). *Home uterine activity monitoring*. Committee Opinion No. 115. Washington, DC: Author.

Allbert, J., Wise, C., Lou, C., et al. (1992). Subcutaneous tocolytic infusion therapy for patients at very high risk for preterm birth. *Journal of Perinatology, XII*(1), 28.

American Diabetes Association. (1987). Position statement on gestational diabetes mellitus. *American Journal of Obstetrics and Gynecology, 156*(2), 488.

Armson, A., Samuels, P., Miller, F., et al. (1992). Evaluation of maternal fluid dynamics during tocolytic therapy with ritodrine hydrochloride and magnesium sulfate. *American Journal of Obstetrics and Gynecology, 167*(3), 758.

Berkowitz, G., Roman, S., Lapinski, R., et al. (1992). Maternal characteristics, neonatal outcome, and the time of diagnosis of gestational diabetes. *American Journal of Obstetrics and Gynecology, 167*(4), 976.

Besinger, R., Niebyl, J., Keyes, W., & Johnson, T. (1991). Randomized comparative trial of indomethacin and ritodrine for the long-term treatment of preterm labor. *American Journal of Obstetrics and Gynecology, 164*(4), 981–988.

Blackburn, S., & Loper, D. (1992). *Maternal, fetal, and neonatal physiology*. Philadelphia: WB Saunders.

Cousins, L., Laxmi, B., Chez, R., et al. (1991). Screening recommendations for gestational diabetes mellitus. *American Journal of Obstetrics and Gynecology, 165*(3), 493.

Creasy, R., & Herron, M. (1981). Prevention of preterm birth. *Seminars in Perinatology, 5*, 297.

Easterling, T., & Benedetti, T. (1989). Preeclampsia: A hyperdynamic disease model. *American Journal of Obstetrics and Gynecology, 160*(6), 1447.

Eronen, M., Pesonen, E., Kurki, T., et al. (1991). The effects of indomethacin and β-sympathomimetic agents on the fetal ductus arteriosus during treatment of premature labor. *American Journal of Obstetrics and Gynecology, 164*(1), 141.

Eskenazi, B., Fenster, L., & Sidney, S. (1991). A multivariate analysis of risk factors for preeclampsia. *Journal of the American Medical Association, 266*(2), 237.

Evans, A., & Benbarka, M. (1991). Endocrine disorders. In K. Niswander & A. Evans (Eds.). *Manual of obstetrics* (4th ed., p. 133). Boston: Little, Brown.

Ferguson, J., Dyson, D., Schutz, T., & Stevenson, D. (1990). A comparison of tocolysis with nifedipine or ritodrine. *American Journal of Obstetrics and Gynecology, 163*(1), 105.

Ferris, T. (1988). Toxemia and hypertension. In G. Burrow & T. Ferris (Eds.). *Medical complications during pregnancy* (3rd ed., p. 1). Philadelphia: WB Saunders.

Fletcher, S., Fyfe, D., Case, C., et al. (1991). Myocardial necrosis in a newborn after long-term maternal subcutaneous terbutaline infusion for suppression of preterm labor. *American Journal of Obstetrics and Gynecology, 165*(5), 1401.

Girz, B., Divon, M., & Merkatz, I. (1992). Sudden fetal death in women with well-controlled intensively monitored gestational diabetes. *Journal of Perinatology, XII*(3), 229.

Graf, R., & Perez-Woods, R. (1992). Trends in preterm labor. *Journal of Perinatology, XII*(1), 51.

Grimes, D., & Schulz, K. (1992). Randomized controlled trial of home uterine activity monitoring in pregnancies at increased risk of preterm labor. Part II. *Obstetrics and Gynecology, 79*(1), 137–142.

Grimes, D., Schulz, K., Hadi, H., & Albazzaz, S. (1989). Cardiac isoenzymes and electrocardiographic changes during ritodrine tocolysis. *American Journal of Obstetrics and Gynecology, 161*(2), 318.

Hankins, G., Hammond, T., & Yeomans, E. (1991). Amniotic cavity accumulation of magnesium with prolonged magnesium sulfate tocolysis. *Journal of Reproductive Medicine, 36*(6), 446.

Harvey, M. (1992). Diabetic ketoacidosis during pregnancy. *Journal of Perinatal and Neonatal Nursing, 6*(1), 1.

Hill, W., Fleming, A., Martin, R., et al. (1990). Home uterine activity monitoring is associated with a reduction in preterm birth. *Obstetrics and Gynecology, 76*(1-Suppl), 13S.

Holcomb, W., Shackelford, G., & Petrie, R. (1991). Magnesium tocolysis and neonatal bone abnormalities: A controlled study. *Obstetrics and Gynecology, 78*(4), 611.

Hollingsworth, D., & Moore, T. (1989). Diabetes and pregnancy. In R. Creasy & R. Resnik (Eds.). *Maternal-fetal medicine* (2nd ed.). Philadelphia: WB Saunders.

Howard, E. (1992). Gestational diabetes mellitus screening tests: A review of current recommendations. *Journal of Perinatal and Neonatal Nursing, 6*(1), 37.

Johnson, J., Egerman, R. & Moorhead, J. (1990). Cases with ruptured membranes that "reseal." *American Journal of Obstetrics and Gynecology, 163*(3), 1024.

Johnston, M., Ramos, L., Vaughn, A., Todd, M., & Benrubi, G. (1990). Antibiotic therapy in preterm premature rupture of membranes: A randomized, prospective, double-blind trial. *American Journal of Obstetrics and Gynecology, 163*(2), 743.

Imanaka, M., Ogita, S., & Sugawa, T. (1989). Saline solution amnioinfusion for oligohydramnios after premature rupture of membranes. *American Journal of Obstetrics and Gynecology, 161*(1), 102.

Khong, T., Sawyer, I., & Heryet, A. (1992). An immunohistologic study of endothelialization of uteroplacental vessels in human pregnancy. *American Journal of Obstetrics and Gynecology, 167*, 751.

Kulb, N. (1990a). Preterm labor. In K. Buckley & N. Kulb (Eds.). *High risk maternity nursing manual* (p. 311). Baltimore: Williams & Wilkins.

Kulb N. (1990b). Cardiac disorders. In K. Buckley & N. Kulb (Eds.). *High risk maternity nursing manual* (p. 89). Baltimore: Williams & Wilkins.

Lewis, D., Major, C., Towers, C., Asrat, T., Harding, J., & Garite, T. (1992). Effects of digital vaginal examinations on latency period in preterm premature rupture of membranes. *Obstetrics and Gynecology, 80*(4), 630–634.

Lucas, M., Leveno, K., & Williams, L. (1989). Early pregnancy glycosylated hemoglobin, severity of diabetes, and fetal malformations. *American Journal of Obstetrics and Gynecology, 161*(2), 426.

Lynam, L., & Miller, M. (1992). Mothers' and nurses' perceptions of the needs of women experiencing preterm labor. *Journal of Obstetric, Gynecologic, and Neonatal Nursing, 21*(2), 126.

Major, C., & Kitzmiller, J. (1990). Perinatal survival with expectant management of midtrimester rupture of membranes. *American Journal of Obstetrics and Gynecology, 163*(3), 838.

Maloni, J., & Kasper, C. (1991). Physical and psychosocial effects of antepartum hospital bedrest. *Image, 23*(3), 187.

Martin, J., Files, J., Blake, P., et al. (1992). Plasma exchange for preeclampsia. *American Journal of Obstetrics and Gynecology, 162*(1), 126.

McGregor, J., French, J., & Seo, K. (1991). Antimicrobial therapy in preterm premature rupture of membranes: Results of a prospective, double-blind, placebo-controlled trial of erythromycin. *American Journal of Obstetrics and Gynecology, 165*(2), 632.

Merkatz, R., & Merkatz, I. (1991). The contributions of the nurse and the machine in home uterine activity monitoring systems. *American Journal of Obstetrics and Gynecology, 164*(5), 1159.

Monahan, P., & DeJoseph, J. (1991). The woman with preterm labor at home. *Journal of Perinatal and Neonatal Nursing, 4*(4), 12.

Mou, S., Sunderji, S., Gall, S., et al. (1991). Multicenter randomized clinical trial of home uterine activity monitoring for detection of preterm labor. *American Journal of Obstetrics and Gynecology,* 165(3), 858–866.

National Commission to Prevent Infant Mortality. (1988). *Infant mortality.* Washington, DC: National Academy Press.

Neal, D., & Bockman, V. (1992). Preterm labor and preterm premature rupture of membranes. In L. Mandeville & N. Troiano (Eds.). *High-risk intrapartum nursing* (p. 57). Philadelphia: JB Lippincott.

Palmer, D., & Inturrisi, M. (1992). Insulin infusion therapy in the intrapartum period. *Journal of Perinatal and Neonatal Nursing, 6*(1), 25.

Plovie, V. (1991). *Diabetes in pregnancy.* Series 2, Prenatal Care, Module 10. White Plains, NY: March of Dimes.

Repke, J. (1991). Prevention of preeclampsia. *Clinics in Perinatology, 18*(4), 779.

Repke, J., & Villar, J. (1989). The role of dietary calcium in pregnancy induced hypertension. *Clinics in Nutrition, 8*, 169.

Repke, J., Villar, J., Anderson, C., et al. (1989). Biochemical changes associated with blood pressure reduction induced by calcium supplementation during pregnancy. *American Journal of Obstetrics and Gynecology, 160*, 684.

Ricci, J., Hariharan, S., Helfgott, A., et al. (1991). Oral tocolysis with magnesium chloride. *American Journal of Obstetrics and Gynecology, 165*(3), 603.

Ridgway, L., Muise, K., Wright, J., et al. (1990). A prospective randomized comparison of oral terbutaline and magnesium oxide for the maintenance of tocolysis. *American Journal of Obstetrics and Gynecology, 163*(3), 879.

Rosenn, B., Miodovnik, M., Kranias, G., et al. (1992). Progression of diabetic retinopathy in pregnancy. *American Journal of Obstetrics and Gynecology, 166*(4), 1214.

Samson, L. (1992). Infants of diabetic mothers. Current perspectives. *Journal of Perinatal and Neonatal Nursing, 6*(1), 61.

Schiff, E., Peleg, E., Goldenerg, M., et al. (1989). The use of aspirin to prevent pregnancy-induced hypertension and lower the ratio of thromboxane A2 to prostacyclin in relatively high risk pregnancies. *New England Journal of Medicine, 321*, 351.

Sibai, B. (1991). Management of preeclampsia. *Clinics in Perinatology, 18*(4), 793.

Sibai, B., Mercer, B., & Sarinoglu, C. (1991). Severe preeclampsia in the second trimester: Recurrence risk and long-term prognosis. *American Journal of Obstetrics and Gynecology, 165*(5), 1408.

Silver, H. (1991). Hypertensive disorders. In K. Niswander & A. Evans (Eds.). *Manual of obstetrics* (4th ed., p. 295). Boston: Little, Brown.

Taylor, R., Casal, D., Jones, L., et al. (1991). Selective effects of preeclamptic sera on human endothelial cell procoagulant protein expression. *American Journal of Obstetrics and Gynecology, 165*(6), 705.

Thorkelsson, T., & Loughead, J. (1991). Long-term subcutaneous terbutaline tocolysis: Report of possible neonatal toxicity. *Journal of Perinatology, XI*(3), 235–238.

Troiano, N. (1992). Cardiac diseases in pregnancy. In L. Mandeville & N. Troiano (Eds.). *High-risk intrapartum nursing.* Philadelphia: JB Lippincott.

Wallenburg, H., Dekker, G., Makovitz, J., et al. (1991). Effect of low-dose aspirin on vascular refractoriness in angiotensin-sensitive primigravid women. *American Journal of Obstetrics and Gynecology, 164*(5), 1169.

White, P. (1978). Classification of overt diabetes. *American Journal of Obstetrics and Gynecology, 130*, 227.

Williams, M. (1991a). Premature rupture of membranes. In K. Niswander & A. Evans. (Eds.). *Manual of obstetrics* (4th ed., p. 430). Boston: Little, Brown.

Williams, M. (1991b). Preterm labor. Premature rupture of membranes. In K. Niswander & A. Evans (Eds.). *Manual of obstetrics* (4th ed., p. 418). Boston: Little, Brown.

Suggested Readings

Austin, D., & Davis, P. Valvular disease in pregnancy. *Journal of Perinatal and Neonatal Nursing, 5*(2), 13.

Eganhouse, D., & Burnside, S. (1992). Nursing and responsibilities in monitoring the preterm pregnancy. *Journal of Obstetric, Gynecologic, and Neonatal Nursing, 21*(5), 355.

Freda, M., Anderson, H., Damus, K., et al. (1990). Lifestyle modification as an intervention for inner city women at high risk for preterm birth. *Journal of Advanced Nursing, 15*, 364.

Friedman, S., Taylor, R., & Roberts J. (1991). Pathophysiology of preeclampsia. *Clinics in Perinatology, 18*(4), 661.

Martin, J., Blake, P., Perry, K., et al. (1991). The natural history of HELLP syndrome: Patterns of disease progression and regression. *American Journal of Obstetrics and Gynecology, 164*(6), 1500.

Mueller-Heubach, E., Reddick, D., Barnett, B., et al. (1989). Preterm birth prevention. *American Journal of Obstetrics and Gynecology, 160*(5), 1172.

Rosas, T., & Constantino, N. (1992). Exercise as a treatment modality to maintain normoglycemia in gestational diabetes. *Journal of Perinatal and Neonatal Nursing, 6*(1), 14.

Rotschild, A., Ling, E., Puterman, M., et al. (1990). Neonatal outcome after prolonged preterm rupture of the membranes. *American Journal of Obstetrics and Gynecology, 162*(1), 46.

Sala, D., & Moise, K. (1990). The treatment of preterm labor using a portable subcutaneous terbutaline pump. *Journal of Obstetric, Gynecologic, and Neonatal Nursing, 19*(2), 108.

Shannon, D. M. (1987). HELLP syndrome: A severe consequence of pregnancy-induced hypertension. *Journal of Obstetric, Gynecologic, and Neonatal Nursing, 16*, 395–402.

Sibai, B. (1990). The HELLP syndrome (hemolysis, elevated liver enzymes, and low platelets): Much ado about nothing? *American Journal of Obstetrics and Gynecology, 162*(2), 311.

Thehaar, M., & Schakenbach, L. (1991). Care of the pregnant patient with a pacemaker. *Journal of Perinatal and Neonatal Nursing, 5*(2), 1.

UNIT V

Adaptation in the Postpartum Period

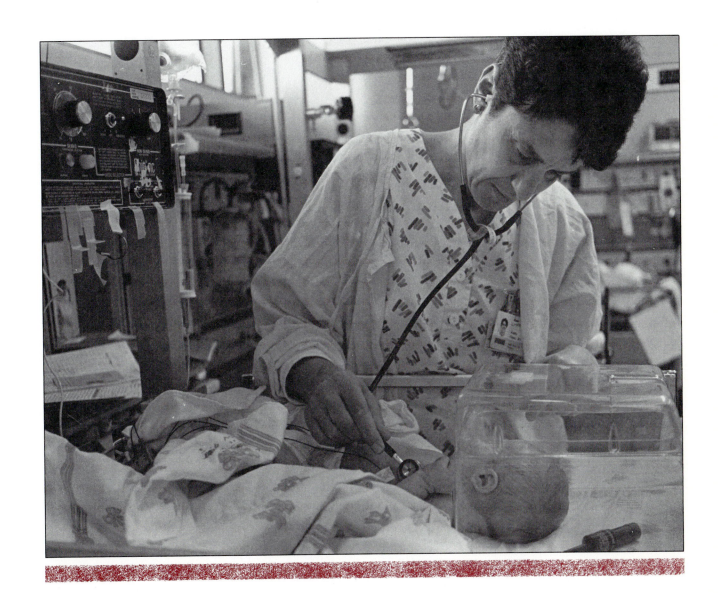

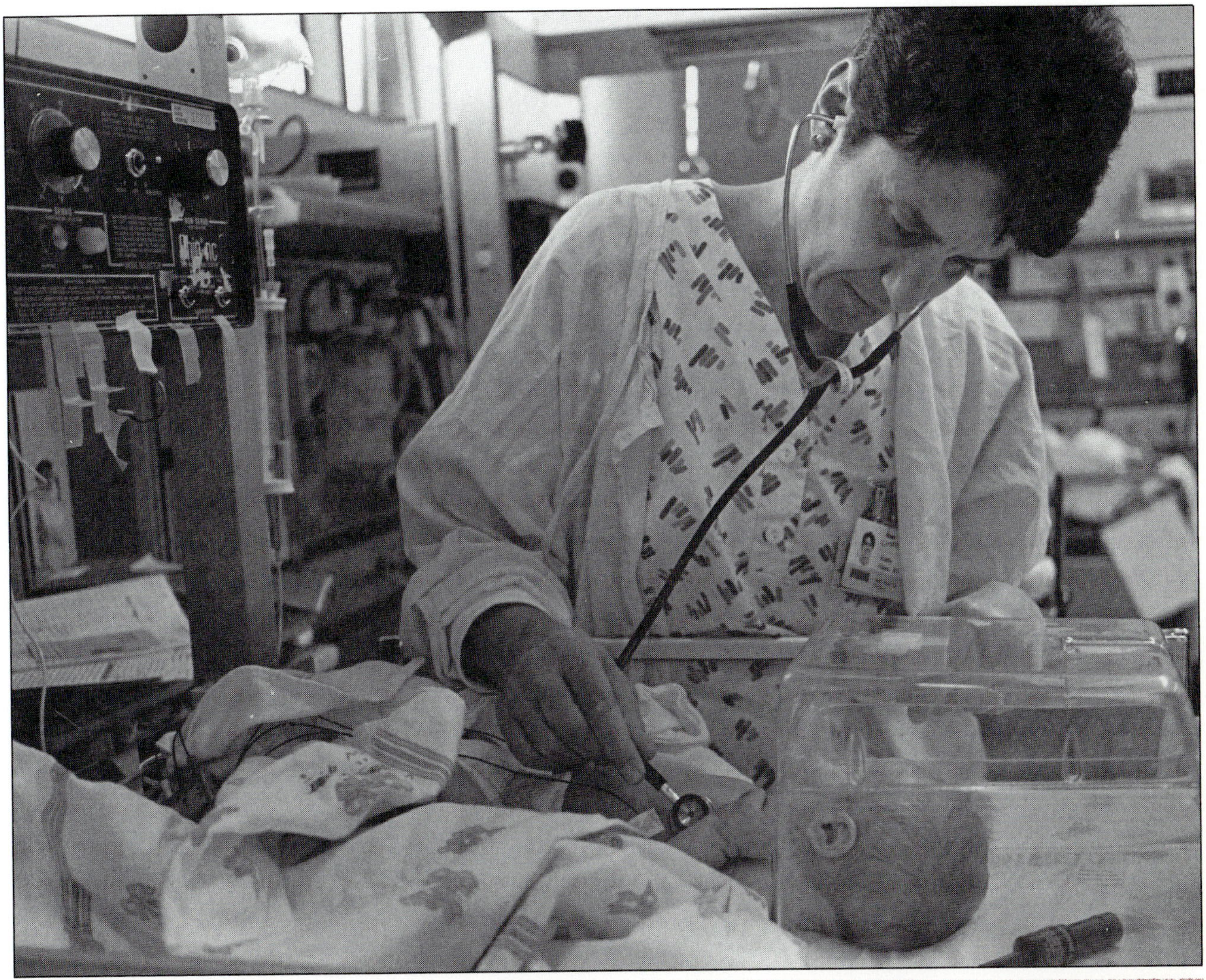

CHAPTER 28

Nursing Care of the Family in the Postpartum Period

Learning Objectives

After studying the material in this chapter, the student will be able to:

- Describe the normal physiologic adaptations occurring in the postpartum period.
- Describe typical psychological adaptations occurring in the parents and family of a newborn.
- Discuss important aspects of the postpartum nursing assessment.
- Identify common nursing diagnoses presented during the postpartum period.
- Describe critical aspects of nursing care for the postpartum woman after vaginal birth and for the postpartum woman after cesarean delivery.
- Develop a nursing care plan for the postpartum woman after vaginal birth.
- Identify common paternal or partner adaptations in the postpartum period.
- Develop a nursing care plan for the postpartum woman after cesarean delivery.
- Discuss important areas of teaching to promote effective self-care and care of the infant.

Key Terms

afterpains
boggy uterus
diastasis recti abdominis
engorgement
fundus
involution
let-down relfex
lochia
micturation
postpartum hemorrhage
thrombosis
uterine atony

Mother–baby care, also known as *couplet* or *dyad care*, is the current trend in nursing care of the postpartum family. It focuses on one nurse caring for the physiologic needs of both mother and neonate, and providing emotional support and education of the new family. Mother–baby care is based on the concept of family-centered maternity nursing illustrated in Figure 28-1. It is based on the acknowledgment that maternal-child health is based not only on physical dimensions, but on psychological, social, and economic dimensions as well (NAACOG, 1989).

Multiple benefits are appreciated for both nursing staff and families when dyad care is implemented. Nursing care is less fragmented, and one nurse is able to assess individual as well as family functioning. Communication between health professionals and parents is better integrated, reducing the potential for confusion and errors. Teaching efforts are also better coordinated because one nurse covers content on both mother and neonate.

The Beginning of a New Family

The postpartum period may seem anticlimactic in comparison with the 9 months of anticipation that accompany pregnancy and the intensity and wonder of the labor and birth experience. In reality, however, the postpartum period is comprised of an amazing variety of complex physiologic and psychological adaptations. The nurse's role is important in assisting new parents through postpartum adjustments and supporting them as they make a fresh start as a new family.

The nursing process is the framework for comprehensive postpartum care. Although most families deliver healthy neonates and progress through the postpartum period without significant difficulty, thorough and accurate assessments will give the nurse the information necessary to provide complete and appropriate care. Systematic assessments will also enable the nurse to identify potential or

May: MATERNAL AND NEONATAL NURSING, 3rd. ed. © 1994 J.B. Lippincott Company.

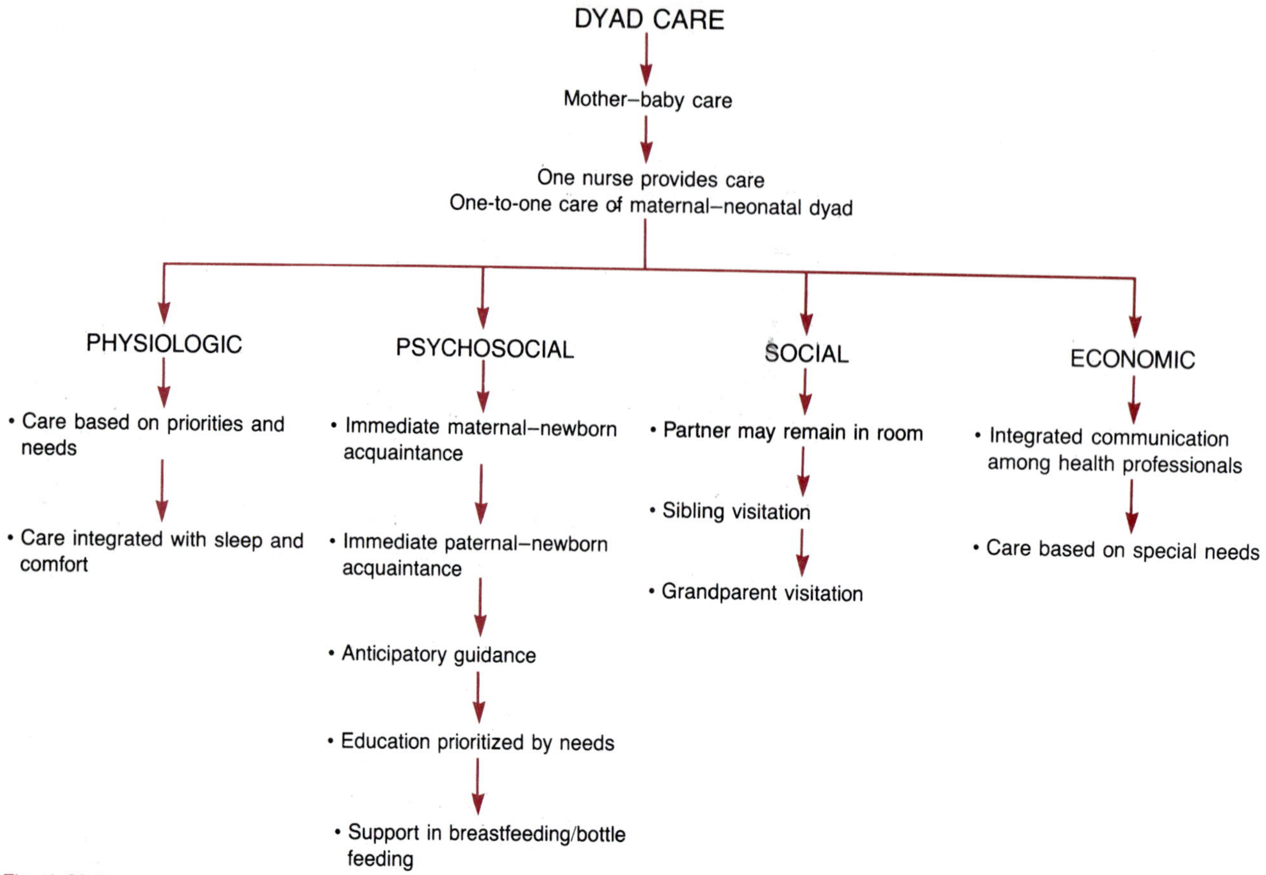

Figure 28-1.
Mother–baby care is based on family-centered maternity nursing.

actual problems early, allowing prompt intervention should it become necessary.

The relatively short postpartum hospitalization of 1 to 3 days requires the nurse to plan effectively for necessary nursing interventions. Interventions include provision of physical care to the woman, emotional support to the new parents, and teaching for effective self-care and neonatal care. Teaching is especially important in the postpartum setting. The postpartum nurse is often the last health professional with whom the woman has personal contact until her visit with the midwife, nurse practitioner, or physician 2 to 6 weeks after the birth. The nurse must identify major teaching needs and provide the information required for successful postpartum adaptations during the first weeks after childbirth.

Maternal Physiologic Adaptations

The postpartum period is usually divided into three phases. The *immediate* postpartum period is comprised of the first 24 hours after birth; the *early* postpartum period, the first week; and the *late* postpartum period the second through sixth weeks. This division reflects the varying character of physiologic changes that occur during this time. The most dramatic and potentially hazardous changes occur in the immediate and early postpartum periods. The rate of change is much more gradual in the late postpartum period.

In the first hours and days after childbirth, the woman undergoes dramatic physiologic adaptations involving nearly every system of the body. Were changes of this magnitude to occur in a person other than a postpartum woman, they would be cause for grave concern. For instance, the postpartum woman typically experiences a weight loss of 6.8 to 7.7 kg (15 to 17 lb) after the infant's birth. Most of this loss 4.5 to 5.4 kg (10 to 12 lb) is the result of the delivery of the neonate, placenta, and amniotic fluid. In addition, 2.2 kg (5 lb) of excess fluid is lost through diuresis, and a blood loss of 500 mL or more may occur. Fluid losses of this degree through diuresis or other mechanisms would probably pose a significant risk of hypovolemic shock to a nonmaternity patient.

Most postpartum women experience relatively little discomfort related to these physical changes and tend to be more concerned about rest, relieving perineal discomfort, and learning about the newborn. Nevertheless, these physiologic changes are significant and must be monitored by the postpartum nurse. Deviations from the normal physiologic changes expected to occur may signal postpartum complications, such as hemorrhage or infection.

Changes in Vital Signs

The woman's oral temperature may range between 36.2°C (98°F) and 38°C (100.4°F). Temporary elevation in the first 24 hours after birth is a result of muscular exertion, dehydration, and hormonal changes. However, the woman should be afebrile after the first 24 hours. After the first 24 hours after birth, elevations over 38°C (100.4°F) on any 2 of the first 10 postpartum days may suggest postpartum sepsis, urinary tract infection (UTI), endometritis, mastitis, or other infections. Breast engorgement on the second or third day was once thought to cause temperature elevations ("milk fever"). This is not a common cause of temperature elevations in newly delivered women. If it does occur, it should not persist more than 24 hours.

It is estimated that approximately 23% of women may experience a shaking chill during or immediately after delivery (Harper, Quintin, Freynin, 1991). This pronounced shivering or shaking chill has been attributed to vasomotor instability and is not thought to be clinically significant when unaccompanied by fever. In a recent study by Harper and associates (1991), over 40% of subjects experienced postpartum shivering, and these shaking chills were associated with lower environmental temperatures. Other researchers suggest that the rapid infusion of cold intravenous (IV) fluids, for instance during epidural anesthesia, may contribute to this phenomenon. Further study is required to determine the causes and significance of postpartum shivering.

Maternal pulse may range from 50 to 90 bpm and respirations from 16 to 24 breaths/min. Blood pressure should be consistent with baseline rates during normal pregnancy. Orthostatic hypotension may occur in the first 24 hours secondary to analgesia, anesthesia, or decreased pelvic vascular resistance.

Neurologic System and Sensory-Motor Adaptations

Many changes in central nervous system (CNS) function are related to the administration of analgesics and anesthesia during childbirth and the immediate postpartum period. Alterations in mentation and sensory-motor function are transient and disappear as the agents used to alleviate pain are metabolized and excreted. Sedation is the most common side-effect of analgesia. Decreased sensory and motor function is common when regional anesthetics such as epidurals or spinals have been administered. Deep tendon reflexes, a sign of CNS integrity, should be normal (1+ to 2+ range). Mild headaches, generally frontal and bilateral, are common in the first postpartum week and may be associated with the dramatic fluid shifts that occur during this period (Blackburn & Loper, 1992). When these headaches are not associated with other signs of pregnancy-induced hypertension (PIH, preeclampsia) and resolve within a week, they are benign. More severe, persistent headaches are sometimes seen after spinal anesthesia and may require special treatment (see Chapter 24).

Sensations of Pain and Discomfort

The level of discomfort or pain that most women have after uncomplicated labor and birth is usually mild. The presence of an episiotomy or perineal lacerations may increase the discomfort. Some women report that the pain associated with severe hemorrhoids is often more intense and unremitting than episiotomy pain and is accompanied by unpleasant sensations of pressure. An additional source of discomfort is nipple soreness related to breastfeeding. It has been described as acutely painful at times, especially when the infant has a strong grasp and suck reflex. If breast engorgement occurs, women may complain of heat, pain, and pressure in the breasts and a temporary, generalized achiness and malaise. Tribotti and associates (1988) found that the most frequently identified nursing diagnosis by women in the early postpartum period was altered comfort. Primigravidas were more likely to report greater levels of discomfort and pain and focus more on unpleasant physical sensations than multiparas.

Alterations in Sleep

Sleep patterns are also altered in the immediate postpartum period. Stage I non-rapid eye movement (non-REM) sleep is longer immediately after birth, with a gradual increase over the next 2 weeks after birth. REM sleep is decreased, and awake time increases. These changes are attributed to the initial excitement and discomforts after delivery. In general, postpartum women have less sleep and are more likely to experience interrupted sleep due to night feedings (Blackburn & Loper, 1992). Lack of sleep remains a major area of concern for women for the first 8 to 12 months postpartum.

Cardiovascular System Adaptations

Perhaps the most dramatic maternal changes in the postpartum period involve the cardiovascular system. Pregnancy-induced hypervolemia, which produces a 50% increase in circulating blood volume at term, allows the woman to tolerate a substantial blood loss at delivery without ill effect. Blood losses of 400 to 500 mL in a vaginal birth and 700 to 1000 mL in a cesarean birth are not uncommon.

Cardiac Output

Immediately after birth, cardiac output is 60% to 80% higher than prelabor levels (Blackburn & Loper, 1992). Several factors may contribute to this rise in cardiac output, including:

- Increased blood return to the vena cava with elimination of the pressure of the gravid uterus on the vena cava and abdominal vessels
- Return of blood from the uteroplacental vascular bed back into the systemic circulation
- Decreased systemic vascular resistance due to contraction and rapid reduction in size of the uterus

- Mobilization of interstitial fluids back into the vascular compartment
- Increase in cardiac stroke volume

This increase in cardiac output persists for at least 48 hours postpartum and then begins to decline gradually over time. By 2 weeks postpartum, cardiac output has decreased by almost 30% from the early postpartum period and has returned to prepregnancy levels by approximately 4 weeks postpartum (Creasy & Resnik, 1989).

Pulse

A heart rate of 50 to 70 bpm is considered normal during the early postpartum period. Bradycardia is a compensatory mechanism for the increased cardiac output and resolves as the cardiovascular system returns to the prepregnant state. Tachycardia is less common and may reflect a greater than normal blood loss, significant postpartum hemorrhage, or infection.

Blood Pressure

Maternal blood pressure should remain stable after delivery. A decrease of 15 to 20 mm Hg or more systolic pressure when the woman moves from a supine to a sitting position probably reflects *orthostatic hypotension*. This condition is caused by a temporary lag in cardiovascular compensation for the decreased vascular resistance in the pelvis. However, any decrease unassociated with position change may reflect continuing blood loss from hemorrhage and requires further assessment at once. An increase of 30 mm Hg systolic or 15 mm Hg diastolic pressure, especially when accompanied by headache or visual changes, may suggest PIH (preeclampsia; see Chapter 27 for a discussion of postpartum PIH.)

Hematologic Adaptations

The postpartum woman's hemoglobin, hematocrit, and plasma volume should remain near prelabor levels. A drop of 1 g in hemoglobin or 4 points in the hematocrit may reflect as much as 500 mL of blood loss during the intrapartum period. During the first 2 to 3 days postpartum, plasma volume decreases further due to the normal diuresis that occurs at this time. If significant edema has developed during pregnancy, hemodilution will occur in the first pospartum week with mobilization of interstitial fluid back to the vascular compartment. A concommitant dilutional drop in hemoglobin, hematocrit, and plasma proteins is observed (Blackburn & Loper, 1992).

The increased red blood cell production that occurs in pregnancy ceases after delivery. Hemoglobin and hematocrit levels should stabilize in the first week after diuresis and mobilization of interstitial fluid. A gradual return to prepregnancy levels occurs by 6 weeks postpartum. Leukocytosis, with an increase in white blood cells of 15,000 to $30{,}000/mm^3$, is common in the immediate postpartum period. Values return to normal within the first week after birth.

The body's blood clotting mechanisms are activated in the immediate postpartum period and may persist for some time after delivery. Significant increases in platelet factor, fibrinogen, and factor V and VIII complex occur. This increase places the woman at higher risk for thromboembolic disorders (Gerbasi, Bottoms, Farag, & Mammen, 1990). A concommitant increase in fibrinolytic activity occurs, peaks at 3 days postpartum, and is reflected in a rise in D-dimer, fibrin–fibrinogen degradation products, and fibrinopeptide. The hemostatic system returns to its prepregnant state by 3 to 4 weeks postpartum.

Respiratory System Adaptations

Rapid changes in respiratory function occur in the immediate postpartum period. A 25% increase in chest wall compliance occurs with relief of pressure on the diaphragm (Blackburn & Loper, 1992). Tidal volume, the amount of air exchanged in a normal breath, returns to normal shortly after birth. A decrease in circulating progesterone levels results in the return of minute volume, the amount of air exhchanged in 1 minute, to normal. Sensations of dyspnea, common in late pregnancy, resolve.

Reproductive System Adaptations

The involution of the uterus begins soon after delivery and proceeds rapidly. After the placenta is expelled, the fundus of the uterus can be palpated midway between the symphysis and the umbilicus in the midline or slightly higher. The contracted uterus in the immediate postpartum period is about the size of a large grapefruit. The uterine walls are closely approximated. The cervix is bruised, soft, and distensible in the first few hours; by 10 to 12 hours after delivery, the cervix has shortened and becomes firmer. Stages in uterine involution are summarized in Table 28-1 and Figure 28-2.

Table 28-1. Stages in Uterine Involution

Time Since Delivery	Position of Fundus	Uterine Weight	Lochia
1–2 h	Midway between umbilicus and symphysis, on midline	1000 g	Rubra
12 h	1 cm above or at umbilicus		Rubra
3 d	3 cm below umbilicus (continues descent at 1 cm/day)		Serosa
9 d	Not palpable above symphysis	500 g	Alba
5–6 wk	Not palpable above symphysis; slightly larger than in nullipara		Not present

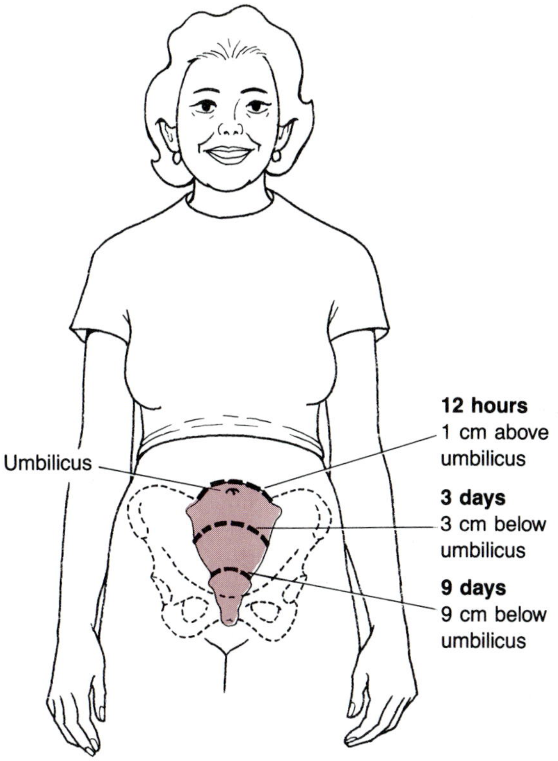

Figure 28-2.
The uterus involutes rapidly after delivery; examples are illustrated here. By 2 weeks, the uterus is once again a pelvic organ and by 6 weeks, it is only slightly larger than its nulliparous size.

Uterine Involution

By 12 hours after delivery, the fundus can be palpated at 1 cm (one finger breadth) above the umbilicus. Uterine contractions continue after delivery of the placenta. In primiparas, uterine tone is usually high, and the uterus remains firm. In multiparas, periodic uterine contraction and relaxation is more common, causing "afterpains" that may be uncomfortable for 2 to 3 days and are likely to be intensified by breastfeeding.

Two days after delivery, the uterus begins to descend and shrink gradually. By the second or third day, the spongy layer of the decidua is sloughed off in the lochia. The outermost layer then becomes necrotic and also sloughs off. The innermost layer remains as the foundation for the new endometrium. By 2 weeks after delivery, the uterus has descended into the true pelvis and is not palpable above the symphysis. Superficial lacerations of the cervix are completely healed, and the external os has regained prepregnant tone. However, the shape of the os itself, now a lateral slit rather than a circular opening, is permanently changed. By 2 to 3 weeks, endometrial glands and stroma from interglandular connective tissue have proliferated, and the entire endometrium is restored, except for the placental site.

By 5 to 6 weeks the uterus has almost returned to its nonpregnant size. This change is due to a decrease in the size of individual cells, not to a reduction in the number of cells.

Lochia

The uterus cleanses itself of debris after childbirth by a vaginal discharge called *lochia* (Table 28-2). *Lochia rubra*, the vaginal discharge of the first 3 days after delivery, is bloody and contains small clots. The presence of numerous large clots suggests unusual bleeding, and the woman should be further evaluated. Contraction of the uterus limits the amount of immediate postpartum bleeding because of compression of blood vessels by muscle fibers. Saturation of one perineal pad in 15 minutes or two in 30 minutes indicates excessive bleeding.

Lochia may appear to be heavier when the woman first stands up because the lochia pools in the vagina while she is recumbent. Once the pooled blood is discharged, lochial flow should return to normal. Flow may also be temporarily increased with the initiation of breastfeeding because oxytocin is released from the posterior pituitary gland, causing

Table 28-2. Characteristics of Lochia

Name	Approximate time Since Delivery	Normal Discharge	Abnormal Discharge
Lochia rubra	Days 1–3	Bloody with clots Fleshy odor Increase in flow on standing up, breastfeeding, or increased physical activity	Numerous large clots Foul smell Saturated perineal pad
Lochia serosa	Days 4–9	Pink or brown with a serosanguineous consistency Fleshy odor	Foul smell Saturated perineal pad
Lochia alba	Day 10	Yellow to white Fleshy odor	Foul smell Saturated perineal pad Persistent lochia serosa Return to pink or red discharge Persistent discharge over 2–3 wk

the uterus to contract. Continuous seepage of bright red blood from the vagina when the fundus is firm suggests bleeding from a cervical or vaginal laceration and requires further evaluation. For a complete discussion of postpartum bleeding, see Chapter 29.

After several days, the blood cell component of the lochia decreases, and the proportion of serous exudate increases. The flow becomes more pink or brown in color and has a serosanguineous consistency. This discharge is called *lochia serosa*. By the tenth day, the lochia (*lochia alba*) has become yellow to white and contains numerous leukocytes and cellular debris.

This progression of the discharge from bloody to pink to white or clear reflects the reestablishment of the uterine lining and the healing of the placental site. Persistent lochia serosa after 2 weeks, or a return to pink or red discharge after it has cleared, indicates subinvolution of the placental site (see the discussion in the following section) or late postpartum hemorrhage. Persistent discharge after 2 to 3 weeks may suggest endometritis, particularly when accompanied by pelvic tenderness or pain and fever. (These complications are dealt with in more detail in Chapter 29.)

Lochia has a fleshy odor similar to that of menstrual flow. A foul smell from the flow or from a used perineal pad suggests infection and the need for further assessment. Vaginal organisms are always present and can be found in the uterus as early as 2 days after delivery. In most cases, however, infection does not occur, perhaps because the organisms are not particularly virulent or because the uterine lining is already protected by a thin layer of granulating tissue.

Involution of the Placental Site

The placental site heals by a different mechanism from the rest of the endometrium. The placental site is an area approximately 8 to 9 cm in diameter. Bleeding from this site is controlled by compression of vessels by the contracted uterine muscle fibers. The site contains thrombosed vessels, some of which will be replaced by new, smaller vessels. The site heals by exfoliation. This process involves the undermining of the site by the growth of endometrial tissue from the margins and the proliferation of endometrial glands in the basal layer of the site. The undermined tissue becomes necrotic and sloughs off, usually around 6 weeks after delivery.

This process results in no fibrous scarring of the endometrium, which would limit the surface available for future implantation. Delay in healing or failure of the placental site to heal completely, called *subinvolution of the placental site*, may result in persistent lochia and episodes of brisk, painless vaginal bleeding.

Vaginal Changes

Immediately after delivery, the walls of the vagina appear edematous and bruised, and small surface lacerations may be present. Vaginal rugae are absent. The hymen may have been torn in several places; the torn edges do not approximate. Small tags called *carunculae myrtiformes* will form along the torn edges. Congestion of the vaginal walls resolves within several days. Vaginal rugae begin to return by 3 weeks. The dimensions of the distended vagina gradually decrease; however, the vagina usually does not return to its previous nulliparous size. The vaginal mucosa remains atrophic until the hormonal cycle regulating menstruation is reestablished. The labia minora and labia majora appear slightly stretched and are less firm after the first vaginal birth.

Perineal Changes

The pressure of the descending fetal head stretches and thins the muscles of the pelvic floor. Common obstetric practice in the United States includes an incision in the perineum called an *episiotomy*. The rationale for this procedure is to prevent overstretching and weakening of the perineal muscles, which predisposes the woman to cystocele and rectocele, to prevent laceration of the perineum, and to expedite the delivery of the fetal head. Recent research indicates that routine episiotomy may not provide these anticipated benefits. Furthermore, women with episiotomies have an increased risk of third and fourth degree lacerations and infection and experience more pain in the postpartum period. See Chapter 21 for a complete discussion of episiotomy.

If an episiotomy has been performed, the edges of the incision should remain approximated. Slight edema or ecchymosis around the incision site is common in the first several days after delivery. Severe edema, erythema, or purulent discharge indicates infection. The discomfort resulting from episiotomy varies according to the type of incision and repair, the length of second stage of labor, and the degree of perineal pressure experienced. Incisional discomfort or pain may persist as long as 5 to 6 weeks in some cases. Regardless of whether an episiotomy was performed, the perineum may become edematous and show some bruising in the early postpartum period. Muscle tone in the perineum will likely be reduced for several weeks and may be improved with specific exercises once the soft tissue has healed.

Adaptations in Breast Tissue

Throughout pregnancy, the breasts are being prepared for lactation under the influence of estrogen and progesterone. Colostrum, a breast fluid that precedes milk production, may appear in the third trimester of pregnancy and continues into the first postpartum week. Breast milk production begins around the third postpartum day. Initial breast engorgement occurs with an increase in the vascular and lymphatic systems surrounding the breast. The breasts become larger, firmer, and tender or painful to touch. These changes will be experienced by most women, unless lactation-suppressant medication has been administered in the immediate postpartum period. If breastfeeding is initiated and occurs frequently (every 2 to 3 hours), the woman will experience milder episodes of engorgement until lactation is well established.

Adaptations of the Urinary Tract and Renal System

Renal plasma flow, glomerular filtration, and plasma creatinine and blood urea nitrogen levels return to normal by 6 weeks postpartum. Urinary excretion of calcium, phosphate, vitamins, and other solutes returns to normal by the end of the first week (Blackburn & Loper, 1992). Return of smooth muscle tone in the ureters may take longer. Dilation of the bladder, ureters, and renal pelvis may persist for several months.

During the birth process, the bladder is subjected to trauma that can result in edema and a diminished sensitivity to fluid pressures. These changes combined with edema of the urethra, meatus, and vulva can lead to incomplete emptying and overdistention of the bladder. The woman may also experience urinary retention during the immediate postbirth period. The risk of bladder distention is exacerbated by the spontaneous diuresis that occurs. The woman may also complain of having to urinate frequently because of increased urine production. The nurse must differentiate urinary frequency caused by diuresis, retention overflow, or infection:

- Frequent voiding due to diuresis is characterized by complete bladder emptying and elimination of 250 to 350 mL or more of urine. The woman feels relieved after voiding.
- Frequent voiding due to retention overflow is distinguished by incomplete bladder emptying (palpable bladder after voiding) and elimination of only 50 to 75 mL urine. The woman feels unrelieved after voiding.
- Frequent voiding due to infection is associated with burning, pain, and possible hematuria. Small amounts of urine (50 to 75 mL) are eliminated. The woman feels unrelieved and may complain of continued bladder pain or spasms.

Hematuria (blood in the urine) in the immediate postpartum period may reflect bladder trauma from delivery. Hematuria after the first 24 hours is most commmonly associated with UTI. A history of bacteriuria in pregnancy, an operative delivery, epidural anesthesia or cesarean delivery requiring placement of a Foley catheter, or even one-time bladder catheterization increase the risk of postpartum infection. Many women with postpartum bacteriuria are asymptomatic for UTI. The physician or midwife may order a urinalysis to rule out infection when the woman is at increased risk for postpartum UTI. Acetonuria and mild proteinuria may also occur in the early postpartum period. Acetonuria may reflect dehydration after prolonged labor, whereas proteinuria reflects catabolic processes involved in uterine involution.

Fluid and Electrolyte Changes

Excess fluid accumulated in tissue during pregnancy is eliminated by diuresis, which usually begins within 24 hours after delivery. This process is due in part to the reduction in level of plasma oxytocin, which has an antidiuretic effect. A urine output of up to 3000 mL/day can be observed, decreasing by the third postpartum day. This diuresis can account for a loss of as much as 2.2 kg (5 lb) in body weight during the early postpartum period. A sustained natriuresis (renal sodium excretion) also occurs during the first 2 to 5 days after birth (Blackburn & Loper, 1992). Sodium and fluid excretions lead to resolution of peripheral edema within the first 2 to 3 weeks. If more than a trace of edema persists beyond this time, it is indicative of disease.

Additonal fluid losses occur with diaphoresis, which can be pronounced during the early postpartum period. Diaphoresis caused by hormonal changes is not clinically significant unless it is accompanied by fever. Fluid and electrolyte balance is achieved by 21 days postpartum.

Adaptations of the Gastrointestinal and Hepatic Systems

Gastrointestinal tone and motility are decreased in the early postbirth period and reestablishment of normal bowel function is delayed into the first postpartum week. This may be exacerbated by fluid losses, the presence of hemorrhoids, and perineal discomfort and can predispose the postpartum woman to constipation. Bowel function is usually reestablished by the end of the first postpartum week as the woman's mobility, appetite, and fluid intake increase and perianal and perineal discomfort is reduced.

Liver function returns to normal within 10 to 14 days after birth and is reflected in normal, nonpregnant levels of liver enzymes and lipids. However, the alkaline phosphatase concentration may remain elevated for up to 6 weeks. Gallbladder contractility is enhanced in the immediate postpartum period, enabling the previously atonic organ to expel microgallstones that developed during pregnancy (Blackburn & Loper, 1992).

Musculoskeletal System Adaptations

In the first postpartum days, the woman may experience generalized muscular fatigue and achiness related to the work of labor and the positions assumed during birth. The abdominal muscles are gradually stretched during pregnancy, causing diminished muscle tone, which is evident in the early postpartum period. The abdomen is often soft, weak, and relaxed.

During pregnancy the rectus muscles may separate, a condition called *diastasis recti abdominis*. When this separation is present, the uterus and bladder can be easily palpated through the abdominal wall when the woman is supine. Muscles and fascia of the abdominal wall and pelvic floor that were stretched during pregnancy gradually regain their tone and approximate their prepregnant length over the late postpartum period. Vigorous exercise is not recommended until this natural healing has occurred. This is usually accomplished by the fourth to sixth pospartum week but will be influenced by the woman's general condition after birth. Cesarean delivery, postpartum hemorrhage, or infection may delay postpartum recovery.

Integumentary System Adaptations

Many of the pigmentation changes that occur during pregnancy will fade during the first postpartum month but may never totally disappear. Persistent hyperpigmentation is more common in women with dark hair or complexions and is evident in darkening of the areolae of the breast, genital skin, and inner aspects of the thighs. Women with fair complexions may note fewer changes in skin pigmentation during pregnancy and are more likely to have fewer changes persisting after birth. Women who experience chloasma (the mask of pregnancy) will also note a dimunition in this skin change by 6 weeks postpartum. Striae gravidarum, stretch marks due to linear tears in dermal collagen, may persist after birth as depressed, irregular white bands over the abdomen and thighs.

Vascular changes including spider nevi, palmar erythema, and superficial varicosities will decrease in prominence by the second to sixth week postpartum. Varicosities in the lower extremities, vulva, and anus may persist and produce ongoing pain and edema. Surgical treatment or injection of sclerosing agents may be indicated if symptoms are severe. Under the influence of estrogen, hair growth slows during pregnancy. After giving birth, many women experience significant hair loss due to a shift in the number of hair fibers, which move from the "slow-growth" into the "no-growth" stage. These hair fibers are subsequently shed from the scalp. Hair loss accelerates between weeks 4 and 20 postpartum. Regrowth begins shortly thereafter, although some women never achieve the abundance of hair possessed before pregnancy.

Trauma to the integumentary system of the perineum is common in the immediate postbirth period. The woman may experience ecchymosis, lacerations, and surgical disruption of the skin and underlying tissues during birth. The time required for healing will depend on the extent of trauma and the degree of edema. The development of infection will also delay healing.

Chafing and cracking of nipples and the development of blisters and fissures on the nipples can occur when women breastfeed. Fair-skinned and red-headed women are particularly prone to breakdown of nipple tissue, even with proper breast care. The development of mastitis, an infection of the breast, is more common when breakdown of nipple integrity occurs.

Endocrine System and Metabolic Adaptations

The woman's endocrine system undergoes abrupt changes during the fourth stage of labor. After delivery of the placenta, estrogen, progesterone, and prolactin levels suddenly decrease. Prolactin levels will continue to decline to normal nonpregnant levels in the nonlactating woman over the first few weeks. Prolactin levels in the lactating woman will increase in response to stimulation from the neonate's sucking. Estrogen in the nonlactating woman gradually increases, reaching follicular phase levels by 3 weeks after delivery. Menstruation usually occurs by the 12th postpartum week in the nonlactating woman and by the 36th postpartum week in the lactating woman. The first menstrual cycle is often anovulatory. Although breastfeeding tends to delay the first ovulatory menstrual cycle, breastfeeding alone is not an effective method of contraception.

The changes in thyroid function that result in relative hyperthyroidism (euthyroid hyperthyroxinemia) during pregnancy are slowly reversed during the the first 4 to 6 weeks after delivery (Blackburn & Loper, 1992). Serum calcium, parathyroid hormone, and calcitonin levels gradually return to pospartum values by 6 weeks postpartum, but hyperplasia of the parathyroid gland persists during lactation to meet the need for increased calcium in milk production.

The postpartum woman is in a state of relative hypopituitarism with decreased production of gonadotropins and growth hormone. The increase in triglyceride synthesis and fat storage, which occur during pregnancy, slows in the postpartum period. However, it may take months for the woman to regain her prepregnancy weight. Adipocytes hypertrophy during gestation to accomodate additional fat, and the rate of postpartum lipolysis and weight loss will depend on the amount of fat stored during pregnancy, the woman's postpartum diet, and her activity level.

The postpartum woman undergoes significant physiologic adaptations during the postpartum period. Most of the changes that occur during pregnancy and the intrapartum period are reversed by the fourth to sixth week after delivery. Most women anticipate these changes with enthusiasm, particularly the elimination of the minor discomforts experienced and the loss of the additional weight gained during gestation. The nurse must have a comprehensive knowledge of postpartum physiologic adjustments to identify normal adaptations and the development of complications. Awareness of physical alterations is also important to prepare the woman for postpartum changes and to teach her about danger signs and symptoms that should be reported to her primary health care provider.

Maternal Psychological Adaptations

Along with the rapid and extensive physiologic changes experienced by the woman during the postpartum period come a myriad of psychological adaptations. The simultaneous occurrence of these emotional changes with the biologic ones makes the woman's adaptation complex. Although the father or partner and other family members do not experience this physiologic reorganization, they must also adjust psychologically to the presence of the newborn. The woman's own psychological well-being depends in large part on how her partner and other family members respond to the birth of the neonate.

The nurse must assess each woman's physical and psychological status and the psychological status of the father or partner and other family members. This must be done to provide appropriate and comprehensive nursing care. Knowledge of the basic psychological characteristics of maternal and paternal or partner adaptation in the postpartum period provides the basis for nursing care.

Behavioral Adaptations

Energy Level and Sleep Patterns

Maternal energy depletion results from physiologic and psychological stressors encountered during pregnancy and the intrapartum period, resulting in the subjective experience of fatigue. Common sources of fatigue are listed in the accompanying display. Fatigue is defined as a generalized decrease in strength and energy. To date, little research has been done on the levels and type of fatigue experienced by women in the postpartum period. Gardner and Campbell (1991) note that reports of postpartum fatigue may be overlooked and underreported.

The ability to sleep and rest is a major factor that influences the woman's energy level and behavioral adaptations. Women usually enter the postpartum period in a sleep-deficit state. During the latter part of the third trimester, the woman's sleep pattern is disrupted because of the physiologic changes of pregnancy. Shortness of breath in a recumbent position and urinary frequency contribute to the woman's inability to rest comfortably. Sleep deprivation is exacerbated by the length of labor, physical energy expanded during childbirth, and intrapartum complications with their attendant emotional impact.

The woman's ability to rest during the day is affected by the number of visitors, the noise level of the unit, the number of nursing procedures, the care of the newborn, and physical discomfort. She is often awakened during the night for evaluation of vital signs and other nursing assessments (Lentz & Killien, 1991); postpartum diruresis can result in the need for frequent trips to the bathroom. Interestingly, nursing research indicates that women who room-in with the newborn do not experience significantly less periods of sleep than women who return the neonate to the nursery at night (Keefe, 1988). Sleep deficits can affect energy levels and mental and social functioning. Women who experience diminished levels of sleep or rest will be less alert and easily fatigued and will have difficulty in learning about and caring for their newborns.

Factors Contributing to Maternal Fatigue in the Postpartum Period

Physiologic Stressors

- Pain level
- Fluid shifts
- Wound healing
- Rapid hormonal shifts
- Changes in hemoglobin
- Sleep cycle disturbances
- Adjustment to breastfeeding
- Intrapartum and postpartum complications

Psychosocial Stressors

- Adjustment to new roles
- Infant care responsibilities
- Housework demands
- Other child care responsibilities
- Paternal adjustment to fathering role
- Social support network
- Economic pressure to return to work

From Gardner, D., & Campbell, B. (1991). Assessing postpartum fatigue. American Journal of Maternal Child Nursing, 16*(9), 264.*

Maternal Functional Status

Nurse researchers have studied the functional status of new mothers and have found that physiologic integrity does not automatically connote the capacity to resume self-care, neonate care, and household responsibilities. As noted, factors such as sleep deprivation itself can reduce the woman's ability to attend to activities of daily living. Tulman and Fawcett (1990b) have summarized the major factors that influence functional status in the postpartum woman:

- Parity
- Health during pregnancy
- Length of labor and type of delivery
- Newborn temperament
- Newborn feeding method
- Education and socioeconomic status
- Satisfaction with motherhood and maternal role
- Nature and extent of social support network

Surprisingly, maternal employment does not appear to strongly influence functional status. In fact, being employed was found to correlate with higher levels of functional status in household, social, community, and self-care activity in a study of postpartum recovery (Tulman & Fawcett, 1990a).

Parental Adaptation

Parental adaptation in the postpartum period involves taking on new role responsibilities and behaviors, readjusting relationships with significant others, and beginning an acquaintance with the long-awaited newborn. This reorganization takes place on many levels and may be either enhanced or inhibited by the woman's physical state, the father's or partner's level of participation, and the nature and quality of their social supports.

Maternal Responses

Patterns have been observed in the progressive adaptation of women in the postpartum period. One of the first maternity nurses to engage in clinical research, Reva Rubin

Rubin's Maternal Phases

Taking In: A Period of Dependent Behavior

- Focus on self
- Verbalization of need for sleep and food
- Reliving of birth experience
- Passive and dependent behavior

Taking Hold: Movement Between Dependent and Independent Behavior

- Widening of focus to include newborn
- Independence in self-care activities
- Verbalized concern about body functions of self and newborn
- Openness to teaching on care of self and newborn
- Lack of confidence (mother is easily discouraged about caretaking skills)

Letting Go: Moving to Independence in a New Role

- Increasing independence in care of self and neonate
- Recognition of newborn as separate from self
- Grief work for relinquished roles, expectations
- Adjustment of family relationships to accommodate newborn

(1963a) observed the behavior of postpartum women as they took on the mothering role. She identified three phases in their behavior, summarized in the accompanying display. The nurse should recognize that many physical, psychological, and cultural factors influence early maternal behavior and the timing of behavioral changes. Moreover, Rubin's work was done in the early 1960s; many aspects of maternity care have changed as have women's expectations about the postpartum period.

Contemporary nurse investigators find that most women progress through these phases much more rapidly today. Ament (1990) discovered that the taking-in phase was noted only in the first 24 hours; taking-in scores were higher for first-time mothers. Both primiparas and multiparas experienced a transition to the taking-hold phase by 24 hours after birth and had similar taking-hold scores by the second postpartum day. These findings are particularly important in light of the move toward early discharge (6 to 24 hours postbirth); most teaching must be accomplished while women are still in the taking-in phase. For further information, the reader is referred to the discussion on teaching self-care found later in the chapter.

Taking In: A Period of Dependent Behavior. The first maternal phase described by Rubin is called *taking in*. During this phase, the woman is primarily focused on herself and dependent on others. The inward focus of labor and birth persists, and the new mother's energy is centered on her own health and well-being, rather than on her newborn. Her behavior may be passive and dependent, and she will readily accept assistance in meeting her physical and emotional needs. Decision-making may be difficult, and assistance and support from care providers are greatly valued. Needs for rest and food are verbalized; the woman may have a large appetite. Emotionally, she is working to integrate the labor and birth process into her life experience. She may relive the events of labor and birth again and again, seeking details and comparing her performance to her expectations, her previous birth experiences, or those of others. In Rubin's early description, the taking-in phase lasted for 1 or 2 days; contemporary clinicians may observe this behavior in the first hours after birth.

Taking Hold: Movement Between Dependent and Independent Behavior. Gradually, the woman's energy level increases. She feels more comfortable, and she is able to focus less on herself and more on her infant. The new mother is now more independent, initiating self-care activities and often voicing concerns about body functions. Control of bowel and bladder function may be one source of worry. The ability to successfully breastfeed, if chosen, may be another. As she regains control of her body, the woman becomes more able to accept responsibility for the care of her newborn. Being successful as caretaker is usually vital to the woman. She responds enthusiastically to instruction and praise regarding her mothering skills.

For this reason, the phase Rubin labels *taking hold* may be ideal for teaching about newborn and self-care. However, the nurse should be careful to avoid assuming the mothering role. The new mother may be anxious and easily discouraged. She may interpret the nurse's competence as a reflection of her own incompetence and see herself as a failure. If, instead, the woman is allowed to assume the care of her newborn with appropriate guidance and frequent reassurance from the nursing staff, she will be more confident.

Letting Go: Moving to Independence in a New Role. The final phase, *letting go*, as described by Rubin, begins near the end of the first week after delivery. Contemporary mothers may progress to this point sooner, but early postpartum discharge still makes it likely that the nurse will not see evidence of this maternal behavior. As the name implies, this is a time of relinquishment for the new mother. She must give up roles that are inconsistent with her new identity, such as that of the childless woman. She now must take on the responsibilities of the new role of mother of a newborn.

The new mother must also adjust to the physical separation of the newborn and recognize that the neonate is no longer a part of her body but a separate and unique individual. She must also give up her fantasized birth and newborn and accept the real versions, as well as dealing with her partner's met and unmet expectations about the birth experience and their newborn. To accomplish this requires some grief work and a readjustment of her relationships with her partner and other family members. Feelings of being "let down" or mild depression in the early postpartum period may be a result of this grief work and reorganization of family ties.

Maternal-Newborn Acquaintance

Along with her observations on maternal phases, Rubin also observed and described development of the early maternal-newborn acquaintance process (1963b). Contrary to common belief, few mothers feel instantly close to their newborns. The relationship between a woman and her neonate must develop over time, as does any relationship between two human beings who do not know each other.

Maternal Touch. The acquaintance process can be observed through maternal and neonate interactions and behaviors. Maternal touch has been described in detail by Rubin (1963b) and Klaus and Kennell (1982). Initially, the mother touches her newborn tentatively, using her fingertips and touching only small portions of the body (Fig. 28-3). Gradually, as she becomes more comfortable with herself as a mother and better acquainted with her neonate, the woman will use her hand to stroke larger areas of the newborn's body. Eventually, as her comfort and familiarity increase, the mother will enfold the neonate in her arms and hold it close to her body.

Many psychological, physical, and cultural factors affect the progression of the maternal-newborn acquaintance process. When Rubin made her first observations over 30 years ago, she noted that it often took a woman several days to fully develop maternal touch. At that time mothers and newborns were routinely separated for hours after birth. Neonates were kept fully clothed and wrapped and mothers often had access to them only at feeding time.

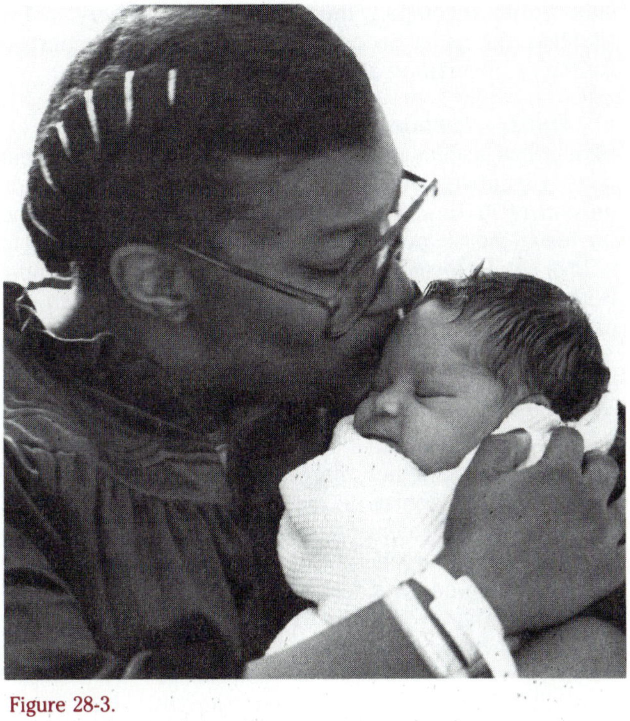

Figure 28-3.
Acquaintance of mother and newborn through visual and tactile sense. (Photo by Kathy Sloane. Courtesy of Alta Bates Medical Center.)

Eye-to-Eye Contact. Eye contact is another behavior that has been studied and described. Cultural studies have confirmed research conducted among American women, which indicate that mothers of full-term newborns spend an increasing amount of time in a face-to-face (*en face*) position with the neonante in the early postpartum period. Biologic mechanisms seem to foster and reward eye-to-eye contact, including the shininess of the neonate's eye, its mobility, and the the capacity of the pupil to vary in diameter (Klaus & Kennell, 1982). Research also suggests that the neonate shows a distinct preference for facial configurations beginning immediately after birth.

Attending to Voice and Cry. As the acquaintace process evolves, both mother and neonate attend to each other's voices. Research indicates that the neonate is able to recognize the mother's voice immediately after birth and will attend to the sound of her voice by alerting behavior and increased sucking (DeCasper & Fifer, 1980). The neonante also demonstrates a preference for the female voice (higher pitch). In turn, the mother becomes skillful in differentiating the meaning among the various cries and vocalizations of the newborn. It is appears that the mother's ability to distinguish among the neonate's cries and respond appropriately to the needs based on interpretation of the cry is one indicator of successful attachment.

Entrainment. The slow-motion analysis of films and videotapes of maternal-newborn interactions indicates that human communication involves a process of "entrainment." When one person speaks, others who are actively listening will move their bodies in a rhythm or in tune to the speaker's voice. Pioneering work by Condon and Sander (1974) revealed that the neonate moves in time to the structure of adult speech, particularly the parent's speech. A synchrony of movement develops between the mother and neonate, which has been described as a "dance of love" (Brazelton, Tronick, Adamson, 1975). A visit to a mother–neonate recovery room in any hospital setting will illustrate that specific behaviors indicative of the acquaintance process are evident in the first hours after birth. This is due in part because of current practices that attempt to promote early contact between parents and their newborn. However, if complications arise for either mother or newborn that delay or interfere with the opportunity for parent–newborn acquaintance, a slower progression in the development of maternal touch can be expected.

Postpartum Blues and Postpartum Depression

The nurse must be aware of the emotional swings commonly experienced by newly delivered women. Research indicates that most healthy women with wanted pregnancies experience a transient state of euphoria and excitement in the immediate postpartum period (Mead-Bennett, 1990). These feelings may persist through the time of discharge, as more women go home within the first 24 to 48 hours.

The terms *postpartum blues* and *baby blues* are used to describe the transient feelings of depression experienced by up to 80% of women in the first 10 days after delivery, after this initial emotional "high." Symptoms may include unexplained tearfulness, sadness, irritability, and disturbances in appetite and sleep patterns.

Many women are unprepared for these let-down feelings because they have been socialized to expect that once the neonate arrives, the family will live "happily ever after." In reality, the adjustment to new parenthood is often difficult, and many factors may combine to bring on these feelings of depression. One stressor, commonly identified as a major contributor to mild depression, is the hormonal fluctuation that occurs after birth. Also contributing are the major psychological adjustments necessary during the transition to parenthood, perineal and breast discomfort, exhaustion, and the mother's disappointment about the appearance of her postpartum body.

The nurse must remember that postpartum or baby blues are self-limiting and recovery is spontaneous. They most frequently occur during the first 6 weeks after delivery but may recur during the first year in response to the ongoing transition to the parental role and adjustments of family life to child care. When depression continues for 2 weeks or more and leads to feelings of despondency and inability to cope with the demands of daily life, the condition is more serious and is accurately described as *postpartum depression*.

Postpartum depression is an affective mood disorder that occurs in approximately 10% of new mothers and responds best to active psychological treatment. In some cases hospitalization and medication are required to treat the disorder. The postpartum nurse plays an important role in the recognition of risk factors for true depression. Beck and associates (1992) discovered that primigravidas who experienced more severe "postpartum blues" in the early postbirth period were at increased risk for true postpartum depression. The nurse should teach the woman and her family about the signs and symptoms suggesting true depression so that they can be reported to the primary health care provider. Postpartum blues and depression are discussed in detail in Chapter 29.

Paternal or Partner Responses

A growing body of knowledge is helping to define the father's adaptation in the postpartum period. Unfortunately, little research has been conducted about the experiences of fathers in unmarried couples and female partners in lesbian couples. It is unwise to speculate about the nature of their postpartum adaptations or to generalize current research findings to these two unique groups. This discussion reviews the research literature as it relates to more traditional fathers' experiences.

Reliving and Integrating the Birth Experience. As men have become more actively involved in childbirth, new postpartum responses have been identified among new fathers. A father may need to relive the birth experience with his partner and with others, yet this need may not always be recognized. Some fathers find that they have little or no opportunity to discuss the birth with anyone other than their partners. This may be troublesome for fathers who had planned to be active participants in the birth but were unable to fulfill that role because of complications during labor.

Physiologic Responses. Research suggests that new fathers also may experience more physical problems, postpartum "baby blues," and even depression during the postpartum period. Ferketich and Mercer (1989) found that men continued to report anxiety, depression, and health problems 8 months after birth of the infant. Upper respiratory tract infection was cited as the most frequent illness. Sleep interruption, concerns about financial responsibilities, insecurity about parenting abilities, and difficulty adapting to the changes in the couple relationship are believed to be contributing factors.

Emotional Responses. Most men have a period of excitement after the birth and may express it in several ways. Some men experience a strong family bond at this time and want to stay close to their partner and the newborn; these men will often take advantage of hospital policies that allow them to stay overnight with the rest of their family. Others will communicate the news to other family members and friends or go out and "celebrate" in traditional ways. The father's immediate postpartum response will depend in large part on his involvement in the birth process. Usually the father experiences fatigue and a need for sleep at about the same time that the mother does but may need to be encouraged to rest. If problems arose during the birth or with the newborn, fathers often accompany the newborn to the nursery; in this situation, the father becomes the mother's most important source of information about the newborn.

Father–Newborn Acquaintance. The father often experiences a fascination with the newborn, just as the mother does. Greenberg and Morris (1974) coined the term "engrossment" to describe the absorption, preoccupation, and interest in the newborn. However, many men are reluctant to hold or handle the newborn and will wait for encouragement from others (see the accompanying Nursing Research display).

Early research suggested that men who were active participants in the birth process developed an earlier and stronger tie to the newborn (Klaus & Kennell, 1982). However, later research shows that although the birth experience is important for the father, many other personality traits and social factors determine his responses to his partner and his newborn. His presence at the birth or early contact with the neonate does not appear to have as significant an effect as was once believed. Significant variables influencing paternal attachment and involvement in newborn care, derived from Mercer and Ferketich (1990), include:

- Infant health status
- Perceived social support
- Relationship with own father
- Sense of competence in parenting
- Readiness for pregnancy and fatherhood

Nursing Research

Father–Newborn Interaction in the Immediate Postpartum Period

Early researchers in human attachment identified a predictable pattern of interaction between new mothers and their infants. A progression in touch from fingertip to palm to full body contact has been documented. Less is known about father–newborn behaviors in the postbirth period. Tomlinson and her associates (1991) videotaped 24 first-time fathers to identify their patterns of interaction.

All newborns were born in traditional delivery rooms and were given to the mothers to hold. Fathers were noted to remain at a physical distance, with gaze behavior (staring at infant and maintaining an en face position) the most frequent activity. Hovering behavior was also common. Touch was not a frequent occurrence, but close proximity and embrace behaviors increased over time with encouragement. As fathers were given the newborns, they immediately used a ventral-to-ventral body position—a "cuddling" hold. An associated behavior was rocking and bouncing.

Fathers were noted to be susceptible to rule setting by the nursing and medical staff and may have been hesitant to touch or hold the newborn because of this lack of freedom in movement. Nurses and midwives should be alert to this factor and regardless of the setting, provide fathers with a sense of control in the environment. Fathers should be encouraged to touch and hold the neonate. Handing the standing partner a newborn, however, while he is still processing the intense sights, smells, sounds, and odors of birth can be a frightening experience. A chair should be provided, and the first contact should be made when the father is seated comfortably at his partner's side.

Thomlinson, P., Rothenberg, M., & Carver, L. (1991). Behavioral interaction of fathers with infants and mothers in the immediate postpartum period. *Journal of Nurse-Midwifery, 36*(4), 232.

- Hospital policies, procedures, classes for new fathers
- Encouragement from partner and nurses to engage in infant care

Nevertheless, *unrestricted access* to their partner and newborn is important to fathers. Opportunities for overnight visiting, particularly when problems occur for the mother or newborn, are essential. Many postpartum rooms now have couches that convert to beds; however, some fathers are even happy to sleep on chairs or makeshift beds consisting of blankets spread on the floor in a safe location, if they are permitted to remain with their family. A father who becomes demanding and angry with hospital staff is often one who has been kept from his partner and neonate by hospital policy or has been made to feel as if he is in the way. Most hospitals now do not consider fathers as visitors on postpartum units; however, many facilities still restrict fathers' access to their partners during postsurgical recovery after cesarean birth or do not welcome them wholeheartedly into the newborn admission nursery.

Paternal Involvement in Parenting. Paternal involvement in neonate care activities during the immediate postpartum period and later varies widely. Jordan (1990) found that many fathers eagerly planned to coparent their newborn, but shortly after birth received strong messages from mates, nurses, and society that their major role was in supporting the woman. Many studies confirm that the new mother has the strongest influence on father involvement and is in essence the "gate-keeper" for access to the infant (Fishbein, 1990).

Family Adaptation

The arrival of a newborn in a family requires that roles and relationships within the family unit be reorganized. Other children now have a younger sibling and parents become grandparents. Although an increasing number of single women now become mothers, many have extended family and partners who are actively involved in the childbearing and childrearing experience. Nurse researchers are beginning to explore the experience of single parenting and the role of unmarried male or female partners in the postpartum adaptation process. In the near future, findings may guide the postpartum nurse in developing family-centered approachers to care, which more effectively incorporate these nontraditional partners. A discussion of possible strategies that may be used now is presented in the following section on nursing care of the postpartum family.

Sibling Responses

Most parents may approach the birth of subsequent children with some trepidation because of concerns about negative sibling reactions and "sibling rivalry." Research indicates that many young children may respond negatively to the birth of a sibling; they may demonstrate some degree of regression, heightened dependency needs, and aggression directed at the newborn. Less research has been conducted on the process of sibling attachment and parental behaviors that facilitate or delay the attachment process.

Anderberg (1988) studied the interaction of children

with new siblings in the immediate postbirth period. She found that most children do demonstrate attachment behaviors including touching, eye contact, and talking to the neonate, although most interacted more with their mothers than with the newborn. Very young children often displayed overtly troubled behavior including expressions of jealousy, rejections of the mother's attempts to give affection, and touching the infant aggressively. Parents who greeted the sibling lovingly, gave the child permission to touch the newborn, and pointed out its special features appeared to facilitate the acquaintance process. Some actions that seemed to delay sibling acquaintance included taking photographs of the infant, forcing the child to touch the newborn, or describing painful elements of the birth.

Grandparent Responses

Many new parents live great distances from their families of origin or do not have close ties with the them. However, grandparents form a vital link between generations and may desire an active role in the new family. The participation of grandparents in the childrearing family can be extremely rewarding for all three generations. Research indicates that when infants and young children are cared for by loving adults who have a vested interest in their well-being, growth and development are fostered and enhanced. The vital role of grandparents in African American families, particularly in the care of infants of adolescent mothers, has been documented (Flaherty, Facteau, & Garver, 1987).

Although grandparents may be well-meaning in their attempts to help the new family, some areas of conflict may arise. Horn and Manion (1985) note that changes in parenting practices over the years may make some child care practices outdated. Today's grandmothers were unlikely to breastfeed and may not be able to offer advice and reassurance to their daughters when they chose to nurse their infants. Issues of discipline may arise and disagreements about issues such as when to pick up a crying infant can result in tension. Many hospitals now offer grandparenting classes that cover information about infant characteristics, feeding, and care.

Readjustments in Role Responsibilities for Family Members

The couple now must share each other's attention with a demanding, dependent newborn. In addition, family routines and living arrangements must be adapted to accommodate the newborn. Even the most organized couple will find that patterns and schedules are totally disrupted during the postpartum period.

Most of this disorganization and reorganization is related to learning to care for and anticipate the needs of the newborn while continuing to meet the other demands of daily life. In family networks where there are many hands to help, this work may be easier and less of a strain on new parents. When no extended network is available, the tasks of caring for a newborn and maintaining work, home, and family life are more difficult. The families who make an easier adjustment are those for whom extended support networks are available and those whose employment and household responsibilities are flexible.

As more women enter the work force and more men become actively involved in child care and household duties, some may assume that the division of labor in childbearing families is now less determined by gender. After the birth of a child, however, families tend to adopt more traditional activities, regardless of their members' previous attitudes toward male and female roles. In families with newborns, women continue to be the primary caretakers and to assume responsibility for household management *regardless of the number of hours they are employed outside of the home*, and men continue to be wage earners with less involvement in child care.

In part, this occurs because the woman requires a period of restoration after birth and because breastfeeding requires close, continuous contact with the newborn, at least for the first several months. However, to a large extent, societal expectations about men's roles may explain the continued unequal burdens in time and work assumed by women. Finally, nurse researchers Rustia and Abbott (1990) note that even when cultural and societal expectations about the conduct of fatherhood begin to change, as they have in the last several decades, actual performance of paternal behaviors lag behind the shifting norms. It may take several decades before more egalitarian redistribution of household and child care tasks occurs.

The woman and her immediate family members undergo significant psychological adaptations in the postpartum period. A major psychological task of both the woman and family members is to make successful adjustments to shifts in roles and responsibilities. Each person's adjustment directly affects the well-being of the family as a unit. For this reason the postpartum nurse assesses the psychological adjustments of the woman and immediate family members. The major goal of postpartum nursing care includes promoting optimal individual and family psychological adaptation. Thus, the nurse's scope of attention and responsibility includes the entire family.

• • Assessment

Although the scope of the nurse's assessment includes the entire family, the immediate nursing priority is to determine the physiologic status of the woman.

Reviewing the Woman's Prenatal and Intrapartum History

The initial assessment begins with a review of the prenatal and intrapartum history, including:

- Significant antepartum complications
- Length of labor and type of delivery
- Length of rupture of membranes
- Presence of episiotomy or perineal lacerations
- Fetal response to labor and condition of neonate at birth

- Analgesia/anesthesia administered during labor and birth
- Other medications received during labor or the immediate postbirth period
- Immediate postbirth complications (ie, uterine atony, retained placenta)

The nurse obtains this information to identify significant risk factors that predispose the woman to postpartum complications. Once the data have been reviewed, the nurse conducts a systematic assessment of the woman's physical and psychological status.

Assessing Maternal Physiologic Status

The nurse must carefully assess and monitor the woman's physiologic status in the immediate postpartum period. The emphasis should be on evaluating vital signs, blood loss, and intake and output. The nurse must have a comprehensive knowledge of the physiologic adaptations that normally occur in the postpartum period to detect deviations from the norm and provide early treatment and supportive nursing care.

Vital Signs

The woman's vital signs must be monitored frequently in the early postpartum period, primarily to assess cardiovascular adaptation and genitourinary function and to screen for infection. Generally, vital signs are taken every 4 hours for the first 24 hours and every 8 to 12 hours thereafter. Fluctuations in vital signs may indicate the development of complications. The following alterations should be noted and reported immediately:

- Temperature: two observations of temperature elevations above 38°C (100.4°F) after the first 24 hours suggest infection.
- Respiration:
  - Bradypnea—a respiratory rate below 14 to 16 breaths/min may be observed with respiratory depression due to the administration of narcotic analgesics or epidural narcotics.
  - Tachypnea—a respiratory rate above 24 breaths/min may suggest excessive blood loss or hypovolemic shock, infection and fever, pain, or respiratory compromise due to pulmonary emboli or pulmonary edema.
- Pulse:
  - Bradycardia—a pulse between 50 to 70 bpm is considered normal in the postpartum period.
  - Tachycardia—a pulse rate over 90 to 100 bpm at rest may indicate excessive blood loss or hypovolemic shock, fever and infection, or pain.
- Blood Pressure:
  - Hypotension—a drop in blood pressure of 15 to 20 mm Hg below normal levels may indicate excessive blood loss and hypovolemic shock. A drop in blood pressure may occur with regional anesthesia (epidural), but should be reversed as sensory and motor function returns in the first 1 to 2 hours postpartum. *Orthostatic hypotension* may be related to excessive blood loss during childbirth, or the administration of analgesia or anesthesia, and is identified by a 15 to 20 mm Hg drop in blood pressure when the woman changes from a recumbent to a sitting position.
  - Hypertension—an increase of 30 mm Hg systolic pressure or 15 mm Hg diastolic pressure over prepregnancy levels or above 140/90 may suggest PIH (preeclampsia). An elevated blood pressure may occur with the use of Methergine, a uterine tonic given to contract the uterus.

Neurologic Integrity

The nurse evaluates the level of consciousness and sensory-motor function during the postpartum period. If the woman has received analgesics or anesthetics during childbirth, the return of sensation and motor function is an integral part of the evaluation. Complaints of dizziness or lightheadedness on sitting upright in bed or standing may preceed a syncopal (fainting) episode secondary to orthostatic hypotension. The woman should be returned to the recumbent position and orthostatic blood pressure checks should be performed before attempting to ambulate. (See the Nursing Procedure below that describes orthostatic blood pressure evaluation.) If PIH was diagnosed antenatally or is suspected in the postpartum period, deep tendon reflexes are assessed for evidence of CNS irritability.

Cardiovascular Status

As noted, significant cardiovascular changes occur in the immediate postpartum period. Maternal pulse rate and quality are assessed and are sensitive indicators of these alterations. Tachycardia and a weak, thready pulse are often the first indicators of complications such as excessive blood loss or hypovolemic shock. The blood pressure is taken with the woman in a supine position and then sitting upright to determine if a significant drop occurs before the first ambulation. Skin color and capillary fill time should be evaluated. Pallor and delayed filling time are observed with postpartum hemorrhage and anemia. The nurse should monitor the postpartum hemoglobin and hematocrit (usually obtained on the first postpartum day) for evidence of blood loss and anemia.

The woman is questioned regarding the presence of pain, heat, or redness in the calf of the leg, a common symptom of deep vein thrombosis. The foot is dorsiflexed to elicit Homans' sign. A positive result is indicated by pain in the calf and suggests deep vein thrombosis (see detailed discussion under Lower Extremities in this section).

Pulmonary Status

The respiratory rate is another sensitive indicator of developing problems; therefore, the respiratory rate and quality of respirations are evaluated. Tachypnea may be observed with infection, hemorrhage, marked pain, or pulmonary embolization. Breath sounds are auscultated. Decreased breath sounds or rales in the lower lobes are associated with surgical birth and the administration of general anesthetics and may lead to the development of pneumonia.

Bradypnea, shallow respirations, and respiratory arrest are rare side-effects of morphine epidural anesthesia or patient-controlled analgesia (PCA). As a result, when PCA or an

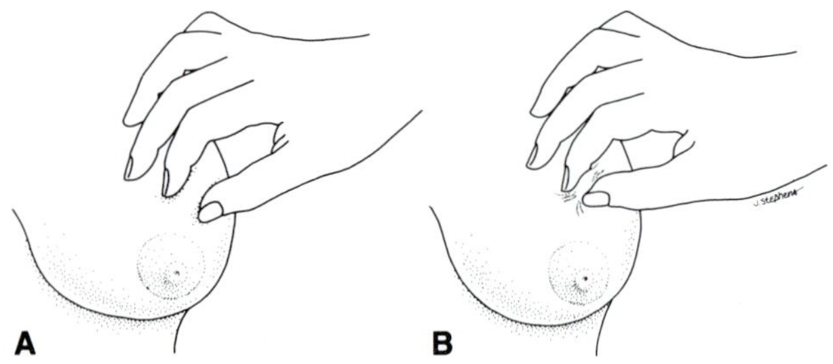

Figure 28-4.
Assessing for elasticity of breast tissue. *A:* Inelastic tissue. *B:* Elastic tissue (Childbirth Graphics).

epidural narcotic is administered for the control of postpartum pain, evaluation of respiratory rate and quality is required every 30 to 60 minutes during the first 24 hours or until the PCA line is discontinued. Refer to Chapter 24 for a detailed discussion of pulmonary assessment and nursing care of the postpartum woman receiving narcotics.

Thrombotic pulmonary embolism is now the leading cause of maternal death after live birth in the United States (Atrash, Koonin, Lawson, Franks, & Smith, 1990). Sudden chest pain and respiratory distress accompanied by cyanosis may signal pulmonary embolism and require immediate and intensive nursing and medical care (see Chapter 29).

Breast Changes

Breast assessment is performed with each physical examination conducted by the nurse. Assessment of the breasts includes inspection and palpation. The breast tissue should be checked for lumps and cysts that may require further medical evaluation. Breast size, shape, and symmetry vary among women and have little affect on lactation. The elasticity of breast tissue also varies. Inelastic tissue feels firmly knitted together, and the overlying skin is taut, firm, and cannot easily be picked up. The elastic breast is looser, and the overlying skin is free and readily picked up (Fig. 28-4). Inelastic breasts are more prone to engorgement.

Examination of the areola and nipple is especially important. The nipple is assessed for evidence of blisters, cracks, or fissures. Early detection and intervention for nipple flatness or inversion will help prevent future feeding problems. The normal and most common nipple type is the *erect everted nipple*. This nipple is easiest for the neonate to draw into its mouth and position properly against the hard palate. The *flat nipple* is smooth and may protrude little or not at all. The *inverted nipple* may partially or completely disappear inside the overlying skin and look like a fold in the skin (Fig. 28-5).

When appearance suggests that protraction of the nipple may be a problem, it is assessed by compressing the areola between the forefinger and thumb just behind the base of the nipple. If the nipple can be made to protrude manually, the flatness and inversion will probably correct itself when the newborn suckles; a truly inverted nipple will stay flat or retract further inward.

The breasts should be soft and nontender during the first 24 to 48 hours after delivery. They will gradually become firmer as they prepare for lactation. The nurse can assess for signs of engorgement by palpating the breast for firmness and questioning the woman about tenderness. Once engorgement has occurred, the nurse should assess the woman's comfort frequently.

Gastrointestinal Function

Assessment of gastrointestinal function includes:

- Inspecting the adomen for evidence of distention
- Auscultating bowel sounds
- Palpating the abdomen for evidence of distention, tenderness, rigidity, or the presence of diastasis recti abdominis
- Percussing the abdomen for evidence and location of gas

The woman is questioned about nausea or vomiting, the ability to pass gas, the presence of flatulence, and bowel movements. These assessments are generally recommended at least twice a day until normal function has been established. Gastrointestinal function may be delayed in women with surgical births or who have received general anesthesia.

Reproductive System Changes

Uterine Tone, Position, and Height. The nurse assesses uterine tone, position, and fundal height by abdominal palpation. In preparing the woman for this assessment, the nurse should explain the procedure and its purpose. The woman should be asked to empty her bladder before the examination to ensure an accurate assessment of uterine tone and position. The head of the bed should be flat and the woman in a supine position.

To identify the location and position of the uterine fundus, the nurse places one hand just above the symphysis pubis to provide support to the lower uterine segment. Support of the lower uterine segment helps to prevent prolapse of

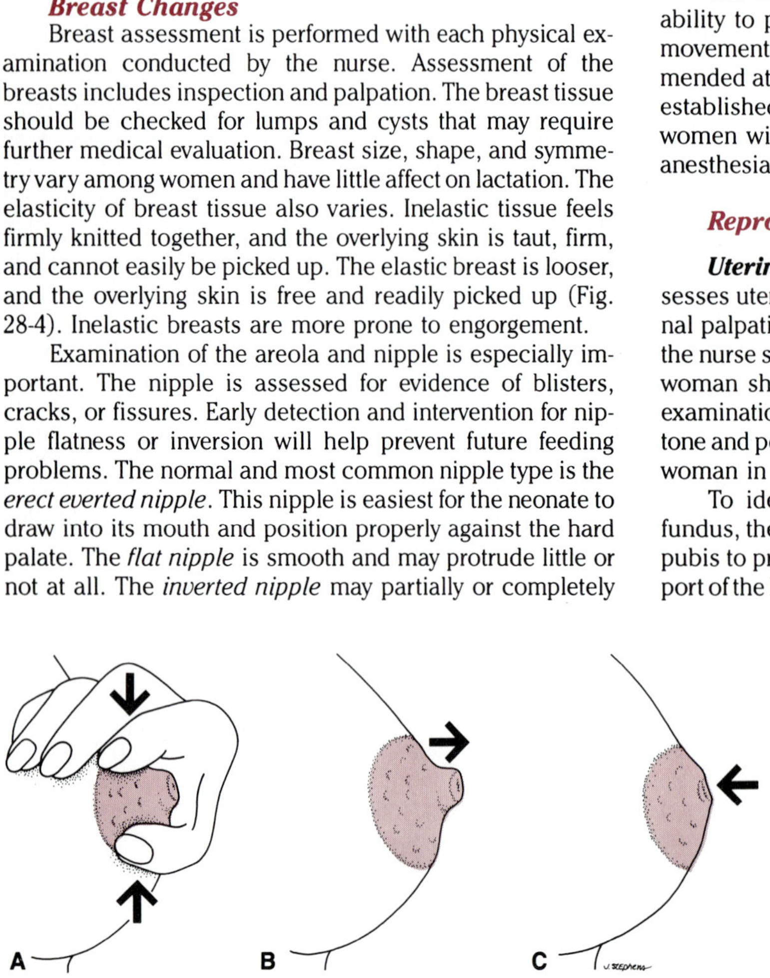

Figure 28-5.
Assessing for nipple flatness or inversion. *A:* The nipple should be assessed before breastfeeding is begun by compressing the areola. *B:* Normally, the nipple will be erect, everted, and protrude. *C:* Flat or inverted nipples or those with little protrusion may require special attention to facilitate breastfeeding (Childbirth Graphics).

the uterus into the vagina should excessive pressure be required to palpate the fundus. Gentle downward pressure (Fig. 28-6) is then applied with the other hand until the fundus is located. The nurse gently palpates the fundus to determine its tone. The involuting uterus will feel rounded and firm, with the consistency of a grapefruit. A boggy uterus feels soft and may be difficult to locate. If the uterus is relaxed, it should be immediately massaged to increase tone. This is essential to prevent excessive bleeding and postpartum hemorrhage.

The position of the uterus in relation to the midline of the abdomen should then be noted. Deviation from the normal midline position may suggest a distended bladder and can predispose the woman to uterine atony and postpartum hemorrhage.

After noting the location, tone, and position of the uterus, the nurse notes the position of the fundus in centimeters or (finger breadths) in relation to the umbilicus. If the nurse can place two fingers between the umbilicus and the fundus, she will chart uterine height as "2 FB below U" or "U/ − 2." If the fundus is one finger breadth above the umbilicus, that would be recorded as "1 FB above U" or " + 1/U." If the fundus is greater than 2 to 3 cm above the umbilicus, it may indicate uterine relaxation or atony, which may result in excessive bleeding or postpartum hemorrahge. The woman's uterine tone, position, and height should be assessed every 4 hours for the first 24 hours after delivery and every 8 to 12 hours thereafter until discharge.

Type and Amount of Lochia. The nurse assesses lochial flow in conjunction with the fundal check. With the woman in a supine position, the nurse removes the perineal pad and assesses lochial flow for amount, color, odor, and presence of clots. The nurse should question the woman to determine how frequently pads have been changed and the degree of saturation.

Lochial flow is described as heavy, moderate, small, or scant. Postpartum hemorrhage is defined as the saturation of one pad within 15 minutes or less. A woman who saturates a pad every 2 hours or more frequently is considered to be experiencing a heavy flow. If the amount of lochia is comparable to menstrual flow experienced during a normal men-

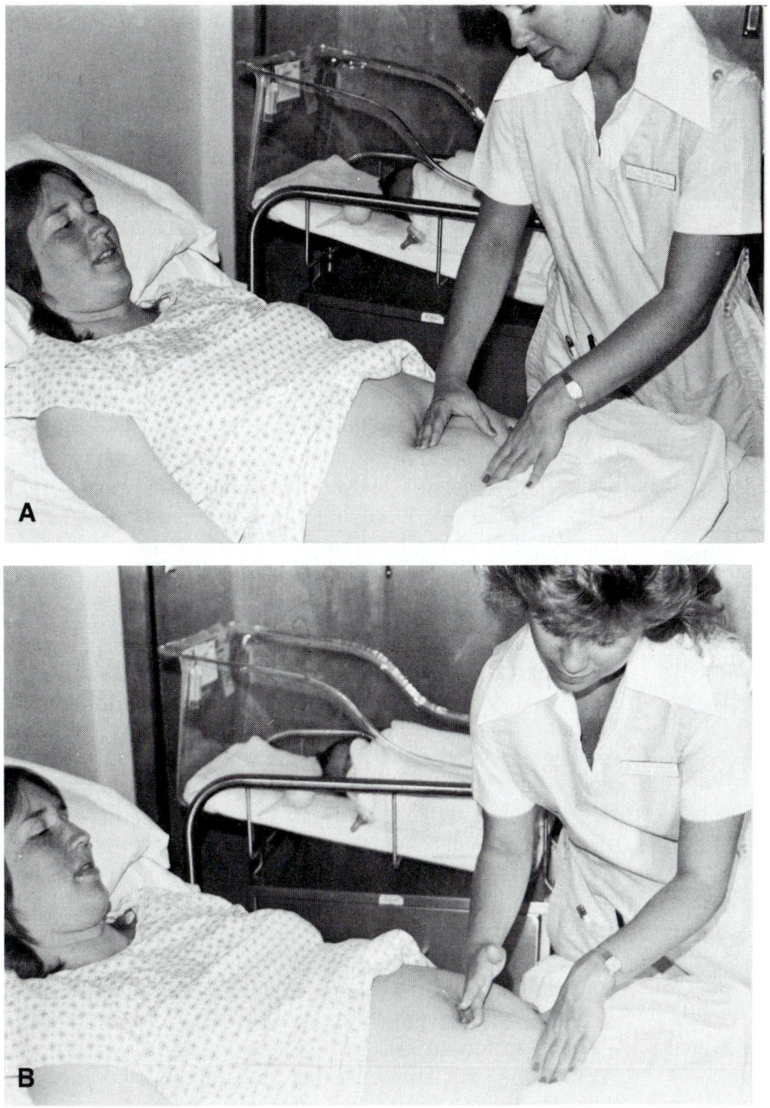

Figure 28-6.
Assessing fundal position and height. *A:* The nurse notes the position of the fundus. *B:* The nurse assesses its height in centimeters from the umbilicus (Samuel Merritt College).

Review of Human Immunodeficiency and Hepatitis Precautions

Latex gloves should be worn *for every patient* when:

- Inspecting the perineum
- Changing or handling perineal pads
- Changing soiled linen
- Starting or discontinuing IV catheters
- Anticipating contact with mucous membranes, blood, body fluids, or nonintact skin

strual period, it is considered moderate, whereas an amount less than that is considered to be scant (see Table 28-2).

Heavy lochial flow always requires further nursing assessment to determine the cause, if possible. The woman will experience what appears to be heavy flow of lochia on rising after several hours in a recumbent position. This is the result of pooling of lochia in the vagina and lower uterine segment. Heavy flow may be related to uterine atony or retained placental fragments. Brisk vaginal bleeding may occur as a result of cervical or vaginal lacerations and may be difficult to distinguish from lochia. Prolonged heavy lochia should be reported to the attending physician or nurse midwife. Refer to Chapter 29 for a discussion of nursing actions when postpartum hemorrhage occurs.

Bladder Function

The nurse should assess urinary output in the postpartum woman to identify potential difficulty in voiding. The first few voidings should be measured. Frequent voiding of small amounts of urine suggests incomplete emptying of the bladder or a bladder infection (cystitis). Urinary retention is verified if a distended bladder is still palpated after the woman urinates and a straight catheterization immediately after a voiding produces 50 mL or more residual urine. Bladder distention without the urge to void is also common in the immediate postpartum period. The nurse should palpate the abdomen to determine whether the uterus is displaced from the midline by a full bladder after the first several voidings. All postpartum women should be instructed to report dysuria, frequency, and burning on urination because these may be early signs and symptoms of UTI.

Condition of the Perineum and Anus

Assessment of the perineum and anus should be performed every 4 hours for the first 24 hours and every 8 to 12 hours thereafter until discharge. The nurse should inspect the perineum by asking the woman to move into a sidelying position and draw the upper knee up toward the chest. The nurse can then gently separate the buttocks and examine both the perineum and the anal area. If the woman has an episiotomy, the nurse assesses for redness, edema, ecchymosis, discharge, and approximation of the wound edges (REEDA). The woman who has not had an episiotomy should be assessed for perineal bruising and edema. The nurse should ask the woman about the degree of discomfort. A bruised, edematous, and painful perineum may suggest a perineal hematoma, and further evaluation by the physician or nurse midwife is needed. The nurse can also assess the anus for hemorrhoids, which are common in the postpartum period and usually resolve without further treatment.

Lower Extremities

The lower extremities should be assessed for sensation, strength, edema, pain, and signs of thromboembolism in the immediate postpartum period. The presence of pain in the upper legs or hip area in women whose legs were placed in stirrups during birth may signal stretching of tendons or ligaments. This can occur with improper positioning of the limbs. The presence of any of the following signs of thromboembolism requires the nurse to restrict the patient to bed rest and notify the midwife or physician immediately:

- Redness, warmth, and pain in the calf area
- Subjective feeling of heaviness in the affected extremity
- Positive Homans' sign: dorsiflexion of foot causes muscles to compress veins, producing pain if thrombosis is present.

Thromboembolism is discussed in more detail in Chapter 29.

Assessing Nutritional Status

Initial assessment of nutritional status in the postpartum period is based on data regarding the woman's prepregnant and pregnant weight, evidence of adequate iron stores, and an adequate dietary history or profile. The nurse also needs to identify any complicating factors that compromise nutritional status, such as unusual blood loss during delivery. If the above factors indicate that the woman is at increased risk for nutritional deficiencies, particularly if she plans to breastfeed, the nurse collaborates with the midwife or physician in initiating a request for a dietary consultation. If the woman is well nourished and at low risk for problems related to nutritional status, the nurse will complete her assessment. This is accomplished by identifying specific areas of postpartum nutritional teaching the woman requires before discharge.

Assessing Energy Level and Quality of Rest

An assessment of the woman's energy level and identification of factors contributing to chronic fatigue should be completed before discharge (see the display on maternal fatigue earlier in the chapter). Appropriate community referrals are initiated by the nurse to aid the woman in reducing physiologic or psychological stressors that may deplete her energy levels and lead to exhaustion. Gardner and Campbell (1991) have developed a postpartum assessment tool that may assist the nurse in the evaluation of maternal fatigue (see the accompanying Assessment Tool).

The nurse should inquire about the amount of rest and sleep the mother is getting and ask what can be done to assist in promoting rest during the woman's hospitalization. Women may not anticipate having difficulty sleeping after the demands of labor and birth. However, excitement, the

Assessment Tool

Postpartum Fatigue Assessment Form
Please circle Yes for only those criteria that apply

Normal Factors

1. Labor longer than 30 h — Yes
Comments:

2. A difficult/high-exertion labor/delivery — Yes
Comments:

3. Perception of a lot of pain — Yes
Comments:

Pathophysiologic Factor

1. Hemoglobin below 10 g/dL on second day postpartum — Yes
Comments:

2. A documented postpartum hemorrhage — Yes
Comments:

3. Any secondary disease (eg, diabetes mellitus or eclampsia) — Yes
Comments:

4. An episiotomy or tear — Yes
Comments:

5. A cesarean birth — Yes
Comments:

6. Alteration in comfort — Yes
Comments:

7. Alteration in mobility — Yes
Comments:

8. A self-care deficit — Yes
Comments:

9. Evidence of substance abuse — Yes
Comments:

Psychological Factors

1. A perception of great fatigue — Yes
Comments:

2. Sleeping difficulties — Yes
Comments:

3. No supportive partner — Yes
Comments:

4. An ill neonate/NICU admission — Yes
Comments:

5. Neonate born with an anomaly — Yes
Comments:

6. Expressions of anxiety — Yes
Comments:

7. A history of depression — Yes
Comments:

Situational Factors

1. Dependent children at home — Yes
Comments: (specify number and age)

2. No help with child care — Yes
Comments:

3. Plans for return to work — Yes
Comments:

4. No household help — Yes
Comments:

5. Problems arranging for babysitter — Yes
Comments:

6. Sleep alterations and deprivation as a result of caring for neonate — Yes
Comments:

7. Family stress/crisis — Yes
Comments:

8. Maternal verbalization of realistic expectations for self and others — Yes
Comments:

9. Poor adjustment to maternal role/lack of attaching — Yes
Comments:

10. Mother an adolescent — Yes
Comments:

11. Prenatal teaching/counseling lacking; knowledge deficit — Yes
Comments:

strange environment, nursing evaluations, and discomfort may seriously disrupt a sleep pattern that was probably already compromised by labor. Mead-Bennett (1990) found that the greater the sleep loss during the intrapartum period, the greater the trend toward hostility and depression scores for women in the first 24 hours postpartum. Women may hesitate to ask for assistance in this area and may not volunteer information because they think it is an unimportant problem.

Assessing Maternal Comfort Level

Recent research indicates that moderate to severe pain levels may interfere with tissue healing (Van de Perre, Simonon, Msellati, et al., 1992). Unremitting pain also interferes with the woman's ability to rest and sleep. Although most women experiencing normal labor and birth usually have minimal discomfort, the nurse frequently assesses the woman's level of comfort and the presence and nature of pain. Pain of moderate intensity may interfere with self-care and newborn care activities and the ability of the woman to process information. The sudden onset of acute pain or a rising level of pain may indicate postpartum complications such as infection or the development of a hematoma.

Assessing Functional Status and Self-Care Abilities

A major goal of nursing care is to promote self-care and newborn care activities before discharge. Therefore, the nurse assesses the functional status of the postpartum woman—the ability to accomplish activities of daily living. Current development of managed care and critical pathways for maternity nursing care lend themselves well to evaluation of functional status (see the Managed Care Plan for the normal postpartum patient). When significant delays occur in return of functional status, further evaluation of physical, psychological, and social factors is indicated to identify underlying problems.

Assessing Maternal Psychological Status

In the first 24 hours after delivery, the nurse assesses the woman's psychological status. This allows the nurse to monitor the woman's mood, her feelings about the birth experience, the responses of significant others to the newborn, and the adequacy of the social support system available.

Immediately after a normal delivery, most women feel great excitement. Even a woman who has just completed a long and difficult labor will feel a rush of energy as she is flooded with joy at the birth of a healthy newborn and relief that she has completed the task of childbirth. Absence of this excitement in the newly delivered woman warrants further assessment.

Maternal Response to Birth

The nurse can use this initial excitement phase to help the woman begin to integrate the birth into her life experience. Reviewing the labor and birth experience with the woman allows the nurse to determine whether she has predominantly negative or positive feelings about the experience. It is appropriate for the nurse to offer praise for a job well done and to convey understanding if the woman expresses disappointment or anger about some aspect of the process. A follow-up visit from the labor and delivery nurse involved in her care further enhances this integration process by allowing the mother to relive the birth with another participant and ask any questions she may have (see the accompanying Nursing Research display).

Body Image Concerns

Although thrilled at the rapid weight loss after birth, most women are dismayed that they cannot fit into prepregnancy clothes and must wear maternity attire for the first month or two or even longer after the birth. Research now indicates that many women may not reattain their prepregnancy weight for up to a year after birth. However, if women are well-conditioned and attend pregnancy and postnatal exercise classes, the recovery period may be accelerated. Feelings of distress about body image may be exacerbated several days after birth when food intake and lax abdominal muscles result in abdominal distention and the renewed appearance of pregnancy for many women. The presence of breast engorgement and uncontrolled leaking of milk, hemorrhoids, varicosities, stretch marks, and other signs of pregnancy and lactation may increase dissatisfaction with body image in some women. A cesarean incision can further add to a woman's concerns about body image.

If the spouse or partner is understanding of the changes in body image and the time needed for full restoration of health, physical functioning, and muscle tone, the woman may feel less unhappy about her body. If her own concerns about weight and body shape are unresolved or if the woman's spouse or partner is critical of the changes wrought by pregnancy and birth, issues surrounding body image may result in depression and delayed postpartum adaptation.

Maternal Perceptions of Family Responses

Another important aspect of the maternal psychological assessment is determining how the mother perceives the response of others to her newborn. The mother's knowledge that the neonate she has delivered is accepted by her mate, family, and friends serves to reinforce their acceptance of her as a woman and a mother. This acceptance seems to be particularly important to successful adaptation to the maternal role. To assess this, the nurse can observe interactions between the mother, father, and other significant persons. The nurse may also ask, "How does your family feel about this baby?" If acceptance of the child by significant others is not clear, the nurse should provide extra support to this mother and observe for potential problems in the parent–newborn relationship.

Finally, the nurse should assess whether the mother is receiving adequate emotional support. Depending on her individual circumstances, such support may come from the woman's mate or the father of the infant, her parents, or friends. Flowers, gifts, phone calls, and visitors are signals of support from others. The woman with no apparent support is at risk for problems in adaptation to motherhood and should receive extra support from the postpartum nurse as well as referral for follow-up on discharge.

Nursing Research

Postpartum Integration

Dyanne Affonso's classic study (1977) of postpartum psychological adaptations revealed that postpartum women could not recall all events that occurred during childbirth. Her subjects indicated a need to recall these "missing pieces." They would spend considerable amounts of time reviewing the events of labor and birth by talking to others, asking questions, and dreaming about their experiences. Affonso postulated that women need to reconstruct their labor and birth experience and fill in these "missing pieces" to continue in their transition to parenthood.

A later study by Stolte (1986) reexamined the concept of "missing pieces." Of 70 women interviewed between 24 and 72 hours postpartum, only 6 identified "missing pieces," for a total of 17% of the sample. The incidence was only a fraction of the percentage Affonso reported in 1977 (90%).

In the most recent examination of "missing pieces," Simkin (1992) found that women in her study had memories of birth that were extremely accurate. Comparisons were made of the woman's accounts about childbirth written immediately after delivery with accounts detailed years later. The majority of subjects could precisely describe even minor details surrounding childbirth that occurred 15 to 20 years previously.

Stolte's findings may differ significantly from Affonso's because mind-altering analgesics and general anesthesiawere used less frequently by the mid 1980s. Simkin's subjects had attended prenatal classes with the goal of "natural childbirth." Important implications for nursing practice arise from these studies. Women retain long-term memories of childbirth including memories about the nursing care they received. The significance attached to both positive and negative experiences remains with them for decades and may take on added importance over time. When women do receive analgesia and anesthesia, they may have gaps in their memory and desire to fill in these "missing pieces."

Nurses should also recognize that most women still wish to recount the story of their childbirth with empathic health professionals, even long after the event. Maternity nurses are ideally suited to listen and reflect with the woman on the meaning of the experience.

Affonso, D. D. (1977). "Missing pieces"—A study of postpartum feelings. *Birth and the Family Journal, 4*, 159.

Stolte, K. (1986). Postpartum "missing pieces:" Sequela of a passing obstetrical era? *Birth, 13*(2), 100.

Simkin, P. (1992). Just another day in a woman's life? Part II. Nature and consistency of women's long-term memories of their first birth experiences. *Birth, 19*(2), 64.

Making Ongoing Assessments of Maternal Psychological Status

The nurse must consider each postpartum woman as an individual. Many factors affect the psychological and emotional responses of a woman after birth. Some of these include the woman's age and parity, her cultural background, and the presence of complications in the intrapartum period. Nurses often assume that primiparas need more assistance and teaching postpartally than do multiparas, because the multipara has been through the experience before and knows what to expect. In reality, however, all new mothers need nursing support. The needs of the multipara are different in that she needs to find the energy to love and care for an additional child, may have lower physical and emotional reserves on which to draw, and must anticipate a greatly increased complexity in her family life.

The emotional mood or affect of each woman is assessed. Does the woman appear elated, excited, or euphoric after the birth or is she quiet, withdrawn, or distant? The nurse listens to the woman's tone of voice and observes her body language and interactions with the infant and other family members to determine her frame of mind or emotional status. The use of open-ended questions, active listening techniques, and a nonjudgmental attitude will encourage the woman to express her feelings.

Assessing Maternal-Newborn Acquaintance

A critical component of the nursing assessment is to observe the early maternal-newborn interactions. Maternal behaviors will be strongly influenced by culture, social class, and educational factors, the woman's physiological status, level of fatigue, the presence of pain, and the course of labor and delivery. The nurse should refrain from making assumptions about the quality of the maternal-newborn acquaintance process from isolated periods of observation. Clues to the nature of early interactions include:

- Progression in maternal touch
- Presence and duration of eye contact
- Evidence of attunement to the infant's cries and vocalizations
- Interest in beginning infant care activities
- Comments about the nature of childbirth
- Comments about the infant such as the resemblance to another family member, the temperament, and response to the mother's efforts to soothe

The nurse assesses and documents evidence regarding these factors as they are observed. Objective language should be used to describe the behavior. When comments are made about the neonate, subjective quotes may be placed in the medical record. These initial notations will provide the basis for future assessment and evaluation of maternal-newborn interaction and referrals for follow-up (see the accompanying Legal/Ethical display).

Assessing Family Adaptation

The nurse may have contact only with the mother and father in the postpartum perod and thus may not be able to assess the process of family adaptation directly. While working with the new mother, however, the nurse should keep in mind the family as the focus of care. The father of the newborn is most often the mother's primary support person. The adaptation of each partner largely depends on that of the other.

Paternal Psychological Status

The nurse must recognize the psychological adaptation required of fathers in the postpartum period. Although men do not experience the profound physiologic changes their partners do, they have similar needs to integrate the birth into their life experience, become acquainted with their newborn, and begin taking on the role of father of a newborn. In addition, most fathers are concerned about their partner's and newborn's physical well-being and need information about their condition. The nurse incorporates evaluation of paternal psychological adaptations into the assessment process.

Father–Newborn Acquaintance

As noted earlier, the father may demonstrate a variety of acquaintance behaviors including gazing, hovering, touching, and holding and may become more engaged in interactions if nursing staff encourage active involvement. The nurse plays a critical role in the identification of potential father–newborn attachment problems and should carefully document negative paternal responses.

Newborn Care Activities

Fathers vary in their comfort with involvement in infant care. Some need encouragement, and others do not see infant caretaking as part of their role as husband and father; the latter view is more common among men from ethnic or cultural groups in which more traditional gender roles are valued. The nurse should assess each father's comfort in assuming caretaking responsibilities, recognizing that families will divide child care duties differently. Regardless of how much actual caretaking the father will provide, however, the nurse should assess his knowledge about the newborn. This knowledge provides part of the basis for the father's interactions with his newborn. If caretaking knowledge or skills are inaccurate or limited, the father may be inhibited in establishing a positive relationship with his infant.

Legal/Ethical Considerations

Documenting Early Maternal–Newborn Attachment Behaviors

Written observations of the woman's interactions with the neonate provide valuable information about the quality of the early maternal–newborn attachment process. This information is critical when there is evidence of impaired parenting, such as in the case of maternal substance abuse, inadequate social support, or a previous history of child abuse. Information contained in the medical record may also be used by psychologists, social workers, child protection workers, and court officials to determine if the newborn should be placed in foster care or with the biologic mother.

The nurse's notes may be used as legal evidence in court proceedings, and the nurse may be asked to testify regarding the observations made during the early postpartum period. It is critical for the nurse to record observations accurately, using objective language or subjective quotes. Placing generalized impressions in the chart such as "poor bonding" or "maternal–newborn attachment absent" are not helpful and fail to reflect professional assessment required of the nurse. Specific details about interactions should be charted such as the following examples:

"Holding infant in an en face position for 30 minutes. Speaking softly to infant, and commenting on the positive aspects of her face including her 'beautiful eyes' and 'pretty mouth'."

"Mother refused to bottle feed infant this morning. States, 'I'll have to feed the brat for the next 6 months.' And she squawks for more milk every couple of hours. I'm too tired to deal with her. You do it this morning."

Recently, nurses who have failed to properly document and report behaviors indicative of problems in parenting have been found negligent if the neonate was injured or died after discharge home with an impaired parent. When delays in the early acquaintance process are noted or alterations in parenting identified, they should be charted in a timely manner, and the midwife or physician should be notified. Social services should be consulted and referrals for follow-up initiated in collaboration with the primary health care provider.

Disappointment and Paternal Adaptation

The nurse should also assess the father's expectations about his partner's postpartum recovery and their mutual roles on returning home. Men are often ill-prepared for the demands of caring for a new infant and for the length of time their partners will require for postpartum recovery. If a man were looking forward to a quick return to his partner's pre-pregnant figure, high energy level, and sexual activity, he may be distinctly disappointed at the restorative time required. This disappointment may contribute to resentment, withdrawn behavior, and potential difficulties in establishing a relationship with the newborn and reestablishing the couple relationship after birth.

Other circumstances may predispose a father to feelings of disappointment in the postpartum period, such as complications in the birth process, maternal complications that delay recovery or threaten the mother's health, or the birth of an infant of the "wrong" sex or with a minor anomaly. Fathers often express a stronger desire than mothers for a newborn of a particular sex and may respond with more shock to a minor physical anomaly, such as a visible birthmark. The nurse should be particularly alert to the father's responses to his newborn and his partner under these circumstances and should carefully assess the father's emotional status as part of overall care.

Family Responses to the Newborn

The responses of other family members are important to the parents, especially the mother. Responses of relatives, grandparents, and other children symbolize acceptance of them as parents and of their new family. The nurse should be especially alert to family responses that imply that there is something unusual about the birth or the newborn. These responses may occur when the newborn has some benign physical variation, such as a molded head or a birthmark. Family responses may also be affected by differences in cultural or religious practices. For example, grandparents may be shocked to see an uncircumcised boy. A sister may disagree with the new mother's decision to bottle feed. In these situations, the nurse can expect the new parents to show some delay in their postpartum adjustment as they attempt to integrate family responses with their own thoughts and feelings about themselves and their newborn.

Assessing Self-Care and Newborn Caretaking Abilities

Because nursing care during the postpartum period is wellness oriented, the nurse assesses the woman's understanding of normal postpartum changes and self-care activities that promote physical and psychological recovery. The nurse also assesses both parent's knowledge of infant characteristics, growth and development, caretaking skills, and health promotion activities. Knowledge of the woman's physical condition and the phase of psychological response to childbirth (taking-in versus taking-hold phase) is essential to develop an effective teaching plan. As an integral part of this process the nurse identifies all primary infant care providers, such as extended family members, so they may be included in teaching session.

In the past, when postpartum women remained in the hospital for longer periods of time, the nurse had time to cover an extensive list of postpartum teaching topics. Today, because many new mothers are discharged within 24 hours of birth, it is essential that the nurse identify knowledge deficits as early as possible and formulate a teaching plan that meets the individualized needs of each woman. Use of a self-administered or nurse-administered assessment tool is essential to identify specific learning needs (see the accompanying Assessment Tool).

Mothers vary considerably in their knowledge of health promotion behaviors and skill in newborn caretaking activities. Some women are complete novices at feeding and caring for neonates, whereas others are experienced and confident. Even an experienced mother, however, may encounter difficulties in caring for a newborn whose behavior is different from that of her previous children. A multipara whose first two children were quiet and easily consoled may become frustrated in caring for a third child who is active and less easily comforted. Fathers are less variable because men usually have less contact or experience with infants. Some experienced fathers may not be confident in their caretaking with small newborns, either because they had little involvement in caretaking when previous children were newborns or because they feel more at ease with older infants.

To assess actual parental caretaking skills, the nurse can observe parents as they provide newborn care and inquire about their previous experience in caring for infants. Providing parents time for return demonstrations of newly acquired skills is an essential aspect of the assessment process. The nurse must also attempt to identify cultural variations in self-care and infant care activities to provide appropriate guidance and teaching.

Assessing Family Support and Assistance After Discharge

The nurse should assess the level of family support and assistance available to the new parents on their return home. Usually such plans are made in advance of the birth and are of some importance to family members. New parents who anticipate no additional assistance in the first few weeks home with their newborn may be at risk for a more difficult adjustment to parenting.

• • Nursing Diagnosis

Nursing diagnosis and planning for care in the postpartum setting are based on the accuracy and completeness of ongoing assessments. Many women and their families will encounter no problems in their postpartum adaptation and will require only supportive care and teaching for effective self-care and infant care. In some families, however, the nurse may identify both existing and potential problems in her physiologic and psychological assessments.

The following nursing diagnoses reflect possible problems in maternal status that may arise in the postpartum

Assessment Tool

Sample: Self-Assessment Checklist of Postpartum Educational Topics

Our nursing staff wish to give you the information you want and need most during your stay with us. Please look over the following list of educational topics and complete the form by putting a check in the column that most applies to you using the following scale:

1 = Most important to learn before I go home
2 = Would like to learn if time permits
3 = Not interested
4 = I already know or am comfortable with

	1	2	3	4	Comments	FOR USE BY NURSING PERSONNEL Date	Signature of nurse providing instruction
Breastfeeding Getting started							
Sore nipples							
Positioning							
Frequency							
Manual expression							
Demand feeding							
Engorgement							
Feeding water							
Nursing for working moms							
Weaning							
Baby Care Bath							
Diaper change							
Axillary temp.							
Cord care							
Jaundice							
Circumcision care							
Uncircumcised baby care							
Care seat							
Crying as communication							
Bottle Feeding Demand feeding							
Types of formulas							
Preparing formula							
Vitamins							
Baby Care after Discharge Solid foods							
Immunizations							
When to call physician or health care provider							
Care of Self Uterine massage							

(continued)

Assessment Tool *(continued)*

Sample: Self-Assessment Checklist of Postpartum Educational Topics

						FOR USE BY NURSING PERSONNEL	
	1	2	3	4	Comments	Date	Signature of nurse providing instruction
Perineal care							
Lochia flow							
Early discharge							
Cesarean Birth Incisional care							
Vaginal birth after cesarean							
Emotions							
Breastfeeding							
After Discharge Signs of infection							
Mastitis							
Episiotomy							
Bladder							
Phlebitis							
Exercise							
Nutrition/diet							
Emotions							
Family planning methods							
Public health referral							
Working mothers							
Day care							
Immunizations							
Single parent issues							
Time out for parents							
Other							

From NAACOG. (1991). *Postpartum nursing care: Vaginal delivery self-assessment checklist.* OGN Nursing Practice Resource. Washington, DC: Author.

period. They may be addressed independently and may be useful in planning postpartum care to new families:

- Decreased Cardiac Output related to postpartum hemorrhage
- Ineffective Breathing Pattern related to epidural narcotic administration
- Altered Urinary Elimination (Retention) related to decreased bladder tone and sensation or edema of urethra and meatus
- Colonic Constipation related to decreased gastrointestinal motility
- Fatigue related to length of labor
- Sleep Pattern Disturbance related to pain or hospitalization
- Pain related to perineal lacerations, episiotomy, or hemorrhoids
- Effective Breastfeeding related to past experience
- Ineffective Breastfeeding related to lack of experience and knowledge
- Altered Role Performance related to birth of the neonate
- Altered Parenting related to separation from nuclear family, lack of knowledge, or change in family unit
- Family Coping: Potential for Growth related to birth of the neonate
- Altered Health Maintenance related to inexperience and lack of information about postpartum self-care and newborn care skills
- Altered Sexuality Patterns related to recovery from childbirth

Nursing Research

Early Postpartum Discharge

Early postpartum discharge is becoming the norm for low-risk women. In a recent study, 131 women were randomly assigned to one of three postpartum discharge times: group 1—12 to 24 hours, group 2—25 to 48 hours, and group 3—4 days postpartum. Subjects were measured for maternal and infant health, breastfeeding incidence, patient satisfaction, confidence in mothering role, and depression and anxiety levels. All the women experienced a relatively healthy postpartum course.

The frequency of infant problems requiring physician referral was 4.3% in groups 1 and 2 and 2.6% in group 3. More of the early discharge group (1), were breastfeeding without supplement at 1 month than women who remained in the hospital for extended time periods. There was no significant difference between the groups at 1 month for anxiety or confidence in mothering roles. Women in the late discharge group (3) were significantly more depressed. Women in the early discharge groups (1 and 2) were more satisfied with their nursing care. The findings indicate that early discharge is safe for low-risk women and does not negatively affect mothering abilities. The nurse caring for the woman who desires early discharge must carefully prioritize discharge teaching, based on the woman's needs and stated goals.

Carty, E., & Bradley, C. (1990). A randomized, controlled evaluation of early postpartum hospital discharge. *Birth, 17*(4), 199.

The nurse must also monitor for and provide supportive care directed at preventing complications and collaborative problems, including:

- Postpartum hemorrhage
- Postpartum mood disturbance (depression)
- Postpartum infection
- Thromboembolic disorders

Such complications require collaboration with other members of the health care team and are discussed in Chapter 29. Some of the interventions in this chapter, however, are directed at preventing complications.

• • Planning and Implementation

With the advent of alternative birth centers and more flexible hospital policies in many areas, healthy mothers and their newborns may now be discharged within the first 24 hours after birth. Most settings have specific criteria for early discharge, such as:

- Uncomplicated pregnancy
- Uncomplicated labor and vaginal delivery
- Vital signs within normal limits
- Firm uterus with moderate lochia
- Voiding without difficulty
- Maternal hemoglobin and hematocrit within normal limits
- Absence of nausea and vomiting
- Healthy newborn
- Positive parent–infant interaction
- Availability of home visit in the first 5 days by a nurse or a representative of a community agency
- Adequate support system

On the basis of identified patient needs, the postpartum nurse plans care, taking into account the following factors:

- Condition of both mother and neonate
- Anticipated length of hospitalization of both mother and neonate
- Availability of the father or partner for involvement in care and teaching

Based on the nurse's assessment of the woman's and family's needs, a plan of care is developed and implemented. Nursing interventions in postpartum care center on monitoring, restoration, and patient education. (See the accompanying Nursing Care Plan for care of the postpartum woman.)

Text continues on page 813

NURSING ALERT

MONITORING THE POSTPARTUM WOMAN FOR COMPLICATIONS

During the early postpartum period, the nurse monitors the woman for complications that may compromise physiologic integrity. Although many problems may be promptly corrected with appropriate care, several postpartum complications are potentially life-threatening. *Postpartum hemorrhage* remains the most serious problem for most woman. The nurse must have a comprehensive knowledge of the predisposing factors and causes of bleeding and be prepared to intervene in *prevention* and immediate *treatment* of hemorrhage until medical help arrives. When abnormal vaginal bleeding is noted or signs of hypovolemia or impending shock occur the nurse must:

- Call for help. Have a staff member notify the midwife or physician.
- Assess the uterine fundus and initiate massage if uterine relaxation (atony) is noted.
- Initiate an IV line with a large-gauge angiocatheter (16 to 18 gauge) or increase the mainline IV infusion if already in place.
- Place the woman in the Trendelenburg position.
- Administer 100% oxygen at 8 to 12 L/min by face mask.
- Assemble drugs required for treatment of uterine atony (oxytocin, Methergine, Prostin).
- Apply a pulse oximeter to monitor oxygen saturation levels.
- Ascertain that a blood sample is available in the lab for type and crossmatch; if not, draw a sample and send for type and crossmatch.
- If signs of hypovolemic shock progress, and the midwife or physician has not yet arrived, place a hospital-wide call for medical assistance.

Nursing Care Plan

The Postpartum Woman After Vaginal Birth

PATIENT PROFILE

History

S.P. is a 32-year-old G2/P1 who experienced a vaginal birth after a 22-h labor. She has a midline episiotomy. She also sustained periurethral lacerations. The estimated blood loss was 450 mL. An infant girl was delivered by vacuum extraction. The Apgar score was 9 at 1 and 5 min. S.P. received narcotic analgesia during labor and a local anesthetic for repair of the perineum. S.P. plans to breastfeed. She spent the first 2 h holding the neonate and attempted to breastfeed, but the infant, although alert, would only lick and mouth the nipple. She would not latch on to the nipple or suck. S.P. has refused breakfast, "I'm just not hungry," but she drank 800 mL of juice.

Physical Assessment

S.P. and the infant remain together in a LDRP room. Her husband has left for work. At 4 h postpartum the nurse conducts an assessment and notes the following: T 37°C (98.6°F), B/P 116/72, p 76 RR 18.

S.P. is quiet and keeps her eyes closed during the examination. Breasts are soft and nipples intact. The fundus is firm, deviates to the right, and is +U/2 FB. S.P. has not voided since delivery. A large bladder is palpable above the symphysis. There is marked perineal edema. Two large, reddish purple hemorrhoids are protruding from the anus. A washcloth covering a perineal ice pack is 50% saturated with rubra lochia 1 h after placement. No clots are noted.

S.P. moves very slowly during the assessment and moans softly as she turns on her side. She says, "My whole bottom is throbbing. But won't drugs for pain affect my baby? I'm so tired, I want to sleep. But I'm worried about the baby not feeding. I don't think I'm going to be any good at breastfeeding. Should I try to nurse her again? It's been 4 hours since she was born. Won't she get sick if she doesn't take some milk soon?"

COLLABORATIVE PROBLEMS/POTENTIAL COMPLICATIONS

- Postpartum hemorrhage
- Retained placenta
- Thromboembolic disorders
- Postpartum PIH
- Bladder trauma
- Infection

(See the accompanying Nursing Alert display and Managed Care Path.)

Assessment	*Nursing Diagnosis*	*Nursing Interventions*	*Rationale*
S.P. has marked perineal edema, has an episiotomy and periurethral lacerations. S.P. has a palpable bladder and the uterus is deviated to the right and is +U/2 FB. S.P. has taken 800 mL of juice. S.P. delivered 4 h ago. S.P. states, "My whole bottom is throbbing."	Altered Urinary Elimination (Retention) related to periurethral lacerations and perineal edema ***Expected Outcome*** S.P. will urinate and completely empty bladder after ambulating to the bathroom and pouring warm water over the perineum, S.P.'s fundus will return to the midline.	After evaluating S.P. for evidence of orthostatic hypotension, assist her to the bathroom to empty her bladder. Use strategies to facilitate voiding: • Pour warm water over the perineum. • Run water in sink. • Give S.P. privacy. • Pour spirits of peppermint into bedpan. Have S.P. sit on bedpan so that peppermint vapors can stimulate micturiation.	Before ambulating S.P., the nurse must ensure that she is not at risk for vertigo and syncope. Warm water may stimulate micturiation. The sound of running water serves as a neuropsychological stimulus to voiding. Some women are unable to urinate in the presence of other people. The vapors released by the spirits of peppermint may relax the urinary meatus and stimulate micturiation.

(Continued)

The Postpartum Woman After Vaginal Birth
(*Continued*)

Assessment	Nursing Diagnosis	Nursing Interventions	Rationale
		If S.P. voids, measure output.	Urinary retention may result in "retention overflow"—the passage of only a small amount of urine (50–75 mL) from the bladder without relief of distention.
		If S.P. is unable to void, notify midwife or physician and obtain order to catheterize bladder.	S.P.'s bladder must be catheterized if she is unable to void or uterine relaxation and bleeding will occur.
		After bladder is emptied, place ice on perineum.	Ice will reduce perineal edema, reduce discomfort, and facilitate voiding.
		Administer analgesics PRN. Continue to monitor S.P. for bladder distention, and measure urine output with next 2 to 3 voidings.	Analgesics will reduce perineal pain and may facilitate voiding. S.P. may continue to have difficulty voiding in the first 24 h until edema is reduced. The nurse must measure the urine output until it is determined that complete bladder emptying occurs.
		If S.P. cannot void after first straight catheterization, Foley catheter may be inserted for first 24 h.	Repeated bladder catheterization is painful and increases risk of UTI.
S.P. has an episiotomy and periurethral lacerations. S.P. has marked perineal edema. S.P. has two large, protruberant hemorrhoids. S.P. states, "My whole bottom is throbbing. But won't drugs for pain affect the baby?" S.P. had local anesthetic for repair of episiotomy but no analgesic since delivery. S.P. moans when moving.	Pain related to episiotomy, lacerations, marked perineal edema, and hemorrhoids ***Expected Outcome*** S.P. will verbalize a decrease in pain sensations and discomfort within 45 minutes of implementing pain-relief strategies.	Apply ice pack to S.P.'s perineum for first 12–24 h.	Ice will reduce swelling, which decreases discomfort. Ice also anesthetizes area, reducing pain.
		Administer analgesics as ordered.	Analgesics are often needed during first 1–2 days when significant edema and perineal trauma have occurred. Postpartum analgesia does not have an adverse effect on the healthy neonate.
		Teach S.P. methods for turning, getting in and out of bed, and sitting down in chair or on toilet. • Use side rails or traction bar to move in bed. • Use pillows to pad chairs. • Press buttocks together when beginning to sit down. • Avoid rubber rings and donuts when sitting.	Use of side rails or traction bar reduce use of perineal and gluteal muscles normally used in turning, sitting up, and standing. Pillows will pad hard surfaces, increasing woman's comfort. Pressing buttocks together reduces tension on perineal suture line.

(*Continued*)

The Postpartum Woman After Vaginal Birth

(Continued)

Assessment	*Nursing Diagnosis*	*Nursing Interventions*	*Rationale*
			Rubber rings or donuts may increase tension on perineal suture lines.
		Initiate sitz baths after first 24 h.	Warm sitz baths stimulate blood flow to perineum to promote healing and prevent infection. Some women find warm sitz bath more effective in relieving discomfort. Cold sitz baths reduce swelling and provide immediate relief of pain. Some women prefer cold sitz baths.
		Administer topical anesthetics to perineum and hemorrhoids as ordered.	Topical anesthetics may provide temporary relief of superficial pain (perineal lacerations and hemorrhoids).
		Administer steroidal or nonsteroidal ointment to hemorrhoids as ordered.	Steroidal ointments may reduce hemorrhoidal swelling. Nonsteroidal ointments reduce local irritation of hemorrhoidal tissues.
		Encourage S.P. to lie on abdomen.	Lying on abdomen reduces pressure on perianal area.
S.P. had a 22-h labor. S.P. states, "I'm so tired, I want to sleep. But I'm worried about the baby not feeding." S.P. verbalizes sensations of pain. S.P.'s husband had to leave to go to work. S.P. keeps eyes closed during assessment	Fatigue related to length of labor, lack of sleep and pain sensations ***Expected Outcome*** S.P. will demonstrate the ability to rest or sleep for several hours. S.P. will verbalize a reduction in her level of fatigue.	Explain to S.P. the causes of her fatigue immediately after birth, and reasons why rest and sleep are necessary at this time.	S.P. must be able to identify causes of fatigue and reasons for rest if she is to participate in plan of care.
		Assist S.P. to identify neonate care activities that can be delegated at this time. Reassure S.P. that newborn will be able to tolerate a short delay in breastfeeding if disinterested in suckling at this time.	Encouraging S.P. to delegate tasks is a central component of family-centered care. It will increase S.P.'s sense of control over situation and may make her more comfortable with decisions made about neonate care.
		Reassure S.P. that neonate can be monitored by nursing staff while she rests.	Reassuring S.P. that nurses will monitor and care for newborn may reduce her anxiety about resting.
		Identify environmental elements that can be altered to promote rest and sleep. • Disconnect telephone. • Limit visitors and delay visiting for several hours.	Rest and sleep will be promoted by reducing environmental stimuli. Pain will reduce ability to rest or sleep.

(Continued)

The Postpartum Woman After Vaginal Birth

(*Continued*)

Assessment	***Nursing Diagnosis***	***Nursing Interventions***	***Rationale***
		• Turn off lights in room and close door. • Delay nonessential nursing activities until S.P. rests. • Administer analgesics to reduce pain.	
S.P.'s infant would not attach to breast and suckle. Infant alert and licking nipple but would not suck. Infant Apgar score 9 at 1 and 5 min. S.P. states, "I'm worried about the baby not feeding. Maybe she doesn't want my breast. Should I try to nurse her again? It's been 4 hours since she was born."	Ineffective Breastfeeding related to infant's disinterest in active breastfeeding. ***Expected Outcome*** After period of rest, neonate will demonstrate readiness cues. After period of rest, neonate will successfully initiate breastfeeding process. S.P. will verbalize satisfaction with progress of breastfeeding.	Permit newborn and mother time to rest, until neonate demonstrates cues of hunger or interest in breastfeeding.	Mother will feel more optimistic and enthusiastic about breastfeeding if level of fatigue is decreased.
		Reassure S.P. that it is common for some newborns to lick and mouth nipple in transition period immediately after birth and does not indicate a dislike or aversion to her breast.	Breastfeeding will be most successful if initiated when newborn demonstrates "readiness" cues (lip smacking, sucking on fists, rooting, alert state).
		Reassure S.P. that neonate can wait another hour or 2 without adverse effects.	Correcting misconceptions and pointing out positive aspects of newborn's behavior may reduce S.P.'s anxiety and concern.
		Reinforce positive aspects of breastfeeding for woman and newborn.	Reinforcing positive aspects of breastfeeding may encourage woman and reduce feelings of discouragement.
		Describe nature and value of colostrum and that neonate takes a small amount of fluid in the form of colostrum in the first day.	
		Reassure S.P. that progress of nursing is slow, unsteady process for many neonates and that her newborn's behavior is normal.	

EVALUATION

After ambulation and nursing interventions to stimulate voiding, S.P. successfully emptied her bladder. Her fundus returned to the midline and was located 2 FB/–U. S.P. verbalized moderate pain relief 50 min after administration of an oral narcotic analgesic and reapplication of an ice pack. The mother and neonate slept for 2 h. When the neonate awoke, breastfeeding was attempted again. The neonate was more alert, latched onto the breast, and nursed for 5–6 min on each breast. S.P. verbalized excitement and pleasure with the breastfeeding experience. She also verbalized a decrease in her level of fatigue.

MANAGED CARE PATH

Vaginal Birth: Postpartum Care

Expected Length of Stay: 2 days

	Day of Delivery	Day 1	Day 2
Key Goals	VS stable, fundus firm, voiding q shift Stable ambulation without assistance Small to moderate lochia. Performs ADL	VS stable, fundus firm, voiding q shift Independent self care and ADL Tolerable discomfort level	Independent self care and ADL Family planning method selected, f/u appts made
Consults	Social work, parent ed, peds prn	→	→
Tests/Labs	Complete blood count, T&S if Rhogam needed	Complete blood count	
Meds	Pain med prn	Pain med prn	Discontinue pain meds. Rubella prn
Treatments	Discontinue IV/prn. Ice to epis × 24 h Measure voidings × 3. VS q 4h. × 12 h, then q 12 h. I&O, cath if distended and no voiding	D/C IV prn. Ice to epis. × 24 h Sitz bath BID/TID Breast care VS q 12 h	Sitz bath BID Tucks pads prn Assess q 12 h Breast care
Teaching	Self-care, unit routine	Self-care review, exercises, role changes, sexuality, nutrition, infant feeding	Review previous topics Infant danger signs, car seat
Equipment	Maternity pack	Breast pump/hit prn	→
Diet	Regular, encourage fluids	→	→
Activity	Up with assistance till stable	Up ad lib	→
D/C Plan	Assess housing, social support	Assess attachment behavior, comfort with infant care, explain birth cert. information	Family plan method chosen Review warning signs Car seat, F/U appts made

Adapted from collaborative paths developed by the Department of Nursing Service, Vanderbilt University Medical Center, Nashville, TN.

Monitoring and Supporting Maternal Physiologic Stability

The postpartum nurse must actively monitor and support the mother's physiologic status in the immediate and early postpartum periods.

Vital Signs

Maternal vital signs are reevaluated every 4 hours during the first 24 hours and every 8 to 12 hours until discharge. Temperature is monitored to screen for the presence of infection. All elevations should be documented and reported; if dehydration is the likely cause, the nurse should recommend an increase in oral fluid intake. If temperature elevation persists, antibiotic therapy is sometimes initiated prophylactically, even before a source of infection is identified. Blood cultures, urine cultures, or cultures of vaginal discharge may be obtained before initiation of antibiotics to document the causative organism and confirm susceptibility to the prescribed antibiotics.

In women experiencing a normal birth, fluctuations in blood pressure can result from pelvic vascular changes that occur with recompression of abdominal contents at the birth of the newborn. Postpartum hemorrhage and the administration of analgesics and anesthetic agents can also influence the blood pressure and predispose the woman to orthostatic hypotension. Tachycardia in the supine woman at rest, without fever or complaints of pain, is a strong indicator of diminished cardiovascular reserve. A history of postpartum hemorrhage or anemia are other indicators of the woman's predispositon to orthostatic hypotension. The nurse should perform orthostatic blood pressure checks before ambulating the at-risk woman (see the accompanying Nursing Procedure). If hypotension is accompanied by rapid pulse, further assessment of uterine tone and lochia is recommended to rule out early postpartum hemorrhage. The midwife or physician should be notified of the findings.

Women experiencing orthostatic hypotension should be instructed to remain in bed, and side rails should be raised to ensure safety, as these patients are susceptible to weakness, dizziness, and falls. Attempts to ambulate should only occur with the assistance of nursing staff. As cardiovascular stability is achieved and the woman is permitted to ambulate, she should be instructed to sit on the edge of the bed for several minutes and then rise slowly before attempting to walk. The nurse should *always* accompany the postpartum mother on her first ambulation to provide assistance.

Uterine Tone

Assessments of uterine tone and fundal position are conducted at least every 4 hours during the first 24 hours postpartum. When the woman has experienced a cesarean

NURSING PROCEDURE
Performing Orthostatic Hypotension Checks in the Postpartum Patient

Failure to ensure patient safety is one of the most frequent allegations of nursing malpractice in the United States, and injuries resulting from falls remains the most common cause of malpractice litigation. Even when the childbirth experience is normal, the postpartum patient is vulnerable to episodes of vertigo, syncope, and falls in the immediate postbirth period. The nurse is responsible for assessing the woman's ability to ambulate after birth by evaluating sensory-motor deficits and the potential for orthostatic hypotension.

Purpose: To identify cardiovascular adaptations to changes in position

To document orthostatic changes in blood pressure the nurse performs the following procedure:

NURSING ACTION	RATIONALE
1. Measure the woman's blood pressure and pulse in the supine position.	To obtain baseline values of cardiovascular status with the woman in a gravity-neutral position
2. Raise the bed to a high Fowler's position, wait 2 to 3 minutes and measure the blood pressure and pulse again.	To determine the effect of elevating the woman's head on the ability of the cardiovascular system to maintain the blood pressure Wait 2 to 3 minutes to permit the cardiovascular system to adapt to a change in position.
3. Monitor the woman for evidence of hypotension including pallor, diaphoresis, symptoms of nausea or lightheadedness.	Hypotension will result in decreased tissue perfusion.
4. Note significant changes in the pulse: • A rise of 20 bpm	Alterations in pulse and blood pressure indicate diminished cardiac reserve.
5. Note significant change in pressure: • A drop of 15 to 20 mm Hg	
6. If no decompensation is noted, the woman is assisted to a sitting position, with legs dangling.	To determine the ability of the cardiovascular system to maintain blood pressure with the legs in the dependent position
7. Wait 2 to 3 minutes and measure the blood pressure and pulse again.	
8. Monitor the woman for signs of hypotension.	
9. If signs of cardiac decompensation or symptoms of hypotension occur in either the high Fowler's or dangling position, return the woman to a supine position.	To improve tissue perfusion and prevent the woman from fainting when ambulating
10. Instruct the woman to remain in bed.	
11. Notify the midwife or physician of the findings.	To make them aware of the abnormal findings and so that medical evaluation can be initiated regarding the cause of hypotension

birth, the fundus is still palpated. The assessment is performed with gentleness because the woman will experience increased discomfort from the surgical incision.

If the fundus feels soft or boggy, the nurse should gently massage it in a slow, circular fashion to avoid overstimulation of the uterine muscle. The nurse should feel the fundal tone increase in a few moments. This may be accompanied by the expulsion of blood or clots from the uterus and vagina. If the uterus does not respond to massage, the physician or nurse midwife should be notified immediately because an oxytocic agent may be required to facilitate restoration of uterine tone and prevent hemorrhage.

Lochia

Heavy lochial flow or the passage of blood clots is usually associated with uterine atony and can be controlled by fundal massage to restore uterine tone. The passage of large clots with voiding should be documented, and if possible, the very large clots should be examined to determine if the woman is expelling fragments of retained placental tissue. If the uterus is firm and lochia remains heavy, the nurse should suspect lacerations of the cervix or vagina and notify the midwife or physician immediately. The nurse also assesses the odor of lochia; the presence of a foul odor is indicative of endometritis. The mother should be taught what normal changes to expect in characteristics and amount of lochial flow and instructed to notify her care provider if symptomatic changes occur after discharge (see the Teaching Considerations display).

Expected Outcomes

- The woman's vital signs remain within normal limits during the pospartum period.
- The woman demonstrates normal uterine involution as evidenced by firm uterine tone, decreasing lochial flow, the absence of clots or tissue, and descent of the uterus at a rate of 1 cm (finger breadth) per day.

Monitoring Renal and Bladder Function

As noted, dehydration can occur as a result of the intense work of labor and a decrease in oral fluid intake during childbirth. The nurse monitors intake and output during the initial postpartum period to identify problems in fluid balance. If the woman has experienced a cesarean birth, intake and output are assessed until the Foley catheter is removed and she is taking oral fluids without difficulty (ie, nausea or vomiting).

The bladder is palpated periodically as uterine tone is assessed, to identify distention. Women who have received IV fluids or regional anesthetics during labor and birth and those with significant perineal edema or periurethral lacerations are at increased risk for bladder distention.

If the woman voids spontaneously, the nurse measures the first voiding to identify retention and residual "overflow" problems as described earlier. The bladder should be palpated immediately after the first void to ensure that emptying has occurred. It is not unusual for the urine to be blood tinged or grossly contaminated with lochia. If the woman is catheterized because she is unable to void and the problem persists, a Foley catheter with urinary drainage bag may be inserted for 24 hours to permit time for reduction in perineal and urethral swelling and restoration of bladder function.

Teaching Considerations

Changes in Lochia to Report

The nurse should instruct every postpartum patient to report the following symptoms to her health care provider immediately:

- Foul-smelling lochia: suggests endometritis
- Heavy lochia: suggests uterine atony, retained placental fragments, or vaginal/cervical laceration
- Lochia rubra after the third postpartum day: suggests delayed involution
- Presence of clots: suggests retained placental fragments or hemorrhage

Expected Outcome

- The woman maintains normal renal function as evidenced by the production of at least 40 to 50 mL of clear, amber urine per hour.

Restoring Cardiovascular Tone and Circulation

Early ambulation in the postpartum period has significantly reduced the incidence of thromboembolic disorders for the postpartum woman. Once normal sensation and strength have returned to the extremities, the woman should be encouraged to begin walking and gentle stretching. The woman who has experienced a cesarean birth may remain in bed for the first 6 to 12 hours, but ambulation is crucially important after surgery to restore muscle tone and prevent thromboembolic disorders. The postsurgical postpartum woman is encouraged to ambulate frequently when she is permitted out of bed.

Pain, warmth, or tenderness in the calf, or a swollen, reddened area that feels thick or knotted are signs of thromboemoblism and must be reported immediately. The extremity involved should be elevated on pillows and the woman confined to bed with movement of the leg minimized, and the midwife or physician should be notified immediately. Early ambulation has many additional benefits including restoration of bladder function and improved muscle tone in the lower extremities.

Expected Outcome

- The postpartum woman establishes normal vascular tone and circulation by 24 hours postpartum (48 hours post-cesarean delivery) as evidenced by the absence of orthostatic hypotension, capillary fill time of less than 3 seconds, and absence of symptoms of thromboemolic disease.

Restoring Respiratory Function

The woman who gives birth vaginally will have few problems related to pulmonary function. The greatest risks are related to respiratory depression secondary to the administration of narcotic analgesics (oral, parenteral, or epidural). The postcesarean patient is at increased risk for respiratory compromise and complications related to abdominal surgery and the use of anesthetics and analgesia for pain control. The nurse initiates a regimen of coughing and deep breathing after cesarean birth. Exercises are performed every 2 hours, and incentive spirometry is highly recommended every 1 to 2 hours while the woman is awake. Close attention to pain control and teaching the patient to splint the abdominal incision will enhance effective deep breathing and coughing efforts. The woman is also encouraged to make frequent position changes while in bed. The reader is referred to the Nursing Care Plan for postpartum care of the woman after cesarean delivery.

Expected Outcome

- The woman establishes normal pulmonary function as evidenced by a normal respiratory rate, unlabored respiratory pattern, and clear breath sounds.

Restoring Bladder Function

The nurse should encourage the woman to void every 3 to 4 hours to avoid overdistention of the bladder. Because the woman usually experiences some decrease in sensation, she may need to be reminded to void. Early ambulation will promote restoration of bladder function. If the woman's condition is stable and no sensory-motor deficits exist as a result of regional anesthesia, the woman should be assisted to the bathroom rather than offered a bedpan for the first voiding. If the woman experiences difficulty in voiding because of her discomfort about urinating with the nurse in the room, privacy should be provided. However, the nurse should remain in the immediate vicinity in case the woman becomes lightheaded or dizzy. Warm water poured over the perineum or the sound of running water may help initiate voiding.

The postpartum woman must void within 6 to 8 hours after delivery or removal of a Foley catheter to prevent overdistention and stasis of urine. If the woman cannot void spontaneously in that time or if bladder distension occurs, the bladder is catheterized. This is essential because a distended bladder contributes to displacement and relaxation of the uterus and predisposes the woman to increased bleeding and postpartum hemorrhage.

Expected Outcome

- The woman maintains normal bladder function as evidenced by absence of bladder distention and spontaneous voiding of urine with complete bladder emptying.

Promoting Hydration and Fluid Balance

Large quantities of fluids are lost from the woman's body during labor and delivery, and dehydration can occur in the immediate postbirth period. The administration of IV fluids diminishes the problem, but fluids by mouth are still indicated. If the woman does not feel nauseated after delivery or is not NPO secondary to cesarean birth, she should be encouraged to drink at least 3000 mL of water and nourishing liquids each day. This will help to restore the body's fluid balance and promote return of bladder and bowel function. When the nurse has encouraged the woman to "force" fluids, or drink liberally, she will want to void often and may need assistance to the bathroom. Adequate hydration also improves blood volume and reduces the risk of orthostatic hypotension.

Expected Outcome

- The woman drinks at least 3000 mL of fluids per 24-hour period.

Restoring Gastrointestinal Function

Nursing care should be directed at promotion of normal gastrointestinal functioning in the postpartum woman. Decreased peristalsis, relaxed abdominal muscle tone, alterations in diet patterns, and concern about discomfort predispose the postpartum woman to constipation.

Early ambulation, especially after cesarean delivery, is important and will accelerate the return of normal peristalsis. A high-fiber diet and fluid intake of 3000 mL/day will aid in decreasing constipation. Stool softeners may be administered to decrease potential perineal discomfort on defecation, particularly when perineal trauma, episiotomy, and hemorrhoids are present.

Anticipated or actual pain associated with an episiotomy can delay the return of normal bowel function. The nurse can help reduce the woman's concern by listening to her fears and providing appropriate information and reassurance. If bowel function is not reestablished by the third or fourth day, an enema may be considered. However, enemas are contraindicated for women with third or fourth degree perineal lacerations because of the risk of trauma and of contamination of the perineal and rectal repair.

Return of gastrointestinal function may be further delayed in the woman who has experienced a cesarean birth because surgery and general anesthesia (if administered) further diminish bowel motility. Abdominal pain due to gas retention is also more common in the postpartum woman

Text continues on page 821

NURSING ALERT

NURSING ASSESSMENT AND CARE OF THE CESAREAN BIRTH PATIENT

The woman who experiences a cesarean birth is also a postoperative patient, with special needs related to the surgical procedure and anesthetic used during delivery. The woman may develop significant postoperative problems that threaten physiologic integrity. The postpartum nurse must be knowledgeable about complications related to surgery and skilled in the implementation of strategies to prevent their development. The nurse must conduct systematic assessments at least q 4 h to identify early signs of complications. Listed below are major complications of cesarean birth, which the nurse must assess for during the postpartum period.

Cardiovascular System

- Hemorrhage
- Hypovolemic shock
- Deep vein thrombosis

Pulmonary System

- Pulmonary embolus
- Pneumonia

Gastrointestinal System

- Paralytic ileus

Genitourinary System

- Renal failure (secondary to hypovelmic or septic shock)
- Hematuria (secondary to bladder trauma)
- Urinary tract infection

Reproductive System

- Infection (endometritis, septic pelvic emboli)

Integumentary System

- Wound infection
- Wound dehiscence and bowel evisceration

Nursing Care Plan

The Postpartum Woman After Cesarean Birth

PATIENT PROFILE

History

C.S. is a 40-year-old G1/P1 who experienced an emergency cesarean birth for fetal distress. A general anesthetic was administered. A healthy baby girl was delivered with Apgar scores of 8 and 9 at 1 and 5 min. The first 24-h postpartum period was uneventful. The Foley catheter was removed at 24 h and a clear liquid diet was initiated. C.S. is receiving 75 mg Demerol intramuscularly every 3–4 h for pain control.

C.S. has been extremely reluctant to turn from side to side, perform deep breathing exercises, or to use her incentive spirometer. C.S. is planning to give her infant formula, but has asked the nurse to feed the infant. "I hurt to much to feed the baby or take care of her yet." C.S.'s partner spent the night in her room and remains at her bedside.

Physical Assessment

At 24 h the nurse performs a physical assessment and notes the following: T. 37.8°C (100°F), B/P 108/76, P 100, RR 24. Faint rales are auscultated bilaterally and there are decreased breath sounds in the lower lobes bilaterally. C.S. has a moist, nonproductive cough. Her respirations are shallow. She refuses to use her incentive spirometer. "It hurts my stitches to take a deep breath. Why are you pushing me to do this?" The abdomen is soft and slightly distended. There are hypoactive bowel sounds. C.S. complains of nausea and has vomited approximately 50 mL of bile-stained fluid at the 3rd and 18th postpartum hour. The abdominal dressing is dry and intact. The fundus is firm in the midline and at the level of the umbilicus. There is scant rubra lochia. C.S. is moving her lower extremities slowly and hesitates to perform leg exercises to stimulate circulation. The Homans' sign is negative.

The nurse prepares C.S. for her first ambulation. She states, "No way! I've just gotten my Demerol and I need to sleep!" C.S. also refuses her clear liquid tray. "I feel nauseated, and I don't want to vomit again."

COLLABORATIVE PROBLEMS/POTENTIAL COMPLICATIONS

- Hemorrhage and anemia
- Thromboembolic disorders
- Pulmonary atelectasis and pneumonia
- Paralytic ileus
- Infection

(See the accompanying Nursing Alert display and Managed Care Path.)

Assessment	*Nursing Diagnosis*	*Nursing Interventions*	*Rationale*
C.S. had a cesarean birth and general anesthesia. C.S. verbalizes reluctance to perform breathing exercises and use the ICS.	Ineffective Airway Clearance related to incisional pain, and position in bed Impaired Gas Exchange related to atelectasis	Encourage and promote deep breathing exercises and use of incentive spirometer q 1 h.	Expansion of lungs is essential to prevent and reverse pulmonary atelectasis and improve gas exchange.
"It hurts my stitches to take a deep breath."	Ineffective Breathing pattern related to pain narcotics, and position	Explain importance of exercises.	C.S. may be more cooperative with pulmonary toilet if she understands postsurgical risks and negative effect of general anesthesia.
Faint rales heard in lower lungs bilaterally. Breath sounds decreased in lower lobes bilaterally.	*Expected Outcome* C.S. will cough and use deep breathing exercises q 1 h.	Elevate head of bed at least 30°.	Elevating HOB increases lung expansion.
T. 37.8°C, P 100; RR 24	C.S. will use ICS q 1 h.	Splint incision area with pillow before having C.S. perform coughing exercises.	Splinting incision will reduce pain associated with coughing and deep breathing.

(*Continued*)

The Postpartum Woman After Cesarean Birth

(Continued)

Assessment	*Nursing Diagnosis*	*Nursing Interventions*	*Rationale*
C.S. favoring supine position with HOB flat. C.S. refuses to ambulate.		Turn C.S. from side to side q 1 h.	Turning promotes expansion of all lobes of lungs and prevents pooling of secretions in one segment of lobe.
		Maintain IV infusion rate until C.S. is taking adequate PO fluids.	Adequate fluid intake is essential to liquify mucous secretions.
		Administer analgesics to control pain.	Analgesics will reduce the pain associated with exercises and ambulation.
		Initiate and encourage frequent ambulation.	Ambulation improves lung expansion and facilitates adequate respiratory pattern.
		Auscultate breath sounds and reassess respiratory pattern q 4 h.	C.S. will remain at risk for pulmonary complication until full restoration of movement and activities.
C.S. has cesarean incision. C.S. states, "It hurts my stitches to take a deep breath." C.S. moans during the assessment. C.S. receives 75 mg Demerol q 3–4 h C.S. must perform coughing deep breathing exercises and ambulate at least QID	Pain related to cesarean incision ***Expected Outcome*** C.S. will verbalize a satisfactory decrease in pain within 45–60 min of administration of the analgesic.	Administer analgesics as ordered and evaluate effectiveness of agent and dose.	The emotional meaning of pain, intensity of pain and C.S.'s weight will influence the amount of pain medication required to relieve pain.
		Notify midwife or physician if analgesic does not effectively reduce pain sensations within 45–60 min after administration.	The nurse must consult with the midwife or physician if pain is not relieved. Severe, unremitting pain may indicate the development of complications such as intra-abdominal bleeding or infection.
		Splint incision site before exercises.	Splinting will reduce tension on the incision site during exercises.
		Provide nonpharmacologic comfort measures such as massage, heat, repositioning, pillows.	Comfort measures will enhance effect of analgesics, convey concern, and may interrupt transmission of pain sensations to CNS, thereby reducing level of pain.
C.S. has 2 episodes of vomiting and states "I feel nauseated and don't want to vomit again." C.S. received general anesthetic. C.S. refuses clear liquids after being NPO for 24 h.	High Risk for Fluid Volume Deficit related to nausea, vomiting, sedation, and pain ***Expected Outcome*** C.S. will verbalize a decrease in sensations to nausea.	Maintain IV infusion at 125 mL/h and encourage increasing oral fluid when nausea and vomiting controlled.	Adequate fluid intake is essential for renal and cardiovascular functioning. IV infusion is only source of intake until C.S. begins taking oral fluids. Fluid requirements are increased after surgery due to fluid and blood losses.

(*Continued*)

The Postpartum Woman After Cesarean Birth

(Continued)

Assessment	Nursing Diagnosis	Nursing Interventions	Rationale
C.S. has hypoactive bowel sounds.		Discuss possible use of antiemetic with physician to reduce nausea.	Demerol may cause nausea and vomiting and can be exacerbated by general anesthesia.
		Monitor intake and output. Assess urine specific gravity. Assess skin turgor. Assess C.S. for signs and symptoms of dehydration: • Decreasing urine output • Increasing thirst • Poor tissue turgor • Dry mucous membranes • High urine specific gravity	The nurse must monitor the woman for evidence of dehydration to prevent renal and cardiovascular compromise.
		Eliminate unpleasant odors and decrease environmental stimuli until nausea and vomiting are controlled.	Environmental stimuli such as food odors or bright light may increase sensation of nausea.
		Notify midwife or physician of negative fluid balance.	The midwife or physician must be notified so that fluid therapy can be revised to meet the woman's needs.
C.S. has been reticent to perform leg exercises, breathing exercises, and ambulation. C.S. says, "No way. I've just gotten my Demerol and I need to sleep." C.S. asks, "Why are you pushing me?"	Noncompliance related to knowledge deficit, pain, and unanticipated cesarean birth ***Expected Outcome*** After reducing her pain and nausea, C.S. will ambulate. C.S. will cough, use deep breathing, and participate in leg exercises q 1 h.	Use open-ended questions to determine level of knowledge about importance of mobility and breathing exercises.	Determine the woman's level of knowledge and understanding before initiating teaching plan.
		Teach C.S. using brief, simple explanations why mobility and exercises are important.	Using brief, simple explanations is important when woman is sedated and in pain as level of comprehension is diminished. Explaining most important reasons for becoming mobile and performing pulmonary toilet may motivate C.S.
		Meet C.S.'s immediate need for pain relief and nausea/vomiting, and then reinforce mobility and pulmonary toilet.	Until the priority needs for relief of pain and nausea. C.S. will not be motivated to cooperate and engage in self-care activities.
C.S. has not fed her neonate since birth. C.S. has asked nurses to feed neonate. This is C.S.'s first child.	Altered Parenting related to pain, nausea, unanticipated cesarean, and sedation ***Expected Outcome*** C.S. will verbalize a desire to increase her participation in newborn care.	Bring neonate to room and encourage C.S. to hold and interact with newborn when pain and nausea are controlled. Report on condition of neonate and progress in feeding.	Early maternal–neonate acquaintance is enhanced by close contact. Having newborn in room may distract C.S. from her pain and nausea and prompt her to begin early interactions with her new-born.

(Continued)

The Postpartum Woman After Cesarean Birth

(*Continued*)

Assessment	Nursing Diagnosis	Nursing Interventions	Rationale
	Expected Outcome C.S. will demonstrate increasing participation in the care of her neonate. C.S.'s partner will assist with care including changing diapers and providing physical support when the newborn cries.	Encourage C.S. to keep newborn in room.	
		Reassure C.S. that nurse will monitor neonate's condition and will assist her in assuming care.	Monitoring neonate frequently may decrease C.S.'s anxiety about having the neonate in her room, and offers the nurse an opportunity to demonstrate newborn care skills.
		Encourage C.S. to verbalize her feelings about her child and the need for a cesarean birth due to fetal distress.	Some women may feel anger or hostility toward the newborn if it is perceived as the cause for the cesarean birth. These feelings usually pass but may require further assessment and referral.
		Inquire about the partner's desires to participate in newborn care and if he desires a role in care, support active participation until C.S. is well enough to begin care of newborn.	Many fathers or partners may be initially reticent to assume neonate care responsibility but are eager to try when encouraged and supported by nursing staff.
		Once pain and nausea are controlled, assist C.S. to assume care and feeding of newborn.	Once C.S.'s priority needs are met, she will be both physically and emotionally more predisposed to begin neonate care.

EVALUATION

After coughing and using deep breathing exercises every 1–2 h, C.S. demonstrated increasing lung volume. Breath sounds became clear and equal bilaterally within 10 h. Her temperature decreased with increased IV and oral hydration and remained within the normal range. When C.S. complained of moderate to intense pain 1 h after administration of Demerol, the physician was notified. The dosage of Demerol was increased and 25 mg Phenergan (IM) was added as an antiemetic and to provide synergistic analgesia. Within 40 min. C.S. verbalized satisfactory pain relief and a cessation of vomiting. One hour after relief from pain and nausea, C.S. ambulated to the bathroom, sat in a chair while her bed was made, and performed breathing and leg exercises every 1–2 h with minimal encouragement. She fed the neonate for the first time and verbalized a desire to have the neonate in the room with her.

MANAGED CARE PATH

Cesarean Birth: Postpartum Care

Expected Length of Stay: 4 days

	Day of Delivery	Day 1	Day 2	Day 3	Day 4
Key Goals	Hemodynamically stable Movement, ambulate prn	Ambulate with assist Tolerates clear liq Voiding q shift	Able to do self-care Ambulate s help Tolerate reg diet	Independent self-care	Select fam plan method Follow-up appts made
Consults	Social work, peds PRN →	→	Lactation consult PRN →	→	
Tests/Labs	Complete blood count, T&S if Rhogam needed				
Meds	Pain med (or epidural narc) per protocol	→	→	→	Discontinue meds Rubella PRN
Treatments	Turning, coughing, and deep breathing q 2 h Foley cath care I+O, IV Assess q 4 h	Turning, coughing, and deep breathing q 2 h while awake I+O till IV d/c Remove abd drsg Assess q 4–8 h Breast care PRN	Discontinue Foley Discontinue epidural Assess q 8 h Breast care PRN	Assess q 8 h Breast care PRN	Staples removed Steristrips to incision Assess q 8 h
Teaching	Pain med use Self care, activity NPO status	Diet progression Self care	Parenting skills Role changes	Exercise, nutrition, sexuality Incision care	Review and reinforce
Equipment	Adm packet Breast pump/kit PRN →	→	Staple remover Steristrips		
Diet	NPO with ice chips	Clear liq	Regular after flatus		
Activity	Up with assistance	Up ad lib →	→	→	
D/C Plan	Assess housing, family life, employment	Assess comfort with self-care, attachment behavior	→	Birth cert info	Family plan Follow-up appts made

Adapted from collaborative paths developed by the Department of Nursing Service, Vanderbilt University Medical Center, Nashville, TN.

after cesarean delivery. Passage of flatus and reduction in abdominal discomfort can be achieved in the postsurgical patient by increased ambulation, the use of an oral simethecone preparation, or a return-flow enema, which stimulates peristalsis and eliminates intestinal gas (see the accompanying Nursing Research display).

Expected Outcomes

- The postpartum woman establishes normal gastrointestinal function as evidenced by presence of bowel sounds, passing flatus, and tolerating a regular diet by the end of the immediate postpartum period (first 24 hours) after a vaginal birth or by 48 hours after a cesarean birth.
- The woman will have a bowel movement by the third to fourth postpartum day.

Promoting Sleep and Rest

The nurse may need to be especially watchful for opportunities to promote rest. After the birth, women usually experience an emotional "high" that can interfere with rest and sleep, as can visitors and phone calls, frequent nursing assessments, time spent with the newborn, and pain. She should be encouraged to limit phone calls and visitors to certain periods so that rest is uninterrupted. The nurse can organize her nursing care to permit unbroken periods for rest and sleep and can suggest use of relaxation techniques or offer comfort measures, such as a warm shower or a back rub, to promote rest. Analgesia and sedatives may also help the mother to achieve restful sleep.

The nurse should also explain the importance of rest once the mother is home with her newborn. She should be encouraged to sleep whenever the newborn does for the first few weeks to help offset the loss of uninterrupted sleep at night. The mother should also be strongly encouraged to plan some relaxation for herself each day, such as reading or a relaxing tub bath if available, or a shower.

Expected Outcome

- The woman verbalizes satisfaction with the amount of rest and sleep obtained during the first postpartum day.

Nursing Research

Nursing Measures to Relieve Postcesarean Gas Pain

Postcesarean women commonly experience abdominal distention and gas pain. An experimental study was conducted by nurse researchers to determine the effects of rocking, diet modification, and antiflatulent medication on the incidence of postcesarean gas pain. Women in the rocking chair group were instructed to actively rock in a rocking chair for 15 to 20 minutes at a time for a total of 60 min/day. The diet modification group received a special diet of low–gas-forming foods started on the first postcesarean day if the woman was tolerating fluids, was afebrile, and bowel sounds were present in two quadrants. Subjects in the medication group received 160 mg simethicone orally after each meal (3 times/day) and one rectal suppository (bisacodyl) twice daily as requested. A combination of regimens was tested.

The investigators found that rocking in combination with either diet modification or antiflatulent medication was the most effective regimen in preventing gas pain. The research findings also indicated that women who simply rocked had less difficulty with intestinal gas, and this may have been due to the fact that they ambulated earlier than women who did not rock. This group was also discharged from the hospital on the average a day earlier than women who did not rock. Investigators note that the act of lowering the body into the rocking chair and holding the newborn on her abdomen while in the rocker also encouraged expulsion of gas.

Rocking and recommendations for a low–gas-producing diet may be implemented safely by nurses for women experiencing uncomplicated postcesarean recovery. Further research is indicated to determine the best combination of rocking, diet modification, and medications. The cost savings appreciated by earlier discharge in the rocking group is a strong incentive to pursue additional studies in this area of nursing practice.

Thomas, L., Ptak, H., Giddings, L., Moore, L., & Opperman, C. (1990). The effects of rocking, diet modifications, and antiflatulent medication of postcesarean section gas pain. *Journal of Perinatal and Neonatal Nursing, 4*(3), 12.

Promoting Comfort and Relieving Pain

Discomfort and pain interfere with the mother's physiologic and psychological restoration and divert energy from other areas, such as learning about her newborn and reestablishing family relationships. Discomfort and pain in the postpartum period are usually associated with the following conditions:

- Perineal lacerations or episiotomy
- Hemorrhoids
- Nipple tenderness
- Breast engorgement
- Uterine contractions (afterpains)
- Cesarean incision
- Gas pains in postcesarean women
- Muscle strain

Analgesics should also be administered if pain is moderate to severe in intensity. Women who plan to breast feed may also receive analgesics and can be reassured that studies indicate they have a minimal effect on the neonate when taken for short periods of time (Lauwers & Woessner, 1990). Antiflatulants such as simethicone tablets may be given for gas pains and abdominal discomfort. Nursing care for uterine, perineal, or rectal pain and breast changes is described in the following sections.

Uterine Contractions

Many women, particularly multigravidas, experience discomfort from uterine contractions, known as afterpains, in the early postpartum period. Afterpains occur when the uterus becomes slightly relaxed and then begins to contract to restore normal tone. Certain conditions predispose the woman to pronounced afterpains and discomfort. Bladder distention displaces the uterus and contributes to uterine relaxation. Physiologic feedback mechanisms then cause contractions of the uterine musculature to restore tone. When this occurs, the woman feels sensations of uterine "cramping" or pain. The woman should be encouraged to empty her bladder frequently to prevent afterpains.

Discomfort from afterpains may also be relieved by analgesics or by positioning the woman on her abdomen for rest, which improves uterine tone. In some cultures, women apply abdominal binders to improve tone, promote uterine involution, and reduce afterpains. There is no evidence that this practice delays healing and may in fact promote contraction of the uterus.

Uterine contractions and cramping may also occur with the initiation of breastfeeding. If afterpains are severe, the woman can take an analgesic before beginning to nurse the newborn. Frequent breastfeeding will improve uterine tone. This will eventually result in a decrease in the relaxation–contraction pattern responsible for afterpains.

Perineal and Rectal Discomfort

Nursing interventions are directed at minimizing perineal discomfort and preventing trauma and infection to the area. Immediately after delivery, perineal ice packs should be applied for 12 to 24 hours to minimize edema and discomfort. The woman should be instructed to rinse the perineal area with warm water after voiding; most postpartum units have special appliances that mothers can use to direct warm, soapy water over the perineal area. The area should be patted dry gently from front to back to avoid contamination from the rectal area.

The woman should be instructed to change perineal pads frequently to maintain cleanliness; saturated pads can be a site for growth of microorganisms. Pads should be worn snugly to avoid friction and irritation. Sitz baths are often advised twice a day, starting 24 hours after delivery. Sitz baths promote healing by increasing circulation to the area and promote comfort by relaxing the tissues and decreasing edema (see the Nursing Research display, Sitz Baths and Perineal Pain).

To minimize the discomfort of sitting down, the woman should be instructed to tighten her buttocks before sitting to decrease the pressure and tension on the perineal area. Analgesics and topical anesthetics are often used to decrease perineal discomfort as well.

Muscle Strain

Some women may experience muscle strain related to positions assumed during the second stage of labor. The nurse can suggest gentle stretching, increasing fluid intake, and early ambulation to reduce discomfort. Warm showers and mild analgesics may be especially helpful.

Breast Engorgement

Treatment of engorgement should include the application of heat, breast massage, and expression of milk. A hot, wet washcloth applied to the breast or a hot shower before massaging the breast decreases the discomfort. The mother should massage by making several gentle but firm stroking movements with the fingertips along the swollen ducts, moving toward the nipple. This should be done around the entire surface of the breast. After massaging, milk should be expressed or pumped until it flows freely. The newborn should then be allowed to nurse from both breasts. However, the best strategy to prevent or reduce breast engorgement is frequent breastfeeding of the neonate (at least every 2 to 3 hours). The mother should be encouraged to wear a nursing bra to provide support for her breasts if they are large or become engorged.

Nipple Soreness

Sore nipples are usually caused by the improper positioning of the neonate on the nipple. The woman should ensure that the newborn is grasping the areola when sucking and not just the nipple. If nipples become sore or cracked, as shown in Figure 28-7, the woman should start feedings on the less affected breast. After feedings, she should air-dry the breasts and expose them to dry heat. Drying the breasts with a hair dryer on low setting or exposing them to an electric

Nursing Research

Sitz Baths and Perineal Pain

The effectiveness of cold sitz baths (rather than the customary warm baths) for relieving perineal episiotomy pain has been evaluated by nurse researchers interested in promoting optimum comfort in postpartum women. In an early study, Ramler and Roberts (1985) measured the degree of pain before and after 40 women had either a warm or cold sitz bath. Patients rated the degree of perineal pain before and after each sitz bath and at 30- and 60-minute intervals after each bath. A 5-point pain scale was used, ranging from no pain to extreme pain. Analysis showed that cold sitz baths were significantly more effective in relieving perineal pain. The greatest amount of pain relief was experienced immediately after the cold sitz baths.

More recently LaFoy and Geden (1989) evaluated the effectiveness of warm versus cold sitz bath to relieve edema and hematomas, as well as reduce the sensation and distress of pain in 20 postpartum patients. Sensation and distress were measured on visual analogue scales. Perineal edema and hematoma formation were graded on a 3-point scale ranging from 0 being none to 3 being extensive edema/hematoma formation. Although cold baths were significantly more effective in reducing edema, both warm and cold baths were found comparable in relieving hematoma formation or pain sensations due to edema.

The investigators suggest that, because both warm and cold sitz baths are comparable with respect to sensation, distress, and hematoma formation, either modality can be considered when reduction of edema is not a consideration. The woman's preference should be a major determinant of water temperature. Some women found cold sitz baths uncomfortable and objected to them. Ongoing research must be conducted to confirm these findings, to determine the optimal time for initiation of either type of sitz bath, and to determine the length of treatment required for best pain relief.

LaFoy, J., & Geden, E. (1989). Postepisiotomy pain: Warm versus cold sitz bath. *Journal of Obstetric, Gynecologic, and Neonatal Nursing, 18*(5), 399.

Ramler, D., & Roberts, J. (1985). A comparison of cold and warm sitz baths for relief of postpartum perineal pain. *Journal of Obstetric, Gynecologic, and Neonatal Nursing, 15*(6), 471.

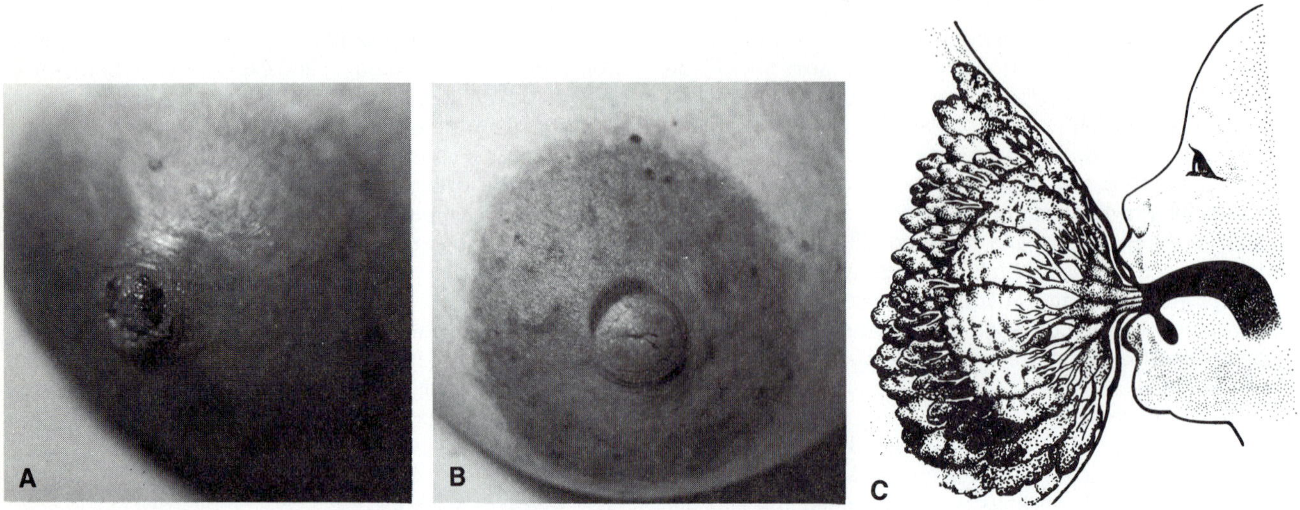

Figure 28-7.
A: Nipples can become sore from improper positioning of the newborn's mouth, for example, if the neonate does not take the entire nipple into the mouth. *B:* Nipples can become cracked and sore because of uneven or repetitive pressure on one area. This can be prevented by varying the position used for nursing. *C:* Nipples may also become sore because the breast are overfull (engorged) and the neonate cannot latch on to the nipple because the breast tissue is too firm (Childbirth Graphics).

lamp with a 60-watt bulb at a distance of 2 to 3 feet for 20 minutes two or three times a day helps to promote healing. Applications of vitamin E, pure aloe vera, or lanolin may be soothing, but these substances should be removed before feeding. Nipple shields or applications of ice just before a feeding may be used if nipples are extremely sensitive; however, the prolonged use of nipple shields should be discouraged because they decrease milk volume production (see the Nursing Research display).

Expected Outcomes

- The postpartum woman verbalizes a decrease in the level of pain or discomfort.
- The woman demonstrates a satisfactory comfort level as evidenced by self-care and neonate care by discharge.
- The woman demonstrates a reduction in the degree of engorgement after initiation as evidenced by soft breasts.
- The woman's nipples remain intact, without evidence of blisters, fissures, or cracks.
- The woman verbalizes a decrease in nipple discomfort after initiation of strategies to reduce discomfort.

Supporting Lactation Suppression

Women who do not wish to breastfeed will need assistance in suppressing lactation. Medications are sometimes freely used for this purpose (Table 28-3). However, the nurse should recognize that medications designed to suppress lactation have side-effects and some risks associated with their use. Mechanical methods of lactation suppression may work almost as well and without the side-effects of commonly used medications.

Even with the use of lactation suppressants, the woman will still experience some degree of engorgement and may require comfort measures. Mechanical methods of lactation suppression, which the woman can be taught, include:

- Wearing a tight-fitting bra or breast binder 24 hours a day until breasts become soft again.
- Avoiding breast and nipple stimulation, such as heat, massage, or pumping breast to remove milk.
- Applying ice packs to the breast.
- Taking analgesics when the intensity of breast discomfort becomes moderate or strong.

Fluid restriction is *not* helpful in suppressing lactation in the postpartum mother. Breast tenderness will decrease in approximately 48 to 72 hours. Complete involution may take up to a month.

Expected Outcome

- The woman verbalizes a decrease in pain related to breast engorgement with the initiation of mechanical methods of lactation supression.

Promoting Breastfeeding

The nurse provides both physical and emotional support for breastfeeding, as well as ongoing education about the process. Physical support includes promotion of comfort, proper positioning, the administration of analgesics, and application of warm moist packs to the breasts should engorgement occur. The woman who has experienced a cesarean birth will require additional assistance, as outlined in the Nursing Procedure display.

Emotional encouragement is as important as physical support. The nurse should remain with the inexperienced mother during early efforts to nurse the newborn. Constant positive feedback is essential, particularly when the initiation of breastfeeding is less than smooth. Teaching should begin with simple instructions and basic facts and proceed with more detail as the woman gains skill and confidence.

Techniques that reduce nipple trauma and soreness

Nursing Research

The Effect of Nipple Shields on Maternal Milk Volume

The nipple shield is a soft rubber or silicon nipple-shaped device that can be placed over the mother's nipple as a breastfeeding aid. Shields are not to be confused with plastic nipple cups that are worn 1 to 2 hours a day during the last trimester of pregnancy to correct inverted nipples. Rubber or silicon nipple shields are used when women have two distinctly different problems related to breastfeeding.

- If the neonate has continued difficulty with latching on to the mother's nipple, the shield may facilitate the latching-on process.
- When the mother's nipples are severely cracked and sore and the latching-on process is extremely painful, the shield may be used to reduce discomfort and further nipple trauma.

Nurses have recommended the use of a nipple shield with the above conditions, but the benefits and disadvantages of its use has only recently been examined. Auerbach (1990) studied the effect of the nipple shield on maternal milk volumes in 25 breastfeeding participants. A comparison was made of milk volumes obtained by pumping the breast with an electric pump, without shields, and milk volumes obtained while pumping the breast with two types of commonly used nipple shields (Cannon silicon (Silastic) shield or rubber Mexican hat model). Significantly larger milk volumes were obtained without the nipple shields. A slightly greater milk volume was obtained using the Silastic shield than the rubber shield. The researcher cautions nurses about routinely recommending the nipple shield. The newborn may develop a nipple shield addiction, and milk supply is reduced. Before suggesting the use of a shield, the nurse should attempt other means of assisting the newborn to latch on (nipple rolling, breast cups, use of breast pump to draw out the nipple, verification of appropriate positioning, and proper nipple care).

Auerback, K. (1990). The effect of nipple shields on maternal milk volume. *Journal of Obstetric, Gynecologic, and Neonatal Nursing, 19*(5), 419.

should be demonstrated with the first feeding. Successful breastfeeding also depends on an adequate diet. The nurse should stress this and review essential aspects of the diet for a lactating woman. Refer to Chapter 34 for a complete discussion of breastfeeding.

Expected Outcome

- By discharge, the breastfeeding mother demonstrates her understanding of breastfeeding techniques that foster newborn feeding and breast integrity.

Promoting Maternal Psychological Adaptation

On the basis of the nurse's assessment of each mother's individual situation, specific nursing support can be offered to facilitate psychological adaptation in the postpartum period. Specific strategies the nurse can use to support the woman include:

- Providing opportunities to review the labor and birth experience. A primary task the woman faces is to "make sense" of the childbirth experience; the nurse serves as an empathetic listener, provides positive feedback about the woman's behavior and efforts during birth, and attempts to fill in "missing pieces" and clarify questions the new mother may have about what transpired during childbirth.
- Providing periods of uninterrupted rest to facilitate spiritual and emotional energy renewal. The nurse plans and organizes care to reduce unncessary interuptions. This provides the woman with an opportunity to rest and regenerate her psychological resources.
- Meeting the woman's physiological needs and providing comfort measures that minimize pain. The woman cannot accomplish psychological adaptations in the immediate postpartum period until the nurse has met overriding physical needs and promotes comfort.
- Reviewing common emotional or psychological reactions in the postpartum period. Anticipatory guidance by the nurse prepares the woman for the emotional lability and psychological changes that occur in the postpartum period.
- Exploring issues of body change and body image with the woman. The current societal emphasis on thinness and perfect body proportions may contribute to the woman's unhappiness with her body.
- Initiating appropriate referrals; providing woman with information about new mother/parent support groups. Early discharge protocols increase the need for ongoing community support. Many new mothers are increasingly isolated on return to the home and benefit psychologically from contact with community health professionals and other women who have recently given birth.

Mothers With Special Needs

Women with special needs include adolescent and older mothers and mothers who experienced complications in the intrapartum period, especially those with cesarean births.

Table 28-3. Drugs Used in Postpartum Care

Drug	Indication/Action	Dosage/Route	Potential Side-Effects	Nursing Implications
Tace	Lactation suppression; inhibits breast stimulation with synthetic estrogen. Not found to be consistently superior to mechanical methods of lactation suppression	72 mg orally b.i.d. for 2 d	Headache, dizziness, lethargy, depression, thromboembolism, nausea, vomiting, diarrhea, uticaria, hyperglycemia, leg cramps	Contraindicated for women with signs of reproductive tract cancer or cardiac, renal, or hepatic disease. Informed consent must be obtained. Woman should wear a tight-fitting bra and avoid breast stimulation.
Parlodel (bromocriptine)	Lactation suppression; prevents secretion of prolactin. Not found to be consistently superior to mechanical methods of lactation suppression	2.5 mg orally b.i.d. for 14 d	Headache, dizziness, drowsiness, confusion, hallucinations, nightmares, burning eyes, visual disturbances, nasal stuffiness, pulmonary infiltrates, hypotension, nausea and vomiting, anorexia, dry mouth, uticaria, leg cramps. Synergistic effect with CNS depressants (ie, narcotic analgesics and antihistamines, alcohol, and hypnotics). Synergistic with drugs that reduce blood pressure.	Assess woman for allergies. Contraindicated in women with hypersensitivity to ergot alkaloids or bromocriptine. Contraindicated in females under the age of 15. Monitor blood pressure and respiratory rate, especially when other medications known to affect blood pressure or cause CNS depression. Take precautions for syncope on first ambulation. Caution woman to avoid driving and other activities requiring alertness as the drug may cause drowsiness. Caution woman to avoid concurrent use of alcohol during course of therapy. Instruct woman to notify midwife or physician if she experiences headache, blurred vision, severe nausea or vomiting, or shortness of breath. Administer at least 4 h after birth and only if vital signs are stable. Administer with food or milk to minimize gastric distress. Patient should wear tight-fitting bra and avoid breast stimulation.
Rubella vaccine live	Indicated for women without signs of rubella or serologically negative (antibody titer 1:8 or less). Attenuated live virus causes antibody response to prevent fetal anomalies due to rubella exposure in future pregnancies.	0.5 mL SC	Temperature elevation, rash, transient arthralgia, polyneuritis, lymphadenopathy; teratogenic during pregnancy	Advise women of need to avoid pregnancy for 3 mo after vaccination. Assess for allergy to neomycin.
HypRho-D, RhoGAM, Gamulin Rh	Indicated for Rh-negative postpartum women who may have had fetal–maternal transfusion of Rh-positive blood cells. Promotes lysis of fetal Rh-positive blood cells in maternal circulation before formation of maternal antibodies that would threaten future pregnancies.	1 vial IM	Mild temperature elevation; soreness at injection site	Must be given within 72 h of birth when following criteria are met: Mother is Rh_0 (D) or D^u negative and without antibodies. Neonate is Rh_1 (D) or D^u positive with negative Coombs test. Verify lot numbers on crossmatched solution and preparation to be administered.

NURSING PROCEDURE
Supporting the Breastfeeding Woman After Cesarean Delivery

The degree of postoperative and incisional pain can affect the woman's comfort levels, interfering with the let-down reflex and pleasure in the breastfeeding experience.

Purpose: To reduce incisional discomfort, promote the let-down reflex, and promote breastfeeding

NURSING ACTION	***RATIONALE***
1. Place the neonate to breast in the recovery room or as soon as possible on woman's transfer to the postpartum unit.	To promote breastfeeding during the period of heightened sensitivity and receptiveness that follow birth To reinforce that the woman is capable of breastfeeding even after surgery To normalize the birth experience for the woman experiencing cesarean birth
2. Avoid bottle feedings, both glucose water and formula, during the immediate postpartum phases.	To prevent development of nipple confusion for the neonate To begin to stimulate the lactation process To emphasize the value of colostrum and to reinforce that the majority of healthy neonates do not need supplemental water or glucose
3. Assist the woman into a sidelying position. Support her back with a pillow. Place two pillows under her head and one pillow between her legs.	The sidelying position in the immediate postsurgical period is usually the most comfortable when the woman is under the influence of analgesia and or anesthesia. The use of pillows will support the limbs, reduce tension on the incision, and enhance comfort.
4. Place a small pillow across the incision site.	To protect the incisional area from the kicking of the baby
5. Encourage the woman to breastfeed 7 to 11 times in a 24-hour period.	To promote rapid advance in the lactation process and development of skill in breastfeeding.
6. If analgesia is needed for pain control, administer the drug 15 to 30 minutes before the beginning of the feeding.	To promote adequate pain relief before the woman is repositioned for breastfeeding, but to minimize the amount of drug passed through the breast milk to the neonate.

Adolescent Mothers. Adolescent mothers typically have greater educational needs than older women, especially in terms of newborn care and effective self-care after discharge. The nurse should discuss with the adolescent mother the arrangements she has made for help and support at home, and if social support seems inadequate, the nurse may initiate referral to community resources. (See Chapter 9 for an in-depth discussion of adolescence during the childbearing cycle.)

Women Over Age 35. First-time mothers over age 35 may also have special needs for nursing support. Frequently the older primipara is well educated and knowledgeable about pregnancy and birth but feels anxious about her knowledge of and skill in child care. Allowing her to express her feelings about the role change she is experiencing may be an important nursing intervention. In many cases, the older primipara has chosen to give up a career to become a mother, and some may find the adjustment difficult. (See Chapter 10 for an in-depth discussion of pregnancy and parenthood after age 35.)

Women with Major Intrapartum Complicatons. Women who experienced long, difficult labors, who were designated high risk, or who developed complications during pregnancy or the intrapartum period need special nursing support in the postpartum period. Obviously, the physical recovery of a woman who has experienced complications or a cesarean birth will be delayed compared to that of a woman with an uncomplicated vaginal birth (see the Nursing Care Plan above for further discussion of parental adaptations after cesarean birth). This delay will affect the woman's psychological adaptation in the early postpartum period. Often her own needs must be met before she can attend to the needs of her newborn and family.

Women Experiencing Cesarean Birth. Women who experience unanticipated or emergency cesarean birth may have additional difficulty with psychological adaptations during the postpartum period. Initial feelings of disbelief and shock may give way to grief as the woman (and her partner) realize they have been deprived of the opportunity to experience a "normal" vaginal birth. The unanticipated delay in recovery, the additional costs of care, and increased pain levels may create feelings of anger and disappointment.

Recent research suggests, however, that many parents have fewer negative feelings after cesarean birth than once suggested. Culp and Osofsky (1989) found no significant difference in levels of depression, marital adjustment, or mother–newborn behavior during feeding. Fortier (1988) discovered that paternal attachment behaviors and paternal caretaking activities did not differ significantly for fathers whose partners experienced a cesarean birth.

However, it is important for the nurse to spend time in the postpartum period with the mother who delivers by cesarean birth to allow her to talk about her birth experience, to express any feelings of loss or inadequacy, and to be reassured that she did the best she could under difficult circumstances. Both parents may have a need to relive the experience by telling it to to others in detail; this should be encouraged as a way of working through what may have been a frightening or unsettling experience. Supportive nursing care will strongly influence the woman's perception of the immediate postbirth period.

The woman may also have gaps in her memory of events. These gaps should be filled in as much as possible by the partner or the nurse to facilitate integration of the birth experience. The nurse should encourage as positive a view of the birth as possible and help the family focus on the newborn and on moving into parenthood. If the newborn's condition is uncertain, the family will need additonal nursing attention and support in the early postpartum period.

Expected Outcome

- The postpartum woman verbalizes concerns, questions, and feelings about the birth experience, changes in body image, and assumption of parenting responsibilities.

Supporting Paternal Adaptation

The father is usually the mother's primary support person throughout the childbearing cycle, yet the father's needs and appropriate nursing interventions have only recently received much attention. In part this reflects the nurse's relatively infrequent or irregular contact with the father. Effective intervention to support the father or partner may require planning for his inclusion in postpartum teaching and newborn care demonstrations as well as taking advantage of opportunities for talking with him about his own feelings, worries, and concerns. The nurse will be most effective in providing family-centered care by remembering that mother, father or partner, and newborn are all her patients, and that family health can be promoted only if all members receive needed support in the adaptation period after childbirth.

Debriefing the Father or Partner About the Birth Experience

The nurse should remember that the father or partner may need to talk about the birth experience as a way of clarifying events in his mind and integrating the birth into his life experience. This need may be especially strong if the father or partner was an active participant in the labor and birth or if unexpected events, such as maternal or neonatal complications, arose. The nurse may be able to include both parents in an unhurried conversation about the birth while monitoring the mother's physiologic status closely in the hours just after birth.

The nurse can offer information to fill in gaps in memory or understanding of birth events. Both parents usually benefit from this, but the father or partner may find it particularly helpful if he or she was absent for periods of time during labor or hesitated to ask questions at the time. The nurse should observe for behavior that suggests that the father or partner has doubts about his effectiveness as the labor support person. Often the woman will express her appreciation of this support, and the nurse can reinforce these positive feelings.

The nurse should be particularly alert to the needs of a father or partner when the woman or newborn develops complications. Fathers or partners sometimes mistakenly believe that they somehow should have prevented complications, the need for medication, or a cesarean birth. The nurse should explore this belief and provide accurate information about the cause of the problem and ways of preventing it. In all cases, the nurse should acknowledge that both parents have completed a difficult task and congratulate them. New mothers are more likely to receive this acknowledgment from family and friends, but fathers or partners may not receive "credit" for having come through a challenging and exciting experience.

Anticipatory Guidance About the Postpartum Period

Another important nursing intervention is providing accurate information about what the father or partner should expect in the early and later postpartum periods. The nurse should begin by asking the father or partner if there are any questions about going home with the new family. After answering the most pressing questions, the nurse can progress to other important areas that should be covered before discharge.

One area often of importance to new fathers that may not be discussed spontaneously is sexual activity after birth. The nurse should approach this area in a sensitive, matter-of-fact way and outline the woman's physiologic recovery in the first month after birth. The nurse should observe carefully to assess whether this information might be most appropriately discussed with the couple together or separately with the woman. In many cases, the nurse can explain the guidelines for resumption of safe and comfortable sexual activity with the couple, reassuring them that this is a common area of concern. If the nurse approaches this topic in a professional manner, appearing comfortable when talking about sexual functioning, new parents are more likely to ask questions and share concerns.

The nurse should also take this opportunity to stress that the couple relationship will require extra attention in the first months of parenthood. Encouraging the father or partner to plan for activities as a couple in the first 2 weeks and pointing out that they were a couple before they were parents can be helpful guidance.

The couple's relationship can be enhanced by encouraging the couple to:

- Allow for open communication between the woman and her mate
- Spend time together without the newborn
- Provide for individual time for relaxation away from the newborn
- Discuss roles and division of household tasks and newborn care
- Develop an awareness of each other's needs and desires for recognition

The nurse should also remind the father or partner that both parents will need time for individual relaxation. It should be stressed that the partner will be the woman's primary support person for the next several weeks. Individual time away from work responsibilities is important for the self-esteem and emotional well-being of both. The nurse may want to reinforce the point that being at home with a newborn is in some ways more demanding than employment outside the home because the duties persist 24 hours a day. The support that the partner provides for the new mother in the early weeks will contribute to a faster physical restoration and will help protect the couple relationship from the inevitable strains posed by new parenthood.

Positive Father (Partner)–Newborn Interaction

The nurse should encourage the father or partner to hold and care for the newborn, while acknowledging the concerns and insecurity most new parents may feel. Research indicates that some men will not ask to hold their newborns but are eager to do so and will respond favorably to sensitive encouragement. If a father or partner seems nervous and unsure, the nurse should take steps to promote confidence. The person should sit comfortably in a chair, and the nurse can then hand him the securely wrapped infant. The nurse should reinforce the fact that newborn care is a learned skill and that many people are uncertain or somewhat anxious initially.

The nurse can also promote positive father (partner)–newborn interaction by pointing out the newborn's unique capabilities and characteristics. Fathers or partners are often "hooked" when they learn that newborns are not simply passive recipients of care but have special abilities and social responses. Some strategies for teaching include demonstrating the newborn's protective reflexes, ability to differentiate voices and follow visual and auditory stimuli, temperamental differences, and states of alertness.

The nurse can assist the father or partner to think about and plan ways that he can routinely participate in care, such as giving baths, bringing the neonate to the mother for breastfeeding at night, or bottle feeding the newborn for a particular feeding each day. Many fathers or partners want to be involved in taking care of the newborn but do not know how to start. They may also lack role models. If the father or partner participates little in early care, this pattern tends to persist. Later, they may experience difficulty matching the mother's well-established competence and routines.

Finally, the nurse may want to encourage the father or partner to seek more information about infant care and parenthood through classes, fathers' support groups, reading, and educational videotapes. Men sometimes assume that parenthood is instinctive or can be learned only through direct experience. The nurse can use the analogy of other learned skills, such as repair work or driving, in which a certain amount of information is acquired before actual practice begins. The nurse working in the postpartum setting should be aware of local resources for fathers such as early parenting courses designed for men. Educational pamphlets that provide practical information for fathers or partners about infant care and infant development should be provided.

Expected Outcomes

- By discharge, the father or partner demonstrates ways to support the woman during the postpartum recovery.
- By discharge, the father or partner demonstrates beginning skill in handling and care of the neonate including holding, diapering, cord care, and initiating safety precautions.

Promoting Parenting

Parent–Newborn Acquaintance

The nurse can facilitate and support the parent–newborn acquaintance process by helping parents to become aware of the individuality of their newborn. Characteristics that indicate temperament can be identified and explained to the parent (see Chapter 30 for a discussion of the behavioral assessment of the newborn). As the nurse points out these characteristics, she can assist the parents in finding ways to respond to their child appropriately, for example, telling parents that the infant is able to see best at a distance of 8 to 10 inches and likes to gaze at the human face. The mother and father or partner can then be encouraged to hold the infant close and to establish eye contact. The nurse's actions increase the parents' knowledge about their newborn and promote the growing parent–newborn relationship (see the Family Considerations display).

Neonatal Care Skills

Teaching sessions should include the father, partner, or other primary caretakers including extended family members who will be involved in neonatal care. The nurse provides information, encouragement, and support to parents as they learn how to care for their neonate. Demonstrating

Family Considerations

Parent–Newborn Acquaintance

Events during the early hours and days following birth can affect the parent–newborn acquaintance. Prolonged neonatal and parent separation, parental health status, and initial contact with the neonate are factors that can have an influence on the parent–newborn relationship. The nurse can foster parent–newborn acquaintance by the following behaviors:

- Encourage the couple to inspect their neonate's body parts
- Compare the neonate's features to other family members
- Encourage parental rest and relaxation
- Encourage early breastfeeding
- Assist the couple in a comfortable position for holding their neonate
- Provide time alone with their neonate
- Provide information on normal newborn characteristics, newborn growth and development, and newborn alertness and sleep patterns
- Praise the couple for their abilities to care for their neonate

basic care skills at the bedside for inexperienced parents is often extremely helpful. This teaching can then be reinforced in a group session on the postpartum unit. Videotapes and cable-access programs on health promotion, self-care, and neonatal care now play an increasingly important role in parent education. Parents may choose when to view the videotapes and the time nurses spend in teaching can be focused on answering parent questions and clarifying important points covered in the presentations.

It is important to give encouragement and praise as new parents attempt newborn care activities. New parents are often insecure about their abilities and will have few opportunities to get direct feedback on their caretaking once they leave the hospital setting. All parents, whether experienced or not, benefit from praise and encouragement about their infant caretaking. (See Chapter 31 for a detailed discussion of parent teaching for newborn care.)

The nurse is the key person in assisting parents with both breastfeeding and formula feeding. Support of the breastfeeding mother as well as the woman using formula is addressed in depth in Chapter 34. The nurse should remember that women who choose formula feeding also need much nursing attention and support.

Expected Outcomes

- By discharge, parents demonstrate beginning acquaintance behaviors, as evidenced by holding the newborn close and in a face-to-face position while feeding or cuddling, making eye contact when the neonate is in quiet alert state, and calling the newborn by name.
- Parents demonstrate correct neonatal care skills including correct techniques for feeding the newborn, changing diapers and clothing, and instituting safety precautions.
- Parents correctly verbalize danger signs in the neonate that require medical attention or assistance.

Promoting Family Adaptation

The nurse should teach other family members as much as possible about newborn care. Siblings, grandparents, and others have great importance in the family unit; if they are prepared for the arrival of the newborn in the home, the parents will be able to devote more of their energy to meeting their own needs and those of their infant (Fig. 28-8).

Sibling Adaptation

The arrival of a new baby brother or sister can stir mixed emotions in other siblings. The response of siblings will vary according to their age, the number of other siblings, and the extent of preparation for the newborn. Even with the best prenatal preparation, older siblings will feel some loss of love and attention and will have periods of unhappiness at sharing parents with the neonate. The nurse should encourage parents to be sensitive to these feelings and to the changes the older children are experiencing.

The parents may wish to take specific steps to ease the transition for older children. The accompanying Family Considerations display lists some ways this might be done.

The nurse should remind parents that young children do not have the judgment or skill to handle a newborn safely without supervision. The parents should not refer to the neonate as "just like a doll," because this might be interpreted by the child as permission to play with it like a doll. Parents should be watchful when the older child is with the newborn. Natural expressions of sibling jealousy may involve rough handling, burying the newborn with toys or throwing them at it, attempting to take the newborn out of a crib or infant seat, and slapping or hitting.

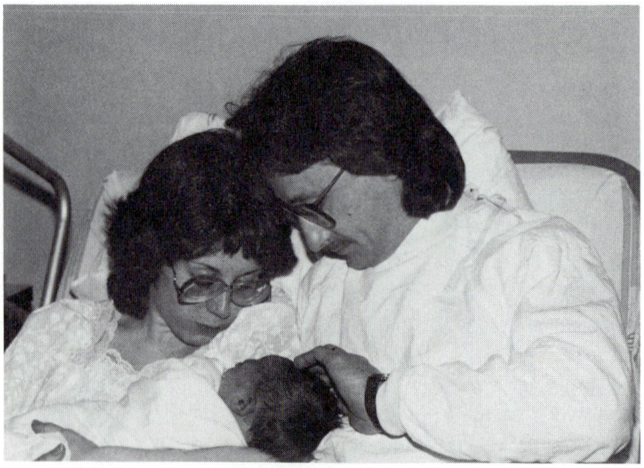

Figure 28-8.
The postpartum period is a time for family closeness and readjustment.

Family Considerations

Easing Adaptation by Older Siblings

The addition of a new member to the family unit can create a disruption to other relationships within the preexisting unit. Older siblings often feel displaced and less loved following the birth of a new sibling. To ease adjustment by older siblings to the birth of a new baby, the mother can take the following measures:

- Let the sibling select a gift for the neonate before delivery, to bring to the hospital after the birth.
- Encourage sibling visitation when hospital regulations allow it.
- Call older children on the phone while she is in the hospital.
- Plan for high-quality, uninterrupted time with the older children.
- Let the father, partner, or another family member carry the neonate on discharge from the hospital so that she can hug and hold other children.
- Give a gift from the neonate to the older children.
- Request that visitors greet older children before focusing on the newborn.
- Allow siblings to care for a doll while she cares for the neonate.
- Celebrate the neonate's arrival with a birthday cake, which the sibling will eat for the newborn.

Expected Outcomes

- Couple discusses the impact of the newborn on older siblings.
- By discharge, couple demonstrates techniques to decrease sibling rivalry.

Promoting Health Maintenance

Before discharge, the nurse should help the family to anticipate and plan for the changes that will occur during their first few weeks at home. The nurse should discuss the changes the couple is likely to experience in the relationship and in the family as a whole. The importance of maintaining the couple bond should be stressed.

The nurse assesses whether a home visit by a community health or home health nurse or referral to a community agency for families with special needs would be helpful. The importance of both the well-baby check and postpartum examination for the health of both woman and newborn is stressed. The nurse should determine if follow-up appointments have been made.

An increasing number of states have passed mandatory infant passenger restraint laws; however, in any setting or location, the nurse should verify that the parents have an infant car seat for use on discharge from the hospital. In circumstances where parents do not have a car seat and cannot afford to purchase one, a community car seat loan program may offer free or low-cost rental. The importance of using an infant car seat for the first ride home and consistently thereafter should be emphasized.

The nurse should verify before discharge that the woman has received any needed immunizations (see Table 28-3) and that the neonate has been screened for inborn metabolic errors (see Chapter 31). The nurse should also emphasize that the woman can call the nursing staff on the postpartum unit or at the newborn nursery at any hour if she has a question or concern.

Expected Outcomes

- The woman states the importance of using a proper neonatal car seat.
- The woman discusses the importance of keeping check-up appointments for both the neonate and herself.
- The woman records a phone number to call if she has any questions or concerns.

Teaching for Effective Self-Care

The new parents' many learning needs must be met for them to care effectively for themselves, their newborn, and their family. Many postpartum units have teaching checklists to guide the nurse (such an example is given earlier in the chapter). Many of these points have already been discussed in detail in this chapter. In addition, each parent should be offered teaching in all aspects of infant care, as described in Chapter 31. Some self-care topics of particular interest and importance to new mothers are discussed here.

Postpartum Rest and Exercise

The postpartum nurse should explain to the woman that going home with a newborn can be exhausting, especially with family and friends flocking to visit. The woman will have more demands than usual placed on her and may find it difficult to rest, particularly if she has other youngsters who need attention and care. She needs increased rest periods because of her increased activity level and the energy requirements for tissue healing. It is important the woman eat nutritious meals and drink adequate quantities of fluids. Without proper nourishment, tissue healing and full postpartum recovery will be delayed.

The nurse should stress that vigorous exercise is to be avoided until after lochia has ceased. An increase in lochial flow or reappearance of lochia after it has ceased is an indication that the activity undertaken may have been too demanding. However, gentle stretching and postnatal exercises, walking, and other physical activities may be introduced in the second or third week. Sample exercises are illustrated in Figure 28-9. Exercise videotapes such as the program created by the American College of Obstetrics entitled "Postnatal Exercise Program" discuss and demonstrate appropriate postpartum exercises.

The general rule should be avoidance of fatigue and

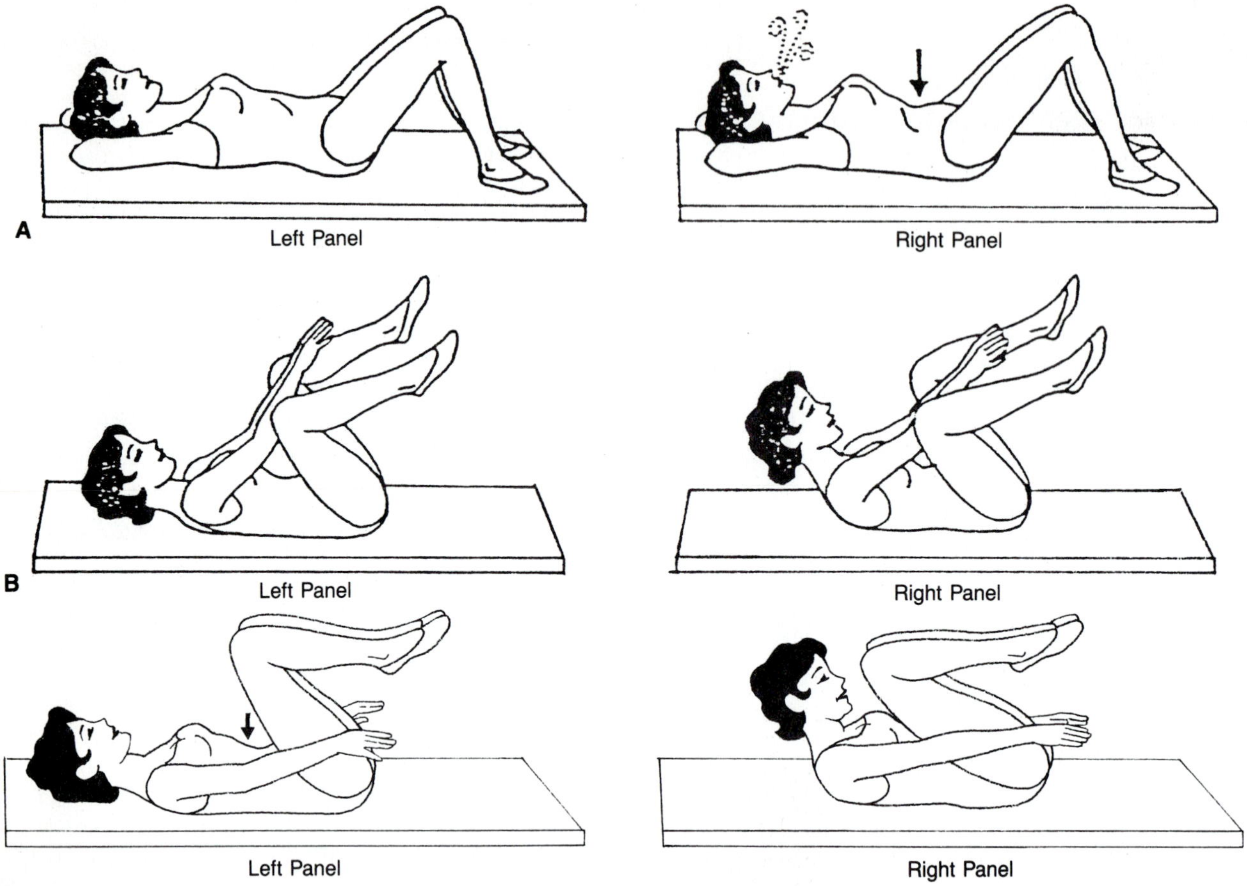

Figure 28-9.
Simple exercises help the postpartum woman strengthen her abdominal muscles and flatten her stomach. They should be done on an exercise mat or a carpeted surface. *A:* The woman lies on her back with her knees bent. Her feet are flat on the floor and placed the same distance apart as her hips (*left panel*). The woman breathes out as she pulls in her stomach hard and presses the small of her back firmly to the floor while raising her buttocks slightly. She breathes in and releases 20 times (*right panel*). *B:* In a second exercise she lies on her back with her knees bent toward her chest. With her knees in a comfortable open position, she raises her arms between her knees (*left panel*). She curls her head and shoulder off the floor and holds for 3 seconds. She lowers and repeats these movements. She may gradually increase the number of times she repeats this exercise (*right panel*). *C:* In a third ecxercise, the woman pulls in her stomach hard with her back pressed firmly to the floor. She brings both bent knees toward her chest and raises her arms slightly at her side (*left panel*). With her chin on her chest, she curls her head and shoulders off the floor, bringing her forehead toward her knees. She rolls back to starting position. Again she starts with a few of these rolls and gradually increases them (*right panel*).

muscle strain. The nurse can provide a brochure that illustrates specific exercises that can be done in the early postpartum period to strengthen the abdominal muscles and promote relaxation and flexibility. These exercises can be started on the first day after delivery. Each should initially be done five times twice a day in a slow, smooth, and relaxing manner and should never make the woman feel sore or tired. The number of repetitions can be gradually increased until the woman feels stronger and, in 4 to 5 weeks, is ready to resume more active exercise. The postcesarean woman should consult her physician regarding an exercise regimen to meet her needs.

Kegel Exercises. Nurses frequently instruct new mothers in the use of Kegel exercises (see Chapter 18) to strengthen pelvic floor muscles after childbirth. It is commonly believed that these exercises increase sexual response, decrease stress incontinence, and speed the recovery of the perineum after vaginal birth. A study by a team of investigators (Samples, Dougherty, Abrams, & Batich, 1988), including two nurses, found that the circumvaginal muscles of women delivered vaginally are significantly weaker that those muscles in nulliparous women or women who had cesarean deliveries. This study of 98 women failed to find improved muscle strength in women who reported doing Kegel exercises. Although there is question as to the reason for this finding and more research is needed, the investigators suggest that nurses recommending Kegel exercises to their patients do so with the understanding that not all women may derive equal benefit from their use.

Rh Immune Globulin (RhIgG)

Trade Name: Rhogam

Dosage: 300–500 μg IM.

Action: Gamma globulin given to Rh negative women who may have been exposed to Rh positive red blood cells. Provides passive immunity by suppressing active antibody response and formation of anti-Rh_O(D) in Rh negative individuals.

Side Effects: Mild temperature elevation, soreness at injection site.

Nursing Implications: Should be given within 72 h of delivery if woman is Rh negative and titer negative, and infant is Rh positive with negative Coombs' test. Should be given prophylactically at 28 weeks of gestation in unsensitized Rh negative woman and following spontaneous or induced abortion or termination of ectopic pregnancy.

Terbutaline sulfate

Trade Name: Brethine, Brethaire

Dosage: 10 μg/min IV titrated up to a maximum of 80 μg/min. Continue at minimum effective dose until uterine activity ceases, then switch to 2.5–5 mg PO q 4–6 h or 0.5 mg/h subcutaneously by continuous infusion.

Action: Synthetic beta-mimetic agent that inhibits myometrial contractility by stimulating beta-adrenergic receptors. Caution is needed in administering this drug to patients with hypertension, cardiac arrhythmias, and diabetes mellitus.

Side Effects: Effects are dose related. CNS: anxiety, nervousness, tremors, headache, lightheadedness. CV: chest tightness, palpitation, maternal and fetal tachycardia, pulmonary edema. GI: nausea, vomiting, diarrhea. May cause sweating, muscle cramps, increased blood glucose, increased free fatty acids.

Nursing Implications: Verify dosages; errors in placement of decimal points can be fatal. Cardiovascular side effects are more common when drug given by SC route. Check pulse and BP before each dose; a pulse rate of >120 bpm requires verification with physician to administer next dose. Monitor I&O closely.

Hydralazine hydrochloride

Trade Name: Apresoline

Dosage: 10–50 mg IM q 4–6 h, or 10–50 mg PO q.i.d., or 5–10 mg IV over 1 minute. Inject at 5- to 10-minute intervals until diastolic pressure is stable between 90 and 100 mm Hg.

Action: Antihypertensive agent that reduces BP by direct effect on vascular smooth muscles or arterial vessels, resulting in vasodilation. Cardiac output and renal and cerebral blood flow are improved. Onset of action in 20–30 min. Crosses placenta readily and is found in breast milk.

Side Effects: Headache, palpitation, tachycardia, orthostatic hypotension, dizziness, difficulty with urination, reduced hemoglobin and red blood cell count, rash, and urticaria.

(continued)

Carboprost tromethamine

Trade Name: Hemabate, Prostin/15M

Dosage: 250 μg (1 mL) IM repeated at 1.5–3.5-h intervals if indicated by uterine responses. Dosage may be increased to 500 μg (2 mL) if contractions are inadequate; maximum total dosage: 12 mg.

Action: Synthetic analogue of prostaglandin F_2-alpha with longer duration. Stimulates myometrial contractions during pregnancy. Used to induce abortion between 13–20 weeks' gestation. May also be used for refractory postpartum bleeding due to uterine atony.

Side Effects: Nausea, vomiting, diarrhea, flushing, cough, fever, chills, headache; all transient and reversible when drug is stopped. May cause bronchospasm and wheezing. Contraindicated in patients with cardiovascular disease, asthma, renal disease, or hepatic disease.

(continued)

Bromocryptine mesylate

Trade Name: Parlodel

Dosage: 2.5 mg tablet, b.i.d. × 14 d.

Action: A dopamine receptor agonist that reduces elevated serum prolactin levels needed for lactation. Used to suppress lactation in the postpartum period.

Side Effect: Orthostatic hypotension, headache, nausea and vomiting, lightheadedness, CVA, acute MI. Contraindicated in women with history of coronary artery disease or CV disease. Patient may have rebound breast engorgement and pain following drug withdrawal.

Nursing Implications: Medication should not be started until 4 h after delivery. Assist patient with first ambulation after medication is begun. Instruct patient to make position changes slowly and to dangle legs 1–2 min before ambulating. Administer medication with meals or milk to reduce GI side effects. Contraindicated in women with hypersensitivity to ergot alkaloids.

Ibuprofen

Trade Name: Advil, Motrin, Nuprin

Dosage: Adult: 400–800 mg PO q.i.d., or t.i.d., to a maximum of 3200 mg/d.

Action: Nonsteroidal antiinflammatory agent with antipyretic and analgesic properties. Blocks prostaglandin synthesis and inhibits inflammatory cell chemotaxis. May increase lithium toxicity. Causes fewer GI side effects than aspirin. Used for relief of discomfort due to postpartum uterine cramping and perineal pain.

Side Effects: Heartburn, nausea, dizziness, occult blood loss, thrombocytopenia, decreased hemoglobin and hematocrit.

Nursing Implications: Absorption rate reduced when administered with food; should be given on an empty stomach 1 h before or 2 after meals. Aspirin or acetaminophen should not be given concurrently with ibuprofen.

Magnesium sulfate ($MgSO_4$)

Trade Name: Epsom Salts

Dosage: Adults: Loading Dose: 4 g in 50 mL D_5W slow IV infusion × 15 to 30 min. Maintenance dose: 1–4 g/h IV (20–40 g in 1000 mL IV solution).

Action: CNS depressant; smooth, skeletal, and cardiac muscle depressant. Decreases circulating acetylcholine and may reduce seizure activity or potential. Is not an antihypertensive agent. Also used as a tocolytic to suppress preterm labor.

Side Effects: Decrease in uterine contractility. Hypermagnesemia and hypocalcemia, as seen in flushing, sweating, extreme thirst, muscle weakness, depressed or absent reflexes, complete heart block, respiratory paralysis.

Nursing Implications: Constant observation required when administering IV. Check BP and pulse q 10–15 min or more often. Test patellar or other reflexes before administering drug. Monitor plasma magnesium levels (normal therapeutic range: 4–7.5 mEq/L). Plasma levels greater than 4 mEq/L associated with depressed tendon reflexes. Check respiratory rate, patellar reflexes, and urinary output carefully. If output $< 40–50$ mL/h, patellar reflexes absent, or respiratory rate < 12 breaths/min, notify physician.

Meperidine hydrochloride

Trade Name: Demerol HCl

Dosage: Postpartum: 25–50 mg IV, 50–100 mg IM, or SC, or 50–100 mg PO q 3–4 h. Obstetric analgesia: 25–50 mg IV; 50–100 mg IM.

Action: Synthetic morphine narcotic that produces analgesia, euphoria, sedation. Relieves moderate to severe pain for 2–4 h. May be used as preoperative sedation, postoperative sedation, and obstetric analgesia.

Side Effects: Euphoria, dry mouth, dizziness, hypotension, nausea and vomiting, sweating, urticaria, constipation, respiratory depression. Toxicity: agitation, hallucinations, convulsions, cardiac arrest.

(continued)

Methylergonovine maleate

Trade Name: Methergine

Dosage: For postpartum bleeding: 0.2–0.3 mg IM or PO. To prevent uterine atony and postpartum hemorrhage and promote uterine involution: 0.2–0.4 mg PO t.i.d. until involution is progressing.

Action: Ergot alkaloid effectively stimulates uterine contractions. IM route primarily used to control postpartum hemorrhage.

Side Effects: May cause painful uterine contractions. Usually produces minimal side effects, but can be toxic if dose is excessive. Toxicity: nausea, vomiting, diarrhea, headache, weak pulse, dizziness. May cause elevation in BP, especially if patient has hypertension, or had regional anesthesia or vasoconstrictor medications before delivery.

(continued)

Oxytocin

Trade Name: Pitocin, Syntocinon

Dosage: May be given IV, IM, SC, or intranasally. Slow IV infusion is most common. For induction of labor: 1 mL (10 U) in 1 L infusion solution, to be infused at a rate starting at 1–2 mU/min. For postpartum bleeding: 10–40 U added to 500–1000 mL infusion solution, or 10 U IM.

Action: Stimulates uterine smooth muscle contractions and can reduce uterine blood flow. Milk ejection reflex stimulated with intranasal route. Can be used to induce or augment labor when contractions are irregular or dysfunctional. May be administered to control postpartum hemorrhage or to stimulate let-down reflex. Is contraindicated in fetal distress, pregnancy-induced hypertension, or women at risk for uterine rupture.

Side Effects: Prolonged therapy may result in water intoxication and possible maternal death from pulmonary edema. Overstimulation of uterus during labor may result in tetanic contractions, uterine rupture, amniotic fluid embolism, and fetal hypoxia.

(continued)

Metronidazole

Trade Name: Flagyl

Dosage: Adult: 2 g once, or 250 mg PO t.i.d., or 500 mg b.i.d. × 7 d.

Action: Synthetic compound with direct trichomonacidal and amebicidal action against *Trichomonas vaginalis* and *Giardia lamblia*. Also used to treat bacterial vaginosis.

Side Effects: Rash, urticaria, pruritus, polyuria, cystitis, nausea, and vomiting. Contraindicated in blood dyscrasias and first trimester of pregnancy.

Nursing Implications: Give before or after meals to reduce GI distress. Therapy in second or third trimester should be given over 7-d period. Advise patient that alcohol ingestion may cause an Antabuse-type reaction for up to 24 h after ingestion of medication.

Hepatitis B Vaccine

Trade Name: Engerix B

Dosage: Infant: 3 doses of 0.5 mL given IM at birth, 1 mo and 6 mo. Adult: 3 doses of 1 mL given IM with 1 mo between first and second dose, and 4 mo between second and third dose.

Action: Recommended 3-dose regimen produces active immunity to hepatitis B infection by inducing protective antibody formation. In healthy individuals, immunity last about 5 y. If given during incubation period after possible exposure, vaccine will not prevent infection. Safety for use during pregnancy and during lactation not established.

Side Effects: Mild, local tenderness at injection site, local inflammatory responses. Fever, malaise, fatigue, headache, dizziness, and faintness, all transient.

(continued)

Nursing Implications: During labor, monitor woman and fetus to detect signs of distress. Woman should never be left unattended during oxytocin infusion. Fetal monitor strip, FHR, and maternal VS should be checked q 10–15 min. Frequency, duration, and strength of uterine contractions should be recorded. Infusion should be discontinued if uterine hyperactivity or fetal distress is evident. During postpartum period, monitor effectiveness of drug by assessing uterine tone. Rate of IV infusion may be increased with physician order if uterine atony occurs.

Nursing Implications: Verify effectiveness by monitoring uterine tone; some patients with calcium deficiencies may not respond to medication. Monitor amount of bleeding, number of pad changes, and presence of clots; inform physician as to status of uterine contraction and bleeding. Contraindicated with hypertension or severe renal or hepatic disease.

Nursing Implications: Offer parents of newborn a pamphlet on medication, and offer explanations as needed. Medication should *not* be administered IV or intradermally. Should be given IM in the anterolateral thigh for infants and deltoid muscle in adults. Epinephrine should be available to treat possible anaphylaxis.

Abdominal Breathing. To perform abdominal breathing, the woman is in a supine position with legs slightly bent. She inhales slowly through her nose, letting her abdomen rise, then slowly exhales through her mouth, flattening her abdomen by contracting her abdominal muscles.

Head and Shoulder Raising. The woman begins head and shoulder raising in a supine position with legs bent and arms outstretched toward knees. She tucks in her chin, lifts her head and shoulders slowly, and holds to a count of five. She then slowly lowers her shoulders and head to the beginning position. The head and shoulders are lifted only as far as needed to clear the shoulder blades from the flat surface.

Arm Raises. For arm raises, the woman is in a supine position with legs bent and arms extended out from her sides at a 90-degree angle. With arms extended, the patient lifts them slowly to the center above the body and then slowly lowers them to the starting position.

Expected Outcome

- The postpartum woman states diet and exercise guidelines appropriate to restoring optimal health and prepregnant appearance.

Supporting Sexuality

The nurse allows the woman to express concerns she may have about sexuality. The nurse may use an opening such as "Most women have concerns about sex after they have had a baby. What are your concerns?" This communicates that the nurse is supportive and willing to listen. During such a discussion, the nurse can provide information as well as allow the patient to express her concerns. Suggested guidelines concerning postpartum sexuality are given in the Teaching Considerations display.

Each woman and her partner should receive teaching about contraception during the postpartum period. Contraceptive teaching should include a review of information about the available methods so that the woman can make an

Teaching Considerations

Sexual Activity During The Postpartum Period

The nurse can use the following points in teaching the postpartum couple

- Sexual intercourse may be resumed around 3 to 4 weeks postpartum for both vaginal and cesarean deliveries.
- Sexual intercourse should not be resumed until vaginal bleeding has stopped, to prevent introduction of infection at the placental site.
- Healing of episiotomy and perineum may be checked by inserting a finger or tampon into the vagina.
- Sexual arousal may cause milk to leak from the breasts. (Nursing the neonate before sexual activity or wearing a bra with absorbent pads during lovemaking may help this problem.)
- Contraceptive cream or a natural vegetable oil (safflower or soy, for example) may be used if additional lubrication is necessary. (K-Y jelly drys out rapidly and turns to little balls of dried lubricant.)
- Longer periods of foreplay will encourage lubrication.
- Couple should communicate openly.
- Alternative forms of sexual expression (mutual masturbation, massage, oral) may be used.
- Baths should not be taken for 2 or 3 weeks to avoid spreading bacteria from other parts of the body to the vaginal opening. (Showers allowed.)
- Kegel exercises may be used immediately after birth, whenever urinating, and frequently during the day.
- Sitz baths 3 times a day help heal the episiotomy scar.
- The perineum is examined with a good light and mirror within a few days of delivery and then again 3 weeks later to reassure yourself that it is healing.
- If something doesn't look right, contact a physician.
- Intercourse and your body do return to "normal."
- A bra is worn 24 hours a day as soon as possible after delivery to help decrease engorgement.
- Partner is advised not to put pressure on breasts while they're sensitive, especially during the night when the infant is sleeping for longer periods without feeding.
- Realistic priorities are set. (Arrange schedule so that you nap when the infant does.)
- Nap or lie down and get off your feet at least 30 minutes every day.
- If you're depressed, help from friends and family is necessary. (Get further help if the depression lasts longer than 3 days.)
- When the infant is weaned, your sex drive will return in full force.
- Feeding should not be rushed just before lovemaking because neonate may sense change in feeding pattern and become irritable or cry.
- The infant can be placed in another room or behind a screen during lovemaking to provide sense of privacy.
- Music will soothe the infant during lovemaking.

informed decision before her postpartum checkup, usually scheduled at 4 to 6 weeks after delivery. Closely spaced pregnancies (1 year or less apart) put a greater stress on the woman's body and place her at slightly higher obstetric risk. The mother may want to consider this if she is planning another pregnancy soon.

Expected Outcome

- By discharge, the postpartum couple understands various methods of contraception, as evidenced by knowledgeable discussion and ability to state one method appropriate to their personal needs and cultural/religious beliefs.

• • Evaluation

Evaluating the effects of specific nursing interventions and the overall quality of postpartum nursing care requires that the nurse identify specific objectives in her plan of care for each patient and then judge outcomes against those objectives. Many interventions in the postpartum period are focused on support and patient teaching. The long-term effects of patient teaching are more difficult to evaluate than are such easily observable outcomes as improved uterine tone or decreased perineal discomfort.

Evaluation of postpartum nursing care is complicated by the fact that postpartum stays have shortened. The postpartum nurse is challenged to deliver more thorough and comprehensive family-centered care in less time. However, maternity nurses continue to meet that challenge and contribute to the health and well-being of new parents and their newborns long after the excitement and change of the postpartum period. Ongoing evaluation by nurses is accomplished in the following ways:

- Community or home health nurse visits
- Early discharge follow-up visits and telephone calls provided by hospital or health maintenance organization
- Early parenting education and support groups
- Nurse midwife postnatal examinations at 4 to 6 weeks
- Pediatric nurse practitioner well-baby assessments (ongoing)
- Postpartum nurse home visits provided as special service of private physician care or a hospital early discharge program

Nursing process during the postpartum period is guided by a family-centered philosophy. The nurse assesses both individual and family adaptations. Although the woman's physiologic status takes priority during the postbirth period, the psychological condition of the new mother and her partner are crucial to the physical and emotional well-being of the neonate. Ongoing assessments aid the nurse in the identification of additional nursing diagnoses and in determining discharge planning. Development of the discharge plan and discharge teaching plan is based on nursing diagnoses. For the healthy woman and well neonate, nursing diagnoses that indicate effective adaptations and appropriate health maintenance may be identified and used in planning care. The postpartum nurse must be skilled in routine physiologic care and knowledge of minor and life-threatening complications. After the woman's condition has stabilized, the focus of care incorporates strategies to facilitate psychological adaptations of the woman, her partner, and the family unit. Nursing activities include both emotional support and hands-on teaching to prepare the woman and new family for neonatal care. Evaluation is focused on whether expected outcomes have been achieved. When stated outcomes are not met, the nurse begins more assessments to identify new diagnoses and interventions.

Chapter Summary

The postpartum period offers a unique opportunity for the nurse to observe individual and family adaptation to the arrival of a new infant. The nurse provides expert knowledge, assistance, and support to the woman, father or partner, and other family members as they learn about the newborn and take on the responsibility of infant care. The mother's physiologic restoration is of particular importance. Nursing assessment and intervention focus on the monitoring of normal physiologic changes, promotion of rest and comfort, and promotion of successful breastfeeding, if the woman so chooses. Nursing assessment and intervention are also directed at identifying and meeting the educational needs of families to promote optimal individual and family adaptation and effective self-care. Teaching is of major importance in postpartum care. The nurse's sensitivity, knowledge, and ability to teach effectively can contribute to a relatively problem-free postpartum transition for most families.

Study Questions

1. *What significant deviations in maternal vital signs indicate complications in the postpartum recovery process?*
2. *What immediate actions must the nurse implement when postpartum uterine atony is identified?*
3. *How can the nurse facilitate restoration of bladder function during the postpartum period?*
4. *How does the treatment of breast engorgement differ between the breastfeeding and bottle-feeding woman?*
5. *What methods are commonly used to suppress lactation?*
6. *What strategies can the nurse use to facilitate the parent–newborn attachment process?*
7. *How can the nurse promote restoration of pulmonary and gastrointestinal function in the post-cesarean patient?*
8. *What are the classic signs of deep vein thrombosis?*
9. *What changes in family roles and relationships can be expected in the postpartum period?*
10. *What are essential components of discharge teaching for self-care in the postpartum period?*

References

Ament, L. (1990). Maternal tasks of the puerperium reidentified. *Journal* of Obstetric, *Gynecologic, and Neonatal Nursing*, *19*(4), 330.

Anderberg, G. (1988). Initial acquaintance and attachment behavior of siblings with the newborn. *Journal of Obstetric, Gynecologic, and Neonatal Nursing*, *17*(1), 49.

Atrash, H., Koonin, L., Lawson, H., Franks, A. & Smith J. (1990). Maternal mortality in the United States 1979–1986. *Obstetrics and Gynecology*, *76*(6),1055.

Beck, C., Reynolds, M., & Rutkowski, P. (1992). Maternity blues and postpartum depression. *Journal of Obstetric, Gynecologic, and Neonatal Nursing*, *21*(4), 287.

Blackburn, S., & Loper, D. (1992). *Maternal, fetal, and neonatal physiology*. Philadelphia: W. B. Saunders.

Brazelton, T. B., Tronick, E., Adamson, L. (1975). *Parent—infant interac*tion. Ciba Foundation Symposium 33. Amsterdam: Elsevier Publishing Co.

Condon, W., & Sander, L. (1974). Neonate movement is synchronized with adult speech: Interactional participation and language acquisition. *Science*, *183*, 99.

Creasy, R., & Resnik, R. (1989). *Maternal-fetal medicine* (2nd ed.). Philadelphia: W. B. Saunders.

Culp, R., & Osofsky, H. (1989). Effects of cesarean delivery on parental depression, marital adjustment, and mother-infant interaction. *Birth*, *16*(2), 53.

DeCasper, A., & Fifer, W. (1980). The fetal sound environment. *Science*, *208*, 1173.

Ferketich, S., & Mercer, R. (1989). Men's health status during pregnancy and early fatherhood. *Research in Nursing and Health*, *12*, 137.

Fishbein, E. (1990). Predicting paternal involvement with a newborn by atitude toward women's roles. *Health Care for Women International*, *11*, 109.

Flaherty, M., Facteau, L., & Garver, P. (1987). Grandmother functions in multigenerational families: An exploratory study of black adolescent mothers and their infants. *Maternal-Child Nursing Journal*, *16*(1), 61.

Fortier, J. (1988). The relationship of vaginal and cesarean births to father-infant attachment. *Journal of Obstetric, Gynecologic, and Neonatal Nursing*, *17*(2), 128.

Gardner, D., & Campbell, B. (1991). Assessing postpartum fatigue. *American Journal of Maternal Child Nursing*, *16*(5), 264.

Gerbasi, F. R., Bottoms, S., Farag, A., & Mammen, E. F. (1990). Changes in hemostatsis activity during delivery and the immediate postpartum period. *American Journal of Obstetrics and Gynecology*, *162*(5), 1158.

Greenberg, M., & Morris, N. (1974). Engrossment: The newborn's impact upon the father. *American Journal of Orthopsychiatry*, *44*, 520.

Harper, R., Quintin, A., Freynin, I., . (1991). Observations on the postpartum shivering phenomenon. *Journal of Reproductive Medicine*, *36*(11), 803.

Horn, M., & Manion, J. (1985). Creative grandparenting. *Journal of Obstetric, Gynecologic, and Neonatal Nursing*, *14*(3), 233.

Jordan, P. (1990). Laboring for relevance: Expectant and new fatherhood. *Nursing Resarch*, *39*, 11.

Keefe, M. (1988). The impact of infant rooming-in on maternal sleep at night. *Journal of Obstetric, Gynecologic, and Neonatal Nursing*, *17*(2), 122.

Klaus, M., & Kennell, J. (1982). *Parent-infant bonding* (2nd ed.). St. Louis: C. V. Mosby.

Lauwers, J., & Woessner, C. (1990). *Chemical agents and breast milk*. Garden City Park, NY: Avery Publishing Group Inc.

Lentz, M., & Killien, M. (1991). Are you sleeping? Sleep patterns during postpartum hospitalization. *Journal of Perinatal and Neonatal Nursing*, *4*(4), 30.

Mead-Bennett, E. (1990). The relationship of primigravid sleep experience and select moods on the first postpartum day. *Journal of Obstetric, Gynecologic, and Neonatal Nursing*, *19*(2), 146.

Mercer, R., & Ferketich, S. (1990). Predictors of parental attachment during early parenthhod. *Journal of Advanced Nursing*, *15*, 268.

NAACOG. (1989). *Mother–baby care*. OGN Nursing Practice Resource. Washington DC: Author.

Rubin, R. (1963a). Puerperal change. *Nursing Outlook*, *9*, 753.

Rubin, R. (1963b). Maternal touch. *Nursing Outlook*, *11*, 828.

Rustia, J., & Abbot, D. (1990). Predicting paternal role enactment. *Western Journal of Nursing Research*, *12*(2), 145.

Samples, J., Dougherty, M., Abrams, R., & Batich, C. (1988). The dynamic characteristics of the circumvaginal muscles. *Journal of Obstetric, Gynecologic, and Neonatal Nursing*, *17*, 194.

Tribotti, S., . (1988). Nursing diagnoses for the postpartum woman. *Journal of Obstetric, Gynecologic, and Neonatal Nursing*, *17*, 410.

Tulman, L., & Fawcett, J. (1990a). Return of functional ability after childbirth. *Nursing Research*, *37*(1), 77.

Tulman, L., & Fawcett, J. (1990b). Functional status during pregnancy and the postpartum: A framework for research. *Image*, *22*(3), 191.

Van de Perre, P., Simonon, A., Msellati, P., Hitimana, D., Vaira, D., Bazubaquira, A., et al. (1992). *Acute pain management in adults: Operative procedures*. Rockville, MD: US Department of Health and Human Services.

Suggested Readings

Affonso, D., Lovett, S., Paul, S., & Sheptak S. (1990). A standardized interview that differentiates pregnancy and postpartum symptoms from perinatal clinical depression. *Birth*, *17*(3), 121.

Bertelsen, C., & Auerbach, K. (1987). Nutrition and breastfeeding: *The cultural connection*. Lactation Consultant Series, Unit 11 LaLeche League International. Garden City Park, NY: Avery Publishing Group Inc.

Jordan, P., & Wall, V. (1990). Breastfeeding and fathers: Illiminating the darker side. *Birth*, *17*(4), 210.

Kearney, M., Cronenwett, L., & Barrett, J. (1990). Breast-feeding problems in the first week postpartum. *Nursing Research*, *39*(2), 90.

Konrad, C. J. (1987). Helping mothers integrate the birth experience. *American Journal of Maternal Child Nursing*, *12*, 268.

Liller, K., Kent, E., & McDermott, R. (1991). Postpartum patients' knowledge, risk perceptions, and behavior pertaining to childhood injuries. *Journal of Nurse-Midwifery*, *36*(6), 355.

NAACOG. (1991). *Facilitating breastfeeding*. OGN Nursing Practice Resource. Washington DC: Author.

Pedersen, B., Blakstad, M., & Bergan, T. (1990). Bacteriuria in the puerperium. *American Journal of Obstetrics and Gynecology*, *162*(3), 792.

Rubin, R. (1984). *Maternal identity and the maternal experience*. New York: Springer Publishing.

Templeton, J., Edgil, A., & Bragg, D. (1988). Reva Rubin revisited. *Journal of Obstetric, Gynecologic, and Neonatal Nursing*, *17*(6), 394.

Walker, M., & Driscoll, J. (1989). Sore nipples: The new mother's nemesis. *Journal of Obstetric, Gynecologic, and Neonatal Nursing*, *18*(4), 260.

Wiley, K., & Grohar, J. (1987). Human immunodeficiency virus and precautions for obstetric, gynecologic and neonatal nurses. *Journal of Obstetric, Gynecologic, and Neonatal Nursing*, *17*, 165.

CHAPTER 29

Postpartum Complications

Learning Objectives

After studying the material in this chapter, the student will be able to:

- Identify the most common complications that occur during the postpartum period.
- Describe predisposing factors for infections of the reproductive and urinary tracts and modes of entry and diffusion of infections.
- Discuss common causes of early and late postpartum hemorrhage.
- Explain treatment modalities and common procedures used in the management of postpartum complications.
- Discuss psychological and social problems encountered in postpartum women experiencing complications.
- Identify the goals of nursing care, appropriate nursing interventions, and their rationale for women with specific postpartum problems.

Key Terms

bacteriuria	oliguria
curettage	parametritis
cystitis	peritonitis
embolus	placenta accreta
endometritis	placenta increta
hematuria	placenta percreta
mastitis	postpartum infection

Most families anticipate the period immediately after birth with enthusiasm and excitement. The woman can put behind her the months of waiting, the minor discomforts of pregnancy, and normal concerns about childbirth. The postpartum period is, however, a time of profound physical and psychological adaptation. Even in ideal circumstances, family members experience some sense of disequilibrium. When problems develop during the postpartum period, people can feel overwhelmed.

Serious medical problems during the postpartum period have an impact on individual coping as well as on early family formation, breastfeeding, and the woman's future health status. The woman's physical problems may make it impossible for her to focus on the needs of the neonate or the early maternal–newborn acquaintance process. Family members may experience acute anxiety because of their concerns regarding the woman's condition, newborn care requirements, and the costs of medical care. These stressors may kindle a family crisis.

This chapter discusses the most common and most life-threatening postpartum complications. The order of the topics reflects the prevalence of the complications: problems discussed in the first section are the most common, and those described toward the end of the chapter represent less frequent complications. Emphasis is placed on nursing care that supports the woman's physiologic and psychological functioning. Nursing care of the high-risk family is discussed in detail in Chapter 25.

Nursing Process

The nurse uses the nursing process to identify postpartum complications, establish appropriate nursing diagnoses, plan and implement individualized care, and evaluate the woman's responses to medical treatment and nursing interventions. The goals of nursing care during this period are to support physiologic integrity when complications arise and to normalize the emotional environment so that successful individual and family adaptations can occur (Long, 1991).

• • Assessment

Assessment of the woman begins with the identification of significant risk factors for postpartum complications. The nurse must review the prenatal and intrapartum records for evidence of preexisting obstetric or medical problems. Table 29-1 lists common postpartum complications associated with prenatal and intrapartum problems. Difficulties that develop in the immediate postbirth period may predispose the woman to ongoing health problems in the later postpartum period. Finally, ongoing assessments until the time of discharge, and in some cases, after the woman returns home, are crucial in the early recognition and appropriate treatment of postpartum complications.

Table 29-1. Risk Factors That May Cause Development of Postpartum Complications

Predisposing Problems	Postpartum Complication
Prenatal Period	
Obstetric Problems	
Placenta previa	Hemorrhage, anemia, UTI
Pyelonephritis	UTI
Medical Problems	
Cardiac disease	Congestive heart failure
Cardiac valve disease	Bacterial endocarditis
Anemia	Anemia, infection
Substance abuse	Depression, parenting disorders
Thromboembolisms	Thrombophlebitis, pulmonary embolism
Depression	Depression
Intrapartum Period	
Abruptio placenta	Hemorrhage, DIC, anemia
PIH	Postpartum PIH, seizures, DIC
Labor dystocia: prolonged labor	Infection, uterine infection, uterine subinvolution
Labor dystocia: precipitous labor	Lacerations, hematomas, uterine atony
Prolonged rupture of membranes	Infection: endometritis, parametritis, uterine subinvolution
Chorioamnionitis	Infection: endometritis, parametritis, uterine subinvolution
Polyhydramnios	Uterine atony, amniotic fluid embolus, postpartum hemorrhage
Multiple fetuses	Uterine atony, lacerations, postpartum hemorrhage
Preterm labor with prolonged bedrest	Muscular weakness, delayed recovery of physical strength
Forceps-assisted delivery	Lacerations, hematomas, infection
Emergency cesarean birth	Pneumonia, paralytic ileus, Thrombophlebitis

DIC, disseminated intravascular coagulation; PIH, pregnancy-induced hypertension; UTI, urinary tract infection.

• • Nursing Diagnosis

Based on assessments the nurse conducts during the postpartum period, appropriate nursing diagnoses are established for the woman with physical or psychological complications.

- Activity Intolerance related to infection, anemia, surgery, or cardiac disease
- Altered Family Processes related to postpartum complications
- Anxiety related to postpartum complication or treatment of problems
- Altered Parenting related to postpartum complications
- Decreased Cardiac Output related to hemorrhage, septic shock, or cardiac disease
- Grieving related to the development of postpartum complications
- Hyperthermia related to infection
- Ineffective Breastfeeding related to mastitis or other postpartum complications
- High Risk for Infection related to prolonged labor, prolonged rupture of membranes, or invasive procedures

• • Planning and Implementation

The nurse plans care to meet the individualized needs of the woman with postpartum complications. The primary focus of care, even in the case of acute psychological disorders, is to achieve and maintain physiologic stability. Close collaboration with the medical team is essential to coordinate nursing care with medical therapy and other services such as respiratory care and physical therapy. Nursing actions that promote rest and physical recovery are of primary importance.

When the woman is too ill to participate in the planning process, the partner or other family members should be included. The contribution of the family to the woman's recovery is frequently overlooked when highly technical nursing care is required. The desires of the father or partner regarding newborn care must be ascertained. Arrangements must be made to accommodate family member involvement with the neonate until the mother is well enough to assume neonatal care activities.

While focusing on the woman's physical needs, the nurse must also plan strategies to provide ongoing emotional support. Anxiety regarding her physical condition and disappointment about the quality of the early postpartum period may precipitate depression in some women. Many women with postpartum complications may demonstrate the classic signs of grieving—emotional shock, denial, anger, and sorrow. A full discussion of the grieving process is described in Chapter 25. The nurse must remain sensitive to the woman's emotional needs and encourage her to express her concerns and feelings.

• • Evaluation

When postpartum complications occur, constant revision of the nursing care plan is essential. Ongoing evaluation of expected outcomes is essential to make appropriate adjustments in the plan. If medical and nursing care is effective, the woman will achieve physiologic stability and demonstrate increasing interest in assuming self-care and newborn care activities. This may take hours, days, or weeks to achieve. In rare cases, the woman may experience permanent disability as a result of severe problems. An essential aspect of the evaluation process includes determining the woman's progress in adapting to the parenting role. This may require follow-up care by a community or home health nurse. The nurse's role in support of parenting is presented in Chapter 25.

Most women with postpartum complications experience threats to physiologic integrity. Others may suffer from profound psychological disequilibrium. Regardless of the nature of the problem, the maternity nurse uses the nursing process to assess the woman's status, identify complications, and provide both immediate and ongoing care. The woman's and family's ultimate perceptions of the postpartum period will be strongly influenced by the quality of nursing care. The skilled nurse can ameliorate the adverse effects of postpartum illness and enhance family adaptations by using a family-centered approach to care.

Postpartum Hemorrhage

Postpartum hemorrhage is classically defined as a blood loss of more than 500 mL after birth. This complication is classified as *early*, occurring within the first 24 hours after birth, or *late*, occurring between 24 hours postbirth and before the sixth week postpartum. Most women enter labor with an expanded blood volume and are able to recover from a limited blood loss at delivery. Other women, however, such as those with anemia or who have preeclampsia accompanied by a decreased intravascular compartment volume, are less able to tolerate this insult.

Etiologic and Predisposing Factors

Knowledge of the risk factors in postpartum hemorrhage helps the nurse and the health care team prevent its occurrence, minimize its magnitude, plan treatment, and focus observation skills. Risk factors for early postpartum hemorrhage include uterine atony, trauma and lacerations, hematoma formation, and inversion of the uterus. Risk factors for late postpartum hemorrhage include retained placental fragments, bleeding disorders, and infection (discussed separately later in this chapter).

Diagnosis

In many cases, frank and profuse bleeding from the vagina is the first indicator of significant blood loss. This may be due to uterine atony or significant lacerations in the genital tract. These problems are discussed in detail later in this chapter. Recent studies suggest that visual estimates of blood loss may be grossly inaccurate (see Chapter 21). For this reason, many clinicians use laboratory data, particularly changes in the hemoglobin and hematocrit level, to make an accurate determination of blood loss (Luegenbiehl, 1991). Generally, a decrease in the hemoglobin value of 1.0 to 1.5 g/dL and a 4-point drop (2% to 4%) reflects a blood loss of 450 to 500 mL (ACOG, 1990; Combs, Murphy, & Laros, 1991). Other data that the nurse or physician may use to determine the extent of blood loss include counting perineal pads and weighing linen and linen protectors.

When postpartum hemorrhage occurs, compensatory mechanisms are initially activated, which result in sympathetic nervous system stimulation. The accompanying display lists signs and symptoms of early hypovolemia and compensated shock.

Less commonly, hemorrhage is concealed. Concealed hemorrhage is suspected when signs and symptoms of hypovolemia and compensated shock appear. Concealed hemorrhage is associated with lacerations in or rupture of the uterus. In this case, vaginal bleeding may be minimal, but large amounts of blood may be lost into the abdominal cavity. In other instances, significant amounts of blood (500 to 1000 mL) may accumulate in perineal, vaginal, or subperitoneal hematomas. Signs of hematoma are discussed later in this chapter.

Maternal Implications

Postpartum hemorrhage is life-threatening and requires immediate emergency treatment. Estimates of mortality from hemorrhagic complications of pregnancy account for approximately 13% of maternal deaths (Cunningham, MacDonald, & Gant, 1989). Postpartum hemorrhage contributes to maternal morbidity whenever it occurs. Uterine/placental blood flow at term is approximately 600 mL/min. For this reason, postpartum hemorrhage can rapidly lead to hypovolemia and shock (Luegenbiehl, 1991). Disseminated intravascular coagulopathy (DIC) may also develop with the loss of clotting factors when bleeding is severe.

Signs of Hypovolemia and Shock in Postpartum Hemorrhage

Early Signs in Compensated Shock

Tachypnea
Tachycardia
Air hunger
Elevation in blood pressure
Cool, clammy, pale skin
Sensations of anxiety or impending doom
Restlessness
Thirst
Decreased urine output

Late Signs in Uncompensated Shock

Tachypnea
Tachycardia
Hypotension
Pronounced pallor
Loss of consciousness
Oliguria

If the woman requires a blood transfusion, she is at increased risk for transfusion-related human immunodeficiency virus (HIV) or hepatitis B infection and transfusion reactions (Combs et al., 1991). Infection of the reproductive or genitourinary system is more likely due to depletion of white blood cells and other humoral immune factors. Although the risk of HIV transmission has been minimized with advances in blood screening, it has become common medical practice to limit transfusions to cases of significant blood loss.

Women with knowledge of transfusion risks may refuse blood replacement unless it is absolutely necessary. As a result, women with pronounced anemia (hemoglobin levels of 9 g/dL or less) will experience a prolonged convalescence. Orthostatic hypotension may occur, resulting in vertigo or syncope. Resumption of self-care and newborn care, breastfeeding, and the acquaintance process are often delayed. After discharge from the hospital, the woman who has had a postpartum hemorrhage commonly experiences greater levels of fatigue.

Treatment

A complete discussion of the treatment of hypovolemic shock is presented in Chapter 26. Major goals of therapy include the following:

- Establish IV access
- Provide blood and fluid replacement
- Improve oxygenation and tissue perfusion
- Correct the underlying problem

Initial treatment of hemorrhage will be determined in part by the underlying cause of bleeding. In cases of uterine atony, fundal massage and the administration of drugs to improve uterine tone is the primary focus of therapy. Ligation of torn vessels is imperative when lacerations cause the hemorrhage. Cervical curettage is necessary when retained placental fragments are responsible for excessive bleeding. A complete discussion of these complications and their treatment is presented later in this chapter.

Implications for Nursing Care

The nurse can provide optimum care and support to the woman by anticipating situations where excessive bleeding can occur. This requires identification of the major risk factors for postpartum hemorrhage. Table 29-1 lists prenatal and intrapartum problems that may result in postpartum bleeding.

The nurse plays a major role in the assessment and management of postpartum hemorrhage. Nursing responsibilities in the management of postpartum hemorrhage are described in Chapter 21. The nurse's role in the identification and treatment of hypovolemic shock is also described in detail in Chapter 26. Major goals of care include:

- Measuring blood loss
- Monitoring intake and output
- Accurately estimating blood loss
- Recognizing early signs of hypovolemia
- Monitoring vital signs and oxygen saturation levels
- Notifying the midwife or physician about bleeding in a timely manner
- Supporting the woman's cardiovascular status until medical help arrives
- Providing equipment, drugs, and other supplies required to treat hemorrhage
- Administering blood products, fluids, and drugs as ordered
- Providing emotional support to the woman

Early Postpartum Hemorrhage

Uterine Atony

Uterine atony accounts for 80% to 90% of cases of immediate postpartum hemorrhage (Cunningham et al., 1989). After delivery the uterus normally contracts, controlling bleeding by clamping severed blood vessels at the site of placental separation. This is referred to as "physiologic ligation." Inadequate myometrial contraction permits patency of the vessels and the free flow of blood.

Etiologic and Predisposing Factors

Predisposing factors in uterine atony include:

- Grand multiparity (five or more births)
- Previous history of uterine atony
- Overdistention of the uterus due to polyhydramnios, a large fetus, or multiple gestation
- Presence of uterine fibroids
- Chorioamnionitis during labor
- Precipitous labor and delivery
- Prolonged first or second stage of labor (or both)
- Oxytocin induction or augmentation of labor
- Magnesium sulfate infusion during labor and delivery
- Use of general anesthesia (halothane)
- Full bladder after delivery

Diagnosis

Vaginal bleeding associated with a soft or "boggy" uterus on abdominal palpation is indicative of uterine atony.

Maternal Implications

When uterine atony is diagnosed, the woman is subjected to firm fundal massage, and it may be necessary for the midwife or physician to perform a bimanual examination and massage. (See the Treatment section for an explanation of bimanual examination.) This is generally painful unless the woman has received an epidural or general anesthetic. Other uncomfortable or painful procedures may further increase her discomfort, such as the initiation of an IV line and the administration of drugs with unpleasant side-effects (such as Prostin/15M).

Pain is usually combined with fear as the woman realizes that complications have occurred. She may see large amounts of her blood on linen, surgical gowns, and sponges, further heightening her fear and distress. If blood loss is severe, the woman will be at increased risk for shock, infection, long-term anemia, and a delayed recovery. Her memory of the event may alter the entire postpartum experience as well as her plans for future childbearing.

Treatment

The physician or midwife will perform a bimanual uterine massage to control hemorrhage and stimulate contraction of the myometrium when uterine atony occurs (Fig. 29-1). A gloved hand is inserted into the vagina and advanced until the fingers make contact with the anterior uterus through the vaginal wall. The hand is then flexed into a fist, and the the anterior uterine wall is massaged with the knuckles. The palm of the other hand is simultaneously placed on the woman's abdomen, and the fundus and posterior uterine wall are massaged. Firm pressure is maintained during the massage so that the uterus is compressed between the hands.

Any accumulated blood clots found in the uterus will be expressed to further facilitate contraction of the myometrium, and uterine tonics will be ordered to promote and maintain uterine tone. Oxytocin, ergot derivatives such as Methergine, and prostaglandins are the most commonly used drugs to combat uterine atony (Table 29-2).

The uterus will be explored manually by the physician or midwife for retained placental fragments or lacerations. If bleeding continues or evidence of hypovolemia or shock develops, blood and additional IV fluids will be ordered.

Surgical intervention will be necessary if uterine atony cannot be reversed. Angiographic embolization and bilateral uterine artery or hypogastric artery ligation may be elected initially, particularly when the woman has indicated a desire for future childbearing. Even when the uterus remains relaxed, bleeding may be controlled in some cases. Hysterectomy may be required when all other measures fail or if the woman's condition does not improve with uterine tonics and fluid and blood replacement.

As soon as possible, analgesia or anesthesia should be administered to control the woman's pain. Bimanual massage and exploration of the uterus may be extremely painful and increases the woman's distress and anxiety. The physician will rely on the nurse to alert the anesthesiologist or nurse anesthetist to assist with pain relief, perform a presurgical evaluation of the woman, and administer anesthesia when required.

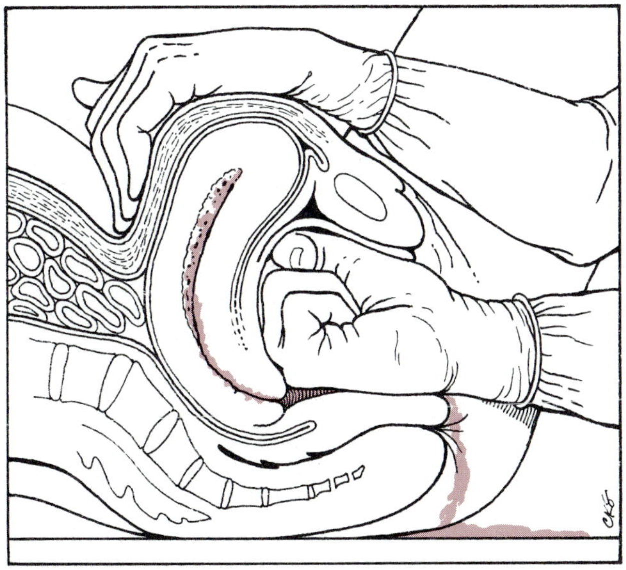

Figure 29-1.
Bimanual compression of the uterus and massage with the abdominal hand usually will control hemorrhage.

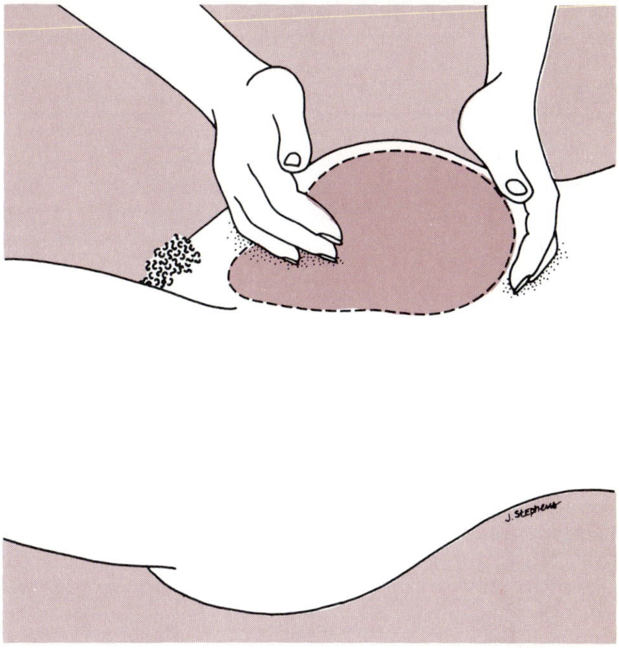

Figure 29-2.
External fundal massage. Shown here are the enlarged uterus immediately after delivery and the maneuvers used to maintain its tone to prevent excessive bleeding and assist its involution. The right hand supports the lower portion of the uterus while the left hand gently palpates and massages the fundus (Childbirth Graphics).

Implications for Nursing Care

Anticipation of possible uterine atony with resultant hemorrhage allows preparatory measures to be taken in advance of the complication. When risk factors are present, the nurse should prepare for delivery by making certain that IV access is initiated with a large-bore angiocatheter (16 or 18 gauge). In addition, the nurse should verify that a sample of the woman's blood is held in the blood bank for possible crossmatching should a transfusion be necessary. Furthermore, the nurse should ensure that uterine tonics, drugs that facilitate contraction of the uterus, are ready for immediate use.

If uterine atony occurs, the nurse calls for immediate help and begins to massage the uterus (Fig. 29-2). It will be necessary to frequently check the consistency of the uterus after bleeding is controlled because uterine relaxation may recur once massage has been discontinued. Vigorous, continuous fundal massage is to be avoided once the uterus contracts because it may result in relaxation of the myometrium. Care must be taken to prevent bladder distention, which may result in uterine displacement and relaxation.

Prompt communication of abnormal findings to the physician or midwife is important so that treatment can be initiated. Hospital protocols often permit the nurse to initiate IV fluids and administer oxytocin before medical help arrives

Table 29-2. Drugs Used to Prevent or Reverse Uterine Atony

Drug	Use	Dosage and Route	Potential Side-Effects and Contraindications
Oxytocin Injection			
(Pitocin, Syntocinon)	To produce uterine contractions and prevent postpartum hemorrhage due to uterine atony	SC, IM, IV: 10 U as necessary IV drip: 10–40 U in 500–1000 mL Ringer's lactate	Seizures, hypotension with IV bolus, nausea, vomiting, hypersensitivity, anaphylactic reaction water retention, and water intoxication (rare with postpartum use)

Implications for Nursing Care

Frequency of fundal checks is determined by physician/midwife orders, the woman's condition, and the status of the fundus: q 10–15 min for the first hour; q 30 min for second postpartum hour; q 4–8 h until discharge.

When oxytocic drugs are used to prevent or reverse uterine atony, a physician or nurse midwife should be immediately available to manage possible complications.

When the drug is administered, the uterus should remain in strong, continuous contraction. The woman may complain of uterine pain or "cramping" as a result of uterine contraction.

Be prepared to administer analgesics for pain relief if cramping is intense.

When the uterus remains atonic (not contracted), the dose of the drug or the rate of IV infusion may be insufficient to effectively control uterine bleeding. Notify the physician or nurse midwife immediately. Be prepared to administer additional doses or increase the IV infusion rate.

Drug	Use	Dosage and Route	Potential Side-Effects and Contraindications
Ergonovine Maleate			
(Ergotrate maleate)	To produce uterine contractions and prevent postpartum hemorrhage due to atony	IM: 0.2 mg q 2–4 h up to a maximum of five doses Oral: 0.2–0.4 mg q 6–12 h to prevent uterine atony for 2–7 days	Dizziness, headache, chest pain, arrhythmias, hypertension, dyspnea, nausea, vomiting, allergic reaction, shock Hypersensitivity or toxicity (ergotism) results in systemic vasoconstriction and is manifested by cold numb fingers and toes, nausea, vomiting, diarrhea, headache, muscles pain, or weakness. Untreated ergotism may result in seizures and gangrene of extremities. Ergonovine is contraindicated in patients with hypersensitivity, infection, hypertension (chronic or due to pregnancy-induced hypertension).

Implications for Nursing Care

Frequency of fundal checks is determined by physician/midwife orders, the woman's condition, and the status of the fundus: q 10–15 min for the first hour; q 30 min for second postpartum hour; q 4–8 h until discharge.

Monitor the patient's blood pressure, pulse, and respirations q 15 min for first h; q 30 min for second postpartum hour.

Report any sudden blood pressure increase, pulse changes, complaints of chest pain or dyspnea.

Assess woman for signs of toxicity (ergotism): cold numb fingers and toes, nausea, vomiting, diarrhea, headache, muscles pain, or weakness. Be prepared to administer vasodilators and heparin to improve circulation. IM injections may cause vigorous contractions for 3 h or more. The woman may have intense pain or uterine cramps and may require analgesia for pain relief.

Notify physician or midwife if severe uterine cramping occurs.

Drug	Use	Dosage and Route	Potential Side-Effects and Contraindications
Methylergonovine Maleate			
(Methergine)	To produce uterine contractions and prevent postpartum hemorrhage due to uterine atony. Also used in management of subinvolution.	IM: 0.2 mg q 2–4 h as necessary Oral: 0.2 mg three to four times daily for a maximum of 1 wk	Dizziness, headache, tinnitus, palpitations, hypertension, hypotension (rare), chest pain, arrhythmias, dyspnea, nausea, vomiting, allergic reactions Contraindicated with known hypersensitivity to drug, hypersensitivity to phenol, with hypertension, severe hepatic or renal disease, sepsis

(continued)

Table 29-2. Drugs Used to Prevent or Reverse Uterine Atony (*Continued*)

Drug	Use	Dosage and Route	Potential Side-Effects and Contraindications
Implications for Nursing Care			
Same as ergonovine maleate			
Prostaglandins			
Prostaglandin $F_2\alpha$ (Prostin/15M)	To control severe hemorrhage secondary to atony when other therapies have failed	0.25 mg IM q 90 min or more for up to five doses	Headache, bradycardia, bronchospasm, wheezing, nausea, vomiting, abdominal cramps, chills, shivering, fever. Contraindicated with known hypersensitivity and in patients with cardiovascular disease, asthma, renal or hepatic disease

Implications for Nursing Care

Frequency of fundal checks is determined by physician/midwife orders, the woman's condition, and the status of the fundus:
Initially q 10–15 min for at least 1.5–2 h after administration; q 30–60 min when woman's condition is stable and until transfer to postpartum unit.
Monitor the woman's blood pressure, pulse, and respirations q 15 min for at least 1.5–2 h after administration; q 30–60 min until transfer to postpartum unit.
Monitor breath sounds frequently. Report any sudden blood pressure increase, pulse changes, complaints of chest pain, dyspnea, or wheezing.
Monitor temperature q 1–2 h and after shaking chill. Administer antipyretic as ordered.
Assess for nausea, vomiting, or diarrhea. Medicate with antiemetic and antidiarrheal as ordered.

when uterine atony cannot be controlled by massage. If hemorrhage and hypovolemia occur, the nurse is often responsible for administering blood products. When uterine atony cannot be reversed, the nurse prepares the woman for angiographic embolization or emergency surgery (bilateral uterine or hypogastric artery ligation or hysterectomy). The anesthesiologist or nurse anesthetist should be notified promptly whenever bleeding cannot be controlled or signs of hypovolemia or shock develop.

The nurse must continue to closely monitor fundal tone and the woman's vital signs after uterine atony is reversed. An important aspect of nursing care is to keep the woman and her family members informed of the changing situation. Communication will minimize fear and apprehension and will maximize cooperation with emergency measures. Nursery personnel should also be alerted so that arrangements can be made to care for the neonate until the woman or another family member is able to do so.

Trauma and Lacerations

Minor lacerations of the perineum, vagina, and cervix occur in most deliveries (see the accompanying display). Periurethral and periclitoral tears are also common problems. Many do not require repair, but all must be inspected. Deep cervical tears may extend into the lower uterine segment and uterine artery or its major branches, resulting in severe postpartum hemorrhage.

Etiologic and Predisposing Factors

Factors predisposing to hemorrhage from lacerations of the genital tract that have been identified (ACOG, 1991; Varner, 1991; Wheeler, 1990) are listed:

- Median episiotomy
- Fetal macrosomatia
- Multiple gestation
- Breech extraction
- Oxytocin use in labor
- Short perineal body
- Friable or tense maternal tissue
- Precipitous labor or delivery
- Use of exaggerated lithotomy position
- Instrumented delivery (forceps or vacuum extraction)
- Abnormal fetal presentation (occiput posterior or face)

Classification of Perineal and Vaginal Lacerations

First degree— involving the skin or vaginal mucosa but not extending into the muscular layers

Second degree— extending from the skin and vaginal mucosa into the muscles of the perineum

Third degree— extending from the skin, vaginal mucosa, and muscle into the anal sphincter

Fourth degree— extending through the rectal mucosa into the lumen of the rectum

Diagnosis

Whenever vaginal bleeding persists in the presence of a firmly contracted uterus, lacerations of the cervix and vaginal vault must be considered. Hemorrhage associated with lacerations of the lower genital tract is frequently bright red and may be severe enough to cause hypovolemia and shock. A constant, slow trickle or oozing of blood may be observed, or frank hemorrhage may occur if a large artery is torn.

Maternal Implications

Lacerations can result in anemia, hypovolemia, and even shock in cases of hemorrhage. The woman may experience acute pain when a laceration occurs, and discomfort may last for days or several weeks depending on the degree of the trauma. Infection at the site of laceration may also occur. These problems will result in a prolonged convalescence and delay in resumption of self-care activities. If the woman has significant edema and pain, her ability to care for the neonate, breastfeed, and engage in the acquaintance process may be impaired. In some instances, scar tissue may form at the site of laceration, distorting the shape of the vagina. This may result in dyspareunia (painful intercourse) when the woman resumes sexual intercourse. Cervical stenosis may also occur with scarring or oversuturing of cervical lacerations (Cunningham et al., 1989).

Treatment

Lacerations must be inspected carefully and the degree of bleeding estimated as soon as possible after birth of the neonate. Treatment will vary depending on the extent of the laceration. In some cases, tamponade (compression pressure to reduce bleeding) with gauze packs must be implemented to reduce hemorrhage while the lacerations are repaired. Suturing is accomplished with a chromic catgut material, which is absorbable and will not have to be removed.

When significant anterior vaginal wall lacerations occur near the urethra or when periurethral lacerations must be repaired, spontaneous voiding may be difficult or impossible for the first 24 hours postpartum. The physician or midwife will insert an indwelling Foley catheter after the repair is completed. The catheter is usually removed after 24 hours or when significant edema is reduced.

Implications for Nursing Care

Nursing care is directed at recognizing predisposing factors for lacerations, monitoring for evidence of hemorrhage, and gathering equipment and drugs needed when significant tears occur. The nurse assists the physician or midwife by providing equipment, supplies, and local anesthetics, and obtaining additional medical help when lacerations are deep and hemorrhage is evident. (See Chapter 21 for further discussion of cervical and vaginal repair.) The woman may need to be repositioned for the repair, or she may be transferred to a surgical unit if deep lacerations must be sutured.

The nurse may be responsible for initiating IV fluids and administering analgesics to control pain during the repair. If significant blood loss occurs, an anesthesiologist or nurse anesthetist may be called to monitor vital signs, support cardiovascular status, and administer blood products or anesthetics. Nursery personnel should be alerted when complications related to lacerations occur so that appropriate infant care can be provided until the woman's condition stabilizes.

As with most emergency situations, communication with the woman to keep her informed and to enhance cooperation is the key to rapid and successful repair of profusely bleeding lacerations. When emergency procedures are instituted, rapport with and confidence in the nurse will help calm the woman.

Hematomas

Hematomas are formed when blood collects in connective tissue of the reproductive tract (Fig. 29-3). This usually occurs after injury to a blood vessel without laceration of the overlying tissue. In the first hours after birth, blood slowly accumulates in the tissue, forming the hematoma. Hematomas can occur anywhere along the birth canal. Most commonly they are found in the perineal or vaginal areas. Less frequent are retroperineal and broad ligament hematomas. However, these latter sites are especially dangerous because massive hemorrhage can occur into the tissues, resulting in hypovolemia and shock. Occasionally hematoma formation is delayed and occurs as late hemorrhage. It results from the sloughing of necrotic tissue in the reproductive tract.

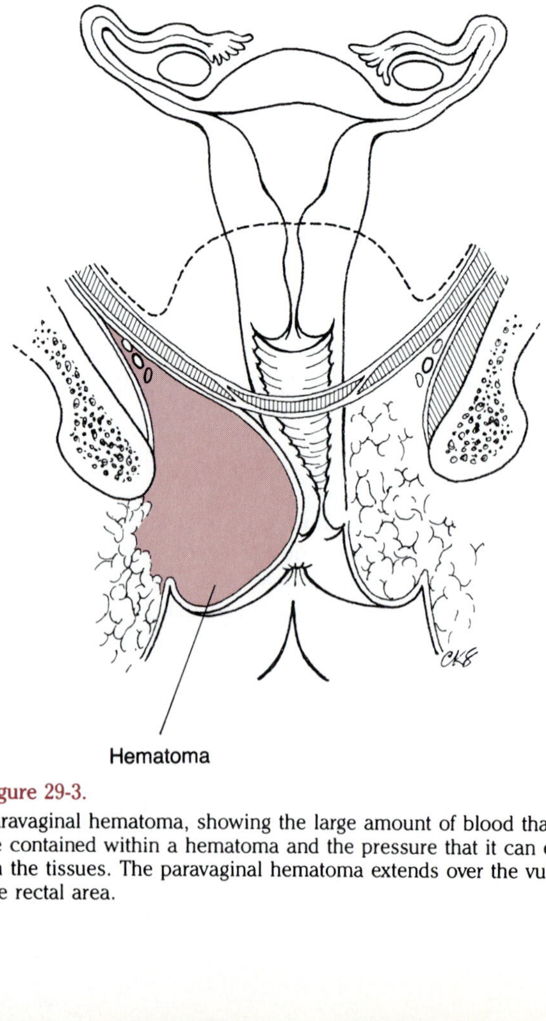

Figure 29-3.
Paravaginal hematoma, showing the large amount of blood that can be contained within a hematoma and the pressure that it can exert on the tissues. The paravaginal hematoma extends over the vulva to the rectal area.

Etiologic and Predisposing Factors

Hematomas occurring in the vaginal wall, often near the ischial spines, may be associated with forceps delivery. They often occur in the perineum or vulva when hemostasis at the time of episiotomy is inadequate. Hematomas are also associated with a difficult and prolonged second stage of labor in which the presenting part exerts pressure on soft tissues and causes local tissue necrosis in the vagina.

Diagnosis

Hematoma formation in the perineum may be anticipated if heavy bruising is present or a traumatic vaginal birth has occurred. The cardinal symptom of hematoma in the unanesthetized woman is severe pain. The pain is often described as a tearing sensation or as intense pressure. If a hematoma forms in the tissues underlying the posterior vaginal wall, sensations of rectal pressure may occur. Pain may be localized at the site of hematoma formation or may radiate down the leg.

Because the bleeding is concealed, hematoma may be suspected when pain or pressure is reported by the woman. Changes in the vital signs indicative of hypovolemia may be the first sign of hematoma formation in the woman who has received an epidural anesthesia for the birth.

A total absence of lochial flow may also suggest vaginal hematoma formation. The enlarging hematoma may occlude the vaginal canal, preventing the flow of blood from the vagina. Vaginal hematomas may be detected by gentle rectal or vaginal examination. This procedure may be done after analgesia has been administered to the woman to reduce sensations of extreme pain.

Maternal Implications

Extreme pain is associated with hematoma formation. The woman is often anxious and restless. In addition, if the hematoma is large, blood loss may be sufficient to produce signs of hypovolemia and shock. The woman may suffer from prolonged anemia and a delayed postpartum recovery. Hematoma sites are susceptible to infection, potentially leading to sepsis and even maternal death. If large hematomas are not treated and infection occurs, calcification and scar tissue will form. Depending on the location, this scarring may permanently distort the reproductive tract anatomy. It may also result in dyspareunia.

Treatment

If the hematoma is large (3 cm or more), it must be incised, drained, and the bleeding vessel(s) ligated. The surrounding area may be packed to promote hemostasis. Small vulvar hematomas may be managed with ice packs or pressure applied to the area. Because the woman with hematoma formation is at increased risk for infection, broad-spectrum antibiotics are often included in the treatment plan. Analgesics are also ordered by the midwife or physician to help control pain associated with this complication.

Implications for Nursing Care

The nurse is responsible for monitoring the woman's condition and vital signs and remaining alert for signs of hematoma formation. The perineal area is examined periodically for evidence of perineal ecchymosis, swelling, or tenseness of the skin overlying perineal tissue. The midwife or physician should be notified if these signs develop, if lochial flow is absent, or the woman complains of vaginal or rectal pressure or pain. When hematoma formation is confirmed, maternal pulse and blood pressure should be assessed at least every 10 to 15 minutes for signs of hypovolemia or early compensated shock.

Uterine Inversion

Inversion or prolapse of the uterus is a rare but dramatic complication occurring in approximately 1 in 15,000 deliveries (Gillogley, 1991). Uterine inversion may occur after delivery of the placenta or in the postpartum period and is evidenced by the uterus turning either partially or completely inside out. Types of uterine inversion are characterized by the degree and the type of force causing the inversion (see the display, Types of Uterine Inversion).

Etiologic and Predisposing Factors

Uterine inversion is more likely to occur with fundal implantation of the placenta. Thinning of the uterine wall at the placental site may allow invagination or prolapse of the myometrium as the placenta separates, initiating the inversion process. Factors that predispose to uterine inversion include:

- Bearing-down efforts after delivery
- Precipitous delivery with the woman in standing position
- Traction on the umbilical cord before placental separation
- Vigorous kneading of the fundus to cause placental separation and expulsion
- Excessive manual pressure on the fundus—for example, during fundal message
- Delivery of a neonate with a short umbilical cord
- Manual separation and extraction of the placenta
- Rapid delivery with multiple gestation or rapid release of excessive amniotic fluid

Diagnosis

A completely inverted uterus will be visible as a bluish gray mass filling the vagina or extending from the vaginal orifice. In rare cases, complete uterine inversion presents

> **Types of Uterine Inversion**
>
> - Complete inversion—collapse of the entire uterus through the cervix into the vagina
> - Incomplete or partial inversion—inversion of the fundus, without extension beyond the external cervical of
> - Forced inversion—inversion caused by excessive pulling of the cord or vigorous manual expression of the placenta or clots from an atonic uterus
> - Spontaneous inversion—inversion due to increased abdominal pressure because of bearing down, coughing, or sudden abdominal muscle contraction

when the placenta delivers still attached to the completely prolapsed uterus. When uterine inversion is partial or incomplete, it may be detected only when profuse vaginal bleeding occurs and the fundus cannot be palpated. A bimanual examination by the midwife or physician will reveal a cup-shaped mass in the vagina (Fig. 29-4).

Maternal Implications

When uterine inversion occurs, the unanesthetized woman will experience severe pain in conjunction with a sensation of extreme fullness in the vagina. She becomes immediately aware that an emergency exists by the responses of the health care team. Acute anxiety or fear are often combined with severe pain. If reinversion is not performed promptly, the uterus becomes atonic and blood loss may be rapid and extreme. The woman may demonstrate signs of hypovolemic shock.

The woman is at increased risk for infection. This results from exposure of the uterine lining and the extensive manipulation required to reverse the uterine prolapse. When hemorrhage occurs, the woman may experience a prolonged postpartum recovery due to anemia. If the prolapsed uterus cannot be replaced, hysterectomy must be performed. The loss of childbearing capacity can be devastating for some women.

Treatment

When uterine inversion is diagnosed, immediate attempts should be made by the midwife or physician to replace the uterus to its normal position. This is done by applying firm, steady pressure on the inverted fundus. If uterine replacement is delayed, the cervix becomes increasingly edematous and constricts around the prolapsed body of the uterus, making reinversion difficult or impossible.

Tocolytic agents such as terbutaline or magnesium sulfate may be administered intravenously to relax the uterus so that replacement is facilitated. In some cases, general anesthesia (halothane) may be needed to relax the uterus sufficiently. When the uterus is replaced, oxytocin and sometimes other uterine tonics (Methergine or Prostin/15M) are administered to stimulate uterine tone and avoid recurring inversion. If hypovolemic shock develops, blood and fluid replacement is essential. In rare instances the uterus cannot be reinverted; emergency hysterectomy is necessary to prevent maternal death from exsanguination. Antibiotic therapy may be initiated after uterine inversion because of the increased risk of infection.

Implications for Nursing Care

The nurse must be alert for symptoms of uterine inversion at delivery and during the postpartum period. If the

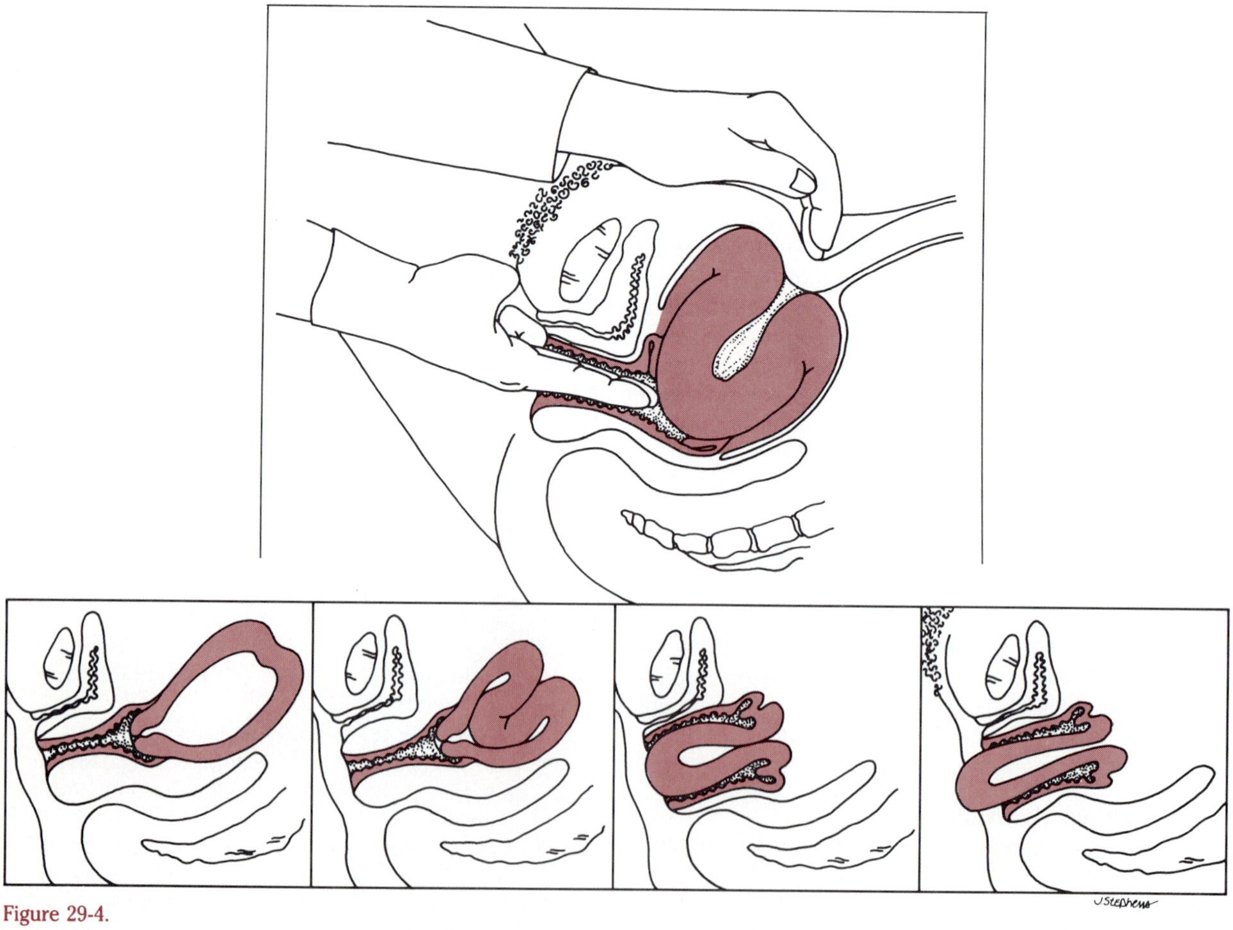

Figure 29-4.

Uterine inversion can be diagnosed by abdominal and vaginal palpation. Lower diagrams show progressive degrees of inversion from slight to complete (Childbirth Graphics).

woman complains of pelvic pain and vaginal fullness or the prolapsed uterus becomes visible through the vaginal introitus, the nurse must call for medical and additional nursing help immediately. The nurse assists in the attempts to replace the uterus as follows:

- Place the delivery table or bed in Trendelenburg position as requested
- Provide additional sterile gloves and supplies required by the physician or midwife
- Administer IV magnesium sulfate or terbutaline as ordered
- Administer uterine tonics after replacement of the uterus

An anesthesiologist or nurse anesthetist should be summoned immediately when uterine inversion is diagnosed. Either can assist the nurse with monitoring the woman's status and administering IV fluids, blood, and drugs. Until help arrives the nurse should remain continuously with the woman. Two large-bore angiocatheters (16 or 18 gauge) should be inserted and a crystalloid solution such as Ringer's lactate initiated. The woman can be placed in the Trendelenburg position and oxygen should be administered at 8 to 12 L/min by face mask. Frequent monitoring of vital signs may be facilitated by use of an electronic blood pressure monitor. A pulse oximeter should be attached to provide data about oxygen saturation levels. A staff person should ascertain that a sample of the woman's blood is available for type and crossmatching should blood replacement become necessary. A sterile red Robinson or Foley catheter and drainage bag should be available in case the midwife or physician wishes to empty the woman's bladder.

If manual replacement is not successful, the nurse must prepare the woman and her family for administration of general anesthesia and possible surgery. The nurse should provide brief, simple explanations of the problem and the care provided. It is helpful to have an additional staff member available to provide emotional support to the woman. When possible, the nursery should be notified so that arrangements can be made to provide neonate care until the woman's condition is stable.

Placenta Accreta, Percreta, and Increta

Placenta accreta, percreta, and increta are anomalies representing progressively more severe degrees of abnormal placental adherence to the underlying uterine wall (Fig. 29-5). *Placenta accreta* occurs when placental tissue is contiguous with and adherent to the myometrium. *Placenta percreta* occurs when placental tissue—specifically, the chorionic villi—invades the myometrium. *Placenta increta* occurs when the villi penetrate the full depth of the uterine wall. These conditions are extremely rare; estimated incidence is 1 in 7000 deliveries.

Abnormal placental adherence cannot be diagnosed until delivery, when spontaneous separation does not occur. Attempts to remove an abnormally adherent placenta manually can result in uterine rupture and severe maternal hemorrhage. Third trimester bleeding with these conditions may occur as a result of a coincident placenta previa.

Etiologic and Predisposing Factors

Placenta accreta, percreta, and increta are believed to result from failure of the decidua (lining of the uterus during pregnancy) to develop in the placental bed, thus allowing placental tissue to have direct contact with the myometrium. The specific cause for this is unknown. Predisposing factors associated with abnormal placental adherence are those that tend to denude or distort the endometrium (lining of nonpregnant uterus) and contribute to abnormal placental implantation, including:

- Uterine scarring from previous cesarean delivery
- History of uterine curettage
- Previous manual removal of the placenta
- Previous uterine sepsis
- Presence of uterine leiomyomas or surgical removal (myomectomy)
- Uterine malformation
- Placenta previa

Diagnosis

The diagnosis of placental accreta, percreta, or increta cannot be made until after delivery. Signs and symptoms will depend on the depths of uterine penetration and the number of cotyledons involved. When placental accreta occurs, the placenta will not separate. The physician or midwife normally determines that a pathologic adherence is the problem when attempts to perform manual separation of the placenta are unsuccessful. If only several placental cotyledons normally separate, but the remainder remain attached, bleeding will occur because the uterus cannot contract adequately while the remaining adherent sections are attached. In most cases, hysterectomy is performed to remove the uterus and stop the bleeding.

Maternal Implications

The presence of placenta accreta, percreta, and increta contributes substantially to maternal morbidity, and the mortality rate may be as high as 10%. Approximately one third of emergency postpartum hysterectomies are performed as a result of abnormal attachments of the placenta. Diagnosis is not possible before delivery because an adherent or penetrating placenta resembles placental tissue that is partially attached. When zealous attempts are made to remove an adherent or penetrating placenta, uterine rupture, hemorrhage, and possibly exsanguination may result.

Fetal/Neonatal Implications

In placenta accreta, percreta, and increta, the placenta functions normally despite its abnormal adherence. In the absence of a concurrent problem, such as placenta previa, the fetus is generally not affected in any way.

Treatment

When minor degrees of placenta accreta exist, adhering tissue may be removed manually or by curettage, usually without further problems. Current research is being conducted to evaluate the effectiveness of injecting oxytocin into the umbilical cord during the third stage of labor to facilitate separation when retained placenta is diagnosed. Further

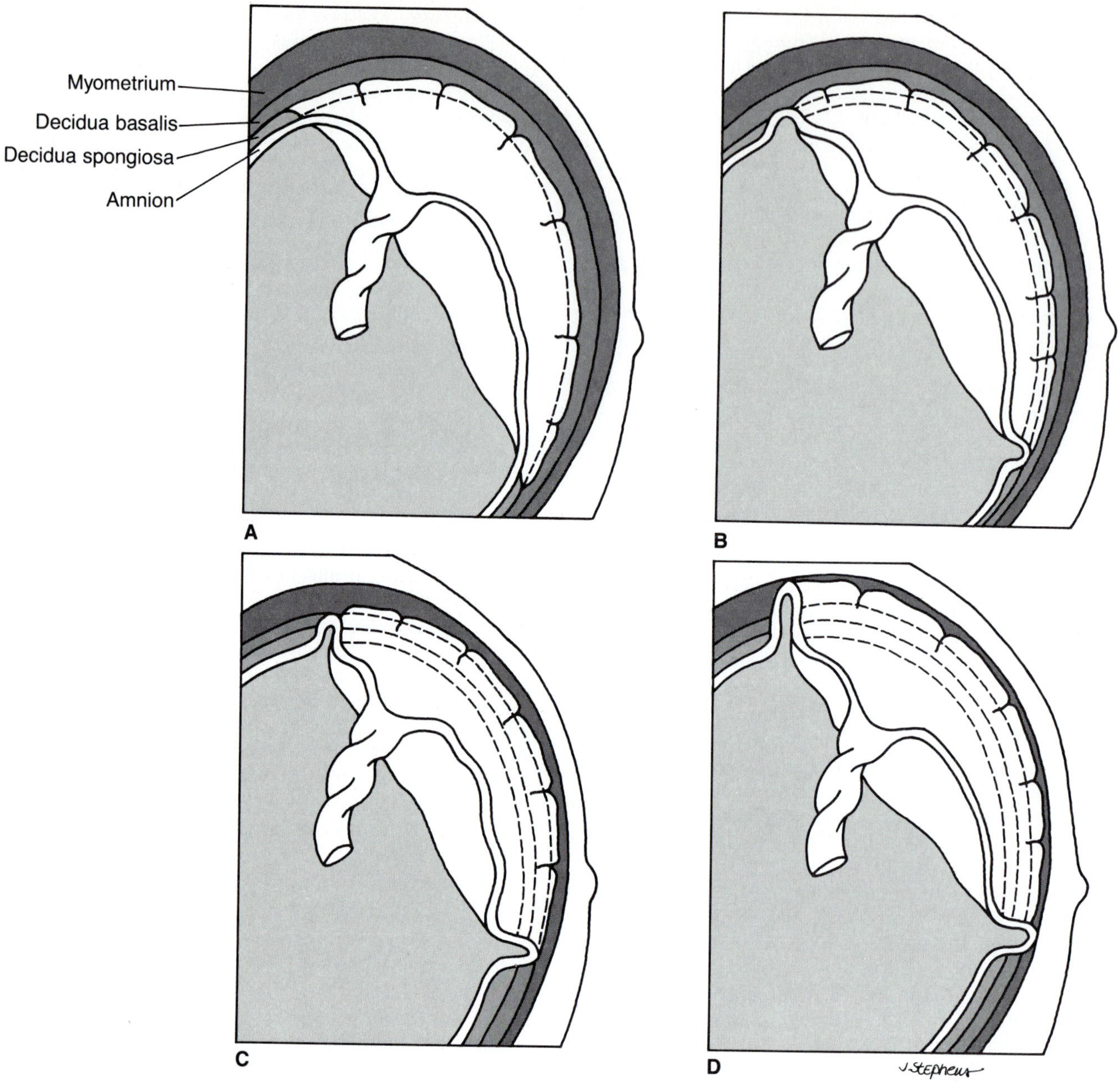

Figure 29-5.

Normal and abnormal placental adherence. *A:* Normal adherence to endometrium. *B:* Placenta accreta: placental tissue is adherent to myometrium. *C:* Placenta increta: placenta has penetrated uterine muscle. *D:* Placenta percreta: placenta has penetrated uterine wall (Childbirth Graphics).

study is indicated before recommendations can be made regarding this procedure.

Hemorrhage or uterine trauma resulting from attempts to remove invasive placentas constitutes a true emergency, and immediate measures are needed to prevent hemorrhagic shock and limit further blood loss. (Shock is discussed later in this chapter.)

If the placenta has invaded the lower uterine segment, which is richly supplied with blood vessels, hysterectomy is performed to save the woman from overwhelming hemorrhage. Placental invasion in other areas of the uterus causes less blood loss but may still require hysterectomy. In rare cases, most placental tissue can be removed and bleeding can be adequately controlled so that hysterectomy is not required. Subsequent pregnancies can result but with an increased risk of placental abnormality.

Implications for Nursing Care

The nurse caring for a woman with possible or diagnosed abnormal placental adherence must focus on monitoring maternal physiologic status and preparing her for surgery. If bleeding is not severe and the woman's condition is stable, uterine exploration and curettage may be attempted; the nurse should provide support and monitor adequacy of maternal analgesia. If bleeding is severe, the nurse must be ready to institute emergency measures for hemorrhagic shock and to prepare the woman for immediate surgery. Because hysterectomy is a distinct possibility, informed consent must be obtained from the woman. The necessity for such surgery must be fully explained and provisions made for contact with a member of the clergy, if the woman desires it and time permits.

Late Postpartum Hemorrhage

Late postpartum hemorrhage occurs after the first 24 hours postdelivery and before 6 weeks postpartum. Although the bleeding can be significant, it does not usually pose the same risk as early postpartum hemorrhage. The usual onset for late postpartum bleeding is 6 to 10 days after birth (Luegenbiehl, 1991).

Etiologic and Predisposing Factors

The three most common causes of late postpartum hemorrhage are infection, uterine subinvolution, and retained placental fragments.

Diagnosis

By definition, late postpartum hemorrhage is the appearance of brisk bleeding or hemorrhage after the first 24 hours of birth. A differential diagnosis must be made to identify the cause of bleeding.

The woman who experiences late postpartum hemorrhage will often present with uterine subinvolution, the delayed return of the postpartum uterus to its normal tone and size. When palpated, the uterus is soft or "boggy." The woman experiences a slow, reddish brown oozing from the vagina over many days, or occasionally, irregular heavy bleeding during the first 6 weeks after birth. She may complain of a low, persistent backache, abdominal pain or tenderness, and fatigue. The diagnosis is confirmed by a bimanual examination of the uterus.

If infection is an underlying cause of subinvolution and bleeding, the vaginal discharge may be foul smelling. The uterus is generally tender on examination, and the woman may have a persistent low-grade fever. Late bleeding may also result from small retained placental fragments. Retention of all or part of the placenta interferes with normal uterine contraction and constriction of the vessels at the placental site. Bleeding will continue until the rest of the placenta is separated and expelled. In some cases, the retained piece of placenta undergoes necrosis. When this necrotic tissue finally separates from the uterine myometrium, hemorrhage can occur. Recently, ultrasonography has been found to be useful in visualizing retained placental fragments and confirming the diagnosis.

Maternal Implications

The woman who experiences late postpartum bleeding often suffers from anemia, persistent abdominal pain, loss of appetite, and fatigue. Feelings of mild depression may occur as a result of these symptoms. Often the woman will report that she cannot get enough rest and is unable to complete self-care and child care activities. These symptoms may be particularly distressing when the woman is responsible for the majority of housekeeping and child care activities or when she must return to work shortly after delivery.

Treatment

Late postpartum hemorrhage is usually treated by a course of oral Methergine, which produces sustained contraction of the uterus. An uncontracted uterus that contains blood clots or placental fragments provides an excellent site for bacterial growth and infection. If infection is suspected or confirmed, a course of oral antibiotics is usually prescribed. The woman is reevaluated in 2 weeks; persistent bleeding after treatment indicates the need for dilatation and curettage of the uterus. When frank hemorrhage occurs and uterine tonics do not reduce the bleeding, curettage of the uterus must be performed immediately. Rest and adequate nutritional intake are also essential to speed the healing process after late postpartum bleeding.

Implications for Nursing Care

Careful examination of the placenta after delivery is a major deterrent to the development of late postpartum hemorrhage due to retained placental fragments. If any areas of tissue appear to be missing, the nurse must bring this to the birth attendant's attention. The nurse is also responsible for monitoring the amount and pattern of bleeding in the early postpartum period. Persistent heavy bleeding in the presence of a firm uterus may indicate retained placental fragments.

Discharge teaching includes specific information regarding signs of uterine subinvolution, infection, and late postpartum bleeding. Most facilities also provide the woman with printed materials that outline signs of abnormal postpartum recovery. The nurse should ascertain that the woman has made arrangements for postpartum evaluation by the midwife or physician. Most women should be reevaluated within several weeks of delivery to confirm uterine involution. If postpartum follow-up care is ordered or provided by the facility, the nurse should assess the woman for signs of late postpartum bleeding or signs of uterine infection or subinvolution.

Postpartum hemorrhage may occur immediately after delivery or in the first several weeks after birth of the neonate. Its causes are varied, but the consequences if left untreated are devastating. The nurse plays a crucial role in the early identification and treatment of hemorrhage. Timely intervention can prevent maternal morbidity or death. The nurse must remain vigilant and supplies must be readily available in the birth setting to initiate immediate emergency management of bleeding.

Postpartum Infection

Postpartum infection (postpartum sepsis) is a major cause of maternal morbidity and mortality. The pelvic cavity is the site of origin for most postpartum infections. Other common sites of infection include the perineum and associated structures, the breasts, the urinary tract, and the venous system.

Current estimates of the incidence of postpartum infection range from 1% to 8% (Silver & Smith, 1991). A number of variables may contribute to this wide range. One is the increasingly common practice of early discharge. If subsequent infection occurs, this problem is not noted in data normally collected after birth regarding postpartum complications. Other variables that influence the reported rate include the increasing administration of prophylactic antibiotics after cesarean delivery and the effectiveness of new broad-spectrum drugs. These changes in management obscure the temperature elevation that is the primary indicator of postpartum infection. Even though the risk during the postpartum period is limited, infection is still one of the primary causes of maternal death.

Etiologic and Predisposing Factors

The most common risk factors predisposing the woman to postpartum infection are shown in the accompanying display. Cesarean delivery has increased the incidence of postpartum infections. Rates of infection after cesarean delivery range from 5 to 30 times greater than vaginal delivery. The types of infection most commonly associated with cesarean deliveries, in order of occurrence, are endometritis, bacteremia, and wound infection.

The bacteria most often responsible for postpartum infection are those normally found in the bowel, which also commonly colonize the perineum, vagina, and cervix (Cunningham et al., 1989). Bacteria most often implicated in genital tract infections are also listed in the display of risk factors.

Diagnosis

Postpartum infection is presumed to be present if the woman has a temperature of 38.0°C (100.4°F) or higher on any 2 of the first 10 days after delivery (exclusive of the first 24 hours). Other signs and symptoms that suggest this complication will depend on the site of infection and may include:

- General malaise
- Uterine tenderness
- Foul or purulent lochia
- Flank pain and hematuria
- Urinary frequency, dysuria, and burning
- Evidence of localized infection (mastitis, infection of episiotomy)

Laboratory tests used for diagnosis include the complete blood count (CBC), venous blood cultures, urine cultures, and in some cases cultures of tissue taken from suspected infection sites, such as the endometrium or wounds.

The CBC yields much information. Hemoglobin, an indicator of the cells' oxygen-carrying ability, may be diminished when infection occurs. Anemia that was not present prenatally or associated with blood loss may suggest infection. More importantly, the CBC includes information about the status of the body's immune system and indicates whether

Postpartum Infection

Risk Factors

Antenatal Factors

- Obesity
- Anemia
- Poor nutritional status
- Low socioeconomic status
- Limited access to health care
- History of pyelonephritis
- History of vaginal infections
- History of susceptibility to infection
- Preexisting medical conditions (diabetes)
- History of smoking or other illicit drug use

Intrapartum Factors

- Urinary catheterization
- Breaks in aseptic technique
- Multiple vaginal examinations
- Labor dystocia
  - Prolonged labor or precipitous birth
  - Prolonged rupture of the amniotic membranes
- Genital tract trauma, lacerations, or hematomas
- Internal electronic fetal and uterine monitoring
- Instrument-assisted deliveries (forceps or vacuum extraction)
- Episiotomy
- Cesarean delivery

Postpartum Factors

- Manual removal of the placenta
- Postpartum hemorrhage and anemia

Organisms Frequently Implicated in Postpartum Genital Tract Infections

Aerobes

- Group A, B, and D streptococci
- Enterococcus
- Gram-negative bacteria: *Escherichia coli, Klebsiella* species, *Proteus* species
- *Staphylococcus aureus*

Anaerobes

- *Peptococcus* species
- *Peptostreptococcus* species
- *Bacteroides bivius, B. fragilis, B. disiens*
- *Clostridium* species
- *Fusobacterium* species

Other

- *Mycoplasma hominis*
- *Chlamydia trachomatis*

there has been a recent challenge to the system. A normal white blood cell count during pregnancy is 15,000 to 18,000/mm^3. With an early infection, this count will rapidly or gradually increase to 20,000/mm^3 or greater, and the differential count of cells will show an early response from the neutrophils or polymorphonuclear leukocytes.

Cultures and Gram stains allow identification of the many microbial agents found with postpartum infection. Gram staining will identify gram-positive and gram-negative organisms and provide immediate direction for treatment. Culturing the infectious agents will later determine the appropriateness of specific antibiotics selected for treatment. It is important to collect specimens for culture before antimicrobial treatment is begun to prevent confusion in the interpretation of clinical data (Dinsmoor & Gibbs, 1988).

Maternal Implications

The physical, emotional, and financial costs of care can be extensive when postpartum infection occurs. Localized infections may spread and can result in involvement of other organs, requiring an extended hospital stay. When infection spreads, septic pelvic thrombophlebitis, pulmonary thromboembolism, pelvic abscess, or septic shock can occur. In rare cases, tissue scarring secondary to a pelvic infection can result in loss of fertility and the capacity to conceive.

When the wound becomes infected (episiotomy, lacerations, or the cesarean incision), necrosis of the fascial tissue layer can occur. Necrotizing fasciitis is a serious complication that can result in loss of tissue, severe scarring, and a prolonged hospitalization. When deep tissue layers of the cesarean incision are infected, spontaneous wound dehiscence (separation of the incision) can also occur. Complete dehiscence of all layers of the incision may result in evisceration (extrusion of the bowel). This is a rare but extremely serious complication.

The woman with a postpartum infection often feels extremely ill and fatigued. Sleep disruption is common due to pain, frequent examinations, wound care, or other required treatments. Significant pain and anxiety can exacerbate sleep deprivation and result in depression and anger. Loss of appetite is also common and retards tissue healing. A prolonged convalescence may be required, and delay in the maternal–newborn acquaintance process and breastfeeding often occurs. A full discussion of the emotional impact of postpartum complications on individual and family adaptations is presented in Chapter 25.

Treatment

In most instances, postpartum infection will require that the woman remain in the hospital for antibiotic therapy. The preferred route for treatment of most soft-tissue infections is IV administration. Furthermore, antibiotics work most effectively when serum concentrations are maintained at a constant level over a specified period of time. If the woman is NPO or experiences nausea and vomiting, gastrointestinal absorption of drugs may be limited, and IV administration will also be necessary. Therapy is continued for 24 to 48 hours after the fever has subsided.

Because many of the infections that develop during the postpartum period are polymicrobial, it is common practice to treat these infections with a combination antibiotic regimen (Dinsmoor & Gibbs, 1988). The drugs of choice for these pathogens are penicillin (or ampicillin), cephalosporin, and aminoglycosides. Table 29-3 presents the antibiotics commonly used to treat postpartum infection.

If infection occurs in the surgical incision (episiotomy or cesarean incision), special wound care will be required. Sitz baths are often ordered for localized infection of the episiotomy. Warm, moist dressings may be applied to a cesarean incision when a superficial skin infection occurs. When deep tissue layers of the incision are infected, the wound must be reopened by the physician. Infected and necrotic tissue are removed (debridement), and a special dressing (wet-to-dry) is applied to keep the exposed tissues clean and moist while healing proceeds. The wound heals by secondary intention. Tissue regenerates from the base of the wound, and it may take weeks before complete healing occurs.

Implications for Nursing Care

Goals of nursing care when the woman is at risk for postpartum infection or when infection has occurred include:

- Identifying the risk factors that predispose the woman to infection
- Maintaining strict medical asepsis to prevent spread of infection
- Teaching the woman about and encouraging the use of medical asepsis
- Monitoring the woman's vital signs and physiologic status
- Encouraging intake of a balanced diet and adequate fluids to support the immune system and medical therapy
- Providing self-care activities for the woman until she is well enough to perform them
- Administering analgesics and providing other support measures to enhance comfort and reduce pain
- Administering antibiotics and other treatments as they are ordered
- Teaching specific procedures such as wound care before discharge
- Providing time for the woman and neonate to interact
- Supporting breastfeeding efforts

The best line of defense against postpartum infections is prevention. The nurse maintains strict medical asepsis and teaches the woman techniques to minimize the risk of infection. Handwashing is the most effective strategy. Other actions are:

- Wiping from front to back after voiding or defecating
- Cleaning the perineum after voiding or defecating using a squirt bottle, portable sitz bath, or other hygiene devices (such as a "surgigator")
- Changing perineal pads with each voiding and at least every 2 to 3 hours
- Encouraging use of sitz bath with perineal lacerations or episiotomy
- Encouraging woman to drink fluids liberally and to empty her bladder frequently (every 2 to 3 hours)

Text continues on page 855

Table 29-3. Antibiotic Drugs Commonly Used to Treat Puerperal Infection

Drug	Use	Dosage and Route	Potential Side Effects
Ampicillin			
(Polycillin)—penicillin group	Treatment of postpartum endometritis, endomyometritis, and parametritis. May be used for treatment of postpartum pneumonia secondary to postoperative atelectasis. May be used for treatment of necrotizing fasciitis and septic pelvic thrombophlebitis.	Orally: 250–500 mg qid IM or IV: 500 mg to 2 g q 6 h	Allergic reaction as seen in penicillin hypersensitivity: rash, nausea, vomiting, dermatitis, anaphylactic reaction. Thrombophlebitis at infusion site. Blood dyscrasias. Superinfection with opportunistic organisms. Seizures have been reported with high doses. May cause false-positive urine glucose (Clinitest) test.

Implications for Nursing Care

Ascertain that specimens for culture and sensitivity have been obtained before starting drug; 30% of hospital strains of *E. coli* are resistant to penicillin drugs.

Assess for history of allergy or hypersensitivity to drug or to penicillin. Drug is not used in patients with penicillin allergy. Observe patient closely for signs of allergy or hypersensitivity. Discontinue drug immediately and notify physician if signs or symptoms of allergy or hypersensitivity occur.

Reconstitute for IM or IV use with sterile water for injection. Must dilute in at least 50 mL or more of IV solution for IV infusion. May give in 5% D/W; 5% D/0.45 NS; lactated Ringers; 0.9 NS. Use within 1 h of reconstituting. Infuse IV over 15–30 min. Faster infusion may cause seizures.

Multiple incompatibilities. Do not infuse with other drugs, or check with pharmacologist before mixing with other agents.

Monitor for opportunistic infections (*Candida* vaginitis).

If urine glucose testing ordered, use glucose oxidase method (ie, Tes-Tape).

Drug appears in breast milk, but does not contraindicate breastfeeding. Neonate should be monitored for rashes, diarrhea, thrush, or vomiting—common side-effects when given directly to newborn.

Drug	Use	Dosage and Route	Potential Side Effects
Cefoxitin			
(Mefoxin)—semisynthetic second-generation cephalosporin and related to penicillin	Treatment of postpartum endometritis and UTIs. May be used to treat wound infections, postpartum pneumonia, and septicemia.	IM or IV: 1–2 g q 6–8 h	Pain, tenderness, induration at IM injection site. Thrombophlebitis at IV site. Rash, fever, allergic reaction, anaphylaxis, nausea, vomiting, diarrhea. Blood dyscrasias, hemolytic anemia. Superinfection with opportunistic organisms. May cause increased BUN, creatinine, AST, ALT, and alkaline phosphatase levels.

Implications for Nursing Care

Ascertain that specimens for culture and sensitivity have been obtained before starting drug.

Assess for history of allergy or hypersensitivity to drug or to penicillin. Drug is not used in patients with penicillin allergy. Observe patient closely for signs of allergy or hypersensitivity. Discontinue drug immediately and notify physician if signs or symptoms of allergy or hypersensitivity occur.

Reconstitute for IM or IV use with sterile water or 0.9 NS for injection. Must dilute each gram or fraction thereof with at least 10 mL of diluent. Dilute in 50 mL of 5% D/W, 5% D/0.45 NS, 5% D/0.9 NS, 0.9 NS of IV solution for IV infusion. When reconstituted, stable at room temperature for 24 hr. Stable for 1 week in refrigerator. Infuse each gram or fraction thereof over 5 min or longer.

Incompatible with all aminoglycosides (eg, gentamycin, tobramycin, amikacin).

Use glucose oxidase method (Tes-Tape) to test urine glucose.

Monitor liver studies and BUN and creatinine.

Insignificant amounts of drug appear in breast milk. May continue to breastfeed.

Drug	Use	Dosage and Route	Potential Side Effects
Clindamycin			
(Cleocin)—semisynthetic antibiotic	Treatment of postpartum *post-cesarean* endometritis, endomyometritis, and parametritis. Drug is reserved for serious infections where less toxic antimicrobials are ineffective. It is the drug of choice in treating *B. fragilis*, a normal inhabitant of genital tract that causes infection when blood clots or necrotic tissue (necrotizing fasciitis) are present.	Orally: 150–600 mg q 6 h IM or IV: 300–600 mg q 6–8 h, up to 4.8 g/day in life-threatening infections	Loose stools, diarrhea, nausea, vomiting, abdominal cramps, pseudomembranous colitis. Rash. Hypotension and arrhythmias. Dizziness, headache. Phlebitis at IV infusion site. May cause abnormal liver function tests or transient decrease in leukocytes and platelets following rapid IV injection.

(continued)

Table 29-3. Antibiotic Drugs Commonly Used to Treat Puerperal Infection (*Continued*)

Drug	Use	Dosage and Route	Potential Side Effects

Implications for Nursing Care

Ascertain that specimens for culture and sensitivity have been obtained before starting drug.

Assess for history of allergy or hypersensitivity. Observe patient closely for signs of allergy or hypersensitivity. Discontinue drug immediately and notify physician if signs or symptoms of allergy or hypersensitivity occur.

Monitor for diarrhea and bloody, mucoid stools and report to physician promptly. May be a sign of pseudomembranous colitis. Instruct patient to report these signs as they may develop up to several weeks following cessation of therapy.

Monitor for opportunistic infections (*Candida* vaginitis).

Dilute each 300 mg or fraction thereof with a minimum of 50 mL of 5% D/W, or 0.9 NS for injection or with any other compatible solution for IV infusion (5% D/W, 5% D/0.45 NS, 5% D/0.9 NS, 0.9 NS, Ringer's lactate, 5% D/Ringer's lactate. Infuse 300 mg or fraction thereof no faster than 10 min. Do not give more than 1200 mg in a single 1-h infusion. Do not give more than 600 mg in a single injection. When diluted, stable for 24 h at room temperature. Crystalizes in refrigerator, but dissolves at room temperature. Do not use if crystalized.

Give oral dose with full glass of water. May give with meals.

Multiple incompatibilities. Do not give with other drugs if possible. Check with pharmacologist before giving with other drugs.

Monitor CBC and liver studies.

Insignificant amounts of drug appear in breast milk. May continue to breastfeed. Monitor infant for bloody stools.

Cefazolin

Drug	Use	Dosage and Route	Potential Side Effects
(Ancef, Kefzol)—first-generation cephalosporin	Treatment of postpartum UTIs. Treatment of postpartum pneumonia secondary to postsurgical atelectasis.	IM or IV: 500 mg to 2 g q 6–8 h	Nausea, vomiting, diarrhea, hypersensitivity, allergy, anaphylaxis, rash. Phlebitis at IV site. Pain with IM injection. Nephrotoxicity, bone marrow depression, and hepatotoxicity.

Implications for Nursing Care

Assess for sensitivity to penicillins or cephalosporins. Observe patient closely for signs of allergy or hypersensitivity. Discontinue drug immediately and notify physician if signs or symptoms of allergy or hypersensitivity occur.

Assess baseline renal and liver function tests and monitor results.

Ascertain that specimens for culture and sensitivity have been obtained before starting drug.

Reconstitute with at least 10 mL of sterile water for injection. Dilute with at least 50 mL of 5% D/W, 5% D/0.45 NS, 5% D/0.9 NS, 5% D in Ringer's lactate, Ringer's lactate, 0.9 NS. Infuse 1 g or fraction thereof slowly over 5 min or slower. When diluted, stable for 24 h at room temperature or 96 h in refrigerator.

Multiple incompatibilities. Do not give with other drugs if possible. Check with pharmacologist before giving with other drugs.

Monitor liver studies.

Use glucose oxidase to test urine glucose (Tes-Tape).

Insignificant amounts of drug appear in breast milk. May continue to breastfeed.

Monitor for opportunistic infections (*Candida* vaginitis).

Amoxicillin and Clavulanate

Drug	Use	Dosage and Route	Potential Side Effects
	Combination of amoxicillin and clavulanate. Clavulanate is a drug that protects amoxicillin from degradation by bacterial enzymes and extends the spectrum of the antibiotic to bacteria normally resistant to amoxicillin. An extended-spectrum antimicrobial used for the treatment of endometritis, endomyometritis, parametritis, and postpartum UTIs.	PO: 250–500 mg amoxicillin with 125 mg clavulanate q 8 h	Hypersensitivity, allergy (risk increased with allergy to penicillin), rashes. Nausea, vomiting, diarrhea. Blood dyscrasias. Superinfection with opportunistic infections. Seizures with high doses. May potentiate the effect of oral anticoagulants.

Implications for Nursing Care

Ascertain that specimens for culture and sensitivity have been obtained before starting drug.

Assess for history of allergy or hypersensitivity to drugs (amoxicillin or clavulanate) or to penicillin. Drug is not used in patients with penicillin allergy. Observe patient closely for signs of allergy or hypersensitivity. Discontinue drug immediately and notify physician if signs or symptoms of allergy or hypersensitivity occur.

May be given with meals.

Use glucose oxidase method (Tes-Tape) to test urine glucose.

Monitor liver studies.

Insignificant amounts of drug appear in breast milk. May continue to breastfeed.

(*continued*)

Table 29-3. Antibiotic Drugs Commonly Used to Treat Puerperal Infection (*Continued*)

Drug	Use	Dosage and Route	Potential Side Effects
Ticarcillin/Clavulanate			
	Combination of ticarcillin and clavulanate. Clavulanate is a drug that protects ticarcillin from degradation by bacterial enzymes and extends the spectrum of the antibiotic to bacteria normally resistant ticarcillin. An extended-spectrum penicillin used for the treatment of skin infections, bacterial septicemia, and postpartum UTIs. Effective against *Klebsiella* species, *E. coli, Pseudomonas aeruginosa*, and *S. aureus*.	IV: 3.1 g ticarcillin (with 125 mg clavulanate) q 6–8 h	Confusion, lethargy. Nausea, diarrhea, colitis. Congestive heart failure, arrhythmias. Hypersensitivity allergy, rash, and uticaria. Hypokalemia, Phlebitis at IV site. May increase effects of oral anticoagulants.

Implications for Nursing Care

Ascertain that specimens for culture and sensitivity have been obtained before starting drug.

Assess for history of allergy or hypersensitivity to drugs (ticarcillin or clavulanate) or to penicillin. Drug is not used in patients with penicillin allergy. Observe patient closely for signs of allergy or hypersensitivity. Discontinue drug immediately and notify physician if signs or symptoms of allergy or hypersensitivity occur.

Dilute each 3.1 g or fraction thereof with 13 mL sterile water for injection. Dilute with 50 mL of 5% D/W or 0.9 NS or Ringer's lactate for IV infusion. Stable at room temperature for at least 6 h once reconstituted or 72 h in refrigerator. Infuse over 30 min.

Multiple incompatibilities. Do not mix with other drugs, or consult with pharmacologist before mixing.

Observe for superinfections (*Candida* vaginitis).

Monitor liver and renal studies and CBC.

Small amounts of drug found in breast milk. May continue to breastfeed. Observe newborn for rash or diarrhea.

Drug	Use	Dosage and Route	Potential Side Effects
Gentamicin			
(Garamycin)—aminoglycoside	Treatment of postpartum endometritis, endomyometritis, and parametritis. Used for treatment of septicemia.	IM or IV: 3–5 mg/kg/daily in three divided doses q 8 h	Ototoxicity, nephrotoxicity. Allergic reactions: rash, pruritus, fever. Burning sensation of skin, local irritation of skin. Phlebitis.

Implications for Nursing Care

Ascertain that specimens for culture and sensitivity have been obtained before starting drug.

Assess for history of allergy or hypersensitivity to drug. Observe patient closely for signs of allergy or hypersensitivity. Discontinue drug immediately and notify physician if signs or symptoms of allergy or hypersensitivity occur.

Dilute each 100 mg with at least 10 mL of 0.9 NS for injection. Dilute with 50 mL of 5% D/W or 0.9 NS or Ringer's lactate for IV infusion. Infuse over 30–60 min.

Administer separately. Inactivated in penicillin solutions and ampicillins.

Observe for superinfections (*Candida* vaginitis).

Monitor blood levels of drug.

Monitor renal studies and urine output.

Keep patient hydrated. Monitor intake, output.

Small amounts of drug found in breast milk. May continue to breastfeed. Observe newborn for rash or diarrhea.

Drug	Use	Dosage and Route	Potential Side Effects
Tobramycin			
(Nebcin)—aminoglycoside	Treatment of postpartum endometritis, endomyometritis, and parametritis. Used for treatment of septicemia.	IM or IV: 3–5 mg/kg/daily, three equal doses q 8 h	Ototoxicity. Nephrotoxicity. Rash. Headache. Nausea, vomiting. Tremor, paraesthesia.

Implications for Nursing Care

Ascertain that specimens for culture and sensitivity have been obtained before starting drug.

Assess for history of allergy or hypersensitivity to drug. Observe patient closely for signs of allergy or hypersensitivity. Discontinue drug immediately and notify physician if signs or symptoms of allergy or hypersensitivity occur. Phlebitis.

Dilute each 40 mg with 1 mL of IV 0.9 NS for injection. Dilute with 50 mL of 5% D/W or 0.9 NS for IV infusion. Infuse over 20–60 min.

Administer separately.

Keep patient hydrated. Monitor intake, output.

Monitor renal function tests.

Small amounts of drug found in breast milk. May continue to breastfeed. Observe newborn for rash or diarrhea.

ALT, alanine aminotransferase; AST, aspartate aminotransferase; BUN, blood urea nitrogen; CBC, complete blood count; D/W, distilled water; NS, normal saline; UTI, urinary tract infection.

- Teaching proper breast care and breastfeeding techniques to prevent breakdown or trauma to nipples
- Using strict surgical asepsis when changing IV tubing and bags or administering IV drugs

Identifying Risks for Infection. The nurse reviews the woman's prenatal and intrapartum records to identify risks for infection. Vital signs and periodic assessments are also conducted to identify early signs of infection. The midwife or physician should be notified in a timely manner when fever or other abnormalities develop.

Monitoring Physiologic Status. When infection occurs, frequent, ongoing assessments (every 4 hours or more often) are essential to determine the woman's response to therapy and identify improvement or deterioration in her condition. Intake and output are monitored closely. The nurse also assesses the woman for evidence of septic shock, a life-threatening complication of postpartum infection (see Chapter 26 for a discussion of septic shock).

Reversing Hyperthermia. The woman with an infection may experience episodes of severe shaking chills followed by elevation in body temperature. The nurse provides extra blankets and should reassure the woman that as her temperature rises, the shaking chill will subside. When the woman's temperature rises above 38°C (100.4°F), antipyretics are administered to reduce the fever and to decrease the muscular aches and headache frequently accompanying pyrexia. In some cases, tepid sponge baths or a cooling blanket may be ordered when the fever is extreme (40°C [104°F]). Care must be taken not to lower the temperature too rapidly because shaking chills may develop.

Promoting Rest and Comfort. The nurse promotes rest and sleep when the woman experiences a postpartum infection to conserve energy, enhance immunologic function, and promote healing. Sleep deprivation can be a serious problem due to the presence of pain, the development of chills and fever, and the requirements of care. The nurse organizes care into clusters of activity to minimize unnecessary disruptions. With the exception of the partner or husband, visitors should be limited, and environmental stimuli should be minimized. The nurse should perform self-care activities for the woman until her condition improves.

The woman's level of discomfort or pain must be monitored closely. Pain may be localized to the site of infection (such as uterus, episiotomy, kidney, bladder), but as noted, general muscular achiness and headache are common. The nurse should administer analgesics liberally and encourage the woman to ask for pain medication before the sensations of pain or discomfort are severe. Other measures are implemented to enhance the woman's comfort such as the use of extra pillows, cool washcloths to the forehead, or a heating pad. Environmental stimuli (light, noise, and unpleasant odors) should be minimized.

The woman with a localized infection (ie, episiotomy or breast) may experience some discomfort or a minor reduction in energy level. But when the infection is severe, with significant inflammation, pain, and fever, generalized malaise and overwhelming fatigue are common. Self-care and newborn care activities will be assumed by the nursing staff or family members until the woman's condition improves. Bed baths and periodic perineal care are essential to promote comfort and conserve the woman's energy level.

Maintaining Fluid and Calorie Balance. If oral intake is permitted, light meals and liberal fluid intake (at least 3000 mL/24 h) should be encouraged. Increased calories are burned when fever occurs. Adequate calories are also required for immunologic function and tissue healing. Fluid requirements are increased with infection due to accelerated insensible water loss secondary to fever. Adequate fluid intake is required to promote excretion of antibiotics, and additional fluids are also required when the site of infection is the genitourinary system.

Administering Antibiotics. When signs and symptoms of infection develop, the nurse assists the midwife in obtaining cultures and blood samples for laboratory analysis.

Once infection has been diagnosed, the nurse is responsible for administering antibiotics and monitoring the woman's response to therapy.

The nurse must inquire about previous drug sensitivities or allergies. If the woman reports symptoms of previous drug reactions, the nurse must clarify the exact nature of the reaction. Before administration of antibiotics, the nurse must ascertain if the physician or nurse midwife is aware of this history of sensitivity. Once an antibiotic has been prescribed, the nurse must instruct the woman to report any symptoms suggestive of a drug reaction, including uticaria (hives); angioedema (swelling); generalized pruritus (rash); itching (eyes, ears, throat); tingling around the mouth; wheezing or shortness of breath; rhinorrhea (clear nasal discharge); or nausea, vomiting, or abdominal bloating.

When therapy is initiated, the nurse must observe the woman for the development of any of these symptoms. The nurse must be alert for anaphylaxis, a life-threatening type I (immediate) hypersensitivity reaction, and be prepared to support the woman until medical help arrives, as described in the accompanying Nursing Procedure.

Many substances can trigger an anaphylactic reaction, particularly antimicrobials such as penicillin and cephalosporins. Typically, the first complaints are of a feeling of uneasiness, apprehension, weakness, or impending doom. The person looks anxious. These sensations are followed, often rapidly, by generalized pruritus or uticarial wheals. Generalized flushing is common, and angioedema of the eyes, lips, and tongue frequently occurs. The person often complains of swelling of the tongue or throat. Dyspnea and shortness of breath are also common complaints, and on auscultation of the lungs, audible wheezing or rales are heard.

Airway obstruction can occur in a matter of seconds. Seventy percent of people who experience an anaphylactic reaction die of respiratory failure (Ignatavicius & Bayne, 1991). The person also becomes hypotensive, with a rapid, weak, and often irregular pulse. Arrhythmias, shock, and cardiac arrest may occur within minutes. Emergency respiratory management is critical, and antihistamines and cardiac

NURSING PROCEDURE

Caring for the Woman When an Anaphylactic Reaction Occurs During the Administration of Antibiotics

Purpose: To support cardiopulmonary function and reverse anaphylaxis

NURSING ACTION	***RATIONALE***
1. Stop the antibiotic if infusing intravenously.	To prevent further reaction to the drug
2. Call for help.	Additional staff will be required to support patient, give emergency drugs, and begin CPR if needed.
3. Initiate a "Code Blue" or CPR page or call.	Full CPR is often required.
4. Open airway.	To facilitate artificial ventilation
5. If patient is able to breathe spontaneously, administer oxygen by mask at 8 to 10 L or by nasal cannula at 5 to 6 L.	To supply supplemental oxygen and support cardiopulmonary function
6. Begin bag and mask ventilation with 100% oxygen if respirations are absent.	To ventilate and oxygenate patient
7. Assess pulse and if absent begin cardiac compression.	To support circulation
8. Administer epinephrine (1 : 1000) (0.2 to 0.5 mL) subcutaneously; repeat every 15 to 20 minutes as needed.	To stimulate cardiac function, promote bronchodilation, and restore blood pressure
9. Be prepared to administer diphenhydramine (Benadryl) 25 to 100 mg intravenously.	To reverse histamine release
10. Be prepared to assist with intubation or emergency tracheostomy.	To permit artificial ventilation when angioedema occludes the patient's airway

stimulants (epinephrine) must be administered to reverse the reaction and support cardiovascular status.

Providing Wound Care. The nurse performs wound care and dressing changes as ordered when infections occur at incision sites or in lacerations. Strict surgical asepsis is maintained during the procedure. Wound care and dressing changes can be painful and extremely traumatic for the woman. The sights and smells can be unpleasant for many people, and significant alterations in body image may occur. Planning for wound care should include the administration of appropriate analgesics and waiting at least an hour after meals before beginning the procedure. The room should be well ventilated, and efforts should be made to provide privacy during dressing changes.

Because the time permitted for hospital stay is limited today by most insurance companies, many women will be expected to perform their own wound care at home after discharge. The nurse must demonstrate the procedure, teach the woman about sterile technique, and supervise her efforts at wound care. This can be a difficult process for some women, and they will require intensive support, reinforcement, and encouragement to accomplish this task.

Promoting Maternal–Newborn Attachment. The neonate is permitted to remain with the woman who experiences a postpartum infection. In most cases, the neonate can continue to breastfeed, even when antibiotics, analgesics, and antipyretics (acetominophen) are administered. Handwashing and medical asepsis are reinforced as the woman assumes infant care activities. If the woman is fatigued, she may desire periods of uninterrupted rest, and the newborn may be placed in the nursery for short periods of time.

If the woman's condition deteriorates and she is unable to care for her newborn, the neonate may remain in the nursery for extended periods of time. The nurse should make a special effort to report on the neonate's condition frequently and to bring the newborn to the woman as often as desired. If breastfeeding is temporarily interrupted because the woman is extremely ill, a breast pump may be used to stimulate milk production. Once her condition stabilizes, breastfeeding can be resumed.

The development of infection during the postpartum period can dramatically alter the woman's physiologic and psychological stability. The nurse plays a central role in identification of postpartum infections and initiation of therapy. Additional nursing care will be required to prevent further complications, promote breast feeding and maternal–newborn attachment, and support family adaptations. The nurse must be skilled in administering IV antibiotics, performing wound care, and beginning immediate emergency support when adverse reactions to treatment, such as anaphylaxis, occur. Family-centered care can foster family formation and reduce the negative consequences of postpartum complications.

Infections of the Reproductive Tract

The pelvic cavity remains the site of infection for most postpartum infections. Bacterial invasion can occur during labor, delivery, or the postpartum period. In some cases, the woman enters the intrapartum period with preexisting problems that predispose her to infection, such as a history of pyelonephritis (see Table 29-1). The woman's physical status, as well as the nature of medical therapy and nursing care, will be determined by the type of postpartum infection. The following section describes common infections of the reproductive tract.

Superficial Endometritis, Endomyometritis, and Parametritis

The most common infection in the postpartum period is an *endometritis* involving the superficial mucous or decidual layer. In its mildest form this infected layer of sloughing cellular material is simply passed away in the form of lochia, and normal involution continues. If for some reason the woman's immunologic resources are compromised and bacterial colonies continue to grow, infections will extend from the endometrium into the muscular layer, or myometrium, of the uterus and result in *endomyometritis*. An undiagnosed or unsuccessfully treated infection of the endomyometrium will progress to involve the entire uterus and may spread to accessory pelvic structures. The main pathway for spread of the infection is the broad ligament, a double fold of peritoneum that encloses the uterus, fallopian tubes, ovaries, and round ligaments and attaches to the lateral walls of the pelvic cavity (Fig. 29-6).

The infection is usually polymicrobial in nature (Silver & Smith, 1991). Commonly isolated pathogens include aerobic gram-negative bacilli (*Escherichia coli* and *Klebsiella*), aerobic gram-positive streptococci (group B streptococcus), anaerobic gram-negative bacilli (*Bacteroides* species), and anaerobic gram-positive bacilli (*Peptostreptococcus* species).

Etiologic and Predisposing Factors

Risk factors for the development of endometritis, endomyometritis, or parametritis include cesarean delivery, prolonged rupture of membranes, or prolonged labor. During the intrapartum period, the use of invasive procedures, such as internal electronic fetal monitoring, fetal scalp sampling, or amnioinfusion, also predispose the woman to infection of the uterus and surrounding tissues.

Diagnosis

Signs and symptoms of a developing endomyometritis include:

- Onset usually 24 hours after delivery
- Foul or purulent lochia
- Uterine tenderness
- Subinvolution of the uterus

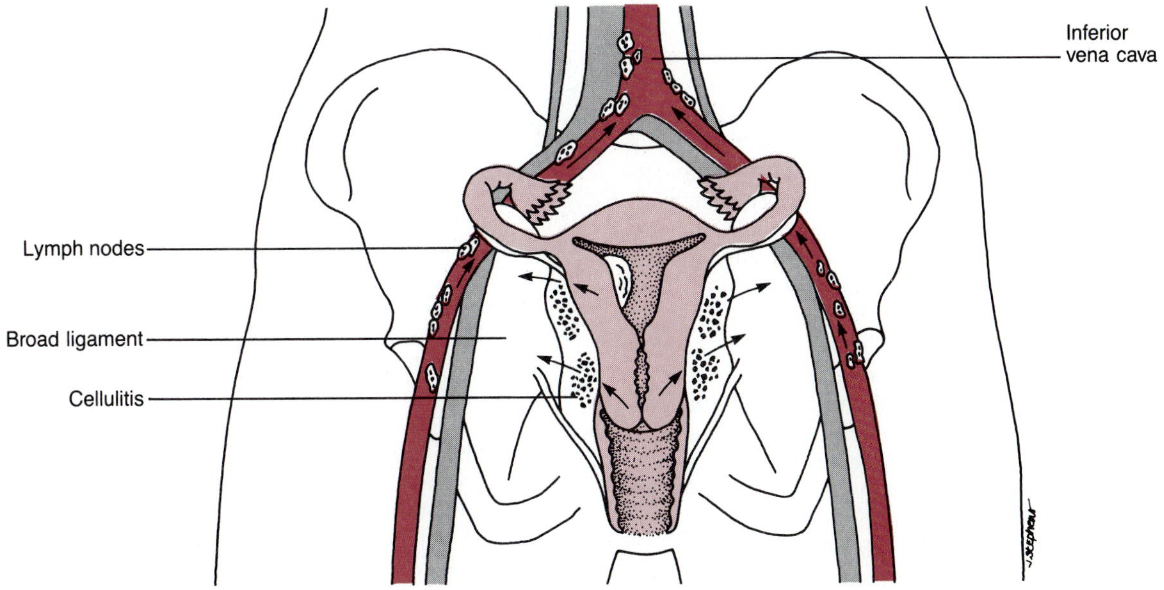

Figure 29-6.

Postpartum infection extends to the structures around the uterus, resulting in pelvic cellulitis (parametritis) (Childbirth Graphics).

- Symptoms of malaise, fatigue, and anorexia
- Tachycardia (averaging 100 to 120 bpm)
- Temperature range 38°C to 38.9°C (100.4°F to 102°F) after the first 24 hours
- Elevation in leukocyte count

Symptoms of parametritis are generally more severe than those of endometritis.

Maternal Implications

The woman may feel quite ill, with fever, generalized muscular aches, headache, and uterine pain and tenderness. Nausea, vomiting, or diarrhea may occur due to pain, antibiotic administration, and the infection. Anorexia is common with high fevers, and in some cases the lochia will be foul or purulent, increasing the woman's general lack of appetite. The woman is often unable to participate in self-care or newborn care activities until therapy is well established. Breastfeeding is permitted and encouraged to facilitate contraction of the uterus and promote maternal–newborn attachment. However, many women may be initially too ill to feed the infant every 2 to 3 hours around the clock. Feelings of depression are common and are often related to the woman's physiologic status.

The woman with an infection of the uterus or surrounding tissues is at risk for life-threatening complications. Unresponsive or refractory infections that do not improve with antibiotic therapy may spread and cause pelvic thrombophlebitis, pelvic abscess, or septic shock. When this occurs, she may be transferred to an ICU for further therapy and invasive monitoring. Individual psychological adaptations to the postpartum period are delayed, and the memories of these complications and events may alter the woman's feeling about the newborn and future childbearing.

Treatment

Treatment consists of aggressive antibiotic therapy. Ninety-five percent of women who have delivered vaginally will respond to a combination of penicillin and an aminoglycoside. The addition of clindamycin to treat anaerobic infections (triple antibiotic therapy) will increase the rate of cure to 98% (Silver & Smith, 1991). When a uterine infection occurs after cesarean birth, the most effective therapy is a combination of an aminoglycoside and clindamycin. Research now indicates that after cesarean delivery, prophylactic administration of a cephalosporin antibiotic such as cefazolin (1 g every 6 hours for three doses) will significantly reduce the incidence of postpartum endometritis (Faro, Martens, Hammill, , 1990).

Antibiotic therapy is continued until the woman has been afebrile for 48 hours. If treatment is unsuccessful, including various combination antibiotic therapies, the physician may consider surgical intervention. The endometrium is cleared using curettage to remove retained infected tissue. Surgical resolution of an abscess is attempted with two methods. If there is a strong suspicion that the abscess is located in the cul-de-sac of Douglas (a recess or cavity created by an extension of the peritoneum between the uterus and vagina anteriorly and the rectum and uterus posteriorly), a colpotomy or incision is made to allow for drainage of purulent material (Fig. 29-7).

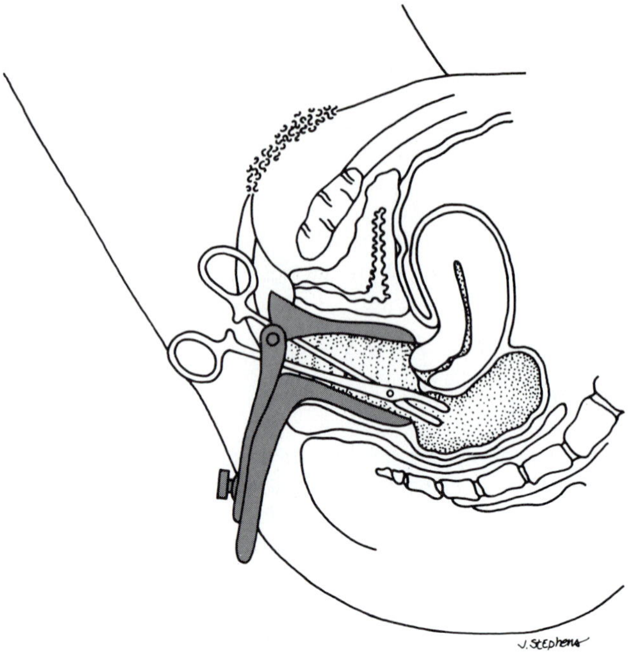

Figure 29-7.
Posterior colpotomy. Draining a collection of localized pus in the cul-de-sac of Douglas (Childbirth Graphics).

The second method involves the use of a laparotomy, or surgical opening of the abdomen, to identify the location and extent of the infection. Once this information has been ascertained, further surgery may be deemed necessary, including removal of the uterus and one or both of the ovaries and fallopian tubes (total abdominal hysterectomy with unilateral or bilateral salpingo-oophorectomy).

Implications for Nursing Care

Nursing responsibilities include those described in the previous sections on general nursing care when postpartum infection occurs. The promotion of recovery through rest, a therapeutic diet, and increased fluid intake is emphasized. The woman is positioned with the head of the bed elevated at 30 to 45 degrees to diminish upward movement of the pelvic infection. Antibiotics are administered as ordered.

Close attention is paid to meeting the woman's hygiene needs, including regular mouth care, perineal care, and bed baths until she is well enough to assume self-care activities. Comfort is promoted through the use of specific strategies including massage, extra pillows, or a cool washcloth to the forehead. Antipyretics are administered to reduce fever, and analgesics are given to maintain comfort, particularly before activities that increase pain, such as ambulation.

The woman's vital signs are monitored every 4 hours or more frequently, depending on her condition. Assessment of intake and output is essential because fluid loss is increased with fever, and oral intake is often limited by nausea, general anorexia, and lethargy. The nurse observes for signs of deterioration in the woman's condition, which occur with spread of infection or septic shock (see Chapter 26). Danger signs include:

- Tachypnea (24 breaths/min or higher)

- Severe tachycardia (greater than 120 bpm)
- Hypotension
- Changes in consciousness including disorientation or agitation
- Decreasing urine output (less than 40 to 50 mL/h)

The woman and her family must be well informed concerning the nature of the infection and its treatment and the risks and benefits of surgery should conventional therapy fail. This is the responsibility of the physician, but frequently the woman will use the nurse to verify her understanding and to further explore the situation. Using active listening as a tool, the nurse can promote optimal adaptation by helping the woman work through her personal reactions to the situation. The nurse also serves as a resource person in referring the woman to other professionals who can provide religious or psychological support or additional medical opinions concerning her condition.

Peritonitis and Adnexal Infections

Etiologic and Predisposing Factors

The peritoneum is a thin membranous tissue that lines the walls of abdominal and pelvic cavities. In some cases, uterine infection extends into the abdominal cavity through the lymphatic system (Fig. 29-8). Infection can also spread to the uterine adnexa, consisting of the ovaries, fallopian tubes, and ligaments of the uterus. Ovarian abscess may develop as well as salpingitis (infection of the fallopian tube).

Diagnosis

Symptoms of peritonitis vary according to the extent of the infection and the type of organisms involved. The most severe symptoms associated with nonlocalized infections that have affected other body systems include:

- Severe shaking chills
- Temperature spikes to 40.5°C (105°F)
- Tachycardia and tachypnea
- Excessive thirst
- Nausea, vomiting, diarrhea
- Acute abdominal pain
- Absence of bowel sounds
- Abdominal distention and rigidity
- Fruity or foul-smelling breath
- Oliguria
- Initial depression in leukocyte count followed by a leukocytosis

Maternal Implications

When infection spreads to the abdominal cavity, the peritoneum produces a fibrous exudate as part of the inflammatory process. This fibrinopurulent exudate binds loops of bowel to one another, creating mechanical obstructions and causing significant alterations in gastrointestinal functioning. Adhesions resulting from peritonitis often disappear with adequate treatment of the infection. If unresolved, the adhesions may harden into fibrous bands that may cause intestinal obstruction later. Another serious complication of peritonitis is paralytic ileus (complete absence of bowel peristalsis). With complete absence of bowel function, abdominal distention, nausea and vomiting, and fluid and electrolyte imbalances can occur.

Fluid and electrolyte imbalances also result from shunting of blood to the abdominal cavity in response to the inflammatory process. Fluid shifts from the vascular compartment to the abdominal cavity, resulting in decreasing circulatory volume, hypotension, and inadequate renal perfusion. Renal failure and severe electrolyte imbalances result. Vomiting and diarrhea also contribute to fluid and electrolyte losses.

The maternal mortality rate associated with peritonitis depends on the success of therapy and the development of

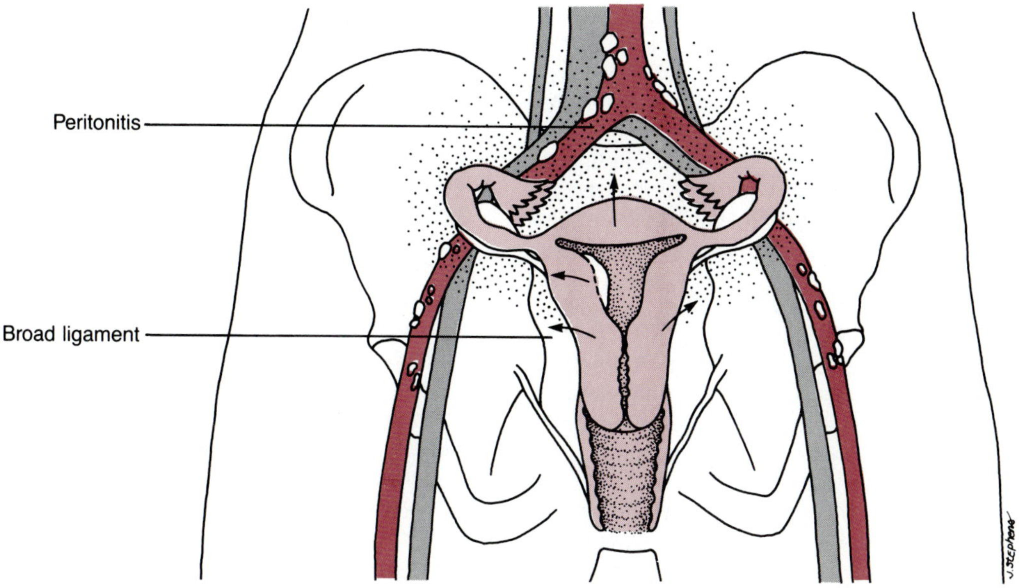

Figure 29-8.

Postpartum infection extends to the peritoneum. Infection is extended by way of the lymph nodes and uterine wall (Childbirth Graphics).

additional complications. When septic shock occurs, mortality rates as high as 81% have been reported. DIC, evidenced by changes in the coagulation profile, may occur in some cases of peritonitis and can lead to hemorrhage and maternal death.

When infection of uterine adnexa occur, the sequelae are usually less serious. However, ovarian abscesses can develop. If the abscess ruptures, peritonitis may result. Salpingitis can lead to scarring and occlusion of the fallopian tube(s), which may cause permanent sterilization in the woman. This complication, although not life-threatening, can greatly alter the woman's life. The prospect of childlessness for a woman who desires more children can be emotionally devastating.

Treatment

Treatment is aggressive and comprehensive. Primary treatment is focused on:

- Diagnosis and treatment of infectious agent
- Replacement of fluid and electrolyte losses
- Maintenance of adequate intravascular volume and blood pressure
- Decompression of the gastrointestinal tract

Once specimens for culture have been obtained, IV antibiotic therapy is begun. The choice of drugs will vary with physicians but often includes a penicillin, an aminoglycoside, and a cephalosporin. IV fluid and electrolyte replacement is initiated. The gastrointestinal tract is decompressed by continuous nasogastric suction. Oral intake is withheld until bowel sounds return and flatus is expelled. If obstruction of the bowel does not resolve with therapy, surgical correction of adhesions or drainage of abscesses will be necessary.

Implications for Nursing Care

Intensive nursing care is required when peritonitis or infection of uterine adnexa is diagnosed. Nursing responsibilities include frequent assessment of vital signs (every hour or more often during the initial period of therapy). Central venous pressure and pulmonary artery pressure monitoring are often implemented to evaluate circulatory status and blood pressure. The nurse monitors and interprets data provided by these methods. Intake and output are measured hourly. The woman will frequently have a nasogastric tube as well as a Foley catheter. Drainage from the nasogastric tube and the amount of emesis are included in the calculation of output.

Complete systems assessments are conducted periodically. Cardiovascular and respiratory status is assessed by frequent checks of vital signs, assessment of skin color, the presence of peripheral edema, capillary fill time, breath sounds, and evidence of respiratory distress. Arterial blood gas readings are obtained when significant alterations in cardiovascular function occur and may herald the onset of adult respiratory distress syndrome. Alterations in mentation may also be indicative of deterioration in the cardiovascular function, circulatory decompensation, or pulmonary dysfunction.

Gastrointestinal function is assessed for the presence of bowel sounds, abdominal contour, the nature of nasogastric drainage, emesis, or stools. Complaints of worsening abdominal pain, increasing abdominal girth, and rigidity are ominous and must be reported immediately. Renal function must also be monitored closely. Fluid volume deficits and hypotension can lead to inadequate renal perfusion. Renal failure (less than 20 mL urine/h) is often a late sign of peritonitis associated with septic shock.

Attention is directed at measures of comfort, oral care, positioning, and providing medications for pain relief and anxiety. Peritonitis is debilitating and will represent a crisis for the new mother and her family. Attention must be paid to keeping the woman's family informed about her condition. If healthy, the newborn may be ready for discharge before the mother. Issues of separation from the newborn may have emotional and psychological impacts on the woman and should be approached carefully. It is of primary importance to determine how the woman feels about the separation and to give reassurance when appropriate.

Infections of the pelvic and abdominal cavities can result in significant morbidity and mortality for the postpartum woman. Because serious complications such as septic shock can occur, the woman's condition must be closely monitored. The nurse must be knowledgeable regarding both subtle and obvious signs of deterioration in the woman's status. Expert nursing care is required to maintain physiologic stability. The nurse is responsible for implementing medical therapy and evaluating the woman's response to treatment. These activities require careful planning. A major goal is to organize care in a manner that reduces unnecessary interruptions and promotes rest and tissue healing.

Infections of the Perineum and Vagina

Infection in the perineum or vagina usually involves the site of a laceration or episiotomy wound. Superficial infections are more common and involve the skin, subcutaneous tissue, and superficial fascial edge. In rare cases, superficial infections may spread to the fascia, the sheet of fibrous tissue that lies below the subcutaneous layer, or to deeper muscle layers.

Superficial or Simple Infections

Etiologic and Predisposing Factors

Infections of soft tissue are defined according to the depth of the infection. A simple or superficial infection involves only the skin, subcutaneous tissue, and superficial fascial edge. Localized infection of the episiotomy is the most common postpartum infection of the external genitalia (Cunningham et al., 1989).

Diagnosis

When a laceration of the episiotomy becomes infected, the wound edges appear erythematous and swollen. The sutures may tear through the infected tissues, permitting the necrotic wound edges to open. Serous, serosanguineous, or purulent material drains from the site. A foul odor is evident, and the woman most often complains of increased pain in the area.

Maternal Implications

Because the infection is localized, the woman may be able to continue activities of daily living, self-care, breastfeeding, and neonate care. Discomfort is often localized to the infected tissues. Because of the pain and edema, the woman will usually have difficulty getting in and out of bed and sitting on the perineal area. Additional discomfort may occur when the woman voids or defecates because of the tension placed on the infected perineum when she bears down.

Hospital discharge may be delayed by several days for antibiotic therapy and wound care. The woman may have fears regarding scarring of the perineal tissue, difficulties with intercourse when sexual relations are resumed, and future problems during labor and birth. Often, however, the woman is reticent about sharing these concerns with others.

Treatment

Treatment includes opening of the wound with exploration for possible hematomas or wall defects between the vagina and rectum, followed by debridement. Cultures are obtained at this time. Drainage alone may be sufficient to promote healing but is usually combined with a broad-spectrum antimicrobial agent. The wound is not sutured and will be allowed to heal by granulation.

Implications for Nursing Care

Nursing care involves close monitoring of the wound for symptoms of spread of the infection. The extent of edema (in centimeters) and the appearance of the tissue must be determined and charted at least once every 8 hours. Once the wound has been debrided, special care is given to promote drainage and provide a clean environment for healing. Perineal care includes sitz baths, exposure to air, and heat lamp treatments in some facilities. Analgesia is offered for pain. If the wound is packed, the physician will write orders for removal of the packing before discharge.

Before discharge the nurse discusses ongoing care at home. Resumption of sexual relations is determined after the physician examines the woman during subsequent office or clinic visits. The nurse should explore the woman's concerns regarding the appearance of the wound and her fears about intercourse. Sensitivity and active listening may reduce the woman's embarrassment about the topic if she is initially uncomfortable talking about these issues.

Necrotizing Fasciitis

Etiologic and Predisposing Factors

A rare but extremely serious complication of perineal or vaginal infection is necrotizing fasciitis. Localized infection extends into deep soft tissues involving the fascia and underlying muscle. Bacteria causing this type of infection are similar to those found in other postpartum infections (both gram-negative and gram-positive aerobic and anaerobic bacteria). *E. coli* and *Clostridium perfringens* are often isolated.

Necrotizing fasciitis of the episiotomy may spread along the fascia to the abdominal wall, thigh, or buttock. By this time the infection frequently involves significant necrosis of the tissue. When the infection involves the muscles below the deep fascia, the condition is called myonecrosis. A differentiating symptom is the existence of severe pain.

Diagnosis

Early symptoms of necrotizing fasciitis may be difficult to distinguish from simple infection of a laceration or episiotomy. As the infection progresses, however, the following signs and symptoms may occur:

- Severe perineal pain
- Pronounced perineal edema
- Onset 3 to 5 days after birth
- Skin overlying infected area becomes blue or brown in color due to occlusion of vessels close to the skin surface
- Formation of bullae (blisters or skin vesicles filled with fluid)
- Tissue hypoesthesia (loss of sensation)
- Leukocytosis

Maternal Implications

The development of necrotizing fasciitis results in prolonged hospitalization, permanent scarring and possibly loss of sensation in the perineal region. The severity of long-term problems will depend on the extent of tissue and muscle dissection required to remove necrotic tissue. Sexual intercourse with penile penetration may be difficult to achieve when scarring is severe and distortion in the anatomy of the vagina and perineum occurs. The ability to have a vaginal birth in subsequent pregnancies may be in question when tissue loss is severe. In many cases, skin grafting will be required later to repair major tissue defects. When infection leads to myofasciitis, capillary leakage, circulatory failure, shock, and death may occur. Mortality is virtually universal without surgical treatment to remove the infected and necrotic tissue.

The woman is extremely ill, requires intensive nursing care, and will be unable to perform self-care or newborn care activities until the healing process is well under way. Alterations in self-concept and body image may occur due to the loss of tissue, scarring, and permanent disability. The woman may manifest signs and symptoms of grief (see Chapter 25), including anger and shock, as she begins to realize the extent of the problem. The partner or husband may also have significant fears about the woman's condition, both during the crisis and afterward. Physical rehabilitation and psychological counseling may be required.

Treatment

Surgical treatment is essential tc remove all infected and necrotic tissue. Debridement is followed by aggressive antibiotic therapy, fluid and electrolyte replacement, and the administration of analgesics. As noted, if significant tissue loss occurs, skin grafts will be required to repair the defects.

Implications for Nursing Care

Nursing responsibilities include those listed previously for superficial infections and those outlined for women with systemic infection. Frequent assessment (every 1 to 4 hours) of the vital signs, the perineum, and all other systems is essential to identify signs or symptoms of deterioration in the woman's condition. Wound care may be an additional area of nursing responsibility and often includes periodic irrigation of the infected area with solutions containing antibiotics.

If extensive debridement or dissection is necessary, the nurse must take the time to help the woman deal with the impact of permanent changes to the anatomy in what is generally considered a sensitive or private area of the body. Such changes may affect the way the woman relates to her own sexuality and may have a lasting impact. Referrals should be made for psychological counseling as indicated or requested by the woman.

Infections of the external genitalia are a common problem in the postpartum period but are usually less serious in nature than those affecting the pelvic or abdominal cavities. Short courses of antibiotic therapy combined with debridement of the wound usually shorten the hospital stay. Nursing care is focused on wound care and the administration of antimicrobial agents.

Although usually less serious in nature, postpartum infections involving the perineum or vagina may be distressing for the woman. Because of the sexual and reproductive functions associated with this area of the body, adverse psychological sequelae may be equal to or greater than negative physical consequences. The nurse must be particularly sensitive to the emotional needs of the woman, while monitoring physiologic status and carrying out medical therapy. Appropriate referrals should be initiated for psychological counseling and support as needed.

Postpartum Urinary Tract Infections

Urinary tract infection (UTI) occurs commonly during the postpartum period and is a frequent cause of morbidity. Cystitis, an infection of the bladder mucosa, and pyelonephritis, an infection of the kidneys, are two common infections documented in postpartum women.

Etiologic and Predisposing Factors

Because of the structure and physiologic processes of the female urogenital tract, bacteriuria is common in many women. Bacteriuria is defined as the presence of 10^5or more bacterial colonies per milliliter of urine on two consecutive, clean, midstream, voided specimens. Normal changes of pregnancy that contribute to an increased risk for UTI include:

- Uterine compression of the ureters at the pelvic inlet
- Dilatation and diminished tone of the ureters as a result of hormonal effects

When these risk factors are combined, urinary stasis promotes bacterial growth. The urogenital tract is made more vulnerable to infection during childbirth by trauma, urinary stasis, and catheterization.

Diagnosis

Signs and symptoms of UTI will depend in part on the location of the infection.

Cystitis is an inflammation of the urinary bladder. Symptoms indicating cystitis include:

- Urinary urgency
- Urinary frequency
- Dysuria
- Suprapubic pain
- Hematuria (not always present)
- White blood cells, red blood cells, and protein in the urine

Pyelonephritis is an inflammation of bacterial origin of one or both of the kidneys. Symptoms of pyelonephritis are:

- Shaking chills and fever
- Flank pain—positive costovertebral angle tenderness
- Nausea and vomiting
- Bacteriuria
- Increased serum white blood cell count
- White blood cells, red blood cells, and protein in the urine

When infection is suspected, a routine urinalysis is done to observe first-line indicators of infection, including an increase in white blood cells, protein, or blood in the urine. A culture of urine obtained by clean-catch technique or sterile catheterization of the bladder is performed to identify the microorganisms. Antibiotic sensitivity tests are also performed so that appropriate drug therapy can be initiated as quickly as possible. The most common offending bacterium is *E. coli*, followed by *Klebsiella* organisms, *Proteus* organisms, streptococci, coagulase-negative staphylococci, and enterococci. Recent research indicates that women with a previous history of bacteriuria who are symptomatic may have UTIs even with lower bacterial counts (10^2 or greater) (Stray-Pedersen, Blakstad, & Bergan, 1990).

Maternal Implications

In many cases, postpartum women are only screened for UTIs when classic symptoms occur. Unfortunately, the consequences of failing to recognize cystitis include progression of the infection along the urinary tract, escalation of symptoms, and ultimately the development of pyelonephritis. Pyelonephritis may result in permanent kidney damage and systemic infection.

With proper treatment, the recovery period is generally short, and long-term adverse sequelae are rare. During the first 24 hours of treatment the woman may need assistance with some self-care or neonate care activities. Breastfeeding should be encouraged, and the newborn can remain with the woman who feels well enough to care for her neonate.

Treatment

Primary treatment includes the use of appropriate antibiotic therapy. If the antibiotic used is appropriate for the organism, symptomatic relief should be obtained within 24 hours (Stamm, 1988). Because many of the gram-negative bacilli implicated in UTIs are resistant to ampicillin, a cephalosporin such as cefazolin should be added to the initial therapy. Further therapy is guided by the results of the culture and sensitivity test. The drugs are given by the IV route until the woman is afebrile for 48 hours. Oral antibiotics are then substituted and administered for 10 to 14 days (Silver & Smith, 1991).

Implications for Nursing Care

Teaching is a primary key to prevention of any UTI and should include the following topics:

- Routine measures for urogenital cleanliness
- Use of cotton underclothing
- Adequate fluid intake
- Frequent voiding
- Voiding before and after intercourse
- Early treatment of vaginitis

Nursing responsibilities of the hospitalized postpartum woman with cystitis include observing for symptoms of an ascending infection and measuring fluid intake and output. The nurse encourages increased fluid intake (at least 1000 mL/8 h) and teaches the woman about proper use of oral antibiotics. Analgesics or agents that reduce bladder spasms may also be given to reduce bladder discomfort and urinary urgency. Once symptoms are relieved, the woman will probably be sent home. The importance of continuing antibiotic therapy and completing the follow-up assessment with a urine culture to test for antibiotic cure should be stressed.

Nursing care of the woman with pyelonephritis includes close observation of vital signs (at least every 4 hours or more often) and monitoring intake and output. The urine is observed for evidence of blood, and a sample may be assessed by urine dipstick once a shift to evaluate effectiveness of therapy. The woman's condition should begin to improve within 24 hours of therapy, and a complete physical assessment is conducted at least every 8 hours to verify effectiveness of treatment.

The nurse supports immune function and tissue healing by encouraging rest, a therapeutic diet, and adequate fluid intake. The woman will have an IV, but if oral fluids are permitted, she should be encouraged to drink liberally (at least 1000 mL every 8 hours). The woman with pyelonephritis often feels extremely ill for the first 24 hours, even with initiation of therapy. She may experience severe chills, high fever, generalized muscular aches, and backache. Relief measures are provided for these discomforts, including the administration of antipyretics and analgesics and the use of a cooling blanket.

Urinary tract infections are a common complication in the postpartum period. The nurse plays a central role in prevention of UTIs and in the early identification of infection when it occurs. A major goal of care is to implement medical therapy in a timely manner so that the risk of ascending infection or the development of systemic infection is minimized. The nurse guides the woman in self-care activities that promote cure and tissue healing, such as maintaining a therapeutic diet and increasing fluid intake. Discharge teaching focuses on the self-administration of antibiotics and prevention of future UTIs.

Infection of the Breast

Mastitis is an infection of the parenchyma of the mammary gland usually occurring within the first 2 to 3 weeks of the postpartum period. Infectious complications involving the breast range from benign inflammations to breast abscesses. During the period of lactation, the breast changes from an essentially nonfunctioning to a complex functioning organ of the body. Because the developing multiductal system necessitates high-volume circulation, the breast becomes a rich environment for the growth of bacteria.

Etiologic and Predisposing Factors

The incidence of mastitis has not been reported definitively, but the probable origins of infection may be divided into two categories. Epidemic mastitis is derived from a nosocomial source. This infection is commonly associated with *Staphylococcus aureus* and localizes in the lactiferous glands and ducts. It occurs among women who have been hospitalized where neonates are cared for in a central nursery. The second source is one of endemic infection, which occurs randomly and localizes in the periglandular connective tissue. This infection is frequently associated with a break in the integrity of the nipple surface (Olsen & Gordon, 1990).

The most common break in the nipple surface is due to a crack or fissure, which may occur as a result of the following factors:

- Improper attachment of the newborn to areola (sucks on nipple and does not compress ducts underlying areola)
- Placing neonate in the same position for each feeding
- Starting the newborn on the same breast at the beginning of each feeding
- Failing to break neonate's attachment to areola and nipple before removing from breast
- Using soap on nipples
- Permitting the nipples to remain wet (using plastic breast shields)

Pronounced breast engorgement results in stasis of blood and lymph and may predispose the woman to mastitis if pathogenic bacteria are introduced through a crack or fissure in the nipple.

Diagnosis

Symptoms that signify mastitis include shaking chills; rapid rise in temperature up to 40°C (104°F); tachypnea and tachycardia; reddened and exquisitely tender breast tissue; and palpable, hard masses in the breast.

Diagnosis and treatment are based on the symptomatology. Under circumstances of persistent infection, white blood cell counts and cultures and sensitivity tests of breast milk are used for a definitive diagnosis of the offending organism. *S. aureus* is the causative agent in 95% of cases. Other organisms implicated in mastitis include group A and B streptococcus, *Haemophilus influenzae*, and *Haemophilus parainfluenzae* (Silver & Smith, 1991).

Occasionally, breast abscesses will develop. Symptoms include all those previously listed for mastitis as well as the following:

- Discharge of purulent exudate from the nipple or breast

- Masses or reddened areas that may develop a bluish hue of the skin over the area of abscess

Maternal Implications

Once glandular breast tissue fills with infectious exudate, circulation within the breast is interrupted, leading to the symptoms of fullness and pain. The woman may feel extremely ill for the first 24 to 48 hours of therapy and may find it difficult to continue breastfeeding, self-care, and newborn care activities. Because engorgement can become severe with inflammation of breast tissue and stasis of blood and lymph, pain in the affected breast can be severe. The woman's level of discomfort is exacerbated by the generalized muscular aches and headache that frequently accompany chills and fever. Breast abscess may develop in rare cases of mastitis and may present a serious threat to the lactating woman. Systemic spread and possible permanent breast tissue damage may result.

For the new mother attempting breastfeeding for the first time, the development of mastitis can be a great disappointment. She may feel discouraged and predisposed to stop breastfeeding. Concerns about the quality of the milk and fear that she may transmit the infection to the newborn may also influence discontinuation of breastfeeding. Alterations in body image and self-concept are common problems associated with mastitis.

Treatment

Treatment of mastitis begins with antibiotic therapy. The drug of choice should be effective against penicillinase-producing *S. aureus* such as dicloxacillin. Antibiotic administration continues for 10 days. Relief of symptoms often occurs 24 to 48 hours after initiation of treatment when effective. Women must be encouraged to complete the entire regimen of therapy. In addition to antimicrobial therapy, breastfeeding should be continued, or the breast should be pumped and emptied on the affected side to relieve engorgement. Ice packs can be applied to reduce pain, and a supportive bra should be worn. Treatment of a breast abscess also includes the use of antibiotics, and surgical incision and drainage of the abscess are indicated.

Implications for Nursing Care

Women must be encouraged to practice personal hygiene measures that will help to protect against mastitis. These measures include:

- Avoidance of soaps on the nipples
- Gentleness when washing breasts
- Breast cleanliness (wash with water, wear clean bra)
- Avoidance of decrusting the nipple of dried colostrum or milk
- Frequent changing of breast pads (especially when wet)
- Intermittent exposure of nipples to the air
- Handwashing before handling breast and before breastfeeding

Once mastitis is diagnosed, the nurse instructs the woman in appropriate self-administration of oral antibiotics. She is encouraged to increase her fluid intake to eight to ten 8-oz glasses per day, mostly of water. Breastfeeding is encouraged at frequent intervals (every 2 to 3 hours) to promote milk flow through the breast. Heat packs or hot showers are used to promote circulation to the area, and mild analgesics are used for the relief of pain. With extreme engorgement, some experts recommend the temporary use of ice packs to reduce sensations of pain.

Opinions vary concerning whether the woman with a breast abscess should continue to breastfeed. Many experts believe that nursing should be discontinued while purulent exudate continues. If the woman is advised by her primary health provider to discontinue breastfeeding, support must be given for suppression of lactation. It should be remembered that breastfeeding is frequently an emotionally laden issue, and support and encouragement may be needed to facilitate continued nursing. If breastfeeding is to be resumed after the infection, a woman will need guidance in the pumping of her breasts and reestablishing lactation (Olsen & Gordon, 1990).

The maternity nurse plays a central role in the prevention and early identification of mastitis. Ongoing teaching and support of the breastfeeding woman will significantly reduce risk factors associated with infection of the mammary glands. When the woman places significant value on breastfeeding, the development of mastitis may be a particularly upsetting event. The pain and engorgement often associated with this infection may exacerbate the woman's level of distress. A major goal of nursing care is to promote and support the continuation of breastfeeding while antibiotic therapy and local treatment of inflammation and engorgement are implemented.

Infection of the Incision From a Cesarean Birth

Wound infections may involve the abdominal incision after cesarean birth. These infections may involve superficial layers of skin and subcutaneous tissue or fascial and muscle layers.

Etiologic and Predisposing Factors

A number of risk factors have been identified that predispose the woman to an abdominal wound infection. They include low socioeconomic status, chorioamnionitis, prolonged surgery, emergency cesarean birth, diabetes mellitus, substance abuse and cigarette smoking, obesity, and malnutrition.

Diagnosis

A wound infection has been defined by the National Academy of Sciences as an incision with signs of inflammation and purulent discharge (Silver & Smith, 1991). Post-cesarean wound infections usually become apparent clinically 3 to 8 days after delivery. The skin surrounding the incision is frequently erythematous and swollen. The site is often tender, and palpable fluctuance occurs under the skin. Drainage of purulent material often occurs but may not become evident until the sutures are removed and the incision is reopened.

Culture of the purulent exudate is performed and antibiotic sensitivity determined. The organisms most frequently isolated from the abdominal incision are those found in the lower genital tract.

The woman may complain of increased tenderness or pain at the incision site, which persists even after the administration of large doses of analgesics. If deep layers of the incision are involved, involuntary muscle rigidity surrounding the incision may be palpated. Fever may be present, but the woman may remain afebrile.

Maternal Implications

Wound infections will prolong the hospital stay, delay postpartum recovery, and may result in significant scarring at the incision site. The woman may be unable to resume activities of daily living as rapidly as is desired after surgical birth, and this may contribute to other postsurgical complications such as pulmonary atelectasis or thrombophlebitis. Significant pain may be experienced, and once the incision is reopened, debridement, wound irrigations, and dressing changes can increase the woman's discomfort.

If the infected incision opens spontaneously (dehiscence), the woman can be extremely frightened. Complete dehiscence may result in evisceration of bowel. This is a medical emergency necessitating return to surgery for return of bowel to the abdominal cavity and debridement of the wound. The woman is exposed to all the risks associated with surgery and will have a prolonged hospital stay.

The incision will not be resutured after it has been debrided, and wound healing will occur by secondary intention. Most women are discharged home before the wound is entirely healed and will be expected to continue wound care and dressing changes at home. This can be a traumatic experience and can result in significant alterations in self-concept and body image. At times, family members will also assist with wound care.

Treatment

The wound must be opened, cleaned, and debrided. Antibiotic therapy is initiated. The physician will order ongoing wound irrigation and dressing changes to be performed several times each day.

Implications for Nursing Care

The nurse caring for the woman with an infection of the abdominal incision is responsible for the ongoing assessment of tissue healing and the effectiveness of therapy. Notations about the presence and size of erythema and edema and the nature of discharge are placed in the medical record after assessment is completed. When dressing changes are performed, the nurse evaluates the condition of the inner layers of tissue. As with other types of postpartum infection, promotion of tissue healing and support of immune function through rest, therapeutic diet, and adequate fluid intake are primary goals of care. Administration of IV antibiotics, antipyretics, and analgesics are an important aspect of nursing care to promote healing, decrease fever, and reduce discomfort. The nurse should be particularly alert to needs for analgesia before ambulation of the woman is planned and before debridement, irrigation, and dressing change procedures.

Removing old packing from the wound and performing irrigations can be an unpleasant experience for the woman. The sights and smells can be upsetting. The nurse should make sure that the room is well ventilated and that these activities take place at least an hour before or after meals.

Abdominal wound infections after cesarean delivery often increase the disappointment a woman may feel when a vaginal birth was anticipated. For the woman experiencing an elective cesarean birth, the development of a wound infection will delay recovery and complicate the postpartum experience. Careful assessment of the incision site is an essential aspect of nursing care. Prompt recognition of infection permits early treatment and may prevent spread of disease to deep tissue levels. The nurse must provide sensitive nursing care, particularly during wound irrigations and dressing changes. The nurse's affect and responses to the condition of the wound during these activities may diminish alterations in body image and self-concept. A major nursing responsibility is to prepare the woman to assume wound care on hospital discharge.

Thrombophlebitis and Thrombosis

Thrombophlebitis is an inflammation of a blood vessel with a possible concurrent development of a thrombus. Thrombus formation results when blood components (cells, platelets, and fibrin) combine to form an aggregated body. Once formed, these thrombi may become detached (emboli), flowing freely through the vascular system until they are either lysed or become lodged in another area (Fig. 29-9).

Etiologic and Predisposing Factors

Circumstances that lead to thrombi formation include injury to the vessel wall, diminished vascular flow, and changes in clotting factors. Pregnancy predisposes a woman to clotting problems through two main mechanisms. First, normal hormonal changes produce a vascular system response of a loss of tone or contractibility in the veins and a state of hypercoagulability. Second, the enlarging uterus imposes a restriction of blood return from the lower extremities, creating a higher incidence of stasis. Stasis is believed to be the strongest single predisposing factor in the development of deep vein thrombosis (Cunningham et al., 1989).

Risk factors associated with thromboembolic disease include prior history of thromboembolic disease, bed rest, obesity, varicosities, cesarean delivery, forceps delivery, older maternal age (over age 40), grand multiparity, recent infection, and lactation suppression with estrogens.

Diagnosis

The definitive tool for diagnosis of deep vein thrombosis of a lower extremity is venography (the use of radiographic dyes to ascertain venous flow). Research suggests, however, that some dyes used in venography may predispose to subsequent development of phlebitis due to local vascular irritation (Williams, 1991). Advances in technology have resulted in newer methods of noninvasive diagnosis. Vascular Dop-

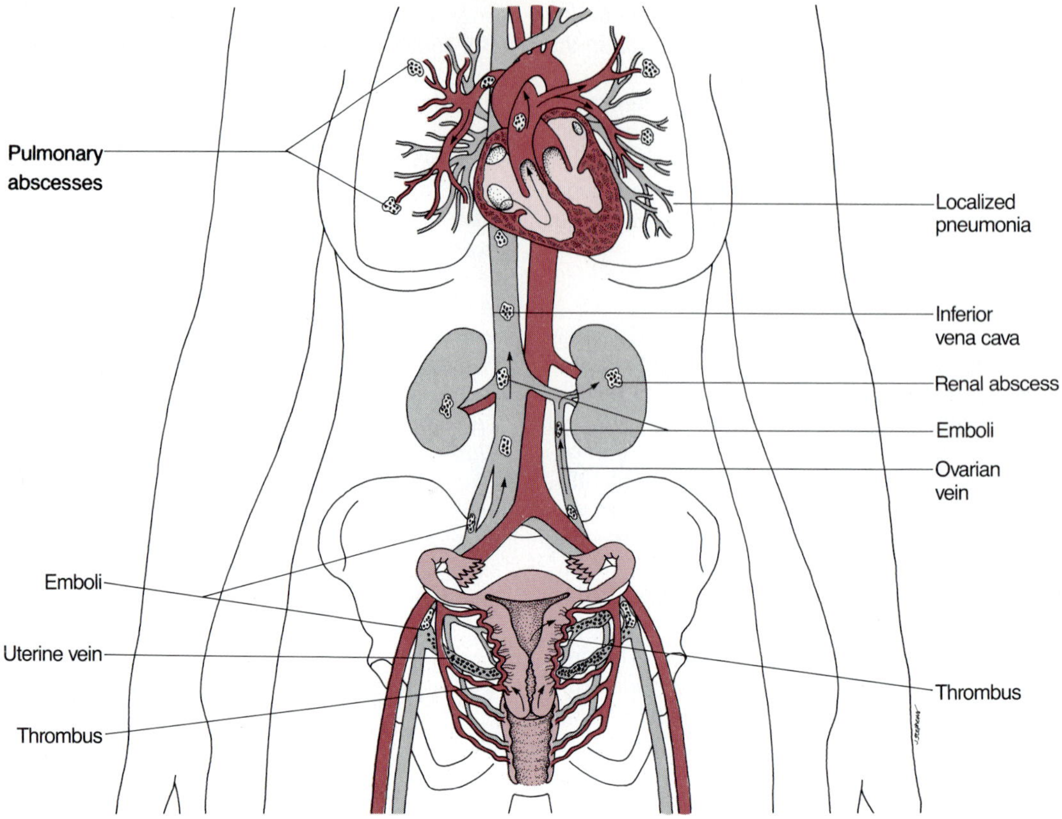

Figure 29-9.
Extension of postpartum infection in pelvic thrombophlebitis (Childbirth Graphics).

pler ultrasound and direct ultrasonic imaging may be used to visualize thrombi in venous structures of the leg. Impedance plethysmography (IPG) is another noninvasive technique that may be useful in diagnosis. IPG permits the measurement of the amount of blood flowing through a vein. These newer modalities are sensitive and specific and are much safer than invasive techniques.

When pulmonary emboli are suspected, chest radiography, arterial blood gases ventilation/perfusion radioisotopic scanning, and pulmonary angiogram are used to confirm the diagnosis.

Maternal Implications

The incidence of postpartum thrombophlebitis is reported to be between 0.1% and 1%. When a thrombosis is not treated, up to 24% of these women will proceed to develop a pulmonary embolism, with an approximate fatality rate of 15%. These statistics stress the importance of early diagnosis and treatment.

Conditions that involve embolisms present the greatest risk to the woman. These conditions include pulmonary emboli, which may cause respiratory distress and cardiac arrest, and emboli to the brain, which may cause cerebral vascular occlusions resulting in death or serious disabilities.

Treatment

Treatment of thromboembolic disease centers on anticoagulation therapy with heparin. In rare cases, surgical removal of the thrombus (thrombectomy) or thrombolytic therapy (streptokinase) may be considered. These latter techniques are generally reserved for life-threatening cases of pulmonary embolism.

Implications for Nursing Care

The nurse plays a major role in the prevention of thromboembolic disease by encouraging and implementing early ambulation for the postpartum woman, particularly after surgical birth. The woman is taught to perform leg exercises (gentle stretching of the calf muscle) while in bed. The woman is also taught other measures to prevent venous stasis including:

- Drinking adequate oral fluids
- Avoiding constrictive pressure in the popliteal area behind the knee
- Avoiding crossing the legs at the knee while sitting
- Elevating the feet when sitting
- Ambulating periodically when sitting for long periods of time
- Wearing antiembolic hose if she has a history of thromboembolic disease of if employed in a job that requires continuous standing

The lower extremities are evaluated during each assessment for signs of inflammation, swelling, and pain. Passive dorsiflexion of the foot is performed. If pain is present (positive Homans' sign), the nurse notifies the midwife or physician promptly.

Peripheral Thrombophlebitis

Thrombophlebitis in the extremities may involve either superficial or deep vascular systems. Superficial venous thrombophlebitis (SVT) may cause significant discomfort but has a favorable prognosis. Conversely, deep venous thrombosis (DVT) can be a life-threatening problem because the larger veins there present more immediate access to the central venous system. If a thrombus is dislodged, an embolus can travel to the lungs, heart, or brain and result in potentially fatal complications.

Etiologic and Predisposing Factors

Risk factors that predispose the postpartum woman to peripheral thrombophlebitis (SVT or DVT) are the same as those listed earlier for thromboembolic disease. In particular, older women with high parity and a previous history of a thromboembolic disorder are at highest risk.

Diagnosis

Signs and symptoms of SVT or DVT include:

- Positive Homans' sign
- Swelling in the affected leg
- Muscle pain in the affected leg
- Tenderness to touch in the affected leg
- Induration along the vein in the affected leg

An extremity diameter 2 cm greater than the opposite leg is considered abnormal and should alert the nurse to the possibility of thromboembolic disease.

Once symptoms develop, one of the noninvasive methods such as IPG, vascular Doppler ultrasound, or direct ultrasonic imaging may be ordered to confirm the diagnosis. Radioisotope venography is reserved for situations in which a definitive diagnosis cannot be made with noninvasive methods.

Maternal Implications

The woman with peripheral thromboembolic disease will be placed on bed rest initially while heparin therapy is initiated. Pain is often present but is rarely severe. Assistance will be needed with completing self-care and newborn care activities. Breastfeeding may continue. Because of its high molecular weight, heparin is not likely to be present in milk. However, if present, it cannot be absorbed from the gastrointestinal tract (Lauwers & Woessner, 1990). If this is the first case of thromboembolic disease for the woman, she will need in-depth teaching regarding predisposing factors and preventive self-care measures.

Treatment

Treatment will depend in part on the location of thrombosis. SVT is generally treated with warm packs to the affected extremity, mild elevation of the involved extremity, and early ambulation. If the woman is unable to ambulate due to local pain and tenderness, physical therapy and range-of-motion exercises for the lower extremities should be instituted (Williams, 1991). Antiembolic support stockings should be applied before initiation of ambulation.

When DVT occurs, anticoagulation therapy is initiated with IV heparin (Table 29-4). As the acute phase of thromboembolic disease resolves, oral anticoagulant therapy with a coumarin derivative (Coumadin) is begun. Bed rest is indicated and the affected extremity is elevated 8 inches above the level of the woman's torso. The bed should be placed in the Trendelenburg position rather than flexing the affected leg at the hip to promote venous drainage. Warm packs are applied to promote blood flow. Flexion and extension of the affected limb should be initiated and ambulation encouraged as soon as pain and inflammation begin to resolve.

Implications for Nursing Care

Nursing responsibilities when SVT or DVT occurs include assessment of vital signs every 4 hours or more frequently and evaluation of the extremity for the degree of inflammation, swelling, and pain. The nurse may be required to measure both legs to determine the difference in circumference of ankle, calf, and thigh. The woman is observed closely for evidence of embolization and the development of life-threatening complications (see pulmonary embolus in the next section).

The nurse is responsible for implementing medical therapy including the administration of IV or oral anticoagulant drugs. Once initiated, the nurse monitors blood coagulation tests and monitors the woman for evidence of unusual bleeding including heavy vaginal bleeding, generalized petechiae, bleeding of the mucous membranes, hematuria, or oozing at venipuncture sites.

The antidote *protamine sulfate* should be readily available in a dosage of 1 mg/100 U heparin.

Analgesics are administered for control of pain. Caution should be taken to make sure that the patient is not given estrogens for lactation suppression because estrogen may encourage the formation of clots.

Support of venous return and blood flow are facilitated by applying warm moist packs and placing the bed in the Trendelenburg position. A hospital-approved aquathermic pad should be used when warm packs are applied. The nurse should supply a footboard when flexion/extension exercises are initiated to facilitate this activity. Antiembolic stockings are also applied.

The nurse assists the woman with self-care and newborn care activities. Breastfeeding should be encouraged and supported. The woman will need special help with positioning the infant for feeding until she is mobile. Before discharge, the woman is taught self-care activities that reduce the risk of thromboembolic disease. (These are listed at the beginning of the section on thrombophlebitis.) She is also taught precautions in self-care activities related to anticoagulant therapy as listed in the Teaching Considerations display.

Pulmonary Embolism

Pulmonary embolism is the condition in which a clot traveling through the venous system becomes lodged within the pulmonary circulatory system, causing an infarction or occlusion. This is a life-threatening complication and requires immediate medical and nursing intervention.

Table 29-4. Anticoagulants Commonly Used in Postpartum Thromboembolic Disease

	Coumadin Derivatives	
Heparin Sodium	Warfarin Sodium (Coumadin, Panwarfin)	Dicumarol
Dose		
IV, SC: 5000–30,000 U May be ordered as a drip over 24 h Prophylactic dose: 5000 U SC q 12 h	IM, IV: 50 mg/vial with diluent Orally: 2.5-, 5-, 7.5-, 10-, 25-mg tablets	Initial, oral: 100 mg; second day: 200 mg; subsequent days: as indicated by prothrombin time Maintenance dose: 25–100 mg/day orally
Use and Mechanism of Action		
Inhibits conversion of prothrombin to thrombin Decreases agglutination of platelets Prolongs clotting time Has no effect on existing clots but prevents extension of old clots and formation of new ones	Inhibits prothrombin synthesis in liver by interfering with the action of vitamin K Acts more quickly than dicumarol, but effects last for a shorter time	Suppresses activity of liver in formation of prothrombin Prolongs clotting Takes 12–14 h to take effect Action persists 24–72 h after drug is discontinued Slower-acting but more prolonged in effect than heparin Used for maintenance
Therapeutic Uses for Postpartum Patients		
Lowering prothrombin time until slower-acting oral anticoagulants can take effect Prophylaxis and treatment of venous thrombosis and its extension Prophylaxis and treatment of pulmonary emboli	Prophylaxis and treatment of pulmonary thrombosis Prophylaxis and treatment of extension of venous thrombosis	Treatment of thrombophlebitis and pulmonary embolism (especially valuable in treatment of thrombosis and embolism)
Contraindications		
Not to be used in patients sensitive to heparin Not to be used in patients with any uncontrolled bleeding Not to be used in patients who cannot be supervised Incompatible with many antibiotics: check before use No IM injections because of risk of hematoma formation	Not to be used in patients with history of coumadin sensitivity Not to be used in patients with any bleeding conditions Not to be used in patients who cannot be supervised Must be used with caution in patients at risk for occupational injury	Same as warfarin sodium
Implications for Nursing Care		
Montior patients constantly for bleeding. Coagulation time determinations should be checked frequently (normal prothrombin time is 11–13 s; levels above this are set for individual patients by physician). Rotate administration sites and check for hemorrhage. Avoid massaging IV site. Observe women for hemorrhage during postpartum period. Breastfeeding may continue; heparin does not appear in breast milk.	Monitor patients constantly for bleeding. Significant decreases in coagulant activity occur in patients taking estrogens, barbiturates, and oral contraceptives. Abdominal or lumbar pain may be due to hemorrhage and thus should be promptly reported. Hemorrhage may be treated with vitamin K or whole blood. Clotting status is monitored by prothrombin time.	Vitamin K should be available as an antidote. Frequent does adjustments are necessary in first 2 weeks of therapy (drug absorption is variable). Patients on maintenance doses may be checked semiweekly, weekly, or at 2- to 4-wk intervals, depending on response to drug.

Etiologic and Predisposing Factors

In many cases, DVT precedes pulmonary embolization. Women who experience pelvic infection with the development of septic pelvic thromboemboli are also at increased risk for this complication. Predisposing factors for thromboembolic disease are listed earlier in the section.

Diagnosis

If the infarction is peripheral, the symptoms observed are pleuritic. A large central embolism causes similar symptoms but may lead to cardiac infarction or right-sided heart failure. A pulmonary embolism is heralded by the symptom of dyspnea and is followed by:

- Tachypnea and tachycardia
- Dyspnea
- Shortness of breath
- Substernal, chest, or pleuritic pain
- Cough
- Hemoptysis

Teaching Considerations

Anticoagulant Therapy

The nurse can use the following points in discharge teaching for a patient on anticoagulant therapy:

- Take the medication at the same time each day.
- Keep follow-up appointments to allow care providers to monitor clotting time and adjust medication.
- Stop taking other medications unless physician approves.
- Be aware of signs of overdose, such as bloody stools, hematomas, widespread bruising, bleeding gums, bleeding into joints.
- If symptoms occur, discontinue the drug and call the physician.
- Avoid trauma or injury that might cause bleeding, such as brushing teeth with hard-bristle toothbrush, contact sports, shaving the legs (use an electric razor).
- Avoid marked changes in eating habits or lifestyle.
- Avoid aspirin and ibuprofen because they inhibit platelet adhesiveness and increase the anticoagulant effect of heparin.
- Understand that stools may change color to pink, red, or black as a result of coagulant use, and change is an indicator of gastrointestinal bleeding.
- Wear a Medic-Alert bracelet or necklace indicating the anticoagulant drug being used.

- Apprehension
- Paleness or cyanosis or both

When a pulmonary embolism is accompanied by a systemic infection, additional symptoms include chills and fever, severe abdominal pain, and hypotension.

Diagnosis of a pulmonary embolus is verified by arterial blood gas studies, chest radiography, ventilation/perfusion radioisotopic scanning, and pulmonary angiogram.

Maternal Implications

Pulmonary embolization can result in a life-threatening event. Complete cardiovascular collapse may occur when the embolus causes extensive disruption of blood flow to the lungs. Fifty percent of cases of fatal pulmonary embolism will have complete cardiovascular collapse as the initial presentation. When less severe symptoms are present, the prognosis is less ominous.

The woman often experiences shortness of breath, dyspnea, chest pain, and impending doom. The initiation of supportive therapy (oxygen, IV fluids, obtaining arterial blood gases) as well as diagnostic tests can increase the woman's level of fear. Many women are transferred to an ICU and are temporarily separated from the newborn and family members. This traumatic event can have long-term effects on postpartum adaptations. It will also delay breastfeeding efforts.

Treatment

The two primary goals of treatment are anticoagulation and immediate cardiorespiratory support. Anticoagulation therapy is most often provided by IV heparin, followed by oral coumarin derivatives as the acute phase resolves. If the woman is conscious and breathing, oxygen should be administered by tight face mask at 8 to 10 L/min. Aminophylline is administered intravenously to improve associated bronchospasm, if present. Hypotension is managed by the initiation of IV fluids and pressor agents such as dopamine. A pulmonary artery catheter may be placed to facilitate fluid and pressor therapy. Morphine is administered for analgesia. When women present with symptoms of cardiovascular collapse, full resuscitative measures are initiated to maintain oxygenation and circulation.

Implications for Nursing Care

When pulmonary embolism is suspected by signs and symptoms of respiratory distress, chest pain, and abnormal vital signs, the nurse initiates emergency supportive care. Additional nursing and medical assistance is summoned. Oxygen is administered by face mask at 8 to 10 L /min. An IV line is initiated if one is not already in place. The head of the bed can be elevated 30 to 45 degrees to facilitate respiratory efforts. The nurse also assembles additional drugs and equipment normally required for treatment (see Treatment section). Vital signs are checked frequently using an electronic blood pressure monitor if one is available. A pulse oximeter should also be used to determine the oxygen saturation level.

Once the woman's condition is stabilized, the nurse is responsible for beginning additional therapy, such as administration of a loading dose of heparin (see Table 29-4). The nurse is also responsible for administering the IV maintenance dose. The woman must be monitored for symptoms of bleeding and allergic reactions. The antidote protamine sulfate should be readily available in a dose of 1 mg/100 U heparin. It is important to note that heparin is incompatible with a number of antibiotics. The nurse should seek clarification about incompatibilities before beginning antibiotic therapy.

Ongoing evaluation of respiratory and cardiovascular status and blood oxygenation is an essential aspect of the nurse's assessment. The nurse supports cardiopulmonary function by administering oxygen, reducing the woman's energy expenditures, and administering drugs such as dopamine or aminophylline. The nurse also prepares the woman for diagnostic tests that may be ordered to evaluate pulmonary blood flow.

The development of thromboembolic disease during the postpartum period poses significant problems for the woman. At best the new mother experiences pain and limited mobility, which reduces her ability to interact with the neonate and assume infant care activities. When pulmonary embolization occurs, the woman is faced with a life-threatening complication that usually requires intensive medical and nursing care. Hospitalization is prolonged, and the woman is often temporarily separated from her newborn and family. The nurse plays a crucial role in the prevention of thromboembolic disease and must assess the woman closely for early signs of this complication. The nurse must also be skilled in the provision of emergency supportive care should embolization occur. The success of postpartum adaptations for the woman and her family will be strongly influenced by the quality of nursing care provided when thromboembolic complications arise.

Postpartum Affective Disorders

At least three separate postpartum affective or mood disorders have been identified: postpartum "blues," postpartum depression, and postpartum psychosis. These mood disorders differ markedly from one another with regard to onset, severity, and the types of medical and nursing care required. They are often associated with interruption of maternal–newborn attachment, disruption of family functioning, or marriage dissolution and can lead to major mental impairment and even suicide if undiagnosed or improperly treated.

Postpartum Blues

Mild postpartum depression, called "postpartum blues" occurs in an estimated 50% to 80% of all women and is usually experienced 3 to 10 days after delivery. It normally resolves with social support and postpartum adaptation. Symptoms lasting more than 2 weeks suggest major depression or postpartum psychosis, requiring pharmacologic treatment and hospitalization (Unterman, Posner, & Williams, 1990). The reader is referred to Chapter 28 for further discussion of postpartum blues.

Postpartum Depression

After the publication of the *Diagnostic and Statistical Manual* by the American Psychiatric Association in 1980, it became fairly well accepted that postpartum depression met the criteria for depressions occurring at other points in life. Recent studies suggest that the depression observed in the postpartum period may, however, be distinct from "major depression" in the general population. Described in psychiatric literature as postpartum major affective disorder, postpartum depression usually presents within 2 weeks to 3 months postpartum. In the United States, the reported incidence ranges from 10% to 26% (Beck, 1992).

Etiologic and Predisposing Factors

It is believed that postpartum depression may be related to psychological, physiologic, and cultural factors. The dramatic hormonal changes experienced during the postpartum period have been suggested as one cause of postpartum depression. However, no confirmed biologic basis has been found for this mood disorder. Social and cultural factors such as role strain and changes in family dynamics have also been suggested as important factors in the development of symp-

Nursing Research

Emotional Disorders and Depression in the Postpartum Period

The nurse plays a crucial role in the early identification and treatment of women with postpartum psychological disorders. Because most women will have returned to their homes and the community when depression or psychosis occurs, assessments by home health or community health nurses are particularly important in the screening process, teaching, and support of new mothers who experience emotional disequilibrium.

Nurse researchers and others interested in postpartum psychological adaptations continue to investigate women's emotional adjustments before and after birth. Gennaro (1988) discovered that even mothers with healthy newborns are likely to experience heightened anxiety and depression in the postpartum period. These feelings are often increased if the neonate is premature or sick. Laizner and Jeans (1990) explored postpartum emotional reactions and found that specific factors were associated with negative psychological experiences including prenatal depression, a previous history of psychological problems, lower health status, and the presence of other problems requiring major life adjustments.

Investigators emphasize the importance of supportive nursing care and patient teaching. Nurses must provide reassurance regarding the emotional reactions experienced after birth and initiate referrals and follow-up when psychological problems are identified.

Gennaro, S. (1988). Postpartal anxiety and depression in mothers of term and preterm infants. *Nursing Research, 37*(2), 82–85.

Laizner, A., & Jeans, M. (1990). Identification of predictor variables of a postpartum emotional reaction. *Health Care for Women International, 11,* 191–206.

toms (Ugarriza, 1992). Research does suggest that the diagnosis of prenatal depression and lack of social support is consistently related to postpartum mood disorder (Pfost, Stevens, & Lum, 1990). Beck and associates (1992) discovered that primiparas experiencing severe postpartum blues in the immediate postbirth period were also at increased risk for true postpartum depression. Extensive research will be required before the etiology of postpartum depression is fully understood.

Diagnosis

Diagnosis of depression remains difficult. Affonso and her associates (1990) discovered that women frequently reported symptoms in the postpartum period that have generally been associated with depression. Many common complaints verbalized by new mothers may result in an inappropriate diagnosis of depression. Conversely, nurses and other health care providers may miss significant indicators of true depression if they attribute reports of profound mood change and somatic complaints to the "postpartum blues" experienced by most healthy women. Further research is essential to identify the major indicators of postpartum depression in the new mother.

Generally, symptoms of postpartum depression occur at least 2 weeks after birth of the neonate. The onset of depression is often insidious and is overlooked by health care providers.

Symptoms of postpartum depression are presented in the accompanying display. These symptoms are far more persistent than normal "postpartum blues" and may never completely resolve without psychological and medical therapy.

Maternal Implications

Beck (1992) interviewed women experiencing postpartum depression, who described this disorder as a "living nightmare" filled with uncontrollable anxiety attacks, consuming guilt, and obsessive thinking. The women contemplated not only harming themselves but also their newborn.

Signs and Symptoms of Postpartum Depression

- Tearfulness
- Mood swings
- Despondency
- Depression
- Insomnia
- Loss of appetite
- Social withdrawal
- Guilt and irritability
- Feelings of inadequacy
- Loss of interest in usual activities
- Impaired memory and inability to concentrate
- Ambivalence about the pregnancy and motherhood

They described extreme loneliness and a loss of interest in all their previous activities.

If postpartum depression is not identified or treated appropriately, the woman may never fully recovery from this mood disorder. The quality of life will be severely compromised, and the other family members will also be adversely affected. Research has consistently demonstrated that maternal depression has negative effects on infant behavior and developmental progress (Beck et al., 1992). Zuravin (1989) reported that moderately depressed mothers were at increased risk for physical aggression against their children, whereas severely depressed women were more likely to verbally abuse them.

Treatment

Medication, psychotherapy, and social support are necessary to promote recovery. Antidepressants are ordered for the woman if symptoms of depression are moderate to severe and physical and emotional functioning have been compromised. Individual and group therapy may be recommended as adjunctive treatment. The woman's partner and immediate family members must be included in counseling sessions so that they develop a full understanding of the disease process, learn how to help the woman appropriately, and have an opportunity to express their own frustrations and concerns. The prognosis for women with postpartum depression depends on the severity of the mood disorder, the woman's prior history, and her support system.

Implications for Nursing Care

Nursing care observations during the immediate postpartum period are valuable in assessing the new mother's general mood. When direct inquiries about mood are ineffective, the nurse may ask questions regarding the newborn's behavior to obtain some clues about how the woman is feeling. Often women who are feeling acutely distressed will answer by stating that the neonate is very fussy, not easily consolable, or irritable. These statements may be viewed as clues needing further exploration.

The nurse should take complaints of sadness, worry, continuing fatigue, and sleeplessness seriously. Abnormal findings should be documented and reported to the health care provider. Once discharge from the hospital has occurred, symptoms may go unrecognized or unreported unless they become extreme enough for the family to communicate them to the health care provider. Some women are not reevaluated by the midwife or physician until the 6-week postpartum visit. For these reasons, nursing assessment of mood or affect must occur during the first postpartum days, so that appropriate interventions can be initiated in the hospital. If concerns about the woman's emotional status persist at the time of discharge or if the woman has a past history of postpartum depression, the health care provider should be notified and appropriate referrals for follow-up care must be initiated. Community or home health nurses may provide follow-up evaluation and care. The woman may also need referrals for psychiatric evaluation. Once postpartum depression is diagnosed, nurses who specialize in care of patients with mood disorders may also be involved in the woman's treatment.

Postpartum Psychosis

The incidence of postpartum psychosis is approximately 1 in 1000 deliveries. Onset is acute and often occurs abruptly after a symptom-free period. Eighty percent of all cases occur between 3 and 14 days postpartum. Incidence rates for postpartum psychosis have remained unchanged since the 1850s even though diagnostic criteria and recording techniques have varied. This seems to indicate relatively stable rates for the complication over the past 130 years.

Etiologic and Predisposing Factors

Of the three types of psychiatric disorders in the postpartum period, psychosis has the strongest genetic ties. Severe hypothyroidism and reaction to ergot alkaloids can also be linked to postpartum psychosis (Unterman et al., 1990). Factors listed in the accompanying display have been proposed to account for the occurrence of postpartum psychosis.

Diagnosis

Two types of postpartum psychosis have been identified: major depression and bipolar depression. Diagnosis is based on presenting signs and symptoms, which are also listed in the display.

Maternal Implications

Postpartum psychosis is a rare but serious illness that may jeopardize the life of the woman and her newborn. Some women experience hallucinations in which voices direct them to kill the neonate or themselves. Hospitalization is often necessary because of the risk of suicide and infanticide. Separation of the woman from her neonate and family can be extremely distressing.

Medications used in psychiatric treatment have some associated risks for the breastfed newborn, and breastfeeding may be contraindicated (Buist, Norman, & Dennerstein, 1990). For the woman whose only source of joy is closeness with her newborn and the act of breastfeeding, separation

Postpartum Psychosis

High-Risk Factors

Hormonal Factors

- Progesterone level declines from 140 ng/mL during pregnancy to 2 ng/mL by postpartum day 10
- Estrogen level drops from 2100 ng/mL during pregnancy to 10 ng/mL by postpartum day 9
- Corticosteroid levels are elevated in pregnancy and fall during the early postpartum period
- Elevation of prolactin level early in postpartum period

Biologic Factors

- Previous history of menstrual cycle distress
- Sleep disorder
- Consanguineous relative with psychiatric disorder
- Labor complications
- Maternal role conflicts

Psychoanalytic Factors

- Unresolved Oedipal conflicts
- Narcissistic personality
- Frustration of oral and dependency needs
- Disturbance of ego control

Psychological Factors

- Poor relationship with own mother
- Inadequate housing
- Reduced social support networks
- Poor marital relationship
- Sexual identity conflict

Other Risk Factors

- Previous history of postpartum psychosis
- History of manic–depressive disorder
- Delirium or hallucinations
- Rapid mood change, agitation, or confusion
- Suicidal ideation

Common Signs and Symptoms

Depression exhibited with either major depression or bipolar depression:

- Tearfulness
- Feelings of guilt
- Feelings of worthlessness
- Insomnia
- Loss of appetite or anorexia
- Delusions
- Hallucinations
- Psychomotor retardation
- Suicidal ideation or attempts
- Self-care or newborn care deficits

The manic phase of a bipolar disorder:

- Irritability
- Hyperactivity
- Euphoria
- Grandiosity
- Insomnia
- Poor judgment
- Confusion
- Self-care or newborn care deficits

and cessation of breastfeeding can cause further psychological disequilibrium.

Women with postpartum psychosis are different from other psychiatric patients. The new mother is faced with the responsibility of caring for her neonate, and she is not able to fulfill that function. She may experience extremely uncomfortable symptoms of insomnia, exhaustion, confusion, frightening hallucinations, and depression. In her mind the sudden onset of illness is unexplained. These women tend to view themselves as inadequate mothers or abnormal because they cannot perform a normal female function. This cluster of symptoms demands the skill and effort of a coordinated, knowledgeable health care team.

Treatment

Women with postpartum psychosis often exhibit suicidal or homicidal ideation or extreme self-care deficits. The woman will often require hospitalization. Management includes hospitalization, chemotherapy (antidepressants, antipsychotics, or lithium), social support, and psychotherapy. A family conference is arranged with the psychiatrist and primary nurses to discuss the woman's condition, diagnosis, plan of medical and nursing care, and prognosis. Intervention by social services or child protective services may be necessary to arrange for ongoing neonatal care if the partner or family members are not available or are unable to meet the neonate's needs.

Prognosis for recovery from postpartum psychosis is good, but the condition may recur after subsequent pregnancies. When the acute phase of the illness has resolved, the woman is permitted home visits. On discharge, outpatient psychiatric care is scheduled. As the patient recovers, she and her family should be informed of the hazard of recurrence of postpartum psychosis with subsequent pregnancy. The risk of recurrence after one episode of postpartum psychosis is approximately one in three or four women.

Implications for Nursing Care

A complete discussion of nursing care of the hospitalized psychiatric patient is beyond the scope of this chapter. The reader is referred to textbooks on psychiatric nursing care for a full discussion of nursing responsibilities. If postpartum psychosis develops before discharge from the postpartum unit, the woman is assigned to a nurse or psychiatric aide or technician with specialized skill in support of psychotic patients. More often, the woman will be transferred to a psychiatric unit for treatment and for her physical safety.

The primary responsibility of the postpartum nurse is to identify abnormalities in mental status and mood that may indicate psychosis and report them immediately to the midwife or physician. Continuous emotional support and physical supervision are required until help arrives (see the accompanying Legal/Ethical Considerations display). Nursery personnel should also be notified about this complication, and arrangements should be made regarding placement and care of the neonate.

Postpartum women may suffer from a variety of mood disorders after childbirth that severely jeopardize individual and family adaptations. Astute observation and differentiation of symptoms are the keys to early recognition, successful treatment, and positive outcomes. The assessment skills of the nurse are crucial in differentiating normal transitory postpartum "blues" from more serious mood disorders. The nurse is also responsible for reporting findings and initiating appropriate follow-up, thereby preventing serious complications. An important aspect of prevention is to alert the woman and her partner or family members to normal and abnormal emotional signs and symptoms during the postpartum period. They should be encouraged to share concerns with the primary health provider early, rather than when severely impaired functioning is evident.

Legal/Ethical Considerations

Nursing Responsibilities When Postpartum Psychosis Is Suspected or Diagnosed

The postpartum nurse conducts periodic assessments of both physiologic and psychological functioning. When signs of mental confusion or disorientation are noted or when the woman's verbalizations indicate delusional thinking or hallucinations, the primary nursing responsibility is to maintain patient safety. The nurse must call for immediate medical assistance. When suicidal ideation is identified or indicators of intention to harm the newborn are noted, a psychiatric emergency exists. If the woman is left unattended and self-injury or newborn injury occurs, the nurse will be held legally accountable for the adverse outcomes.

A staff member should be assigned to remain *constantly* with the woman who verbalizes hallucinations or delusional thinking until the midwife or a physician arrives. Because of the risk of suicide or harm to the newborn, *the woman should never be left alone* until arrangements have been made for continuous attendant care or transfer to the psychiatric unit. Additional protection may be needed if a disoriented woman is extremely agitated, attempts to hurt herself or the newborn or attempts to leave the unit. Hospital policy and procedures should guide the nurse in the application of physical restraints until a physician arrives and a complete evaluation of risk is completed. If restraints are applied, it does not relieve the nurse of the responsibility of remaining continuously with the woman. If nurses with psychiatric expertise are available, the nurse may consult with them regarding the implementation of appropriate safeguards until the physician or midwife arrives.

Chapter Summary

Although most women experience an uneventful postpartum recovery, complications do arise that interrupt successful adaptations. Most problems are resolved quickly with appropriate medical and nursing management, but life-threatening complications do occur. In these situations, the nurse plays a primary role in the early identification of physiologic and or psychological decompensation and must initiate emergency supportive care until medical help arrives. The nurse relies on the nursing process to plan and implement care and to evaluate the effectiveness of treatment. A family-centered approach will reduce the emotional distress that normally accompanies postpartum complications and increases satisfaction with care.

Study Questions

1. *What factors predispose the postpartum woman to hemorrhage?*
2. *What are signs of hypovolemia and compensated shock in the postpartum woman? What are primary nursing responsibilities when signs and symptoms of shock are identified?*
3. *What are the primary nursing responsibilities when uterine atony is identified?*
4. *What signs indicate the possibility of lacerations as the source of postpartum hemorrhage?*
5. *What are the most common signs and symptoms of perineal and vaginal hematoma formation?*
6. *What factors predispose a woman to postpartum infection?*
7. *What signs and symptoms indicate the possibility of a postpartum urinary tract infection?*
8. *What self-care activities can the postpartum woman perform to reduce the recurrence of a urinary tract infection?*
9. *What factors predispose the woman to mastitis? What preventive measures can the nurse teach the breastfeeding woman to reduce the risk of mastitis?*
10. *What factors predispose the postpartum woman to thromboembolic disease?*
11. *What self-care activities can the postpartum woman perform to reduce the development of thromboembolic disease?*
12. *How can the nurse differentiate between postpartum "blues" and postpartum affective mood disorder (depression)?*
13. *What strategies can the nurse use to effectively assess the postpartum woman's mood or emotional status?*

References

ACOG. (1990). *Diagnosis and management of postpartum hemorrhage* (No. 143). ACOG Technical Bulletin. Washington, DC: Author.

Affonso, D., Lovett, S., Paul., S., & Sheptak, S. (1990). A standardized interview that differentiates pregnancy and postpartum symptoms from perinatal clinical depression. *Birth*, *17*(3), 121–130.

Beck, C. (1992). The lived experience of postpartum depression: A phenomenological study. *Nursing Research*, *41*(3), 166.

Beck, C., Reynolds, M., & Rutkowski, P. (1992). Maternity blues and postpartum depression. *Journal of Obstetric, Gynecologic, and Neonatal Nursing*, *21*(4), 287.

Buist, A., Norman, T., & Dennerstein, L. (1990). Breastfeeding and the use of psychotropic medication: A review. *Journal of Affective Disorders*, *19*, 197.

Combs, C., Murphy, E., & Laros, R. (1991). Factors associated with postpartum hemorrhage with vaginal birth. *Obstetrics and Gynecology*, *77*(1), 69.

Cunningham, F. G., MacDonald, P., & Gant, N. (1989). *Williams Obstetrics* (18th ed.). Norwalk, CT: Appleton & Lange.

Dinsmoor, M. J., & Gibbs, R. (1988). The role of the newer antimicrobial agents in obstetrics and gynecology. *Clinical Obstetrics and Gynecology*, *31*(2), 423.

Faro, S. (1990). Ticarcillin/clavulanate: An alternative to combination antibiotic therapy for treating soft tissue pelvic infections in women. *Journal of Reproductive Medicine*, *35* (Suppl. 3), 353.

Gillogley, K. (1991). Abnormal labor and delivery. In K. Niswander & A. Evans (Eds.), *Manual of obstetrics* (4th ed.). Boston: Little, Brown.

Ignatavicius, D., & Bayne, M. (1991). *Medical-surgical nursing*. Philadelphia: W. B. Saunders.

Lauwers, J., & Woessner, C. (1990). *Chemical agents and breast milk*. Garden City Park, NY: Avery Publishing Group Inc.

Long, P. (1991). Bleeding and the third stage of labor. *NAACOG Clinical Issues in Perinatal and Women's Health Nursing*, *2*(3), 391.

Luegenbiehl, D. (1991). Postpartum bleeding. *NAACOG Clinical Issues in Perinatal and Women's Health Nursing*, *2*(3), 402.

Olsen, C., & Gordon, R. (1990). Breast disorders in nursing mothers. *American Family Physician*, *41*(5), 1509.

Pfost, K., Stevens, M., & Lum, C. (1990). The relationship of demographic variables, antepartum depression, and stress to postpartum depression. *Journal of Clinical Psychology*, *46*(5), 588.

Silver, H., & Smith, L. (1991). The puerperium. In K. Niswander & A. Evans (Eds.), *Manual of obstetrics* (4th ed.). Boston: Little, Brown.

Stamm, W. E. (1988). Dysuria: Establishing a diagnostic protocol. *Contemporary Obstetrics and Gynecology*, *32*(4), 81.

Stray-Pedersen, B., Blakstad, M., & Bergan, T. (1990). Bacteriuria in the puerperium: Risk factors, screening procedures, and treatment program. *American Journal of Obstetrics and Gynecology*, *162*(3), 792.

Unterman, R., Posner, N., & Williams, K. (1990). Postpartum depressive disorders: Changing trends. *Birth*, *17*(3), 131.

Ugarriza, D. (1992). Postpartum affective disorders: Incidence and treatment. *Journal of Psychosocial Nursing*, *30*(5), 29.

Varner, M. (1991). Postpartum hemorrhage. *Critical Care Clinics*, *7*(4), 883.

Wheeler, D. (1991). Intrapartum bleeding. *NAACOG Clinical Issues in Perinatal and Women's Health Issues*, *2*(3), 381.

Williams, M. (1991). Thromboembolic disease and vascular complications. In K. Niswander & A. Evans (Eds.), *Manual of obstetrics* (4th ed.). Boston: Little, Brown.

Zuravin, S. (1989). Sererity of maternal depression and three types of mother-to-child aggression. *American Journal of Orthopsychiatry*, *59*, 377–389.

Suggested Readings

Cosico, J., & Rothlauf, E. (1992). Indications, management, and patient education: Coagulation therapy. *American Journal of Maternal Child Nursing*, *17*(3), 130–135.

Gerbasi, F., Bottoms, S., Farag, A., & Eberhard, M. (1990). Changes in hemostasis activity during delivery and the immediate postpartum period. *American Journal of Obstetrics and Gynecology*, *162*(5), 11580.

Hampson, S. (1989). Nursing interventions for the first three postpartum months. *Journal of Obstetric, Gynecologic, and Neonatal Nursing*, *18*(2), 116.

Faro, S., Martens, M., Hammill, H., . (1990). Antibiotic prophylaxis: Is there a difference? *American Journal of Obstetrics and Gynecology*, *162*(4), 900.

Lennon, M., Wasserman, G., & Allen, R. (1990). Infant care and wives' depressive symptoms. *Women and Health*, *17*(2), 1.

Long, P. (1991). Bleeding and the third stage of labor. *NAACOG Clinical Issues in Perinatal Women's Health Nursing*, *2*(3), 385.

Lowe, T. (1990). Hypovolemia due to hemorrhage. *Clinical Obstetrics and Gynecology*, *33*(3), 454.

Luegenbiehl, D., Brophy, G., Artigue, G., . (1990). Standardized assessment of blood loss. *American Journal of Maternal Child Nursing*, *15*, 242.

Mead-Bennett, E. (1990). The relationship of primigravid sleep experience and select moods on the first postpartum day. *Journal of Obstetric, Gynecologic, and Neonatal Nursing*, *19*(2), 146.

Milligan, K. (1991). Use of halogenated anesthesia with maternal hemorrhage. *NAACOG Clinical Issues in Perinatal Women's Health Nursing*, *2*(3), 396.

Neugebauer, R., Kline, J., O'Connor, P. (1992). Depressive symptoms in women in the six months after miscarriage. *American Journal of Obstetrics and Gynecology*, *166*(1), 104.

Peyser, M., & Kupkerminc, J. (1990). Management of severe postpartum hemorrhage by intrauterine irrigation with prostaglandin E_2. *American Journal of Obstetrics and Gynecology*, *162*, 694.

Schmidt, J., & Schimpeler, S. (1990). Obstetric and gynecologic abdominal wound infections: A comprehensive nurse-managed program. *Journal of Perinatal and Neonatal Nursing*, *4*(3), 25.

CHAPTER 30

Assessment of the Neonate

Learning Objectives

After studying the material in this chapter, the student should be able to:

- Describe the major physiologic adaptations required of the neonate in the first 24 hours of life.
- Describe the major behavioral adaptations required of the neonate in the first 24 hours of life.
- Outline essential steps in the process of newborn assessment.
- Describe normal physical and behavioral findings in the newborn.
- Explain the purpose of a gestational age assessment and describe the components of this assessment.

Key Terms

acrocyanosis
caput succedaneum
cephalhematoma
erythema toxicum
frenulum linguae
full-term infant
habituation
hypoglycemia
icterus neonatorum
infant
jaundice
meconium
milia
molding
mongolian spots
Moro reflex
neonate
nonshivering thermogenesis
plethora
polycythemia
pseudomenstruation
reactivity
rugae
vernix caseosa
webbing

Major physiologic and behavioral adaptations must be made before the neonatal period is safely concluded at the 28th day of life. The extrauterine adjustments made during the first 24 hours are particularly critical to the neonate's chances for survival.

This chapter discusses the major physiologic and behavioral adaptations the neonate must undergo after birth. Normal newborn characteristics and common variations in physical appearance and behavior are also described. Essential aspects of the nursing assessment of the newborn are delineated to assist the beginning practitioner.

Neonatal Adaptation to Extrauterine Life

The nurse is in a unique position to aid the neonate in the stressful transition from a warm, dark, fluid-filled environment to an outside world filled with light, sound, and novel tactile stimuli. Depending on the type of birthing facility the woman chooses, a certified nurse midwife or delivery room nurse may actually present the woman and her partner with the new family member. The nurse performs an initial assessment to evaluate the neonate, its immediate postbirth adaptations, and the need for further support. Later, a pediatric or neonatal nurse practitioner or nursery nurse will conduct a comprehensive assessment to determine the infant's status and to identify internal and external stressors that might jeopardize successful adaptation.

Physiologic Adaptations

Respiratory Adaptations

The major adaptation to extrauterine life required of the neonate is the ability to breathe. This ability depends on a variety of factors related to fetal growth and development. In preparation for the tremendous demands placed on its respiratory system at the moment of birth, the fetus normally begins breathing movements in utero. To facilitate full expansion of alveoli with air when the first breath is taken, fetal alveoli are filled with fetal lung fluid. Fetal lung fluid distends alveoli and improves the ability of these air sacs to stretch and remain open when air is inspired. The ability of lung tissue to expand with inspiration and partially relax to permit exhalation of carbon dioxide during expiration is known as lung compliance.

Fetal lungs must also be developed sufficiently to produce surfactant, a complex of phospholipids that reduces surface tension in the alveoli and prevents their collapse on expiration. Surfactant is produced by type II alveolar cells, which begin to produce this phospholipid in limited amounts at about 24 to 26 weeks' gestation. Secretion of pulmonary surfactant becomes extensive after 35 to 36 weeks' gestation, permitting successful inflation of the lungs and preventing collapse or atelectasis during the expiration phase of the respiratory cycle.

The pulmonary vascular bed must be developed and in proximity to lung tissue for gas exchange to occur. Finally, the newborn must possess an intact central nervous system (CNS) to initiate and coordinate respiratory efforts.

Initiation of Respiration

Many stimuli during labor and delivery contribute to the initiation of respiration in the newborn. Four major categories of stimuli have been identified. Figure 30-1 illustrates how these stimuli interact to influence the onset of respiration.

Chemical Stimuli. The fetus experiences a transient asphyxia. This is a result of interruptions in placental blood flow during uterine contractions and with compression and severing of the umbilical cord at birth. Chemoreceptors in the carotid artery and aorta are stimulated by the lowered arterial oxygen tension (Pao_2), the elevated arterial carbon dioxide tension ($Paco_2$), and the decrease in arterial pH

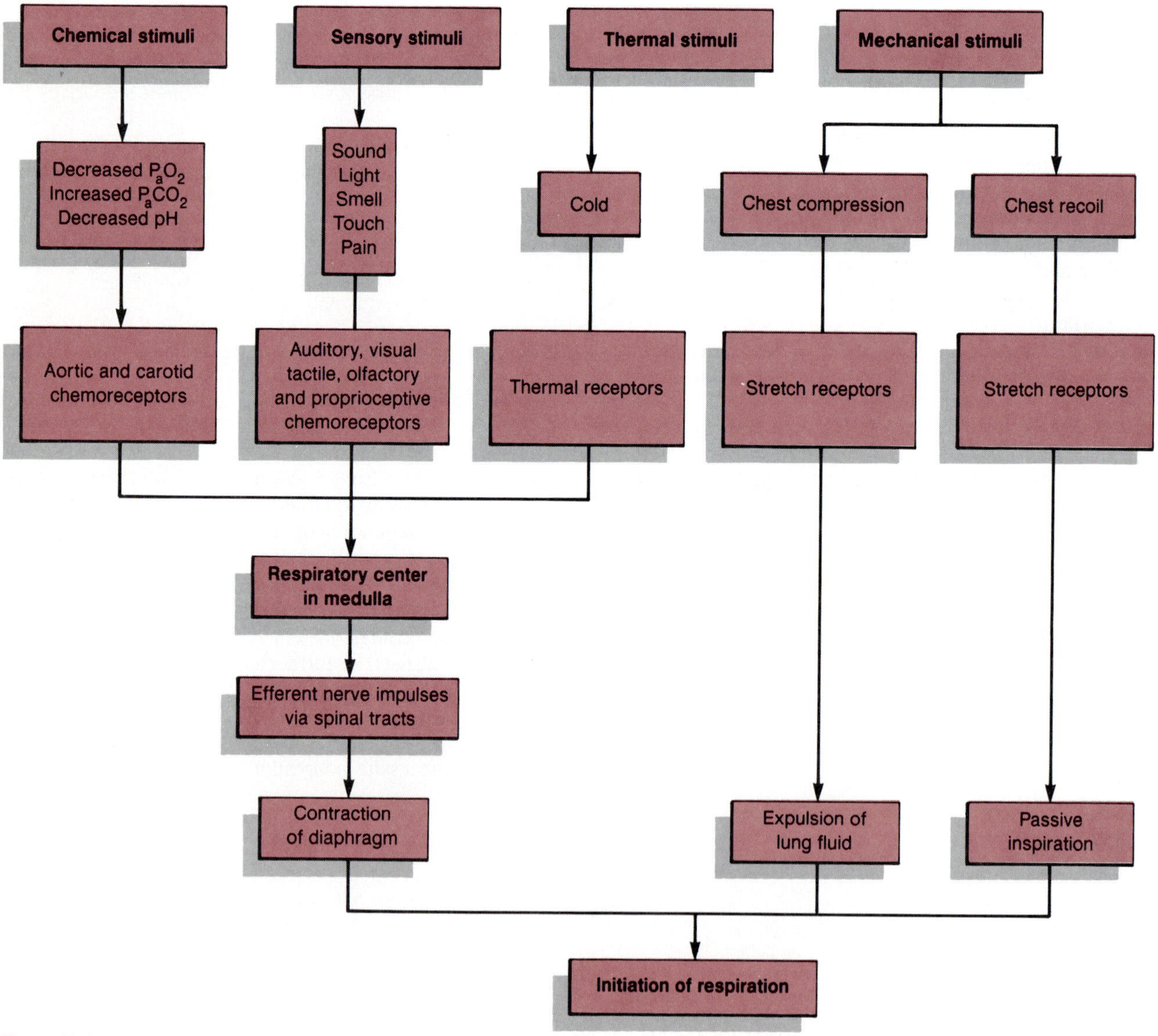

Figure 30-1.
Interaction of stimuli in the initiation of neonatal respiration.

below 7.35. Impulses triggered by these chemoreceptors stimulate the respiratory center in the medulla.

Sensory Stimuli. The neonate is bombarded with a variety of new stimuli during labor and delivery. Even when the tactile, visual, auditory, and olfactory stimuli are reduced, as in gentle birthing environments, their combined effects still contribute to the initiation of respiration.

Thermal Stimuli. Cold appears to be a powerful stimulus to the initiation of breathing in the neonate. When the newborn's warm, wet body is delivered, evaporation causes an immediate drop in the skin temperature. Thermal receptors, particularly on the face and chest, relay impulses to the medulla, triggering the first breath. Profound cooling can cause a drop in the core temperature and lead to respiratory depression and acidosis.

Mechanical Stimuli. During the passage through the birth canal, approximately 30% of the fetal lung fluid filling the airways and alveoli is squeezed out. It is estimated that up to 30 mL of tracheal fluid is expelled through the oropharynx before birth. During vaginal birth, as the chest is delivered, recoil of the chest wall occurs, drawing air into the partially cleared passages. Infants born by cesarean delivery do not experience this compression of the thorax and may suffer from transient respiratory distress caused by retained fetal lung fluid.

Factors Opposing the First Breath

Several factors inhibit the neonate's efforts to take the first breath, including alveolar surface tension, lung fluid viscosity, and lung compliance. The diaphragm must descend forcefully to create a negative intrathoracic pressure powerful enough to overcome these forces (40 to 80 cm H_2O pressure). Air then rushes in, expanding the alveoli, reducing surface tension, and forcing the remaining lung fluid out through the pulmonary capillaries and lymphatic system. A functional residual capacity is established so that alveolar sacs remain partially expanded on expiration. Thus, subsequent breaths require less effort and lower pressure (6 to 8 cm H_2O). Figure 30-2 illustrates the effects of the first breath on pulmonary circulation and gas exchange in the lungs.

The pulmonary vascular bed, which was constricted during fetal life, must now dilate to allow adequate perfusion of lung tissue and effective gas exchange. With the first breath, the rise in alveolar oxygen tension (PaO_2), decrease in arterial pH, and an increase in the level of blood bradykinin, a vasoactive peptide protein, results in dilatation of the pulmonary arteries. The pulmonary vascular resistance decreases, permitting a greater flow of blood through the pulmonary vessels. This increased pulmonary perfusion facilitates oxygen and carbon dioxide exchange. Persistent hypoxemia and acidosis constrict the pulmonary arteries; this decreases pulmonary perfusion and can reverse those critical pulmonary adaptations in the newborn, resulting in respiratory distress. Figure 30-3 illustrates the changes in pulmonary vascular resistance after initiation of respiration and the resulting cardiovascular adaptations. Table 30-1 illustrates changes in blood gas and pH values during the first hour of life.

Pulmonary artery pressure normally decreases to approximately 50% of systemic arterial pressure within 24 hours of birth. Persistent elevation in pulmonary artery pressure may occur in infants born with an abnormal thickening of the medial muscle layer of pulmonary arterioles. Chronic intrauterine hypoxemia has been implicated in hypertrophy or abnormal thickening of pulmonary artery musculature.

Cardiovascular Adaptations

With clamping of the umbilical cord and initiation of the first breath, dramatic changes occur in the cardiovascular system of the neonate.

Closure of the Foramen Ovale

As the pulmonary arteries dilate in response to oxygenation of lung tissue, pulmonary vascular resistance decreases and pressure drops in the right side of the heart. Simultaneously, pressure rises in the left side of the heart. This leads to functional closure of the foramen ovale within several hours of birth. Permanent closure of this bypass is not accomplished for several months. Right-to-left shunting of blood may occur until that time, and this accounts for the nonpathologic murmurs heard in some neonates.

Closure of the Ductus Arteriosus

The ductus arteriosus is sensitive to changes in arterial oxygen tension. As blood oxygen tension (PaO_2) levels rise with the first breath, the ductus arteriosus constricts. Functional closure usually occurs within 15 hours of birth, and permanent closure is accomplished by 3 weeks. Hypoxemia leads to continued patency of the ductus and shunting of blood through this fetal circulatory bypass. Research indicates that sustained crying may result in reopening of the ductus in some infants (see the accompanying Nursing Research display).

Closure of the Ductus Venosis

The clamping of the umbilical cord results in closure of the ductus venosus. Fibrosis of this fetal circulatory bypass occurs within a week.

Systemic blood pressure rises with the clamping of the umbilical cord because elimination of the large placental vascular bed results in increased systemic resistance. Concomitantly, the severing of the placental circulation and the consequent decreased blood return via the inferior vena cava contribute to a lowered venous blood pressure.

Endocrine and Metabolic Adaptations

The endocrine system is a master system that coordinates the newborn's adjustments to extrauterine life. Hormones synthesized and released by endocrine glands support major metabolic functions and mediate responses to internal and external stressors. Endocrine activity is linked with the nervous system in a complex arrangement of feedback loops. Three major neuroendocrine pathways supporting neonatal adaptations are the hypothalamic–anterior pituitary axis, the hypothalamic–posterior pituitary axis, and the parasympathetic–adrenal medulla path. Major neurohormonal systems are intact at birth, and hormones essential for

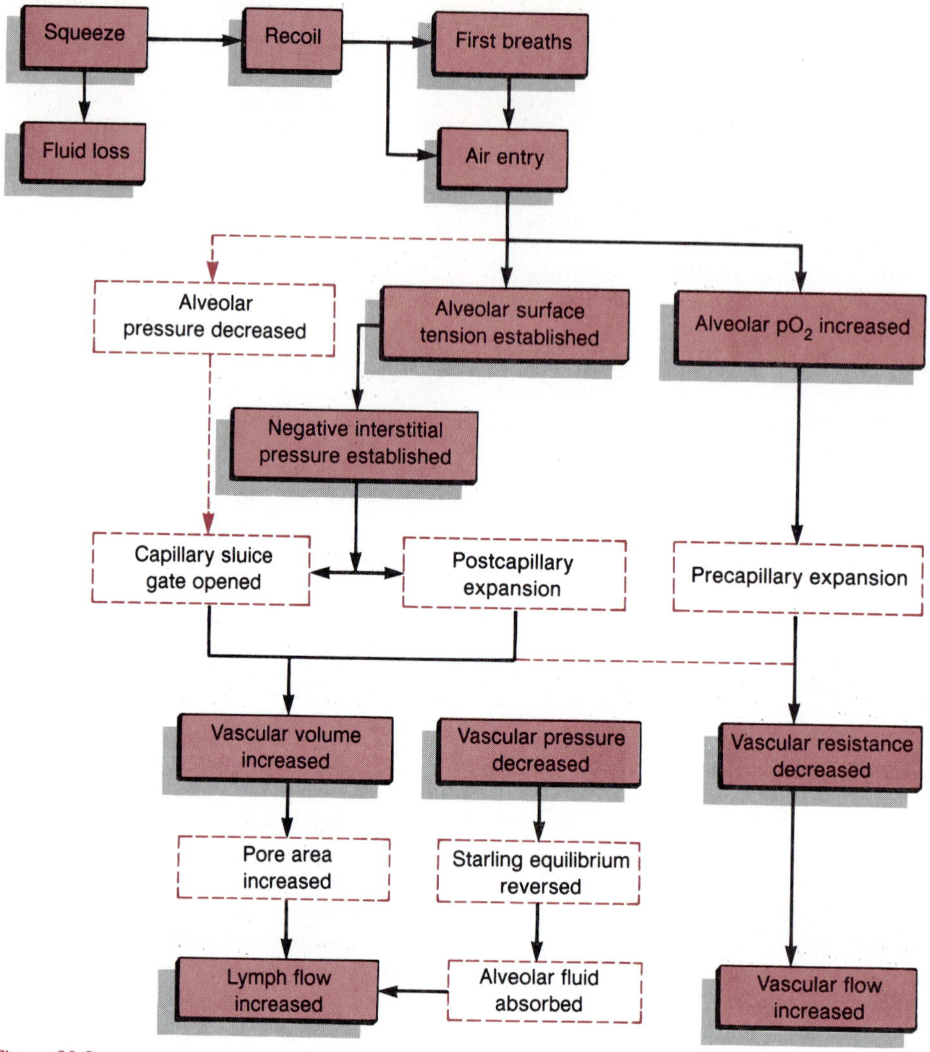

Figure 30-2.

Effect of first breath on neonatal pulmonary circulation and gas exchange. Broken lines indicate hypothesized mechanisms involved in the transition to extrauterine pulmonary function. (From Smith, C., & Nelson, N. [1976]. *The physiology of the newborn infant* [4th ed.]. Springfield, IL: Charles C. Thomas.)

neonatal adaptations, including growth hormone, thyroid-stimulating hormone, adrenocorticotropic hormone, cortisol, and catecholamines, are secreted.

Thermoregulation

Thermoregulation, the ability of the neonate to produce heat and maintain a normal body temperature, is a vital metabolic function mediated by the neuroendocrine system. Neonates are especially susceptible to heat loss because of a combination of unique anatomic features and environmental factors surrounding birth.

Factors Contributing to Heat Loss. Neonates are prone to heat loss because they have a large surface area in relation to their body weight. In addition, because they have less adipose tissue for insulation, thinner skin, and blood vessels in closer proximity to the skin surface, newborns experience a greater transfer of heat to the external environment. The neonate's skin is wet at birth, and the ambient room temperature at birth is much cooler than that of the intrauterine environment. The low humidity and fast air currents found in many delivery rooms as a result of air-conditioning systems also increase heat loss. Table 30-2 describes the four major mechanisms of heat loss and heat transfer to which the newborn is susceptible. It also describes environmental factors contributing to hypothermia.

Neonatal Responses to Hypothermia. The infant responds to cold stress in various ways, as illustrated in Figure 30-4. Heat loss is decreased by vasoconstriction of vessels. Shivering, a major mechanism of heat production in adults, is rarely seen in newborns. Heat production occurs through an increase in metabolic rate and muscular activity. *Nonshivering thermogenesis is the primary method of heat production in neonates.*

When skin temperature begins to drop, thermal receptors transmit impulses to the CNS. The sympathetic nervous system is stimulated. Norepinephrine is released by the adre-

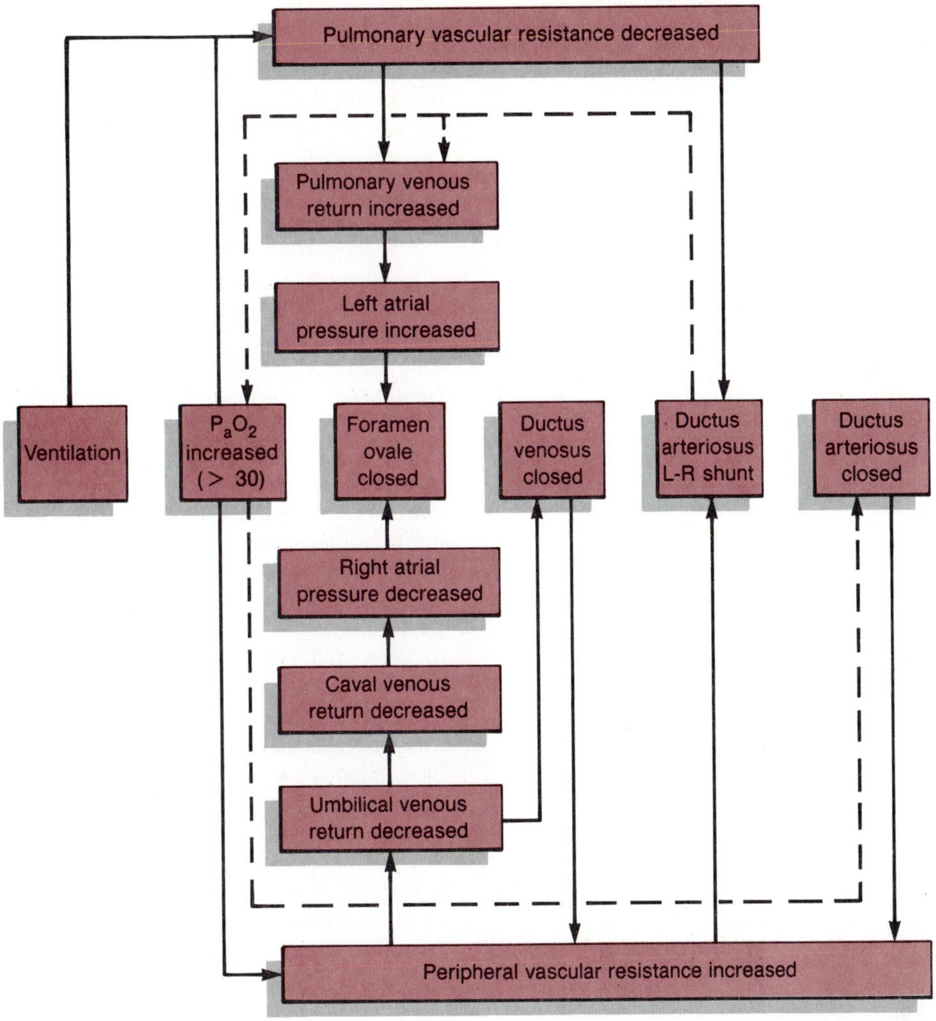

Figure 30-3.

Alterations in pulmonary vascular resistance and neonatal circulation following initiation of respiration. Broken lines indicate hypothesized mechanisms involved in alterations in pulmonary vascular resistance. (From Smith, C., & Nelson, N. [1976]. *The physiology of the newborn infant* [4th ed.]. Springfield, IL: Charles C. Thomas.)

nal gland and at nerve endings located in a special type of adipose tissue known as brown fat. Brown fat is extremely dense, highly vascular adipose tissue that is metabolized to produce heat. Found only in infants, brown fat is located in the intrascapular area, the neck, thorax, and axilla, and around the kidneys and adrenal glands.

Although nonshivering thermogenesis and an increased metabolic rate are effective means of heat production in the neonate, both result in increased demands for oxygen and glucose. Healthy full-term neonates will have no difficulty in meeting these demands initially by increasing the respiratory rate and releasing liver stores of glucose. With pro-

Table 30-1. Oxygen Tension, Carbon Dioxide Tension, pH, and Base Excess Values in Cord Blood and Arterial Blood During the First 24 Hours of Life

	Birth					
	Umbilical Vein	Umbilical Artery	**5–10 Minutes**	**30 Minutes**	**60 Minutes**	**24 Hours**
Pa_{O_2} (mm Hg)	27.5	16	50	54	63	73
Pa_{CO_2} (mm Hg)	39	49	46	38	36	33
pH	7.32	7.24	7.20	7.29	7.33	7.36
Base excess	−5.5	−7.2	−9.8	−7.8	−6.5	−5.2

Nursing Research

Postnatal Adaptations and Crying in Neonates

Although crying in neonates during the transitional period has been regarded traditionally as a normal behavior, physiologic research suggests that crying may actually be harmful, particularly in high-risk or sick neonates. Studies have demonstrated reestablishment of fetal circulation with shunting of unoxygenated blood through the foramen ovale secondary to increased intrathoracic pressure during crying. Other studies have discovered adverse effects on cerebral blood flow resulting in intraventricular bleeding in premature infants.

Nurse scientists are now studying crying behaviors and strategies to prevent or reduce the duration of crying episodes in the neonate. Crying was reduced when neonates received nurturing support between 0.5 and 4 hours after birth. They also achieved physiologic stability more rapidly. The newborn exhibits precry cues that may alert caregivers to crying (grimace, red face, body tension, and clenched fists). Crying generated by some painful procedures can be reduced by simple interventions such as the use of a glucose-sweetened pacifier. Further research is indicated, but it appears appropriate at this time to recommend that clinicians observe neonates for crying cues and attempt to reduce the intensity and duration of crying episodes.

Gill, N. E., White, M. A., & Anderson, C. G. (1984). Transitional newborn infants in a hospital nursery: From first oral cue to first sustained cry. *Nursing Research, 33*(4), 213–217.

Shapiro, C. (1989). Pain the neonate: Assessment and intervention. *Neonatal Network, 8*(1), 7.

longed cold stress or in compromised neonates, brown fat sources and glucose stores may be depleted, which can result in hypothermia and hypoglycemia. These infants must rely on external sources of heat to maintain their body temperatures.

Neonatal Responses to Hyperthermia. The newborn infant will respond to an elevation in temperature by dilating blood vessels to dissipate heat. Sweat glands are less active than in an adult, but a full-term infant is capable of perspiring and may lose some heat through evaporation. Metabolic rate, oxygen consumption, and insensible water loss increase significantly with hyperthermia in the newborn (Te Pas, 1988). Figure 30-5 illustrates the rise in oxygen consumption with hyperthermia.

Hepatic Adaptations

Normal development of liver tissue and the biliary ducts is essential for hepatic function at birth. Although the neonatal liver is immature, it is capable of performing vital functions, including carbohydrate metabolism, production of coagulation factors, bilirubin conjugation, and iron storage.

Carbohydrate Metabolism

The fetus stores glycogen during the last weeks of gestation, and at birth the neonate must maintain glucose homeostasis by producing and regulating its own glucose supply. This requires activations of gluconeogenesis and glycolysis. Gluconeogenesis occurs in neonatal hepatic cells immediately after birth although less efficiently than in adults. Glucose is the major energy source in the first hours after birth before feedings begin. The brain is an obligate glucose user, as are peripheral nerves, red and white blood cells, and the medulla of the kidney. As blood glucose levels drop, glycogenolysis occurs and glucose is released into the neonate's bloodstream to maintain a blood glucose level of approximately 60 mg/dL. Glycogen stores can be rapidly depleted in the presence of stressors such as birth asphyxia or hypothermia. Ninety percent of hepatic glycogen stores may be consumed by the third to fourth hour of life, resulting in hypoglycemia (Fig. 30-6). Hypoglycemia is defined as a blood glucose level of less than 30 mg/dL during the first 72 hours of life. The reader is referred to Chapter 31 for an in-depth discussion of hypoglycemia.

Insulin, glucagon, and growth hormone, the three major hormones involved in glucose homeostasis, are present at birth. Normal serum insulin levels in fasting neonates range from 6 to 24 μU/mL. Neonatal insulin secretion is sluggish during the first 2 weeks of life because of the immaturity of the endocrine system; thus, effective glucose utilization is limited.

Blood Coagulation

Coagulation factors are essential elements in the process of hemostasis. Maternal coagulation factors do not cross the placenta. Immaturity of the liver at birth causes a temporary deficit in liver-synthesized coagulation factors and a prolonged blood coagulation time in the neonate. Four of the factors (II, VII, IX, and X) are activated under the influence of vitamin K produced by bacteria in the gut (Fig. 30-7). However, because the gastrointestinal tract is sterile until birth and normal intestinal flora are not established until the neonate begins to ingest milk, vitamin K levels remain low until approximately postnatal day 8. The newborn is therefore at special risk between the second and fifth days of life for a bleeding disorder referred to as hemolytic disease of the newborn. For this reason, vitamin K is given prophylactically to protect the newborn.

Bilirubin Conjugation

Indirect (fat-soluble) bilirubin is a breakdown product of red blood cell lysis. It is converted by a liver enzyme, glucuronyl transferase, into a water-soluble form (direct bilirubin) that can be excreted in urine and stool. In the newborn, because the liver is immature, the ability to conjugate (convert) indirect bilirubin is somewhat limited. This, cou-

Table 30-2. Environmental Factors Contributing to Neonatal Heat Loss

Major Mechanisms	Environmental Factors
Evaporation	
Loss of heat when water on the neonate's skin is converted to a vapor	Wet blankets or diapers in contact with skin Water or urine on skin
Convection	
Transfer of heat when a flow of cool air passes over the neonate's skin	Drafts from open windows Drafts from open portholes on isolette Drafts from air-conditioning ducts Flow of unheated oxygen over face
Conduction	
Transfer of heat when the neonate comes in direct contact with cooler surfaces and objects	Cold mattresses, cold sidewalls in crib or isolette Cold blankets, shirts, diapers Cold hands of caregiver Cold weight scale Cold stethoscope
Radiation	
Transfer of heat from the neonate to cooler surfaces and objects not in direct contact with the neonate	Cold sidewalls of crib or isolette Cold outside building walls and windows Cold equipment in neonate's environment

pled with the high red blood cell count in the neonate and the increased hemolysis resulting from the shorter life span of fetal red blood cells, accounts for the frequent appearance of physiologic jaundice between 48 and 72 hours after birth. Serum bilirubin levels range from 4 to 12 mg/dL at 3 days of age; the average peak serum level is 6 mg/dL followed by a rapid decline to 3 mg/dL by the fifth day of life (Fig. 30-8).

A more serious consequence of high levels of indirect bilirubin can be its accumulation in brain tissue, a condition called kernicterus, which can cause permanent brain damage and retardation. For this reason, the neonate's bilirubin levels are monitored closely. If necessary, steps are taken to facilitate the conversion of indirect bilirubin to direct bilirubin, which can then be excreted by the kidneys. (See Chapter 31 for a discussion of the treatment modalities for hyperbilirubinemia.)

Iron Storage

The neonate is born with iron stores accumulated during fetal life. If the mother's iron intake was adequate, the infant will have sufficient iron to produce red blood cells until about 3 to 5 months of age. As fetal red blood cells are lysed after birth, iron is recycled and stored in the liver until needed for new red blood cell production. If the mother's iron intake was deficient during pregnancy, supplemental iron should be administered to the infant as a medication or in iron-fortified formula during the first year of life (American Academy of Pediatrics, 1976).

Gastrointestinal Adaptations

Normal rapid growth and development demands that the neonate ingest, digest, and absorb sufficient nutrients. Although both structurally and functionally immature, the gastrointestinal tract is capable of digesting and absorbing breast milk and modified cow's milk and eliminating waste products. The mouth is shaped to facilitate breastfeeding. Ridges and corrugations on the hard palate, strong sucking muscles in the mouth and jaw, and fat pads in the cheeks assist the newborn to grasp the nipple and compress the areola of the breast during breastfeeding. Taste buds located primarily on the tip of the tongue can distinguish between sweet and sour. Salivary glands are immature and saliva production is scant.

Gastric capacity is limited in the first day of life to approximately 40 to 60 mL. Because the stomach distends easily, capacity increases when feedings are introduced, and reaches 90 mL in many infants by 3 to 4 days of age. Pepsinogen is present and begins the digestion of milk when it enters the stomach. Stomach emptying time is approximately 2 to 4 hours. The cardiac sphincter is immature, and slight regurgitation of milk after feedings is common in the newborn.

The neonate's intestinal tract is proportionately longer than that of an adult and has a large absorption surface. Enzymes essential for protein digestion are present in the newborn. Fats are digested and absorbed less effectively because the amount of pancreatic lipase is inadequate. The fats in breast milk are more easily digested than those found in cow's milk because of the lipase in breast milk.

Renal Adaptations

Although urine is produced and excreted into the amniotic fluid by the fetus from the fourth month of gestation, the kidney is still immature at birth. Nephrons continue to develop in the first years of life. The neonate is extremely susceptible to dehydration, acidosis, and electrolyte imbalance if normal fluid intake is restricted or vomiting or diarrhea occur.

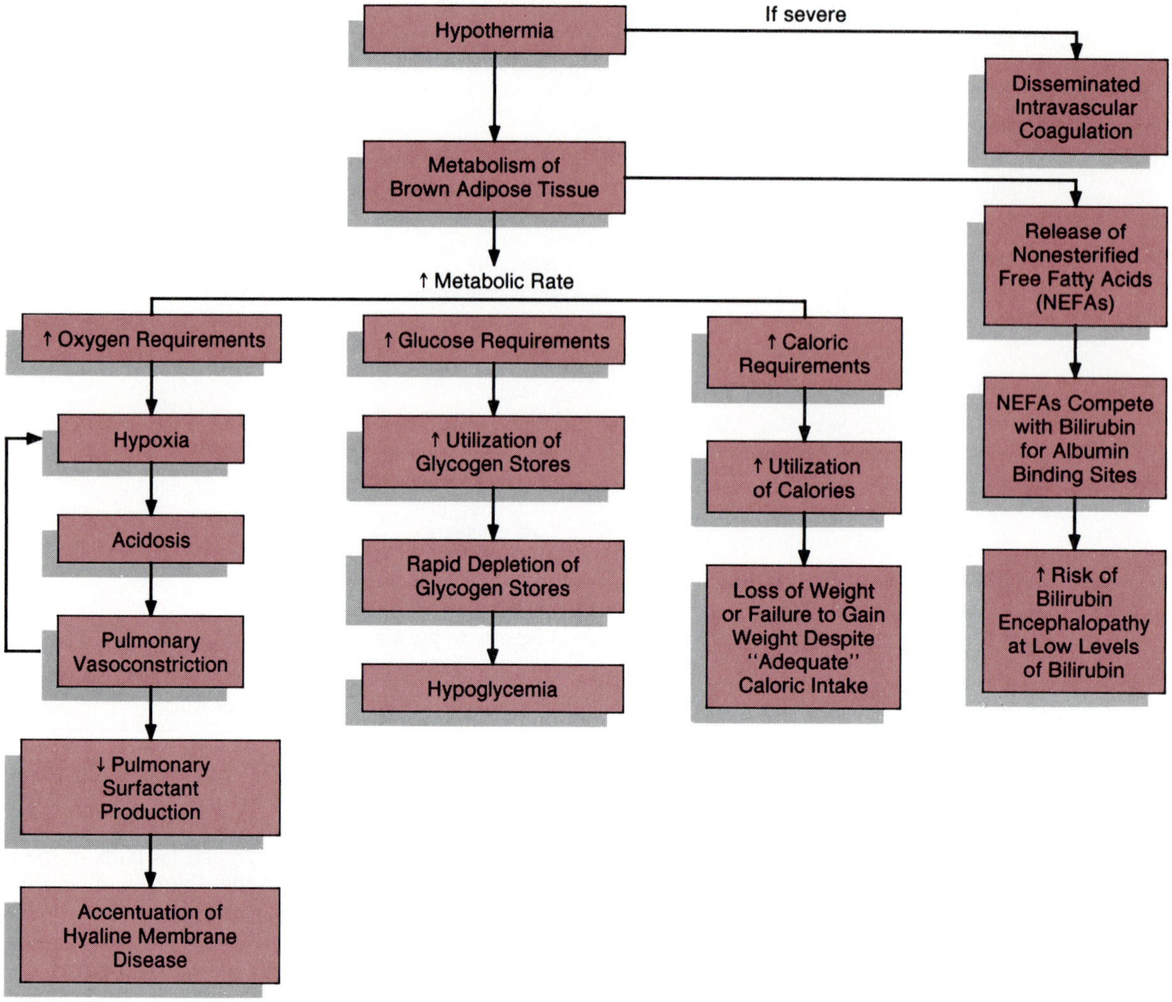

Figure 30-4.
Deleterious effects of hypothermia in the neonate. (From Streeter, N. [1986]. *High-risk neonatal care* [p. 101]. Rockville, MD: Aspen Publishers.)

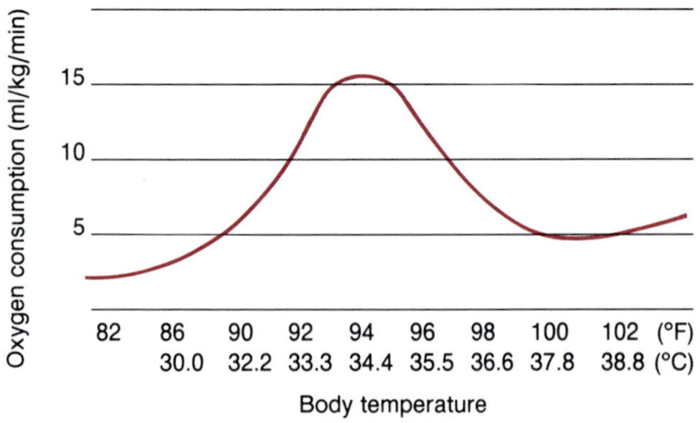

Figure 30-5.
Alterations in neonatal oxygen consumption related to body temperature. (From Graven, S. [1976]. Heat and body temperature. In N. Dahl, S. Frazier, & M. Duxbury [Eds.]. *Neonatal thermoregulation.* White Plains, NY: The National Foundation/March of Dimes.)

Most newborns (92%) void within 24 hours after birth. The first voiding may be dark amber and cloudy because of the mucous and urate content. Uric acid crystals excreted in the urine leave peach-colored crystals or "brick-dust" stains in the diaper, a sign with no clinical significance. The urine will become clear, straw colored, and less concentrated with increased fluid intake. Urine output may be scant during the first few days of life as the newborn adjusts to feedings. Urine output in the full-term neonate ranges from 15 to 30 mL/kg per 24 hours. Approximately 30 to 60 mL urine is produced in the first day of life depending on fluid intake and the solute load of feedings. Frequency increases from 2 to 6 voidings the first day to up to 20 voidings per day once the neonate's intake improves.

Specific gravity is low in the neonate due to the immature concentrating ability of the nephron. Values range from 1.006 to 1.012 (Richardson, 1991). The glomerular filtration rate is also low. The tubules are short and narrow, which limits the effectiveness of tubular reabsorption and urine concentration mechanisms. Amino acids and bicarbonate

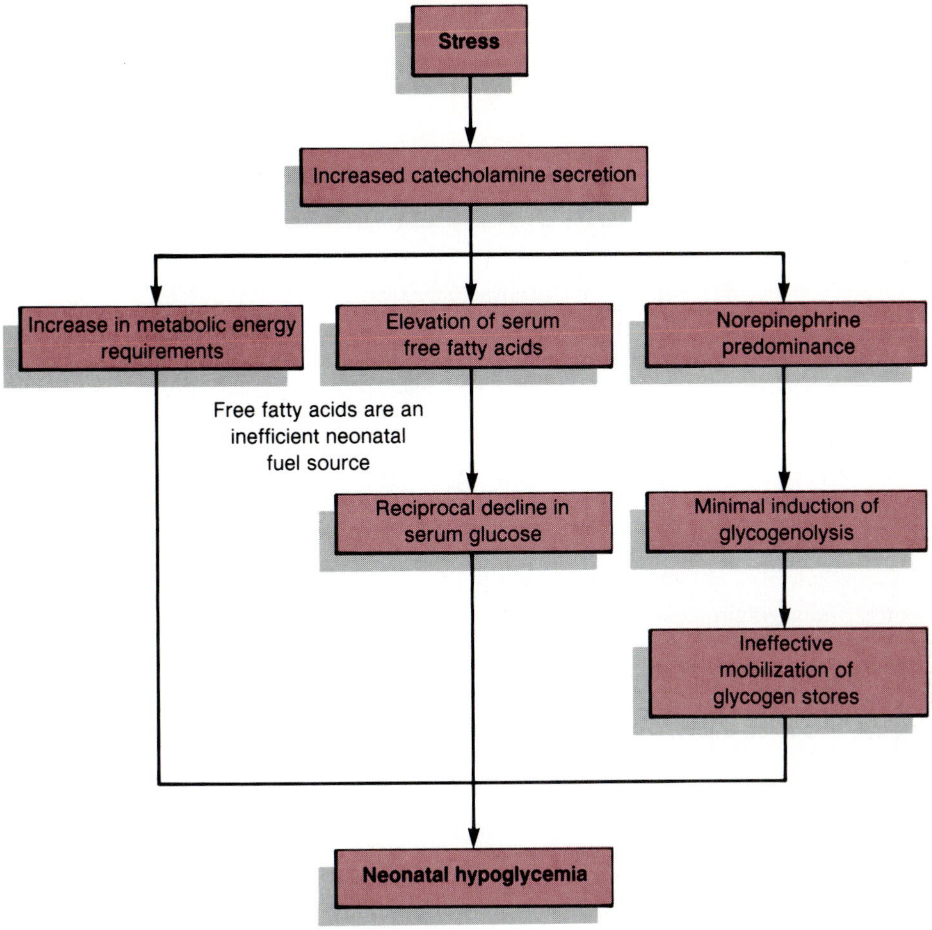

Figure 30-6.
The effects of stress on neonatal serum glucose levels. (From Fantazia, D. [1984]. Neonatal hypoglycemia. *Journal of Obstetric and Gynecologic Nursing, 13*, 298.)

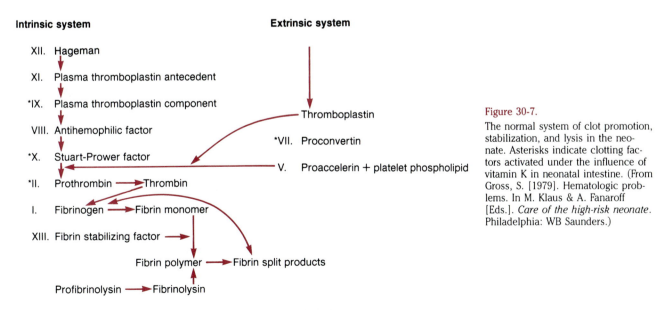

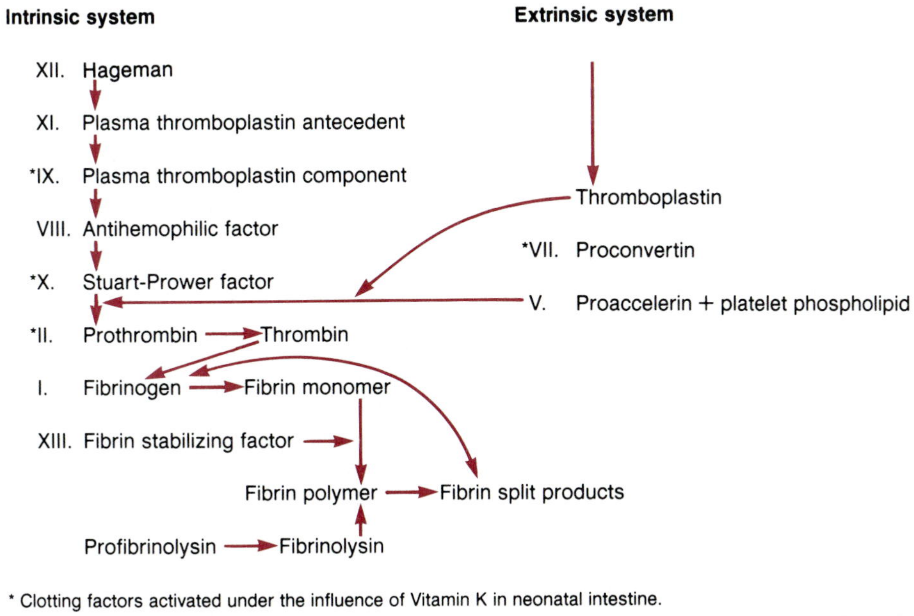

Figure 30-7.
The normal system of clot promotion, stabilization, and lysis in the neonate. Asterisks indicate clotting factors activated under the influence of vitamin K in neonatal intestine. (From Gross, S. [1979]. Hematologic problems. In M. Klaus & A. Fanaroff [Eds.]. *Care of the high-risk neonate*. Philadelphia: WB Saunders.)

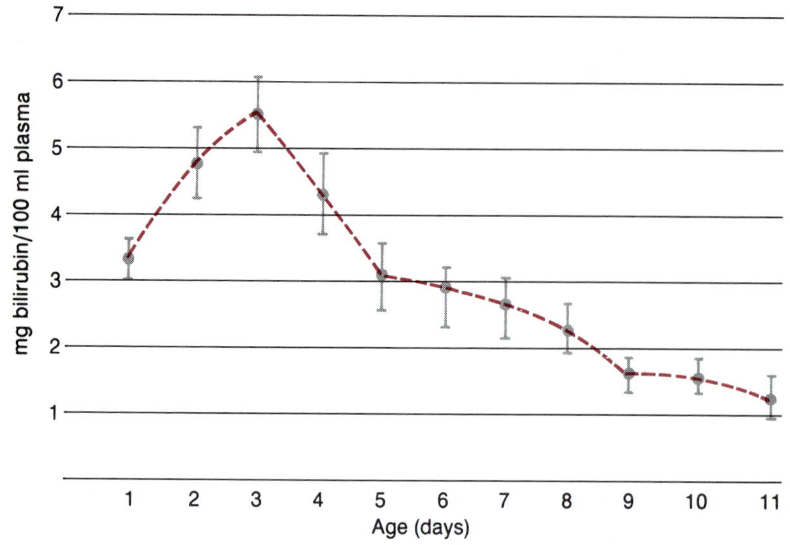

Figure 30-8.
Average serum unconjugated bilirubin levels in full-term neonates. (From McMillan, J., Stockman, J., & Oski, F. [1982]. *The whole pediatrician catalog*. Philadelphia: WB Saunders.)

may be lost in the urine. Transient proteinuria (trace to +3) is not uncommon. Protein excretion is highest in the first day of postnatal life and rapidly decreases thereafter (Portman, 1989). Persistent proteinuria occurs with severe asphyxia, urinary tract infections, and renal injury.

Neurologic Adaptations

Although the sophisticated physiologic functioning and behavioral capabilities of the neonate are evidence of an intact neurologic system, the system is immature at birth. The brain is only 25% of its adult size and myelinization of nerve fibers is incomplete. The newborn exhibits many primitive reflexes, discussed later in the chapter. These reflexes disappear as the nervous system develops. Transient tremors, frequent startles, and incoordinate motor activity can also be observed.

Although the nervous system is immature, it is sufficiently integrated to support neonatal adaptations at birth. The autonomic nervous system and brain stem coordinate vital respiratory and cardiac functions, and sensory capabilities are well developed. Protective, feeding, and social reflexes are present and provide the neonate with a repertoire of behaviors that greatly improve chances of survival. Painful stimuli, which can be perceived by the neonate, alter physiologic functioning and neurobehavioral functioning, including sleep cycles (see the Nursing Research display, Neonatal Pain Perception and Adaptation). Growth occurs in a cephalocaudal, proximal–distal fashion. Gross motor skills are mastered before those requiring fine motor coordination.

Immunologic Adaptations

Although some controversy exists over the extent to which the immune system of the neonate is impaired, it is generally accepted that the infant's response to infection is limited at birth. Phagocytosis and localization of infection appear limited and low levels of a particular antibody, IgM, may be responsible for the infant's susceptibility to gram-positive infections.

The fetus is capable of synthesizing small amounts of certain immunoglobulins by the 20th week of gestation (IgM, IgG, and IgE), and passive immunity is acquired against many bacterial and viral diseases to which the mother has developed antibodies, including diphtheria, poliomyelitis, tetanus, measles, and mumps. This is accomplished by the passage of IgG across the placenta in the third trimester.

IgM is the largest immunoglobulin. It does not cross the placenta, and elevated levels in the newborn may indicate a fetal response to such intrauterine infections as toxoplasmosis, syphilis, rubella, cytomegalovirus (CMV) infection, or herpes. These infections are often referred to as the TORCH infections. The infant born with one of the TORCH infections may show signs of chronic intrauterine infection (small brain size, retardation, and hepatomegaly) and may continue to shed live virus for months.

IgA does not cross the placental barrier in appreciable amounts. It is not normally produced in utero, but increased levels of IgA are found in neonates with CMV infections. IgA is secreted in colostrum, and research indicates that IgA confers passive immunity to certain gastrointestinal and respiratory infections in the breastfed infant (Quie, 1990).

Hematopoietic Adaptations

At birth the bone marrow constitutes the major hematopoietic organ. Changes in red blood cell count, white blood cell count, and hemoglobin concentration occur slowly during the first 6 months of life.

Red Blood Cell Production. To compensate for the relatively low blood oxygen concentration in utero, the fetus has a much higher erythrocyte and hemoglobin count than an adult. The newborn's erythrocyte count ranges from 5.0 to 7.5 million/mm^3. The hematocrit count is also high, with a range of 45% to 65%. Immediately after birth, as the lungs assume responsibility for tissue oxygenation, blood oxygen saturation rises and erythropoietic activity is suppressed. Erythropoietin, the renal hormone that mediates red blood cell production, is barely detectable for 8 to 12 weeks. By the first week of life, red blood cell production is less than one

Nursing Research

Neonatal Pain Perception and Adaptation

Many health care professionals previously did not believe that neonates could feel pain (or perceive pain to the same degree as adults). This was based on the false assumption that pain impulses could not be carried by unmyelinated nerve fibers. It is now recognized that pain impulses may be transmitted by unmyelinated c-polymodal fibers, although at a slower rate.

Nurse researchers have begun to explore the pain behaviors and responses of neonates. Alterations in respiratory rate, systolic blood pressure, blood oxygenation, serum cortisol levels, and behavioral capacities have been observed in infants exposed to activities that are considered painful, such as circumcision and heel sticks. Physiologic changes induced by painful procedures adversely affect both physiologic and behavioral adaptive processes in the neonate and place the already compromised infant at greater risk.

The goals of current neonatal pain research are: (1) identifying signs of pain, (2) enhancing the nurse's ability to recognize pain-invoked behaviors, and (3) establishing safe and effective treatment of pain in infants. Further research is required; however, current findings have begun to alter practice. Clinicians are attempting to ameliorate and limit painful experiences for the neonate through both pharmacologic and nonpharmacologic interventions.

NAACOG. (1991). Prevention, recognition, and management of neonatal pain. *OGN Nursing Practice Resource. Washington, DC: Author.*

tenth the level in utero. Furthermore, the life span of fetal erythrocytes (80 to 100 days) is shorter than that of an adult (approximately 120 days), and the red blood cell count begins to decline shortly after birth. This decline continues to a low of 3 to 4 million/mm^3 by the eighth to tenth week after birth, when erythropoietic activity increases.

Hemoglobin Concentration. Several types of hemoglobin are detectable in the neonate. Fetal hemoglobin (Hgb F), which has a greater oxygen-carrying capacity than adult hemoglobin (Hgb A), is the predominant form (70% to 80%). After birth, the concentration of Hgb A slowly increases as the production of Hgb F ceases. The newborn's hemoglobin level ranges between 15 and 20 g/dL. As the red blood cell count drops, the hemoglobin level also decreases, reaching 10 to 11 g/dL at its nadir, or lowest point.

White Blood Cell Concentrations. In the neonate, white blood cells, or leukocytes, function as the body's internal defense against infection. Polymorphonuclear cells (neutrophils) are the predominant form of leukocyte (40% to 80%) found in the newborn. The lymphocyte count (approximately 30%) slowly rises from birth and surpasses the neutrophil count by 1 month of age. The total white blood cell count is high (9000 to 30,000/mm^3). Leukocytosis is a normal response to the stress of birth; however, the white blood count does not always rise in response to infection. Leukocytes in neonates have a significant deficiency in chemotactic factors generated by *Staphylococcus aureus* and *Escherichia coli*. This may increase susceptibility to infections caused by these organisms if the neonate is compromised by birth asphyxia, prematurity, or other problems at birth. An increase in the number of immature leukocytes and neutropenia (a decrease in the number of neutrophils) is not uncommon in neonatal sepsis.

Platelet Count. Platelet function is adequate in the newborn (range, 150,000 to 400,000/mm^3). Thrombocytopenia may be found in the presence of neonatal sepsis.

Reproductive and Sexual Adaptations

Physical signs of sexual–reproductive adaptation in the neonate may appear several days after birth. The uterus in the female neonate, which has been stimulated by maternal estrogens during pregnancy, involutes and may produce a blood-tinged mucoid vaginal discharge (pseudomenstruation) several days after birth. Both male and female newborns may exhibit temporary breast engorgement, a result of fetal estrogen stimulation. Fluid, sometimes called "witch's milk," may be discharged from the neonate's nipples. The testes normally descend into the scrotal sac in 90% of full-term male neonates by the time of birth.

Research suggests that neonates are born with the potential for sexual pleasure and expression. Penile erection, vaginal lubrication, and pelvic rocking have been observed in young infants, and it has been suggested that infants may experience orgasm. Self-pleasuring activity appears in conjunction with the development of other motor skills in the older infant and remains a more or less observable behavior throughout childhood, depending on parental response to the activity.

Behavioral Adaptations

Periods of Reactivity

In the period immediately after birth the neonate progresses through a series of predictable behavior patterns known as periods of reactivity. These distinct stages, which begin at birth, are characterized by waking and sleep states and by rapid changes in physiologic functioning (Fig. 30-9). The infant may need specialized nursing care during each period because adaptations, especially respiratory and temperature adjustments, are not always accomplished smoothly.

First Period of Reactivity. This period, which lasts 15 to 30 minutes immediately after birth, is characterized by a

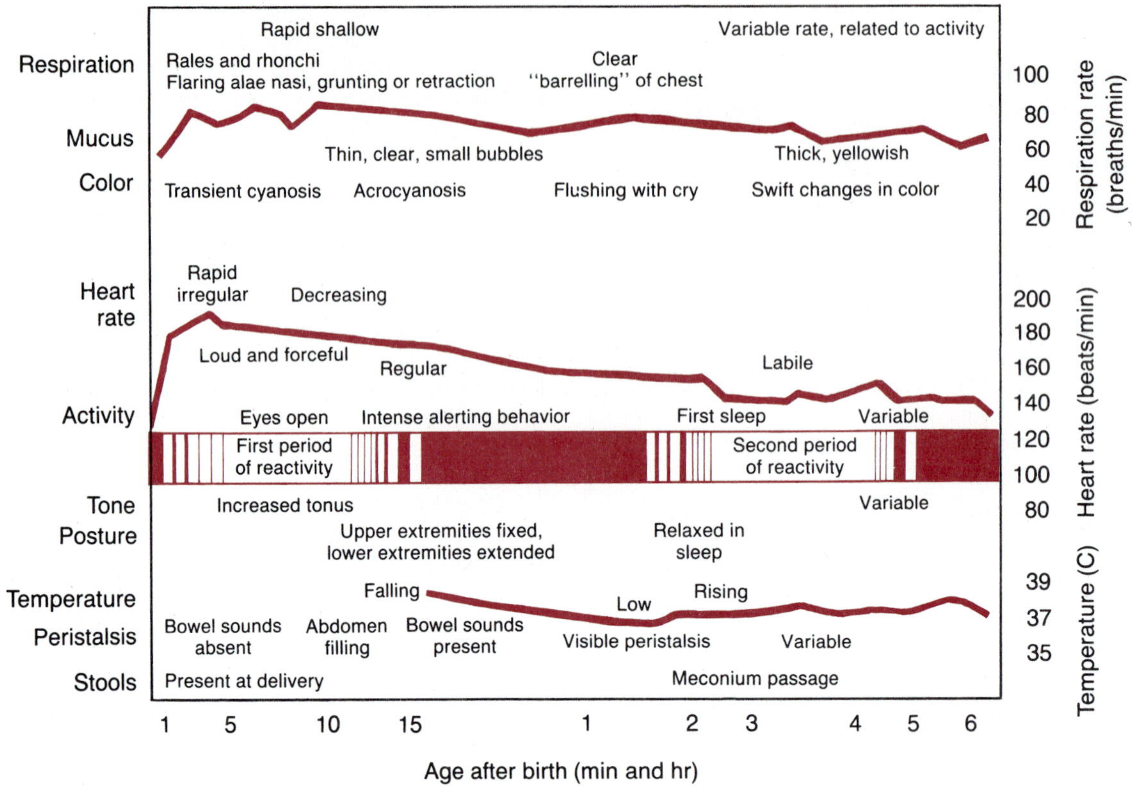

Figure 30-9.
Neonatal periods of reactivity. (Adapted from Arnold, H. W., Putnam, N. J., Barnard, B. L., et al. [1965]. Transition to extrauterine life. *American Journal of Nursing, 65*[10], 78.)

state of alert awareness alternating with episodes of vigorous activity, crying, and rapid irregular respirations and heart rate. Because the neonate's eyes are open at times and a strong sucking reflex is frequently present, this is an excellent time for the nurse to assist the parent–newborn acquaintance process. It is also an ideal time to initiate breastfeeding. Although bowel sounds are normally still absent, breastfeeding at this time is often successful and satisfying to both mother and infant.

Period of Inactivity. After approximately half an hour, the neonate becomes progressively quieter and eventually enters a sleep phase. This period of inactivity lasts 2 to 4 hours, and difficulty may be encountered in waking the infant or initiating breastfeeding during this period. Respiratory and cardiac rates slow to resting or baseline rates. The temperature may drop to its lowest point and bowel sounds become audible.

Second Period of Reactivity. Gradually the neonate awakens and enters the second period of reactivity, which lasts from 4 to 6 hours. Although the neonate attempts to reach physiologic stability during this period, this phase may show the most variability in behavioral responses. Respiratory and cardiac rates may change rapidly. There may be periods of tachypnea, gagging, regurgitation of mucus, and transient cyanosis, alternating with episodes of quiet sleep. The neonate may even experience apnea. Bowel sounds increase, meconium may be passed, and the newborn again demonstrates interest in feeding.

By about 6 to 8 hours after birth, most healthy full-term infants have achieved a state of equilibrium. The transition from the intrauterine to the extrauterine environment is successfully accomplished. The newborn settles into a less dramatic routine of sleep followed by wakefulness interspersed with periods of crying. The development of circadian and diurnal rhythms begins but is strongly influenced by the newborn's environment (Anders & Keener, 1985). The need for careful, frequent monitoring usually ends at about 8 hours after birth. The infant is normally then ready to move into the mother's room or a central nursery.

The neonate undergoes dramatic physiologic and behavioral changes during the immediate postbirth period. Although most healthy neonates make these adjustments with minimal difficulty, appropriate supportive care is required when maladaptations occur. Therefore, the nurse must possess a comprehensive knowledge of normal neonatal adaptations to identify significant deviations and to plan and implement appropriate care. In addition, one of the most effective strategies for promoting early parent–newborn attachment is to teach the new parents about these extraordinary adjustments and their infant's unique abilities to accomplish them.

Neonatal Admission Assessment

The nurse is often the first health care professional to perform a thorough assessment of the newborn. Although an immediate evaluation is made by the birth attendant (certified nurse midwife or physician), the nurse is usually responsible for monitoring the infant during the 6- to 8-hour transition period. It is also necessary to perform a complete systems assessment and the estimation of gestational age. The nurse then monitors the continuing adaptations to extrauterine life while the neonate remains in the hospital or birthing center. Nursing responsibility for the newborn assessment is being extended to the community as the number of home births and early hospital discharges continues to rise.

Neonatal Health History

The neonatal assessment should be completed in an organized manner. Before beginning the actual physical examination of the neonate, the nurse should collect pertinent historical data about the mother's pregnancy, labor, and delivery. The delivery room nurse should provide a verbal report of the birth, the 1-minute and 5-minute Apgar scores (see Chapter 21), and any significant findings (birth injuries, anomalies, or abnormal umbilical cord blood gas/pH results). It is also important to determine if any resuscitative measures were performed. Table 30-3 lists significant data to be included in the initial health history of the neonate. Arm and leg identification bands are rechecked against the identifying data on the birth record to verify the newborn's identity before the assessment is conducted or care is initiated.

Neonatal Physical Assessment

Once the nurse has an adequate data base from which to start, the physical assessment is begun. The physical examination is performed in a cephalocaudal manner or by systems and includes the four major components of assessment in the following order: inspection, auscultation, palpation, and percussion. The nurse usually uses a neonatal assessment tool provided by the health care facility to complete the admission examination and document the findings (see sample Assessment Tool).

Subsequent assessments are conducted in the same organized fashion. Documentation of the neonate's condition varies among health care facilities and can include flow sheets, checklists, graphs, and problem-oriented nurse's notes.

The nurse should conduct the assessment in a warm, well-lit environment that is free of drafts. The admission examination is often completed under an overhead radiant warmer to minimize cold stress during the transition period. It may be possible to perform the admission assessment at the mother's bedside if the hospital provides alternative birthing rooms or has a mother–infant recovery room. If the newborn is transferred to a central admission nursery, encouraging the father or support person to accompany the newborn and observe the assessment is an excellent way to initiate the father–newborn acquaintance process. An effort should be made to conduct subsequent daily evaluations at the mother's bedside. This provides an excellent opportunity for parent teaching and support.

General Appearance

The nurse begins the assessment by inspecting the infant's posture, color, respiratory effort, and skin appearance. This inspection gives information about the neurologic, cardiac, respiratory, and nutritional status of the neonate. The general appearance of the newborn can change dramatically in response to stress. Pink, healthy neonates with well-flexed extremities can suddenly become cyanotic and flaccid if they are unable to clear the airway of mucus or if they aspirate regurgitated milk. Such changes are indications that immediate help is required. The nurse must become skilled in making rapid appraisals of the neonate's general appearance.

Posture

The posture of the neonate is influenced by the position maintained in utero, oxygenation status, neurologic status, and gestational age. The healthy full-term newborn assumes a flexed posture. Muscle resistance is evident when attempts are made to extend the extremities and there is rapid recoil to the flexed position. Neonates who have been in a breech presentation in utero may exhibit temporary full extension of the lower extremities or assume a "frog-leg" appearance, depending on the type of breech presentation. However, the normal state of flexion will be assumed in several days.

Neonates who have sustained neurologic injury at birth as a result of trauma or asphyxia will demonstrate varying degrees of muscle flaccidity and extension of extremities. These neonates are often described as "floppy" newborns. Decreased muscle tone will also be evident in hypoxemic and premature infants. Decreased muscle tone correlates with the degree of prematurity and is a result of incomplete neuromuscular development.

Color

Because of the large number of red blood cells present at birth, white and Asian newborns will have a pale pink skin tone. When the neonate cries or passes stool, the color changes to bright pink or beefy red. African American newborns have a warm brown skin color at birth and also become obviously ruddy with crying. Variations in skin color are observed in the newborn and are due to physiologic instability and immaturity of organ systems.

Acrocyanosis, localized cyanosis of the hands and feet, is common in the neonate. It is a result of the sluggish peripheral circulation and is exacerbated when the newborn is cold. *Circumoral cyanosis*, localized transient cyanosis around the mouth, is sometimes observed in the infant during the transition period. Circumoral cyanosis that persists or occurs with feeding or crying is abnormal and may indicate cardiac anomalies. *Mottling*, a transient pattern of pink and white lacelike blotches on the skin (seen especially when the infant is cold), is a result of vasomotor instability.

Table 30-3. Essential Elements of the Neonatal Health History

Major Categories of Data Obtained	Specific Elements of Health History
Maternal prenatal care	Extent of prenatal care:
	Number of visits
	Degree of compliance with care plan
	Type of facility (clinic, health department, private practice)
	Type of prenatal education
Maternal prenatal history	Last menstrual period (LMP)
	Estimated due date (EDD)
	Weight gain in pregnancy
	Obstetric complications
	Medical complications
	Types of treatment received
	Types of medication received
	History of hospitalization
	Amniocentesis
	Ultrasonography
Maternal blood type and Rh factor	History of isoimmunization (Rh or ABO incompatibilities)
	Antibody titers
Maternal screening test results	Rubella titer
	Hepatitis antigen screening
	Chlamydia screening
	VDRL
	Gonorrhea cultures
	Herpes cultures
	HIV screening
	β-Streptococcus cultures
	Maternal serum α-fetoprotein
Labor history	Onset of labor
	Length of labor
	Length of gestation at time of labor
	Obstetric complications
	Medication administration
	Types and amount
	Time of last medication
	Anesthesia received in labor
Rupture of membranes	Length of time between rupture of membranes and onset of labor
	Color of fluid
	Amount of fluid
	Presence of meconium
Fetal monitoring record	Indication for monitoring
	Internal or external monitoring
	Abnormal fetal heart rate patterns
	Evidence of fetal distress
	Fetal scalp sampling
	Blood gas analysis results
Delivery history	Length of second stage
	Type of delivery
	Vaginal
	Cesarean
	Place of delivery
	Delivery room
	Alternate birthing room
	Labor room
	Home birth
	Planned
	Unplanned
	Nuchal cord
	Anesthesia administered
	Medication administered
	Use of forceps/vacuum extractor
	Fetal heart rate pattern in second stage

(*continued*)

Table 30-3. Essential Elements of the Neonatal Health History ***(continued)***

Major Categories of Data Obtained	Specific Elements of Health History
	Fetal position at birth
	Shoulder dystocia
	Compound presentation
	Breaks in sterile technique
Postnatal history	Delay in cord clamping
	Respiratory effort at birth
	Assisted
	Unassisted
	Need for resuscitation
	Type and extent of 1- and 5-min Apgar scores
	Medications administered to neonate
	Cord blood gas analysis
	Parent–newborn interaction
	Quality
	Extent
	Evidence of birth injury
	Evidence of narcosis
	Passage of urine or stool
	Other significant physiologic or behavioral responses
	Other significant procedures performed
	Gastric aspiration
	Laryngoscopy and tracheal suctioning
	Other
Significant social history	Family structure
	Anticipated versus actual birth experience
	Presence of significant others at birth
	Evidence of social support system
	Significant cultural variables
	Ethnic background
	Primary language
	Religious practices related to infant care
	Plans for feeding neonate
	Plans for rooming-in
	Anticipated length of hospital stay
	Early discharge
	Traditional length for recovery
	Significant social problems
	Lack of social support system
	Language barrier
	History of substance abuse
	Lack of adequate housing
	Financial distress
	Others

In *harlequin sign*, a distinctive color pattern caused by vasomotor instability, one side of the body is pink while the other side is pale. *Plethora*, a deep red coloration of the skin, often exaggerated with crying, is caused by the increased number of red blood cells in the neonate (polycythemia).

Jaundice. *Jaundice* (icterus neonatorum) is a yellow cast to the skin and sclera. Because it is fat soluble, indirect bilirubin has an affinity for certain types of body tissue. Accumulation of indirect bilirubin in subcutaneous tissue gives the skin the characteristic yellow color observed when hyperbilirubinemia occurs. It is often more observable in the sclera and in skin surfaces or mucous membranes that have been blanched.

Physiologic jaundice occurs in approximately 50% of full-term neonates, appearing on the head first, and then progressing caudally. Physiologic jaundice is differentiated from pathologic jaundice by the time at which the jaundice appears. Physiologic jaundice occurs after the first 24 hours of life and usually resolves with hydration and frequent feedings, which promote elimination of direct, water-soluble bilirubin. Pathologic or nonphysiologic jaundice occurs within the first 24 hours of life and can be caused by a variety of problems, including blood incompatibilities, inherited metabolic disorders, and severe birth asphyxia.

Jaundice associated with breastfeeding appears, generally, in breastfed neonates. They have slightly higher serum

Text continues on page 894

Assessment Tool

Newborn Admission History

Name		
Sex Male Female Amb.	Birthdate	Admission Date
Admitting Diagnosis		
Inborn	UC Setup	Outborn

II. INFANT HISTORY

Apgars 1'' ________ 5'' ________

G.A. ________ Birthweight ________

Delivery Complications

- ☐ None
- ☐ FHR Abnormality
- ☐ Meconium
- ☐ Nuchal Cord/Prolapse
- ☐ Other ________

III. MATERNAL HISTORY

Age	Gravida	Para	AB

Delivery ☐Vaginal ☐Cesarean section—reason:

Pregnancy Complications:

- ☐ None
- ☐ Preclampsia/Toxemia
- ☐ No Prenatal Care
- ☐ Suspected sepsis
- ☐ PROM > 24°
- ☐ Pre/Post-term labor
- ☐ Abruptio/Placenta previa
- ☐ Other: ________

IV. PHYSICAL ASSESSMENT

Instructions: Check the appropriate descriptive term for all the following items. Asterisked items need not be completed for infants in Admit Nursery. Please describe all abnormal findings objectively; use comment column if necessary.

1. Reflexes (Check if present and normal)
   Moro ________ Grasp ________ Suck ________
2. Tone/Activity
   a. Active ________ Quiet ________ Lethargic ________
   Flaccid ________ Paralyzed ________ Tremors ________
   Seizure Activity ________
   b. Cry Vigorous ________ Weak ________
   High Pitched ________ Difficult to elicit ________
3. Head/Neck
   a. Anterior Fontanelle soft ________ firm ________
   flat ________ bulging ________ depressed ________
   b. Sagittal Suture: approx. ____ sep. ____ overriding ____
   c. Facial Features: symmetrical ____ assymetrical ____
   d. Scalp molding ________
   caput succedaneum ________ cephalohematoma ________
4. Eyes
   clear ________ drainage ________
5. ENT
   a. Ears normal ________ abnormal ________
   b. Nares patent bilaterally ____ obstructed ____ flaring ____
   c. Palate normal ________ abnormal ________
6. Abdomen
   a. soft ____ firm ____ flat ____ distended ____
   *girth ________ cm.
   *b. liver down ≤ 2 cm. Ⓡ CM ________
   down > 2 cm. Ⓡ CM ________

IV. PHYSICAL ASSESSMENT

7. Thorax a. symmetrical ________ assymetrical ________
   b. retractions 0-1 ________ 1+ ________
   1-2+ ________ 2+ ________
   c. clavicles normal ________ abnormal ________
8. Lungs
   a. Breath sounds equal bilat. ____ Br. Sounds unequal ____
   b. Breath sounds audible in all lung fields ________
   inaudible ________ diminished ________
   c. Breath sounds clear ________ rhonchi ________
   rales ____ wheezing ____ secretions ____ grunting ____
   d. Respirations: spont. ____ rate ____ FIO_2 ____ hood ____
   Assisted ventilation CPAP ________ MV ________
   FIO_2 ________ PIP/PEEP ________ Rate ________
9. Heart a. Sounds NSR ________ Ectopics ________
   Murmur ________ PMI ________
   b. Rate ________
   c. Capillary Filling Time: Trunk ____ Extremities ____
10. Extremities a. moves all extremities ________
    limited range of motion ________ unable to assess ________
    b. Periferal Pulses

	STRONG	WEAK	ABSENT
Ⓡ brachial			
Ⓛ brachial			
Ⓡ femoral			
Ⓛ femoral			
Ⓡ			
Ⓛ			

Upper & lower extremities equal ________ unequal ________
   c. hips normal ________ abnormal ________
   unable to assess ________
11. Umbilicus normal ________ abnormal ________
    inflamed ________ drainage ________
    number of cord vessels ________
12. Genitals
    normal female ________ normal male ____ ambiguous ____
13. Anus patent ________ imperforate ________
14. Spine normal ________ abnormal ________
15. Skin
    a. color pink ________ plethoric ________ pallor ________
    jaundice ________ cyanosis trunk ________ nailbeds ________
    circumoral ________ periorbital ________
    b. rash ________
    c. birthmarks ________
16. Temperature
    a. environment
    radiant warmer ________ temperature set ________
    incubator ________ abmient temperature ________
    open crib ________
    b. skin temperature ________

(continued)

Assessment Tool *(Continued)*

Comments:

V. SOCIAL HISTORY

Parents — Ages

Address

Phone: where parents can be reached

Employment

Parent/Infant Bonding

Mother		Father
	touched	
	held	
	spoke to	
	visited	
	named	
	eye contact	

Other significant social information

Parents response to prior experiences of illness &/or hospitalizations

Other children

Other children

Support systems (or significant others) for parents:

Introduction to Unit

Instruction Booklet

Tour of Unit

Parent Support Group Info

Photo of Infant Given

Date_______________ Signature____________________

bilirubin levels in the first 3 to 4 days of life than formula-fed neonates. This phenomenon has no clinical significance, and generally resolves when the neonate is breastfed every 2 to 3 hours to facilitate the passage of urine and stool. In contrast, true breast milk jaundice is associated with significant elevations in serum bilirubin levels, which may require temporary cessation of breastfeeding and the implementation of phototherapy.

True breast milk jaundice occurs in only 1% of infants and appears around the third or fourth day of life when the woman begins producing greater amounts of breast milk (Cloherty, 1991). Although the etiology is unknown, several factors have been implicated in the development of true breast milk jaundice. Pregnanediol, an enzyme that interferes with the release of conjugated bilirubin from neonatal liver cells, has been suggested as a possible contributing factor. More recent research has also implicated the presence of elevated lipase levels in the breast milk of mothers of infants exhibiting breast milk jaundice. Increased lipase activity may result in the accelerated release of free fatty acids, which may inhibit bilirubin conjugation in the newborn.

Dangerous elevations in serum bilirubin rarely occur, and kernicterus has not been reported in the case of true breast milk jaundice. Serum bilirubin levels may reach 20 to 30 mg/dL by 14 days of age if breastfeeding is continued. In most cases, however, when the serum bilirubin level exceeds 16 to 18 mg/dL, breastfeeding is usually stopped for 12 to 48 hours, and phototherapy may be initiated if the bilirubin level reaches 20 mg/dL (Cloherty, 1991). The mother is instructed in the manual expression or hand pumping of breast milk so that her milk supply does not diminish. If the hyperbilirubinemia is solely related to breastfeeding, the serum bilirubin levels fall rapidly within 48 hours. Nursing can usually be resumed when the neonatal bilirubin level falls below 15 mg/dL. An alternative therapy to the total cessation of breastfeeding that promotes maternal efforts to nurse her newborn is to alternate breast milk with formula until bilirubin levels decrease.

Respiratory Effort

At rest, the normal neonate's respiratory pattern is quiet, shallow, and irregular. The mouth remains closed and air moves in and out of the nose without flaring of the nares. Respiratory movements are abdominal, and chest expansion, while shallow, is synchronous with the rise and fall of the abdomen. There is no retraction of the chest wall (collapse of sternum or intercostal muscles toward the spine) with inspiration although transient or intermittent retraction may be observed during the neonatal transition period. Expiratory grunting, a high-pitched peeping noise, should not be evident or audible on auscultation of the chest with a stethoscope. A complete discussion of normal respiration is presented later in this chapter.

Appearance of the Skin

The skin provides a visible record of the neonate's intrauterine history, birth experience, and gestational age. The full-term newborn with an uneventful gestation has pink, smooth, intact skin with good turgor at birth. *Turgor* is the natural elastic rebound characteristic of healthy tissue that can be observed when it is pinched and then released. Some loss of turgor and superficial peeling of skin occurs after several days as a result of limited fluid intake, fluid shifts, and continued elimination of wastes. Greenish yellow staining of the skin and nails indicates passage of meconium in utero related to hypoxia and fetal distress.

A full-term neonate's skin is relatively opaque. Few veins are visible and many creases cover the soles of the feet. Thick parchment-like skin that is peeling at birth is indicative of postmaturity. Premature neonates have a transparent skin with many visible veins, and the skin on the soles is shiny with few creases. Loose, wrinkled skin with poor turgor occurs with chronic intrauterine malnutrition.

Ecchymoses and *petechiae* are visible when labor has been precipitous or delivery difficult. Forcep marks (facial bruising) may be evident when forceps are used during delivery. Small scalp lacerations are common when an internal fetal monitor has been applied during labor or capillary blood samples have been obtained from the scalp. There may be a bright red, circular, raised mark over the presenting part if a vacuum extractor was applied to the head to facilitate delivery of the fetus.

A variety of unique skin characteristics and birth marks in the neonate can be observed. The major characteristics follow.

Vernix caseosa is the white, cream-cheeselike substance that serves as a protective skin covering in utero. It may form a thick covering between 36 and 38 weeks of gestation. By 40 weeks, vernix is usually found only in skin folds of the axilla and groin of the neonate. Vernix is gradually absorbed by the skin and may be gently removed during bathing.

Milia are small white papules on the nose, chin, and cheeks that are formed by plugged sebaceous glands. They are commonly mistaken for blemishes by parents. They should not be squeezed and will disappear spontaneously within the first few weeks of life.

Lanugo is the fine, downy hair that covers the fetus in utero. It begins to thin before birth and by 40 weeks of gestation is normally found only on the shoulders, back, and upper arms. It is gradually removed by the friction of clothing and bed linen (see Fig. 30-20*B*).

Erythema toxicum is a benign maculopapular rash with an erythematous base and a pale yellow papule. It may appear on any part of the skin surface except the palms and the soles. This rash occurs in 30% to 70% of neonates and peak incidence is the second and third day of life. It usually resolves in 48 to 72 hours. Its cause is unknown and no treatment is indicated.

Birthmarks

Birthmarks fall into two categories: pigmented and vascular nevi. *Pigmented nevi* are lesions containing cells colored by melanin. They range from yellow to black in color. *Vascular nevi* are lesions containing enlarged blood vessels. They are usually reddish or purplish in color. Mongolian spots are bluish gray pigmented nevi found primarily on the skin of the sacrum and buttocks of Asian and African American babies. They are frequently mistaken for bruises by concerned parents. Mongolian spots slowly fade and disappear in childhood. Moles are pigmented nevi. They have no clinical significance in the neonate.

Nevus flammeus (*port-wine stain*), a vascular nevus, is a capillary angioma located below the dermis. It is a flat, sharply demarcated purple red birthmark commonly found on the face. This birthmark does not enlarge after birth nor will it fade. Recent advances in laser technology make removal of the birthmark possible. Although normally an isolated finding, nevus flammeus may be associated with a life-threatening genetic disorder known as Sturge-Weber syndrome and spinal anomalies found in Cobb syndrome (Tallman et al., 1991).

Nevus vasculosus (*strawberry mark*), a vascular nevus, is a capillary angioma located in the dermal and subdermal layers of the skin. It is a raised, sharply demarcated, rough-surfaced birthmark. Strawberry marks continue to grow after birth and then recede after the first year of life. They may completely disappear by 10 years of age.

Vital Signs and Measurements

After the general inspection, the nurse proceeds to take vital signs and obtains important measurements.

Respiratory Rate

Normal rate ranges from 30 to 60 breaths per minute. Respirations are counted for 1 full minute by observing the abdomen. Auscultation of breath sounds is discussed later in the chapter.

Heart Rate

Normal heart rate ranges from 120 to 160 bpm. The rate may drop to 100 bpm during sleep and rise to 180 bpm with crying. The heart rate should be auscultated for 1 full minute over the cardiac apex, which is normally located at the third or fourth intercostal space in the midclavicular line (Fig. 30-10). Auscultation of heart sounds is discussed later in this chapter.

Pulses

The brachial, radial, femoral, popliteal, and dorsalis pedis pulses are palpated in the neonate. The pulses are assessed for equality, amplitude, and rhythmicity. Simultaneous palpation of right and left pulses and lower and upper pulses assists the nurse in evaluating structural integrity of the cardiovascular system. The quality of pulses is normally documented using a numeric scale. Although several different scales have been devised to assist clinicians in the assessment of pulses, the scale recommended by the American Association of Critical Care Nurses is described here because it recognizes the full range of pulse amplitude that may be palpated in the neonate: 0 = absent pulse, 1+ = palpable pulse, 2+ = normal pulse, 3+ = full pulse, and 4+ = bounding pulse.

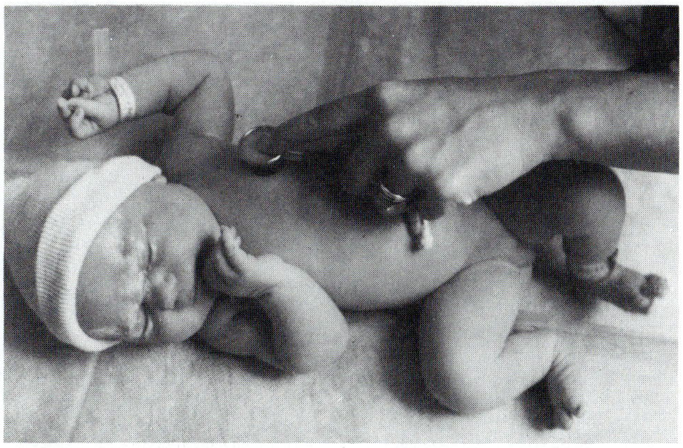

Figure 30-10.
Auscultation of heart rate. After the admission bath, gloves need not be worn during auscultation.

Capillary Fill Time

The skin on the infant's trunk is blanched for assessment of central capillary fill time (CFT), an indirect evaluation of tissue perfusion. Central CFT is normally 3 seconds or less. Peripheral CFT may be inaccurate due to the normally sluggish peripheral perfusion of the newborn.

Temperature

Accurate monitoring of the neonatal temperature is essential to determine the adequacy of postbirth adaptations (see the accompanying Nursing Research display). Normal temperature ranges from 36.4°C to 37.2°C (97.5°F to 99°F) in the neonate.

Nursing Research

Assessment of Neonatal Axillary Temperature

Nurse researchers have evaluated optimal neonatal thermometer placement time, defined as the duration of time required for the temperature to be accurately recorded in 90% of neonates. Hunter examined optimal placement times when obtaining an axillary temperature in the neonate for a mercury thermometer and an IVAC electronic thermometer. For both types of thermometer, stabilization occurred within 3 minutes for 100% of the sample. Other researchers have reported 90% stabilization in axillary temperature in 5 minutes. Until further research resolves these contradictions in findings, it may be more appropriate to place the thermometer for the longer period of time (5 minutes). To use nursing time effectively, the nurse may conduct other bedside activities such as counting the respiratory rate or auscultating the apical heart rate while obtaining accurate temperature readings.

Hunter, L. (1991). Measurement of axillary temperatures in neonates. *Western Journal of Nursing Research, 13*(3), 324.

Stephens, S. B., & Sexton, P. R. (1987). Neonatal axillary temperature: Increases in readings over time. *Neonatal Network, 5*(6), 25.

Axillary measurement is preferred because of the risk of traumatizing or perforating the rectal mucosa when a rectal temperature is taken. Previously some facilities permitted an initial rectal temperature to assess the patency of the anal opening. This is no longer recommended as a safe method for identifying an imperforate anus. Another advantage of measuring axillary temperature is that it permits early identification of heat loss and hypothermia. This is possible because the axillary temperature is a measure of the skin temperature, which will decrease before the core temperature begins to drop. The thermometer is held in the axillary fold for 5 minutes to obtain an accurate reading (Fig. 30-11).

When a rectal temperature must be taken, the nurse must take care to stabilize the infant's lower extremities with one hand while inserting the lubricated thermometer bulb to a depth no greater than 0.25 to 0.5 inch or 1 cm. The neonate must never be left unattended while the thermometer remains in the rectum.

Infrared technology has been used to measure tympanic membrane temperature in adults. It involves placing a portable sensor probe with a disposable cover in the external auditory canal. The device measures the temperature of blood flowing through the internal carotid artery in several seconds. Because it is accurate, rapid, and noninvasive, infrared thermometry has been proposed as a measurement of temperature in full-term and preterm newborns. The need to disturb the infant and the risk of heat loss, common problems when obtaining temperature readings in a neonate, are eliminated. Early research findings (Weiss, 1991) suggest that tympanic temperature is as accurate an estimation of body temperature in the neonate as axillary temperature. However, further studies are indicated to confirm initial results.

Weight

Average full-term weight is 3400 g (7 lb 8 oz); 95% of neonates weigh between 2500 and 4250 g (5 lb, 8 oz to 9 lb, 6 oz). The neonate should be weighed at the same time each day, preferably before feeding. The infant should be undressed completely, including diaper, and placed on the prebalanced or calibrated scale in the supine position. A

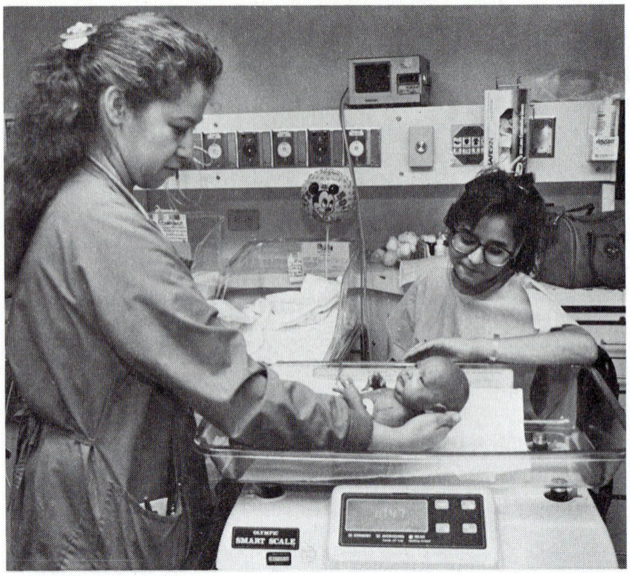

Figure 30-12.
Weight measurement.

protecting hand should be placed just above the infant while reading weight (Fig. 30-12).

A weight loss of between 5% and 10% of birth weight may occur in the newborn during the first 4 to 5 days. This weight loss results from continued voidings and stool passage, limited intake, insensible water loss, and a high metabolic rate. Weight loss should stabilize by about the fifth day, and a weight gain of approximately 30 g (1 oz) per day will occur with adequate fluid and caloric intake.

Length

Average full-term length is 49.5 cm (19.5 inches). The length from bregma (anterior fontanelle) to heel should be measured. The neonate should be placed on a flat surface. Care is taken to extend the legs fully before measuring length (Fig. 30-13).

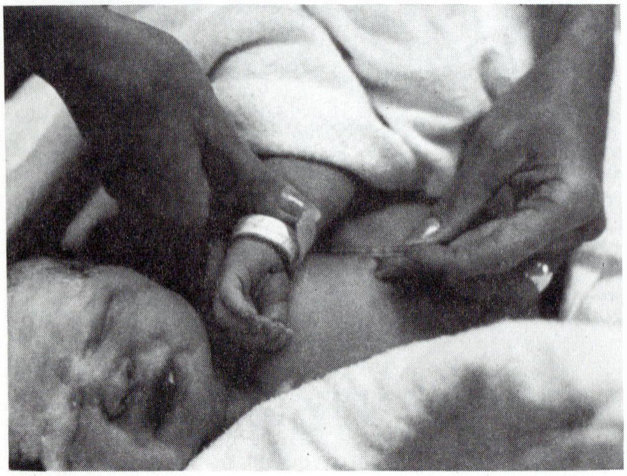

Figure 30-11.
Axillary temperature measurement.

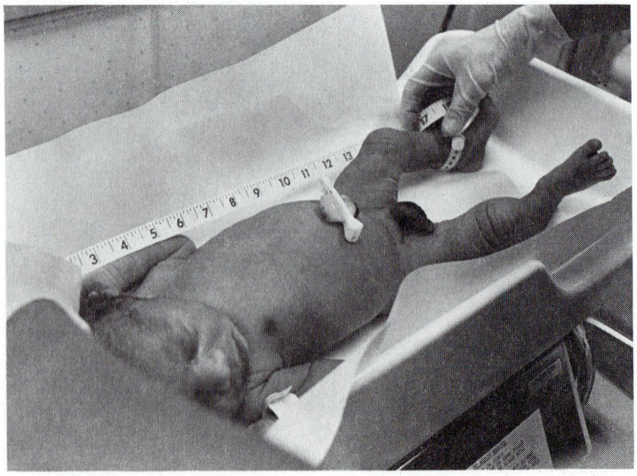

Figure 30-13.
Length measurement.

Head Circumference

Average head circumference is 35.5 cm. Normally it is approximately 2 cm larger than the chest. The tape measure should be placed above the eyebrow, directly above the top of the ears and around the fullest part of the occiput (Fig. 30-14).

Chest Circumference

The tape measure should be placed across the lower border of the scapulae and over the nipples. Average chest circumference is 33 cm. It is approximately 2 to 3 cm smaller than the head.

Blood Pressure

Average blood pressure at birth is 80/46 mm Hg. The mean value in neonates 1 to 3 days of age is 65/41 mm Hg (Park & Da-Hae, 1989). The ultrasound (Doppler) method is the most accurate and most commonly used method of blood pressure measurement in neonates. It uses a Doppler device on an inflatable cuff attached to the neonate's arm or leg. This device allows the nurse to obtain an electronic reading of systolic, diastolic, and mean arterial pressure. Several cuff sizes imprinted with arm circumference measurements or weight guidelines are available so that the appropriate cuff is used. This is essential to obtain accurate blood pressure measurements. Infant movement can also affect the accuracy of the blood pressure measurement, so the Doppler device should be used when the neonate is quiet. Routine blood pressure monitoring is not generally performed in healthy neonates. Most experts recommend an initial assessment of the blood pressure to identify abnormally low readings (shock, asphyxia, hypovolemia) or levels in the hypertensive range (coarctation of the aorta).

Detailed Physical Assessment

A detailed physical assessment gives the nurse important information about the neonate's progress in adapting to extrauterine life and about the infant's particular capabilities and level of maturity. Table 30-4 summarizes normal and unusual physical findings in the neonatal assessment. Normal variations are rarely charted in the neonatal record but should be explained to parents if they have questions or concerns. The nurse should note any unusual findings and ascertain if they have been recorded by other examiners in the neonate's chart. If not, the nurse should chart his or her findings according to that setting's protocol and bring them to the physician's attention.

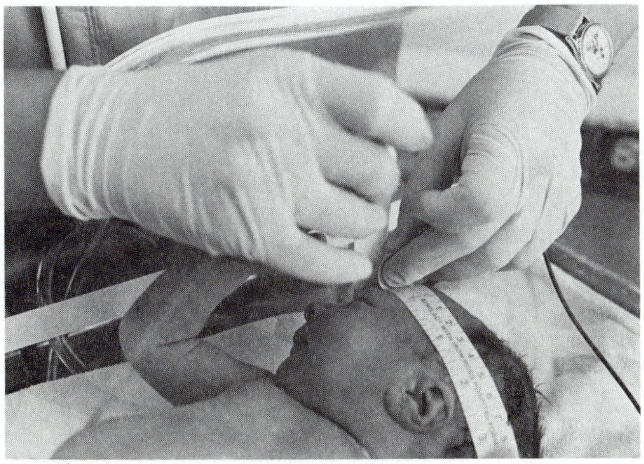

Figure 30-14.
Measurement of head circumference.

Head and Face

The nurse inspects the size and shape of the head first. The newborn head is large (approximately 25% of the total body size), with a prominent cranium and forehead. The face appears small in comparison and has a receding chin. The shape of the head may be asymmetrical or elongated. This is due to molding, an overlapping of the cranial bones that occurs as the fetus moves through the birth canal. Molding is temporary and the head will assume a rounded appearance several days after birth.

The general appearance of the face is evaluated. The nurse inspects for signs of asymmetrical movement and facial paralysis (best assessed when the neonate is crying). The distance between the eyes is noted. Ocular hypertelorism is the excessive spacing of the eyes. It is defined as a distance of greater than 3 cm between the inner canthi of the eyes in full-term infants. The size and shape of the nose are assessed. The bridge of the nose normally is low, and the nose may appear flat as a result of labor and delivery. The presence of birth marks, bruising, petechiae, lacerations, or edema is noted. Plagiocephaly, or facial asymmetry, may also be noted. It occurs with persistent positioning of the fetal head against the maternal pelvis and results in premature closure of a cranial suture. The face and head usually resume a symmetrical appearance when pressure is relieved after birth and concomitant molding resolves.

Palpation

Palpation of the cranium follows inspection. The cranium is composed of seven bones (two parietal, two temporal, two frontal, and one occipital), which are not fused together at birth. Palpation of the suture lines, the separating lines between the bones, may reveal overlapping due to molding. The cranial bones are pliable. Palpation may reveal the presence of craniotabes, a rare abnormal localized softening of the bones.

Fontanelles

The fontanelles are the membranous openings at the juncture of three cranial bones. The largest is the anterior fontanelle, or bregma, which is located at the junction of the frontal bone and the parietal bones. It is diamond-shaped and measures approximately 3 to 4 cm long by 2 to 3 cm wide. It remains open for 12 to 18 months. The posterior fontanelle is smaller, triangular in shape, and located at the junction of the occipital bone and parietal bones. The posterior fontanelle may actually be closed at birth due to molding but can be palpated again after several days. It closes within 8 to 12 weeks.

The nurse palpates the anterior fontanelle to assess changes in intracranial pressure and the degree of hydration. A sunken fontanelle may indicate dehydration, whereas a tense or bulging fontanelle suggests increased intracranial pressure. The neonate should be in a sitting position and

Text continues on page 904

Table 30-4. Physical Findings in the Assessment of the Neonate*

Normal Findings and Common Variations	Unusual Findings and Significant Deviations	Possible Causes and Potential Problems
Integument		
General Appearance and Texture		
Skin smooth and pliant, with good turgor and visible layer of adipose tissue below	Skin thick and leathery, cracked with generalized peeling Long nails	Postmaturity
Superficial peeling after first 24 h Veins rarely visible Milia over nose, chin, and forehead Vernix only in skin creases or absent Lanugo patchy or absent Nails soft and pliant but well formed	Skin thin and transparent with minimal adipose tissue, and many visible veins Thick layer of vernix or lanugo Nails thin and incompletely developed	Prematurity
	Skin wrinkled with poor turgor and minimal adipose tissue Umbilical cord thin Skin, umbilical cord, and nails stained with meconium	Intrauterine growth retardation Chronic maternal malnutrition
	Generalized edema	Severe erythroblastosis fetalis
Color		
Skin pink, with incomplete pigmentation in dark-skinned races at birth Acrocyanosis	Pallor	Anemia Asphyxia Shock Sepsis Hypothermia Congenital heart disease
Mottling Harlequin sign Jaundice (after first 24 h)	Cyanosis	Asphyxia Anoxia Congenital heart anomaly Hypoglycemia
	Plethora	Polycythemia
	Jaundice (within first 24 h)	Blood incompatibilities Sepsis Biliary obstruction Drug reactions
Integrity		
Skin intact, with petechiae over presenting part	Lacerations or punctures	Accidental incision of skin with surgical scalpel during cesarean delivery Application of fetal scalp electrode during labor Fetal scalp sampling
	Generalized petechiae	Clotting disorders Sepsis
Ecchymosis secondary to application of forceps	Ecchymosis secondary to birth trauma or manipulation during delivery of infant	Cephalopelvic disproportion Shoulder dystocia Breech presentation at birth Precipitous delivery
Rashes		
Erythema toxicum Diaper rash	Skin pustules	Staphylococcal or β-hemolytic streptococcal skin infection
	Vesicles	Congenital syphilis Herpesvirus infection
	Perianal eruptions	Yeast infection (*Candida albicans*)
	Spreading diaper rashlike skin eruption	Congenital rubella
	Generalized scaling	Genetic disorders
Vascular and Pigmented Nevi		
Nevus vasculosus	Nevus vasculosus	Genetic disorders (Sturge-Weber syndrome)
	Nevus flammeus Cavernous hemangiomas	Genetic disorders
Mongolian spots	Café-au-lait spots	Neurofibromatosis
	Hypopigmentation	Genetic disorders

(*continued*)

Table 30-4. Physical Findings in the Assessment of the Neonate* (*continued*)

Normal Findings and Common Variations	Unusual Findings and Significant Deviations	Possible Causes and Potential Problems
Head		
Size		
	Microcephaly	Intrauterine growth retardation Genetic disorders Fetal alcohol syndrome
	Macrocephaly	Hydrocephalus
Shape		
Head rounded, with mild to moderate molding Plagiocephaly	Severe molding	Cephalopelvic disproportion
Caput succedaneum	Brachycephaly with flat occiput	Down syndrome
	Cephalhematoma	Head trauma secondary to labor dystocia, cephalopelvic disproportion, or forceps application
	Craniotabes	Postmaturity
Fontanelles		
Anterior fontanelle diamond-shaped, 3–4 cm by 2–3 cm wide (closes by 12–18 mo)	Bulging, tense fontanelle	Hydrocephalus Meningitis
Posterior fontanelle triangular-shaped; may be closed at birth due to molding (closes by 8–12 wk)	Abnormally large, flat open fontanelle	Hypothyroidism Intrauterine growth retardation Prematurity
	Depressed fontanelle	Dehydration
Sutures		
Sutures slightly separated or overlapping at birth due to molding	Widely separated sutures	Hypothyroidism Hydrocephalus Prematurity Intrauterine growth retardation
	Premature closure of sutures (craniosynostosis)	Genetic disorders
Hair		
Hair silky; may be curly or kinky based on familial and racial traits	Fine and wooly, sparse	Prematurity
	Coarse, brittle	Endocrine disorders Genetic disorders Intrauterine growth disorders
	Low-set hairline, low forehead	Genetic disorders
Eyes		
Appearance and Position		
Eyes symmetrically spaced, less than 3 cm apart, clear, with transient discharge secondary to chemical conjunctivitis	Agenesis (failure to develop) Hypertelorism (abnormal width in eye spacing)	Genetic disorders Teratogenic injury
Pseudostrabismus	Persistent purulent discharge	Ophthalmia neonatorum Chlamydia conjunctivitis
Cornea and Lens		
Eyes clear, without clouding	Large or uneven cornea	Congenital glaucoma
	Corneal ulcerations	Herpesvirus infection
	Clouding or opacity of lens	Cataracts (rubella infection)
Sclera and Conjunctiva		
Sclera white or with faint blue tinge	True blue sclera	Osteogenesis imperfecta
Icteric after first 24 h	Icteric within first 24 h	Pathologic jaundice
Chemical conjunctivitis	Persistent purulent eye discharge	Ophthalmia neonatorum Chlamydia conjunctivitis
Subconjunctival hemorrhage		
Iris		
Slate gray or brown in color	Pink iris	Albinism
	Colobomas (lesions or clefts in structures)	May be benign or may be associated with genetic disorders
	Brushfield's spots	Down syndrome

(*continued*)

Table 30-4. Physical Findings in the Assessment of the Neonate* (continued)

Normal Findings and Common Variations	Unusual Findings and Significant Deviations	Possible Causes and Potential Problems
Pupils		
Pupils equal and reactive to light	Anisocoria (unequal pupil size) Nonreactive, fixed	Neurologic injury
Retina		
Presence of red reflex	Absence of red reflex	Congenital cataracts
Eyelids and Lacrimal Glands		
Eyelids close completely	Eyelids fused closed	Genetic disorders
Transient edema		Severe prematurity
Transient erythema and petechiae	Ptosis	11th cranial nerve injury
Epicanthal folds in Asian infants and in 15%–20% of non-Asian infants	Shortened palpebral fissures Epicanthal folds in non-Asian infants Absence of eyelashes	Fetal alcohol syndrome Down syndrome in conjunction with other physical findings Genetic disorders
Eyelashes		
Absence of tears, scant tearing	Excessive tearing	Plugged lacrimal duct
Neuromuscular Function		
Transient tracking and fixation ability	Persistent strabismus	Neuromuscular disorder
Transient strabismus	Vertical nystagmus	Seizure disorder
Doll's eye movement	Setting sun sign	CNS injury/disorders
Blink reflex	Blink reflex absent	CNS injury Neuromuscular disorders
Ears		
Ears normally placed with pinna at or above level of line drawn from canthus of eye	Low-set ears	Genetic abnormalities
Ears well formed and firm with good recoil if folded against head	Soft, unformed ear with little cartilage	Prematurity
Auricular skin tags	Preauricular sinus	Failure of embryonic closure of branchial cleft; may lead to infection
Nose		
Nose in midline with wide flat bridge	Short, upturned with hypoplastic philtrum	Fetal alcohol syndrome
Infant is obligate nose breather	Nasal flaring, grunting	Nasal obstruction, choanal atresia
Scant nasal discharge	Copious nasal discharge	CNS anomalies Tracheoesophageal fistula Infection
Occasional sneezing	Frequent sneezing Snuffles	Drug withdrawal Congenital syphilis
Mouth and Chin		
Mouth moist and pink with scant saliva production	Fusion of lips, atresia, or agenesis of oral structures	Genetic disorders Teratogenic injury
Symmetrical movement with crying and sucking	Asymmetry of mouth with sucking or crying	Facial nerve injury
Inclusion cysts, Epstein's pearls		Genetic disorders
Lips intact; labial tubercles present	Cleft lip	Teratogenic injury
Tongue mobile with short frenum	Macroglossia (hypertrophied tongue)	Genetic disorders Prematurity
Sucking fat pads in cheeks	White plaques on tongue, gums, buccal cavity	*C. albicans* infection
	Hypertonic suck	Drug withdrawal
	Weak, uncoordinated suck	Prematurity Neuromuscular disorders Asphyxia
Palates intact	Cleft palate Uvula not in midline	Genetic disorder Teratogenic injury
Presence of rooting, sucking, swallowing, gagging reflexes	Absence of reflexes	Prematurity Asphyxia CNS injury/disorders

(continued)

Table 30-4. Physical Findings in the Assessment of the Neonate* (*continued*)

Normal Findings and Common Variations	Unusual Findings and Significant Deviations	Possible Causes and Potential Problems
Vigorous cry	High-pitched cry	CNS disorders
	Crowing cry	Laryngeal disorder
	Natal teeth	Potential for aspiration if dislodged
Neck and Shoulder		
Neck short, in midline, with head maintained in midline	Abnormally short	Genetic disorders (Turner's syndrome)
	Deviation from midline	Congenital torticollis
	Lateral flexion	
Range of motion normal	Limited range of motion	Meningitis
	Nuchal rigidity	
Ability to raise head momentarily	Inability to control head	Prematurity
	Severe head lag	Asphyxia
		CNS injury
		Neuromuscular disorders
Trachea in midline	Trachea deviated	Neck mass
Thyroid not palpable	Enlarged thyroid	Hyperthyroidism
		Hypothyroidism
	Lump or crepitus over clavicle	Fracture of clavicle
Chest		
Lung		
Normal respiratory rate	Tachypnea	Sepsis
		Respiratory distress
		Hypothermia
		Hypoglycemia
Symmetrical respiratory excursion	Seesaw breathing	Diaphragmatic hernia
	Retractions	Respiratory distress
	Grunting	Prematurity
Breath sounds clear and equal bilaterally	Rales	Atelectasis
Transient rales at birth	Rhonchi	Meconium aspiration
	Decreased breath sounds	Atelectasis
		Pneumothorax
	Hyperresonance	Air trapping
Shape		
Chest rounded, symmetrical	Asymmetrical chest	Pneumothorax
Transient breast engorgement and nipple discharge (nonpurulent)	Unilateral chest bulging	Air trapping
	Supernumerary nipples	Benign finding, but potential cosmetic concern in later life
Heart		
Heart rate normal	Tachycardia	Prematurity
		Anemia
		Shock
		Sepsis
		Congenital heart anomalies
Sinus rhythm with transient arrhythmias	Persistent arrhythmias	Congenital heart anomaly
Transient murmurs	Persistent murmur	Persistent fetal circulation
		Congenital heart anomaly
		Fluid overload
Quiet precordium	Active precordium	Persistent fetal circulation
		Congenital heart anomaly
		Fluid overload
		Congestive heart failure
Back, Hips, and Buttocks		
Back straight, spine intact, posture slightly flexed	Pilonidal dimple	Possible CNS anomaly
	Pilonidal sinus	Possible CNS anomaly
		Possible infection
	Hairy nevus at base of spine	Possible CNS anomaly

(*continued*)

Table 30-4. Physical Findings in the Assessment of the Neonate* (*continued*)

Normal Findings and Common Variations	Unusual Findings and Significant Deviations	Possible Causes and Potential Problems
	Meningomyelocele	CNS anomaly
	Hip clicks	Congenital hip dysplasia
Symmetrical buttock folds	Asymmetrical buttock folds	Congenital hip dysplasia
Mongolian spots on buttocks		
Transient ecchymosis of buttocks after breech delivery		
Anus patent	Absence of stools after 24 h	Imperforate anus, GI obstruction
	Anal fissures	Potential infection
Abdomen		
Abdomen full, rounded, and soft	Scaphoid abdomen	Diaphragmatic hernia
	Flat abdomen with horizontal wrinkles	Intrauterine growth retardation Chronic malnutrition
Bowel sounds	Hyperactive bowel sounds	Drug withdrawal Bowel obstructions
	Visible peristaltic waves	Pyloric stenosis
	Hypoactive bowel sounds	Sepsis
	Abdominal distention at birth	Abdominal masses GI obstruction Malrotation of bowel Hydronephrosis
	Development of abdominal distention after birth; no passage of stools	GI obstruction Meconium plug Meconium ileus Hirschsprung's disease Imperforate anus
	Presence of fecal smears in diaper without passage of stool through anus	Rectovaginal fistula
Liver palpable 1–2 cm below right costal margin	Hepatosplenomegaly	Intrauterine infection
Linea nigra		
Umbilical cord		
Umbilical cord white with Wharton's jelly	Thin, meconium-stained cord	Fetal distress Intrauterine growth retardation
	Urine drainage around umbilical cord	Patent urachus
	Oozing of blood at base of cord	Premature detachment of cord stump Trauma to base of cord
	Purulent discharge at base of cord, foul odor, red streaking from base of cord across abdomen	Omphalitis
Two arteries, one vein	One artery, one vein	Congenital heart anomaly
	Intestine palpated in abdominal area at base of umbilical cord	Umbilical hernia
	Protrusion of abdominal contents on surface of abdomen at umbilicus	GI anomaly (omphalocele)
	Protrusion of abdominal contents on surface of abdomen, but not involving umbilicus	GI anomaly (gastroschisis)
	Bladder distention	Meatal stenosis
Presence of helix or twist; majority twist to left	Absence of helix or twist	Multiple gestation Single umbilical artery
Genitals		
Female		
Labia majora large (may be slightly edematous), covering clitoris and labia minora	Ambiguous genitalia	Genetic disorder
Transient mucoid vaginal discharge		
Pseudomenstruation		
Hymen tag visible		

(*continued*)

Table 30-4. Physical Findings in the Assessment of the Neonate* *(continued)*

Normal Findings and Common Variations	Unusual Findings and Significant Deviations	Possible Causes and Potential Problems
First void within 24–48 h	Absence of full stream	Meatal stenosis
	Absence of urination	Meatal stenosis
		Renal disorder
Uric acid crystals present		
Male		
Penis with foreskin intact (if no circumcision)	Ambiguous genitalia	Genetic disorder
Foreskin covers glans	Inability to retract foreskin to any degree	True phimosis
Meatus in center of glans at tip of penis	Meatus located on dorsal surface of penis	GU anomaly (epispadias)
		GU anomaly (hypospadias)
	Meatus located on ventral surface of penis	
Full urine stream	Spurts or dribbling of urine	Meatal stenosis
Glans clean, erythematous, with nonpurulent serous membrane postcircumcision	Purulent discharge and foul odor	Infection
Uric acid crystals present in urine		
Scrotum large, pendulous, many rugae	Small, shiny scrotum with few or absent rugae	Prematurity
Testes descended	Testes undescended	Cryptorchidism
Transient edema of scrotal sac after birth		Prematurity
		Genetic disorder
	Fluid in testes	Hydrocele
	Presence of intestine in inguinal canal	Inguinal hernia
Extremities		
Arms		
Posture of flexion at rest	Extension of arm from shoulder or elbow	Brachial plexus injury
Symmetrical movement	Asymmetrical movement of arms or guarding of extremity	CNS injury
		Fracture of long bone
		Brachial plexus injury
	Repetitive rowing motions	Seizure disorder
Strong muscle tonus and good recoil with extension of arm	Weak or absent tonus	Prematurity
		CNS injury
		Neuromuscular disorders
		Genetic disorder
Palpable brachial and radial pulses	Bounding pulses	Fluid overload
	Absence of radial pulse	Congenital absence
		Spasm or obstruction
Hands and Fingers		
Fingers flexed at rest	Hand relaxed	CNS injury
Strong grasp reflex	Absence of grasp reflex	Neuromuscular disorder
		Brachial nerve injury
Symmetrical hand movement	Asymmetrical hand movement	Fracture, soft tissue injury, CNS injury
Multiple palmar creases	Simian crease	Down syndrome (in conjunction with other findings)
Five fingers, flexed but straight and separate	Polydactyly	Familial trait
	Syndactyly	Familial trait
		Genetic disorder
	Incurving of little finger	Down syndrome
Nails firm, pliant, well formed	Thin, incompletely formed nails	Prematurity
	Meconium-stained nails	Fetal distress
Moro reflex symmetrical	Asymmetrical Moro	CNS injury
		Brachial nerve injury
		Fracture of long bone or clavicle
Legs		
Legs well flexed at rest	Amelia or phocomelia	Genetic disorder
		Teratogenic injury
Slightly bowed appearance	Shortened long bones	Genetic disorder (dwarfism or achondroplasia)
Muscle tonus strong with good recoil when legs are extended	Weak or absent muscle tone	Prematurity
		Neuromuscular disorder
		CNS injury

(continued)

Table 30-4. Physical Findings in the Assessment of the Neonate* ***(continued)***

Normal Findings and Common Variations	Unusual Findings and Significant Deviations	Possible Causes and Potential Problems
	Asymmetrical movement or guarding of extremity	Fracture of long bone Soft-tissue injury CNS injury
Femoral pulses palpable	Differential between pulses in upper and lower extremities	Coarctation of aorta
	Blanching of one extremity	Thrombosis, arterial spasm
Feet and Toes		
Feet have fat pad on sole	Rocker-bottom soles	Genetic disorder
Sole crease over at least anterior two thirds of foot	Absence of creases or few sole creases	Prematurity
Ankle mobile, with full range of motion	Abnormal positioning or rigid fixation of ankle or heel	Congenital clubfoot (talipes deformity)
	Deformity of arch of foot	Congenital clubfoot (talipes deformity)
Pedal pulses palpable	Differential in pulses between upper and lower extremities	Coarctation of aorta
Five toes	Polydactyly	Familial trait
	Syndactyly	Familial trait Genetic disorder
Toenails well formed	Thin, poorly developed nails	Prematurity
Presence of plantar grasp	Absence of grasp	CNS injury
Positive Babinski reflex	Negative Babinski reflex	Neuromuscular disorder

quiet when the fontanelles are palpated because they may bulge slightly with crying. It is normal to feel pulsations through the membrane, especially when the infant is lying down.

A hand is passed over the scalp to assess the location, degree, and extent of any swellings. A localized soft-tissue edema of the scalp, *caput succedaneum*, may be present. Caput, which results from sustained pressure of the presenting part against the cervix during labor, feels spongy and may cross suture lines. It is usually present at or soon after birth and resolves within 24 to 48 hours of birth.

Cephalhematoma is a collection of blood between the periosteal membrane and the cranial bone. It will produce a soft, fluctuant, localized swelling on the head that does not cross suture lines. It may take up to several months for all the blood in a cephalhematoma to be reabsorbed. If the cephalhematoma is large, a considerable number of red blood cells will be hemolyzed, contributing to the development of jaundice in the neonate. Table 30-5 outlines and illustrates the differences between caput succedaneum and cephalhematoma.

The scalp is inspected carefully for bruising, redness, or lacerations. If an internal fetal scalp electrode was attached to monitor the fetal heart rate (FHR) or if fetal scalp sampling was performed, small lacerations will be present on the neonate's head. The texture and amount of hair is noted. Whether the hair is curly or straight, it should have a silky texture without coarseness or brittleness.

Eyes

It may be difficult to inspect the eyes of the newborn immediately after birth because of edema of the eyelids. The sclera has a bluish tinge due to the relative thinness of the membrane. The iris is normally slate gray or blue. (The permanent color cannot be ascertained until the infant is approximately 3 months of age.) Small subconjunctival hemorrhages may appear in the sclera as a result of changes in ocular pressure during birth. An ophthalmoscope is used to examine the pupil, lens, cornea, and retina. Bringing the infant to a sitting position often causes the eyes to open and assists the nurse with assessment. The pupillary and blink reflexes are present at birth and should be symmetrical. The pupil and cornea are round. When light is directed at the pupil, it should appear clear of opacities or cloudiness (cataracts). A red-orange flash of light will be observed (red reflex) as the light reflects off the retina. Not all nurses possess the level of skill required to examine the neonate's eyes with an ophthalmoscope. In this case, a pediatric nurse practitioner, nurse midwife, or pediatrician will complete this aspect of the assessment. Sensory perception and neuromuscular coordination are limited, but recent research has revealed greater visual capabilities in newborns than was once recognized. They have binocular vision and can fixate for up to 10 seconds on near objects. Acuity, or clarity, of vision is best within a distance range of 9 to 12 inches. Neonates seem most interested in the human face but also show interest in geometric shapes (circles, squares, and dots) at least 2 to 3 inches tall, in patterns of medium complexity, and with sharp black and white contrast. They fixate longest on colors of medium intensity (medium pinks, yellows, and greens). Accommodation, the ability of the eyes to adjust for distance, is absent for the first month; however, conjugation, the ability of the eyes to move together, is present.

Muscular control of ocular movement is imprecise, and transient strabismus and nystagmus are common. Transitory strabismus is due to immature neuromuscular control. Pseudostrabismus or "cross-eyed" appearance is an illusion. This

Table 30-5. Comparison of Caput Succedaneum and Cephalhematoma

Caput Succedaneum	Cephalhematoma
Localized soft-tissue edema	Soft, fluctuant, localized swelling
Appears at birth	Appears several hours after birth
Does not increase in size	Increases in size for 2–3 days
Disappears several days after birth vague, poorly defined outline	Disappears approximately 6 wk after birth
Has crosses suture lines	Has well-defined outline
Caused by diffuse, edematous swelling involving the soft tissues of the scalp	Never crosses suture lines
Complications; rarely, anemia	Caused by subperiosteal hemorrhage
	Complications: jaundice, underlying skull fracture, intracranial bleeding, shock

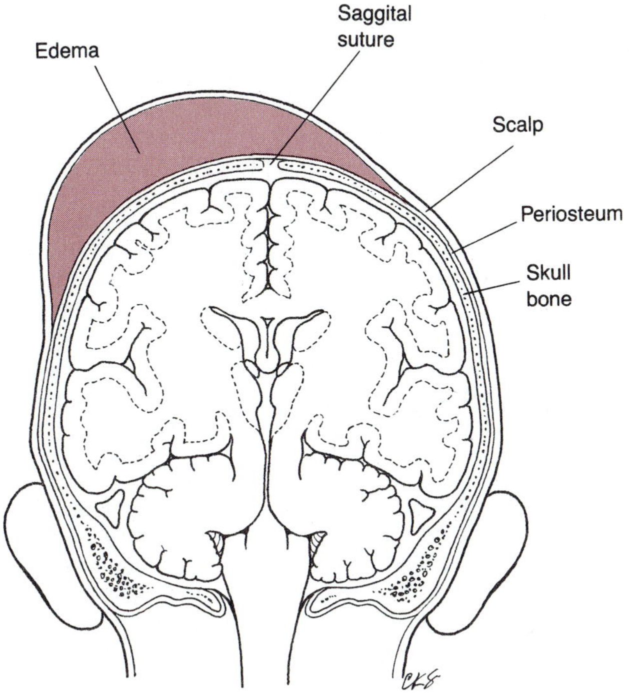

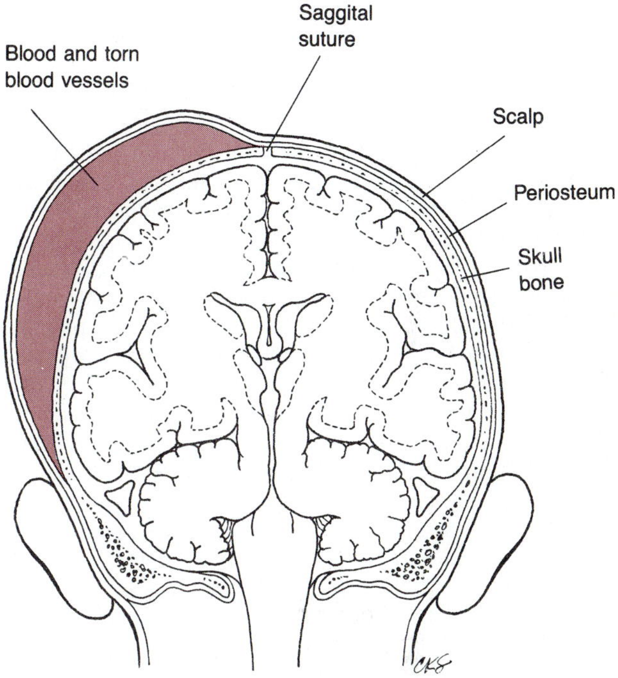

is created by the large epicanthal fold many infants have covering the inner canthus of the eye. This skinfold narrows the visible width of the sclera medial to the iris, creating the impression of strabismus. Doll's eye phenomenon may also be observed when the head is turned quickly from side to side and eye movement lags behind.

Nose and Mouth

The nasal passages in the neonate are narrow and have a delicate mucosal lining. The infant is an obligate nose breather. Any obstruction in the nose (such as mucus or edema) can lead to respiratory distress. The nurse checks for choanal atresia, a rare congenital blockage of the nasal passage. Patency of the nasal passage is evaluated by closing the infant's mouth and compressing one naris at a time. A wisp of cotton or a mirror can be placed at the open naris to check for movement of air. Routine passage of catheters to assess patency is not recommended because of risk of trauma to the mucosa with resultant bleeding and swelling. Sneezing occurs occasionally and is the neonate's means for clearing the nose of mucus, milk, or lint particles.

Although the neonate should have moist, pink mucous membranes, salivary glands are immature and saliva production is scant. Heavy drooling or constant bubbling of oral mucus is abnormal and may indicate a tracheoesophageal fistula. The lips are sensitive to touch, and stimulating them causes the infant to suck. Labial tubercles, or sucking calluses, may actually be present at birth as a result of strong sucking activity in utero.

Next, the gums, hard and soft palate, and tongue are assessed. Firm, rounded inclusion cysts may be found on the gums and are benign. Occasionally, precocious teeth are discovered at birth. If they are loose, they may be removed at this time to prevent accidental aspiration. If they are true primary teeth and not loose, they may be left in place. The tongue is short but mobile. The frenulum attached from the base of the tongue to the base of the mouth is also short, giving the newborn the appearance of being "tongue-tied." The frenulum should not be clipped and will lengthen with growth and development of the infant. The tongue and cheeks should be examined for evidence of thrush. Thrush is a yeast infection caused by *Candida albicans*, which can be acquired by the neonate during passage through an infected vagina. The infection is characterized by white, adherent, curdlike patches on the tongue and cheeks.

Using a good light source and a tongue blade, the nurse

should carefully examine the hard and soft palate. Cleft palate may extend the entire length of the hard palate or may involve only the soft palate or uvula. Small, firm, white inclusion cysts (Epstein pearls) may be found on the palate and are considered benign.

Ears and Neck

The full-term neonate's ears (pinna) are soft and pliable but recoil readily when bent toward the head. The nurse must inspect the ears for placement, size, shape, and firmness of ear cartilage. The top of the ear should be at or above the level of an imaginary line drawn from the inner and outer canthus of the eye to the ear. Low-set ears may be indicative of certain chromosomal abnormalities or organ anomalies (particularly renal anomalies, since the ears and kidneys develop concurrently in utero). Preauricular skin tags or dermal sinuses may be found immediately in front of the ear. They are often isolated findings and can be removed or repaired. Visualization of the tympanic membrane with an otoscope is not usually attempted immediately after birth. The ear canal is normally obliterated with vernix and blood, making accurate assessment difficult. The nurse may not possess the skills necessary to perform an examination with the otoscope. In this case the pediatric nurse practitioner, nurse midwife, or pediatrician will complete this part of the assessment.

Hearing is well developed once the eustachian tube is aerated and the outer ear is free of blood, vernix, and mucus. The infant will show a startle reflex to a sudden loud noise. In the alert awake state, the neonate will attend to auditory stimuli, such as the ringing of a bell or the parent's voice by diminishing activity, or reducing sucking (Letko, 1992). Studies of newborn auditory capacity suggest that neonates prefer high-pitched voices (high frequency range) to low-pitched voices.

Many nurseries are now screening infants to identify those at risk for hearing loss. The following risk factors are associated with hearing loss

- Defects in the ears, nose, or throat
- History of hearing loss before age 50 in a family member
- Suspected maternal rubella infection during pregnancy
- Birth weights of less than 1500 g (3 lb, 5 oz)
- Maternal exposure to industrial noise greater than 65 to 75 dB during pregnancy

The neck is short and has several thick folds of skin. The muscles that control and support head movement are not fully developed. The head lags when the neonate is pulled from a supine to a sitting position. When placed on the abdomen, the full-term infant can raise its head momentarily and turn it from side to side. The nurse must evaluate the neck for evidence of webbing, a connecting tissue or membrane extending from the base of the skull to the shoulder, and for range of motion. Webbing is associated with chromosomal abnormalities. Nuchal rigidity may suggest damage to the sternocleidomastoid muscle (congenital torticollis) or CNS disorder, including meningitis.

Because the clavicle is the bone most frequently fractured during delivery, the nurse must carefully palpate both clavicles for evidence of a lump or crepitus (a snapping or crackling feeling). The nurse should also elicit the Moro (startle) reflex at this point. If a clavicle is fractured, the Moro reflex is absent or diminished on the affected side. The assessment of reflexes is discussed in detail later in this chapter.

Chest

The nurse now places the neonate in a supine position on a flat surface and inspects the chest. The infant's chest is round, slightly smaller than the head, and symmetrical. The sternum is midline and the xiphoid cartilage is visible under the skin as a nodule. The nipples and areola are pigmented in the full-term infant. Buds of breast tissue approximately 10 mm in size can be palpated below the nipple (see Fig. 30-19). Breast engorgement may be evident 2 to 3 days after birth due to the effects of withdrawal of maternal estrogen, and a cloudy fluid discharge (witch's milk) may be secreted from the nipple. Accessory nipples (supernumerary nipples) may be noted below and medial to the nipples. Accessory nipples are fairly common and are benign.

Shallow symmetrical chest expansion is noted with respirations (30 to 60/min). This should be synchronous with abdominal movement. The sternum and intercostal muscles should not retract (collapse in toward the spine) with inspiration.

The intensity of heart action is estimated by placing a hand on the precordium and feeling the heart impulse through the chest wall. Slight chest movement over the point of maximum impulse may be observed and is normal.

Breath Sounds. Auscultation of the breath sounds requires practice. This assessment may have limited usefulness in neonates because sound emanating from one lung may be transmitted to the other. Bowel sounds and upper airway noises (created by the movement of air over the soft tissues of the upper airway and mouth) are heard over the chest wall and may make auscultation difficult. However, with experience, the nurse will be able to distinguish normal variations in breaths sounds caused by crying, vibration of soft palate tissue, and bowel sounds from abnormal breath sounds.

The nurse auscultates the breath sounds over the anterior and posterior chest. Rales, identified as crackling noises predominantly on inspiration, may be heard in the transition period immediately after birth, indicating retained fetal lung fluid and areas of atelectasis. Rales should be absent within several hours of birth as lung fluid is absorbed through the lymphatics. Clearing of fluid can be facilitated by chest percussion and suctioning in the full-term neonate. However, chest physical therapy must be performed carefully and cautiously in preterm neonates. There is an increased association of this procedure with systemic blood pressure changes and intraventricular hemorrhage in preterm infants. Rhonchi, identified as coarse rattling noises, are less frequently heard. Rhonchi indicate fluid, mucus, or meconium in the larger bronchi and may be associated with more life-threatening conditions, such as meconium aspiration syndrome. (Meconium aspiration syndrome is discussed in Chapter 33).

Heart Sounds. Heart sounds should be auscultated when the infant is quiet. Auscultation begins at the point of maximum impulse (normally the apex). The stethoscope is then moved slowly over the entire precordium, below the left axilla, and posteriorly over the left scapula. If a murmur is auscultated, the nurse determines whether it occurs after the first heart sound (caused by closure of the mitral and tricuspid valves) or the second heart sound (caused by the closure of the pulmonic and aortic valves). In neonates, 90% of all murmurs are transient and are related to incomplete closure of the foramen ovale or ductus arteriosus.

The nurse listens for the presence of the splitting of heart sounds, thrills, and gallops. Any irregularity in heart rhythm is noted, as well as any shift in the point of maximum impulse. This might indicate pneumothorax or diaphragmatic hernia (displacement of intestinal contents into the thoracic cavity through a defect in the diaphragm). However, many full-term health neonates experience some dysrhythmia during the first 6 to 12 hours of life, including sinus tachycardia and premature ectopic beats of supraventricular and ventricular origin. They are generally asymptomatic and require no treatment but should be monitored carefully.

Abdomen

The inspection of the abdomen is begun with the infant in a supine position and quiet. The shape is rounded and protuberant because of the weakness of the abdominal musculature. The skin should be smooth with few visible veins. It should not appear stretched or shiny. A shrunken or scaphoid abdomen may indicate diaphragmatic hernia. A flat abdomen covered by loose, wrinkled skin is suggestive of chronic intrauterine malnutrition.

The umbilical cord normally appears white and gelatinous in the first few hours of life. It is clamped about an inch from the surface of the skin, and the three vessels (one vein and two arteries) may be visible at the cut edge. The umbilical cord begins to dry after a few hours, shrinks in size, and turns brownish black. If kept clean and dry, it begins to separate from the skin, and usually falls off between the sixth and tenth day of life. Oozing of blood or purulent discharge from the cord is abnormal and may indicate loosening of the cord clamp, trauma to the cord, or omphalitis. In a small percentage of infants (especially black infants), an umbilical hernia may be noted. This is due to incomplete closure of the abdominal muscles and requires no special care at birth. Most umbilical hernias close without surgical intervention within the first 2 years of life.

Unless immediately indicated, auscultation and palpation of the abdomen can be deferred until the period of inactivity. This is approximately 30 minutes after birth, when the infant is relaxed and less responsive to external stimuli and bowel sounds are audible. Auscultation should be done first because palpation may cause a transient decrease in the intensity of bowel sounds.

The abdomen feels soft, without distention or tenderness. The edge of the liver may be palpated 1 to 2 cm below the right costal margin. The spleen may be palpated 1 to 2 cm below the left costal margin. The kidneys, most easily identified before the intestines fill with air and digested milk, feel like firm oval masses about the size of walnuts. They are located by deep palpation 1 to 2 cm above and slightly lateral to the umbilicus. The bladder is also an abdominal organ in the newborn because of the smallness of the pelvis. It may be palpated when filled with urine.

Genitalia

Female Genitalia. The external genitalia of the female infant reflect gestational age. In the full-term neonate the labia majora are large, may be swollen as a result of the influence of maternal hormones, and completely cover the labia minora. By contrast, the preterm female infant has little adipose tissue in the labia majora. The labia minora are visible but are small and incompletely developed. The clitoris is prominent and the urinary meatus is located just below it (see Fig. 30-22). The vaginal opening should be identified. Many female neonates have a mucoid vaginal discharge, which may be blood-tinged (pseudomenstruation) as a result of withdrawal of estrogen at birth. A hymenal tag may protrude from the vaginal opening. Vernix and smegma may be found in the creases of the labia and are gently washed away with bathing. The urine stream should be observed to eliminate the possibility of meatal stenosis. In the female neonate, a full stream should be observed although it does not project more than 1/4 to 1/2 inch beyond the labia majora.

Male Genitalia. The male genitalia also reflect the degree of maturity at birth. The penis is relatively small and the foreskin covers the glans. The prepuce (foreskin) may not retract easily from the glans, but true phimosis, the inability to retract the foreskin at all, is rare. The foreskin may be removed surgically by circumcision. In circumcised infants, the glans will be exposed, slightly edematous, and erythematous for the first few days after the procedure. A yellow exudate may be formed over the glans after circumcision, but bleeding or the presence of purulent discharge is abnormal.

The nurse locates the meatal opening, which is normally on the tip of the glans. Hypospadias is a congenital anomaly in which the urethral meatus is located on the ventral surface of the penis. Epispadias occurs when the meatal opening is on the dorsal surface. Both may be repaired surgically. The urine stream should be observed to eliminate the possibility of meatal stenosis. The bladder empties when approximately 15 mL urine is collected. In the male neonate, the stream is forceful and can project 6 to 8 inches upward in an arc.

In the full-term male infant, the scrotum is large and pendulous and the skin is rugous. The nurse palpates the scrotum gently. The testes are normally descended (in 90% of males) and palpable in the scrotal sac (see Fig. 30-21). Cryptorchidism, failure of the testes to descend into the scrotal sac of the full-term neonate, is rare but requires medical attention to identify the cause and, if possible, correct the condition. Edema and hydrocele, a collection of fluid in the testis, are common and usually benign findings that resolve spontaneously. By contrast, the scrotal sac of the preterm infant is small, smooth, and shiny and the skin is smooth. The testes, which do not normally descend until the 36th week, may not be palpable.

Back and Buttocks

The neonate is placed in a prone position so that the back and buttocks can be examined. The back appears rounded because of the normal flexed posture, but the spine is straight and does not develop the lumbar and sacral curves until the infant begins to sit upright and walk. The finger is passed slowly along the spine to ascertain its shape. The spine is both inspected and palpated for masses and openings. The sacrum and base of the spine are examined for tufts of hair or small indentations, which may indicate spina bifida occulta (incomplete closure of the vertebral column). If a pilonidal dimple is present (a fold of skin located in the midline of the sacrococcygeal area), it should be inspected for evidence of a sinus tract.

The buttocks should be separated and the anal opening inspected for patency. No membrane should be evident over the opening. This would indicate an imperforate anus. Anal fissures may be present. They are often identified by the presence of slight, bright red bleeding from the rectum. Small fissures often heal quickly if the anal area is carefully cleansed after each bowel movement and periodically exposed to air. The anal area should also be examined for fistulas, which appear as small openings or dimples in the skin.

Hips

While the neonate remains in a prone position the hips are examined. The skinfolds of the buttocks are assessed for symmetry, which is a normal finding. Uneven folds may indicate congenital hip dysplasia, which is a congenital deformity of the pelvis that is often accompanied by hip dislocation. The neonate is then placed in a supine position and the Ortolani maneuver is performed, as illustrated in Figure 30-15.

In this maneuver the infant's knees are flexed. The thighs are held with the examiner's thumbs on the inner aspect of the thighs and the fingers along the outer thighs from the knees to the greater trochanters. The thighs are adducted, internally rotated, and then abducted at least 175 degrees so that the thighs lie almost flat against the mattress. If a jerk is felt or a clunking sound heard, it is a result of the head of the femur moving into the acetabulum and is a significant indication of hip dysplasia. A "click" unassociated with a sense of movement may be felt in approximately 25% of neonates and is a result of minor joint incongruities. Finally, the hips and knees are flexed and the infant's feet are placed flat on the mattress. If hip dislocation is present, the knee on the affected side will be higher (Allis sign).

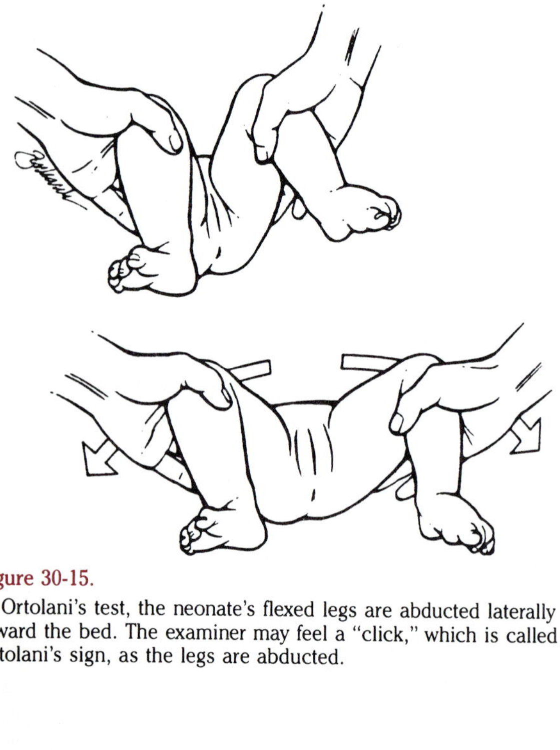

Figure 30-15.
In Ortolani's test, the neonate's flexed legs are abducted laterally toward the bed. The examiner may feel a "click," which is called Ortolani's sign, as the legs are abducted.

Upper Extremities

The arms are normally well flexed and should move symmetrically in the full-term neonate. When the arms and hands are fully extended, the fingertips should reach to approximately the midthigh. The hands are plump and the fingers are tightly flexed. The fingernails are soft and extend beyond the tips of the fingers and should not be stained. Three palmar creases normally extend across the palm at a slight angle.

The symmetry and strength of muscle resistance to extension of the arms are assessed, as is the range of motion of the joints. The arm is palpated for lumps, evidence of trauma, or limitation in movement because the humerus is the second most frequently fractured bone during delivery. The brachial and radial pulses are palpated and their strength is assessed. Partial or complete flaccidity of the arm may indicate trauma to the brachial plexus, which also occurs during delivery. Erb-Duchenne paralysis, a result of injury to the fifth and sixth cranial nerves, is characterized by partial paralysis of the arm. In this condition, the elbow is extended and the forearm pronated. The Moro reflex cannot be elicited on the affected side. Complete paralysis of the arm results from injury to the entire plexus and is rare. Return of function in either type of paralysis depends on the severity of injury.

The grasp reflex is elicited by placing a finger in each palm and then slowly raising the infant toward a sitting position. The normal newborn can hold onto the examiner's finger long enough to achieve a momentary upright position. The palms should be inspected for evidence of a single simian crease, which runs straight across the hand, and an incurving of the small finger. These signs are frequently present in infants with Down syndrome. Polydactyly, extra digits, may occur as a benign inherited phenomenon or may be associated with genetic disorders. Syndactyly (webbing) is the presence of a membrane between fingers and is rare.

Lower Extremities

The legs are short, appear bowed, and are usually well flexed. In a prone position the knees are flexed and the thighs are tucked up against the abdomen. The feet also appear plump and in the full-term infant at least two thirds of the anterior sole is creased. An inward turning of the foot (varus deviation) may be evident and is frequently the result of a position maintained in utero. If the foot can be brought to the midline without force, no orthopedic correction is necessary. Talipes deformity (clubfoot) requires surgical correction.

After the lower extremities are inspected, muscle tone and symmetry of movement are assessed. Strength of resistance to extension of the legs and range of motion of the joints are evaluated. The toes are examined for polydactyly and syndactyly. Unusual spacing of the big toe from the others may indicate a chromosomal abnormality. Finally, pulses (femoral and pedal) are palpated and their strength is assessed.

Assessment of Neuromuscular Integrity

A general evaluation of neurologic status is conducted at the outset when posture, head size, and the fontanelles are being assessed. A more thorough systematic assessment of neuromuscular integrity should be performed before the examination of the newborn is completed. A readily apparent sign of neuromuscular status in the neonate is the sound of the cry. The full-term newborn has a loud, lusty cry. A shrill, high-pitched cry is indicative of CNS injury or abnormality.

Neonatal Reflexes

Although several reflexes may already have been elicited during the assessment, a complete evaluation of reflexes should be done at this time. Blink, cough, sneeze, and gag reflexes are present at birth and remain unchanged into adulthood. Some reflexes reflect the neurologic immaturity of the neonate and disappear in the first year of life. Table 30-6 lists these neonatal reflexes and how to elicit them, and Figure 30-16 illustrates common neonatal reflexes.

Assessment of Gestational Age

A major determinant of a neonate's ability to survive is the degree of maturity at birth. Historically, the estimation of gestational age was based on the mother's estimated due date (EDD) calculated from her last menstrual period (LMP). In the past, the infant's birth weight was used to classify the newborn as premature, mature, or postmature. These methods were unreliable. Many women are unable to provide precise dates for their LMP, and the infant's birth weight can be significantly above or below the norm for a particular gestational age as a result of maternal nutritional status, disease processes, exposure to environmental hazards, and inherited disorders in the fetus. The following are terms used in gestational age assessment.

- *Premature infant*: an infant born before 37 weeks of gestation
- *Mature (full-term)*: an infant born between 38 and 42 weeks of gestation
- *Postmature infant*: an infant born after 42 weeks of gestation
- *Small-for-gestational-age (SGA)*: a newborn whose weight is below the 10th percentile for estimated week of gestation or two standard deviations below the mean
- *Appropriate-for-gestational-age (AGA) infant*: a newborn whose weight falls between the 10th and 90th percentile for estimated gestational age or within two standard deviations from the mean
- *Large-for-gestational-age (LGA) infant*: a newborn whose weight is above the 90th percentile for estimated gestational age or two standard deviations above the mean

Objective tools for assessing gestational age have been developed to address the need for accurate assessment of gestational age. The Dubowitz scale allows a detailed, systematic assessment of physical signs and neurologic traits. It can be used by skilled examiners to accurately estimate gestational age in infants between 28 and 42 weeks of gestation. It takes 15 to 20 minutes to complete.

The Ballard Scale

When a prompt assessment of gestational age is needed on a neonate requiring immediate care, a modified, simplified version of the Dubowitz scale, the Ballard scale, is used (Ballard, Novack, & Driver, 1979). The Ballard scale is more commonly used by nurses to estimate the gestational age of the neonate. The neonate is given a score ranging from 0 to 4 on each of 13 traits. The score is totaled, and a maturity rating in weeks of gestation is determined using the scoring guide, as shown in the accompanying Assessment Tool. The following sections discuss the assessment.

Physical Characteristics

Skin. The skin is inspected for thickness, integrity, color, and the presence of visible veins. The skin of the preterm infant is thin, red or pink, and smooth, with veins quite visible. The full-term newborn has a thicker skin that is opaque and has few visible veins. Superficial peeling may be evident. After 42 weeks of gestation, the skin becomes thick and leathery with deep cracking and significant peeling (Fig. 30-17). Veins are not visible.

Lanugo. The presence and amount of lanugo is assessed (see Fig. 30-20). The very premature infant (under 28 weeks) has a fine, barely visible covering of lanugo. Lanugo becomes thickest between 28 and 30 weeks of gestation and slowly disappears so that the full-term infant has only small amounts along the shoulders and scapular area.

Plantar Creases. The creases on the soles are examined. Sole creasing develops first at the anterior portion of the foot and proceeds to the heel. The full-term infant has plantar creases over the entire sole (Fig. 30-18). The sole creases must be assessed in the first 12 hours of life because superficial cracking and peeling occur as the skin begins to dry after birth.

Breast Tissue. The amount of breast tissue (not adipose tissue) is evaluated. The presence of a nipple and development of the areola are checked. The breast tissue under the nipple is placed between the forefinger and the middle finger to assess the size of the breast bud. The premature infant has no perceptible breast bud. A small bud (1 to 2 mm) is felt at approximately 36 weeks of gestation, and this increases to approximately 5 mm in size by 40 weeks of gestation. It continues to increase in size with increasing gestational age. The nipple and areola are not

Table 30-6. Assessment of Neonatal Reflexes

Reflex	Category	How Elicited	Normal Response	Abnormal Response	Duration of Reflex
Rooting and sucking (Fig. 340-16*A*)	Feeding	Touch cheek, lip or corner of mouth with finger or nipple.	Infant turns head in direction of stimulus, opens mouth, and begins to suck.	Weak or absent response seen with prematurity, neurologic deficit or injury, or CNS depression secondary to maternal drug ingestion (*eg*, narcotics)	Diminished by 5th to 6th mo; disappears by 1 y
Swallowing	Feeding	Place fluid on back of tongue.	Infant swallows in coordination with sucking.	Gagging, coughing, or regurgitation of fluid; possibly associated with cyanosis secondary to prematurity, neurologic deficit, or injury Often seen after laryngoscopy	Does not disappear
Extrusion	Feeding	Touch tip of tongue with finger or nipple.	Infant pushes tongue outward.	Continuous extrusion of tongue or repetitive tongue thrusting seen with CNS anomalies and seizures	Disappears by about 4th mo
Moro (Fig. 30-16*B*)	Postural	Change infant's position suddenly or place on back on flat surface.	Bilateral symmetrical extension and abduction of all extremities, with thumb and forefinger forming characteristic "C," followed by adduction of extremities and return to relaxed flexion.	Asymmetrical response seen with peripheral nerve injury (brachial plexus) or fracture of clavicle or long bone of arm or leg No response with severe CNS injury	Diminished by 4th mo; disappears by 6th mo
Stepping	Postural	Hold infant in upright position and touch one foot to flat surface.	Newborn will step with one foot and then the other in walking motion.	Asymmetrical response seen with CNS or peripheral nerve injury or fracture of long bone of leg	Disappears within 1–2 mo
Prone crawl	Postural	Place infant on abdomen on flat surface.	Infant will attempt to crawl forward with both arms and legs.	Asymmetrical response seen with CNS or peripheral nerve injury or fracture of long bone	Disappears within 1–2 mo
Tonic neck or "fencing" (Fig. 30-16*C*)	Postural	Turn infant's head to one side when infant is resting.	Extremities on side to which head is turned will extend and opposite extremities will flex. Response may be absent or incomplete immediately after birth.	Persistent response after fourth month May indicate neurologic injury Persistent absence in CNS injury, neuromuscular disorders	Diminishes by 4th mo
Startle	Protective	Expose infant to sudden movement or loud noise.	Infant abducts and flexes all extremities and may begin to cry.	Absence of response may indicate neurologic deficit or injury. Complete, consistent absence	Diminishes by 4th mo

(*continued*)

Table 30-6. Assessment of Neonatal Reflexes ***(continued)***

Reflex	Category	How Elicited	Normal Response	Abnormal Response	Duration of Reflex
				of response to loud noises may indicate deafness. Response may be absent or diminished during deep sleep.	
Crossed extension	Protective	Place infant in supine position and extend one leg while stimulating bottom of foot.	Infant's opposite leg will flex and then extend rapidly as if trying to deflect stimulus to other foot.	Weak or absent response seen with peripheral nerve injury or fracture of long bone	Disappears by 4–6 mo
Glabellar "blink"	Protective	Tap bridge of infant's nose when eyes are open.	Infant will blink with first four or five taps.	Persistent blinking and failure to habituate Suggestive of neurologic deficit	
Palmar grasp (Fig. 30-16*D*)	Social	Place finger in palm of infant's hand.	Infant's finger will curl around object and hold momentarily.	Diminished response with prematurity Asymmetry with peripheral nerve damage (brachial plexus) or fracture of humerus No response with severe neurologic deficit	Diminishes by 4th mo
Plantar grasp (Fig. 30-16*E*)	Social	Place finger against base of toes.	Infant's toes will curl downward.	Diminished response with prematurity No response with severe neurologic deficit	Diminishes by 4th mo
Babinski (Fig. 30-16*F*)	Not categorized	Stroke one side of foot upward from heel and across ball of foot.	Infant's toes will hyperextend and fan apart from dorsiflexion of big toe.	No response with CNS deficit	Disappears by 1 y

visible in the very premature infant. The areola becomes raised at approximately 34 weeks of gestation and increases in size as the nipple bud increases (Fig. 30-19).

Ears. The degree of cartilage distribution and the resulting ear form are assessed. The external ear is relatively shapeless and flat before 34 weeks of gestation (Fig. 30-20). If the ear is bent forward against the side of the head, it will remain in that position. By 34 to 36 weeks some cartilage formation is present and slight incurving of the upper pinna is noted. By 40 weeks there is incurving over two thirds of the pinna, and if the ear is bent forward, it quickly recoils to its original position. The firmness of the ear increases after 40 weeks, and the ear stands erect and away from the head.

Male Genitalia. The male genitalia are assessed to determine the size of the scrotum and degree of rugation and whether the testes have descended (Fig. 30-21). In the premature infant the scrotum is small and has very few rugae, and the testes remain high in the inguinal canal. Rugation increases with gestational age. By 40 weeks of gestation, the scrotum is large, pendulous, and heavily rugous, and the testes have descended into the lower scrotum.

Female Genitalia. The female genitalia are examined to determine the amount of subcutaneous fat deposition in the labia majora and the prominence of the labia minora and clitoris (Fig. 30-22). Because the amount of adipose tissue also depends on the provision of adequate nutrients in utero, the size of the labia majora will be affected by factors other than gestational age. Before 36 weeks of gestation, the labia majora are small and widely separated and the labia minora and clitoris are prominent. After 36 weeks the labia majora begin to cover the internal structures, and by 40 weeks the labia minora and clitoris are completely covered.

Neuromuscular Characteristics

After the assessment and scoring of physical characteristics has been completed, the neurologic evaluation is conducted. The degree and strength of muscle tonus and flexion is assessed. The Ballard scale lists six neuromuscular traits.

Text continues on page 914

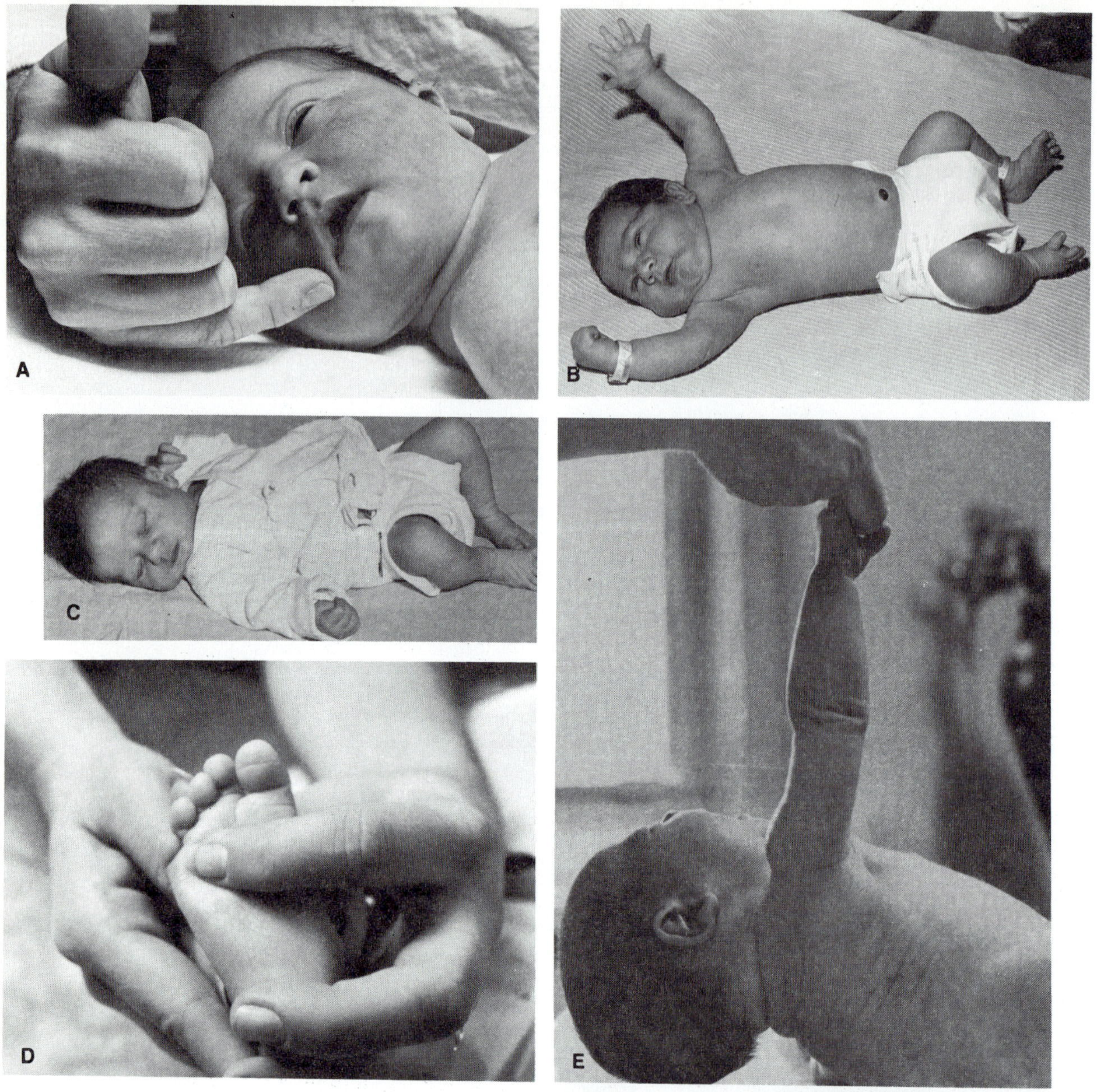

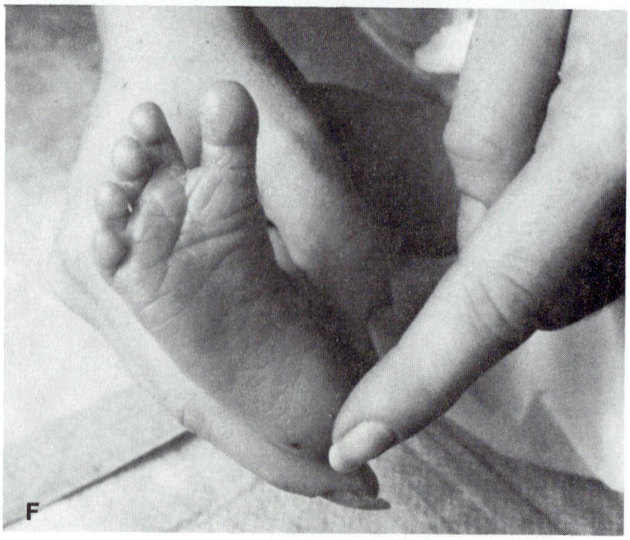

Figure 30-16.

Neonatal reflexes. *A:* Rooting reflex. (From Sullivan, R., Foster, J., & Schreiner, R. L. [1979]. Determining a newborn's gestational age. *American Journal of Maternal Child Nursing*, Jan/Feb, pp. 38–45.) *B:* Moro reflex. *C:* Tonic neck reflex. *D:* Plantar grasp reflex (Childbirth Graphics). *E:* Palmer grasp reflex (From Mead Johnson). *F:* Babinski reflex (Childbirth Graphics).

Assessment Tool

Estimation of Gestational Age by Maturity Rating

NEUROMUSCULAR MATURITY

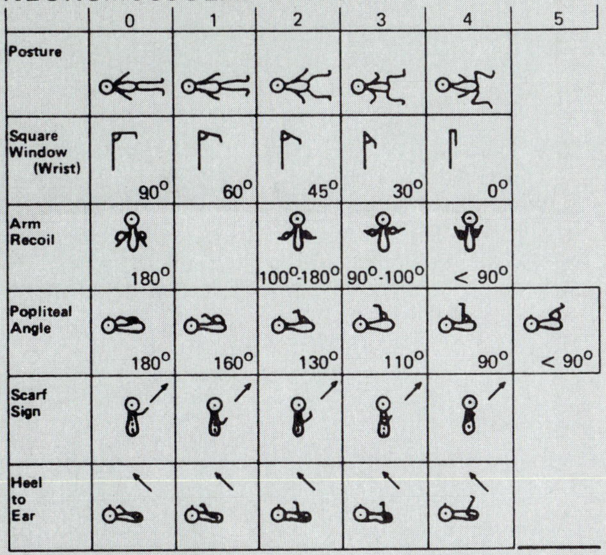

	0	1	2	3	4	5
Posture						
Square Window (Wrist)	90°	60°	45°	30°	0°	
Arm Recoil	180°		100°-180°	90°-100°	< 90°	
Popliteal Angle	180°	160°	130°	110°	90°	< 90°
Scarf Sign						
Heel to Ear						

PHYSICAL MATURITY

	0	1	2	3	4	5
SKIN	gelatinous red, trans-parent	smooth pink, visible veins	superficial peeling &/or rash, few veins	cracking pale area, rare veins	parchment, deep cracking, no vessels	leathery, cracked, wrinkled
LANUGO	none	abundant	thinning	bald areas	mostly bald	
PLANTAR CREASES	no crease	faint red marks	anterior transverse crease only	creases ant. 2/3	creases cover entire sole	
BREAST	barely percept.	flat areola, no bud	stippled areola, 1–2 mm bud	raised areola, 3–4 mm bud	full areola, 5–10 mm bud	
EAR	pinna flat, stays folded	sl. curved pinna, soft with slow recoil	well-curv. pinna, soft but ready recoil	formed & firm with instant recoil	thick cartilage, ear stiff	
GENITALS Male	scrotum empty, no rugae		testes descend-ing, few rugae	testes down, good rugae	testes pendulous, deep rugae	
GENITALS Female	prominent clitoris & labia minora		majora & minora equally prominent	majora large, minora small	clitoris & minora completely covered	

Gestation by Dates ________________ wks

Birth Date __________ Hour __________ am / pm

APGAR __________ 1 min __________ 5 min

MATURITY RATING

Score	Wks
5	26
10	28
15	30
20	32
25	34
30	36
35	38
40	40
45	42
50	44

SCORING SECTION

	1st Exam=X	2nd Exam=O
Estimating Gest Age by Maturity Rating	______ Weeks	______ Weeks
Time of Exam	Date ______ am Hour ______ pm	Date ______ am Hour ______ pm
Age at Exam	______ Hours	______ Hours
Signature of Examiner	______ M.D.	______ M.D.

Scoring system from Ballard, J. L., et al. (1977). A simplified assessment of gestational age. Pediatric Research, 11, 374. Figures adapted from Sweet, A. Y. (1977). Classification of the low-birth-weight infant. In M. H. Klaus & A. A. Fanaroff (Eds.), Care of the high-risk infant. Philadelphia: WB Saunders.

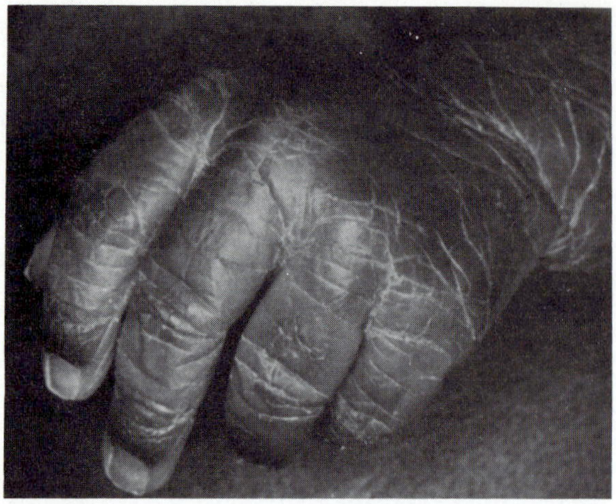

Figure 30-17.

Postterm newborn's hand. Note dry, peeling, cracked skin. (From Sullivan, R., Foster, J., Schreiner, R. L. [1979]. Determining a newborn's gestational age. *American Journal of Maternal Child Nursing* Jan/Feb, pp. 38–45.)

Posture. The resting posture of the neonate is assessed (Fig. 30-23). In the very premature infant (under 30 weeks of gestation), the extremities are in full extension. By approximately 34 to 36 weeks, partial flexion of both upper and lower extremities is evident. The full-term neonate assumes a posture of complete flexion of all extremities.

Wrist Flexion ("Square Window"). The extent of wrist flexion is evaluated (Fig. 30-24). The nurse flexes the infant's wrist down toward the ventral forearm. The angle between the hypothenar eminence and the forearm is measured. A 90-degree angle is observed in infants below 32 weeks of gestation. A 30-degree angle is noted in infants between 38 and 40 weeks. The palm and forearm can be

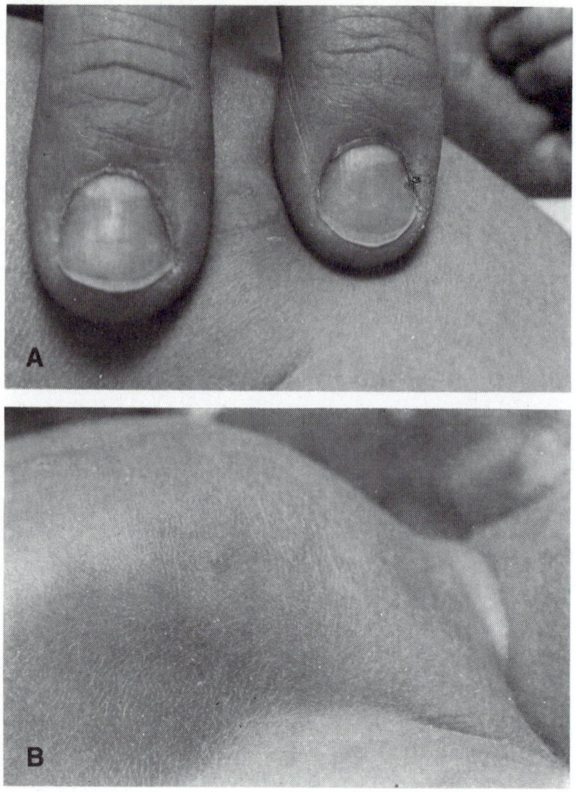

Figure 30-19.

Note the relatively distinct areola and underlying breast bud of the term neonate (*A*) when compared to the preterm neonate (*B*). (From Sullivan, R., Foster, J., & Schreiner, R. L. [1979]. Determining a newborn's gestational age. *American Journal of Maternal Child Nursing*, Jan/Feb, pp. 38–45.)

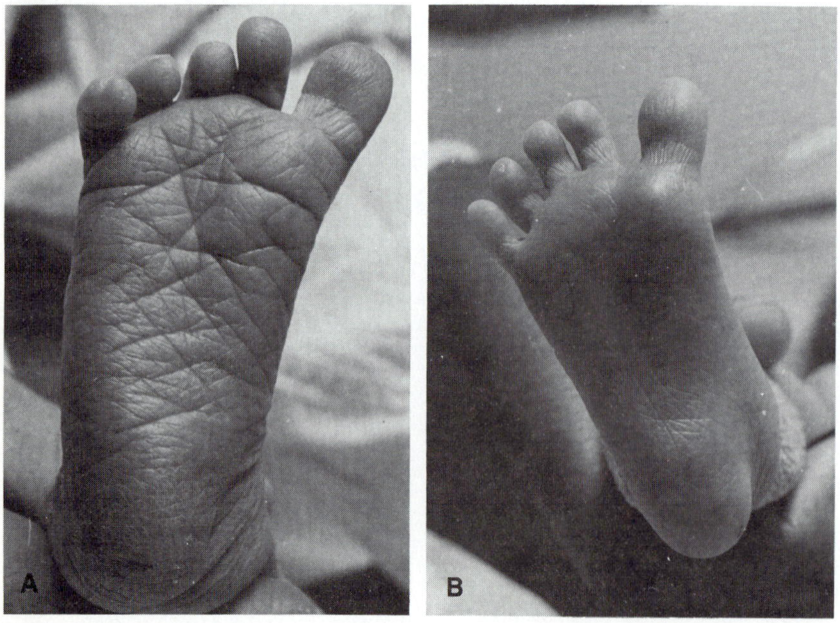

Figure 30-18.

A comparison of the sole creases on the foot of a term neonate (*A*) with those of a preterm neonate (*B*). At 40 weeks of gestation, the entire foot, including the heel, is crisscrossed with creases. (From Sullivan, R., Foster, J., & Schreiner, R. L. [1979]. Determining a newborn's gestational age. *American Journal of Maternal Child Nursing*, Jan/Feb, pp. 38–45.)

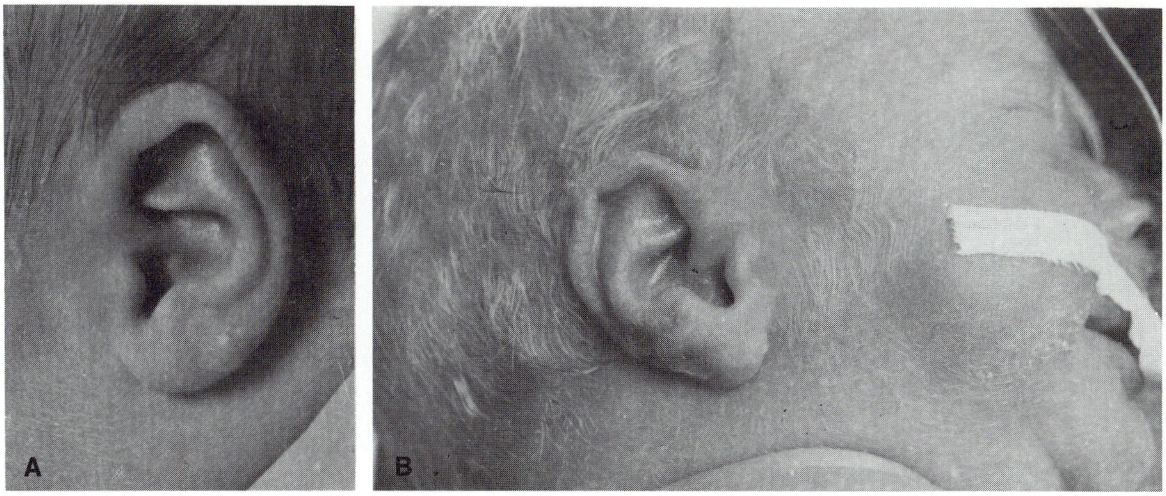

Figure 30-20.

Cartilage is well developed in the term neonate (*A*) and the ear is erect, away from the head, whereas the ears of the preterm neonate (*B*) lie flat against the head. Also note the matted hair and the presence of lanugo on the face of the preterm neonate. (From Sullivan, R., Foster, J., & Schreiner, R. L. [1979]. Determining a newborn's gestational age. *American Journal of Maternal Child Nursing*, Jan/Feb, pp. 38–45.)

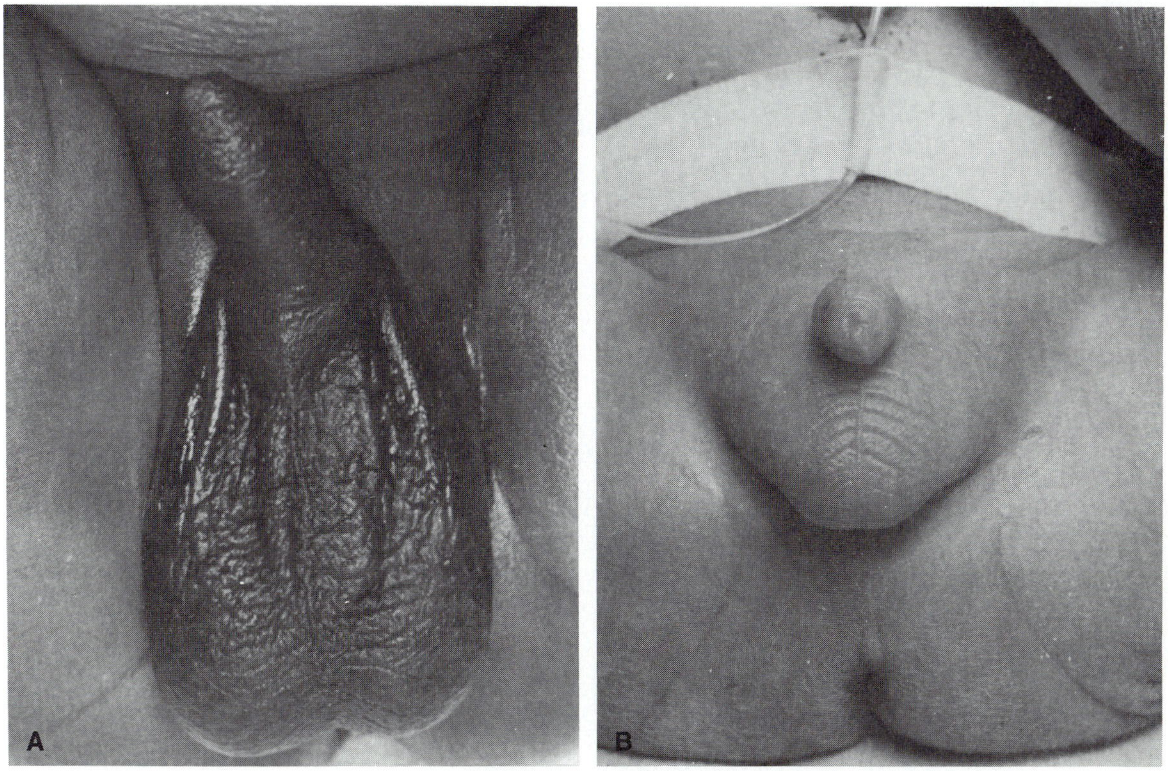

Figure 30-21.

In the term neonate (*A*) the testes are well descended into the scrotal sac and the scrotum is covered with numerous rugae. In the preterm neonate (*B*) the testes remain high in the inguinal canal and the rugae are largely underdeveloped. (From Sullivan, R., Foster, J., & Schreiner, R. L. [1979]. Determining a newborn's gestational age. *American Journal of Maternal Child Nursing*, Jan/Feb, pp. 38–45.)

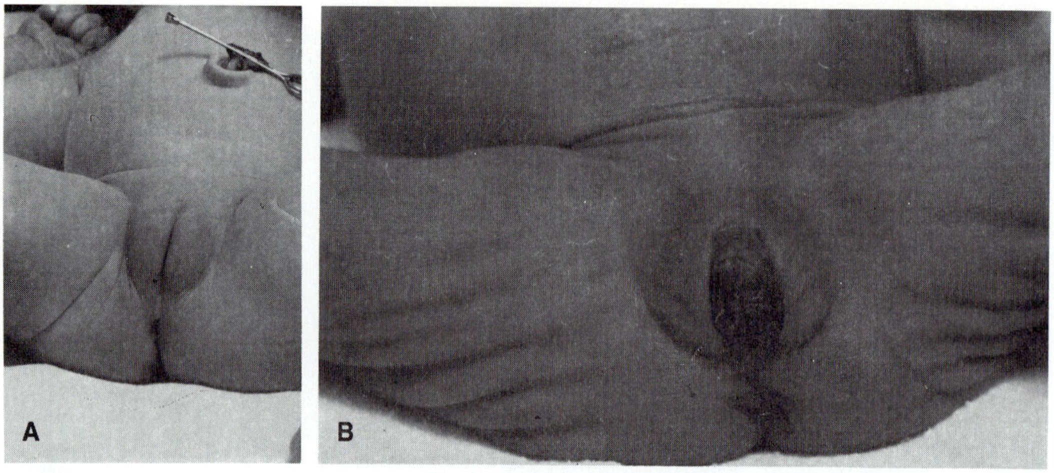

Figure 30-22.

The labia majora of the term neonate (*A*) completely cover the labia minora and clitoris while they are small and widely separated in the preterm neonate (*B*). Also note the loose skin folds on the posterior thighs of the preterm neonate. (From Sullivan, R., Foster, J., & Schreiner, R. L. [1979]. Determining a newborn's gestational age. *American Journal of Maternal Child Nursing*, Jan/Feb, pp. 38–45.)

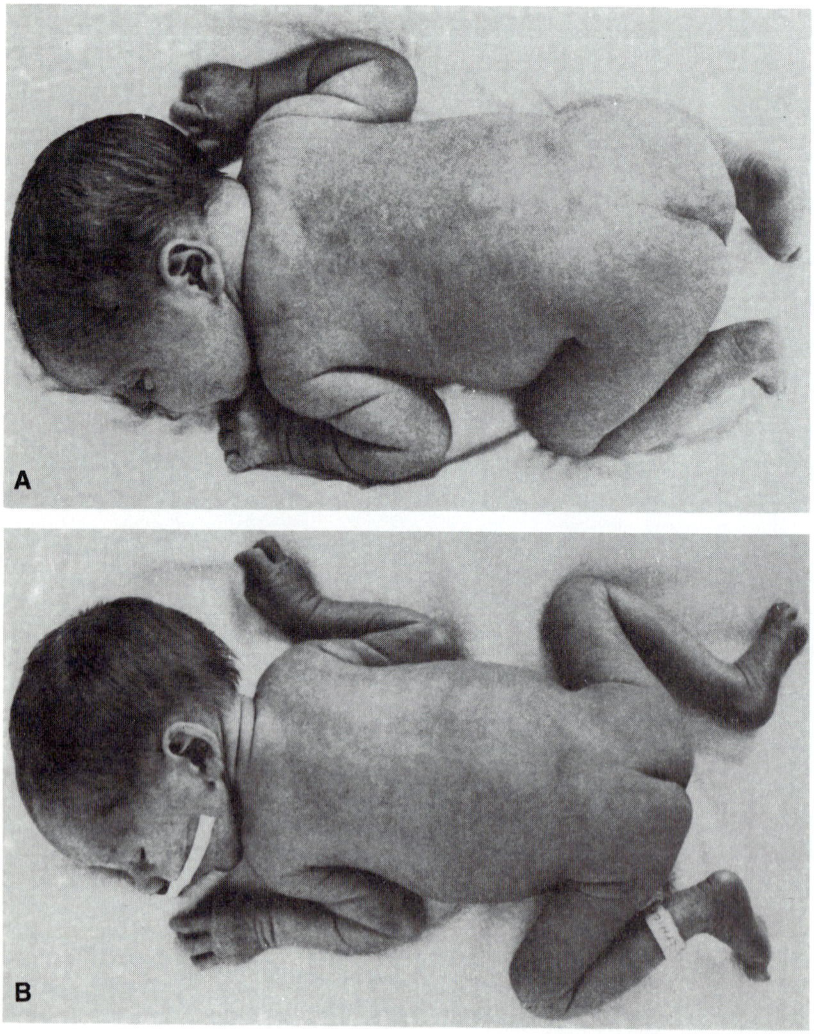

Figure 30-23.

Resting posture. Note the flexion of the extremities in the term neonate (*A*) compared to the partial flexion in the preterm neonate (*B*), resulting in a froglike resting posture.

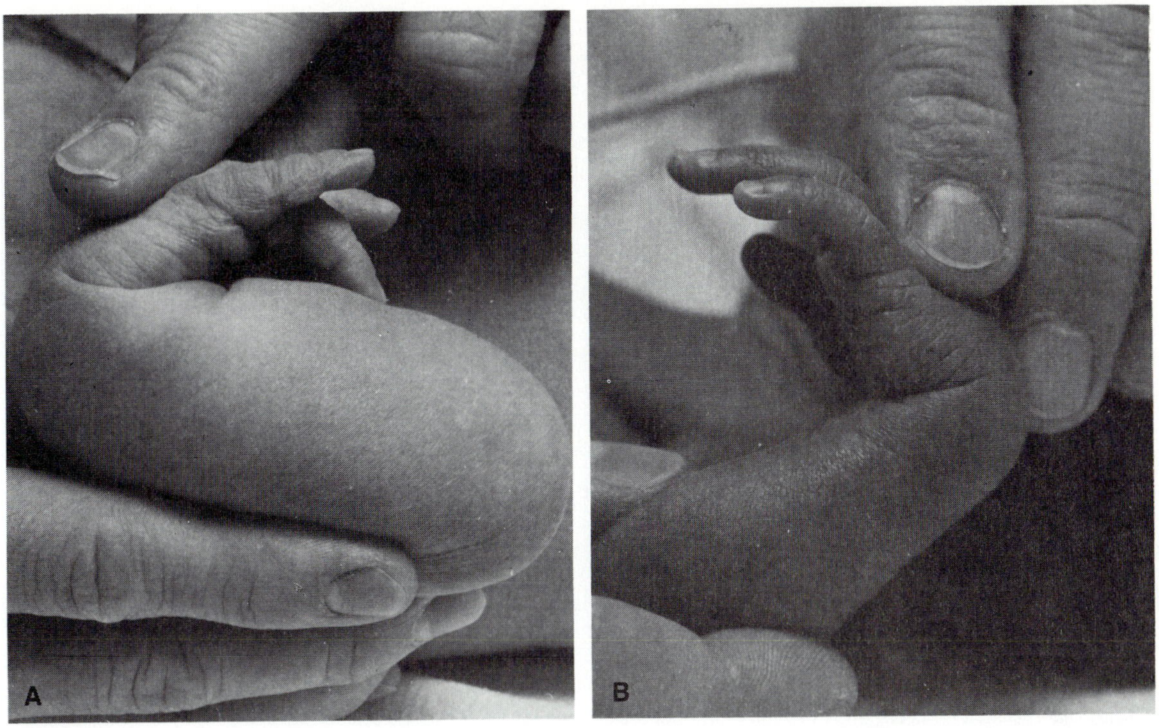

Figure 30-24.
Wrist flexion. In the term neonate (*A*) the wrist can be flexed onto the arm, but the wrist can only be flexed to an angle of about 90 degrees in the preterm neonate (*B*). (From Sullivan, R., Foster, J., & Schreiner, R. L. [1979]. Determining a newborn's gestational age. *American Journal of Maternal Child Nursing*, Jan/Feb, pp. 38–45.)

approximated (0 degrees) in the infant after 40 weeks of gestation.

Arm Recoil. The degree of elbow flexion is assessed. The neonate is placed in a supine position. The nurse completely flexes both elbows, holds the position for 5 seconds, fully extends the arms, and then releases them. In the full-term infant, rapid recoil to flexion is the normal response to this maneuver. The angle formed at the elbow on recoil is less than 90 degrees. The premature infant demonstrates slow recoil and a greater angle with flexion (greater than 90 degrees).

Popliteal Angle. The degree of knee flexion is evaluated. The neonate is placed in a supine position. The nurse flexes the thigh on the abdomen. While holding the thigh against the abdomen with one hand, the nurse places the index finger of the other hand behind the infant's ankle and extends the lower leg until resistance is met. In the full-term newborn, resistance to extension of the knee is strong and the angle formed behind the knee is less than 80 degrees. In the premature newborn the angle is increased (greater than 90 degrees) and there is less resistance to extension.

Scarf Sign. The extent of shoulder flexion is assessed (Fig. 30-25). The infant is placed in a supine position. The arm is drawn across the chest as far as possible until resistance is met. It is permissible to lift the elbow across the body as the arm is extended. The location of the elbow is noted. In the premature infant (before 36 weeks of gestation), the elbow can be drawn past the midline. Between 36 and 40 weeks of gestation the elbow reaches the midline and after 40 weeks the elbow cannot be drawn to the midline.

Heel-to-Ear Extension. The degree of knee extension and the ability to draw the foot to the head are assessed (Fig. 30-26). The neonate is placed in a supine position. While stabilizing the hips on the mattress, the nurse draws the foot toward the ear on the same side. The distance between the foot and head is noted as well as the degree of extension at the knee. There will be marked resistance in the full-term neonate. The popliteal angle will be 90 degrees or less. The foot cannot be drawn much farther toward the head than the umbilicus. The premature infant will demonstrate less resistance and the foot can be drawn closer to the head. This maneuver may be less accurate in neonates delivered in frank breech presentation.

Obtaining and Interpreting the Ballard Score

Once the nurse obtains a score for the neuromuscular assessment, it is added to the score calculated for the physical assessment portion of the rating scale. The sum of the two scores is matched against a column listing gestational age. Once the gestational age is determined, the neonate can be identified as premature (preterm), mature (full-term), or postmature (postterm). A determination can then be made

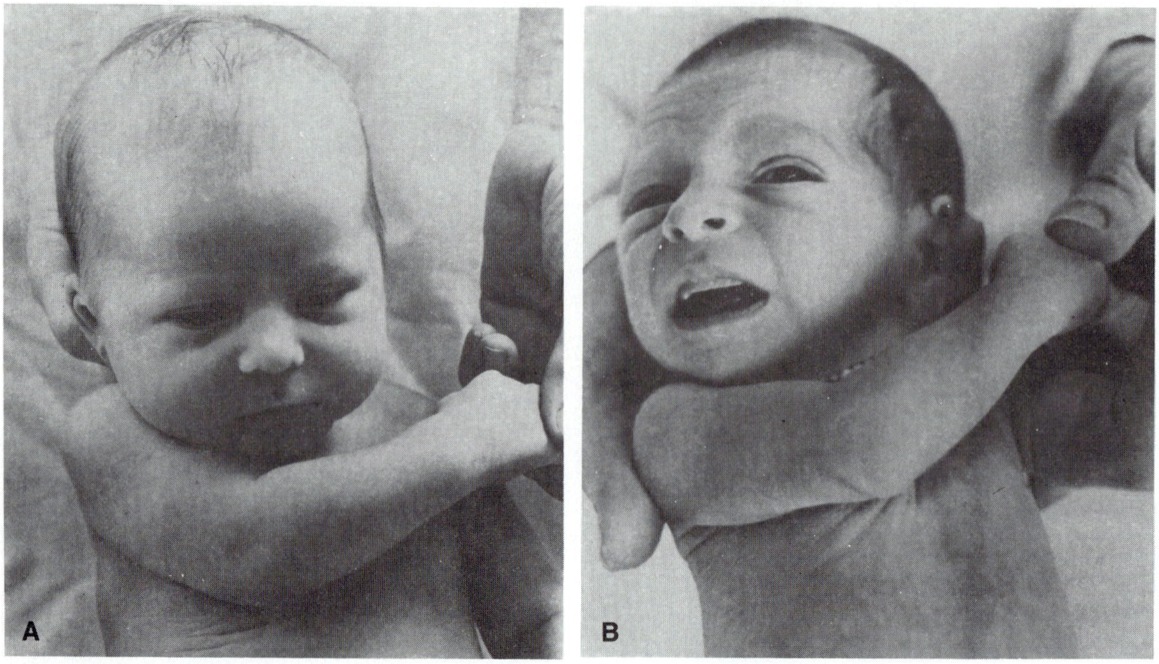

Figure 30-25.
Scarf sign. In the term neonate (*A*) the elbow will not reach the midline, but in the preterm neonate (*B*) the elbow will reach across the midline (Mead Johnson.)

about whether size (birth weight, head circumference, and length) is appropriate for estimated gestational age (Fig. 30-27). This determination is important because SGA or LGA neonates have special needs and problems. Because of the major adaptations required of the neurologic system during the first days of life, the gestational age rating should be performed twice to fully evaluate the neuromuscular component. The first evaluation should be performed within the first 6 hours of life, before the skin begins to dry and crack. If the infant is sick, has sustained neurologic injury, or is heavily sedated as a result of medication given to the mother during labor and delivery, the neurologic assessment is postponed. A skilled examiner may still be able to estimate gestational age by evaluating only the physical characteristics; this type of assessment is essential if the neonate is sick and requires immediate treatment. In some cases, a second assessment is conducted between 24 and 48 hours after delivery to determine changes in the neurologic status of the neonate.

Assessment of Behavioral Capabilities

Researchers have shattered the assumption that the neonate is merely a passive recipient of care with limited sensory perception and behavioral capabilities. Each newborn is now known to possess unique behavioral competencies that

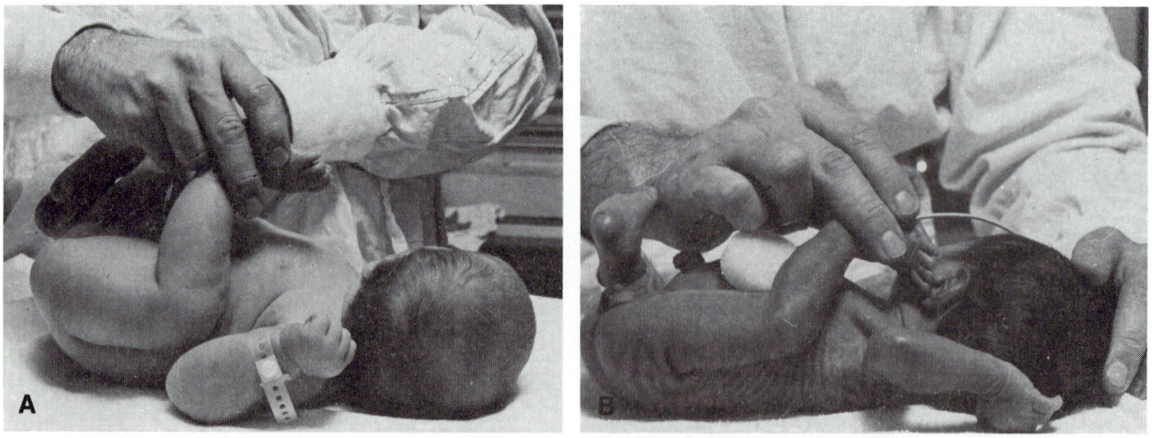

Figure 30-26.
Heel to ear test. In the term neonate (*A*) there is a marked resistance in the leg as the foot is gently drawn toward the ear. *B:* In the neonate very little resistance is noted. (From Sullivan, R., Foster, J., & Schreiner, R. L. [1979]. Determining a newborn's gestational age. *American Journal of Maternal Child Nursing*, Jan/Feb, pp. 38–45.)

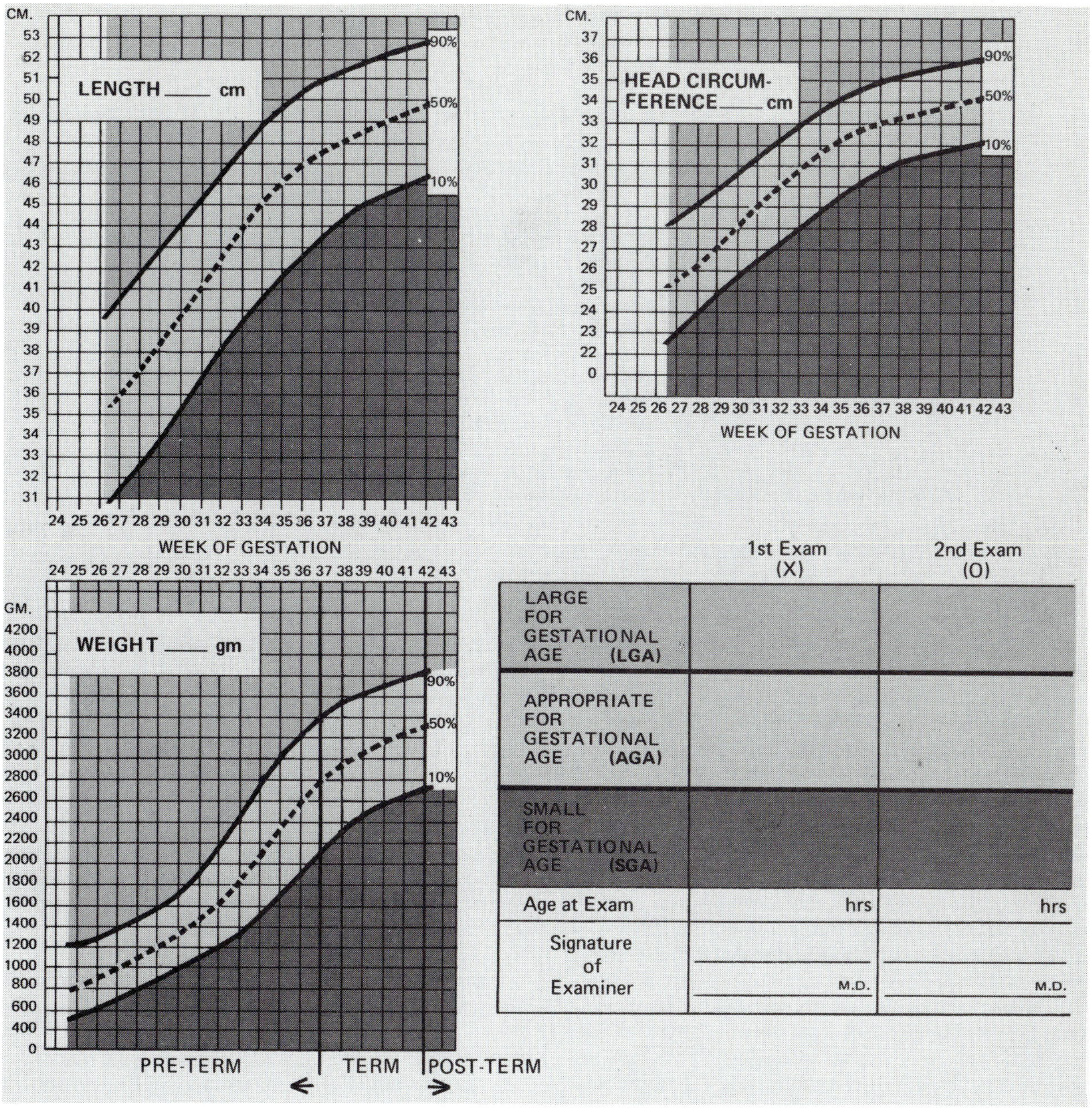

Figure 30-27.

Classification of newborns based on maturity and intrauterine growth. (From Lubchenco, L. C., Hansman, C., & Boyd E. [1966]. *Pediatrics, 37*, 403. Battaglia, F. C. & Lubchenco, L. C. [1967]. *Journal of Pediatrics, 71*, 159, copyright American Academy of Pediatrics.)

exert a powerful effect on parent–newborn interactions and increase the neonate's chance of survival by engaging the caretaker's attention. The mature neonate has behavioral competencies that reflect intact CNS structure, neurologic maturity, and appropriate functioning. Table 30-7 summarizes behaviors reflecting neonatal CNS integrity.

Temperamental differences are reflected in differing reactions to external events. Two major infant temperament types ("easy" and "difficult") have been described (Thomas, Chess, & Korn, 1982). The "easy" infant is characterized by regular body functions, a positive mood, and quick adaptability in new situations, whereas the "difficult" infant shows irregular body rhythms and intense, generally negative responses to new situations. More recent research confirms these earlier findings. Furthermore, these personality traits demonstrate considerable stability over time (Green, Bax, & Tsitsikas, 1989). While the terms "easy" and "difficult" are commonly used by health care professionals, the word "difficult" may have negative connotations for parents and alter their attitude toward the infant. Other less value-laden terms may be used to describe the temperament and adaptability of neonates at birth.

Table 30-7. Behaviors Reflecting CNS Integrity in the Neonate

CNS Capability	Specific Behavior
Reliable social interactions	Fixates on faces
	Follows faces moving in 180-degree arc
	Shows interest in patterns
	Alert to voices
	Responds preferentially to parental voices
	Demonstrates cuddling behavior
	Demonstrates physiologic stability with exposure to soothing sounds
State regulation	Moves smoothly from state to state
	Expends minimal energy during state transitions
	Habituates to stimuli
	Demonstrates self-consoling behaviors
Muscle control	Maintains flexor tone at rest and with position change
	Demonstrates brisk reflex response with stimuli
	Sustains strong suck
	Moves extremities in smooth, controlled, tight arcs
Autonomic nervous system control	Maintains physiologic stability with stimulation (physical or social)

Adapted from Belling, L. (1989). A window on the neonate's brain. *Neonatal Network, 7*(4), 13.

Brazelton Neonatal Behavioral Assessment Scale

Terry Brazelton, a pediatrician, created an assessment tool to assist in the evaluation of newborn behavioral competencies. The scale is composed of 27 behavioral items and 20 measures of reflexes that are elicited during the evaluation to determine the newborn's capabilities. For each item, if the first response is less than optimal, the test is repeated. The infant is scored on the best performance rather than on an average response to each test. Because the infant passes through periods of behavioral disorganization during the first few days after birth, it is recommended that the assessment be done on the third day after delivery. This creates a problem in many settings because of increasing numbers of normal neonates being discharged before 72 hours of age. The assessment, which takes approximately 30 minutes, should be conducted in a quiet, dimly lit area. The examiner must complete training in the use of the Brazelton tool before performing the assessments. Brazelton and associates have also developed an instrument for the assessment of the preterm infant's behavior, the APIB.

The behaviors on the Brazelton assessment scale are divided into the following six categories: habituation, orientation, motor maturity, self-quieting ability, social behaviors, and sleep–wake states. Each is briefly discussed here.

Habituation. Habituation is the ability of the newborn to diminish a response to specific repeated stimuli. In response to sound, light, or a pinprick to the heel, a normal newborn will startle. As the stimulus is repeated, the newborn will shut it out and stop responding. Immature neonates and those with CNS anomalies or injury may respond in an erratic or unpredictable manner to stimuli. They may never fully habituate, thus making it difficult for parents to anticipate or predict their response to specific care-giving activities.

Orientation. Orientation refers to the newborn's ability to attend to visual and auditory stimuli. When alert, normal newborns will attend to voices and fixate and follow visual stimuli. By the third day of life, they can turn their head toward the light or sound and follow faces moving in 180-degree arcs. Preterm infants have a limited ability to orient and attend to visual stimuli and a limited attention span. Attempts to attract the preterm neonate's attention for even short periods may lead to episodes of bradycardia or apnea. Parents and caregivers must minimize environmental stimuli and plan periods of interaction and stimulation that recognize the individual neonate's limitations.

Motor Maturity. Motor maturity is reflected in the newborn's ability to control and coordinate motor activities. Normal full-term newborns demonstrate smooth, free movements within restricted arcs. Occasional tremors and startles can also be noted. Preterm infants and those with CNS anomalies or injury may move their extremities in wide, uneven arcs. Movements are frequently jerky.

Self-Quieting Ability. Self-quieting ability is the ability of neonates to use their own resources to quiet and comfort themselves. The normal newborn demonstrates a variety of self-consoling behaviors, such as hand-to-mouth movements, sucking on fist or tongue, and attending to external stimuli. Infants with neurologic injury or anomalies may be unable to engage effectively in self-quieting activities and require more frequent comforting from caregivers when aroused.

Social Behaviors. Social behavior in neonates refers to the extent to which infants need and respond to cuddling and how often they smile. Newborns vary in their need for and response to being held. Some infants are "cuddlers" who seek and enjoy being held. Others are less tolerant of restraint and stiffen when attempts are made to cuddle them.

Neonates with CNS injury or anomalies may resist any form of cuddling or comforting behavior initially. These infants require consistent caregivers who can assist them in gradually developing tolerance to close physical contact.

Sleep–Wake States. Two sleep states and four awake states have been identified in neonates. Most infants move smoothly between these states, as if moving up and down a ladder, one step at a time (Blackburn & Kang, 1991). Figure 30-28 demonstrates this process of state change. Recognizing these states and their patterns, how long newborns remain in a state, and how frequently they move from one state to another is critical to understanding individual neonatal behavioral capacities. It is also important in helping new parents become acquainted with the unique characteristics of their infant. Identification of the neonate's state of consciousness (sleep or awake) is an essential component of Brazelton's scale.

When the infant is in *deep sleep*, eyes are closed, there is no eye movement, breathing is regular, and there is no spontaneous activity except for occasional startles. Startles are not easily elicited by external stimuli and are quickly suppressed. Even very loud noises may not disturb the infant, and attempts at arousal (eg, for feeding) may be met with frustration. State changes are less likely during deep sleep than in any other state.

In *light sleep*, the neonate's eyes are closed, there is rapid eye movement, and respirations are irregular. Random movements, occasional sucking, and startles can be noted. Startles can be elicited with less difficulty and often result in state changes.

When the neonate is in the *drowsy state*, eyes can be open or closed, and eyelids may flutter. Intermittent motor activity and occasional startles can be noted. The infant is reactive to sensory stimuli but response is delayed. State changes can frequently be noted after stimulation. Movements are usually smooth.

When in the *quiet alert state*, the neonate has a bright look and focuses attention on the source of stimulation. This is an ideal state for parent–infant interactions because the infant is able to attend to vocal and visual stimuli for relatively long periods. Other stimuli may eventually interrupt concentration, but response is delayed. Motor activity is minimal.

In the *eyes open state*, the neonate demonstrates considerable motor activity with thrusting movements of the extremities and occasional startles. The infant reacts to external stimulation with increased startles and motor activity. Discrete reactions are difficult to distinguish because of the generally high activity level.

In the *crying state*, the neonate cries loudly and does not respond to outside stimuli readily. It may take some time to calm the infant so that it will attend to other activities, such as feeding.

By performing ongoing physical assessments of the neonate, the nurse is in a unique position to identify behavioral competencies and abnormalities (see the Nursing Research display, Neonatal Assessment). The nurse uses knowledge about neonatal behavioral capabilities in planning and providing care for the newborn. Interventions can focus on

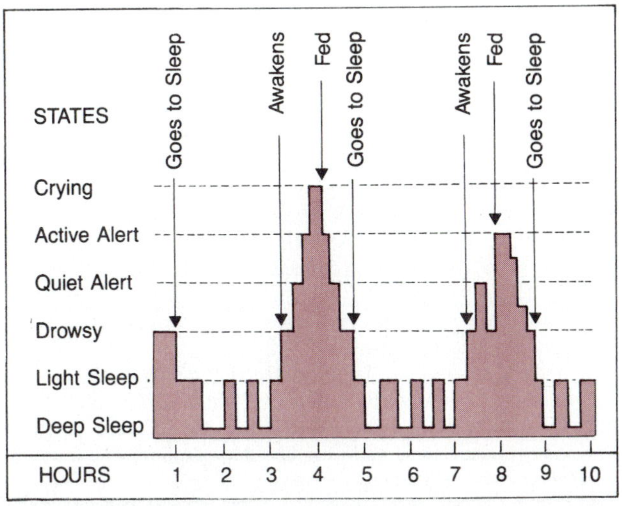

Figure 30-28.

Steplike pattern of change in state during the neonatal period. (Adapted from Blackburn, S., & Kang, R. [1991]. *Early parent–infant relationships* (2nd ed.). Series 1: The first six hours after birth. Module 3. White Plains, NY: March of Dimes Birth Defects Foundation. Reprinted with permission of the copyright holder.)

Nursing Research

Neonatal Assessment

Traditional pediatric evaluation instruments identify gross problems, but they may fail to detect behavioral dysfunction or very early signs of physiologic destabilization. Skilled nurse clinicians often identify subtle signs of dysfunction in neonates before obvious illness or neurologic abnormality is evident. These infants are labeled as "unusual," "funny-looking," "funny-acting," or "different." Nursing research indicates that, while nurses often have difficulty articulating their suspicions of dysfunction, they do posses the ability to accurately identify problems. Nurses focus on interactive competencies (responsiveness, irritability, and posturing); repeated contact with neonates provides nurses with opportunities to note subtle changes in functioning. Nurses using the Brazelton Neonatal Behavioral Assessment Scale (BNBAS) to assess behavioral traits should persist in alerting physicians when they suspect problems, even if they are not able to clearly articulate their impressions.

Maloni, J. A., Stegman, C. E., Taylor, P. M., & Brownell, C. A. (1986). Validation of infant behavior identified by neonatal nurses. *Nursing Research, 35*(3), 133–138.

acquainting parents with the unique behavioral competencies and state patterns of their neonate. They can be taught when and how best to interact with the neonate. The nurse supports early parenting efforts in this manner, thus facilitating parent–newborn attachment.

Before appropriate nursing care can be planned and implemented, the nurse must conduct a comprehensive physical assessment of the neonate. Once the neonate's condition is stabilized after birth, and the woman and her support person have had time to interact with the newborn, the nurse can begin the general assessment. The nurse must be skilled in physical assessment techniques, have a thorough knowledge of normal newborn characteristics, and normal adaptations made after birth. Encouraging the woman and her partner to observe this examination is an excellent method for acquainting them with the unique characteristics and specialness of their infant. It is also a strategy that supports family-centered nursing care.

Chapter Summary

Extrauterine adjustments made during the first 24 hours after birth are critical to the neonate's chances for survival. The nurse is in a unique position to aid the newborn in these adjustments. The nurse must develop a sound knowledge base for assessing the normal neonate and identifying problems.

Definite physiologic and behavioral adaptations are made by the normal neonate. Various stimuli work together to initiate respiration, which begins a chain of cardiovascular events and other physiologic adaptations. Each system begins functioning independent of the maternal support provided while the fetus is in utero. Periods of reaction can be noted, and general characteristics for the normal neonate can be observed.

Comprehensive nursing assessment of the neonate's physical status and behavioral capabilities forms the foundation for subsequent nursing care of the normal neonate. Because the neonate is unable to express needs except through crying, the nurse must be skilled in assessment to collect the data needed for planning and implementing care.

Study Questions

1. *What factors are responsible for initiation of respiration in the neonate?*
2. *What are the four major mechanisms of heat loss/heat transfer in the neonate?*
3. *What is the significance of cold stress in the neonate, and how can the nurse prevent it?*
4. *What is physiologic jaundice, and how is it distinguished from pathologic jaundice in the newborn?*
5. *What is the difference between true breast milk jaundice and jaundice associated with breastfeeding?*
6. *How are the neonate's behavioral responses affected by the periods of reactivity/inactivity?*
7. *What is the significance of the gestational age assessment for the neonate?*
8. *What is the Brazelton Neonatal Behavioral Assessment Scale, and what is its significance?*
9. *How do the sleep–wake states influence parent–newborn interactions?*

References

American Academy of Pediatrics Committee on Nutrition. (1976). Iron supplementation for infants. *Pediatrics*, *58*, 765.

Anders, T. F., & Keener, M. (1985). Developmental course of nighttime sleep-wake patterns in full-term and premature infants during the first year of life. I. *Sleep*, *8*(3), 173–192.

Ballard, J. L., Novak, L. K., & Driver, M. (1979). A simplified score for assessment of fetal maturation of newly born infants. *Journal of Pediatrics*, *95*, 769.

Blackburn, S., & Kang, R. (1991). *Early parent–infant relationships* (2nd ed.). Series 1: The first six hours after birth. Module 3. White Plains, NY: March of Dimes.

Cloherty, J. (1991). Neonatal hyperbilirubinemia. In J. P. Cloherty & A. Stark (Eds.), *Manual of neonatal care* (pp. 298). Boston: Little, Brown.

Gerhardt, K. (1990). Prenatal and perinatal risks of hearing loss. *Seminars in Perinatology*, *14*(4), 309.

Green, J., Bax, M., & Tsitsikas, H. (1989). Neonatal behavior and early temperament. *American Journal of Orthopsychiatry*, *59*(1), 82.

Letko, M. (1992). Detecting and preventing infant hearing loss. *Neonatal Network*, *11*(5), 33.

Park, M., & Da-Hae, L. (1989). Normative arm and calf blood pressure values in the newborn. *Pediatrics*, *83*(2), 240.

Portman, R., Browder, S., & Destefano, S. (1989). Neonatal nephrology. In G. Merenstein & S. Gardner (Eds.), *Handbook of neonatal intensive care* (2nd ed.). St. Louis: CV Mosby.

Quie, P. (1990). Antimicrobial defenses in the neonate. *Seminars in Perinatology*, *14*(Suppl. 1), 2.

Richardson, K. (1991). Renal function in the preterm neonate. *Neonatal Network*, *10*(4), 17.

Tallman, B., Tan, T., Morelli, J., Piepenbrink, J., Stafford, T., Trainor, S., & Weston, W. (1991). Location of port-wine stains and the likelihood of ophthalmic and or central nervous system complications. *Pediatrics*, *87*(30), 323.

Te Pas, K. E. (1988). *Thermoregulation in newborns*. Module 1. White Plains, NY: The National Foundation/March of Dimes.

Thomas, A., Chess, S., & Korn, S. (1982). The reality of difficult temperament. *Merrill-Palmer Quarterly*, *28*, 1.

Weiss, M. (1991). Tympanic thermometry for full-term and preterm neonates. *Clinical Pediatrics*, *30*(Suppl) 42.

Suggested Readings

Bellig, L. (1989). A window on the neonate's brain. *Neonatal Network*, *7*(4), 13.

Brown, L. (1987). Physiologic responses to cutaneous pain in neonates. *Neonatal Network*, *6*(3), 18–22.

Cole, M. (1991). New factors associated with the incidence of hypoglycemia: A research study. *Neonatal Network*, *10*(4), 47.

Hulman, S., Edwards, R., Chen, Y., Polansky, M., & Falkner, B. (1991). Blood pressure patterns in the first three days of life. *Journal of Perinatology*, *XI*(3), 231.

Johnson, K., Ghatia, P., & Bell, E. (1991). Infrared thermometry of newborn infants. *Pediatrics*, *87*(1), 34–38.

NAACOG. (1991). Physical assessment of the neonate. *OGN Nursing Practice Resource*. Washington, DC: Author.

Thoman, E. (1990). Sleeping and waking states in infants: A functional perspective. *Neuroscience and Biobehavioral Reviews*, *14*(1), 93.

CHAPTER 31

Nursing Care of the Low-Risk Neonate

Learning Objectives

After studying the material in this chapter, the student will be able to:

- Discuss how hospital environments influence neonatal adaptation.
- Describe specific nursing interventions that facilitate stabilization of physiologic functions in the transitional period.
- Describe specific nursing interventions that promote the parent–newborn interaction.
- Discuss common nursing interventions used to prevent potential neonatal complications.
- Formulate a nursing care plan for daily care of the neonate.
- Develop an appropriate parent-teaching discharge plan.
- Describe newborn screening tests and discuss their importance in preparation for discharge.
- Discuss the risks and benefits of circumcision.

Key Terms

aspiration	hypothermia
attachment	omphalitis
circumcision	ophthalmia neonatorum
cradle cap	polycythemia
demand feeding	prophylaxis
diurnal rhythm	regurgitation
hyperbilirubinemia	rooming-in
hypoglycemia	

The nurse can make the neonate's adjustment to extrauterine life less traumatic by adapting the environment, providing individualized nursing care, and facilitating the parent–newborn attachment process. These interventions are best accomplished by adherence to principles of family-centered maternity care and use of the nursing process in organizing the care. These two factors remain regardless of the variety of settings and the duration of care.

Assessment of the newborn has been discussed in Chapter 30. This chapter deals with nursing care designed to support physiologic and behavioral adaptation and to facilitate the parent–newborn attachment process during neonatal transition and during ongoing care in a variety of settings. Suggestions for discharge teaching are delineated.

Environmental Considerations in Neonatal Nursing Care

Of particular importance in planning and implementing effective nursing care is an understanding of how the various environments influence neonatal adaptation and the provision of neonatal nursing care. Table 31-1 outlines the advantages and disadvantages of the major sites of care.

Birthing Room or Labor–Delivery–Recovery–Postpartum (LDRP) Room

The birthing room may offer the low-risk family the optimal environment for birth and the immediate postdelivery period within the hospital setting. This private, homelike room introduces the neonate to a quiet, dimly lit extrauterine environment. Parents and the neonate can get acquainted at leisure in comfortable surroundings, and this process is not interrupted by transfer to another room or unit. Siblings or other family members may be allowed to participate in the experience. The nurse should recognize the nature of this intimate family event, providing parents with guidance and support, as needed, but also offering opportunities for privacy.

The birthing room simulates the home environment

Table 31-1. Environmental Factors That Influence the Quality of Family-Centered Neonatal Nursing Care

Type of Environment	Advantages	Disadvantages
Birthing center (separate from hospital)	Homelike environment Elimination of "high-tech" atmosphere Low-stress environment for staff and client Good opportunity for personalized nursing care Mother and neonate may remain together during sensitive alert period right after birth Low exposure to pathogens found in hospital environment Cost effectiveness for low-risk women Good opportunity for mother to breastfeed when neonate demonstrates readiness More opportunities to practice neonatal care Faster establishment of 24-h circadian rhythm	Absence of advanced life-support equipment Little opportunity for frequent monitoring of neonate Potential separation of parents from neonate if neonatal transport is necessary Not universally available for women with limited income
Birthing room or labor–delivery–recovery room	Homelike environment Elimination of "high-tech" atmosphere Low-stress environment for staff and client Advanced life-support equipment available in mot facilities Good opportunity for family privacy Good opportunity for early discharge Mother and neonate may remain together during sensitive alert period right after birth Good opportunity for mother to breastfeed when neonate demonstrates readiness	Life-support equipment frequently not in room if needed Less than optimum conditions for immediate resuscitation of neonate (oxygen, adequate light) Potential for disruptions in bonding due to interruptions by hospital staff Exposure to hospital pathogens Little opportunity for close monitoring of infant (poor lighting, request for privacy, bundling of infant)
Maternal–neonatal recovery room	Resuscitation and life-support equipment in room Good opportunity for frequent monitoring of neonate Mother and neonate remain together during sensitive alert period right after birth Good opportunity for mother to breastfeed when neonate demonstrates readiness	New family remains in "high-tech" environment Few opportunities for family privacy Sensory stimuli may decrease or otherwise alter neonatal behavioral responses Exposure to hospital pathogens Little opportunity for personalized nursing care
Admission nursery or central nursery	Resuscitation and life-support equipment available in room Continual monitoring of neonate possible Efficient use of nursing staff Nursing staff can care for neonate if mother ill or fatigued	Parents and neonate are separated during sensitive alert awake period right after birth Sensory stimuli may decrease or otherwise alter neonatal behavioral responses Little opportunity for personalized nursing care Exposure to hospital pathogens Little opportunity for mother to breastfeed when neonate demonstrates readiness Risk of iatrogenic illness due to invasive monitoring Lack of privacy for family

and, therefore, equipment used for resuscitation and monitoring of the neonate is placed out of sight or outside the room but must be immediately available. Birthing room light sources used for inspection of the neonate may be inadequate. Because the neonate is usually placed against the mother's skin and covered with blankets directly after birth in a birthing room, it is difficult for the nurse to assess subtle changes in skin color and respiratory effort. The nurse must be skillful in balancing the need to monitor vital signs and physiologic adaptations against the family's need for a personal experience free from interruption and unnecessary technologic intervention.

Maternal–Neonatal Recovery Room

The maternal–neonatal recovery room provides the family with an opportunity to remain together during the first 4 to 6 hours after birth. Parents or other family members can become acquainted with their neonate while the neonate is awake and particularly alert to external stimuli. Because the neonate may be placed under a radiant warmer and attached to an electronic temperature probe in this setting, the nurse can easily monitor skin temperature, respiratory status, and color. Adequate light sources are available for inspection of the neonate and resuscitation equipment is readily at hand should it be needed.

Because the recovery room is a more institutional, less intimate environment than a birthing room, effort must be made to foster a meaningful family-centered experience. Curtains should be drawn around the family to provide privacy. Noise levels should be minimized. Care should be taken to limit interruptions of the family–newborn acquaintance process. The nurse may also use the opportunity provided by the neonatal assessment to educate the parents about the unique characteristics of their infant.

Admission Nursery

An admission nursery is frequently used when the mother or neonate is ill and requires special care immediately after birth. A normal newborn may also be placed in the nursery after delivery by cesarean birth while the mother remains in the postsurgical or postanesthesia recovery room. The admission nursery has special resuscitation and monitoring equipment that may be required during the transition period. The newborn is usually placed under a radiant warmer and a temperature probe is attached to the skin. The nurse monitors the neonate and is responsible for the neonate's care and emotional support.

The nurse must be creative in planning family-centered care for the neonate placed in an admission nursery. The father or another family member may accompany the neonate to the nursery. The admission procedures can be explained and teaching can be done during the admission assessment. If the father of the newborn is present, these strategies may facilitate the father–neonate acquaintance process. The father or support person can be encouraged to hold the newborn while the infant is awake, alert, and receptive to external stimuli. A continual effort must be made to provide the mother with information about her newborn. It is important that both parents feel that the nurse caring for their newborn is sensitive to the neonate's needs for comfort and love as well as the parents' concern for their newborn.

Rooming-In

Most hospitals in the United States and Canada provide mothers with the opportunity to keep their newborns with them in the postpartum unit. This arrangement, known as *rooming-in*, allows mother and infant to become acquainted through continuous contact 24 hours a day. In a recent study, Norr and Roberts (1991) found a strong association between rooming-in and maternal attachment scores in both adult and adolescent mothers. New parents have greater opportunities to practice neonatal care skills and become familiar with their neonate's personality. Furthermore, recent research indicates that newborns who room-in more quickly establish a 24-hour circadian sleep–wake pattern because light and dark sequencing is similar to that found at home (McMillen, Adamson, Deayton, & Nowak, 1991) (see the accompanying Nursing Research display, Neonatal Rooming-In and Maternal Sleep Patterns).

The nurse caring for the newborn plans to perform as much of the care as possible at the mother's bedside. This is a good time to teach parents and to facilitate the acquaintance process. The nurse can also help build the mother's self-confidence in her new role by guiding her initial efforts in neonatal care and providing her with frequent positive feedback. The father should be welcome in this environment. He should be included in teaching sessions and encouraged in his efforts to learn parenting skills.

Central Nursery

Hospital personnel frequently provide parents with a central nursery where the neonate can be cared for if the mother is ill during the postpartum period. A mother who is rooming-in may also use the central nursery during visiting hours or when she desires a period of uninterrupted rest or sleep before returning home with her newborn. The nurse is responsible for the physical care and emotional support of the newborn while the neonate remains in the nursery (Fig. 31-1). Care should be organized to allow the neonate periods of quiet sleep between feedings and assessments. If the mother is ill, the nurse should make every effort to incorporate maternal visits with her neonate into the plan of care. The nurse must keep the mother informed of her neonate's condition; she should also encourage the father to visit the nursery and support him in his efforts to care for the neonate.

Nursing Research

Neonatal Rooming-In and Maternal Sleep

Recent nursing research has examined the impact of rooming-in on maternal sleep. Self-reports by the subjects in a study by Keefe (1988) found no significant differences in the number of hours slept or the perceived quality of sleep between woman who roomed-in and those who returned their neonates to a central nursery at night. In a recent study by Lentz and Killien (1991), women reported that the most frequent reason for interruption of sleep was not due to the needs of the newborn but due to the nurse's awakening them for assessments and care. Weiss and Armstrong (1990) found that all participants preferred to have their newborns in the room at night, regardless of the care delivery system, but wished the option of sending the neonate to the nursery if desired. Further research is indicated to support these findings, particularly with groups of women from varying socioeconomic and cultural backgrounds.

Keefe, M. R. (1988). The impact of infant rooming-in on maternal sleep at night. *Journal of Obstetric, Gynecologic, and Neonatal Nursing 17*(2), 122–126.

Lentz, M., & Killien, M. (1991). Are you sleeping? Sleep patterns during postpartum hospitalization. *Journal of Perinatal Neonatal Nursing, 4*(4):30.

Weiss, M., & Armstrong, M. (1990). Postpartum mothers' preferences for nighttime care of the neonate. *Journal of Obstetric, Gynecologic, and Neonatal Nursing, 20*(4), 290.

Maintaining a Secure Environment

Abduction of a neonate from the hospital is a rare event, yet it receives national attention when it occurs. It is one of the most serious crises a new family may encounter and may represent the most distressing event in the career of a maternity nurse. Although only 12 to 18 infants are taken from birthing centers or hospitals each year (Rabun, 1991), the

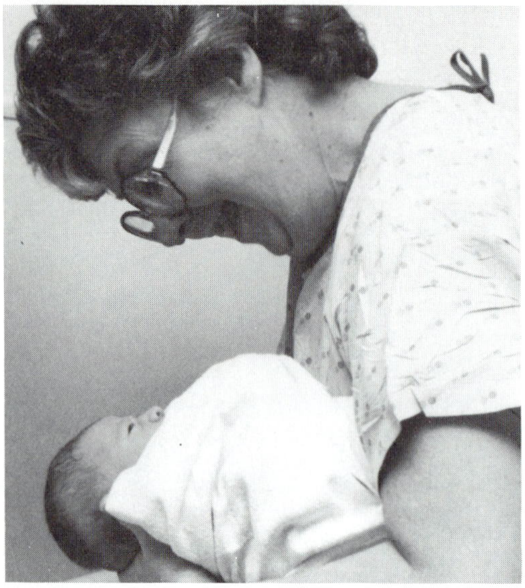

Figure 31-1.
The nurse provides individualized care, comfort, and stimulation for the neonate. (Photo by BABES, Inc.)

number is increasing and has caused significant changes in hospital security systems.

A profile of the "typical" abductor has been developed by law enforcement agencies, and every maternity nurse should be familiar with it. The kidnapper is usually a woman, who most often uses one of two methods to obtain the infant (Beachy & Deacon, 1992). She may impersonate a nurse and remove the neonate from the room, using the excuse that an examination or procedure must be performed. A less commonly used method is simply to take the infant from the nursery when the staff is not in the immediate environment. This rarely happens today because most nurseries require at least one nurse to be in attendance in the nursery at all times when infants are in the unit.

Hospital and unit-based strategies have been developed to prevent neonatal kidnapping. They are listed in the accompanying display. Although sophisticated technologies are available to deter abductions, including electronic identification bracelets, diapers with electronic sensors, and videocamera surveillance systems, most security experts agree that vigilance on the part of parents and nursing staff is the first line of defense against kidnapping. Parents should be cautioned never to allow the newborn to leave with anyone who does not have proper hospital identification. If the parent is not familiar with the individual requesting to take the neonate or is unsure about the reason for the neonate's removal, the best action for the parents is to personally transport the newborn to the nursery or call the nursery for clarification.

Prevention of Neonatal Kidnapping

Profile of the Typical Abductor *

- 15 to 44-year-old female
- May have lost an infant or incapable of having one
- Usually married or cohabiting; partner's desire for a child may be motivating factor
- Usually a resident of community when abduction occurs
- Frequently visits the nursery before the abduction
- Asks detailed questions about hospital procedures and layout of maternity floor
- Plans abduction but does not necessarily target the infant
- Takes infant as opportunity presents itself
- Frequently impersonates a nurse or other hospital personnel
- Often acquainted with hospital personnel or victim's parents

Strategies to Prevent Abduction†

- Report unusual behavior to hospital security.
- Wear picture identification at all times.
- Develop and enforce visiting policies.
- Never leave neonate unattended in nursery.
- Identify all neonates by using bracelets and taking footprints or photographs.
- Post patients' names and room numbers away from areas of public traffic.
- Orient parents to all unit security policies.
- Teach parents to confirm identity of anyone wanting to take the neonate from the room.
- Teach parents never to leave neonate unattended in room.
- Examine maternity unit layout and offer suggestions for improvement in security.
- Train staff in procedure to follow when a neonate is discovered missing.

** There is no guarantee that a newborn abductor will fit this description. Adapted from Mead Johnson. The "typical" abductor.* Safeguard Their Tomorrows. *Evansville, IN: Author.*

† Adapted from Beachy, P., & Deacon, J. (1992). Preventing neonatal kidnapping. Journal of Obstetric, Gynecologic, and Neonatal Nursing, *21(1), 12.*

Neonatal adaptations and parent–newborn interaction are best supported in an environment that facilitates close, sustained maternal-newborn contact. The setting should be conducive to privacy, breastfeeding, and periods of uninterrupted interaction between parent(s) and neonate. The childbearing family has a variety of settings available that foster a family-centered experience. Nursing care of mother and neonate can be accomplished as effectively in this environment as in a traditional nursery. If problems require the neonate's placement in a central nursery, the nurse makes every effort to bring the mother to her neonate. When the neonate's condition stabilizes, parents decide the arrangements for contact.

Care of the Neonate During Transition to Extrauterine Life

In most postpartum health care settings the nurse is the health team member who provides direct care immediately after birth. Although most newborns successfully accomplish the transition to extrauterine life, the first hours after birth are a critical period of adjustment.

• • Assessment

The nurse must know the mother's prenatal history and the course of her labor and delivery to support the neonate's extrauterine adaptation effectively. Maternal illness, poor nutrition, and even psychosocial problems during pregnancy may have a direct effect on the newborn's condition at birth. Obstetric complications and drugs administered during labor and delivery will also affect the newborn's immediate responses. (The reader is referred to Table 30-3 for a review of the essential elements of the initial fetal–neonatal history.) The nurse should know the neonate's 1- and 5-minute Apgar scores, umbilical cord blood gas results if done, and the type of delivery room care the mother received (see Chapter 21). It is particularly important for the nurse to note if there was any evidence of asphyxia or need for any type of resuscitation at birth.

The neonate is weighed and measured, and the first set of vital signs is taken soon after birth. Temperature, apical heart rate, and respiratory rate are recorded and reassessed at least every 30 minutes for the first hour and then once an hour for the next 4 to 6 hours. A blood pressure reading is usually included in the initial assessment.

Once the nurse has completed an assessment of the neonate and identified any problems, a nursing care plan is initiated. Many institutions have standardized care plans that can be adapted to the individual needs of each newborn.

• • Nursing Diagnosis

Based on review of the antepartum and labor and delivery records as well as other elements of the nurse's assessment on admission (see Chapter 30), the nurse formulates applicable nursing diagnoses. The following are nursing diagnoses that reflect possible problems that may arise in transitional care of the newborn and may be addressed independently. Priorities in care may be established based on these diagnoses.

- Ineffective Thermoregulation related to limited shivering ability or fluctuating environmental temperatures
- Ineffective Airway Clearance related to oropharynx secretions
- Impaired Skin Integrity related to susceptibility to nosocomial infection secondary to lack of normal skin flora
- Altered Nutrition: Less than Body Requirements related to diminished sucking
- High Risk for Infection related to vulnerability of infant, lack of normal flora, or open wound (umbilical cord or circumcision)
- Ineffective Breastfeeding related to lack of knowledge regarding care
- Altered Health Maintenance related to insufficient parental knowledge of infant care skills
- Altered Parenting related to change in family unit or new infant

Complications requiring collaboration with other members of the health care team may arise during transitional care. Such complications include infection, hypoglycemia, hemorrhage, and hyperbilirubinemia. Thus, in addition to routine care, the nurse is responsible for monitoring for and preventing potential complications. Monitoring for these specific complications is discussed at the end of this section on transitional care.

• • Planning and Implementation

When planning nursing care to meet identified neonatal needs, the nurse must consider the length of time the mother and newborn are likely to be hospitalized, the mother's physical condition, the emotional state and learning needs of parents and other family members, and the physiologic adaptations required of the newborn. Nursing interventions during the transitional period focus on prevention and early identification of physiologic complications, assessment of extrauterine adaptation, establishment of a feeding pattern, and support of parent–newborn attachment. Preparation for discharge is begun early by initiating the teaching plan shortly after birth.

The nurse implements a variety of actions to support physiologic adaptation. Agency policies and procedures or protocols often guide the nurse in the initiation of specific interventions such as obtaining blood samples for hematocrit determination or neonatal screening tests. Until the first bath is completed, the nurse wears gloves in compliance with universal body substance precautions while performing specific nursing care activities (see the accompanying Nursing Procedure).

Supporting Thermoregulation

Neonatal thermoregulation is discussed in detail in Chapter 30. Nursing strategies to prevent heat loss and support thermoregulation begin *before* birth. Warm blankets and a stockinette cap are prepared when birth is imminent. If special procedures (intubation and laryngeal suctioning or resuscitation) are anticipated, a radiant warmer should be turned on before delivery to permit prewarming of the mattress and linen. NAACOG guidelines for managing thermoregulation indicate that the room should be free of drafts and suggest that the temperature of the delivery room maintained at 71°F (22°C) with a relative humidity of 60% to 65% (NAACOG, 1990).

The nurse must carefully dry the newborn at birth to prevent heat loss by evaporation. Particular attention should

NURSING PROCEDURE

Using Universal Precautions in Newborn Care

Purpose: To prevent transmission of the human immunodeficiency virus.

Because the prenatal history, physical examination, and laboratory tests cannot reliably identify all women infected with the human immunodeficiency virus (HIV) or other blood-borne pathogens, such as hepatitis, the United States Department of Health and Human Services has recommended the following universal body substance precautions be established in *ALL* settings for *ALL* patients.

NURSING ACTION	*RATIONALE*
1. Carry a clean pair of gloves in the pocket of the uniform at all times.	To permit quick application of gloves in emergency situations or when gloves are *not* readily available
2. Wear gloves and protective skin coverings when handling the neonate before and during procedures.	To prevent skin and mucous membrane exposure to blood and body fluids
3. Wear gloves during the following procedures: venipunctures, heel sticks, IV insertion procedures, when applying pressure to accomplish hemostasis after venipuncture, IV removal, and suctioning newborn.	To prevent skin exposure to blood or body fluids
4. Wear gloves when changing diapers and when collecting and testing urine or stool samples.	To prevent skin exposure to urine or stool
5. Wear goggles or face masks during procedures that are likely to generate splashing, such as the neonate's first bath and a circumcision procedure.	To prevent eye contamination with blood or other body fluids
6. Wash hands, skin surfaces, eyes, and mucous membranes immediately if contaminated with body fluids.	To reduce the length of skin exposure to pathogen
7. Take precautions to prevent injuries caused by needles or other sharp instruments.	To prevent accidental needle sticks
• Needles should not be recapped or purposely bent or broken after use. They should be placed directly into a puncture-resistant container.	
• Heel stick lancets should be disposed of immediately after use in a puncture-resistant container.	To prevent accidental puncture with the lancet
8. Place reusable sharp instruments in a puncture-resistant instrument container for transport to the reprocessing area.	To prevent accidental puncture or laceration with the instruments
9. Place resuscitation bags and infant masks in all infant care areas for quick availability. Manual suction devices, such as the De Lee Mucus Trap, should no longer be used to aspirate mucus, blood, or meconium from the neonate's airway.	To avoid mouth-to-mouth resuscitation and to minimize exposure to blood or mucus and the need for mouth-to-mouth resuscitation. (To prevent exposure to blood, mucus, or meconium when suctioning the infant's airway)
10. Have meconium aspirators and mechanical suction equipment available in all infant care areas. (Adaptors are available to connect mucous-trap catheters to wall suction if aspiration is needed.)	
11. Ensure that all health care workers who have exudative lesions or weeping dermatitis refrain from all direct patient contact and patient equipment contact until the condition resolves.	To prevent transmission of HIV across broken skin surfaces

be paid to drying the head, which is 25% of the total body surface. Recent research (Vaughans, 1990) indicates that fostering skin-to-skin contact with the mother or double-wrapping the neonate in warm, dry blankets works equally well to prevent evaporative heat loss. A dry stockinette cap should be placed on the newborn's head. In the immediate postbirth period, a diaper is not always placed on the newborn. Blankets should therefore be changed immediately if the neonate urinates or passes meconium.

The neonate's temperature is taken at the beginning of the initial assessment and at least every hour for the first 4 to 6 hours of life. During the measurement procedure, the nurse prevents heat loss by keeping the neonate well covered. The nurse can hold the thermometer in place under the blanket. The neonate can also be temporarily placed under a radiant warmer to prevent heat loss while the temperature is measured and the nurse performs the initial physical assessment. The normal newborn temperature range is 36.4°C to 37.2°C (97.5°F to 99.0°F). If the first temperature is below 36.4°C (97.5°F), the neonate should be placed (or remain) in an incubator or under the radiant warmer to prevent further heat loss and support thermoregulation. See the Nursing Procedure for the safe use of infant radiant warmers.

Care should be taken to prevent hypothermia during the initial bath. The bath should be delayed until the neonate's temperature is stabilized in the high range of normal (37.0°C to 37.2°C or 98.6°F to 99.0°F). The infant should be bathed quickly in a draft-free environment. As noted, the head constitutes 25% of the total body surface and should be bathed last to prevent significant heat loss. The head and body should be thoroughly dried—preferrably while the infant is under a radiant warmer. Warm dry blankets and a stockinette cap should be applied immediately afterward. The neonate's temperature is measured again after the bath. If it has not dropped below 36.4°C (97.5°F), the neonate remains double-wrapped in warm blankets with the stockinette cap on its head and may be given to the mother. If the temperature is lower than 36.4°C (97.5°F), the newborn is placed back in an incubator or under the radiant warmer until its temperature reaches the normal range and has stabilized. While under the radiant warmer, all clothing and the stockinette cap are removed for optimum heat transfer from the radiant heat infrared element to the neonate's body. If the neonate is placed in an incubator, a diaper may be applied after the bath. A shirt or blanket is generally not placed on the newborn so that the nursery staff can continue to monitor color, tone, and respiratory pattern until the neonate's temperature stabilizes.

Ongoing nursing care is conducted in draft-free environments. The neonate's clothing and diapers should be changed as soon as possible when they become wet. The nurse should not completely undress the neonate for periodic assessments. Each body area to be assessed is exposed for evaluation and then re-covered before proceeding to the next body part or system. In cold weather the neonate should not be placed directly next to a window because significant heat loss can occur by conduction and convection. Conversely, the neonate should not be placed directly under air-conditioning vents during the summer months. These methods of heat loss were outlined in Table 30-2. The accompanying display lists nursing actions that support neonatal thermoregulation and prevent heat loss.

Expected Outcome

- Newborn maintains a stable temperature as evidenced by axillary temperature of 36.4°C to 37.2°C (97.5°F to 99.0°F) within 2 to 4 hours of birth.

Promoting Respiratory Adaptation

The neonate may need assistance with respiratory adaptations immediately after birth because regurgitation of mucus and swallowed amniotic fluid may lead to obstruction of the airway or aspiration. A bulb syringe should be available for clearing the nose and mouth (Fig. 31-2). An 8 or 10 French catheter attached to wall suction (low-pressure setting) should be available for gastric suctioning if the stomach contents are to be suctioned. Directions for using the bulb syringe are given in the section on promoting health maintenance at the end of the chapter.

Immediately after delivery the newborn may be placed in Trendelenburg's position (supine, with the head tilted down) to facilitate drainage of fluids. The use of Trendelenburg's position is controversial, and a sidelying position without a tilt may be just as effective. The head-down position may cause increased intracranial pressure and may increase the risk of intraventricular hemorrhage, especially in preterm newborns, or if there was cephalopelvic disproportion, prolonged labor, or forceps or vacuum extraction. If this position is used, the incline should not be more than 15 degrees. Once stabilized, the newborn should be positioned on his or her side. The newborn should never be left unattended in a supine position during the postbirth transition period because in this position the danger of aspiration of mucus or fluid regurgitated from the stomach is always present.

Respiratory function is directly affected by body temperature. Neonates who are chilled are most likely to suffer respiratory complications for several reasons. First, hypothermia leads to increased oxygen consumption and tachypnea. Second, cold drafts over the neonate's face and chest can cause apnea. Finally, cold stress leads to a decrease in surfactant production with resultant atelectasis of pulmonary alveoli.

Neonates may regurgitate mucus or milk at any time but are particularly likely to do so during the second period of reactivity. This is because the gastrointestinal system and central nervous system (CNS) are in a state of hyperactivity during this period. (Periods of reactivity are discussed in Chapter 30.) As a result of their physiologic and anatomic immaturity, neonates are at risk of aspiration when they suddenly regurgitate large amounts of fluid. The nurse is responsible for implementing actions to maintain a patent airway and to minimize the risk of aspiration if regurgitation occurs (see the accompanying Nursing Procedure display).

Expected Outcomes

- Neonate breathes without assistance as evidenced by normal respiration between 30 and 60 breaths/min within 2 to 4 hours of birth.
- Neonate maintains a patent airway.

NURSING PROCEDURE

Observing Safety Measures in the Use of the Infant Radiant Warmer

Purpose: To support thermoregulation and prevent hypothermia in the neonate. To prevent hyperthermia or thermal burns during use of the radiant warmer.

NURSING ACTION	***RATIONALE***
1. Remove neonate's clothes and stockinette cap.	To permit optimum transfer of heat from infrared heating element to neonate's body
2. Remove plastic diaper.	To prevent thermal skin burn where plastic comes in contact with skin
3. Place neonate in center of mattress.	To ensure that infrared ray directed to center of mattress covers neonate's body
4. Attach skin probe and turn the control to servo control on automatic if neonate is to remain under the radiant warmer for more than 10 minutes.	To prevent hyperthermia
5. Attach skin probe with a foam-backed, the self-adhesive, reflective shield.	To provide insulation of the probe from heat of the infrared heating element
6. Place probe flush on the skin surface.	To ensure direct skin contact so that servomechanisms can accurately measure skin temperature
7. Place probe on the upper surface of neonate's skin—facing the radiant heater infrared element. (Use only probe designed by manufacturer.)	To ensure proper functioning servocontrol mechanisms cannot function when probe is underneath the neonate's body. (Probes from other radiant warmer units may fit unit, but may not function properly.)
8. Set temperature control point between 36°C to 37°C (96.8°F to 98.6°F).	To prevent hypothermia or hyperthermia
9. Keep side walls of radiant warmer up.	To ensure infant safety and to prevent heat loss by convection
10. Inspect infant's skin every 30 minutes for evidence of: • Redness • Probe adherence and attachment to skin	To identify early changes indicative of thermal burn
11. Measure axillary skin temperature every 30 to 60 minutes.	To prevent hypothermia or hyperthermia

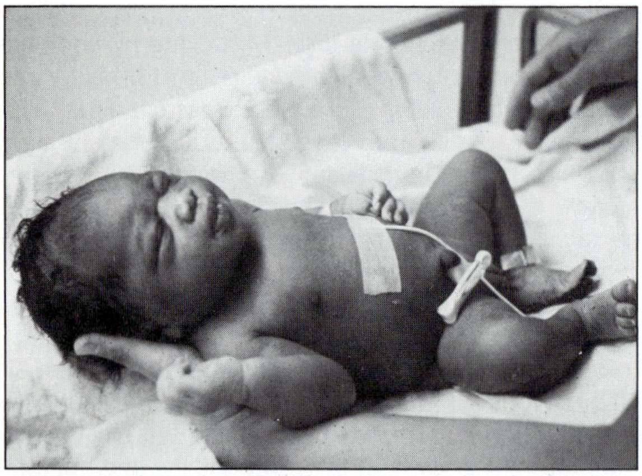

Step 11. Monitoring skin temperature with a heat sensor (Childbirth Graphics).

12. Document: • Temperature control set point • Power output • Setting and operation of alarm system • Neonate temperature	To provide permanent record of nursing actins and infant response to radiant heat

Adapted from Te Pas, K. (1988). Thermoregulation in newborns. *Series 1. The first six hours after birth. Module 1. White Plains, NY: The National Foundation/March of Dimes.*

Nursing Interventions to Support Neonatal Thermoregulation and Prevent Heat Loss

Support of thermoregulation is a priority nursing responsibility of the neonatal nurse. An understanding of the mechanisms of heat transfer and loss is essential to implement rational strategies to prevent hypothermia in the neonate.

Evaporation

- Dry the neonate's body and head.
- Remove wet blankets and diapers.
- Place dry stockinette cap on head immediately after birth and after bath.
- Wash head last and dry immediately after bath. (When sponge-bathing neonate, wash one body part at a time, dry and cover before bathing another part of the body.)
- Keep humidity in delivery room between 60% and 65% to reduce rate of evaporation at birth.
- Do not bathe infant until temperature is stable at 37.0°C or 98.6°F.

Conduction

- Preheat radiant warmer before use.
- Warm blanket and stockinette cap before use.
- Warm hands and stethoscope before use.
- Place neonate in skin-to-skin contact with mother's body.
- Place a warm pad on weight scale before weighing neonate.
- Preheat restraint board or place warm blanket on restraint board before circumcision.

Convection

- Place crib out of direct line of window, fan, or air-conditioning vent.
- Raise the side walls of the radiant warmer to reduce neonate's exposure to air currents.

Radiation

- Use a radiant warmer when neonate's body must be exposed for procedures or during drying after bath.
- Use double-walled incubator or plastic heat shields to prevent heat loss in low-birth-weight neonates.
- Remove neonate from areas with cold surfaces such as outer walls of building or windows.
- Preheat incubator before placing the neonate into it.

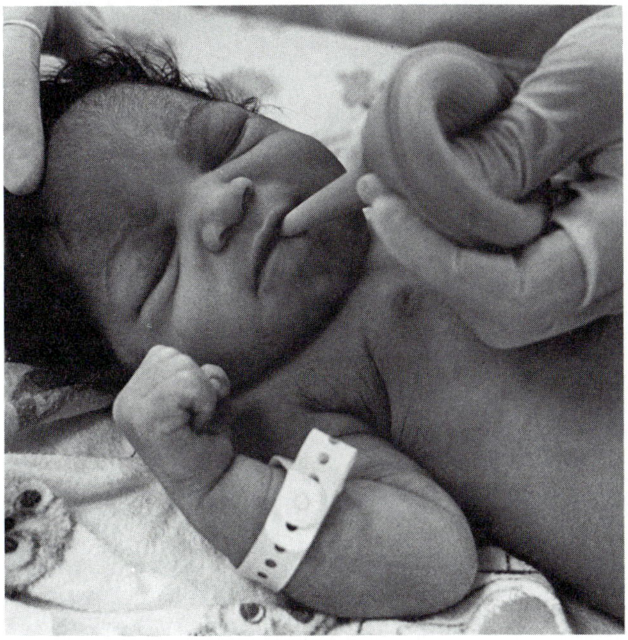

Figure 31-2.
A bulb syringe is used to suction mucus from the neonate's nose and mouth. The bulb is compressed before insertion into the nares or mouth and then slowly released to create suction. (Photo by Kathy Sloane.)

Promoting Circulatory and Cardiac Adaptation

The nurse can best support circulatory and cardiac adaptation by maintaining the neonate's temperature within normal limits and clearing all mucus from the airways so that effective gas exchange and oxygenation of tissues occurs. It is important to examine the umbilical cord to make sure that the cord clamp is secure and that no bleeding is occurring from its base. The nurse conducts ongoing assessments of the infant's color to detect cardiac dysfunction, which may be indicated by generalized or circumoral cyanosis.

The brachial, radial, femoral, popliteal, and dorsalis pedis pulses are palpated. The skin on the infant's trunk is also blanched periodically for assessment of central capillary fill time (CFT), an indirect evaluation of tissue perfusion. A capillary hematocrit is obtained to identify anemia or an excess of red blood cells (polycythemia). Both conditions constitute additional stress to the cardiac system as the transition from fetal to neonatal circulation occurs in the first hours after birth.

Expected Outcome

- Neonate demonstrates normal cardiac output as evidenced by a regular heart rate of 120 to 160 bpm within 2 hours of birth, central CFT under 4 seconds, and hematocrit between 45% and 65%.

NURSING PROCEDURE
Minimizing the Risk of Aspiration and Preventing Aspiration

Purpose: To minimize the risk of aspiration of gastric contents and obstruction of the neonate's airway.

NURSING ACTION	***RATIONALE***
1. Have emergency resuscitation equipment, including wall suction and oxygen available.	To prevent delays in the implementation of airway clearance and oxygen delivery
2. Have 8 and 10 French feeding tubes available.	To permit gastric suctioning if stomach is to be emptied
3. At the time of admission place a bulb syringe in the neonate's crib, where it is easily visible and readily available.	To permit rapid aspiration of secretions from the neonate's nose, mouth, and oropharynx should regurgitation occur
4. Evaluate the sucking and swallowing reflexes of the neonate before the first feeding.	To determine the integrity of the suck and swallow reflex before attempting to initiate oral feedings, thus reducing the risk of aspiration
5. Test the patency of the esophagus and rule out esophageal and tracheal anomalies by giving a small amount of sterile water before the first bottle feeding if the neonate is to be formula fed.	To prevent aspiration of formula through a tracheoesophageal fistula into the lungs
6. Avoid overfeeding the formula-fed neonate and carefully burp the newborn after each feeding.	To prevent gastric distention and resultant regurgitation of stomach contents
7. Always position the newborn in the sidelying position after feedings or when under the radiant warmer.	To prevent backflow of regurgitated stomach contents into the oropharynx, reducing the risk of aspiration To facilitate the drainage of secretions and fluids from the mouth
8. Demonstrate proper feeding and burping techniques to the mother and other neonate care providers	To prevent stomach distention and regurgitation
9. Demonstrate proper use of the bulb syringe	To promote proper airway clearance

If the neonate begins to gag or choke or becomes suddenly cyanotic.

NURSING ACTION	***RATIONALE***
10. Turn the neonate on side or abdomen with the head slightly lower than the feet (10–15-degree angle)	To facilitate drainage of fluids from the neonate's mouth and nose
11. Pat the neonate firmly on the back.	To facilitate drainage of fluids from the mouth and nose
12. Insert a bulb syringe or suction catheter attached to wall suction (on low pressure) into the mouth first and remove all secretions.	To prevent stimulation of gasping activity, which can occur when the nose is suctioned first and which can lead to aspiration of secretions
13. If using a bulb syringe, be sure to compress the bulb first before inserting the tip into the neonate's mouth.	To prevent blowing secretion deeper into the neonate's airway
14. Suction both nares.	To remove secretions from nose
15. If the neonate is apneic or remains cyanotic after secretions are removed from the mouth and nose, apply 100% oxygen by resuscitation bag and mask apparatus and begin ventilation at 40 breaths/min until color improves and breathing is resumed.	To provide oxygen To follow next step in CPR: • Open airway • begin breathing

Promoting Skin Integrity

If vital signs remain stable, the infant is usually bathed to remove amniotic fluid, dried blood, and mucus from the skin and hair, which constitute a medium for bacterial growth. A 3% hexachlorophene solution may be used once to decrease the risk of staphylococcal skin infection; however, this is not done routinely because the solution is absorbed through the skin and is neurotoxic. In most cases Neutrogena soap, Lowila Cake, or Moisturel cleanser should be used. Ivory soap is no longer recommended (Cetta, Lambert, & Ros, 1991). The umbilical cord is often treated with an iodine solution, triple dye, or an antibiotic ointment after the first bath to reduce bacterial colonization and the risk of omphalitis.

Expected Outcomes

- Neonate maintains skin integrity as evidenced by absence of skin rashes or infection.
- Neonate remains free of signs of omphalitis.

Promoting Newborn Nutrition

The neonatal nurse assists the newborn with the initial intake of fluids and nutrients. Safety and comfort are foremost considerations and are guided by a thorough knowledge of gastrointestinal structure and function. Once physiologic stability is achieved, the nurse is alert for feeding cues that indicate the neonate is ready for the first feeding experience. Breastfeeding, formula feeding, and nursing care related to maternal and infant nutrition are discussed in detail in Chapter 35. The following sections on feeding considerations apply to both breastfed and bottle-fed neonates in the hospitalization period.

Safety Considerations

Oral intake is initiated only when the neonate demonstrates successful transition to the extrauterine environment. Cardiorespiratory and temperature-regulating systems must be intact and functioning. The nurse assists the mother with initiation of the feeding process. The neonate should be observed closely for evidence of choking or cyanosis during the first feeding.

The bottle-fed neonate may be given a small amount of sterile water before the introduction of formula to assess the integrity of the suck, swallow, and gag reflexes. If the infant has difficulty with this feeding and aspiration occurs, the use of sterile water minimizes potential lung damage. Glucose water is not an acceptable test fluid for the first feeding because it is as traumatic to lung tissue as is formula. A small amount of water is sufficient; if the neonate has no problem, formula can be substituted immediately, thereby preventing a delay in feeding.

The patency of the esophagus is assessed during the initial sterile water feeding. A small number of newborns have an abnormal connection between the esophagus and trachea (tracheoesophageal fistula, or TEF). The esophagus itself may end in a blind pouch. Neonates with this condition are often identified by excessive drooling or episodes of cyanosis even before the introduction of formula or breast milk. If any newborn presents with these signs or gags and becomes cyanotic during the first feeding, a thorough examination of the upper gastrointestinal tract must be performed to rule out TEF.

A neonate who is breastfed may not receive the preliminary sterile water feeding. The small amount of colostrum obtained during the initial feeding would not constitute a major hazard should aspiration occur. Furthermore, the use of a rubber nipple is strongly discouraged by some experts who believe this may cause nipple confusion for the infant and delay successful initiation of breastfeeding.

Basic rules of safety to be observed during and after feeding should be discussed with the mother. She should be instructed in the use of the bulb syringe to clear the nose and mouth if milk is regurgitated. Proper positioning of the newborn on his or her side after feeding to facilitate drainage and avoid aspiration of milk should also be demonstrated. The nurse should discuss with the mother the dangers of "bottle propping," laying an infant on his or her back with the bottle propped in the mouth. Bottle propping deprives the infant of close physical contact essential for normal growth and development and increases the risk of aspiration. It is particularly important that the nurse stress the danger of aspiration and caution the mother never to leave her infant unattended during a feeding.

Breastfeeding

Ideally, the first episode of breastfeeding should occur in the immediate postbirth period when the infant is in an alert, awake state. The neonate's behavior during and responses to the breastfeeding experience are assessed (NAACOG, 1991a). The critical role of the nurse in promoting successful breastfeeding has led to the development of a position statement by NAACOG (1991b) and is presented in the accompanying display.

Recent research has revealed the significant contribution of the infant to the success of breastfeeding. Each infant will exhibit a pattern of feeding characteristics that shape future nursing interventions and parent teaching. Matthews (1991) found that the higher the neonate scored on a breastfeeding competence scale scored by the mother, the greater was the mother's satisfaction with the infant and the breastfeeding experience.

A tool recently developed to assist the nurse is the Systematic Assessment of the Infant at Breast (Shrago & Bocar, 1990). The instrument consists of four components of infant behavior that influence the success of the breastfeeding experience: alignment, areolar grasp, areolar compression, and audible swallowing. Additional research is required to establish reliability of the instrument and its utility in a variety of birth settings.

Other factors to consider when evaluating the infant's contribution to breastfeeding include physical characteristics that impede success. If any of these problems are identified, the nurse must report them to the physician, midwife, or nurse practitioner. Appropriate referrals should be initiated to provide the woman and infant with appropriate support.

Formula Feeding

The nurse should also assist the mother who is formula feeding with the first feeding. Principles of positioning for comfort are similar to those used for breastfeeding mothers. The mother is usually helped to a sitting position and the infant placed in her arms with the back at approximately a 45-degree angle. She is then guided in eliciting the rooting reflex and placing the nipple well into the neonate's mouth. The bottle is positioned so that the nipple is on the top of the tongue and the nipple and neck of the bottle are always filled with formula. This prevents the infant from swallowing excessive amounts of air.

The amount of formula to be given at the first feeding should be discussed with the mother. Immediately after birth the newborn may take only 20 to 30 mL (1 oz) of formula because of a limited stomach capacity. Burping techniques should be demonstrated. The newborn can be placed in a sitting position with head and neck supported while the back is gently patted and massaged; alternatively, the newborn

NAACOG Position Statement

Issue: Breastfeeding

Background

Breast milk is the ideal food for infants and is the standard against which all commercially prepared formulas are measured. The protein content of breast milk is digested more easily than the protein in infant formulas. The fatty acid and cholesterol content of breast milk is perfectly suited to the development of the infant's central nervous system. In addition, the carbohydrate content of breast milk helps to control the growth of bacteria and improves the absorption of important minerals. Epidemiologic studies have demonstrated that breastfeeding may reduce the incidence of certain bacterial and viral infections and allergic disorders. The immunologic protection provided by human milk cannot be duplicated in commercially prepared formulas. Breastfeeding is economical, is convenient, promotes maternal uterine involution, and promotes synchrony between mother and infant, and may provide maternal protection against the development of breast cancer.

Position

NAACOG recognizes the many benefits of breastfeeding and advocates breastfeeding as the optimal method of infant feeding. NAACOG supports the belief that the public should be informed about the advantages of breastfeeding. Ideally, this information should be shared during pregnancy and in the immediate postpartum period so that the mother can make an informed decision about infant feeding. However, if the mother chooses not to breastfeed, she should be supported in her decision, and appropriate instruction and assistance should be provided. NAACOG maintains that support should be provided regardless of the method of infant feeding that is selected. NAACOG recognizes the unique role of nurses in the provision of patient and family education and support in the initiation and maintenance of lactation. NAACOG encourages nurses to pursue professional educational opportunities regarding the benefits of breastfeeding, the anatomy and physiology of lactation, initiating lactation, managing common problems, using support equipment, nutrition in lactation, drugs in breast milk, and lactation in special circumstances such as relactation and breastfeeding multiples and preterm infants. NAACOG also supports efforts to change employment policies and working conditions to make breastfeeding practical for working mothers. NAACOG supports the belief that the promotion of breastfeeding will contribute to the reduction of infant morbidity and mortality rates. Members may obtain complimentary copies of position statements on AWHONN letterhead from Marsha Shaw, Department of Practice and Health Policy, 1-800-673-8499 (U.S.) or 1-800-245-0231 (Canada), ext. 2435, or collect, 202-863-2435.

Approved by the Executive Board November, 1991.

may be placed against the mother's shoulder or across her lap in a prone position.

All questions should be answered and positive reinforcement and praise given frequently during the feeding. The amount of information given to the mother at this time should be confined to basic instructions so that she is not overwhelmed and can enjoy this special time with her new infant. Instruction regarding methods for sterilization of bottles and nipples when indicated should be planned for subsequent feedings as part of the nurse's discharge teaching (discussed later in this chapter).

Evaluating Satiety—Demand Feeding

A frequent question is "How will I know when my baby has had enough milk?" The concept of demand feeding should be discussed with both breastfeeding and formula-feeding mothers. The normal newborn stops sucking and frequently falls asleep when full and satisfied. The neonate can be expected to wake as often as every 2 hours, especially in the first few days after birth while the lactation process is being established. Breastfeeding is most successful and mothers experience fewer engorgement and nipple problems when they nurse their infants frequently (every 2 to 3 hours).

The formula-fed neonate normally remains satisfied for longer (4 hours or more) than the breastfed newborn because of slower digestion of formula than breast milk. When feeding her neonate, the mother should watch for signs of satiety. The newborn will slowly cease sucking and may actually let his or her mouth drop open slightly or push the nipple forward with his or her tongue. If the newborn is full, small amounts of formula may drool from the corner of the mouth as he or she relaxes and stops sucking. As the infant begins to drift off to sleep, efforts to stimulate further feeding by jiggling or pumping the nipple should be avoided. By the third day of life most full-term neonates are taking 2 to 4 oz (60 to 120 mL) of milk per feeding (Fig. 31-3).

Expected Outcomes

- Mother demonstrates ability to feed newborn by discharge.
- Newborn takes nourishment within 2 to 4 hours of birth.

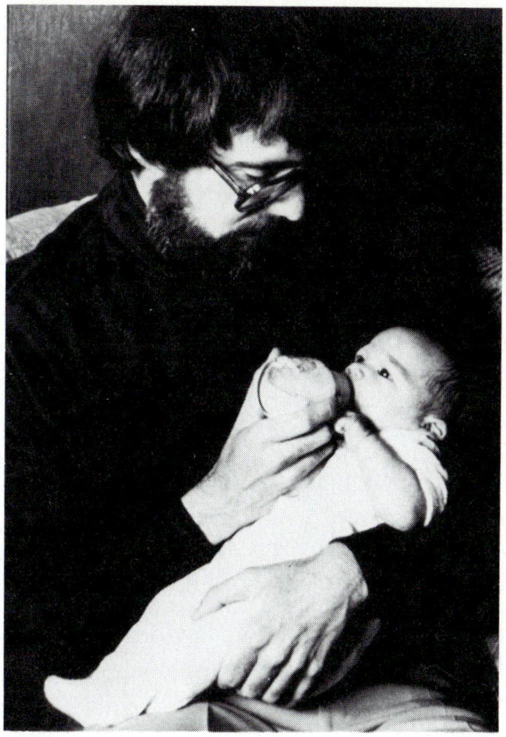

Figure 31-3.
If the newborn is to be bottle fed, the nurse can encourage the father's involvement by assisting him in feeding. (Photo by BABES, Inc.)

Minimizing the Newborn's Risk for Infection

The nurse caring for the neonate is responsible for minimizing the newborn's exposure to pathogenic organisms. Each person coming in contact with the newborn must observe principles of asepsis. *Handwashing is the single most important preventive measure* (see the accompanying display, Recommendations for Handwashing).

Recommendations for Handwashing

Health personnel providing direct infant care should take the following steps:

- Remove all rings, bracelets, and wristwatches, which act as fomites.
- Wash hands, wrists, forearms, and elbows for 2 minutes with an antiseptic preparation.
- Clean fingernails and wash hands again.
- Wash hands for 15 seconds with soap and vigorous scrubbing before and after handling infants or contaminated objects.

Adapted from NAACOG. (1992). Neonatal skin care. *OGN Nursing Practice Resource. Washington, DC: Author.*

Other procedures in addition to handwashing to be followed in the prevention of infection include the following:

- Providing separate supplies for each infant (eg, cotton balls, diapers, blankets)
- Limiting the number of infants placed in the nursery to allow adequate space between cribs (at least 18 inches apart and aisles at least 3 feet wide)
- Limiting the number of personnel who may enter the nursery
- Following established guidelines regarding the restriction of personnel with infections (respiratory tract infections, diarrhea, open wounds, infectious skin rashes, herpesvirus, and other communicable diseases)
- Encouraging frequent and prolonged contact between mother and newborn (eg, rooming-in, skin-to-skin contact, and breastfeeding)
- Teaching handwashing to family members

It is recommended that cover gowns be provided for nonnursing personnel who handle newborns (ie, phlebotomists or other technicians who perform diagnostic tests). However, the practice of having all nursery staff wear cover gowns has been eliminated in most settings (see the accompanying Nursing Research display).

Nursing Research

The Use of Cover Gowns: A Nursery Ritual

The majority of studies have concluded that the risk of transmission of infectious agents to the newborn by the clothing of nurses or the newborn's parents is negligible (less than 2/10,000 newborns). It was also discovered that while the gowning policy is scrupulously adhered to, nursery staff often fail to wash their hands before and after contact with the neonates. Handwashing is the single most important preventive measure in controlling infection.

Further research to confirm preliminary findings regarding gowning policies is required, but it appears appropriate at this time to revise policies regarding who should gown and when. Several medical centers have eliminated the requirement of cover gowns for personnel who enter the well-baby nursery but do not come in direct contact with the neonate. This has resulted in the savings of thousands of dollars per month in gown supplies and laundry costs.

Rush, J., Chiovitti, R., Kaufman, K., & Mitchell, A. (1990). A randomized controlled trial of a nursery ritual: Wearing cover gowns to care for healthy newborns. *Birth, 17*(1), 25.

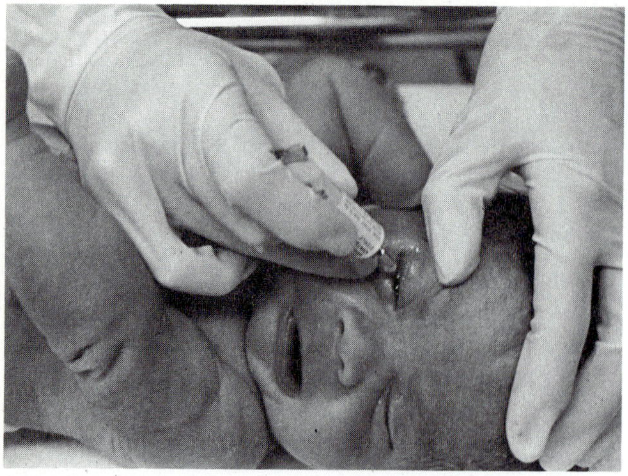

Figure 31-4.
The nurse administers either silver nitrate solution or erthromycin ophthalmic ointment to prevent ocular infection. Administration may be delayed several hours after birth to allow the neonate to see clearly during its first period of reactivity immediately after birth. (Photo by Kathy Sloane. Courtesy of Alta Bates Medical Center.)

Eye Prophylaxis

Before the practice of instilling silver nitrate drops in newborns' eyes, thousands of infants suffered permanent blindness as a result of gonococcal eye infections. *Ophthalmia neonatorum*, a severe ocular infection within the first month of life, may be caused by *Chlamydia trachomatis* (the most common cause of conjunctivitis), *Neisseria gonorrhea*, and less commonly by staphylococci, streptococci, *Escherichia coli*, and other gram-negative bacteria. Today all states require the administration of a prophylactic agent in the eyes of all neonates to prevent infection and blindness (Fig. 31-4). Acceptable agents for prevention and treatment of ophthalmia neonatorum include silver nitrate solution (1%), erythromycin (0.5%) ophthalmic ointment or drops, and tetracycline (1%) ophthalmic ointment or drops.

Silver nitrate solution is a caustic chemical that can cause irritation of ocular mucous membranes and, in a small percentage of cases, a severe conjunctivitis with purulent eye drainage. As a result, many health care facilities have begun using a less irritating erythromycin or tetracycline for eye prophylaxis. Because use of these drugs temporarily interferes with the infant's ability to see clearly, it is recommended that instillation be delayed for 1 to 2 hours after birth to allow the neonate unimpaired eye contact with the parents.

Hepatitis B Vaccination

With the development of an effective vaccine, the serious health and economic consequences of both acute and chronic hepatitis B infection are now preventable. In 1991, the Centers for Disease Control issued new guidelines that recommend the universal vaccination of all infants born in the United States regardless of the hepatitis B surface antigen (HBsAg) status of the mother. The first dose of 0.5 mL vaccine is to be given intramuscularly within 12 hours of birth. Infants born to mothers who are HBsAg positive should concurrently receive 0.5 mL hepatitis B immunoglobulin (HBIG) prophylaxis. The nurse also administers HBIG intramuscularly to the neonate, but at a different site than the vaccine. The second dose of vaccine is administered at 1 month of age and is followed by a final dose when the infant is 6 months old (Centers for Disease Control, 1991).

Cord Care

Another aspect of preventive nursing care is special treatment of the umbilical cord (Fig. 31-5) during the transition period. Many nurseries apply an antibiotic ointment (eg, bacitracin) or an antibacterial solution (such as betadine) to the umbilical cord after birth and each day thereafter to reduce the chance of omphalitis. In birthing units, this practice is frequently abandoned because infection is much less likely to develop in a rooming-in setting than in a central nursery with a large number of newborns.

In most health care facilities, the umbilical cord is swabbed with alcohol at each diaper change to remove urine and stool and to facilitate the desiccation process. The diaper should be folded below the cord to promote air drying.

Although no method of cord care has been proved to effectively prevent omphalitis, there is general agreement that the umbilical area should be kept clean and exposed to air to promote healing and drying (Mugford, Somchiwong, & Waterhouse, 1986).

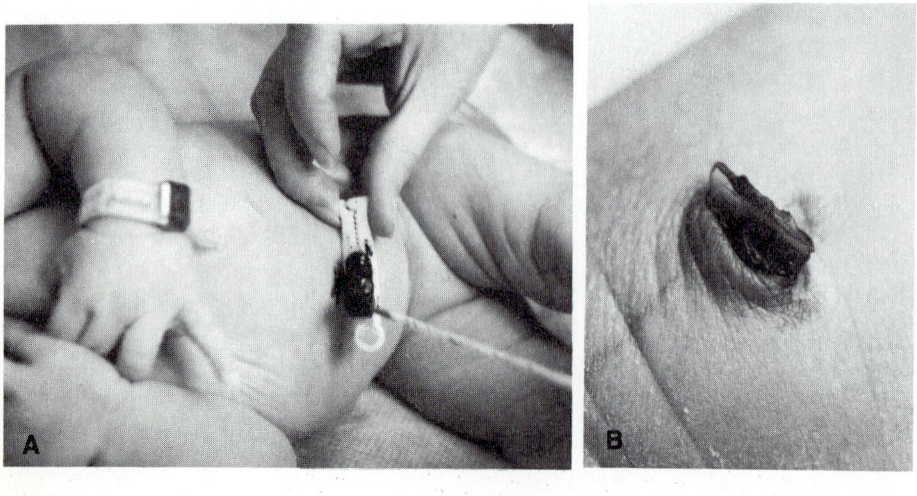

Figure 31-5.
The umbilical cord stump may be painted with antibacterial solution after birth. *A:* Special care must be taken to avoid risk of infection until the clamp has been removed and the cord stump has dried *B* (Childbirth Graphics).

Promoting Parent–Newborn Interaction

Because the infant is awake and particularly alert to visual and auditory stimuli during the first period of reactivity (up to 1 hour after birth), this is an ideal time for the nurse to foster parent–newborn interaction (Fig. 31-6). Eye prophylaxis can be delayed up to 2 hours to enhance the quality of early contact with parents. The new family should be offered privacy but with the understanding that a nurse is close by if needed.

From their studies of early parent–infant interaction and an extensive review of related research, Klaus and Kennell (1982) concluded that the first few hours after birth may be a particularly sensitive period for the formation of bonds between parents and neonate. Subsequent research findings indicate that a sequence of *reciprocal* interactions occur between mother and newborn, which "lock" them together and ensure the further development of attachment. Of critical importance is the newborn's role in this process. The infant's contribution to interactions is based on neurobehavioral capacities and is altered by the physical status at birth. Vocalizations and cry, soothability, state control, habituation, "cuddliness"—all components of newborn temperament—strongly influence the parent's continued desire to initiate and participate in ongoing interactions (Green & Bax, 1989).

Certain types of nursing interventions may facilitate the formation of these ties. Encouraging skin-to-skin contact between mother and infant immediately after birth may enhance the quality of early interaction and can be combined with breastfeeding if the mother plans to breastfeed. The nurse reduces environmental stimuli so that parents and infant can focus on this first encounter without distraction. Dimming lights and delaying the instillation of eye ointment for neonatal prophylaxis of gonorrheal or chlamydial conjunctivitis encourages the neonate to open its eyes and make eye contact with parents. Health professionals should reassure concerned parents who do not have an opportunity for early contact that newborns are adaptable and that the parent–infant relationship evolves over time as a result of repeated, mutually satisfying encounters.

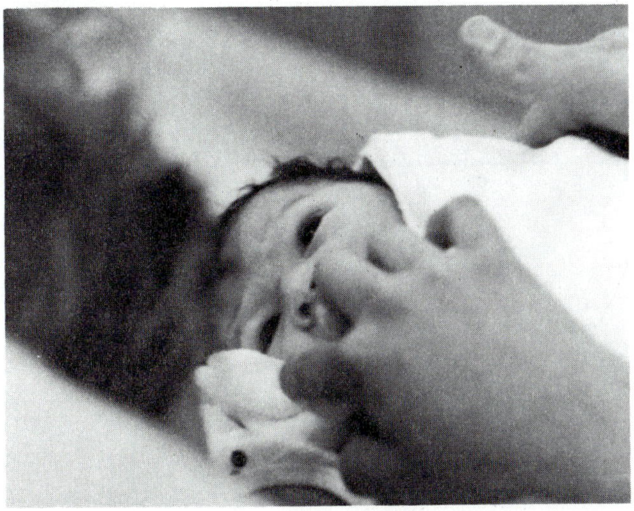

Figure 31-6.

An alert newborn sucks on his mother's finger and gazes at her face only minutes after delivery. The nurse should facilitate this type of close contact in the first hour of life as the parents wish and as the newborn's condition allows. (Photo by BABES, Inc.)

Once the neonate's condition is stabilized, the nurse should provide the parents and their newborn with further opportunities to become acquainted; for example, rooming-in or extended periods of contact during the day can be encouraged. Norr and associates (1988) found that economically disadvantaged women who experienced rooming-in scored higher on maternal attachment scores.

An important nursing activity that promotes the parent–newborn attachment process is teaching about newborn characteristics and each neonate's unique capabilities. An excellent strategy is to have the parents present when the neonate is examined by the nurse practitioner or pediatrician. Parents can also be invited to observe the Brazelton Neonatal Behavioral Assessment of their neonate if it is done in the nursery. Nursing research indicates that teaching parents about the neonate's unique behaviors makes a positive difference in sensitivity to the newborn's cues and responses to the infant's distress signals (Tedder, 1991). Including the father in teaching activities has also been shown to influence future paternal-infant interactions (Beal, 1989).

Instructing parents in infant care tasks is another nursing intervention used to foster attachment. As much infant care as possible should be done at the mother's bedside to increase opportunities for teaching and reinforcement of parenting skills. Using principles of adult learning, the nurse begins with simple tasks that can be easily accomplished by new parents and moves on to more complex activities as the parents gain confidence in their ability to care for the newborn. The subjects of cord care and diaper changing thus precede taking and reading the infant's temperature or bathing the infant. The nurse who is expert in handling and caring for newborns must be especially patient with first-time parents and avoid taking over when parents are slow and uncertain. Positive reinforcement is offered to enhance the parents' sense of competency in new infant care tasks. Parent–neonate interactions should be observed and significant findings recorded in the newborn's chart. Nursing documentation forms the basis for appropriate referrals and follow-up after the family is discharged from the hospital or birthing center.

Expected Outcome

- Newborn and parents demonstrate interaction as evidenced by touching, eye contact, and responding to each other.

Monitoring for and Preventing Complications

Optimum physiologic adaptation to extrauterine life is the primary goal of the transitional period. The nurse has the responsibility of monitoring the newborn for potential complications. In addition to recognizing complications related to dysfunction in the pulmonary and cardiac systems and in thermoregulation described in the previous section, the nurse caring for the normal neonate during the transition period is responsible for monitoring and preventing, as far as possible, complications.

Potential Complication: Polycythemia

Many nurseries obtain a heel stick capillary blood sample for hematocrit determination. The accompanying Nursing Procedure describes the appropriate site and procedure for the heel stick.

The normal neonatal hematocrit range is 45% to 65%. A hematocrit above 65% to 70% may be indicative of polycythemia. A venous blood sample is obtained in this instance to confirm the diagnosis of true polycythemia, defined as a central hematocrit value greater than 65%.

Potential Complication: Hypoglycemia

Because the newborn's brain is almost entirely dependent on glucose for its metabolic functioning, early detection of hypoglycemia is essential for prevention of neurologic impairment and injury. *Hypoglycemia* is defined as a blood glucose level under 30 mg/dL whole blood during the first 72 hours of life in the full-term neonate. In many facilities, a heel stick blood sample is routinely obtained to screen blood glucose concentrations within the first 4 hours of birth. In many birthing centers with low-risk neonates, blood glucose sampling is only performed when indicated by the development of signs of hypoglycemia (jitteriness, lethargy, or temperature instability) or when existing conditions predispose the neonate to low glucose levels (low or high birth weight, asphyxia, respiratory distress, newborn of a diabetic mother). A glucose-sensitive strip is saturated with a drop of blood (see heel stick procedure) and after a specified period of time is visually read or is determined by using a portable glucose analyzer. If the blood glucose level is less than 40 to 45 mg/dL, a venous sample is drawn to confirm the finding.

Early feeding and prevention of cold stress reduce the risk of hypoglycemia. Immediate intervention is necessary when hypoglycemia is diagnosed to prevent depression of vital functions controlled by the CNS. Seizures and apnea are potential complications of untreated hypoglycemia. Treatment is initiated when the blood glucose is less than 40 to 45 mg/dL. Treatment may consist of 5% glucose in water or formula feedings (oral or gavage) if the neonate's condition is stable, or a slowly administered IV bolus of 10% to 25% glucose followed by administration of a continuous IV infusion of 10% glucose until blood glucose levels are stabilized. Further discussion about hypoglycemia can be found in Chapter 33.

Potential Complication: Hemorrhage

Because intrauterine circulating stores of vitamin K are depleted and enteric production is still low at birth, the neonate experiences a transient deficiency in the vitamin. This places the newborn at risk for hemorrhage from 2 to 5 days after birth, with bleeding problems most common on the second or third day of life. To prevent bleeding, a 0.5- to 1-mg dose of vitamin K (phytonadione) is administered intramuscularly after birth. The vastus lateralis or rectus muscle of the anterior thigh is the preferred site of injection, as shown in Figure 31-7.

• • Evaluation

The nurse is responsible for the ongoing evaluation of the appropriateness and effectiveness of transitional care during the neonate's adaptation to extrauterine life. Many units have standards of care to which the nurse is accountable in determining a neonate's readiness for transfer to the mother's room or central nursery. Such evaluation criteria include the following: absence of signs of respiratory distress; evidence of adequate thermoregulation; absence of signs of infection, hypoglycemia, or hyperbilirubinemia (including completion of laboratory work, as ordered); administration of prophylactic antibiotics and vitamin K, as ordered; and provision of support for early parent–neonate interaction. When these criteria are met, the nurse implements the plan for daily care of the newborn awaiting discharge.

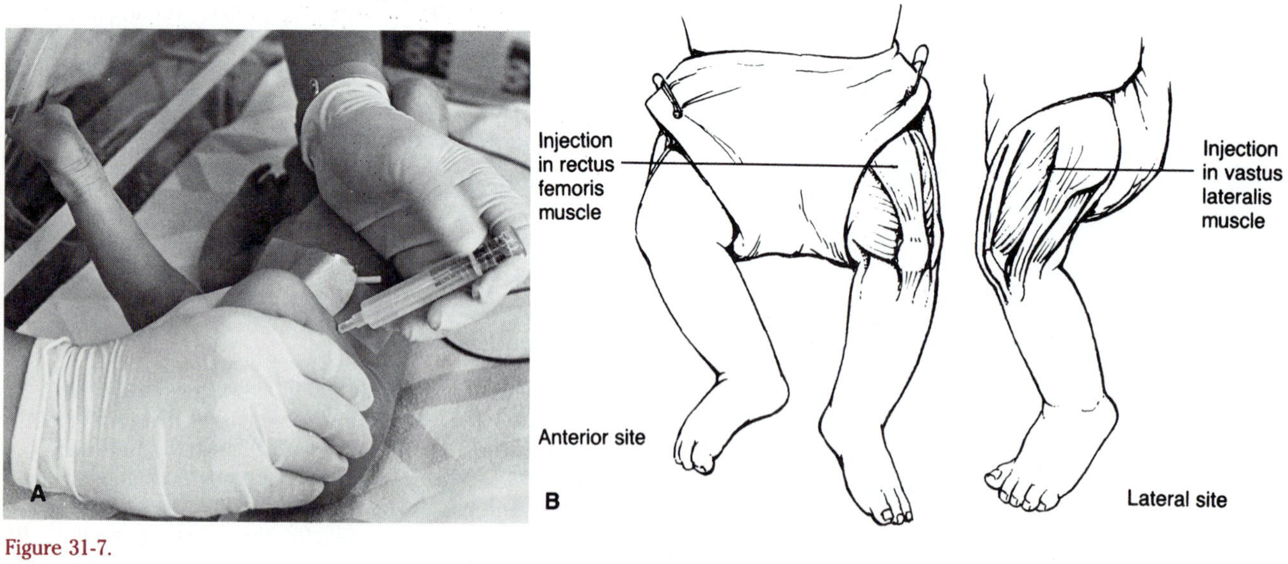

Figure 31-7.

A: Intramuscular injection of vitamin K prevents excessive bleeding in the neonatal period when endogenous production of the vitamin is still low. *B:* Sites for intramuscular injection in neonates (Childbirth Graphics).

NURSING PROCEDURE
Performing a Heel Stick Procedure

Purpose: To obtain a capillary blood sample. This permits avoidance of the more invasive venipuncture procedure, which increases the risk of infection.

NURSING ACTION	***RATIONALE***
1. Warm neonate's heel for about 10 minutes, using a warm, moist wrap or a specially designed chemical heat pad.*	To facilitate blood flow to the surface of the neonate's skin and promote blood flow when the puncture is made
2. Stabilize the neonate's foot by placing your thumb behind the heel and dorsiflexing the foot against the shin.	To prevent the infant from a reflex withdrawal from painful stimuli, which could result in laceration of the foot or ineffective puncture

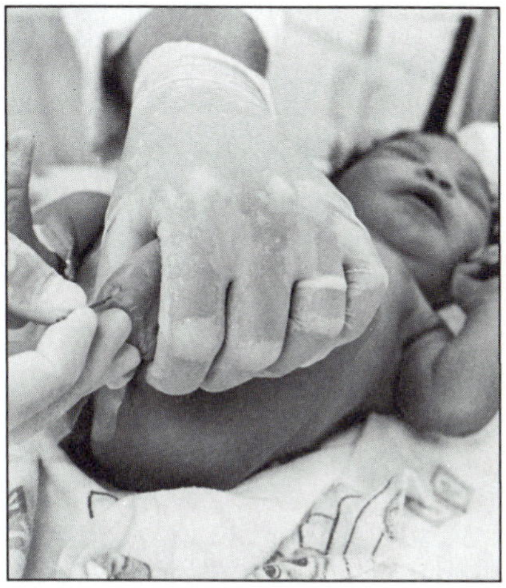

Step 2. Stabilizing the neonate's foot.

3. Circle the heel stick site firmly with hand but do not squeeze.	To prevent dilution of the sample with interstitial fluid
4. Cleanse selected heel stick site with alcohol and blot dry with sterile gauze. The best site is the lateral aspect of the heel, but the medial aspect of the heel is also acceptable.	To prevent infection To prevent stinging at puncture site

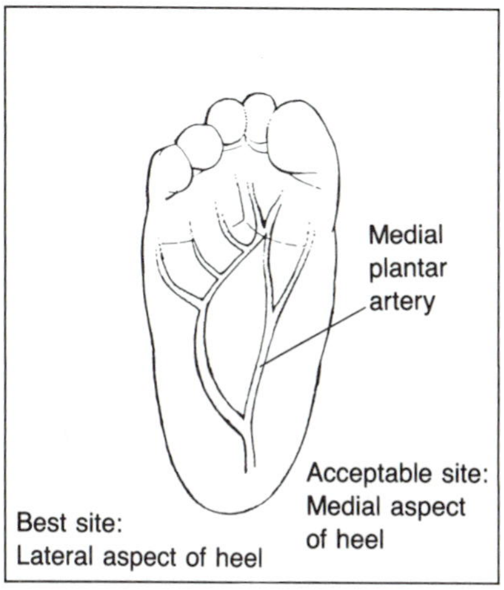

Step 4. Best sites for heel stick.

5. Using microlancet (pediatric size), puncture skin with one quick downward movement toward the heel.	To achieve a clean incision and minimize tissue trauma

NURSING PROCEDURE
Performing a Heel Stick Procedure (continued)

NURSING ACTION	*RATIONALE*
6. Allow small drops of blood to form and then wipe away with sterile gauze.	To remove skin cells from puncture site
7. Allow second large drop to form (avoid squeezing) and fall onto the glucose-sensitive strip.	
8. Follow manufacturer's direction for timing of test and interpretation of results.	To determine correct results

**Severe burns have occurred when plastic diapers have been saturated with water and heated in a microwave oven before application to the heel. If a chemical heat pad is not available,* do not microwave *moist compresses. Use warm tap water only when applying moist compresses to the neonate's foot.*

Photo by Childbirth Graphics.

The neonatal transition period is characterized by rapid alterations in the newborn's condition. Dramatic changes in cardiac and pulmonary function require supportive nursing care during this postbirth period. The neonatal nurse must be alert to the development of common problems such as airway obstruction, hypothermia, and hypoglycemia. Swift action is often required, and the nurse must be skilled in performing basic life-support functions as well as routine infant care activities. A major goal is the promotion of family-centered maternity care, while monitoring the neonate for complications that can occur at this time. Support of breastfeeding and early parent–newborn interaction aid in creating a family-centered environment. Respect for other family preferences and cultural practices will also greatly enhance the early postnatal experience for the expanding family.

Ongoing Neonatal Care

The internal regulatory mechanisms of normal neonates are able to maintain physiologic adaptations made in the first hours of life with little if any support from caregivers. Neonates begin to eat, sleep, and eliminate wastes with amazing regularity, and a watchful observer can see an impressive range of newborn reflexes demonstrated throughout the day, including rooting, sucking, sneezing, blinking, and the fencing and Moro reflexes.

• • Assessment

The nurse continues to evaluate the neonate periodically throughout the day, monitoring vital signs, fluid and caloric intake, elimination patterns, and weight gain or loss. Most institutions use a combination flow sheet–graphic record to note neonatal parameters of healthy adaptation. In addition, the newborn is observed for evidence of the development of regular behavioral patterns (feeding, sleeping, and elimination) and for indications of temperament. Table 31-2 describes the standard of care for assessment of neonatal vital signs.

• • Nursing Diagnosis

Ongoing nursing care of the normal neonate focuses on supporting ongoing physiologic and behavioral adaptations as well as monitoring and supporting the neonate during procedures that may be done before discharge. The following nursing diagnoses reflect priorities useful in directing care:

Table 31-2. Standard of Care for Assessment of the Vital Signs in the Normal Neonate

	Transition Period (Birth to 4 h)	First Postnatal Day (4–24 h)*	Second Postnatal Day (24–48 h)†
Temperature	q 30–60 min	q 8 h	q 8–12 h
Respirations	q 30–60 min	q 8 h	q 8–12 h
Apical pulse	q 30–60 min	q 8 h	q 8–12 h

*Many low-risk newborns are discharged from the hospital or birthing center by the end of the first postnatal day.
†In many units, the 24-h day is divided into two 12-h shifts. Vital signs are taken once on each shift by the primary nurse.

- Fluid Volume Deficit related to decreased oral intake
- Altered Nutrition: Less than Body Requirements related to decreased intake of formula or breast milk
- Altered Nutrition: Less than Body Requirements related to diminished sucking
- Diarrhea related to infection or formula imbalance
- Impaired Skin Integrity related to susceptibility to nosocomial infection secondary to lack of normal skin flora
- High Risk for Infection related to vulnerability of infant, lack of normal flora, or open wound (umbilical cord or circumcision)
- Altered Health Maintenance related to insufficient parental knowledge of infant care skills
- Ineffective Breastfeeding related to lack of knowledge
- Altered Parenting related to change in family unit or new infant
- Health Seeking Behaviors related to parents' desire to learn about neonatal care
- Ineffective Thermoregulation related to limited shivering ability or fluctuating environmental temperatures

Although the newborn may be normal in all aspects, monitoring for and preventing potential complications remains a priority in care. Potential complications or collaborative problems for which the nurse monitors are hypothermia, hypoglycemia, infection, maladaptation of other body systems, phenylketonuria (PKU) or other inborn errors in metabolism, and congenital hypothyroidism.

• • Planning and Implementation

The nurse implements a plan of ongoing care for the normal neonate, recognizing that discharge may occur as soon as 6 hours after birth. Furthermore, because the neonate will ideally spend much of that time with the parents, the nurse must plan care to include ongoing assessment of the neonate's status, involvement of parents in care, and discharge teaching. Plans must also be initiated at this time if home follow-up is desirable. A written discharge plan is completed as necessary.

Promoting Hydration and Nutrition

The neonate is weighed at the same time each day, usually in the morning before an early feeding, so that an accurate estimate of weight gain or loss can be made. All clothing and the diaper are removed before the newborn is weighed, and lightweight barrier paper (scale paper) is placed between the newborn and the scale to prevent cross-contamination. The nurse must be careful to keep one hand just above the neonate during the weighing process to prevent an accidental fall.

The neonate can be expected to lose between 5% and 10% of its body weight in water during the first 4 to 5 days of life. A 1-oz or 30-g weight gain should occur each day thereafter if the newborn ingests a sufficient amount of fluids and calories. Daily caloric requirements for the neonate are approximately 115 to 120 kcal/kg body weight per 24 hours. Daily water requirements are approximately 105 mL (3.5 oz)/kg body weight per 24 hours. Parents should be reassured that the initial weight loss is normal; a mother who is breastfeeding for the first time may be concerned that she does not have sufficient breast milk.

Careful monitoring of the neonate's fluid and caloric intake will assure both nurse and parents that the infant is healthy and receiving adequate nutrients. A formula-fed infant can be expected to take between 2 and 4 oz (60 to 120 mL) of formula every 3 to 4 hours in a 24-hour period for a total of approximately 24 oz (720 mL)/day.

The breastfed infant will nurse vigorously for 15 to 20 minutes and then will fall asleep for 2 to 3 hours. Both breastfed and formula-fed newborns should produce six to eight wet diapers per day after the first 24 to 48 hours of life, have normal skin turgor, and moist mucous membranes. If the physician or nurse practitioner is concerned about whether the fluid intake of a breastfed infant is adequate, the newborn can be weighed before and after each feeding, in which case the diapers should also be weighed.

Expected Outcome

- Newborn regains birth weight by 7 to 14 days of life.

Promoting Normal Elimination Patterns

Newborns demonstrate a wide variation in elimination patterns during the first few days after birth. Urine output slowly increases with increasing fluid intake so that by the end of the first week of life, a neonate may void as frequently as 20 or 30 times a day. Parents are often amazed by the number of wet diapers they discover. However, as noted, six to eight wet diapers per 24-hour period indicates adequate hydration.

Stool patterns also vary, depending on the type and frequency of feeding and amount taken. The thick, greenish black, viscous meconium stool slowly gives way to the yellowish green transitional stool within 2 to 3 days of birth. Some infants pass very large stools with much force and vocalization after each feeding, soiling themselves and their clothes from head to toe. Others pass few stools initially and show a slower, more gradual change to formula or breastfed stools after 3 or 4 days. New parents may be initially alarmed by their infant's redness and the straining that accompanies passage of stool and need reassurance that this is normal.

The nurse monitors the neonate closely for the passage of the first stool, which normally occurs within the first 24 to 48 hours of life. The absence of stools, or the presence of only small stool streaks on the diaper, may indicate intestinal blockage. If there is no evidence of meconium passage by 24 hours of age, the physician, midwife, or nurse practitioner should be notified and close attention paid to bowel sounds, abdominal girth, and contour. The passage of blood or mucus in the stool is abnormal. Diarrhea, which can result from bacterial infection or formula intolerance, is an extremely dangerous sign in the neonate because it can lead to rapid depletion of fluid and electrolytes. Whenever diarrhea occurs, all diapers should be weighed to determine the extent of fluid loss. The newborn should be placed under isolation precautions as well until infection is eliminated as a cause of the diarrhea.

Expected Outcome

- Newborn demonstrates urinary and bowel elimination patterns within normal limits for mode of feeding.

Maintaining Skin and Mucous Membrane Integrity

The skin serves as a major barrier against the entry of pathogenic organisms. Any disruption in the skin may predispose the neonate to infection. The nurse inspects the skin daily for evidence of erythema, excoriation, or rash. Although a sponge bath may be given, cleansing soiled areas with warm water and drying the skin thoroughly is usually adequate to meet the infant's hygiene needs during the first few days of life. The parent teaching section of this chapter has an in-depth description of infant bathing.

Occasionally, skin lacerations are noted at birth secondary to the insertion of a fetal scalp electrode or capillary blood sampling from the fetal scalp during labor. These areas should be inspected frequently for evidence of edema, erythema, or prurulent discharge. The primary health care provider may order the application of a topical antibiotic ointment to reduce the risk of infection.

The eyes are assessed for evidence of redness or prurulent discharge, common signs of conjunctivitis. The administration of erythromycin or tetracycline ophthalmic ointment is the first line of defense against conjunctivitis. Scrupulous handwashing before touching or examining the infant reduces the risk of iatrogenic eye infection. The oral mucous membranes are examined for neonatal thrush (patchy white, adherent lesions on the gums or tongue), which is due to a *Candida albicans* infection. A topical antifungal agent is ordered if oral candidiasis occurs.

The umbilical cord and surrounding skin are examined with each diaper change. The base of the cord should be assessed for evidence of omphalitis (edema, erythema, and prurulent discharge). Once the umbilical cord is cut and clamped, thrombosis of the vessels ensues. Desiccation (drying) of the cord stump occurs and by 24 hours of age, the cord clamp can be removed in most neonates. Occasionally, the cord will decompose and detach through a process known as moist gangrene. Proteolytic decomposition of the cord occurs by bacterial action. The cord remains soft, moist, and may have a foul odor. It is distinguished from omphalitis by the absence of erythema or prurulent discharge at the base of the cord. If the cord remains moist after 24 hours the nurse should report this condition. The primary health care provider may order a culture of the umbilical area to rule out infection.

The nurse can support the desiccation process and prevent infection by folding the front of the diaper down below the cord to permit circulation of air around the umbilical area. The cord stump and base of the cord are wiped with 70% isopropyl alcohol with each diaper change to cleanse the area and promote drying. (See a further discussion of cord care later in this chapter.)

The genitalia, anal area, and buttocks are assessed for evidence of redness, erythematous macular rash, or skin breakdown. Diaper rash (diaper dermatitis) is less commonly observed by the nurse with the growing trend for early discharge. When the neonate remains in the hospital beyond 24 hours, for example after cesarean birth, diaper dermatitis may be identified. Skin irritation can develop within 2 to 3 days of birth as the neonate begins to void and pass stool with regularity. Frequent diaper change, exposure to air after meticulous cleansing of the skin, and the application of a barrier ointment such as A and D ointment or zinc oxide are effective for the prevention or treatment of diaper rash.

Expected Outcome

- The neonate's skin and mucous membranes remain intact and free of infection or irritation.

Legal/Ethical Considerations

Role of the Nurse in the Parental Decision Regarding Circumcision

Nurses have a moral obligation to promote the physical and psychologic well-being of the neonate. A growing ethical dilemma for many clinicians centers around the issue of circumcision. Researchers have discovered altered sleep patterns and circadian rhythms in circumcised infants. Recognition of the infant's ability to perceive pain and evidence in some newborns of posttraumatic behaviors further support arguments against circumcision. Finally, each year a small percentage of newborns suffer major complications from this procedure, including infection, hemorrhage, permanent disfigurement of the penis, and in rare instances even death.

Another moral principle observed by nurses is that infants have rights but cannot speak for themselves. What would they choose? When the parents' choice is motivated by religious convictions, nurses may feel less conflict but in other circumstances to what extent should the nurse be involved in the decision-making process? An early study found that comprehensive disclosure of circumcision risks precipitated a crisis in parental confidence regarding their decision to permit the procedure and created dissatisfaction with their physician's behavior (Christensen-Szalanski, 1987).

It is the responsibility of the practitioner to fully inform parents, answer all questions, and provide them with all available resources in making their decision. Finally, the nurse must respect and support the parents' ultimate decision.

A nurse who strongly opposes circumcision, with the support of professional organizations, can educate parents and physicians and can attempt to influence legislators and insurance companies to reduce or eliminate financial reimbursement for circumcisions.

Christensen-Szalanski, J., Boyce, T., Harrell, H., & Gardner, M. (1987). Circumcision and informed consent. Medical Care, *25(9), 856.*

Care of the Circumcised Male

A common focus is skin care of the male neonate after circumcision, which is the surgical removal of the foreskin of the penis (Fig. 31-8). The procedure has its origins in religious tradition or the cultural practice of rite of passage to manhood. It is more common in certain socioeconomic, ethnic, and religious groups. Jews and Muslims are circumcised after birth for religious reasons. The procedure is less common among the poor and Hispanic Americans (Poland, 1990). The practice of routine circumcision in United States hospitals is based on commonly held beliefs about penile hygiene and the relationship between the uncircumcised penis and a variety of diseases. Many parents choose circumcision when the father has been circumcised so that the male child's penis will "look like daddy's."

In 1989 the American Academy of Pediatrics' Task Force on Circumcision reviewed all research literature on this issue and published a new position statement. Circumcision has potential medical benefits and advantages as well as disadvantages and risks. It prevents phimosis, paraphimosis, and balanoposthitis; reduces the risk of cancer of the penis; and reduces urinary tract infections in infants. It has been suggested that uncircumcised men exposed to HIV during heterosexual intercourse appear more susceptible to infection (Simonsen, 1988; Cameron, 1989).

One in 500 infants has complications related to circumcision including bleeding, infection, and although very rare, death. Gangrene of the penis, sloughing of the skin surrounding the surgical site, and accidental removal of a part of the penis have been reported (Tedder, 1989). Research has demonstrated adverse physiologic responses in neonates who were circumcised, including agitation and changes in sleep patterns and serum cortisol levels (NAACOG, 1985).

Although fewer parents request elective circumcision today than in the past, more than 60% of all male newborns in the United States are still circumcised. Although the process of obtaining informed consent remains a responsibility of the primary health care provider, the nurse often plays a role in the decision-making process. The nurse is often asked about circumcision by parents and may contribute to the discussion and debate about this issue when teaching prenatal classes for expectant parents. It is essential that the nurse possess accurate and current information about this procedure and be able to discuss the benefits and risks in a nonjudgmental manner. Parents can then make a final decision without undue distress or guilt.

Circumcision Methods. Two methods are commonly used for circumcision: Gomco clamp and Plastibell. They are briefly described here.

In the *Gomco (Yaellen) clamp method*, the adherent prepuce is separated from the glans with a surgical probe. The prepuce is then stretched and drawn over a metal cone, and a clamp is applied with sufficient pressure to ligate blood vessels and prevent bleeding. After 3 to 5 minutes the prepuce above the clamp is removed with a surgical scalpel.

In the *Plastibell method*, the prepuce is separated from the glans and the Plastibell is positioned over the glans. Next a suture is tied around the prepuce at the rim of the Plastibell, and the prepuce above the area of ligation is then removed with a scalpel. The plastic rim of the bell remains in place 2 to 3 days and falls off with healing of the tissues.

Assisting at the Procedure. The neonate who is to be circumcised is not fed for 2 to 4 hours before surgery to reduce the risk of vomiting and aspiration during the procedure. The nurse must verify that the consent form has been signed before preparing the newborn for circumcision. In many facilities, the nurse witnesses the signing of the consent form and may be asked to clarify specific aspects regarding the procedure and recovery process. The nurse prepares the neonate for the procedure, assists the physician, assesses the neonate during the procedure, and supports the neonate afterward.

Usually the nurse is responsible for positioning the newborn on a specially designed molded plastic board (circumcision board), where the limbs are restrained (Fig. 31-9). Care is taken to prevent cold stress during the procedure.

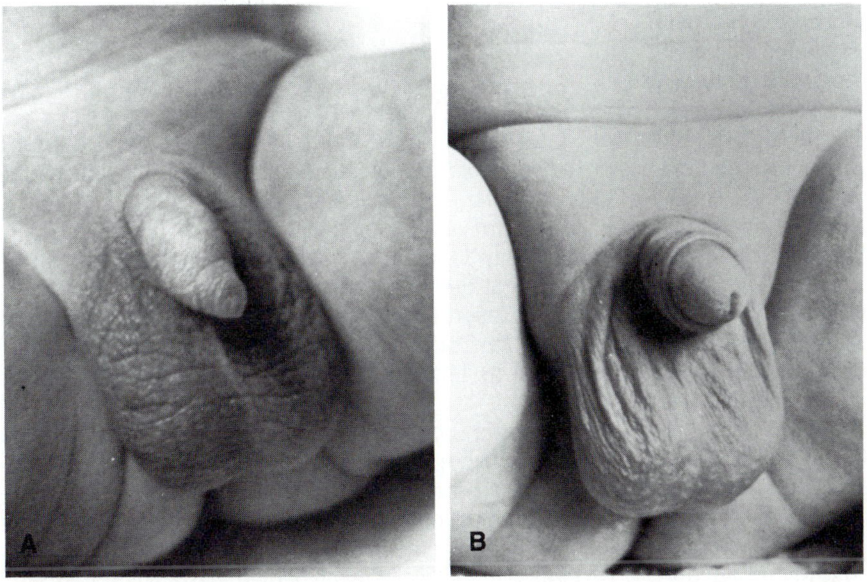

Figure 31-8.
A: Uncircumcised male neonate. *B:* Circumcised neonate. (Childbirth Graphics.)

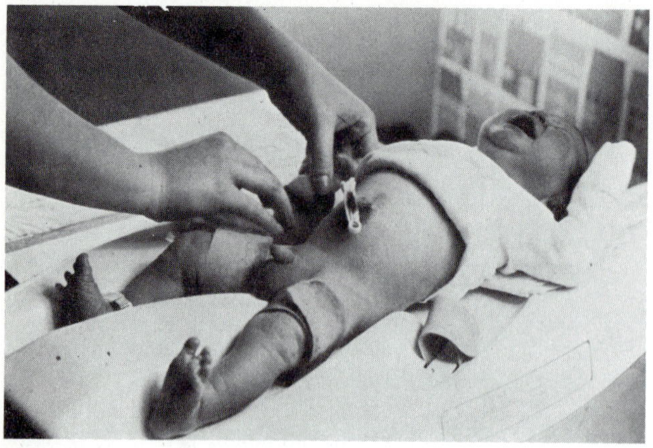

Figure 31-9.
The neonate is restrained in a specially designed circumcision board during the procedure (Childbirth Graphics).

Warm blankets can be placed on the cool plastic surface of the circumcision board before securing the neonate to it, or a radiant warmer can be placed over the neonate during the procedure. The nurse assists the physician by preparing equipment and placing necessary supplies on the circumcision tray.

Nursing diagnoses that might result from the circumcision procedure are:

- High Risk for Infection related to disruption of the skin at the incision site
- Pain related to the surgical procedure and tissue edema
- Altered Urinary Elimination Pattern related to tissue edema or clot formation at meatal opening

Hemorrhage is a potential complication.

The nurse is responsible for promoting comfort and reducing pain during and after the procedure. Current guidelines from the United States Department of Health and Human Services (1992) state that the obligation to manage pain and relieve an infant's suffering is a crucial element of a health professional's commitment to health care. Circumcision is still performed without the benefit of anesthesia in most settings. A belief that neonates cannot experience pain and concerns about the complications associated with analgesia and anesthesia have resulted in this practice. However, research findings indicate that neonates can and do experience pain and that pain has many negative physiologic and behavioral effects. These data have led to new suggestions for pain control during circumcision.

Traditionally, the neonate has been soothed by use of a pacifier or strokes on his cheek. However, Marchette and associates (1991) and Marrone (1990) found no significant effect of nonnutritive sucking on the neonate's pain level (measured by physiologic variables). More effective methods are now being studied. The benefits of offering the infant a sucrose-flavored pacifier during circumcision was investigated by Blass and Hoffmeyer (1991). Crying was reduced by 49% when infants were allowed to suck on a nipple into which a sucrose-saturated gauze pad was placed. Dorsal penile nerve block with 1% lidocaine for relief of pain during circumcision has reduced evidence of physiologic stress and behavioral changes associated with the pain during circumcision (Arnett, Jones, & Horger, 1990; Marrone, 1990). Administration of a penile block may become a common practice if it is found to be a safe, effective method of pain control. After the circumcision, parents should be encouraged to support and comfort the newborn by holding and rocking him and by offering him the mother's breast or formula.

The nurse monitors the neonate for complications related to circumcision. Postoperative checks for bleeding and hemorrhage are performed by the nurse every 15 minutes for the first hour and then every 30 minutes for the next 3 to 4 hours. The first voiding is also noted. Petroleum jelly gauze may be applied to the glans when the foreskin is removed to prevent soiling and trauma at the surgical site. It is replaced by clean gauze and a liberal amount of petroleum jelly with each diaper change.

Expected Outcomes

- Neonate remains free of complications related to the circumcision procedure.
- Neonate urinates within 4 to 6 hours after the circumcision.
- Neonate demonstrates physiologic and behavioral signs of decreased pain sensation after implementation of pain control techniques.

Promoting Behavioral Adaptation

The nurse plans and implements care that supports behavioral adaptations in the neonate. The establishment of circadian rhythm can be fostered by simulating the cycle of darkness and light experienced during a 24-hour day. Rooming-in is one strategy to support the development of a diurnal pattern; reducing light intensity at night if the infant remains in the nursery is another. The nurse avoids disturbing the neonate during periods of deep sleep whenever possible, and fosters parent–newborn interactions when the neonate is in the quiet, alert state.

Expected Outcomes

- Neonate initiates a circadian rhythm and diurnal pattern.
- Neonate makes smooth transitions between behavioral states.

Obtaining Newborn Screening Tests

Most states require that all infants be screened for the presence of PKU before being discharged from the hospital. PKU is an inborn error of metabolism in which the infant is unable to metabolize phenylalanine, an amino acid common in many foods. If an infant with PKU is fed normally, a biochemical buildup leads to progressive mental retardation. If the disorder is diagnosed by a simple blood test done shortly after birth, brain damage and retardation can be prevented by limiting the amount of phenylalanine in the diet.

The newborn must have 2 to 3 days of milk or formula ingestion before the blood sample for the serum phenylalanine screening test is obtained. If initial feeding of the neonate has been delayed or early discharge is planned for the infant, arrangements must be made for the PKU test to be performed in a clinic or in the pediatrician's office after 3 full days of milk feedings. Performance of the screening test before adequate amounts of milk have been ingested may lead to a false-negative test result.

When the PKU screening is done, the newborn can also be tested for other inborn errors of metabolism, including galactosemia, maple syrup urine disease, and homocystinuria. Because congenital hypothyroidism occurs with greater frequency than PKU and can also lead to permanent neurologic impairment, many states now require that neonates also be screened for this disorder.

Expected Outcome

- Newborn continues to make physiologic and behavioral adaptations.

Promoting Health Maintenance Through Discharge Teaching

Responsible neonatal nursing care involves the creation and implementation of an individualized discharge teaching plan that will prepare parents to meet the physical and emotional needs of their newborn when they return home. Discharge planning is initiated in the traditional hospital setting when the neonate is admitted to the newborn unit. It is completed by the traditional discharge date 24 to 48 hours after delivery. In birthing units where early discharge (6 to 24 hours after birth) is possible, discharge teaching is initiated in the unit but completed in the community during follow-up care of the family.

Individualized Education

Nursing research supports the need for individualized teaching. The first step in this process is to determine the parent's level of knowledge regarding infant characteristics, behavior, and caretaking activities, and to identify their primary concerns. The nurse must also determine the educational level and primary language of the new family. Fifty-five percent of American adults are either functionally or marginally illiterate (read or write at fourth or fifth grade level). In a recent study by DeFlorio (1991) less than half the terms commonly used by nurses in teaching parents were correctly explained by the new mothers.

The nurse also evaluates the mother's sense of competence in performing infant care skills. Studies indicate that a woman's level of confidence will influence the time required to attempt and master newborn care activities. Anxiety and poor self-esteem interfere with the learning process. Furthermore, observing a skillful nurse's effortless performance can weaken the new mother's sense of confidence (Froman & Owen, 1990).

Having parents assume an increasingly large share of the care is the nurse's ultimate goal. By discharge the parents should feel comfortable with their newborn, be aware of the newborn's capabilities and limitations, and be able to meet the basic physical and emotional needs. The new mother's tentative efforts at infant care should be encouraged, and positive reinforcement should be given frequently. The nurse should refrain from "taking over" if parents are having difficulty completing care tasks. Rather they should be guided in appropriate techniques to successfully master the activity. Written material given to parents should be age appropriate (ie, in the case of an adolescent mother) and at a reading level that matches their abilities. Simple diagrams, audiovisual aids, and verbal instructions are given when the woman is unable to read (Barnes, 1992).

However, the mother who has several children may wish to spend more time resting and simply enjoying her newborn. She will not be anxious to be shown skills with which she is already familiar. Nursing staff should recognize and respect her desire for assistance with the routine day-to-day care of the neonate and help her enjoy a short reprieve from her busy routine at home.

The neonatal nurse will inevitably encounter parents who are unreceptive to information about infant care and safety. This may present the clinician with an ethical dilemma: patient autonomy versus the professional nurse's responsibility to promote health and safety. After the nurse completes a comprehensive assessment, the individual's right to autonomy may be overridden if the nurse concludes that the neonate is at risk for injury or abuse. This decision must be supported by objective documentation that can withstand the scrutiny of representatives of the legal system. The nurse must discuss concerns with the primary health care provider. A referral for evaluation and follow-up (social service, psychiatric service, or public health nurse) should be made as soon as possible.

Discharge Planning

Family-centered maternity care guides the nurse in development of the teaching plan. The nurse should attempt to identify the family member or support person who will be providing neonatal care. In many cultures, such as traditional Chinese, women living in extended families are encouraged to rest for a specified period of time and allow others to care for the newborn.

The father or partner should be included as much as possible in demonstrations of neonatal care skills and discharge teaching sessions. Men's attitudes toward fathering have changed, but the extent of participation varies by age, ethnic background, and socioeconomic status. The father's involvement is also determined in part by the mother's attitudes about parenting roles. In a recent study, Beal (1989) discovered that fathers who were allowed to observe the Brazelton Neonatal Behavioral Assessment Scale performed on their newborns demonstrated a higher quality of interaction with the infant at 8 weeks postnatally.

Although nurses are encouraged to include fathers in the discharge teaching plan and to support their participation in infant care, this may not be an appropriate intervention with all men. Until models evolve, clinicians should carefully assess the individual father's interest in and desire to care for his newborn before they develop and initiate the discharge teaching plan.

Most postpartum settings have organized parent-teaching procedures, including classes, demonstrations, and discharge teaching guides. Topics of common concern to most parents, such as the subjects listed in the accompanying Teaching Considerations display, are often addressed. Some subjects have also been discussed in prenatal classes, and the nurse should build on those, where applicable. Parents can obtain additional information from child care reference books, videotapes, community health nurses, and parent

Teaching Considerations

Common Concerns of New Parents

The nurse is responsible for instructing parents on the following points:

- Bathing and skin care
- Cord care
- Circumcision care
- Uncircumcised male care
- Diapering and clothing
- Crying and sleeping–wake patterns
- Feeding
- Formula preparation
- Sterilization methods
- Burping
- Elimination patterns
- Prevention/care of diaper rash
- Swaddling and wrapping
- Handling and carrying
- Taking a temperature
- Safety considerations
  - Use of a bulb syringe
  - Accident prevention
  - Positioning
  - Poisoning prevention
  - Cigarette smoking
  - Infant car seat use
- Infant stimulation
- Signs/symptoms of illness
- Newborn day care

education groups. Companies marketing infant care products and formula have also developed pamphlets and parent-teaching aids that are available to families without charge; many of these are available in more than a dozen languages to assist parents when English is not read or spoken.

Bathing and Skin Care

Current research indicates that many health care providers and parents have incomplete and inaccurate information regarding appropriate bathing and infant skin care techniques (Cetta, Lambert, & Ros, 1991). Most newborns do not need daily baths. Routine bathing can strip the epidermis of essential lubricants, alter the acid mantle, and destroy normal flora. Until the infant begins to crawl and eat solid foods, sponge baths with plain water are usually adequate. The head should be shampooed only once or twice per week. However, the face, neck, genitalia, and perianal area should be washed *daily*.

The bath should be a pleasant, relaxing time for parent and neonate. Some newborns require time to get used to the bathing routine, but as both parent and child become comfortable with the activity, it becomes a time for loving interaction and play. All necessary equipment is collected beforehand to avoid having to carry a wet infant around while gathering forgotten supplies. The infant should never be left unattended during the bath—on the countertop or in the water. The room should be draft-free and warm—75°F to 80°F (24°C to 26.5°C) and the water comfortable when tested with the elbow—98°F to 100°F (36.5°C to 37.8°C). A mild soap such as Neutrogena, Lowila Cake, a soapless soap, or Moisturel should be used on both the body and scalp (Cetta et al., 1991). Ivory soap is no longer recommended for infants because it alters the acid mantle of the skin and may serve as a medium for bacterial growth.

First the infant's eyes should be washed with clear water from the inner to the outer canthus. A new area of the washcloth or a new cotton ball should be used with each wipe to prevent cross-infection of the eye. The nares and the outer ear should be cleaned with the tip of the washcloth or a cotton-tipped swab. Nares and ear canals should never be probed with swabs, which can damage fragile tissues. While the infant is still clothed, the head can be shampooed. The scalp should be washed every other day and then brushed with a soft-bristled brush to prevent the development of "cradle-cap," a grayish white, crusty scalp disorder (seborrheic dermatitis). The "football hold" is recommended for washing the head because it provides the parent with a free hand to massage and rinse the scalp (Fig. 31-10).

Once the infant's head is dried, he or she can be undressed and placed in the water. Soap should be used *sparingly* and may be applied before the infant is placed in the water to be rinsed. New parents may find the infant slippery. Wrapping the infant in a towel and then placing him or her in the water is an easy way to prevent slipping. The towel then

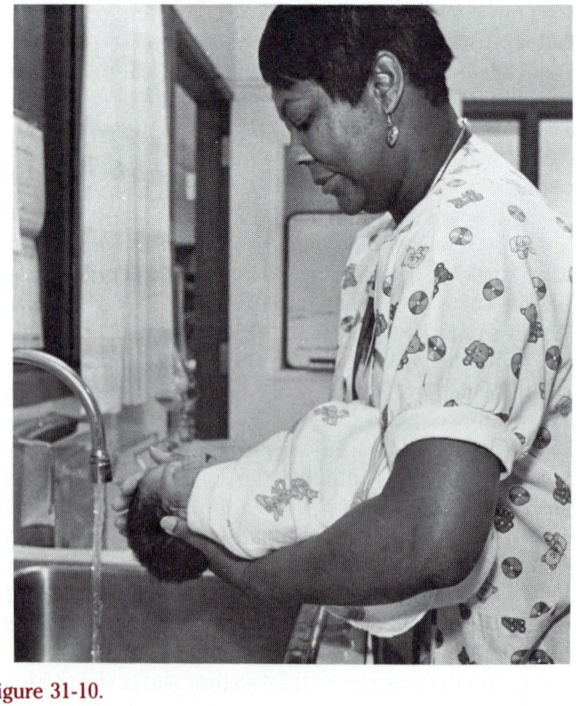

Figure 31-10.
Using the football hold while washing the infant's head. (Photo by Kathy Sloane.)

serves as an additional cushion in the bottom of the sink or tub.

The bath should proceed from the cleanest (eyes and then face) to the most soiled areas, with the genitals and perianal area being washed last. Special care should be taken to clean and dry skin folds. Female genitals should be washed from front to back. In an uncircumcised male infant, it is not necessary to retract the foreskin for the first 3 to 6 months. The infant may be bathed at any time during the day; many mothers like to give the bath when the father is at home so that he may participate in this activity. A variety of infant tubs are available commercially, but a clean kitchen sink padded with a towel is adequate.

Infants are routinely exposed to skin-care products containing potentially toxic chemicals. Application of hazardous chemicals to the skin may result in systemic toxicity. Research is lacking on the effects of many of these commercial products; however, recent studies suggest that infant rashes, which are very common in the first year of life, are due in some instances to over-the-counter infant skin products. The incidence of skin rashes caused by allergic reactions, blocked oil glands, and yeast and bacterial infections can be reduced by eliminating the use of powders, lotions, and oils. Baby lotions frequently contain dyes and fragrances that may produce allergic reactions. Baby oils are not recommended because they may clog pores. Infant deaths have been reported with the inhalation of baby powder, which should *not* be used.

Family Considerations

Care of the Umbilical Cord

Cultural beliefs regarding appropriate postnatal care of the umbilical cord vary widely. In some cultures a "belly band," a tight swaddling cloth often colorfully embroidered, encircles the abdomen over the cord area. This practice is believed to prevent umbilical hernias or infection. Other groups place a coin or flat stone over the umbilical stump and secure it with a swaddling band. Some families desire to keep the desiccated cord when it separates from the abdomen as a memento or to prevent evil spirits from obtaining any part of the infant's body.

The nurse must recognize and respect these cultural beliefs. Usually there is no contraindication to family practices. The nurse should encourage families to use clean fabrics and coins and to visually inspect the umbilical cord area daily for signs of healing or infection.

Cord Care

The umbilical cord stump will usually dry and fall off 7 to 10 days after birth. Parents are encouraged to keep the diaper folded down away from the area of the cord, and they may apply a small amount of 70% isopropyl alcohol on a cotton ball at the base several times a day to keep the cord clean and dry (see the accompanying Family Considerations display). Parents can sponge-bathe the newborn until pink granulation tissue covers the site of detachment (usually after 7 to 10 days).

Circumcision Care

The nurse must prepare parents to observe for bleeding and signs of infection in their circumcised sons. They should be aware that a yellow exudate often forms naturally over the surgical site but that a foul-smelling purulent exudate is abnormal and should be reported to the nurse practitioner or pediatrician at once. Petroleum jelly gauze is often placed on the circumcision site to keep the mucous membrane moist and prevent urine and stool from soiling the area. Before it is removed, it can be soaked with warm water to prevent trauma to tissues that have adhered to it. Each time a diaper is changed, the penis should be washed with clear, warm water gently squeezed from a cotton ball. Alcohol should never be used on the site; this would be extremely painful to the infant. A large dab of petroleum jelly may be placed in the diaper over the area that comes in contact with the penis. If the Plastibell method is used, no special gauze dressing or ointments are applied to the site; however, warm water may be used for cleansing, as described above. This special care should continue until the site is completely covered with clean, pink granulation tissue.

Care of the Uncircumcised Male

Daily bathing of the uncircumcised male should include washing of the external genitalia without efforts to retract the foreskin or expose the glans. Although natural loosening of the foreskin from the glans begins at birth, the foreskin is retractable in only 50% of all 1-year-old infants. Parents should be advised against vigorously or forcefully retracting the infant's foreskin because it may be difficult to return it to its normal position owing to swelling of the glans. If the foreskin remains too tight as the infant grows, a surgical incision in the foreskin may be necessary to loosen the retracted tissue.

Diapering and Clothing

The neonate voids and defecates with amazing frequency. Diapers should be checked often and changed when wet or soiled. It is not necessary to cleanse with soap and water after each voiding; clear warm water is adequate. Soap and water washings can be reserved for when the infant defecates. Premoistened wipes, which are convenient to use and save time for busy parents, are commercially available for perianal cleansing. They may be an unnecessary expense for families with limited resources. These wipes also frequently contain chemicals and fragrances that may irritate the neonate's skin.

Diaper rash, which results from ammonia irritation, develops rapidly if the area is not cleansed. A and D ointment or zinc oxide may be applied after washing and careful drying if the infant's skin is especially sensitive. Exposure to air is recommended. If cloth diapers are used, they should be laundered with a nondetergent soap and rinsed twice to eliminate all traces of ammonia. Many parents use disposable diapers. Occasionally an infant develops a rash where the skin comes in contact with the plastic on these diapers. If this occurs, the parents should switch to cloth diapers. Because of environmental concerns, many parents now consider the use of cloth diapers and will ask nurses to discuss the pros and cons of "cloth versus plastic." The nurse should be prepared to review current information about diapers or provide literature about the topic (see the accompanying Legal/Ethical display).

Parents often ask about their neonate's need for clothing. As a general rule neonates are comfortable with several layers of light, loose clothing (diaper, T-shirt, and medium-weight neck-to-toe coverall) in an environment with an ambient temperature of 68°F to 75°F (20°C to 24°C). If a parent feels cold and requires a sweater, the infant should also be dressed in an additional layer of clothing. Hats or caps should be worn outdoors in cool or cold weather. In hot weather babies feel most comfortable in a lightweight T-shirt and diaper. A sun hat should be worn in the sun, and care should be taken to protect the skin from sunburn.

Legal/Ethical Considerations

The Role of the Nurse in the Diaper Debate

More than 16 billion disposable diapers are sold each year. Disposable diapers account for approximately 3% of waste in landfills and $300 million dollars is spent annually to discard soiled diapers. Additionally, a public health hazard is created when diapers are improperly handled in the refuse disposal system. As a result of the crisis of enormous garbage volume and the potential infection risk, the American Public Health Association has issued a policy statement on the health and environmental hazards of disposable diapers. It recommends ongoing research on the health, safety, and handling of various types of diapers to reduce the threat to public health.

Conversely, laundering facilities for cloth diapers require the use of water, detergents, and a waste treatment system. Diaper delivery services are not available in all communities, particularly poor, urban areas. Furthermore, poor families may not have regular access to laundry facilities. Families in which both parents work full-time may believe that the use of cloth diapers is not feasible or is simply too inconvenient.

Nurses are at the center of environmental ethics and activities aimed at reducing the impact and hazards of garbage and waste products generated by the health care industry. Nurses are viewed as content experts by environmentally conscious parents considering diaper alternatives.

American Public Health Association. (1990). Policy Statement 8910. Health and environmental hazards of disposable diapers. American Journal of Public Health, *80(2), 230.*

Wong, D., Brantley, D., Clutter, L., DeSimone, D., Lammert, D., Nix, K., et al. (1992). Diapering choices: A critical review of the issue. Pediatric Nursing, *18*(1), 41–54.

Crying and Sleep–Wake Patterns

Parents, particularly women planning to return to work, are extremely interested in the topic of crying and infant sleep–wake patterns. Infants less than 3 months of age sleep on average 15 hours a day. Quiet alert, active, and fussy periods occur for varying periods of time during waking hours. Continuous nighttime sleep for at least 6 hours is rare in most newborns who wake to hunger cues every 2 to 4 hours. Some parents are tempted to introduce solid foods very early to encourage longer periods of nighttime sleep. This practice is not recommended; the early introduction of solid foods has been associated with gastrointestinal disorders, allergies, and hematologic problems in the infant.

Crying is the infant's only means of communication. Most infants cry an average of about 2 hours each day, but some cry more often in response to discomfort, boredom, or exposure to new experiences. Research has indicated that the infant cries less and sleeps more when the diurnal cycle develops in the first months of life. Establishing a daytime light/nighttime dark pattern immediately after birth by having the mother room-in with the infant promotes quiet sleep and may facilitate the earlier development of the diurnal rhythm (Keefe, 1988). Another study found that infants fell asleep faster when exposed to white noise such as recordings of intrauterine sounds (Spenser, Moran, & Talbert, 1990).

Physical, psychological, environmental, and genetic factors influence crying behavior. When the infant cries, the parents should try to discover the source of distress. It is perfectly acceptable to pick the infant up and offer comfort; neonates will not be spoiled if they are picked up when they cry. Newborns need a tremendous amount of loving attention, and crying is their request for it. However, an exhausted mother who has spent hours trying to soothe a healthy but irritable infant should not feel guilty about laying the infant down in a crib, closing the door, and spending some time in the next room recouping her energy. Parents should be advised to find someone who can occasionally relieve them of caretaking to decrease their stress levels in this situation. An in-depth discussion of infant crying and sleep pattern is presented in Chapter 36.

A serious health hazard for infants, which has only recently been identified, is "shaken-baby syndrome." Shaking may occur during the process of play but is more often a response of an angry, fatigued, or frustrated caregiver to a crying infant (see the accompanying display). The nurse must educate parents about the permanent and debilitating effects that even one episode of shaking can have on neurologic development.

Feeding

The nurse will continue to provide appropriate information regarding nutrition and feeding techniques to women

Shaken-Baby Syndrome: A Preventable Tragedy

Shaken-baby syndrome may result in permanent neurologic injury, mental retardation, and death. The neck cannot provide stability for the neonatal head, because the neck muscles are not fully developed and the head is proportionately large in relation to the body. The highest incidence of the syndrome is in infants under 6 months of age. Shaking causes an acceleration/decleration-type injury in the brain. Even small shakes can result in subdural and subarachnoid hemorrhages. Blindness, hearing loss, behavior and seizure disorders, psychological disturbances, cerebral palsy, and spinal cord injuries can be experienced. It is estimated that 10% of mentally retarded children were shaken in infancy (Hines, 1992).

Shaking injuries can occur during play. Research indicates that boys are twice as likely to incur injury in this manner as girls because parents more often engage in vigorous or rough play with male infants. However, the majority of infants experiencing shaken-baby syndrome are shaken by parents, older children, or other caregivers in response to crying behavior.

Nurses should encourage parents to ask for help when the crying infant cannot be consoled. If someone cannot temporarily relieve the parent, the mother or father should take a short break. Parents should be given the names and phone numbers of parenting support groups and telephone "hot-lines" should feelings of hostility build to a desire to physically injure the infant.

Hines, C. (1992). Nurses join new campaign against shaken-baby syndrome. Nurseweek, *5(20), 1.*

who plan to bottle feed and those who are nursing their infants. In-depth information regarding breastfeeding is reviewed in Chapter 35. Research suggests that nurses may play a central role in the continuation of breastfeeding after the woman is discharged from the birthing unit.

A major factor implicated in breastfeeding failures is the distribution of formula gift packs by nurses during discharge procedures. Critics of the practice argue that nurses who distribute the gift packs are unpaid promoters of formula companies. Nurses may inadvertently convey a message in support of bottle feeding. Nurses can also positively influence the success of breastfeeding and avoid sending mixed messages when they refrain from giving or even offering formula samples to nursing women.

Burping. All infants swallow air as they feed (bottle-fed infants swallow more than breastfed infants), and burping allows the swallowed air to escape from the stomach. When the infant is bottle feeding, the nipple should be kept full of fluid so the infant does not take in air with each swallow. Feeding the infant in a nearly upright position allows air naturally to rise to the top of the stomach, where it can readily be brought up without much milk being brought up with it.

Newborns may not always burp after a feeding; if after 3 minutes of gentle patting and rubbing, an infant has not burped, he or she may not need to. Burping the infant is best done with the child held upright against the adult's shoulder. Holding the infant on the stomach on the adult's lap for burping is likely to bring up milk when air escapes. Holding the infant in a sitting position may also not work well because air may not be able to escape from the stomach.

Elimination Patterns

The nurse should discuss expected changes in stool consistency and frequency of elimination in the neonate. This is especially important with new parents who are unfamiliar with normal newborn stool characteristics and patterns of elimination. If the mother is encouraged to change the infant's diapers during her hospital stay, she will gain confidence in her ability to recognize normal variations in her infant's stools and habits.

Prevention and Care of Diaper Rash

Diaper rash is a localized cutaneous reaction caused primarily by the ammonia found in urine as well as by detergents used in the laundering of cloth diapers. The best preventive measures include frequent diaper changes and thorough rinsing of the skin and skin folds with warm water with each diaper change. If cloth diapers are used, a non-detergent soap specifically created for laundering diapers should be used, and the diapers should be rinsed twice to remove any soap residue.

Even with the best care, some infants are prone to diaper rash. If a rash occurs, the infant should be placed in cloth, not plastic disposable, diapers. The buttocks should be exposed to air and sunlight several times a day for 20 minutes or so, and an ointment specifically formulated for diaper rash protection (such as A and D ointment) should be used on the tender area to decrease exposure of the skin to urine. At no time should a skin powder and ointment be used together; this combination cakes on the skin surface and exacerbates the irritation of delicate skin tissues.

Swaddling and Wrapping

Wrapping the infant securely can help meet the need for contact comfort and provide a relaxing arrangement for sleep. Wrapping the infant also prevents his or her own jerky movements from disturbing sleep and keeps the infant warm. The infant can be wrapped in a soft baby blanket, with the edges of the blanket tucked smoothly under the infant to secure the blanket in place. A wrapped infant may also be easier for new parents to lift and carry because the blanket helps support the extremities and limits the infant's movements.

Handling and Carrying

Newborns have an inborn fear of being dropped; this is apparent in their distress when their heads or extremities are

NURSING PROCEDURE
How to Use the Bulb Syringe

Purpose: To quickly and safely clear the neonate's airway when regurgitation of milk or mucus occurs. The nurse teaches the following steps in suctioning the mouth and nares with the bulb syringe.

NURSING ACTION	***RATIONALE***
1. Place the neonate in a football hold.	To free one hand to use the bulb syringe
2. Place the head downward.	To facilitate drainage of fluids
3. Compress the bulb syringe quickly before placing into mouth and nares.	To prevent blowing the fluids deeper into oropharynx or trachea
4. Insert tip of bulb syringe *first* into mouth in area between cheek and gums.	Placing tip of syringe into nares first may stimulate gasp, drawing fluids deeper into oropharaynx or trachea
5. Slowly release compression of bulb.	To create vacuum and to aspirate fluids from mouth
6. Remove tip of syringe from mouth, compress bulb, and reinsert in mouth to remove remaining liquids.	To expel aspirated fluids from bulb To remove remaining fluids
7. Repeat steps 4, 5, and 6 until mouth is clear.	
8. Compress bulb and gently place tip of syringe in nares. Slowly release compression of bulb.	To remove any fluids regurgitated into nares
9. Repeat procedure until nares are clear.	

left unsupported or their position is suddenly changed. To avoid startling the newborn when picking him or her up, talk to the newborn and put your hands under his or her body for a second or two before lifting. The newborn may also feel more secure if securely wrapped in a blanket while being carried or held close to the caregiver's body.

Parents should be advised to carry the newborn in a "football" hold (infant's head supported by adult's hand, infant's body supported on adult's lower arm and securely held against adult's body) or securely braced against the shoulder with the hand supporting the infant's head when going up and down stairs; this leaves one hand free to manage doors or use handrails.

Taking a Temperature

If the nurse takes the neonate's vital signs at the mother's bedside as part of the daily assessment, she can then teach both axillary temperature-taking techniques described earlier in this chapter. The mother should be able to state the normal temperature range and demonstrate correct temperature-taking and reading techniques before she leaves the hospital. Some parents have never used a thermometer. If they are unable to consistently read a temperature accurately, the nurse might suggest that they purchase plastic temperature strips. These strips are placed on the skin surface and provide an approximate temperature reading; these are an acceptable alternative if parents cannot read a mercury thermometer accurately. Digital thermometers are also available and are slightly more expensive than the plastic temperature strips.

Safety Considerations

An important safety factor is the use of the bulb syringe when regurgitated milk or mucus occurs in the infant's airway. Parents should be taught how to perform this safety feature (see the accompanying Nursing Procedure and Fig. 31-2).

Accidents. Because accidents are the leading cause of death in children from 1 month of age through adolescence, the nurse should cover the topic of accident prevention in depth and reinforce information at every opportunity.

The importance of using a passenger restraint system designed for infants should be stressed. Automobile accidents are the leading cause of infant death, and some neonates are injured or even killed during their first car ride on the way home from the hospital. Most states have enacted mandatory auto passenger restraint laws requiring that all infants and children be placed in federally approved auto restraint devices (not infant carriers). The nurse should encourage parents to obtain and use an infant car seat. Many local public health departments and hospitals offer car seat rental or loan programs for parents with limited economic resources. Some nurseries require the nurse to teach proper placement of the newborn in the carseat before discharge.

Other areas of accident prevention the nurse should discuss with parents are prevention of falls, aspiration, and electric shock. All electrical outlets should have covers, and cords should be out of sight and out of reach as much as possible. The nurse should stress that an infant must never be left unattended on any unguarded surface; newborns can roll over and fall with amazing speed. Choking and aspiration are other major causes of death in infancy. To prevent this, bottle propping should be avoided, and the infant should be placed on his or her side or abdomen after being fed. Because the neonate is capable of random hand-to-mouth movements, all objects small enough to fit into the mouth should be kept out of reach. Parents should be encouraged to attend first aid courses with a specific focus on infants.

The infant's sleep environment should be discussed with the parents. Pillows should not be used for infants because they can cause suffocation. Infants should *never* sleep on adult waterbeds; there have been reports of infant asphyxiation in newborns placed in or rolling to a prone position on adult waterbeds. Makeshift plastic covers should not be placed over the mattress to protect it from moisture. If parents intend to purchase an old or antique crib, they should be told that such cribs do not always meet contemporary safety standards, which require use of a nonlead paint. Guidelines for the distance between slats should be provided. Other types of older infant furniture such as high chairs may also be hazardous to the infant and should be used with caution.

Controversy exists about the safety of having an infant sleep in the parents' bed. In many cultures infants automatically sleep with their mothers until they are no longer nursed or are old enough to sleep with siblings. A relatively new approach to parenting endorses a "family bed," in which all children sleep with parents until they indicate a desire for their own bed. However, some health professionals fear that infants may be accidentally suffocated by the weight of their sleeping parents. Parents should be particularly cautious about using alcohol or any type of CNS depressant that would render them unresponsive to the infant's presence or needs. While respecting the mother's cultural values, the nurse should nevertheless suggest that the mother provide her infant with a simple sleeping crib with sides. Such a crib can be placed next to the mother's bed so that she can nurse the infant easily.

Positioning. Parents have been taught that the infant should be placed in the prone or sidelying position after feeding and for sleep. However, a recent analysis of research findings on the causes of sudden infant death syndrome (SIDS) found a strong statistical association between the prone sleeping position in infants and an increased risk of SIDS (Guntheroth & Spiers, 1992). As a result, the investigators recommend avoidance of the prone position for sleep in infants under 6 months of age. The American Academy of Pediatrics is currently reviewing these data and the recommendation made by Guntheroth and Spiers. Until a final analysis of the data is completed, parents should be encouraged to place the infant in the sidelying position for sleep during the first 6 months of life. The nurse should demonstrate how diapers or blankets can be fashioned into bed rolls to support the back and abdomen to prevent the infant from rolling into the supine or prone position.

Poisoning. Parents should begin to "childproof" their home before their infant is old enough to crawl and begin to explore the environment. Cleaning solutions, medications, cosmetics, and other toxic substances should be placed in locked cabinets. Specially designed easy-to-install locks are available as part of a "childproofing" kit that can be purchased in hardware and infant specialty stores. Many houseplants are also poisonous.

Local poison control centers have information on plants and can help parents identify those that are harmful. Parents should have with them the phone number of the local poison control center when they leave the hospital and should place it near their phone along with other emergency numbers.

Lead poisoning remains a significant public health problem, particularly for poor infants and children living in deteriorating housing in large, inner urban areas. Before the 1980s, lead was widely used in the preparation of paints and solder for repair of water pipes. Lead poisoning can result in permanent CNS damage. The most common sources of lead poisoning (plumbism) in newborns and young infants include:

- Lead dust created by sanding lead-containing paints
- Lead fumes released when heat guns are used to remove lead-containing paints
- Lead fumes released into the air from autos and trucks (higher in housing that abuts major highways)
- Lead-contaminated water used for formula preparation (leached from lead pipes in older homes or cooking vessels containing lead)

Boiling water before adding it to powdered or concentrated formula may increase lead concentration of tap water, amplifying the risk of lead intoxication (Shannon & Graef, 1992). Additionally, some neonates may have toxic blood levels caused by prenatal lead exposure. Cases of lead dust importation into the home by working mothers or fathers, or direct toxic exposure of pregnant women employed in industries where contact with lead occurs have been documented (Brown, Bellinger, & Matthews, 1990). Nurses are in an excellent position to teach parents about the risks of lead exposure and make appropriate referrals to public health agencies or lead poisoning prevention programs.

Infant Cardiopulmonary Resuscitation (CPR). Infant resuscitation classes have become an integral part of discharge teaching in the neonatal intensive care unit. Today, parents of healthy infants are also interested in and committed to learning infant CPR. Although hospitals may provide parents with information about CPR classes available in the community, the time required for teaching CPR usually precludes covering this material before discharge. However, some community hospitals are now offering infant CPR classes as part of expectant or new parent classes. A recent report by Donaher-Wagner and Braun (1992) described the successful development of a 3-hour class in infant resuscitation. Parents were overwhelmingly in support of the program and described an increase in self-confidence. More hospitals may be expected to offer infant CPR classes as part of the

the total program of classes available to expectant and new parents.

Exposure to Cigarette Smoke

The negative effects of second-hand or passive cigarette smoking for neonates and older infants are now well documented. This information should be shared with parents, and information about smoking cessation programs provided for the new mother or other family members who smoke and will come in contact with the neonate. The nurse should use a supportive and nonjudgmental approach. Parents should be encouraged to provide a healthy, safe environment for the infant, and the positive benefits of smoking cessation for all family members should be emphasized (see the accompanying display).

Infant Stimulation

Research indicates that specific types of sensory stimulation may produce highly specific beneficial effects on infant growth and development. Audio tapes, mobiles, murals, cribs, hammocks, and toys have been specifically designed to stimulate one or more sensory organ. Infant stimulation equipment such as mobiles and age-appropriate toys are often expensive and may not offer significant advantages to infants reared in middle class homes. Further research is indicated to evaluate the effect of multimodal stimulation in high-risk populations.

Nurses should be cautious about recommending any specific sensory stimulation device because beneficial effects in healthy, full-term infants have not been established. Simple, inexpensive mobiles or hand-drawn, bold black and white patterns and faces attached to the crib or walls in the infant's room may be just as effective in stimulating the infant's interest. Counseling should be directed toward helping parents recognize and use their own abilities to interact with their infants and provide appropriate infant stimulation.

Signs and Symptoms of Illness

First-time parents may be especially concerned about being able to recognize signs and symptoms of illness in their infant. The nurse can provide them with a simple but descriptive list of significant signs:

- Lethargy—difficulty in waking the infant
- Fever—temperature above 100°F (37.2°C)
- Loss of appetite—refusal of two feedings in a row
- Vomiting—spitting up of a large part or all of a feeding two or more times
- Diarrhea—three or more green, liquid stools in succession

If parents observe any of these signs or symptoms, they should call their nurse practitioner or physician. If they are unable to contact their health care provider and the infant's condition is getting worse, they should take the child to a clinic or emergency room.

Evaluating Newborn/Infant Day Care Options

In the past 10 years, the fastest growth of women in the work force has been among those with new infants. Many women return to work within 6 weeks to 3 months after birth. Unlike most other industrialized nations, the United States has failed to develop a rational and comprehensive child care system for the millions of infants and children who require day care services. The nurse, therefore, plays a key role in assisting parents to find a safe, nurturing day care environment for the newborn.

The nurse should review with the parents the types of day care services available and explore the benefits and advantages of each. Health and safety factors that parents must consider before making a final decision should be described. The value of close, individualized attention from day care workers should be stressed. Although research suggests that growth and development are not adversely affected by early day care, consistent attention from caring individuals knowledgeable about the unique needs of infants is essential.

Expected Outcomes

- Parents perform return-demonstrations of techniques that were covered in discharge teaching.
- Parents demonstrate growing comfort and ease in handling the newborn by time of discharge.
- Parents state correctly signs of illness and sources of injury in newborns by time of discharge.

The Effects of Tobacco Smoke Exposure on Neonates

Infants and young children chronically exposed to tobacco smoke have a higher risk of developing acute respiratory illnesses such as bronchitis and pneumonia. Hospitalization is more often necessary to manage these conditions when they occur. Several studies have linked cigarette smoking to reduced lung function, reactivity to aeroallergens, and childhood asthma. Current research is also investigating the link between tobacco smoke exposure and childhood cancer.

Referrals can be made to smoking cessation programs. Family members who continue to smoke should be strongly advised not to smoke in the home, automobile, or in any setting when neonates, infants, or children are present. Furthermore, eliminating adult roles models who smoke from the home may reduce the likelihood of children imitating parents in their smoking behavior.

Chilmonczyk, B., Knight, G., Palomaki, G., Pulkkinen, A., William, J., & Haddow, J. (1990). Environmental tobacco smoke exposure during infancy. American Journal of Public Health, 80*(10), 1205.*

Martinez, F., Cline, M.; & Burrows, B. (1992). Increased incidence of asthma in children of smoking mothers. Pediatrics, 89*(1), 21.*

Monitoring for and Preventing Complications

The newborn should continue to make physiologic adaptations to extrauterine life. The nurse assesses the neonate for danger signals indicative of illness or ineffective postnatal adaptations. The nurse is in a position to detect specific signs of complications in the earliest stages. Table 31-3 discusses presenting signs of complications, potential disorders, and ineffective adaptation.

Text continues on page 956

Table 31-3. Danger Signs in the Neonate

Affected System	Presenting Signs	Potential Neonatal Disorder
Central nervous system	Jitteriness	Hypoglycemia, hypocalcemia, hypomagnesemia, drug withdrawal (maternal use)
	Diaphoresis	Chromosomal anomalies (cri du chat) Drug withdrawal
	Abnormal cry	Asphyxia
	Excessive irritability	Intracranial hemorrhage
	Twitching	Brain edema
	Convulsions	Neuromuscular anomalies Asphyxia Drug withdrawal
	Hypotonia	Sepsis Chronic intrauterine infection Chromosomal anomalies
	Small head size	Fetal alcohol syndrome
	Bulging fontanelle, large head size	Hydrocephalus
Cardiovascular and respiratory systems	Apnea	Congenital heart anomaly
	Rapid, slow, or irregular pulse	Persistent fetal circulation
	Cyanosis	Hypoplastic lung
	Rapid respiration, chest retraction	Respiratory distress syndrome (type I or type II)
	Grunting	Meconium aspiration syndrome
	Flaring	Tracheal malacia
	Stridor	Aspiration
	Pallor	Pneumothorax
	Plethora	Polycythemia
	Single umbilical artery	Congenital heart anomaly
Gastrointestinal system	Vomiting	Gastrointestinal obstruction Drug withdrawal
	Abdominal distention	Gastrointestinal obstruction
	No meconium stool (beyond 48 h after birth)	Imperforate anus, gastrointestinal obstruction
	Diarrhea	Sepsis
	Jaundice (within first 24 h of life)	Hemolytic disease of newborn, biliary atresia
	Excessive salivation	Tracheoesophageal fistula
Genitourinary system	Delayed/inadequate voiding (beyond 48 h after birth)	Genitourinary anomalies, renal failure secondary to hypoxia
Musculoskeletal system	Hypotonia	Congenital neuromuscular anomaly
	Hypertonia	Asphyxia
	Uneven thigh or buttock folds	Congenital hip dysplasia
	Facial asymmetry with crying	Facial nerve injury
	Limited movement of arm	Brachial palsy
Integumentary system	Purulent discharge from cord	Omphalitis
	Skin pustules	Staphylococcal skin infection
	Rash	Congenital rubella, congenital syphillis
Hematologic system	Bleeding or oozing from cord, petechiae	Hemorrhage
Immunologic system	Hypothermia	Sepsis
	Fever	Intracranial hemorrhage

Nursing Care Plan

The Full-Term Newborn Who Is Receiving Phototherapy for Hyperbilirubinemia

PATIENT PROFILE

History

Baby B, a 4100 g (9 lb, 3 oz) full-term male infant was born by forceps extraction after 40 h of labor. His mother received oxytocin for labor dystocia. At birth Baby B was noted to have marked facial bruising. His hematocrit at 4 h of age was 68%.

At 30 h of age the nurse performed an assessment of Baby B and noted the following abnormalities:

- Cephalhematoma over the right parietal bone
- Marked jaundice over his entire body
- Serum bilirubin 16.2 mg/dL (drawn at 29 h of age)

An order was given by the pediatrician to initiate phototherapy. A cavitron high-intensity tungsten lamp was used for the phototherapy treatment.

Physical Assessment

At 40 h of age Baby B remains in an incubator for phototherapy with a serum bilirubin level of 15.8 mg/dL. His mother is being treated for a uterine infection and is receiving IV antibiotics. She has requested the nursing staff feed her baby. "I'm sick and feel exhausted. I don't know how I'm going to take care of him. I can't do anything right."

The nurse measures the vital signs before feeding Baby B who is receiving formula: temperature 37.4°C, pulse 156, respirations 58.

Baby B is taken from the incubator for the feeding. He is lethargic and takes 25 minutes to ingest 40 mL formula. (He took 35 mL at his last feeding).

The nurse changes his diaper and notes that the infant has passed a large, liquid, dark green stool. His perianal area is reddened and a small area of excoriated skin is noted on his right buttock.

COLLABORATIVE PROBLEMS/POTENTIAL COMPLICATIONS

- Dehydration
- Priapism
- Bronze baby syndrome
- Retinal damage

(See the Nursing Alert display and the Managed Care Path following the Care Plan.)

Assessment	*Nursing Diagnosis*	*Nursing Interventions*	*Rationale*
Bilirubin level remains at 15.8 mg/dL	High Risk for Injury related to hyperbilirubinemia	Place infant nude under cavitron light.	To expose all skin surfaces to the phototherapy light
Infant lethargic and is a "poor feeder"	***Expected Outcome***	Turn infant every 2 h.	
Ingested 35 mL last feeding and 40 mL this feeding	Baby B's serum bilirubin will continue to fall over period of 24h.	Cover eyes with patches or "Bili" mask.	High-density light may cause corneal or retinal damage
	Baby B's serum bilirubin will remain below 12 mg/dL.	Place infant in incubator.	To provide neutral thermal environment
	Baby B's eyes will remain protected from light.	Measure energy delivered and record in watts/cm^2.	Adequate light energy must be delivered for photo-oxidation of bilirubin in skin.
		Obtain and monitor serum bilirubin q 4–8 h.	To determine if therapy is effective and when to discontinue phototherapy

(*Continued*)

The Full-Term Newborn Who Is Receiving Phototherapy for Hyperbilirubinemia

(*Continued*)

Assessment	***Nursing Diagnosis***	***Nursing Interventions***	***Rationale***
		Encourage frequent feedings and supplement with water if indicated by fluid deficit.	Promotes excretion of conjugated bilirubin
Neonate in incubator Use of cavitron light Temp 37.4°C	Hyperthermia related to use of cavitron light and placement of infant in incubator	Reduce incubator temperature.	Temperature inside incubator can contribute to hyperthermia.
	Expected Outcome Baby B's temperature will decrease to a normal range within an hour.	Increase fluid intake (supplement feedings with sterile water).	Dehydration can increase body temperature.
		Monitor neonate's temperature q 2–3 h.	Identify swings in temperature related to phototherapy and inability to wear clothing during the procedure.
		Monitor incubator temperature q 2 h.	Temperature setting of incubator can drift.
Neonate is lethargic Took 35 mL last feeding Took 40 mL this feeding Birthweight 4100 g Passing liquid stool	High Risk for Fluid Volume Deficit related to phototherapy, hyperthermia, and decreased fluid intake	Report condition of lethargy and decreased fluid intake to primary health care provider.	To obtain order for increasing fluid intake and supplement with water
	Expected Outcome Baby B will maintain a normal fluid balance as evidenced by: • Bottle feeding q 3 h • Intake of 60–90 mL/feeding • Urine output of 6–8 diapers daily • Normal weight loss/gain pattern in first week • Normal tissue turgor	Calculate fluid needs and replace. Maintain normal body temperature.	Hyperthermia will increase insensible water loss.
		Monitor intake and output q 8 h	To detect negative fluid balance and evaluate need for additional fluids
		Monitor consistency and frequency of stools.	
		Monitor weight daily.	
		Assess tissue turgor q 4–8 h.	Poor tissue turgor is an indicator of fluid loss and dehydration.
Redness around perianal area Excoriation of right buttock Passing loose green stools	Impaired Tissue Integrity related loose, frequent stools "Bili" stools	Keep diaper area clean and dry.	Loose stools and urine will predispose skin to breakdown.
	Expected Outcome Baby B's skin will remain intact without evidence of increasing redness or excoriation.	Avoid oil-based ointments.	Oils can cause thermal burns when phototherapy implemented.
		Monitor skin condition q 4–8 h.	Skin can breakdown with exposure to urine, stool, and phototherapy light increasing the risk of infection.
Verbalization of guilt, anxiety Verbalization of inadequacy in parenting skills Maternal illness Distressed affect	Alteration in Parenting related to anxiety, illness, and impaired acquaintance process	Inform mother about neonate's status, and progress in therapy at frequent intervals.	Reduces maternal anxiety
	Expected Outcome Mother will be able to visit Baby B.	Provide opportunity for mother to verbalize feelings.	

(*Continued*)

The Full-Term Newborn Who Is Receiving Phototherapy for Hyperbilirubinemia
(*Continued*)

Assessment	Nursing Diagnosis	Nursing Interventions	Rationale
	Mother will interact with Baby B.	Encourage the mother to visit the nursery when she feels better.	Facilitates maternal–infant acquaintance process
	Mother will verbalize a decrease in anxiety and distress related to infant and parenting role.	Encourage father or other family member to visit neonate until mother well.	May reduce anxiety if mother knows that family member is acting as newborn advocate
		Provide mother with opportunities to care for neonate when condition of both neonate and mother permits.	Facilitate enhanced competence in parenting skills and promotes maternal–infant acquaintance and bonding
		Remove eye patches when mother is to feed neonate.	Eye contact enhances maternal–infant acquaintance process.

EVALUATION

Phototherapy for Baby B was discontinued when two consecutive serum bilirubin levels measured 11 mg/dL. Baby B's temperature stabilized between 36.8°C and 37.2°C with a reduction in the incubator temperature.

Baby B took between 60 mL and 90 mL fluid every 3 h with an output of 6–8 weight diapers in 24 h. Normal tissue turgor was noted. There was a weight loss under 10% in 24 h. Temperature remained within normal range. Redness and excoriation of skin in the perianal region resolved and there was no further skin breakdown.

As the mother's condition improved, she began to visit the nursery for each feeding. Baby B's mother fed him and demonstrated increasing competence with parenting skills. She verbalized decreased anxiety about Baby B's condition and in her ability to provide care and increased satisfaction as Baby B's condition improved.

Potential Complication: Hyperbilirubinemia and Jaundice

Nursing care is also directed at monitoring the infant for jaundice and reducing the incidence and severity of neonatal hyperbilirubinemia. Approximately 9% of healthy neonates will suffer from hyperbilirubinemia greater than 15 mg/dL, and many of these neonates will receive phototherapy in the hospital or home setting for at least 24 hours. Bilirubin conjugation and jaundice are discussed in Chapter 30. Because artificial lighting and colored walls in the nursery hinder accurate evaluation of skin color, detection is best accomplished by careful inspection of the neonate in natural light. Jaundice first appears on the head and over the face and then spreads toward the lower extremities. In fair-skinned neonates the face and sclera should be inspected first. The skin over the bridge of the nose should be blanched to reveal underlying jaundice. In newborns with dark skin pigmentation, the gums and buccal mucosa should be examined. The nurse should then proceed toward the toes, blanching the skin over bony prominences to determine the extent of icterus.

Research, however, indicates that visual estimates of bilirubin concentration are not always accurate. A noninvasive method for estimating serum bilirubin levels has been developed to assist nurses in assessing the severity of hyperbilirubinemia. Transcutaneous bilirubinometry can be used as a screening device to identify newborns with abnormally high levels of serum bilirubin. A probe attached to a jaundice meter is placed flat against the neonate's skin, and a reading is obtained. High levels should be reported and follow-up laboratory analysis of serum bilirubin obtained (Schumacher, 1990).

Specific nursing actions that aid in the prevention of jaundice and decrease serum bilirubin levels are:

NURSING ALERT

NURSING RESPONSIBILITIES WHEN CARING FOR THE NEONATE WHO REQUIRES PHOTOTHERAPY

When the neonate requires phototherapy, the nurse is responsible for maintaining a *safe environment* during the course of the treatment. The nurse monitors the neonate for complications of therapy and must intervene in a timely manner to *prevent injury*. Major nursing actions include:

- Monitor incubator and neonate's temp at least q 3–4 h to prevent hyperthermia.
- Ensure that eye patches are secure and properly positioned to prevent eye damage or obstruction of the nose.
- Remove eye patches for each feeding and assess eyes to identify early signs of infection.
- Monitor intake and output carefully to identify negative fluid balance and prevent dehydration.
- Shield genitalia by placing face mask or small diaper over genitalia to prevent exposure of skin over gonads and genitalia to beam of light.
- Observe skin color in natural light to identify early signs of skin bronzing so that therapy can be discontinued in a timely manner.
- Ensure that locks of incubator door are engaged, so that neonate cannot accidentally push door open.

These nursing actions should be documented periodically in the nurse's notes.

- Prevention of cold stress
- Promotion of adequate hydration
- Initiation of early and frequent feedings

Controversy still exists about whether breastfed infants characterized as "slow" or "poor" feeders should receive formula or sterile water supplementation when jaundice develops. Inadequate fluid intake in the first 2 to 3 days of life delays excretion of conjugated bilirubin and may contribute to hyperbilirubinemia. The nurse should make every effort to support the breastfeeding mother who desires to meet her newborn's fluid and nutritional needs through breast milk alone. The frequency of breastfeeding can be increased in this case.

When serum bilirubin levels rise above 13 mg/dL in the first 24 to 48 hours of life in the normal newborn, or above 15 mg/dL after 48 hours, phototherapy is generally recommended (Tan, 1991). The nurse is responsible for implementation of the procedure and monitoring the neonate's responses to the therapy including the following:

- Reinforcing information provided by the primary health care provider
- Preparing equipment required for phototherapy
- Preparing the newborn for treatment
- Monitoring vital signs
- Monitoring serum bilirubin levels

MANAGED CARE PATH

Term Infant

Expected Length of Stay: 1–2 days

	Day of Delivery	Day 1
Key Goals	Chemstrip WNL Temp WNL in open crib Feeding begun Pediatric care provider identified	Parent able to feed infant Parent performs care Discharge within 48 h of birth
Consults	Social work, lactation and parent ed consult PRN →	→
Test/Labs	Heelstick hematocrit and glucose	PKU, daily weight
Meds	Aquamephyton 1 mg IM Illotycin oint OU within 1 h of birth Triple dye to cord	
Treatments	Admit weight, VS q 30 min × 2 h; q/h × 3; then q 4 h Measurements: length, head and chest Cord, circumference care	Cord, circumcision care per protocol Assess VS PRN
Teaching	Feeding, diaper care Use of bulb syringe, safety, security	Bath, skin, use of car seat Warning signs, normal behavior Elimination
Equipment	Warmer, suction kit Admission kit, bath kit, bassinet	Bassinet, circ tray PRN Heel warmer, car seat, gift packs
Diet	Sterile water × 1, breast or bottle per protocol →	→
Activity	Mother's room at lib →	→
D/C Plan	Notify ped care provider, check circ preference Home health, WIC referral PRN	Videos on parenting PRN F/U appointments made

Adapted from collaborative paths developed by the Department of Nursing Service, Vanderbilt University Medical Center, Nashville, TN.

- Monitoring the neonate for complications related to phototherapy
- Promoting parent–infant interactions and caretaking activities

In some cases home phototherapy may be implemented to treat physiologic jandice. Home health nurses are responsible for daily assessment of the neonate, evaluation of the serum bilirubin level, and communication with the pediatrician until therapy is discontinued.

The accompanying Nursing Care Plan for the low-risk neonate with hyperbilirubinemia provides further information. Treatment and care of the high-risk newborn with hyperbilirubinemia and jaundice are discussed in Chapter 33.

• • Evaluation

The nurse is responsible for evaluating the neonate's physiologic and behavioral adaptations as well as progress in the parent–newborn acquaintance process in preparation for discharge. In general, evaluation criteria include the following: stabilization of physiologic and behavioral functioning, successful establishment of feeding, and initiation of the parent–neonate acquaintance process. The nurse must ascertain that newborn screening tests have been completed or provisions to complete these tests after discharge have been made. The parents should be able to describe normal behavior and developmental needs during the neonatal period as well as signs and symptoms of infant illness. They should also be able to perform basic infant care practices safely.

The neonate may be discharged shortly after birth when physiologic and behavioral adaptations are successful. Until the new family is ready to leave the hospital or birthing unit, the nurse is responsible for ongoing assessment of neonatal physiologic status and behavioral competencies. The data obtained provide the basis for further nursing care as well as individualized parent teaching. Because the time from birth to discharge is often short, the nurse must be skilled in rapid identification of the infant's unique needs and the new parent's desires regarding discharge teaching. Specifics of the teaching plan are presented in the next section.

Chapter Summary

Nursing care of the normal neonate is based on knowledge of the major physiologic and behavioral adaptations of the newborn to extrauterine life and parents' needs to learn about and care for their infant in preparation for their life together. Nursing interventions focus on supporting the neonate's physiologic adaptation, preventing potential neonatal complications, and facilitating parent–infant interaction. A major focus of nursing interventions relates to parenting education so that families can competently assume the care for their new family member. The nursing process is used to ensure systematic assessment, appropriate nursing diagnoses, careful planning, relevant intervention, and accurate evaluation of the newborn and family.

Study Questions

1. *How do different neonatal environments influence the type of nursing care provided the newly formed family?*
2. *What are major nursing considerations in the prevention of aspiration in the neonate?*
3. *What specific nursing actions can be implemented to prevent hypothermia?*
4. *What are major nursing considerations in the promotion of breastfeeding and bottle feeding?*
5. *What is the major nursing action performed to prevent infection in the neonate?*
6. *What is hypoglycemia and how can it be detected in the neonate?*
7. *What is hemorrhagic disease of the newborn and how is it prevented?*
8. *What vaccines and drugs does the neonate receive at birth for the prevention of infection?*
9. *How does early feeding reduce the likelihood of hyperbilirubinemia in the newborn?*
10. *What are the normal fluid and caloric requirement of the newborn, and how does the nurse determine the individual neonate's requirements?*
11. *What are major nursing responsibilities in the care of the circumcised neonate?*
12. *What are the major complications of phototherapy and what nursing actions can be implemented to prevent them?*
13. *How does the nurse support or foster parent–newborn attachment in provided daily neonatal care?*
14. *What are major topics to be included in the discharge teaching plan for parent education?*
15. *What actions can the nurse take to prevent neonatal abduction?*

References

Arnett, R., Jones, S., & Horger, E. (1990). Effectiveness of 1% lidocaine dorsal penile nerve block in infant circumcision. *American Journal of Obstetrics and Gynecology*, *163*(3), 1074.

Barnes, L. (1992). The illiterate client: Strategies in patient teaching. *American Journal of Maternal Child Nursing*, *17*(3), 127.

Beachy, P., & Deacon, J. (1992) Preventing neonatal kidnapping. *Journal of Obstetric, Gynecologic, and Neonatal Nursing*, *21*(1), 12.

Beal, J. (1989). The effect on father–infant interaction of demonstrating the neonatal behavioral assessment scale. *Birth*, *16*(1), 18.

Blass, E. M., & Hoffmeyer, L. B. (1991). Sucrose as an analgesic for newborn infants. *Pediatrics*, *87*(2), 215.

Brown, J., Bellinger, D., & Matthews J. (1990). In utero lead exposure. *American Journal of Maternal Child Nursing*, *15*(2), 94.

Cameron. D., Simonson, J. & DiCosta, L. (1989). Female to male transmission of human immunodeficiency virus type I. *Lancet*, *2*, 403–407.

Centers for Disease Control. (1991). Hepatitis B virus: A comprehensive strategy for eliminating transmission in the United States through universal childhood vaccination. *Morbidity and Mortality Weekly Report*, 40(RR-13).

Cetta, F., Lambert, G., & Ros, S. (1991). Newborn chemical exposure from over-the-counter skin care products. *Clinical Pediatrics*, *30*(5), 286.

DiFlorio, I. (1991). Mothers' comprehension of terminology associated with the care of a newborn baby. *Pediatric Nursing*, *17*(2), 193.

Donaher-Wagner, B., & Braun, D. (1992). Infant cardiopulmonary resuscitation for expectant and new parents. *American Journal of Maternal Child Nursing*, *17*(1), 27.

Froman, R., & Owen, S. (1990). Mothers' and nurses' perceptions of infant care skills. *Research in Nursing and Health*, *13*, 247.

Green, J., & Bax, M. (1989). Neonatal behavior and early temperament. *American Journal of Orthopsychiatry*, *59*(1), 82.

Guntheroth, W., & Spiers, P. (1992). Sleeping prone and the risk of sudden infant death syndrome. *Journal of the American Medical Association*, *267*(17), 2359.

Keefe, M. R. (1988). The impact of infant rooming-in on maternal sleep at night. *Journal of Obstetric, Gynecologic, and Neonatal Nursing*, *17*(2), 122–126.

Klaus, M. H., & Kennell, J. J. (1982). *Parent–infant bonding* (2nd ed.). St. Louis: CV Mosby.

Marchette, L., Main, R., Redick, E., Bagg, A., & Leatherland, J. (1991). Pain reduction interventions during neonatal circumcision. *Nursing Research*, *40*(4), 241.

Marrone, B. (1990). The effect of anesthesia or comforting on the infant's response to pain during circumcision. *Neonatal Network*, *8*(4), 73.

Matthews, M. K. (1991). Mother's satisfaction with their neonate's breastfeeding behaviors. *Journal of Obstetric, Gynecologic, and Neonatal Nursing*, *20*(1), 49.

McMillen, C., Kok, J., Adamson, M., Deayton, J., & Nowak, R. (1991). Development of circadian sleep-wake rhythms in preterm and full term infants. *Pediatric Research*, *29*(4), 381.

Mugford, M., Somchiwong, M., Waterhouse, I. (1986). Midwifery treatment of umbilical cords: A randomised trial to assess the effect of treatment methods on the work of midwives. *Midwifery*, *2*(4), 177–186.

NAACOG. (1991a). *Facilitating breastfeeding*. OGN Nursing Practice Resource. Washington, DC: Author.

NAACOG. (1991b). Issue: Breastfeeding. NAACOG Position Statement. Washington, DC: Author.

NAACOG. (1990). *Neonatal thermoregulation*. OGN Nursing Practice Resource. Washington, DC: Author.

NAACOG. (1985). *Nurses' role in neonatal circumcision*. OGN Nursing Practice Resource. Washington, DC: Author.

Norr, K., & Roberts, J. (1991). Early maternal attachment behaviors of adolescent and adult mothers. *Journal of Nurse-Midwifery*, *36*(6), 334.

Norr, K., Roberts, J., & Freese, U. (1988). Early postpartum rooming-in and maternal attachment behaviors in a group of medically indigent primiparas. *Journal of Nurse-Midwifery*, *33*(5), 411.

Poland, R. (1990). The question of routine neonatal circumcision. *New England Journal of Medicine*, *322*(18), 1312.

Rabun, J. (1991). *Guidelines on preventing abduction of infants from hospitals*. Arlington, VA: National Center for Missing & Exploited Children.

Rush, J., Chiovitti, R., Kaufman, K., & Mitchell, A. (1990). A randomized controlled trial of a nursery ritual: Wearing cover gowns to care for healthy newborns. *Birth*, *17*(1), 25.

Schumacher, R. (1990). Noninvasive measurements of bilirubin in the newborn. *Clinics in Perinatology*, *17*(2), 417.

Shannon, M., & Graef, J. (1992). Lead intoxication in infancy. *Pediatrics*, *89*(1), 87.

Shrago, L., & Bocar, D. (1990). The infant's contribution to breastfeeding. *Journal of Obstetric, Gynecologic, and Neonatal Nursing*, *19*(2), 209.

Simonsen, J. Cameron, D., & Gakinya, M. (1988). Human immunodeficiency virus infection among men with STDs. *New England Journal of Medicine*, *319*, 274–278.

Spenser, J., Moran, D., & Talbert, D. (1990). White noise and sleep induction. *Neuroscience Biobehavioral Review*, *14*(1), 93.

Tan, K. (1991). Phototherapy for neonatal jaundice. *Clinics in Perinatology*, *18*(3), 423.

Task Force on Circumcision. (1989). Report of the task force on circumcision. *Pediatrics*, *84*(4), 388.

Tedder, J. (1991). Using the Brazelton Neonatal Assessment Scale to facilitate the parent–infant relationship in a primary setting. *Nurse Practitioner*, *16*(3), .

Tedder, J. (1989). Circumcision considerations. *Journal of Obstetric, Gynecologic, and Neonatal Nursing*, *18*(4), 277.

United States Department of Health and Human Services Public Health Service. (1992). *Acute pain management in infants, children, and adolescents: Operative and medical procedures*. Rockville, MD: Author.

Vaughans, B. (1990). Early maternal-infant contact and neonatal thermoregulation. *Neonatal Network*, *8*(5), .

Walker, M. (1989). Functional assessment of infant breastfeeding patterns. *Birth*, *16*(3), 140.

Suggested Readings

Anderson E., & Geden, E. (1991). Nurses' knowledge of breastfeeding. *Journal of Obstetric, Gynecologic, and Neonatal Nursing*, *20*(1), 58.

Conte, L. (1992). Factors that influence the use of universal precautions by neonatal nurses. *Neonatal Network*, *11*(1), 27.

Downey, J., & Bidder, R. (1990). Perinatal information on infant crying. *Child: Care, Health and Development*, *16*, 113.

Eidelman, A. (1992). Early discharge-early trouble. *Journal of Perinatology*, *XII*(2), 101.

Hubbard, F., & Ijzendoorn, M. (1991). Maternal unresponsiveness and infant crying across the first 9 months. *Infant behavior and Development*, *14*, 299.

Jones, L., Heerman, J. (1992). Parental division of infant care: Contextual influences and infant characteristics. *Nursing Research*, *41*(4), 228.

Kimble, C. (1992). Nonnutritive sucking: Adaptation and health for the neonate. *Neonatal Network*, *11*(2), 29.

Meyers, D. (1991). Preventing neonatal hepatitis B virus infection. *Neonatal Network*, *10*(2), 11.

NAACOG. (1992). *Neonatal skin care*. OGN Nursing Practice Resource. Washington, DC: Author.

Newman, T., & Maisels, J. (1992). Evaluation and treatment of jaundice in the term newborn. *Pediatrics*, *89*(5), 809.

Pedersen, F. (1989). *The father–infant relationship*. New York: Praeger Special Studies.

Rasmussen, L., Weatherstone, K., & Leff, R. (1992). Efficacy and safety of topical anesthesia for circumcision of the newborn. *Neonatal Network*, *11*(3), 64.

Wandel, J. C. (1991). Pain perception in the neonate: Implications for circumcision. *Journal of Professional Nursing*, *7*(3), 188.

CHAPTER 32

Assessment of the At-Risk Neonate

Learning Objectives

After studying the material in this chapter, the student will be able to:

- Identify major goals and objectives in the assessment of neonatal risk factors.
- Demonstrate the use of the Apgar score to assess the neonate's need for resuscitation after birth.
- Describe the use of umbilical cord blood pH and gas analysis in medical treatment and nursing care of the neonate.
- Demonstrate the prescribed steps in resuscitation of the neonate.
- Describe danger signals or signs in the neonate that indicate actual or potential problems.
- List signs of behavioral disorganization in the high-risk neonate.
- Describe the phases in recovery of behavioral capacities in the sick or injured neonate.

Key Terms

apnea	low–birth-weight neonate
asphyxia	morbidity
cyanosis	mortality
decerebrate posture	neonatology
decorticate posture	perinatal
hypoxemia	postterm neonate
hypoxia	preterm neonate
intrauterine growth retardation	resuscitation
	small-for-gestational age neonate

Modern technology makes it possible to save neonates who would have died in the past. These newborns, however, are at greater risk for complications. As a result nurses have had to create a new standard of care for high-risk neonates. This is done by following assessment protocols and using sophisticated equipment that enhances the nurse's ability to recognize illness early. Neonatal nursing as an emerging specialty is the result. Neonatal nurses have advanced theoretical preparation and clinical training to function in their specialized role.

The scope of practice, once narrowly defined by the walls of the neonatal intensive care unit, has expanded. Neonatal nurses provide professional outreach to the parents of the high-risk neonate after the infant is discharged from the hospital. They also serve as consultants to nurses who work in community hospitals. They are involved in long-distance transportation of sick newborns to facilities offering specialized care and services.

This chapter defines the concept of risk assessment in the neonatal period and demonstrates how nursing assessment can be used systematically in the early recognition and treatment of potential or actual problems. The nurse's role in the resuscitation, stabilization, and support of the high-risk newborn is described.

Identification of Perinatal Risk Factors

Optimal care is best provided when the health care team is prepared for the birth of a high-risk neonate. The proper equipment and supplies needed for resuscitation of the newborn can be assembled ahead of time, and essential members of the team can be present in the delivery room to begin immediate evaluation and support of the newborn.

Identification of Prenatal Risk Factors

Approximately 60% of neonates requiring special care and treatment at birth can be identified through careful evaluation of the mother's prenatal history. Table 32-1 lists exam-

Table 32-1. Prenatal Risk Factors and Potential Fetal and Neonatal Complications

Risk Factors	Potential Complications
Demographic Factors	
Maternal age	
Under 16 or over 35 y	Small-for-gestational-age (SGA); genetic abnormalities
Primigravida over 30 y	Labor dystocia; birth trauma
Parity	
Grand multiparity (over five pregnancies)	Fetal malposition/malpresentation
Substance abuse	
Drug addiction	SGA; neonatal withdrawal syndrome; neonatal HIV
Alcoholism	Fetal alcohol syndrome
Smoking	SGA; polycythemia
Multiple sex partners, prostitution	Neonatal HIV; sexually transmitted diseases; hepatitis B
Sex partner IV drug abuser or bisexual	Neonatal HIV; sexually transmitted diseases; hepatitis B
Maternal Nutritional Status	
Maternal malnutrition	
Weight less than 100 lb (45.4 kg)	SGA
Weight more than 200 lb (91 kg)	SGA, large-for-gestational-age (LGA)
Previous Pregnancy Complications	
Fetal loss at over 28 wk of gestation	Fetal loss
Premature delivery	Prematurity
Abnormal fetal position/presentation	Fetal malposition and potential birth trauma
Bleeding in second or third trimester	Recurrent bleeding in subsequent pregnancy
Pregnancy-induced hypertension	Recurrent hypertension
Rh sensitization	Erythroblastosis and jaundice
Fetal distress of unknown origin	Fetal distress
Birth of neonate with anomalies	Congenital anomalies
Birth of neonate over 10 lb	Birth of LGA neonate
Birth of post-term neonate	Post-term neonate; intrauterine growth retardation (IUGR)
Neonatal death	Neonatal death
Central Nervous System (CNS) Disorders	
Hereditary CNS disorders	Inherited CNS disorder
Seizure disorders requiring medication	Congenital anomalies (as a result of Dilantin use)
Cardiovascular Disease	
Chronic hypertension	IUGR; asphyxia; SGA neonate
Congenital heart disease with congestive heart failure	Prematurity; inherited defects
Hematologic Disorders	
Anemia (Under 10 g)	Prematurity; low birth weight
Sickle cell disease	IUGR; fetal demise
Hemoglobinopathies	IUGR; inherited hemoglobinopathies
Idiopathic thrombocytopenic purpura (ITP)	Transient ITP
Renal Disease	
Chronic glomerulonephritis	IUGR; SGA; prematurity; asphyxia
Renal insufficiency	IUGR; SGA; prematurity; asphyxia
Reproductive Disorders	
Uterine malformation	Prematurity; fetal malposition
Cervical incompetence	Prematurity

(*continued*)

Table 32-1. Prenatal Risk Factors and Potential Fetal and Neonatal Complications ***(Continued)***

Risk Factors	Potential Complications
Metabolic Disorders	
Diabetes	LGA; hypoglycemia and hypocalcemia; anomalies; respiratory distress syndrome
Thyroid disease	Hypothyroidism; CNS defects Hyperthyroidism, goiter
Current Pregnancy Complications	
Pregnancy-induced hypertension	IUGR; SGA
Maternal infections:	
TORCH infections	IUGR; SGA; active infection; anomalies
Sexually transmitted disease	Ophthalmia neonatorum; congenital syphilis
Acute cystitis, pyelonephritis	Prematurity
Hepatitis	Hepatitis
AIDS or HIV seropositive	Neonatal HIV
Multiple gestation	Prematurity; asphyxia; IUGR; SGA
Fetal malposition	Prolapsed cord; asphyxia; birth trauma
Rh sensitization	Erythroblastosis fetalis
Prolonged pregnancy	Postmaturity; meconium aspiration; IUGR; asphyxia

ples of prenatal maternal conditions and obstetric complications that place the fetus at risk for increased morbidity and mortality. This table clarifies the need for the nurse to have access to the prenatal history to appreciate the potential problems confronting the newborn when the mother has experienced problems in the present or in a previous pregnancy. If a woman is referred to a level II or level III perinatal regional center for prenatal care when complications arise, maternity and neonatal nurses can be alerted before the birth and will be prepared to meet the special needs of the infant.

Some prenatal risk factors, such as the hemoglobinopathies, are rarely seen and require nurses to consult with nurse specialists and physicians on the health care team to identify potential problems and to plan care. Other disorders, such as maternal diabetes and chronic hypertension, are frequently encountered. Standardized nursing care plans are available to assist nurses in identifying problems and in planning and implementing appropriate care.

Identification of Intrapartum Risk Factors

Using the prenatal history alone, it is not possible to predict with complete accuracy which neonates will require special assistance and care after birth. Approximately 10% to 20% of all women who experienced normal pregnancies will develop intrapartum problems that place the newborn at increased risk for neonatal complications. Obstetric emergencies, such as abruptio placentae and prolapse of the umbilical cord, can occur without warning. The administration of analgesia or anesthesia and the use of forceps or a vacuum extractor to assist in delivery may place the infant at greater postnatal risk.

Electronic fetal monitoring is now used extensively to assess fetal well-being during labor and delivery. Monitoring of maternal vital signs, evaluation of the progress of labor, and inspection of amniotic fluid after rupture of the membranes are all essential aspects of assessment and aid the nurse in identifying risk factors.

Table 32-2 lists major intrapartum factors that contribute to neonatal morbidity and mortality. Some of these factors, such as severe intrapartum hemorrhage or infection, can result in life-threatening complications that require immediate intervention. Others merely increase the risk of injury or illness. The nurse attending the birth must report all pertinent information about the delivery to the nurse assuming responsibility for the neonate.

Research findings suggest that the 5-minute Apgar score may predict immediate postnatal organ dysfunction, as well as the long-term neurologic status of the full-term neonate (Portman, Carter, Gaylord, et al., 1990). This is particularly true when the 5-minute Apgar score is 3 or less, and the neonate experiences seizures in the neonatal period (ACOG, 1991). The association between neonatal depression and neurologic abnormalities in low–birth-weight infants is unclear. Recent studies suggest that the value of Apgar scoring, particularly in very low–birth-weight premature infants 3 lb, 4 oz to 3 lb, 14 oz (1500 to 1800 g) may be limited (Behnke, Eyler, Carter, et al., 1989). The nurse who assumes care for the neonate should be aware of the Apgar scores assigned at 1 and 5 minutes. Additionally, it is imperative that the nurse be cognizant of any resuscitation efforts used to support the neonate immediately after delivery.

Umbilical cord blood gas and acid–base analysis have been suggested as tools to diagnose hypoxia and metabolic acidemia during the intrapartum period (ACOG, 1991). Research findings indicate that cord blood gas and pH analysis may be useful in *excluding* intrapartum asphyxia as the cause for neonatal neurologic problems when the neonate is

Table 32-2. Intrapartum Risk Factors and Potential Fetal and Neonatal Complications

Risk Factors	Potential Complications
Umbilical Cord	
Prolapsed umbilical cord	Asphyxia
True knot in cord	Asphyxia
Velamentous insertion	Intrauterine blood loss; shock; anemia
Vasa previa	Intrauterine blood loss; shock; anemia
Rupture or tearing of cord	Blood loss; shock; anemia
Membranes	
Premature rupture of membranes	Infection; RDS; prolapsed cord; asphyxia
Prolonged rupture of membranes	Infection
Amnionitis	Infection
Amniotic Fluid	
Oligohydramnios	Congenital anomalies
Polyhydramnios	Congenital anomalies; prolapsed cord
Meconium-stained fluid	Asphyxia; meconium aspiration syndrome
Placenta	
Placenta previa	Prematurity; asphyxia
Abruptio placentae	Prematurity; asphyxia
Placental insufficiency	IUGR; SGA; asphyxia
Abnormal Fetal Presentations	
Breech delivery	Asphyxia; birth injuries (CNS, skeletal)
Face or brow presentation	Asphyxia; facial trauma
Transverse lie	Asphyxia; birth injuries; cesarean delivery
	Umbilical cord prolapse
Labor Dystocias	
Prolonged labor	Asphyxia; birth trauma; infection
Uterine inertia	Complications of prolonged labor
Uterine tetany	Asphyxia
Precipitate labor	Asphyxia; birth trauma
Delivery Complications	
Forceps-assisted delivery	CNS trauma; cephalhematoma; asphyxia; facial trauma
Vacuum extraction	Cephalhematoma
Manual version or extraction	Asphyxia; birth trauma; prolapsed cord
Shoulder dystocia	Asphyxia; brachial plexus injury; fractured clavicle
Precipitate delivery	Asphyxia; birth trauma (CNS)
Undiagnosed multiple gestation	Asphyxia; birth trauma
Administration of Drugs	
Oxytocin	Complications of uterine tetany (asphyxia)
Magnesium sulfate	Hypermagnesemia; CNS depression
Analgesics	CNS and respiratory depression
Anesthetics	CNS and respiratory depression; bradycardia

depressed at birth (Winkler, Hauth, Tucker, et al., 1991). Further research is needed to define normal and abnormal acid–base and blood gas parameters and the usefulness of the cord blood gas and pH test in predicting long-term neurologic outcomes. Umbilical cord blood analysis and the nurse's role in obtaining blood samples is described in Chapter 21.

Identification of Neonatal Risk Factors

Another useful instrument the nurse can use to identify infants at greatest risk for neonatal morbidity and mortality is the neonatal mortality rate chart (Fig. 32-1). The chart relates the mortality rate to the gestational age and birth weight of the neonate. The chart shows that the risk is greatest for premature neonates whose weight and gestational age fall to the lower left corner of the graph. The causes of death in these infants are related to the extreme immaturity of all systems and include respiratory distress syndrome, intracranial hemorrhage, and infection. The presence of congenital anomalies is another major contributing factor to the high rate of morbidity and mortality in these neonates.

The nurse caring for the high-risk neonate must identify all risk factors that could influence successful adaptation in the immediate postnatal period. This requires extensive knowledge of the mother's prenatal history, including the preexistence of disease states that affect fetal growth and development, such as diabetes or chronic hypertension. Life-style variables, including nutritional status, diet, drug use, and exposure to organisms or substances that may be hazardous to the fetus, should be reviewed. Obstetric and medical problems that occurred during the pregnancy also should be known to plan appropriate care. The progress of labor and the development of intrapartum complications may jeopardize the infant's postnatal adjustment. The nurse should be well informed about any maternal or fetal problems that have occurred during the critical hours before delivery. The presence of factors that may prevent immediate cardiovascular and pulmonary adaptations are of particular importance, such as the administration of analgesia or the diagnosis of fetal distress distress shortly before birth. Finally, the infant's status at delivery, including the Apgar scores, biochemical analysis of umbilical cord blood samples, and the need for resuscitation, must be known. Planning and implementation of care cannot proceed until the nurse has identified all significant perinatal risk factors.

Initial Assessment and Support

A neonatal nurse and physician (pediatrician or neonatologist) often collaborate in the initial assessment of the high-risk neonate at birth. Level II and level III perinatal regional centers have been created to care for high-risk women, fetuses, and neonates (discussed in Chapter 31). In these

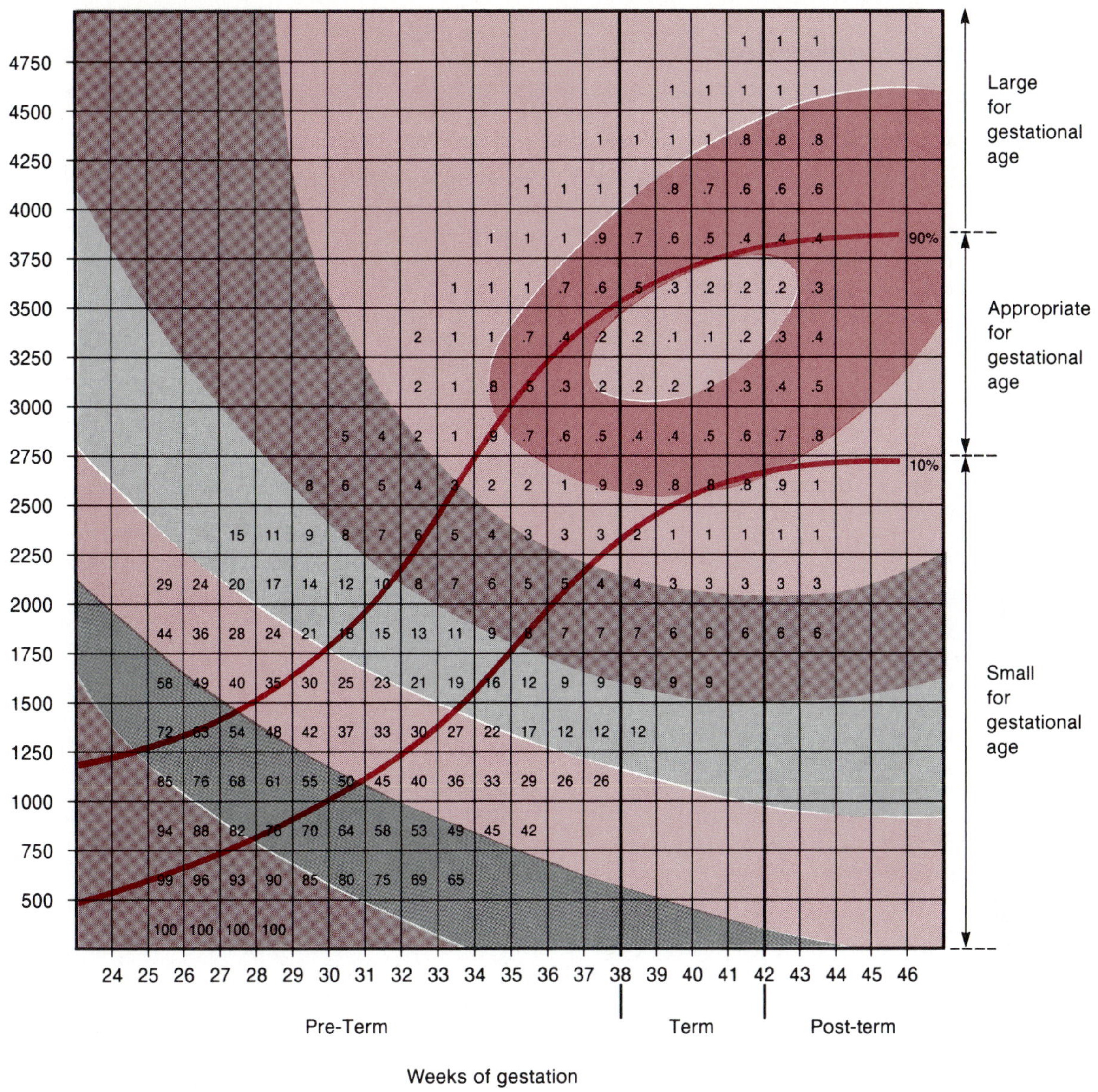

Figure 32-1.
Neonatal mortality rate chart. The chart shows the relationship between neonatal mortality, shown in percentages by numbers in boxes, and birth weight and gestational age. Note the dramatic decrease in mortality as age and weight increase. Shaded zones are areas of similar mortality. (Original data from University of Colorado Medical Center, redrawn from Mead Johnson Laboratories.)

centers neonatologists, nurses, and other personnel skilled in the evaluation and stabilization of neonates are usually present at the delivery of a high-risk infant. The accompanying Legal/Ethical Considerations display lists health care providers frequently responsible for neonatal resuscitation.

In level I hospitals, where low-risk women give birth, the nurse must be prepared to assess the neonate, initiate resuscitation, and provide immediate supportive care until help arrives. It is estimated that approximately 85,000 neonates suffer some degree of birth asphyxia each year, and 90% of them are delivered in level I facilities (Paxton & Harrell, 1991). All delivery units must have the equipment and drugs required to perform resuscitation. All nurses caring for neonates at birth or during the postnatal period must be skilled in performing neonatal resuscitation and should have completed the American Heart Association's (AHA) program to certify neonatal resuscitators. The American Academy of Pediatrics (AAP) has mandated that at least one person skilled in neonatal resuscitation be in attendance at every delivery (AHA/AAP, 1990).

Assigning an Apgar Score

One-Minute Apgar Score

Although the first Apgar score is not assigned for 60 seconds, evaluation of the neonate begins *immediately* after birth. The newborn is quickly dried to prevent heat loss, and

Legal/Ethical Considerations

The Nurse's Responsibilities in Planning for and Initiating Neonatal Resuscitation

In today's medicolegal climate, claims of negligence may be leveled against health professionals involved in the birth and neonatal resuscitation process when a diagnosis of birth asphyxia is made. Each hospital or birthing facility must have a formal policy and procedure to guide nurses and other health care providers in preparing for and implementing neonatal resuscitation. The most frequent allegations of negligence leveled against the nurse when birth asphyxia occurs include the following:

- Failure to notify neonatal staff in a timely manner
- Failure to have essential equipment, supplies, and drugs available and ready for the resuscitation procedure
- Failure to initiate CPR in a timely manner
- Failure to perform CPR correctly

When the nurse anticipates the need for neonatal resuscitation, designated support personnel must be notified well in advance of the birth whenever possible. If conflicts arise between the obstetrician or midwife and the nurse regarding the need for neonatal support staff at delivery, the chain of command should be used to obtain timely consultation with managers or other health care providers with expertise in neonatal care.

A variety of professionals qualified to perform neonatal resuscitation include the following:

Nurses

Delivery room nurse
Certified nurse midwife
Neonatal nurse practitioner
Neonatal nurse
Nursery nurse
Nurse anesthetist

Physicians

Obstetrician
Pediatrician
Neonatologist
Anesthesiologist

Others

Respiratory therapist

The professionals designated to initiate CPR must complete the American Heart Association/American Academy of Pediatrics' course in Neonatal Resuscitation (1990). The nurse is responsible for documenting the resuscitation process including:

- Time of request for assistance
- Time of arrival of support staff
- Names of professionals involved in resuscitation
- Procedures performed (suctioning, ventilating, chest compression)
- Drugs administered
- Apgar scores
- Umbilical cord blood gas and pH values

Fisher, C. (1990). The abnormal infant: Protecting yourself against blame. RN, *53(4), 69.*
Mahlmeister, L., & Mahlmeister, M. (1991). Professional accountability and the respiratory care practitioner. AARC Times.

the neonate's mouth and nose are suctioned to clear the airway. The nurse then observes respirations, notes the color, and determines the heart rate by auscultating the apical rate or palpating pulsations in the umbilical cord. These initial steps should be accomplished within 20 seconds of birth (AHA/AAP, 1990). By 30 seconds after birth the nurse must begin appropriate resuscitation of the neonate based on this initial assessment.

At 1 minute the first Apgar score is assigned (determination of the Apgar score is discussed in Chapters 21 and 32). The infant's condition at that time provides evidence of the effectiveness of initial resuscitation efforts during the first 60 seconds of life. The primary value of the 1-minute Apgar score is to guide the nurse in determining the need for continued resuscitation and appropriate interventions (Epstein, 1991; AHA/AAP, 1990; Table 32-3).

Five-Minute Apgar Score

The 5-minute score reflects the neonate's changing condition and the adequacy of resuscitative efforts. Persistence of a low Apgar score indicates the need for further therapeutic efforts. As noted, a 5-minute Apgar score of 3 or less may predict short-term organ dysfunction in the neonate secondary to asphyxia and long-term neurologic dysfunction (Epstein, 1991).

Differences in Apgar Scores

Neonates with Apgar Scores of 8 to 10. The neonate who receives an Apgar score of 8 to 10 has a strong, regular heart rate of over 100 bpm; has an adequate respiratory effort; and responds quickly to stimulation. Major interventions are unnecessary. The mouth and pharynx are suc-

Table 32-3. Management of Neonatal Resuscitation Based on the Neonate's Condition and Assigned Apgar Score

Apgar Score	Neonate's Condition	Nursing Interventions
8 to 10 (No evidence of asphyxia)	Pink, active, responsive to stimuli, crying, heart rate over 100 bpm	Suction mouth and nares Dry thoroughly, including head Maintain body temperature Perform brief physical examination Unite with parents Assign 5-min Apgar score
5 to 7 (Mild asphyxia)	Cyanotic, moving with decreased muscle tone, breathing shallow, decreased respiratory effort, heart rate above 100 bpm	Suction mouth, nares, and larynx if amniotic fluid is meconium stained Dry quickly Maintain body temperature Stimulate gently by rubbing body dry Provide 100% oxygen using bag and mask set-up by placing over neonate's nose and mouth Call for help if alone in case neonate's condition deteriorates As soon as possible, assign someone to support parents
3 to 4 (Moderate asphyxia)	Cyanotic, minimal movement, decreased muscle tone, breathing shallow, poor respiratory effort, heart rate below 100 bpm	Suction mouth, nares, and larynx if amniotic fluid is meconium stained Dry quickly Maintain body temperature Provide 100% oxygen using bag and mask Call for help if alone Continue ventilating at 40 to 60 times/min until heart rate is above 100 bpm, color is pink, and spontaneous respirations begin As soon as possible, assign someone to support parents
0 to 2 (Severe asphyxia)	Deeply cyanotic, no muscle tone, absent respiratory effort or periodic gasps, heart rate slow or absent	Clear airway quickly; call for help Insert endotracheal tube Initiate bag ventilation with 100% oxygen at 40 to 60 breaths/min at pressures great enough to move chest wall Perform cardiac massage at a rate of 120 times/min If heart rate is under 80 bpm despite adequate ventilation and cardiac massage, for a minimum of 30 seconds, insert umbilical venous catheter and administer drugs (see Table 31-4) As soon as additional personnel arrive, ensure maintenance of body temperature Assign someone to support parents

tioned with a bulb syringe, the skin is dried quickly, the neonate is wrapped with warm blankets to prevent hypothermia, and it is given to the parents as quickly as possible to promote early parent–newborn acquaintance. The nurse continues to observe the newborn closely for signs of maladaptations but allows the new family to become acquainted, keeping distractions and interruptions to a minimum.

Neonates with Apgar Scores of 5 to 7. The neonate with an Apgar score of 5 to 7 is mildly depressed and requires immediate assistance to establish and maintain effective respirations. The neonate appears cyanotic, with a decreased muscle tone and diminished respiratory effort. Heart rate is usually above 100 bpm. Gentle stimulation can then be accomplished by briskly drying the neonate. The infant's mouth and nose are suctioned to clear the airway. An oxygen-enriched atmosphere should be provided by placing the mask of a bag-and-mask device with continuous flow over the neonate's nose and mouth. The goal is to elevate the level of arterial oxygen (Po_2) by delivering more oxygen to the alveoli with each breath. A laryngoscope should be inserted by a trained professional and the larynx suctioned if the amniotic fluid is meconium stained. This is done to clear the airway and prevent meconium aspiration. The process of laryngoscopy requires special training and may be performed in some settings by a nurse who has completed an advanced neonatal life support course.

Neonates with Apgar Scores of 3 to 4. The neonate with an Apgar score of 3 to 4 is moderately depressed. The neonate appears cyanotic and flaccid and has weak, ineffectual respirations. The heart rate is under 100 bpm. Immediate support is necessary to reverse the newborn's deteriorating condition. After the neonate is quickly dried, the mouth and nose are suctioned. If meconium is present in the amniotic fluid, a laryngoscope should be inserted for suctioning, followed by the administration of 100% oxygen through a tightly fitting face mask. The face mask is attached to a flow-inflating bag.

Ventilation is initiated by compressing the bag 40 to 60 times per minute, using pressures of 15 to 20 cm H_2O. High pressures (30 to 40 cm H_2O) may be required initially to expand the lungs adequately, but continued application of excessive pressures may result in pneumothorax (AHA/AAP, 1990). Use of a ventilation bag with a pressure "pop-off" valve reduces the risk of overinflation of the lungs. Generally, the moderately depressed neonate will respond to these measures with an increased heart rate, improved color, and spontaneous respirations. If there is no improvement or the neonate's condition deteriorates, the resuscitation team advances to the next stage of resuscitation, which is described below.

Neonates with Apgar Scores of 0 to 2. The neonate with an Apgar score of 0 to 2 is severely depressed and requires maximum resuscitation efforts and support. The neonate is cyanotic and flaccid. There may be no respiratory effort or heart rate. Stimulation will not effect an improvement in the neonate's condition, and precious time should not be wasted flicking the soles of the feet or otherwise attempting to stimulate the infant. The newborn is quickly dried, the mouth and nose suctioned, and resuscitative efforts initiated. A laryngoscope should be inserted by a trained professional and an endotracheal tube passed immediately after the airway is cleared by suctioning. A flow inflating bag is attached to the end of the endotracheal tube, and 100% oxygen is administered using the rate and pressure guidelines listed previously. (Higher rates or pressures may be required with severe meconium aspiration.) If maternal overmedication with narcotics is identified as a contributing factor in the neonate's depressed state, narcotic antagonists are administered.

If the heart beat is absent or the heart rate remains low (under 80 bpm) after 1 minute of ventilation, external cardiac massage is begun at a rate of 120 compressions per minute (AHA/AAP, 1990). Drugs may be administered to correct metabolic acidosis (sodium bicarbonate), hypoglycemia (glucose), or bradycardia (epinephrine or atropine).

Managing Neonatal Resuscitation

Resuscitation efforts are conducted with a recognition of the unique anatomic and physiologic characteristics of the neonate, a knowledge of neonatal emergency drugs, and an understanding of the special equipment required for neonatal resuscitation.

Airway Management

Initially the newborn is placed on a flat surface in a Trendelenburg position (15- to 30-degree tilt) to facilitate mucus drainage. Once the airway is cleared and ventilation is established, the examining table is returned to a horizontal position (unless an injury or anomaly requires a different position). If ventilation is necessary, the infant's head is placed in a "sniffing position" to open the airway fully. A folded towel may be placed under the shoulders to bring the head into correct alignment. Care must be taken not to hyperextend or underextend the neck because this will decrease air entry (Fig. 32-2).

When the neonate is placed in a supine position, the tongue does not usually fall back and obstruct the airway as it does in older children and adults. Many neonatologists skilled in resuscitation of the newborn believe that a pharyngeal airway, a plastic hollow tube placed into the mouth to maintain a patent upper airway, is unnecessary. High-risk neonates with chromosomal disorders, characterized by a large protruding tongue or those with congenital anomalies of the face and neck, may require pharyngeal airways.

Suctioning and Suction Equipment

Because the neonate is an obligate nose breather, once the mouth and pharynx are suctioned, the nose should be cleared. If the newborn is moderately to severely depressed, a laryngoscope is inserted, and the larynx is carefully suctioned (Fig. 32-3). When in utero meconium passage has occurred, a suction catheter is inserted past the vocal cords under direct visualization by the laryngoscope, and deep suctioning is used to remove all meconium before it is inhaled into terminal bronchioles and alveoli and results in meconium aspiration syndrome. The procedure of laryngoscopy requires specialized training and is only performed by nurses and other health care providers after they complete advanced life support training. Hospital policies and procedures also govern who may perform laryngoscopy.

Bulb Syringe. A bulb syringe is adequate only for removing secretions from the mouth and nose. Usually it is used by the birth attendant after the head is delivered but before the thorax emerges from the birth canal. If the infant receives an Apgar score of 7 to 10 and no meconium was passed in utero, the nurse can complete the suctioning process with the bulb syringe after the infant is delivered. The bulb must be compressed fully before the syringe tip is inserted into the mouth or nares (see Fig. 31-2). Compressing the bulb after it is inserted will force fluids deeper into the airway. Care must be taken to avoid stimulation of the posterior pharynx because it may elicit a reflex vagal response, which can result in bradycardia or apnea.

Suction Catheter. With the introduction of universal body substance precautions to prevent the transmission of human immunodeficiency virus, the equipment and procedures recommended for suctioning have been revised (see the display and illustrations on suctioning the neonate delivered through meconium). In the past a manually operated suction catheter with mucus trap (De Lee Mucus Trap) was used to suction meconium from the neonate's mouth and nares. The practitioner applied negative mouth pressure to the end of this catheter to suction secretions. The danger of accidentally aspirating contaminated body fluids into the operator's mouth has rendered this equipment unsafe for

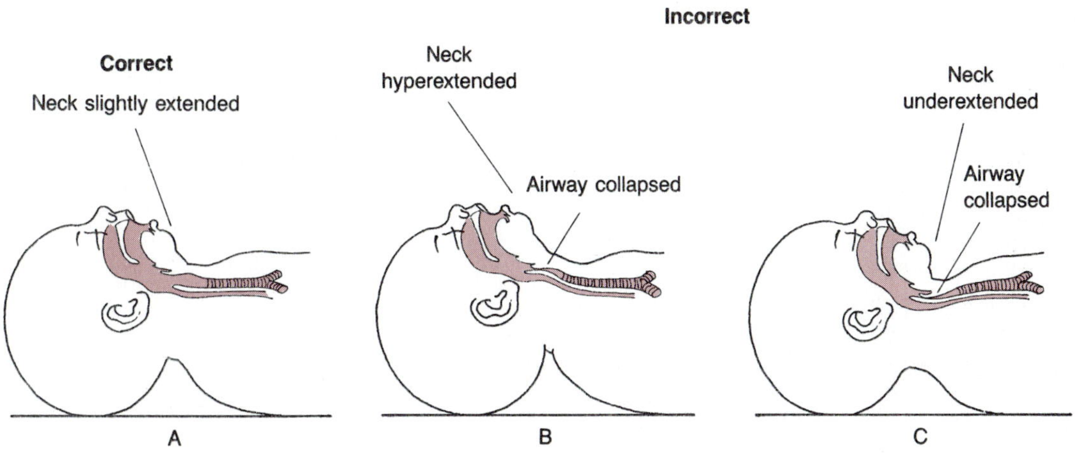

Figure 32-2.

Neonatal resusitation. *A:* The neonate should be placed on the back with neck slightly extended. This is known as the "sniffing" position. *B:* Hyperextension of the neck will cause decrease in air entry. *C:* Underextension of the neck also will decrease air entry.

use today. An 8 to 12 French catheter is now attached to a mechanical suction device to remove meconium from the mouth, oropharynx, and nares.

When the amniotic fluid is meconium stained, laryngoscopy and tracheal suctioning are performed to aspirate meconium from the lung. The endotracheal tube is first inserted below the level of the vocal cords. The upper end of the endotracheal tube is connected to a "meconium trap." Mechanical suction is then applied to aspirate secretions.

Ventilating the Neonate

The nurse must ventilate the neonate using the correct rate, pressures, oxygen concentration, and equipment. Improper technique or equipment can lead to injury or permanent damage.

Ventilation Rate. The normal ventilation rate is 30 to 50 times per minute. Exceptions to the rule exist, such as the presence of severe meconium aspiration, when higher rates may be necessary for the adequate exchange of gases.

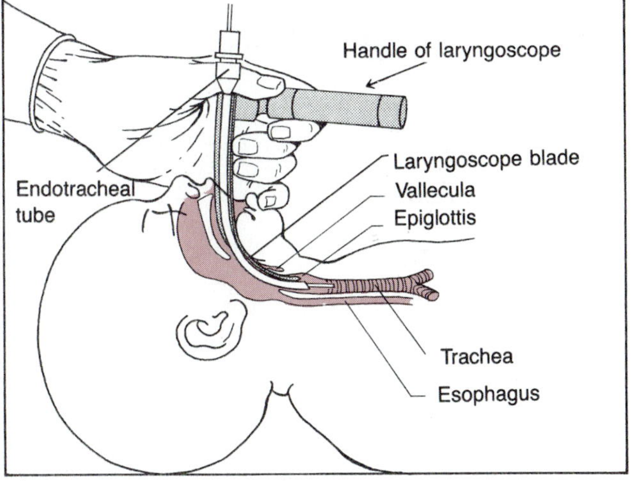

Figure 32-3.

Laryngoscopy allows visualization and suctioning of meconium and mucus from the airway and is necessary for placement of an endotracheal tube if ventilation is required.

Ventilation Pressures. The initial pressure required to inflate the lungs may be quite high (more than 40 cm H_2O). Subsequent pressures of 25 to 35 cm H_2O or lower should be sufficient. The nurse should carefully note the rise and fall of the chest to make sure correct ventilation technique is being used.

Hand Ventilation. With hand ventilation an inflatable bag is compressed to deliver a breath to the infant. The preferred ventilation bag is a flow-inflating anesthesia-type with a safety pressure release (pop-off valve) (Fig. 32-4*A*). This prevents the buildup of excessive pressures within the bag and decreases the risk of pneumothorax. A manometer should be attached to the ventilation system to assist the nurse in monitoring the pressures applied during hand ventilation (see Fig. 32-4*B*).

The flow-inflating anesthesia bag (Fig. 32-5*A*) has several advantages. It has the ability to deliver continuous positive airway pressure, which decreases the risks of alveoli collapsing during expiration. This feature is especially important in premature neonates who lack surfactant and whose alveoli are predisposed to collapse with each expiration. An additional advantage of the flow-inflating bag is the ability to deliver 100% oxygen. A disadvantage of this bag is that it does not have a preset pop-off valve that automatically limits the amount of pressure. The risk of pneumothorax is increased when the bag is used by a person inexperienced in hand ventilation if excessive pressures are used to inflate the lungs.

A second type of resuscitation bag is self-inflating (see Fig. 32-5*B*) and does not need to be attached to flowing oxygen to function. Many of these bags have a preset pressure limit, which reduces the risk of pneumothorax. However, the concentration of oxygen delivered by this unit is limited to approximately 40%. A special adaptor may be attached to increase the concentration to 90% or slightly higher.

Suctioning of the Neonate Delivered Through Meconium

Evidence of the passage of meconium by the fetus prior to delivery requires attendance of personnel at the delivery who have advanced training and skills in newborn intubation and resuscitation. When the neonate's head is delivered at the perineum (or in cesarean birth, at the level of the abdomen) and before delivery of the rest of the body, the nares, mouth, and pharynx should be suctioned an 8 to a 12 French catheter attached to mechanical suction. This helps to remove meconium the neonate could inhale with the first gasping respiration when the thorax is delivered.

After delivery is complete, the neonate should be placed quickly on the radiant warming table with as little stimulation as possible to prevent vigorous crying. This could increase aspiration of meconium. The nursery nurse, nurse anesthetist, or physician skilled in intubation should then quickly intubate the neonate orally.

A meconium aspirator is attached to the end of the tube, and mechanical suction is applied to aspirate meconium present below the level of the vocal cords. This is done as the endotracheal tube is removed. Reintubation may be required several times for repeated suctioning until meconium is cleared. This method of intubation and suctioning provides more efficient removal of very thick meconium and is preferred to using the suction catheter alone.

The practice of placing one's mouth directly over the end of an endotracheal tube to suction meconium from the trachea after intubation is no longer permissible. It has been discarded with the institution of universal body precautions to prevent transmission of HIV.

Even if the neonate appears quite asphyxiated with a heart rate as low as 40–60 bpm, at least one quick intubation with suctioning should be performed. This is done before the oxygen bag is applied to the endotracheal tube and preceeds further resuscitation efforts. After endotracheal suctioning and resuscitation in the delivery room, the neonate should be taken to the admission or intensive care nursery as the infant's condition warrants. Additional interventions, including postural drainage, percussion, and other care directed at consequences of possible meconium aspiration, should be performed.

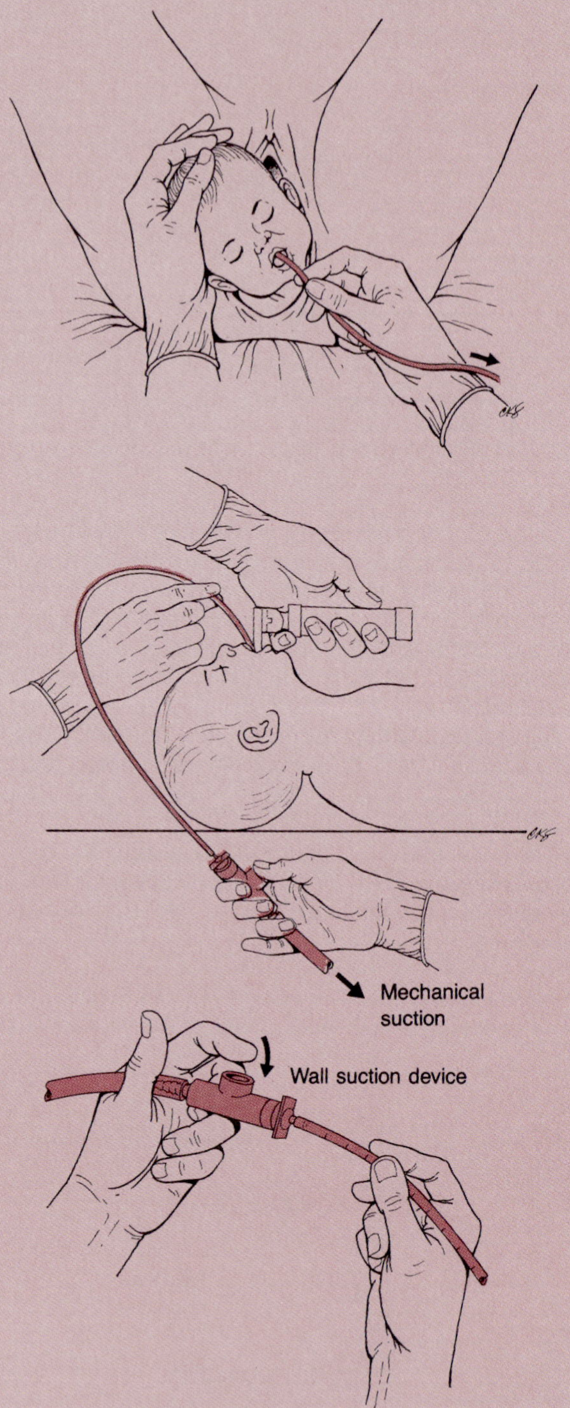

Administering Oxygen to the Neonate

During the initial resuscitation efforts, a 100% oxygen concentration is administered to the neonate. As soon as the neonate's condition is stabilized, the concentration is adjusted with an oxygen blender to maintain the Pao_2(partial pressure of oxygen in the blood) within acceptable limits. The Pao_2 is determined by obtaining and analyzing arterial blood gas samples. Adjustment of the arterial oxygen concentration is essential, because elevated Pao_2 levels (caused by administration of oxygen in high concentrations) can cause irreparable damage to retinal vessels (retrolental fi-

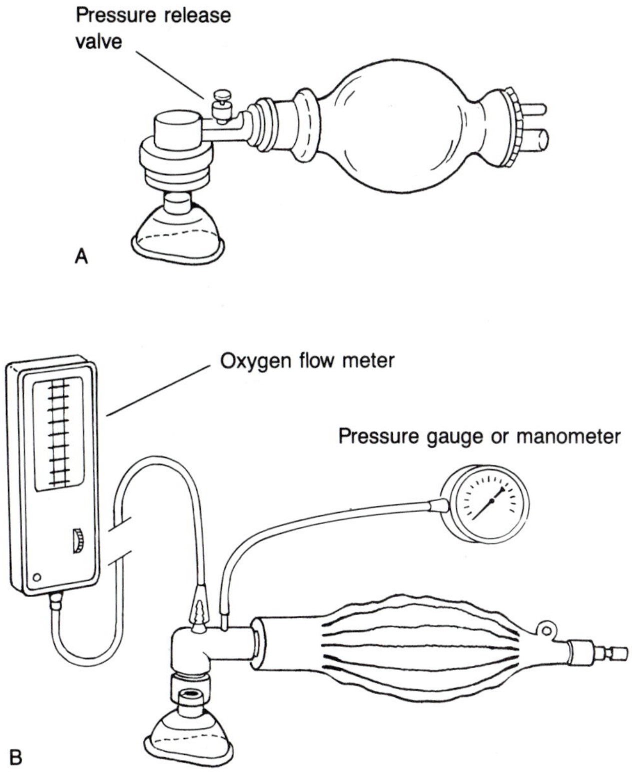

Figure 32-4.
Preventing hyperinflation of the neonates lungs. *A:* A pressure-release valve, otherwise known as a pop-off valve, is a feature most commonly found on self-inflating bags. Pressure-release valves are generally set at 30 to 35 cm H_2O on self-inflating bags. *B:* A manometer, used with a flow-inflating bag, is attached to the bag to measure pressures generated when the bag is compressed. The manometer allows the person using the bag to more precisely control the pressure of gas delivered to the neonate. Pressure is measured in centimeters of water.

broplasia), particularly in preterm infants. Furthermore, high oxygen concentrations can directly injure lung tissue. Generally, adequate oxygenation of tissue can be achieved by maintaining a Pa_{O_2} of 50 to 80 mm Hg. The actual Pa_{O_2} level to be maintained will be determined by the infant's gestational age and conditions (Richardson, 1991). (See Chapter 33 for further discussion.)

Oxygen Mask. Oxygen masks are used only as a temporary method for delivering oxygen to the neonate during resuscitative efforts. If a newborn is mildly (Apgar score of 5 to 7) to moderately (Apgar score of 3 to 4) depressed at birth, oxygen is administered through a tight-fitting mask specifically designed for neonates. The nurse must be certain to use the correct size mask to avoid oxygen leaks (Fig. 32-6). Care must be taken to prevent pressure on the neonate's eyeballs, because this can cause tissue ischemia and blindness. The use of soft-edged masks to deliver oxygen will minimize the risk of trauma to the face and eyes.

Endotracheal Tube. When the neonate is severely depressed (Apgar score 0 to 2), oxygen is administered through an uncuffed endotracheal tube (see Fig. 32-2). The end of the tube is attached to a ventilation bag or to a mechanical ventilator if the neonate requires extended ventilatory assistance. The nurse must be familiar with the varying sizes of endotracheal tubes designed for neonates. During resuscitation the nurse often is responsible for providing the appropriately sized endotracheal tube, which is determined by the neonate's gestational age and weight.

External Cardiac Massage

If the heartbeat is absent or below 60 bpm or remains between 60 to 80 bpm after breathing is established, external

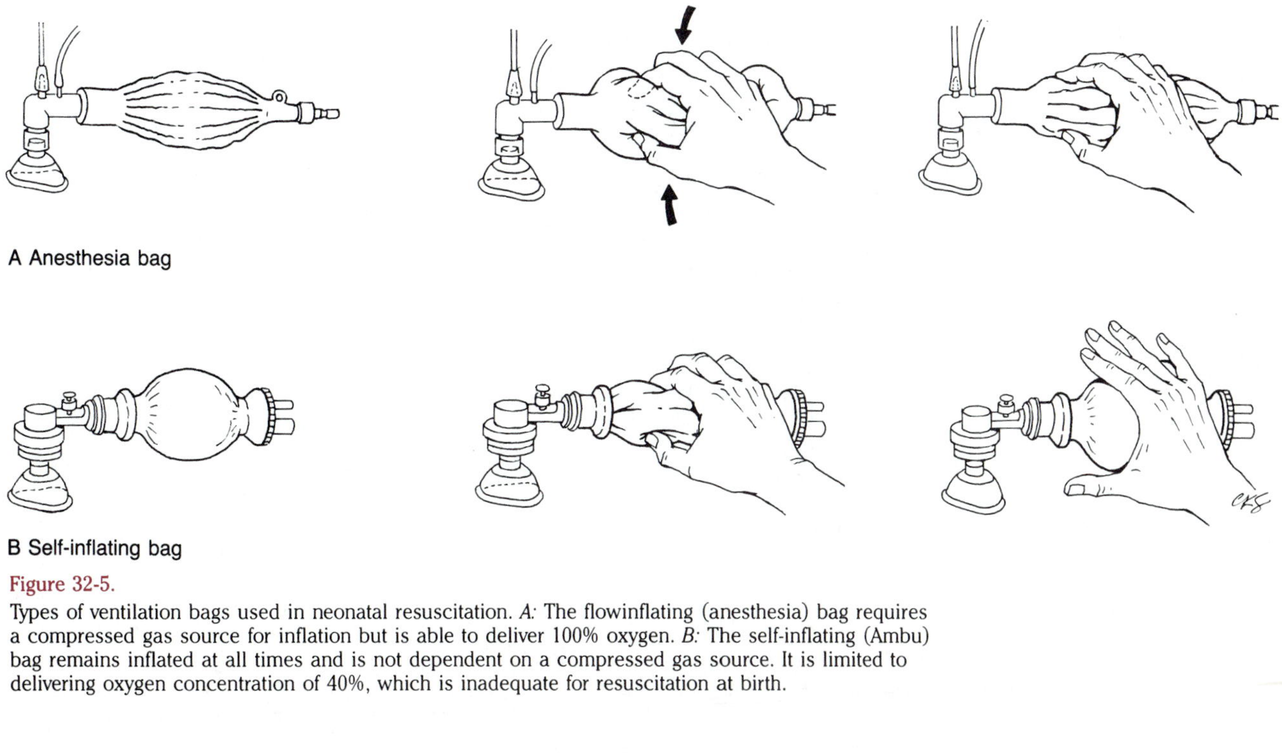

Figure 32-5.
Types of ventilation bags used in neonatal resuscitation. *A:* The flowinflating (anesthesia) bag requires a compressed gas source for inflation but is able to deliver 100% oxygen. *B:* The self-inflating (Ambu) bag remains inflated at all times and is not dependent on a compressed gas source. It is limited to delivering oxygen concentration of 40%, which is inadequate for resuscitation at birth.

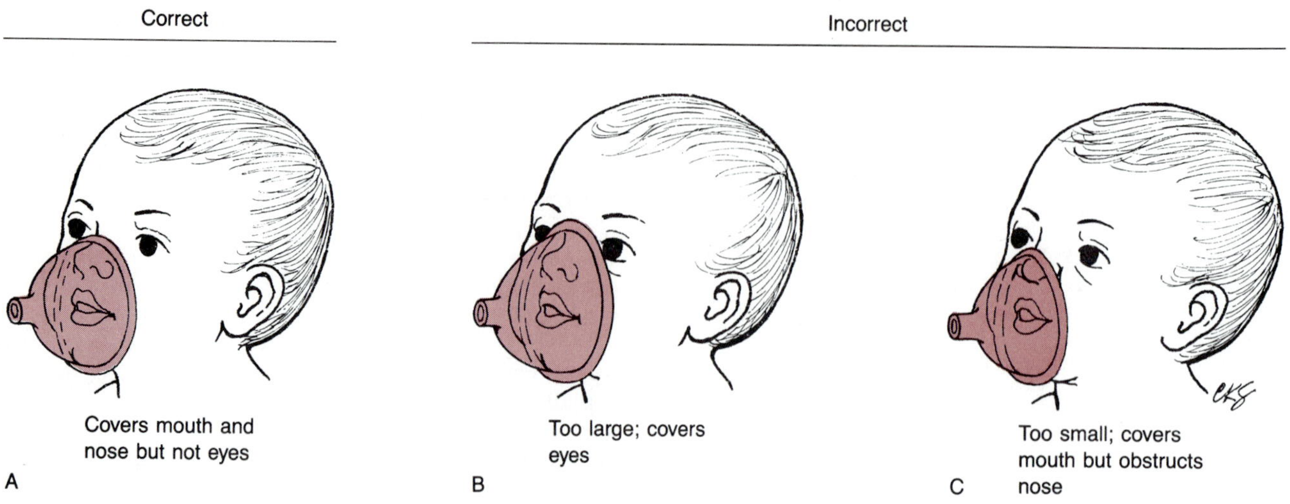

Figure 32-6.

Correct placement of the neonatal oxygen mask. Neonatal oxygen masks are made in several sizes suitable for infants weighing less than 1000 g to those over 4000 g. *A:* Correct placement of mask allows for complete coverage of nose and mouth. *B:* If the mask is too large, the eyes may be injured and an incomplete seal results in inadequate ventilation. *C:* If the mask is too small, the nose is compressed and an incomplete seal results in inadequate ventilation.

cardiac massage should be initiated. The following are guidelines established by the AHA and the AAP (1990):

1. The neonate is placed in a supine position on a flat, firm surface.
2. The index and middle finger are placed on the middle third of the sternum (Fig. 32-7*A*). An alternative method is to stand at the foot of the infant and place both thumbs on the middle third of the sternum (Fig. 32-7*B*).
3. The sternum is depressed 1 to 2 cm at a rate of 120 times per minute.
4. The effectiveness of massage is evaluated by palpating the femoral pulse or the umbilical cord.
5. The pulse rate should be checked 30 seconds after initiation of chest compression.
6. The heart rate should be checked for no longer than 6 seconds.
7. The heart rate is checked periodically (as often as 30 seconds) thereafter. Heart rate checks may be performed at less frequent intervals in neonates requiring prolonged cardiopulmonary resuscitation.

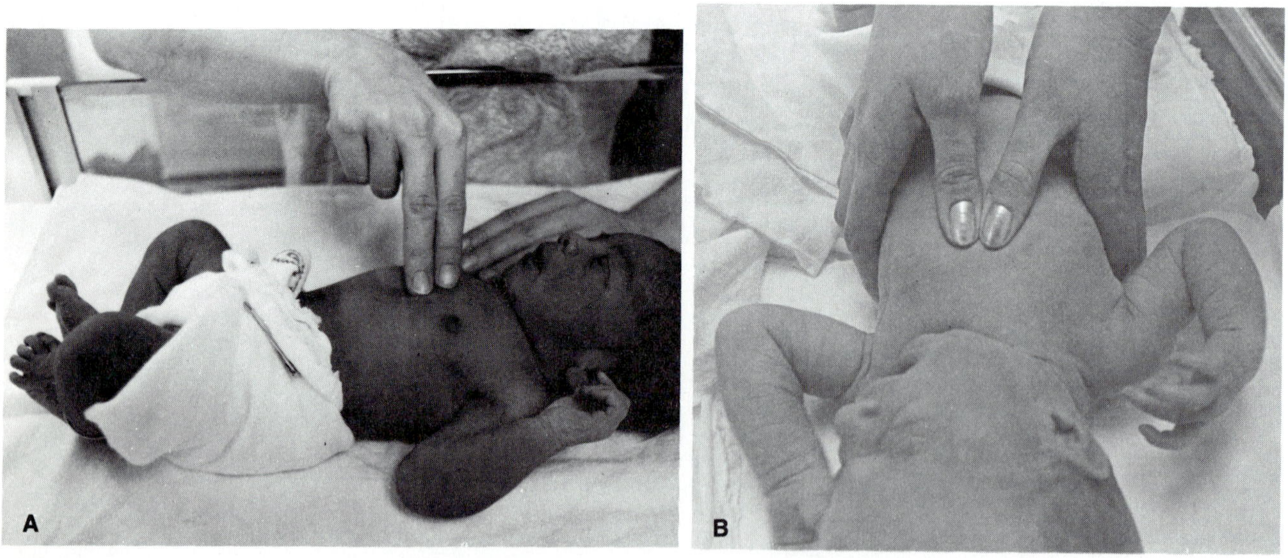

Figure 32-7.

External cardiac massage of the neonate. *A:* In the two-finger method, the fingertips are placed over the middle third of the sternum. The sternum is compressed 1 to 2 cm at a rate of 120 times per minute. *B*: The two-thumb method requires the nurse to stand at the foot of the neonate and encircle the chest with her hands. Thumb placement and compression rate are similar to the two-finger method.

8. Chest compression is discontinued when the spontaneous heart rate reaches 80 bpm or greater.
9. Compressions (at a rate of 40 to 60 per minute) should always be accompanied by positive pressure ventilations with 100% oxygen. No data permit a recommendation regarding the coordination of ventilation and chest compressions. Research is yet to determine if interposed ventilations have an advantage or disadvantage over simultaneous ventilations and chest compressions (AHA/AAP, 1990).

Use of Orogastric Tube

Because air may enter the stomach during prolonged bag and mask ventilation, an orogastric tube should be passed into the stomach to prevent gastric distention (Fig. 32-8). Coordinated efforts should result in rapid, smooth passage of the tube (5 to 10 seconds) with minimal interruption in ventilation or cardiac compressions. Use of an endotracheal tube is the most effective ventilation method and eliminates the introduction of air into the stomach.

Adjunctive Drug Therapy

If a spontaneous heart rate of at least 80 bpm has not been established despite effective ventilation with 100% oxygen and chest compressions for a minimum of 30 seconds or if the heart rate is zero, adjunctive drug therapy is initiated (AHA/AAP, 1990). Medications are administered by the following routes: umbilical vein, endotracheal instillation, and peripheral veins.

The umbilical vein is the most common route for administration of drugs during the initial resuscitation in the delivery room. It is easily located and cannulated by a trained professional, usually a neonatologist or pediatrician. Drugs administered through an umbilical venous catheter are given to correct metabolic acidosis, hypoglycemia, and poor cardiac output (Table 32-4).

Several selective drugs may be given through the endotracheal tube. Epinephrine may be injected directly into the bronchial tree to stimulate cardiac function. Naloxone, a narcotic antagonist, also may be given. Synthetic surfactant is given in special cases to preterm infants to prevent collapse of the pulmonary alveoli and development of respiratory distress syndrome.

Peripheral veins may be used for administering drugs or solutions but are generally difficult to access during the immediate resuscitative efforts in the delivery room.

The most important assessment of neonatal status is made in the first minute of life. In this first 60 seconds the nurse and other health care providers must determine the appropriate level of support required by the neonate to make successful postbirth adaptations. Based on this immediate evaluation the nurse will establish priority needs and initiate timely interventions to maintain neonatal cardiopulmonary function. This may include basic and advanced life-support measures.

The nurse is guided in the assessment of the neonate's condition and response to supportive care by established guidelines. The AHA and the AAP have established recommendations for evaluation of the neonate and appropriate steps in resuscitation. All nurses who participate in the birth and immediate assessment of the neonate must be skilled in the basics of resuscitation developed by the AHA and AAP.

Ongoing Assessment

Once the neonate's condition has stabilized after birth, it may be possible to reunite infant and parents and provide the new family with extended contact in a rooming-in arrangement. Ongoing assessment occurs at the mother's bedside and provides the nurse with opportunities for teaching and support.

A neonate who requires additional support and observation after delivery will be placed in an admission or observation nursery or may be transferred to an intensive care unit. Technologic advances permit the use of many types of monitors to increase the nurse's data base when observing or conducting the assessment of a high-risk infant. Table 32-5 lists equipment commonly used to monitor specific components of neonatal physiologic functioning. If the neonate must be taken to the nursery immediately after birth, the father or partner can accompany the infant and remain in the unit to provide emotional support during the admission procedures. When the neonate must remain in the nursery, the parents should be encouraged to visit the infant as soon as possible. Further discussion of the nurse's role in support of the parent and high-risk newborn acquaintance process is discussed in Chapter 25.

Identifying Danger Signs

The neonate is usually placed in an incubator or under a radiant warmer to support thermoregulatory control. If necessary, the neonate may be attached to a cardiorespiratory monitor and pulse oximeter for continuous assessment of cardiopulmonary function and blood oxygen saturation. Because the newborn is unable to articulate problems and needs, the nurse must be alert for signs of change in condition. Often the first signs of morbidity are subtle and barely perceptible. Because the neonate is physiologically immature, many signs of illness are nonspecific. A thorough physical examination, laboratory analysis of body fluids, and other tests may be required to identify the exact cause the problem. Major danger signals that may identify the high-risk neonate are shown in the accompanying display.

Central Nervous System Signs

The neurologic system is particularly sensitive to external and internal stressors. Chromosomal anomalies and chronic intrauterine infection associated with mental retardation often are characterized by central nervous system (CNS) aberrations. Decreases in blood oxygen concentration and serum glucose levels result in CNS dysfunction. This is manifested by altered states of consciousness, seizure activity, or even coma. The nurse is frequently first alerted to illness in the neonate by alterations in CNS functioning.

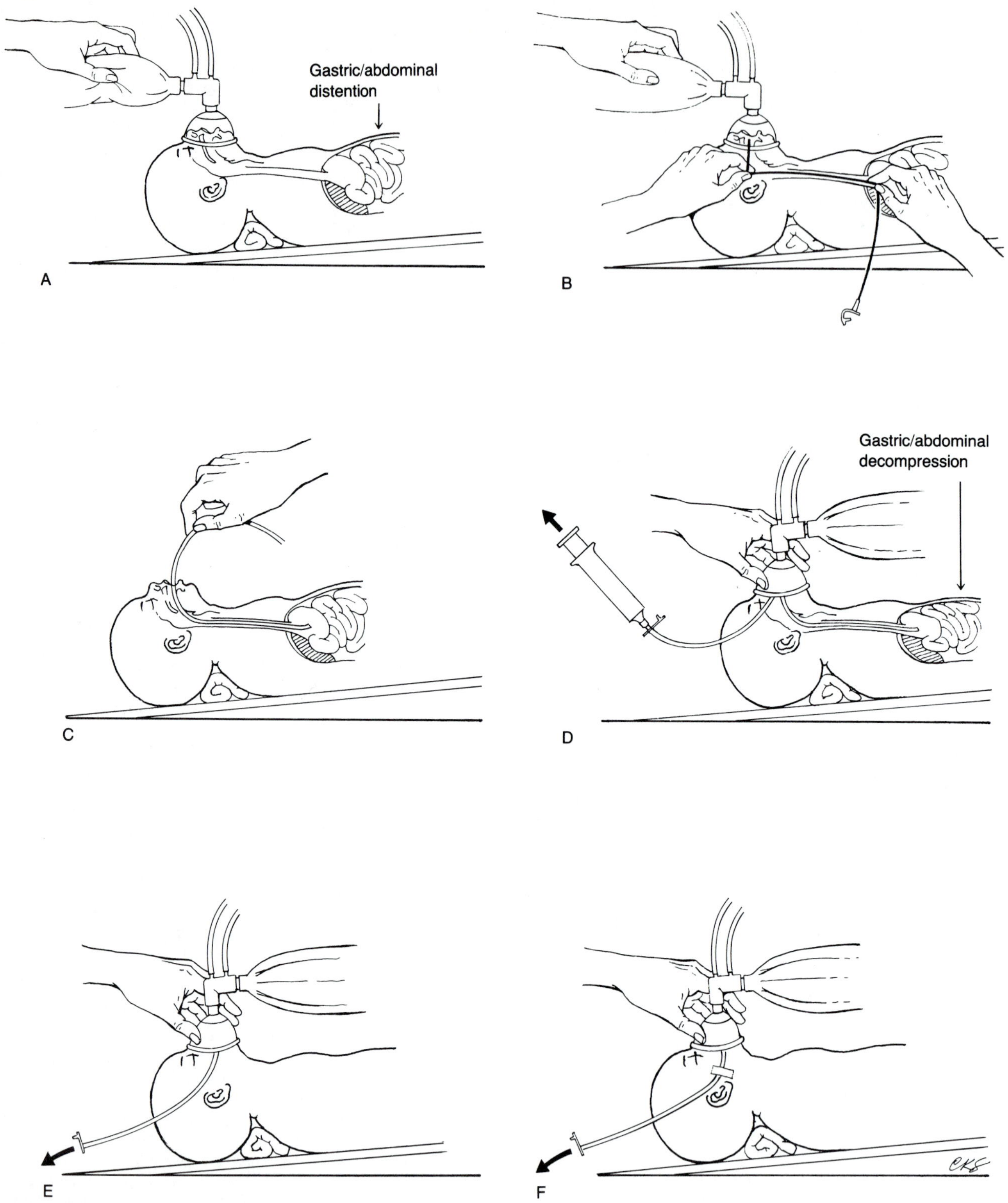

Figure 32-8.

Prevention of stomach distention. *A* and *B:* The problems related to gastric or abdominal distention and aspiration of gastric contents can be prevented by inserting an orogastric tube. *C:* Insert the catheter *through the mouth* rather than the nose. The nose should be left open for ventilation. Ventilation can be resumed as soon as the catheter is placed. *D:* Once the catheter is inserted the desired distance, attach a 20 mL syringe and quickly, but gently remove the gastric contents. *E:* Remove the syringe from the catheter, and leave the end of the catheter open to provide a vent for air entering the stomach. *F:* Tape the catheter to the neonate's cheek to ensure that the tip remains in the stomach and is not pulled back into the esophagus.

Table 32-4. Adjunctive Therapy Used During Resuscitation

Agent	Dosage and Concentration	Route and Rate of Administration
Epinephrine	0.1–0.3 mL/kg of a 1:10,000 solution	Inject directly into the umbilical vein infusion rapidly or diluted 1:1 with normal saline into the endotracheal tube to correct asystole or severe bradycardia
Sodium bicarbonate	2 mEq/kg of a 0.5 mEq/mL (4.2% solution)	Infuse slowly for 2 to 4 min through the umbilical vein to correct metabolic acidosis only if the infant is being effectively ventilated
Naloxone	0.1 mg/kg of a 0.4 mg/mL (pediatric) concentration	Inject intravenously or into endotracheal tube (preferred routes) or give by intramuscular or subcutaneous route to reverse narcosis
Dopamine	40 mg/mL	Begin continuous intravenous infusion at 5 μg/kg/min as needed to maintain blood pressure. May increase up to 20 μg/kg/min if necessary
Dextrose	0.5–1.0 g/kg (2–4 mg/kg) of a 25% solution	Infuse slowly through umbilical vein to correct hypoglycemia
Whole blood	10–20 mL/kg	Infuse slowly for 5–10 min intravenously to correct blood loss and hypotension
Albumin	10–15 mL/kg of 5%	Infuse slowly for 5–20 min intravenously as volume expander to correct hypotension and improve perfusion
Ringer's lactate	10 mL/kg	Infuse slowly for 5–20 min intravenously to improve perfusion

When physical assessment is conducted in a systematic manner, neurologic status is evaluated first.

Lethargy. A change in the neonate's state of consciousness may be the first indication of illness. The infant may become listless or lethargic and difficult to rouse for feedings. The nurse must review the intrapartum record to determine if maternal analgesia or anesthesia could be a possible cause of sleepiness or lethargy. Persistent lethargy is a significant finding that must be documented and reported to the physician.

High-Pitched Cry. A high-pitched or shrill cry may indicate CNS injury or abnormality in the newborn. It is often found in neonates with brain defects caused by chromosomal abnormalities, such as *cri du chat* syndrome; with drug withdrawal (neonatal abstinence syndrome); or with fetal alcohol syndrome.

Pupillary Abnormalities and Unusual Eye Movement. The neonate who has a CNS abnormality or injury or is experiencing drug withdrawal or postasphyxial brain damage will often demonstrate unusual eye movement, including the following:

- Vertical and horizontal nystagmus (jerky, rapid eye movements)
- Tonic eye deviations (gaze fixed to one side of the head)
- Setting sun sign (bottom part of the iris sinking below the rim of the lower eyelid)
- Marked, repetitive blinking or fluttering of the eyelids

With brain stem injury the pupils may be fixed and dilated. This is a very poor prognostic sign.

Jitteriness. Transient jitteriness (fine rhythmic motor tremors) is observed in normal infants when they are hungry or irritable. Persistent jitteriness is common when the brain has sustained injury, as in hypoxic encephalopathy and intracranial hemorrhage or with drug and alcohol withdrawal. Jitteriness also occurs with hypoglycemia, hypocalcemia, and hypomagnesemia when brain cells are depleted of glucose, the essential fuel for metabolic activities. Neonates of addicted mothers may demonstrate severe tremulousness during postnatal withdrawal from drugs the mother ingested prenatally (Parker, Zuckerman, Bauchner, et al., 1990). The experienced nurse easily recognizes marked tremors. Tremors can be stopped by gently flexing or touching the affected extremity and distinguishes jitteriness from true seizure activity, which is not stopped by holding the limb. An immediate evaluation of the serum glucose level should be obtained, because untreated hypoglycemia can result in permanent neurologic injury. The nurse discusses observations and the results of the serum glucose test with the physician. If glucose levels are normal, further diagnostic tests are ordered to determine the cause of the jitteriness.

Seizure Activity. Seizure activity also is a nonspecific sign of disease and injury in the neonate. It most frequently presents as subtle signs difficult for the untrained observer to recognize. The signs include nystagmus (involuntary and rapid movement of the eye from side to side or up and down).

Table 32-5. Equipment Commonly Used to Assess and Monitor Neonatal Status

Equipment	Function	Nursing Implications
Vital Signs Measurement		
Automated blood pressure and pulse monitor (noninvasive)	Measures pulse rate; systolic, diastolic, and mean arterial blood pressure. Uses traditional limb cuff, which is attached to the monitor.	Correct size cuff must be used for circumference of neonate's limb. Infant must be quiet during the reading because movement and crying will prevent measurement of vital signs. Current technology may not permit measurements in very low–birth-weight neonate (below 600 g).
Cardiorespiratory monitor (noninvasive)	Provides continuous measurement of pulse rate and respiratory rate. Provides continuous paper readout of EKG on graph paper during episodes of bradycardia or apnea. Permits invasive arterial blood pressure monitoring (see Intra-arterial blood pressure monitoring).	Placement of EKG leads is important for proper functioning of monitor and to obtain visual display of respiratory pattern. Adhesive used to secure EKG leads to skin may damage epidermis in preterm neonate. Reports of fungal infection on skin under EKG leads have been noted if not changed periodically.
Intra-arterial blood pressure monitor (invasive)	Provides continuous measurement of pulse rate, systolic, diastolic, and mean arterial blood pressure. Fluid filled catheter inserted into umbilical, radial, or dorsalis pedis artery; pressure in artery transmitted through fluid-filled catheter to a transducer attached to the monitor. Provides visual display on videoscreen of arterial pressure (waveform). Intra-arterial catheter permits sampling of blood for pH and gas analysis.	Invasive method can result in infection, emboli formation, and subsequent tissue necrosis due to interruption of blood flow distal to the clot. Nurse must be competent in assembly of equipment, troubleshooting monitor, and calibrating transducer. EKG leads must be changed on a regular basis to prevent skin breakdown and infection.
Temperature probe (noninvasive)	Measures skin temperature through attachment of probe to neonate's skin. Probe is connected to a servocontrol heating unit that permits automatic adjustment in the environmental temperature (radiant warmer or incubator) to maintain neonate's temperature within normal range.	Placement of probe is important to proper functioning of monitor. Probe must not be attached to the neonate's extremities, or over bony areas. Probe must not be placed on skin surface in contact with mattress. Adhesive used to secure probe to skin can traumatize the epidermis in preterm neonate. Axillary temperature must still be monitored to determine that the servocontrol unit is functioning properly.
Transcutaneous oxygen and carbon monitor $TcPo_2$ monitor (noninvasive)	Provides continuous reading of skin surface Po_2 (partial pressure of oxygen) and Pco_2 (partial pressure of carbon dioxide). Heated electrode, which is attached to skin, arterializes capillary blood flow in skin. Some machines have the capability to provide a hard copy (graph paper) of the $TcPo_2$ and $TcCo_2$ levels with time.	Temperature required to heat skin 107.6°F to 113°F (42°C to 45°C) may cause thermal burns, particularly in preterm neonate. Adhesive used to secure probe to skin may damage epidermis in preterm neonate. Probe may not be attached to skin over bony prominence. Skin surface to which probe is attached must be flat. Site must be changed every 3–4 hours. Nurse must be competent in attaching trouble-shooting and calibrating equipment.
Pulse oximeter (noninvasive)	Measures percentage of arterial blood oxygen saturation (Spo_2). Some machines have the capability to provide a hard copy (graph paper) of oxygen saturation level with time (trend data).	Proper placement of sensor is essential to obtain an accurate reading of neonatal sensor. Neonatal sensor may not function properly if infant is active. Poor skin perfusion may result in sensor inability to read O_2 saturation concentration. Adhesive required to secure probe may damage epidermis in very preterm neonate. There have been reports of burns at the sensor site in very preterm infants. Adhesive strip used to attach probe should be applied so that circulation is not impeded.

Major Danger Signs of Neonatal Morbidity

Central Nervous System Signs

Lethargy
High-pitched cry
Jitteriness
Abnormal eye movement
Seizure activity
Abnormal fontanelle size or bulging fontanelles

Respiratory Signs

Apnea
Tachypnea
Nasal flaring
Chest retractions
Persistent rales and rhonchi
Asynchronous breathing movements
Expiratory grunting

Cardiovascular Signs

Abnormal rate and rhythm
Murmurs
Changes in blood pressure
Alterations and differentials in pulses
Changes in perfusion and skin color

Gastrointestinal Signs

Refusal of two or more feedings
Absent or uncoordinated feeding reflexes
Vomiting
Abdominal distention
Changes in stool patterns

Genitourinary Signs

Hematuria
Absence of urine production
Failure to pass urine

Metabolic Alterations

Hypoglycemia
Hypocalcemia
Hyperbilirubinemia and jaundice

Temperature Instability

Other signs are repeated blinking, sucking motions, or tongue thrusting. Vasomotor instability with mottling of skin and apnea also have been associated with seizures. More obvious indicators include rhythmic rowing movements of upper extremities, bicycling motions of lower extremities, and assumption of a rigid posture. Classification of neonatal seizures is based on clinical descriptors (Ballweg, 1991).

- *Subtle seizures* occur most frequently. They are characterized by repeated blinking, staring, or tonic horizontal or vertical eye deviations; repetitive sucking or tongue protrusions; swimming, rowing, bicycling, or stepping movements; or tonic posturing of a single limb.
- *Tonic seizures* occur most frequently in preterm infants who exhibit tonic extension or flexion of upper or lower limbs, which resembles decerebrate or decorticate posturing. Apnea may occur.
- *Multifocal clonic seizures* occur in term infants and are expressed as clonic jerking movements that migrate randomly from extremity to extremity.
- *Focal clonic seizures* are seen most often in term neonates and are characterized by localized, repetitive clonic jerking of a muscle group, such as a single extremity, one side of the face, or a finger.

The nurse must distinguish jitteriness from seizure activity. Tremors, as noted previously, can be stopped by gently flexing or holding the extremity. Neonates at greater risk for developing seizures include those who sustained severe asphyxia or intracranial hemorrhage at birth and those who have meningitis. Neonates experiencing acute drug withdrawal also are susceptible. Other known causes of seizure activity include hypoglycemia, hypocalcemia, electrolyte imbalances, sepsis, kernicterus, and familial and genetic seizure disorders. The nurse takes note of risk factors associated with the development of seizures and closely observes the neonate for evidence of seizure activity.

Abnormal Fontanelle Size or Bulging Fontanelles. The anterior fontanelle may normally pulsate or bulge slightly when the infant cries vigorously, especially in a supine or prone position. The fontanelle should be assessed with the infant in an upright position. True bulging or palpable tenseness of the fontanelles is associated with increased intracranial pressure resulting from hemorrhage or hydrocephalus (an abnormal accumulation of cerebrospinal fluid in the ventricles of the brain). Enlarged fontanelles are associated with chromosomal anomalies, such as trisomies; skeletal disorders, including osteogenesis imperfecta; and congenital hypothyroidism. Small fontanelles are observed in preterm infants and in small-for-gestational-age infants and neonates who have microcephaly.

The nurse must report and document findings of abnormal fontanelle size or shape and obtain daily measurements of head circumference to determine the rate of head growth. Hydrocephalus may be obvious at birth or can develop rapidly within the first several months of life. Early detection will assist in the diagnosis and treatment of the disorder.

Respiratory System Signs

Any alterations in cardiac or respiratory function will result in observable changes in respiratory effort. Early signs of distress, such as mild nasal flaring or an increased respiratory rate, may be missed if the nurse is not alert to these subtle signs of dysfunction. Marked respiratory distress is obvious and is manifested by cyanosis, tachypnea, tachycardia, chest retractions, stridor, or grunting. It may appear suddenly with acute airway obstruction or pneumothorax.

The neonate may present with immediate signs of respiratory distress at the time of birth or develop symptoms at any time during the neonatal period. Close observation and frequent monitoring of respiratory function are essential for preventing life-threatening compromise in high-risk neonates. Prematurity, birth asphyxia, meconium aspiration, pneumonia, pneumothorax, and diaphragmatic hernia are associated with respiratory distress.

Apnea. The neonate may experience episodes of apnea immediately after birth and at any time thereafter. True apnea is defined as a cessation of respiration for 15 seconds or longer and is accompanied by bradycardia (heart rate less than 100 bpm) or cyanosis (Epstein, 1991).

Primary apnea occurs immediately after delivery. A severely depressed neonate will take several gasping breaths in an effort to initiate respirations and then stop breathing. After a pause ranging from several seconds to 1 to 2 minutes, weak and ineffectual breathing efforts begin again. Quick response and appropriate management by the nurse include maintenance of the airway, oxygenation and ventilation, and mild stimulation, which generally results in improved respiratory effort and stabilization of the neonate. The accompanying Nursing Procedure gives steps for using free-flow oxygen to improve the neonate's color.

If measures are not initiated to assist the severely depressed neoante during the initial gasping and apnea episode, secondary apnea ensues. Progressive hypoxia and brain stem depression will make subsequent attempts to resuscitate the neonate difficult. Tactile stimulation and directing free-flowing oxygen over the neonate's nose (blow-by oxygenation) will not be sufficient to stimulate respirations. Immediate endotracheal intubation and ventilation with 100% oxygen are essential if the infant is to have any chance to survive.

In addition to primary and secondary birth apnea, apneic episodes are associated with a variety of conditions, including hypoxia, sepsis, gastroesophageal reflux, choanal atresia, seizures, and fatigue. Premature infants may suffer from episodes of apnea for many weeks after birth until the CNS matures. Obstructive apnea, defined as absent airflow with inspiratory effort, occurs less frequently. Passive neck flexion in the preterm infant may obstruct the airway and impede airflow.

An apneic episode is frequently preceded by "periodic breathing," which consists of shorter periods of apnea lasting 5 to 15 seconds followed by rapid and often shallow respirations. The nurse must be alert to alterations in respiratory patterns. The use of pulse oximetry and cardiorespiratory and transcutaneous oxygen monitors can document apnea and changes in oxygenation. Recurrent episodes of apnea indicate the need for further evaluation. A four-channel pneumocardiogram is a diagnostic tool that measures heart rate, respiratory effort, nasal airflow, and oxygen saturation to assess the nature of apneic episodes. Once a diagnosis is made, appropriate treatments, such as drug therapy or continuous positive airway pressure, can be initiated.

Signs of respiratory distress are evident as the neonate struggles to improve oxygen intake. The degree of distress may be graded using the Silverman-Andersen index, shown in Figure 32-9.

Tachypnea. One of the earliest signs of illness in the neonate and a common indicator of respiratory distress is a rapid respiratory rate (over 60 breaths per minute). Transient tachypnea of the newborn (TTN) is a mild, self-limited respiratory disorder. It is characterized by a respiratory rate of more than 60 breaths per minute, usually without retractions, and mild cyanosis. The requirements for supplemental oxygen do not exceed 40% (Stark & North, 1991). It is suggested that TTN is due to delayed resorption of fetal lung fluid and is commonly observed in neonates born by cesarean delivery at or near term.

Nasal Flaring. The neonate is an obligate nose breather. With respiratory distress the neonate will dilate the nares with each inspiration in an attempt to increase the inflow of air.

Chest Retractions. Pulmonary atelectasis and noncompliant lung tissue increase the amount of negative intrathoracic pressure experienced on inspiration. As the rib cage expands with each inspiration, the soft tissues of the thorax and weak intercostal muscles are pulled in toward the spine, giving rise to intercostal retractions. Breathing is difficult and labored.

Asynchronous Breathing Movements. As respiratory distress increases in severity, chest and abdominal breathing movements become asynchronous. The chest flattens, and the abdomen protrudes with each inspiration. Respirations that follow this pattern are called seesaw respirations.

Expiratory Grunting. The neonate in respiratory distress exhales against a partially closed glottis in an effort to increase intrapulmonary pressure and keep alveoli open during exhalation. This prevents atelectasis. The result of exhalation against a partially closed glottis is a peeping noise, which may be audible without a stethoscope in severe respiratory distress. Intermittent grunting may be heard in the normal neonate during the first 1 to 2 hours after birth, but persistent grunting is associated with respiratory distress.

Rales and Rhonchi. Abnormal respiratory sounds may be auscultated in some high-risk newborns. *Rales* are characterized as crackling noises similar to those heard

NURSING PROCEDURE

Using Free-Flow Oxygen to Improve the Neonate's Color

Purpose: To relieve cyanosis in infants with adequate respirations and a heart rate above 100 bpm.

NURSING ACTION	***RATIONALE***
1. Attach oxygen tubing to 100% oxygen.	A neonate who has central cyanosis after respirations are established should receive a high concentration of oxygen.
2. Position neonate's head in a neutral or "sniffing" position.	To permit maximal entry of air into the lungs.
3. Adjust flow meter to deliver oxygen at 5 L/min.	To provide an adequate flow of oxygen.
4. If using end of oxygen tubing, place it 1/2 inch from neonate's nose.	To provide infant with maximum concentration of oxygen (approximately 80%).
5. Hold tubing steady and aimed at nares.	Waving the end of the tubing back and forth in front of nares decreases oxygen concentration.
6. If using oxygen mask attached to mask, hold mask firmly on neonate's face.	To deliver high concentration of oxygen (approximately 100%).
7. Once the neonate is pink, withdraw the oxygen gradually until the infant remains pink on room air.	To permit neonate time to compensate for decreased oxygen concentration.

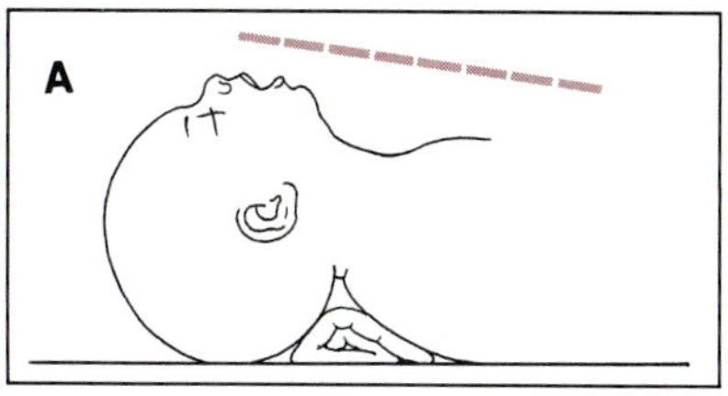

Step 2. Sniffing position.

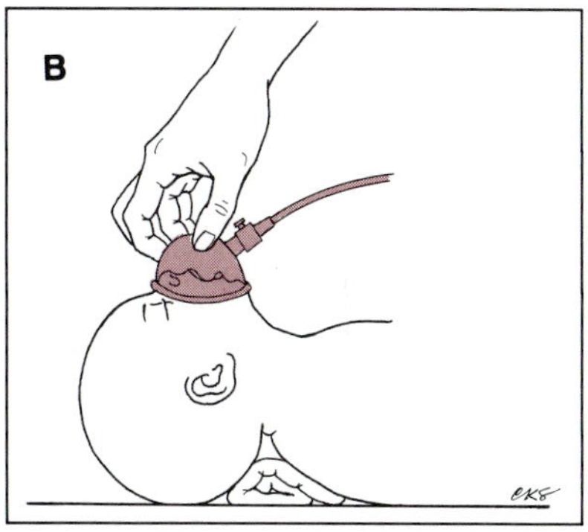

Step 6. Mask held firmly.

From American Heart Association/American Academy of Pediatrics. (1990). Textbook of neonatal resuscitation. *Elk Grove Village, IL: American Academy of Pediatrics.*

when a piece of cellophane is crumpled. They may be fine (crepitant) or course (moist) depending on the amount and location of secretions in the lungs. Rales are commonly heard over areas of partially collapsed alveoli (atelectasis). They can be auscultated when meconium aspiration or delayed resorption of lung fluid (transient tachypnea of the newborn) occur. *Rhonchi* are very coarse, moist rales due to the presence of secretions in the bronchioles. Rhonchi also may be auscultated with meconium aspiration.

Decreased or Absent Breath Sounds. In certain conditions breath sounds may be diminished or absent. Pneumothorax is the presence of air in the thoracic cavity and results from the leakage of air from ruptured alveoli into the thoracic space. Gradual buildup of air in the thoracic cavity will eventually cause collapse of the lung on the affected side. A skilled clinician may be able to auscultate decreased breath sounds over the area of lung collapse. Diaphragmatic hernia is the displacement of abdominal contents into the thoracic cavity through a defect in the diaphragm. Decreased or absent breath sounds are common on the side affected by the hernia due to compression of the lung by abdominal organs.

Cardiovascular System Signs

Congenital heart anomalies, pulmonary disease, and severe asphyxia affect cardiovascular function. The nurse assesses color, skin perfusion, heart rate and rhythm, and peripheral pulses for evidence of alteration in cardiovascular status. Because the nurses caring for the neonate conduct systematic evaluations of heart function at least once per shift, the nurse often initially identifies cardiovascular abnormalities.

Changes in Perfusion and Skin Color. The nurse should evaluate skin perfusion and color in a well-lit environment. Subtle color changes may be one of the first signs of illness in the neonate. A pale or gray color or circumoral cyanosis, particularly when associated with feeding or crying, may indicate a cardiac problem or the presence of a tracheoesophageal fistula. Generalized mottling and poor peripheral perfusion (capillary filling time greater than 3 seconds) may be an early sign of disease or distress.

Abnormal Blood Pressure. The neonate with compromised cardiac function, congenital anomalies of the

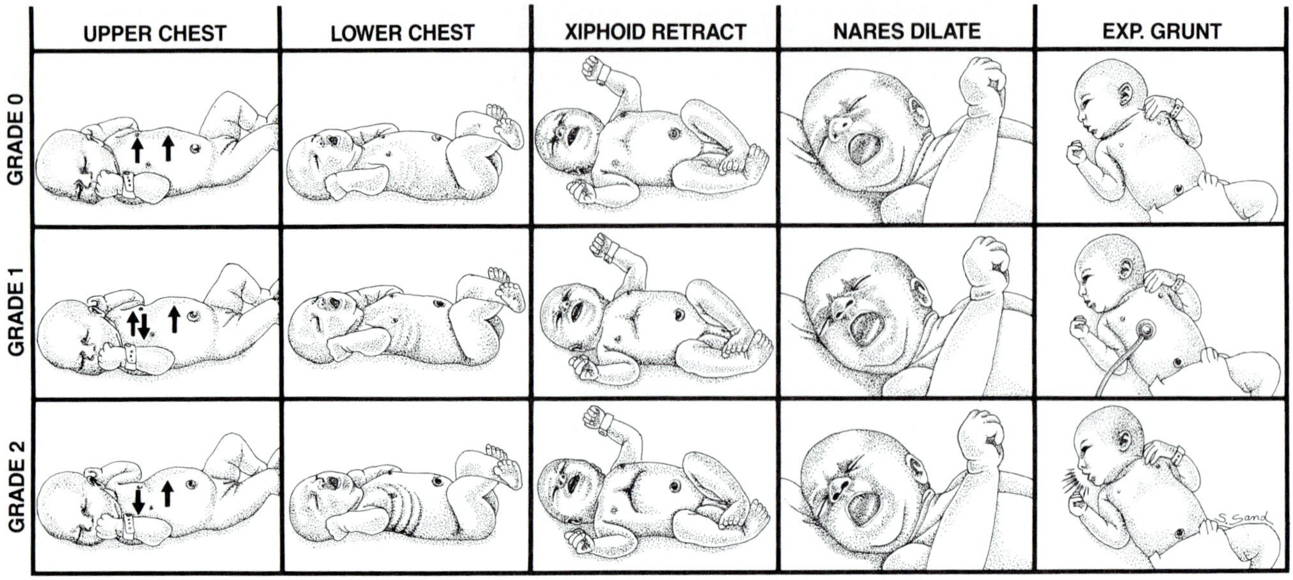

Figure 32-9.

The Silverman-Andersen index of neonatal respiratory distress. Observation of retractions. An index of respiratory distress is determined by grading each of five arbitrary criteria. Grade 0 indicates no difficulty; grade 1 indicates moderate difficulty; and grade 2 indicates maximum respiratory difficulty. The retraction score is the sum of these values; a total score of 0 indicates no dyspnea, whereas a total score of 10 denotes maximal respiratory distress.

heart and aorta, persistent fetal circulation, or pulmonary hypertension often demonstrates significant changes in blood pressure. Initially, transient adaptive rises in blood pressure may be noted in the neonate in response to cardiovascular or pulmonary complications. Hypotension will then occur as the workload of the heart increases beyond the capacity of the myocardium. Hypotension also is observed with hypovolemia and shock. Neonates with coarctation of the aorta (see Chapter 33) will demonstrate differential blood pressures. Blood pressure will be very low in the legs, and hypertension is common in the upper extremities. Many high-risk infants with compromised cardiovascular function will have a central hemodynamic monitoring line inserted into the umbilical or radial artery. This invasive technique permits continuous blood pressure assessment, as well blood sampling for biochemical and gas analysis.

Abnormal Rate and Rhythm. Dysrhythmias may be found in the normal neonate (sinus tachycardia, paroxysmal atrial tachycardia (PAT), and ectopic beats), but they also occur with cardiomyopathies, certain drug therapies, electrolyte imbalance, and congenital anomalies. The neonatal heart responds to mild to moderate stress with an increase in heart rate. Premature infants normally have a high baseline rate (above 160 bpm). Transient tachycardia also is common in normal newborns in the first several hours after birth and during episodes of crying. Persistent tachycardia is associated with respiratory distress in the high-risk neonate and is observed with hypovolemic shock.

If stressors placed on the cardiovascular system are severe, such as profound hypoxia or massive brain hemorrhage, bradycardia will occur. Sinus bradycardia, a heart rate 2 standard deviations below the mean for the neonate's gestational age, is found with hypoxemia, acidosis, and elevated intracranial pressure. It also occurs with congenital heart block, digitalis toxicity, and hypothyroidism. Transient bradycardia can be induced by stimulating the vagus nerve during suctioning or endotracheal intubation. Premature infants also may experience bradycardia in association with apnea or fatigue.

Murmurs. Murmurs can be heard in up to 60% of normal neonates after the first 2 hours of life. They result from the incomplete closure of fetal circulatory bypasses. Most are grade 1 and 2 systolic ejection murmurs, which are best auscultated at the second left intercostal space. Pathologic murmurs frequently are associated with other cardiovascular findings, such as cyanosis, diminished or bounding pulses, hypotension, hypertension, and abnormal cardiac size or shape. Holosystolic murmurs coupled with thrills or with an active precordium (easily palpated movement of the chest wall over the heart associated with systole) also indicate pathology. Pathologic murmurs also are associated with congenital heart anomalies, such as ventricular septal defect.

Premature infants are at high risk for developing murmurs associated with persistent patent ductus arteriosus. It is suggested that lack of muscular development in ductal tissues in very immature neonates contributes to persistent patent ductus. The ductus is extremely sensitive to blood oxygen concentrations and normally closes with rising Pao_2 levels after birth. Both preterm and full-term neonates with severe hypoxia may develop murmurs with the reopening of the ductus arteriosus secondary to lowered Pao_2 levels.

Alterations and Differentials in Pulses. Weak or thready pulses (charted as 1+) are evident with hypovolemia and shock. Bounding (3+) pulses may be palpated with congestive heart failure. Differential pulses (that is, pulses in which the amplitude or volume is different between left and right upper extremities or upper and lower extremities) may be found with shunting and with certain cardiac anomalies. The nurse palpates the peripheral pulses (brachial, femoral, dorsal pedal, and posterior tibial) at regular intervals to detect alterations in rate, regularity, amplitude, volume, rhythm, and symmetry. Cardiac monitors and pulse oximeters are frequently used by the nurse to assist in continuous monitoring of heart rate and rhythm and blood oxygen saturation in the high-risk or sick neonate. Alarms may be set on these electronic monitors to alert the nurse to episodes of tachycardia, bradycardia, and decreasing blood oxygen saturation. Electrocardiograph strips can be generated during periods of abnormal heart activity to assist physicians in diagnosing cardiac abnormalities.

Gastrointestinal System Signs

The feeding and elimination patterns of the healthy neonate are remarkably predictable. Many neonates are alert and stable enough to breastfeed almost immediately after birth. The passage of meconium stools should occur in the first 24 to 48 hours of life and frequently within several hours of birth. The neonate who refuses two or more feedings is a sick infant. This is often an early sign of neonatal complications. The nurse observes the neonate closely for deviations from these norms in behavior.

Absent or Uncoordinated Feeding Reflexes. A neonate who feeds slowly with weak and uncoordinated suck, swallow, or gag reflexes is characterized as a "poor feeder." This pattern is encountered with prematurity. It also is common in cases of congenital cleft lip or palate, oropharyngeal trauma secondary to endotracheal intubation, maternal narcotic administration in labor and delivery, and as a sequela of birth asphyxia or injury. The neonate with a weak suck and uncoordinated feeding reflexes is at risk for aspiration and pneumonia. The neonate also may have calorie and fluid deficits secondary to inadequate oral intake. Careful assessment of the neonate's ability to suck and swallow effectively is therefore essential.

Vomiting. Although some degree of regurgitation is normal in neonates because the cardiac sphincter is immature and weak, vomiting is an abnormal sign associated with overfeeding, sepsis, metabolic disorders such as galactosemia, increased intracranial pressure, and intestinal atresia and stenosis. It also may be a nonspecific indicator of illness in the neonate. It is essential that the nurse differentiate between regurgitation and vomiting. Regurgitation most frequently occurs within the first hour after feeding and commonly occurs in conjunction with burping or spontaneous eructation of air. Simple regurgitation is not normally associated with disease and does not cause fluid and electrolyte imbalances. In contrast vomiting is often projectile in nature, can occur at any time, and results in the loss of significant amounts of body fluids and electrolytes.

The nurse assesses the nature of the emesis. The vomitus may be mixed with a large amount of mucus, suggesting an obstruction proximal to the stomach; it may be bile stained, suggesting an obstruction distal to the ampulla; or it may be fecal, indicating a lower gastrointestinal tract obstruction. Hematemesis also occurs and may be caused by swallowed maternal blood during labor or organic disease in the neonate. A laboratory test called the Apt test is available to differentiate between maternal and fetal blood.

Abdominal Distention. An increase in abdominal girth is associated with a variety of neonatal complications. These complications include necrotizing enterocolitis, meconium plug and ileus, and congenital atresia or stenosis of the bowel. Abdominal distention may be present at birth or can develop within the first 24 to 48 hours of life. The abdomen becomes tense and protuberant, the skin appears taut and shiny, and superficial veins become prominent over the abdomen. Respiratory distress occurs if distention becomes severe. Bowel sounds may be absent, or peristaltic waves strongly suggestive of obstruction may be visible.

The nurse must obtain serial measurements of abdominal girth at the level of the umbilicus when the neonate is at risk for the development of gastrointestinal disorders or when abdominal distention is suspected. Continued frequent inspection, palpation, and auscultation of the abdomen are essential aspects of nursing assessment. Routine palpation is contraindicated if the abdomen is distended or tight.

Changes in Stool Patterns. Diarrhea may be a sign of intestinal infection or intolerance to cow's milk. An absence of stools after birth may indicate imperforate anus or congenital intestinal atresia or stenosis. Meconium ileus or meconium plug will result in diminished or absent stooling and may be due to cystic fibrosis. Blood in the stools (gross or microscopic) occurs with necrotizing enterocolitis and is a grave sign. Altered stool patterns, including loose stools, can follow antibiotic therapy and can occur with a neonate receiving phototherapy.

The nurse documents the passage of all stools, noting the amount, color, consistency, and odor. In high-risk or sick neonates, fecal material is tested for the presence of blood or glucose, both of which are early warning signs of gastrointestinal dysfunction. When blood is detected in the stool, the Apt test can be performed to determine if the source is maternal or neonatal.

Genitourinary System Signs

Renal dysfunction may be evident in the neonate as a result of congenital malformations, such as renal hypoplasia or agenesis or meatal stenosis. Many syndromes that are due to chromosomal abnormalities, including Beckwith-Wiedemann, prune-belly, VATER, trisomy 13, and Down syndromes, have associated renal anomalies. Acute renal failure can occur with birth asphyxia, hypovolemic shock, septic shock, congestive heart failure, and the administration of nephrotoxic drugs. Signs of neonatal renal problems follow.

Hematuria. The presence of gross blood in the neonate's urine is very uncommon. Hematuria can occur with hemorrhagic disease of the newborn. This cause has been greatly reduced with the prophylactic administration of vitamin K shortly after birth. Congenital neoplasms, such as neuroblastoma, infection, renal artery thrombosis, and birth trauma, also may cause hematuria. The nurse assesses the color of the neonate's urine and uses a chemical strip to test for the presence of blood in the urine. In some cases orange-red staining of the urine may be due to the presence of uric acid crystals. This is a normal variation and resolves in several days with adequate hydration.

Failure to Pass Urine. The normal full-term neonate has between 6 and 44 mL of urine in the bladder at birth but may not void for the first 24 to 48 hours of life (Ingelfinger, 1991). The failure to pass urine is due to one of two major problems:

- Failure to produce urine
- Obstruction to urinary flow

The inability to produce urine may be due to birth asphyxia, which results in renal tissue necrosis and kidney failure. Hypovolemia and hypotension in the neonate will reduce renal perfusion and urine production. Decreased urine output may occur due to dehydration secondary to a weak or discoordinate suck. The use of radiant warmers and phototherapy will increase insensible water loss in the newborn and reduce urine production. If no urine is passed after the first 24 hours, a urine collection bag may be placed over the genitalia to ensure that any urine voided is collected and assessed.

Obstruction to urinary flow is observed less frequently and is due to a variety of anomalies, including urethral strictures, diverticulum, and tumors. A neonate with a neurogenic bladder will not spontaneously void. Infants born with lesions or deformities in the spinal column, such as spina bifida, may have neurogenic bladder problems, which lead to distention and the inability to pass urine. The nurse observes the neonate during voiding for the quality of the urine stream (see Chapter 30 for a full discussion).

Metabolic Alterations

The high-risk or sick neonate is at risk for a variety of metabolic disorders that can be lethal if left untreated. These disorders occur as a result of stressors that deplete the neonate's energy reserves and injure cells essential to major metabolic functions. Responsibility for early detection of these metabolic abnormalities lies primarily with the nurses who are caring for the infant.

Hypoglycemia. One of the major complications of disease or injury in the neonate is hypoglycemia. Hypoglycemia is defined as a glucose level of less than 30 mg/dL of whole blood during the first 72 hours after birth in the full-term infant and less than 40 mg/dL after the first 72 hours. Normal blood values are slightly lower in low–birth-weight neonates (less than 20 mg/dL of whole blood with two consecutive blood samples).

Many high-risk neonates are born with limited or depleted stores of liver glucose, including small-for-gestational age, preterm, and postterm infants. Neonates who are stressed at birth (from asphyxia or cold) quickly use all available glucose stores and become hypoglycemic. Infants of diabetic mothers may experience profound hypoglycemia shortly after birth as a result of rebound hyperinsulinism. Another group of neonates at risk for the development of hypoglycemia includes those whose mothers received tocolytic therapy with beta-sympathomimetic agents, such as terbutaline. Cole (1991) found a much higher rate of hypoglycemia even in normal newborns without potential risk factors, which suggests that all neonates must be screened carefully for hypoglycemia.

Hypoglycemia is frequently manifested by jitteriness, lethargy, and poor feeding. The nurse who identifies signs of hypoglycemia must determine the serum glucose level immediately. A glucose oxidase (Chemstrip) test can be used to determine the blood glucose level in 60 seconds when a capillary blood sample is obtained by heel prick. When the level is determined to be 40 mg/dL or less, a venous blood sample is drawn for a more accurate laboratory determination. The glucose strip test can be used as a guide for immediate therapy until laboratory results are obtained.

Hypocalcemia. Hypocalcemia is defined as a total serum calcium level of less than 7 mg/dL and an ionized calcium concentration of less than 4 mg/dL. It is found in preterm neonates with immature parathyroid function, in neonates of diabetic women with hypertrophy of the parathyroid gland, and in neonates who have sustained birth asphyxia. Any high-risk neonate who receives intravenous fluids containing low levels of calcium also is at risk for hypocalcemia. Signs of hypocalcemia include jitteriness, twitching, hyperreflexia, and heightened sensitivity to sensory stimuli. If untreated, the infant may develop carpopedal spasms, laryngospasm, and convulsions. Vomiting and hematemesis may occur. The nurse observes infants at risk for hypocalcemia for signs of increased neuromuscular irritability and monitors serum calcium levels closely.

Early neonatal hypocalcemia occurs within the first 2 to 3 days of life and is related to the previously mentioned conditions. *Late hypocalcemia* often occurs between the sixth and tenth day of life, but onset is seen as late as several weeks after birth. It can result from the ingestion of formula with an inappropriate calcium–phosphorus ratio. With recent advances in the development of feeding formulas for preterm and high-risk neonates, late hypocalcemia is encountered less frequently. Other specific problems associated with delayed onset include congenital absence of the parathyroids, maternal hyperparathyroidism, hypoalbuminemia, lipid infusions, sepsis, and shock.

Hyperbilirubinemia and Jaundice. Many sick neonates are at risk for the development of hyperbilirubinemia and jaundice. Preterm neonates and infants of diabetic mothers have an immature liver enzyme system. Asphyxiated infants are at increased risk because acid metabolites compete with bilirubin for albumin binding sites. Other conditions predisposing to the development of jaundice are congenital obstruction of the intestinal tract, urinary tract infections, enclosed hemorrhage, hypoglycemia, hypothermia, and extreme ecchymosis secondary to traumatic delivery. The nurse examines the infant (in natural light if possible) for evidence of jaundice and closely monitors serum bilirubin levels. See Chapter 31 for further discussion of hyperbilirubinemia and evaluation of jaundice.

Temperature Instability

The elevation in temperature that normally accompanies bacterial infections in adults may be absent in the newborn. Hypothermia and wide swings in temperature are more common and may be an early sign of sepsis. The rapid depletion of brown fat and liver glucose stores that often accompanies severe stress contributes to hypothermia in the high-risk neonate. Neonates who have sustained severe head injuries and intracranial hemorrhage also suffer from temperature instability. Because high-risk infants are so susceptible to temperature swings or hypothermia, they are frequently placed in an incubator or under a radiant warmer to support their thermoregulatory function. A temperature probe may be attached to the skin surface to assist the nurse in monitoring changes in skin temperature. When the probe senses changes in skin temperature, the heating element used to warm the infant is adjusted automatically to maintain the neonate's body temperature within normal limits.

Identifying Behavioral Abnormalities

The high-risk or sick neonate may have limited behavioral capacities during the stabilization period after birth. Internal and external stressors may render the infant incapable of organizing its responses into adaptive behavior patterns that support social interaction with caregivers and parents. Attempts at stimulation may actually worsen the infant's condition if they are improperly timed or inappropriate for the level of neurobehavioral development. Gorski (1979) identified three stages of behavioral organization unique to the high-risk neonate. Recently, researchers (Ballard, Khoury, Wedig, et al., 1991; Tronick, Scanlon, & Scanlon, 1990) have expanded on Gorski's initial work, examining behavioral adaptations in extremely premature infants. Once the neonate has achieved physiologic stability, it is essential for the nurse to conduct an assessment of the high-risk infant's behavioral capacities.

Physiologic Stage

During the first critical days after birth, the high-risk infant may be unable to participate reciprocally with caregivers or parents in establishing mutually satisfying interactions. All of the neonate's energies are focused inward on the development of physiologic stability. During this acute phase the infant may lie motionless for long periods, remaining primarily in an undifferentiated sleep state. Response to painful stimuli may range from a generalized startle or uneven and intermittent focal reactions to no observable response. The nurse may be unable to rouse the infant to the alert state of consciousness, or extreme stress reactions may be noted when the infant is in the alert state. The neonate is incapable of organizing behaviors for any type of social response.

First Active Response Stage

As a state of physiologic stability is achieved, the neonate begins to respond to external stimuli in an organized manner. The neonate is able to provide caregivers with some indication of behavioral capacities and unique temperament. During the active response stage, the neonate is capable of moving to an alert, awake state of consciousness for short periods. The extremely premature sick infant, however, may remain in a state of "protective apathy," unavailable to stimulation and easily stressed by it (Tronick, 1990). This behavior represents a protective mechanism that conserves the neonate's energy and aids in recovery.

During this recovery phase caregivers can significantly affect the physical and emotional well-being of the neonate by responding appropriately to cues. Feeding schedules can be adjusted to emerging sleep–wake cycles. Eliminating nonessential stimuli (noise and light) from the environment and providing time for cuddling and eye contact also have a positive impact on the neonate's condition. The nurse guides and supports parents with initial interactions at this time. Nursing interventions are discussed further in Chapter 33.

Reciprocity Stage

The neonate is now strong enough to respond to caregiver behaviors in specific and predictable ways. Brazelton (1989), a pioneer in research on neonatal behavioral states found that the developing relationship between parents and the infant plays a key role in this final stage of development. A critical factor is the parents' ability to identify and respond to the neonate's cues in an appropriate manner. Infants who are overstimulated or who are stimulated at the wrong times are at risk for physical and emotional disorders. Nursing interventions are aimed at acquainting parents with the unique behavioral capacities of their infant and supporting appropriate reciprocal interactions. The nurse's role in support of behavioral adaptations is discussed in Chapter 33.

Some high-risk neonates continue to suffer from behavioral disorganization and do not provide consistent cues (Schraeder & McEvoy-Shields, 1992). They may have a diminished capacity for social interaction. Infants who have suffered permanent damage to the lungs or intestinal tract may display prolonged agitation, a condition initially defined by nurse researchers (Frank, 1987). Agitated infants are irritable, may not habituate to environmental stimuli, and remain inconsolable when aroused. Parents of these infants also require continued assistance and support. Further research is needed to identify specific behaviors that differentiate agitation from other behavioral problems.

Identifying Parenting Risk Factors

An integral aspect of risk assessment is an ongoing evaluation of the parents' responses to the birth of the high-risk or sick neonate. The nurse must be familiar with current theories regarding psychologic reactions to this stressful event to understand observations and analyze the data collected. Refer to Chapter 25 for a review of crisis and grieving theory and a discussion of the childbearing couple's response to high-risk pregnancy and birth of a high-risk neonate.

The nurse must be skilled in the assessment of the high-risk neonate and have a comprehensive knowledge of danger signs. The development of problems in the high-risk neonate may be manifested by subtle signs of dysfunction. The nurse must be alert to these first indicators of maladaptation. Ongoing assessment is necessary to identify changes in the neonate's condition with time. Many of these initial subtle cues will become marked with continuing decompensation. The goal of assessment is the early recognition of problems so that timely interventions can be initiated. A complete systems assessment, including physiologic and behavioral functioning, is essential to accomplish this goal.

Chapter Summary

Nursing assessment and identification of the neonate at risk for complications in the neonatal period are essential aspects of neonatal care. The nurse identifies health risks to the fetus during the prenatal period, assists in the immediate resuscitation and stabilization of the infant in the delivery room, and assumes responsibility for ongoing nursing assessment and diagnosis after birth. This chapter has discussed the components of neonatal risk. It describes how the nursing process begins with assessment to identify potential or actual problems that lead to the development of nursing diagnoses. Nursing care of the high-risk neonate and family is presented in Chapters 25 and 33. Interventions are based on accurate assessment and continuous monitoring of the high-risk infant.

Study Questions

1. *What is the purpose of identifying perinatal risk factors for the neonate?*
2. *What is the significance of the Apgar score for immediate and long-term neonatal outcome?*
3. *What is the role of the nurse in immediate stabilization and resuscitation of the neonate at birth?*
4. *What are the recommended steps in resuscitation of the neonate?*
5. *What drugs are commonly used in neonatal resuscitation, and what is their therapeutic function?*
6. *What are danger signs of potential illness in the high-risk neonate?*
7. *What are the phases of behavioral adaptation in the high-risk or sick neonate?*

References

ACOG Committee on Obstetrics: Maternal and Fetal Medicine. (1991). *Utility of umbilical cord blood acid-base assessment*. ACOG Committee Opinion Number 91 (February). Washington, DC: Author.

American Heart Association/American Academy of Pediatrics. (1990). *The textbook of neonatal resuscitation*. Elk Grove Village, IL: American Heart Association.

Ballard, J., Khoury, J., Wedig, K., et al. (1991). New Ballard Score, expanded to include extremely premature infants. *Journal of Pediatics*, *119*(3), 417.

Ballweg, D. (1991). Neonatal seizures: An overview. *Neonatal Network*, *10*(1), 15.

Behnke, M., Eyler, F., Carter, R., et al. (1989). Predictive value of Apgar scores for developmental outcome in premature infants. *American Journal of Perinatology*, *6*(1), 18.

Brazelton, B. (1989). The infant at risk. *Journal of Perinatology*, *9*(3), 307.

Cole, M. (1991). New factors associated with the incidence of hypoglycemia: A research study. *Neonatal Network*, *10*(4), 47.

Epstein, M. F. (1991). Resuscitation in the delivery room. In J. P. Cloherty & A. R. Stark (Eds.). *Manual of neonatal care*. Boston: Little, Brown & Co.

Frank, L. (1987). A national survey of the assessment and treatment of pain and agitation in the neonatal intensive care unit. *Journal of Obstetric, Gynecologic, and Neonatal Nursing*, *16*(6), 387.

Gorski, P., Davison, M., Brazelton, B. (1979). Stages of behavioral organization in the high-risk neonate: Theoretical and clinical considerations. *Seminars in Perinatology*, *3*(1), 61.

Ingelfinger, J. (1991). Renal conditions in the newborn period. In J. P. Cloherty & A. R. Stark (Eds.). *Manual of neonatal care*. Boston: Little, Brown & Co.

Parker, S., Zuckerman, B., Bauchner, H., et al. (1990). Jitteriness in full-term neonates: Prevalence and correlates. *Pediatrics*, *85*(1), 331.

Paxton, J., & Harrell, H. (1991). Delivery room management of the asphyxiated neonate. *NAACOG's Clinical Issues in Perinatal and Women's Health Nursing*, *2*(1), 35.

Portman, R., Carter, B., Gaylord, M., et al. (1990). Predicting neonatal morbidity after perinatal asphyxia: A scoring system. *American Journal of Obstetrics and Gynecology*, *162*(1), 174.

Richardson, D. (1991). Mechanical ventilation. In J. P. Cloherty & A. R. Stark (Eds.). *Manual of neonatal care*. Boston: Little, Brown & Co.

Schraeder, B., & McEvoy-Shields, M. (1992). Development and longitudinal follow-up of low-birth weight infants. *NAACOGs Clinical Issues in Perinatal and Women's Health Nursing*, *3*(1), 147.

Stark, A., & North, J. (1991). Transient tachypnea of the newborn. In J. P. Cloherty & A. R. Stark (Eds.). *Manual of neonatal care*. Boston: Little, Brown & Co.

Tronick, E., Scanlon, K., & Scanlon, J. (1990). Protective apathy, a hypothesis about the behavioral organization and its relation to clinical and physiologic status of the preterm infant during the newborn period. *Clinics in Perinatology*, *17*(1), 125.

Winkler, C., Hauth, J., Tucker, M., et al. (1991). Neonatal complications at term as related to the degree of umbilical artery acidemia. *American Journal of Obstetrics and Gynecology*, *164*(2), 637.

Suggested Readings

Bowen, F. (1992). Neurologic evaluation of the preterm infant. *NAACOGs Clinical Issues in Perinatal and Women's Health Nursing*, *3*(1), 75.

Carroll, P. (1991). Pneumothorax in the newborn. *Neonatal Network*, *10*(2), 27.

Fox, M. (1992). Measurement of urine output volume. *Neonatal Network*, *11*(3), 11.

Graff, M., Goldie, E., Lee, G., et al. (1991). The four-channel pneumogram in infants with recurring apneas and bradycardias. *Journal of Perinatology*, *11*(1), 10.

Gunderson, L. P., Kenner, C. (1987). Neonatal stress: Physiologic adaptation and nursing implications. *Neonatal Network*, *6*(1), 37.

Harbold, L. (1989). A protocol for neonatal use of pulse oximetry. *Neonatal Network*, *8*(1), 41.

Headrick, C. (1992). Hemodynamic monitoring of the critically ill neonate. *Journal of Perinatal and Neonatal Nursing*, *5*(4), 58.

Mitchell, A., Watts, J., Whyte, R., et al. (1991). Evaluation of graduating neonatal nurse practitioners. *Pediatrics*, *88*(4), 789.

Lansdown, L., & Spitz, L. (1989). Factors associated with developmental progress of full term neonates who required intensive care. *Archives of Diseases in Childhood*, *64*, 333.

Rios, A., Goyal, M., & Kresch, M., et al. (1992). Magnetic resonance imaging in full-term infants with repetitive focal seizures. *Journal of Perinatology*, *12*(3), 252.

Seguin, J. (1992). Effects of transcutaneous monitor electrode heat on skin servo-controlled environments. *Journal of Perinatology*, *12*(3), 276.

Sobel, D. (1992). Burning of a neonate due to a pulse oximeter: Arterial saturation monitoring. *Pediatrics*, *89*(1), 154.

Tolentino, M. (1990). The use of Orem's self-care model in the neonatal intensive-care unit. *Journal of Obstetric, Gynecologic, and Neonatal Nursing*, *19*(6), 496.

CHAPTER 33

Nursing Care of the High-Risk Neonate

Learning Objectives

After studying the material in this chapter, the student will be able to:

- Describe the implications of perinatal regionalization for families and health care providers.
- Identify nursing interventions in the care of the neonate with altered respiratory function.
- Demonstrate nursing interventions when providing neonatal nutritional needs.
- Identify principles of infection control in the special care nursery.
- Discuss nursing actions in support of parents of the high-risk neonate.
- Describe therapeutic interventions used in the prevention of hyperbilirubinemia and kernicterus.
- Identify predisposing factors in birth asphyxia.
- Explain problems of the neonate with complications related to gestational age.
- Describe care of the neonate with effects of maternal substance abuse.
- Discuss prevention of neonatal infection.
- Describe birth trauma and its results.

Key Terms

apnea
asphyxia
intrauterine growth retardation
large-for-gestational age neonate
low–birth-weight neonate
neonatal abstinence syndrome
postterm neonate
preterm neonate
respiratory distress syndrome
sepsis
small-for-gestational age neonate

When complications arise, the nurse, while sharing in the family's sadness, also must create a climate to support the new parents. At the same time the physical needs of the sick neonate must be met with the use of an increasingly complex array of technologic devices. The nurse must possess the basic skills and knowledge required to recognize major neonatal complications, initiate resuscitation, and assist in stabilizing the neonate's condition. The outcome of the neonate's condition is influenced by the care received immediately after birth.

Regardless of gestational age, the high-risk neonate's extrauterine existence is compromised by events occurring before, during, or after birth and is in need of specialized nursing and medical care. High-risk newborns fall into three broad categories:

- Newborns with alterations in gestational length and intrauterine growth (eg, preterm or postterm infants or small- or large-for-gestational age [LGA] infants)
- Newborns with acquired disorders (eg, respiratory distress syndrome [RDS], Rh incompatibility, birth injuries, neonatal sepsis)
- Newborns with congenital anomalies, including chromosomal alterations and genetic defects

These categories are not mutually exclusive, and a newborn may fall into more than one category of risk.

A major goal of nursing care of the high- or at-risk neonate is to provide optimal family-centered care, that is, to recognize the inherent worth and unique characteristics of each newborn, to facilitate parent–newborn attachment, and to support parents during the grieving process that occurs with the loss of the "perfect child" or with the actual death of a severely ill neonate. The nursing process can serve as a basis for meeting these needs.

This chapter describes how the nursing process can used to accomplish the goals of nursing care in a rational and systematic manner. Nursing interventions to meet the basic life-support needs of the high-risk neonate, as reflected in nursing diagnoses, are discussed in the first section of this

Legal/Ethical Considerations

Responsibilities of the Nursery Head Nurse or Charge Nurse in Preparation for the Birth of the High-Risk Neonate

The courts have begun to scrutinize the response time of the nursery staff to the birth of a compromised newborn. The nursery head nurse or charge nurse must implement a formal plan for ongoing communication with labor and delivery personnel. Hourly calls or rounds should be made to the unit to update nursery staff on the status of women in labor. A list of all women in labor and delivery should be maintained so that staff and equipment are prepared for the birth of an at-risk neonate. It may even be appropriate to alert other personnel, such as radiologists, on-call neonatologists, and respiratory therapists, to ensure a rapid response when the neonate is born.

Conversely, the labor and delivery head nurse or charge nurse must alert nursery personnel immediately when a woman is admitted in an advanced state of labor, and the potential for newborn compromise is identified. A list should also be developed, identifying all instances when nursery staff should be notified and present for the birth. If a woman has not received prenatal care prior to labor, it is advisable that at least one member of the nursery team be present to assist with the evaluation and support of the newborn, in case problems arise after birth.

chapter. Specific neonatal disorders and congenital anomalies are discussed with nursing implications in the second half of this chapter.

Specialized Neonatal Care

Perinatal Regionalization

Although all nurses caring for the newborn should possess knowledge and skills to recognize neonatal risk factors and should be capable of functioning competently in emergency situations, continuing care of the high-risk neonate requires specialized services provided by a limited number of health care professionals and facilities. There often is inequity in the distribution of these essential services. In rural and impoverished areas health care facilities may be limited in their ability to provide the equipment and personnel necessary. In large urban settings services may be duplicated unnecessarily.

In an effort to solve these problems, a coordinated system for the provision of care within a designated area or region has been developed. Three levels of perinatal care have been defined with functions and goals for each. An additional goal of perinatal regionalization is to limit the spiraling rise in health care costs resulting from the development of subspecialties within the field of neonatology and the use of complex technology. Table 33-1 describes the types of care provided and the roles and responsibilities of nurses at each level.

Level I Facilities

A level I facility offers services to low-risk clients. It has three major functions:

- Management and care of mothers and newborns in normal births
- Early identification of high-risk pregnancies or high-risk neonates
- Provision of emergency care during unanticipated obstetric or neonatal emergencies

Women or newborns requiring more sophisticated care are referred or transported to level II or level III facilities.

Nurses in level I facilities are prepared through basic nursing education to care for healthy mothers and infants and must be skilled in assessment of risk factors and the stabilization of sick clients for transport when unexpected complications arise.

Level II Facilities

A level II facility offers services to low- and medium-risk clients. Its major function is to be able to provide competent care in 75% to 90% of maternal or neonatal complications. Women and newborns requiring care beyond the capability of the facility are referred or transported to a Level III center.

Nurses in level II facilities have advanced training or graduate education in the care of high-risk and sick clients. They must be skilled in the use of electronic monitoring equipment and other devices designed to support the delivery of medical and nursing care (Fig. 33-1).

Level III Facilities

A level III facility offers services to high-risk clients who require the most sophisticated level of care. Full-time specialists and state-of-the-art equipment are available to handle complex perinatal disorders (see Fig. 33-1). Additional functions of the level III facility include continuing education for level I and level II health team members through perinatal outreach programs and the development of a system of referral and transport so that other facilities can move high-risk clients to an appropriate high-risk center.

Nurses in a level III facility must have advanced training or graduate education in the care of clients with complex disorders. They also must be knowledgeable about community outreach and health education because preparation and support of the families of sick mothers and infants and continuing education of health care professionals are major functions of a level III institution.

Neonatal Transport

Highly skilled nurse–physician or nurse–nurse transport teams are on call 24 hours a day to move the sick neonate

Table 33-1. Levels of Care, Functions, and Nursing Roles in Regionalization of Perinatal Care

Level I	Level II	Level III
Management and care of low-risk clients Normal pregnancy, labor, delivery Normal newborns Identification of high-risk clients Referral of high-risk clients to level II or III facility Provision of emergency care and stabilization of client for transport to level II or III facility	Management and care of low-risk clients using facility Management and care of medium- and high-risk clients Pregnancy, labor, and delivery High-risk or sick neonates Emergency care and stabilization of clients Referral of high-risk clients (clients requiring care beyond the facility's capability—eg, fetal surgery, neonatal cardiac surgery) to level III facilities	Management and care of high-risk clients Pregnancy, labor, and delivery Fetal surgery Neonatal care Neonatal surgery Long-term care of high-risk infants with multiple medical problems who remain acutely ill (eg, extreme prematurity) Provision of continuing education programs for staffs of level I and level II facilities Inhouse programs Community outreach Development and provision of both short- and long-distance transport system for high-risk clients
Staff Nurse		
Assessment, diagnosis, planning, and implementation of care for low-risk families Childbirth preparation Discharge teaching and parent education Identification of high-risk clients Consultation with other health team members in planning care Referral of clients with special needs (to nutritionists, social workers, clinical nurse specialists) Preparation of high-risk clients for referral to level II or III facility Emergency care and stabilization of high-risk client prior to transport	Assessment, diagnosis, planning, and implementation of nursing care for low-risk clients (see level I) Assessment, diagnosis, planning, and implementation of nursing care for medium- and high-risk clients Provision of special education and orientation of clients with special health care needs (eg, diabetes management) Childbirth education Initial emergency care and stabilization of clients Neonatal resuscitation Use of electronic monitors and diagnostic devices to assist in assessment and care of clients Consultation with other health team members in planning care of clients with special needs (eg, with nutritionists, respiratory therapists) Referral of clients with special needs to appropriate resources: physical therapy, clergy, community agencies, financial counselor Parenting education for parents of normal and high-risk infants	Assessment, diagnosis, planning, and implementation of nursing care for high-risk clients (see level II)
Clinical Nurse Specialist		
Clinical nursing consultation for patients with complex care needs; primary nursing care for selected patients. Staff education and development Consultation with nursing staff and other health team members in planning care for clients Client education Referral of clients to level II or III facility Nursing research Assistance with emergency care and stabilization of high-risk clients for transport	Staff education and development Consultation with nursing staff and other members of health team in planning care for clients with special needs Patient education for clients with special needs Referral of clients to level III facilities Nursing research Direct patient care of selected high-risk clients Participation in transport of high-risk clients from level I facility Development and implementation of nursing care plans and procedures to meet the needs of high-risk clients	(See level II) Development and implementation of educational programs for level I and II staff nurses within the designated perinatal region Direct supervision and training of level I and II nurses who are in training at the level III facility

(continued)

Table 33-1. Levels of Care, Functions, and Nursing Roles in Regionalization of Perinatal Care (*Continued*)

Level I	Level II	Level III
Neonatal Nurse Practitioner		
Management and care of low-risk neonates and their families Neonatal resuscitation Emergency care and stabilization of ill neonates prior to transport to level II or III facility Referral of newborns to level II or III facility Management of neonates during transport Staff education Parent education Consultation with nursing staff and other members of the health care team Nursing research	Management and care of • low-risk neonates and their families • high-risk neonates born in institution or transported from level I facility • intermediate care of neonates return transported from level III facility Neonatal resuscitation Emergency care and stabilization of ill neonates prior to transport to level III facility Referral of neonates to level III facility Management of neonates during transport Staff education Parent education Consultation with nursing staff and other members of health care team Nursing research	Management and care of • high-risk neonates and their families • newborns with chronic health problems • Newborns requiring intermediate care Neonatal resuscitation Emergency care and stabilization of ill neonates at birth Referral of neonates back to level I and II facility Comprehensive management of neonates during transport Consultation with nursing staff and other members of health care team Staff education Parent education Nursing research

from the place of birth. A telephone call or radio message from the referring physician or nurse midwife activates the transport system. A specially designed mobile transport unit (ambulance, helicopter, or airplane), containing all the equipment required to support the infant, can be dispatched within minutes. Telephone consultation with neonatologists and nurses at the level III facility will assist the staff at the referring hospital to stabilize the neonate and prepare him or her for transport.

Implications for Nursing Care

Only a few dozen neonatal nurses in a large geographic area may be trained to provide specialized nursing care to critically ill newborns. Consequently, the neonates cared for at level I and II facilities are less acutely ill, which alters the focus of newborn nursing within these hospitals. Although many level II hospitals are providing more comprehensive care, the more premature or critically ill newborns and those

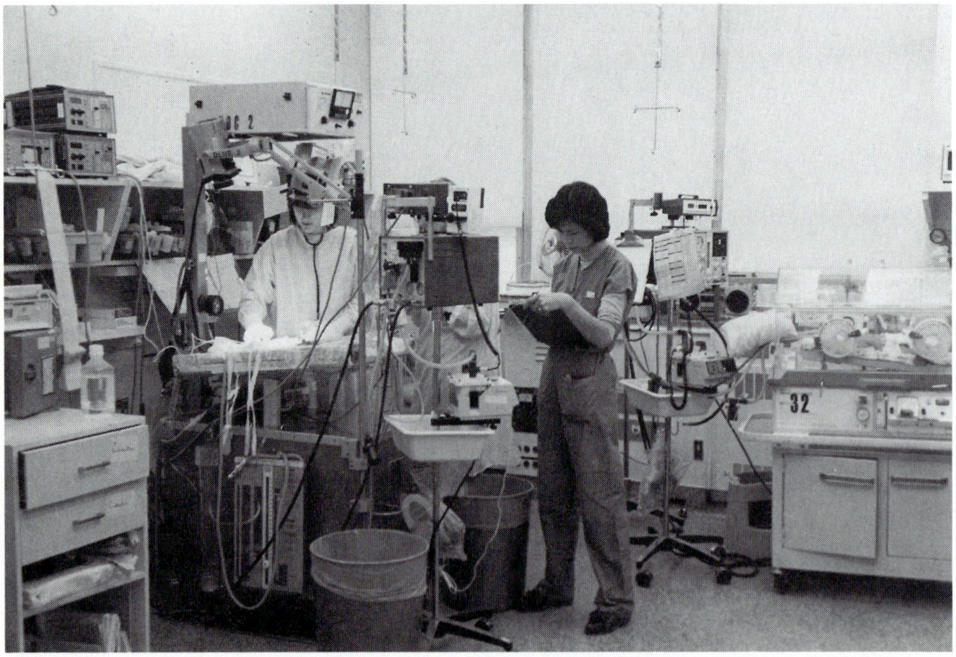

Figure 33-1.

Nurses working in level II and level III facilities are specialists in neonatal care and are expert in managing complex nursing problems with the use of sophisticated technology. (Photo by Colleen Stainton, University of California, San Francisco.)

requiring surgical or high-tech interventions continue to be transported to level III facilities.

In light of this change in nursing roles and responsibilities for most maternal–newborn nurses, this chapter provides only basic information about major complications and congenital anomalies.

All nurses caring for these high-risk neonates in level I and II facilities must be familiar with major categories of defects. They must have a basic understanding of how the neonate is affected, the types of treatment available, immediate nursing interventions required, and prognosis to care for the infant's immediate needs after birth and to support the parents.

Common Elements in the Care of a High-Risk Neonate

Neonates with the following complications are discussed in this chapter: birth asphyxia, gestational age and growth, hemolytic disease, and maternal substance abuse.

Many elements in the planning and implementation of nursing care for these high-risk neonates are similar, regardless of the specific disorder. The following section discusses these common elements of high-risk neonatal nursing care as they relate to frequently used nursing diagnoses. This section is followed by a more detailed discussion of specific neonatal disorders and appropriate nursing care.

• • Assessment

Initial assessment of the neonate is discussed in Chapter 30, and further assessment of the at-risk neonate is discussed in Chapter 32. Data are gathered from the maternal and neonatal health histories, and a systematic physical, gestational, and neurobehavioral assessment is made.

Assessing for Murmurs

Murmurs are nothing more than audible turbulence of blood flow, encountered when blood within the heart chambers is trying to flow where it should not. The greater the turbulence, the louder the murmur. Auscultation and interpretation of murmurs is best performed by skilled clinicians. The student nurse may be able to appreciate a loud, "machinery-like" murmur over the lower left sternal border, indicating a closing ductus arteriosus. Murmurs usually are graded on a scale of I to VI, from barely audible to appreciable when the stethoscope is inches off the neonate's chest.

The nurse often may be the first person to detect a murmur. The subsequent workup might include a comparison of blood pressures of all four limbs (to detect coarctation of the aorta), chest x-ray studies (to observe the cardiac shadow and to determine if the newborn is demonstrating signs of cardiac failure), and a 12 lead electrocardiogram (to assess for abnormal electrical impulses within the heart). The neonate with a potentially lethal cardiac anomaly will need to be transferred to a tertiary facility for echocardiography, cardiac catheterization, or surgery.

Assessing the Cardiac System

A quiet, well-lit area with adequate warmth (overhead warmer) is provided. The neonate should be relatively free of distractions (fed, dry diaper, pacified) and (ideally) in a quiet alert state. Activity, state, and temperature of the neonate will greatly affect the assessment, so care must be taken to provide optimal conditions.

The cardiac system examination can be divided into three major components: *look*, *listen*, and *feel*. The "look" component involves observation or inspection of the neonate. The color, mucous membranes, precordium, and the presence of edema are evaluated. Figure 33-2*A* outlines the normal or normally abnormal findings (in uppercase lettering) and the abnormal findings (in lower case). The "listen" component is the parameters assessed with a stethoscope and includes apical pulse for rate, rhythm, and murmurs and the point of maximal impulse (PMI). Figure 33-2*B* provides the possible findings. The "feel" component is components of the cardiac examination assessed by palpation. These include pulses, perfusion, temperature, turgor, the precordium, and the liver. Figure 33-2*C* indicates the normal, normally abnormal (in capitals), and abnormal findings.

Assessing for Cardiac Anomalies

Detection of cardiac anomalies, especially those that are life-threatening, may be the most crucial element of the assessment process after the delivery of the high-risk neonate. The advent of fetal echocardiography and ultrasonography has improved the diagnostic certitude with which lethal anomalies are detected before delivery. This allows for delivery of potentially compromised infants in not only a timely fashion, but in the facility most capable of meeting the neonate's immediate needs (including cardiac surgery if indicated). Other cardiac anomalies will be detected based on compromised circulation, oxygenation, cardiac rhythm, or respiratory status, and need to be further evaluated by skilled clinicians and highly technical diagnostic equipment.

Assessing for Behavioral Adaptation

All newborns go through a period of behavioral adaptation as neurologic and behavioral processes are reorganized for the neonate to interact and respond appropriately. The nurse must understand neonatal behavioral capabilities and responses, including recognition of signs of stress and overstimulation (see the display on neonatal behavior in the intensive care nursery [ICN]). The display also lists signs of stability in the high-risk neonate. Using this knowledge, the nurse assesses the neonate's response to the neonatal intensive care unit (NICU) environment and caregiving actions, reduces stressful aspects of the NICU environment, and implements protocols that minimize routine handling of fragile and unstable neonates.

• • Nursing Diagnosis

Based on the initial assessment of neonatal status, the nurse formulates diagnoses that direct subsequent nursing care. Nursing diagnoses focus on continued support of phys-

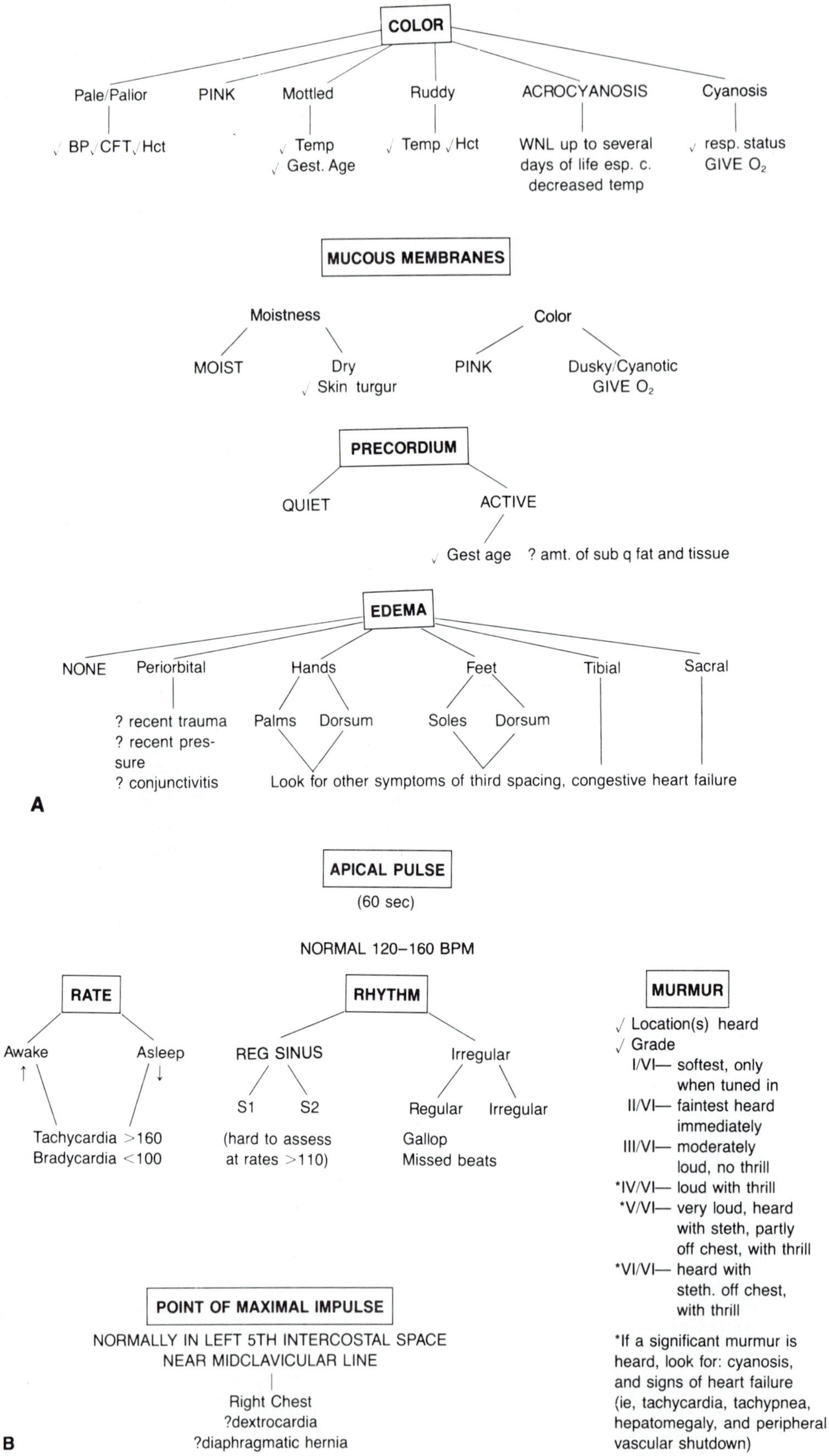

Figure 33-2.

Three major components of examining the cardiac system of a high-risk neonate. *A:* Observation and inspection: LOOK. *B:* Auscultation: LISTEN.

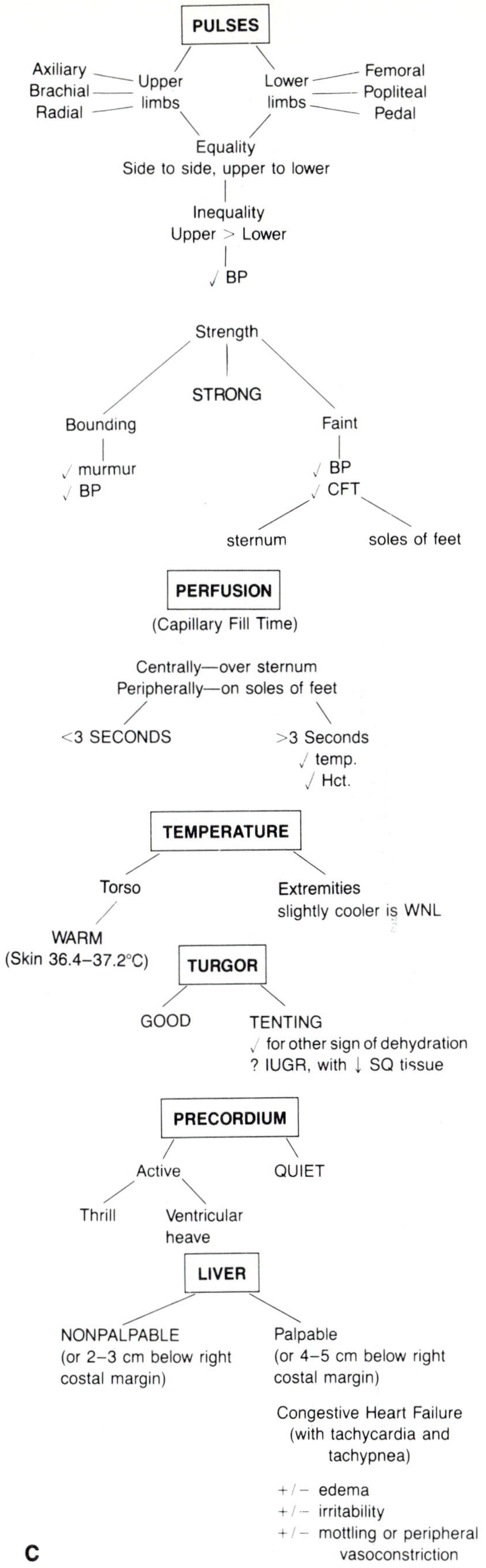

Figure 33-2 (*continued*) *C:* Palpation: FEEL. *Note:* Normal or normally abnormal findings are printed in upper case letters; abnormal findings are printed in lower case letters. (From Timm, K. [1991]. Unpublished paper. Cardiovascular assessment of the neonate. Used with permission, © K. Timm.)

iologic functions and promote optimal family adaptations. The following possible nursing diagnoses are applicable to direct independent nursing care of the high-risk neonate and family:

- Impaired Gas Exchange related to meconium aspiration or RDS
- Altered Tissue Perfusion related to inadequate chest excursion
- Fluid Volume Deficit related to impaired renal function
- Altered Nutrition: Less than Body Requirements related to severe perinatal asphyxia
- High Risk for Infection related to intrapartum bacterial exposure
- High Risk for Altered Body Temperature related to ineffective thermoregulation
- Sleep Pattern Disturbance related to neonatal abstinence syndrome
- Sensory-Perceptual Alterations related to prematurity
- Altered Parenting related to prolonged hospitalization of neonate
- Family Coping: Potential for Growth related to adaptive tasks used in providing care
- Dysfunctional Grieving related to birth of a "less than perfect" neonate

The neonatal nurse continues to observe and monitor for early, often subtle, signs of serious complications that result from the neonate's condition or the therapeutic modalities used.

• • Planning and Implementation

Once nursing diagnoses have been established, the nurse plans and implements appropriate interventions to support physiologic functions and neurobehavioral adaptations. Nursing interventions for the high-risk neonate are similar to those for the normal neonate, but the possibility of complications is increased. Interventions include preventing and identifying physical complications, assessing extrauterine adaptation, establishing a feeding pattern, promoting neurobehavioral adaptation, and supporting parent–infant attachment.

The nurse, when planning care, takes into account the degree of seriousness of the newborn's condition, the emotional and physical status of family members, the physiologic adaptations required of the newborn, and neonatal responses to the nursery environment and caregiving. When complications arise, regardless of the etiology of the disorder, the principles on which care is based remain the same. Those common elements of care are discussed in this section. Nursing interventions are organized to minimize physiologic stress, disturbance of the neonate, disruption of sleep patterns, and sensory overload.

Promoting Pulmonary Adaptation

Because cold stress and unnecessary stimulation increase the newborn's metabolic requirements and hence the need for oxygen, the nurse must minimize energy requirements and support thermoregulatory function for the new-

Neonatal Behavior in the Intensive Care Nursery

Signs of Stress

Autonomic System	*Motor System*	*State System (range)*	*Attention-Interaction System*	*Self-Regulatory System*
Respiration Pauses, tachypnea, gasping *Color Changes* Paling around nostrils, perioral duskiness, mottled, cyanotic, gray, flushed, ruddy *Visceral* Hiccups, gagging, grunting, spitting up Straining as if actually producing a bowel movement *Motor* Seizures Tremoring/startling Twitching Coughing Sneezing Yawning Sighing	*Fluctuating Tone* Flaccidity of • Trunk • Extremities • Face *Hypertonicity* • Leg extensions • Salutes • Airplaning • Sitting on air • Arching • Finger splays • Tongue extensions • Fisting *Hyperflexions* • Trunk • Extremities • Fetal tuck *Frantic, diffuse activity*	*Diffuse states* Sleep: • Twitches • Sounds • Jerky moves • Irregular respirations • Whimpers • Grimacing • Fussy in sleep *Awake* • Eye floating • Glassy eyed • Strained fussy • Staring • Gaze aversion • Panicked, worried or dull look • Weak cry • Irritability • Abrupt state changes	*May demonstrate stress signals of other systems* • Irregular respirations • Color changes • Visceral responses • Coughing, twitches • Sneezing • Yawning • Sighing • Eye floating • Glassy eyed • Staring • Straining • Gaze aversion • Panicked, worried, or dull look • Weak cry • Irritability • Abrupt state changes • Fluctuating tone • Frantic, diffuse activity • Becomes stressed with more than one mode of stimuli	*May use the following to attempt to gain balance* • Lowers state • Postural changes • Motoric strategies leg or foot bracing, hand clasping, foot clasping, finger folding, hand to mouth, sucking, grasping, hand holding, tucking • Good self-quieting and consolability • Rhythmic, robust crying • Clear sleep state • Focused alertness with shiny eyed and focused attention, animated expression, frowning, cheek softening, "ooh" face, cooing, smiling

Intervention Strategies to Reduce Stress

Modified environment (light, noise, traffic) Positioning Minimal handling Swaddling or covering	Positioning Handling to contain limbs Handling slow/gentle Blanket rolls Containment, nesting	Clustering care Primary nursing to accurately read infant cues Appropriate timing of activities and daily routines Autonomic and motoric subsystems must have reached stability	Interactions modulated to infant's tolerance level Supports necessary to bring out best alertness One mode of stimulation at a time Modulated voice, face, rattle, face and voice together (Baby responds best to animate stimuli)	Provision of support • hand holding • foot holding Modified interactions Modified environment Swaddling Organize daily routine to infant's best times

Signs of Stability

Autonomic System	*Motor System*	*State System*	*Attention System*	*Self-Regulatory System*
Smooth, regular respirations Pink, stable color Stable viscera with no evidence of: • Seizures • Gagging • Emesis • Grunting • Tremors • Startles • Twitches • Coughing • Sneezing • Yawning • Sighing	Smooth, controlled posture Smooth movements of extremities, head seen in: • Hand clasp • Leg or foot bracing • Foot clasp • Finger folding • Hand to mouth • Grasping • Sucking • Tucking • Hand holding Good consistent tone throughout body	Clear, well-defined sleep states Good self-quieting and consolability Robust crying Focused, clear alertness with animated expressions such as: • Frowning • Cheek softening • "Ooh" face • Cooing • Smiling	Responsivity to auditory and visual stimuli bright and of long duration Actively seeks out auditory and shifts attention smoothly on own from one stimulus to another Face demonstrates bright-eyed purposeful interest varying between arousal and relaxation	Neonate has sophisticated, well-differentiated repertoire of successful strategies to maintain each system: autonomic, motor, state, and attention, such as: *autonomic:* sucking, grasping *motor:* tucking, foot bracing *state:* visual locking, sucking *attention:* hand to mouth, hand holding

Interventions

Interventions not necessary to reduce stress but to enhance and facilitate normal development.

From Van den Berg, K., & Franck, L. S. (1990). Behavioral issues in infants with BDD. In C. H. Lund (Ed.), Bronchopulmonary dysplasia *(pp. 124–125). Petaluma, LA: Neonatal Network.*

born. After initial resuscitation and stabilization at birth, newborns requiring continuing respiratory support will be placed in an incubator or under a radiant warmer. Equipment essential for pulmonary support must be at hand. The nurse, in conjunction with the medical team, assists the neonate to maintain an adequate airway and when indicated provides an enriched oxygen atmosphere.

Open Airway

The potential for accidental aspiration is present in all newborns. Because of immature cardiac sphincter function, regurgitation or vomiting of gastric contents occurs. Weak neck muscles prevent quick repositioning of the head for drainage of these fluids. A sick or compromised neonate can be at greater risk for airway obstruction as a result of mucus or meconium in the airways; congenital anomalies of the mouth, pharynx, and neck; or a weak or absent gag reflex.

Positioning

If not contraindicated, neonates should be positioned on their side to facilitate drainage of fluids from the mouth and nares. Many sick neonates are initially placed in a supine position on an open bed to facilitate the placement of umbilical artery or venous lines or to perform such procedures as chest x-rays, ultrasonography, or chest tube placement. The nurse can provide small blanket roll supports behind the newborn's back and turn the newborn's head in the same direction to encourage drainage of fluids. When the newborn is extremely flaccid or hypotonic, the nurse may need to place a small towel roll under the scapulae to bring the head into proper alignment ("sniff" position) to prevent airway obstruction. Oropharyngeal airways, although available in infant sizes, are rarely indicated or used in newborns. Once the neonate is stabilized, he or she may be repositioned to prone, sidelying, and so forth. Preterm neonates often are placed prone to stabilize the chest wall, thereby facilitating respiration and oxygenation.

Suctioning

Although a bulb syringe may be adequate for clearing the mouth and nares of the newborn with normal gag and swallow reflexes, the sick or compromised neonate often needs additional assistance. A suction catheter (5 to 10 French) attached to a portable suction machine or a wall outlet can be used to clear the airway of mucus. This method is most often used with neonates who have secretory disease processes (meconium aspiration syndrome [MAS], bacterial pneumonia) or who are attached to a mechanical ventilator and require intermittent suctioning.

For endotracheal (deep) suctioning, sterile technique should be used. It should last no longer than 5 seconds with a low-pressure setting to decrease the amount of oxygen removed from the airways. Negative pressure is applied only after the catheter has been inserted into the airway to the designated depth and is being withdrawn. Applying negative pressure while the catheter is being passed, using too much pressure, or inserting the suction catheter too far can cause trauma to the airway mucosa. The newborn's heart rate must be monitored closely during suctioning of the oropharynx, nasopharynx, or trachea, because bradycardia can occur due to stimulation of the vagus nerve. Components of endotracheal suctioning are summarized in the accompanying display. Also see the display on suctioning of the neonate delivered through meconium in Chapter 32.

Chest Physiotherapy

Another method for facilitating the drainage of mucus and maintaining a patent airway involves gentle chest percussion or vibration and postural (gravity) drainage, followed by suctioning. These procedures are used with newborns who have meconium aspiration, pneumonia, or severe atelectasis and hypercapnia. These procedures are associated with complications such as hypoxia, rib fractures, bruising, and dislodged tubes. In addition there is continuing controversy regarding the efficacy of chest physiotherapy in the neonate, especially in preterm newborns. Because of this controversy, many level III facilities are no longer performing postural drainage, and nurses perform vibration or percussion only when clinically indicated. Due to the increased risk of intracranial hemorrhage in the premature neonate, Trendelenburg positioning (with the concomitant rise in intracranial blood pressure and blood flow) is contraindicated.

Expected Outcomes

- The neonate maintains a sidelying position for drainage.
- The neonate's airway remains open.

Supporting Ventilation

The high-risk neonate may require assistance with ventilation to oxygenate tissues adequately. Neonates with depressed central nervous system function or congenital anomalies of the chest or abdomen and premature neonates with RDS frequently need ventilatory assistance. Four forms of ventilatory support are used: continuous positive airway

Components of Endotracheal Suctioning

Oxygen: Increase 10% to 15% over baseline

Pressure: Baseline

Rate: Additional breaths prior to and following suctioning

Irrigant: Normal saline, 0.25–0.50 mL

Catheter size: 6 French for endotracheal tube size 3.0 or less

8 French for endotracheal tube sizes 3.5 and 4.0

Negative pressure: 75–80 mm Hg

Suction duration: 5 sec applied intermittently only during withdrawal of catheter

Suction depth: Length of endotracheal tube or length of endotracheal tube plus 1 cm

From Turner, B. (1991). Nursing procedures. In J. Nugent (Ed.), Acute respiratory care of the neonate. p. 88.

pressure (CPAP), conventional mechanical ventilation, high-frequency ventilation, and extracorporeal membrane oxygenation (ECMO).

CPAP

CPAP is applied to the lungs during the respiratory cycle in an effort to prevent alveolar collapse and atelectasis. Neonates may be able to breathe without assistance and yet require CPAP to ease the work of breathing by preventing alveolar collapse with each expiration. CPAP may be applied through a face mask, nasal prongs, nasopharyngeal tube, or endotracheal tube attached to a mechanical ventilator. CPAP also has been used to decrease the frequency of apnea of prematurity.

Conventional Mechanical Ventilation

Conventional mechanical ventilation is used most frequently. Many machines are available that operate on volume cycle, time cycle, or pressure limited principles. Pressure-limited, time-cycled, continuous flow ventilators are used most often (Fig. 33-3). Conventional ventilation generally is applied through an endotracheal tube. Positive end expiratory pressure usually is applied to the lung at the end of the expiratory cycle to prevent alveolar collapse.

High-Frequency Ventilation

High-frequency ventilation, a newer technique of mechanical ventilation, was developed in an effort to reduce the barotrauma that occurs in neonates who require assisted ventilation at high mean airway pressures and tidal volumes. High-frequency ventilation is a technique for delivering small volumes of gas at very high rates (150 breaths per minute, up to 3000 cycles per minute). Several types of high-frequency ventilation are now available, including high-frequency oscillation, flow interruption, or jets. These ventilators are being used with neonates with severe respiratory problems in a limited number of institutions.

ECMO

ECMO is a recently developed technique to provide lifesaving cardiopulmonary support for critically ill neonates who have not responded to conventional ventilatory therapy, such as conventional ventilation with 100% oxygen. ECMO centers have been developed in some level III units with a specially trained ECMO team. ECMO is a temporary substitute for the heart and lungs using a cardiopulmonary bypass circuit with a membrane oxygenator (Fig. 33-4). ECMO is used primarily for large preterm and term neonates with MAS, congenital diaphragmatic hernia, persistent pulmonary hypertension, pneumonia, and RDS. ECMO is generally not used with preterm neonates younger than 34 to 35 weeks' gestation because of the high rate of complications, especially intercranial hemorrhage.

Neuromuscular Blocking Agents

Neuromuscular blocking agents may be used to improve ventilation and oxygenation. For example, full-term neonates with normal muscle tone may struggle against the respiratory phases of the ventilator, disrupting gas exchange. Skeletal muscle paralysis is achieved by administration of a drug, such as Pavulon (pancuronium bromide), which blocks

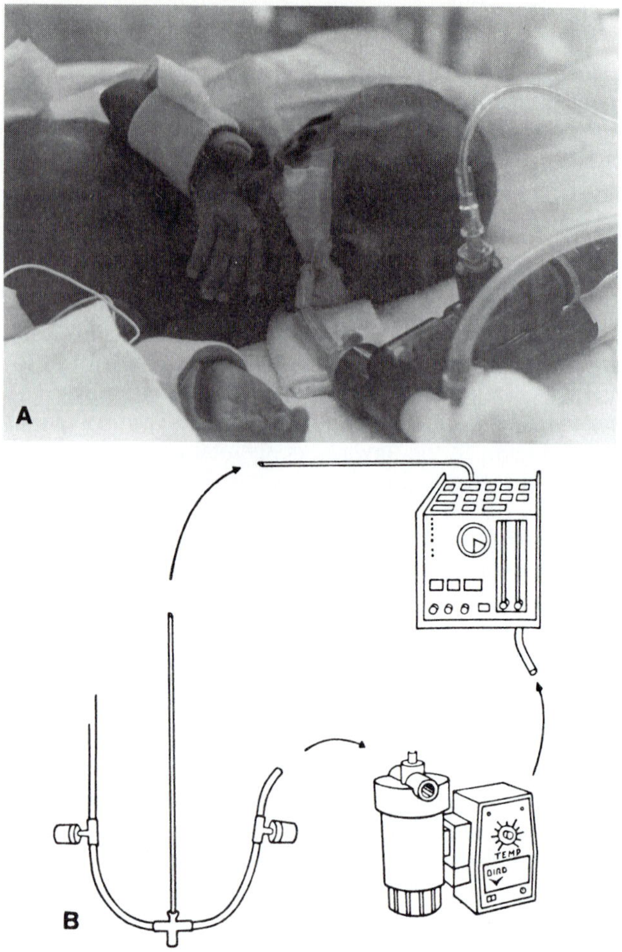

Figure 33-3.
Mechanical ventilation assists the sick neonate by preventing collapse of alveoli with expiration and by reducing the work needed to maintain effective respiration. *A:* Baby on ventilation. *B:* Typical ventilator circuit used with neonates. (Photo by Colleen Stainton.)

transmission of acetylcholine across the neuromuscular synapse. Therefore, the neonate remains fully conscious and perceptive to pain stimuli. Morphine, fentanyl (a synthetic narcotic), or similar agents also should be administered to relieve pain and sedate the neonate. The nurse must remain at the bedside at all times to assess significant changes in the neonate's respiratory status. He or she also should be prepared to initiate ventilation with a bag and mask if the neonate's condition suddenly deteriorates while on mechanical ventilation or if the ventilator fails.

Administering Oxygen

During the initial resuscitaiton efforts, a 100% oxygen concentration is administered to the neonate. As the neonate's condition stabilizes, the concentration is adjusted to maintain the Pa_{O_2} (partial pressure of oxygen in the blood) within acceptable limits. This adjustment is essential, because elevated Pa_{O_2} levels (caused by administration of oxygen in high concentrations) can cause irreparable damage to retinal vessels. Furthermore, high oxygen concentrations can directly injure lung tissue. Premature neonates with

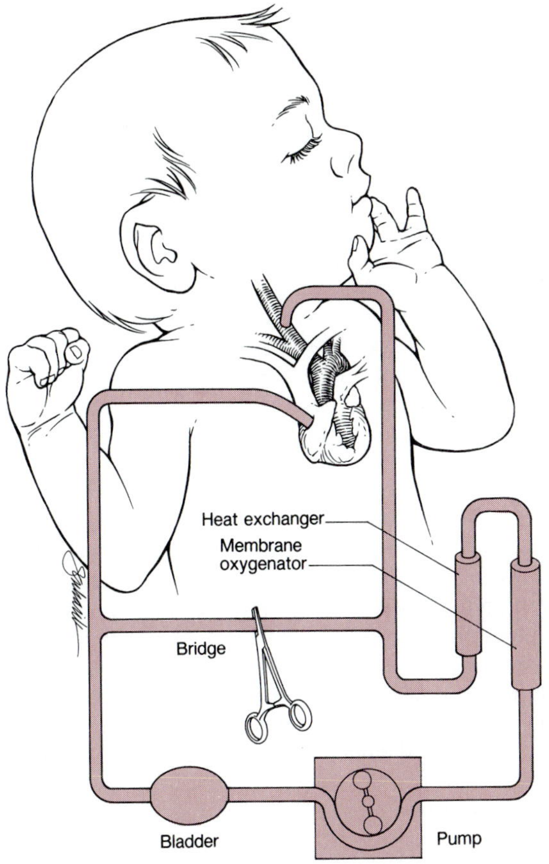

Figure 33-4.
Components of the ECMO circuit. Unoxygenated blood drains out of the right atrium. Blood passes through a bladder that monitors volume. A pump pushes the blood up toward the oxygenator. Blood passes through the oxygenator and warmer, then flows into the right carotid artery.

immature lungs and eye vessels are at particular risk for two conditions that are associated with hyperoxia: retinopathy of prematurity (ROP) and bronchopulmonary dysplasia (BPD). These complications are discussed later in this chapter.

Oxygen Mask

An oxygen mask is used only as a temporary method. If a neonate is moderately depressed at birth, oxygen and CPAP can be administered through a tight-fitting mask specifically designed for neonates. The nurse must be certain to use the correct size to avoid oxygen leaks. Care also must be taken to prevent pressure on the neonate's eyes, because this can cause tissue ischemia and blindness. Correct placement of a neonatal oxygen mask is illustrated in Figure 32-6. Short-term "blow-by" oxygen therapy may be administered by placing the mask in close proximity to the neonate's face, it is an imprecise means of oxygen supplementation and should be used only during initial stabilization until a determination is made as to the efficacy of the neonate's own respiratory efforts.

Endotracheal Tube

When the infant is severely depressed at birth, oxygen is administered through an uncuffed endotracheal tube. The end of the tube is attached to a ventilation bag or to a mechanical ventilator if the neonate requires extended ventilatory assistance. Placement of the endotracheal tube is illustrated in Figure 32-3.

Oxygen Hood

If the neonate requires continuing oxygen therapy after the initial resuscitation but can breathe without assistance, a clear plastic oxygen hood is frequently used (Fig. 33-5). It fits over the neonate's head and is connected to oxygen tubing. This noninvasive delivery system allows for exposure of the neonate's body for essential procedures and treatments, while permitting an oxygen-rich environment concentrated around the neonate's airway. Oxygen can be delivered directly into an incubator, but this method usually is reserved for lower supplemental oxygen concentrations (chronic therapy) when the neonate requires minimal interventions and can tolerate the slight fluctuations in oxygen concentration that occur when the portholes are opened to permit access to the neonate. Furthermore, direct supply to the ambient air in the incubator allows for greater movement on the part of the neonate.

Nasal Prongs

Nasal prongs may be used to deliver oxygen to the neonate who is fairly stable and breathing on his or her own but requires an oxygen concentration higher than room air (21%) for extended periods of time. Growing preterm neonates with BPD or neonates with cardiac disease may be administered oxygen using nasal prongs to allow the neonate to be placed in an open crib, thereby altering the spectrum of external stimuli available to the neonate. This method also allows the parents and staff to hold and cuddle the neonate for longer periods without disconnecting him or her from the source of oxygen.

Expected Outcome

- The neonate maintains an effective respiratory pattern and an adequate gas exchange.

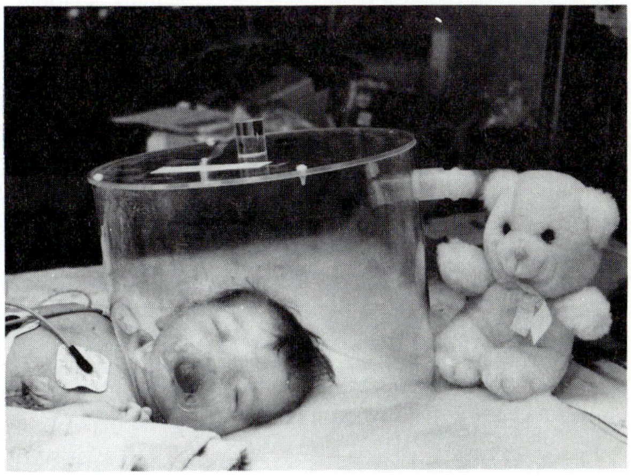

Figure 33-5.
The oxygen hood is used for neonates who require oxygen administration but who can breathe without mechanical assistance. (From Skale, N. [1992]. *Manual of pediatric nursing procedures*. Philadelphia: JB Lippincott.)

Supporting Cardiac Adaptation and Tissue Perfusion

Adequate oxygenation of the neonate is intrinsically tied to adequate circulation and blood volume. In the moments after delivery, all neonates must convert from a "parallel" method of circulation to one that operates "in series." Those newborns who are unable to establish adequate chest excursion to physically open the pulmonary vascular bed (thereby decreasing pulmonary vascular resistance and promoting blood circulation to the lungs) will maintain fetal circulation, as will those newborns who have defective hearts. The various cardiac lesions and anomalies found in newborns are discussed later in this chapter. Promotion of appropriate blood volume begins with timely clamping of the umbilical cord. For the high-risk neonate, inappropriate placental transfusion can further complicate adaptation. An increase in blood volume can cause relative desaturation and sluggish perfusion, while hypovolemia can quickly lead to organ compromise and multisystem failure.

Expected Outcome

- The neonate's blood volume remains stable.

Maintaining Circulatory Volume

Circulating blood volume usually is adequate unless there has been placental abruption, twin-to-twin transfusion, or rupture of and exsanguination through the umbilical cord. In these instances personnel and supplies must be prepared in the delivery suite to establish and maintain adequate circulating volume.

Adequate blood volume can be assured by administration of volume expanders, such as whole blood, packed red blood cells (RBCs), 5% albuminated saline, or normal saline. Intravenous (IV) access can be obtained quickly by a skilled clinician through the umbilical vein. Once position of the catheter tip below the liver or above the portal venous system in the inferior vena cava is established, relatively large amounts of fluids may be instilled.

Cardiac compromise as a result of cyanotic heart lesions usually occurs as a late sign in neonates. Until the closing of the ductus arteriosus, neonates with even lethal anomalies may appear "normal." For this reason prostaglandin E_1 may be administered to the neonate suspected of having a ductus-dependent lesion to maintain patency of the ductus arteriosus. This will ensure continued fetal circulation in the neonate until corrective surgery (if indicated) can be performed. Although technically hypoxic, the neonate is relatively hyperoxic when compared with the fetal state and can tolerate $Pa{O_2}$ levels in the 35 to 45 range for a while.

Expected Outcome

- The neonate maintains normal cardiac output and adequate tissue perfusion.

Promoting Fluid and Electrolyte Balance

The sick neonate is at special risk for fluid and electrolyte imbalances. Oral fluid intake frequently is limited or impossible as a result of anomalies, injury, or disease. Sick neonates often are lethargic or poor feeders. Congenital anomalies of the face may interfere with the neonate's ability to suck and swallow, and preterm and small-for-gestational age (SGA) neonates have a limited stomach capacity. Oral intake may be absolutely contraindicated after severe asphyxia with severe respiratory distress or with major congenital anomalies of the gastrointestinal or respiratory tracts.

Fluid losses also may be greater for the sick neonate. Vomiting, diarrhea, and drainage of body fluids from open wounds, cysts, or exposed organs deplete water and essential electrolytes. Insensible water loss also is greatly increased in neonates with rapid respiratory rates and in those placed under radiant warmers or phototherapy lights. These factors are complicated by the immature kidney function normally present in the newborn, which limits the capacity to conserve fluids and electrolytes.

Nursing care focuses on the prevention and correction of fluid volume deficits and electrolyte imbalances. Careful monitoring of fluid intake and output alerts the nurse to excessive losses. Placing the neonate in a neutral thermal environment prevents the elevation in metabolic rate and minimizes the concomitant water loss that occurs when cold stress activates nonshivering thermogenesis (see the section "Neutral Thermal Environment" later in this chapter). Because insensible water losses are greatly increased when the neonate is placed under a radiant warmer, a transparent barrier, such as plastic wrap, is stretched across the neonate between the warmer's side guards. The neonate should be placed in an incubator with a double wall or a heat shield as soon as possible. The nurse also carefully limits the amount of blood withdrawn to the absolute minimum necessary to obtain blood gas studies and other tests.

Intravenous Therapy

IV therapy may be instituted to meet the infant's basic fluid requirements when oral intake is limited. Fluid requirements during the first few days of life are approximately 60 to 75 mL/kg per day. This figure may be adjusted upward when sensible and insensible water losses are excessive. The nurse must evaluate the newborn carefully for signs of dehydration or fluid overload during IV therapy. Table 33-2 lists the major indicators of fluid imbalance in the neonate.

Peripheral Intravenous Lines. Peripheral veins may be used for the infusion of fluid and electrolytes and are preferred to the umbilical artery or central veins, because the risk of serious complications is lower. Veins on the scalp and dorsal aspects of the hand and foot frequently are chosen (Fig. 33-6). Many needles and catheters are available for peripheral IV infusions, and the type chosen depends on the neonate's size, the purpose for which the line is to be used, and the sites available for insertion. Teflon angiocatheters often are preferred to stainless steel needles, because the risk of infiltration is lower, and the line can normally be maintained for a longer period.

The nurse often is responsible for inserting the IV line and should be skilled in proper venipuncture technique, securing the line, and protecting the site. He or she must carefully restrain the neonate before the procedure. Tightly swaddling the neonate is an effective way of preventing

Table 33-2. Signs of Fluid Imbalance in the Neonate

Dehydration	Overhydration
Early Signs	
Lower urine volume (less than 1 mL/kg/h)	Higher urine volume (more than 3 mL/kg/h)
Higher urine osmolality (more than 400 mOsm)	Lower urine osmolality (less than 10 mOsm)
Higher urine specific gravity (more than 1.012)	Lower urine specific gravity (less than 1.008)
Signs of Decompensation	
Weight loss (5%–15% a day)	Weight gain (5%–15% a day)
Higher serum sodium (more than 150 mEq/L)	Lower serum sodium (less than 130 mEq/L)
Higher serum osmolality (more than 300 mOsm)	Lower serum osmolality (less than 270 mOsm)
Dry mucous membranes	Subcutaneous edema
Sunken fontanelles	
Poor skin turgor	
Higher hematocrit (10% or more)	Lower hematocrit (≤10%)
Higher serum protein (>6 g/dL)	Lower serum protein (less than 4 g/dL)
Lower blood volume	Higher blood volume
Late Signs	
Shock	Pulmonary edema and rales Cardiac failure

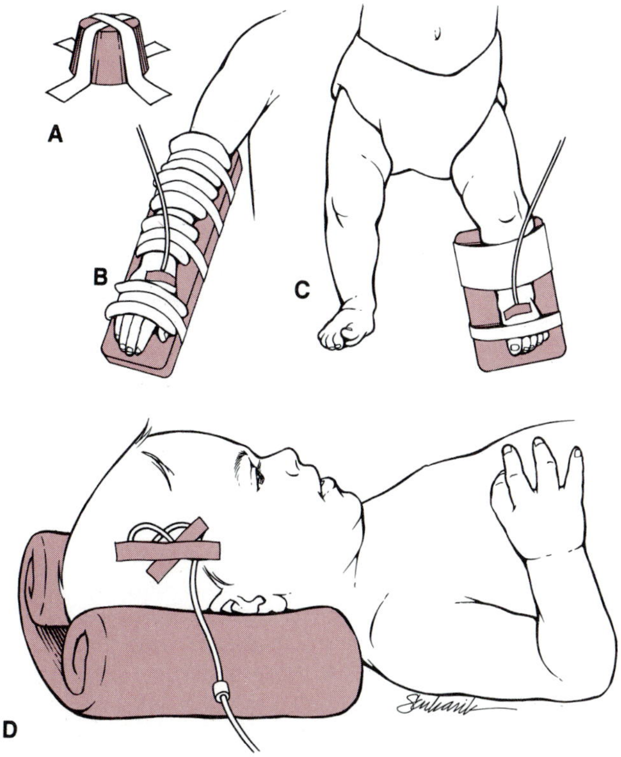

Figure 33-6.

Intravenous sites in neonates with proper restraints. *A:* Paper cup tapes over insertion site. *B:* Arm restraint for protecting dorsal hand IV site. *C:* Leg restraint for protecting dorsal foot IV site. *D:* Positioning and protection of scalp vein site.

movement during the insertion and accidentally dislodging the needle. If an arm vein is used, the limb should be restrained on a padded armboard before insertion of the line. A fiberoptic transilluminator may be held against the skin to locate veins and facilitate successful venipuncture.

Tape must be applied to secure the IV line, but the fragile condition of the neonate's skin and the need to observe the insertion site closely must be taken into account when applying adhesives. Clear, porous tape allows the nurse to inspect the site and is less adherent, thus minimizing injury to the skin when removed. Even clear porous tape may damage the skin of very premature newborns, and special skin adhesives and barriers must be used with them (see the section "Preventing Infections" later in this chapter). The application of tincture of benzoin to provide a protective layer between tape and skin is not recommended, because it may be absorbed and potentiates epidermal stripping.

Once the line is secured, the nurse must take care to prevent accidental removal. Often secure taping to prevent stress or pull on the line can achieve this goal. Some newborns, especially term neonates, may require additional restraints. Usually, however, allowing free movement of the extremity will keep the stronger neonate from pulling against the restraining device and dislodging the catheter.

Because small amounts of fluid are administered at very slow rates (as slow as 2 mL/h or less), a special infusion pump must be used. All solutions should be infused through minidrip tubing (60 drops/mL) attached to a fluid reservoir (Volutrol) that contains no more than several hours' worth of fluid. This prevents accidental infusion of a large and potentially lethal volume. Meticulous measurement of all fluid intake and output is essential with IV therapy, as is evaluation of urine specific gravity at least once per shift.

The nurse must examine the IV site hourly for signs of

infiltration or irritation of the vein. Circulation distal to the site also must be evaluated. The infusion pump is checked for proper functioning and the tubing for kinks or obstruction. If the limbs are restrained, they should be released at least every 2 hours for passive range of motion exercises (see the accompanying Legal/Ethical Considerations display).

Central Intravenous Lines. Neonates requiring prolonged IV therapy or hyperalimentation may have a special central IV catheter inserted. The procedure is normally performed by a skilled practitioner using sterile technique. The catheter may be introduced through a peripheral vein in the arm and then slowly threaded into a central vein (percutaneous insertion), or less commonly in current practice, it may be inserted into the scalp, passed into the jugular vein, and finally placed in the superior vena cava. Clinical experience with both techniques suggests there is a lower incidence of thrombophlebitis with prolonged vessel catheterization when the distal cutaneous site is used. Percutaneous radial artery catheterization may be used as an alternative to umbilical artery catheterization as a means for monitoring blood gas levels and blood pressure.

The nurse caring for the neonate with a central IV line must be alert to common complications, including infiltration, phlebitis, and systemic infection; accidental fluid overload; and air embolus. All tubing and IV solution must be replaced every 24 hours or per unit protocol using strict sterile technique. Care must be taken when disconnecting lines to prevent the accidental introduction of air into the system. The nurse must inspect the skin at the site of insertion for evidence of erythema, edema, or leakage of solution. He or she must observe for edema in the neck and chest area,

Legal/Ethical Considerations

When the Neonate Requires Intravenous Therapy

When the neonate requires an intravenous (IV) line, the nurse is responsible for hourly assessment of the IV site, IV infusion, and equipment used to deliver IV fluids. The nurse may be found negligent for failure to maintain the IV site and prevent injury related to intravenous therapy.

The neonate can suffer scarring and permanent motor impairment in an arm or leg as a result of the infiltration of intravenous fluids. The smaller the neonate, the greater the risk of injury. Infiltration can result in excessive buildup of fluid in the surrounding tissues, known as *compartment syndrome.* Impairment of blood flow and pressure on nerves can lead to tissue ischemia, necrosis, and neurologic impairment. In the worst case, surgical intervention is required to relieve pressure in the affected extremity to prevent permanent damage.

Infiltration can also result in extravasation of drugs and electrolytes into tissues, leading to inflammation, full-thickness tissue burns, and tissue necrosis. Severe scarring of the skin and underlying fascia and muscles may require serial plastic surgeries to correct the damage and restore use of the extremity.

Inappropriate use of adhesive tape or limb restraints used to secure the IV line can result in damage to the epidermis or impairment of circulation in an extremity. The use of make-shift devices to protect the IV insertion site have been implicated in claims of negligence. In a recent case, the nurse was found negligent for using a plastic medication cup to protect an IV site. The cup, which had been split in half, caused significant damage when the cut edges lacerated the neonate's skin.

The nurse must evaluate the IV site at least once an hour and evaluate the following:

- Color, consistency, and temperature of tissue surrounding the IV site
- Evidence of swelling at IV site or in the extremity
- Capillary fill time of nailbeds in the extremity distal to the IV site
- Evidence of leaking or purulent discharge at insertion site

All of these observations should be recorded hourly using the appropriate chart form provided by the agency. Charting by exception permits check-marking a line or box on a flowsheet that indicates that all of the above assessments were performed and that there is no indication of problems. The nurse should follow agency policies and procedures to secure IV lines, using only approved skin tape and soft limb restraints.

When infiltration occurs, the nurse must notify the physician immediately. The type and approximate amount of fluid that has infiltrated the tissue should be reported. The nurse should be prepared to follow physician orders regarding treatment such as elevation of the extremity, use of warm moist soaks to the affected site, or use of an agent such as hyaluronidase to limit the extent of chemical damage.

——. *(1992). Plastic cup on I.V. site: Nurse–expert testimony.* Regan Report on Nursing Law, *33(7), 2.*
Raszka, W., Kueser, T., Smith, F., & Bass, J. (1990). The use of hyaluronidase in the treatment of intravenous extravasation injuries. Journal of Perinatology, *X(2), 146–149.*

which would suggest infiltration. The occurrence of sudden respiratory distress and cyanosis suggests infiltration of the central line, air embolus, or fluid overload.

Umbilical Artery Catheterization. The umbilical artery frequently is used for the administration of drugs and fluids in sick neonates. A radiopaque catheter is inserted into one of the arteries and passed into the abdominal aorta. Catheterization is considered a surgical procedure requiring strict aseptic technique. Once placement of the catheter is confirmed by radiographic examination (either above or below the level of the renal arteries), it is secured in place with suture and tape. The catheter allows arterial blood samples to be obtained for blood gas analysis, and a special electronic monitor can be attached to the catheter to monitor systemic blood pressure.

Several major complications have been associated with umbilical artery catheterization: infection, thrombosis, vasospasm, and hemorrhage. The nurse caring for the neonate with an umbilical artery line must use scrupulous aseptic technique when opening the system to prevent infection and the introduction of air emboli. The nurse also must be alert for signs of compromised blood flow below the level of the catheter, including blanching and coolness of the skin in the perineal area, over the buttocks, and in the lower extremities and absence of femoral and pedal pulses.

Electrolyte Supplementation. Electrolytes (sodium, chloride, potassium, and calcium) are frequently added to the IV solution and are essential if the neonate remains unable to take food by mouth for more than 24 to 48 hours. Electrolyte values are monitored closely, and the nurse must be familiar with norms and daily maintenance requirements. Table 33-3 lists daily electrolyte requirements and normal blood values for the neonate. When calcium and potassium are infused, it is essential that the neonate be placed on a cardiac monitor because of their effect on myocardial function. Furthermore, because infiltration of calcium-containing solutions can cause severe sloughing of tissues, the IV site must be observed closely for evidence of infiltration.

Expected Outcomes

- The neonate achieves fluid and electrolyte balance.
- The neonate achieves normal urine output.

Providing for Nutritional Needs

Meeting the nutritional needs of the high-risk neonate and preventing caloric and nutrient deficits are major challenges. Many complications make it difficult or impossible for the neonate to breastfeed or bottle feed or to digest the standard formulas prescribed for the healthy full-term newborn. Many formulas and solutions have been developed to provide calories and essential nutrients to the high-risk neonate, and special equipment is available to deliver them through the gastrointestinal tract or IV routes.

The nurse must carefully monitor responses to the substances ingested or infused. Vital signs are taken before each feeding, and the abdominal girth is measured on a regular basis if nutrients are given by the gastrointestinal tract. The urine is tested periodically for the presence of sugar and protein and the stools for blood. When nutrients are infused intravenously, the newborn's blood is tested frequently for evidence of protein, carbohydrate, or fat intolerance.

Table 33-3. Maintenance of Electrolyte Balance

Electrolyte	Normal Blood Value*	Daily Requirement
Sodium	148 mEq/L (134–160)	2–3 mEq/kg/d†
Chloride	102 mEq/L (92–114)	2 mEq/kg/d
Potassium	6.0 mEq/L (5.2–7.3)	2 mEq/kg/d
Calcium	8.0 mg/100 mL (6.9–9.9)	150–200 mg/kg/d

*24–48 h after birth.
† Extremely preterm infants may require higher amount due to renal immaturity.
Cloherty, J. Stark, A. (1991). *Manual of neonatal care.* Boston: Little, Brown & Co.

If the newborn can tolerate oral feedings, there are several ways to provide the necessary nutrients.

Nipple Feedings

Special care and patience are required if the neonate is allowed to nipple feed. The sick neonate often is characterized as a "poor feeder" who sucks weakly. Preterm and asphyxiated neonates in particular may have an uncoordinated suck–swallow reflex. Energy reserves may be low, and sucking efforts can easily exhaust the neonate. The nurse must allot extra time for the feeding and carefully note the neonate's response (heart, respiratory rate, and color). Breastfeeding may be possible, and the host-resistance factors contained in breast milk are especially beneficial to the sick neonate. When bottle feeding is selected, special soft nipples can be used to assist and decrease the work of feeding. There also are specially designed nipples for neonates with cleft lip or palate.

Gavage Feedings

Nipple feeding is contraindicated for some high-risk neonates. Preterm neonates born before 33 to 34 weeks of gestation lack a gag reflex and the ability to coordinate sucking, swallowing, and breathing, so they might aspirate a breastfeeding or bottle feeding. Neonates with very rapid respiratory rates (above 70 per minute) and those with severe cardiac disease may not tolerate nipple feedings because of their diminished energy reserves. They may experience increased respiratory distress when attempting to suck. Gavage feeding may be the method of choice in these circumstances, or the infant may be kept NPO until the respiratory status is stable.

Orogastric feedings

An orogastric tube (5 or 8 French) is passed, and milk flows into the stomach from a syringe or feeding funnel by gravity drainage. Before beginning the gavage feeding, proper placement of the tube must be confirmed (most commonly by injecting a small amount of air into the tube and auscultating over the stomach and by aspirating stomach contents) to rule out passage of the tube into the trachea. The nurse must secure the tube before the feeding so that it is not accidentally pulled out. If necessary, the vigorous neonate may be gently restrained (see the Nursing Procedure, Inserting a Gavage Tube).

The amount of milk remaining in the stomach from the

NURSING PROCEDURE
Inserting a Gavage Tube

Purpose: An oral gavage tube is used to provide enteral nutrients when the neonate is unable to ingest formula due to prematurity, facial anomalies, or illness.

NURSING ACTION	*RATIONALE*
1. Obtain a feeding tube, syringe, skin tape, stethoscope, breast milk or formula, and graduated measuring bottle. Use correct size feeding tube for neonate's weight and size (usually 8 or 10 French catheter for oral gavage feeding).	To have all equipment ready before beginning the procedure. To increase comfort and permit adequate flow of milk or formula.
2. Obtain the neonate's vital signs.	To identify changes in the neonate's status that would preclude the procedure such as respiratory distress.
3. Measure the neonate's abdominal girth as ordered. Auscultate bowel sounds in all 4 quadrants.	To identify abdominal distention and GI dysfunction such as necrotizing enterocolitis.
4. Place the neonate in a supine position with the head in the midline and in a neutral position.	Proper placement of the neonate's head facilitates accurate measurement of the GI tract.
5. Place the tip of the feeding tube at the corner of the neonate's mouth and measure to the earlobe of the same side of head. Then measure from the earlobe to a point midway between the xiphoid process and the umbilicus (indicated by arrows).	To permit an accurate estimate of the length of tube that must be advanced to reach the stomach. To ensure that the tip of the feeding tube is placed in the stomach, preventing aspiration of milk or formula.
6. Place a piece of tape on the feeding tube that marks the point to which it should be advanced.	To ensure that the tip of the feeding tube has been advanced far enough to rest in the stomach.
7. Swaddle the neonate if active or agitated.	To restrain the arms and prevent accidental dislodgement of the tube during the procedure
8. Pour the correct amount of formula into a graduated container such as a Volutrol bottle.	To ensure administration of the correct fluid volume.
9. Stabilize the neonate's head, gently squeeze the cheeks, and gently pass the feeding tube into the mouth and down the esophagus.	Smooth, gentle passage of the tube will reduce the neonate's discomfort.
10. If the neonate experiences respiratory distress, apnea, bradycardia, or cyanosis remove the tube immediately.	Accidental intubation of the trachea will result in respiratory distress. Stimulation of the vagus nerve can occur and may result in bradycardia.
11. Attach the syringe and aspirate gastric contents. Notify the physician if a residural is greater than 25% of the previous feeding and then return gastric content to stomach.	Large gastric residual may indicate retention due to formula intolerance or illness. To prevent loss of fluid and electrolytes.
12. If no gastric residual or stomach contents are obtained, place a stethoscope over the stomach and insufflate 0.5 mL of air from the syringe into the feeding tube.	To verify placement of the tube's tip in the stomach.
13. Tape feeding tube to neonate's cheek. Remove plunger from syringe, and add correct amount of formula from Volutrol into syringe barrel.	To secure feeding tube during the procedure. To permit introduction of formula.
14. Permit formula to enter stomach slowly by gravity drip (approximately 10 to 15 minutes depending on amount of formula).	To prevent rapid distention of stomach.

last feeding (gastric residual) is measured at this time. Physicians' directives often are provided to guide the nurse as to whether or not to subtract the residual amount from the next feeding. Stomach contents are rarely discarded, because this would cause the loss of hydrochloric acid and lead to alkalosis. Increasing residuals or the sudden presence of a large residual may indicate intolerance of the formula or the development of a severe and life-threatening intestinal disorder, known as necrotizing enterocolitis (NEC), which is frequently encountered in very premature infants. For this reason the nurse reports unusual gastric residuals immediately.

When the feeding is begun, the milk reservoir is held no

higher than 12 inches above the neonate. Force should not be applied with a syringe plunger to speed the flow of milk. This can lead to regurgitation of fluid and aspiration. The tube is clamped before it is withdrawn to prevent milk remaining in the tube from dripping into the pharynx and being aspirated. If not contraindicated by a gastrointestinal or respiratory anomaly, the neonate may be offered a pacifier during and immediately after the gavage feeding to satisfy non-nutritive sucking needs and to stimulate the flow of saliva and digestive juices. The neonate is burped in the same manner as a breastfed or bottle fed newborn after the feeding.

Continuous Nasogastric or Transpyloric Feeding

Other methods of feeding are continuous nasogastric and transpyloric feeding. These may be indicated with problems of gastric retention or regurgitation and in very low–birth-weight neonates. For continuous nasogastric feeding a 5 French polyethylene feeding tube is threaded slowly through the naris and passed until it enters the stomach. Formula or breast milk is administered at a constant slow rate by a pump after placement is confirmed. If transpyloric feeding is desired, a Silastic feeding tube is threaded through the naris and allowed to pass through the pylorus into the jejunum or duodenum. Proper placement of the tube is tentatively verified by a pH reading of over 5 in aspirated contents and confirmed by radiographic examination. Formula or breast milk is then administered at a constant rate by infusion pump.

Gastric residuals are checked at least every 4 hours (or with each bolus feeding) to monitor gastric emptying; presence of residuals may indicate malposition of the tube, intestinal obstruction, or ileus.

With continuous nasogastric or transpyloric feeding, the nurse must guard against bacterial growth in the tubing or other equipment. For this reason syringes and connector tubing should be changed regularly and the nasogastric tube changed every 48 to 72 hours to prevent bacterial growth and possible sepsis.

Total Parenteral Nutrition

If the introduction of nutrients through the gastrointestinal tract is contraindicated, they can be provided through IV infusion of specially prepared parenteral solutions. Total parenteral nutrition (TPN) is the delivery of fluid, calories, minerals, and vitamins by the IV route. Energy sources available for TPN include carbohydrates (dextrose), protein (protein hydrolysates and free amino acid solutions), and fats. Fats are delivered in a separate solution (intralipids) piggybacked to the TPN infusion. TPN may be infused peripherally or through a central percutaneous line threaded through the antecubital vein into the superior vena cava. The central venous route requires placement by a skilled clinician and is becoming more common. The reduced rate of mechanical complications coupled with a reduced rate of infiltration and the ability to deliver higher glucose concentrations outweigh the potential risk of systemic infection.

The nurse must monitor the TPN infusion closely. The site should be examined at least every hour for evidence of infiltration or inflammation. TPN solution is an excellent medium for the growth of bacteria and will cause severe damage to tissues (necrosis, sloughing, and scarring) if infiltration occurs. If intralipids are administered, the neonate is observed for such complications of lipid infusion as respiratory distress, vomiting, and diarrhea. Because of the high dextrose concentration found in TPN, the neonate is at risk for hyperglycemia, osmotic diuresis, and dehydration. The nurse must be alert for signs of fluid imbalance, keep meticulous intake and output records, and test the urine for the presence of glucose and protein at least once every 8 to 12 hours. The specific gravity of the urine also is measured. The neonate is evaluated for potential hyperbilirubinemia secondary to cholestasis, a complication of TPN.

If hyperglycemia persists, the glucose concentration in the hyperalimentation solution is decreased. Continuous intravenous infusion of insulin may be initiated if plasma glucose levels remain higher than 250 mg/dL (Shannon, 1988).

Expected Outcome

- The neonate maintains nutritional requirements for growth and development.

Preventing Infection

The high-risk newborn is susceptible to infection. The skin is the first line of defense against infection. If the neonate is born with an injury or anomaly that disrupts this natural barrier or is so premature that the skin is thin and permeable, pathogenic bacteria and viruses can gain entry to the body. Because neonates are unable to localize infection due to immaturity of host defense mechanisms, this can quickly lead to a generalized septicemia. Severe birth asphyxia, especially in preterm neonates, can lead to ischemia and necrosis of intestinal tissue and invasion of the damaged mucosa by enteric bacteria, a condition known as NEC. Many life-sustaining procedures and diagnostic tests are invasive and thus become routes for the transmission of pathogens.

Handwashing

Handwashing is the most important preventive measure against infection. Because hands are the most common vehicle for the spread of pathogens, it is essential that they be washed after contact with an neonate before touching another neonate or his or her equipment. Parents should be taught to wash their hands before holding their newborn. The nurse also must monitor other health team members and remind them to observe good handwashing technique before they come in contact with the neonate. Most neonatal intensive care nurseries also require an initial 2- to 3-minute wash, from fingertips to elbows, with an antibacterial detergent for nursing staff. Iodinated solutions are preferred because of their action against gram-positive cocci and gram-negative rods.

Nursery Attire and Procedures

Attire. Nurses caring for the sick neonate should wear scrub suits or uniforms with short sleeves, which allow them to wash up to the elbows. Family or health team members who handle the neonate should wear long-sleeved gowns that cover street clothes or other hospital attire. Research indicates that the use of caps, hairnets, or masks is not necessary.

Policies on Illness. A parent, other family member, health team member, or other hospital employee who experiences any of the following illnesses or signs of illness should not have contact with the neonate:

- Cold, sore throat, or fever
- Infectious skin rash or lesions (eg, impetigo, herpesvirus)
- Diarrhea
- Hepatitis
- Other communicable diseases (eg, chickenpox, tuberculosis)

Isolation. Routine isolation of neonates born out of asepsis (eg, precipitous home or automobile birth) or after prolonged rupture of membranes is no longer advocated. Even neonates with bacterial meningitis, septicemia, or pneumonia need not be isolated. Similarly, the routine separation of mother and neonate when there is a postpartum infection is not always necessary, because many infections are not spread by maternal–neonatal contact. Only neonates with diarrhea or draining infections must be moved to a separate nursery. Neonates with active or presumed disseminated herpesvirus, congenital rubella, or varicella (chickenpox) also should be handled with strict isolation. Placing them in an incubator is not adequate protection for other newborns who are in open cribs in the same environment. The air circulating in the interior of the incubator is expelled into the room when ports are opened. The practice of observing universal body substance precautions with all newborns is the most effective method for preventing transmission of pathogens and should be routinely implemented.

Care of Equipment. The newborn is exposed to numerous pieces of equipment that can serve as fomites for the transmission of pathogenic organisms. Care must be taken to clean all equipment coming in contact with the neonate. All IV bags and tubing and oxygen equipment must be changed every 24 hours. Periodic culturing of nursery equipment and plumbing fixtures to identify potential sources of contamination is an essential aspect of infection control.

Skin Care. Because the skin is the newborn's first line of defense against infection, skin care practices are of special importance. Alkaline soaps have been found to temporarily disrupt the protective acid mantle of the skin; thus, infrequent baths, using only water, are recommended. When more thorough cleansing is necessary, a less alkaline soap (Neutrogena, Lowila, or Oilatum) should be used. When adhesive tape is removed from the skin, the epidermis can be removed with it. Hollihesive, a porous adhesive described as a "skin blanket," can be applied first and the tape needed to secure equipment placed on top of it. This will help prevent denuding of skin surfaces. Alcohol, tincture of benzoin, and adhesive removers should be avoided. The skin can be prepped adequately for heel sticks and injections with sterile water and cotton balls. Iodinated solutions should be used sparingly when used to prepare the skin for drawing blood cultures or starting IV lines.

Expected Outcomes

- The neonate's skin and mucous membranes remain free of infection.
- The neonate's temperature remains between 36.4°C and 37.2°C (97.7°F to 99.0°F).

Supporting Thermoregulation

Many of the interventions in this section disclose the importance of supporting the newborn's body temperature. This intervention begins immediately after birth and is important through the newborn period. It is especially important in the high-risk newborn.

Prevention of Cold Stress

The effects of cold stress on the neonate have been well documented. They include an increase in the metabolic rate, an increase in oxygen consumption, a decrease in surfactant production, and hypoglycemia. Cold stress initiates the breakdown of brown fat stores for heat production, releasing acid metabolites into the bloodstream. High-risk neonates are particularly susceptible to cold stress because interventions, beginning with resuscitation in the delivery room, require exposing body surfaces. The nurse's first step in resuscitation is to place the neonate under a radiant warmer and quickly dry the skin and head as other health team members establish an airway.

The neonate must be able to produce and conserve heat to maintain a normal body temperature and prevent hypothermia. The high-risk neonate is at a distinct disadvantage. The neonate's ability to accomplish nonshivering thermogenesis depends on his or her stores of brown fat tissue. Newborns who are preterm and SGA have limited amounts of brown fat. They also lack the thermal insulation adipose tissue provides, and thus experience a more rapid dissipation of heat from the blood vessels underlying skin surfaces. To some extent a flexed posture decreases heat loss by decreasing the amount of skin surface exposed. Neonates who are severely depressed and flaccid are therefore at greater risk for heat loss and may need the nurse's assistance in assuming a flexed position.

Neutral Thermal Environment

The high-risk neonate initially is placed in a neutral thermal environment, which minimizes the work of maintaining the body temperature. The radiant warmer is preferred when the neonate requires frequent evaluations, tests, and procedures that require exposure (Fig. 33-7*A*). An incubator is used when the neonate can be left undisturbed for long periods of time and requires less intensive care (see Fig. 33-7*B*). The ambient temperature is adjusted to maintain the infant's temperature in the range of 36.4°C to 37.2°C (97.7°F to 99.0°F).

Ideally, all oxygen administered to the neonate should be warmed. Cold air blown across the face can stimulate thermal receptors and induce apnea. Wet towels or clothing should be replaced, and care should be taken to cover the infant's head (25% of the total body length) with a stockinette cap when it is feasible to do so. The hands of the nurse should be warmed before she handles the neonate, especially a very low–birth-weight neonate, to decrease heat

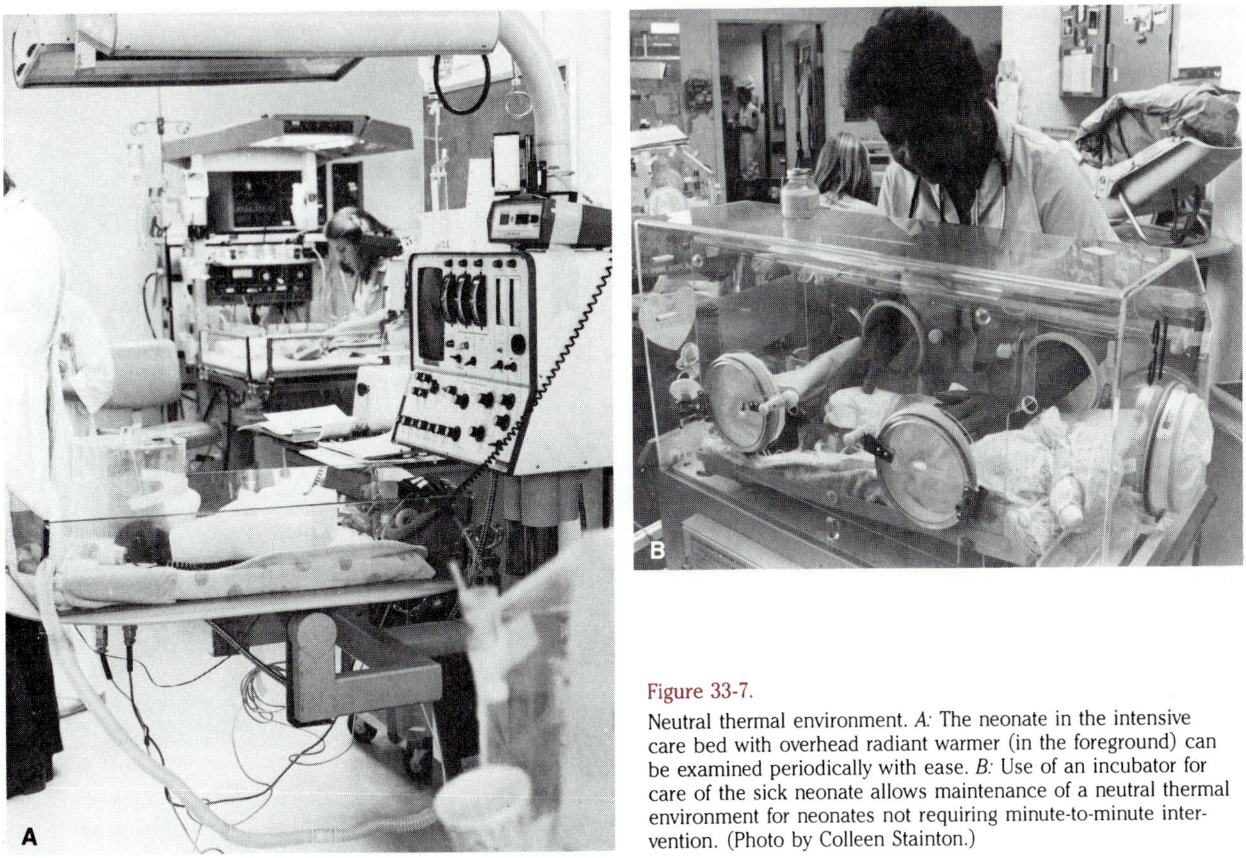

Figure 33-7.

Neutral thermal environment. *A:* The neonate in the intensive care bed with overhead radiant warmer (in the foreground) can be examined periodically with ease. *B:* Use of an incubator for care of the sick neonate allows maintenance of a neutral thermal environment for neonates not requiring minute-to-minute intervention. (Photo by Colleen Stainton.)

transfer by conduction. If the newborn is in an incubator, the portholes should be kept closed between procedures, and work should be organized to minimize entry.

Rapid swings in temperature must be avoided. Neonates who are hypothermic must be warmed slowly and cautiously, because a rapid rise in temperature may cause apnea. The newborn who has been in a neutral thermal environment for an extended time must be weaned from it slowly to prevent hypothermia and cold stress. The neonate's temperature-regulating center needs time to assume the total work of temperature maintenance.

Expected Outcomes

- The neonate maintains an axillary temperature of 36.4°C to 37.2°C (97.7°F to 99.0°F).
- The neonate demonstrates a stable temperature.

Promoting Neonatal Behavioral Adaptation

Promoting behavioral adaptation involves providing an environment and caregiving that reduces stress, promotes growth and development, and provides opportunities for the organization of state, behavior, and social responsiveness. This task is more difficult for high-risk neonates in the intensive care nursery, coping with a variety of health problems, and deprived of normal parental care in the home environment. High-risk neonates, therefore, are both dependent on and vulnerable to this early environment.

Strategies to promote neurobehavioral development in high-risk neonates include altering caregiving patterns to respond to neonatal cues, providing routine care only after the neonate has awakened spontaneously, using state modulation techniques to arouse (alert) the neonate before feeding or other caregiving activities, soothing (or quieting) the neonate after caregiving, and providing stimuli (visual, auditory, tactile, or proprioceptive) appropriate to the neonate's maturity and health status.

The nurse also assists parents in understanding their neonate's unique abilities and in interacting with their newborn in ways appropriate to the neonate's health status, state, and level of maturity (Blackburn & VandenBerg, 1993).

This approach to care is known as developmentally supportive care or developmental intervention and has replaced an earlier focus on infant stimulation. The developmental intervention approach is based on the synactive theory (Als, 1986). Intervention strategies are individualized for each neonate and based on ongoing assessment. An underlying assumption is that the high-risk neonate is vulnerable to sensory overload. The focus is on supporting emerging behaviors and organization while reducing stress. Sensory input (stimulation) is provided only when appropriate physiologic and neurobehavioral status are individualized to the needs and abilities of the neonate at that time (Blackburn & VandenBerg, 1993).

Expected Outcomes

- The neonate develops habituation behaviors to environmental stimuli.

- The neonate establishes recognized sleep and awake states.
- The neonate acquires increasingly sophisticated self-quieting behaviors.

Encouraging Parent–Newborn Attachment and Interaction

The parent–newborn attachment process is seriously threatened when the newborn is taken to the neonatal intensive care unit. The neonate may even be transported to a tertiary care center located many miles from the hospital, making visiting by parents difficult or impossible.

When a complication arises at birth, parents must be informed as soon as possible about the nature and extent of the problem. A brief statement may be all that is possible if immediate resuscitation or emergency care is required: "Your newborn is having difficulty breathing and the doctor is helping him. We will let you know how he is doing as soon as we can."

If the neonate is stable but has an obvious congenital anomaly, the parents should be prepared for what they will see and given a simple explanation of what the anomaly is, how it will affect the neonate, and what can be done about it. The physician often imparts this information in the delivery room. The nurse then reinforces the information and answers any questions the parents may have.

Once the neonate has been transferred to the special care nursery, parents should be kept closely informed of the neonate's condition and progress. Initially they may be overwhelmed by the sounds, lights, and equipment of the intensive care nursery (Fig. 33-8). They may not hear what is being said, so information will have to be repeated. Explanations should be simple but complete. An individualized discharge plan is developed to allow parents to assume increasing responsibility for the neonate's care. If this is accomplished by discharge time, they are more likely to feel capable of recognizing and meetings his or her needs. Additionally, studies indicate advantages for the newborn and mother if skin-to-skin holding is permitted as soon as the infant stabilizes and no longer requires oxygen therapy.

The special care nursery should have open visiting hours. Even when the neonate is critically ill, parents should be given an opportunity to touch and talk to him or her. As the neonate's condition stabilizes, the parents can be encouraged to spend an increasing amount of time caring for, feeding, bathing, and holding him or her. The parents may at first be afraid to handle the neonate, especially the premature neonate who appears extremely fragile. The nurse must reassure them, guide and support their initial efforts, and praise their successes. Patience is required of the skilled nurse, who knows he or she could accomplish a task with greater speed and proficiency. Most NICUs also provide opportunities for siblings, grandparents, and other significant family members to visit.

If possible, the neonate should be assigned a primary care nurse, who then becomes the consistent contact between parents and the unit. Parents should have the nursery telephone number and be encouraged to call day or night with questions and concerns. Parents also should be made to feel that they are the most important people in the newborn's life and feel supported in the care they provide. Parents should be actively involved in providing developmentally supportive care and as the infant recovers and matures, provide as much of the sensory input as possible. A special care unit that attempts to implement these suggested interventions will effectively facilitate the parent–newborn attachment process.

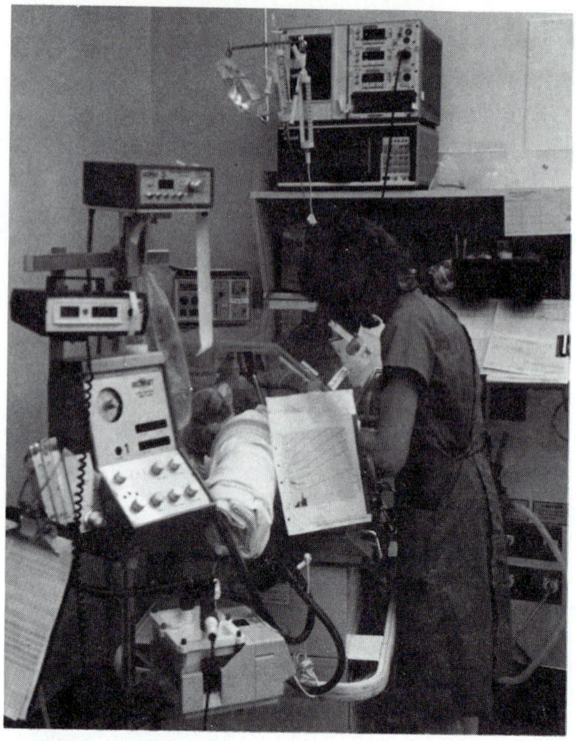

Figure 33-8.
Parents may be overwhelmed by the sights, sounds, and busy staff in the intensive care nursery. (Photo by Colleen Stainton.)

Expected Outcomes

- The neonate demonstrates orienting behaviors toward parents and caregivers while maintaining physiologic stability.
- The neonate engages in social behaviors with parents and caregivers.

Supporting Parental Coping and Grieving

The nurse is in an excellent position to observe coping mechanisms. She can alert the health team to potential or actual problems that arise as a result of ineffective coping. Many intensive care nurseries have clinical nurse specialists, social workers, or psychologists with expertise in family therapy to support and guide parents. A support group may be formed for all parents with neonates in the special care unit. The sharing of experiences, fears, and frustrations can help parents realize they are not alone.

First and foremost, the nurse must understand the dynamics of the grieving process and accept the parents' expression of grief, whether it is denial, anger, guilt, or sadness. Although parents must have privacy and time to be alone with their feelings of sadness and loss, they also should feel

Family Considerations

Using Guilt Constructively to Affirm Parental Coping

Guilt is one of the primary and often most intense reactions of parents to the birth of a sick neonate. Whetsell and Larrabee (1988) note that it is common practice for health care providers to attempt to diffuse guilt feelings, although they are a functional response to the shock of a negative birth experience and have the potential for stimulating positive family response. While guilt may have destructive effects, the nurse can intervene therapeutically to foster positive outcomes.

Whetsell and Larrabee have developed an affirmation model, a strategy that assists parents to channel guilt feelings into constructive goal-setting. The nurse accomplishes this by affirming the parents' experience; exploring the negative outcomes of guilt; negotiating a time for parental care giving; redirecting the parents' focus to the present; aiding parents in goal setting and caretaking plans; implementing the parental caretaking plan; and reinforcing parents' actions and encouraging self-evaluation.

Whetsell, M. V., & Larrabee, M. J. (1988). Using guilt constructively in the NICU to affirm parental coping. Neonatal Network, *6(4), 21–27.*

that a caring staff is available to support them. The nurse who hurries in and out of the mother's room, attending only to her physical needs, is failing to meet the equally important psychological needs. It is important to avoid phrases such as "It's God's will" or "You're young and can have another baby." These statements convey a lack of understanding about the extent of the parents' grief at this time. A sincere expression of sorrow by the nurse, followed by silence and an opportunity for the parent to verbalize his or her feelings, is an appropriate therapeutic approach.

Staff should not be surprised if anger is directed toward them. Anger is a normal phase of the grieving process, and parents must be allowed to vent their feelings of frustration, disappointment, and helplessness. Tranquilizers and sedatives have limited therapeutic value at this time and should never take the place of supportive nursing care. Crying also has therapeutic value, and parents should be given permission to cry if they appear to be fighting back tears: "It's OK to cry. What's happening with your newborn is very upsetting." Putting an arm around the parent and staying with him or her at this time conveys a sense of acceptance and caring.

Expected Outcomes

- The parents demonstrate normal expressions of grief.
- The parents participate in a unit support group.

Administering Medications

Medication therapy depends on the specific condition of the high-risk neonate. It is beyond the scope of this chapter to discuss drug therapy in high-risk conditions. Some of the common drugs used to support cardiac function are furosemide (Lasix), prostaglandins, tolazoline (Priscoline), sodium nitroprusside, digoxin, dopamine, and indomethacin (Fuller, 1989).

Monitoring for Complications

General screening tests for such metabolic alterations as phenylketonuria, galactosemia, branched-chain amino acid defects (maple syrup urine disease), homocystinuria, and congenital hypothyroidism were discussed in Chapter 30. Care of the infant with such conditions is a specialized field and is not discussed in this text.

While performing independent interventions, the nurse also is responsible for preventing potential complications related to therapy. Oxygen toxicity is a major complication of oxygen therapy in the neonate. Hyperbilirubinemia and kernicterus also are potential complications.

Potential Complication: Oxygen Toxicity

Conditions Related to Hyperoxia. Two conditions have been associated with oxygen toxicity: ROP and BPD.

ROP is a disease of the eye that usually is associated with high $Pa{O_2}$ levels and the incompletely vascularized retina of preterm neonates. Hyperoxemia often is the event associated with the initial vasoconstriction of the retinal arteries, although it is also postulated that the relative hyperoxic state of the extrauterine environment is all that is required to arrest development of the vessels. This leaves some vessels permanently constricted and necrotic, while others proliferate in an attempt to revascularize the retina.

ROP may resolve spontaneously or proceed to later stages. These later stages include dilation of retinal vessels and rapid proliferation. Hemorrhage and edema from damaged vessels may lead to scarring and detachment of the retina, causing permanent blindness. Although the incidence of ROP is highest in preterm neonates with the highest $Pa{O_2}$ levels, the disease has been reported in full-term neonates maintained at lower $Pa{O_2}$ levels during oxygen therapy and in preterm infants who received minimal oxygen therapy. Because the disease also has been documented in neonates (including preterm and full-term) who have not received oxygen, it is difficult to determine a completely safe therapeutic $Pa{O_2}$ range for all neonates, especially preterm infants.

The following factors have been associated with the development of ROP (Carlson, 1991):

- Very low birth weight or prematurity
- Hyperoxia or hypoxia
- Blood and exchange transfusions
- Intraventricular hemorrhages
- Apnea requiring bag and mask ventilation
- Infection
- Hypercarbia or hypocarbia
- Patent ductus arteriosus (PDA)

- Prostaglandin synthetase inhibitors
- Lactic acidosis
- Prenatal complications
- Genetic factors
- Light

A classification system has been developed to describe the extent of injury (staging or grading) and the location of the disease in the retina. Three methods of surgical treatment have been attempted in the treatment of retrolental fibroplasia (RLF), with varying degrees of success:

- Laser therapy to reattach the retina
- Cryotherapy to freeze selected areas of the retina to prevent abnormal vasoproliferation. (This technique has been demonstrated to be effective and is used for many infants with ROP.)
- Cryotherapy with scleral buckling to support retinal reattachment.

BPD is a disease of the lungs associated with prolonged oxygen therapy (more than 30 days), barotrauma from positive-pressure mechanical ventilation, and exposure to high oxygen concentrations. Injury to the lung is not due to a high blood oxygen tension as may occur with ROP, but rather to the direct effect of high oxygen concentrations on lung tissue and to changes caused by pressure (barotrauma). Oxygen toxicity results in thickening and necrosis of the alveolar walls and bronchiolar epithelial lining. The neonate becomes oxygen- and ventilator-dependent, and weaning him or her from oxygen therapy is prolonged and difficult. Respiratory acidosis and right-sided heart failure secondary to pulmonary changes are common complications. The infant often remains in the hospital for months during the weaning process and may be discharged home with oxygen. A mortality rate between 30% and 40% has been documented in affected infants.

Monitoring Oxygen Therapy. To minimize the risk of oxygen toxicity, it is essential that the nurse continuously assess the oxygen delivery system and intermittently monitor arterial blood gases. The use of transcutaneous oxygen monitors and pulse oximeters also enables the nurse to evaluate the neonate's blood oxygenation status.

The percentage of oxygen (FIO_2 = fraction of inspired oxygen) administered to a neonate is monitored by an *oxygen analyzer*. The oxygen analyzer is placed within the neonate's environment as close to the airway as possible to measure the concentration of oxygen the neonate inspires. If the newborn is placed on a mechanical ventilator, the oxygen analyzer is usually connected directly to the airway tubing through which the oxygen flows.

Neonates receiving oxygen therapy also require frequent determinations of Pao_2 levels. In arterial blood gas analysis, a direct monitoring technique, a small arterial blood sample (usually less than 1 mL) is obtained directly from the umbilical, temporal, pedal, or radial artery. The pH, Pao_2, and $Paco_2$ can be measured as well as the HCO_3 (bicarbonate) level and base excess (amount of base buffer available to neutralize acid metabolites). The most accurate blood gas measurements are obtained by the invasive technique of withdrawing and analyzing arterial blood samples. Repeated withdrawal of blood, however, increases the risks of infection and anemia.

Transcutaneous oxygen ($TcPo_2$)/*carbon dioxide* *($TcPco_2$) monitoring* is an indirect, noninvasive method for measuring Pao_2 and $Paco_2$ levels in the neonate. A heated electrode attached to the neonate's skin surface measures the oxygen and carbon dioxide tension of blood flowing past the skin site. A constant "readout" or measurement of the Pao_2 and $Paco_2$ is possible, allowing the nurse to evaluate the effects of nursing care and procedures on the neonate's blood oxygen levels. For less critically ill neonates this method also eliminates the risks of invasive monitoring. For more seriously ill neonates for whom precise monitoring of blood gases is needed, $TcPo_2$/$TcPco_2$ monitoring will be used in combination with intermittent arterial blood gas analysis, often using blood drawn from umbilical artery catheters.

A minor complication encountered with noninvasive monitoring is the development of skin blisters and pitting at the site of electrode placement. The electrode is heated (42°C to 44°C) to increase blood flow to the skin and may cause superficial injury if the site is not changed frequently (every 2 to 3 hours) or if the probe is too hot (premature infants cannot tolerate higher settings).

Another noninvasive method of assessing the blood oxygenation status of the neonate is *pulse oximetry*. The pulse oximeter sensor contains two light-emitting diodes (LED) and a photodetector. The sensor is wrapped around a finger, toe, hand, foot (Fig. 33-9), or wrist so that the LED is aligned directly opposite the photodetector. The tissue bed interposed between the two sides of the probe is transilluminated by the LED, and the photodetector measures the heart rate and oxygen saturation of arterial hemoglobin (Sao_2).

Significant complications have not been reported with the use of pulse oximetry. The most notable problem is the potential for damage to the fragile skin of preterm neonates from the adhesive tape used to secure the sensor to the extremity. This can be avoided by wrapping a small piece of gauze around the probe and securing it with tape. No adhesive needs to be attached to the skin (Comer, 1992).

The accuracy of Sao_2 readings is influenced by bright ambient light, movement of the extremity to which the sen-

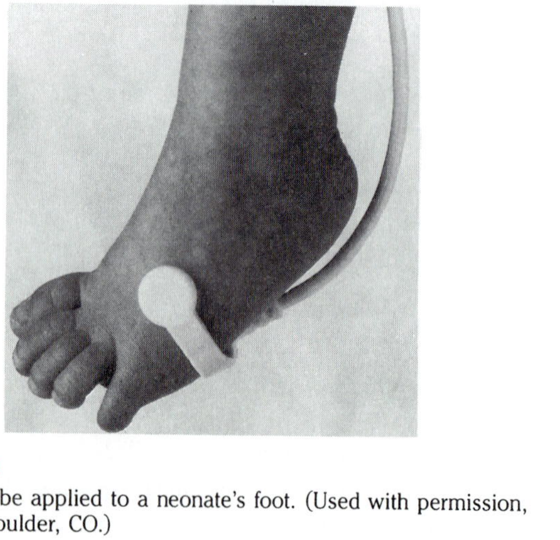

Figure 33-9.
Flexible probe applied to a neonate's foot. (Used with permission, Ohmeda, Boulder, CO.)

sor is applied, and the presence of abnormal hemoglobin. Finally, the accuracy of the pulse oximeter is not reliable at saturations above 90%. Hyperoxia may thus be missed. It is therefore imperative to monitor the Pa_{O_2} directly with blood gas analysis when oxygen is administered to the neonate.

Expected Outcome

- The neonate's arterial blood gas (Pa_{O_2}) values are normal.

Potential Complications: Hyperbilirubinemia and Kernicterus

The sick or compromised newborn is at greater risk for development of hyperbilirubinemia and jaundice. Major disorders associated with pathologic jaundice are listed in the display. The goal of therapeutic nursing interventions in the care of infants with hyperbilirubinemia is to prevent kernicterus, an encephalopathy caused by the deposition of unconjugated and unbound bilirubin in brain cells. Kernicterus has been associated with serum bilirubin levels approaching 20 mg/dL in the full-term neonate and with much lower levels in the extremely premature neonate. Recent studies suggest that there is no evidence that healthy term neonates are at risk for kernicterous at bilirubin levels in the 20 to 24 mg/dL range (Cloherty & Stark, 1991). The student is referred to Chapter 30 for a discussion of bilirubin conjugation and jaundice.

The classic signs of kernicterus, including lethargy, diminished reflexes, hypotonia, and seizures, are seen less frequently today as a result of advances in medical treatment and nursing care. Preterm neonates weighing less than 1500 g and who are ill appear to be at greatest risk for developing kernicterus and sustaining permanent neurologic damage (deafness, cerebral palsy, or mental retardation). Other factors that appear to contribute to the development of kernicterus are hypothermia, asphyxia, acidosis, hypoalbuminemia, and sepsis.

When the newborn develops pathologic jaundice, the nurse supports the conjugation and excretion of bilirubin by the following measures:

- Preventing hypothermia and reducing energy expenditures by placing the neonate in a neutral thermal environment
- Supporting frequent feedings to facilitate adequate hydration and excretion of wastes (if oral feeding is not contraindicated)
- Supporting adequate caloric intake to meet energy requirements and maintain adequate serum albumin levels

The nurse also will initiate phototherapy when it is ordered by the physician.

Phototherapy. Phototherapy is the exposure of the newborn's skin to high-intensity light. The process by which phototherapy reduces serum bilirubin involves the photoisomerization of unconjugated bilirubin deposited in the skin to a polarized compound. This compound diffuses into the bloodstream bound to albumin and is transported back to the liver. Figure 33-10 illustrates guidelines for the management of hyperbilirubinemia and indicates when phototherapy and exchange transfusions should be initiated to prevent kernicterus where hepatic cells secrete it in unconjugated form into the biliary tract. The bilirubin is then excreted into the duodenum with bile salts and removed from the body with fecal wastes. Oxidation products also are formed in the skin when bilirubin is exposed to light, and these photodegradation products are excreted in the urine. Several types of phototherapy lights are available today. A bank of eight to ten fluorescent lights with a wavelength of 425 to 475 nm; banks of daylight lamps, blue light, and high-intensity quartz holide lamps; and woven fiberoptic blankets

Major Disorders Associated With Pathologic Jaundice

- Intravascular hemolysis
  - Hemolytic disease of the newborn
    - Rh incompatibility
    - ABO incompatibility
  - Acquired hemolytic disorders secondary to infection
  - Chemical hemolysis related to drugs
  - Inherited defects of red cell metabolism
    - Hereditary spherocytosis
    - G6PD deficiency
    - hemoglobinopathies
  - Polycythemia
- Extravascular hemolysis (extravasation of blood)
  - Petechiae
  - Ecchymoses
  - Hemorrhage
  - Hematomas
- Swallowed blood
- Impaired hepatic function
  - Glucoronyl transferase deficiency
    - Familial nonhemolytic jaundice (type I, II)
    - Transient familial neonatal hyperbilirubinemia (Lucey–Driscoll syndrome)
  - Sepsis
    - Bacterial
    - Nonbacterial (TORCH)
  - Abnormal metabolic function
    - Infants of diabetic mothers
    - Galactosemia
    - Hypothyroidism
    - Hypopituitarism
    - Tyrosinosis
    - Cystic fibrosis
- Increased enterohepatic circulation of bilirubin
  - Intestinal obstruction
  - Pyloric stenosis
  - Meconium ileus
  - Paralytic ileus
  - Hirschsprung's disease
- Biliary obstruction
  - Biliary atresia

<table>
<tr><th>Serum bilirubin (mg/100 ml)</th><th>Birth weight</th><th><24 hrs</th><th>24–48 hrs</th><th>49–72 hrs</th><th>>72 hrs</th></tr>
<tr><td><5</td><td></td><td></td><td></td><td></td><td></td></tr>
<tr><td>5–9</td><td>All</td><td>Phototherapy if hemolysis</td><td></td><td></td><td></td></tr>
<tr><td rowspan="2">10–14</td><td><2500g</td><td rowspan="2">Exchange if hemolysis</td><td colspan="3">Phototherapy</td></tr>
<tr><td>>2500g</td><td></td><td colspan="2">Investigate if bilirubin > 12 mg</td></tr>
<tr><td rowspan="2">15–19</td><td><2500g</td><td rowspan="2" colspan="2">Exchange</td><td colspan="2">Consider exchange</td></tr>
<tr><td>>2500g</td><td colspan="2">Phototherapy</td></tr>
<tr><td>20 and +</td><td>All</td><td colspan="4">Exchange</td></tr>
</table>

☐ Observe ☐ Investigate jaundice

Use phototherapy after any exchange

In presence of:

1. Perinatal asphyxia
2. Respiratory distress
3. Metabolic acidosis (pH 7.25 or below)
4. Hypothermia (temp below 35°C)
5. Low serum protein (5g/100 ml or less)
6. Birth weight < 1500 g
7. Signs of clinical or CNS deterioration

} Treat as in next higher bilirubin category

Figure 33-10.
Guidelines for management of hyperbilirubinemia.

specifically designed for phototherapy are all available to provide the proper irradiance.

The neonate's clothes are removed and patches placed over the eyes to protect them from the light source. The newborn is then placed in an incubator or under a radiant warmer, which provides a neutral thermal environment (Fig. 33-11). The light source is positioned above the neonate, and a photometer is used to measure the light intensity. Light flux should normally range between 6 to 8 W/cm^2/nm. The distance of the light source from the neonate should be based on the photometric reading. Light bulbs should be changed at preset intervals to ensure appropriate light output. It is suggested that Cavitron bulbs be changed after 150 hours of use and fluorescent lights before 2000 hours (Cloherty & Stark, 1991). The neonate is turned approximately every 2 hours to expose all body surfaces to the light. Phototherapy is continued until serum bilirubin levels fall to within normal limits.

Nursing care of the jaundiced neonate who remains under the "bili lights" focuses on preventing complications of phototherapy, educating parents about this therapy, and providing emotional support and opportunities for them to hold and feed their newborn. The nurse checks vital signs every 2 to 4 hours, because hyperthermia can occur under the lights. Because insensible water loss is increased with phototherapy and copious loose green "bili stools" are common sequelae of the treatment, the neonate is observed for signs of dehydration. Intake and output are monitored closely, and fluid intake is increased by at least 25% (10 to 15 mL/kg increase). Breastfeeding is not contraindicated, although the neonate needs to receive adequate hydration. The skin is inspected for evidence of excoriation resulting from the passage of bili stools. Care must be taken to keep the skin clean and dry. Surgical face masks may be used as "bikini diapers" for neonates who are urinating or stooling frequently and changed when soiled to prevent skin breakdown. A benign bronzing or tanning of the skin or the development of a diffuse maculopapular rash occurs in some neonates as a response to phototherapy. No treatment is necessary, and no long-term adverse effects of bronzing or rashing have been documented.

Protection of the eyes is an essential aspect of care. The

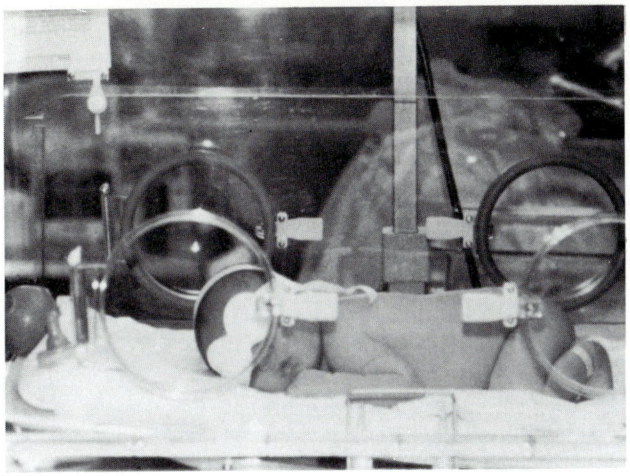

Figure 33-11.
A full-term newborn receiving phototherapy in a closed isolette for hyperbilirubinemia. (Photo by BABES, Inc.)

nurse should observe the neonate frequently to be sure the patches are correctly positioned and the eyes remain closed. Phototherapy is discontinued and eye patches removed for feedings and when the parents hold and interact with their newborn. The patches should be changed every 12 to 24 hours to reduce the possibility of iatrogenic eye infection. Phototherapy lights also must be turned off or redirected each time a blood specimen is drawn for serum bilirubin determination (usually every 12 hours) to prevent photoisomerization of the specimen. The reader is referred to Chapter 31 for a complete discussion of phototherapy and a nursing care plan for an infant undergoing phototherapy.

If home therapy is to be used, the nurse teaches the family how to use the equipment and what precautions to take (see the display on home phototherapy).

Exchange Transfusion. In an exchange transfusion the neonate's blood is withdrawn to remove serum bilirubin and is replaced with donor blood to maintain normal blood volume and provide free albumin binding sites for bilirubin. This procedure is rarely used because of the use of phototherapy and decreased incidence of hemolytic disease of the newborn.

Exchange transfusions also are used in the treatment of Rh isoimmunization to remove RBCs that will be hemolyzed by maternal antibodies, thus elevating serum biliribin levels and to correct severe anemia caused by hemolysis of sensitized RBCs. The reader is referred to the section "The Neonate With Hemolytic Disease" (later in this chapter) for further information on blood incompatibilities and their treatment.

Expected Outcomes

- The neonate responds to phototherapy with reduction of hyperbilirubinemia.
- The newborn receiving exchange transfusion remains free of complications.
- The newborn maintains serum bilirubin levels within normal limits.

Family Considerations

Home Phototherapy

Home phototherapy has been instituted in some family-oriented maternity centers in the United States. Portable equipment is available, and the American Academy of Pediatrics has developed guidelines to help health care providers establish a home phototherapy program. It is recommended that home phototherapy be limited to neonates with the following characteristics: (1) term gestation, 48 hours old but otherwise healthy; (2) serum bilirubin levels greater than 14 mg/dL but less than 18 mg/dL; (3) no elevation in direct bilirubin levels; and (4) negative diagnostic evaluation.

Before phototherapy is instituted outside of the hospital setting, the home environment and the parents' ability to care for the newborn and follow phototherapy guidelines should be evaluated. A visiting nurse, in collaboration with a physician, must be available to assess the neonate every 12 to 24 hours, check equipment, and measure serum bilirubin levels. Findings are documented and the physician contacted by phone or messenger service. Program evaluations have demonstrated the success of home therapy and its acceptance by families, nurses, and physicians.

• • Evaluation

The quality of nursing care for the high-risk and sick neonate cannot necessarily be measured by complete recovery and discharge of the newborn to the care of his or her parents. Very premature newborns and those with severe physiologic insults of congenital anomalies present medical and nursing problems of tremendous complexity. Neonatal outcomes cannot be predicted with confidence, and nurses in the field of neonatal care often must intervene when knowledge and time are limited. However, the nurse in neonatal care functions as part of an expert team of professionals; through the collaborative efforts of physicians, social workers, health science researchers, and others, the frontiers of knowledge are constantly being expanded.

Evaluation of family-centered nursing care in the environment of the neonatal intensive care unit also is difficult. Nursing interventions to support parents and assist them in establishing a meaningful relationship with their newborn must take into account the conflicting forces of hope and grief. The neonatal nurse may never see the results of her sensitive care for parents. The evidence of effective nursing care may only be apparent in the resolution of parental grief and the reintegration of family life. However, the most valued sign of expert and effective nursing care remains the "graduation" of a recovered and thriving neonate or infant to the care of happy parents and the reunion of a new family.

Regardless of the specific disorder of the high-risk neonate, many elements in the provision of nursing care are similar. Major points in the planning and implementation include promoting pulmonary adaptation, supporting ventilation, administering oxygen, supporting cardiac and tissue perfusion, maintaining circulatory volume, promoting fluid and electrolyte balance, providing for nutritional needs, preventing infection, supporting thermoregulation, promoting behavioral adaptation, encouraging parent–newborn attachment and interaction, and supporting parental coping and grieving. These nursing actions are independent. The nurse also monitors for potential complications and provides therapy as needed. Potential complications for the high-risk newborn include oxygen toxicity, hyperbilirubinemia, and kernicterus. The nurse also teaches the parents to provide therapy, such as phototherapy, at home.

The Neonate With Birth Asphyxia

Birth asphyxia is a condition characterized by hypoxemia (decreased PaO_2), hypercarbia (increased $PaCO_2$), and acidosis (lowered blood pH and increased base deficit). Respiratory effort may be minimal or absent due to brain stem hypoxia, or the neonate may exhibit signs of distress (especially tachypnea) in an effort to correct the low pH by blowing off large amounts of CO_2. With severe asphyxia, cardiac function is also depressed due to hypoxia of the myocardium.

Asphyxia is a progressive process that can be reversed in its initial stages with proper medical and nursing management. The initial drop in PaO_2 leads to a selective shunting of blood to the vital organs (brain, myocardium, and adrenals). The newborn may be observed to gasp in an attempt to inflate the lungs. If efforts at ventilation fail and resuscitation is not initiated, the myocardium is eventually affected by the lowered PaO_2 level, and cardiac output decreases. This then affects all organ systems. Conversion to anaerobic metabolism and the burning of brown fat stores for energy lead to metabolic acidosis. The hypoxemia further causes vasospasm of the pulmonary vasculature, promotes maintenance of fetal circulation, and thereby inhibits oxygenation of the blood.

A vicious downward spiral in the newborn's condition can then ensue. The myocardium and brain rely on glucose for energy; once glycogen stores are depleted, both brain and myocardial function deteriorate further. Unless vigorous resuscitation is started immediately, irreversible changes in brain and myocardial function will result, leading to permanent brain damage or death.

Etiologic and Predisposing Factors

A variety of maternal, fetal, and neonatal conditions can lead to neonatal asphyxia at birth.

Impaired Maternal Blood Flow Through the Placenta. Asphyxia occurs when the flow of oxygenated maternal blood to the intervillous spaces of the placenta is diminished or when maternal oxygenation is impaired. Any condition that leads to a decrease in the mother's blood pressure will impair blood flow to the intervillous spaces. Vena cava syndrome (supine hypotension) and conduction anesthesia are two common causes of maternal hypotension, but it also may result from hemorrhage and hypovolemic shock. Maternal vascular disease may lead to birth asphyxia. The severe vasospasm found in pregnancy-induced hypertension leads to a decreased blood flow to the intervillous spaces. Vascular changes of chronic hypertension also interfere with placental perfusion, as do placental accidents, such as infarcts and premature separation. Additionally, maternal hypoxemia decreases the amount of oxygen available to the fetus. Conditions such as cigarette smoking, acute opiate withdrawal, or carbon monoxide poisoning can impede oxygenation to the fetus. This hypoxemia in utero diminishes the neonate's reserves and promotes intolerance of labor and birth asphyxia in the neonate.

Impaired Blood Flow Through the Umbilical Cord. Compression of the umbilical cord prevents oxygen transport through the fetal bloodstream. Compression occurs when the cord is trapped between a fetal part and the maternal pelvis or cervix (occult or prolapsed cord). Partial or total compression also can occur when the cord is tightly wrapped around a part of the fetal body, for example the neck (nuchal cord) or the body (bandolier cord), or when there is a true knot in the cord.

Impaired Fetal Circulation. Any condition that decreases the efficiency of fetal circulation will lead to asphyxia. Trauma that produces fetal hemorrhage and hypovolemic shock, severe anemia (Rh disease with hydrops fetalis), and congestive heart failure all diminish cardiac output and lead to fetal hypoxia.

Impaired Respiratory Effort. Whereas asphyxia leads to impaired respiratory effort, several conditions present at birth prevent the initiation of respiration and lead to asphyxia. Severe neonatal narcosis caused by maternal overmedication (eg, narcotics, general anesthesia, and magnesium sulfate) and an obstructed airway (meconium aspiration, hyaline membrane disease) will both lead to asphyxia unless quickly corrected.

Diagnosis

During labor the fetal heart tracing is the best indicator of fetal well-being. As discussed in Chapter 22, efforts are made to maintain maternal circulation and placental perfusion through hydration and position in a lateral recumbant fashion. Maternal and fetal oxygenation is promoted through the use of supplemental oxygen using a face mask. In the event that these interventions are insufficient and ominous fetal heart rate tracings continue (severe variable decelerations, persistent late decelerations), a direct sampling of fetal blood may be obtained to document fetal blood pH. Fetal scalp sampling, performed under aseptic conditions, approximates the venous blood gas of the fetus. Normal fetal blood pH ranges from 7.25 to 7.35. A value of < 7.15 indicates immediate delivery. Serial scalp samplings may be performed if the fetus is determined to have some reserve or if the fetal heart tracing becomes more reassuring.

After birth, direct sampling of arterial blood from a peripheral or umbilical artery provides definitive measurement of acid–base status. Supplemental oxygen may be delivered by numerous routes. Hyperventilation using a bag and mask or endotracheal tube and bag may be performed to raise the blood pH by blowing off CO_2 and excess hydrogen atoms.

Perinatal asphyxia is diagnosed by assessment of the neonate's respiratory and circulatory status. A mottled, grayish coloring combined with respiratory distress in a listless, limp neonate often indicates perinatal asphyxia. Often, a vacant, wide-eyed, glassy stare is seen in neonates immediately after birth when there has been an anoxic insult or periods of hypoxia.

Neonatal Implications

If resuscitation efforts result in a newborn with sustained respiratory and cardiac function, the neonate is transferred to a special care unit for continued observation and treatment. This is essential because hypoxia can lead to necrosis of tissues in major organ systems and profound metabolic alterations.

Postasphyxial syndrome is the resultant condition and is characterized by a constellation of signs. The neonate with postasphyxial syndrome can exhibit seizure activity, resulting from cerebral edema, within the first 12 to 24 hours after birth. More severely affected neonates will have seizures sooner. Edema is caused by the death of brain cells and the increased permeability of cerebral vessels secondary to increased $Paco_2$ levels. Intracranial hemorrhage also can occur as a result of increased capillary fragility secondary to metabolic acidosis or the too rapid infusion of sodium bicarbonate during neonatal resuscitation.

Necrosis of both renal and intestinal tissues is a result of the protective shunting of blood to the brain, heart, and adrenals that occurs with hypoxia. Renal failure, characterized by either high or low output urine volume, is observed. Hypoxic injury to the neonatal gut leads to a condition known as NEC. Areas of necrotic tissue in the intestinal lumen may perforate, spilling intestinal contents into the peritoneal cavity and causing peritonitis. Preterm neonates are particularly susceptible to NEC, and the mortality rate remains very high.

Metabolic alterations are associated with postasphyxial syndrome. Glucose stores are rapidly depleted during asphyxial episodes, and this leads to hypoglycemia. An initial high serum glucose level may be obtained if the neonate is delivered shortly after exhibiting signs of distress, but this merely represents mobilization of glycogen stores, and the level will soon drop dramatically if supplemental glucose is not initiated. Hypocalcemia occurs, and although its etiology is unclear, changes in parathyroid function and increased cell permeability secondary to hypoxia appear to alter the calcium–phosphorus ratio. Potassium is released into the vascular compartment from cells damaged by hypoxia and causes hyperkalemia.

The major concern after an asphyxial episode and oxygen deprivation to the neonate's brain is the long-term neurologic outcome. Recent research suggests that the previous cause–effect relationship presumed between asphyxia and cerebral palsy is inaccurate. In fact the asphyxia must be nearly lethal to be considered a possible cause of the chronic neuromuscular disability. There continues to be an "association" between asphyxia and chronic neurologic impairment (seizures, mental retardation, or cerebral palsy), but a stronger indicator appears to be the development of postasphyxial seizures in the neonate. Although statistical evidence is available to assist physicians in determining prognosis, it is often difficult to predict accurately an individual newborn's neurologic status.

Treatment

If the delivery of a potentially compromised newborn is suspected, personnel experienced in the immediate stabilization and resuscitation of neonates should be in attendance at the birth. During the first 60 seconds the airway is cleared and the newborn is quickly dried and stimulated. The heart rate, respiratory effort, color, muscle tone, and reflex irritability are all rapidly evaluated. Oxygen may be given, and ventilation and cardiac compression are begun if the infant is severely depressed (see Immediate Resuscitation of the Neonate in Chapter 32).

Once the condition is stabilized, the newborn is transferred to the special care unit, where medical and nursing care are directed at supporting vital functions (eg, cardiac, respiratory, and thermal regulation), avoiding or minimizing potential complications (intraventricular hemorrhage, NEC), and further assessing the degree of compromise for the infant. The accompanying Nursing Care Plan outlines care of an asphyxiated neonate.

In cases of airway obstruction or impaired respiratory effort, the neonate is supported with mechanical ventilation. When hypovolemia or severe anemia is present, the neonate can receive volume expanders or a blood transfusion using type O Rh negative blood (universal donor). Initiation of venous and arterial access lines are crucial to the maintenance of circulation. All attempts are made to avoid wide swings in blood pressure, due to the increased friability of the cerebral arteries. This helps lessen the possibility of intracranial, specifically intraventricular, hemorrhages. In severe cases of asphyxia, multisystem complications or postasphyxial syndrome may result.

Implications for Nursing Care

The newborn is monitored closely for signs of increased intracranial pressure, including bulging fontanelles, "setting sun" eyes (a condition in which the sclera are visible above the iris), decreased or absent reflexes, and seizures. All of these signs are extremely difficult (or impossible) to assess in the newborn who is ventilated and receiving neuromuscular blocking agents and sedatives. The nurse must carefully assess the neonate's response to the environment through physiologic indicators (heart rate, blood pressure, pulse pressure) instead. Seizures can be detected in the paralyzed neonate using episodes of desaturation in an otherwise stable neonate, wide swings in blood pressure, and a widening pulse pulse pressure. Due to the subtlety of these signs, it is often difficult to prove seizure activity, so an electroencephalogram may need to be performed. The neonate is

Text continues on page 1019

Nursing Care Plan

The Asphyxiated Neonate

PATIENT PROFILE

History

Baby B is a 3670 g male neonate. He was born by forceps-assisted delivery at 40 weeks' gestation when the FHR dropped to 60 BPM for 4 min during the second stage of labor. Baby B's mother had a normal pregnancy. Labor was prolonged, and the membranes were ruptured for 26 hours. Severe variable decelerations were noted during the last 20 minutes of labor before the sudden drop in the FHR.

Apgar scores were 5, 7, and 9 at 1, 5, and 10 minutes, respectively. Umbilical cord blood analysis revealed the following data:

Vein: pH 7.28; pO_2 24; pCO_2 42 **Artery**: pH 7.18; pO_2 14; pCO_2 50

The base deficit was −10, which indicated fetal metabolic acidosis. Baby B was placed in an observation nursery. An IV line was initiated, and a solution of 10% dextrose was infused to provide 50 mL/kg per day of fluid. The neonate was made strictly NPO, and IV fluid intake has been limited to 50 mL/kg/per day. Prophylactic antibiotics were started after a partial septic workup, and then Baby B was placed in an incubator.

Physical Assessment

The nurse performed an assessment of Baby B 4 h after birth and noted the following data:

T. 37.0 C (98.6F); P 146; R 54. Lethargic, with a generalized, slight decrease in tone. Suck, cry, and Moro reflex are weak when elicited. The pupils are dilated but responsive to light. There is marked molding of the head. The anterior fontanelle is open and soft. The heart rhythm is irregular with frequent ectopic beats. There is a soft systolic murmur, and peripheral pulses are palpated as normal (+2). Respirations are shallow and irregular. Breath sounds are clear and equal bilaterally. The abdomen is soft, and there are bowel sounds in all four quadrants. Baby B has not voided.

As the assessment is completed, the nurse notes a 20- to 30-sec episode of rapid eyelid blinking and vertical nystagmus of the eyes. Repetitive lip-smacking also is noted, coupled with rhythmic tongue thrusting movements. Baby B then has a 20-sec period of apnea, during which he becomes cyanotic.

COLLABORATIVE PROBLEMS/POTENTIAL COMPLICATIONS

- Seizures
- Cerebral edema
- Congestive heart failure
- Persistent pulmonary hypertension
- Necrotizing enterocolitis
- Renal tubular necrosis
- Hypoglycemia

(See the accompanying Nursing Alert display.)

Assessment	*Nursing Diagnosis*	*Nursing Interventions*	*Rationale*
Baby B experienced asphyxia at birth with 1-min Apgar of 5 and 5-min Apgar of 7. Baby B has shallow, irregular respirations at 54/min. At 4 h of age, neonate has 20-sec period of apnea with skin color changing from pink to cyanotic.	Ineffective Breathing Pattern related to seizure ***Expected Outcome*** Baby B will maintain a respiratory rate of 30 to 60 breaths per minute, oxygen saturation (SaO_2) of >90%, and normal arterial blood gases.	Call for help.	To obtain additional assistance and supplies
		Place neonate's head in neutral or "sniffing" position.	To open airway by bringing head and neck into correct alignment
		Suction mouth and oropharynx with 10 French catheter.	To clear mucus or gastric fluids from airway

(*Continued*)

The Asphyxiated Neonate
(*Continued*)

Assessment	Nursing Diagnosis	Nursing Interventions	Rationale
	Baby B will demonstrate no further episodes of apnea.	Administer 100% oxygen using a bag and mask.	To facilitate maximum oxygenation of tissues because persistent hypoxia can result in permanent tissue damage, opening of ductus arteriorsus, or lead to persistent pulmonary hypertension
		Begin ventilating neonate at 30 to 50 breaths per minute until spontaneous respirations begin.	To facilitate gas exchange
		Notify physician.	To obtain medical assistance and further orders
		Apply cardiorespiratory monitor and pulse oximeter. Set alarm limits and turn alarms on.	To permit continuous monitoring of cardiorespiratory status, percentage of oxygen saturation of hemoglobin (SaO_2), and determine effectiveness of therapy
		Obtain electronic blood pressure reading.	To obtain baseline blood pressure reading.
		Assist with obtaining arterial blood gases by positioning and holding Baby B.	To facilitate rapid assessment of blood pH and gas status. To prevent need for additional needle sticks, which may be necessary if neonate is agitated or moving
		Place resuscitation bag and mask inside incubator or on treatment bed if neonate is placed under radiant warmer.	To have resuscitation equipment readily available in the event of continued episodes of apnea
		Maintain close observation of neonate.	To permit prompt identification and treatment of further seizure activity or apnea
		Note and record vital signs every hour.	To identify significant changes in Baby B's vital signs
		Monitor Baby B for further evidence of ineffective breathing patterns including: • tachypnea • grunting • flaring • retracting • apnea • central cyanosis	

(*Continued*)

The Asphyxiated Neonate

(Continued)

Assessment	*Nursing Diagnosis*	*Nursing Interventions*	*Rationale*
		Suction Baby B only when secretions must be cleared from airway.	Suctioning has been shown to cause significant decreases in oxygenation and increases in acidosis and bradycardia.
Baby B had severe variable decelerations during the last 20 min of labor followed by a 4-min period during which the FHR was 60 BPM. Apgar scores were 5, 7, and 9 at 1, 5, and 10 minutes. UV and UA pH and gases indicated metabolic acidosis. Baby B has decreased tone and dilated pupils that are responsive to light. Suck, cry, and Moro reflex are weak. Period of rapid eyelid blinking, vertical nystagmus, rhythmic lip-smacking, and tongue-thrusting are noted. Baby B has 20-sec period of apnea with cyanosis.	High Risk for CNS Injury related to birth asphyxia and episode of apnea *Expected Outcome* Baby B will remain free of further seizure activity. Baby B will maintain a flat, soft anterior fontanelle, normal level of consciousness, reflexes, and muscle tone.	Assess level of consciousness and reflexes q 4–8 h. (Suck, swallow, gag, Moro, blink)	Level of consciousness and reflexes are two of the most sensitive indicators of neurologic function. Decreased muscle tone may indicate severity of asphyxia and IIP.
		Measure size of fontanelle from bone edge to bone edge q 8–12 h. Assess sutures for evidence of splitting. Measure width of sutures q 8–12 h when evidence of increased intracranial pressure is present.	Cerebral edema and IIP will result in bulging fontanelle and splitting sutures as brain edema develops.
		Assess size and responsiveness of pupils to light q 4–8 h.	With IIP, pupils may become dilated and fixed.
		Monitor Baby B for evidence of increasing intracranial pressure: • Increasing size or bulging of anterior fontanelle • Decreasing muscle tone • "Setting sun" sign in eyes	Early recognition of IIP facilitates prompt treatment and may improve long-term condition of neonate.
		Monitor Baby B for evidence of seizure activity: • Tonic eye deviations • Blinking or eyelid fluttering • Rhythmic sucking or lip-smacking • Rhythmic rowing movements of arms • Rhythmic bicycling of legs • Apnea	Recognition of seizure activity permits treatment and may prevent further apnea episodes.
		Obtain heel stick blood sample, and determine glucose level.	Glucose stores may be depleted during asphyxial episode resulting in hypoglycemia, which will exacerbate CNS injury.

(Continued)

The Asphyxiated Neonate

(*Continued*)

Assessment	Nursing Diagnosis	Nursing Interventions	Rationale
			Hypoglycemia is a cause of seizures.
			There is an increase in the metabolic rate during seizure activity, and glucose stores may be depleted.
		Maintain fluid restrictions as ordered.	Cerebral edema and IIP will be exacerbated by fluid overload.
		Administer antiepileptic drugs as ordered.	Seizure activity will worsen CNS injury by causing further hypoxia and hypoglycemia.
Apical pulse of 146 is irregular with ectopic beats. Soft systolic murmur +2 peripheral pulses. Skin is pink.	Decreased Cardiac Output related to asphyxial injury to myocardium	Assess heart rate and rhythm 1 h	Myocardial ischemia may occur with asphyxia resulting in cardiac dysfunction.
	Expected Outcome Baby B will maintain a regular heart rate between 120 and 160 BPM. Baby B will maintain a normal cardiac output as evidenced by a blood pressure within normal limits, a central capillary fill time <3 seconds, and +2 peripheral pulses.	Auscultate heart for murmurs	Murmurs may result from myocardial asphyxial damage, such as tricuspid valve insufficiency. The ductus arteriorsus may reopen or remain open with hypoxia, causing a pathologic murmur.
		Apply cardiac monitor and pulse oximeter.	Permits continuous monitoring of cardiac rate and rhythm. Permits continuous assessment of oxygen saturation.
		Obtain electronic blood pressure reading q 4–8 h.	Provides baseline data regarding blood pressure level and will alert nurse to changes in cardiac output.
		Assess central capillary fill time q 4–8 h.	Perfusion changes reflect the status of cardiac output.
		Palpate peripheral pulses for equlaity and pressure q 4–8 h.	Hypotension will occur with decreased cardiac output and cardiogenic shock.
			A decrease in peripheral pulses will be noted when cardiac output is compromised.
		Administer oxygen per protocol if cyanosis is noted, until medical help arrives.	To facilitate oxygenation of tissues and prevent hypoxic tissue damage
		Notify physician of findings if abnormalities noted.	To obtain medical help and further orders

(*Continued*)

The Asphyxiated Neonate

(Continued)

Assessment	Nursing Diagnosis	Nursing Interventions	Rationale
		Administer cardiogenic drugs and agents to improve blood pressure as ordered.	Drugs may be needed to improve cardiac contractility and improve cardiac output and blood pressure.
Baby B has not voided since birth. Fluid intake has been limited to 50 mL/kg per day.	High risk for Fluid Volume Excess related to asphyxial damage to renal system and excessive ADH secretion ***Expected Outcome*** Baby B will excrete at least 1 to 3 mL/kg per hour urine.	Monitor intake and output closely.	Baby B with renal damage may develop oliguria in the first postnatal day. Oversecretion of ADH may occur after asphyxial episode causing further fluid retention. Early recognition of renal compromise will prevent fluid overload and permit early treatment.
		Place urine bag over external genitalia.	Collecting urine permits more accurate assessment of urine output than simply weighing diapers.
		Weigh neonate daily. Weigh all diapers. Measure urine-specific gravity.	Weighing infant daily permits a more accurate estimation of fluid retention.
		Restrict fluids as ordered.	Excessive fluid intake will exacerbate fluid overload and development of cerebral edema.
		Administer all IV fluids with an infusion pump.	To prevent accidental fluid bolus.
		Obtain and monitor serum electrolytes.	Serum hyponatremia and hyperkalemia may occur with asphyxia and may result in further cerebral edema and cardiac irregularities.
		Assess Baby B for evidence of peripheral edema.	To determine the extent of fluid retention
		Administer diuretics as ordered.	Diuretics may be ordered with oliguria to relieve severe fluid overload.

EVALUATION

Baby B was given a loading dose of phenobarbital (15 mg/kg) intravenously and was then placed on a maintenance dose of 3 mg/kg per day. No further seizure activity or episodes of apnea occurred. The heart rate and rhythm stabilized by 36 hours. Urine output remained within normal limits. Within 48 hours the neonate was more alert and responsive to stimuli. Strong suck, swallow, gag, and Moro reflexes were established, and muscle tone was normal. The CBC and blood cultures that were obtained after admission to the nursery were negative. Baby B was discharged home on the fifth postnatal day and was scheduled for pediatric follow-up care.

NURSING ALERT

NURSING RESPONSIBILITIES IN THE ADMISSION CARE OF THE ASPHYXIATED NEONATE

The nurse must be prepared to initiate supportive care for the asphyxiated neonate who is admitted to the nursery until the physician (pediatrician or neonatologist) arrives. Standardized protocols, preprinted physician orders, or hospital policies and procedures often guide the nurse in the provision of care. When the neonate experiences moderate to severe asphyxia, the muscle tone and protective reflexes often are depressed or absent. The pupils may be dilated and the neonate lethargic. When these signs are present, the nurse must initiate emergency measures that will sustain the neonate's vital functions. The neonate is placed in a neutral thermal environment. A treatment bed and radiant warmer permit access to the neonate and are preferred. The head and neck are positioned to maintain a patent airway. If respiratory efforts are weak or cyanosis persists, 100% oxygen should be administered by bag and mask ventilation. (The concentration may be decreased for the preterm neonate.) The neonate should be made strictly NPO, and gastric contents should be suctioned to prevent regurgitation and aspiration. (The contents should be saved in a sterile container for possible Gram staining or culture.)

A heel stick blood sample should be obtained for assessment of serum glucose and hematocrit level. A peripheral intravenous (IV) line should be initiated or a heparin or saline lock placed for IV access. If the neonate is hypoglycemic, glucose should be administered by the IV route. It is unsafe to administer glucose by the oral route (nipple or gavage) in the asphyxiated neonate.

closely monitored for myocardial ischemia (arrhythmias), intestinal ischemia, and NEC. Sloughing of the bowel wall, observed by bloody, mucous discharge from the gut, may occur. Signs of NEC, including increasing residuals, increasing abdominal girth, visible bowel loops, decrease or absence of bowel sounds, and the presence of a reddened, shiny abdomen, only occur after the initiation of feedings. In an attempt to "rest" the gut, an asphyxiated neonate will remain NPO for up to 1 week and can receive venous hyperalimentation instead. The nurse is responsible for monitoring gastrointestinal status and function before and during feedings.

Intake and output are meticulously recorded to evaluate renal function and rule out renal failure. The urine is checked with each voiding for the presence of blood and protein, an indication of renal injury, and the stools are tested for heme, a danger sign suggesting the development of NEC. Serial blood glucose determinations are made by obtaining heel stick blood samples to detect hypoglycemia or hyperglycemia, and serum electrolytes are checked once or twice each day for evidence of hypocalcemia, hyperkalemia, and hyponatremia.

Intravenous therapy is administered to meet immediate needs for fluid, calories (dextrose), and electrolytes (calcium, sodium, and potassium), and antibiotic therapy usually is implemented when risk factors for infection are present, including invasive monitoring devices (umbilical artery or vein lines or endotracheal intubation).

If seizure activity is noted, the neonate will be placed on phenobarbital or phenytoin (Dilantin). Diuretics and agents that relieve cerebral swelling and edema also may be incorporated into the therapeutic regimen. The nurse is responsible for administering the medications and for observing for potential side effects.

Most parents are well aware of the impact of asphyxia on mental functioning. The wait-and-see policy often maintained by physicians is extremely difficult for parents to accept. They may bombard the nurse with questions regarding signs of possible brain damage and press for concrete predictions regarding neurologic function. It is important that parents receive consistent messages regarding their newborn's condition and prognosis. Parents will need ongoing support and counseling to deal with the uncertainties regarding current status and expected neurologic capabilities. Long-term follow-up of the newborn will be necessary, and it may be years before the child's maximum neurologic capabilities can be determined.

Birth asphyxia is a high-risk condition characterized by hypoxemia, hypercarbia, and acidosis. Asphyxia is a progressive process resulting from a variety of maternal, fetal, and neonatal conditions. The fetal heart tracing is the best indicator of fetal well-being during labor. When the delivery of a potentially compromised neonate is suspected, experienced personnel should be present to stabilize and resuscitate the newborn immediately. Asphyxia can be reversed in its initial stages with proper medical and nursing management. If immediate resuscitation is not begun, irreversible changes in brain and myocardial function will lead to permanent brain damage or death.

The Neonate With Complications Related to Gestational Age and Growth

The Preterm Neonate

The preterm or premature neonate is one born before 37 weeks of gestation. The etiologic factors of preterm labor are poorly understood, although variables associated with premature delivery have been identified. Table 33-4 discusses complications that may be involved in prematurity. Preterm newborns suffer from anatomic and physiologic immaturity in all systems, preventing them in many instances from making major adaptations without continuous medical and nursing care. It is no longer possible to describe a typical preterm newborn.

Although technologic advances have made it possible for newborns under 500 g and between 24 to 26 weeks of gestation to survive, the mortality rate is highest among these "micronates" (Hack, Hobar, Mallory, Tyson, Wright, & Wright, 1991). Their physical characteristics and physiologic capabilities are quite different from those of the preterm neonate born at 36 weeks of gestation. Although a description of these differences is beyond the scope of this chapter, it is possible to discuss the problems and requirements for nursing care that preterm newborns have in common.

Table 33-4. Factors Associated With Prematurity

Obstetric Complications	Medical Complications	Socioeconomic Factors
Uterine malformation	Maternal diabetes	Absence of prenatal care
Multiple gestation	Chronic hypertensive disease	Low socioeconomic status
Incompetent cervical os	Urinary tract infection	Malnutrition
Premature rupture of membranes and chorioamnionitis	Other acute illnesses	Early adolescent pregnancy
Pregnancy-induced hypertension		
Placenta previa		
History of previous premature birth		
Rh isoimmunization		

Neonatal Implications

High Risk for Impaired Gas Exchange. The preterm neonate is at risk for respiratory complications because the lungs and the regulatory centers of the central nervous system are immature at birth. Terminal air sacs (primitive alveoli) begin to differentiate and increase in number at 24 weeks of gestation, but the surface for exchange of gases is limited, and air sacs tend to collapse because of minimal surfactant production. The regulatory center for respiration located in the brain is also immature, and the preterm neonate can suffer from serious episodes of apnea and bradycardia.

Respiratory Distress Syndrome. RDS is a disorder of the lungs characterized by pulmonary hypoperfusion, hypoxemia, metabolic and respiratory acidosis, and classic changes in lung tissue, including decreased compliance, capillary damage, and alveolar necrosis. RDS is primarily due to immaturity and inadequate surfactant production, leading to progressive atelectasis and decreased perfusion of lung tissue.

Newborns with RDS exhibit rapid, labored respirations as they attempt to re-expand collapsed alveoli with each inspiration. Classic signs of distress, including cyanosis or pallor, retractions, nasal flaring, grunting, and see-saw breathing, are evident. The neonate is hypotonic and inactive, focusing all energy on the effort to sustain respiration. Mechanical ventilation is frequently used. If adaptations are successful, respiratory distress diminishes within 3 to 5 days as surfactant production increases and alveoli expand. Death is rare after 72 hours in cases of uncomplicated RDS.

Surfactant replacement therapy through an endotracheal tube has been demonstrated in recent clinical trials to improve survival and reduce the severity of RDS (Dunn, Shennan, Zayack, & Possmayer, 1991). Surfactant replacement therapy may be given before the newborn's first breath (still in clinical trials), within a few minutes of birth (preventive therapy), or after signs of RDS have developed ("rescue" or treatment therapy). Doses may be repeated up to three times.

Apnea. Preterm neonates may suffer from apneic episodes, even in the absence of identified disorders, as a result of immature neurologic and pulmonary function. Continued severe apnea will result in decreased PaO_2, increased $PaCO_2$, and acidosis. Theophylline or caffeine, both respiratory stimulants and bronchodilators, are used in the treatment of apnea with good results.

High Risk for Altered Cardiac Output. The major cardiovascular adaptation in full-term and preterm neonates is the change from fetal to neonatal circulation. Fetal circulatory bypasses close as a result of an increase in systemic blood pressure, lung expansion, and the shift in pressure gradients from the right side of the heart to the left. A rise in blood oxygen concentration also facilitates closure of the ductus arteriosus. Incomplete development of the pulmonary system in the preterm infant significantly affects major cardiovascular adaptations.

Patent Ductus Arteriosus. In the full-term neonate the ductus arteriosus is sensitive to oxygen and constricts with rising PaO_2 levels. It is hypothesized that immature muscular development of the ductus arteriosus in the preterm neonate results in the incomplete constriction and closure of this fetal shunt. As systemic blood pressure rises, primarily due to umbilical cord clamping and the removal of the low pressure placenta from the circulatory system, and pressure in the right side of the heart decreases, left-to-right shunting occurs. Shunting results in an increased blood volume entering the pulmonary vessels and leads to pulmonary congestion, decreased lung compliance, and increased respiratory effort. Pulmonary congestion, in turn, impairs adequate gas exchange and results in hypoxia. The accompanying Nursing Care Plan discusses the preterm neonate with PDA.

The vicious cycle initiated with PDA and shunting of blood is difficult to reverse. In some newborns PDA can be managed successfully by fluid restriction. Indomethacin, a prostaglandin-inhibitor, has been used with moderate success to constrict the ductus arteriosus, but it has severe side effects, including renal failure and gastrointestinal bleeding. Surgical ligation of the ductus is used in the treatment of PDA, but surgery poses major risks for the unstable preterm neonate. Despite the potential untoward effects, PDA must be treated. The persistent hypoxic perfusion of the gut promotes ischemia and necrosis of the mucosal lining, eventually resulting in perforation.

High Risk for Fluid Volume Deficits. Immaturity in the structure and function of the renal system produces fluid

Text continues on page 1025

Nursing Care Plan

The Preterm Neonate

PATIENT PROFILE

History

Baby P is a 7-day-old preterm, appropriate for gestational age neonate born at 32 weeks' gestation. Her weight was 1750 g (3 lb 14 oz) at birth. The Apgar scores were 7 and 8 at 1 and 5 minutes. Umbilical cord blood pH and gases were within normal limits. This female neonate experience mild respiratory distress syndrome (RDS) of prematurity. There were no complications related to oxygen therapy and mechanical ventilation or the umbilical artery line that was inserted for ABG analysis. They were discontinued on the fourth postnatal day.

Baby P initially received parenteral nutrition through a peripheral IV line. Intermittent oral gavage feedings were initiated 2 days ago. She is receiving 20 mL of a 24 calorie/oz premature infant formula q3h. The neonate remains in an incubator in a neutral thermal environment. This morning Baby P weight 1520 g (3 lb 6 oz). She gained 5 g during the last 24 h.

Baby P has been diagnosed with a patent ductus arteriosus (PDA). She has had two apnea episodes lasting approximately 25 to 30 sec with bradycardia to 90 BPM during the night and one time this morning. They resolved with gentle tactile stimulation. She has not experienced apnea prior to this.

Physical Assessment

The nurse assesses Baby P at 12 noon prior to a gavage feeding and notes the following data:

T 36.3 C, P 168, RR 50. Incubator temperature is 29.5 C. The neonate's tone is appropriate for her gestational age, and no change in tone is noted from the last assessment. The skin is pink. Baby P is in a quiet drowsy state. The heart rate is regular, and there is a loud systolic murmur. The oxygen saturation (SaO_2) is 95%. Peripheral pulses are +3 (strong but not bounding). The breath sounds are clear and equal bilaterally. The abdomen is soft, and there are bowel sounds in all four quadrants. A 2-mL gastric residual is aspirated, and there is no increase in abdominal girth since the morning feeding. The liver is palpable 1 cm below the right costal border. She has passed a small, formed yellow stool, which is heme negative. Clear, pale yellow urine is noted on the diaper, which weighs 10 g on the diaper scale.

COLLABORATIVE PROBLEMS/POTENTIAL COMPLICATIONS

- Intraventricular hemorrhage
- Patent ductus arteriosus
- Respiratory distress syndrome
- Anemia
- Retinopathy
- Necrotizing enterocolitis
- Hypolycemia
- Congestive heart failure
- Kernicterus

(See the accompanying Nursing Alert display).

Assessment	*Nursing Diagnosis*	*Nursing Interventions*	*Rationale*
Baby P is a 7-day-old preterm neonate born at 32 weeks' gestation. She was appropriate for her gestational age.	Ineffective Breathing Pattern related to prematurity and patent ductus arteriosus *Expected Outcome* Baby P establishes effective respiratory function as evi-	Maintain continuous cardiorespiratory monitor and pulse oximetry. Set alarms, and turn alarm system on.	To alert the nurse to alterations in cardiorespiratory function or oxygen desaturation.

(*Continued*)

The Preterm Neonate

(Continued)

Assessment	*Nursing Diagnosis*	*Nursing Interventions*	*Rationale*
She weighs 1520 g. She experienced mild RDS. She has had three episodes of apnea since midnight lasting 25 to 30 sec with bradycardia to 90 BPM, which resolved with gentle tactile stimulation.	denced by a respiratory rate between 30 and 60 breaths per minute. Baby P remains free of apnea and bradycardia episodes.	Position neonate to facilitate chest expansion (prone may be best).	The preterm neonate with weak chest and abdominal muscles may have difficulty with chest expansion in the supine or sidelying position.
		Place suction and ventilation equipment inside incubator.	To facilitate prompt treatment of apnea.
		Maintain neutral thermal environment.	Hypothermia and hyperthermia can precipate.
		Use gentle tactile stimulation. Place neonate on a rocker or water bed. Use audio device that simulates maternal heart beat.	Tactile and auditory stimulation may break apnea or bradycardia episodes and facilitate regular respiratory efforts.
		Implement bag and mask ventilation if gentle stimulation is not successful in restoring respirations.	If gentle stimulation does not result in respiratory efforts, positive pressure ventilation is necessary to prevent hypoxia.
		Assess serum glucose level as ordered with apnea episode.	Hypoglycemia may cause apnea.
		Assess neonate for evidence of necrotizing enterocolitis (NEC) or worsening of PDA.	The development of complications such as NEC or PDA may precipitate apnea.
		Administer theophylline as ordered.	Theophylline is a CNS stimulant, which may decrease the frequency of apnea episodes.
Baby P is a preterm neonate born at 32 weeks' gestation. Pulse 168; +3 pulses Loud systolic murmur three episodes of apnea Baby P has a PDA.	Decreased Cardiac Output related to patent ductus arteriosus *Expected Outcome* Baby P will demonstrate normal cardiac function as evidenced by heart rate range of 120 to 160 BPM, regular rhythm, quiet precordium, +2 peripheral pulses. Baby P's PDA will close with advancing gestational age or treatment.	Strictly monitor intake and output. Weigh diapers. Weigh neonate daily.	Early identification of fluid imbalance permits timely intervention and may prevent PDA. Fluid overload may facilitate reopening of PDA or precipitate congestive heart failure (CHF) with PDA.
		Assess neonate for evidence of peripheral edema.	Peripheral edema is an indicator of fluid retention or overload.
		Assess pulses q 3–4 h for quality and pressure.	Bounding pulses and rising blood pressure are indicators of fluid overload and may indicate PDA or CHF.
		Auscultate heart sounds and breath sounds q 3–4 h. Assess blood pressure q 4–8 h.	Pulmonary edema may occur with fluid overload, PDA, or CHF. Murmur may be indicator of PDA. Systolic murmur

(Continued)

The Preterm Neonate

(*Continued*)

Assessment	*Nursing Diagnosis*	*Nursing Interventions*	*Rationale*
			may be loudest when PDA is opening or closing.
		Observe chest wall for evidence of heart action.	Visible heart action (active precordium) may indicate PDA or CHF.
		Use infusion pump to administer IV fluids.	To prevent accidental bolus of IV fluid.
		Restrict fluid intake as ordered.	To prevent fluid overload.
		Administer diuretics (Lasix) or cardiotonics (digoxin) as ordered.	To facilitate fluid excretion and prevent or decrease symptoms of PDA.
		Administer indomethacin as ordered.	Cardiotonics may be necessary to treat CHF. Indomethacin is a prostaglandin synthetase inhibitor used to promote closure of PDA.
		Organize care to decrease periods of activity.	Neonate with PDA or CHF has minimal reserves and requires extended periods of rest to prevent deterioration in condition.
		Maintain neutral thermal environment.	To reduce energy expenditure required to maintain body temperature.
		Administer preoperative drugs or IV fluids if surgical ligation of PDA planned.	Surgical ligation of PDA may be required if drug therapy is unsuccessful.
Baby P's temperature is 36.3°C (97.3°F). Incubator temperature is 29.5°C.	Ineffective Thermoregulation related to prematurity. ***Expected Outcome*** Baby P will maintain a temperature between 36.4°C (97.5°F) and 37.2°C (99.0°F).	Monitor neonate's temperature q 3–4 h or before each feeding.	To facilitate early identification and treatment of hypothermia.
Baby P has had three episodes of apnea since midnight.		Maintain neutral thermal environment.	To promote normal temperature range in neonate, thus preventing hypothermia.
Weight is 1520 g and neonate was born at 32 wk 7 days ago.		Place heat shield or insulating blanket over neonate.	To prevent heat loss by convection and conduction
		Keep incubator away from air vents or outside walls.	To prevent heat loss by radiation
		Warm hand and stethescope before touching neonate.	
		Warm linen and other equipment before placing on neonate.	To prevent heat loss by evaporation
		Keep skin and linens dry.	

(*Continued*)

The Preterm Neonate

(Continued)

Assessment	*Nursing Diagnosis*	*Nursing Interventions*	*Rationale*
		Place cap on neonate's head.	Head is largest surface (25% of total surface) and results in significant heat loss.
		Use skin temperature (servo-control) device.	To alert nurse to temperature swings
		Assess serum glucose level when hypothermia occurs.	Hypoglycemia may cause or result from hypothermia or temperature instability.
Oral gavage feedings started 2 days ago. Baby P is a 7-day-old preterm neonate born at 32 weeks' gestation. Weight is 1520 g. Abdomen is soft and nondistended. Bowel sounds in all four quadrants. Passed small, formed, yellow stool. No increase in abdomen girth since last feeding. 2 ml gastric residual.	High Risk for Altered Bowel Elimination: NEC related to prematurity and PDA ***Expected Outcome*** Baby P will not develop NEC.	Assess vital signs q 3–4 h or before each feeding.	To facilitate early identification and treatment of NEC.
		Measure and record abdominal girth before each feeding.	Abnormal increase in girth may indicate NEC.
		Palpate abdomen before each feeding.	Distended, tender, or erythematous abdomen are indicators of NEC.
		Assess neonate for gastric residual before each oral gavage feeding. Hold oral feedings if gastric residual is greater than 25% of previous oral intake, and notify physician.	To obtain medical evaluation and further physician orders.
		Auscultate bowel sounds before each feeding.	Absent bowel sounds may indicate development of NEC.
		Test all stools for occult blood or heme.	Presence of blood may indicate NEC.
		Promptly respond to apnea episodes.	Hypoxia may cause shunting of blood from bowel and contribute to the development of NEC.
Baby P has lost 230 g since birth (approximately 14% of birth weight). Neonate has gained 5 g in past 24 h. Neonate is receiving 20 mL of 24 cal/oz premature infant formula. Neonate receives oral gavage feedings q 3 h. Neonate has 3 mL gastric residual.	High risk for Altered Nutrition: Less than Body Requirements related to prematurity ***Expected Outcome*** Baby P will gain 10 to 15 g/day. Baby P's stool will remain free of glucose. Baby P takes feedings without becoming fatigued.	Weigh daily and record weight gain or loss.	To identify inadequate growth
		Assess for gastric residual before each feeding.	Presence of residuals may indicate intolerance to formula.
		Observe and evaluate for evidence of fatigue or exhaustion with feedings.	Excessive expenditure of energy when the neonate feeds will prevent weight gain.
		Observe for development of suck, swallow, and gag reflexes.	Development of feeding reflexes will permit advancing neonate to bottle feeding or breastfeeding.
		Test stools for presence of glucose.	Presence of glucose may indicate intolerance to formula.
		Maintain neutral thermal environment.	Excessive expenditure of calories to maintain temperature results in poor weight gain.

(Continued)

The Preterm Neonate

(Continued)

Assessment	*Nursing Diagnosis*	*Nursing Interventions*	*Rationale*
		Test serum glucose levels as ordered or with jitteriness.	Inadequate intake may result in hypoglycemia.
		Place neonate on right side after feeding.	To promote stomach emptying.
		Elevate HOB 10–30 degrees after feeding.	To prevent regurgitation of formula through weak cardiac sphincter.

EVALUATION Baby P gained 10 to 15 g/d during the following 2 weeks and remained free of signs and symptoms of formula intolerance. She progressed to bottle feeding within 10 days when the suck, swallow, and gag reflexes developed. Baby P was discharged 30 days after birth weighing 1950 g.

NURSING ALERT

NURSING RESPONSIBILITIES WHEN PHYSIOLOGIC DECOMPENSATION OCCURS IN THE PRETERM NEONATE

Rapid deterioration may occur in the preterm neonate due to the development of life-threatening complications, such as sepsis, necrotizing enterocolitis, or pneumothroax. Sudden changes in the neonate's status that require immediate emergency care include the following:

- Apnea
- Bradycardia
- Hypotension
- Hypoxia or hypercapnia

When the neonate exhibits any of these signs, the nurse should call for assistance and initiate supportive measures. In some cases the neonate may be removed from the mechanical ventilator, and hand ventilation with a anesthesia bag may be indicated to establish more effective gas exchange. The nurse may be asked to assist the physician with rapid evaluation of pleural air associated with a pneumothorax by providing equipment and positioning the infant. Vasopressors such as dopamine may be initiated to sustain the neonate's blood pressure.

The nurse caring for the preterm neonate must be prepared to act promptly and at times independently until medical help arrives to maintain the neonate's vital functions. The neonatal nurse is guided by standardized protocols, preprinted physician orders, and hospital policy and procedure when initiating emergency measures such as those described.

and electrolyte imbalances in the preterm neonate. The diminished ability to concentrate urine or excrete fluids efficiently increases the risk for dehydration and overhydration. There is an increased risk for metabolic acidosis because of excessive bicarbonate loss. The preterm neonate is susceptible to fluid volume deficits and dehydration as a result of increased frank and insensible fluid losses and the inability to conserve water.

High Risk for Altered Nutrition. The preterm neonate's immature gastrointestinal tract prevents ingestion, digestion, and absorption of essential nutrients. Suck, swallow, and gag reflexes are often absent, requiring the delivery of nutrients by alternative routes. The stomach capacity is greatly reduced and requires that nutrients be introduced in very small volumes. Liver glycogen stores are minimal, so the neonate is at risk for development of hypoglycemia. Digestive enzymes and bile salts also may be deficient, resulting in inadequate digestion of nutrients. Neonates who are capable of nipple feeding are easily exhausted by sucking efforts and may experience episodes of apnea, bradycardia, and cyanosis during feeding. Finally, commercial formulas available for the full-term neonate do not provide sufficient calories and minerals for growth nor the appropriate proportions of casein and whey for the preterm neonate.

Necrotizing Enterocolitis. The preterm newborn is at great risk for the development of NEC, a disorder in which necrosis of the bowel is associated with mucosal injury from asphyxia and ischemia. It is hypothesized that hypoxia leads to shunting of blood from the kidney, intestines, and muscles to the brain, heart, and adrenals to sustain essential neurologic, cardiac, and metabolic functioning. Cell death follows this "gut shunting," allowing entrance of enteric bacteria into the mucosal lining of the gut. Gases created by proliferation of the bacteria accumulate and eventually cause bowel wall necrosis. Perforation of the intestinal wall also can occur. Localized infection and septicemia frequently complicate the condition. Figure 33-12 illustrates the possible etiology and consequences of NEC.

Surgical intervention often is necessary to remove necrotic sections of the bowel, and a temporary colostomy may be performed. A small percentage of neonates develop "short gut syndrome" after surgery. The neonate suffers from chronic malnutrition and failure to thrive secondary to removal of large sections of the intestines and incomplete absorption of nutrients. The mortality rate for NEC is high, ranging between 30% and 40% (Cloherty & Stark, 1991).

Intraventricular Hemorrhage. Intraventricular hemorrhage is the most common type of central nervous system hemorrhage in preterm neonates. It is associated with asphyxia and resultant hypoxia and hypercapnia; immaturity; infusion of hyperosmotic substances, such as sodium bicarbonate; and impaired cerebral autoregulation (Dietsch, 1993).

Hemorrhage occurs in tissue surrounding the ventricles. The blood then enters the brain cavities, circulating in the cerebrospinal fluid. The neonate who sustains a catastrophic intraventricular hemorrhage experiences a sudden deterioration in his or her condition. There is shock with depressed or absent vital signs. Seizures may be evident. Bulging fontanelles, falling hematocrit, hypothermia, and hypotonia also are observed. Prognosis and long-term neurologic sequelae depend on the extent of the bleeding.

Hypothermia. Preterm neonates have little ability to generate heat or prevent heat loss. Heat production is limited by minimal brown fat and glycogen stores and the immaturity of the thermoregulatory center. Heat loss is greater than in the full-term neonate because the preterm neonate has little subcutaneous fat, has a much larger ratio of body surface to mass, and remains in a more relaxed, less flexed posture.

Infection. Maternal antibodies cross the placenta after 32 to 34 weeks of gestation, and the very premature neonate is deprived of these immunoglobulins and becomes more susceptible to infection. Preterm neonates also are at increased risk for infection because their immunity is depressed, and the skin is immature. The invasive nature of diagnostic procedures and treatments, such as mechanical ventilation and umbilical catheters, place the neonate at further risk for infection.

Hyperbilirubinemia. Because the liver is immature and the number of albumin-binding sites is decreased, the preterm neonate is at greater risk for hyperbilirubinemia and jaundice. Hemolysis associated with sepsis, acidosis, and bleeding disorders also increases the incidence of jaundice in preterm infants. Kernicterus and irreversible brain damage can occur at much lower blood levels of bilirubin than in the full-term newborn. As a result, blood exchange transfusions and phototherapy are initiated earlier.

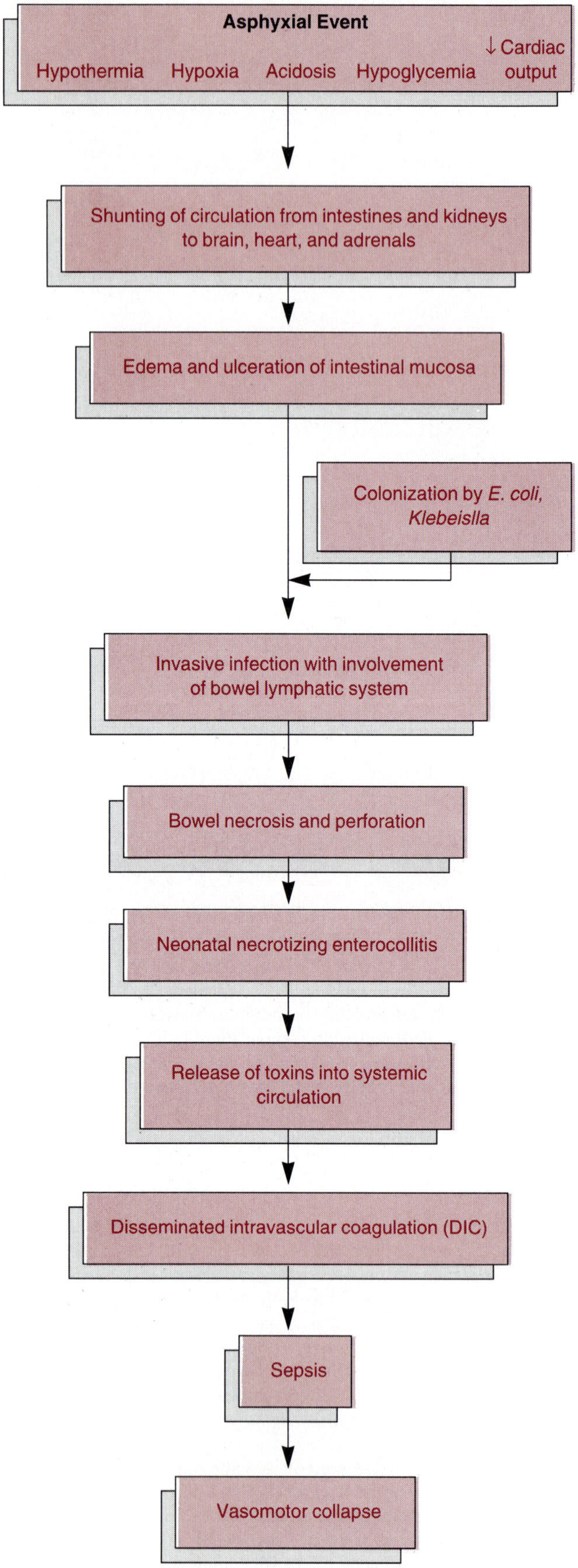

Figure 33-12.
Possible causes and consequences of neonatal NEC.

Impaired Mobility. Flexion is essential for the development of normal body movement and control, but most preterm neonates are born before physiologic flexion has developed. Preterm newborns are at risk for impaired mobility later in life as a result of postural problems and improper body mechanics in the nursery rather than from neurologic impairment. For instance some neonates eventually exhibit rigid posturing, arching of the back, and other abnormal motor patterns, such as toe walking, the inability to place the heel of the foot flat on the floor. Excessive hypotonia and muscle flexibility in the preterm neonate, coupled with improper positioning and handling by nursery personnel result in these nursery-acquired mobility problems.

High Risk for Altered Parenting and Behavioral Adaptation. The preterm neonate is exposed to numerous environmental stimuli and physical insults in the neonatal intensive care unit. A premature birth causes separation from the comforting world of the womb, and immaturity often limits cuddling or comforting by the parents for a prolonged period. After the neonate has achieved physiologic stability, an incubator is used until adequate growth and development permit transfer to a crib or bassinet. Social isolation and further distortion of external stimuli occur in incubators. Under these conditions the development of sensory-perceptual capabilities can be adversely affected.

Implications for Nursing Care

Supporting Physiologic Functioning. Nursing care of the preterm neonate is focused on supporting major physiologic adaptations, preventing complications, and supporting the parents. Encouraging behavioral implementation of this care is discussed earlier in this chapter.

Apneic episodes can be decreased or eliminated in many preterm neonates by nursing care aimed at maintaining body temperature, reducing adverse environmental stimuli, ensuring minimal handling, and placing the neonate in a prone position to stabilize the chest wall.

Promoting Neuromuscular Development. The infant is positioned to promote flexion, avoid excessive extension, and maintain symmetric positioning (Fig. 33-13). Placing the newborn in a prone position with its arms and legs flexed and close to the body is the optimum position. If the neonate must be supine to accommodate equipment and procedures, blanket rolls can be placed around the body to encourage as much flexion as possible and to prevent later arching behaviors. Providing the neonate with boundaries that contain his or her movements also supports flexion, promotes comfort, and may assist in optimal neuromuscular development as the neonate learns to control muscles and body parts by pushing against firm surfaces.

Supporting Behavioral Adaptation. Initially the preterm neonate will demonstrate periods of behavioral disorganization related to neurologic immaturity and illness and will be unable to respond in predictable and appropriate ways to stimuli. Routine nursing care activities and interaction can result in rapid neonatal physiologic deterioration. Sleep patterns are different from those demonstrated in the full-term neonate. As the condition stabilizes, the neonate will be able to engage in very short periods of reciprocal interaction with caregivers but will become quickly exhausted by these encounters.

It may take many months before the preterm neonate begins to exhibit the behavioral patterns of full-term neonates. Parents may be unable to reconcile their fantasized image of their child with the preterm newborn presented to them. They may become discouraged when their attempts to communicate do not produce the expected response. Furthermore, if the neonate actually experiences physiologic decompensation during interaction with parents, they may become frightened and withdraw from future efforts at interation.

Caution must be taken in providing stimulation to preterm infants and in protecting them from sensory overload and overstimulation. The preterm infant may become exhausted or overwhelmed by positive and negative stimuli.

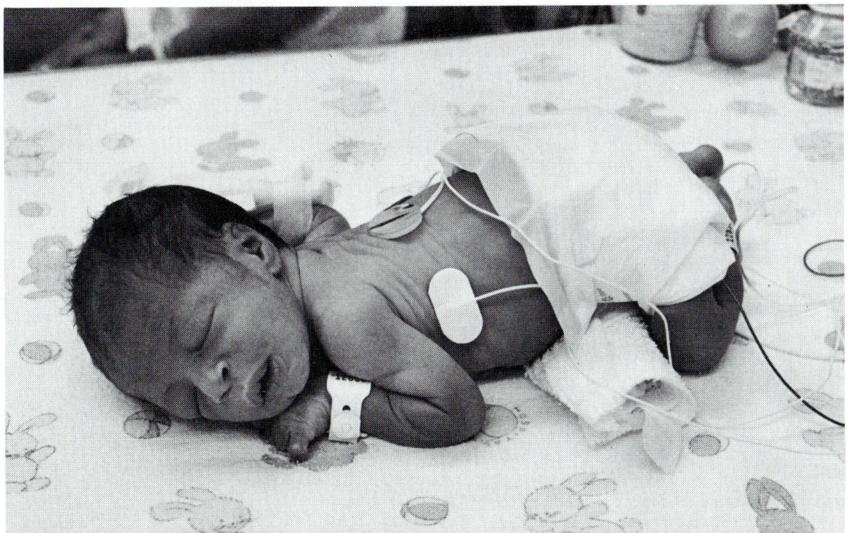

Figure 33-13.
Correct flexion can be encouraged in the neonate by bringing knees up to the chest, placing arms close to the body, and placing a small roll under the hips when the neonate is in the prone position. (Adapted from Fry, M. [1988]. The positive effect of positioning. *Neonatal Network*, 6[5], 23–28.)

Signs of sensory overload are listed in the display on neonatal behavior in the intensive care nursery in the assessment section earlier in the chapter.

Once overloaded, the preterm infant tends to recover best if left alone. In general the preterm infant needs stimuli presented in small amounts, at slower rates and may require greater exposure to derive optimal benefit from the stimulus. Initially the infant may find a single stimulus modality (ie, experiencing only visual or only auditory stimuli rather than auditory and visual stimuli together) less stressful.

Nursing interventions with parents include teaching regarding neonatal behavioral abilities, states, and alerting and consoling (or soothing) maneuvers; their neonate's unique behavioral characteristics and signs of overload; anticipatory guidance regarding developmental changes; and opportunities for positive interactions with their neonate. Teaching guidelines concerning neonatal sensory stimulation for the stabilized preterm neonate are given in the display.

Teaching Considerations

Sensory Stimulation Techniques for Stable Preterm Neonates

The nurse can use the following points about sensory stimulation when teaching parents with stable preterm neonates.

Touch

- Gently stroke skin in head-to-toe direction at a rate of approximately 12 strokes per minute.
- Expose to a variety of texture, including cotton, satin, and silk.

Taste

- Allow neonate to such on a pacifier (if not contraindicated by a gastrointestinal or respiratory anomaly) to stimulate salivary glands and digestive enzymes.

Vision

- Place black and white schematic faces in an *en face* position within visual range (19 to 22 cm).
- Provide time for eye-to-eye contact.
- Periodically reduce intensity of lights.

Smell

- Introduce different pleasant-smelling odors, including the smell of the mother's breast milk if she intends to breastfeed.

Hearing

- Play a tape recording of the parents' voices
- Play soft classical music
- Eliminate loud and unnecessary noises.

Kinesthetics

- Place the neonate on an oscillating bed
- Periodically rock the neonate or place him or her in a swing.

The Small-for-Gestational Age Neonate

Although the SGA neonate resembles the preterm neonate in size, the physical characteristics and physiologic capabilities are quite different. The SGA neonate is any neonate (regardless of gestational age) whose weight falls below the tenth percentile or is 2 standard deviations below the mean.

Intrauterine Growth Retardation

The low birth weight and subsequent physiologic adaptations are a result of intrauterine growth retardation (IUGR) caused by a variety of prenatal conditions. Table 33-5 provides an expanded list of disorders and other factors associated with inadequate intrauterine growth. (See Chapter 27 on chronic maternal disease, especially diabetes, and its effects on placental functioning.)

Two types of IUGR have been identified. These affect the general appearance of the neonate and the potential for normal growth and mental development after birth.

Symmetric IUGR occurs when the fetus has experienced early and prolonged nutritional deprivation caused by severe chronic maternal malnutrition, intrauterine infection, fetal congenital malformations, chromosomal anomalies, or genetic disorders. Hypoplastic cell growth and development occur, and there is a generalized deficiency in cell numbers throughout the body and in the size of all organ systems. The neonate's body and head appear small (proportional growth retardation). Head circumference often falls below the tenth percentile. This condition is associated with diminished brain size and permanent mental retardation. The neonate never catches up with other neonates of the same gestational age whose birth weights fall within the mean.

Asymmetric IUGR, in contrast, results from nutritional deficits and placental insufficiency in late pregnancy. Atrophy of preexisting cells occurs, resulting in diminished cell size, but cell numbers are not reduced. The neonate appears to have a disproportionately large head in relation to his or her body (disproportional growth retardation). The body is long and emaciated, with little subcutaneous fat. There is evidence of generalized muscle wasting, and the abdomen is wrinkled and scaphoid in shape. The skin has very poor turgor, the hair on the scalp is coarse and sparse, and underlying sutures are widely separated. Although these neonates fall below the tenth percentile for birth weight, head circumference approaches the norm on the growth curve. Postnatal growth and development are rapid, and the potential for normal intellectual functioning is excellent.

Neonatal Implications

High Risk for Impaired Gas Exchange. Perinatal asphyxia is increased in the SGA newborn. These neonates

Table 33-5. Maternal Factors Associated With Intrauterine Growth Retardation

Obstetric Complications	Medical Complications	Socioeconomic Factors	Environmental Factors
History of infertility History of abortions Grand multiparity Pregnancy-induced hypertension	Heart disease Renal disease Chronic hypertension Sickle cell disease Phenylketonuria Diabetes mellitus (class D, E, F, or R) Other chronic diseases	Low socioeconomic status Maternal age (extremes of youth and age) Absence of prenatal care Marital status (single)	Poor living conditions High altitude Use of therapeutic drugs: Antimetabolites Anticonvulsants Substance abuse Alcohol Drugs Cigarettes Malnutrition

may experience chronic hypoxia in utero due to altered placental function with diminished oxygen transfer. As a result the neonate may be unable to tolerate the additional stresses of labor and delivery. Aspiration of meconium in utero is associated with asphyxia and results from relaxation of the anal sphincter and respiratory gasping secondary to hypoxia. The presence of meconium in the airways and alveoli at birth prevents adequate gas exchange after birth (see the section "Meconium Aspiration Syndrome" later in this chapter). Meconium aspiration is seen only in term or near-term SGA neonates.

High Risk for Hypoglycemia, Hypothermia, and Polycythemia. IUGR results in minimal stores of liver glycogen. The SGA neonate is therefore at risk for hypoglycemia in the period immediately after birth.

All low–birth-weight neonates are at risk for hypothermia because limited stores of brown fat and liver glycogen prevent adequate heat production. Heat loss is increased as a result of the SGA neonate's large surface area in relation to mass and the lack of adipose tissue to serve as insulation.

Chronic intrauterine hypoxia appears to cause increased RBC production (polycythemia). When the neonate's hematocrit rises above 65% to 70%, problems related to increased blood viscosity (thick blood syndrome), including respiratory distress, cyanosis, renal vein thrombosis, hypoglycemia, and congestive heart failure, occur. A partial exchange transfusion is performed to remove some of the RBCs. The RBCs are replaced with fresh frozen plasma or 5% albumin.

Implications for Nursing Care

Nursing care is aimed at supporting physiologic adaptations after birth and preventing major complications associated with this disorder. Because IUGR is frequently associated with maternal disease or life-style (eg, alcoholism, smoking, or absence of prenatal care), the mother may experience overwhelming feelings of failure and guilt and will require ongoing emotional support. Newborns frequently require referrals for continued care and evaluation at discharge. See the accompanying Nursing Care Plan for the SGA neonate.

The Large-for-Gestational Age Neonate

The LGA neonate belies the maxim "a fat baby is a healthy baby." LGA infants are at risk for a variety of complications. Birth injuries, including fractures and intracranial hemorrhage, are more common, as are hypoglycemia, polycythemia, and perinatal asphyxia. Major physiologic adaptations are related to these complications. The predisposing factors for excessive size (defined as birth weight over 4000 g [8 lb, 13 oz], above the 90th percentile, or 2 standard deviations above the mean for gestational age) include genetic predisposition, excessive maternal weight gain during pregnancy, and maternal gestational diabetes.

Infant of a Diabetic Mother

The infant of a diabetic mother (IDM) is often LGA as a result of the high levels of maternal glucose that cross the placenta during pregnancy and the effect of fetal hyperinsulinism on cell growth. (Women with severe or long-standing diabetes with vascular changes, which in turn cause decreased placental functioning, usually deliver neonates who are growth retarded or SGA.) The IDM is at risk for the classic complications of the LGA infant.

Neonatal Implications

Transient Tachypnea of the Newborn. Transient tachypnea of the newborn (TTN) is the most common form of respiratory distress seen in IDMs. TTN may be related to the IDM's decreased level of surfactant production and to delayed clearance of fetal lung fluid. TTN is seen more frequently in infants delivered by cesarean (who are frequently LGA), probably due to insufficient thoracic "squeeze" resulting in retained fetal lung fluid.

Hypoglycemia. The IDM's blood glucose levels are high at birth because of maternal hyperglycemia (which readily crosses the placenta). Pancreatic insulin production is also high because the neonate's islet cells are hypertrophied. The neonatal blood glucose level begins to drop

Text continues on page 1034

Nursing Care Plan

The Large-for-Gestational Age Neonate of a Diabetic Mother

PATIENT PROFILE

History

Baby Girl H is a 5300 g (11 lb 11 oz) large-for-gestational age (LGA) neonate born at 39 weeks' gestation by cesarean delivery. The L/S ratio was 2:1, and phosphatidyl glycerol (PG) was detectable. The surgical birth was scheduled due to fetal macrosomia, a sudden decrease in maternal insulin requirements, and a deteriorating biophysical profile. Baby H's mother, G1/P1, is a gestational diabetic who was unable to comply with dietary restrictions. She gained 75 lb during pregnancy and required insulin by the 30th week of gestation. There was difficulty extracting the neonate from the uterus during the cesarean delivery due to her size. The right clavicle appeared fractured, and chest x-ray confirmed the diagnosis.

Physical Assessment

Baby H was admitted to the observation nursery 20 minutes after birth and is noted to be markedly jittery. She was placed under a radiant warmer after she was weighed, and the following data is obtained: T 36.9°C (98.4°F), P 156, RR 76. The skin is pink with acrocyanosis. There is normal muscle tone, and an asymmetric Moro reflex that is decreased in the right arm. Baby H is alert and exhibits rooting and strong suck. She has a vigorous cry. The heart rate is regular and +2 peripheral pulses are palpated. There is marked nasal flaring, audible grunting, and intermittent intercostal retraction. Rales are auscultated bilaterally in right and left lower lobes. The abdomen is protuberant and soft. There are no bowel sounds. No stool or urine has been passed yet.

There is ecchymosis over the midportion of the right clavicle, and crepitus is noted on palpation of this area of the bone. The neonate begins to cry when the assessment of the clavicles is performed. Baby H demonstrates instant, symmetric recoil of the forearms when they are extended at the elbow. A strong palmar grasp is elicited in both right and left hand.

A heel stick capillary blood sample is obtained. The Chemstrip glucose reading is 20 mg/dL. The hematocrit is 56%.

COLLABORATIVE PROBLEMS/POTENTIAL COMPLICATIONS

- Birth trauma
- Transient tachypnea of the newborn
- Respiratory distress syndrome
- Congenital anomalies
- Hypoglycemia
- Hypocalcemia
- Polycythemia

(See the accompanying Nursing Alert display.)

Assessment	*Nursing Diagnosis*	*Nursing Interventions*	*Rationale*
Baby H is 38 weeks' gestation and a neonate of a diabetic mother. RR is 72. Rales are auscultated in lower lobes of lung bilaterally. Neonate exhibits flaring, grunting, and intermittent intercostal retraction.	Impaired Gas Exchange related to possible incomplete surfactant production or retained lung fluid. *Expected Outcome* Baby H will establish a normal respiratory pattern as evidenced by a respiratory rate of 30 to 60 breaths per min-	Assess respirations, respiratory efforts, and breath sounds q 30 min or more frequently until stable Then q 1 h for 4 h, then q 3–4 h as ordered and indicated by Baby H's condition. Attach cardiorespiratory monitor and pulse oximeter.	To alert nurse to alterations or deterioration in cardiorespiratory status and permits prompt treatment

(*Continued*)

The Large-for-Gestational Age Neonate of a Diabetic Mother

(Continued)

Assessment	Nursing Diagnosis	Nursing Interventions	Rationale
L/S ratio is 2:1 with PG is detectable.	ute and absence of flaring, grunting, and retractions.	Attach transcutaneous o_2 and Co_2 ($TcPo_2/Co_2$) monitor as ordered.	A $TcPo_2$ and Co_2 monitor is usually used when oxygen therapy is ordered to monitor blood oxygen and carbon dioxide levels.
			The neonate of a diabetic woman is at increased risk for RDS due to slower surfactant production.
			The neonate born by cesarean delivery may experience transient tachypnea and signs of respiratory distress because of retained lung fluid.
		Position neonate to maintain head in neutral or "sniffing" position and in supine position with head of bed	Hyperextended or flexed neck may cause airway obstruction.
			Macrosomia neonate may experience greater difficulty with respiratory excursions when the abdominal contents expert pressure on the diaphragm.
		(HOB) elevated 10%.	Elevating the HOB will displace abdominal contents downward, relieving pressure on diaghragm.
		Aspirate air and gastric contents from stomach.	Stomach distention prevents full respiratory excursion.
		Withhold oral feedings until respiratory status is stable.	Neonate with respiratory distress can become rapidly exhausted when attempting to bottle feed or breastfeed, leading to further deterioration in respiratory status.
		Administer oxygen as ordered.	Hypoxia can lead to persistent pulmonary hypertension and reestablishment of fetal bypasses.
		Monitor oxygen contraction with oxygen analyzer.	To verify that neonate is receiving correct percentage of oxygen
Baby H is a 5300-g (11 lb 11 oz) neonate of a diabetic mother.	High Risk for Injury related to hypoglycemia	Assess Chemstrip on admission to nursery and q 30 min until stable, then q 1 h until feedings initiated.	To promptly identify and treat hypoglycemia, which may result CNS injury or death.
Neonate is markedly jittery.	***Expected Outcome*** Baby H will maintain a stable plasma glucose level between 40 mg/dL and 120 mg/dL.		
Chemstrip glucose test is 20 mg/dL.		Repeat Chemstrips before meals until plasma glucose	Jitteriness is a classic sign of hypoglycemia.

(Continued)

The Large-for-Gestational Age Neonate of a Diabetic Mother

(*Continued*)

Assessment	Nursing Diagnosis	Nursing Interventions	Rationale
Infant is tachypenic, and flaring, grunting, and retractions are noted.		level are stable, if neonate is jittery, and as ordered. If neonate's condition is unstable, initiate an IV line and administer 10% D/W (2 ml/kg/ per minute) followed by maintenance dose of 8 mg/kg/per minute.	To rapidly stabilize the glucose level Continuous IV infusion is required when glucose levels are fluctuating, neonatal condition is unstable, or oral feedings are contraindicated.
		When neonate is stable, initiate oral feeding of 5% D/W, formula, or breast milk as ordered.	Formula or breast milk should be initiated as soon as possible because they help to stabilize plasma glucose levels over several hours due to slower digestion and absorption than glucose.
Baby H is an LGA neonate who weighs 5300 g (11 lb 11oz). There was difficulty extracting the neonate during delivery due to macrosomia. Diagnosed with fracture of right clavicle. Neonate has asymmetric Moro but symmetric forearm recoil and strong palmar grasp in both hands.	High Risk for Injury related to macrosomia. ***Expected Outcome*** Baby H will be able to rest comfortably with positioning and stabilization of arm.	Assess neonate for evidence of trauma, such as ecchymosis, petechia, or skin lacerations. Skull fracture: • Palpable depression in skull • Scalp lacerations • Cephalhematoma Intracranial hemorrhage: • Severe head molding • Lethargy • Seizures • Apnea • Hypotonia Fractured clavicle: • Crepitus over area of fracture • Deformity over clavicle • Hematoma formation • Asymmetric Moro Erb-Duchenne or brachial plexus palsy: • Asymmetric or absent Moro • Flaccid arm • Weak or absent palmar grasp	To permit prompt identification and treatment of injuries Macrosomia may result in birth trauma due to difficult passage through birth canal or at time of delivery (shoulder dystocia). Soft-tissue damage, fractures, hematomas, and nerve injury are the most common injuries. The clavicle is the most commonly fractured bone due to its perpendicular angle in relation to the birth canal.

(*Continued*)

The Large-for-Gestational Age Neonate of a Diabetic Mother

(Continued)

Assessment	Nursing Diagnosis	Nursing Interventions	Rationale
		Bell's palsy (facial hemiparesis): • Asymmetry of facial movement • Drooping eyelid or lip on affected side • Lack of forehead wrinkling on affected side Phrenic nerve injury: • Respiratory distress • Decreased breath sounds in lower lung lobes • Absent rise in abdomen with inspiration	
		When fractured clavicle is diagnosed, keep neonate on unaffected side.	To promote comfort and healing of fracture
		Pin shirt sleeve on affected side to opposite shoulder.	Callus forms, and pain subsides in 7 to 10 days.
		Observe neonate for signs of jaundice.	If hematoma formation occurs with injury, hyperbilirubinemia and jaundice may occur.
Baby H is newborn of a diabetic woman.	High Risk for Injury related to hypocalcemia ***Expected Outcome*** Baby H will establish a calcium level greater than 7 mg/dL and less than 11 mg/dL	Assess neonate for evidence of hypocalcemia: • Jitteriness • Irritability • Seizures • Apnea • Chvostek's sign	The neonate of the diabetic woman is at increased risk for the development of hypocalcemia. To identify and facilitate prompt treatment of hypocalcemia. Signs and symptoms of hypocalcemia may be clinically indistinguishable from those of hypoglycemia.
		Obtain and monitor serum calcium levels as ordered. Notify physician is calcium level is below 7 mg/dL.	Laboratory tests are required to determine calcium and glucose levels.
		If level is less than 7 mg/dL, prepare for and administered IV calcium as ordered.	To restore normal calcium level
Baby H's mother is a G1/P1. Baby H requires special care of right arm and clavicle.	Knowledge Deficit related to care of fractured clavicle	Identify parent's knowledge level about fracture and caretaking skills.	Obtaining baseline data regarding parents' knowledge level and skills is the first step in formulating a teaching plan.

(Continued)

The Large-for-Gestational Age Neonate of a Diabetic Mother

(*Continued*)

Assessment	Nursing Diagnosis	Nursing Interventions	Rationale
	Expected Outcomes Baby H's parent(s) will demonstrate correct technique for positioning of the neonate and stabilization of the right arm.	Demonstrate proper positioning of Baby H on unaffected (left) side.	Providing information and role modeling skills is the first step in teaching parents special care.
	Baby H's parent(s) will verbalize satisfaction with their skill level before discharge.	Demonstrate stabilization techniques, such as pinning right sleeve to left side of shirt to form sling.	
		Provide parents with opportunities to practice skills before discharge.	Repeated opportunities for practice are essential for parents to become skilled and comfortable with providing specialized care.
		Offer positive reinforcement and encouragement of parental efforts at caregiving.	Positive feedback will increase parental self-esteem and feelings of competence with neonate care.

EVALUATION

A tentative diagnosis of "transient tachypnea of the newborn" was made. Baby H was placed in an oxygen hood, and oxygen therapy was initiated after arterial blood gas and pH analyses were performed. An FIO_2 of 0.30 was delivered. A radial artery line was inserted to assess arterial blood pH and gases. An IV line was initiated and the neonate received an infusion of 10% D/W. The glucose level stabilized in 4 h at 80 mg/dL. The respiratory rate slowly decreased to 45 breaths per minute. Flaring, grunting, and retractions ceased 12 hours after birth, and the ABGs were within normal limits. Oxygen therapy was then discontinued.

Oral feedings were initiated 24 hours after birth. The plasma glucose levels remained within normal limits. No signs of hypocalcemia developed. The parents demonstrated appropriate skill in stabilizing Baby H's right arm and positioning her for comfort. The neonate was discharged on the fourth postnatal day with breastfeeding well established.

after the umbilical cord is clamped, due to elimination of the glucose supply, but pancreatic activity (insulin production and release) remains high. Severe hypoglycemia can rapidly ensue unless glucose supplementation is given.

Congenital Anomalies. The incidence of congenital anomalies is higher in IDMs and is associated with the severity of the maternal diabetes. The most common defects seen are the central nervous system anomalies, congenital heart defects, and tracheoesophageal fistula. The basis for the increased risk of anomalies is thought to be maternal hyperglycemia during critical stages of fetal organ development in the first 2 months of gestation. Programs emphasizing metabolic control and intensive management of diabetic women before pregnancy and in the early weeks after conception have reduced the incidence of congenital anomalies in these newborns.

Polycythemia. The exact etiology of increased numbers of RBCs is not clearly understood, but IDMs are at greater risk than other neonates for polycythemia. Because IDMs may be delivered early to prevent fetal demise or the complications related to excessive size, they also fall prey to the complications of the premature neonates, one of which is polycythemia. Additionally, the increased hemolysis of fetal RBCs (due to the increased number) can lead to clinical jaundice and hyperbilirubinemia.

Perinatal Asphyxia. The IDM neonate is at greater risk for perinatal asphyxia for two primary reasons: (1) ex-

NURSING ALERT

NURSING CARE OF THE LARGE-FOR-GESTATIONAL-AGE NEONATE

The large-for-gestational age (LGA) neonate may suffer from significant trauma as well as metabolic alterations such as hypoglycemia. The nurse must complete a systematic assessment in a timely manner and implement more frequent monitoring of the neonate's vital signs, glucose levels, and postnatal adaptations. Signs of complications in the LGA neonate include the following:

- Head trauma (bruising, forceps marks, cephalhematoma)
- Facial asymmetry (facial nerve injury)
- Crepitus and bruising overlying clavicle (fracture)
- Decreased tone or flaccidity of arm (brachial palsy injury)
- Bruising or edema overlying humerus (fracture)
- Generalized hypotonia (asphyxia)
- Jitteriness, lethargy, temperature instability (hypoglycemia)
- Respiratory distress—tachypnea, flaring, grunting, retracting (surfactant deficiency)

If the nurse notes any of the above signs, the physician should be notified immediately. Continued close observation and supportive care of the neonate is maintained until a medical evaluation is completed and additional orders are written.

Hypoglycemia, indicated by a heel stick glucose reading of less than 40 mg/dL, should be treated immediately. The nurse is often guided by printed protocols that indicate the route of glucose administration and the type and amount of fluid to be administered. This permits timely treatment of hypoglycemia before the physician arrives.

cessive size resulting in prolonged descent through the birth canal, and (2) relative lack of surfactant resulting in impaired establishment of an air–liquid interface and resultant alveolar collapse. See the section of this chapter on the neonate with birth asphyxia, which examines perinatal asphyxia in depth.

Birth Injuries. The excessive size of IDM and LGA neonates, primarily neonates who weigh more than 4000 g (8 lb, 13 oz) at birth, places them at greater risk for birth injuries. Often a clavicle is intentionally broken to facilitate delivery when shoulder dystocia occurs. The nurse's responsibilities then focus on pain control and positioning the neonate to avoid impairing tissue perfusion or impeding the proper realignment of the fractured bone (see the section "Neonate With Fractures" later in this chapter).

Implications for Nursing Care

Nursing care of the IDM (and affected LGA) neonate is primarily aimed at preventing hypoglycemia through periodic monitoring of blood glucose levels using heel stick samples. Early oral feeding or an IV glucose infusion is initiated to maintain blood sugar levels, depending on the severity of the hypoglycemia. The nurse monitors the neonate closely for signs and symptoms of hypoglycemia, RDS, and hyperbilirubinemia. The neonate is assessed carefully at birth for signs of birth trauma (see the preceding Nursing Care Plan for the SGA neonate).

The Postterm Neonate

The postterm neonate is born after 42 weeks of gestation. Many of this neonate's problems are related to the compromised placental functioning and starvation associated with prolonged pregnancy. The newborn is long and very thin. The head appears disproportionately large because of the wasted appearance of the body. The skin is thick, wrinkled, and parchment-like, and there may be generalized peeling of the epidermis. There may be meconium staining of the skin, nails, and umbilical cord as a result of intrauterine hypoxia. The neonate has a wide-eyed, alert look and may suck hungrily at his or her hands.

The etiology of postmaturity is poorly understood. Fetal and maternal factors associated with postmaturity are the following:

- First pregnancy
- Grand multiparity (five or more pregnancies)
- History of prolonged pregnancy
- Anencephaly (congenital absence of cranial vault and underlying cerebral hemispheres)
- Trisomy 16 to 18 (chromosomal anomaly)

The mortality rate for postterm neonates is more than twice as great as that for full-term neonates, and they are at risk for the development of complications related to compromised uteroplacental perfusion and hypoxia.

Neonatal Implications

Meconium Aspiration Syndrome and Persistent Pulmonary Hypertension of the Newborn. Intrauterine hypoxia leads to relaxation of the anal sphincter and increased intestinal peristalsis with passage of meconium in utero. The asphyxiated fetus engages in gasping movements, which draw meconium into the large airways. At birth, meconium is inhaled into the distal airways and alveoli when the infant takes the first breath. The thick, viscous meconium creates a ball-valve effect in the alveolus. Inspired air is trapped in the alveolous by the meconium plug, distending the alveolar sac but preventing adequate gas exchange. This condition is known as MAS. Chemical pneumonitis occurs as a response to meconium aspiration and leads to thickening of alveolar walls and interstitial tissues. This rigid, noncompliant lung tissue also prevents adequate gas exchange.

MAS is often complicated by *persistent pulmonary hypertension of the newborn* (PPHN). PPHN, also called persistent fetal circulation, is caused by elevated pulmonary vascular resistence. PPHN may occur alone, possibly due to abnormal development of the pulmonary vessels, or as a complication of other disorders such as MAS. In MAS vasoconstriction and vasospasm occur in pulmonary vessels in response to hypoxia. The resultant pulmonary vascular hypertension leads to elevated pressures in the right side of the heart, reopening of fetal cardiac shunts (eg, the ductus arteriosus and foramen ovale), and right-to-left shunting of blood. Blood exiting the right side of the heart bypasses the lungs, increasing systemic hypoxemia and exacerbating pulmonary vasoconstriction (Fig. 33-14).

Mechanical ventilation at very high rates and pressures

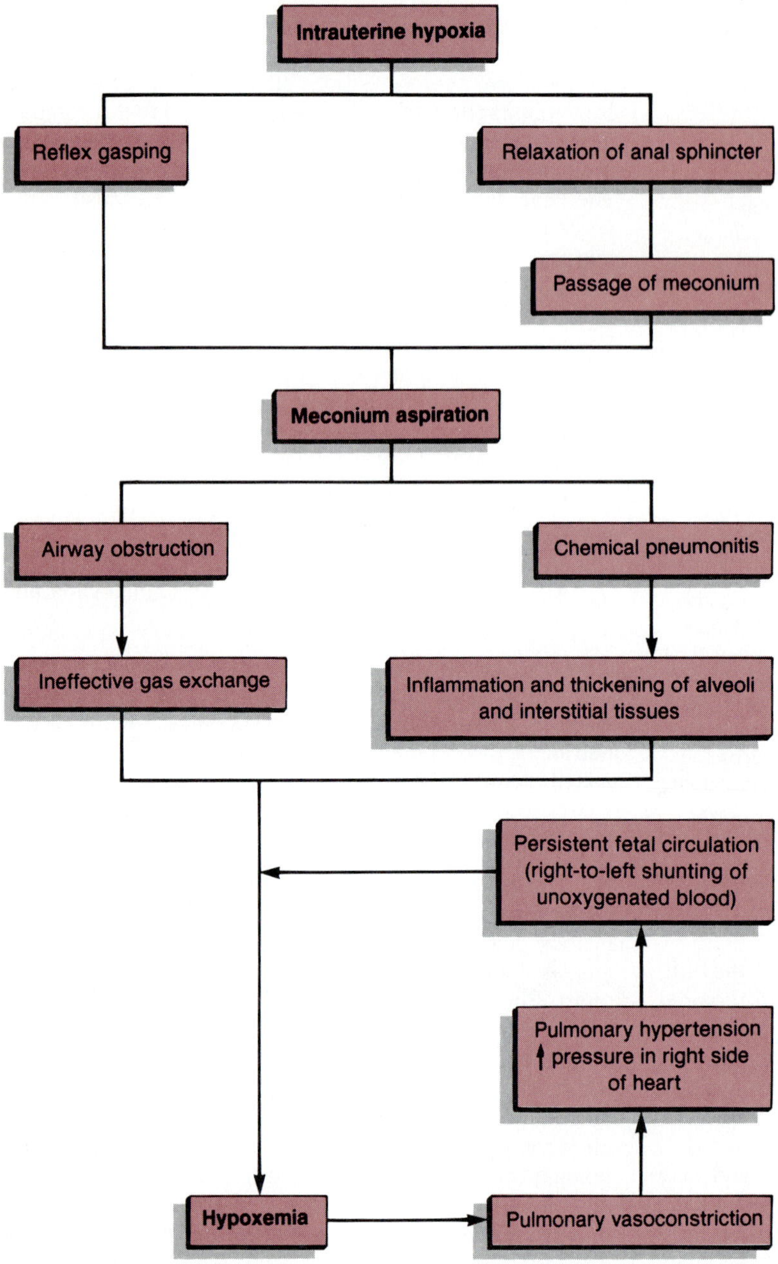

Figure 33-14.
Causes and consequences of meconium aspiration syndrome.

often is necessary to ventilate the lungs adequately, but even very high concentrations of oxygen may not correct the hypoxemia that occurs with hypertension and shunting. A potent vasodilator, tolazoline, may be used in an attempt to correct pulmonary hypertension. Its significant side effects, including gastrointestinal hemorrhage and severe hypotension, limit the use of the drug to select groups of neonates. Other drugs, such as dopamine, may be used to improve cardiac output.

One of the newest therapies used to treat neonate's suffering from PPHN or MAS is ECMO. Discussed previously in this chapter, ECMO is an invasive treatment in which a cardiopulmonary bypass is established to allow the lungs to rest and heal. The neonate's blood is rerouted to a machine that functions as a lung, removing carbon dioxide and reoxygenating the blood (see Fig. 33-4).

Pneumothorax. Pneumothorax is a major complication of MAS secondary to the pathologic changes in lung tissue and the high ventilator pressures required to treat the disease. Sudden, acute respiratory distress is the classic sign of pneumothorax, but a constellation of systemic signs and symptoms often is evident (see the display on signs and symptoms of pneumothorax). With rupture of alveoli, air enters the pleural space, causing lung tissue to collapse. Breath sounds may be diminished on the affected side, and as air accumulates in the pleural space, mediastinal shifting toward the uninvolved side of the chest occurs. The PMI of cardiac activity may also shift to the unaffected side.

Once pneumothorax is suspected, transillumination of the chest wall with a high-intensity fiberoptic light source can be performed immediately to assist the physician in a correct diagnosis. With pneumothorax transmission of light

Signs and Symptoms of Pneumothorax

Sudden acute respiratory distress:
- Tachypnea
- Flaring
- Grunting
- Retraction

Cyanosis or pallor

Mottling of the skin

Decreased PaO_2

Decreased pH

Possible diminished breath sounds on affected side

Asymmetric chest expansion

Hyperresonance with chest percussion

Cardiovascular changes:
- Tachycardia (initially)
- Bradycardia
- Arrhythmias
- Distant heart sounds
- Shift in heart sounds
- Shift in point of maximal impulse
- Decreased arterial blood pressure
- Pressure in right side of heart
- Right-to-left shunting of unoxygenated blood

across the affected side of the chest is increased. Diagnosis is confirmed by chest x-ray. Because pneumothorax is a life-threatening complication, immediate intervention may be required before a chest x-ray study is performed. A small-gauged scalp-vein needle, connected to a stopcock and a 20-mL syringe, is inserted through the chest wall into the pleural space, and air is aspirated. Emergency aspiration is associated with complications, including hemorrhage, lung perforation, and phrenic nerve injury and must be performed by a skilled practitioner.

Chest tubes are inserted to remove air and fluid from the pleural space and to allow the collapsed lung to re-expand. The tubes are connected to a closed-drainage system, which prevents air from reentering the pleural space. The system is then connected to a suction source to aid in the removal of air and fluid from the chest cavity.

High Risk for Hypoglycemia, Polycythemia, and Hypothermia. The postterm newborn is at increased risk for the development of hypoglycemia as a result of depletion of liver glycogen stores. Polycythemia is hypothesized to occur in the postterm neonate in response to intrauterine hypoxia. The neonate may be born with a hematocrit of 65% or higher and is at risk for the development of complications associated with hyperviscosity, including hypoglycemia, cerebral ischemia, thrombus formation, and respiratory distress. The loss of subcutaneous tissue in the last weeks of a prolonged pregnancy deprives the postterm neonate of insulating adipose tissue and puts the neonate at risk for hypothermia.

Implications for Nursing Care

An immediate and essential aspect of nursing care when assisting at the birth of a postterm neonate with meconium-stained amniotic fluid is to aid the physician in suctioning the trachea to remove any meconium present in the airway. As soon as the neonate is delivered, an endotracheal tube is passed, and deep tracheal suctioning is performed by the pediatrician until the neonate's airway is clear. The neonate's chest may be swaddled to prevent him or her from taking the first breath until the airway is adequately suctioned. (See Chapter 21 for a discussion of delivery room management of the neonate delivered through meconium.)

Ongoing nursing care focuses on support of respiratory function and prevention of complications associated with postmaturity. (The Nursing Care Plan for the respiratory care of the SGA infant also is applicable to the postterm neonate with potential MAS.) A hematocrit is obtained by 4 hours of age to determine whether polycythemia is a complicating factor. A partial exchange transfusion may be necessary to prevent such impairment of tissue perfusion, renal damage, and seizures. Serial glucose determinations are made to monitor blood glucose levels. Postterm neonates can be voracious eaters, and early feedings often are initiated (if not contraindicated by respiratory complications) to prevent hypoglycemia. Although the neonate may possess little adipose tissue and thus may be at risk for hypothermia, the thermoregulatory center is mature, and careful attention to bundling and avoiding drafts is usually adequate to prevent cold stress. When meconium aspiration complicates the postnatal course, the postterm neonate will be placed in a neutral thermal environment.

Continuous monitoring of the neonate who sustained a pneumothorax is essential. The nurse must be familiar with the closed-drainage system used in the evacuation of fluid and air from the pleural space.

The newborn may be at risk because of complications related to gestational age. A preterm or premature neonate is born before 37 weeks of gestation. All systems of preterm neonates are immature anatomically and physiologically. This usually prevents the neonate from making major adaptatins without continuous medical and nursing care. An SGA neonate is any neonate whose weight falls below the tenth percentile or is 2 standard deviations below the mean. The low birth weight is a result of IUGR. An LGA neonate is one whose weight is above the 90th percentile or 2 standard deviations above the mean. The infant of a diabetic mother is often LGA. The postterm neonate is born after 42 weeks' gestation. This newborn is long and very thin.

The Neonate With Infection

The neonate is susceptible to infection as a result of immature immunologic functioning at birth. Susceptibility is increased when the neonate is preterm or suffering from other complications, such as asphyxia or trauma. Infection can be the result of maternal disease during pregnancy (eg, rubella, syphilis, or chlamydia). The neonate also can come in contact with pathogens during passage through the birth canal (eg, herpesvirus, gonococci, or beta-hemolytic streptococci). The increasing use of invasive procedures and diagnostic tests places the neonate at risk for iatrogenic infection during the neonatal period.

Signs of Infection

Early signs and symptoms of infection often are subtle and nonspecific. The neonate may become lethargic, refuse feedings, or vomit. Temperature instability, hypothermia, and subtle color changes (cyanosis, mottling, or grayish tone) also may be noted. Less frequently, apnea may occur as a sign of infection. Other signs, while possibly indicating the source of infection, are nonspecific and may indicate the presence of other disorders. Jitteriness and seizure activity may be observed with central nervous system infections, or they may be signs of neonatal abstinence syndrome. Respiratory distress is exhibited with pulmonary infections and cold stress. Diarrhea is seen with intestinal infections or with bilirubin excretion while under phototherapy.

Once an infection occurs, regardless of its primary site, it can spread quickly through the bloodstream, and generalized sepsis will ensue. Because of the subtlety of symptoms and the dire consequences of fulminant sepsis, a workup to rule out sepsis is frequently performed on high-risk neonates who demonstrate signs of and who are at risk for an infection.

The neonate also may demonstrate signs of viral infection transmitted during the prenatal period from mother to fetus. Evidence of chronic intrauterine infection at birth includes growth retardation, microcephaly, and hepatosplenomegaly. Central nervous system involvement is common (microcephaly, cerebral calcification, and mental retardation). The neonate is frequently SGA and suffers from problems common to this group of infants (see the section "Small-for-Gestational Age Neonate" in this chapter), including hypoglycemia and hypothermia.

Once infection is suspected, a septic workup is performed. Blood and spinal fluid cultures are obtained, and a latex agglutination study is performed on urine; a complete blood count with differential also is obtained. A chest x-ray study is performed on neonates exhibiting signs of respiratory distress. Viral studies may be included in the evaluation of infants suspected of suffering from intrauterine or postnatal viral infection, especially those with microcephaly. The level of immunoglobulin M (IgM) is measured in the cord blood or the neonate's serum. IgM does not cross the placenta, and elevated levels (over 20 mg/100 mL) indicate intrauterine infection. TORCH screening and antibody tests also can be performed on the neonate's serum to determine the presence of this group of prenatal viral infections (see the section "Viral and Protozoan Infections" later in this chapter). Viral cultures for cytomegalovirus (CMV) and herpesvirus and a urine sample for CMV also may be obtained if indicated.

Bacterial Infections

Bacterial infections in the neonate can result in permanent disability and accounts for 10% to 20% of all infant mortality. Most bacterial infections are acquired prenatally (by movement of microorganisms through the mother's vagina and cervix) and during passage of the fetus through the birth canal at the time of delivery. The most significant bacterial infections are discussed in the following sections.

Group B Beta-Hemolytic *Streptococcus*

The group B beta-hemolytic streptococcal (GBS) microorganism is the most common cause of neonatal infection today. Many pregnant women are silent carriers of this potentially lethal pathogen, harboring the bacteria in the cervix or vagina. The neonate is colonized with the microorganism during labor and delivery and may develop the infection in the neonatal period. Although preterm neonates are at greatest risk for developing GBS infections, it is not possible to identify all neonates at risk. Even apparently healthy full-term neonates develop infections.

Two varieties of GBS infection occur in the newborn. The *early onset form* develops within the first 24 hours of life and is often fatal. The neonate is hypotonic, hypothermic, and presents with acute respiratory distress and pneumonia. Cardiovascular collapse and death can occur within hours of the first indication of infection. The *late onset form* usually occurs after the first 2 weeks of life as a meningeal infection. The neonate presents with fever, lethargy, and signs of increased intracranial pressure (bulging fontanelle, nuchal rigidity, and high-pitched cry). The late onset form is associated with a much lower mortality rate than early onset GBS infection, but permanent neurologic disability secondary to meningitis can be a complicating factor. Both forms of the disease are treated with antibiotics (gentamicin, ampicillin, or penicillin) administered intravenously.

Listeria

Listeria, a gram-positive organism, is an intracellular parasite recently implicated in the etiology of neonatal sepsis. Most affected newborns contract the disease during passage through a maternal birth canal colonized with the organism. An early onset and a late onset form have been identified. The neonate with an *early onset Listeria* infection frequently demonstrates diffuse granulomatous skin papules over the trunk and on the pharynx. The neonate appears very ill and may experience respiratory distress and cyanosis.

As with GBS infection, the *late onset* form of *Listeria* infection usually occurs around the second week of life. The disease usually is manifest as a meningitis that appears to be associated with a different strain of the organism (type IV B) found in the environment. Ampicillin and gentamicin (or kanamycin) are recommended for treatment of both forms of the disease.

Escherichia coli

One strain of *Escherichia coli* (K1 antigen-positive) is an extremely virulent gram-negative organism recognized as a major cause of neonatal meningitis and septicemia. *E. coli* is transferred from mother to neonate in a manner similar to the transmission of GBS. The neonate is colonized during labor and delivery and develops signs of infection within several days. *E. coli* infections also can be acquired from nursery personnel who are colonized with the pathogen. It has been suggested that neonates susceptible to this pathogen have a decreased circulating antibody level against *E. coli* K1 antigen (Oellrich, 1985). Treatment consists of IV antibiotic administration.

Neisseria gonococcus

Ophthalmia neonatorum is a severe infection of the conjunctiva caused by the pathogen *Neisseria gonococcus*. The mother who has gonorrhea transmits the microorganism to her newborn as he or she passes through the birth canal during labor and delivery. The instillation of a 1% silver nitrate solution or erythromycin ointment into the neonate's eyes will prevent gonococcal conjunctivitis. An untreated neonate will exhibit signs of eye infection (copious purulent discharge) by the third or fourth day of life. Corneal ulceration and blindness occur rapidly, if appropriate treatment is not initiated. Therapy consists of saline eye irrigations followed by topical and systemic administration of penicillin. In rare cases the gonococcal organism will invade joint capsules, causing a septic arthritis that requires prolonged systemic antimicrobial therapy for 4 weeks or more.

Tuberculosis

Congenital tuberculosis is rare and is seen only when the mother has advanced, untreated pulmonary disease. The tubercle bacillus is transmitted through the placenta and umbilical vein. The focus of the disease is usually the liver, although tuberculosis meningitis has been diagnosed in newborns. The neonate is lethargic, may be febrile, and is a poor feeder. Hepatomegaly and splenomegaly often are evident. The chest x-ray study may be normal. Treatment of active disease consists of the administration of isoniazid (INH) with rifampin for 1 year.

The neonate also can acquire tuberculosis during birth by aspiration of infected secretions or during the neonatal period through contact with infected parents. The neonate is separated from the mother until she is no longer contagious. Prophylaxis for the newborn is a 1-year course of INH administration. If evaluation of the family and home environment indicates a high probability of noncompliance with INH therapy, bacillus Calmette-Guérin vaccine may be administered.

If the mother has an inactive infection at birth, is receiving treatment, and has negative sputum and a negative x-ray study, the mother–newborn dyad is not separated. The nursery should have a carefully delineated policy and procedure regarding care of the newborn when tuberculosis is suspected in the mother or newborn.

The incidence of tuberculosis is high among recent immigrants from Southeast Asia and is increasing in the United States as a result of the rise in homelessness and human immunodeficiency virus (HIV). When mother and neonate are separated at birth, intense anxiety may be generated in parents who suffer from language barriers, lack of understanding regarding the disease, or who fear that the neonate is being taken away from them because they lack living accomodations. Parents should be reassured that the separation is temporary. Social services, interpreters, and child welfare workers can assist in supporting the new family and planning for discharge.

Viral and Protozoan Infections

The neonate also is susceptible to more than 12 known viral infections contracted either in utero or in the postnatal period. *TORCH* is an acronym for a group of infections that can attack the fetus and result in permanent physical disability or mental retardation in the neonate: *T*—toxoplasmosis; *O*—other viruses known to attack the fetus, including syphilis; *R*—rubella; *C*—CMV; and *H*—herpesvirus type 2.

Toxoplasmosis

Toxoplasmosis is a protozoan infection caused by *Toxoplasma gondii*. Raw meat and infected feces appear to be the vehicles for transmission of this infection. The cat is the most common carrier of the pathogen in the United States. The pregnant woman may have a silent infection that is undiagnosed and untreated. Placental transmission of the organism occurs, and the neonate is born with serious disease. Signs of toxoplasmosis include microcephaly, cerebral calcifications, chorioretinitis, hepatosplenomegaly, and jaundice.

Treatment consists of drug therapy, which appears to limit further central nervous system injury but does not reverse the prenatal damage already sustained by the neonate. Repeated courses of pyrimethamine, an antimalarial drug, sulfadiazine, and folinic acid are administered within the first year of life. Corticosteroids also may be administered to infants with chorioretinitis.

Syphilis

Transmission of the organism responsible for syphilis (*Treponema pallidum*) can occur during the second half of pregnancy. If the mother does not receive treatment for this sexually transmitted disease, the neonate will be born with congenital syphilis and is usually infectious. Clinical signs of the disease include IUGR, ascites (fluid in the peritoneal cavity), persistent rhinitis (snuffles), jaundice, anemia, hepatosplenomegaly, and lymphadenopathy. The classic chancre observed in adult first-stage syphilis does not appear in the neonate, but a copper-colored rash may develop over the face, the palms of the hands, and the soles of the feet within the first week of life.

A fluorescent-labeled IgM specific for antitreponemal IgM antibodies is available as a diagnostic tool. A positive serologic test necessitates immediate treatment with procaine penicillin G for 10 to 14 days. Nasal secretions and open syphilitic lesions are extremely infectious; the neonate is, therefore, initially placed in isolation. After 24 hours of penicillin therapy, the neonate is no longer infectious.

Rubella

The rubella virus is another pathogen that attacks the fetus in utero. The severity of damage apparent in the neonate born with congenital rubella reflects the length of intrauterine infection and the time of first exposure to the virus. Approximately 30% to 50% of fetuses who acquire rubella in the first month of gestation suffer cardiac anomalies. Neural deafness is a common sequela when infection occurs in the second gestational month. Other signs of rubella infection in the neonate include congenital cataracts, glaucoma, microphthalmia, and blindness. The neonate may exhibit other signs of chronic infection, such as IUGR and hepatosplenomegaly. Central nervous system involvement is reflected in microcephaly and mental retardation.

The neonate born with congenital rubella is often highly infectious and should be isolated and cared for only by nursery personnel with immunity to the disease. It is possible to isolate the mother and neonate together, if the neonate does not require special care. No specific drug therapy is effective in limiting the disease process postnatally, and the neonate may continue to shed the virus for 1 year or longer. He or she remains a source of infection during this time.

Cytomegalovirus

CMV disease is a poorly understood infection that causes severe central nervous system injury in neonates who acquire the infection prenatally. The neonate is born with a constellation of signs characteristic of many other intrauterine viral infections (microcephaly, IUGR, cerebral calcifications, and hepatosplenomegaly). The diagnosis can be confirmed by isolating the virus in the urine. Recently, more sophisticated tests allow identification of specific CMV antibodies in serum. Many neonates who harbor the virus are asymptomatic, but develop central nervous system injury (eg, blindness and mental retardation) later in childhood. Neonates with a symptomatic CMV infection have a very poor prognosis. Approximately 30% die in infancy, and 90% of survivors suffer from CNS, visual, and auditory handicaps (Modlin, 1985). At present, there is no effective means of preventing or treating CMV. Nursing care of the neonate with this infection is supportive.

Herpesvirus Type 2

The neonate with herpesvirus type 2 infection usually contracts the disease during passage through the birth canal. Prenatal infection is rare. The risk of developing a neonatal infection after vaginal delivery, when the membranes have been ruptured for longer than 6 hours before delivery or when the mother has an active genital lesion is as high as 50%. Neonates born to mothers with primary herpes infections develop a more severe, systemic form of the disease (hepatitis, pneumonia, encephalitis, and disseminated intravascular coagulopathy). Death can occur within hours of birth. The mortality rate of neonates presenting with neonatal herpes infection approaches 50%. An additional 30% will experience major neurologic sequelae, including seizures, mental retardation, and hydrocephalus (Samson, 1988).

Newborns of mothers with recurrent infections often have a milder disease process. Vesicular skin lesions, lethargy, hypothermia, and hypotonia are frequently present, but severe systemic infection does not occur. Viral cultures are obtained and blood samples are drawn to identify specific IgM antibodies. The neonate is highly contagious and is isolated. Treatment with antiviral drugs such as acyclovir or vidarabine has been attempted but with limited success. Nursing care in the milder form of the disease is primarily supportive. Life support systems are used in the care of critically ill neonates, and intensive nursing care is required 24 hours a day.

Hepatitis B

The transmission of hepatitis B virus and surface antigen (HBsAg) occurs transplacentally during pregnancy and during passage through the birth canal when women have a hepatitis B infection of either a chronic (carrier state) or acute nature. Although the neonate rarely presents with classic signs of the disease, prematurity and low birth weight are frequently observed. Jaundice, hepatomegaly, abdominal distention, and a poor feeding pattern develop some time (usually 4 to 6 weeks) after birth. Significantly, most neonates who become HBsAg positive due to transmission of the virus in the perinatal period suffer from the chronic (carrier state) form of the disease and never demonstrate signs and symptoms of acute infection.

Neonates at risk for the development of hepatitis B include those born to mothers who are intravenous drug users and refugees from Southeast Asia and the Far East, where the incidence of the disease is very high. Currently, recommended prophylaxis for the neonate born to a woman found to be positive for HBsAg consists of the intramuscular administration of 0.5 mL of hepatitis B immunoglobulin intramuscularly as soon as possible after birth (at least within 12 hours). Hepatitis B vaccine, 0.5 mL, is given intramuscularly within 7 days of birth, at 1 month, and at 6 months of age. Current Centers for Disease Control (CDC) recommendations include vaccinating *all* infants against hepatitis B (CDC, 1991).

Chlamydia

Chlamydia is an intracellular parasite found in the vagina of 2% to 13% of women in this country. It has only recently been identified as a causative agent in neonatal infection. It is the most frequently occurring sexually transmitted disease in the United States today (approximately three times as common as gonorrhea) and is the most common cause of blindness in the world. *Chlamydia* is transmitted from mother to neonate during the passage through the birth canal and can result in neonatal conjunctivitis, pneumonia, and otitis media. It also may infect the genital tract.

Prenatal diagnosis of chlamydia is possible, and screen-bottle nipple and neck of bottle full of formula to prevent air ingestion. Never prop a bottle; this can cause regurgitation, aspiration of formula, ear infections, and cavities in older children. Avoid feeding rapidly; burp infant frequently to avoid regurgitation and gas pains. • Infants should be placed on their side after feeding to avoid aspiration. • Stomach capacity is very small; therefore, avoid overfeeding or forcing infant to finish a bottle. When satiated, infant usually ceases sucking slowly and may push nipple out of mouth. Do not stimulate infant to feed further. • If clean water source not available, formula and equipment should be sterilized using the aseptic technique or terminal heat method.

Storage of formula

Large cans provide enough formula for 24-h period, but any unused portion should be discarded after 24 h. A partially emptied bottle of formula should be discarded after feeding (microorganisms can be introduced to milk during feeding and may grow later in remaining milk).

Burping

Burp infant frequently by holding against shoulder, in sitting position with head or neck supported or across lap in prone position. Massage or pat back gently. Burp prior to feeding if infant has been crying.

(continued)

Potential Complications

Hemorrhage, infection, shock, sepsis, acute pain, preterm labor, pregnancy-induced hypertension, dehydration, proteinuria, fetal compromise, anemia

Intrapartum nursing diagnosis

Pain related to uterine contractions • High Risk for Injection related to intrapartum procedures • Fear related to threat to maternal or fetal status

Potential complications

Hemorrhage, fetal distress, hypertension

Postpartum nursing diagnoses

Pain related to trauma to perineum • High Risk for Infection related to delayed uterine involution • Effective Breastfeeding related to support sources • Ineffective breastfeeding related to engorgement, lack of knowledge • Interrupted Breastfeeding related to employment • High Risk for Altered Parenting related to inadequate social support • Altered Health Maintenance related to lack of knowledge • Ineffective Thermoregulation related to immaturity (newborn) • High Risk for Infection related to immaturity (newborn)

Potential complications

Hemorrhage, infection, hyperbilirubinemia, thrombophlebitis, deep vein thrombosis

neonates are obligate nose breathers. • Teach mother to observe sucking pattern. When sucking movements are rhythmic and jaw movement is observable, nutritive sucking is occurring. Neonates usually empty each breast in 5–7 minutes. • Nursing sessions of 10 minutes per breast should satiate the newborn. If both breasts are suckled at one feeding, the mother should begin her next feeding on the last breast suckled. A safety pin can be put on the bra to indicate which breast was last suckled, serving as a reminder to mother. • Mother should slip her finger into side of neonate's mouth to break suction and avoid nipple trauma when removing newborn from breast. • Changing positions during nursing can help empty all lactiferous sinuses and avoid clogged ducts. • Neonate should be awakened q 3–4 h during day to feed to help coordinate sleep cycles. Emphasize the importance of supply and demand; explain the more the mother nurses, the more milk she will make. Important to stress that it usually takes 2–3 wk to establish breastfeeding patterns. • Breast milk can be pumped from breasts (using manual or electric pumps) and stored in sterile baby bottles in the freezer 2–3 mos. Frozen milk should be rewarmed under warm running water, *not* in microwave (can create "hot spots" in milk and burn infant).

Teaching Considerations: Formula Feeding

Advantages
Infant may be fed by different caregivers; feedings occur every 3–4 h.
Disadvantages
Formula does not provide immunologic factors, not as easily digested as breast milk.
Types of formula
Powdered—must have water added to correct concentration per manufacturer's instructions. Concentrated—must be diluted according to manufacturer's instructions. Ready-to-use, and ready-to-use prepackaged—ready to feed in multiple or individual serving sizes. Evaporated milk or cow's milk mixtures are usually not recommended for infant feeding.
Preparation
Care must be taken to avoid overdilution and underdilution. If formula is not iron fortified, iron supplement may be added after 4 mo. • Cleanliness in preparation is important. If clean water source is available, sterilization is not necessary. Wash equipment well in soapy water, rinse and store in a clean area. • When feeding, keep

(*continued*)

Formula Feeding (*continued*)

Typical Pattern of Infant Feedings

Age	Number of feedings	Volume (oz)	Total (oz)
Birth–2 wk	6–10	2–3	12–30
2 wk–1 mo	6–8	3–4	18–32
1–3 mo	5–6	5–6	25–36
3–7 mo	4–5	6–7	25–36
7–12 mo	3–4	7–8	25–36

Teaching Considerations: Breastfeeding

Advantages
Breast milk more easily digested, contains immunologic factors that decrease infection rate and offer protection against allergies. Meets entire nutritional needs for 4–6 mos. Ideal activity for mother–infant attachment.
Disadvantages
Sore nipples, potential for engorgement or mastitis; time consuming; feedings q 2–3 h for first several months.
Procedure
• Mother should hold neonate in a comfortable position with her thumb placed above the nipple and remaining fingers cupped under the breast. • Stroke neonate's upper lip with nipple until neonate opens mouth, then bring neonate straight into breast. • Cover as much of areola areas as possible in neonate's mouth. The neonate needs to compress at least an inch of tissue around the nipple. This stimulates milk ejection reflex and prevents "chewing" on the nipple, which leads to nipple abrasion and soreness. Care should be taken not to occlude nostrils during breastfeeding because

(*continued*)

North American Nursing Diagnosis (NANDA)-Approved Nursing Diagnoses (1992)

An actual diagnosis is made according to the presence of specific signs and symptoms. *High risk for (diagnosis)* is based on assessment that an individual is more vulnerable than others in a similar situation. *Possible (diagnosis)* is based on suspicion that a problem may be present, but more data are needed to confirm the diagnosis. *Collaborative problems* are patient problems for which care must be ordered by the physician but which are managed by nurses; often they are listed as *potential complications*.

Prenatal nursing diagnoses
Pain related to physiologic changes • Altered Sexuality Patterns related to discomforts of pregnancy • Constipation related to decreased gastric motility • Activity Intolerance related to fatigue, dyspnea • Altered Oral Mucous Membrane related to vomiting • Fear related to possibility of pregnancy loss or complication • Fatigue related to increasing metabolic demands of pregnancy • Health Seeking Behavior: (seeking prenatal care) • High risk for Infection related to altered urinary patterns • Body Image Disturbance related to biophysical effects of pregnancy • Grieving related to loss of pregnancy, role loss • High Risk for Altered Nutrition: Less than Body Requirements related to nausea, vomiting, lack of knowledge

(*continued*)

Teaching Considerations: Common Infant Care Concerns

Bathing
Collect all necessary equipment before beginning bath. Water temperature should feel warm to elbow test. Use nonperfumed mild soap and bathe from head to toe, covering areas not being bathing with a soft towel. Do not put soap on infant's face. Do not probe ear canals or noses with cotton swabs. Head may be shampooed while infant is fully clothed. Avoid use of baby oil because it clogs pores. Powder is not necessary; if used, avoid face because it can be inhaled and may cause aspiration pneumonia. Infants do not need complete bath daily, but face, hands, neck, genitalia, and rectal area should be washed daily. May want to wait until partner can be present to bathe and have special time with infant. Initiate tub bathing only after cord has fallen off.

Cord care
Cord stump usually dries and falls off after 7–10 d. Until that time, fold diaper down away from cord and clean base of cord with alcohol several times a day. Continue

(*continued*)

Common Infant Care Concerns (*continued*)

Stool patterns
Infant stools change from tarry, dark green (meconium) to thin, brownish green (transitional) to pale or golden yellow, depending on how the infant is fed. Breastfed infants tend to have looser stools than formula-fed infants. Soap and water on rectal area should be used after each defecation.

Diaper rash
If diaper rash occurs, A & D ointment or zinc oxide ointment may be applied. Exposure to air hastens healing. If using disposable diapers, switching to cloth diapers may help.

Teaching Considerations: Signs of Newborn Illness

Symptoms to Report

Significant signs and symptoms of illness
- Lethargy—Listless behavior or difficulty rousing newborn
- Loss of appetite—Refusal of two feedings in a row
- Fever—Axillary temperature above 100°F (37.3°C) or below 97°F (36.1°C), or rectal temperature above 101°F (38.3°C) or below 98°F (36.6°C)
- Vomiting—Spitting up large amount of feeding two or more times
- Diarrhea—Three or more green, liquid stools in succession
- Oliguria—Fewer than 6 wet diapers a day

(*continued*)

Teaching Considerations: Newborn Safety Factors

Importance
Accidents are the leading cause of death in children from age 1 mo until adolescence. Accident prevention should be discussed in detail with parents.

Infant car seat
All states have mandated child restraint laws. Parents should be instructed to purchase a car seat, and use it *every time* infant is in the car. Car seats should be placed on the back seat and turned toward the rear of the car with the seat belt attached to the car seat. Used car seats should be carefully inspected to ensure the restraint device works properly.

Poisoning
Second leading cause of death in older infants and children. Teach parents to "childproof" their home. Electrical outlets should have covers. Cleaning solutions, medications, and toxic substances should be in locked cabinets or cabinets where doors cannot be opened by infants or children. Household plants may be poisonous.

(*continued*)

Teaching Considerations: Complications of Pregnancy

Symptoms to Report

Vaginal bleeding
May indicate threatened abortion, ectopic pregnancy in first trimester, placenta previa or abruptio placentae in second or third trimester.
Leakage of fluid from vagina
May indicate premature rupture of membranes.
Dizziness or pelvic uterine pain
May indicate ectopic pregnancy (especially with shoulder pain), or abruptio placentae.
Uterine/pelvic cramping or low backache
May indicate preterm labor, especially when associated with rhythmic tightening of uterus or leakage of fluid from vagina.

(continued)

Teaching Considerations: Early Postpartum Care

The lining of the uterus is a perfect site for infection to occur following delivery. Meticulous hygienic care is imperative.
Bathing
Daily baths or showers should be taken and perineal area washed with soap and water and patted dry.
Perineal pads
Pads should be applied from front to back, being careful not to touch the side of the pad that covers the perineum. Pads should be changed with each voiding, defecation, or when soiled with lochia. Lochia is usually a moderate flow with small clots (6–8 pads used daily on average). If clots larger than a quarter are passed, they should be saved and the health care provider notified. Any foul odor to lochia should be reported to the health care provider.
Lochia changes
Lochia rubra lasts 1–3 days and looks and smells like menstrual blood. Lochia serosa is light pink to brownish color and last 2–3 days. Lochia alba is a whitish discharge, which may last for several weeks.

(continued)

Teaching Considerations: Postpartum Complications

Symptoms to Report

Infection
Temperature of 100.4°F (38°C) for 2 consecutive days may indicate uterine infection.
Lochia changes
When lochia changes from alba to serosa or rubra or has foul odor, uterus may be relaxed or infection present.
Uterine tenderness
Indicative of uterine infection.
Breast engorgement
If breastfeeding, encourage feeding on demand, warm showers, and breast massage. Warm moist heat before nursing will facilitate emptying of breasts. If not breastfeeding, apply ice packs PRN, wear tight bra or binder for 24 h and avoid breast stimulation. Take analgesics as needed.

(continued)

Teaching Considerations: Emotional Changes

Symptoms to Report

Postpartum blues
Woman may feel "blue" or depressed with labile emotions for several weeks. May cry for no reason. Family members should be counseled about postpartum mood swings. Hormonal changes may contribute to mood swings. New mothers may also feel isolated and lonely, and may have little family support or no extended family available. Irritability, unexplained tearfulness, sleep and appetite disturbances are within normal limits in first 2 wk after delivery.
Warning signs
If these symptoms continue for more than 2 wks, and woman is having difficulty with activities of daily living, is despondent or exhibits poor attention span, she may be experiencing significant postpartum depression. Woman with history of depressive episodes may be at increased risk.

(continued)

Universal Precautions: Prevention of Transmission of Human Immunodeficiency Virus, Hepatitis B Virus, and Other Blood-Borne Pathogens in Health Care Settings

Human immunodeficiency virus (HIV), the virus that causes acquired immunodeficiency syndrome (AIDS), is transmitted during sexual contact, through the sharing of intravenous drug needles and syringes while "shooting" drugs, through exposure to infected blood or blood components, and perinatally from mother to neonate. Currently there is neither a cure for nor an immunization to prevent AIDS. The increasing prevalence of HIV increases the risk that health care workers will be exposed to blood from patients infected with HIV.

The Centers for Disease Control in Atlanta has developed "Universal Precautions" (formerly called "Universal Blood and Body Fluid Precautions") as recommendations to all health care workers. Under universal precautions, blood and certain body fluids of **all** patients are considered potentially infectious for HIV, hepatitis B virus (HBV), and other blood-borne pathogens. Universal precautions are intended to prevent parenteral, mucous membrane, and nonintact skin exposures of health care workers to blood-borne pathogens. In addition, immunization with HBV vaccine is recommended as an important adjunct to universal precautions for health care workers who have been exposed to blood. (The implementation of control measures for HIV and HBV does not obviate the need for continued adherence to general infection-control principles and general hygiene measures.) Below is a summary of the CDC's recommendations.

Body Fluids to Which Universal Precautions Apply

Universal precautions apply to blood and other body fluids containing visible blood. **Blood is the single most important source of HIV, HBV, and other blood-borne pathogens in the health care facility**. Infection control efforts for HIV, HBV, and other blood-borne pathogens must focus on both preventing exposures to blood and delivering HBV immunization. Universal precautions also apply to semen and vaginal secretions, tissues, and the following fluids: cerebrospinal, synovial, pleural, peritoneal, pericardial, and amniotic.

Body Fluids to Which Universal Precautions Do Not Apply

Universal precautions *do not* apply to feces, nasal secretions, sputum, sweat, tears, urine, and vomitus unless they contain visible blood. The risk of transmission of HIV or HBV from these fluids is extremely low or nonexistent.

General Precautions

- Use universal precautions for **all** patients.
- Use appropriate barrier precautions routinely when contact with blood or other body fluids of any patient is anticipated.
  - Wear gloves when touching blood and body fluids, mucous membranes, or nonintact skin; when handling items or surfaces soiled with blood or body fluids; and when performing venipuncture and other vascular access procedures.
  - Change gloves after each contact with patients.
  - Wear masks and protective eyewear or face sheilds during procedures that are likely to generate drops of blood or other body fluids to prevent exposure of mucous membranes of mouth, nose, and eyes.
  - Wear gowns or aprons during procedures that are likely to generate splashes of blood or other body fluids.
- Wash hands and other skin surfaces immediately and thoroughly if contaminated with blood or other body fluids.
- Wash hands immediately after gloves are removed.
- Take precautions to prevent injuries caused by needles, scalpels, and other sharp instruments or devices during procedures; when cleaning used instruments; during disposal of used needles; and when handling sharp instruments after procedures.
  - Discard needle units uncapped and unbroken after use.
  - Place disposable syringes and needles, scalpel blades, and other sharp items in puncture-resistant containers.
  - Place puncture-resistant containers as near as practical to the area of use.
- Although saliva has not been implicated, to minimize the need for emergency mouth-to-mouth resuscitation, make mouthpieces, resuscitation bags, or other ventilation devices available for use in areas where the need for resuscitation is predictable.
- If you have exudative lesions or weeping dermatitis, refrain from all direct patient care and from handling patient care equipment until the condition resolves.

Precautions for Invasive Procedures

- If you participate in invasive procedures, use appropriate barrier methods: gloves, surgical masks, protective eyewear, face shields, gowns, and aprons.
- If you perform or assist in vaginal or cesarean deliveries, wear gloves and gowns when handling the placenta or the infant until blood and amniotic fluid have been removed from the infant's skin and during postdelivery care of the umbilical cord.
- If a glove is torn or a needlestick or other injury occurs, remove the gloves and use a new glove as promptly as patient safety permits; remove the needle or instrument used in the incident from the sterile field.

Environmental Considerations

- Standard sterilization and disinfection procedures currently recommended for use in health care settings are adequate.
- Sterilize instruments or devices that enter sterile tissue or the vascular system before reuse.
- Clean and remove soiled surfaces on walls, floors, and other surfaces routinely; extraordinary attempts to disinfect or sterilize are not necessary.
- Use chemical germicides approved as hospital disinfectants (and tuberculocidals) to decontaminate spills of blood and other body fluids.

Precautions With Soiled Linen

- Observe hygienic and common-sense storage and processing of clean and soiled linens.
- Handle soiled linen as little as possible and with minimum agitation.
- Bag all soiled linen at the location where it is used.
- Place and transport linen soiled with blood or body fluids in bags that prevent leakage.

Infective Waste

- It is practical to identify those wastes with the potential for causing infection during handling and disposal and for which some special precautions seem prudent (eg, microbiology laboratory waste, pathology waste, and blood specimens or blood products).
- Incinerate or autoclave infective waste before disposal in a sanitary landfill.
- Carefully pour bulk blood, suctioned fluids, excretions, and secretions down a drain connected to a sanitary sewer.

From *Guidelines for Prevention of Transmission of Human Immunodeficiency Virus and Hepatitis B Virus to Health-Care and Public-Safety Workers.* U.S. Department of Health and Human Services, Centers for Disease Control, Atlanta, GA, February 1989; *Update: Universal Precautions for Prevention of Transmission of Human Immunodeficiency Virus, Hepatitis B Virus, and Other Blood-borne Pathogens in Health-Care Settings. Morbidity and Mortality Weekly Report,* 1988; *Recommendations for Prevention of HIV Transmission in Health-Care Settings. Morbidity and Mortality Weekly Report,* 1987.

ing of pregnant women is practiced to aid in the identification of *Chlamydia trachomatis* and to prevent infection in the neonate.

Chlamydial Conjunctivitis

An infection of the neonate's eyes, chlamydial conjunctivitis or inclusion blennorrhea results in inflammation of the conjunctiva, edema of the eyelids, and copious purulent discharge. A pseudomembrane may form over the eye. The disease is usually bilateral. Instillation of a 1% silver nitrate ophthalmic solution does *not* provide prophylaxis against chlamydial conjunctivitis. Treatment consists of the topical application of erythromycin ointment or tetracycline combined with the systemic administration of oral erythromycin. The nurse caring for the neonate with chlamydial conjunctivitis must observe scrupulous aseptic technique, because the disease is highly contagious. Prophylactic treatment against opthalmia neonatorum (due to gonorrheal exposure) and chlamydial conjunctivitis is accomplished by instilling erythromycin ophthalmic ointment in the neonate's eyes shortly after delivery. Due to this dual coverage, hospitals have discontinued use of 1% silver nitrate solution, and use erythromycin instead.

Chlamydial Pneumonia

Chlamydial infection of the lungs results in the development of a late onset pneumonia (around 6 weeks of age). The neonate usually is afebrile and presents with a severe, often paroxysmal cough. Diffuse lung involvement is common, and rales often can be auscultated. The pneumonia is frequently preceded by a chlamydial conjunctivitis that has been ineffectively treated with topical antibiotics alone. Treatment with systemic antibiotics, including erythromycin, is recommended. Recovery is often slow and may take up to 2 months.

HIV Infection and Acquired Immunodeficiency Syndrome

Acquired immunodeficiency syndrome is an immune disorder that destroys the neonate's defenses against infection. The etiologic agent is a retrovirus, HIV, that primarily infects T lymphocytes. The virus is able to replicate by altering the T cell's genetic makeup. Immunologic evidence of the disease includes B-cell abnormality and elevated immunoglobulins (IgG, IgA, and IgM). The neonate is unable to develop antibodies in response to infection or immunization. The exact mode of perinatal HIV transmission is unknown. Possible modes of infection include transplacental transmission, intrapartum contact with contaminated maternal secretions, or through breast milk. Because at least one case of transmission from breast milk has been documented (Ziegler et al., 1985), it is suggested that breastfeeding be avoided by women with HIV. While the exact risk of perinatal transmission is unknown, currently quoted rates range from 13% to 30%.

Neonates who are truly infected with HIV usually show clinical evidence (opportunistic infections) within several months of birth. The classic signs and symptoms of HIV in adults may not be present in neonates. Newborns exhibit chronic lymphadenopathy, hepatosplenomegaly, recurrent salivary gland enlargement, oral candidiasis, bacterial infections, and failure to thrive. Many infants with HIV are premature or SGA, with microcephaly. Fever, diarrhea, dehydration, lethargy, encephalitis, spasticity, and recurrent eczema also are frequently observed (Bastin, Tamayo, Tinkle, Amaya, Trejo, & Herrera, 1992).

There is no cure for HIV, and the prognosis remains poor. All treatment modalities are experimental. Intravenous gamma globulin with HIV-specific or anti-CMV antibody, interleukin-2, and acyclovir have been used with varying degrees of success. Current clinical trials include administering zidovudine (AZT) to women during pregnancy and delivery and then to their newborns. The major focus of nursing care is supportive.

Fungal Infections

In recent years there has been an increase in the incidence of fungal infections in neonates. At particular risk are very low–birth-weight, preterm newborns. The most common fungal organism implicated in topical and systemic infections is *Candida albicans*, but *Candida tropicalis, Aspergillus*, and *Cryptococcus* are other species implicated in neonatal sepsis. Colonization may occur during birth with passage of the neonate through infected vaginal secretions. Candidal infection is also spread by direct contact with infected people.

Impaired host factors in preterm neonates, including impaired cellular and humoral immune responses and poor skin and gastrointestinal mucosal barriers, predispose the neonate to fungal infections. Iatrogenic causes contributing to *Candida* sepsis include the administration of broad-spectrum antibiotics, which inhibit normal microbial flora, the use of central indwelling arterial or venous catheters, and TPN.

While the most common neonatal candidal infections are cutaneous (thrush and diaper dermatitis), disseminated systemic infections are estimated to occur in up to 10% of neonates weighing less than 1000 g (2 lb, 2 oz). Neonates may present with nonspecific signs of deterioration, including temperature instability, episodes of apnea, feeding intolerance, carbohydrate intolerance, and generalized erythematous rash. Diagnosis is often difficult. Sites of infection include the urinary tract, central nervous system, heart, lungs, joints, and eyes.

Implications for Nursing Care

The nurse caring for a neonate with an infection places him or her in a neutral thermal environment to support thermoregulatory function and decrease energy expenditures. Antibiotic therapy is normally instituted immediately when bacterial infection is suspected and will be discontinued after 72 hours if cultures and tests prove negative, after 5 days if the mother was treated for an infection during labor, and after 7 to 14 days if pneumonia or meningitis is documented. An IV infusion or heparin or saline lock is normally started to provide a route for the administration of antibiotics, because they are poorly absorbed by the gastrointestinal tract or

muscle. An enriched oxygen atmosphere may be provided if the neonate demonstrates signs of respiratory distress or if the lung is the site of infection. The neonate's vital signs are monitored closely, and a cardiorespiratory monitor is attached to assist the nurse in continuous evaluation of cardiopulmonary function. If diarrhea or vomiting occurs or if respiratory distress is evident, oral feedings are discontinued, and fluids and electrolytes are provided intravenously until the neonate's condition is stabilized.

Because the neonate with an infection may be separated from his or her parents, the nurse must provide special loving support and comfort when they are not present. Parents should be encouraged to visit the nursery frequently and at any time convenient for them. They should be made to feel that their presence is particularly important for the neonate's care and recovery.

To prevent the transmission of neonatal infections to other newborns or staff members, universal body substance precautions are observed with *every* neonate. This procedure eliminates the need for the isolation category "Blood and Body Fluid Precautions" previously recommended for patients infected with blood-borne pathogens. Each unit also should have established policies and procedures for the care and treatment of infants with specific infectious diseases, such as herpesvirus or tuberculosis.

Normal nursing care of the neonate at risk for hepatitis B includes administration of the hepatitis B immunoglobulin and hepatitis B vaccine and scrupulous but gentle removal of all maternal blood, mucus, and amniotic fluid from the neonate's skin as soon as possible after birth. Care is taken to remove excess secretions from the nares and oropharynx. Stomach contents also may be aspirated to remove maternal body fluids swallowed during passage through the birth canal. If the neonate is born with problems, immediate supportive care is provided.

When the neonate's condition has stabilized and the temperature is within normal limits, he or she may remain with the mother. She is instructed in proper handwashing techniques, and reinforcement is provided as needed. There is some controversy about breastfeeding. Hepatitis B virus is found in breast milk, but many experts believe that this route of contamination is rare, and nursing should be allowed. Other neonatologists suggest that breastfeeding should be discouraged when the mother has the acute form of the disease.

Nurses caring for newborns with HIV should observe universal body substance precautions. Current data indicate that occupational exposure to patients with HIV poses little threat to health care workers if CDC guidelines are observed (NAACOG, 1992). There is a tendency to avoid neonates with HIV and their parents. This places the neonate at risk for sensory deprivation. Daily sensory stimulation and interaction with nurturing caregivers is essential. Special support services (social workers, counselors, and child welfare agencies) should be used to support parents and assist the nurse with discharge planning. Boland and Czarniecki (1991) note that some nurses may blame parents for the infant's health problems. Nurses who work intensively with HIV-positive neonates often need to seek professional support to overcome negative feelings.

Nursing care in fungal infections is directed first and foremost at preventing infection by using scrupulous handwashing and maintaining aseptic technique when handling equipment and TPN solutions and during blood-drawing procedures. Preventing skin trauma is critical. The drug of choice in the treatment of candidiasis is amphotericin B. Other agents used with limited effectiveness include fluorocytosine and miconazole nitrate. Because of the potentially toxic side effects of these drugs, close monitoring of vital signs and the neonate's general response to the infusion of these agents is essential.

Because of immature immunologic functioning at birth, the neonate is susceptible to infection. If the neonate is preterm or has other complications, the susceptibility is increased. Early signs and symptoms often are subtle and nonspecific. Once the infection occurs, it can quickly spread through the blood. Frequently a workup to rule out sepsis is performed on high-risk neonates. Universal body substance precautions are observed with every neonate to protect other newborns and staff members from transmission of the infection.

The Neonate With Fractures

Fractures occur in the neonate as a result of traction, manipulation, or compression of body parts during delivery or from the use of forceps. Certain neonates are at greater risk for fractures. The increased chest circumference of LGA infants may lead to shoulder dystocia at the time of birth. Neonates with abnormal presentations at delivery, such as breech or arm presentations, also are at increased risk for skeletal injury. Preterm neonates whose bones are especially fragile may sustain fractures with very little manipulation at birth.

Both complete fractures of the bone and greenstick fractures, in which one side of the bone is broken while the other side is intact or slightly bent, may occur. When fractures occur in the long bones (clavicle, humerus, ulna, and femur), edema, erythema, or ecchymosis may be evident over the injury. There may be diminished movement or "guarding" of the affected extremity, and if nerve damage accompanies the fracture, partial or complete flaccidity of the extremity may be observed. Skull fractures and fractures of the vertebrae may have more serious sequelae because they can result in injury to the central nervous system and permanent impairment in function.

Fracture of the Clavicle

Clavicular fracture is the most common fracture during vaginal birth. It can result in the development of ecchymosis or hematoma over the injured site and diminished movement of the extremity on the affected side. The Moro reflex may be asymmetric. A snapping noise or crepitus (a crackling sound produced by the rubbing together of bone fragments) may sometimes be heard with movement or "felt" with palpation. Fracture of the clavicle is painful, and guarding of the extremity on the affected side often will be noted.

Fracture of the Humerus or Femur

Fractures of the humerus or femur occur less frequently and are often associated with assisted breech deliveries. Edema, ecchymosis, hematoma, and even hemorrhage can occur over the fracture site, and marked restriction of the extremity is noted. It may be necessary to manipulate the bone to accomplish realignment; casts, slings, or splints may be indicated to maintain correct positioning of the extremity.

Skull Fracture

Because the neonate's skull is quite pliable at birth, as a result of incomplete mineralization, skull fractures are less common than those involving long bones. Skull fractures may, however, occur during labor or delivery, and neonates delivered by forceps are at increased risk for this type of birth injury. The two types of skull fracture seen are linear and depressed. Simple linear fractures are frequently benign and normally heal without treatment. They may be associated with cephalohematoma and are discovered when an x-ray study is performed.

Depressed skull fractures may be palpated under the scalp as a depression in the bone. They may result in an actual break in the bone and can cause tears in the meninges, rupture of blood vessels, and damage to brain tissue underlying the fracture. If brain tissue is injured, neurologic signs and symptoms, including increased intracranial pressure and seizures, may be evident, and permanent neurologic impairment can occur. Depressed fractures, sometimes called ping pong ball fractures because of their configuration and sensation with palpation, may require surgical elevation.

Implications for Nursing Care

Some birth injuries may be visibly or easily identified by the nurse during the assessment of the neonate. Other injuries may be internal or so minor at birth that they are missed until the neonate shows evidence of trauma. The nurse who is aware of the major types of trauma to which the neonate is susceptible during labor and delivery can more quickly recognize them and implement appropriate care.

A fractured clavicle normally heals quickly and without special treatment. Nursing interventions are aimed at minimizing pain. This is accomplished by gentle handling and positioning the neonate on the abdomen or the unaffected side as much as possible. If a long-sleeved shirt is worn, the sleeve can be pinned to the infant's shirt to stabilize the arm on the affected side, but the use of splints is not recommended.

If a cast is applied, the nurse must carefully assess the tissues for adequate circulation by blanching the fingers or toes. If the tissue does not blanch, congestion may be present; if blanching persists for more than 3 seconds, circulation may be impaired. Either finding should be documented and reported to the physician. The nurse must be sure that there is adequate room around the edges of the cast to prevent pressure sores. The condition of the skin also must be evaluated frequently. The rough edges of the cast can excoriate the skin, and moleskin should be placed along the edges to prevent trauma.

Because a plaster cast is porous and will absorb urine and liquid stools, it is important that it be waterproofed once it has completely dried. Diapers should be changed frequently to prevent excessive soiling of the cast. The neonate should not be lifted by the legs to change diapers when a leg has been casted, because this can place pressure on the tissue surrounding the cast edges and can distort bone alignment or place undue tension on leg ligaments above the level of the cast.

Nursing interventions are aimed at minimizing pain by gentle handling of the infant and immobilization of the extremity. Pain medications are not normally prescribed, because they will make the infant lethargic, depress feeding reflexes, and increase the risk of aspiration. Support of the parents and preparation for discharge are essential aspects of care when the infant will go home with a splint or cast or will require special swaddling. Parents should be provided with ample opportunities to handle and care for the neonate in the hospital so that they will feel comfortable and confident about their ability to meet the newborn's needs. Appointments for follow-up care should be made before discharge, and parents should be given the names and telephone numbers of health professionals to contact if questions or problems arise at home.

The neonate suspected of or diagnosed as having a skull fracture is assessed closely for evidence of increased intracranial pressure secondary to hemorrhage or brain edema. Such evidence includes seizure activity, hypotonia, bulging fontanelles, unusual posturing, depressed cardiac or respiratory function, and hypothermia. A cardiorespiratory monitor is attached for continuous evaluation of vital signs, and the neonate is placed in an incubator to support thermoregulatory function and minimize energy requirements.

Because the neonate who has sustained neurologic injury as a result of skull fracture is at risk for the development of seizures, oral feedings are normally discontinued, and an IV fluid is infused until the newborn's condition stabilizes. If hypotonia or paralysis is present, the neonate is positioned to maintain a patent airway and to align extremities correctly so that contractures may be prevented.

Sandbags, mattress rolls, hand rolls, or recently developed "nesting devices" will aid the nurse in positioning the neonate. Frequent turning of the neonate and placement of a sheepskin mattress beneath him or her help prevent skin breakdown. Anticonvulsants will be administered to control seizure activity.

As with asphyxia, the parents usually are primarily concerned about the long-term neurologic sequelae of the injury. It is impossible at present to predict accurately the eventual intellectual capacity and neuromuscular function of a child in the neonatal period. Physicians are encouraged to be truthful with parents about the extent of the injury but to remain hopeful about the eventual outcome.

Nurses should be supportive of parents, taking time to answer questions about the infant's current condition and to reinforce information that the physician has imparted. Even

when the infant is totally unresponsive or comatose, the parents should be allowed to spend as much time as they desire and, as is possible at the bedside, touch and talk to him or her. Allowing them to participate in skin care and range of motion exercises can help dispel some of the sense of helplessness and hopelessness parents experience, supporting the early attachment process.

Neonatal fractures may be the result of traction, manipulation, or compression during delivery. Some neonates are at greater risk than others for fractures. Both complete fractures and greenstick fractures may occur. Nerve damage may accompany the fracture. Especially serious are skull fractures and fractures of the vertebrae. An experienced nurse will recognize birth injuries during the neonatal assessment, although some injuries may be minor or internal and will not be evident until the neonate shows evidence of trauma. If a cast is applied, the nurse performs cast care. The cast must be kept dry as the neonate voids and has bowel movements. The nurse also provides the family with opportunities to handle the neonate and arranges for follow-up care after discharge.

The Neonate With Central Nervous System Injuries

Intracranial Hemorrhage

Rupture of cerebral vessels resulting in intracranial hemorrhage is one of the most serious complications of the neonate. It may result in permanent neurologic impairment or death. Intracranial hemorrhage can occur with prolonged labor and severe molding of the fetal skull, a difficult vaginal birth that requires rotation of the fetal head or forceps extraction, or a precipitous labor or delivery that causes a sudden, severe increase in intracranial pressure. Tears in the dura mater may cause hemorrhage and an accumulation of blood in the subdural space (subdural hematoma).

The type and extent of neurologic injury depend on the location of the hemorrhage. Hemorrhage within the posterior fossa results in compression of the fourth ventricle and obstruction in the flow of cerebrospinal fluid. Signs of increased intracranial pressure will occur, including seizures; decreased or absent reflexes; hypotonia; bulging fontanelles; enlarged head circumference; "setting sun eyes"; a high, shrill cry; hypothermia; and episodes of apnea or bradycardia. Hemorrhage is confirmed by computed tomography scan.

The outcome of intracranial hemorrhage depends on the extent and location of the hemorrhage. In severe hemorrhage when minimal brain activity is recorded by electroencephalogram and decerebrate posturing occurs, the prognosis is very guarded. With milder hemorrhages minimal neurologic dysfunction is evident in later years.

Nerve Injury

A variety of nerve injuries can result from excessive pressure or traction on areas of the neonate's head and neck or in association with fractures.

Brachial Plexus Injury

The brachial plexus is a major network of nerves that arises from the spinal column (C-5 through T-7). The plexus is located in the base of the neck above the clavicle. The nerves in the plexus innervate the muscles of the arm and upper extremities. The plexus may be injured as a result of the stretching or torsion of the neck or extremities during a difficult delivery (breech or vertex). Nerve trauma also can occur in conjunction with fractures. The resultant limitation in movement may be a transient phenomenon or a permanent disability.

In approximately 80% of affected neonates, injury to the brachial plexus involves the nerves emanating from the upper spinal roots (C-5 and C-6) and leads to a loss of motor function in the upper arm. In Erb-Duchenne palsy the arm assumes a characteristic position, tightly adducted with internal rotation of the shoulder, extension of the elbow, and pronation of the forearm. The Moro reflex cannot be elicited on the affected side. There is usually no loss of sensory function. If injury to the plexus involves nerves emanating from the lower spinal roots (C-7 and T-1), the muscles of the lower arm are affected. There is a rare injury that leads to loss of motor function in the muscles of the hand (Klumpke's paralysis). The grasp reflex cannot be elicited. The entire brachial plexus also can be damaged, resulting in complete paralysis of the arm and hand.

Phrenic Nerve Injury

Paralysis of the diaphragm occurs when the phrenic nerve is injured. It is most frequently associated with brachial plexus injury when lateral hyperextension of the neck occurs during delivery. The diaphragm on the affected side is elevated and fixed (eventration). Lung tissue is displaced upward and fails to expand completely, resulting in diminished respiratory excursion on the affected side. The infant is tachypneic and evidences signs of respiratory distress. Atelectasis and pneumonia are common complications. The diagnosis of diaphragmatic paralysis is confirmed by fluoroscopy or ultrasonography. Often the condition is temporary, with eventual complete return of function.

Facial Nerve Injury

Facial paralysis frequently occurs when pressure is applied to the facial nerve by the blade of the obstetric forceps during delivery. The affected side of the face remains flaccid when the infant cries. The eyelid on the affected side may not close completely, and the lips do not grasp the nipple effectively for sucking. Facial paralysis usually is transient.

Implications for Nursing Care

Nursing care revolves around the particular injury. Nursing interventions for the neonate with intracranial hemorrhage are aimed at supporting vital functions and reducing energy requirements to a minimum. The neonate is placed in a neutral thermal environment, and using a cardiorespiratory monitor, vital signs are observed constantly. The head is

elevated slightly above the hips, and its circumference is measured daily to determine the presence and extent of head enlargement. If flaccidity or paralysis is evident, care is taken to maintain a patent airway, correctly align extremities, and turn the infant routinely to prevent skin breakdown.

Because the neonate may demonstrate depressed reflexes and diminished responsiveness, oral feedings are suspended and IV therapy is instituted. The nurse keeps an accurate intake and output record. Anticonvulsants may be administered to control seizure activity. Emotional support of the parents is the same as for an infant who has sustained brain injury secondary to skull fracture (see the nursing interventions described in the section "Skull Fracture" previously in this chapter).

The primary nursing responsibility in the care of a neonate with brachial plexus injury is to prevent contractures of the affected muscles by placing the arm in a neutral position and performing passive range of motion exercises. Rigid immobilization of the extremity and corrective positioning (external rotation of the shoulder, flexion of the elbow, and supination of the forearm) are no longer recommended, because they may actually result in contractures and deformities. The arm is immobilized in a natural position by pinning the sleeve to the shirt or by swaddling. After approximately 7 to 10 days, gentle passive range of motion exercises are initiated. Before discharge, the parents are instructed in the correct positioning of the arm and range of motion exercises and should be given ample time and opportunities to practice care.

In phrenic nerve injury nursing care is aimed initially at alleviating respiratory distress. The neonate is placed in a neutral thermal environment, and an enriched oxygen atmosphere is frequently ordered by the physician. The neonate is placed on the affected side to allow for full expansion of the opposite lung. Oral feedings may be withheld initially to decrease energy expenditures and prevent the risk of aspiration. Gavage feedings may be performed, but as the neonate's condition stabilizes, breastfeeding or bottle-feeding will be allowed. Parents will need encouragement and support in their efforts to feed and hold the neonate. They must feel fully competent to care for the neonate before discharge.

Nursing responsibilities when the neonate has facial nerve injury include protecting the eye on the affected side by applying artificial tears and keeping the eyelid closed with a dressing until the paralysis disappears. Additional support also may be needed during feeding to prevent drooling of formula or aspiration. Support and education will provide parents with the skills needed to meet their newborn's needs.

Central nervous system injuries range from permanent neurologic impairment or death to transient conditions. One of the most serious complications of the neonate is intracranial hemorrhage. Intracranial hemorrhage may result in permanent impairment or death. The type and extent of injury depends on the location of the hemorrhage. A variety of nerve injuries may result from excessive pressure or traction on the neonate's head or neck during birth or in association with fractures. The resultant limitation in movement from brachial plexus nerve injury may be transient or permanent. Paralysis of the diaphragm occurs when the phrenic nerve is injured and lung and respiratory complications result. Often the condition is temporary. Facial paralysis from injury to the facial nerve usually is transient.

The Neonate With Hemolytic Disease

Hemolytic disease of the newborn is a disorder in which the neonate's RBCs are destroyed or hemolyzed with resultant hyperbilirubinemia and jaundice. It may be caused by maternal antibodies that cross the placenta and enter the fetal bloodstream. Other causes of RBC hemolysis include infection and enzymatic deficiencies in the RBC (eg, glucose-6-phosphate-dehydrogenase deficiency, or G6PD). Two of the most frequently occurring hemolytic diseases of the newborn are ABO incompatibility and Rh disease.

At birth, the neonate with Rh incompatibility has a positive direct Coombs' test, indicating the presence of circulating maternal antibodies in the bloodstream. The neonate is anemic and has a falling hematocrit; the number of circulating immature RBCs is increased. A rapidly rising serum bilirubin level occurs with continued hemolysis of RBCs, and pathologic jaundice develops soon after birth. Phototherapy is initiated, and an exchange transfusion may be performed to prevent kernicterus when serum bilirubin reaches dangerously high levels.

Rh Incompatibility (Erythroblastosis Fetalis)

Rh disease occurs when the mother is Rh negative and the fetus is Rh positive. When fetal Rh positive RBCs gain access to the maternal bloodstream, which contains Rh negative RBCs, an antigen–antibody response is stimulated. The maternal immune system becomes primed and ready to attack fetal RBCs in subsequent pregnancies when the fetus is Rh positive. Conditions that increase the likelihood of fetal RBCs having entered the maternal circulation from a previous pregnancy include previous abortions, placental accidents, amniocentesis, and separation of the placenta at birth. Rh positive antibodies are produced, pass through the placenta, attach to the fetal RBCs, and destroy them. The fetus reacts by producing large numbers of immature RBCs to replace those that were hemolyzed (thus the name *erythroblastosis fetalis*).

Hydrops Fetalis

In the most severe form of the disease, known as hydrops fetalis, the fetus becomes severely anemic. Hepatosplenomegaly is evident at birth. Fluid leaks out of the intravascular compartment (due to decreased oncotic pressure), resulting in hydrothorax (fluid in the pleural space) and ascites. Generalized edema also is evident. Eventually, severe cardiomegaly and hypoxia lead to cardiac failure and death if the fetus is not treated by intrauterine transfusion of RBCs and delivered before term.

ABO Incompatibility

ABO incompatibility is a much milder form of hemolytic disease. It involves group A or B infants born to group O mothers and less frequently group B infants born to group A mothers. Because anti-A and anti-B antibodies naturally exist in the bloodstream of group O mothers, senitization can occur with the first pregnancy. Stillbirths and the severe hydrops seen in the Rh disease almost never occur. The neonate becomes jaundiced after birth, but massive hemolysis and resultant anemia are rare.

Implications for Nursing Care

If the neonate with a blood incompatibility develops pathologic jaundice, phototherapy is instituted. The nurse initiates the therapy and monitors the neonate closely for common complications of the procedure, including hyperthermia, dehydration, skin excoriation, rashes, and bronzing. An exchange transfusion may be performed to remove sensitized RBCs and serum bilirubin and correct severe anemia, but because of the risk of transmission of hepatitis and HIV with blood transfusion, lower RBC and hematocrit levels may be tolerated in neonates today (see the section "Hyperbilirubinemia and Kernicterus" previously in this chapter.)

Nursing care is organized to allow extended periods of rest for the anemic neonate who is hemolyzing RBCs and is jaundiced. A neutral thermal environment is used to reduce energy expenditures until the neonate's condition stabilizes. Vital signs are monitored frequently. Tachycardia may be evident with severe anemia. Parents are encouraged to visit frequently and are given the opportunity to hold and care for the neonate each day. Phototherapy should be discontinued (even if only for short periods of time) to allow parents to have eye-to-eye contact with their neonate.

Hemolytic disease of the newborn is a disease in which the neonate's RBCs are destroyed or hemolyzed with resultant hyperbilirubinemia and jaundice. Two of the most frequently occurring hemolytic diseases are Rh disease and ABO incompatibility. Rh incompatibility, also called erythroblastosis fetalis, occurs when the mother is Rh negative and the fetus is Rh positive. The most severe form of the disease is hydrops fetalis, and death may occur if the fetus is not treated by intrauterine transfusion of RBCs and delivered before term. ABO incompatibility is a milder form of hemolytic disease.

The Neonate With Effects of Maternal Substance Abuse

The woman who abuses drugs, alcohol, or other substances delivers a newborn with many physical and neurobehavioral characteristics that reflect the direct effect of the substance on fetal growth and development (Fig. 33-15). Additionally,

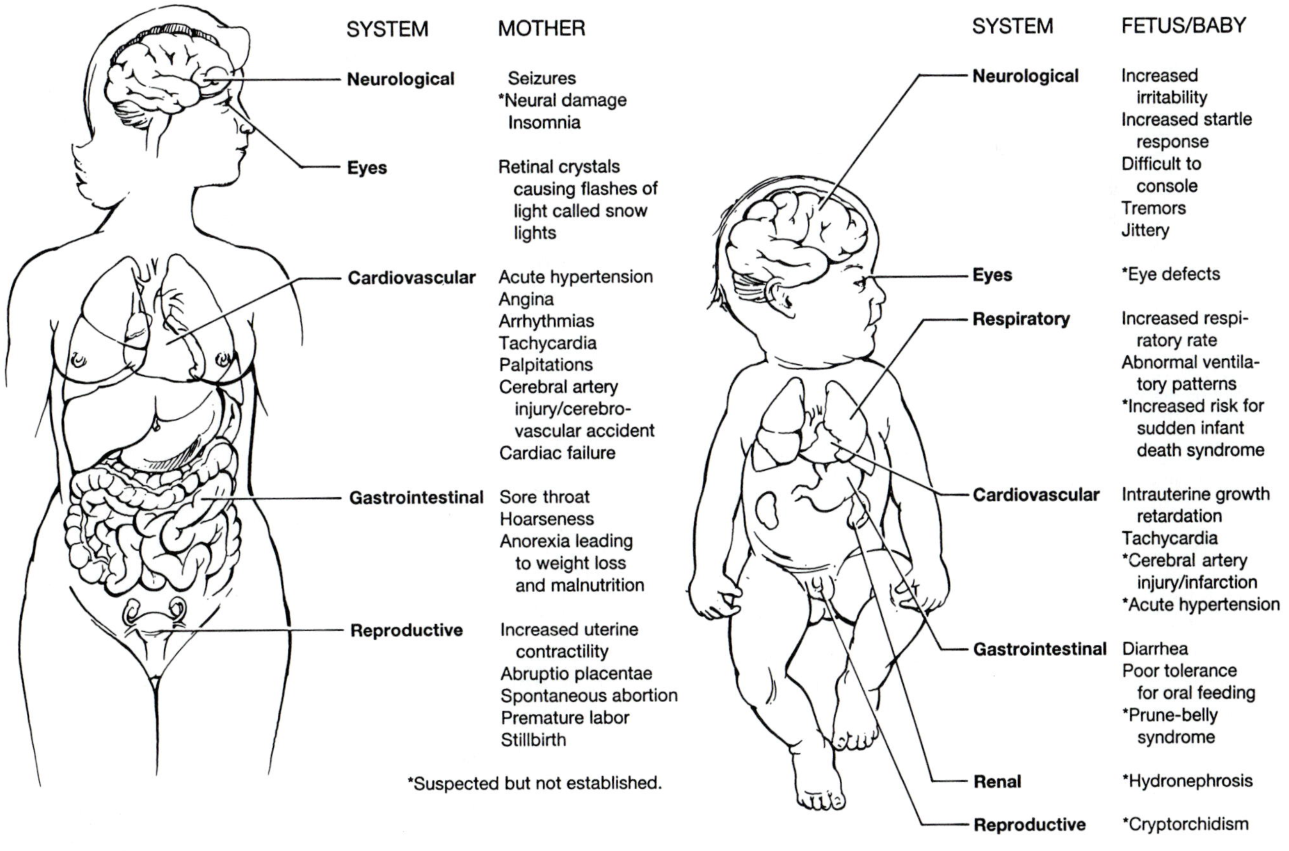

Figure 33-15.
Substance abuse affects the systems of both the mother and fetus-neonate.

neonates may suffer from neonatal abstinence syndrome (formerly referred to as narcotic withdrawal) after birth. The infant of a substance abusing mother (ISAM), formerly called the infant of an addicted mother, is likely to suffer from the effects of maternal malnutrition (ie, to be SGA) and from disease processes associated with drug abuse (eg, sexually transmitted diseases and hepatitis). These newborns are considered high risk. For a variety of reasons alcohol, cocaine, and opiates are the most prevalent substances abused in Western society, so the effects of these substances on the fetus and neonate are discussed in this chapter. Neonatal abstinence syndrome is discussed also.

Maternal Alcohol Abuse

Fetal Alcohol Syndrome

Fetuses of mothers who ingest more than 3 oz of 100% alcohol per day are at risk for being born with *fetal alcohol syndrome* or *fetal alcohol effects*, a milder configuration of the syndrome. Affected newborns present with a number of physical signs that aid in the diagnosis of the disorder:

- Microcephaly
- Facial anomalies: short palpebral fissure; epicanthal folds; short, upturned nose, micrognathia; thin upper lip
- Cardiac defects (primarily septal)
- Minor joint and limb anomalies, especially joint malformations
- Altered palmar crease patterns
- Postnatal growth retardation (failure to thrive)
- Mental retardation

These newborns experience withdrawal symptoms somewhat similar to those of neonates of narcotic abusing mothers (see the section "Neonatal Abstinence Syndrome").

Maternal Cocaine Abuse

Cocaine use and abuse in the general population has been exponentially increasing since the mid-1970s; however, researchers did not begin looking at the effects on the developing fetus and on the neonate until the mid-1980s. Longitudinal studies are now comparing children who were exposed to cocaine in utero with unexposed and opiate-exposed children. The findings are alarming but as yet inconclusive. More research needs to be conducted to further describe the long-term effects of cocaine exposure in utero and to describe interventions that assist these children to maintain state and behavioral control.

The fetal effects most often associated with maternal cocaine abuse include lower birth weights, lower gestational ages due to preterm labor and birth (frequently as a result of placental abruption), decreased head circumference, anemia, and IUGR (Peters & Theorell, 1991). Table 33-6 lists the potential neonatal effects. Additionally, there is a slightly higher risk for sudden infant death syndrome among cocaine-exposed infants (5.7 in 1000 versus 4.9 in 1000 for nonexposed infants).

Table 33-6. Potential Neonatal Effects of Maternal Cocaine Use

Physical	Behavioral
Decreased gestational age	Irritability
Decreased birth weight	Tremors
Decreased length	Poor feeding
Decreased head circumference	Frantic fist sucking
Prematurity	Abnormal sleep patterns
Intrauterine growth retardation	Sneezing
Anemia	Yawning
Ileal atresia	High-pitched cry
Prune belly syndrome	Increased startles
Cryptorchidism	State disorganization
Hypospadius	State lability
Hydronephrosis	Poor visual processing
Hypertonia	Decreased spontaneous activity
Seizures	Dull alert periods
Tachycardia	Difficult to console
Fever	
Tachypnea	
Congenital heart disease	
Skull defects	
Hypertension	
Cerebral infarction	
Absent digits	
Vomiting	
Diarrhea	

From Kennard, M. J. (1990). Cocaine use during pregnancy: Fetal and neonatal effects. *Journal of Perinatal and Neonatal Nursing, 3*(4), 53–63, with permission of Aspen Publishers, Inc., © 1990.

The behavioral effects of cocaine observed in neonates are probably due to effects of the drug itself (whether from fetal exposure or from direct effects of the drug ingested just before delivery) than from an abstinence syndrome. Many of the neurobehavioral signs are similar to those exhibited by neonates withdrawing from opiates but are not as severe nor as protracted. Further research will more accurately define the neonatal and childhood effects of cocaine exposure.

Maternal Opiate Abuse

Newborns who seem to be most distressed (and distressing to nursing staff) are those born to narcotic- or opiate-abusing women (primarily heroin and methadone). Their acute withdrawal symptoms may last for several months and pose numerous challenges for the caregivers. The following section discusses these symptoms and the nursing care of these neonates. Unlike cocaine and alcohol, opiates seem to have minimal long-term effects (such as mental retardation, seizure disorders, and learning disabilities). The immediate neonatal period is the crucial period.

Neonatal Abstinence Syndrome

The neonate exposed to opiates in utero begins to experience acute abstinence syndrome shortly after birth. The severity and length of time that symptoms are experienced depend on the type and amount of drug the mother was

abusing during pregnancy and the timing of the last ingestion before delivery.

Symptomatology

Abstinence syndrome symptoms involve primarily the central nervous, respiratory, and gastrointestinal systems.

Central Nervous System. The newborn is irritable, tremulous, hypertonic, and has a high-pitched cry. State control is affected, so the neonate moves abruptly from sleep to a hyperactive state. Sleep cycles are significantly shortened. The slightest noise, light, or movement will startle the ISAM into an escalating pattern of disorganization and frenzy. Constant activity leads to excoriation of the skin at pressure points over bony prominences (primarily knees, elbows, and nose). Seizure activity may be demonstrated with severe abstinence syndrome.

Respiratory System. Tachypnea and tachycardia are common, and the neonate may be incapable of nipple feeding (due to discoordination) when symptoms are most severe. Nasal stuffiness, which results from vasomotor instability, exacerbates the neonate's tachypnea and can lead to respiratory distress.

Gastrointestinal System. Gastrointestinal signs and symptoms often are marked and interfere with ingestion of adequate calories and fluid. Although the newborn has an unusually strong, hyperactive nonnutritive suck, he or she is a very poor feeder with an uncoordinated suck–swallow reflex. Frequently, the ISAM's jaws merely clamp down on the nipple, frustrating the neonate and caregiver. Persistent regurgitation of feedings (whether from crying or intolerance of feedings) may lead to severe fluid and electrolyte imbalances. It may be necessary to discontinue oral feedings until the crisis has passed.

Other Systems. Hyperthermia frequently accompanies other symptoms and is related to increased metabolic rate, physical activity, dehydration, central nervous system involvement, and environmental causes. The neonate also experiences vasomotor instability as reflected by sweating, flushing, and stuffy nose.

Implications for Nursing Care

Supporting the Neonate. Nursing care of the ISAM requires great patience and skill. (The accompanying Nursing Care Plan for the Small-for-Gestational Age Neonate experiencing narcotic abstinence syndrome outlines nursing implications.) ISAM newborns cry frequently, often for no apparent reason, and attempts to soothe them are to no avail. They are hypertonic and resist cuddling or holding; they are most comfortable when tightly swaddled (thereby preventing startle reflexes to maintain sleep states) and placed in a "rocker bed." The rhythmicity of the rocking motion, along with the uterine sounds emitted by the bed, provide a comfort that cannot be matched by the nurse.

Because of the neonate's inability to habituate, a quiet, dimly lit environment is necessary. To keep the environment quiet the nurse places the neonate away from doors, garbage pails (although the lids may be padded to reduce the noise), and other newborns, whose monitors may alarm them.

Seizures may occur, in which case the neonate will require anticonvulsants (phenobarbitol or phenytoin [Dilantin]). All attempts are made, however, to treat symptomatology, even pharmacologically if necessary, to avoid seizures. Valium may be administered for several days to relax the neonate enough for sleep and nipple feedings. Paregoric (camphorated tincture of opium) may be administered if the gastrointestinal motility is resulting in weight loss, cramping, gastrointestinal distress, or skin excoriation of the buttocks. Extra time is required during feedings, because the neonate may gag and be uncoordinated or may vomit the milk. Volunteer programs have been extremely beneficial in providing unhurried, caring personnel who are able to spend time with these neonates. Intravenous therapy may be initiated when fluid and electrolyte imbalances occur. Because of the constant rubbing of extremities against the mattress and increased incidence of diarrhea, meticulous care of the skin is required to prevent its breakdown.

The nurse must monitor vital signs closely and observe for evidence of seizure activity (which may be subtle and not tonoclonic in nature), respiratory distress, and hyperthermia. Several instruments have been developed that aid the nurse in a systematic assessment of neonatal narcotic abstinence syndrome. The nurse completes the assessment tool at least once each shift (see the accompanying display on the Lewis Protocol). A cardiorespiratory monitor and pulse oximeter may be attached to assist in continuous surveillance of cardiopulmonary function. Fluid intake and output

NURSING ALERT

RESPIRATORY SUPPORT OF THE NEONATE EXPERIENCING ABSTINENCE SYNDROME

Neonatal abstinence syndrome (NAS) can precipitate sudden life-threatening complications that require prompt emergency measures. The neonate may experience seizure activity related to the withdrawal phenomenon or secondary to infection that is transmitted by the mother during pregnancy or birth. Seizures may be accompanied by apnea episodes. Gastrointestinal symptoms may result in regurgitation, projectile vomiting, and airway obstruction. Nasal stuffiness is common with NAS and may cause respiratory distress. If the neonate is treated with diluted tincture of opium or other central nervous system depressants to reduce the severity of withdrawal symptoms, lethargy and respiratory depression may occur.

The nurse must monitor the neonate closely for evidence of respiratory compromise. The neonate should be positioned to reduce the risk of regurgitation and aspiration after feeding (sidelying with head of crib elevated). Suction, oxygen, and ventilation equipment should be readily available. A bulb syringe should be used to remove mucus and formula as needed from the nares. If persistent tachypnea, and signs of respiratory distress (flaring, grunting, and retractions) develop, a cardiorespiratory monitor and pulse oximeter should be applied for continuous monitoring.

Text continues on page 1052

Nursing Care Plan

The Small-for-Gestational Age Neonate Experiencing Narcotic Abstinence Syndrome

PATIENT PROFILE

History

Baby Boy S is a 2325-g neonate born at approximately 37 weeks' gestation. His mother, a daily heroin user, did not receive prenatal care, and her EDD was uncertain. The neonate was born after a rapid, uneventful labor. Apgar scores were 7 and 9 at 1 and 5 minutes. Umbilical cord blood gases were within normal limits. Postnatal examination revealed a stable small-for-gestational age (SGA) neonate.

Baby S is placed on prophylactic antibodies while blood cultures and other tests for infection are analyzed. There are no physical signs of infection. Oral feedings are implemented. A special 24 calorie/oz formula is given every 3 hours. Baby S initially has strong, coordinated suck and swallow reflexes and ingests 25 to 30 mL per feeding by 24 hours postbirth.

At 48 hours Baby S begins to exhibits a high-pitched cry and is agitated for prolonged periods. The tone becomes markedly increased, and he arches his back and neck intermittently. There are frequent startles and marked jitteriness. He must be tightly swaddled to prevent self-perpetuated agitation and jitteriness. Sucking and swallowing becomes discoordinated, and it takes Baby S 30 to 40 minutes to ingest 15 to 20 mL or formula. A diagnosis of neonatal abstinence syndrome is made.

Physical Assessment

At 72 postnatal hours the nurse performs an assessment and notes the following data: Weight is 2170 g (decreased 40 g from previous day). T. 37.5°C (99.5°F), P 166, RR 72. The neonate has marked hypertonia and jitteriness. The skin is pink, diaphoretic, and the skin turgor is decreased (recoil of tissue 3–4 seconds). Small excoriations are evident on the bony prominences of the ankles, knees, elbows, chin, and nose. The cry remains high pitched, and the suck is hypertonic. There are crusts of formula and mucus in the nares and there is marked nasal flaring. The heart rate is regular, +2 peripheral pulses are palpated, and the precordium is quiet.

Breath sounds are clear bilaterally. The abdomen is flat and soft, and there are hyperactive bowel sounds. A large, liquid, yellow–green stool has been passed. The skin in the perianal area is erythematous and excoriated. There is no urine in the diaper, and the neonate has not voided for 4 hours.

COLLABORATIVE PROBLEMS/POTENTIAL COMPLICATIONS

- Hypoglycemia
- Seizures
- Infection
- Polycythemia

(See the accompanying Nursing Alert display).

Assessment	*Nursing Diagnosis*	*Nursing Interventions*	*Rationale*
Respirations 72 min Crusts of dried mucus and formula in nares Marked nasal flaring Baby S is experiencing neonatal abstinence syndrome.	Ineffective Airway Clearance related to developmental level (neonate) and mechanical obstruction (mucus and formula)	Suction nares gently with bulb syringe.	To remove mucus and formula from nares. Use of suction catheter should be avoided to suction nares because it may traumatize delicate nasal mucous and cause swelling.
	Expected Outcome Baby S's airway, including nares, will remain patent and free from mucus and formula.	Administer saline nasal drops as ordered.	To soften dried crusts for easier removal.

(*Continued*)

The Small-for-Gestational Age Neonate Experiencing Narcotic Abstinence Syndrome

(Continued)

Assessment	Nursing Diagnosis	Nursing Interventions	Rationale
			To reduce nasal stuffiness associated with NAS.
		Elevate head of bed (HOB) after feedings, and place neonate on right side.	To reduce risk of regurgitation Placing neonate on right side promotes stomach emptying, thus reducing risk of regurgitation.
Temperate is 37.5°C (99.5°F). Skin is diaphoretic. Neonate is hypertonic and exhibits agitated movement and crying. Neonate is tightly swaddled to reduce agitation.	Hyperthermia related to hypertonicity, agitation, and crying ***Expected Outcome*** Baby S's airway, including nares, will remain patent and free from mucus and formula.	Monitor temperature q 3–4 h.	To permit early identification and treatment of hyperthermia.
		Remove extra clothing (shirts, cap).	To reduce body temperature.
		Gives sponge bath with warm water.	To permit controlled heat loss by evaporation when the neonate is hyperthemic.
		Use thin cotton blanket to swaddle neonate.	
		Use rolled blankets to "nest" neonate.	"Nesting" neonate, by placing blanket rolls around body may reduce self-perpetuating movement and agitation, thus reducing heat generation.
Temperature is 37.5°C (99.5°F). Decreased skin turgor (3–4 sec recoil). Baby S ingests 15 to 20 mL in 30 to 40 min. Passed large liquid stool. No urine passed in 4 h.	Fluid Volume Deficit related to hyperthermia Altered Nutrition: Less than Body Requirements related to decreased intake ***Expected Outcome*** Baby S will gain at least 15 to 20 g each day. Baby S will ingest 100 to 120 Kcal/kg/d without regurgitation or diarrhea.	Strictly monitor intake and output. Weigh diapers. Weigh neonate daily. Measure (weigh) regurgitated formula. Assess tissue turgor. Measure specific gravity of urine.	To permit early identification of fluid and calorie deficits. Significant loss of fluid may occur when the neonate experiences NAS. To identify fluid deficits and dehydration.
		Assess glucose levels as ordered.	Hypoglycemia may occur with inadequate calorie intake and with excessive activity. The SGA neonate has limited glycogen stores. The SGA neonate has a small stomach capacity and may need special formula, in small amounts, at frequent intervals.
		Maintain body temperature within normal limits.	Hyperthermia will increase insensitive fluid loss.

(Continued)

The Small-for-Gestational Age Neonate Experiencing Narcotic Abstinence Syndrome

(*Continued*)

Assessment	***Nursing Diagnosis***	***Nursing Interventions***	***Rationale***
		Administer dilute tincture of opium or other drugs as ordered.	To reduce GI abnormalities (diarrhea and vomiting) associated with NAS.
		Administer IV fluids or provide enteric feedings by oral gavage route as ordered.	Additional IV fluids may be needed if the neonate is unable to ingest or retain formula. Gavage feedings may be required if the suck and swallow reflexes are discoordinated.
Baby S has decreased tissue turgor (3–4 sec recoil). Excoriations noted on bony prominences. Perianal excoriations noted. Loose yellow–green stool noted.	Impaired Skin Integrity related to agitation, diaphoresis, diarrhea. ***Expected Outcome*** Baby S will exhibit a resolution of skin excoriations and perianal irritation.	Assess skin integrity q 4–8 h.	To identify and treat skin breakdown promptly.
		Keep skin and linens dry. Change diapers when soiled.	Moisture will contribute to skin breakdown and the growth of bacteria and yeast.
		Expose perianal area to air. Use heat lamp Use 25-w bulb and focus 18–20 in from skin for 15 min	Air will facilitate healing of tissue. Heat promotes blood flow to tissues and accelerates healing. To prevent burns.
		Apply moisture barrier, such as zinc oxide, to perianal area.	To reduce exposure of skin to urine and stool.
		Swaddle neonate to reduce agitation-caused excoriations.	To reduce self-perpetuating limb movement, jitteriness, and agitation.
		Maintain temperature within normal range.	To reduce diaphoresis and moisture on skin.
		Maintain fluid balance.	To improve skin turgor.
		Place sheep skin mattress pad to crib.	To reduce friction-generated skin trauma
Baby A is 37-wk SGA neonate who was exposed to heroin in utero. Neonate is experiencing NAS: • Hypertonia • Arching of back and neck • Jitteriness • High-pitched cry • Frequent startles • Agitation	Sleep Pattern Disturbance related to in utero exposure to heroin and NAS Altered Growth and Development related to prenatal heroin exposure ***Expected Outcome*** Baby S will demonstrate decreased periods of agitation and increased periods of sleep.	Assess neonate for evidence and severity of NAS, and document q 4–8 h.	To facilitate identification and treatment of NAS.
		Tightly swaddle neonate.	To reduce self–perpetuating agitation and jitteriness.
		Place neonate on rocker or water bed.	To promote sleep and reduce agitation. To provide appropriate kinesthetic stimulation.
		Offer pacifier.	To provide support for non-

(*Continued*)

The Small-for-Gestational Age Neonate Experiencing Narcotic Abstinence Syndrome

(Continued)

Assessment	*Nursing Diagnosis*	*Nursing Interventions*	*Rationale*
			nutritive sucking and to reduce tension.
• Hyperthermia • Discoordinate suck and swallow • Regurgitation • Loose stools	Baby S will exhibit decreasing signs and symptoms of narcotic abstinence as evidenced by normal muscle tone, coordinated reflexes, and feeding patterns.	Reduce environmental stimuli. • Dim lights • Reduce noise level Develop infant stimulation plan as NAS resolves.	To promote normal growth and development of neuromuscular system.
		Initiate physical therapy consult if available.	To prevent neurobehavioral and motor dysfunction and disability.
		Teach caregiver about the neonate behavioral cues and appropriate interaction and stimulation activities.	To foster neonatal caretaking skills appropriate for the drug-exposed neonate and to support caretaker–neonate acquaintance and attachment

EVALUATION

Baby S was placed on an electric rocker bed in a quiet corner of the observation nursery. Lights were dimmed and a schedule was established that organized nursing care activity into clusters to reduce stimulation. The neonate was given dilute tincture of opium (neonatal opium solution) 0.05 mL/kg q 6 h for 1 week.

Signs and symptoms of NAS were gradually reduced. After 2 days of drug therapy, Baby S was able to ingest 30 to 40 mL of formula q 3 h. The diarrhea stopped 24 hours after administration of the first dose of opium. Skin turgor improved and urine output increased. The neonate's temperature remained between 36.8°C and 37.2°C (97.3°F to 99°F). The mother was discharged from the hospital on the third postpartum day and did not return to the nursery to visit the neonate. A social worker made arrangements for placement of the neonate in foster care with a family skilled in caring for an infant with NAS.

are measured. Skin turgor and the condition of mucous membranes are evaluated frequently to alert the nurse to signs of dehydration.

Supporting the Parents. Pregnant women who abuse heroin may be able to enter methadone maintenance programs, which then continue into the postpartum period. The goals of these programs are the following:

- Altering the life-style and drug-seeking behaviors that would otherwise occur
- Preventing fetal seizures and pregnancy loss that occurs with abstinence and inconsistent drug use
- Decreasing the fetal exposure to unknown and possibly toxic substances that are used to "cut" street heroin

Methadone "withdrawal" is not any easier than heroin withdrawal for newborns and in fact may be more difficult, but the neonates of mothers in these programs stand a better chance of being born at term, thereby avoiding the complications of prematurity.

These mothers need extra support and encouragement during the early neonatal period. They may experience overwhelming remorse and guilt and avoid being around their newborn. Other mothers with fewer resources may not have insight into the cause-and-effect relationship between their drug abuse and the abstinence experience of their newborn. Nurses working with mothers and family members must meet the challenge of maintaining an accepting, nonjudgmental attitude in the face of life-styles that they may find objectionable.

The nurse should focus his or her energies on supporting appropriate efforts at parenting, allowing mothers to

Lewis' Protocol
Behaviors of Prenatal Drug-Exposed (PDE) Infants 0 to 12 Months

Infant Name/No. ________ Date of Birth ________ Age ________ Date ________

Birth Wt. ________ Present Wt. ________ Birth Length ________ Present Length ________

Birth Head Circ. ________ Present Head Circ. ________ 1—Male 2—Female (Circle #) CODE: ________ - ________

Ethnicity (Circle #): 1—White 2—Black 3—Hispanic 4—Asian Clinician ________

Circle: # 1—Own Home 2—Foster Home 3—Hospital # Foster Home Placements ________

Diagnosis: ________

Legend: 0 = Never 1 = Rare 2 = Moderate 3 = Frequent PB = Previous Behavior

I. State Systems
1. Passivity ____
2. Irritability ____
3. Dull alert state ____
4. Frequency or rapidity of state changes ____
5. Difficult to comfort ____

Subscale Total: ____

Comments: ________

II. Neurobehavioral System
6. Lethargy ____
7. High-pitched cry ____
8. Frequent startle response ____
9. Increased sucking ____
10. Tremors ____
11. Hyperactivity ____

Subscale Total: ____

Comments: ________

III. Visual System
12. Jerky eye movement ____
13. Eye muscle imbalance ____
14. Difficulty tracking horizontal and vertical ____
15. Difficulty initiating eye contact ____
16. Difficulty maintaining eye contact ____
17. Limited visual monitoring of hands ____

Subscale Total: ____

Comments: ________

IV. Autonomic System
18. Sweating ____
19. Frequent yawning ____
20. Hiccupping ____
21. Unexplained fevers ____
22. Gaze aversion ____
23. Increased respiration ____
24. Sneezing ____

Subscale Total: ____

Comments: ________

V. Respiratory System
25. Nasal stuffiness ____
26. Labored breathing ____

Subscale Total: ____

Comments: ________

VI. Gastrointestinal System
27. Regurgitation ____
28. Difficult feeding ____
29. Loose stools ____

Subscale Total: ____

Comments: ________

VII. Muscle Tone
30. Low muscle tone ____
31. High muscle tone ____
32. Fluctuating muscle tone ____
33. Tone difference in extremities ____

Subscale Total: ____

Comments: ________

VIII. Movement Pattern
34. Jerky movements ____
35. Widespread arms ____
36. Intolerance to cuddling ____
37. Head lag over 4 months when pull-to-sit ____

Subscale Total: ____

Comments: ________

IX. Communications
38. Undifferentiated cries ____
39. No social laugh ____
40. No social smile ____
41. Limited vocalizations ____
42. Limited intonation ____
43. Limited vocalization to caregiver's response ____

Subscale Total ____

X. Play
44. Limited banging, shaking, squeezing of objects ____
45. Excessive banging, throwing, or mouthing of objects ____
46. Limited functional use of toys ____
47. Limited imitating with objects, people ____
48. Limited initiation of play ____
49. Distractible ____
50. Easily frustrated ____

Subscale Total: ____

Comments: ________

TOTAL SCORE: ____

ventilate feelings of guilt and anxiety, and answering questions as they arise. Before discharge the parents should be given every opportunity to care for their neonate so they are confident of their ability to recognize and meet special needs. Signs of central nervous system disturbance may persist for many months after the acute phase of abstinence, and the family will need concrete suggestions for dealing with a hyperactive, irritable neonate. Referrals for follow-up by a social service agency and a visiting nurse or a public health nurse are essential.

Sometimes temporary foster care placement is made if conditions in the home are hazardous to the neonate's welfare. The final decisions made by the court regarding parental rights and neonatal placement are often based, in part, on nursing documentation. It is essential that the nurse document all telephone calls and visits made by the parents, and chart subjective and objective data regarding maternal–newborn interactions. Regardless of the ultimate disposition of the neonate, the parents should have every opportunity to visit the nursery and provide care until the neonate is discharged.

Newborns of mothers who abuse substances have many physical and neurobehavioral characteristics that reflect the direct effect of the substance on fetal growth and development. Additionally, the ISAM is likely to suffer from the effects of maternal nutrition and drug-associated disease processes. Fetal alcohol syndrome can be recognized in newborns of mothers who ingest more than 3 oz of 100% alcohol per day. Neonatal abstinence syndrome is a condition in which the neonate suffers from withdrawal of substances after birth. Nurses must support the neonate and parenting skills in neonatal abstinence syndrome.

The neonate experiencing maladaptations secondary to prenatal drug exposure poses many challenges for the nurse. Both physiologic and behavioral problems may complicate the immediate postbirth period and the infant's early years. The nurse plays a key role in the early identification of problems and support of the neonate. The goal of care is to aid the neonate in achieving physiologic stability and behavioral competence. Once this goal is met, the nurse assists the parents in establishing ties with their neonate and guides them in appropriate care.

Chapter Summary

Provision of family-centered care occurs in less-than-ideal circumstances when complications occur in the neonatal period. Innovative approaches to care must be devised to support neonates and parents. This can best be accomplished using the nursing process in assessing needs, diagnosing problems, planning interventions, and evaluating outcomes of care. The nurse must be skilled in promoting pulmonary adaptation and ventilation, supporting cardiac adaptations, promoting fluid and electrolyte balance, providing nutritional needs, preventing infection, supporting thermal regulation, and monitoring and preventing complications, in addition to providing routine care of the newborn. The nurse must be adept at handling neonatal emergencies and must possess a comprehensive knowledge of theories about attachment, behavioral adaptation, parental grieving, and crisis prevention to support the new family.

Study Questions

1. *What therapeutic techniques can be used to maintain a patent airway in the high-risk neonate?*
2. *What are the major risks of oxygen therapy for the neonate?*
3. *What are preventive measures against infection in the nursery?*
4. *What is the significance of a "neutral thermal environment" for the high-risk or sick neonate?*
5. *How can the nurse prevent altered parenting for a neonate in the intensive care nursery?*
6. *By what mechanism does phototherapy reduce serum bilirubin levels? What are the major complications of phototherapy?*
7. *Why is the infant of a diabetic mother at increased risk for the development of hypoglycemia?*
8. *What is meconium aspiration syndrome? Which groups of infants are at increased risk for the development of this complication?*
9. *What are the major nursing interventions in the care of the neonate who has been casted after a long bone fracture at birth?*
10. *How can the nurse best support the neonate experiencing neonatal abstinence syndrome?*

References

Als, H. (1986). A synactive model of neonatal behavioral organization: Framework for the assessment of neurobehavioral development in the premature infant and for the support of infants and parents in the neonatal intensive care environment. *Physical and Occupational Therapy in Pediatrics*, *6*, 3–53.

Bastin, N., Tamayo, O., Tinkle, M., Amaya, M., Trejo, L., & Herrera, C. (1992). HIV disease and pregnancy. Part 3. Postpartum care of the HIV-positive woman and her neonate. *Journal of Obstetric, Gynecologic, and Neonatal Nursing, 21*(2), 105–111.

Blackburn, S., & VandenBerg, K. (1993). Assessment and management of neonatal neurobehavioral development. In Kenner, C., Gunderson, L., & Brueggemeyer, A. (Eds.), *Comprehensive neonatal nursing care: A physiologic perspective*. Philadelphia: W. B. Saunders.

Boland, M., & Czarniecki, L. (1991). Start life with HIV. *RN, 54*(1), 54–59.

Carlson, G. E. (1991). Retinopathy of prematurity: Nursing interventions. *Pediatric Nursing*, 17(4), 348–351.

Centers for Disease Control, (1991). Hepatitis B virus. A comprehensive strategy for eliminating transmission in the United States through universal childhood vaccination. *Morbidity and Mortality Weekly Report, 40*(RR13), 1–25.

Cloherty, J. P., & Stark, A. (1991). *Manual of neonatal intensive care* (3rd ed.). Boston: Little, Brown.

Comer, D. M. (1992). Pulse oximetry: Implications for practice. *Journal of Obstetric, Gynecologic, and Neonatal Nursing, 21*(1), 35–41.

Dietch, J. (1993). Periventricular-intraventricular hemorrhage in the very low birthweight infant. *Neonatal Network, 12*(1), 7–16.

Dunn, M. S., Shennan, A. T., Zayack, D., & Possmayer, F. (1991). Bovine surfactant replacement therapy in neonates of less than 30 weeks' gestation: A randomized controlled trial of prophylaxis versus treatment. *Pediatrics, 87*(3), 377.

Grippi, C., Wand, L., Roncoli, M. (1988). The case of baby Alice: AIDS/ARC in infancy. *Neonatal Network*, *6*(5), 9–14.

Hack, M., Horbar, J., Malloy, M., Tyson, J., Wright, E., & Wright, L. (1991). Very low birth weight outcomes of the national institute of child health and human development neonatal network. *Pediatrics*, *87*(5), 587–596.

NAACOB. (1992). Issue: The HIV-infected health care worker. *NAACOG position statement*. Washington, DC: NAACOG.

Perez-Woods, R., & Malloy, M. D. (1992). Positioning and skin care of the low-birth-weight neonate. *NAACOG's Clinical Issues in Perinatal and Women's Health Nursing*, *3*(1), 97–113.

Peters, H., & Theorell, C. J. (1991). Fetal and neonatal effects of maternal cocaine use. *Journal of Obstetric, Gynecologic, and Neonatal Nursing*, *20*, 121–126.

Samson, L. (1992). Infants of diabetic mothers: Current perspectives. *Journal of Perinatal and Neonatal Nursing*, *6*(1), 61–70.

Shaw, N. (1990). Common surgical problems in the newborn. *Journal of Perinatal and Neonatal Nursing*, *3*(3), 50–65.

Samson, L. F. (1988). Perinatal viral infections and neonates. *The Journal of Perinatal and Neonatal Nursing*, *1*(4), 56–65.

Short, B. L., & Avery, G. B. (1993). Venipuncture. In M. A. Fletcher & M. G. MacDonald (Eds.), *Atlas of procedures in neonatology* (2nd ed.). Philadelphia: J.B. Lippincott.

Ziegler, J. B., Johnson, R. O., Cooper, D. A, et al. (1985). Postnatal transmission of AIDS-associated retrovirus from mother to infant. *Lancet*, *330*, 896–897.

Suggested Readings

Affonso, D., Hurst, I., et al. (1992). Stressors reported by mothers of hospitalized premature infants. *Neonatal Network*, *11*(6), 63–70.

Bass, L. (1991). What do parents need when their infant is a patient in the NICU. *Neonatal Network*, *10*(4), 25–33.

Becker, P. T., Grunwald, P. C., Moorman, J., & Stuhr, S. (1991). Outcomes of developmentally supportive nursing care for very low birthweight infants. *Nursing Research*, *40*, 150–155.

Blackburn, S., & Patteson, D. (1991). Effects of cycled lighting on activity state and cardiorespiratory function in preterm infants. *Journal of Perinatal and Neonatal Nursing*, *4*(4), 47–54.

Boeckling, A. (1992). Exogenous surfactant therapy for premature infants. *Journal of Neonatal and Perinatal Nursing*, *6*(2), 59–66.

Damato, E. G. (1991). Discharge planning from the neonatal intensive care unit. *Journal of Neonatal and Perinatal Nursing*, *5*(1), 54–63.

Fuller, R. (1989). Cardiac function and the neonatal EKG: Part VI: Nursing responsibilities. *Neonatal Network*, *8*(2), 45–48.

Gunderson, L. P., & Kenner, C. (1990). *Care of the 24–25 week gestational age infant (small baby protocol)*. Petaluma, CA: Neonatal Network.

Haney, C., & Allingham, T. U. (1992). Nursing care of the neonate receiving high-frequency jet ventilation. *Journal of Obstetric, Gynecologic, and Neonatal Nursing*, *21*(3), 187–195.

Harrison, L. et al. (1991). Effects of hospital-based instruction on interactions between parents and preterm infants. *Neonatal Network*, *9*(7), 27–33.

Krause, K. D., & Youngner, V. J. (1992). Nursing diagnoses as guidelines in the care of the neonatal ECMO patient. *Journal of Obstetric, Gynecologic, and Neonatal Nursing*, *21*(3), 169–176.

Kuhnly, J. E., & Freston, M. S. (1993). Back transport: Exploration of parents' feelings regarding the transition. *Neonatal Network*, *12*(1), 49–57.

Ladden, M. G., & Damato, E. (1992). Parenting and supportive programs. *NAACOG's Clinical Issues in Perinatal and Women's Health Nursing*, *3*(1), 174–187.

LeBlanc, M. (1991). Thermoregulation: Incubators, radiant warmers, artificial skins, and body hoods. *Clinics in Perinatology*, *18*(3), 403–421.

Nugent, J. (Ed). (1991). *Acute respiratory care of the neonate*. Petaluma, CA: Neonatal Network.

Roncoli, M., & Medoff-Cooper, B. (1992). Thermoregulation in low-birth-weight infants. *NAACOG's Clinical Issues in Perinatal and Women's Health Nursing*, *3*(1), 25–33.

Shapiro, C. (1993). Nurses' judgments of pain in term and preterm newborns. *Journal of Obstetric, Gynecologic, and Neonatal Nursing*, *22*, 41–47.

Schlomann, P. (1992) Ethical considerations of aggressive care of very low birth weight infants. *Neonatal Network*, *11*(4), 31–36.

Urrutia, N. L. (1991). Sorting the complexity of respiratory distress syndrome. *MCN: American Journal of Maternal Child Nursing*, *16*, 308–311.

VandenBerg, K., & Franck, L. S. (1990). Behavioral issues for infants with BPD. In C. H. Lund (Ed.), *Bronchopulmonary dysplasia*. Petaluma, CA: Neonatal Network.

Whitclow, A., Heisterkamp, G., Sleath, K., Acoiet, D., & Richards, M. (1988). Skin to skin contact for very low birth weight infants and their mothers. *Achives of Disease in Childhood*, 63, 1377–1381.

CHAPTER 34

Congenital Anomalies in the Neonate

Learning Objectives

After studying the material in this chapter, the student will be able to:

- Discuss immediate care of the parents on the birth of a neonate with a congenital anomaly.
- Discuss legal and ethical dilemmas related to providing or withholding care to the newborn with a congenital defect.
- Identify the most common types of congenital anomalies detected in the neonatal period.
- Describe the physical characteristics of a neonate with Down syndrome.
- Explain the importance of screening for phenylketonuria

Key Terms

anomaly	congenital
atresia	hereditary

One of the most distressing situations health team members face is the birth of a neonate with a congenital anomaly. In most instances the anomaly was undiagnosed and unexpected. Despite the frequent use of ultrasonography during pregnancy, defects may be missed.

Parents are sensitive to nonverbal cues from the health care team. When a neonate is born with an anomaly, there is a sudden change in the behavior of the team members. Communication patterns are altered, and silence often ensues. Rather, the birth attendant should inform the parents at once that there is a problem. If the newborn requires immediate emergency care, a member of the health team should be available to support the parents and provide them with basic information until the pediatrician can speak with them.

It is difficult to tell parents their newborn has a physical defect. Parents may view even a minor anomaly, which poses no threat to the neonate's health, as a major crisis, especially when the defect involves the face or genitalia. Parents differ in their responses, but the health team should be prepared for reactions commonly observed in the early stages of the grieving process. The partner, in particular, may be overwhelmed if the mother also is ill or has had a cesarean delivery. He or she is often the parent who accompanies the sick neonate to the intensive care nursery, who is asked to sign consent forms, and who must make immediate decisions about life-sustaining procedures. This places a heavy burden of responsibility on the partner during a time of disorganization and crisis.

A number of anomalies may occur in the neonate. This chapter does not begin to cover this specialized field. It discusses the most common abnormalities found and summarizes appropriate nursing care.

Legal and Ethical Issues

Ethical concerns related to quality of life and financial concerns, including the need to contain spiraling health care costs, are involved in the decision to provide or withhold care from the newborn with a congenital defect. Tertiary care

Legal/Ethical Considerations

Ethical Dilemmas and Decision-Making in the Nursing Care of Sick Neonates

As survival rates for smaller and sicker neonates improve each year, neonatal intensive care nurses are confronted with greater numbers of complex moral and ethical dilemmas. Some of the most commonly faced issues include resuscitation, withdrawal of life support systems, hydration and feeding of severely handicapped neonates, parent participation in treatment decisions, and the rights of newborns as research subjects.

The American Nurses Association Code for Nurses (1976) provides a mandate for nursing participation in ethical decision making. Several bioethical decision-making models have been developed to facilitate moral reasoning in nursing practice. Thompson and Thompson (1985) list 10 steps, that may be used to explore an ethical issue:

1. Review the situation to determine the ethical dilemma, decisions to be made, and individuals involved.
2. Gather any additional data needed to clarify the issue.
3. Identify the key ethical issue.
4. Define the professional moral responsibilities.
5. Identify the moral values of the individuals involved.
6. Identify value conflicts.
7. Determine who should be responsible for decision making.
8. Identify a range of actions and possible outcomes.
9. Decide on a course of action and carry it out.
10. Evaluate the results.

Chally, P. (1992). Moral decision making in neonatal intensive care. JOGNN, 21*(6), 475–482.*

Gehl, M. B., & Erlen, J. (1993). An ethical dilemma in the neonatal intensive care unit: Providing due care. Journal of Perinatology, 13*(1), 50–55.*

Thompson, J. E., & Thompson, H. O. (1985). Bioethical decision-making for nurses. *Norwalk, CT: Appleton-Century-Crofts.*

centers, discussed in Chapter 33, have ethics committees to help parents and health team members deal with the problems surrounding birth defects. Genetic counselors are available to discuss with the family the known causes of the defect and the probability of the anomaly occurring in subsequent pregnancies.

In recent years the federal government became involved in the decision-making process through the "Baby Doe" regulations intended to ensure that neonates with serious congenital anomalies receive needed care, even if there are doubts as to their viability and expected quality of life. The United States Supreme Court has since struck down the "Baby Doe" rules, stating that the federal government cannot force hospitals to treat severely handicapped newborns over the objections of their parents. The appropriate roles for parents, health care professionals, and the government in the decision-making process concerning the treatment of the impaired child are being heatedly debated. The Supreme Court decision does leave intact the traditional role of states in regulating these matters. State courts can appoint guardians when parents make decisions the court considers "against the best interests of the child." All hospitals are encouraged to establish review committees composed of medical, legal, and ethics specialists. Professional nurses take their place on these committees to provide input and sustain excellence in practice.

Nurses caring for neonates with congenital anomalies must examine and understand their own values and belief system before attempting to care for families with high-risk neonates. There are no easy answers to the questions being raised. Current technologic capabilities have pushed ahead of the current legal and moral codes; such codes were established by society during an era when most critically ill babies died because there were no medical solutions.

Regardless of personal convictions, the nurse must convey respect for the parents' feelings and beliefs. The major objective of care should be to provide the neonate with the highest level of nursing care possible, regardless of the elected course of medical treatment or prognosis.

Implications for Nursing Care

The nurse involved in the care of a family whose neonate is found to have congenital anomalies must be prepared for a complex situation with emotional, ethical, technologic, medical, and nursing factors that influence outcomes. Such families often are in need of the most technologically sophisticated medical and nursing care and the most sensitive emotional care. In addition to providing necessary care for the neonate, the nurse also must provide caring and knowledgeable support as parents come to grips with the perceived threat to their newborn's health and well-being. The field of genetics and congenital anomalies is increasingly specialized. The nurse who provides labor and birth care is responsible not only for providing initial nursing care to the neonate, but also for interacting effectively with a team of neonatal care providers to ensure that family needs are met.

Common elements in the nursing care of the high-risk neonate are discussed in Chapter 33. The neonate with a congenital anomaly has the same basic needs of other high-risk neonates. Care can best be accomplished using the nursing process in assessing needs, diagnosing problems, planning interventions, and evaluating outcomes of care. The nurse must possess a comprehensive knowledge of theories about attachment, parental grieving, and crisis to support the family. Specific nursing implications for congeni-

tal anomalies are discussed with the particular system and condition.

Congenital Anomalies of the Body Systems

There are periods of fetal development in which particular body systems are susceptible to environmental influences. Any disturbance in the normal course of events may lead to a congenital defect. Some defects are mild enough to corrected with surgery or therapy, while others are incompatible with life.

Central Nervous System Anomalies

Congenital anomalies of the central nervous system (CNS) usually are obvious at birth or shortly thereafter. Some anomalies are accompanied by mental retardation. Defective closing of the neural tube of the CNS can result in mild defects, while other defects are life-threatening.

Spina Bifida Occulta

Spina bifida occulta is the absence or incomplete closure of one or more of the vertebral arches. The skin covering the defect may be dimpled or covered with a tuft of hair. If there is no extrusion of meninges or spinal cord through the opening, the condition usually is asymptomatic, and repair may not be required.

Meningocele and Myelomeningocele

A meningocele is a cyst outpouching of the meninges and cerebrospinal fluid, through a defect in the vertebral column, without associated anomalies of the spinal cord (Fig. 34-1). Because the sac may rupture, and infection can occur, surgical repair usually is indicated. The prognosis is good when the spinal cord is not involved.

A myelomeningocele is a cystic outpouching of the meninges, cerebrospinal fluid, and spinal cord through a defect in the posterior wall of the vertebral column (see Fig. 34-1). The neonate has no motor or sensory function below the level of the defect. Surgical repair can prevent rupture of the cyst and infection. Prognosis depends on the degree of spinal cord involvement and the level of the defect. The higher the defect, the greater the degree of neurologic impairment the neonate will sustain. Even with surgical correction, the child may never be able to walk and may suffer from incontinence of both urine and stool.

The primary nursing responsibility when a cyst is present is to prevent rupture and subsequent CNS infection. The neonate is positioned on the side to eliminate pressure on the defect. If leakage of cerebrospinal fluid is evident, the sac should be covered with a sterile pad and strict asepsis maintained when the dressing is being changed. There must be meticulous attention to skin care to prevent breakdown of delicate tissues. The bladder may need to be emptied by Credé massage at regular intervals.

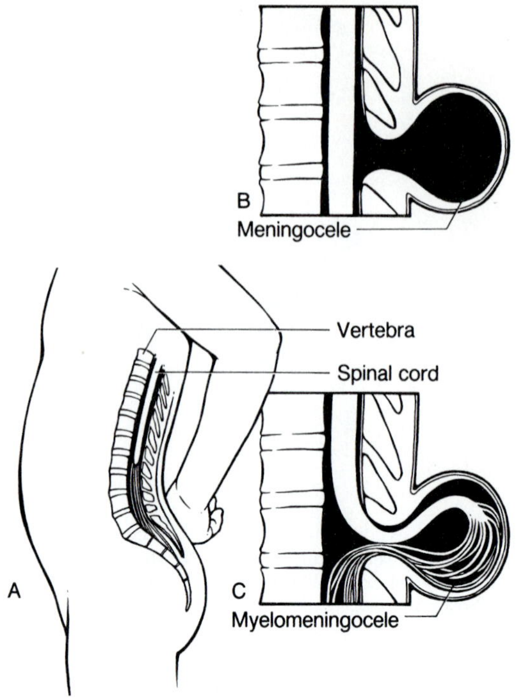

Figure 34-1.
Cross section of a normal spine (*A*) compared to a meningocele (*B*) and a myelomeningocele (*C*).

Anencephaly

Anencephaly is the congenital absence of part of the cranial vault and underlying brain tissue. It is incompatible with life. The neonate may be born with a heart rate and respiration but dies within hours of birth.

Hydrocephalus

Hydrocephalus is an abnormal accumulation of cerebrospinal fluid in the ventricles of the brain. It is frequently associated with myelomeningocele due to blockage in the flow of fluid. The neonate's head circumference increases with the accumulation of fluid. Suture lines in the cranium separate, and the fontanelles bulge and feel tense. The neonate exhibits "setting sun eyes" and has a high-pitched cry (Fig. 34-2). If the buildup of fluid has been extensive prenatally, the neonate may suffer permanent brain damage.

Surgical repair involves placing a polyethylene shunt between the ventricles and peritoneum to drain excess fluid from the ventricles. Prognosis depends on the success of the shunt procedure and the degree of brain damage sustained before surgery.

The nurse must support the head carefully when handling the neonate and position the neonate to maintain a patient airway. A waterbed and sheepskin mattress pad can be used to prevent the skin from breaking down when the head is very large and neurologic impairment is present. The head circumference is measured daily. If the neonate is fed orally, care must be taken to prevent aspiration and to watch for projectile vomiting, which may occur with increased intracranial pressure.

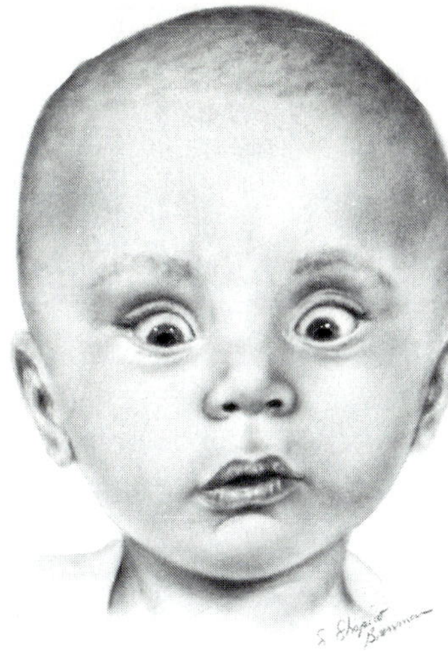

Figure 34-2.
Typical facial expression of hydrocephaly. The eyes deviate downward, creating the "setting sun" sign. (Redrawn from Paine, R. S. [1960]. Neurological examination of infants and children. *Pediatric Clinics of North America, 7*, 476.)

Respiratory System Anomalies

Many factors influence embryonic development of the respiratory tract. Genetic or environmental conditions may interrupt or distort structure development. Biochemical maturation of the respiratory system also can be affected by interference with surfactant.

Choanal Atresia

Choanal atresia is the unilateral or bilateral blockage of the posterior nares. Because the neonate is an obligate nose breather, he or she will suffer from immediate respiratory distress at birth if both nares are occluded. Surgical intervention is then essential, and the prognosis is excellent if there are no associated anomalies. Unilateral blockage may not require any intervention.

Diaphragmatic Hernia

Diaphragmatic hernia is a congenital defect in the diaphragm, which allows herniation of abdominal contents into the thoracic cavity and displacement of the heart and lung tissue. The neonate has a scaphoid-shaped abdomen, and bowel sounds may be heard over the chest wall. Birth asphyxia and respiratory distress are common with severe herniation.

Surgical intervention is essential to remove abdominal organs from the thoracic cavity and relieve pressure on the lungs. The prognosis depends on the adequacy of ventilation and support before surgery and the extent of the herniation. If the defect is large, severe herniation prenatally leads to incomplete development of lung tissue, which is incompatible with extrauterine life. Immediate endotracheal intubation and hand ventilation are essential to establish respiration.

The nurse assists the physician with resuscitation efforts. The neonate is placed on the affected side to let the normal lung expand fully, and the head is elevated. The gastric contents are aspirated to decompress the stomach, and an orogastric tube is passed and secured in place to prevent distention of the gastrointestinal (GI) tract with air. An umbilical artery catheter is inserted, and the nurse administers the intravenous (IV) drugs and fluids required for stabilization. If assisted ventilation is required, the neonate is intubated and placed on a mechanical ventilator. Small tidal volumes and a rapid respiratory rate are preferred to reduce the risk of pneumothorax. Surgery to repair the herniation is performed as soon as possible. Some experimental fetal surgery has been performed with limited success. Initial attempts at defect correction involved returning the abdominal contents to the abdomen and placing a Dacron patch over the "hole" in the diaphragm. Current surgery involves creating a gastroschisis, patching the diaphragm, and repairing the gastroschisis after delivery. Either method is extremely complicated, invasive, and has limited success.

Pulmonary Hypoplasia Agenesis

Pulmonary agenesis, the underdevelopment or complete absence of one or both lungs, is a rare but often fatal congenital defect. One third of newborns die within the first year of life, often secondary to recurrent pulmonary infections. Approximately 50% of cases are associated with anomalies of the cardiovascular, GI, urogenital, and skeletal systems. This defect may result when a diaphragmatic hernia occurs, caused by the limited space available for growth and development of the lung. Pulmonary agenesis also has been associated with oligohydramnios, and it is postulated that lack of amniotic fluid in the fetal alveoli prevents normal lung expansion and growth in utero.

The neonate with pulmonary agenesis may exhibit signs of acute respiratory distress, including dyspnea, tachypnea, stridor, diminished breath sounds and chest asymmetry, and respiratory lag on the affected side. In some instances the newborn may be asymptomatic. Chest x-ray studies will demonstrate a homogeneous density or complete opacification on the involved side.

Maintaining a patent airway and supporting pulmonary function are critical aspects of nursing care. The neonate's oropharynx or endotracheal tube may need to be suctioned frequently. Preventing pulmonary infection is another objective of care, and scrupulous sterile technique, as well as chest physiotherapy to prevent stasis and encourage drainage of pulmonary secretions, is essential.

Oral feedings are initiated only after the newborn is stabilized, and the nurse proceeds slowly to prevent respiratory distress or aspiration of formula. Breastfeeding may be permitted if the neonate tolerates nipple feedings. Discharge planning must begin early. Parents will require extensive teaching regarding pulmonary toilet and suctioning. The neonate may be discharged home with an apnea monitor, and families must understand how to apply the monitor and respond to system alarms. A visiting nurse referral is essential.

Cardiovascular System Anomalies

Congenital heart disease (CHD) involves structural or functional heart anomalies present at birth, although symptoms may not be detected at birth. The incidence of CHD is

reported to be between 4 and 10 in every 1000 live births (Hoffman, 1990). The number of aborted or stillborn fetuses with CHD is thought to be significant.

Congenital cardiac anomalies are a significant cause of neonatal morbidity and mortality in the first year of life. Traditionally conditions were grouped related to the presence or absence of cyanosis (Bayne, 1988). However, neonates with acyanotic defects may eventually develop cyanosis, and neonates who have what are called cyanotic defects may have normal skin coloring at times (Jackson & Saunders, 1993). Additionally, congenital cardiac anomalies may be categorized further in relationship to increased or decreased pulmonary blood flow. (Jackson & Saunders, 1993).

The primary goal of nursing care of the neonate with a cardiac anomaly is to decrease the workload of the heart. The neonate may be placed in a neutral thermal environment. To reduce cyanosis and maintain an adequate blood oxygen tension, oxygen is administered as indicated. The neonate may be given cardiotonics and diuretics.

Feeding can be stressful and tiring. Gavage feedings may be ordered to decrease energy requirements, and small frequent feedings are given to prevent overdistention of the stomach and respiratory embarrassment. Care is taken to calm the neonate and anticipate needs if crying episodes increase cyanosis. Positioning the neonate in a cardiac chair or infant seat with the head and shoulders elevated can help to alleviate respiratory distress. Prevention of infection also is essential to reduce stress on the heart.

Although prognosis has greatly improved, parents may be overwhelmed with feelings of anxiety and guilt. Nursing interventions are focused on repeating necessary explanations as needed, promoting initial interactions, and encouraging parental caregiving as feasible. Parents may become particularly anxious when their neonate turns blue. Parents are taught specific techniques that may alleviate the cyanotic episode. Cardiopulmonary resuscitation training is provided. A discharge planning team should meet with parents well in advance of discharge to prepare them for home care.

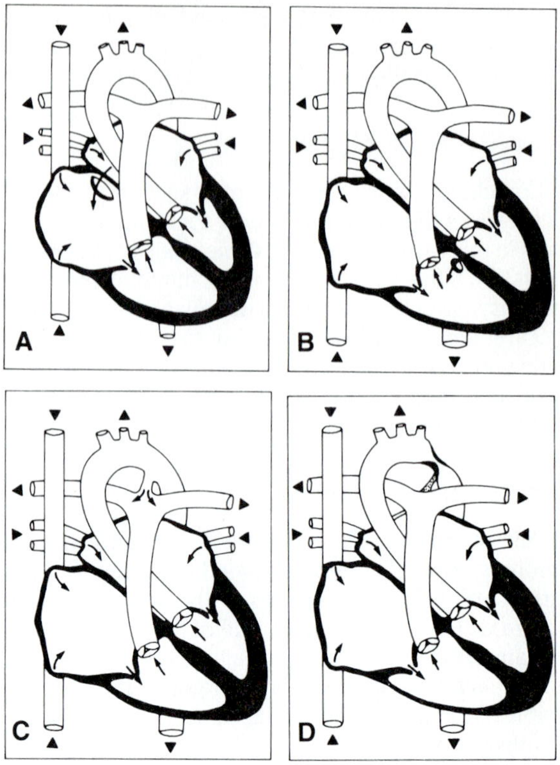

Figure 34-3.
Major congenital anomalies that result in acyanotic heart disease. *A:* Atrial septal defect is an abnormal opening between the left and right atria that leads to left-to-right shunting of blood. *B:* Ventricular septal defect is a condition in which abnormal openings occur between the right and left ventricles. *C:* Patent ductus arteriosus is the abnormal persistence of a vascular connection that, during fetal life, short circuits the pulmonary vascular bed and directs blood from the pulmonary artery to the aorta. *D:* In coarctation of the aorta, an abnormal narrowing of the lumen of the aorta causes an increased left ventricular pressure and workload (Ross Laboratories).

Atrial Septal Defect

An atrial septal defect is an opening in the septum between the atria of the heart, as shown in Figure 34-3*A*. Because of the higher pressure in the left side of the heart (systemic pressure is greater than pulmonary pressure), blood is shunted from left to right. Blood circulates through the pulmonary vasculature and, thus, there is no cyanosis. Atrial septal defect is most frequently asymptomatic. The defect is closed by a surgical procedure to prevent possible development of subacute bacterial endocarditis later in life.

Ventricular Septal Defect

A ventricular septal defect (VSD) is an opening in the septum between the ventricles of the heart (see Fig. 34-3*B*). It is the most frequently occurring cardiac anomaly, accounting for more than 20% of all defects. A VSD may be totally asymptomatic or may be severe enough to cause pulmonary edema and congestive heart failure. When the opening between the left and right ventricles is large, blood is shunted into the right ventricle, increasing its workload and eventually leading to right-sided heart failure. Pulmonary congestion also is seen and is the result of the increased amount of blood flowing from the right ventricle into the pulmonary vasculature. Surgical correction is possible using a Dacron patch. Prognosis is good if the VSD is not associated with other cardiac anomalies.

Patent Ductus Arteriosus

Patent ductus arteriosus (PDA) is the persistent opening of the fetal bypass that connects the aorta to the pulmonary artery (see Fig. 33-3*C*). Any newborn who suffers from hypoxemia and preterm neonates under 1500 g may experience a reopening of the ductus. A PDA is often diagnosed by a harsh grade 2 or 3 systolic murmur auscultated at the upper left sternal border. A left-to-right shunting of blood occurs and can lead to right-sided heart failure and pulmonary congestion. Medical management, including oxygen therapy and blood transfusions to maintain adequate oxygenation of tissue, is sufficient to prevent problems in many of the neonates. Fluid restriction and the administration of cardiotonics and diuretics may also be necessary. Indomethacin, a

prostaglandin inhibitor, has been used with moderate success to close the bypass pharmacologically. The ductus can be ligated surgically if medical management fails.

Coarctation of the Aorta

Coarctation is a narrowing of a section of the aorta, which causes the backup of blood above the stricture and results in increased pressure in the left side of the heart (see Fig. 34-3*D*). If the extent of stenosis is minimal, the anomaly may be asymptomatic except for diminished femoral pulses. Surgical intervention is required but may be postponed for several months if there are no immediate problems. The prognosis is very good if the coarctation is not associated with other cardiac defects.

Pulmonary Stenosis

Pulmonary stenosis is a stricture or narrowing of the pulmonary artery that prevents blood from leaving the right ventricle and entering the lungs. If the stenosis is severe, pressure will build in the right side of the heart, reopening the foramen ovale and causing a right-to-left shunt with mild cyanosis. Surgical intervention to remove the stricture is possible. Prognosis is good if the stenosis is not associated with other anomalies.

Tetralogy of Fallot

Tetralogy of Fallot is an anomaly composed of four separate defects: pulmonary stenosis, a VSD, an overriding aorta, and hypertrophy of the right ventricle (Fig. 34-4*A*). The pulmonary stenosis prevents blood from leaving the right ventricle and entering the lungs. Pressure builds up in the right side of the heart, leading to right ventricular hypertrophy and shunting the blood to the left side of the heart through the ventricular septal defect. Cyanosis can occur with the left-to-right shunt because blood circulates inadequately through the pulmonary vascular system. Any stressors, such as crying or feeding, cause an increase in cyanosis and respiratory distress. Surgical intervention to correct the defects is possible but usually is performed later in childhood.

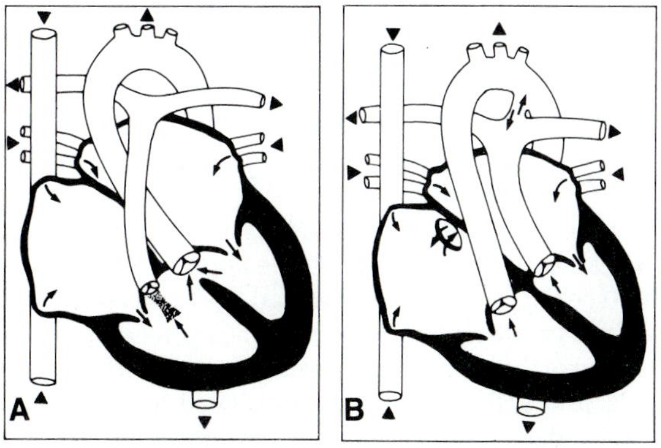

Figure 34-4.
Major congenital anomalies resulting in cyanotic heart disease. *A:* Tetralogy of Fallot is characterized by the combination of four defects: pulmonary stenosis, ventricular septal defect, an overriding aorta, and hypertrophy of the right ventricle. *B:* In transposition of the great vessels, the aorta originates from the right ventricle and the pulmonary artery from the left ventricle (Ross Laboratories).

Transposition of the Great Vessels

In transposition of the great vessels (see Fig. 33-4*B*) the aorta arises from the right ventricle and the pulmonary artery from the left ventricle. Blood enters the right side of the heart, exits the right ventricle, and enters the aorta. It then circulates through the body, completely bypassing the lungs and the oxygenation process. Blood entering the left side of the heart passes through the atrium, the ventricle, and then the pulmonary artery, where it enters the pulmonary vascular bed. It circulates through the pulmonary vasculature and then returns to the left side of the heart. There are two totally separate and nonfunctional circulatory systems. Unless there is a congenital opening between the right and left sides of the heart or one is created surgically, this defect is incompatible with life. Surgery is performed as soon as possible to create an opening if none exists, and major repairs are completed later. The prognosis is poor because of the nature of the defect and the current limitations of the surgical procedure.

Tricuspid Atresia

Tricuspid atresia is a cardiac anomaly characterized by VSD, hypoplastic right ventricle, and enlarged left ventricle. It may be associated with transposition of the great arteries, pulmonary stenosis, or both. It results from the failure of the right atrioventricular valve to develop. Blood entering the right atrium cannot pass into the right ventricle, and both a patent foramen ovale and some type of passage between the right side of the heart and the lungs are necessary for survival. The newborn usually is very cyanotic shortly after birth, and surgery is required to construct an adequate shunt from the right heart to the lungs (Blalock-Taussig shunt). With surgery, a 50% survival rate at 1 year has been demonstrated in some newborns.

Truncus Arteriosus

The truncus arteriosus is an embryonic arterial structure that normally divides during fetal growth and development into the aorta and pulmonary artery. Failure of separation results in the presence of a single great artery, originating from the base of the heart, which supplies both the systemic and pulmonary circulation. A VSD also is associated with this defect. Pulmonary congestion and congestive heart failure develop within the first month of life, and prognosis is very poor without medical and surgical treatment. Recent advances in pediatric cardiac surgery, however, have greatly improved outcome and long-term survival.

Anomalous Venous Return

In anomalous venous return one or more pulmonary veins empty into the right atrium. Frequently the neonate is cyanotic shortly after birth. If all pulmonary veins return to the right side of the heart, surgical correction to permit an

arterial connection is essential to provide the systemic circulation with adequate amounts of oxygenated blood.

Gastrointestinal System Anomalies

The first 10 weeks of fetal life are crucial in normal GI development. Abnormalities may occur anywhere along the GI tract.

Cleft Lip and Cleft Palate

Cleft lip is a result of the incomplete fusion of the nasomedial or intermaxillary process. The extent of the defect ranges from a slight dimpling in the lip area to a unilateral cleft lip combined with cleft palate (Fig. 34-5), large bilateral clefts associated with cleft of the palate. With recent advances in facial cosmetic surgery, cleft lip repairs are very successful. Surgery may now be performed relatively soon after birth, which greatly improves neonatal ability to nipple feed and gain weight.

Cleft palate results from incomplete fusion of the palatal process. The extent of the defect ranges from a small unilateral groove on the uvula to bilateral clefts that extend the entire length of the hard and soft palates and involve the nasal cavity. Because there is an opening in the palate, the neonate cannot create a vacuum in the mouth when sucking on a nipple. When the neonate feeds, milk is often forced upward into the nasal cavity and expelled through the nose. There may be problems with speech development and dentition if the defect is extensive. Surgical repair is undertaken between 12 and 18 months of age, when further development of the palate and jaw has occurred. Current techniques can produce excellent results, but multiple surgical procedures and orthodontia may be necessary before the repair is completed.

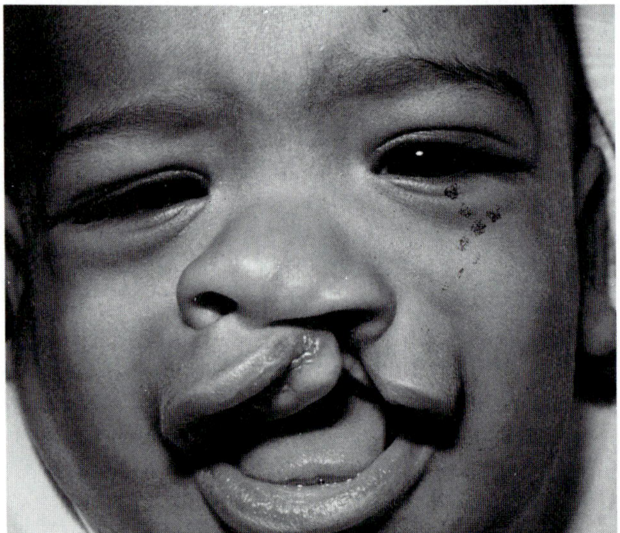

Figure 34-5.
Unilateral cleft lip and palate. (Krause, C. J. et al. [1991]. *Aesthetic facial surgery*. Philadelphia: JB. Lippincott.)

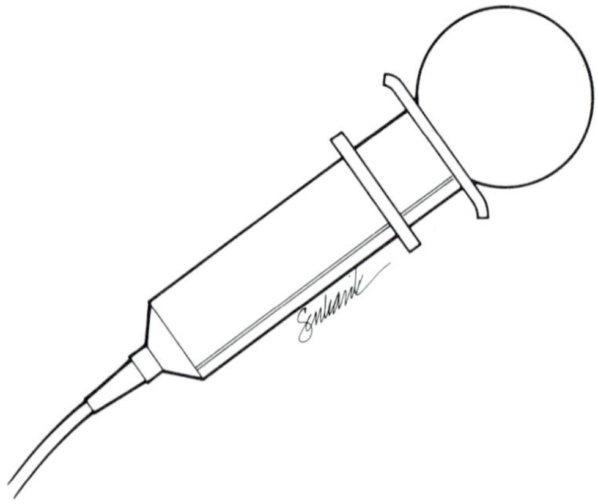

Figure 34-6.
A Brecht feeder allows formula to pass directly to the neonate's posterior oropharynx.

Nursing care immediately after birth is focused on assisting the neonate to ingest nutrients without aspirating the milk or regurgitating it through the nose. Neonates differ in their ability to feed. Some will be able to breastfeed or take formula from a bottle with little difficulty; others will require special equipment. A variety of special nipples and feeding systems are available. Some have special phalanges that fit over the opening in the palate and improve the neonate's ability to suck. A small percentage of infants will fare better when fed with a spoon or a syringe with a soft tip. A Brecht feeder (Fig. 34-6), an asepto syringe attached to rubber tubing, is useful in neonates with very large cleft palate. It allows formula to pass directly to the posterior oropharynx. The newborn's position during feeding also will make a difference. Once a satisfactory method is found, the nurse helps the parents become comfortable with feeding their neonate before discharge.

Esophageal Atresia and Tracheoesophageal Fistula

A variety of defects involving the trachea and esophagus occur when the two structures do not develop normally, as shown in Figure 34-7. The most frequently occurring anomaly results in the esophagus ending in a blind pouch (atresia) with a fistula that connects it to the trachea. Episodes of cyanosis and drooling of saliva are experienced. If the neonate is fed sterile water or milk, the blind pouch will fill up, fluid will enter the trachea through the fistula, and the neonate will suffer acute respiratory distress and cyanosis. Immediate surgical intervention is essential. Although aspiration pneumonia is a frequent sequela, prognosis is excellent if the defect is not associated with other major anomalies.

Nursing care is aimed at preventing aspiration until surgery is performed. Nothing is ingested orally, and a nasogastric catheter is passed into the blind pouch and attached to intermittent low suction to prevent the accumulation of mucus in the esophagus. The nurse supports the neonate's vital functions in a neutral thermal environment and administers IV fluids to prevent hypoglycemia.

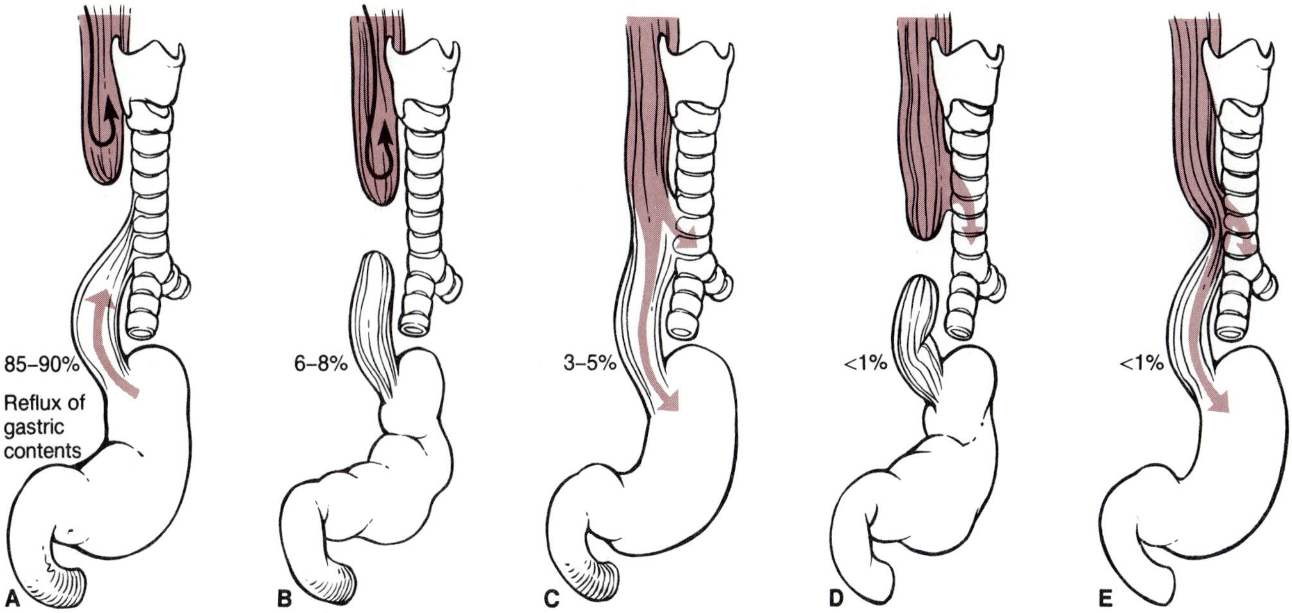

Figure 34-7.

Tracheoesophageal abnormalities. Colored areas and arrows indicate path of feedings or oral secretions. *A:* Blind pouch of the upper esophageal segment with a fistula between the lower segment and trachea. *B:* Blind pouches of both upper and lower segments. *C:* Intact esophagus with tracheoesophageal fistula. *D:* Blind pouches of both esophageal segments with a fistula between the upper segment and trachea. *E:* Esophageal atresia with fistulas between both segments.

Pyloric Stenosis

Pyloric stenosis is the congenital obstruction of the pylorus, the distal opening of the stomach through which gastric contents empty into the duodenum. Males are affected three to four times more frequently than females. The classic signs of this anomaly include vomiting, observable gastric peristaltic waves, and constipation. The condition is rarely diagnosed in the newborn nursery, unless the neonate has an extended stay as a result of other problems. Most neonates with pyloric stenosis begin to vomit in the third to fifth week of life. Surgical correction is indicated and consists of incision of the muscles of the pylorus. The prognosis is excellent after the defect is corrected.

Omphalocele and Gastroschisis

Omphalocele is the protrusion of abdominal contents through a defect in the ventral abdominal wall with herniation of abdominal viscera through an open umbilical ring. The protruding bowel is normally covered by a thin membrane composed of amnion and peritoneum. The umbilical cord inserts into this membrane with the umbilical arteries and vein contained within the sac. Omphalocele occurs in approximately 1 in 6000 live births. The protruding sac may contain small and large intestine, stomach, liver, spleen, bladder, uterus, and ovaries. Many other anomalies and syndromes are associated with omphalocele (ie, meningomyelocele, intracardiac defects, and trisomy syndromes) and complicate treatment and prognosis.

Gastroschisis is a much rarer anomaly, occurring in approximately 1 in 30,000 to 50,000 live births. The neonate is frequently premature. The disorder is characterized by evisceration of abdominal contents (intestines, stomach, gallbladder, uterus, fallopian tubes, bladder, undescended testes, and liver) through a full-thickness defect in the abdominal wall, usually located to the right of the umbilical cord. Associated anomalies are rare.

Immediate surgery is required to reduce the bowel. If the defect is large, it may be impossible to reduce abdominal contents at one time. Several repairs may be needed. Prognosis is guarded if the defect is associated with other congenital anomalies or is very large and includes all major abdominal organs. Nursing interventions immediately after birth are aimed at protecting abdominal contents. The protruding organs are covered with a sterile gauze moistened with warm sterile saline. A nasogastric tube is passed and attached to suction to prevent the intestines from becoming distended with air. No nourishment is given by mouth, and IV therapy is initiated to prevent fluid and electrolyte imbalance and to supply needed calories for metabolic activity. The prevention of hypothermia, strict sterile technique to prevent infection, and maintenance of fluid and electrolyte balance are major nursing goals.

The physical appearance of the anomaly and the life-threatening nature of omphalocele or gastroschisis may result in shock and disbelief in parents. They may hesitate to form initial bonds with the neonate because of the guarded prognosis. Nursing interventions are aimed at reinforcing information provided by physicians, identifying grief responses, and functioning as a liaison between parents and the tertiary level hospital where the newborn is transported. Before the neonate is transferred, the nurse may take photographs of the newborn for the mother.

Intestinal Obstructions and Imperforate Anus

Intestinal obstructions in the neonate may range from a narrowing of the lumen to complete atresia. Twisting of a part of the intestine (volvulus) also can occur and will result in obstruction. The neonate may fail to pass meconium and experiences increasing abdominal distention. Vomiting occurs and may be bilious or fecal in nature. Surgical intervention is essential. If the obstruction is due to a simple defect, prognosis is good.

Imperforate anus is an anomaly of the lower rectum or anus. The extent of the defect ranges from a transparent membrane at the anal opening, which can be surgically incised, to a major obstruction in which the rectum ends in a blind pouch some distance from the anal orifice. Fistulas connecting the intestine with the bladder or vagina are frequently associated with imperforate anus. Surgical repair is essential and may require a temporary colostomy if the defect is some distance from the perineum. Prognosis is good.

Signs of intestinal obstruction are not immediately evident. When obstruction is suspected, nursing care is focused on the assessment of GI function and supportive care that diminishes neonatal energy requirements. Abdominal girth is measured frequently, and bowel sounds are auscultated. The newborn's stooling pattern is monitored closely, and the nature and amount of vomitus are assessed. Nothing is given by mouth, and an orogastric tube is passed and attached to low intermittent suction or gravity drainage. IV therapy is administered to prevent fluid and electrolyte depletion and to meet the neonate's energy requirements.

Genitourinary System Anomalies

Abnormal growth of the embryonic genitourinary system causes significant congenital defects anywhere in the reproductive and urinary systems.

Hypospadias and Epispadias

Hypospadias is a condition in which the urethral opening is found on the ventral side, or underside, of the penis or on the perineum in males (Fig. 34-8). In females born with hypospadias, the meatal urethra opens in the vagina. It is a fairly common anomaly in males; approximately 1 in 300 male neonates may have clinically significant hypospadias (Jackson & Saunders, 1993). The condition usually is corrected surgically shortly after the first year of life. Nurses should be aware that circumcision is contraindicated when the male has hypospadias, because the foreskin is frequently useful in the later surgical correction of this anomaly.

Epispadias, a rare anomaly, is the congenital absence of the anterior wall of the urethra. It is more common in males and ranges in severity from a small meatal opening on the dorsal surface of the penis to a deep furrow or groove that extends its entire length. Epispadias often is associated with other major genitourinary anomalies, including exstrophy of the bladder. Surgical repair is indicated with this defect.

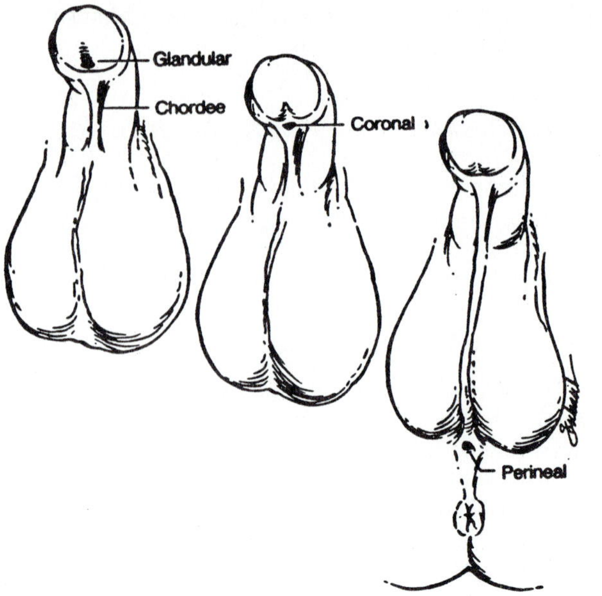

Figure 34-8.
Typical hypospadias. The defect is described by the anatomic location of the aberrant urethral meatus and its association with the chordee.

Ambiguous Genitalia

A small proportion of neonates are born with anomalies of the genitalia, which make it impossible to identify their sex merely by observing the external genitalia. These anomalies may be associated with defects in the internal reproductive organs. Chromosomal studies determine biologic sex, and reconstructive surgery is performed as soon as possible to prevent gender identity problems. Because of their concerns about sexuality, gender identity, and reproductive functioning, parents of neonates with genitourinary anomalies require special support and counseling. Health team members skilled in the repair and treatment of these anomalies are best prepared to discuss the long-term consequences of the particular defect.

Exstrophy of the Bladder and Patent Urachus

Exstrophy of the bladder results from incomplete closure of the abdominal wall and pubic arch. The bladder is exposed on the surface of the abdomen, and the anterior wall of the bladder is absent, exposing its inner surface. As urine enters the bladder, it drains directly onto the skin surface surrounding the defect. Surgical repair is essential. Results are often poor because of associated anomalies of the ureters, and an ileal conduit may have to be constructed connecting the ureters to the small intestine.

Patent urachus is the persistence of a fetal opening between the bladder and the base of the umbilical cord. Urine constantly drains onto the surface of the abdomen. Surgical repair is performed early.

Nursing care of neonates with anomalies of the bladder is aimed at preventing infection. With exstrophy of the bladder a sterile covering is placed over the bladder to protect it.

Meticulous skin care is essential to prevent breakdown from the constant drainage of urine.

Musculoskeletal System Anomalies

Any environmental, teratogenic, or genetic interruption of normal development during the prenatal period can cause problems with ambulation or activities of daily living. Fortunately most of these abnormalities can be treated.

Congenital Hip Dysplasia

The newborn with congenital hip dysplasia has an abnormally formed acetabulum. Usually the acetabulum is shallow and imperfectly rimmed with cartilage so that the head of the femur does not fit snugly into the hip capsule. The femoral head may ride on the lateral edge of the acetabulum in a state of partial dislocation (subluxation), or it may be completely dislocated above the acetabular rim (luxation). This anomaly is found approximately six times more frequently in females than in males and is a potentially crippling disorder associated with degenerative arthritis in adult life.

Congenital hip dysplasia is detected by inspecting the dorsal gluteal folds for asymmetry in appearance and performing Ortolani's maneuver (see Chapter 31) to identify hip instability. A significant "clunking" noise may be heard or an appreciable sudden movement or "jerk" in the upper thigh can be felt when it is abducted and when the dislocated femoral head is reduced and moves back into the acetabulum.

Treatment consists of reducing the femoral head into the acetabulum and maintaining its position while muscle and cartilage develop and a stable hip capsule forms. This is accomplished through use of an appliance that causes abduction and external rotation of the femur, such as a Frejka pillow splint or Pavlik harness. In some cases the use of triple diapers may be sufficient to reduce the head of the femur into the acetabulum.

A thorough assessment of hip stability by the nurse will aid in the early diagnosis of the anomaly. Once the neonate is fitted with the appropriate orthopedic device, care is directed toward preparing the parents for home care and helping them feel comfortable holding and caring for the neonate in the appliance. Meticulous skin care also must be performed to prevent skin breakdown around the edges of the appliance and accumulation of urine and feces because of inadequate cleansing.

Talipes Equinovarus

Talipes, commonly known as "clubfoot," is a congenital deformity of the ankle and foot. A variety of talipes deformities occurs, as summarized in Table 34-1 Their characteristic appearance is determined by the degree and extent to which the muscles and tendons of the foot, ankle, and leg are shortened or atrophied. In talipes equinovarus, the most common form, the heel is turned toward the midline of the body (inversion), and the foot is fixed in a position of plantar flexion. In valgus deformities the heel is turned outward from the midline of the body.

Treatment of talipes deformity consists of correcting the position of the foot and heel by applying successive plaster casts during infancy. Denis-Browne splints may be used. The device consists of foot plates attached to a rigid crossbar. When the child begins to walk, he or she is fitted with specially designed orthopedic shoes or may merely wear shoes on the appropriate feet to maintain the foot in the correct position. Prognosis is favorable if treatment is initiated in the neonatal period.

Nursing care is directed toward supporting the parents and educating them about the anomaly. Most neonates with talipes are placed in plaster casts before they are discharged from the nursery. The nurse prepares the parent for home care, explaining why the cast is applied, how to keep it clean, and the signs of complication (ie, compromised circulation and pressure sores). Many parents may be afraid to hold or cuddle the neonate in a cast, and the nurse must demonstrate proper handling and support parents in their initial attempts to hold their neonate.

Chromosomal Abnormalities

Genetic code and fetal development are discussed in Chapter 12. The normal neonate is born with 46 chromosomes in 23 pairs. An aberration in the number or pairs of chromosomes will result in an abnormality.

Trisomies

The presence of a third chromosome in a neonate results in a trisomy. The extra chromosome can be found attached to different chromosome pairs and results in identifiable syndromes frequently associated with mental retardation and multiple congenital anomalies.

Down syndrome results from the presence of an extra chromosome at pair 21 or 22 or a translocation usually involving pairs 15 and 21. Newborns with Down syndrome present with a variety of signs that aid in the initial tentative diagnosis; the diagnosis is confirmed by chromosomal studies. The neonate may have close-set, slanting eyes with narrow palpebral fissures. The nose is flat, and the tongue appears large and protruding. The fingers are short and thick, and there is incurving of the fifth finger. A simian crease may be apparent on the palmar surfaces. The posterior aspect of the neck is thickened or "webbed," and the occiput is flattened. The neonate's mental capacity is impaired to some degree. The multiple congenital anomalies frequently associated with the syndrome include cardiac and GI tract defects. Recent advances in surgical repair of cardiac and GI anomalies have improved the life expectancy of newborns with Down syndrome, but mental capacity is still limited.

Some Down syndrome neonates will be stable at birth and free of life-threatening anomalies. In such cases nursing interventions are aimed at supporting parents and helping them work through the grieving process. If major anomalies are evident, nursing care is focused on providing the specific support required by the congenital defects. Genetic counseling is indicated to assist parents in understanding the extent

Table 34-1. Common Foot and Ankle Disorders

Type	Description	Type	Description
Metatarsus varus (adductus)	"Toeing in." The forefoot turns toward the midline of the body, and the heel remains straight. 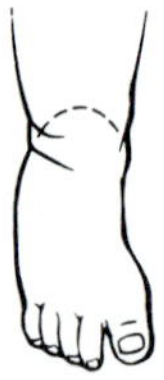	Talipes calcaneovalgus	The foot is dorsiflexed at the ankle. Toes point upward and outward—type of "clubfoot." 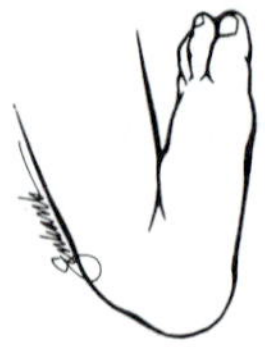
Metatarsus valgus	"Toeing out." The forefoot turns away from the midline of the body, and the heel remains straight. 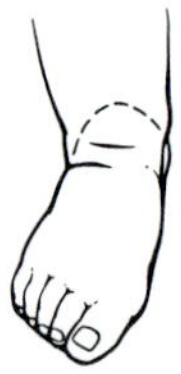	Talipes varus	Foot and ankle bend toward the midline of the body. 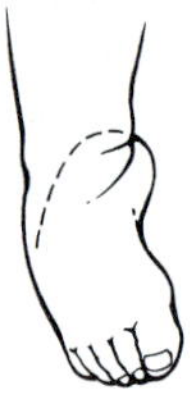
Talipes equinovarus	The foot and ankle deviate toward the midline of the body and plantar flexion of the forefoot; most severe type of "clubfoot" deformity. 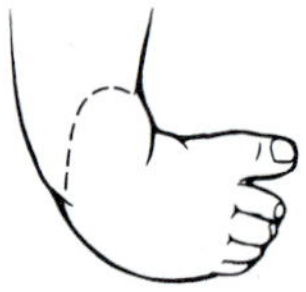	Talipes valgus	Foot and ankle bend away from the midline of the body. 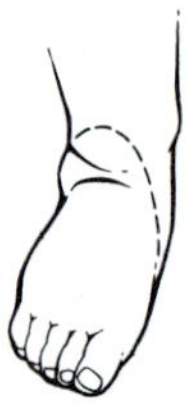

From Jackson, D. B., & Saunders, R. B. (1992). *Child health nursing: A comprehensive approach to the care of children and their families* (p. 1692). Philadelphia: J.B. Lippincott.

of the anomaly and the probability of recurrence with future pregnancies. A social worker may be involved in discharge planning to assist parents who choose to place the neonate in a special care facility. If the neonate is discharged home to the parents, referrals to a public health nurse or visiting nurse will be made.

Inborn Errors of Metabolism

The neonate with an inborn error in metabolism has an enzyme deficiency that results in aberrations in protein, fat, or carbohydrate metabolism. Accumulation of toxic metabolites may cause permanent brain damage or death in the severest forms of this disorder. An inborn error of metabolism is an inherited defect usually transmitted by an autosomal recessive gene (two heterozygous parents who carry the trait produce a homozygous neonate with the disease). Recent advances in detection make it possible to screen neonates for many of the disorders within several days of birth before the abnormal metabolites in the bloodstream and brain reach toxic levels.

Phenylketonuria

One of the first inborn errors in metabolism to be recognized and treated was phenylketonuria (PKU). Neonates with PKU lack the enzyme phenylalanine hydroxylase and are unable to convert the amino acid phenylalanine to tyrosine. Phenylalanine is an essential amino acid found in breast milk and most formulas. Phenylpyruvic acid and phenylacetic acid, abnormal metabolites of phenylalanine, begin to accumulate in the body if the neonate with PKU ingests milk. If untreated, the neonate will show symptoms of failure to thrive, including vomiting, listlessness, and poor weight gain. Signs of CNS damage and mental retardation are evident as early as 6 months of age.

Most states require a neonatal screening test in all newborn nurseries. Because screening equipment may not detect the disorder when abnormal metabolites are present in

very low concentrations in the neonate's bloodstream, it is essential that the test be delayed for at least 24 hours after milk feedings are initiated. Ideally, testing should occur 6 days after initiation of feeding, but the fear of losing neonates to follow-up prompts the current practice.

Treatment consists of dietary restriction of foods high in phenylalanine. The neonate with PKU is placed on a special formula, low in this essential amino acid. Because phenylalanine is found in most animal and vegetable products, parents require ongoing support and instruction regarding food restrictions. The long-term prognosis for normal brain growth and development is excellent if PKU is detected and treatment is begun in the neonatal period. For optimum effectiveness the diet should be started before 3 weeks of life.

Nursing intervention in the detection of PKU involves careful notation regarding the initiation of feeding so that screening tests can be performed at the proper time. Nurses perform the screening tests, and the blood specimen must be collected accurately. Parent education is particularly important if the neonate is sent home before the neonatal screening tests can be performed. The nurse must be sure that parents understand the importance of returning to the hospital, clinic, or pediatrician's office for the test after milk feedings are established.

Branched-Chain Ketoaciduria and Homacystinuria

Recent research has led to the discovery and understanding of other metabolic disorders in which aberrations in enzyme pathways lead to the accumulation of toxic metabolites. Two rare disorders of protein metabolism that can now be detected by neonatal screening tests are maple syrup urine disease and homocystinuria.

Newborns with branched-chain ketoaciduria, or *maple syrup urine disease* (MSUD), have an enzyme defect that prevents the metabolism of three amino acids: leucine, isoleucine, and valine. The untreated neonate shows signs of CNS injury within several days after milk feedings have been started. The urine of an untreated neonate has a characteristic maple syrup odor. A special formula (MSUD formula) low in the three amino acids has been developed. Dietary restrictions are observed throughout early childhood. The prognosis for normal neurologic development of the child in whom MSUD is diagnosed and treated within the first weeks of life appears promising.

Homocystinuria is a rare metabolic disorder in which an enzyme defect prevents the conversion of the amino acid methionine to cystine. The newborn with homocystinuria exhibits signs of CNS damage, which, if untreated, results in mental retardation. Dietary restriction of methionine is the required treatment for this inborn error in metabolism. Long-term neurologic prognosis is good when the disorder is detected early and treated promptly.

Galactosemia

Galactosemia is an inborn error of carbohydrate metabolism, which is detected by neonatal screening tests. The neonate with galactosemia is unable to convert galactose into glucose. As galactose levels rise in the bloodstream, signs of CNS involvement (lethargy, poor feeding, seizures) appear. The early diagnosis and treatment of galactosemia (removal of galactose from the diet) reverses the CNS signs. Prognosis for normal neurologic development is excellent.

Congenital Hypothyroidism

One cause of congenital hypothyroidism is an inherited enzymatic deficiency that prevents the normal synthesis of thyroid hormone. The neonate may appear normal at birth but soon develops early signs of thyroid insufficiency, including failure to thrive (poor feeding, poor weight gain, and lethargy), neonatal jaundice, and constipation. If untreated, the neonate will demonstrate an arrested growth pattern and mental retardation. Neonatal screening tests can now detect congenital hypothyroidism. Prompt treatment with the appropriate dosage of thyroid medication reverses early signs and prevents retardation.

Chapter Summary

Provision of family-centered care occurs in less-than-ideal circumstances when congenital anomalies, chromosomal abnormalities, and errors of metabolism occur in the neonatal period. Innovative approaches to care must be devised to support both neonate and parents. Legal and ethical dilemmas arise over providing or withholding care. Nurses also must examine and understand their own beliefs and values related to technologic advances in the care of compromised neonates.

Study Questions

1. *How can the nurse best support parents of a newborn with a congenital anomaly immediately after birth?*
2. *What strategies can the neonatal nurse use to deal effectively with legal and ethical dilemmas?*
3. *What is the major goal of nursing care of the neonate with a cardiac anomaly?*
4. *What is the primary form of treatment for neonates who have inborn errors of metabolism?*

References

Bayne, E. J. (1988). Etiology, diagnosis, and management of congenital cardiac disorders. *Comprehensive Therapy, 14* (8), 31–40.

Hoffman, J. I. (1990). Congenital heart disease; Incidence and inheritance. *Pediatric Clinics of North America, 37*(1), 25–43.

Jackson, D. B., & Saunders R. B. (1993). *Child health nursing: A comprehensive approach to the care of children and their families*. Philadelphia: J.B. Lippincott.

Suggested Readings

Avery, G. B. (Ed.). (1993). *Neonatology: Pathophysiology and management of the newborn* (4th ed.). Philadelphia: J.B. Lippincott.

Bass, L. (1991). What do parents need when their infant is a patient in the NICU? *Neonatal Network*, *10*(4), 25–33.

Brentner, S. (1987): Abdominal defects: Omphalocele and gastroschisis. *Neonatal Network*, *6*(3), 29–41.

Castanada, A. R., Mayer, J. E., Jonas, R. A., Lock, J. E., Wessel, D. L., & Hickey, P. R. (1989). The neonate with critical congenital heart disease: Repair—A surgical challenge. *Journal of Thoracic and Cardiovascular Surgery*, *98*(5), 869–875.

Fuller, R. (1989). Cardiac function and the neonatal EKG: Part VI: Nursing responsibilities. *Neonatal Network*, *8*(2), 45–48.

Ladden, M., & Damato, E. (1992): Parenting and supportive programs. *NAACOG'S Clinical Issues in Perinatal and Women's Health Nursing*, *3*(1), 174–187.

Medelin, G. J., et al. (1989). Interventional catheterization in congenital heart disease. *Radiologic Clinics of North America*, *27*(6), 1223–1240.

Oski, F. A., DeAngelis, C. D., Feigin, R. D., Warshaw, J. B. (Eds.). (1990). *Principles and practice of pediatrics*. Philadelphia: J.B. Lippincott.

CHAPTER 35

Maternal and Infant Nutrition

Learning Objectives

After studying the material in this chapter, the student will be able to:

- Explain the nutritional requirements of the lactating and nonlactating mother during the fourth trimester.
- Discuss the effects of nutrition on the quality and quantity of breast milk produced.
- Explain the nutritional requirements of the infant from birth to 6 months of age.
- Identify factors that affect maternal weight loss after childbirth.
- Advise mothers about dietary recommendations for themselves and their infants during the fourth trimester.

Key Terms

casein
colostrum
epidermal growth factor
fluoride
lactalbumin
lactation
renal solute load
whey

The perinatal nurse is in a unique position to assess the nutritional status of women in the fourth trimester and to support optimal newborn feeding practices. New parents require information and support as they take over the responsibility for neonatal and infant feeding. Mothers who choose to breastfeed require special support and teaching as they learn the necessary skills. New mothers often are motivated to return to their nonpregnant physical state as quickly as possible. They are frequently open to suggestions about nutrition and exercise that will expedite the process. They welcome the nurse's teaching about nutrition.

The postpartum nurse is able to assess the concerns, eating habits, and activities of new mothers. Observations of new parents' behaviors provide insight into individual needs for counseling, teaching, self-help, and financial or social services. In the area of nutrition, one of the most important parameters of health, the nurse—in conjunction with the nutritionist—can have a significant effect on comprehensive care in the fourth trimester.

This chapter provides the information necessary to assess and plan appropriate nursing actions to meet the nutritional needs of women and their neonates. Breastfeeding versus formula feeding, nutritional requirements for lactating and nonlactating women, and nutrition for newborn and infant health are discussed. In addition nursing diagnosis, intervention, planning, and evaluation are presented to guide nutritional care in the postpartum setting. Specific nursing support of breastfeeding and formula feeding during the postpartum hospitalization period is discussed in Chapter 28.

Maternal and Infant Fourth-Trimester Nutritional Needs

The new mother and the infant have special nutritional needs in the first 3 to 6 months after birth. The following section discusses the nutritional comparison between breast milk and formula and the nutritional needs of the infant and mother.

Nursing Research

Mothers' Perceptions of Breastfeeding and Breast Milk

A qualitative study conducted in Canada examined mothers' perceptions of breast milk and breastfeeding and the factors that mothers believed influenced the quality and quantity of breast milk. Nine middle-class mothers were interviewed in-depth. Subjects had breastfeeding experience ranging from 4 months to one mother who had breastfed four children sequentially for approximately 9 years.

Mothers believed that breast milk was an important infant food but knew little about how it was produced in the body. When mothers had concerns or problems with breastfeeding, they generally viewed other women who had successfully breastfed as the experts with whom they should consult.

While mothers viewed breast milk as a nutritious infant food, its appearance did not meet their expectations of a rich, wholesome food; mothers often compared it to skim milk and expressed surprise that something so "watery" could nourish an infant for 6 months or more. While they recognized that breast milk was easily digestible and saw this as a positive attribute, they also saw it as "less filling" than formula. These mothers hoped that their infants would establish feeding patterns more like those of formula-fed infants, even though they knew that breastfed infants required more frequent feedings throughout the day and night.

Some mothers made decisions to introduce formula to their infants when they believed that their milk was not "good enough" to meet the infant's needs or that their milk supply was insufficient. Others regarded milk quality and quantity as under the mother's control to some extent. These mothers worked hard to ensure breastfeeding success and felt responsible when breastfeeding problems occurred.

This study suggests that patients should be given an opportunity to see breast milk, to discuss changes in breast milk appearance, and to discuss factors that influence breast milk production. Mothers should be encouraged to discuss how breastfeeding can be a demanding task at times but that it is also convenient and inexpensive. Future research into the beliefs and attitudes of other groups of breastfeeding mothers would be useful in understanding how beliefs and attitudes affect breastfeeding behavior.

Bottorff, J., & Morse, J. (1990). Mothers' perceptions of breast milk. *Journal of Obstetric, Gynecological and Neonatal Nursing, 19*(6), 518–527.

Rediscovery of Breastfeeding

Throughout most of human history, breastfeeding was the only means of feeding newborns. If biologic mothers were unable to nurse their infants, other lactating mothers (called *wet nurses*) took over the feeding. In the 20th century, however, the baby bottle became a symbol of women's freedom and of the "modern" way of childrearing. The popularity of formula feeding was helped by the availability of a number of "ready-to-feed" infant formulas, which made formula preparation easy and safe. In the 1950s and 1960s formula feeding became quite common and well accepted in the United States. Breastfeeding was largely forgotten in a culture in which women's breasts were either hidden or displayed as sexual objects.

Breastfeeding increased significantly during the 1970s. This trend peaked in the early 1980s and has since reversed itself. Data show that the woman who breastfeeds her infant is generally well educated, older, and white. Data on the incidence and duration of breastfeeding are limited, but it is known that the decision to breastfeed is based on a number of social, cultural, economic, and psychological factors (Institute of Medicine, 1991). Infants who are not breastfed usually are given one of the many commercially prepared infant formulas. In the United States whole cow's milk and home-prepared evaporated milk formula are no longer considered to be appropriate for infant feeding.

Scientific investigation has demonstrated that breastfeeding offers greater immunologic and nutritional advantages to newborns and infants and physiologic benefits to the mother. In its 1991 report entitled *Nutrition During Lactation*, the Institute of Medicine of the National Academy of Sciences stated among its conclusions that "Women living under a wide variety of circumstances in the United States and elsewhere are capable of fully nourishing their infants by breastfeeding. Breastfeeding is recommended for all infants in the United States under ordinary circumstances."

Nutritional Comparison of Breastfeeding and Formula Feeding

The positive effects of breastfeeding include health benefits and often psychologic benefits for the infant and the mother. Breast milk is ideally suited to the human infant. It contains the nutrients, minerals, and other substances needed for optimal growth. When the digestibility, absorption, and metabolism of breast and cow's milk are compared, breast milk is found to be superior. In addition to its biochemical, nutri-

tional, antibacterial, and immunologic value, breastfeeding also maximizes physical interaction between mother and infant and may provide optimal conditions for infant social and cognitive development (Lawrence, 1989).

Production of infant formulas has reached a high degree of sophistication. There are many different types of formula, some based on cow's milk protein and others on protein from sources such as soybeans. Protein hydrosylates also may be used. The fat in commercial formulas may be cow's milk fat or vegetable fat. Various carbohydrates are used, including lactose, sucrose, glucose, and corn starch. Some formulas contain combinations of these ingredients. Specific vitamins and minerals also may be added. Several formulas come very close to breast milk in content and are called *humanized* by their manufacturers. However, these formulas are not completely equivalent to breast milk. A comparison of mature breast milk and various types of commercial infant formulas is found in Table 35-1.

Protein, Fat, and Carbohydrate Comparison

The protein in breast milk is more easily digested and more readily absorbed than the protein in any other infant food. Cow's milk has more protein than breast milk, but 80% of cow's milk protein is in the form of casein. This milk protein forms a large, tough curd in the human stomach, may be poorly digested by infants, and may cause intestinal obstruction. Cow's milk must, therefore, be treated chemically or mechanically to reduce the curd tension so that it can be digested readily by human infants. The whey protein lactalbumin constitutes the other 20% of cow's milk protein; in contrast, it constitutes 60% of breast milk protein. Whey proteins such as lactalbumin form a smaller, softer, easily digestible curd in the stomach than casein.

Breast milk contains enzymes that, when activated by bile salts in the intestine, help digestion of the lipid or fat component of milk. Breast milk fat is better absorbed than cow's milk fat; as a result the calcium in breast milk has a higher rate of absorption as well. Excess dietary fat (or poor fat absorption) results in an excess of fat in the intestine. This causes excessive excretion of calcium in the stool. Despite the fact that cow's milk is higher in calcium than breast milk, only 17% of cow's milk calcium is absorbed, in contrast to the 51% absorption rate of calcium from breast milk.

The carbohydrate content of breast milk is 7%. Cow's milk has a carbohydrate content of 4.8%. The higher carbohydrate content of breast milk provides a favorable intestinal environment for the growth of beneficial microorganisms and is thought to enhance the absorption of calcium, magnesium, and other minerals. With respect to the metabolism and use of nutrients, the high protein, calcium, phosphorus, magnesium, sodium, potassium, and chloride levels of cow's milk result in a renal solute load about two thirds greater than that resulting from the ingestion of breast milk. The renal solute load consists of metabolic end products, especially nitrogenous compounds and electrolytes. These end products must be excreted by the kidneys. Young infants have a limited ability to concentrate urine. Some cow's milk formulas can place a strain on an infant's immature kidneys because the solutes it contains may require three to four times as much water for excretion as the solutes in breast milk. Generally, the increased renal solute load resulting from formula is not a problem for healthy infants.

Breast milk is a rich source of cholesterol, and infants who consume breast milk develop serum cholesterol levels similar to or slightly higher than the levels found in infants fed formulas containing fat from vegetable sources. Because high serum cholesterol levels have been associated with coronary heart disease, there has been interest in lowering serum cholesterol levels for all groups, including infants. Research is needed to determine if limiting dietary cholesterol in infants is harmful. Cholesterol is used in the synthesis of myelin, bile salts, and steroid hormones. Ingestion of cholesterol early in life may be necessary to trigger the enzyme systems that regulate the biosynthesis and catabolism of cholesterol later.

Immunologic and Biochemical Properties of Breast Milk

Another benefit of breastfeeding is the protection it provides against infections and allergies. Breast milk also includes epidermal growth factor (EGF), which may have an effect of neonatal growth.

Prevention of Infection. Because of the immunologic value of breast milk, breastfed infants have lower rates of infection than formula-fed infants. The incidence of necrotizing enterocolitis, diarrhea, respiratory infections, and gastroenteritis is very low in breastfed infants. This suggests that breastfeeding in the early months of life may offer protection against infections.

Prevention of Allergies. In addition to protecting against infections, breastfeeding may help protect against the development of allergies. It is believed that prolonged breastfeeding (longer than 6 months) may be associated with a low incidence of obvious allergic disease. This is particularly true in infants with a family history of allergies. Specifically, prolonged breastfeeding decreases the incidence of allergic dermatitis (eczema) in all infants up to 1 year of age. Breastfeeding also decreases the incidence of food allergies in infants with a family history of such allergies.

Growth-Promoting Factors. As more sophisticated methods became available to analyze the composition of breast milk, it was discovered that the milk contains a substance with growth-promoting activity. This substance, a polypeptide called EGF, has been found in breast milk and in human plasma, serum, urine, and amniotic fluid. This growth factor has significant biologic effects in mammals, particularly in the fetus and neonate. Effects on the fetus and neonate include enhanced proliferation and differentiation of the epidermis, increased growth and maturation of fetal pulmonary epithelium, and stimulation of DNA synthesis in the digestive tract. Researchers have concluded that the demonstrated ability of breast milk to stimulate DNA synthesis and cell multiplication in cell cultures is probably due to the presence of EGF. Breast milk is actually more potent in producing this effect than purified EGF itself, leading to speculation that breast milk may contain substances that

Table 35-1. Nutritional Comparison of Human Milk and Commonly Used Commercial Infant Formulas

	Cow's–Milk-Based Formula*	Human Milk	Soy Isolates†
Components			
Protein	Nonfat milk	—	Soy isolate
Fat	Vegetable oils	—	Vegetable oils
Carbohydrate	Lactose	—	Corn syrup or sucrose
Major Constituents			
Protein	1.5–1.55	1.05–1.35	1.8–2.5
Fat	3.6–3.7	3.5–4.3	3–3.6
Carbohydrates	7.0–7.2	6.95–7.45	6.4–6.8
Ash (minerals)	0.3–0.37	0.19–0.21	0.4–0.5
Cal‡	20/oz (0.6/mL)	20–23/oz (0.6–0.76/mL)	20/oz (0.6/mL)
Percent of Calories			
Protein	9	6	12–15
Fat	48–50	52	45–48
Carbohydrate	41–43	42	39–40
Minerals per Liter			
Sodium (mEq)	6.5–11	6.0–9.5	9–24
Potassium (mEq)	14.3–19	12.5–14.3	15–28
Chloride (mEq)	10–17	10.1–13.5	7–15
Calcium (mg)	445–600	254–306	700–950
Phosphorus (mg)	300–454	118–162	500–690
Magnesium (mg)	40–43	33–37	50–80
Copper (mg)	0.4–0.6	0.22–0.28	0.4–0.6
Zinc (mg)	3.2–5	1.0–1.4	2–5.3
Iodine (μg)	40–69	70–150	70–160
Iron (mg)§	Trace–1.5	0.2–0.4	8.5–12.7
Vitamins per Liter			
A (IU)	1650–2650	2230	2100–2500
D (IU)	400–423	22	400–423
E (IU)	9.5–15	2	9–11
K (μg)	—‖	2.0–2.2	0.09–0.15
C (mg)	52–58	30–50	50–55
Thiamine (μg)	510–710	175–245	400–700
Riboflavin (μg)	620–1060	325–375	600–1060
Niacin (mg)	7–8.25	1.3–1.7	5–8.4
Pyridoxine (μg)	400–423	175–235	400–530
Folacin (μg)	32–100	45–55	50–100
B_{12} (μg)	1.1–2	0.3–0.7	2–3
Pantothenate (mg)	2.1–3.1	1.6–2.0	2.6–5

* Enfamil, Similac, SMA.
† Prosobee, Isomil, Nursoy, Neo-mulsoy, i-soyalac (contains tapioca starch).
‡ Diluted per manufacturer's specifications.
§ Iron-fortified formula 12–12.7 mg/L.
‖ Vitamin K not added because milk base supplies ample amounts.

enhance the effect of EGF. Potency of EGF in breast milk appears to be highest shortly after birth and decreases thereafter.

Psychophysiologic Advantages of Breastfeeding

Psychological advantages of breastfeeding are more difficult to document clinically than immunologic or nutritional advantages. Breastfeeding provides a synchronous reciprocal interaction, with mother and infant simultaneously giving and receiving physical and emotional pleasure. If the infant associates the comfort of suckling and feeding with the mother, a strong infant-to-mother attachment may develop. Formula-feeding mothers also can develop strong feelings of attachment to their infants; however, breastfeeding may enhance such an attachment.

Breastfeeding also is beneficial to the mother's physical restoration after birth. Infant suckling stimulates the produc-

tion of oxytocin, which causes the uterus to contract, thereby promoting good uterine tone. The high energy demands of lactation lead to the use of fat reserves, which may help the mother regain her prepregnant figure. (See chapter 28 for a more complete discussion of the process and management of lactation.)

The nurse must remember that breastfeeding will not be successful if the mother does not want to breastfeed. The nurse can answer the mother's questions, discuss any concerns the mother may have, and provide encouragement for breastfeeding if the mother has not made a firm decision about how to feed her infant. However, if the mother has considered her own feelings and situation and decided to formula feed, the nurse should support this decision and provide appropriate nursing care. Potential reasons mothers may not choose to breastfeed and counseling about breastfeeding are included in Chapter 28.

Infant Nutritional Needs

The physical growth and development of infants largely depends on the nutritional status of the mother before, during, and after (if she is breastfeeding) pregnancy, as well as on the adequacy of the infant's diet. Hereditary, cultural, and environmental factors also play a role and must be considered in any evaluation of an infant's nutritional status. Generally, the following characteristics are considered to indicate a well-nourished infant:

- Steady increase in weight and length
- Regular sleeping and elimination patterns
- Vigorous activity and generally happy disposition
- Firm muscles and moderate amount of subcutaneous fat
- Teething at 5 to 6 months

The infant undergoes more rapid growth during the first year of life than in any other period. Most infants double their birth weight by 4 to 6 months and triple their birth weight by the end of the first year. During the first 6 months the weekly weight gain normally averages 140 to 230 g (5 to 8 oz); in the second 6 months it decreases to 110 to 140 g (4 to 5 oz). A neonate whose birth length is 50.8 to 55.8 cm (20 to 22 in) adds another 22.8 to 25.4 cm (9 to 10 in) in the first year of life.

In general as the infant grows, the number of daily feedings decreases, and the volume of feedings increases. A typical pattern of feedings for the first year of life is shown in Table 35-2. This pattern may be disrupted during growth spurts, which commonly occur at 6 and 12 weeks of age, at which time the infant may demand more frequent feedings.

A variety of factors affect the physical growth and development of the infant. A child who does not receive minimal levels of each needed nutrient will not reach his or her full physical and intellectual potential. Brain growth is not complete until the child reaches the age of 2. It has been postulated that malnutrition during early infancy and this period of brain growth may result in a decrease the number of brain cells, causing permanent impairment of brain development (Institute of Medicine, 1991).

Nutritional Needs of Breastfed Infants

Breast milk is sufficient to meet most of the nutritional needs of the infant for the first 4 to 6 months of life, although some supplementation for particular nutrients is necessary for the breastfed infant, as discussed in the following section. After 6 months the nutrients from breast milk are insufficient, and the infant's diet should be supplemented with other foods.

Nutritional Supplementation for Breastfed Infants

Recommendations for nutritional supplementation of breastfed infants are made to prevent the development of nutrient deficiencies. The specific nutrient supplements recommended are vitamin K, vitamin, D, fluoride, and iron.

Vitamin D is produced in the skin of humans when exposed to the ultraviolet rays of the sun. Various factors influence the amount of vitamin D synthesis, including the latitude at which an infant lives, the time of year, the total exposure to sunlight, and skin pigmentation. Because breast milk does not contain adequate amounts of this vitamin, it is important to evaluate the infant's exposure to sunlight. If there is doubt about the adequacy of sunlight exposure, the infant should be given supplemental vitamin D.

The term infant's iron stores last approximately 4 months. The concentration of iron in breast milk is approximately 0.5 mg/L, 50% of which is absorbed by the infant. The average 4- to 5-month-old infant consumes approximately 1 L of breast milk a day and therefore receives approximately 0.25 mg of iron daily. The recommended daily iron requirement from birth to age 6 months is 7.5 mg/d, and from 6 months to 12 months it is 10 mg/d. (Breast milk does not provide the infant with an adequate supply of iron.) Iron can be provided to the older breastfed infant through supplements or more often through food sources such as iron-fortified infant cereals.

There has been much discussion about the need for fluoride supplementation for the breastfed infant. Fluoride is a dietary mineral necessary for the developmental of dental

Table 35-2. Typical Pattern of Infant Feedings

Age of Infant	Number of Feedings	Volume per Feeding	Total
Birth–2 wk	6–10	2–3 oz (60–90 mL)	12–30 oz (360–900 mL)
2 wk to 1 mo	6–8	3–4 oz (90–120 mL)	18–32 oz (540–960 mL)
1–3 mo	5–6	5–6 oz (150–180 mL)	25–36 oz (750–1080 mL)
3–7 mo	4–5	6–7 oz (180–210 mL)	25–36 oz (750–1080 mL)
7–12 mo	3–4	7–8 oz (210–240 mL)	25–36 oz (750–1080 mL)

enamel. The current recommendation of the Institute of Medicine and the American Academy of Pediatrics (Committee on Nutrition, 1985) is to supplement fluoride for breastfed infants if the household drinking water contains less than 0.3 ppm of fluoride. Adequate intake of fluoride based on water supplied to the household from public sources should not be assumed. Although most public water sources are fluoridated, many people use commercially bottled water for personal consumption.

Nutritional Needs of Formula-Fed Infants

Commercially prepared infant formulas also are sufficient to meet the infant's nutritional needs for the first 4 to 6 months of life. However, if the infant formula is purchased in the "ready to use" form, it may have insufficient fluoride. Supplementation of this mineral might be necessary. If either concentrated or powdered commercial formula is mixed with water from a fluoridated public water supply, additional fluoride is not indicated. Bottled water varies in fluoride content. If bottled water is used to prepare infant formula from powder or concentrate, information on the fluoride content should be obtained from the manufacturer to determine if supplementation is needed.

Commercial formulas are available with or without iron fortification. Iron fortification is not necessary during the first 4 months of life. After 4 months iron supplements are needed. The American Academy of Pediatrics advocates the use of iron-fortified formula to meet the iron needs of infants between the ages of 4 and 12 months. Infants often are started on this formula from birth. This practice prevents having to change from one formula to another, a difficult task for some parents to accomplish. If iron-fortified formulas are not well tolerated, the infant can get supplemental iron from iron-fortified infant cereals after age 4 months.

Adding Solid Food to the Diet

From 6 months to the end of the first year, breast milk or formula continues to be the most important part of the infant's diet. However, solid foods in the form of iron-fortified infant cereals, fruits, vegetables, and meats should be introduced during this period to help meet the infant's increasing demands and to provide the infant with the opportunity to learn about different flavors and textures. Positive feeding experiences will begin to establish healthy food habits. The infant is ready for supplemental foods between 4 and 6 months of age, when they have developed sufficiently to swallow nonliquid foods. It is inappropriate to introduce solid foods before the infant has reached this developmental stage, although parents may feel significant social pressure to do so. Dietary requirements for infants up to 1 year of age are listed in Table 35-3.

Table 35-3. Recommended Dietary Allowance for Infants

Nutrient	Recommended Dietary Allowance: Birth to 6 Mo	6 Mo to 1 Y
Calories	kg × 108	kg × 98
*Protein (g)	kg × 2.2	kg × 1.6
Vitamin A (μg RE)†	375	375
*Vitamin D (μg, cholecalciferol)	7.5	10
Vitamin E (mg, α TE)‡	3	4
*Vitamin C (mg)	30	35
Folacin (μg)	25	35
Niacin (mg, NE)§	5	6
Riboflavin (mg)	0.4	0.5
Thiamin (mg)	0.3	0.4
*Vitamin B_6 (mg)	0.3	0.6
Vitamin B_{12} (μg)	0.3	0.5
*Calcium (mg)	400	600
Phosphorus (mg)	300	500
Iodine (μg)	40	50
Magnesium (mg)	40	60
Zinc (mg)	5	5
*Iron (mg)	6	10

*Only these nutrients have been discussed in this chapter.
† RE = retinol equivalents
‡ TE = tocopherol equivalents
§ NE = niacin equivalents
Adapted from National Research Council. (1989). *Recommended dietary allowances*, (10th ed.). Washington, DC: National Academy Press.

Maternal Nutritional Needs in the Fourth Trimester

The nutritional status of the mother in the fourth trimester is important to her own and to her infant's well-being. All new mothers need adequate nutrients to promote healing of tissues traumatized by labor and delivery. The breastfeeding woman has an increased need for fluids, nutrients, and calories to produce sufficient amounts of milk for her neonate.

The woman who has a chronic illness, such as diabetes or heart disease, or the woman who experienced complications during pregnancy or delivery may have special dietary needs. These needs are best evaluated by a registered dietitian. It is the nurse's responsibility to recommend the intervention of a registered dietitian when appropriate and to ensure that all postpartum women receive nutritional counseling that meets their needs.

Replacement of Iron Stores

Many women have iron deficiency anemia when they become pregnant. This means that iron stores in the body have been depleted because of an iron-poor diet, a previous pregnancy, loss of blood through hemorrhage, or excessive loss of blood during menstrual periods. Iron deficiency anemia reduces the oxygen-carrying capacity of the blood. It may produce a variety of symptoms, including paleness of the skin, weakness, shortness of breath, lack of appetite, and a general slowing of vital body functions.

The nurse should explain to the postpartum woman some of the possible causes of her iron deficiency anemia. Once the woman learns the cause of the disorder or experiences symptoms, she may realize the importance of replenishing her iron stores and become consistent about taking her iron pills if she was not during her pregnancy.

The woman should be counseled about iron-rich foods, such as lean meats, leafy dark green vegetables, whole grain products, legumes, and molasses to include in her daily diet and should be given a prescription for supplemental iron to be taken daily. The nurse should be sure to explain that reversing iron deficiency is a slow process, and iron pills must be taken every day. If diet without supplementation is used to treat iron deficiency anemia, it takes 2 years to replace the iron lost during pregnancy.

Nutritional Requirements of Lactating Mothers

Lactation is a physiologic part of the reproductive process and may be influenced by maternal nutrition during pregnancy and after childbirth. The weight gain recommended during pregnancy, 11.5 to 16 kg (25.3 to 35.2 lb), provides adequately for fetal growth and the accumulation of maternal reserves. In some respects lactation makes even greater demands on the maternal organism than pregnancy. Nutritional requirements for pregnant, lactating, and nonlactating women are shown in Table 35-4. Due to the difference in the composition and volume of breast milk during various phases of lactation, it should be noted that the nutrient requirements for the mother decrease slightly in the second 6 months of lactation. A lactating woman can meet the energy requirement for milk production through an adequate dietary intake of calories and protein and through the catabolism of body tissue (fat or lean tissue).

Calcium Requirements

Lactating mothers produce 850 mL of breast milk per day on the average. The fat reserve accumulated during pregnancy can provide an additional 200 to 300 kcal/d for 100 days to assist in breast-milk production. These factors, and the efficiency with which breast milk is produced, were considered when the current recommended dietary allowances for energy for lactating women was proposed; that is, an additional 500 kcal/d above the normal dietary intake level is recommended. Women with low weight gain during pregnancy have less energy reserve and therefore may require more than this additional 500 kcal a day to meet their energy needs without causing the catabolism of lean tissue. Women who engage in heavy activity or who breastfeed beyond 6 months require a higher caloric intake.

Protein Requirements

Protein needs for the lactating woman are an additional 15 g/d during the first 6 months of lactation; this drops to 12 g of protein per day over usual requirements for the second 6 months of lactation (Institute of Medicine, 1991).

Fluid Requirements

Although there is no recommended dietary allowance for fluid, the lactating woman needs extra fluid to support lactation. She should drink a minimum of 2 L of fluid per day, half to provide adequate fluid for breast milk and half to meet her own needs. More fluid can be taken as desired.

Table 35-4. Recommended Dietary Allowances for Adult Women

	Woman's Condition			
Nutrients	Nonpregnant	Pregnant	Lactating First 6 Months	Lactating Second 6 Months
Calories	*	* + 300	* + 500	* + 500
Protein (g)	†	† + 10	† + 15	† + 12
Vitamin A (μg RE)‡	800	800	1300	1200
Vitamin D (μg cholecalciferol)	5	10	10	10
Vitamin E (mg α TE)§	8	10	12	11
Vitamin C (mg)	60	70	95	90
Folacin (mg)	180	400	280	260
Niacin (mg NE)‖	15	17	20	20
Riboflavin (mg)	1.3	1.6	1.8	1.7
Thiamine (mg)	1.1	1.5	1.6	1.6
Vitamin B_6 (mg)	1.6	2.2	2.1	2.1
Vitamin B_{12} (μg)	2.0	2.2	2.6	2.0
Calcium (mg)	800	1200	1200	1200
Phosphorus (mg)	800	1200	1200	1200
Iodine (μg)	150	175	200	200
Iron (mg)	1.5	30	15	15
Magnesium (mg)	280	320	355	340
Zinc (mg)	12	15	15	16

* See Table 17-1.
† See Table 17-2.
‡ RE = retinol equivalents.
§ TE = tocopherol equivalents.
‖ NE = niacin equivalents.
Adapted from National Research Council, National Academy of Sciences. (1989). *Recommended dietary allowances,* (10th ed.) Washington, DC: National Academy Press.

Vitamin and Mineral Requirements

The lactating woman needs extra amounts of most vitamins and minerals for milk production, as shown in Table 35-4. It is believed that the content of water-soluble vitamins in breast milk is directly related to the maternal intake of those vitamins. In contrast, concentrations of fat-soluble vitamins and minerals in breast milk appear to be unrelated to maternal diet. If calcium is not ingested by the mother in sufficient quantities for breast-milk production, the needed amount will be mobilized from her bone stores.

Effects of Maternal Nutrition on Lactation

It was once thought that the process of lactation was unaffected by nutritional deficits. However, increasing evidence shows that suboptimal maternal nutrition adversely affects lactation. The problem of maternal depletion has not been well researched. Milk production and infant well-being have been of greater interest, so studies have usually emphasized three criteria in the evaluation of lactational performance: milk volume, milk composition, and rate of infant growth.

Most women are unaware of the extra energy demands imposed by lactation. However, studies of well-nourished women indicate that successful lactation is associated with increased food intake. One classic study compared lactating and nonlactating women with respect to dietary pattern and weight loss. Both groups lost an average of 3 kg (6.6 lb) during the first 3 months postpartum. The lactating women ingested an average of 2930 kcal per day, whereas the nonlactating women ingested an average of 2070 kcal/d (Whichelow, 1975).

The same study observed that the intake of women who were successfully breastfeeding ranged from 2460 to 3060 kcal/d. All of the women studied were losing weight at a modest rate, except for those whose intakes exceeded 2950 kcal/d. Women who consciously restricted their intake to 1950 kcal/d did not produce sufficient milk for their infants and had to use supplemental feedings. Whichelow also reported two cases of lactational failure, both of which were attributed to inadequate weight gain during pregnancy (4.5 and 5 kg [9.9 to 11 lb], respectively). These women failed to produce a sufficient volume of milk despite dietary intakes of 2400 kcal/d or more. This suggested that mobilization of body fat and catabolism of lean tissue to support lactation may be more limited than was previously believed. Nutritional status during pregnancy may be of some importance in determining lactational success.

Poor lactational performance in poor women may be caused by substandard diets. Failure also may be related to the combined stresses of maternal disease, chronic undernutrition, and difficult living conditions. In general, lactational performance in undernourished women is less than optimal. Milk composition may be normal because maternal stores of essential nutrients, such as iron and calcium, are used. However, milk volume often is less than 500 mL/d, resulting in poor infant growth. When the diets of undernourished women are supplemented with protein and additional calories, milk production increases and is sustained for a longer period.

Dietary Recommendations for the Breastfeeding Mother

The lactating mother has an increased need for fluid, energy, protein, minerals, and vitamins. These nutrients are necessary to provide sufficient calories to produce milk and to protect against a nutritional deficit. Energy requirements vary depending on the amount of milk being produced. An infant weighing 4990 g (11 lb) needs 600 kcal/d, which requires 850 mL of milk. As the amount of milk needed for the infant increases, so does the need for additional calories in the mother's diet. Women who gain sufficient weight during pregnancy have body fat reserves that can be mobilized for extra milk production.

The amounts of essential nutrients required during lactation are greater than those needed in pregnancy. The breastfeeding mother's diet should contain at least three servings of milk products a day. Adequate milk intake protects against calcium and phosphorus drain. When maternal calcium intake is low, calcium supplements should be provided. Large amounts of fluid are essential for providing water to the breast milk in addition to meeting the mother's needs for fluid. Each day 2 L (1.07 qt) of various liquids should be consumed; vegetable and fruit juices (which provide vitamins and minerals), water, and milk are good choices. Table 35-5 shows suggested servings of food groups for lactating and nonlactating mothers. Breastfeeding requires extra energy, so the lactating woman needs to ingest 500 kcal more than her normal maintenance diet to sustain adequate milk production.

Although the United States Department of Agriculture's (USDA's) food guide pyramid, published in the fall of 1992, has not drawn up specific recommendations for lactating women, some advice is given. For instance the following number of servings are suggested for adolescent girls and active women. The bulletin (USDA, 1992) advises pregnant or breastfeeding women to use "somewhat more:"

Table 35-5. Daily Food Guide for Woman

	Minimum Number of Servings		
Food Group	Nonpregnant 11–24 years	Nonpregnant 25–50 years	Pregnant/ Lactating 11–50 years
Protein foods	5*	5*	7†
Milk products	3	2	3
Breads, cereals, grains:	7	6	7
Whole	4	4	4
Enriched	3	2	3
Fruits and vegetables:			
Vitamin C-rich	1	1	1
Vitamin A-rich	1	1	1
Other	3	3	3
Unsaturated fats	3	3	3

* Equivalent in protein to 5 oz of animal protein; at least three servings per week should be from the vegetable protein list.

† Equivalent in protein to 7 oz of animal protein; at least one of these servings should be from the vegetable protein list daily.

California Department of Health Services, Maternal and Child Health Branch. (1990). Nutrition during pregnancy and the postpartum period: A manual for health care professionals. Sacremento, CA: Author.

- 9 bread group servings
- 4 vegetable group servings
- 3 fruit group servings
- 3 milk group servings
- 6 meat group servings (ounces)
- 73 total fat (grams)
- 12 total added sugars (teaspoons)

Foods eaten by the mother have nutrients and other components that are passed on to the infant through breast milk. Over the years anecdotal information about specific foods producing coliclike symptoms in infants (fussiness, bouts of unexplained crying after feeding) has been passed along to new mothers. Foods implicated range from chocolate to legumes to fresh fruit; even some herbs and spices have been thought to cause symptoms in the breastfed infant. These reactions are often real and are usually infant specific; there is no evidence that intolerance to food components in the mother's diet is consistent between siblings.

There is no definitive list of foods that should be avoided during lactation. However, if an infant develops symptoms after maternal consumption of a particular food, the mother should intentionally try the same food a second time and note the infant's response. If the symptoms recur, the food should be avoided for 1 to 2 months and then tried again. Because symptoms are frequently "dose related" (the amount of the offending component in the food per kg of infant weight), the food may not cause problems when the infant's body size increases. One food that frequently causes symptoms in the infant is the cow's milk consumed by the mother. In this case the symptoms can be relieved by reducing the total volume of milk consumed or by replacing milk with other dairy products, such as yogurt or cheese.

Nutritional Requirements of Formula-Feeding Mothers

The nutritional status of a woman affects not only her own health, but also that of her family. A woman of reproductive age who already has children usually has a basic knowledge of and understanding about the need for specific nutrients, food groups, and a well-rounded diet. If the family plans their meals with these concepts in mind, they will benefit from the positive effects of good nutrition. However, the nurse cannot assume that every woman has this knowledge.

A formula-feeding mother has special dietary needs. While adjusting to her neonate and her higher than normal energy requirements, the mother should be particularly aware of her own nutrient intake. Her nutrient stores may have been lost during pregnancy and must be replaced to provide the energy and stamina she requires for her physical and mental health. Table 35-5 gives a fourth-trimester food guide for the nonbreastfeeding woman. The number of servings in the USDA's pyramid (USDA, 1992) were listed in the previous section.

Additional information in the Teaching Considerations display later in this chapter provides guidance about how to reduce caloric intake to assist the nonlactating mother to return to her prepregnant weight. If the woman has other children and pregnancies have been close together, the store of nutrients expended during the previous pregnancy may not have been fully replenished. This is particularly true if the pregnancies occurred within 1 year of one another, so healthy food choices may be especially important. Women should be conscious of the need to improve their nutritional status during the postpartum and interconceptual periods. The woman who follows the recommended dietary allowances with careful food purchasing and meal planning can be assured of adequate nourishment that will benefit her health and that of her family.

Nutritional Requirements of Adolescent Mothers

When the postpartum mother is an adolescent, her nutritional deficits are compounded. Adolescence is a period of rapid growth, when nutritional needs for body metabolism are greatly increased. As described in Chapter 17, the pregnant adolescent must consume an unusually large number of calories to meet her own growth requirements, as well as the nutrient demands of her fetus. The increased amounts of protein, iron, calcium, and other essential nutrients are important. During pregnancy, when her nutritional status is closely monitored to assure proper weight gain and dietary intake, the adolescent may become relatively well nourished. However, her only postpartum contact with a health professional may occur at her 6-week checkup or when she seeks contraception.

The nurse should give adolescent mothers special attention and must be realistic in developing a nutritional plan. Adolescents generally are very active, may be dependent financially, are subject to peer pressure, and will feel the urgent need to get their bodies back in shape. Early postpartum referral to a public health nurse may be helpful in following the adolescent at home; this nurse can reinforce and encourage good eating habits and offer support if the young mother is feeling stressed.

The perinatal nurse assesses the nutritional status of women and supports optimal infant-feeding practices. The new mother and the infant have special nutritional needs in the first 3 to 6 months after birth. Breast milk is sufficient to meet most of the nutritional needs of the infant for the first 4 to 6 months of life. Commercially prepared infant formulas also are sufficient to meet the infant's nutritional needs for the first 4 to 6 months of life. The nutritional status of the mother in the fourth trimester is important to her own and to her infant's well-being. All new mothers need adequate nutrients to promote healing of tissues traumatized by labor and delivery. The breastfeeding woman has an increased need for fluids, nutrients, and calories to produce sufficient amounts of milk for her neonate. A formula-feeding mother has special dietary needs. While adjusting to her newborn and her higher than normal energy requirements, the mother should be particularly aware of her own nutrient intake. The nurse can assist the new mother to establish and maintain good nutritional practices.

Implications for Nursing Care

Promoting optimal maternal–infant nutrition is a significant part of nursing care for childbearing families. The following sections briefly address the process of assessment, identification of potential and actual problems in relation to maternal–infant nutrition, and the nurse's role in providing care.

• • Assessment

Initial assessment of maternal nutritional status in the postpartum period is based on data regarding maternal prepregnant and pregnant weight, evidence of adequate iron stores, an adequate dietary history or profile, and the recognition of any complicating factors, such as unusual blood loss during delivery. The assessment of infant nutritional status usually is carried out in routine pediatric care and thus is not an area of responsibility of the perinatal nurse. However, the perinatal nurse is directly responsible for assessing the parents' knowledge and skills related to infant feeding and for providing essential teaching in the early postpartum period. This teaching is detailed in Chapter 28.

• • Nursing Diagnosis

Problems related to maternal–infant nutrition in the first 3 months after birth usually are diagnosed by standard indicators, such as infant weight gain and feeding patterns, maternal weight loss or gain, restoration of maternal iron stores, maternal energy levels, and maternal patterns of elimination. The perinatal nurse's most consistent contact with childbearing women and their neonates usually occurs in too short a time frame to pick up such problems. However, the postpartum nurse can anticipate common concerns among new mothers about infant feeding and self-care and may identify particular patient needs for teaching and support. The following are some nursing diagnoses that may be useful in providing nursing care related to maternal–infant nutrition:

- Altered Nutrition: More than Body Requirements related to stressful life circumstances
- Altered Nutrition: Less than Body Requirements related to maternal weight reduction attempts
- High Risk for Activity Intolerance related to fatigue and increased family responsibilities
- Ineffective Breastfeeding related to inadequate knowledge

• • Planning and Implementation

Major concerns shared by most new mothers include weight loss and reestablishing prepregnant weight, maintaining energy levels, and establishing and maintaining breast-milk supply if the mother chooses to breastfeed. The perinatal nurse is responsible for early instruction regarding breastfeeding and formula feeding and for assisting parents in their first attempts to feed their neonate.

Promoting Optimal Maternal Nutrition

The nurse can anticipate that the new mother will have concerns about reestablishing her normal patterns quickly in the postpartum period. Postpartum women may need nutritional guidance in relation to their own physical restoration. The nurse should guide the woman in her food choices, as shown in the accompanying Teaching Considerations display on healthy food choices.

Expected Outcome

- The postpartum woman constructs several sample healthful menus for herself and her family.

Advising Regarding Weight Loss

One of the primary concerns of the new mother is her weight; she would like to return to her prepregnant shape. Delivery causes a weight loss of approximately 5.5 to 7.7 kg (12 to 17 lb) due to expulsion of the infant, placenta, amniotic fluid, and to some degree other body fluid. Another small weight loss occurs during the first 2 to 5 days postpartum, when fluid accumulated in the body during the prenatal period is eliminated through diuresis and diaphoresis. The nurse should reassure the mother that by her 6-week checkup she will have lost approximately 9 to 11 kg (20 to 25 lb) and should not attempt a weight-loss diet until after this visit.

The breastfeeding mother should be advised not to try to lose weight until her infant is weaned. To avoid fatigue and anemia she needs to reestablish and maintain her nutritional reserves. The weight of breast tissue, stored milk, and additional fluid all contribute to the weight of the lactating mother. Weaning is usually accompanied by a spontaneous 1.8 to 2.7 kg (4 to 6 lb) weight loss. The mother who is formula feeding should receive information about healthy food choices that allow her to reduce her caloric intake while maintaining adequate intake of nutrients.

Expected Outcomes

- The lactating woman maintains dietary intake sufficient to support breastfeeding until she decides to wean her infant.
- The postpartum woman achieves desired weight loss within 6 to 8 months after childbirth while maintaining a healthy dietary intake.

Promoting Energy

During the postpartum period the new mother's energy level is normally low. The mother will have more demands than usual placed on her and may find it difficult to rest. This is particularly true if she has other children who need attention and care. Because of her increased activity level and the need for postpartum healing, it is important that the mother eats nutritious meals and drinks quantities of fluids. Without proper nourishment, she will soon become exhausted.

The nurse may reassure the mother that by her 6-week checkup she and her infant will have their feeding and sleep schedules established. Her body will be back to a more normal state at this time. The new mother may be more rested and adjusted to her new routine. An anemic woman

Teaching Considerations

Healthy Food Choices

The nurse can use the following points when teaching patients about healthy food choices for themselves and their families.

Protein Foods

- Choose poultry and fish often. Remove skin before eating.
- Avoid breaded and fried varieties (like fish sticks, fish cakes, chicken nuggets).
- Choose only the leanest cuts of meat, and trim away any visible fat before eating.
- Bake, broil, poach, or simmer instead of frying.
- Avoid high-fat processed meats (like hot dogs, luncheon meats, sausages).
- Limit peanuts, peanut butter, nuts, and seeds.

Milk Products

- Use nonfat or lowfat milk.
- Limit use of cheese and use part-skim milk cheeses (like farmer, ricotta, mozzarella) as much as possible.
- Limit sweetened milk products (like fruited yogurt, chocolate milk, custard, ice cream, pudding).

Breads, Cereals, Grains

- Emphasize whole-grain breads, cereals, and grains (like whole-wheat bread, oatmeal, and brown rice).
- Limit sweetened breads and cereals.
- Limit products made with added fat (like granola, crackers, croutons, muffins, pancakes, waffles).

Fruits and Vegetables

- Choose fruits rather than juices (for more fiber).
- Limit sweetened fruits and juices.
- Limit those with added sauces, butter, or margarine.
- Avoid fried vegetables (like french fries, hashed browns).

Fats and Sweets

- Limit visible fats (like butter, margarine, oil, mayonnaise, salad dressings).
- Limit fried snack and fast foods (like chips, burgers).
- Limit sweets (like candy, cake, cookies, pie).
- Limit sodas and other sweetened beverages.

California Department of Health Services. (1990). Nutrition during pregnancy and the postpartum period. A manual for health care professionals. *Sacramento, CA: Author.*

may need longer to regain her former energy level (see the section on replacement of iron stores in this chapter).

Expected Outcomes

- The postpartum woman reports an understanding of the relationship between adequate dietary and fluid intake and energy levels.
- The postpartum woman reports increasing energy levels within 3 months of childbirth.

Promoting Successful Breastfeeding

The perinatal nurse is responsible for early instruction regarding breastfeeding and for assisting parents in their first attempts to feed their neonate. Assisting with breastfeeding is discussed in Chapter 28.

• • Evaluation

Evaluation of the effectiveness of nursing care in regard to maternal–infant nutrition is sometimes difficult. This is because outcomes can be observed only after discharge, when most perinatal nurses no longer have contact with families. Evaluation of care by necessity focuses on the consistency and quality of teaching in the early postpartum period. Outcomes of effective nursing care in the postpartum period may include a rising incidence of successful breastfeeding up to and beyond 6 months and evidence of maternal physical restoration. Satisfactory weight loss and adequate iron stores and energy levels also are outcomes the nurse can evaluate.

Promoting optimal maternal–infant nutrition is a significant part of nursing care for childbearing families. Initial assessment of maternal nutritional status in the postpartum period is based on data regarding maternal prepregnant and pregnant weight, evidence of adequate iron stores, an adequate dietary history or profile, as well as the recognition of any complicating factors, such as unusual blood loss during delivery. Postpartum women may need nutritional guidance in relation to their own physical restoration. Major concerns shared by most new mothers include weight loss and reestablishing prepregnant weight, maintaining energy levels, and establishing and maintaining breast-milk supply if the mother chooses to breastfeed.

Chapter Summary

Breastfeeding is the method of feeding infants recommended by health professionals in the United States and worldwide. It has many advantages for the infant and mother. The lactating woman will need more foods and more nutrients and will probably lose weight more readily than the mother who chooses to formula feed her infant. The nurse should provide information and assistance as needed and should support the mother's chosen infant-feeding method. Mothers differ in their nutrient needs depending on whether or not they choose to breastfeed their infant.

Nutrient needs of the breastfed and the formula-fed infant are the same, but different supplementation is needed, depending on the type of feeding used. The nurse plays a vital role in teaching new parents about breastfeeding and formula feeding. Thus, it is essential that the nurse understands the principles that are the basis for teaching about maternal and infant nutrition in the first year after birth.

Study Questions

1. *Why is breastfeeding desirable for the neonate and the mother?*
2. *What nutritional supplementation is recommended for breastfed and formula-fed infants and at what age(s)?*
3. *How does breast milk of poorly nourished populations differ from that of well-nourished groups? What implications does this have for infant growth?*
4. *How does the recommended dietary intake of calories and protein for the lactating mother compare with that for the nonlactating mother?*
5. *What are good sources of protein, iron, calcium, and calories for all women?*

References

Committee on Nutrition, American Academy of Pediatrics. (1985). *Pediatric nutrition handbook*. Elk Grove, IL: Author.

Institute of Medicine, National Academy of Sciences. (1991). *Nutrition during lactation*. Washington, DC: National Academy Press.

Lawrence, R. (1989). *Breastfeeding: A guide for the medical profession* (3rd ed.). St. Louis, MO: C.V. Mosby.

United States Department of Agriculture. (1992). *USDA's Food Guide Pyramid*. Washington, DC: Human Nutrition Information Service.

Whichelow, M. (1975). Calorie requirements for successful breastfeeding. *Archives of the Diseases of Children*, *50*, 669–675.

Suggested Readings

Lawrence, R. (1989). *Breastfeeding: A guide for the medical profession* (3rd ed.). St. Louis, MO: C.V. Mosby.

Satter, E. (1991). *Child of mine: Feeding with love and good sense*. Palo Alto, CA: Bull Publishing.

CHAPTER 36

Individual and Family Adaptation in the Year After Childbirth

Learning Objectives

After studying the material in this chapter, the student will be able to:

- Describe changing roles in families during the year after childbirth.
- Describe unanticipated stressors encountered by families during the year after childbirth.
- Discuss myths about parenthood.
- Relate family characteristics to ease of transition to the parental role.
- Assess family adaptation.
- Identify nursing objectives for families during the year after childbirth.
- Identify families at risk for difficulties in adaptation.
- Describe nursing actions that facilitate healthy family adaptation.
- Develop teaching care plans that foster self-care in the family during the year after childbearing.

Key Terms

blended family
behavioral cues
colic
failure to thrive (nonorganic)
family development
irritable infant syndrome
role taking

Ongoing adaptations are required of families during the first year of life with an infant. Changes occur in roles, communication among family members, family health practices, and family–community interactions. Family relationships must be realigned, and many developmental tasks must be accomplished. Professional nurses play an increasingly important role in the ongoing care of the family within the community setting. Community and home health nurses, nurse midwives, and family and pediatric nurse practitioners offer a wide range of services that support the family as it adjusts to the presence of a new member or members.

Throughout the first year of parenthood, the nurse monitors individual and family responses to the birth of the infant. The primary goal of nursing care of new families is to facilitate achievement of developmental tasks and support the complex adjustments required. Focusing on family strengths will foster healthy family adaptations and promote infant growth and development. Providing anticipatory guidance and professional advice and initiating appropriate referrals when problems occur in family functioning are important aspects of nursing care.

This chapter discusses family adaptations during the first year of an infant's life and describes effective nursing care to promote a positive and healthy transition. The major developmental tasks, processes of parent–infant attachment, and family role taking are described. Major factors affecting successful family functioning and the nurse's role in assuring positive adjustments are reviewed. The impact of family composition and structure and culture on family adaptations is discussed.

Family Development

The nurse can use family developmental theory with its concept of developmental task attainment to assess family functioning and adaptation. The transition to parenthood is

typically defined as encompassing two phases: the expectancy phase and the expanding phase. The *expectancy phase* begins during pregnancy and involves the accomplishment of the developmental tasks inherent in the process of pregnancy and birth, such as giving of self and ensuring safe passage of the fetus. As discussed in Chapter 8, the tasks faced by the individual and family during this phase are biologically triggered. Family members must readjust their relationships with each other and prepare for the birth of the neonate. Progress through the expectancy phase is influenced by factors such as age and maturity of the family members and the family's strengths and weaknesses.

The *expanding phase* encompasses the developmental task of incorporating the new family member (or members when a multifetal conception occurs) into the preexisting family unit. During the first year after birth, the woman must make physical and psychological adjustments. Other family members also must adapt and reorganize their life-styles to meet the needs of the newborn. Life-style changes, such as sleep deprivation, alterations in daily routine, and a decrease in the amount of time available for interpersonal interaction, may cause adverse physical and emotional reactions. Expectancy and expanding phase developmental tasks are reviewed in the accompanying display.

Implications for Nursing Care

Information about achievement of developmental tasks can be collected from health records, interviews with family members, or direct observation of behavior. Data obtained through the assessment process aid the nurse in determining whether individual family members adjust successfully during the first year after birth of the infant. Ongoing assessment provides evidence of family developmental task attainment such as providing infant care, mobilizing support systems, and reorganzing finances.

During the process of adaptation and reorganization, family members may experience disequilibrium and stress. Although stress is an essential ingredient of healthy reorganization, many individual and family stressors, such as maternal physiologic complications, altered patterns of sexual expression, sibling distress, or an infant with a health problem, may surpass the adaptive capacity of the family. Even when families are well prepared for the many changes precipitated by the birth of a newborn, when unexpected complications arise, family decompensation may occur (see Chapter 25).

The nurse must determine whether individual family members are adequately prepared for the reality of parenthood, siblinghood, or grandparenthood. Myths about parenting abound in every society. These myths are perpetuated by the media and folklore but also arise from experiences within one's own family. Families often are bombarded with information that bears little resemblance to the realities of parenting and family life in contemporary North American society. In the past television depicted a romanticized image of an urban, affluent, two-parent family. More recently, programs have been created that reflect a more realistic diversity in family structure, such as blended families and family units with same-sex parents. Although new parents' expectations of parenting vary widely, some common misconceptions remain constant. The accompanying display lists common myths about parenting.

Parent–Infant Attachment

A major developmental task to be accomplished during the first year of the infant's life is the process of parent–infant attachment. Attachment is an interactive process between parent and infant, resulting in satisfying experiences and an emotional bond that motivates the parent to care for the infant (Mercer & Ferketich, 1990). This process evolves slowly with time. The physical and emotional survival of the infant depends on successful accomplishment of this task. Attachment occurs within a framework of beliefs, values, and expectations about the infant, the parent role, and how smoothly the individual will move into the role.

The transition to parenthood is a challenging process in the family life cycle. Much study has been devoted to delineating maternal–infant attachment and interaction. Less is known about paternal attachment. Recent studies suggest that new fathers go through a similar process of attachment when compared with new mothers. There are, however, observable differences between men and women as they work through this process.

Acquaintance

Acquaintance is the natural beginning of all human relationships and the first stage of the attachment process. The acquaintance process begins when parents gather information about and form impressions of their fetus and later about the infant. When questioned about the fetus, many pregnant women describe unique attributes, such as activity level, temperament, and even fetal reactions to specific foods or beverages that she eats.

After the neonate's birth the woman and her partner continue this process of acquaintance. Gazing at the newborn, touching, and talking to and about the neonate are behaviors that have been described by researchers in both mothers and fathers in the immediate postpartum period (Tomlinson, 1990; Tomlinson, Rothenberg, & Carver, 1991). These behaviors are thought to indicate the early acquaintance process and are described in Chapter 28. Parents compare the "real" newborn to the expected or fantasized newborn with respect to such characteristics as gender, size, overall appearance, and temperament. In some cases prenatal expectations are confirmed; in others parents may be surprised by the differences that become evident after the birth.

Ongoing interactions between parent and infant after discharge from the hospital or birthing unit provide the opportunity for reinforcement or change in the initial perceptions of the infant. This is the next phase in the attachment process. Normally, parents grieve the loss of the anticipated or fantasized newborn as they come to know the "real" newborn. When successful adaptation occurs the parents recognize and come to appreciate the individual characteristics, cues, rhythms, and personality of their infant. However,

*Developmental Tasks for Families**

Expectancy Phase

- Anticipates providing for the physical care of the expected neonate
- Adapts family financial pattern
- Defines evolving role patterns
- Adjusts patterns of sexual expression to pregnancy
- Expands communication systems to meet present and anticipated emotional needs
- Reorients relationships with relatives
- Adapts relationships with friends and community at large to realities of pregnancy
- Acquires knowledge and plans for specifics of pregnancy, childbirth, and parenthood
- Maintains morale and philosophy of life

Expanding Phase

- Reconciles conflicting concepts of roles
  - Demonstrates parental role taking
  - Reconciles fantasized expectations with reality
- Accepts and adjusts to the strains and pressures of parenthood
  - Exhibits intrafamily cooperation
  - Demonstrates mutual parental support by sharing infant caretaking and family maintenance tasks
  - Describes realistic perception of stressors
  - Demonstrates appropriate active problem-solving behavior
  - Mobilizes support systems to augment family resources
- Learns to care for infant with confidence and competence
  - Demonstrates appropriate identification of infant cues
  - Demonstrates appropriate caretaking behaviors
  - Expresses positive regard for characteristics of infant and pleasure in his or her thriving
- Establishes and maintains a family wellness lifestyle
  - Demonstrates appropriate postpartum physiologic restoration
  - Demonstrates awareness of and compliance with basic health concepts of nutrition, hydration, rest, hygiene, exercise, reaction, and stress reduction
- Nurtures development of infant and young child
  - Demonstrates appropriate verbal and tactile communication
  - Provides appropriate sensory stimulation
  - Demonstrates knowledge of age-specific safety hazards and realistic protection of infant
  - Exhibits awareness of unique temperament of child, and modifies nurturing behavior accordingly
- Promotes marital relationship
  - Reestablishes satisfactory sexual, emotional, and recreational interaction
  - Maintains open, effective patterns of communication
- Adjusts to practical realities of expanding family life
  - Adapts to limits of time, space, and privacy
  - Develops appropriate priorities for use of family resources
- Maintains personal autonomy of family members
  - Encourages expression of sense of self with personal values and interests
  - Promotes expression of and respect for individuality of members
  - Promotes individual growth and development of members
- Explores and develops sense of family identity
  - Establishes sense of family cohesion, affection, and shared goals
  - Demonstrates positive regard for peer group and community at large
  - Exhibits traditions and values reflecting cultural heritage and family identity

**The nurse needs to confirm the appropriateness of these tasks with various cultural groups.*

After Duvall, E. (1979). In Donaldson, N. E. The postpartum follow-up clinician role—a design for extending the scope of nursing practice. Master's project, 1979, California State University at Los Angeles.

when prenatal expectations differ greatly from the "real" infant, the parent may experience unresolved grief and impairment in the attachment process. Specific verbal cues that may indicate problems with parent–infant attachment are listed in the accompanying display.

Implications for Nursing Care

The nurse fosters the immediate postbirth acquaintance process by uniting the newborn with his or her parents as quickly as possible. During assessments and physical examinations, the nurse should take time to acquaint parents with the unique characteristics and behavioral capacities of their infant. The nurse monitors progress in the acquaintance process and identifies obstacles in the environment or parental problems that may interfere with their growing awareness of the neonate and infant. A more complete discussion of immediate postbirth nursing interventions to support the acquaintance process is presented in Chapter 31.

Common Myths About Parenthood

- Childrearing is fun.
- Children are sweet and cute.
- Children will turn out "well" if they have "good" parents.
- Girls are harder to rear than boys.
- Today's parents are not as good as those of the past.
- Childrearing today is easier.
- Children appreciate all the advantages their parents are able to give them.
- The hard work of rearing children is justified because parents are going to make a better world.
- There are no "bad" children, only "bad" parents.
- Two parents are always better than one.
- Modern science has been helpful to parents.
- Love is enough to sustain good parental performance.
- All married couples should have children.
- Children can improve a marriage.

Verbal Cues That Indicate a Potential Problem With Parent–Infant Attachment

Disappointment With Gender

"I wish he was a girl," or "I wish she was a boy."

"I don't like boys (girls)."

"This was my last try for a boy (girl). I wanted a boy (girl) so badly."

"I only bought clothes for a boy (girl)."

Infant Characteristics Remind Parent of Relative Who Is Disliked, Hated, or Feared

"She looks just like my mother. She was so cold and judgmental."

"He looks like his father. The guy took off when he found out I was pregnant."

"I had an aunt with a chin like hers. She was a bitch."

Unexpected Infant Characteristics Associated With Negative Traits

"He doesn't look at all like me. Could someone else be the father?"

"I was never sure I was really the father."

"Her face is really ugly. They said she'd look pretty after a few days, but she doesn't."

"That birthmark means she's cursed."

"She always crying and grabbing for my breast. She's greedy and selfish."

"He knows when I sit down to rest and starts screaming. He does it on purpose."

Bonding

In the 1970s and early 1980s the process of parent–infant attachment was studied in depth by researchers. The term *bonding* was coined by researchers and was described as a process of rapid attachment occurring immediately after birth. It was theorized that bonding occurred when the new mother and infant were permitted to touch and interact during a hypothesized sensitive period immediately after birth. Some researchers theorized that when the woman and her infant missed the opportunity to bond during this period of heightened receptivity, future attachment could be jeopardized.

Pioneering studies by Klaus and Kennell (1982) examined the effects of maternal–infant separation on the attachment process. The concept of bonding caught the attention of the media and expectant parents. Dissemination of research findings in the popular literature had widespread positive effects on the development of family-centered maternity care. Unfortunately, misinterpretation of data also resulted in unfounded fears among many parents that attachment would not occur when initial contact between parent and infant was limited due to obstetric complications or the birth of a sick neonate.

Later studies conducted by Klaus and Kennell, as well as other researchers, suggest that limited early contact may be a potential risk to future attachment only for select groups of high-risk women. At particular risk are women with a history of child abuse, chemical dependency, or severe emotional problems. In reality the process of human attachment is complex and is characterized by great adaptability. In most cases the nature of ongoing interactions *with time*, rather than immediate postbirth contact, determines the quality of parent–infant attachment.

Implications for Nursing Care

With a greater understanding of the acquaintance process, the concept of bonding as a critical phenomenon has changed. The nurse must appreciate the full range of attachment behaviors and have a sound understanding of the process. Although a critical time or "sensitive" period may exist during which close contact between parent and infant facilitates later attachment, all is not lost when this is not possible. Anxious parents should be reassured that irreparable harm is not done if they are unable to hold and remain with the infant immediately after birth. Efforts should be made, however, to reunite parent and infant as quickly as possible. When separations are prolonged due to illness of the mother or infant, ongoing assessment and support is essential when

the family returns to the home and community to determine if problems with attachment occur.

Attachment and Its Stressors

The nature and extent of prenatal attachment is not clearly understood. Many factors are believed to influence the timing, progress, and process of attachment. Some women exhibit behavioral and verbal cues suggesting a close attachment to the fetus. Others remain less engaged with the growing fetus. Results of recent research by nurse scientists and others interested in attachment before and after birth may delineate the process in the future. Some of the predictors of parental attachment are described in the Nursing Research display. Three factors in attachment are discussed in the following sections.

Infant Temperament and Behaviors

One factor that may affect parent attachment is the newborn's temperament as evidenced by neonatal behaviors. Research findings indicate that the neonate has a unique personality or temperament, which may strongly influence family adjustment during the first postpartum year (see Chapter 31). The ease with which the infant adapts to new stimuli is one indicator of temperament. In studies of neonatal temperament, parents have described the newborn who adjusts smoothly to novel situations, new foods, and strange environments as "easy." Conversely, the newborn who reacts negatively (rigid posture, crying, irritability) to these situations has been termed "difficult."

When the newborn has difficulty adapting to new settings or other situations, parents may feel they are in some way to blame. The difficult neonate's responses to the same stimuli often are inconsistent. A parental response to cries of distress may work one time when used to soothe the newborn but not the next. Parents may experience an extreme sense of inadequacy or incompetence in the parenting role in this situation. Individual and family maladaptation may occur. The process of attachment may be delayed or adversely affected.

Implications for Nursing Care

Infant behaviors encompass a wide range of responses to caretaking activities by parents. Current teaching often places the emphasis on maternal competence without adequate consideration of the role of infant temperament in successful caretaking. Incorporation of neonatal behavioral assessments, particularly in relation to consolability, habituation, and response to stimulation, will assist mothers to identify newborn characteristics that affect maternal–newborn interaction.

Timely nursing interventions to assist parents in understanding the difficult infant's strengths and weaknesses may reverse feelings of inadequacy. The nurse must be careful to

Nursing Research

Predictors of Parental Attachment During Early Parenthood

Parents begin the attachment process during pregnancy, and the process continues in the months following birth. The process, an interactive one between parents and newborn, creates in parents an enduring emotional commitment. Researchers have attempted to measure attachment by observing parental behaviors. Behavioral cues that may indicate the process of attachment include maintaining close proximity, holding the newborn, and aligning the parent's face with the newborn's face (*en face* position).

Mercer and Ferketich (1990) have developed a model that identifies significant variables associated with attachment. Both high-risk and low-risk women and their partners were interviewed over time to better understand the evolution of the process. Measurements were taken at 6 weeks and at 8 months following the birth. The investigators measured the degree of perceived stress (stressful life events and pregnancy and childbirth stress), self-esteem, perceptions of health status, and social support to determine their influence on attachment. Sense of mastery in the parent role, parental competence, anxiety and depression, readiness for pregnancy, and family functioning also were measured. Parental competence was a major predictor of attachment. Early parent–infant contact was not found to be a positive predictor of parental attachment. There was evidence of stronger attachment in the group of high-risk women than in low-risk women at 6 weeks, but by 8 months the difference was not significant. Attachment also was associated with perceived support, particularly in the high-risk group.

The study gives direction for further research concerning how nurses can positively affect parent–newborn attachment by promoting feelings of competence in parents. For example nurses may enhance self-esteem and a sense of competence by role modeling neonatal care behaviors, encouraging parents to practice skills, and providing positive feedback as they successfully achieve mastery. Nurses also need to assess carefully the family's support system and make appropriate referrals when families lack the help of family or friends.

Mercer, R. T., & Ferketich, S. L. (1990). Predictors of parental attachment during early parenthood. *Journal of Advanced Nursing, 15*, 268–280.

avoid labeling the infant as "difficult" and should guide parents in the development of strategies that support the infant in smooth adjustments to new situations.

Colic

Colic is another factor in parent–infant attachment behaviors. Colic has dramatic effects on family adaptation during the first year postpartum. This disorder is characterized by abdominal spasms and rigidity that result in abdominal pain. Infants with colic exhibit persistent unexplained and inconsolable crying and move rapidly in and out of sleep. They demonstrate irritable behaviors while feeding and excessive activity (Cervisi, Chapman, Niklas, & Yamaoka, 1991). Parents find these behaviors stressful despite other signs that the infant is thriving (eg, weight gain). A parent may react by crying with the infant; becoming fatigued, depressed, or angry; or resenting the infant. Physical abuse of the infant may occur when crying is prolonged and parents have inadequate resources to cope.

Colic or irritable infant syndrome occurs in approximately 15% to 25% of all infants regardless of ethnicity, gender, birth order, gestational age, or socioeconomic status (Keefe & Froese-Fretz, 1991). This syndrome emerges when neonates are approximately 2 weeks old, peaks at approximately 6 weeks, and may persist for up to 6 months. Research has never conclusively identified a cause for colic, and many interventions are based on hypothesized causes, such as immature gastrointestinal function, milk allergy, and maternal anxiety (Keefe & Froese-Fretz, 1991).

Parents often are bombarded with a variety of explanations, myths, and advice about colic. Families' stresses can be increased by these contradictory suggestions. Parents also can become distressed when physiologic problems are ruled out, and no specific cause of the problem can be identified (Cervisi et al., 1991). Stressed families may be affected on multiple levels. Parent–infant interactions, marital relationships, and family dynamics in general all can be disturbed. Parents have described experiencing stress, fatigue, and role ambivalence. In one small sample, parents in Britain reported shaking and hitting their infants during crying episodes (Mortimer & Kevill, 1985).

Implications for Nursing Care

Families require assistance in coping with colic. Parents generally call health care providers when infant crying has become unbearable and stressful. A team approach with the active involvement of parents, extended family, physicians, and nurses is most effective. A thorough physical examination should be conducted to reassure families that the infant is normal. The infant's diet and feeding pattern should be reviewed to rule out any feeding or organic problems. The family can be given objective data that support the diagnosis of colic. This information provides the family with evidence of infant developmental problems and not problems with parenting skill. Family members should not be made to feel that they are responsible for their infant's difficulties but rather that this developmental problem will resolve with time.

Crying and Sleep Disturbances

Even infants who do not exhibit colic may cry for prolonged periods of time (20 to 30 minutes or longer) during a 24-hour period. Concerns about infant crying and sleep disturbances cause parents a great deal of emotional distress and sleep deprivation. They also can become very frustrated and angry when their sleep is disturbed repeatedly. Sleep disturbances in infancy commonly take two forms: sleeplessness and arousal. Sleeplessness can occur as struggles at bedtime not to fall asleep or nighttime awakenings. Arousal disorders include nightmares and night terrors.

Although by 6 months most infants sleep through the night, sleeplessness can occur with frequent awakenings; this may occur when parents return to work or school or when an infant is teething. Arousals are common when infants move between different sleep cycles. Many infants return to sleep without parent intervention. However, when falling back to sleep becomes routinely associated with parental interventions, such as rocking or taking the infant into the adult bed, infants may rely on parents to go back to sleep (Balsmeyer, 1990).

Night arousals, such as nightmares and night terrors, occur when infants move from non-REM sleep to REM sleep. The infant may scream, appear terrified, breathe heavily, or cry and not respond to parental consolation. Episodes often last for a few minutes, followed by a normal sleep. These episodes may frighten parents. Interruptions in routines, illness, or losses such as a change in child care arrangements can increase the number of night arousals (Balsmeyer, 1990).

Implications for Nursing Care

The nurse, who requires data in relation to the infant's crying and sleep patterns before recommending specific strategies, can request families to keep diaries regarding crying and sleep. The family's reaction to sleep disturbances also must be evaluated. Information should be obtained about the infant's developmental stage and sleep behaviors, as well as characteristics of the sleep environment (eg, type of room, temperature, and location). Events such as teething and daytime separation may be linked to sleep disorders. Knowledge of these relationships may enable the family to respond appropriately by setting firm guidelines for nighttime behavior and a "getting to sleep" routine. The goal of treatment is to foster the infant's ability to get to sleep without parental help. The infant must learn self-quieting behaviors and gain confidence in his or her ability to develop successful self-consoling activities.

Small manageable steps should be recommended to ensure success. The family should be consistent about its actions. Effective behavioral modification techniques have been developed to stop crying behavior at bedtime. Conditions in the infant's room should remain as constant as possible. The infant who has come to rely solely on the parent(s) to get to sleep may initially resist parental efforts to withdraw consoling behaviors by screaming and crying loudly. The infant may appear extremely distressed, and parents often are so disturbed by this behavior that initially they find it impossible not to revert to maladaptive behaviors

(picking the infant up or taking the infant into the adult's bed). The infant can be introduced to gradual withdrawal of the parent's presence. When the infant cries, the parent can enter the room, embrace the infant in his or her crib, offer verbal support, and then leave the room. The parent remains out of the infant's room for longer and longer periods of time until the crying behavior stops. Infants may take several days before their behaviors are changed. Dramatic videotapes have captured the eventual development of self-consoling behaviors that permit the infant to get to sleep without parental intervention. Many parents are astounded that successful sleep patterns can be established in a matter of hours or days.

The physical and emotional survival of the infant depends on accomplishment of the parent–infant attachment process, which is a major developmental task to be accomplished in the first year. The process is complex, evolves over a period of time, and is characterized by great adaptability. Acquaintance is the first step in this process and begins in the fetal period. The nurse helps in this process by uniting the newborn and parents as quickly as possible after birth. Several factors affect attachment: infant temperament and behaviors, colic, and crying and sleeping disturbances. The nurse should assess the parents' relationship to the newborn and encourage the parents in their attachment process.

Family Role Taking

Role taking is a complex and lengthy process in which family members adopt new roles within the framework of the family structure. Parental role taking is influenced by parental attachment. Parenting, sibling, and grandparenting roles require continuous adaptation as the infant exhibits changes associated with growth and development. The arrival of each neonate provides new uncharted territory that must be negotiated on an ongoing basis. Parenthood, siblinghood, and grandparenthood begin abruptly and are irrevocable. Although research has focused more on maternal role taking, some preliminary work also has described paternal, sibling, and grandparent role taking. The following sections describe each of these areas.

Maternal Role Attainment

A woman experiences many changes in her life during the first year after birth. The woman must reorganize her life and add motherhood to a preexisting set of roles. If she is a multipara, she must modify the preexisting maternal role to include the new offspring. Maternal role definition or redefinition occurs in relation to the newborn, the situational context, values about motherhood, culture, and self-concept. To some extent maternal role behaviors will reflect societal norms, the woman's role models, and others such as her partner or extended family members (Mercer, 1985). However, each woman develops her own personal style in the maternal role.

Perceptions of Competence

A woman attains the maternal role as she gains a sense of competence as a caregiver and nurturing parent. During the early postpartum period, a new mother learns to care for her newborn through a process of trial and error. Even skilled mothers must experiment to some extent to determine how the newborn will respond to her caretaking activities. By 2 to 3 days after birth, a woman's estimate of her parenting abilities is an early indicator of maternal role attainment. Women who verbalize satisfaction with early parenting efforts are more likely to achieve the maternal role in a smooth, predictable manner.

When the newborn responds positively to initial caretaking activities and expressions of affection, the woman is generally reassured about the appropriateness of her developing maternal role behaviors. As the woman deals successfully with neonatal needs and problems, such as hunger, wet diapers, or crying, estimates of her competence will grow, and the maternal role is reinforced. With time, if the infant thrives, actively engages in play, and gives and takes affection, the maternal role is further validated and developed. If the infant responds to maternal efforts negatively or unpredictably, the woman's role competence is reduced, and role attainment is delayed.

Implications for Nursing Care

The nurse caring for the family once they return to the community must appraise the woman's mastery of neonatal care skills and confidence in the evolving maternal role. The mother should be praised as she initiates and achieves skill in neonatal care tasks. Persistent difficulties with identifying neonatal needs and emotional states and the inability to meet basic physical and emotional needs of the newborn must be addressed immediately. Early signs of failure to thrive, a delay in normal growth and development, are a common indicator of failure to attain the maternal role. Referrals must be made to social service agencies, a child psychologist, or other health professionals skilled in the treatment of mothering disorders.

Maternal Characteristics

Even when the woman rapidly develops competence with neonatal care activities, maternal role attainment is a challenging process. In one study, at 6 months postpartum, 45% of women indicated their transition to the maternal role was more difficult than expected (Tulman & Fawcett, 1991). Ease of role attainment is influenced by such personal characteristics as age, education, socioeconomic status, ethnic background, and previous experience with infants. For example a single adolescent mother with limited education and financial supports may have more difficulty during the transition to the maternal role than a well-educated woman with adequate resources.

Implications for Nursing Care

Nursing interventions to support maternal role attainment must be altered according to the woman's age, developmental level, and education. Teaching plans and specific

recommendations for health promotion are based on these factors and must take into account the financial situation of the family. Very young mothers (younger than age 18) and those older than age 35 have special needs that alter the speed and ease of maternal role attainment. The reader is referred to Chapters 9 and 10 for a full discussion of maternal role attainment in these two groups of women.

Support System

The quality and extent of the woman's social support system has a significant impact on maternal role attainment. During normal adaptation after birth some support usually is offered by the partner or extended family. This support may or may not be considered helpful. For example in a study by Pridham and Zavoral (1988), women who received help with neonatal care and household tasks from their parents did not always report that help as supportive. In other instances help with household tasks and child care is strongly desired but is not forthcoming from fathers. Research clearly indicates that few fathers carry an equal burden in terms of child care and household responsibilities. Grandparents also have been identified as supportive but often only for limited periods of time.

The nature of social support does appear to be important. Most women desire and value emotional support from their partners or important family members after the birth. Women who are in less close, supportive partnerships have greater difficulty in adjusting to the maternal role (Cox, Owen, Lewis, & Henderson, 1989; Flagler, 1990). However, research indicates that many women are uncomfortable with accepting physical help from their partners, friends, or other family members. They may feel obligated to return favors received, and this increases their burden in the after the birth. Other women derive a sense of control in performing all neonatal care activities themselves. Male partners of new mothers have described the woman as a gatekeeper to parenting activities. These women decide how much and what type of assistance they will accept from the father of the infant (Jordan, 1990).

Even when women desire support from female friends or female relatives it often is unavailable because most women of childbearing age are employed, and many women are separated from female family members. Driscoll (1990) suggests that early discharge from the hospital, lack of family support, and limited community resources may produce crises for parents, especially new mothers, during the first year after childbirth. Lack of support is linked with impaired physiologic and emotional recovery and potential impairment in maternal role attainment.

Implications for Nursing Care

A critical aspect of the nursing assessment is to identify the nature and quality of the woman's social support network. The ease of maternal role attainment will in great part depend on the woman's physical and emotional resources. The single mother with limited help from family or friends generally will require more intensive nursing care and support during the first postpartum year than the woman with a close partner relationship and a loving extended family. The nurse must make appropriate community referrals for professional assistance when support networks are limited or absent. Many organizations have been established to assist new mothers with parenting skills and child care when they are without social support.

Perceived Loss

The ability to attain the maternal role also is affected by the extent of real and perceived losses experienced by the woman after the birth. Losses during the year after childbirth may not be clearly articulated, partially because of myths about motherhood and parenting. Demands experienced with motherhood, such as decreased personal time for work, recreation, and sexual intimacy; sleep deprivation; loss of employment; and loss of freedom, complicate the process of role attainment. Changes in body image may result in a profound sense of loss. All mothers must engage in grief work to restore themselves and to promote integration and acceptance of their losses.

Implications for Nursing Care

Demands experienced by the woman during the process of maternal role attainment challenge nurses to engage in anticipatory guidance for the woman and her family. However, research data indicate that women often are not receptive to information about parenting during the prenatal period. Furthermore, physiologic and emotional changes experienced in the early postpartum period may reduce the amount of energy available for education and anticipatory guidance. These factors coupled with an increasing emphasis on early discharge require nurses to shift their interventions to a community context.

Community and home health nurses, nurse midwives, and nurse practitioners all have an excellent opportunity to support the woman coming to grips with the losses and tremendous demands experienced during the transition to parenting. Support groups led by the nurse can offer opportunities for parents to ventilate their feelings about parenting. Parents, particularly mothers, need an opportunity to acknowledge losses associated with taking on a nurturing role without feeling like disloyal or "bad" parents. Parenting support groups and classes also provide opportunities for families to examine changes (perceived as another loss) in the couple relationship and in communication. Communication between partners appears to facilitate a close, sharing relationship and that has implications for women's childrearing practices (Cox et al., 1989; Flagler, 1990).

The nurse can reassure the woman that the perceived sense of loss and ambiguities about parenthood are normal experiences during the first postpartum year. Anticipatory guidance may be offered to smooth the transition to the new role of mother or to mother of more than one child. When the woman demonstrates unresolved difficulties during the role transition and is unable to resolve her grief over the loss of other roles, the nurse makes appropriate referrals for counseling or psychological assistance.

Cultural Influences

The woman's ethnic background and culture will influence maternal role attainment in very powerful but often

subtle ways. Culture profoundly affects the following aspects of parenthood for the woman:

- Maternal status and prestige
- Infant care and infant feeding practices
- Relationship with parents and in-laws
- Input and power in family decision making
- Resumption of sexual intimacy with father of infant
- Infant care activities during the first 4 to 6 weeks postpartum

The impact of culture will in part depend on the woman's educational level, social class, the presence of family members, and exposure to other cultures. For instance the woman who has recently emigrated from her country of origin may more closely adhere to maternal role behaviors prescribed by her culture than a woman who has lived and worked in another country for a long period of time. Even when the woman has assimilated the dominant values and norms of this country, she may be expected to adopt the traditional maternal role behaviors espoused by her culture when she becomes a mother.

Implications for Nursing Care

Before the nurse can develop an appropriate plan of care to meet the needs of the new mother, an assessment must be completed to identify cultural influences on maternal role attainment. Various resources, including other family members, health professionals from the woman's culture, and written resources, may be used to develop a full appreciation of the woman's ethnic background. Consideration must be given to the woman's belief system regarding infant care and maternal role behaviors when making recommendations about health promotion.

Paternal Role Attainment

A father experiences major changes in his life during the first postpartum year. However, there appears to be less opportunity for flexibility and variation in how men interpret fathering than in how women interpret mothering. Recent research indicates that men desire more involvement with their infant and are assuming less traditional roles as fathers (see the Nursing Research display). Many men want to be more active physically and psychologically in the life of the infant. However, there continues to be a lag between intention and actual paternal role performance (Bowen & Orthner, 1990).

Societal Values Regarding Fathering

Many men still place a greater emphasis on the work role than on fathering (Tripp-Reimer & Wilson, 1990). Men's

Nursing Research

Predicting Paternal Role Enactment

Research findings on fathering indicate an increase in the number of involved, nurturing fathers. However, there is little explicit theory on how or why men select a specific pattern of paternal behaviors. Rustia and Abbott (1990) sought to determine whether fathers' normative expectations, personal expectations, and prior learning about parenting predict paternal role performance across a 2-year period.

The researchers hypothesized that: (1) fathers' perceptions of appropriate paternal behaviors (normative expectations) would be positively related to role performance; (2) fathers' personal expectations (or what they believe they will do) would be positively related to role performance; (3) mothers' perceptions of appropriate paternal behaviors would be positively related to role performance; and (4) fathers who had more prior learning experiences regarding paternal role would perform more paternal role behaviors.

Fifty-three white middle class father–mother dyads were studied. Data were collected at seven points spanning a 2-year period following birth. Results indicated that 75% of the fathers were participating in as many play activities with the infant (vocalizing, playing, cuddling, and holding) as the mothers. However, 70% of the fathers reported that mothers were doing more or all of the infant caretaking activities, such as diapering, bathing, dressing, and comforting. At all time periods fathers appeared to do less than they said they intended to do. Men's willingness to help their partners and actual performance of child care tasks did increase over time. During the first year, women consistently reported that their partner's performance behaviors lagged behind their expectations.

The results appear to confirm that the cultural expectations for fatherhood have changed more rapidly than the actual conduct of fatherhood. Men may feel ambivalent and guilty about their failure to live up to the new image of fatherhood portrayed in society. New fathers require some assistance to acquire new paternal behaviors. Anticipatory guidance by nurses can occur prenatally and in the early postpartum period. Assistance also can be offered during community contacts with fathers. Nurses need to explore teaching techniques that facilitate the learning of child caretaking behaviors by fathers.

Rustia, J., & Abbott, D. A. (1990). Predicting paternal role enactment. *Western Journal of Nursing Research, 12*(2), 145–160.

work roles generally have been given more status and recognition than their family roles (Bowen & Orthner, 1990). Men continue to be judged primarily on their work performance and not on their contributions as parents (Hall, 1991). However, there is some evidence that work organizations are beginning to change their attitudes toward paternal responsibilities. Changes have been made, such as paternity leave, flexible work hours, and on-site child care for men with children. Nevertheless, underlying attitudes about the value of fathering have not changed for most men, and few new fathers take advantage of extended paternity leave after the birth of the infant, even when paid release time is offered.

Paternal Role Models

Some new fathers do not have clear role models; they remember their own fathers as distant and disengaged from their family (Jordan, 1990). As a consequence, they are searching for new parenting roles (Jordan, 1990; Sayers, 1991). Some fathers are particularly moved by the newborn's recognition of their presence and positive responses to direct caregiving activities. They delight in becoming acquainted with the newborn and experiencing a growing sense of attachment (Jordan, 1990). However, the primary paternal role enacted by most men continues to place a strong emphasis on play rather than caretaking (Fig. 36-1).

Expectations of the Woman

The woman may disagree with her male partner about an appropriate fathering role. She may desire more direct involvement in caretaking activities or prefer a more traditional approach to fathering. When disagreement arises, there must be open discussion and eventual compromise about essential aspects of parenting. The couple must work together to establish agreement on parenting issues so that closeness is maintained between them and the infant experiences consistency in care and nurturing (Jurich, White, White, & Moody, 1990). If successful adaptation occurs, the parent role becomes incorporated with others, such as spouse, provider, son, and so forth for the new father.

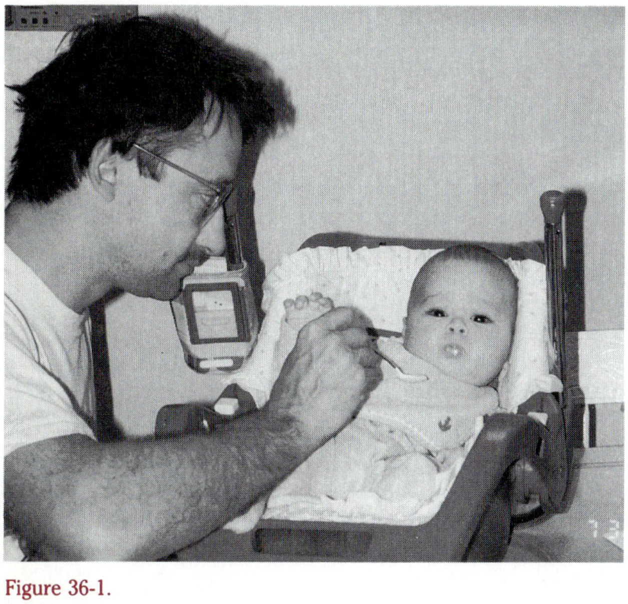

Figure 36-1.
The father's role in parenting is expanding in many families to include caretaking activities.

Cultural Influences

Cultural variations in paternal roles cannot be ignored. Ethnicity affects the way fathers perceive and enact the parenting role. In African American families women continue to assume the primary caretaker role, but fathers may participate in parenting activities. Research findings suggest that some African American fathers are actively involved in the care and socialization of their children and that historic images of absent, disinterested fathers are not accurate. When enacting parental roles, African American fathers have demonstrated an authoritative, parental pattern that emphasized control, support, strict childrearing, and egalitarian family roles. Generally, African American fathers report a positive perception of fathering and of shared parenting. Some have indicated that daily contact with their children is important, because children have needs that only a father can meet (Mirandé, 1990).

Hispanic American fathers traditionally have been viewed as dominant, authoritarian figures. Although Hispanic Americans are a diverse group, some shared values affect the paternal role. The cold, distant, father figure has retreated and has been replaced by a more egalitarian, sharing figure. Hispanic Americans highly value the paternal role and believe that the father's presence significantly affects the child's development. A crucial aspect of the fathering role includes providing for the financial needs of the family (Mirandé, 1990).

In Asian American families fathers also have been depicted as dominant, authoritarian figures. Asian American families are in transition, and fathers are faced with tensions between traditional values and current demands made by contemporary American society. Traditionally, power and authority were vested in both parents, although in different spheres: the woman inside the home and the father outside of the home. Regulation of the family was based on senior–junior relationships (ie, grandparents having more power than new parents).

The Asian woman's mother-in-law is a particularly powerful influence in the development and expression of the maternal role when she is present in the family unit. The grandfather often plays a less central role in the development of paternal role. As Asian American women have increased their labor force participation and their power in the family, some alteration has occurred in traditional paternal roles. Shifts to greater father involvement have occurred in some families, but childrearing activities are still regarded primarily as women's work (Mirandé, 1990). The maternal or paternal grandmother often remains the primary infant caretaker when the new mother returns to work.

Paternal roles of Native American fathers have not been studied by researchers. Native American families have been characterized as extended families involving entire villages. These connections were often destroyed in the past by U.S. government policies that supported the systematic removal

of Native American children from their families. Where traditional native societal values continue, childrearing is shared by a number of adults, both male and female. Ultimate power is vested in communities rather than individual fathers (Mirandé, 1990).

Despite the cultural diversity in paternal roles, individual and family values define the father's role for a particular family. A man's relations with his own father, his father's approach to the parenting role, and the influence of other role models, such as grandfathers and peers' fathers, societal pressures, and a man's own personality will affect his performance as a father (Seward, 1990). Men may try to duplicate the fathering they received, father in a totally different way, or choose aspects of their father's role while rejecting others.

Implications for Nursing Care

Nurses are in a powerful position to acknowledge and support involved fatherhood. Men can be encouraged to participate in parenting classes where they can learn about infant behaviors and appropriate caregiving activities. At that time open communication about parenting roles should be encouraged between partners. This is important because as noted, women can serve as gatekeepers to childrearing and may discourage their partners from becoming actively involved in caretaking. Men can be assisted to define their roles more broadly and examine their values and attitudes in relation to shared parenting. Involving men in infant caretaking may assist them to remove attitudinal blocks or develop new attitudes about infant care.

Nurses must continue to explore and develop creative programs and interventions to foster paternal recognition and involvement in expanding families. Parenting support groups specifically designed for new fathers either in the community or at work would be important interventions. Parenting support groups in the community may need to be organized around specific content, such as cardiopulmonary resuscitation courses for infants, so that men initially can be brought together in a group format. Nurses need to advocate male support for a man's nurturing capabilities.

Sibling Role Taking

Sibling responses to changing roles after the birth of a newborn greatly affect the well-being of all family members. The newborn's arrival creates stress and anxiety for siblings during what is an exciting but also a potentially traumatic time. The sibling is required to shift roles during this complex event. With increasing numbers of alternate family life-styles, such as single parent and blended families, sibling relationships have become even more important. When there are already several children, siblings can offer each other security, comfort, and continuity (Nelms, 1991). When the child has no other brothers or sisters, the parents must be very sensitive to the unique needs of this older sibling when a newborn is introduced into the family.

After the birth, family attention may be shifted from the older sibling(s) to the newborn, who may receive many gifts. Siblings may feel rejected, neglected, and displaced by the newborn's arrival. They may react by clinging, withdrawing, crying, or regressing to earlier adaptive behaviors. Temper tantrums, sleep problems, and hyperactivity also may occur. Adults may grieve the loss in intensity of relationships with older sibling(s) (Fortier, Carson, Will, & Shubkagel, 1991).

A sole sibling acquires a new role as brother or sister (Nelms, 1991). When there are several siblings, the place of the child in the family is changed (eg, one of three children, one of four children). Older children often are involved in discussions of changing family roles and are encouraged to take on additional responsibility at home. Siblings presented with new roles in caregiving may demonstrate developmental progress or regress. The response of an individual child will depend on the following factors:

- Age
- Development maturity
- Prebirth preparation for sibling role
- Presence of support persons (father and other relatives) during birth and early postbirth period
- Parents' relationship with the child after the birth of the infant
- Parents' expectations about the child's role as sibling and family member

Implications for Nursing Care

The family must be assessed to identify sibling roles and the sibling's level of involvement in neonatal care. The nurse can then facilitate the child's development of realistic expectations of the newborn sibling. Assisting the child to recognize and express feelings regarding the newborn also is a nursing responsibility (Johnsen & Gaspard, 1985). Parents, grandparents, and friends can be encouraged to formulate strategies that will enable the older children to develop realistic expectations of the neonate and to express feelings about the newborn's arrival. Role playing with a doll can assist children to develop safe behaviors when handling newborns. A discussion of appropriate behavior with newborns and ways of expressing anger that are not harmful to the newborn is helpful.

Expression of negative and positive feelings toward the newborn can occur through discussion with older children. Younger children may express their ideas and feelings more readily through art. Omission of the newborn or self or use of figure size and color to delineate family relationships can provide valuable information about their feelings about the situation (Johnsen & Gaspard, 1985). Family members also can be encouraged to describe how they will cope with specific sibling reactions at home. These can include acting out by older children, demands by older children for increased time, hostile actions by older children toward the newborn, and regressive behaviors from older children. Family members should be encouraged not to compare children but to treat each child as a valued individual (Nelms, 1991).

Parents can stress the consistency in their children's lives by identifying people, places, and things that have not changed. They can identify special people, such as grandparents, friends, or baby-sitters who will spend special time with older children. These activities enable children to develop positive feelings about their sibling. They may encourage active role taking in caregiving and enhance the child's transitions into siblinghood by promoting cognitive and

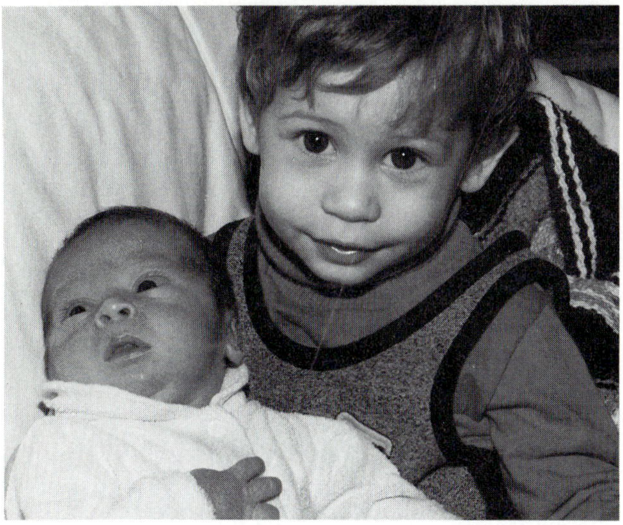

Figure 36-2.
Under close supervision, parents should promote interaction between the older sibling and the newborn.

emotional growth and a loving and durable sibling bond (Fig. 36-2).

Grandparent Role Taking

Developmental changes occur in grandparents at the time that their children become parents. Many adults may have ambivalent feelings about the transition to the role of grandparent. They may feel their advice is old-fashioned or unwelcomed. They may feel that the aging process has accelerated with the transition to grandparenting, and they may not be ready to accept that change. It may signify a closer proximity to death. They may be employed and have role conflict in relation to their availability for their children and grandchildren. While some grandparents strongly desire to babysit for their grandchildren, others do not desire to be active participants in the care or the rearing of their grandchildren. Finally, generational relationships shift with the arrival of the first child. The adult child is now a parent also, and this may put him or her on equal footing with their parent for the first time (Maloni, McIndoe, & Rubenstein, 1987).

Grandparents serve as a vital link between generations, and the period after childbearing provides an ideal time to strengthen these relationships (Horn & Manion, 1985). Changes in childrearing practices can widen communication gaps between parents and grandparents. Such areas as changes in styles of infant care, feeding, and use of pacifiers may be new to grandparents. They may disapprove of certain infant care practices that the new parents demonstrate. At a time when family members feel vulnerable about their childrearing knowledge and skills, casual or critical remarks from grandparents can be viewed as interference and stimulate anger and conflict (Maloni et al., 1987). When family members choose to ignore or challenge grandparents' advice, they may feel hurt or rejected. Parents may fear that by disregarding grandparents' advice, they will loose their support or become engaged in open conflict.

Grandparents are a repository of the family's rituals and histories. They provide a framework of values and traditions that can give the family stability. They have accumulated life experiences that can place events in perspective. Grandparents may be willing and able to provide resources, such as time and money. Grandparents can pass on the family's legacy and nurture family members during times of crisis and transition. The grandparent role is very important during the first year after childbirth. With the widespread problems of chemical dependence in women of childbearing age and the acquired immunodeficiency syndrome epidemic, foster grandparenting has become common across the United States. Hundreds of thousands of grandparents have assumed responsibility for the rearing of their grandchildren when parents are unable or unavailable to do so. These individuals need special attention and assistance from professional nurses.

Implications for Nursing Care

Initially the nurse must assess the presence, role, and participation of grandparents in the new family. The nurse must take every opportunity to acquaint grandparents with recent childbearing and childrearing practices so that the communication between generations can occur from the same parenting framework. Teaching can be provided about the capabilities of the newborn and contrasts between current and past methods of infant care, feeding, and safekeeping. Grandparents can be encouraged to share their feelings about childrearing (Maloni et al., 1987). Emphasis should be placed on changes in information rather than right and wrong ways to parent. The nurse can suggest references grandparents can use to learn about effective and creative grandparenting. If the grandparent(s) will assume primary responsibility for neonatal care, community referrals should be initiated to provide ongoing support and assistance.

The importance of the grandparents' supportive relationships with all family members and especially older siblings should be stressed. This is especially true in dual-earner families in which assistance with childrearing is at a premium. Grandparents should be offered opportunities to explore their own expectations about their role responsibilities and to communicate these to their families. Nurses can assist them and their families to develop an appreciation of their special contributions. In some communities nurses have developed classes for grandparents that focus on infant growth and development, infant care (including cardiopulmonary resuscitation), and the grandparenting role.

At birth family members adopt new roles within the framework of the family structure. Parental role taking is influenced by parental attachment. Women attain the maternal role by gaining competence as a caregiver and nurturing parent. Ease of maternal role attainment is influenced by personal characteristics, such as age, education, socioeconomic status, ethnic background, and previous experiences with child care. The nature of the mother's social support in this role is important. Although fathers are making major changes in their lives during this same period, there appears to be less oppor-

tunity for flexibility and variation for men. Men have fewer paternal role models in caretaking than women. Further, cultural variations cannot be ignored for either parent. A newborn's arrival creates stress and anxiety for siblings, also affected by the sibling's placement in the family as an only child or in a larger family. The role of the sibling shifts with the new arrival. Grandparents serve as a vital link between generations, although changes in childrearing practices can create communication gaps. The nurse plays an important role in assessing and intervening in adaptations to family roles. Many of these interventions focus on teaching and anticipatory guidance.

Diversity in Families

Because changes have affected the American family, nurses will encounter a variety of families in terms of family structure, life-style, and cultural influences. Changing societal attitudes to divorce, remarriage, and single parenthood continue to affect family structure. Medical advances and techniques of assisted reproduction have resulted in the possibility of childbearing and parenthood for people who previously may not have had this choice. Continuing immigration, including influxes of refugees, presents challenges for nurses in providing culturally sensitive care for families of different ethnic and cultural backgrounds.

The following section of this chapter describe a number of variations in families that nurses may encounter. These include lesbian families, families in which the mother is affected by a chronic illness or disability, families with multiple infants, families from a variety of ethnic or cultural groups, adoptive families, dual-earner families, and single-parent families.

Lesbian Families

In stable, committed relationships, the biologic mother and her lesbian partner frequently see themselves as coparents or comothers of the newborn. Involvement of the biologic father is uncommon. Involvement of the biologic mother's lesbian partner, sometimes referred to as the *nonbiologic* mother, may pose problems if health care policies are restrictive. When both women intend to take on parenting roles, attachment and role assumption is important for both, not just for the biologic mother.

Regardless of the method of conception, fear about child custody and negative reactions of health care providers are areas of concern for the new parents. Many lesbians are reluctant to publicly identify themselves as lesbian mothers because of widespread homophobia. Research indicates that some lesbians fear that their physical well-being may be jeopardized by health care providers who disapprove of the lesbian life-style. Many lesbian couples therefore do not reveal their situation.

Implications for Nursing Care

The nurse caring for new families will observe much diversity. To promote optimum family adaptations, it is essential to maintain a nonjudgmental approach to care. The nurse must convey respect for the person, regardless of his or her own moral or religious belief systems. The lesbian woman may have legitimate concerns about child custody and harassment or less than optimum care by judgmental health care providers. The woman must therefore give permission before any documentation of her sexual orientation is made in the medical record (Harvey, Carr, & Bernheine, 1989). Because they are not always revealed or evident, many lesbian families remain unrecognized by nurses. Without recognition the needs of these families cannot be identified or met by professional nurses. The family will not benefit from services available for childbearing families in the year after the infant's birth. They may feel isolated unless they reside in a community with other lesbian families. When the nurse approaches each family with an open, nonjudgmental approach, a sense of trust will develop, and family members may reveal their true concerns and needs.

Families Coping With Chronic Illness or Disability

Technologic and medical advances and changing societal attitudes toward people with disabilities make childbearing a choice for some women who in the past would not have considered or attempted this option. Nurses will increasingly encounter women (or the partners of women) who have a chronic illness or disability. Little is known of the special needs and concerns of parents who are significantly disabled or who have a chronic illness. Some researchers and clinicians have, however, begun to explore the needs of women who are physically challenged (Carty, Conine, & Hall, 1990).

In adapting to parenthood these women share many concerns with able bodied women, but they have additional challenges. Carty et al. (1990) have described their experiences working with women who have physical and sensory disabilities, such as hearing and visual impairments, spinal cord injuries, and rheumatoid arthritis. They found that coordination of services to enable these women to become confident parents is lacking.

Many health care professionals have little or no experience caring for such women and may be pessimistic about their ability to care for an infant. Some health care professionals or social service agencies have participated in court proceedings to remove infants from the care of disabled women.

Implications for Nursing Care

Because each woman will have a unique set of abilities, limitations, and coping strategies, her involvement in the development of a nursing care plan for care after discharge is central. A team approach involving coordination of the contributions of nurses, physiotherapists, occupational therapists, social workers, and physicians is crucial to provide quality care and anticipating needs. The goal of care is to prepare the woman to provide the aspects of care she is capable of performing and helping her develop a support system to meet the other aspects of care. Ideally, one of the

team members is designated as the case manager and acts as a liaison between team members.

A discharge planning conference that involves the woman and other support people, as she wishes, can be effective for planning ongoing care. Carty et al. (1990) identify some areas that need particular attention. These are needs related to rest, exercise, and comfort; sexuality and family planning; and environmental adaptations and aids to enable the mother to care for her infant. Some examples of environmental adaptations are cribs that open from the front and raised playpens that allow access for women in wheelchairs. Aids that facilitate infant feeding and holding also are described by Conine, Carty, and Safarik (1988).

The nurse can play a particularly helpful role by fostering the woman's confidence as she takes on her parenting role and by optimistically acknowledging the challenges ahead for these families. Carty et al. (1990) emphasize that effective care requires full involvement of a woman in identifying her special needs and planning care that will meet those needs.

Families With Multiple Infants

If the first year of parenting is challenging but joyous for families who have one infant, to have twins or more newborns provides even more challenges and more joy. Because the prematurity rate is five to seven times greater with twins than with singletons and because the risk rises as the number of fetuses increases, many parents of multiple neonates have experienced a period of stress and separation from their neonates (Noble, 1991). The stress and separation surrounding twin births can result in an increased incidence of child abuse and neglect. However, it may not be the multiples who are abused; some families abuse the older siblings.

Many families are able to leave the hospital at the same time as their newborns. When they are unable to do so, they often face feelings of emptiness and loss. Parents report receiving little guidance about the challenges they will face when caring for their newborns at home. They also report concerns about financial management, more housing space, reactions of family members, difficulties with feeding and rest, and increased time demands (Theroux, 1989). The predominant challenge faced by families with multiple neonates is the unrelenting mental work. Parents must learn to interpret their neonates' cues. Furthermore, they must coordinate neonatal care activities and plan and make decisions about the day. They are constantly evaluating themselves against their own ideal of what constitutes a good parent.

Parents often feel their lives are in chaos. They feel overloaded and isolated from family and friends. They suffer from chronic sleep deprivation, lack time for intimacy with their partner, and lack time to assist siblings with adjustments to the newborns' arrival (Sollid, Evans, McClowry, & Garrett, 1989; Theroux, 1989). Parents who feel overwhelmed by the demands of neonatal care often neglect their own needs for nutrition, rest, and relaxation. Personal time can be at a premium.

Implications for Nursing Care

The nurse must assess the family's need for community services. Appropriate referrals to community agencies and support groups can be crucial to facilitate adjustment (Theroux, 1989). The family can be encouraged to draw on support people, accept offers of help, and organize time for themselves to achieve a healthy adjustment. The nurse can offer practical suggestions to simplify care, such as sharing the neonates' equipment.

Some parents report that strollers designed specifically for multiple infants are crucial for mobility during the first 2 years after birth. Because the neonates often provide a sense of comfort for each other, sleeping in one crib may decrease fussiness. Feeding equipment, such as bottles and spoons, often are shared but may increase the transmission of common infant and childhood illnesses. Modified demand feeding may be used, wherein one infant is fed on awakening, and once the first is fed, the next infant is awakened and fed (Sollid et al., 1989). An increasing number of parents successfully breastfeed their twins and even triplets. They require assistance from family members and nurses who are fully supportive of breastfeeding multiple infants and knowledgeable about feeding more than one infant.

Another area in which the nurse can encourage the parents is learning to recognize each infant as an individual. Many months may be required for parents to form attachments with each infant (Theroux, 1989). Development of individuality is fostered by referring to each infant by name, rather than as "the twins" or "the triplets." Another strategy that may be suggested is spending some time with each infant separately, to identify the differences and similarities of each infant. Often the best help and support for these families comes from parents who have had personal experience caring for multiple infants. In many communities there are informal groups of parents of multiple infants. Such groups offer practical suggestions and share used equipment with new members, and they provide social and emotional support (Theroux, 1989). There also are many excellent books available for parents and professionals about parenting multiple infants.

Families From Ethnic or Cultural Minorities

All cultures regard the early period after birth as a special time—a time for certain rituals and a period of adaptation with an accompanying set of expectations or rules. As noted, many culturally based beliefs and customs exist regarding the recovery period for women after childbirth, neonatal care, and family roles. Although the specifics vary, there are some common themes.

The first step in providing culturally sensitive care to families from different cultural or ethnic minorities is the nurse's recognition of the influence of her or his own ethnicity and culture (Waxler-Morrison, Anderson, & Richardson, 1990). Nurses need to be aware of the values they hold not only as a result of their personal backgrounds, but also as a result of their professional education and participation in the health care system—a system that favors

the biomedical model of health and illness. Kleinman (1986) cautions that even when the nurse and patient share common cultural backgrounds, value conflicts may arise from other factors, such as social class, religion, gender, and age.

Implications for Nursing Care

The nurse needs to explore the influence of the parents' ethnicity on beliefs about recovery from childbirth, infant care, sexuality, family planning, and family roles (Waxler-Morrison et al., 1990). Awareness of differences between the nurse and the family in beliefs about these matters is fundamental to delivering culturally sensitive health care. Some areas to explore are how recently the family has settled in the host country, the place of birth of family members and whether it was urban or rural, and the occupation of the family members at present and in the country of origin. Having the family recount their story, in addition to such specific facts, can promote an understanding of their unique perspective.

Beliefs About Rest and Confinement to the Home

It is common for cultures to define a time period after childbirth when women are expected to remain at home, restrict their activity level, and rest. This is considered a time for physical, emotional, and spiritual regeneration. Women often receive special foods and herbs that are believed to promote recovery. In other cultures where women's work is essential for survival of the family, especially agricultural communities, the woman may work until the onset of labor, give birth in the fields, and then complete her work before returning home to observe a ritual period of reduced activity or rest. For some women this special time is the only period in their adult lives when others attend to their needs, and they do not have to perform the combined arduous burdens of household tasks, neonatal care, breastfeeding, and food gathering and preparation. The extent of the woman's education and the degree of acculturation to the dominant American culture, her social class, and the presence of family members will influence how rigidly she adheres to cultural prescriptions regarding rest and activity.

For example some groups of women from China and Southeast Asia (ie, Laos and Cambodia) view the first month after birth as a period of time for relative confinement and rest. This behavior often is referred to as "doing the month." Female family members, often the mother-in-law if she is available, perform household and neonatal care activities. Mexican American women and those from Central America may observe a slightly longer (40 days) period of confinement, during which extended female family members assist with housekeeping tasks and neonatal care. In contrast in the American culture, women often are out of the hospital or birthing center 6 to 12 hours after delivery and may perform light tasks or leave the house to visit family and friends in the first few days after discharge. An increasing number of American women return to their jobs in the first postpartum month either by choice or economic necessity.

Most cultures also establish appropriate environments for recovery. The home often is the preferred site for rest and rejuvenation; however, some societies have special buildings or shelters that house postpartum women during the first 4 to 6 weeks after delivery. Cold air and drafts are to be avoided in many cultures during this time, because they are believed to delay recovery or cause chronic health problems later in life. For instance Chinese American women may be cautioned by older relatives that such exposure will cause rheumatism or arthritis later in life. Some groups, such as Laotian women, may keep the head covered (Waxler-Morrison et al., 1990). Bathing practices that expose the woman to cold air are avoided; however, all cultures have evolved special activities related to hygiene.

Implications for Nursing Care

In caring for the woman from another culture, the nurse must attempt to determine what self-care and neonatal care activities are permitted in the immediate postbirth period. Some women may be extremely distressed when the nurse encourages or demands early ambulation, resumption of self-care activities such as grooming, and responsibility for her infant's care. The woman may resist these efforts when she believes they may harm her eventual recovery or invalidate the rest she has earned after accomplishing the tremendous feat of giving birth.

While scientific knowledge indicates that ambulation is essential to prevent the negative effects of bed rest, particularly for postsurgical women after cesarean birth, care must be taken to respect cultural practices related to rest. The nurse should try to explain the purpose of ambulation or other self-care activities, while acknowledging the value of rest and reduced strenuous activity.

The nurse also must determine who will have primary responsibility for neonatal care during the immediate postpartum period and during the time of rest. It is essential to include these individuals in the plan of teaching and convey respect for their special knowledge about care of the postpartum woman and her infant. Most folk customs, rituals, and care may be safely used by the woman and her family and may actually speed recovery. The nurse should demonstrate respect for these practices and incorporate them into her teaching plan as knowledge is gained about the culture of the women cared for in the hospital or birthing unit.

Hygiene Practices and Beliefs About Body Secretions

Many cultures have ritual purification practices that meet the hygiene needs of the woman and express beliefs about the nature of menstrual or lochial flow. Some groups bathe the external genitalia with water, oil, or sand as part of the hygiene and ritual purification process in the immediate postbirth period. The cloths used to absorb lochia may be burned or buried when lochia is considered a contaminant or is endowed with special powers, while other groups simply wash and reuse perineal cloths.

In some cultures it is considered improper for men to come in contact with lochial secretions or to live in the same room or house with the postpartum woman until lochial flow ceases. At the end of the special period of rest, some cultures perform a ritual purification bath that prepares the woman to re-enter society and resume contact with men. Although exposure to cold air or drafts precludes full showers or baths

in some cultures, all have prescribed practices that meet the hygiene needs of the woman and promote healing of the external genital region.

Implications for Nursing Care

To meet the hygiene needs of the postpartum woman in the immediate and later postpartum period, the nurse must identify the important practices related to bathing and perineal care. Forcing the woman to shower or wash her hair may be a very frightening or frustrating experience for her when she believes this is extremely harmful to her health or delays the postpartum recovery. It may be viewed as a sign of extreme disrespect or demonstrate a lack of basic consideration for the woman's health and well-being. The nurse may be seen as lacking basic information about essential health practices, undermining his or her ability to teach the woman and her family about health-promoting behaviors.

Recommendations for Special Foods in the Postpartum or Lactation Diet

Most cultural groups, including middle-class, white, North Americans, have some beliefs about food in the early period after childbirth. For example some foods are believed to promote effective lactation or to upset the breastfeeding infant. Thus, almost all women will get some advice about what they should or should not eat, especially if they are breastfeeding. Many cultures prohibit the ingestion of foods that are thought to be harmful to the woman's health or delay recovery in the vulnerable period after birth.

The concept of *hot* and *cold* foods influences the diets of those whose roots are in the Chinese, Mexican, Central American, or southern Asian cultures. Many Chinese American women eat a special soup in the belief that it speeds involution. Soups that contain a large amount of ginger root may actually cause excessive bleeding because of their vasodilating effects. Large quantities of these should be avoided. Chinese American women also may avoid tap water, especially cold water, preferring hot water that has been boiled. Laotian women may avoid soups and other fluids, preferring dry foods. Iranian women may take special preparations of rice and barley to promote lactation.

Implications for Nursing Care

To promote adequate nutritional intake to speed recovery and support lactation, the nurse must assess the woman's dietary habits. The nurse may need to consult with a registered dietician or with an appropriate nutrition text to determine if the culturally prescribed foods provide the necessary nutrients, vitamins, minerals, and calories. Whenever possible, the woman should be encouraged to meet nutritional needs through ingestion of foods that are culturally acceptable and permissible during the postpartum period. Some foods have ritual, rather than nutrititive, value, and their consumption should be respected.

Neonatal Care Practices

Newborns receive care based on beliefs about their special needs and vulnerabilities. Bathing routines, umbilical cord care, perineal hygiene, dressing, and circumcision practices (male *and* female) are all culturally defined. Bathing and clothing practices often are focused on protecting the infant from physical or spiritual dangers. For instance, Asian babies often are dressed in several layers to keep them warm. Clothing also provides obvious cues about the infant's gender. For example in American society the color blue has been associated with boys and pink with girls, although these distinctions are blurring. Special amulets, charms, or religious medals may be attached to clothing to protect the infant or confer spiritual benefits. In some cultures oil is used to moisturize and clean the infant's scalp rather than soaps and lotions. Umbilical cord care varies greatly within American society and cultures around the world. A special belly band may be seen on Mexican American babies and those from other cultures. It is believed to prevent umbilical hernias. Many American mothers are taught to apply alcohol to the umbilical cord to speed drying and detachment.

Implications for Nursing Care

Once the family's cultural practices are identified, the nurse must adapt teaching regarding bathing and clothing to reflect a respect and understanding of the family's belief system. While the use of oils on neonatal skin has been discouraged by dermatologists, the greatest concern is with scented products derived from petrochemicals. Families who use naturally occurring vegetable oils in moderation to bathe or moisturize the newborn's skin may continue this practice but should be encouraged to keep applications to a minimum and to change soiled linen and clothing promptly. The belly band and other devices (stones, coins) that are applied to the umbilicus should be cleaned, and the nurse can teach parents how to assess the area daily for evidence of infection.

Neonatal Feeding Beliefs and Practices

In the past, in most cultures around the world, breastfeeding was the accepted and most valued infant feeding method. With the development of formula, some groups now view bottle feeding as the preferred method. Bottle feeding may be selected because it is believed to be scientific or the modern approach to infant nutrition. Formula may be erroneously assumed to contain vitamins and other desired nutrients that breast milk does not provide. Bottle feeding may be considered a status symbol; families that can afford to buy formula may do so as an expression of their wealth or financial means.

When breastfeeding is selected as the method of infant feeding, the mother may initiate the process immediately after birth or may delay feeding. Delays in breastfeeding may be based on a belief that the breasts do not contain milk or that there is no value in giving the neonate colostrum. In some cultures colostrum may even be considered nonbeneficial. Female relatives with experience in breastfeeding most often guide the new mother during the early postpartum period and at times when problems arise. Breastfeeding may be continued for several years or longer in many cultures, and women may continue to nurse older children, even after the birth of another neonate.

Implications for Nursing Care

An important aspect of nursing care is to educate all parents to the superior value of breastfeeding. Underlying cultural practices that favor breastfeeding should be strongly reinforced. Scientific information that demonstrates that breast milk is better for newborns should be provided to family members. If the woman wishes to delay initiation of breastfeeding until the milk supply is established and basic information about the value of colostrum is not accepted, her decision should be respected. The cultural practice of delaying breastfeeding is fairly common in some cultural groups and does not discourage eventual breastfeeding success for most of the women in those societies.

Naming and Acknowledging the Newborn

Naming the neonate, announcing the birth, and permitting viewing of the newborn are strongly influenced by culture. Some groups name the neonate well before birth; others wait for several weeks or longer. A delay in naming may be influenced by high infant mortality rates in some cultures. The newborn does not achieve personhood or merit a name until he or she survives the first month of life, during which most neonates who die succumb to illness. In other cultures a name is given based on characteristics or temperament the newborn exhibits in the first days or weeks after birth.

Announcing the birth of a neonate who is perceived as vulnerable or defenseless may be prohibited in some cultures when there is an underlying belief in evil spirits. In this case acknowledging the newborn or giving compliments is to be avoided for fear of attracting the "evil eye." Many Mexican Americans, for instance, fear the evil eye if the newborn is admired too openly. Parents may avoid taking the newborn out of the house, even to see a doctor in some cases when they believe in the evil eye. Visiting the newborn is an expectation in some cultures, however, such as Arab American families, and the neonate may be taken out quite early to visit.

Implications for Nursing Care

An essential component of the nursing assessment is to determine the family's practices in acknowledging and naming the neonate. The nurse should not assume that failure to assume all neonatal care activities in the first month postbirth or to provide a name immediately indicates a problem in parent–newborn attachment. If a general belief is held by the group regarding the "evil eye," the nurse must adapt his or her behaviors to minimize attention to the neonate. Verbally acknowledging and complimenting the neonate should be avoided until the parents bring the neonate out into the community or permit visiting. A baptism or christening ceremony in Christian cultures often is a symbolic rite of passage in the naming and acknowledging of the neonate, and the nurse can use this as a cue to alter the interaction process with the family during visits to the home or office.

Circumcision Practices

Circumcision practices vary around the world and are based on religious and cultural belief systems. The timing of circumcision and the decision about who performs the ritual also are based on culture. Female circumcision is a common practice in parts of Africa and the Middle East. The labia majora, and at times the labia minora and clitoris, are excised, and the remaining edges of skin are sewed together to conceal the vaginal introitus and urinary meatus. A small opening is left for passage of menstrual flow and urine.

Female circumcision may be performed in infancy or later childhood and is used to control female sexual activity. It causes severe mutilation of the external female genitalia and may result in death from hemorrhage or infection when performed by unskilled practitioners. Anesthesia is rarely administered during the procedure, although herbs or naturally occuring opiates and mood-altering drugs may be used to diminish awareness. At the time of marriage the scar tissue is partially incised to permit sexual intercourse with the husband. During labor, the scar tissue is further resected to permit vaginal delivery. After delivery, tissues usually are resutured to conceal the vaginal opening.

Implications for Nursing Care

While respecting the family's belief system regarding circumcision, the inherent risks and disadvantages of the procedure should be stressed. When male circumcision is performed for religious reasons, the nurse must respect the family's decision. Female circumcision is a particularly dangerous procedure and is strongly discouraged. It is not performed in the United States in any medical setting; however, some families will return to their country of origin when financial means permit and have the female infant circumcised there. The nurse can work with other health professionals from the family's community to educate them about the extreme risks and disadvantages of female circumcision.

The nurse must assess the role of culture in neonatal care practices before providing anticipatory guidance and making ongoing recommendations for health-promoting behaviors. When practices appear to be harmless or beneficial to the neonate's well-being, they may be incorporated into the teaching plan developed by the nurse. If a specific practice appears to be harmful, the nurse must be careful to approach the issue with respect for cultural values and family members who recommend it. When possible, enlisting the assistance of a health professional from the family's culture who speaks their language may be particularly useful when the nurse must attempt to alter a particular behavior or practice.

Sexuality and Family Planning

The period of abstinence after birth, resumption of sexual relations, and the use of specific methods of birth control are strongly tied to culture and associated religious beliefs. With global concerns regarding population control, many cultures incorporate modern forms of contraceptive control into traditional family planning practices (such as abstinence and breastfeeding). Government-funded family planning programs have been implemented around the world. However, in many cultures discussion of sexuality and contraception does not properly occur in "mixed" company. Furthermore, responsibility for contraception rests with

women in most societies. Most women, therefore, want information about controlling their fertility.

The typical period of abstinence varies greatly among women. For example Chinese American women may refrain from sexual relations for up to 100 days after birth. In some cultures the woman is considered unclean while she is bleeding, and as noted, cleansing or purification rituals may be used before sexual relations are resumed with the partner at approximately 4 to 6 weeks postpartum. The traditional 6-week period of abstinence among American women is rarely observed today. Sexual relations often are resumed when the woman desires to do so, and there is no physical discomfort with sexual activity.

Implications for Nursing Care

The nurse often is the primary provider of information about family planning, contraception, and resumption of sexual activity in the United States. The work of nurse practitioners is central to family planning clinics across the country, and women and their partners look to nurses for guidance, education, and contraceptive services. In all settings (hospital, birthing unit, ambulatory care unit, home) the nurse should assess each woman's family planning needs.

In 1990 the American Nurses Association took an official position regarding women's reproductive services. *All women, regardless of income, should have access to a full range of reproductive health and family planning services*. Nurses in all settings that provide care to new families must be educationally prepared to discuss basic information about family planning. There should be no legal hindrance ("gag rules") to the discussion of a woman's full range of options for reproductive control, including the availability of abortion services, when abortion is a legal option.

The nurse must identify the woman's preferences in relation to contraception and family planning and how her cultural background may influence the acceptance of certain contraceptive methods. The woman's concerns and questions regarding individual methods should be addressed, and she should be given ample time to consider her options before making a final decision about family planning. The nurse must recognize that in many cultures, the woman must still have permission and acceptance from the partner regarding the contraceptive method, if it is to be used. Issues related to human immunodeficiency virus, however, make it imperative that the woman be aware of her risks of not using one of the available barrier devices when she is unsure of her partner's sexual behavior.

Adoptive Families

Adoptive parents share many concerns about becoming parents. They may worry about developing close relationships with their adoptive infants. They may believe that society regards the biologic relationship as paramount in developing parent–infant attachment. A study that compared European-American adoptive mothers with the birth mothers revealed that adoptive mothers generally saw their infants for the first time and took them home later than birth mothers (Koepke, Austin, Anglin, & Delesalle, 1991).

Adoptive parents often are older simply because they have usually first dealt with diagnosis and treatment of fertility problems and then have often waited a considerable time for the adoption process to be completed. Some adoptive parents may have difficulty acknowledging the adoptive relationship because of their feelings of stigma associated with their infertility. Some members of society may still convey the message to adoptive parents that they are not *real* parents. Grandparents may indicate that these children will not really be their grandchildren. These reactions may make adoptive parents feel that their children are second best or not as valued as biologic children (Miall, 1987). Although adoptive parents may worry about forming attachments to their infants, some women do report feelings of love on first contact with the infant (Koepke et al., 1991) Similar to biologic mothers, they experience fatigue, positive emotions, and changes in their marital relationships. They also must deal with feelings of sadness for the birth mothers who have surrendered the neonate to their care. In the study by Koepke and associates, adoptive mothers reported that their spouses experienced love for their adoptive infants but did not always receive physical assistance from their spouses with infant care. Few studies have been conducted on this subject, however.

Families currently choose between two forms of adoption: open and closed. In open adoptions adoptive parents meet the birth parents or mother. Identities and addresses are known. Adoptive and birth parents participate in the separation and placement process. Birth parents retain the right to continuing contact and knowledge of the child's location and welfare. Communication in the form of letters, phone calls, and visits are negotiated by the adoptive parents and birth parents. In closed adoption birth mothers and adoptive parents are provided with background information, but identities usually are not known and contact often is not encouraged (Dewarle, 1992).

Each of these options has advantages and disadvantages for adoptive families and the relinquishing parents. Families must explore and choose the option best suited for them. The accompanying Legal/Ethical Considerations display describes many of the advantages and disadvantages of the open option for adoptive and birth parents and their infants and indicates some of the dilemmas nurses face when assisting families during this time.

Implications for Nursing Care

Nurses can assist adoptive families who have a history of infertility to deal with their feelings in this area before pursuing an adoption. Reassurance and support for their roles as parents are important. In addition nurses can design parenting classes to enable adoptive parents to feel comfortable with child care and behavioral cues. Counseling also may be necessary if the adoptive parents feel stigmatized by others. Some individual counseling also may be necessary to assist adoptive parents to deal with any feelings of sadness and with changes in their spousal relationship, as well as to seek out and use other sources of support. Nurses can assist in the development of adoptive parent support groups.

Legal/Ethical Considerations

Open Adoption

Concerns have been expressed about open adoption in relation to the birth parents, the adoptive parents, and the child. For the birth parents concerns include unresolved grief with lack of closure to adoption, anger over disapproval of adoptive parents' childrearing techniques, and guilt over possible declining levels of participation in the relationship. For the adoptive parents concerns include interference with the attachment process, continual reminders of their status as adoptive parents, and fear of intrusion into family life by the birth parents. Concerns for the child include identity confusion in relation to parents, exposure to two sets of parental values, and feelings of rejection if the birth parents diminish their level of contact.

The potential benefits of open adoption also must be considered. For birth parents benefits include a less overwhelming sense of loss, less guilt because the home is chosen, and less concern about the child feeling rejected. For adoptive parents benefits include a more open relationship with the child, more detailed information about the birth parent (health and social facts), and an acknowledgment of the contribution of the two families. For the child benefits include a more realistic understanding of the adoption, an enhanced sense of identity, and fewer feelings of abandonment.

Nurses will encounter birth families and adoptive families following completion of the adoptive process. Nurses may be involved in supporting both groups and in advocating for their rights. This may present legal, moral, and ethical dilemmas, because during this highly emotional time, both adoptive and biologic parents experience conflicting needs and make conflicting demands on health professionals. There may even be open conflict at times, which requires the support and guidance of social workers, the court system, and child-protection workers.

Nurses must clarify their own values and not permit them to affect the support they offer to birth and adoptive parents. Nurses need to assess carefully both adoptive and biologic parents' needs. Families may require assistance to work out satisfactory visiting arrangements. In the event of serious conflicts, legal advice should be sought. The infant should be protected from any unreasonable acts from either set of parents. Open communication should be encouraged among family members. The nurse must try to remain objective and not become committed to one set of parents or the other.

Dewarle, B. K. (1992). Open adoption. Canadian Nurse, *88(3), 14–16.*

Dual-Earner Families

In a growing number of two-parent families, both adults are employed during the first postpartum year. Many women who are employed now return to work before the infant is 1 year old due to limited maternity leave, a desire to be employed, or financial pressures (Tulman & Fawcett, 1990). Increasingly, women's earnings are crucial to the economic survival of their families, and this serves as the impetus to retain a work role (Eggebeen & Hawkins, 1990). When both parents are employed outside the home, it often adds additional stress (Avant, 1988) due to the reduction in time available for household tasks, infant care, and interpersonal interaction (Eggebeen & Hawkins, 1990).

Although greater demands are placed on both parents when the woman is employed outside the home, many women benefit from working outside of the home. Employment has been associated with positive effects on psychological well-being for women. However, women employed full time in physically demanding work experience more injuries than those who are employed part time or are not employed (Walker & Best, 1991). Furthermore, women employed in convenience stores, restaurants, and taverns are increasingly at risk for work-related injury and death secondary to crime (armed robbery and assault). In addition women with children often take additional sick time to care for sick infants or children (see the Nursing Research display).

Role strain has been linked to a deterioration in employed women's physical and mental health. Families' attitudes and perceptions have been linked to the effect of multiple roles on parents' well-being and health. As noted, most women continue to assume primary responsibility for household tasks and child care in addition to employment. The demands are overwhelming at times. Generally, women who express satisfaction with employment, have adequate child care, and higher levels of social support experience less role strain (Hemmelgarn & Laing, 1991).

When both parents are employed, they often expect and seek assistance from each other to cope with multiple roles (Tulman & Fawcett, 1990). Support also may be provided by family and friends or by paid employees, such as babysitters, gardeners, and housekeepers (Hall, 1991). Women

Nursing Research

Employed Mothers and Homemaking Mothers' Well-Being

In general, studies have demonstrated that employment has a positive or neutral effect on women's physical and mental health. There may, however, be stressors that are unique to employed mothers that diminish their well-being. Walker and Best (1991) compared women's stress levels and their health-promoting life-styles in a sample of full-time employed mothers and homemaking mothers. The researchers predicted that full-time employed mothers with infants would report greater stress, less health-promoting life-styles, and less positive self-evaluations in the maternal role than homemaking mothers with infants. One hundred and seventy-three mothers with infants age 2 to 11 months old responded to questionnaires, which included items about perceived stress and maternal role and health-promoting behaviors.

Full-time employed mothers reported significantly more stress and fewer health-promoting behaviors than homemakers. Full-time employed mothers also reported less positive self-evaluations of themselves as mothers than did homemakers. Homemakers reported that their two greatest stressors were fatigue or sleep disturbance and work overload. Employed mothers reported their two greatest stressors were conflicts about going back to work and lack of time.

The researchers discovered that one way employed mothers managed parenting and employment was by paying less attention to their own personal health and well-being. The authors suggested a need for programs focused on facilitating the integration of work and family roles among employed women with infants. Other possible solutions that evolve from the study's findings include the following: Occupational health nurses can advocate on-site clinics for women's (and men's) health promotion. Health providers offering women's health services also should offer infant health care services so that the health needs of both can be met at the same time on the same premises.

Walker, L. O., & Best, M. A. (1991). Well-being of mothers with infant children: A preliminary comparison of employed women and homemakers. *Women and Health, 17*(1), 71–89.

continue to bear the greatest burden of responsibility in most two-parent families. In many studies of employed mothers, subjects frequently indicate that they had no time for themselves or their spousal relationships and that they felt exhausted. In contrast men report feeling less overwhelmed than their spouses, in part because of accepting less responsibility for child care and household management and maintaining different views about the importance of household tasks (Hall, 1992).

Implications for Nursing Care

Community or home health nurses who perform postpartum follow-up visits must begin with an assessment of the division of family labor, family attitudes and values, and the extent of role strain experienced by family members. Involving fathers in infant caregiving early in the first childbearing year is a strategy that can reduce familial role strain. Other issues contributing to familial role strain also must be addressed. Outside sources of support could help to ease the burdens associated with sharing multiple responsibilities (Hemmelgarn & Laing, 1991). Nurses can offer suggestions for use of outside services when they are available and economically feasible for the family.

Nurses have developed a number of valuable professional roles to assist parents when both are employed. Nurses have created home-help services, which provide professional child care workers or household helpers for busy new mothers. Because most day care facilities do not accept sick infants, nurses have developed day care facilities for sick infants and children. Where these agencies have opened, they have experienced immediate success (Fig. 36-3).

Single-Parent Families

The difficulties and challenges faced in two-parent families are magnified in single-parent families. Role changes and attachment must occur without support and advice from a partner. A single parent may have the responsibility for infant caretaking 24 hours a day. The number of single-parent families continues to rise in all ethnic and minority groups; however, the incidence of single parenting is highest among African American women (Duncan & Rodgers, 1987).

Despite the increasing number of single-parent families, two-parent families are still highly valued. Consequently, single parents may feel reduced self-esteem. Being a single father may be viewed as even more stigmatizing than being a single mother, because generally societies expect women to nurture children (Weinberg, 1985). Stigmatization of either single female or male parents can lead to isolation, especially if no extended family members are nearby. For that reason social support has been one of the most consistent predictors of maternal role behavior for adult single women.

Research about single fathers is less common and often has focused on adolescent parenting for young men. Recent studies of single mothers have found many negative consequences of parenting alone. When single parenting results in maternal stress and social support is lacking, it has been

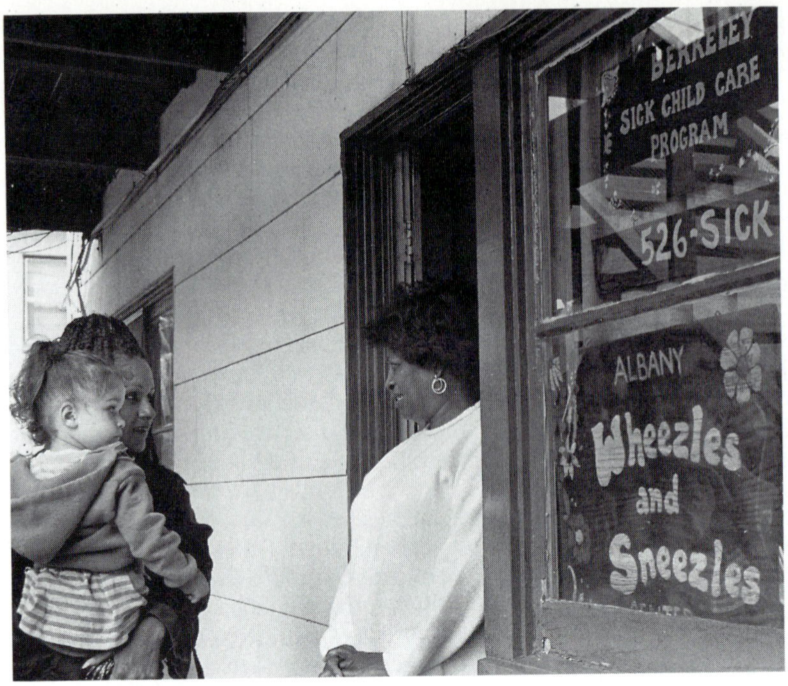

Figure 36-3.
A day care facility specializing in sick infants and children. (Photo by Kathy Sloane.)

linked to sleep disturbances in the infant (Becker, Chang, Kameshima, & Bloch, 1991). Stresses and concerns that single-parent families face include financial difficulties, lack of emergency and back-up child care arrangements, scheduling and time management problems, and difficulties with separated or divorced spouses if they have been married (Weinberg, 1985).

Financial difficulties arise when there is only one employed parent. However, single fathers enjoy higher incomes than single mothers. In addition fathers seldom experience the ongoing court battles to secure child support payments from an employed spouse that many women in American society face (Weinberg, 1985).

Caring for a sick infant when the woman or man is employed and does not have child care is a major problem. Arranging emergency and back-up child care may be very difficult or impossible (Weinberg, 1985). As noted, most day care agencies do not accept sick infants or children. The single parent often is reduced to taking a sick day or a day without pay to stay home with the infant. If they do have child care and go to work, they may feel guilty about leaving the infant. Increasingly, single parents without adequate child care, fearing they will loose their jobs, leave very young children home alone when they are too ill to be placed in day care. If discovered, they may face criminal charges of child abandonment.

Role flexibility (or the ability to alter schedules and routines) appears to ease the difficulties of balancing work and parenting responsibilities (Semchuk & Eakin, 1989; Weinberg, 1985). High incomes, good child care arrangements, sympathetic supervisors, and access to social support through social networks improve role flexibility. Semchuk and Eakin (1989) reported that single mothers with the least flexibility in jobs and child care indicated they experienced the most stress and used the least desirable health options for their children. Scheduling and balancing time demands also are important issues for single parents. They must be extremely efficient to meet all their expectations and responsibilities associated with multiple roles. This can be particularly stressful for single fathers who have traditionally relied on others to nurture infants and complete household chores. Usually, single parents must place themselves on tight schedules and accomplish many tasks simultaneously (Weinberg, 1985).

Dealing with separated or divorced spouses can cause additional stress for single parents. The single parent may still feel anger, resentment, and suspicion toward a former partner, and those feelings can make visitation periods or shared custody difficult. Single parents may worry that any lapse on their part could result in visits from child welfare authorities or complaints from a former partner. Infants and young children are sensitive to these tensions and may demonstrate behavioral changes that further compound a parent's guilt. Energy must be directed into developing new rules and relationships for a changed family unit (Weinberg, 1985). Even single never-married parents may have difficulties with demands from the biologic mothers or fathers of their infants.

Implications for Nursing Care

Nurses can offer practical advice about stress reduction. They can assist parents to balance schedules and time demands. Parents can be linked to community resources that would serve them in emergency situations. Occupational nurses in the workplace can serve as advocates for flexible work schedules and routines to assist single parents. Also, less expensive forms of sick care for infants should continue to be developed by nurses working in the community.

Because support appears to be an important mediator for stress, creative solutions need to be sought to provide

these parents with support. Single-parent support groups and baby-sitting cooperatives, volunteer grandparents, and networks among single-parent and dual-parent families could all serve as sources of support that would ameliorate the social isolation of single-parent families.

Nurses can assist single parents to identify behavioral cues indicating that their infants are responding to stressful situations. Sleep disturbances and increased infant fussiness and irritability could be indicators. These alterations in behavior should not be dismissed as transitory aspects typical of the first year after birth.

Finally, professional nurses can work for passage of laws that facilitate improved collection of absent fathers' income for child care and maintenance of the single-parent female-headed household. Single-parent fathers must be recognized as legitimate caregivers, and their particular concerns also should be be addressed.

Most nurses will encounter a diverse range of family structures, life-styles, and cultural influences. These may include lesbian families, families coping with chronic illness or disability, families with multiple infants, families from ethnic or cultural minorities, adoptive families, dual-earner families, and single-parent families. Each type of family affects nursing implications. Above all, the nurse must not be judgmental of these diversifications. The nurse's responsibility is to accept these families as they are and give them guidance in adapting good child care principles to their uniqueness.

Major Factors Affecting Infant Well-Being and Family Functioning

Two major factors affecting infant survival and family adaptations during the first year after childbirth are postpartum depression (PPD) and child abuse. The following sections discuss the effect of these factors on family functioning and individual family members. This information will help the nurse recognize signs and symptoms and diagnose, plan, intervene, and evaluate family adjustment.

Postpartum Depression

A significant and often unrecognized problem affecting family adjustment in the first year after childbirth is PPD. Although the *baby blues* or *postpartum blues*, which are common in the first few days postpartum, may be seen, the community nurse is more likely to see PPD. Nurses can play a role in early recognition and treatment of this problem by assessing women; informing them, their families, and the public about PPD; and informing about the community resources available for sufferers. The reader is referred to Chapter 29 for a complete discussion of PPD.

Interaction between the mother and newborn is negatively affected when the mother is depressed. The depressed mother is less responsive and less emotionally available to her newborn (Karl, 1991). Neonates of depressed mothers are at risk of being neglected and abused. Recent research has illustrated that cognitive, emotional, and behavioral development of the child is adversely affected when the mother has PPD and when there is family discord (Caplan et al., 1989). Family discord invariably occurs in association with maternal depression. It is unclear whether dissatisfaction with the marriage is a precipitating factor or a result. Nevertheless, women who are depressed distance themselves physically and emotionally from their partners.

Implications for Nursing Care

Women who are experiencing PPD must be identified and must receive supportive care. Nurses who have contact with families during the first year after childbirth can watch for signs of PPD. Observing a mother's lack of enjoyment in her infant may alert the nurse to the need for more in-depth assessment.

All families can be given information about resources, such as crisis telephone lines. For women who are depressed postpartum support groups may be the only intervention necessary if the PPD is mild and identified early. In some communities, groups specifically designed for women with PPD may be available. These organizations offer "buddy" or peer support, as well as self-help support groups. Other women will benefit from individual or couple counseling. With severe PPD, interventions that include modeling effective parenting skills may be required. Social services referrals are indicated when abuse or neglect is suspected.

Alerting families to the possibility of PPD will help in early identification. Postpartum units and community health units can provide materials (posters, educational television segments, and pamphlets) to educate all families. Such materials can highlight the prevalence, signs, and consequences of PPD and inform parents of local resources.

Child Abuse

Child abuse is universal and crosses all cultural and socioeconomic barriers. In 1990 2.5 million cases of child abuse were reported in the United States, a 4% increase from 1989 (Brucker, 1991). Although child abuse has received growing recognition by health care professionals, often the more obvious forms of physical abuse are identified, while the subtler forms of abuse go unrecognized. Types of abuse include emotional abuse and neglect, physical abuse and injury, and sexual abuse.

Emotional abuse refers to the habitual verbal harassment of a child by disparagement, criticism, threat, and ridicule. Rejection and withdrawal are substituted for love. *Neglect* comprises a lack of physical caretaking and supervision and a failure to engage in the developmental needs of the child through stimulation. This can include failure to seek proper medical treatment and failure to meet the physical and emotional needs of the child. Failure to thrive that develops from nonorganic sources would be considered a form of neglect (Castiglia, 1988; Meehan, 1991). *Physical abuse* can be defined as harm or threatened harm suffered by a child through nonaccidental injury or poisoning as a result of acts or deliberate omission by the person responsible for the care of the child. *Sexual abuse* is the involvement

of dependent, developmentally immature children in sexual activity or offenses as a result of acts or omissions of the person responsible for the care of the child (Meehan, 1991; Rhodes, 1987). These generally violate social taboos or acceptable family roles.

Many social, familial, and individual factors have been associated with parental or caretaker abuse of children. These include financial pressures, substandard housing, caretaker immaturity, unrealistic developmental expectations of the child, poor caretaker self-esteem, unstable or unsatisfactory adult relationships, a history of familial abuse, feelings of caretaker incompetence, social isolation, chemical dependency, high levels of caretaker stress, and severe disciplinary action during childhood, leading to overuse of discipline (Anderson, 1987; Brucker, 1991; Meehan, 1991). Specific infant characteristics also have been associated with child abuse, including being an unwanted child or labeled "difficult" in temperament, prematurity, chronic illness, congenital defects, or mental disability (Brucker, 1991).

Implications for Nursing Care

Current state laws mandate that nurses report suspected or confirmed child abuse. Nurses who fail to fulfill this obligation may suffer criminal or civil penalties (Brucker, 1991). Nurses must be knowledgeable about risk factors for child abuse and be alert for subtle and overt signs of negligence or abuse. A neglected infant may demonstrate a flat affect, lack of motor activity and vocalization in response to a stimulus, neglected physical appearance, reduction in weight, height, and head circumference when compared with expected norms, developmental delay, and possibly an extended prior period of hospitalization (Brucker, 1991; Castiglia, 1988; Meehan, 1991).

A physically abused infant may present with burns and scalds, nonaccidental poisoning, severe and closed head injuries accompanied by retinal hemorrhage, rib and lower-extremity fractures, and abdominal injuries. These serious injuries generally indicate abuse in infants up to 1 year of age (Rivara, Kamitsuka, & Quan, 1988). Signs of sexual abuse usually are local trauma, including perineal soreness, vaginal discharge, and anal pain and bleeding (Meehan, 1991).

Awareness of factors associated with abuse and overt signs of abuse will permit nurses to assess families effectively and to identify vulnerable families. The outcomes of abuse for children run the gamut from emotional scarring, to learning and physical disabilities, to death (Anderson, 1987). Comprehensive assessments also will assist nurses to identify necessary supports and to provide supports to prevent abusive situations. If a nurse identifies an abusive situation, he or she is legally and morally bound to report it to the authorities.

Current limitations in funding of health care services have hindered efforts to support new families so that factors associated with abuse, such as poverty and chemical dependence, can be eliminated. Funding cuts have lead to staffing cuts. Professional nurses may not be available to assess and intervene when child abuse occurs. Factors alerting nurses to a potentially abusive situation may not be considered significant enough by supervisors to warrant a second visit.

Nurses can refer parents at high risk for abusive behavior to community support groups and family agencies, such as Parents Anonymous, crisis counseling, and homemaker or foster care assistance. Alternatives to physical discipline that are age appropriate can be used. Parents must receive praise and support when parenting effectively. Evaluation of interventions is crucial because ineffective interventions or familial responses can place vulnerable children at significant risk (Anderson, 1987).

Nurses must not only be aware of community resources that are in place, but also must advocate for the development of resources, such as multidisciplinary child protection teams (Mogielnicki, Chandler, Weissberg, & Mogielnicki, 1988). In addition, advocacy for basic social change, such as improving employment, housing, and social support, will assist in preventing situations that stress vulnerable families and tip the balance toward child abuse.

Two factors that can profoundly affect the health and well-being of childbearing families are postpartum depression and child abuse. Both of these problems affect families from all walks of life. The nurse is responsible for assessing the families in his or her care for these problems, and for ensuring that the family receives appropriate assistance. Specifically in the case of child abuse, the nurse is morally and legally bound to report cases of suspected child abuse to the appropriate authorities. The nurse also plays an important role in prevention of these conditions by assessing families carefully for factors that put them at risk, and encouraging families to use available community resources to help them cope with the stressors associated with the first months of parenthood.

Chapter Summary

The first postpartum year lays the foundation for successful infant and child growth and development. Families require ongoing support from relatives, friends, health professionals, and the community to achieve successful adaptation. Societal factors have lead to a disruption in the support systems of most families (Donaldson, 1991; Rush & Kitch, 1991).

The role of the nurse is central in the provision of family-centered care to new and expanding families. The goal of nursing care is to support the strengths of the family unit and to offer appropriate education, guidance, and referrals. Changes in American society have challenged nurses to create new ways of helping families. The development and expansion of community, home health, and ambulatory care nursing are essential to meet the needs of new parents. Because more than 50% of American women are now employed at least part time within the first postpartum year, occupational health nurses must continue to develop work site child care and parenting programs. Nurses must develop new approaches to providing information, such as telephone advice and "hot-line" services. Community-based parenting programs also must have expanded hours, so employed parents can take advantage of them after work hours.

Study Questions

1. *What are the developmental tasks of the expanding family? What nursing interventions will promote a family's achievement of each of these tasks?*
2. *What role does infant behavior play on parent–infant attachment?*
3. *What nursing actions will support parental, sibling, and grandparent role taking?*
4. *What cultural and ethnic practices may the nurse encounter in the postpartum period?*
5. *What are signs of PPD? How does PPD affect family members?*
6. *What factors could alert a nurse to infant physical abuse? What are the nursing responsibilities associated with identified child abuse?*
7. *What are the implications for the family in early discharge? What preparations can be beneficial for families anticipating early discharge?*
8. *What community programs might benefit families during the first year after childbirth?*

References

Anderson, C. L. (1987). Assessing parenting potential for child abuse risk. *Pediatric Nursing, 13*(5), 323–327.

Avant, K. C. (1988). Stressors on the childbearing family. *Journal of Obstetric, Gynecologic, and Neonatal Nursing, 17*(3), 179–185.

Balsmeyer, B. (1990). Sleep disturbances of the infant and toddler. *Pediatric Nursing, 16*(5), 447–452.

Becker, P. T., Chang, A., Kameshima, S., & Bloch, M. (1991). Correlates of diurnal sleep patterns in infants of adolescent and adult single mothers. *Research in Nursing and Health, 14*, 97–108.

Bowen, G. L., & Orthner, D. K. (1990). Effects of organizational culture on fatherhood. In F. W. Bozett & S. M. H. Hanson (Eds.), *Fatherhood and families in cultural context* (pp. 187–217). New York: Springer Publishing.

Brucker, J. M. (1991). Battered child syndrome: Educating the pediatric nurse. *Journal of Pediatric Nursing, 6*(6), 428–429.

Caplan, H. L., Cogill, S. R., Alexander, H., Robson, K. M., Katz, R., & Kumar, R. (1989). Maternal depression and the emotional development of the child. *British Journal of Psychiatry, 154*, 818–822.

Carty, E., Conine, T., & Hall, L. (1990). Comprehensive health promotion for the pregnant woman who is disabled. *Journal of Nurse Midwifery, 35*(3), 133–142.

Castiglia, P. T. (1988). Failure to thrive. *Journal of Pediatric Health Care, 2*(1), 50–51.

Cervisi, J., Chapman, M., Niklas, B., & Yamaoka, C. (1991). Office management of the infant with colic. *Journal of Pediatric Health Care, 5*(4), 184–190.

Conine, T., Carty, E., & Safarik, P. (1988). *Aids and adaptations for parents with physical or sensory disabilities* (2nd ed). Vancouver: School of Rehabilitation Medicine, University of British Columbia.

Cox, M. J., Owen, M. T., Lewis, J. M., & Henderson, V. K. (1989). Marriage, adult adjustment and early parenting. *Child Development, 60*(5), 1015–1024.

Dewarle, B. K. (1992). Open adoption. *Canadian Nurse, 88*(3), 14–16.

Donaldson, N. E. (1991). A review of nursing intervention research on maternal adaptation in the first 8 weeks postpartum. *Journal of Perinatal and Neonatal Nursing, 4*(4), 1–11.

Driscoll, J. W. (1990). Maternal parenthood and the grief process. *Journal of Perinatal and Neonatal Nursing, 4*(2), 1–10.

Duncan, G. J., & Rodgers, W. (1987). Single parent families: Are their economic problems transitory or persistent? *Family Planning Perspectives, 19*(4), 171–178.

Eggebeen, D. J., & Hawkins, A. J. (1990). Economic need and wives' employment. *Journal of Family Issues, 11*(1), 48–66.

Evans, C. J. (1991). Description of a home follow-up program for childbearing families. *Journal of Obstetric, Gynecologic, and Neonatal Nursing, 20*(2), 113–118.

Flagler, S. (1988). Maternal role competence. *Western Journal of Nursing Research, 10*(3), 274–290.

Flagler, S. (1990). Relationships between stated feelings and measures of maternal adjustment. *Journal of Obstetric, Gynecologic, and Neonatal Nursing, 19*(5), 411–416.

Fortier, J. C., Carson, V. B., Will, S., & Shubkagel, B. L. (1991). Adjustment to a newborn: Sibling preparation makes a difference. *Journal of Obstetric, Gynecologic, and Neonatal Nursing, 20*(1), 73–79.

Hall, W. A. (1991). The experience of fathers in dual-earner families following the births of their infants. *Journal of Advanced Nursing, 16*, 423–430.

Hall, W. A. (1992). A comparison of the experience of women and men in dual-earner families following the birth of their first infant. *Image, 24*(1), 33–38.

Harvey, S. M., Carr, C., & Bernheine, S. (1989). Lesbian mothers: Health care experiences. *Journal of Nurse-Midwifery, 34*(3), 115–119.

Hemmelgarn, B., & Laing, G. (1991). The relationship between situational factors and perceived role strain in employed mothers. *Family and Community Health, 14*(1), 8–15.

Honig, J. C. (1986). Preparing preschool-aged children to be siblings. *American Journal of Maternal Child Nursing, 11*, 37–43.

Horn, M., & Manion, J. (1985). Creative grandparenting, bonding the generations. *Journal of Obstetric, Gynecologic, and Neonatal Nursing, 14*(3), 233–236.

Johnsen, N. M., & Gaspard, M. E. (1985). Theoretical foundations of a sibling preparation class. *Journal of Obstetric, Gynecologic, and Neonatal Nursing, 14*(3), 237–241.

Jordan, P. (1990). Laboring for relevance: Expectant and new fatherhood. *Nursing Research, 39*(1), 11–16.

Jurich, A. P., White, M. B., White, C. P., & Moody, R. A. (1990). Internal culture of the family and its effect on fatherhood. In F. W. Bozett & S. M. H. Hanson (Eds.), *Fatherhood and families in cultural context* (pp. 237–262). New York: Springer Publishing.

Karl, D. (1991). The consequences of maternal depression for early mother–infant interaction: A nursing issue. *Journal of Pediatric Nursing, 6*(6), 384–389.

Keefe, M. R., & Froese-Fretz, A. (1991). Living with an irritable infant: Maternal perspectives. *American Journal of Maternal Child Nursing, 16*, 255–259.

Klaus, M., & Kennell, J. (1982). *Parent–infant bonding*. St. Louis: C. V. Mosby.

Kleinman, A. (1986). *Culture in the clinic: A cultural framework for assessing cultural problems in patient care*. Paper presented at the University of British Columbia. Vancouver, British Columbia.

Koepke, J. E., Austin, J., Anglin, S., & Delesalle, J. (1991). Becoming parents: Feelings of adoptive mothers. *Pediatric Nursing, 17*(4), 333–336.

Mackenzie, J.C. (1989) Parenting multiples: The first year. *Great Expectations, 2*(1), 46–50.

Maloni, J. A., McIndoe, J. E., & Rubenstein, G. (1987). Expectant grandparents class. *Journal of Obstetric, Gynecologic, and Neonatal Nursing, 16*(1), 26–29.

Meehan, F. (1991). Suffer the little children. *Nursing, 4*(27), 16–17.

Mercer, R. T. (1985). The process of maternal role attainment over the first year. *Nursing Research, 34*(4), 198–203.

Mercer, R. T., & Ferketich, S. L. (1990). Predictors of parental attachment during early parenthood. *Journal of Advanced Nursing, 15*, 268–280.

Miall, C. A. (1987). The stigma of adoptive parent status. *Family Relations, 36*(1), 34–39.

Mirandé, A. (1990) Ethnicity and fatherhood. In F. W Bozett & S. M. H.

Hanson (Eds.), *Fatherhood and families in cultural context* (pp. 53–82). New York: Springer Publishing.

Mogielnicki, P., Chandler, J. E., Weissberg, M. P., & Mogielnicki, N. P. (1988). Parents about to abuse. *Emergency Medicine*, *20*(9), 85–88.

Mortimer, P., & Kevill, F. (1985). Frustration and despair. *Community Outlook*, *May*, 19–22.

Nelms, B. C. (1991). Sibling relationships, more important now than ever. *Journal of Pediatric Health Care*, *4*(2), 57–58.

Noble, E. (1991). *Having twins* (2nd ed.). Boston: Houghton-Mifflin.

Pridham, K. F., & Chang, A. S. (1991). Mothers' perceptions of problem-solving competence for infant care. *Western Journal of Nursing Research*, *13*(2), 164–180.

Pridham, K. F., Lytton, D., Chang, A. S., & Rutledge, D. (1991). Early postpartum transition: Progress in maternal identity and role attainment. *Research in Nursing and Health*, *14*, 21–31.

Pridham, K. F., & Zavoral, J. H. (1988). Help for mothers with infant care and household tasks: Perceptions of support and stress. *Public Health Nursing*, *5*(4), 201–208.

Pritchard, P. (1986). An infant crying clinic. *Health Visitor*, *59*, 375–377.

Rhodes, A. M. (1987). Identifying and reporting child abuse. *American Journal of Maternal Child Nursing*, *12*(6), 399.

Rivara, F. P., Kamitsuka, M. D., & Quan, L. (1988). Injuries to children younger than 1 year of age. *Pediatrics*, *81*(1), 93–97.

Rush, J. P., & Kitch, T. L. (1991). A randomized controlled trial to measure the frequency of use of a hospital telephone line for new parents. *Birth*, *18*(4), 193–197.

Sayers, R. (1991). Male parenting: Beyond the female agreement, a psychological perspective. In Y. Ornstein (Ed.), *From the hearts of men* (pp. 289–293). Woodacre, CA: Harmonia Press.

Semchuk, K. M., & Eakin, J. M. (1989). Children's health and illness behavior: The single working mother's perspective. *Canadian Journal of Public Health*, *80*(5), 346–350.

Seward, R. R. (1990). Determinants of family culture: Effects on fatherhood. In F. W. Bozett & S. M. H. Hanson (Eds.), *Fatherhood and families in cultural context* (pp. 218–236). New York: Springer Publishing.

Sollid, D. T., Evans, B. T., McClowry, S. G., & Garrett, A. (1989). Breastfeeding multiples. *Journal of Perinatal and Neonatal Nursing*, *3*(1), 46–65.

Theroux, R. (1989). Multiple birth: A unique parenting experience. *Journal of Perinatal and Neonatal Nursing*, *3*(1), 35–45.

Tomlinson, P. S. (1990). Verbal behavior associated with indicators of maternal attachment with the neonate. *Journal of Obstetric, Gynecologic, and Neonatal Nursing*, *19*(1), 76–77.

Tomlinson, P. S., Rothenberg, M. A., & Carver, L. D. (1991). Behavioral interaction of fathers with infants and mothers in the immediate postpartum period. *Journal of Nurse-Midwifery*, *36*(4), 232–239.

Tulman, L., & Fawcett, J. (1990). Maternal employment following childbirth. *Research in Nursing and Health*, *13*, 181–188.

Tulman, L., & Fawcett, J. (1991). Recovery from childbirth: Looking back after 6 months. *Health Care for Women International*, *12*, 341–350.

Tripp-Reimer, T., & Wilson, S. E. (1990). Cross-cultural perspectives on fatherhood. In F. W. Bozett & S. M. H. Hanson (Eds.), *Fatherhood and families in cultural context* (pp. 1–27). New York: Springer Publishing.

Walker, L. O., & Best, M. A. (1991). Well-being of mothers with infant children: A preliminary comparison of employed women and homemakers. *Women and Health*, *17*(1), 71–89.

Waxler-Morrison, N., Anderson, J., & Richardson, E. (1990). *Cross-cultural caring: A handbook for health professionals in Western Canada*. Vancouver, British Columbia: University of British Columbia Press.

Weinberg, T. S. (1985). Single fatherhood: How is it different? *Pediatric Nursing*, *11*(3), 173–175.

Suggested Readings

Collins, C., Tiedje, L. B., & Stommel, M. (1992). Promoting positive well-being in employed mothers: A pilot study. *Health Care for Women International*, *13*(1), 77–85.

Holden, J. M., Sagovsky, R., & Cox, J.L. (1989). Counselling in a general practice setting: Controlled study of health visitor intervention in treatment of postpartum depression. *British Medical Journal*, *298*, 223–226.

Brazelton, T. B. (1985). *Working and caring*. Reading MA: Addison-Wesley.

Mercer, R. T. (1986). *First-time motherhood experiences from teens to forties*. New York: Springer.

Rubin, R. (1967). Attainment of the maternal role: 1. Processes. *Nursing Research*, *16*, 237–245.

APPENDIX A

The Maternity Patient's Bill of Rights

The woman has a right to participate in decisions regarding her well-being and that of her fetus or neonate, except in emergency situations that prevent her participation.

The woman has the following rights:

1. To have access to affordable, prenatal services that facilitate optimum maternal, fetal, and neonatal well-being.
2. To have access to and receive information about available pregnancy, childbirth preparation, and parenting classes.
3. To know the name and professional qualifications of the persons providing nursing and medical care during pregnancy, childbirth, and the postpartum period.
4. To be informed of any potential benefits and risks to herself, fetus, and neonate that may result from a diagnostic test, procedure, or a drug prescribed by the nurse midwife or physician during the pregnancy, childbirth, postpartum, or lactation period, *prior* to its implementation.
5. To be informed of known alternative therapies *prior* to implementation of a proposed procedure, therapy, or drug.
6. To be informed if a specific procedure or drug is medically indicated or is an elective therapy performed for the convenience of the health care staff or for teaching purposes.
7. To be informed in a timely manner of problems that arise and may cause maternal, fetal, or neonatal difficulties.
8. To determine without pressure from health care providers, partner, or family members whether she will accept the risks inherent in a proposed diagnostic test, therapy, or drug.
9. To receive information about proposed diagnostic tests, therapy, or drugs in her language of origin, when language barriers exist.
10. To have access to specialized perinatal care and services should complications arise during pregnancy, labor, or the postpartum period.
11. To give birth in a family-centered maternity setting that permits the presence and participation of the woman's partner and other family members.
12. To choose a position for labor and birth that is most comfortable, after consultation with her nurse midwife or physician.
13. To have her neonate remain with her after birth, and cared for at her bedside when the infant's condition is stable.
14. To have 24 hour per day visiting rights when the neonate is ill and must remain in the nursery or neonatal intensive care unit.
15. To receive clear and complete explanations about events that occur during pregnancy, childbirth, and the postpartum period.
16. To receive detailed and current information about the benefits of breastfeeding *prior* to childbirth.
17. To breastfeed her neonate according to the infant's needs, rather than according to hospital regimen.
18. To receive ongoing education and physical and emotional support for breastfeeding from qualified health care providers, and appropriate resources and referrals for breastfeeding mothers on discharge from the hospital.
19. To receive care that is culturally sensitive and respects variations in health care and parenting practices based on the woman's cultural beliefs.
20. To have access to her complete medical record in accordance with state laws, and to have present an impartial advocate who can explain the record when she chooses to read it.

Adapted from: Haire, D. B. (1975). The pregnant patient's bill of rights. *Journal of Nurse Midwife, 20*, Winter, 29; Organization for Obstetric, Gynecologic, and Neonatal Nurses. (1991). Standards for the nursing care of women and newborns. (4th ed). Washington, DC: AWOHNN (formerly NAACOG); ANA Report of Consensus Conference. (1987). Access to prenatal care: Key to preventing low birthweight. Consensus Conference on Access to Prenatal Care and Low Birthweight. Washington, DC: American Nurses Association.

APPENDIX B

Normal Values and Reference Tables

TABLE B-1. Normal Peripheral Blood Values at Different Ages

Age	Hemoglobin (g/dL)	Hematocrit (%)	MCV (fl)	WBC ($10^3/mm^3$)	Neutrophils (%)	Lymphocytes (%)	Platelets ($10^3/mm^3$)
Birth	13.5–21	42–65	100–140	9–30	60	30	100–300
1 wk	13.5–21	42–65	95–135	5–21	40	50	100–300
1 mo	10–16	30–48	85–125	5–21	35	55	100–300
Adult:							
Male	14–18	42–54	80–100	4–11	0	30	100–300
Female	12–16	36–48	80–100	4–11	60	30	100–300
Pregnancy	11.5–12.3	32–39	80–95	12–15	60 ± 10	34 ± 10	100–300

TABLE B-2. Blood Chemistries

Determination	Specimen	Age/Sex	Normal Value	
Acetone	Serum/plasma			
Qualitative			Negative	
Quantitative (acetone and acetoacetic acid)			0.3–2.0 mg/dL	
Albumin (see Protein electrophoresis)				
Aldolase	Serum	Newborn	4 × adult value	
		Adult	<11 IU/L	
Alpha fetoprotein	Serum		<10 mg/dL	
Amylase	Serum	Newborn	5–65 U/L	
		>1 y	25–125	
Ascorbic acid	Serum		0.6–2.0 mg/dL	
Bicarbonate	Serum	Arterial	21–28 mmol/L	
		Venous	22–29	
	Serum	Pregnancy	20.5–26	
Base excess	Whole blood	Newborn	(−10)–(−2) mmol/L	
		Adult	(−3)–(+3)	
			Premature (mg/dL)	**Full-term (mg/dL)**
Bilirubin, total	Serum	Cord	<2	<2
		0–1 d	<8	<6
		1–2 d	<12	<8
		2–5 d	<16	<12
		Adult	<2	0.2–1.0
		Pregnancy	Unchanged	
Bilirubin, direct (conjugated)	Serum		0.8–0.2 mg/dL	
Calcium, ionized	Serum, plasma, whole blood	Cord, newborn	5.5 ± 0.3 mg/dL	
		3–24 h	4.3–5.1	
		24–48 h	4.0–4.7	
		Adult	4.48–4.92	

(continued)

Table B-2. Blood Chemistries *(continued)*

Determination	Specimen	Age/Sex	Normal Value
Calcium, total	Serum	Cord, newborn	9–11.5 mg/dL
		3–4 h	9–10.6 mg/dL
		24–48 h	7–12
		4–7 d	9–10.9
		Adult	8.4–10.2
		Pregnancy	7.8–9.3
Carbon dioxide, partial pressure (P_{CO_2})	Whole blood, arterial	Newborn	27–40 mm Hg
		Infant	27–40
		Pregnancy	27–32
		Female adult	32–45
Carbon dioxide (total CO_2)	Serum, venous	Cord	14–22 mmol/L
		Premature (1 wk)	14–27
		Newborn	13–22
		Infant	20–28
		Adult	23–30
		Pregnancy	23–30 at term
Carbon monoxide	Whole blood		0.5–1.5% saturation of Hgb (children and nonsmokers); symptoms >20%
Carboxyhemoglobin (See Carbon monoxide)			
β-Carotene	Serum	Infant	20–70 mcg/dL
		Adult	60–200
Chloride	Serum or plasma	Cord	96–104 mmol/L
		Newborn	97–110
		Adult	98–106
		Pregnancy	Slight elevation
	Sweat	Normal	0–35 mmol/L
		Marginal	30–60
		Cystic fibrosis	60–200
Cholesterol, total	Serum	Cord	45–100 mg/dL
		Newborn	53–135
		Infant	70–175
		Adult	140–220
		Pregnancy	Elevated
Copper	Serum	Newborn–6 mo	20–70 mcg/dL
		Adult: M	70–140
		F	80–155
Cortisol	Plasma or serum	8 AM specimen	5–23 mcg/dL
		4 PM specimen	3–15
Creatine kinase, CK (creatine phosphokinase, CPK; 30°C)	Serum	Newborn	68–580 U/L
		Adult: M	12–70
		F	10–55
			(higher after exercise)
Creatinine	Serum or plasma	Cord	0.6–1.2 mg/dL
		Infant	0.2–0.4
		Adult: M	0.6–1.2
		F	0.5–1.1
		Pregnancy	(0.47–0.7)
Creatinine clearance (endogenous)*	Serum or plasma and timed urine	Newborn	40–65 mL/min/1.73 m^2
		Under 40 y	
		M	97–137
		F	88–128
			(decreases 6.5 mL/min/decade)
		Pregnancy	Decreased
Disaccharide tolerance (dose: twice oral glucose tolerance test dose)	Serum		>20 mg/dL change in glucose concentration
Ethanol	Blood		0.0%
			Toxic: 50–100 mg/dL; CNS depression: >100 mg/dL
Fatty acids, free	Serum or plasma	Adults	8–25 mg/dL
		Children and obese adults	<31

(continued)

Table B-2. Blood Chemistries *(continued)*

Determination	Specimen	Age/Sex	Normal Value		
Fibrinogen	Whole blood	Newborn	125–300 mg/dL		
		Adult	200–400		
		Pregnancy	450		
Folate	Serum	Newborn	7–32 ng/mL		
		Adult	1.8–9 ng/mL		
		Pregnancy	1.9–14		
Follicle-stimulating hormone (FSH)	Serum/plasma	Birth–7 y M	<1–12 mU/mL		
		F	<1–20		
		Adult F	5–30		
		Premenopause	4–30		
		Midcycle peak	10–90		
Galactose	Serum	Newborn/Infant	0–20 mg/dL		
		Adult	<5		
Glucose	Serum	Cord	45–96 mg/dL		
		Premature	20–60		
		Neonate	30–60		
		Newborn, 1 d	40–60		
		Newborn, >1 d	50–90		
		Adult	70–105		
	Blood	Adult	65–95		
	Urine		<0.5 g/d		
Glucose tolerance	Serum		**Time**	**Normal**	**Diabetic**
Dosages:			Fasting	70–105	>115
Child 1.75 g/kg of ideal weight, maximum 75 g			60 min	120–170	≥200
Adult 75 g total dose			90 min	100–140	≥200
			120 min	70–120	≥140
Growth hormone (HGH), fasting	Serum or plasma	Cord	10–50 ng/mL		
		Newborn	10–40		
		Adult: M	<5		
		F	<8		
Immunoglobulin levels	Serum		**IgA (mg/dL)**	**IgG (mg/dL)†**	**IgM (mg/dL)**
		Cord	0–5	760–1700	4–24
		Newborn	0–2.2	700–1480	5–30
		Adult	60–380	600–1600	40–345
IgD	Serum	Newborn		None detected	
		Adult		0–8 mg/dL	
IgE	Serum	M		0–230 IU/mL	
		F		0–170	
Insulin, (12 h, fasting)	Serum, plasma	Newborn		3–20 mcIU/mL	
		Adult		7–24	
			IgA (mg/dL)	**IgG (mg/dL)†**	**IgM (mg/dL)**
Insulin with oral glucose tolerance test	Serum			0 min:	7–24 mcIU/mL
				60 min:	18–276
				120 min:	16–166
				180 min:	4–38
Iron-binding capacity (TIBC)	Serum	Infant	100–400 μg/dL		
		Adult	250–400		
		Pregnancy	300–450		
Iron	Serum	Newborn	100–250 μg/dL		
		Infant	40–100		
		Adult: M	50–160		
		F	40–150		
		Pregnancy	Decreased		
Lactate	Whole blood, venous		0.50–2.2 mmol/L		
	Whole blood, arterial		0.50–1.6		

(continued)

Table B-2. Blood Chemistries ***(continued)***

Determination	Specimen	Age/Sex	Normal Value
Lactate dehydrogenase (LDH)	Serum	Newborn	160–450 U/L
		Infant	100–250
			60–170
		Adult	45–90
Lead	Whole blood	Child	<30 mcg/dL
		Adult	<40
		Acceptable for industrial exposure	<60
		Toxic	≥100
Lipase (Tietz method; 37°C)	Serum		0.1–1.0 U/mL
		Child	1–6 mIU/mL
		Adult:	4–14
		F, premenopause	4–25
		F, midcycle	25–250
		F, postmenopause	25–200
Magnesium	Serum	Newborn	1.2–1.8 mEq/L
		Adult	1.3–2.1
Methemoglobin	Whole blood		0.06–0.24 g/dL
Osmolality	Serum		275–295 mOsm/kg H_2O
Oxygen capacity	Whole blood, arterial		1.34 mL/g hemoglobin
Oxygen, partial pressure (Po_2)	Whole blood, arterial	Birth	8–24 mm Hg
		5–10 min	33–75
		30 min	31–85
		>1 h	55–80
		1 d	54–95
		Adult	83–108 decreases with age
Oxygen, % saturation	Whole blood, arterial	Newborn	40–90%
		Thereafter	95–99%
pH (37°C)	Whole blood, arterial	Premature (48 h)	7.35–7.50
		Birth, full term	7.11–7.36
		5–10 min	7.09–7.30
		30 min	7.21–7.38
		>1 h	7.26–7.49
		1 d	7.29–7.45
		Mid pregnancy	7.40–7.45
Phenylalanine	Serum	Premature/low birth weight	2.0–7.5 mg/dL
			1.2–3.4
		Full-term newborn	0.8–1.8
		Adult	
Phosphatase, acid prostatic, 37°C	Serum		<3.0 ng/mL
			0.11–0.60 U/L
Phosphatase, alkaline SKI method		Infant	50–155 U/L
		Child	20–150
		Adult	20–70
		Pregnancy >50% rise	
Phospholipids (lipids P × 25)	Serum and plasma	Newborn	75–170 mg/dL
		Infant	100–275
		Adult	125–275
Phosphorus, inorganic	Serum	Cord	3.7–8.1 mg/dL
		Premature (1 wk)	5.4–10.9
		Newborn	4.3–9.3
		Adult	3.0–4.5
		Pregnancy	Unchanged
Potassium	Serum	Newborn	3.9–5.9 mmol/L
		Infant	4.1–5.3
		Adult	3.5–5.1
		Pregnancy	3.5–5.3
Protein, total	Serum	Premature	4.3–7.6 g/dL
		Newborn	4.6–7.4
		Adult, recumbent–0.5 g higher in ambulatory patients	6.0–7.8

(continued)

Table B-2. Blood Chemistries *(continued)*

Determination	Specimen	Age/Sex	Total Protein (g/dL)	Albumin (g/dL)	α_1-glob (g/dL)	α_2-glob (g/dL)	β-glob (g/dL)	γ-glob† (g/dL)
Protein, electrophoresis, (cellulose acetate)	Serum							
		Premature	4.3–7.6	3.0–4.2	0.1–0.5	0.3–0.7	0.3–1.2	0.3–1.4 g/dL
		Newborn	4.6–7.4	3.6–5.4	0.1–0.3	0.3–0.5	0.2–0.6	0.2–1.0
		Infant	6.2–8.0	4.0–5.0	0.2–0.4	0.5–0.8	0.5–0.8	0.3–1.2
			6.0–7.8	3.5–5.0	0.2–0.3	0.4–1.0	0.5–1.1	0.7–1.2
		Pregnancy		decreased 2nd and 3rd trimester	increased 2nd trimester	increased 2nd trimester	increased 2nd trimester	decreased 3rd trimester

Determination	Specimen	Age/Sex	Normal Value
Salicylates	Serum, plasma		Negative: <2.0 mg/dL Therapeutic: 15–30 Toxic: >30
Sodium	Serum	Newborn	134–146 mmol/L
		Infant	139–146
		Adult	136–146
		Pregnancy	Increased retention >500 over normal
T_3 resin uptake (T_3RU)	Serum	Newborn	26–36%
		Adult	26–35
		Pregnancy	Decreased
Testosterone	Serum	Adult: M	572 ± 135
		F	37 ± 10
Thiamine (vitamin B_1)	Serum		2.0 mcg/dL
Thyroid-stimulating hormone (TSH)	Serum, plasma	Cord	3–12 mcU/L
		Newborn	3–18
		Adult	2–10
Transferrin	Serum	Newborn	130–275 mg/dL
		Adult	200–400

Determination	Specimen	Age/Sex	Male (mg/dL)	Female (mg/dL)
Triglycerides (TG)	Serum, after 12-h fast	Cord blood	10–98	10–98
		0–5 y	30–86	32–99
		6–11	31–108	35–114
		12–15	36–138	41–138
		16–19	40–163	40–128
		20–29	44–185	40–128
		Recommended (desirable) levels for adults:	Male 40–160	Female 35–135

Determination	Specimen	Age/Sex	Normal Value
Tyrosine	Serum	Premature	7.0–24.0 mg/dL
		Newborn	1.6–3.7
		Adult	0.8–1.3
Urea nitrogen	Serum/plasma	Cord	21–40 mg/dL
		Premature (1 wk)	3–35
		Newborn	3–12
		Adult	7–18
Uric acid	Serum	Child	2.0–5.5 mg/dL
		Adult: M	3.5–7.2
		F	2.6–6.0
Vitamin A	Serum	Newborn	35–75 mcg/dL
		Adult	30–65
Vitamin B_{12}	Serum	Newborn	175–800 pg/mL
		Adult	140–700
Vitamin C	Plasma		0.6–2.0 mg/mL
Vitamin E	Serum		5–20 mcg/mL
Volume	Whole blood	Premature	90–108 mL/kg
		Newborn	80–110
		Adult	72–100
	Plasma	Adult	49–59

* Endogenous creatinine clearance is expressed in mL/min and is corrected to average adult surface area of 1.73 m^2.

$$\frac{UV}{P} \times \frac{1.73}{A} = \text{mL/min}$$

† Higher in African Americans.

TABLE B-3. Urine Chemistries

Determination	Age/Sex	Normal Value
Catecholamines (24 h)	Infant	
	Norepinephrine	0–10 μg/d
	Epinephrine	0–2.5
	Adult	15–80
	Norepinephrine	
	Epinephrine	0.5–20
Chloride (24 h)	Infant	2–10 mmol/d
	Adult	110–250
	(varies greatly with Cl intake)	
Creatinine (24 h)	Infant	8–20 mg/kg/d
	Adult	14–26
	Pregnancy	Elevated
Homovanillic acid (HVA) (24 h)	Child	3–16 μg/mg creatinine
	Adult	<15 mg/d
17-Hydroxycorticosteroids (24 h)	0–1 y	0.5–1.0 mg/24 h
	Adult: M	3.0–10.0
	F	2.0–8.0
17-Ketogenic steroids (17-KGS) (24 h)	0–1 y	<1 mg/d
	Adult: M	5–23
	F	3–15
17-Ketosteroids (17-KS) (24 h)		
Zimmerman reaction	Infant	<1 mg/d
	Adult: M 18– 30 y	9–22
	>30 y	8–20
	F	6–15
	(decreases with age)	
Lead (24 h)		<80 μg/L
Osmolality (random)		50–1400 mOsmol/kg H_2O depending on fluid intake. After 12 h fluid restriction
		>850 mOsmol/kg H_2O
Porphyrins		34–234 μg/d
Coproporphyrin (24 h)		0–2.0 mg/d
Porphobilinogen (24 h)		1–14 mg/dL
Protein, total 24 h		50–80 mg/d (at rest)
		<250 mg/d after intense exercise
		<150 mg/dL (as glucose)
Reducing substances		
Specific gravity		
Random void		1.002–1.030
After 12-h fluid restriction		>1.025
24 h		1.015–1.025
Vanillylmandelic acid	Newborn	>1.0 mg/d
VMA	Infant	>2.0
(24 h)	Adult	2–7

From Fischbach, F. (1992). *A manual of laboratory and diagnostic tests.* (4th ed). Philadelphia: J. B. Lippincott.

APPENDIX C

Laboratory Data and Procedures to Assess the Prenatal Patient

Laboratory Test	Normal Nonpregnant Value	Normal Pregnant Value	Comments
Blood Tests			
Complete Blood Count (CBC)			
White blood cell count (WBC)	4500–10,000/mm^3	12,000–15,000/mm^3 (during pregnancy); 18,000–25,000/mm^3 (during delivery and immediate postpartum period)	WBCs are elevated during an infectious process, eclampsia, following hemorrhage, and in response in physiologic stress. Additional tests to detect infection should be performed to avoid unnecessary antibiotic therapy.
Red blood cell count (RBC)	4,000,000–5,000,000/mm^3	Increased 25–30%	By 6–8 wk of gestation there is progressive increase in blood plasma and RBC volume. It peaks at 28–32 wk and remains constant until delivery. Plasma volume increases 40–50% whereas red cell mass increases only 25–30%, resulting in dilutional (physiologic) anemia of pregnancy.
Hemoglobin	1–16 g/100 mL	11–13 g/100 mL at term; 11.5 g/100 mL mean in midpregnancy; 12.3 g/100 mL mean in late pregnancy	Hemoglobin value measures the body's capacity to transport oxygen. Anemia is diagnosed when the form value is 10.5 g/100 mL or under. The most common form is iron deficiency anemia.
Hematocrit	36–46%	32–39%	The percentage expresses the portion of the total blood volume occupied by the RBCs. This test is also used in the detection of anemia; a value of under 32% indicates anemia.
Red Cell Indices			
Mean corpuscular volume (MCV)	80–95 μm^3	Same	This index describes the size of the cell. A value under 80 is *microcytic*, or smaller than normal, as found in iron deficiency anemia, parasite infestation, or thalassemia. A value over 95 is *macrocytic*, or larger than normal.
Mean corpuscular hemoglobin concentration (MCHC)	32–36 g/dL	Same	This test measures the portion of each cell occupied by hemoglobin. A reading of over 39 g/dL occurs in only one condition, hereditary spherocytosis, a congenital abnormality of the cell wall. A decreased reading may indicate anemia.
Red cell morphology			This test measures variability in cell size and shape; the amount of blueness in the cells (amount of retained RNA); the presence of central pallor in the cells; other cells such as sickle cells, spherocytes, cells seen in thalassemia.
Platelets	140,000–450,000/mm^3	Same	
Coagulation factors Fibrinogen factor (I)	300 mg/dL	450 mg/dL	
Factors II, VII, VIII, IX, and X		Increased	Platelet counts are unchanged, but certain coagulation factors are altered as shown. Also called thrombocytes, the platelets contribute to hemostasis by forming platelet plugs at bleeding sites and promoting thrombin formation. They are formed in the bone marrow. A decrease in their production is never benign. Low levels are found in leukemia, disseminated intravascular coagulation (DIC), uremia, severe systemic infection, and bone marrow hypofunction.
Factors XI and XIII		Decreased	
Prothrombin time	11–12 s	Same	Despite alterations in blood factors II, VII, VIII, IX, X, XI, and XIII, prothrombin and bleeding times remain within the normal nonpregnant range.
Bleeding time	1–5 min	Same	

(continued)

Laboratory Data and Procedures to Assess the Prenatal Patient *(continued)*

Laboratory Test	Normal Nonpregnant Value	Normal Pregnant Value	Comments
Blood Tests			
Reticulocytes	0.5–1.5%	Increased	Reticulocytes are immature red blood cells that are released from the bone marrow in response to hemolysis, hemorrhage, or iron therapy for anemia. Reticulocytosis (increased production) may reach 3% in response to iron therapy in anemic pregnant women.
Erythrocyte sedimentation rate (ESR)	0–15 mm/h	Not valid in pregnancy	ESR is elevated during infection and helps to document chronic inflammatory processes in patients with vague symptoms. Higher levels of fibrinogen and plasma globulins in pregnancy make this test invalid.
Iron			
Serum iron	50–150 μg/dL	60–150 μg/dL	Low serum values usually result from insufficient intake of iron (iron deficiency anemia). Causes include repeated pregnancies, low-iron diet (especially in adolescents), heavy menses, pregnancy (600–900 mg iron is drained from the mother by the fetus), and IUD use.
Total iron-binding capacity (TIBC)	280–400 μg/dL	300–450 μg/dL	The ability of the RBCs to bind iron is increased in pregnancy because of maternal and fetal needs for iron. A simple formula to rule out iron deficiency anemia is: Serum iron ÷ TIBC = % saturation A result of ≤ 16% is diagnostic of iron deficiency anemia; such a result, in conjunction with mean corpuscular volume < 80, requires further study.
Serum Folate	1.9–14.0 ng/mL		Folate is essential for production of RNA and DNA. The fetus parasitizes large quantities from the mother. Combined iron and folate deficiency is common in pregnancy. Most prenatal vitamins now supply a folate supplemental dose of 1 mg.
Electrolytes			
Sodium	135–148 mEq/L	Increase in retention of 500–900 mEq/L over the norm	Aldosterone is the sodium-conserving hormone of the adrenal cortex. Its excretion is increased throughout pregnancy, causing cumulative total sodium retention. Urinary loss of sodium in late pregnancy is normal.
Potassium	3.5–5.3 mEq/dL	Same	Aldosterone is also potassium depleting. However, the increase in its production during pregnancy does not cause potassium wastage.
Chloride	102.7–107.0 mEq/L	98–108 mEq/L	There is no significant change.
Calcium	3.5–5.0 mg/dL	Increased	Increased intake is necessary to meet fetal requirements along with increased vitamin D to promote intestinal calcium absorption.
Phosphorus	2.5–4.5 mg/dL	Same	
Blood Chemistry			
Albumin	3.5–5.0 g/dL	3.0–4.2 g/dL	Albumin concentration falls quickly in the first 3 mo, then more slowly until late pregnancy. Decline in serum albumin below normal pregnancy levels is associated with preeclampsia.
Cholesterol		Desirable range 140–220 mg/dL Values vary with age, diet, exercise	Increased Double the prepregnancy level by 3rd trimester
Human chorionic gonadotropin (HCG)	None (placental hormone of pregnancy)	50,000–100,000 mIU/mL (early); 10,000–20,000 mIU/mL (late)	Concentration peaks at 10 wk of gestation, then declines and remains at this lower level until delivery. HCG sustains progesterone secretion in early pregnancy and is necessary for growth and preparation of endometrium for implantation. Levels that far exceed normal in conjunction with exaggerated pregnancy symptoms, large-for-dates uterus, bleeding, and absent fetal heart tones may indicate trophoblastic disease.

(continued)

Laboratory Data and Procedures to Assess the Prenatal Patient *(continued)*

Laboratory Test	Normal Nonpregnant Value	Normal Pregnant Value	Comments
Blood Tests			
Serum creatinine	0.8–1.4 mg/dL	0.9–2.0 mg/dL	Elevated levels may indicate kidney disease or pre-eclampsia.
Thyroid hormone T_3	100–200 ng/dL	25–35% decrease	T_3 is in lower concentrations than T_4 but is biologically more active and has a shorter serum half-life.
Thyroid hormone T_4	5.0–12.0 mcg/dL	5–10% increase	T_4 levels directly measure the thyroxine in serum. Increased T_3 levels and decreased T_4 levels may indicate hyper- or hypoactivity of the thyroid gland.
Hemoglobin electrophoresis (% of total hemoglobin)	Hgb A 95–97% Hgb A_2 2.0–3.5% Hgb F < 2%	Same	This test identifies hemoglobinopathies, such as sickle cell trait of disease, hemoglobin C disease, and thalassemia, by the changed ratios of the three types of normal hemoglobin. (*eg*, Hgb A_2 level > 3.5% is diagnostic of thalassemia.)
Glucose-6-phosphate dehydrogenase (G6PD) (IU/g)			G6PD is an enzyme that protects hemoglobin from denaturation. When activity of this enzyme is less than 25% of normal, hemolysis occurs. Drugs that can precipitate anemia are acetaminophen, aspirin, sulfa drugs, vitamin K, thiazides, Furadantin, and Macrodantin, and patients should be warned against their use. In pregnancy, when serum iron is normal but the patient is anemic, G6PD disease must be ruled out. Pregnancy complications include urinary tract infections, neonatal jaundice, hydrops fetalis, anemia.
Creatinine Blood urea nitrogen (BUN) Uric acid	0.6–1.2 4 mg/dL 13.0 ± 3.0 mg/dL 2.6–6.0 mg/dL	0.46–0.13 mg/dL 8.7 ± 1.5 mg/dL 2.5–4.0 mg/dL	Increase in GFR by 40–50% results in increased excretion of creatinine blood urea nitrogen and a decrease in uric acid.
Blood Sugar Levels Fasting 2-h postprandial	 75 mg/100 mL 120 mg/100 mL (upper limit)	 65 mg/100 mL 145 mg/100 mL (upper limit)	Screening for diabetes mellitus is done in pregnancy for all patients and is especially important when there is consistent spilling of glucose in the urine (glucosuria) or there is a family history of the disease or some other indicator of diabetes.
The normal values for this test are as follows: Oral glucose tolerance test	(see below)		Values that are abnormal in any two specimens constitute a positive test.

Hour	*Whole Blood* (mg/dL)	*Plasma* (mg/dL)	*Serum* (mg/dL)
0	90	103	100
1	165	188	200
2	145	165	150
3	125	143	130

Laboratory Test	Normal Nonpregnant Value	Normal Pregnant Value	Comments
Blood Group and Rh Factor	O, A, B, AB Rh+ Rh−	Same Same Same	If the mother has type O blood and her partner has type A, B, or AB, an ABO incompatibility may exist in the infant. The incidence of clinically significant incompatibility resulting in hemolytic disease in the infant is small. To prevent Rh immunization, screening will identify that 15% of the population that is Rh−. The presence of anti-D serum identifies the Rh immunized woman. All Rh negative women are given anti-D globulin after abortion, amniocentesis, or delivery of an RH+ infant and, prophylactically, in pregnancy in unsensitized women.
Rubella Titer	Depends on sensitization	Same	A result of less than 1.8 indicates that the patient is *not* immune to rubella. Such a patient should be advised to avoid exposure to the disease. If she is exposed, a titer should be obtained in 3–4 wk.
Serology or VDRL Test	Negative	Negative	A serology test is done to detect syphilis in the pregnant woman at the first prenatal visit. When positive, the VDRL screen is confirmed by an FTA-ABS test specific for syphilis.

(continued)

Laboratory Data and Procedures to Assess the Prenatal Patient *(continued)*

Laboratory Test	Normal Nonpregnant Value	Normal Pregnant Value	Comments
Urine Tests			
Urinalysis			
pH	4.5–7.5	Same	The pH test measures acidity or alkalinity of the urine. Levels below the norm indicate high fluid intake; levels above the norm indicate inadequate fluids and dehydration.
Color	Yellow	Same	
Specific gravity	1.010–1.020	Same	
Protein	Negative	Negative	Small amounts may occur from vaginal contamination and dehydration. Amounts of 2+ to 4+ may indicate urinary tract or kidney infection or preeclampsia.
Glucose	Negative	Negative or 1+	Urine that registers 1+ may result from decreased renal threshold and increased glomerular filtration rate in pregnancy. High levels of glucose may indicate high levels of blood sugar, gestational diabetes, or diabetes mellitus.
Ketones	Negative	Negative	Ketone bodies are products of fatty acids and fat metabolism. Fasting causes breakdown of fat when carbohydrates and protein are not available. Ketones may be deleterious to the fetus and should be avoided in pregnancy by regular eating habits.
Bilirubin	Negative	Negative	Bilirubin is a product of RBC destruction. Its presence in urine suggests liver or gallbladder disease.
Blood	Negative	Negative	Blood in urine suggests urinary tract infection, kidney disease, or vaginal contamination.
White Blood Cells	Negative	Negative	>5–10/high power field (HPF) may indicate urinary tract or vaginal infection.
Bacteria	Negative	Negative	Trace = rare; 1+ = 1–10/HPF; 2+ = 10–12/HPF; 3+ = innumerable; and 4+ = closely packed. Result greater than 4/HPF indicates urinary tract infection.
Casts	Negative	Negative	Casts are molds of the kidney tubules and may indicate kidney disease or excessive exercise.
Crystals	Few	Few	These compounds of various chemicals are found in most specimens.
Epithelial Cells	None	None	These are found when the specimen is contaminated by vaginal discharge. A clean-catch specimen should be obtained.
Urine Culture and Sensitivity	Negative	Negative	Specimens for urine cultures should be obtained by clean-catch only. The test cannot be accurately read and reported when contaminated with vaginal secretions. A colony count >100,000 (10^5) represents a positive culture and indicates urinary tract infection. The sensitivity of the infecting organism to various antibiotics is also reported.

From Blackburn, S., & Loper, D. (1992). *Maternal, fetal, and neonatal physiology.* Philadelphia: W. B. Saunders, and Fischbach, F. (1992). *A manual of laboratory and diagnostic tests.* (4th ed.). Philadelphia: J. B. Lippincott.

APPENDIX D

Conversion Tables

Table D-1. Temperature Conversion Table (Centigrade to Fahrenheit)

Celsius (C°)	Fahrenheit (F°)	Celsius (C°)	Fahrenheit (F°)
34.0	93.2	38.6	101.4
34.2	93.6	38.8	101.8
34.4	93.9	39.0	102.2
34.6	94.3	39.2	102.5
34.8	94.6	39.4	102.9
35.0	95.0	39.6	103.2
35.2	95.4	39.8	103.6
35.4	95.7	40.0	104.0
35.6	96.1	40.2	104.3
35.8	96.4	40.4	104.7
36.0	96.8	40.6	105.1
36.2	97.1	40.8	105.4
36.4	97.5	41.0	105.8
36.6	97.8	41.2	106.1
36.8	98.2	41.4	106.5
37.0	98.6	41.6	106.8
37.2	98.9	41.8	107.2
37.4	99.3	42.0	107.6
37.6	99.6	42.2	108.0
37.8	100.0	42.4	108.3
38.0	100.4	42.6	108.7
38.2	100.7	42.8	109.0
38.4	101.0	43.0	109.4

Conversion of Celsius (Centigrade) to Fahrenheit: 9/5 × temperature) + 32
Conversion of Fahrenheit to Celsius (Centigrade): (Temperature − 32) × 5/9

Table D-2. Pounds and Ounces to Grams Conversion Table

	Ounces															
Pounds	0	1	2	3	4	5	6	7	8	9	10	11	12	13	14	15
0	—	28	57	85	113	142	170	198	227	255	283	312	340	369	397	425
1	454	482	510	539	567	595	624	652	680	709	737	765	794	822	850	879
2	907	936	964	992	1021	1049	1077	1106	1134	1162	1191	1219	1247	1276	1304	1332
3	1361	1389	1417	1446	1474	1503	1531	1559	1588	1616	1644	1673	1701	1729	1758	1786
4	1814	1843	1871	1899	1928	1956	1984	2013	2041	2070	2098	2126	2155	2183	2211	2240
5	2268	2296	2325	2353	2381	2410	2438	2466	2495	2523	2551	2580	2608	2637	2665	2693
6	2722	2750	2778	2807	2835	2863	2892	2920	2948	2977	3005	3033	3062	3090	3118	3147
7	3175	3203	3232	3260	3289	3317	3345	3374	3402	3430	3459	3487	3515	3544	3572	3600
8	3629	3657	3685	3714	3742	3770	3799	3827	3856	3884	3912	3941	3969	3997	4026	4054
9	4082	4111	4139	4167	4196	4224	4252	4281	4309	4337	4366	4394	4423	4451	4479	4508
10	4536	4564	4593	4621	4649	4678	4706	4734	4763	4791	4819	4848	4876	4904	4933	4961
11	4990	5018	5046	5075	5103	5131	5160	5188	5216	5245	5273	5301	5330	5358	5386	5415
12	5443	5471	5500	5528	5557	5585	5613	5642	5670	5698	5727	5755	5783	5812	5840	5868
13	5897	5925	5953	5982	6010	6038	6067	6095	6123	6152	6180	6209	6237	6265	6294	6322
14	6350	6379	6407	6435	6464	6492	6520	6549	6577	6605	6634	6662	6690	6719	6747	6776
15	6804	6832	6860	6889	6917	6945	6973	7002	7030	7059	7087	7115	7144	7172	7201	7228
16	7257	7286	7313	7342	7371	7399	7427	7456	7484	7512	7541	7569	7597	7226	7654	7682
17	7711	7739	7768	7796	7824	7853	7881	7909	7938	7966	7994	8023	8051	8079	8108	8136
18	8165	8192	8221	8249	8278	8306	8335	8363	8391	8420	8448	8476	8504	8533	8561	8590
19	8618	8646	8675	8703	8731	8760	8788	8816	8845	8873	8902	8930	8958	8987	9015	9043
20	9072	9100	9128	9157	9185	9213	9242	9270	9298	9327	9355	9383	9412	9440	9469	9497
21	9525	9554	9582	9610	9639	9667	9695	9724	9752	9780	9809	9837	9865	9894	9922	9950
22	9979	10007	10036	10064	10092	10120	10149	10177	10206	10234	10262	10291	10319	10347	10376	10404

APPENDIX E

Known Teratogens That Cause Human Malformations

Teratogen	Classification	Effects on Embryo/Fetus
Drugs		
Testosterone	Male hormone	• May cause virilization of female fetus; ambiguous genitalia with hypertrophy of clitoris and fusion of labia
Estrogens diethylstilbestrol (DES), stilbestrol	Female hormone	• Cause a variety of genital malformations in female fetuses and some possible changes in males. Genital cancer may occur in female offspring of mothers who took DES during their pregnancy
Cyclophosphamide (Cytoxan, Endoxana)	Antineoplast and immunosuppressant (folic acid antagonist)	• Blocks synthesis of DNA, RNA, and protein. During first trimester of pregnancy, it is used only when potential benefits to mother outweigh hazards to fetus because it causes many major congenital deformities
Busulfan (Myleran)	Antineoplast (tumor-inhibiting)	• May cause skeletal deformities, corneal opacities, cleft palate, hypoplasia of organs, and stunted growth
Methotrexate (Amethopterin, Mexate)	Antineoplast	• Multiple skeletal deformities of face, skull, limbs, and vertebral column
Aminopterin	Antineoplast	• May result in death of conceptus during embryonic period. Multiple skeletal and other congenital malformations may occur if fetus survives
Phenytoin (Dilantin)	Anticonvulsant	• Causes fetal hydantoin syndrome: IUGR, mental retardation, microcephaly, inner epicanthic folds, ptosis of the eyelids, depressed nasal bridge, phalangeal hypoplasia
Warfarin (Coumadin)	Anticoagulant	• Nasal hypoplasia, mental retardation, microcephaly, optic atrophy, chondroplasia punctata
Lithium carbonate (Cibalith, Eskalith, Lithane, Lithobid)	Psychotropic drug (used to control manic episodes of manic–depressive psychosis)	• May cause a variety of malformations, particularly involving heart and great vessels
Thalidomide	Antiemetic in early pregnancy (no longer available)	• Absence of one or more limbs, meromelia and other limb deformities; and malformations of heart, gastrointestinal system, and external ear
Alcohol	Drug	• Fetal alcohol syndrome: IUGR, mental retardation, microcephaly, ocular anomalies, joint abnormalities, short palpebral fissures
Isotretinoin (Accutain)	Antiacne agent	• Causes a wide range of anomalies (CNS, CV, craniofacial defects, thymus gland abnormalities and microcephaly, hydrocephaly) and blindness
Ribavirin (Virazole)	Antiviral	• Malformation of skull, palate, eye, jaw and GI tract
Tetracycline	Antibiotic (Antiinfective)	• Hypoplastic tooth enamel; bone and tooth anomalies
Maternal Disease		
Herpesvirus	Infection	• Microcephaly, microphthalmia, retinal dysplasia, mental retardation
Rubella virus (German measles)	Infection	• Cataracts, cardiac malformations, deafness, glaucoma, chorioretinitis
Cytomegalovirus	Infection	• Abortion during embryonic period, IUGR, microphthalmia, chorioretinitis, blindness, microcephaly, mental retardation, deafness, cerebral palsy, cerebral calcifications, hepatosplenomegaly (enlargement of liver and spleen)
Toxoplasma gondii (contracted by eating raw or poorly cooked meat; infects cats; causes toxoplasmosis)	Protozoan infection (intracellular parasite)	• Oocyst of contaminated cat crosses human placenta, causing microcephaly, microphthalmia, hydrocephaly
Treponema pallidum (causes syphilis)	Spirochete infection	• Hydrocephaly, deafness, mental retardation, Hutchinson's teeth, saddle nose, poorly developed maxilla
Syphilis	Infection	• Deformed nails; osteochondritis at joints of extremities; abnormal epiphyses
Varicella zoster (chickenpox)	Infection	• Skin and muscle defects; limb abnormalities; eye anomalies
Diabetes mellitus	Carbohydrate intolerance	• CNS and cardiac defects
Phenylketonuria	Inborn error in metabolism	• Microcephaly; mental retardation
Chemical Agents		
Lead	Heavy metal	• CNS anomalies; mental retardation
Methyl mercury	Metal compound	• CNS anomalies; microcephaly blindness
Radiation		
High-level radiation therapy, radioiodine, atomic weapons	Radiation	• Microcephaly, mental retardation, skeletal deformities

APPENDIX F

Medications in Breast Milk

Drug or Agent	Contra-indicated	Prescribe With Caution	No Apparent Harm	Insufficient Information	Comment
Analgesics					
Acetaminophen			X		Small amounts excreted
Aspirin			X		Infant salicylate plasma level should be monitored if mother is on high chronic doses
Codeine			X		Small amount excreted
Propoxyphene (Darvon)			X		Small amount secreted
Morphine			X		Small amount secreted
Meperidine			X		Small amount secreted
Oxycodone			X		Small amount secreted
Methadone			X		Avoid breastfeeding 3–4 h after dose during peak level
Anticoagulants					
Ethyl biscoumacetate	X				Bleeding in infant
Phenindione	X				Bleeding in infant
Heparin			X		No passage into milk
Warfarin sodium (Coumadin)			X		
Bishydroxycoumarin (Dicumarol)		X			
Anticonvulsants					
Ethosuximide (Zarontin)			X		Milk levels close to maternal serum level. Do infant level
Phenobarbital			X		Accumulation may occur. Infant levels should be done
Primidone (Mysoline)			X		Possible drowsiness
Carbamazepine			X		Possible drowsiness; significant infant levels: no reported effects
Diphenylhydantoin (phenytoin, Dilantin)			X		Low levels in infant methemoglobinemia, one case Monitor level of infant sedation
Valproic acid			X		Small amounts excreted
Methimazole	X				Thyroid suppression
Bronchodilators					
Aminophylline (Theophylline)			X		Irritability, one case; rapidly absorbed
Iodides	X				Thyroid suppression
Sympathomimetics				X	Inhalers probably safe. Observe for excessive irritability, tremors, and tachycardia
Cardiovascular Agents					
Atenolol (Tenormin)			X		Secreted in small to moderate amounts
Digoxin			X		Insignificant levels
Propranolol			X		Insignificant levels
Reserpine	X				Nasal stuffiness, lethargy
Guanethidine (Ismelin)				X	Insignificant levels
Methyldopa (Aldomet)				X	
Quinidine				X	Insignificant levels; potential accumulation and thrombocytopenia
Verapimil (Isoptin)		X			Insignificant levels

(continued)

Medications in Breast Milk *(continued)*

Drug or Agent	Contra-indicated	Prescribe With Caution	No Apparent Harm	Insufficient Information	Comment
Cathartics					
Anthraquinones	X				Diarrhea, cramps
Aloe, senna		X			Safe in moderate doses
Bulk agent, softeners			X		
Contraceptives, Oral					
Diethylstilbestrol	X				Possible vaginal cancer
Depo-Provera		X			May affect lactation at 300 mg IM, not at 150 mg
Noresthisterone		X			May affect lactation
Ethyl estradiol		X			May affect lactation
Levonogestrel (NORPLANT)				X	Insufficient data on infants in first 6 weeks of life. Steroids are not considered first choice of contraception for lactating women.
Diuretics					
Chlorthalidone				X	Low levels, but may accumulate
Thiazides		X			May affect lactation; low levels in milk
Spironolactone			X		Insignificant levels
					Avoid in first month of lactation
Ergot Alkaloids					
Bromocriptine	X				Lactation suppressed
Ergot	X				Vomiting, diarrhea, seizures
Ergotamine	X				Vomiting, diarrhea, seizures
Ergonovine	X				Brief postpartum course may be safe; insignificant levels
Methylergonovine	X				Brief postpartum course may be safe, insignificant levels
Hormones					
Corticosteroids				X	Low levels with short-term prednisone or prednisolone
					Avoid feeding for 4 h after dose
Sex hormones (see Contraceptive, Oral above)					
Thyroid (T_3, T_4)			X		Levels too low to interfere with neonatal thyroid screening; excreted in milk
Insulin			X		Not absorbed in breast milk
ACTH			X		Not absorbed in breast milk
Epinephrine			X		Not absorbed in breast milk
Antihistamines					
Diphenylhydantoin (Benadryl)		X			Small amounts excreted; increased sensitivity of newborn to antihistamines
Trimeprazine (Temaril)			X		Small amounts secreted
Tripelennamine (Pyribenzamine)			X		Small amounts secreted
Clemastine (Tavist)	X				Neck stiffness, irritability in neonate when combined with phenytoin
Antiinfective Agents					
Most antiinfective agents can cause (1) modification of bowel flora, (2) possible allergic sensitization, (3) interference with culture results, and (4) potential drug accumulation owing to infant's immature liver enzymes systems and renal elimination pathways.			X		

(continued)

Medications in Breast Milk *(continued)*

Drug or Agent	Contra-indicated	Prescribe With Caution	No Apparent Harm	Insufficient Information	Comment
Antiinfective Agents					
Aminoglycosides (kanamycin, gentamicin)					Significant secretion in milk; not absorbed
Chloramphenicol	X				Bone marrow depression; gastrointestinal and behavioral effects
Clindamycin			X		Small amounts secreted
Erythromycin			X		No adverse effects
Penicillins and cephalosporins			X		Possible sensitization
Sulfonamides		X			Hemolysis, G6PD deficiency; bilirubin displacement, avoid premature infants
Tetracyclines			X		Limited absorption by infant
Nalidixic acid		X			Hemolysis in G6PD; low levels in milk
Nitrofurantoin		X			Possible G6PD hemolysis
Metronidazole (Flagyl)		X			Give single 2-g dose for trichomonas and continue breastfeeding for 24–48 h. Low absorption but potentially toxic
Isoniazid		X			High levels in milk, possible toxicity
Pyramethamine	X				Vomiting, marrow depression, convulsions
Chloroquine			X		Not excreted
Trimethoprim		X			Thrombocytopenia; avoid in G6PD deficiency
Aspirin			X		Perform infant salicylate plasma levels if mother is on high chronic doses
Indomethacin		X			Seizures, 1 case
Phenylbutazone		X			Low levels, possible blood dyscrasia
Gold	X				Found in infant: nephritis, hepatitis, hematologic changes
Ibuprofen			X		Small amounts secreted
Naproxen			X		Small amounts secreted
Naproxen sodium			X		Small amounts secreted
Steroids				X	Low levels with prednisone and prednisolone; avoid feeding for 4 h after the dose
Antineoplastic Agents					
Azathioprine		X			Low levels of mercaptopurine in milk when mothers took 75–100 mg in 3 infants
Cisplatin	X				Potentially carcinogenic
Cyclophosphamide	X				Neutropenia
Doxorubicin	X				Possible immune suppression
Methotrexate	X				Very small excretion; may accumulate
Antithyroid Agents					
Radioactive iodine	X				Thyroid suppression
Propylthiouracil	X				Thyroid suppression
Narcotics					
Codeine			X		In usual doses
Meperidine (Demerol)			X		Small amounts excreted
Morphine			X		Low infant levels on usual dosage
Heroin	X				Addiction and withdrawal in infants
Methadone		X			Minimal levels
Oxycodone			X		Small amount excreted
Psychotherapeutic Agents					
Alprazolam (Xanax)				X	If used, monitor infant for poor feeding and drowsiness

(continued)

Medications in Breast Milk *(continued)*

Drug or Agent	Contra-indicated	Prescribe With Caution	No Apparent Harm	Insufficient Information	Comment
Psychotherapeutic Agents					
Lithium	X				High levels in milk (40% of maternal serum level)
Phenothiazines		X			Drowsiness; chronic effects uncertain
Tricyclic antidepressants				X	Low levels; effects uncertain
Diazepam (Valium)	X				Lethargy, weight loss, EEG changes; may accumulate
Meprobamate (Equanil)	X				High levels in milk; 2–4 times that of maternal plasma
Chlordiazepoxide (Librium)	X				Low levels in milk but can accumulate, especially in neonates
Radiopharmaceuticals					
^{131}I	X				No breastfeeding for 72 h
Technetium (Tc-99^{M})	X				No breastfeeding for 48 h
^{131}I albumin	X				No breastfeeding for 10 d
Sedatives–Hypnotics					
Barbiturates		X			Short-acting, some drowsiness
Chloral hydrate		X			Drowsiness; 50–100% of maternal blood level
Bromides	X				Depression, rash
Diazepam (Valium)	X				Depression, weight loss
Flurazepam	X			X	Chemically related to diazepam
Nitrazepam				X	
Social–Recreational Drugs					
Alcohol			X		Milk levels equal plasma; moderate consumption apparently safe; high levels inhibit lactation; may cause sedation
Caffeine			X		Jitteriness with very high intakes
Nicotine			X		Low levels in milk
Marijuana (dronabinol)			X		Minimal passage in milk; THC can reach high levels with heavy use
Phencyclipine	X				Concentrates in milk
Cocaine	X				One case of cocaine intoxication
Miscellaneous					
Atropine		X			May cause constipation or inhibit lactation
Cyclosporine	X				May cause immunosuppression
Dihydrotachysterol		X			Renal calcification in animals; hypercalcemia in infant
Etretinate	X				Manufacturer considers use contraindicated owing to potential adverse effects
Isotretinoin (Accutane)	X				Manufacturer considers use contraindicated owing to potential adverse effects
Tretinoin (Retin-A)				X	Minimal topical absorption

From Committee on Drugs. (1989). Transfer of drugs and other chemicals into human milk. *Pediatrics, 84*(5), 924–936, and Lauwers, J., & Woessner, C. (1990). *Chemical agents and breast milk.* Garden City Park, NY: Avery Publications.

APPENDIX G

Nursing Diagnoses, North American Nursing Diagnosis Association, 1992 to 1993

Activity Intolerance
Activity Intolerance, High Risk for
Adjustment, Impaired
Airway Clearance, Ineffective
Anxiety
Aspiration, High Risk for
Body Image Disturbance
Body Temperature, High Risk for Altered
Breastfeeding, Effective
Breastfeeding, Ineffective
Breastfeeding, Interrupted*
Breathing Pattern, Ineffective
Cardiac Output, Decreased
Caregiver Role Strain*
Caregiver Role Strain, High Risk for*
Communication, Impaired Verbal
Constipation
Constipation, Colonic
Constipation, Perceived
Coping, Defensive
Coping, Ineffective Individual
Decisional Conflict (Specify)
Denial, Ineffective
Diarrhea
Disuse Syndrome, High Risk for
Diversional Activity Deficit
Dysreflexia
Family Coping: Compromised, Ineffective
Family Coping: Disabling, Ineffective
Family Coping: Potential for Growth
Family Processes, Altered
Fatigue
Fear
Fluid Volume Deficit
Fluid Volume Deficit, High Risk for
Fluid Volume Excess
Gas Exchange, Impaired
Grieving, Anticipatory
Grieving, Dysfunctional
Growth and Development, Altered
Health Maintenance, Altered
Health-Seeking Behaviors (Specify)
Home Maintenance Management, Impaired
Hopelessness
Hyperthermia
Hypothermia
Incontinence, Bowel
Incontinence, Functional
Incontinence, Reflex
Incontinence, Stress
Incontinence, Total
Incontinence, Urge
Infant Feeding Pattern, Ineffective*
Infection, High Risk for
Injury High Risk for
Knowledge Deficit (Specify)
Noncompliance (Specify)
Nutrition, Altered: Less than Body Requirements
Nutrition, Altered: More than Body Requirements
Nutrition, Altered: Potential for More than Body Requirements
Oral Mucous Membrane, Altered
Pain
Pain, Chronic
Parental Role Conflict
Parenting, Altered
Parenting, High Risk for Altered
Peripheral Neurovascular Dysfunction, High Risk for*
Personal Identity Disturbance
Physical Mobility, Impaired
Poisoning, High Risk for
Post-Trauma Response
Powerlessness
Protection, Altered
Rape Trauma Syndrome
Rape Trauma Syndrome: Compound Reaction
Rape Trauma Syndrome: Silent Reaction
Relocation Stress Syndrome*
Role Performance, Altered

Self-Care Deficit
- Bathing/Hygiene
- Feeding
- Dressing/Grooming
- Toileting

Self-Esteem, Chronic Low
Self-Esteem, Situational Low
Self-Esteem Disturbance
Self-Mutilation, High Risk for*
Sensory-Perceptual Alterations (Specify) (visual, auditory, kinesthetic, gustatory, tactile, olfactory)
Sexual Dysfunction
Sexuality Patterns, Altered
Skin Integrity, High Risk for Impaired
Skin Integrity, Impaired
Sleep Pattern Disturbance
Social Interaction, Impaired
Social Isolation
Spiritual Distress
Suffocation, High Risk for
Swallowing, Impaired
Therapeutic Regimen, Ineffective Management of*
Thermoregulation, Ineffective
Thought Processes, Altered
Tissue Integrity, Impaired
Tissue Perfusion, Altered (Specify Type) (renal, cerebral, cardiopulmonary, gastrointestinal, peripheral)
Trauma, High Risk for
Unilateral Neglect
Urinary Elimination, Altered
Urinary Retention
Ventilation, Inability to Sustain Spontaneous*
Ventilatory Weaning Response, Dysfunctional*
Violence, High Risk for: Self-Directed or Directed at Others

* New diagnoses from 1992 conference.

Glossary

abortion Termination of pregnancy before viability of the fetus (which begins between 20 and 24 weeks)
complete Abortion in which all the products of conception have been expelled
habitual Spontaneous abortion occurring in third or subsequent consecutive pregnancies
incomplete Abortion in which some portions of the products of conception are retained in the uterus
induced Intentional abortion by consumption of drugs, removal of the products of conception by suction, or injection of drugs into the amniotic sac
inevitable Impending abortion in presence of bleeding, pain, and dilatation and effacement of the cervix
missed Condition in which the embryo dies in utero and the products of conception are retained in the uterus
septic Infected abortion in which infective organisms disseminate into the maternal circulatory system
spontaneous Spontaneous expulsion of the products of conception before the 20th week of gestation
therapeutic Legally and medically sanctioned interruption of pregnancy before the 20th week of gestation
threatened Condition in which intrauterine bleeding occurs in early pregnancy; the cervix does not dilate and the products of conception are not necessarily expelled

abortus A fetus that spontaneously delivers at less than 21 weeks gestational age and weighs less than 600 g

abruptio placentae Complete or partial separation of the normally implanted placenta from the uterine wall (synonym: abruption)

abruption See **abruptio placentae**

abscess Localized collection of pus resulting from disintegration of tissue in any part of the body

abstinence Abstention from sexual intercourse

acetonuria Presence of acetone bodies in the urine from ketosis of diabetes or starvation

acidosis Excessive acidity of body fluids due to accumulation of acids or loss of bicarbonate, resulting in lowered pH

acini cells Milk-secreting cells of the breast

acquaintance Process of getting to know the newborn; includes bonding and initial attachment

acrocyanosis Cyanosis of the extremities in most infants at birth; may persist for 7 to 10 days

acrosome Head of the spermatozoon

adnexa Accessory parts of the uterus: fallopian tubes and ovaries

aerobes Microorganisms that live and grow in oxygen

afibrinogenemia A blood disorder that results from the absence or decrease of fibrinogen in the blood plasma, which becomes incoagulable; the acquired type may occur in obstetric practice when abruptio placentae or retention of a dead fetus occurs

afterbirth Placenta and membranes that are expelled after birth of a child

afterpains Uterine contractions that cause pain during the first few days after childbirth

AGA Appropriate (weight) for gestational age

agenesis Absence of an organ

AIDS Acquired immunodeficiency syndrome; see **HIV**

albuminuria Presence of albumin in the urine

alkalosis Increase in pH of the body fluids

alleles Different forms of a gene that can occupy the same locus on homologous chromosomes

alveolar surface tension Cohesive force exerted by intermolecular attraction in the surface layer of fluid lining the alveolar walls; the force exerted results in a constant tendency for contraction of the surface fluid layer and collapse of alveoli

amenorrhea Absence of menstruation, primary or secondary

amniocentesis Insertion of a needle through the abdominal wall into the uterus and amniotic cavity to withdraw amniotic fluid by syringe

amnion Membrane that forms the lining of the amniotic sac; fetal membranes

amnionitis Inflammation of the inner layer of the fetal membranes

amniotic fluid Transparent fluid contained in the amnion that protects the fetus and maintains its temperature

amniotomy Artificial rupture of the amniotic sac or bag of waters

anaerobic Pertaining to microorganisms that can live and grow in the absence of oxygen

androgen Male hormone; the substance that produces or stimulates male characteristics

android pelvis Male type of the bony pelvis

anemia Condition in which number of red blood cells and hemoglobin concentration are reduced

anencephaly Congenital absence of brain and spinal cord

anesthesia Partial or complete loss of sensation with or without loss of consciousness

general anesthesia Pharmacologic pain relief measures that produce progressive central nervous system depression, loss of consciousness, and thus loss of sensation from the entire body

local anesthesia Pharmacologic pain relief measures that block sensory nerve pathways at the organ level, producing loss of sensation in that organ only

regional anesthesia Pharmacologic pain relief measures that block sensory nerve pathways along large sensory nerves from an organ and surrounding tissue, providing loss of sensation in that organ and the surrounding area

anomaly Marked deviation from the norm; a malformation in an organ or structure

anorexia Loss of appetite

anovulatory cycle Menstrual cycle in which menstrual flow was not preceded by discharge of an ovum

anoxia Deficiency of oxygen

anteflexion Bending forward of the uterus

antenatal Occurring before birth

antepartal Occurring before the onset of labor

antibody titer Level of circulating antibody, measured per designated volume

antidiuresis Suppression of urine secretion

antiemetic Substance that prevents or alleviates nausea and vomiting

antigen Foreign substance introduced into the body that stimulates the immune system to form antibodies

antipyretic Agent that reduces fever

antiseptic Agent that prevents the growth or arrests the development of microorganisms

anuria Failure of the kidney to produce urine

anus Distal end of the large intestine and the outlet of the rectum

Apgar score System of numerical evaluation of neonate's condition at 1 minute and 5 minutes after birth; the maximum score is 10, and the higher the score the better the condition of the neonate

apnea Cessation of respirations

ARC AIDS-related complex; a cluster of severe physical symptoms that may occur in individuals who have been infected by HIV

areola Ring of dark pigment surrounding the nipple

ascites Accumulation of serous fluid within the abdominal cavity

asepsis Absence of infective organisms

aseptic technique Method used to prevent transmission of pathogenic organisms

asphyxia Condition caused by a lack of oxygen in the blood

aspiration Act of inhaling; in the neonate, aspiration of mucus, meconium, or stomach contents into the lungs may result in atelectasis or pneumonia

atelectasis Incomplete expansion of the lung or a portion of the lung

atony Lack of normal muscle tone or strength (eg, in uterine musculature)

atresia Congenital absence or closure of a normal body opening

atrial septal defect Congenital cardiac defect in which there is an abnormal opening between the atria of the heart

attachment Affiliative tie formed after a period of mutual stimulation and response

attitude Relationship of fetal parts to each other; the most common fetal attitude in utero is flexion, where the fetal head is bent onto the chest, the back is curved forward, and the arms and legs are folded in front of the body (fetal position)

auscultation Listening for sounds within the body, that is, listening for fetal heart tones with a fetoscope

autosome Any of the 22 ordinary paired chromosomes, that is, a chromosome other than either of the two sex chromosomes

azoospermia Absence of spermatozoa in the semen

bacteremia Presence of bacteria in the blood

bacteriuria Presence of bacteria in the urine

bag of waters Amnion, or the membranes enclosing the amniotic fluid and the fetus

ballottement Technique of palpation used to detect a floating object in the body; in pregnancy it is the rebound of a fetal part when displaced by a light tap of the finger through the abdominal wall or vagina

Bandl's ring Abnormal, ringlike thickening at the junction of the upper and lower uterine segment that may obstruct delivery of the infant

Barr body Material in the inactivated one of the two female (X) chromosomes in each body cell of normal females

Bartholin's glands Small, mucous-secreting glands located at either side of the base of the vagina

basal body temperature Temperature when body metabolism is at its lowest; used as an indirect method of determining whether ovulation has occurred (measurement in tenths of degrees is used to determine slight differences in temperature)

baseline fetal heart rate Average fetal heart rate within a

10-minute interval in the absence of or between contractions; normal baseline rate is 120 to 160 beats per minute

bearing down Reflex effort on the part of the woman to coordinate activity of the abdominal muscles with the uterine contractions

bicornuate uterus Uterus in which the fundus is divided into two parts

bilirubin Yellowish pigment in bile produced from the hemoglobin of the red blood cells

bilirubinemia Presence of an abnormal amount of bilirubin in the blood when red blood cells are broken down from a pathologic cause

bimanual examination Pelvic examination performed with both hands; the first two fingers of one hand are placed in the vagina while the other hand is placed on the abdomen

biophysical profile Prenatal surveillance of the fetus at risk by use of tests of fetal well-being, such as nonstress test, contraction stress test, fetal movement

biparietal diameter Largest transverse diameter of the fetal head; usually about 9.5 cm

birth Passage of the fetus from the uterus

birth defect Congenital anomaly

birth rate Number of live births per year for each 1000 individuals in the population

bisexuality Sexual attraction to members of both sexes

blastocyst Structure that results when fluid accumulates within the morula, producing a cavity with the inner cell mass at one pole

blastomere Cell that results from the cleavage of a fertilized ovum

blastula Stage of the fertilized ovum in which the cells are arranged in a hollow ball

blighted ovum Ovum with abnormal development

bloody show Blood-tinged mucous discharge from the vagina that accompanies dilatation of the cervix in early labor

bonding Initial phase in a relationship thought to be characterized by strong attraction and desire to interact

brachial palsy Paralysis of the arm from injury to the brachial plexus during birth

bradycardia Heartbeat slower than 60 beats per minute

Braxton Hicks contractions Painless intermittent contraction of the uterus during pregnancy that may be noticeable on abdominal palpation; may be perceived by the pregnant woman as painless tightening of the uterus

breakthrough bleeding Vaginal bleeding or spotting occurring between periods. In women using oral contraceptives, a result of the estrogen in the pill being inadequate to maintain the endometrium

breast pump Electric or manual pump used to extract milk from the lactating breast

breech birth Birth in which the buttocks or feet present first

broad ligament Fibrous sheath covered by peritoneum extending from each side of the uterus to the lateral wall of the pelvis

bulbourethral glands Two small glands lying along the membranous urethra of the male, just above the bulb of the corpus spongiosum (synonym: Cowper's glands)

Caldwell-Moloy classification Classification of pelves into four types: anthropoid, gynecoid, android, and platypelloid

calorie Unit of heat

Candida Yeastlike fungus that is common inhabitant of the skin, nails, mouth, and vagina; susceptibility to vaginal candidiasis increases during pregnancy because of changes in vaginal pH and increased levels of glycogen in the vaginal epithelium

capacitation Process in which the surface characteristics of sperm cells change and enzymes are released, particularly hyaluronidase; these surface changes contribute to the sperm's ability to penetrate the ovum

caput succedaneum Swelling produced on the fetal head during labor

cardiomegaly Pathologic enlargement of the heart

carrier Person who has two different forms of a particular gene (one normal and one mutant) at a given locus on a pair of homologous chromosomes (synonym: heterozygote)

caudal Pertaining to a taillike structure

cephalad Toward the head

cephalhematoma Localized collection of blood beneath the periosteum of the newborn skull caused by disruption of blood vessels during birth

cephalic Pertaining to the head, or directed toward the head

cephalopelvic disproportion (CPD) Condition in which the infant's head is of a shape, size, or position that prevents it from passing through the mother's pelvis; the most common indication for cesarean delivery

cerclage Encircling of the cervix with a suture

cervical intraepithelial neoplasia (CIN) Abnormal condition of cell growth in the cervix, formerly called dysplasia, which is the precursor to carcinoma

cervical mucus Secretion of the columnar cells lining the endocervical canal

cervicitis Inflammation of the uterine cervix

cervix Lower portion of the uterus extending from the internal to the external cervical os

cesarean delivery Extraction of the fetus, placenta, and membranes through an incision in the abdominal wall

Chadwick's sign Bluish discoloration of the vaginal wall and vestibule; a presumptive sign of pregnancy

cheilosis Reddened appearance and fissures at the angles of the lips; seen frequently in vitamin B deficiency

chlamydia Caused by the organism *Chlamydia trachomatis*, this sexually transmitted disease is the most preva-

lent STD in the United States; as a sexual pathogen it is associated with a wide variety of adverse reproductive consequences

chloasma Skin change in pregnancy characterized by the appearance of irregular brownish patches on the face (synonym: mask of pregnancy)

chorioamnionitis Inflammation of the chorion and amnion

chorion Outer wall of the amniotic sac; composed of trophoblast and mesenchyme

chorionic plate The portion of the chorion attached to the placenta

chorionic villi Slender, branching projections of the chorion containing capillaries that are the means by which all substances (nutrients, gases, waste products) are exchanged between the maternal and fetal circulation

chorionic villi sampling (CVS) Aspiration of chorionic villi from the uterus during the first trimester for testing of chromosomal and medical disorders

chorioretinitis Inflammation of the choroid and retina of the eye

chromosome One of several microscopic rod-shaped bodies within the nucleus of a dividing cell that contain the hereditary material (genes) of the organism; the total chromosome number in human beings is 46: females have 44 autosomes plus two X chromosomes; males have 44 autosomes plus one X and one Y chromosome

chromosome disorder Abnormality of chromosome number or structure

circumcision Removal of all or part of the prepuce, or the foreskin, in the male infant

cleavage Process by which the zygote divides into blastomeres

cleft lip Congenital fissure of the lip

clinical nurse specialist A registered nurse who has become expert in a defined area of knowledge and practice in nursing at the graduate level

clitoris Small, cylindrical, erectile body in the female that is homologous to the male penis

clonus Spasmodic contraction and relaxation

coitus Sexual intercourse; copulation

colostrum Breast fluid secreted 2 or 3 days after childbirth and before the onset of true lactation

colposcope Magnifying instrument inserted into the vagina to view the tissues of the vagina and cervix

colpotomy Incision into the wall of the vagina

conception Fertilization of the ovum by the sperm

conceptus Products of conception

condom Thin, flexible sheath worn over the penis during sexual intercourse to prevent deposition of sperm into the vagina

condyloma Sexually transmitted, viral, wartlike growth on the skin of the genitals

confidentiality Implies that a private and personal relationship exists between the provider and the client

congenital Present at birth

congenital anomaly Abnormality present at birth

consanguinity Blood relationship to another person

constipation Difficult defecation

contraception Prevention of conception

contraction Periodic, rhythmic tightening of the uterine musculature during labor that effaces and dilates the cervix and, in concert with maternal pushing effort, expels the fetus

contraction stress test Stimulation of the uterine muscles by use of oxytocin to assess fetal oxygen reserves before labor

contracture of the pelvis Reduction in size of the bony pelvis so that a fetus of normal size cannot pass through; contracture may be general or at the inlet, midpelvis, or outlet

convulsion Paroxysm of involuntary muscle contractions and relaxations

Coombs' test Test used to detect sensitized red blood cells in erythroblastosis fetalis

copulation Sexual intercourse

cord prolapse Obstetric emergency in which the umbilical cord descends into or through the cervix ahead of the presenting fetal part, making it vulnerable to compression and resulting in diminished fetal oxygenation

coronal suture Membrane-occupied spaces between the bones of the infant's head that extend transversely from the anterior fontanelle and lie between the parietal and frontal bones

corpus luteum Solid yellow body that develops within a ruptured ovarian follicle; an endocrine structure, it primarily secretes progesterone

cotyledon Segment or subdivision of the uterine surface of the placenta

Couvelaire uterus Uterus with blood forced within the uterine walls between the muscle fibers; the condition may accompany premature separation of the placenta

Cowper's glands Two small glands lying along the membranous urethra of the male, just above the bulb of the corpus spongiosum (synonym: bulbourethral glands)

cradle cap Seborrheic dermatitis of the newborn that appears on the head, scalp, and face of the newborn

crisis Sudden change in condition; a turning point during which disorganization occurs because normal coping mechanisms fail

crowning Distention of the perineum by the largest diameter of the presenting part; in a normal vertex presentation, this would be the biparietal diameter

crown–rump length An estimate of fetal gestational age based on measurement from the top of the head (crown) to the buttocks

cryptorchidism Condition in which testicles are undescended

cues Signals expressed behaviorally and verbally

cul-de-sac Extension of the peritoneal cavity lying be-

tween the rectum and the posterior wall of the uterus (synonym: pouch of Douglas, rectouterine pouch)

culdocentesis Aspiration of fluid from the pouch of Douglas by puncture of the posterior vaginal fornix

culdoscopy Visual examination of the female pelvic viscera through the posterior vaginal fornix by means of an endoscope

cultural relativism Practice of judging a group or its traits by its own or similar standards

cunnilingus Oral sexual stimulation of the female genitals

curettage Scraping of the inner surface of the uterus with a curet to remove its lining or contents

cystitis Infection of the urinary bladder

cystocele Bladder hernia protruding into the vagina; usually occurs after repeated childbirth

cytomegalovirus (CMV) Group of herpesviruses that may cause disease in the newborn if the mother is infected

cytotrophoblast Inner layer of trophoblast cells that is bathed in maternal blood for passage of nutrients, oxygen, and gases to the fetus and for removal of its waste products

decidua Endometrium of the uterus enveloping the impregnated ovum

delivery Expulsion of the fetus, placenta, and membranes at birth

demand feeding Practice of allowing the infant to determine the frequency of feeding and amount of milk ingested, as opposed to the imposition of rigid time schedules for feeding by adult caregivers

descent Passage of the presenting part of the fetus into and through the birth canal; begins at the onset of labor and proceeds during effacement and dilatation of the cervix

development Gradual advance in the process of total human growth with emphasis on behavioral aspects of functioning

developmental task Step, stage, or phase in the process of growth that is sequential and prerequisite to further growth

dextroversion Deviation of the uterus from its normal position to the right side

diagonal conjugate measurement Chief internal pelvic measurement made to determine the approximate diameter of the pelvic passage; it is the distance between the sacral promontory and the lower margin of the symphysis pubis

diaphoresis Profuse perspiration

diaphragm, pelvic Muscles and fascia providing primary support to the pelvic viscera

diastasis recti Separation of the abdominal recti muscles; may occur during pregnancy because of stretching of the abdominal wall

dilatation Opening or enlargement; the cervical canal dilates from a few centimeters to 10 cm in diameter during labor (synonym: dilation)

dilatation and curettage Procedure in which the uterine cervix is dilated and the endometrium of the uterus is scraped away; performed for diagnostic or therapeutic purposes, to remove the products of conception after incomplete abortion, and for therapeutic abortion

disseminated intravascular coagulation (DIC) A pathologic form of coagulation, diffuse throughout the body, in which certain clotting factors are consumed to the extent that generalized bleeding occurs

diuresis Increased secretion of urine

dizygotic twins Twins resulting from two fertilized ova; dizygotic twins have different genetic constitutions and may be of the same or different sex

Doderlein's bacillus Normal inhabitant of the vagina that helps to maintain its acidic pH (synonym: *Lactobacillus acidophilus*)

dominant trait Trait that is clinically expressed in both homozygous and heterozygous individuals

Doppler ultrasound sensor Device used to monitor fetal heart rate

Down syndrome Congenital condition characterized by mental retardation and multiple physiologic defects

Dubowitz tool Method of estimating gestational age of a newborn based on 21 strictly defined clinical signs

ductus arteriosus Channel between the fetal aorta and the main pulmonary artery; it is usually closed by normal neonatal respiratory function and may be medically or surgically treated if it remains open after birth

ductus venosus Fetal blood vessel that connects the umbilical vein and the inferior vena cava

dysgenesis Abnormal or defective development of the embryo

dysmenorrhea Painful menstruation

dyspareunia Painful intercourse

dysplasia Abnormal development of tissue

dyspnea Labored breathing

dystocia Difficult labor resulting from fetal or maternal causes

dysuria Painful urination

early withdrawal bleeding Vaginal bleeding or spotting associated with oral contraceptives that begins during active pill taking and continues into the inactive or pill-free interval

ecchymosis A form of macula that appears in large, irregularly formed hemorrhagic areas of the skin and results from extravasation of blood into the skin's mucous membrane; a bruise

eclampsia Toxemia of pregnancy accompanied by high blood pressure, albuminuria, oliguria, tonic and clonic convulsions, and coma; may occur before, during, or after childbirth

ectoderm Outer layer of the embryo; it develops into the epidermis and neural tube

ectopic pregnancy Implantation of the ovum outside of the uterine cavity (eg, in the fallopian tube or abdomen)

ectopy Displacement or placement in an abnormal position

edema Excessive accumulation of fluid in the tissues

effacement Softening, thinning, and shortening of the cervical canal as it is drawn up into the body of the uterus by labor contractions

effleurage Light, rhythmic stroking of the abdomen during labor; useful for enhancing relaxation

ejaculation Sudden emission of semen from the urethra that occurs during sexual intercourse or masturbation

embolus Clot or other plug carried by a blood vessel and blocking a smaller one

embryo Stage of human development occurring between the ovum and the fetal stages, or from 2 to 8 weeks after conception

emesis Vomiting

en face Position in which mother and infant are face-to-face with eye-to-eye contact

endemic disease Disease with a low mortality rate occurring continuously in a particular population

endocervix Membrane lining the canal of the uterine cervix

endocrine Pertaining to an organ or gland that secretes a hormone into the bloodstream to induce a specific effect on another organ

endogenous Pertaining to anything produced by or arising from within a cell or organism

endometrial biopsy Diagnostic procedure in which a sample of endometrial tissue is obtained

endometrial cycle An integrated evolutionary process of endometrial growth and regression that is repeated up to 300 to 400 times during a woman's adult life

endometriosis Pathologic condition in which normal tissue that lines the uterus (endometrial tissue) grows outside of the uterus, often around the fallopian tubes, contributing to infertility

endometritis Inflammation of the endometrium

endometrium Mucous membrane lining the uterus (during pregnancy it is known as the decidua)

endoscope Illuminated optical instrument used to visualize the interior of a body cavity or hollow organ

endotoxin Toxin confined within bacteria and freed when the bacteria are broken down

engagement Point in labor at which the widest diameter of the fetal presenting part passes through the pelvic inlet

engorgement Hyperemia; local congestion; excessive fullness, for example, of the breast

epididymis Organ made up of long, coiled seminiferous tubules; it provides for storage, transit, and maturation of sperm

epidural anesthesia Anesthesia of the pelvis, abdomen, or genital area achieved by injection of a local anesthetic into the epidural space of the spinal column

episiotomy Incision into the perineum and vagina during delivery to enlarge the vaginal opening to prevent tearing of the underlying fascia and muscle as the neonate's head is born

Erb's palsy Partial paralysis of the upper brachial plexus caused by traumatic injury during childbirth, often from forcible traction during delivery

erectile tissue Vascular tissue, such as that in the penis, clitoris, and nipples, that becomes erect when filled with blood

erotic Tending to arouse sexual desire

erythema Inflammation of the skin or mucous membrane resulting from the dilatation and congestion of superficial capillaries

erythroblastosis fetalis Hemolytic anemia of the fetus and newborn occurring when the blood of the fetus is Rh positive and the blood of the mother is Rh negative

escutcheon Pattern of hair growth over the genitalia and lower abdomen; considered a secondary sexual characteristic

estrogen Female hormone that promotes development of female secondary sexual characteristics, affects the menstrual cycle, and prepares the female genital tract for fertilization and implantation of a fertilized ovum each month

ethnocentrism Belief in the natural superiority of the group to which one belongs; tendency to judge a group by standards appropriate to another group

exsanguination Extensive, severe blood loss that is so extreme that it is incompatible with life

extrinsic coagulation factors Blood factors V, VII, and X

fallopian tube Oviduct

false labor Irregular uterine contractions felt in late pregnancy that do not cause dilatation or effacement of the cervix (synonym: Braxton Hicks contractions)

fecundity Ability to produce offspring (synonym: fertility)

fellatio Oral stimulation of the penis

ferning Fernlike pattern seen microscopically when cervical mucus is thinly applied to a glass slide and allowed to dry; the pattern, which results from crystallization of sodium chloride in the mucus, confirms the presence of estrogen at midcycle

ferritin Protein containing iron; it is the form of iron stored in the liver, spleen, and bone marrow and is essential for hematopoiesis

ferrous Containing iron

fertilization Union of the male sperm and the female ovum to form a zygote, from which the embryo develops

fetal alcohol syndrome Set of birth defects in infants whose mothers ingest excessive amounts of alcohol during pregnancy

fetal dystocia Difficulty in labor caused by fetal size, malposition, or abnormality or by a multiple pregnancy

fetal heart rate (FHR) Number of fetal heartbeats in a given time; normal FHR is 120 to 160 beats per minute

fetal hydrops Extreme edema of the fetus or newborn

occurring in severe hemolytic disease (synonym: hydrops fetalis)

fetal membranes Membranes consisting of an outer chorionic and an inner amniotic membrane that adhere to each other during the fifth month of fetal life and form the amniotic sac

fetal souffle Sound of blood racing through the umbilical artery that is synchronous with the fetal heartbeat (synonym: funic souffle)

fetopelvic disproportion Inability of the fetus to pass through the maternal pelvis

fetoscope Stethoscope used for auscultating the fetal heartbeat through the maternal abdomen

fetus Infant in utero after completion of the embryonic stage at 8 weeks of gestation; major development occurs from this time until birth

fibrocystic breast disease A condition in which there are palpable lumps in the breasts, usually associated with pain and tenderness, that fluctuate with the menstrual cycle and become progressively worse until menopause

fimbria Fingerlike projections of the infundibular portion of the fallopian tube

flaccid Flabby, soft, lacking normal muscle tone

flexion Normal bending forward of the fetal head in the uterus or birth canal

fluctuance Wavy impulse felt during palpation of a fluid-filled space that is produced by vibration of body fluid

fontanelles Unfused areas between fetal skull bones that are covered with strong connective tissue, which allows movement of bones and molding of fetal head during birth

football hold Method of holding a newborn, which is known as the safety hold in nurseries; the neonate's back is supported on the nurse's lower arm, while its bottom is tucked securely between the elbow/upper arm of the nurse and its head rests in nurse's hand

foramen ovale Opening between atria in the fetal heart that normally closes within hours after birth; when the opening remains patent it can be closed surgically

forceps Two-bladed instrument used to assist delivery of the fetus after the cervix is fully dilated and the fetal head is engaged

foreskin Prepuce, or loose fold of skin, covering the penis or clitoris

fornices Anterior and posterior spaces into which the upper vagina is divided

fourchette Fold of mucous membrane at the posterior junction of the labia minora

frenulum linguae Fold of mucous membrane extending from the floor of the mouth to the inferior portion of the tongue and restraining its movement

friable Easily broken, for example, blood vessels of the cervix

Friedman curve Graph showing the progress of labor that facilitates detection of dysfunctional labor

full-term infant Infant born between 38 and 42 weeks of gestation

functional residual capacity Volume of gas that remains in the lung after a normal exhalation

fundus Upper portion of the uterus lying between the points of insertion of the fallopian tubes

galactorrhea Lactation or flow of milk not associated with childbirth or nursing; may be a symptom of a pituitary gland tumor

gamete Mature male or female germ cell; a spermatozoon or ovum

gametogenesis Maturation of gametes through the process of meiosis

gavage The feeding of liquid nutrients through a tube passed into the stomach through the nose or mouth

gene Segment of a DNA molecule that codes for the synthesis of a single product; the smallest unit of heredity

genitalia Organs of reproduction

genitourinary Pertaining to the genital and urinary organs

genome The complete set of chromosomes of an organism

genotype Fundamental, hereditary makeup of a person's genes

germ layers Three primary cell layers of the embryo that develop into organs and tissues: ectoderm, mesoderm, and endoderm

gestation Time from conception to birth, approximately 280 days

gestational age Estimated age of the fetus calculated in weeks from the first day of the last menstrual period

gestational sac Amnion and its contents (products of conception)

gestational trophoblastic disease Disorder in cellular growth that results in the destruction of the embryo and abnormal growth of the outer layer of the blastocyst, causing benign disease (hydatidiform mole) or invasive carcinoma

gingivitis Condition in which the gums become inflamed and spongy and bleed easily; common in pregnancy, but with good oral hygiene and a balanced diet, will clear shortly after delivery

glucogenesis Formation of glucose in the liver from sources that are not carbohydrates, such as fatty or amino acids

glucose-6-phosphate dehydrogenase Enzyme of the liver and kidney that plays an important role in the conversion of glycerol to glucose; a hereditary deficiency of the enzyme causes hemolytic anemia in persons who ingest certain drugs

glucosuria Presence of glucose in the urine

goiter Enlargement of the thyroid gland

gonadotropins Hormones having a stimulating effect on the gonads; FSH (follicle-stimulating hormone) causes ovarian follicles to grow and secrete estrogen, and LH (luteinizing hormone) causes formation of the corpus luteum following ovulation and produces progesterone during the second half of the menstrual cycle

gonads Male and female sex organs (testes and ovaries)

gonorrhea A sexually transmitted infection of the genital mucous membrane of the male and female

Goodell's sign Softening of the cervix and vagina as determined by bimanual examination; an indication of pregnancy

graafian follicle Ovarian sac that contains an ovum

gravida Woman who is or has been pregnant, regardless of pregnancy outcome

G6PD See **glucose-6-phosphate dehydrogenase**

gynecoid pelvis Type of pelvis that is characteristic of the normal female and is the ideal pelvic type for childbirth

haploid cell Cell containing only one member of each pair of homologous chromosomes; the haploid number in human beings is 23

heel stick A pin or lancet prick performed on an infant's heel to assess the blood for hematocrit, glucose levels, or other tests as indicated

Hegar's sign Softening of the lower uterine segment felt on bimanual examination; a probable sign of pregnancy

hematocrit Volume percentage of red blood cells in whole blood; the normal range in women is between 38% and 46%

hematoma, puerperal Collection of blood in the soft tissue of the pelvis caused by the trauma of childbirth

hematuria Blood in the urine

hemoconcentration Decrease in plasma volume, resulting in increased concentration of red blood cells

hemodilution Increase in blood plasma volume, resulting in reduced concentration of red blood cells

hemoglobinopathy Disease caused by or associated with forms of abnormal hemoglobin

hemolysis Destruction of red blood cells

hemolytic anemia Anemia due to the premature destruction of red blood cells (synonym: hemolytic disease)

hemorrhage Rapid loss of large amounts of venous or arterial blood; bleeding may be external or internal

hemorrhoid Dilatation of one or more of the hemorrhoidal plexus of veins; an external hemorrhoid is the dilatation of rectal veins beneath the skin of the anal canal; it may occur during labor due to pushing and distention of the anal tissues

hepatosplenomegaly Pathologic enlargement of the liver and spleen

hereditary Genetically transmitted from parent to offspring

herpesvirus Family of viruses causing herpes simplex, herpes zoster, and varicella (chickenpox)

HIV Human immunodeficiency virus; causes AIDS, a virulent infection that causes collapse of the body's immune system and eventual death from opportunistic infection

Homans' sign Pain in the calf on dorsiflexion of the foot; an indicator of thrombosis or thrombophlebitis

homeostasis State of equilibrium in the internal environment of the body that is naturally maintained by adaptive body responses

homologous chromosomes Matched pairs of chromosomes, one from each parent, having the same gene loci in the same order

homosexuality Sexual attraction to members of the same sex

homozygote Individual who has two matching alleles at a given locus on a pair of homologous chromosomes

hot flush (flash) A symptom of menopause, characterized by sudden sensation of heat and profuse sweating, directly related to decreasing estrogen circulation

human papilloma virus (HPV) A sexually transmitted infection that may play a role in the development of cervical cancer

hydramnios Excessive amniotic fluid inside the uterus leading to overdistention

hydrocephaly Accumulation of cerebrospinal fluid within the ventricles of the brain

hydrops fetalis See **fetal hydrops**

hymen Fold of mucous membrane that partially covers the vaginal orifice

hyperbilirubinemia Excessive concentrations of bilirubin in the blood that may lead to jaundice

hypercapnia Excessive carbon dioxide in the blood

hyperemesis gravidarum Abnormal condition of pregnancy where protracted vomiting, weight loss, and fluid and electrolyte imbalance occur

hyperemia Increased blood flow to a part as evidenced by redness of the skin

hyperglycemia Excessive glucose in the blood

hyperplasia Excessive proliferation of normal cells in the normal arrangement in a structure or organ

hyperreflexia Increased action of the reflexes

hypertonicity State of greater than normal muscle tension

hypertrophy Increase in size of an organ or structure not resulting from an increase in the number of cells

hypoplasia Defective tissue development

hypospadias Developmental anomaly in which the male urethra opens on the undersurface of the penis

hypotonia Failure of the muscles to contract and retract with normal strength and frequency

hypoxemia Deficiency of oxygen in the blood

hypoxia Reduction to below physiologic levels in the supply of oxygen to tissues

hysterectomy Surgical removal of the uterus

hysterosalpingogram Diagnostic procedure in which radiopaque dye is injected into the cervix, uterus, and fallopian tubes to determine their patency

iatrogenic Pertaining to any adverse mental or physical condition unintentionally induced by treatment by a physician or surgeon

icteric Pertaining to jaundice

icterus neonatorum Physiologic jaundice in the newborn

imperforate hymen Hymen with no opening

implantation Process by which the conceptus attaches to the uterine wall and penetrates both the uterine endometrium and the maternal circulatory system

implantation bleeding Slight endometrial oozing of blood at implantation; may be noted as "spotting" by the woman

impotence Inability of the male to achieve or maintain an erection

impregnation Fertilization of an ovum

inborn error of metabolism Hereditary disease caused by deficiency of a specific enzyme

incest Sexual intercourse between those of near relationship

incontinence Inability to control the excretion of urine or feces

incubator Enclosed crib in which the temperature can be controlled; used in caring for premature infants

induction of labor Deliberate initiation of uterine contractions

infant Child under 1 year of age

infant mortality rate Number of deaths in the first year of life per 1000 live births

infertility Inability to produce offspring

in situ In position

insulin Hormone secreted by the beta cells of the islets of Langerhans of the pancreas

internal rotation Mechanism of labor characterized by rotation of the presenting part of the fetus within the birth canal

international unit (IU) Internationally accepted amount of a substance; the form in which quantities of fat-soluble vitamins, some hormones, enzymes, and vaccines are expressed

interstitial Referring to spaces within a tissue or organ

intractable Unrelenting

intrapartum Occurring during labor or birth

intrauterine device (IUD) Small metal or plastic form placed in the uterus to prevent implantation of fertilized ovum

intrauterine growth retardation (IUGR) Fetal condition characterized by failure to grow at the expected rate

introitus Vaginal opening

invagination Insertion of one part of a structure within a part of the same structure; to ensheathe (synonym: intussusception)

inverted nipple Deformity of the nipple that causes it to recede rather than to become erect when stimulated

in vitro fertilization Process whereby ova are extracted surgically from a woman, fertilized in a test tube, and implanted in the uterus

involution Reduction in the size of the uterus following delivery (total involution takes 6 weeks)

ischemia Temporary obstruction of circulation to a part

isthmus Constriction on the uterine surface between the uterine body and the cervix

jaundice Yellow discoloration of the skin, whites of the eyes, mucous membranes, and body fluids caused by excessive bilirubin in the blood

joule Work done in 1 second by current of an ampere against a resistance of 1 ohm; 1 kilocalorie is equal to 4185.5 joules

karyotype Chromosomal makeup of the nucleus of a human cell; also, the photomicrograph of chromosomes arranged in an organized way

Kegel exercise Conscious tightening and relaxing of the pubococcygeal muscles, which strengthens the muscles of the vagina and perineum

kernicterus Abnormal toxic accumulation of bilirubin in the brain due to hyperbilirubinemia

ketoacidosis Acidosis accompanied by excessive ketones in the body and resulting from faulty carbohydrate metabolism; primarily a complication of diabetes mellitus

ketones End products of fat metabolism

ketosis Accumulation of abnormal amounts of ketones in the body resulting from inadequate ingestion of carbohydrates; seen in starvation, in diabetes, and, rarely, in pregnancy

kick count A maternal check of fetal health after 38 weeks by counting the number of times the fetus kicks each day

kilocalorie (kcal) Unit of measure for heat; in nutrition it is known as a large calorie and written with a capital C

labor Rhythmic contraction and relaxation of the uterine muscles with progressive effacement and dilatation of the cervix (synonym: parturition)

lactalbumin Important constituent of whey

lactation Postpartum production of milk

Laminaria Genus of moisture-absorbing seaweed used to dilate the cervix before elective abortion; it is placed in the cervix at least 12 hours before the procedure and is used as a physiologic means of dilating the cervix

lanugo Downy hair that covers the body of the fetus, especially preterm

laparoscopy Examination of the abdominal cavity by introduction of a laparoscope through a small abdominal incision; organs of the abdomen and pelvis can be visualized and such procedures as sterilization performed

large-for-gestational-age (LGA) infant Infant of any weight who falls above the 90th percentile on the intrauterine growth curve

latent phase of labor Period from initiation of true labor contractions through 3 to 4 cm of cervical dilatation

lecithin/sphingomyelin (L/S) ratio Ratio of lecithin to sphingomyelin in the amniotic fluid; a ratio of 2:1 is used as an indicator of fetal lung maturity

let-down A reflex caused by increased oxytocin from the pituitary gland in the brain and resulting in contractions

of muscles of the breasts that force milk into the ducts leading to the nipple

leukocytosis Increase in number of leukocytes (white blood cells) to more than 10,000/mm^3

leukorrhea White or yellowish mucous discharge that normally drains from the cervix or vagina

LGA See **large-for-gestational-age infant**

libido Sexual drive

lie Relationship of the long axis of the fetus to the long axis of the mother

lightening Descent of the uterus into the pelvis occurring 2 to 3 weeks before labor in primigravidas, just before or during labor in multigravidas

linea nigra Dark line of pigmentation extending from the pubis to the umbilicus during pregnancy

lithotomy position Position in which the patient lies on her back with thighs flexed on the abdomen and legs abducted on the thighs

lochia Discharge of blood, mucus, and tissue that flows from the uterus in the postpartum period

locus Location of a gene on a chromosome

lordosis Abnormal anterior convexity of the spine

low-birth-weight infant Infant weighing 2500 g or less at birth, regardless of gestational age

lunar month 28 days

macrosomia Unusually large body, as in infants of diabetic mothers

malpresentation Faulty or abnormal fetal presentation

mammogram An x-ray study of breast tissue used in the diagnosis of breast disease or cancer

manual rotation Obstetric maneuver that is used to turn the fetal head by hand from a transverse to an anteroposterior position to facilitate delivery

mastitis Acute inflammation of the breast caused by bacteria entering a cracked nipple during lactation

masturbation Induction of sexual excitement to self through manipulation of the genitals or other body parts

maternal mortality rate Number of maternal deaths from any cause during the pregnancy and postpartum period per 100,000 live births

meconium Fecal material discharged by the newborn, green black in color and consisting of mucus, bile, and epithelial shreds; its presence in amniotic fluid during labor may indicate fetal distress

megaloblastic anemia Pernicious anemia characterized by megaloblasts, or large abnormal red blood corpuscles

meiosis Cell division occurring in germ cells and leading to the production of gametes containing half the usual number of chromosomes, that is, one chromosome of each pair and one sex chromosome

menarche First menstruation that marks the beginning of cyclic menstrual function

menopause Cessation of menstruation; it is considered complete when menses has not occurred for a year

menstrual cycle A hallmark of reproductive function in females associated with endocrine changes and cyclic menstruation

menstruation Physiologic cyclic bleeding that, in the absence of pregnancy, normally occurs monthly in women of reproductive age

metritis Inflammation of the uterus

metrorrhagia Bleeding from the uterus at any time other than the menstrual period; may be caused by lesions of the cervix

microcephaly Abnormal smallness of the head with underdevelopment of the brain

microphthalmia Abnormally small size of one or both eyes

milia Minute white cysts on the skin of newborns caused by obstruction of hair follicles; milia are commonly facial, appear over the bridge of the nose, chin, and cheeks, and disappear within a few weeks

miscarriage Lay term for spontaneous abortion

mitosis Cell division leading to the production of two daughter cells, each containing the same chromosomal makeup as the parent cell

mittelschmertz Abdominal pain on the side of ovulation that some women experience in the middle of the menstrual cycle

molar pregnancy Abnormal condition in which cells forming the placenta continue to invade the uterine lining after the fetus has died (synonym: hydatidiform mole)

molding Normal process by which the fetal head is shaped during labor as it passes through the tight birth canal; the head often becomes elongated and the bones of the head may overlap slightly at the suture lines

mongolian spots Benign bluish pigmentation over the lower back and buttocks that may be present at birth, especially in dark-skinned races

monosomy Chromosome disorder in which one chromosome of a pair is missing

monozygous twins Two offspring originating from a single fertilized ovum; the offspring are of the same sex and have identical genetic characteristics

mons veneris Pad of fatty tissue lying over the symphysis pubis, which becomes covered with short, curly hair after puberty

Montgomery's glands Sebaceous glands in the areola; they secrete a lubricant that protects the nipple during nursing

morbidity The condition of being diseased or sick; pertaining to the sickness rate

morning sickness Symptoms of nausea and vomiting occurring in some women in early pregnancy; it usually clears after the third month but may continue to some degree throughout pregnancy

Moro reflex Defensive reflex present from birth to 3 months of age that causes the infant to draw its arms across the chest in an embracing manner when startled

mortality Condition of being mortal; pertaining to the death rate

mosaicism Condition of an individual with at least two cell lines with differing karyotype

mucous plug Plug developing in the endocervical canal during pregnancy that blocks the entrance of substances or bacteria into the uterus; the mucous plug becomes the "bloody show" in early labor when it breaks loose from its capillaries and is expelled

multifactorial Pertaining to the interaction of genetic and nongenetic (ie, environmental) factors

multigravida Woman who is pregnant and has been pregnant before

multipara Women who has completed two or more pregnancies to the stage of viability

mutagen Agent that causes permanent genetic variation

mutation Permanent change in the genetic code

myelomeningocele Spina bifida with protrusion of the cord and membranes

Nagele's rule Method of estimating the expected date of delivery; add 7 days to the last menstrual period and count back 3 months

narcosis State of profound unconsciousness produced by a drug

natal Pertaining to birth

nausea Sensation that usually leads to the urge to vomit

navel Umbilicus

neck webbing Presence of a membrane connecting the lateral aspects of the neck with the shoulder

necrosis Death of areas of tissue, surrounded by healthy tissue

necrotizing enterocolitis Acute inflammatory bowel disorder that may occur in preterm or low-birth-weight neonates

neonate Infant from birth through the first 28 days of life

neonatologist Physician with special training in the care of the neonate

neonatology Art and science of diagnosis and treatment of disorders of the neonate

neural tube defect Group of congenital malformations that involves defects of the spinal column caused by failure of the neural tube to close during embryonic development

neuropathy Abnormal condition characterized by inflammation and degeneration of peripheral nerves

nidation Implantation of a fertilized ovum into the endometrium

nipple shield Soft latex shield used by lactating women to protect the nipples when they become sore and cracked from infant nursing; the infant nurses from the nipple of the shield

nonstress test Evaluation of fetal heart rate as it relates to fetal movement; performed late in pregnancy

nonviable fetus Immature fetus that is incapable of surviving outside the uterus

nulligravida Woman who is not now and never has been pregnant

nullipara Woman who has never carried a pregnancy to the stage of viability

nurse midwife Certified nurse midwife (CNM) who holds a license as a registered nurse and has completed a specialized course of training accredited by the American College of Nurse Midwives in the care of the woman and her family during pregnancy, childbirth, and the postbirth and interconceptional periods

obstetric forceps Metal forceps that may be used to assist in the delivery of the fetal head

oligohydramnios Abnormal decrease in the amount of amniotic fluid within the uterus

oliguria Diminished production of urine

omphalic Pertaining to the umbilicus

omphalocele Congenital herniation of the abdominal viscera through a defect in the abdominal wall at the umbilicus; surgical closure is performed after birth

oocyte Early primitive ovum before it has completely developed

oogenesis Formation and development of the ovum

ophthalmia neonatorum Purulent conjunctivitis of the newborn; gonorrheal conjunctivitis

organogenesis Formation of body organs from embryonic tissue

orgasm Culmination of sexual excitement; in females, contractions of the outer third of the vagina at the apex of sexual arousal

orgasm restriction Specific direction not to have orgasm by any means because it is deemed threatening to the pregnancy

os Any opening in the body, but particularly the cervical opening

ossification Formation of bone or conversion of other tissue into bone

osteoporosis A serious disorder, partly due to estrogen decline, that increases porosity of bone as women age

ovarian cycle A series of events controlled by the hypophysial hormones in which the ovaries produce reproductive cells and female hormones, maintain the secondary sexual characteristics, prepare the uterus for pregnancy, and stimulate the mammary glands

ovulation Periodic ripening and rupture of the mature ovarian follicle with discharge of the ovum into the abdomen near the fallopian tube; occurs approximately 14 days before the beginning of the next menstrual period

ovum Female germ cell

oxytocics Drugs used to stimulate uterine contractions to assist childbirth and prevent postdelivery hemorrhage; during lactation they increase the let-down reflex

oxytocin challenge test (OCT) Tests the response of the

fetus to uterine contractility stimulated by oxytocin (Pitocin) and assesses placental function

Papanicolaou smear Cytologic test of cervical cells used as a screening test for cervical cancer (synonym: Pap smear)

paracervical block Injection of local anesthetic into the paracervical nerve for pain relief in active labor

parametritis Inflammation of the parametrium (synonym: pelvic cellulitis)

parametrium Connective tissue around the uterus

parity Number of pregnancies reaching viability—not the number of fetuses delivered (synonym: para)

parturient Woman in labor

parturition Act of giving birth (synonyms: childbirth, delivery)

patent ductus arteriosus Congenital abnormal opening between the pulmonary artery and the aorta that does not close after birth; the defect allows recirculation of arterial blood through the lungs, increasing the workload of the left side of the heart

pelvic inflammatory disease (PID) Bacterial infection of the pelvic organs, often caused by the presence of an IUD or venereal disease; a common cause of tubal adhesions, scar tissue, and consequent infertility

pelvimetry Clinical measurement of the pelvis to determine its adequacy for passage of the fetus during labor and delivery

perimenopausal period Period of years during which women experience gradual transition from reproductive to nonreproductive physiologic processes; generally thought to be from age 35 to age 60.

perinatal period Period from the 28th week of gestation through the 28th day of life

perinatologist Obstetrician with special interest and experience in the perinatal period, particularly with high-risk mothers and infants

perineum Floor of the pelvis; the tissues between the lower end of the vagina and the anal canal and lower rectum

peritonitis Inflammation of the peritoneum

petechiae Small, purplish hemorrhagic spots on the skin

phenotype Physical appearance of a person

phenylketonuria Congenital disease caused by defective metabolism of the amino acid phenylalanine; if early treatment is not instituted, severe mental retardation will result

phototherapy Therapeutic use of light to treat hyperbilirubinemia and jaundice in the newborn

pica Craving during pregnancy to eat substances that are not food, such as chalk, clay, starch, glue, toothpaste

placenta Oval, flat, vascular structure in the uterus through which the fetus derives its nourishment

placenta previa A placenta that is implanted in the lower uterine segment

podalic version Internal manual version of the fetus; the infant's feet are grasped inside the uterus and turned to a footling breech; version is complete when the feet are brought through the introitus for delivery

polycythemia Excessive number of red blood cells

polyhydramnios Excessive amount of amniotic fluid

position Relation of the fetal presenting part to the maternal pelvis

postcoital test Diagnostic procedure in which a sample of cervical mucus is extracted within about 6 hours of sexual intercourse at the presumed time of ovulation; the mucus is examined microscopically for the presence of live, motile sperm as well as for adequate ferning (indicating that estrogen levels are optimal for conception)

postpartum hemorrhage Loss of 500 mL or more of blood from the uterus after completion of the third stage of labor

postpartum period Period from birth to 6 weeks (42 days) after birth

postprandial Following a meal

post-term infant Infant born after the onset of the 42nd week of gestation

precipitate labor Labor that terminates in delivery of the infant in less than 3 hours

preeclampsia Disorder of pregnancy or the postpartum period characterized by hypertension, edema, and proteinuria

premature infant Infant born before the end of the 37th week of gestation (synonym: preterm infant)

premature rupture of membranes Rupture of the amniotic sac before the onset of uterine contractions

presentation Position of the fetus as described by the fetal part that appears first at the pelvic outlet, for example, vertex (head), breech, arm, or face

preterm labor Labor that occurs before the 37th week of gestation

primary infertility Inability to conceive or carry a pregnancy to viability with no previous history of pregnancy carried to live birth

primigravida Woman pregnant for the first time (synonym: gravida 1)

primipara Woman who has delivered one fetus who reached the stage of viability

proband A person presenting with a mental or physical disorder whose heredity is studied to determine if other members of the family have had the same disease or are carriers

prodromal labor Period preceding labor when lightening occurs and increased pressure in the pelvis is felt

progesterone Hormone secreted by the corpus luteum that prepares the endometrium to receive the fertilized ovum

prolactin Pituitary hormone that in association with estrogen and progesterone promotes breast development and the formation of milk during pregnancy and lactation

prolonged labor Active labor that continues more than 20 hours

prolonged rupture of membranes Rupture of the amniotic sac that occurs 24 hours or more before the onset of labor

prophylaxis Protection from or prevention of a disease or event

prostaglandin (PG) Fatty acid found in many body tissues that affects smooth muscles and the cardiovascular system; one of its properties is to stimulate the uterus to contract

proteinuria Presence of protein in the urine

prothrombin time Test of clotting time used to evaluate the effect of anticoagulant therapy

pruritus Intense itching

pseudocyesis False pregnancy

ptosis Drooping of a part or organ, for example, the eyelid

puberty Point at which a person is first capable of reproduction; also the phase marked by first development of secondary sex characteristics

puerperal sepsis Infection during the puerperium originating in the pelvic organs

puerperium Period of 42 days following childbirth

quickening Perception of the first fetal movements by the mother, generally between the 18th and 20th weeks of pregnancy

RDA (recommended daily allowances) Standards by age and sex group for intake of major nutrients; serve as guidelines for maintaining health through nutrition

recessive Trait or gene that is clinically expressed only when homozygous

rectocele Protrusion of the posterior vaginal wall from pressure of the anterior wall of the rectum against the vagina

rectouterine pouch (pouch of Douglas) Pouch formed from the parietal peritoneum, bounded anteriorly by the posterior fornix of the vagina and posteriorly by the rectum

respiratory distress syndrome (RDS) Disease of the newborn who is delivered before full lung maturity has occurred; symptoms include cyanosis, grunting, abnormal respiratory pattern, and retraction of the chest wall during inspiration

retraction ring Physiologic area of constriction at the junction of the upper, or contracting, portion and the lower, or dilating, portion of the uterus; Bandl's ring is pathologic constriction of the retraction ring

Rh (D) immunoglobulin Passive immunizing solution of gamma globulin that contains anti-Rh; when given within 72 hours after delivery of an Rh positive neonate to an Rh-negative mother, it prevents the maternal Rh immune response

round ligaments Fibromuscular bands extending from the superior lateral surface of the uterus down and forward through the inguinal canal to terminate in the labia majora; they stretch during pregnancy and may cause discomfort

rubella Acute infectious disease (synonym: German measles)

Rubin's test Insufflation of the fallopian tubes with carbon dioxide to test their patency

rupture of membranes Breaking of the amniotic sac spontaneously or mechanically before or during labor

saddle block anesthesia Injection of an anesthetic agent into a spinal subarachnoid space

salpingitis Inflammation of the fallopian tubes

salpinx Fallopian tube

scotoma Blind spot in the visual field

sebum Fatty secretion of sebaceous glands

secondary infertility Inability to conceive or carry a pregnancy to a live birth after one or more successful pregnancies

secundigravida Woman pregnant for the second time (synonym: gravida 2)

semen Viscid, sperm-containing secretion that passes from the male urethra at sexual climax

sensitized Having developed a susceptibility to a specific substance

sepsis Presence of pathogenic microorganisms or their toxins in blood or other tissues

septum Wall dividing two cavities

Sertoli's cells Cells of the seminiferous tubules that nourish spermatids

sex chromosome Chromosome responsible for sex determination; in human beings, females have two X chromosomes (XX), males have one X and one Y (XY)

SGA A small-for-gestational-age infant weighing less than 2500 g but not premature by calculation of dates

Sheehan's syndrome Hypopituitarism caused by infarct of the pituitary gland following postpartum shock or hemorrhage

Shirodkar cerclage Operative procedure that sutures an incompetent cervix to ensure that it cannot dilate until removal of sutures in early labor

shunt Passage that diverts flow from one main route to another

Skene's glands Glands whose ducts open into the female urethra; in gonorrheal infections these glands are always infected

small-for-gestational-age infant Infant of any weight who falls below the tenth percentile on the intrauterine growth curve; infant weighing less than 2500 g at term

spermatogenesis Formation of mature, functional spermatozoa

spermicide Agent that kills spermatozoa

spina bifida Congenital defect in which the spinal canal fails to close at the lumbar region; protrusion of the cord and meninges occurs

spinnbarkeit Cervical mucus that has the property of elasticity at the time of ovulation

spontaneous rupture of the membranes Rupture of the amniotic sac without medical interference

spotting Spotting of blood from the vagina between periods or during pregnancy

squamocolumnar junction Location on the endocervix or on the ectocervix where transition from squamous to columnar epithelium occurs

station Measurement of fetal descent into the bony pelvis in relation to the ischial spines

stenosis Narrowing or stricture of a duct or canal

sterilization Complete removal or destruction of all microorganisms; process rendering a person unable to produce children

stilbestrol Diethylstilbestrol, an estrogenic compound

stillbirth Birth of a dead fetus

striae gravidarum Whitish or reddish lines seen on parts of the body where skin has been stretched; in pregnancy, they occur primarily on the abdomen, thighs, and breasts

stroma Foundation or supporting tissues of an organ

subinvolution Incomplete return of a body part to its normal size after physiologic hypertrophy; may occur in the uterus following childbirth as an abnormal condition

supine hypotensive syndrome Lowered blood pressure and bradycardia in the supine position due to compression of the inferior vena cava by the weight of the pregnant uterus

surfactant Substance that lowers surface tension in the lungs and maintains expansion of its small air sacs; abnormalities in surfactant in premature infants cause respiratory distress syndrome

sympathomimetics Drugs that mimic the stimulation of the sympathetic nervous system

syncytiotrophoblast Outer layer of cells covering the chorionic villi of the placenta that is in contact with the maternal blood

syphilis A sexually transmitted disease that is transmitted by the spirochete *Treponema pallidum*; it is characterized by lesions that may involve any organ or tissue and may exist without symptoms for many years

Tanner staging A standard method for measuring and classifying the development of sexual characteristics of the maturing reproductive system; stages progress from 1 to 5

teratogen Substance that causes abnormal development of embryonic structures

term Normal end period of pregnancy, occurring between 38 and 42 weeks

testes Two male reproductive glands, located in the scrotum, that produce testosterone, the male hormone, and spermatozoa, the male reproductive cells

tetanic contraction Abnormally long uterine contraction, lasting more than 70 seconds; usually in response to hyperstimulation from oxytocin infusion

thalassemia A genetic disorder that affects hemoglobin in red blood cells and causes chronic anemia; it primarily affects people of Mediterranean, Asian, and African ancestry

thelarche The beginning of breast development at puberty

thrombocytopenia Abnormal decrease in the number of platelets in the blood

thrombophlebitis Formation of a thrombus in conjunction with inflammation of a vein

tocolytic agent Drug that diminishes the force of uterine contractions

toxemia Complication of pregnancy of unknown cause characterized by elevation of blood pressure, proteinuria, and edema (preeclampsia); when convulsions occur, condition is called eclampsia

toxoplasmosis An infection caused by the protozoa *Toxoplasma gondii*

transition The last segment of active phase of labor from 8 to 10 cm of cervical dilatation, which may be characterized by particularly intense maternal discomfort

trichomoniasis Vaginal infection caused by the parasite *Trichomonas vaginalis*

trimester One of three periods into which pregnancy is divided; the first trimester is from the first day of the last menstrual period until 12 weeks; second trimester is from 13 weeks to 27 weeks; third trimester is from 28 weeks to 40 weeks or delivery

trisomy Chromosome disorder in which three copies of homologous chromosomes are present rather than two

ultrasound Use of sound waves to produce an outline of the shape of body organs and tissues; used in fetal assessment

umbilical cord Cord containing two arteries and one vein that connects the fetus with the placenta

uterine prolapse Downward displacement of the uterus that sometimes causes it to protrude from the vagina

vacuum aspiration Method of first trimester abortion in which the products of conception are extracted from the uterus by suction

vaginitis Infection of the vaginal mucosa, usually accompanied by itching, increased discharge, and burning

varicocele Varicose vein of the spermatic cord, more often the left; a common cause of male infertility

vasa praevia Anomaly of insertion of the umbilical cord in which the umbilical blood vessels traverse the lower uterine segment and present at delivery in advance of the head

vasectomy Method of male sterilization in which the vasa deferens are cut and ligated to prevent sperm from entering the ejaculate

vasocongestion Congestion of blood vessels

velamentous insertion Insertion of the umbilical cord where the blood vessels leave the placenta, course between the amnion and chorion, and unite to form the

umbilical cord at some distance from the edge of the placenta

vernix caseosa Gray white, cheeselike sebaceous material that covers the skin of the fetus to protect it from the amniotic fluid

version Manipulation to alter presentation of the fetus

vertex presentation Cephalic presentation

viable Capable of living outside the uterus; the age of viability was previously considered to be 28 weeks, but many states now prepare birth certifications for pregnancy at 20 weeks of gestation or more, or for a fetus weighing 500 g or more

weaning Discontinuing breast milk and substituting other nourishment for the infant

whey Liquid that remains after the cream and curd are separated from the milk

witch's milk Lay term for milk secreted by the newborn infant's breast as a result of stimulation by circulating prolactin in the mother

withdrawal bleeding Vaginal bleeding that occurs after the last oral contraceptive pill of the cycle has been taken

X-linked transmission Transmission of characteristics by genes on the X chromosome

zygote Cell produced by union of the sperm and egg; the fertilized egg

Spanish Phrases Helpful in Maternal and Neonatal Nursing

ENGLISH-TO-SPANISH PHRASES

Prepared by Judith Chavez, RN, BSN, Staff Nurse and Translator, San Francisco General Hospital

A woman and her family will be more at ease and feel relaxed if someone on the staff speaks their language. Some health-care facilities provide interpreters. When an interpreter is not available the nurse can use a few phrases that have been learned. The following table presents English phrases with the corresponding words in Spanish. The third column is a key to pronunciation, given in phonetics. The syllable to be accented is in *italic* type.

English	**Spanish**	**Pronunciation**
Please*	Por Favór	Por Fah-*vor*
Thank You	Grácias	*Grah*-see-ahs
Good Morning	Buénos Días	*Bway*-nos *Dee*-ahs
Good Afternoon	Buénas Tárdes	*Bway*-nas *Tar*-days
Good Evening	Buénas Nóches	*Bway*-nas *Noh*-chays
My Name is	Mi Nómbre Es	Me *Nohm*-bray Ays
Yes/No	Si/No	See/No
I Am A Student Nurse	Soy Estudiénte Enferméra	Soy Ays-stoo-dee-*ayn*-tay Ayn-fay-*may*-rah
Remove Your Clothing	Quítese Su Ropa	*Key*-tay-say Soo *Roh*-pah
Put On This Gown	Pongáse La Bata	Pohn-*gah*-say Lah *Bah*-tah
Need A Urine Specimen	Es Necesário Una Muéstra De Su Orina	Ays Nay-say-*sar*-ee-oh Oo-nah Moo-*ay*-strah Day Oh-*ree*-nah
Be Seated	Siéntese	See-*ayn*-tay-say
Recline	Acuestése	Ah-cways-*tay*-say
Sit Up	Siéntese	See-*ayn*-tay-say
Stand	Parése	Pah-*ray*-say
Bend Your Knees	Dóble Las Rodíllas	*Doh*-blay Lahs Roh-*dee*-yahs
Relax Your Muscles	Reláje Los Músculos	Ray-*lah*-hay Lohs *Moos*-koo-lohs
Try To	Aténte	Ah-*tayn*-tay
Try Again	Aténte Ótra Vez	Ah-*tayn*-tay *Oh*-tra Vays

*You should begin or end any request with the word PLEASE (POR FAVOR).

English	Spanish	Pronunciation
Do Not Move	No Se Muéva	Noh Say Moo-*ay*-vah
Turn On (Or To) Your Left Side	Voltése A Su Ládo Izquiérdo	Vohl-*tay*-say Ah Soo *Lah*-doh Is-key-*ayr*-doh
Turn On (Or To) Your Right Side	Voltése A Su Ládo Derécho	Vohl-*tay*-say Ah Soo *Lah*-doh Day-*ray*-choh
Take a Deep Breath	Respíra Profúndo	Ray-*speer*-rah Pro-*foon*-doh
Hold Your Breath	Deténga Su Respiración	Day-*tayn*-gah Soo Ray-speer-ah-see-*ohn*
Don't Hold Your Breath	No Deténga Su Respiración	Noh Day-*tayn*-gah Soo Ray-speer-ah-see-*ohn*
How Long?	¿Hace Cuánto?	¿*Ah*-say *Kwahn*-toh?
How Much?	¿Cuánto?	¿*Kwahn*-toh?
How Do You Feel?	¿Como Se Siénte?	¿*Koh*-moh Say See-*ayn*-tay?
Do You Have Allergies?	¿Tiéne Alérgias?	¿Tee-*ay*-nay Ah-*layr*-hee-ahs?
Are You Warm?	¿Tiéne Calór?	¿Tee-*ay*-nay Kahl-*or*?
Are You Warm Enough?	¿Esta Suficiénte Caliénte?	¿*Ay*-stah Soo-fee-see-*ayn*-tay kahl-ee-*ayn*-tay?
Are You Cold?	¿Tiéne Frío?	¿Tee-*ay*-nay *Free*-oh?
Do You Have Pain?	¿Tiéne Dolór?	¿Tee-*ay*-nay Doh-*lorh*?
Where Is The Pain?	¿Adónde Es El Dolór?	¿Ah-*Dohn*-day Ays Ayl Doh-*lorh*?
Do You Want Medication For Your Pain?	¿Quiére Medicación Para Su Dolór?	¿Key-*ay*-ray May-dee-kah see-*ohn* *pak*-rah Soo Doh–*lorh*?
Are You Comfortable?	¿Está Comfortáble?	¿Ay-*stah* Kohm-for-*tah*-blay?
Your Membranes Have Ruptured?	¿Sus Membránas Se Rupturarón?	¿Soos Maym-*brah*-nahs Say Roop-too-*rah*-rohn?
Has Your Bag of Water Ruptured?	¿Se Rómpio La Bólsa De Agua?	¿Say *Rohm*-pee-oh Lah *Bohl*-sah Day *Ah*-gwah?
Are You Feeling Contractions?	¿Siénte Contrácciones?	¿See-*ayn*-tay Cohn-*trahc*-see-ohn-nays?
Is There Vaginal Bleeding?	¿Hay Sangrádo Vagínal?	¿I Sahn-*grah*-doh Vah-*hee*-nahl?
Breathe Slowly—Like This (In This Manner)	Respíre Despácio—Asi	Ray-*speer*-ray Day-*spah*-see-oh Ah-*see*
This Is Oxygen	Este Oxigéno	*Ah*-stay Ohx-ee-*hay*-noh
Push Like This (In This Manner)	Púje Asi	*Pooh*-hay Ah-*see*
Push Now	Púje Ahora	*Pooh*-hay Ah-*or*-ah
Don't Push	No Púje	Noh *Pooh*-hay
Pant/Blow Like This (In This Manner)	Jadé/Sóple Asi	Yah-*day*/*Soh*-play Ah-*see*
Look	Míre	*Meer*-ray
An Operation Is Necessary	Una Operación Es Necesária	*Oo*-nah Oh-payr-ah-see-*ohn* Ays Nay-say-*sayr*-ee-ah
You Should (Try To):	Tráte De:	*Trah*-tay Day:
Call For Help/Assistance	Llamár Para Asisténcia	Yah-*marh* Pah-rah Ah-sees-*tayn*-see-ah
Empty Your Bladder	Orínar	Oh-*ree*-narh
Feed Your Baby	Dárle De Comér A Su Bébe	*Dahr*-lay Day Koh-*mayr* Ah Soo *Bay*-bay
Change The Diaper	Cambiár El Pañal	Kahm-bee-*arh* Ayl Pahn-*yahl*
Ambulate	Caminár	Kah-mee-*narh*

English	Spanish	Pronunciation
It Is Important To:	Es Importánte De:	Ays Eem-por-*tahn*-tay Day
Walk (Ambulate)	Caminár	Kah-mee-*narh*
Drink Fluids	Bebér Líquidos	Bay-*bayr Lee*-key-dohs
Feed Your Baby Now	Dárle De Comér A Su Bébe Ahora	*Dar*-lay Day Koh-*mayr* Ah Soo Bay-bay Ah-*or-ah*
Place (Position) The Baby On Its Side	Posicionár El Bébe En Su Ládo	Poh-zee-see-oh-*narh* Ayl Bay-bay Ayn Soo *Lah*-doh
You Will Feel Pressure	Vá A Sentír Presión	Vah Ah Sayn-*teer* Pray-see-*ohn*
I Am Going To:	Voy A:	Voy Ah
Count (Take) Your Pulse	Tomár Su Púlso	Toh-*marh* Soo *Pool*-soh
I Am Going To:	Voy A:	Voy Ah
Take Your Temperature	Tomár Su Temperatúra	Toh-*marh* Soo Taym-pay-rah-*too*-rah
Take Your Blood Pressure	Tomar Su Presión	Toh-*marh* Soo Pray-see-*ohn*
Examine Your Cervix	Examinár Su Cervíz	Ayx-ah-mee-*narh* Soo Sayr-*veez*
I Am Going To:	Va A:	Vah-Ah
Start An IV Line	Comensár Una Intravenósa	Koh-mayn-*sarh Oo*-nah Een-trah-vayn-*oh*-sah
Give You Pain Medicine	Dárle Medicación Para Dolór	*Darh*-lay May-dee-kah-see-*ohn* Pah-rah Doh-*lohr*
Empty Your Bladder With A Small Tube	Vaciár Su Vejíga Con Una Túbo Pequeño	Vah-see-*arh* Soo Vee-*hee*-gah Kohn *Oo*-nah *Too*-boh Pay-*kay*-nyoh
Give You An Enema	Dárle Un Lavádo	*Darh*-lay Oon Lah-*vah*-doh
Clean The Umbilical Cord Like This (In This Manner)	Limpiár El Cordón Umbílical Así	Leem-pee-*arh* Ayl Korh-*dohn* Oom-*bee*-lee-kahl Ah-see
Clean The Baby Like This (In This Manner)	Limpiár El Bébe Asi	*Leem*-pee-arh Ayl Bay-bay Ah-see
Fold The Diaper Like This (In This Manner)	Dóblar El Pañal Asi	*Doh*-blarh Ayl Pahn-*yahl* Ah-see
Fasten The Diaper Like This (In This Manner)	Segúre El Pañal Asi	Say-*gurh*-ay Ayl Pahn-*yahl* Ah-see
Place The Soiled Diapers Here	Pónga El Pañal Súcio Aquí	*Pohn*-gah Ayl Pahn-*yahl Soo*-see-Ahoh-*key*
Are You Hungry?	¿Tiéne Hámbre?	¿Tee-*ay*-nay *Ahm*-bray
Are You Thirsty?	¿Tiéne Sed?	¿Tee-*ay*-nay Sayd
You May Not Eat/Drink	No Cóma/Béba	Noh *Koh*-mah/Bay-*bah*
You Can Only Drink Water	Solo Puéde Tomár Água	Soh-loh *Pway*-day Toh-mar *Ah*-gwah
You Can Only Take Ice Chips	Solo Puéde Tomár Pedazítos De Hiélo	Soh-loh *Pway*-day Toh-*marh* Pay-dah-*zee*-tohs Day Eee-*ay*-loh
It Will Be Uncomfortable	Séra Incomódo	*Say*-rah Een-koh-*moh*-doh
It Will Sting	Va Ardér	Vah Ahr-*dayr*

Index

Note: Page numbers in italics *indicate illustrations; page numbers followed by t indicate tables; page numbers followed by b indicate boxed material.*

Nursing Procedures Appearing in This Text

Other recurring displays are listed in the front matter following the Expanded Contents. Universal Precautions and Cervical Dilatation appear on endpapers at the back of the book.

THIRD EDITION

Maternal and Neonatal Nursing

Family-Centered Care

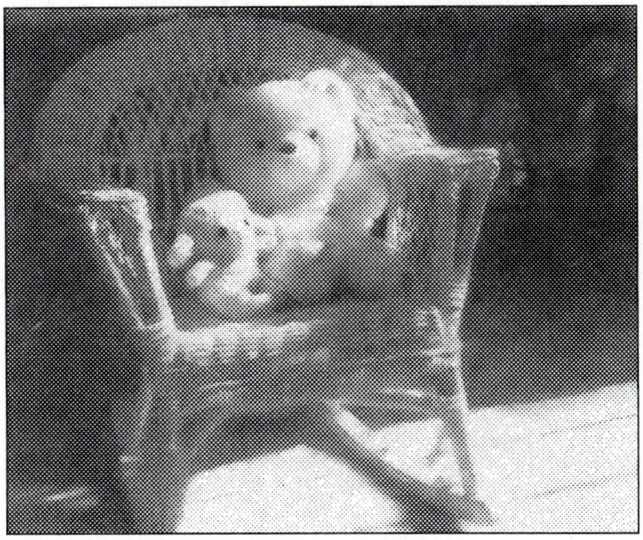

THIRD EDITION

Maternal and Neonatal Nursing

Family-Centered Care

Katharyn A. May, RN, DNSc, FAAN

Professor and Associate Dean for Research
Vanderbilt University School of Nursing
Nashville, Tennessee

Laura R. Mahlmeister, RN, PhD

Professor
Loewenberg School of Nursing
Memphis State University
Memphis, Tennessee

1792

J.B. Lippincott Company   Philadelphia

Assistant Editor: Jennifer E. Brogan
Developmental Editors: Rhonda M. Kumm, RN, MSN; Eleanor D. Faven
Project Editor: Mary Rose Muccie
Indexer: Ellen Murray
Design Coordinator: Kathy Kelley-Luedtke
Interior Designer: Susan Blaker
Cover Designer: Jerry Cable
Production Manager: Helen Ewan
Production Coordinator: Nannette Winski
Compositor: Circle Graphics
Printer/Binder: Courier Book Company Westford

Third Edition

Previous editions of this book were published under the title *Comprehensive Maternity Nursing*.

1 3 5 6 4 2

Library of Congress Cataloging in Publications Data

Maternal and neonatal nursing : Family-centered care / [edited by]
Katharyn A. May, Laura R. Mahlmeister. — 3rd ed.
p. cm.
Rev. ed. of: Comprehensive maternity nursing. 2nd. ed. c1990.
Includes bibliographical references and index.
ISBN 0-397-54953-9
1. Maternity nursing. 2. Infants (Newborn)—Care. I. May, Katharyn A. II. Mahlmeister, Laura Rose. III. Comprehensive maternity nursing.
[DNLM: 1. Obstetrical Nursing. 2. Perinatology—nurses' instruction. WY 157 M425 1994]
RG951.C66 1994
610.73'67—dc20
DNLM/DLC
for Library of Congress 93-26479
CIP

The following figures have been illustrated by Childbirth Graphics®, a Division of WRS Group, Inc. (P.O. Box 21207, Waco, Texas 76702-1207): 4-2, 4-4, 4-5, 4-6, 4-7, 4-9, 4-10, 4-11, 4-12, 4-13, 4-14, 4-15, 4-16, 4-17, 4-18, 4-19, 4-20, 4-21, Table 5-1, 7-6, 7-7, 11-1, 11-2, 11-5, 12-6, 12-7, 12-8, 12 DE: Major Events of the Embryonic Period, 13-1, 13-2, 13-3, 14-4, 16-1, 16-2, 16-3, 18-3, 18-4, 19-1, 19-2, 19-4, 19-5, 19-8, 19-9, 19-10, 19-11, 19-12, 19-13, 19-15, 19-16, 19-18, 19-19, 21-11, 21-15, 22-3, 22-6, 22-7, 23-1, 23-2, 23-3, 23-5, 24-3, 24-5, 26-1, 26-2, 26-3, 26-4, 26-5, 26-8, 26-10, 26-12, 26-14, Table 26-3, 28-4, 28-5, 28-7, 29-2, 29-4, 29-5, 29-6, 29-7, 29-8, 29-9, 30-16E, 30-16F, 31-5, 31-7A, 31-8, 31-9, 31 DE: Using the Infant Radiant Warmer.

Photos for Unit I, II, IV, V by Kathy Sloane.

Any procedure or practice described in this book should be applied by the health-care practitioner under appropriate supervision in accordance with professional standards of care used with regard to the unique circumstances that apply in each practice situation. Care has been taken to confirm the accuracy of information presented and to describe generally accepted practices. However, the authors, editors, and publisher cannot accept any responsibility for errors or omissions or for any consequences from application of the information in this book and make no warranty, express or implied, with respect to the contents of the book.

Every effort has been made to ensure drug selections and dosages are in accordance with current recommendations and practice. Because of ongoing research, changes in government regulations and the constant flow of information on drug therapy, reactions and interactions, the reader is cautioned to check the package insert for each drug for indications, dosages, warnings and precautions, particularly if the drug is new or infrequently used.

To my dear friends Jake, Nicole, and David, who taught me a lot about families. · To J. Benjamin Smith of Duke University, who influenced so many lives through his fiery and inspired teaching, for showing me that passionate commitment to excellence was the only path worth taking, and whose own life was well and truly lived on that path. · To my wonderful husband Michael, for his love, encouragement, and calm faith, and for never once complaining. · To my father, who taught me to use my heart and my head, and to my mother, who always wanted to be a maternity nurse, and who would have been the best ever.

K.A.M.

To Michael Mahlmeister, my mainstay through the course of work on this book.

L.R.M.

To the memory of Deanna Tomlinson Sollid, our friend who never realized how truly extraordinary she was and whose influence is interwoven here like a shining thread—in her philosophy of childbirth education, her emphasis on parent support and independent nursing practice, and in the many beautiful BABES photos that enliven the pages of this text. Her energy, intelligence, and compassion worked miracles and changed the world, one family at a time.

And to Dr. Ramona T. Mercer, Professor Emerita of Nursing, University of California, San Francisco. RTM guided us as graduate students, welcomed us as colleagues, and by her own brilliant example, continues to show us how to discover, how to teach, and how to make a difference in the lives of students and families.

K.A.M., L.R.M.

Contributors

Linda L. Chapman, RN, DNSc
Associate Professor, Nursing
Samuel Merritt College
Oakland, California
Chapter 28: Nursing Care of the Family in the Postpartum Period

Martha Eakes, RNC, MSN, CNA
Lecturer, Maternal–Newborn Nursing
University of North Carolina at Greensboro
Greensboro, North Carolina
Chapter 5: Human Sexuality

Wendy A. Hall, RN, MSN
Assistant Professor
School of Nursing
University of British Columbia
Vancouver, British Columbia, Canada
Chapter 9: Adolescent Childbearing and Parenting
Chapter 36: Individual and Family Adaptation in the Year After Childbirth

Nancy R. Hudson, MS, RD
Program Director, Dietetics
University of California
Berkeley, California
Chapter 17: Nutrition During Pregnancy
Chapter 35: Maternal and Infant Nutrition

Mary Dirr Kostenbauder, CNM, MEd, MSN
Lecturer
University of Florida
Gainesville, Florida
Professor
Seminole Community College
Sanford, Florida
Chapter 13: Nursing Assessment of the Pregnant Woman
Chapter 15: Nursing Care of the Expectant Family

Kathleen Lagana, RN, MSN, PCNS
Lecturer; Clinical Instructor
Department of Nursing
San Francisco State University
Lecturer; Clinical Instructor
School of Nursing
University of San Francisco
San Francisco, California
Chapter 29: Postpartum Complications

Janie Capps Macey, MSN, PhD
Associate Professor for the Practice of Nursing
Vanderbilt University
School of Nursing
Nashville, Tennessee
Teaching Cards

Laura Rose Mahlmeister, RN, PhD
Professor
Loewenberg School of Nursing
Memphis State University
Memphis, Tennessee
Staff Nurse
Labor and Delivery Unit
San Francisco General Hospital
San Francisco, California
Chapter 10: Childbearing and Parenting After Age 35
Chapter 19: The Process of Labor and Birth: Maternal and Fetal Adaptations
Chapter 20: Nursing Care in Normal Labor: First Stage
Chapter 21: Nursing Care in Normal Birth: Second Stage of Labor Through Recovery
Chapter 22: Monitoring the At-Risk Fetus
Chapter 23: Modifying Labor Patterns and Mode of Delivery
Chapter 24: Managing Pain During the Intrapartum and Postpartum Periods
Chapter 25: Nursing Care of the At-Risk Family in the Perinatal Period
Chapter 26: Intrapartum Complications
Chapter 27: Perinatal High-Risk Challenges
Chapter 30: Assessment of the Neonate
Chapter 31: Nursing Care of the Low-Risk Neonate
Chapter 32: Assessment of the At-Risk Neonate

Lisa K. Mandeville, RN, MSN
Director of Perinatal Services
Associate
Department of Obstetrics and Gynecology
Vanderbilt University Medical Center
Nashville, Tennessee
Chapter 14: Assessment of Fetal Well-Being

Katharyn Antle May, RN, DNSc, FAAN
Professor and Associate Dean for Research
Vanderbilt University
School of Nursing
Nashville, Tennessee
Chapter 1: Contemporary Maternal and Neonatal Care
Chapter 2: Conceptual Foundations of Maternal and Neonatal Nursing
Chapter 3: Challenges in Maternal and Neonatal Nursing
Chapter 8: Individual and Family Adaptations to Pregnancy

Royanne A. Moore, RNC, MSN
Associate Professor for the Practice of Nursing
Vanderbilt University
School of Nursing
Nashville, Tennessee
Chapter 6: Women's Health Across the Life Span

Mary E. Muller, RN, PhD
Perinatal Consultant
Columbus, Ohio
Chapter 4: Normal Reproductive Anatomy and Physiology
Chapter 11: Physiologic Adaptations in Pregnancy

Deborah Narrigan, MSN, CNM
Assistant Professor in the Practice of Nursing
Vanderbilt University
School of Nursing
Nashville, Tennessee
Chapter 7: Fertility Management
Chapter 16: Complications of Pregnancy

Pamela Pletch, RN, PhD
Associate Professor
School of Nursing
University of Wisconsin—Milwaukee
Milwaukee, Wisconsin
Chapter 12: The Genetic Code and Fetal Development

J. Alison Rice, RN, BSN, MS
Assistant Professor
University of British Columbia
School of Nursing
Vancouver, British Columbia, Canada
Chapter 18: Comprehensive Education for Childbirth
Chapter 36: Individual and Family Adaptation in the Year After Childbirth

Kathleen Gaines Timm, RN, MS, CNS
Women's and Children's Services Nurse Educator
San Francisco General Hospital
San Francisco, California
Chapter 33: Nursing Care of the High-Risk Neonate
Chapter 34: Congenital Anomalies in the Neonate

Reviewers

Janet Carroll Brookman, RN, DSN
Clinical Assistant Professor
College of Nursing
The University of Alabama in Huntsville
Huntsville, Alabama

Barbara L. Calder, RN, BSN, MCEd
Associate Professor and Assistant Dean
College of Nursing
University of Saskatchewan
Saskatoon, Saskatchewan, Canada

Harriet W. Ferguson, RNC, MSN, EdD
Associate Professor
Temple University
Philadelphia, Pennsylvania

Helen Jacobson, MSN, CNM
Seton Hall University
South Orange, New Jersey
Nurse Midwife
Planned Parenthood of Essex County
Essex County, New Jersey

Christabel A. Kaitell, RN, BN, MPH, SCM
Assistant Professor
School of Nursing
Faculty of Health Science
University of Ottawa
Ottawa, Ontario, Canada

Celesta Carty Kirk, RN, CS, MA, MSN, FNP
Assistant Professor
East Tennessee State University College of Nursing
Department of Family Community Nursing
Johnson City, Tennessee

Cecilia M. Tiller, RN, DSN
Assistant Professor
Department of Parent–Child Nursing
Medical College of Georgia
Augusta, Georgia

Beth M. Wagner, RN, MSN
Nursing Staff Development Instructor for Obstetrics and Pediatrics
Pocono Medical Center
East Stroudsburg, Pennsylvania

Deirdre L. Waywell, RN, SCM, MSN, IBCLC
Childbirth Educator
Department of Family Medicine
Queen's University
Kingston, Ontario, Canada

Patricia E. Zander, RNC, MSN
Assistant Professor—Nursing
Viterbo College
LaCrosse, Wisconsin

Preface

Health care is changing dramatically. New knowledge and technology develop so quickly they push the boundaries of professional practice forward at an astonishing pace. In no other specialty is this change as obvious as in maternal–neonatal care. The professional nurse of today and tomorrow faces an almost overwhelming array of technologic applications to care and is called on to assume increasing responsibilities. At the same time, the human aspect is still of the utmost importance in such an overwhelming life event.

As if these challenges were not enough, into this environment has come a more disturbing element: *so many women and their children and families are at significant health risk that society's future will be compromised unless the basic needs of women, children, and families are met.* The truth is inescapable. The major sources of health risk to women and their families are preventable conditions: poverty; lack of access to primary care; and a health care system that demonstrates attributes of sexism, racism, and ageism, and that fails to use effectively the resources of all its expert care providers. This textbook, then, attempts to bring these elements to the attention of the student and to make the student aware of these concerns as they develop their nursing skills.

It is a challenge to build a textbook that will help nursing students understand contemporary health care problems and will guide them into their future professional practice. *Maternal and Neonatal Nursing* brings together the scientific and humanistic foundations of maternal–newborn nursing care and reemphasizes a philosophy of nursing: *it is a privilege to share in the wonder of life; to assist, counsel, and care for women and their families; and to improve the lives of those who come to us for care.*

Nursing can be a powerful force for change. We hope *Maternal and Neonatal Nursing* stimulates thinking and discussion, thus providing a useful foundation from which to build professional nursing practice.

Organization

The chapters are divided into two types: knowledge-base chapters and nursing care chapters. Knowledge-base chapters present scientific foundations and focus on the emphasis of adaptation. Nursing care chapters have headings related to adaptation and the nursing process. Nursing diagnoses are used to organize the content, where appropriate.

The textbook is organized into four units, all of them employing the family-centered approach to nursing care. **Unit 1, Introduction to Maternal and Neonatal Nursing**, lays the foundation for the text, emphasizing the place of maternal–neonatal nursing within the larger health care system and the nursing profession as a whole. Provision of optimal maternal and perinatal care, emerging roles in maternal nursing, and legal and ethical issues are discussed.

Unit 2, Dynamics of Human Reproduction, addresses the physiologic, genetic, and psychosocial factors of human reproduction and the areas of sexuality, women's health, and fertility and fertility control, all important to clinical nursing care. Family-centered care builds on this scientific base.

Unit 3, Adaptation in the Prenatal Period, continues to build on the scientific and humanistic approach of the previous chapters. The following are emphasized: the physiologic processes that prepare the woman's body to support the growing fetus; the development of the fetus from conception; the family's psychosocial adaptation to the many changes pregnancy brings; nutrition as a primary factor influencing perinatal outcome; the teaching and counseling of the expectant family; and common pregnancy-related problems.

Unit 4, Adaptation in the Intrapartum Period, provides the student with detailed knowledge of current practices in preparation for childbirth, the process of labor and birth, and the basis of nursing care in low-risk, moderate-risk, and high-risk situations.

Unit 5, Adaptation in the Postpartum Period, encompasses the critical transitions experienced by the woman, her newborn, and her family in the first hours, days, and year after birth.

Three new chapters have been added to this edition. **Chapter 6, Women's Health Across the Life Span**, discusses the effects of sexism on women's health, major health concerns of women, and common health concerns at various stages of the life cycle. **Chapter 10, Childbearing and Parenting after Age 35**, addresses this increasingly common phenomenon and complements the revised chapter on adolescent childbearing and parenting. **Chapter 27, Perinatal High-Risk Challenges**, is devoted exclusively to the discussion of major perinatal challenges of this decade: preterm labor, diabetes, and pregnancy-induced hypertension (PIH).

As nurses and authors, we are aware of the growing

discomfort with sexist and prejudiced language. In this edition we have made a special effort to avoid it. We have diligently avoided referring to the nurse as "she." We have tried to use the term "mother" and "father" only when specifically referring to parenting functions and have tried to use the terms "partner" and "spouse" where appropriate.

Integrated Nursing Process

The use of the nursing process as a conceptual foundation of maternal nursing care is explained in Chapter 2. Consistent use of the nursing process forms the framework for the nursing care chapters. Each step of the process builds on the others.

Assessment includes physiologic and behavioral adaptations of the woman, her fetus or newborn, and the family. An emphasis is placed on parent–neonatal attachment throughout. A variety of *Assessment Tools* help the student assess the woman and family's condition. The section on NANDA **nursing diagnosis** includes the most current and commonly used diagnoses in maternal and neonatal care. They are identified along with potential complications for which the nurse monitors. The **Planning and Implementation** section addresses each diagnosis. Each of these interventions is followed by **Expected Outcome(s)** that correspond with the original nursing diagnosis. The section ends with interventions to monitor, prevent, or give care for potential complications. At the end of the section or chapter, the **Evaluation** section ties together all the previous elements.

Nursing Care Plans strengthen and further integrate application of the nursing process. A *Patient Profile*, with history and physical assessment, first describes a client or patient with a specific problem. A *Collaborative Problems and Potential Complications* section lists other factors to be addressed and refers to a *Nursing Alert* display that further discusses collaborative problems that may occur with that specific condition and to a *Managed Care Path* that shows expected progress of the patient. The actual nursing care plan presents assessment factors, specific nursing diagnoses, nursing interventions with rationale, and expected outcomes. An Evaluation section at the end of the care plan sums up the results of the interventions for that specific person.

Special Displays

Continuing the well-received practice of the first two editions, in which displays and figures were used for instruction, the third edition has further developed the use of art and displays. Many new photos and line drawings with color have been added to the book. In addition to Assessment Tools, Nursing Care Plans, and Nursing Procedures (explained with the new features of the book), four additional displays are used throughout the textbook.

Family Considerations highlight concerns of diverse family types and sibling involvement.

Teaching Considerations focus on learning needs of a particular type of patient. The displays list points the nurse can use in teaching these patients.

Nursing Research exposes students to the relationship of research to practice.

Legal/Ethical Considerations describe issues, discusses implications for nursing care, and suggest some appropriate nursing actions.

New Features

There are several features new to the third edition. They complement the scientific and humanistic knowledge base and its clinical application.

- **Nursing Procedures**. Thirty-six nursing procedures appear in 2-column format giving step-by-step interventions and rationale. In many procedures a third column includes figures that illustrate major points of the procedure.
- **Managed Care Paths**. The newest tool in nursing care is managed care paths, which show the expected progression of the client from initiation of care through discharge. Examples of these paths accompany various nursing care plans in the text. They list important expected outcomes as benchmarks, interventions to achieve those outcomes, and specific time frames in which these outcomes should be achieved.
- **Spanish Phrases Helpful in Maternal and Neonatal Nursing**. A list of English-to-Spanish phrases that the nurse can use in providing quality care follows the Glossary at the end of the book. As part of its humanistic emphasis, the text helps health care workers adapt to the changing ethnic and cultural face of society.
- **In-Text Summaries**. Short summaries appear in color type throughout the chapters. These in-text summaries reinforce major points in the chapter and help the student understand and retain key information.
- **Perforated Drug Cards** and **Teaching Considerations Cards**. Twenty-four cards are inserted in the book. Half the cards comprise common medications used in maternal–neonatal care. The other half are significant teaching topics in maternal and neonatal nursing care. The cards are sized for the nurse to carry to clinical areas.

Other Pedagogic Aids

As in the first two editions, Learning Objectives and Key Terms appear at the beginning of each chapter. The objectives are behavioral goals to guide the student while studying the material in the chapter. Instructors may use them as teaching or testing features. The key terms are defined in the Glossary at the back of the book.

In addition to the in-text summaries, each chapter has a final summary at the end. These chapter summaries tie together the major discussions and points of the chapter. Study questions at the end of every chapter help the student review the chapter information. References and Suggested Readings supply additional resources for further reference and study.

Appendices include the Maternity Patient's Bill of Rights, a table of normal values and references, laboratory data and procedures to assess the prenatal woman, conversion tables, a table of known teratogens that cause human malformations, medications in breast milk, and the list of NANDA-approved nursing diagnoses.

Teaching–Learning Package

To underscore this text's presentation of humanistic and scientific foundation of maternal–newborn nursing care, a comprehensive teaching–learning package has been developed. These ancillaries are designed to assist students and faculty.

Two supplemental books are available for the student. *Study Guide to Accompany Maternal and Neonatal Nursing* provides an opportunity for study, learning, and self-evaluation corresponding chapter-by-chapter with text. *Pocket Guide to Maternal and Neonatal Nursing* summarizes important points and facts helpful in the clinical area. The size is convenient for the student to carry in a pocket.

Supplemental materials for the faculty include an *Instructor's Manual to Accompany Maternal and Neonatal Nursing, 52 Color Overhead Transparencies to Accompany Maternal and Neonatal Nursing*, and a 1,000-question *Computerized Test Bank*.

Katharyn A. May, RN, DNSc, FAAN
Laura R. Mahlmeister, RN, PhD

Acknowledgments

We want to acknowledge the assistance of our valued colleagues in the preparation of this edition.

First, thanks to the Department of Nursing Service, Vanderbilt University Medical Center, Nashville, Tennessee for their expert consultation on the use of managed care paths in maternal–newborn nursing, and for allowing us to adapt the products of their hard work for this edition.

Thanks to Kathy McCarthy, RN, MSN, Jeanne Youngkins, RN, MSN, Bonnie Pilon, RN, DSN, Mimi Jones, RN, MSN, Sheron Salyer, RN, MSN, Cheryl Glass, RN, MSN, and the many other expert perinatal nurses who gave us constructive criticism and creative encouragement.

Thanks to Judith Chavez, RN BSN, of San Francisco General Hospital for her meticulous work in translating the English-to-Spanish phrases and terms at the back of the book.

Thanks to the nurses at San Francisco General Hospital Maternal–Newborn Division. They provided the role models for perinatal nursing practice that guided the development of the nursing care plan profiles, and to Kathleen Timm, RN MSN, for her timely contributions to the chapters on the high-risk neonate.

Thanks to Rhonda M. Kumm, RN, MSN, whose energy, enthusiasm, and hard work helped create this superb third edition. And to Susan Blaker, whose creative ideas encompassed the book through her design and are seen in the development of the art program.

Finally, thanks to the folks at J.B. Lippincott, who worked so hard with us and whose good work is visible on every page, especially to Jennifer E. Brogan, Eleanor D. Faven, Nannette Winski, and Mary Rose Muccie.

K.A.M., L.R.M.

Contents

Expanded Contents

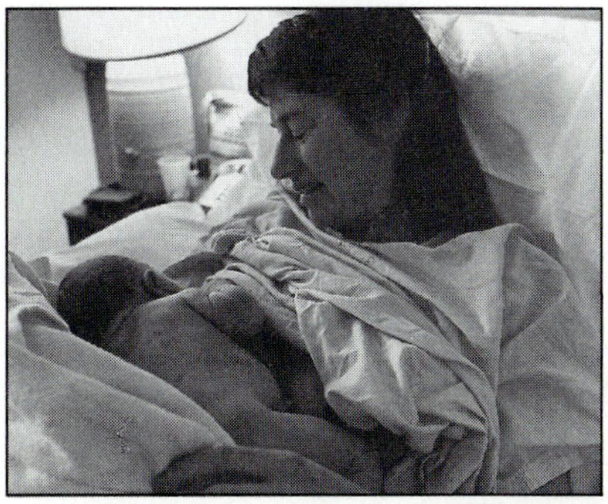

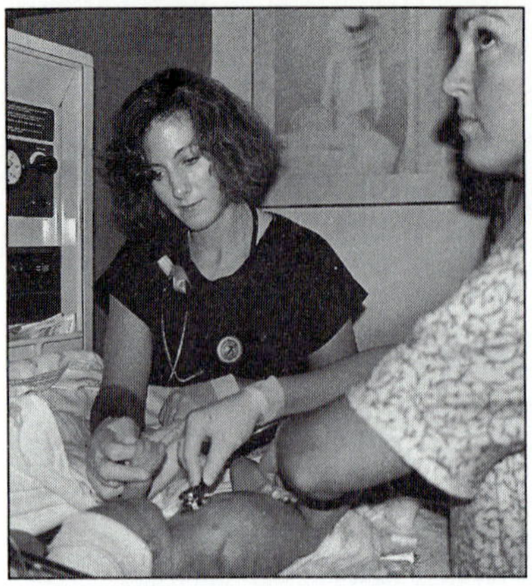

CHAPTER 5
Human Sexuality 81

CHAPTER 6
Women's Health Across the Life Span 95

CHAPTER 7
Fertility Management 129

UNIT III
Adaptation in the Prenatal Period 161

CHAPTER 8
Individual and Family Adaptation to Pregnancy 163

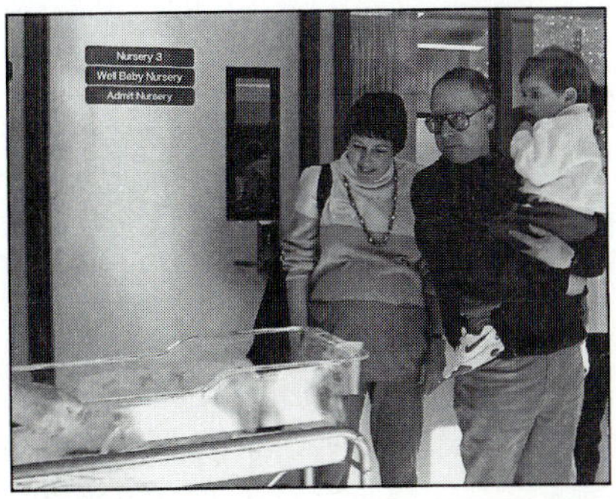
Nursery 3
Well Baby Nursery
Admit Nursery

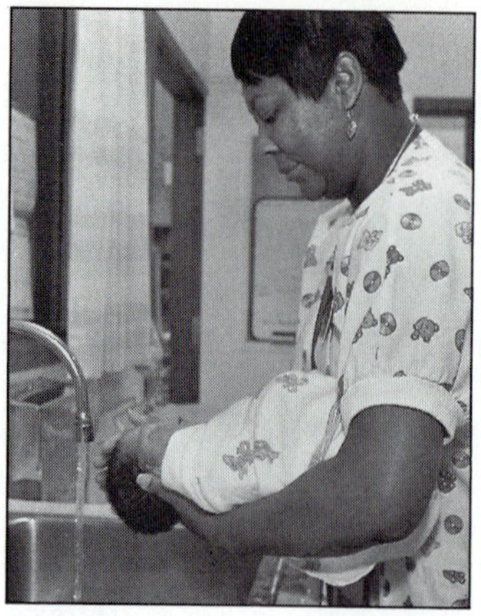

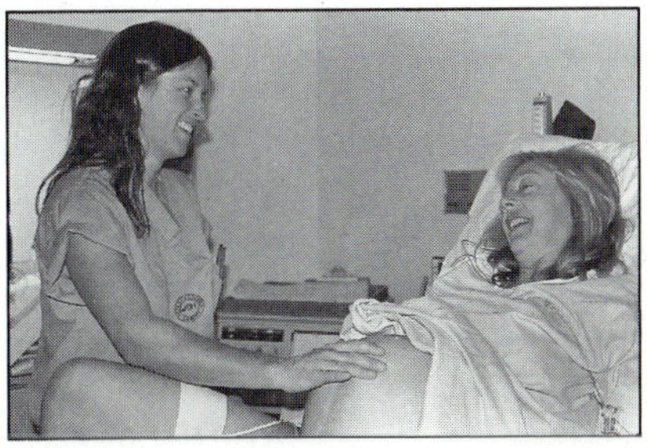

CHAPTER 22
Monitoring the At-Risk Fetus 547

CHAPTER 23
Modifying Labor Patterns and Mode of Delivery 569

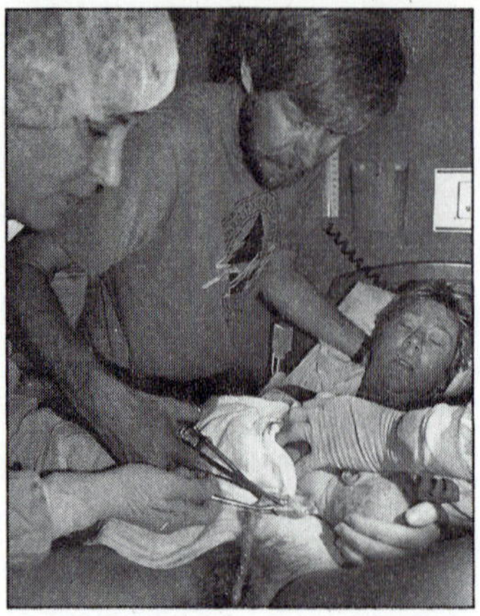

CHAPTER 24
Managing Pain During the Intrapartum and Postpartum Periods 599

CHAPTER 25
Nursing Care of the At-Risk Family in the Perinatal Period 637

CHAPTER 26
Intrapartum Complications 661

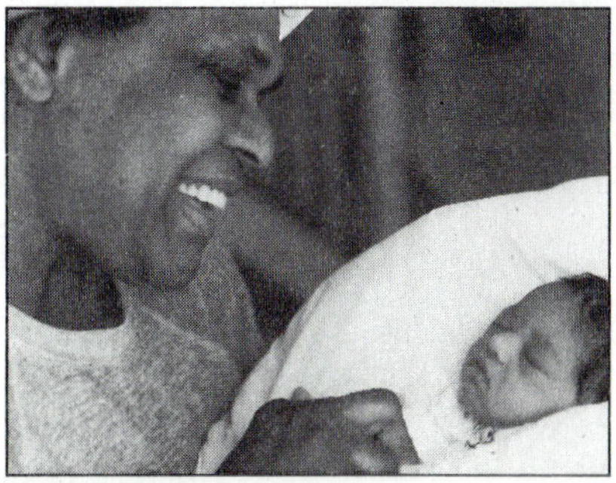

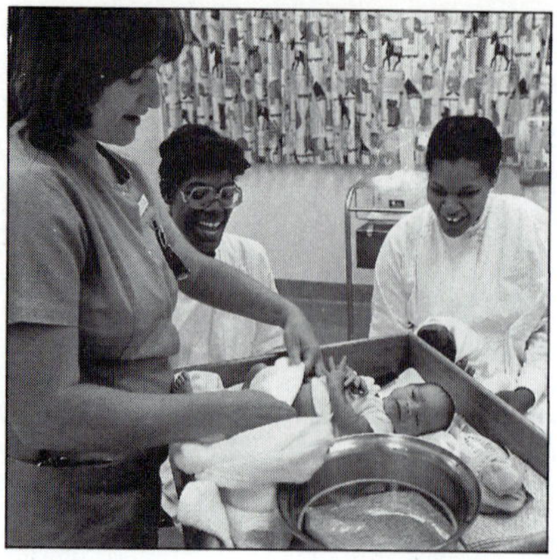

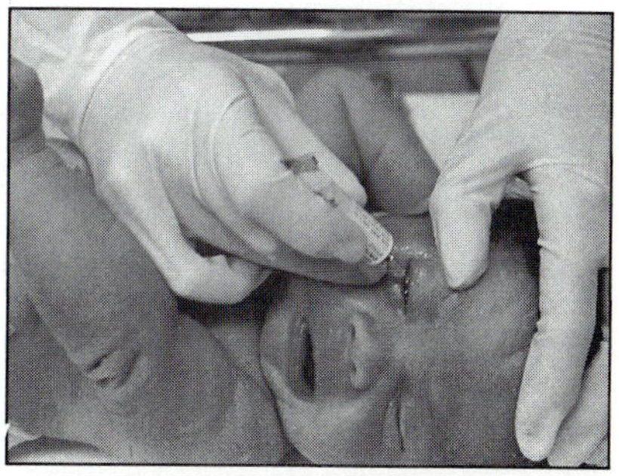

Recurring Displays Appearing in This Text

Nursing Care Plans

A list of Nursing Procedures appears on the front endpaper.

Assessment Tools

Legal/Ethical Considerations

Nursing Research

Family Considerations

Teaching Considerations

Problem Solving Tactics